Principles and Practice of Anesthesia for Thoracic Surgery

Peter Slinger
Editor

Randal S. Blank · Javier Campos
Jens Lohser · Karen McRae
Associate Editors

Principles and Practice of Anesthesia for Thoracic Surgery

Second Edition

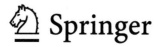

Editor
Peter Slinger
Department of Anesthesiology
University of Toronto
Toronto, ON
Canada

ISBN 978-3-030-00858-1   ISBN 978-3-030-00859-8   (eBook)
https://doi.org/10.1007/978-3-030-00859-8

Library of Congress Control Number: 2018965487

This Springer imprint is published by the registered company Springer Nature Switzerland AG
The registered company address is: Gewerbestrasse 11, 6330 Cham, Switzerland

The Editor would like to thank the members of his family for their never-ending support and patience.
Photo Left to right:
Back row: Colin (son-in-law), Eric (baby, grandson), Lee (daughter), Peter (editor), Rusty (wife), Robyn (daughter-in-law), Luke(son).
Front row: Reagan (grand-daughter,) Jake (grandson), Bruce (Luke's dog)

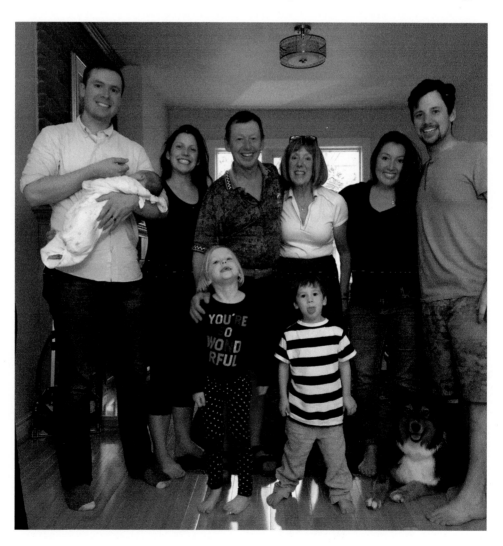

Preface

It has been 8 years since the Associate Editors (Randall Blank, Javier Campos, and Karen McRae) and I assembled the first edition of *Principles and Practice of Anesthesia for Thoracic Surgery*. In this time period, there has been considerable evolution in the anesthetic management of patients requiring anesthesia for non-cardiac intrathoracic diagnostic and therapeutic procedures. We felt that it would be useful to update and expand the original text for practitioners of thoracic anesthesia at all levels including Staff Anesthesiologists, Residents, Fellows, Nurse Anesthetists, Nurse Practitioners, Anesthesia Assistants, and other Allied Health Professionals. We welcome the addition of Jens Lohser, from the University of British Columbia, as an Associate Editor for this second edition.

Among the major advances that we address in this new edition, we include the expanded role of ultrasound beyond transesophageal echocardiography (Chap. 30): Lung ultrasound has evolved from a curious pattern of artifacts to an essential clinical role in chest trauma and management of pleural effusions (Chap. 28). Ultrasound is now an established tool for the placement of many types of central and peripheral vascular access (Chap. 29). And, ultrasound has permitted the development of several new regional anesthetic blocks (e.g., serratus anterior and erector spinae, Chap. 59) that are useful modalities for management of postoperative pain.

Also new in this edition is the role of extracorporeal membrane oxygenation (ECMO) (Chap. 27) in thoracic anesthesia. Veno-venous ECMO is becoming an established therapeutic option for management of intraoperative hypoxemia in complex types of lung and airway surgery and in whole lung lavage. Venoarterial ECMO is rapidly replacing cardiopulmonary bypass as the main method of extracorporeal lung support in lung transplantation (Chap. 47).

There have been major advances in postoperative pain management for thoracic surgery in this decade. In addition to the new blocks mentioned above, the book covers the expanded use of paravertebral blocks and the use of long-acting local anesthetics (Chap. 60). Also, there have been a variety of new bronchial blockers and modified double-lumen tubes developed that facilitate lung isolation in patients with difficult airways (Chaps. 16, 17, and 18).

We would like to welcome the first Authors of new chapters.

Among these are:

- Daniel Sellers (University of Toronto, Intraoperative Extracorporeal Lung Support for Pulmonary and Airway Surgery, Chap. 27)
- Rebecca Klinger (Duke University, Perioperative Fluid Management in Thoracic Surgery, Chap. 21)
- Danielle Shafiepour (McGill University, Trouble-Shooting One-Lung Ventilation, Chap. 26)
- Nathan Ludwig (University of Western Ontario, Lung Ultrasound, Chap. 28)
- Natalie Silverton (University of Utah, Ultrasound for Vascular Access, Chap. 29)
- Alexander Huang (University of Toronto, Pulmonary Resection in the Patient with Pulmonary Hypertension, Chap. 34)
- Helen Lindsay (New Zealand, Anesthesia for Open Descending Thoracic Aortic Surgery, Chap. 41)

- Andrew Levin (Stellenbosch University, Cape Town, South Africa, Bronchopleural Fistula, Chap. 43)
- Maureen Cheng (Cambridge University, Anesthesia for the Patient with a Previous Lung Transplant, Chap. 48)
- Emily Teeter (University of North Carolina, Enhanced Recovery After Thoracic Surgery, Chap. 52)
- Hadley Wilson (University of North Carolina, Trouble-Shooting Chest Drains, Chap. 58)
- Wendell H. Williams III (MD Anderson Cancer Center, Long-Acting Local Anesthetics for Post-Thoracotomy Pain, Chap. 60)

We would also like to welcome several new first Authors of previous chapters, including Drs. Amanda Kleiman (University of Virginia, Non-respiratory Functions of the Lung, Chap. 7), Javier Lasala (MD Anderson Cancer Center, Intravenous Anesthesia for Thoracic Procedures, Chap. 12), Lorraine Chow (University of Alberta, Anesthesia for Patients with Mediastinal Masses, Chap. 14), Daniel Tran (Yale School of Medicine, Lung Isolation in Patients with Difficult Airways, Chap. 18), Jennifer Macpherson (University of Rochester, Intraoperative Ventilation Strategies for Thoracic Surgery, Chap. 22), Florin Costescu (McGill University, Anesthesia for Patients with End-Stage Lung Disease, Chap. 31), George Kanellakos (Dalhousie University, Thoracic Surgery for Morbidly Obese Patients and Patients with Obstructive Sleep Apnea, Chap. 33), Valerie Rusch (Memorial Sloan Kettering Cancer Center, Pancoast Tumors and Combined Spinal Resections, Chap. 37), Swapnil Parab (Tata Memorial Hospital, Mumbai, India, Thoracic Anesthesia in the Developing World, Chap. 42), Timothy Maus (UC San Diego, Anesthesia for Pulmonary Thromboendarterectomy, Chap. 49), Michael Hall (University of Pennsylvania, Anesthetic Management of Post-Thoracotomy Complications, Chap. 53), and Wendy Smith (UC San Francisco, Postoperative Respiratory Failure and Treatment, Chap. 54).

New to the second edition is the incorporation of video. Relevant video clips will be available online to readers of the print text. For the online text, streaming video clips will allow the reader to point and click to see techniques as they are described. This is particularly useful for ultrasound-guided procedures and lung isolation.

Personally, I would like to thank the returning Authors and Coauthors from the first edition for the thorough updates of their previous chapters. Thank you to the Associate Editors for their hard work and support. And, thank you to the Editors at Springer Clinical Medicine, Daniel Dominguez and Becky Amos, for their encouragement.

Toronto, ON, Canada   Peter Slinger
March 2018

Contents

Contributors

David Amar, MD Department of Anesthesiology and Critical Care Medicine, Memorial Sloan Kettering Cancer Center, New York, NY, USA

Dalia Banks, MD Department of Anesthesiology, University of California San Diego Health, La Jolla, CA, USA

Cassandra Bailey, MB, BCh Department of Anesthesiology, University of Cincinnati, Cincinnati, OH, USA

Mark Bilsky, MD Department of Neurosurgery, Memorial Sloan Kettering Cancer Center, New York, NY, USA

Randal S. Blank, MD, PhD Department of Anesthesiology, University of Virginia Health System, Charlottesville, VA, USA

Jay B. Brodsky, MD Department of Anesthesia, Perioperative and Pain Medicine, Stanford University Medical Center, Stanford, CA, USA

Jean S. Bussières, MD, FRCPC Department of Anesthesiology, Institut Universitaire de Cardiologie et de Pneumologie de Quebéc – Université Laval, Quebéc City, QC, Canada

Javier Campos, MD Department of Anesthesia, University of Iowa Health Care, Roy and Lucille Carver College of Medicine, Iowa City, IA, USA

Maria D. Castillo, MD Department of Anesthesiology, Mt. Sinai College of Medicine, New York, NY, USA

Tzonghuei Herb Chen, MD Department of Anesthesiology, Warren Alpert Medical School of Brown University, Rhode Island Hospital, Providence, RI, USA

Maureen Cheng, MBBS, MMED Anesthesia Department of Anesthesia and Intensive Care, Papworth Hospital, Papworth Everard, Cambridge, UK

Lorraine Chow, MD, FRCPC Anesthesiology, Perioperative and Pain Medicine, University of Calgary, Foothills Medical Center, Calgary, AB, Canada

Edmond Cohen, MD Department of Anesthesiology, Mount Sinai Hospital and School of Medicine, New York, NY, USA

Stephen R. Collins, MD Department of Anesthesiology, University of Virginia Health System, Charlottesville, VA, USA

Ian Conacher, MB ChB, MD, FFARCS, FRCP(Ed) Department of Cardiothoracic Anesthesia, Freeman Hospital, Newcastle upon Tyne, Tyne and Wear, UK

Florin Costescu, MD, FRCPC Department of Anesthesia, McGill University Health Centre – Montreal General Hospital, Montreal, QC, Canada

Etienne J. Couture, MD, FRCPC Department of Medicine, Critical Care Division, University of Montreal, Montreal, QC, Canada

Gail Darling, MD, FRCSC Department of Surgery, Division of Thoracic Surgery, Toronto General Hospital, University Health Network, Toronto, ON, Canada

Marc de Perrot, MD, MSc Department of Thoracic Surgery, University of Toronto, Toronto General Hospital, Toronto, ON, Canada

Maria Deja, MD Department of Anesthesiology and Intensive Care Medicine, Charité-University Medicine Berlin, Berlin, Germany

Chris Durkin, MD FRCPC Department of Anesthesiology, Pharmacology and Therapeutics, University of British Columbia; Vancouver General Hospital, Vancouver, BC, Canada

Gordon N. Finlayson, BSc, MD, FRCP (C) Department of Anesthesiology, Division of Critical Care, Vancouver General Hospital, University of British Columbia, Vancouver, BC, Canada

Alan Finley, MD Department of Anesthesia and Perioperative Medicine, Medical University of South Carolina, Charleston, SC, USA

Marili Frenette, MD Department of Anesthesiology and Critical Care, Université Laval, Quebec City, QC, Canada

John Granton, MD, FRCPC Division of Respirology, Department of Medicine, University of Toronto and University Health Network, Mount Sinai Hospital, Women's College Hospital, Toronto, ON, Canada

Benjamin Haithcock, MD Department of Surgery, Department of Anesthesiology, University of North Carolina at Chapel Hill, Chapel Hill, NC, USA

Michael A. Hall, MD Anesthesia Services, P.A., Department of Anesthesiology, Christiana Care Health System, Newark, DE, USA

Paul M. Heerdt, MD, PhD Department of Anesthesiology, Yale University School of Medicine, New Haven, CT, USA

Ahmed F. Hegazy, MB BCh, MSc, FRCPC Departments of Anesthesiology and Critical Care Medicine, Western University, London Health Sciences, London, ON, Canada

Jagtar Singh Heir, DO The University of Texas MD Anderson Cancer Center, Department of Anesthesiology and Perioperative Medicine, Houston, TX, USA

Alexander Huang, MD, FRCPC Department of Anesthesia and Pain Management, Toronto General Hospital, University Health Network and University of Toronto, Toronto, ON, Canada

Julie L. Huffmyer, MD Department of Anesthesiology, University of Virginia Health System, Charlottesville, VA, USA

William E. Hurford, MD Department of Anesthesiology, University of Cincinnati, Cincinnati, OH, USA

J. Michael Jaeger, PhD, MD, FCCP Department of Anesthesiology, University of Virginia Health System, Charlottesville, VA, USA

George W. Kanellakos, MD FRCPC Department of Anesthesia, Pain Management & Perioperative Medicine, Dalhousie University, Halifax, NS, Canada

Cengiz Karsli, BSc, MD, FRCPC Department of Anesthesiology, The Hospital for Sick Children, Toronto, ON, Canada

Amanda M. Kleiman, MD Department of Anesthesiology, University of Virginia Health System, Charlottesville, VA, USA

Rebecca Y. Klinger, MD, MS Department of Anesthesiology, Duke University Medical Center, Durham, NC, USA

Lavinia M. Kolarczyk, MD Department of Anesthesiology, University of North Carolina at Chapel Hill, Chapel Hill, NC, USA

Karen Lam, MD FRCPC University of Toronto, Department of Anaesthesia, Toronto, ON, Canada

Javier D. Lasala, MD Department of Anesthesiology and Perioperative Medicine, The University of Texas MD Anderson Cancer Center, Houston, TX, USA

Ilya Laufer, MD Department of Neurosurgery, Memorial Sloan Kettering Cancer Center, New York, NY, USA

James P. Lee, MD Department of Anesthesiology, University of Utah School of Medicine, Salt Lake City, UT, USA

Andrew Ian Levin, MBChB, DA, Mmed, FCA, PhD Department of Anaesthesiology and Critical Care, University of Stellenbosch, Tygerberg Hospital, Cape Town, WC, South Africa

Alexandra Lewis, MD Department of Anesthesiology, Memorial Sloan Kettering Cancer Center, New York, NY, USA

Helen A. Lindsay, MBChB Department of Anesthesia & Perioperative Medicine, Auckland City Hospital, Auckland, New Zealand

Keith E. Littlewood, MD Department of Anesthesiology, University of Virginia Health System, Charlottesville, VA, USA

Jens Lohser, MD, MSc, FRCPC Department of Anesthesiology, Pharmacology, and Therapeutics, University of British Columbia, Vancouver General Hospital, Vancouver, BC, Canada

Jason Long, MD, MPH Department of Surgery, University of North Carolina Hospitals, Chapel Hill, NC, USA

Nathan Ludwig, BSc, MD, FRCPC Department of Anesthesiology, Western University, London Health Sciences, London, ON, Canada

Martin Ma, MD, FRCPC Department of Anesthesia and Pain Management, University Health Network, Toronto General Hospital, Toronto, ON, Canada

Peter MacDougall, MD, PhD, FRCPC Department of Anesthesia and Family Medicine, Queen Elizabeth II Health Sciences Centre, Halifax, NS, Canada

Jennifer A. Macpherson, MD Department of Anesthesiology and Perioperative Medicine, The University of Rochester Medical Center, Rochester, NY, USA

Katherine Marseu, BSc, MD, FRCPC, MSc (HSEd) Department of Anesthesia and Pain Management, Toronto General Hospital, University Health Network and University of Toronto, Toronto, ON, Canada

Timothy M. Maus, MD, FASE Department of Anesthesiology, University of California San Diego Health, La Jolla, CA, USA

William T. McGee, MD, MHA Critical Care Division, Department of Medicine and Surgery, University of Massachusetts Medical School, Baystate Medical Center, Springfield, MA, USA

Sean R. McLean, MD, FRCPC Department of Anesthesiology, Pharmacology, and Therapeutics, University of British Columbia, Vancouver General Hospital, Vancouver, BC, Canada

Karen McRae, MDCM, FRCPC Department of Anesthesia and Pain Management, Toronto General Hospital, University Health Network, Toronto, ON, Canada

Massimiliano Meineri, MD Department of Anesthesia, Toronto General Hospital, University of Toronto, Toronto, ON, Canada

Gabriel E. Mena, MD Department of Anesthesiology and Perioperative Medicine, The University of Texas MD Anderson Cancer Center, Houston, TX, USA

Sheila Nainan Myatra, MD, FCCM Department of Anesthesiology, Critical Care and Pain, Tata Memorial Hospital, Mumbai, Maharashtra, India

Ju-Mei Ng, FANZCA Department of Anesthesiology, Perioperative and Pain Medicine, Brigham and Women's Hospital, Boston, MA, USA

E. Andrew Ochroch, MD, MSCE Department of Anesthesiology and Critical Care, University of Pennsylvania, Philadelphia, PA, USA

Maral Ouzounian, MD PhD FRCSC Division of Cardiovascular Surgery, Department of Surgery, Toronto General Hospital, Toronto, ON, Canada

Stephen V. Panaro, MD Department of Anesthesia, Hartford Hospital, Hartford, CT, USA

Swapnil Yeshwant Parab, MD Department of Anesthesiology, Critical Care and Pain, Tata Memorial Hospital, Mumbai, Maharashtra, India

Kalpaj R. Parekh, MBBS Department of Cardiothoracic Surgery, University of Iowa Hospitals and Clinics, Iowa City, IA, USA

Alessia Pedoto, MD Department of Anesthesiology and Critical Care Medicine, Memorial Sloan Kettering Cancer Center, New York, NY, USA

Stephen H. Pennefather, MRCP, FRCA Department of Anesthesia, Liverpool Heart and Chest Hospital, Liverpool, Merseyside, UK

Jean Y. Perentes Department of Thoracic Surgery, University of Toronto, Toronto General Hospital, Toronto, ON, Canada
Department of Thoracic Surgery, University Hospital of Lausanne, Lausanne, Switzerland

Wanda M. Popescu, MD Department of Anesthesiology, Yale School of Medicine, New Haven, CT, USA

Jeffrey Port, MD Department of Cardiothoracic Surgery, Weill Medical College of Cornell University, New York, NY, USA

Ron V. Purugganan, MD Department of Anesthesiology and Perioperative Medicine, The University of Texas MD Anderson Cancer Center, Cardiothoracic Anesthesia Group, Unit 409, Faculty Center, Houston, TX, USA

Clare Paula-Jo Quarterman, MBChB, BSc, FRCA Department of Anaesthesia, Liverpool Heart and Chest NHS Foundation Trust, Liverpool, Merseyside, UK

Karthik Raghunathan, MD, MPH Department of Anesthesiology, Duke University, Durham, NC, USA

Jesse M. Raiten, MD Department of Anesthesiology and Critical Care, Perelman School of Medicine at the University of Pennsylvania, Philadelphia, PA, USA

James Ramsay, MD Department of Anesthesia and Preoperative Care, University of California San Francisco, San Francisco, CA, USA

Cara Reimer, MD, FRCPC Department of Anesthesiology and Perioperative Medicine, Kingston Health Sciences Centre, Kingston, ON, Canada

Bernhard J. C. J. Riedel, MD, MBA, FANZCA, PhD Department of Anesthesiology, Perioperative and Pain Medicine, Peter MacCallum Cancer Centre, Melbourne, VIC, Australia University of Melbourne, Melbourne, VIC, Australia

Andrew Roscoe, MB ChB, FRCA Department of Anesthesia, Papworth Hospital, Cambridge, UK

Valerie W. Rusch, MD Thoracic Service, Department of Surgery, Memorial Sloan Kettering Cancer Center, New York, NY, USA

Travis Schisler, MD, FRCPC Department of Anesthesiology, Pharmacology, and Therapeutics, University of British Columbia, Vancouver General Hospital, Vancouver, BC, Canada

Robert Schwartz, HBSc, MD, FRCPC Department of Anesthesia, Children's Hospital of Eastern Ontario, Ottawa, ON, Canada

Anupamjeet Kaur Sekhon, MD Detar Family Medicine Residency Program, Texas A&M University College of Medicine, Victoria, TX, USA

Daniel Sellers, MBBS, FRCA Department of Anesthesia and Pain Management, Toronto General Hospital, University Health Network, Toronto, ON, Canada

Danielle Sophia Shafiepour, BSc, MD CM, FRCPC Department of Anesthesiology, Montreal General Hospital, Montreal, QC, Canada

Tawimas Shaipanich, MD, FRCPC Interventional Pulmonology, Respiratory Medicine, and Integrative Oncology, St Paul's Hospital, BC Cancer Agency and University of British Columbia, Vancouver, BC, Canada

Natalie A. Silverton, MD Department of Anesthesiology, University of Utah, Salt Lake City, UT, USA

Peter Slinger, MD, FRCPC Department of Anesthesia, Toronto General Hospital, Toronto, ON, Canada

Wendy Smith, MD Department of Anesthesiology and Perioperative Care, University of California at San Francisco, San Francisco, CA, USA

Claudia Spies, MD Department of Anesthesiology and Intensive Care Medicine, Charité-University Medicine Berlin, Berlin, Germany

Coimbatore Srinivas, MD, FRCA, FRCPC Department of Anesthesia, Toronto General Hospital, Toronto, ON, Canada

Erin A. Sullivan, MD, FASA Department of Anesthesiology, UPMC Presbyterian Hospital, University of Pittsburgh Medical Center, Pittsburgh, PA, USA

Emily G. Teeter, MD, FASE Department of Anesthesiology, University of North Carolina at Chapel Hill, Chapel Hill, NC, USA

Brian J. Titus, MD, PhD Department of Anesthesiology, University of Virginia Health System, Charlottesville, VA, USA

Daniel Tran, MD Department of Anesthesiology, Yale School of Medicine, New Haven, CT, USA

Vera von Dossow, MD Department of Anesthesiology, Ludwig-Maximilians Universität München, Klinikum Großhadern, Munich, Germany

Marcin Wąsowicz, MD, PhD Department of Anesthesia and Pain Management, Toronto General Hospital, University Health Network and Department of Anesthesia University of Toronto, Toronto, ON, Canada

Cardiovascular Intensive Care Unit, Toronto General Hospital, Toronto, ON, Canada

Wendell H. Williams III, MD The University of Texas MD Anderson Cancer Center, Department of Anesthesiology and Perioperative Medicine, Houston, TX, USA

Hadley K. Wilson, MD, MS Department of Surgery, Division of Cardiothoracic Surgery, UNC Hospitals, Chapel Hill, NC, USA

Paul J. Wojciechowski, MD Department of Anesthesiology, University of Cincinnati, Cincinnati, OH, USA

Gavin Michael Wright, MBBS (Melb), FRACS, PhD Department of Cardiothoracic Surgery, Royal Melbourne Hospital, Parkville, VIC, Australia

Department of Surgery, University of Melbourne, Melbourne, VIC, Australia

Joshua M. Zimmerman, MD, FASE University of Utah School of Medicine, Salt Lake City, UT, USA

Bernhard Zwissler, MD Department of Anesthesiology, Ludwig-Maximilians Universität München, Klinikum Großhadern, Munich, Germany

Part I

Introduction

History of Thoracic Anesthesiology

Ian Conacher

Key Points

- Because of the concern relating to the natural history of pneumothorax, the development of a thoracic surgery discipline comparatively was late.
- Tuberculosis was the stimulus to overcome concern and caution.
- Control of contaminating secretions was an early anesthesia objective.
- Rigid bronchoscopy, lung separation, and positive-pressure ventilation are milestones of significance.
- Modern materials have enabled considerable advances in essentially early ideas.
- The anesthesia challenge of surgery of respiratory failure is to counteract the negative effects of positive-pressure ventilation.
- Surgery for lung cancer remains the bulk of workload.

Introduction

Infantry in disciplined armies like those of the Romans were trained to inflict a penetrating stab injury to the chest wall. Early depictions capture the paradox of a small and bloodless injury inevitably being fatal: and a dignity to a transition into another world as deep to the wound the lung collapses, respiration becomes paradoxical, and carbon dioxide retention and hypoxia ease the passing. In the nineteenth century, as surgery was advancing apace because of antisepsis and anesthesiology, it was opined that the surgeon's knife would for these old reasons inevitably lead to the death of the patient: surgically attempting to incise into the thorax was something of a taboo, only to be breached by *Ferdinand*

Sauerbruch (1875–1951) little more than a century ago (Fig. 1.1).

The late beginning to the thoracic surgery discipline is overlooked. The author occasionally assisted the distinguished *Phillip Ayre (1902–1979)* who had worked with a surgical collaborator of Sauerbruch. This was *Laurence O'Shaugnessy (1900–1940)*. A casualty of the Second World War, he left to posterity one of the earliest surgical methods of treatment for angina and distinctive forceps that graced thoracic surgical instrument trays for 60 years and has been modified for minimal access use (Fig. 1.2).

The fatal process – wound, pleural penetration, lung collapse, respiratory, and cardiac arrest – was interrupted with construction of an operating environment that counteracted the elastic force that paralyzes respiratory function. With encasement of the surgeon and patients' torso in a negative-pressure chamber, atmospheric pressure (now positive in physiological terms) operated at the patient's exposed mouth and prevented the lung collapsing as soon as parietal pleura was breeched. Expired tidal ventilation and gas exchange can continue to counter the toxic effect, described as "pendelluft," of moving physiological dead space gas back and forth between the lungs. Accumulation of carbon dioxide in the self-ventilating patients was delayed and albeit limiting operating time was enough to open the historical account of thoracic surgery.

The Sauerbruch technique was replaced by more efficient methods to reverse intrapleural dynamics and based on supra-atmospheric pressures applied to the airway – a move recognizable in modern day practices of tracheal intubation and positive-pressure ventilation. The change is typical of an early phenomenon: the thoracic discipline attracted inspired minds, with ingenious ideas to build on templates of pioneers. Here are to be found stories of great physiologists, physicians, surgeons, and anesthesiologists without whom, for instance, the groundwork for a diversification into cardiac surgery would have been significantly delayed. Indeed in many countries, the latter services still are rooted in establishments that once were sanatoriums, serving the needs of early patients for chest surgery.

I. Conacher (✉)
Department of Cardiothoracic Anesthesia, Freeman Hospital,
Newcastle upon Tyne, Tyne and Wear, UK

© Springer Nature Switzerland AG 2019
P. Slinger (ed.), *Principles and Practice of Anesthesia for Thoracic Surgery*, https://doi.org/10.1007/978-3-030-00859-8_1

Fig. 1.1 A diagram of Sauerbruch's negative-pressure chamber for thoracic anesthesia. The animal or patient's torso and the surgeons were enclosed in an airtight chamber evacuated to −10 cm H_2O pressure. The subject was then anesthetized breathing air-ether spontaneously from a mask. When the thorax was opened, the lung did not collapse and hypoxemia was averted, although hypercarbia would gradually develop due to pendelluft. This marked the beginnings of elective thoracic anesthesia and surgery. (From Mushin W, Rendell-Baker L. The principles of thoracic anaesthesia. Oxford: Blackwell Scientific Publications; 1953.)

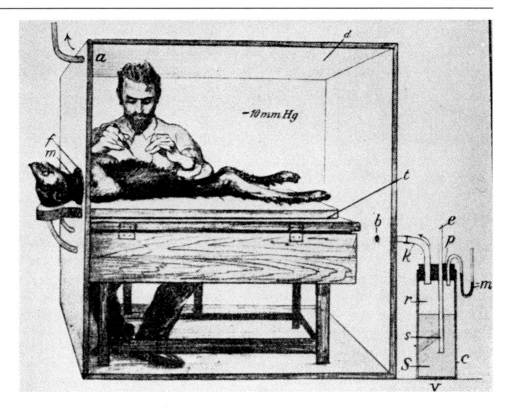

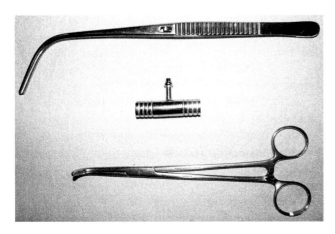

Fig. 1.2 Thoracic ephemera. From top to bottom: Krause's Forceps, Ayres "T" piece, O'Shaughnessy Forceps

In each development, an anesthesiologist of the day has had to innovate, adapt, and change with new ideas, materials, and advances being presented to him or her. A formative beginning with candle power disappeared with antimicrobial therapy but leaves a legacy of thoracoscopy, lateral thoractomy, lung separators, and pain relief techniques that are but little modified.

Paradigm shifts are usually marked by the two World Wars of the twentieth century. Though these are defining elements of any historical analysis, and certainly colored the individuals who are part of the story, developments in thoracic surgery that now govern modern practice are better seen in the light of changes in the medical challenges of disease which changed coincidentally at the same time points.

Ages of Thoracic Surgery

Surgery for Infective Lung Disease

The nineteenth century, a time of great population and societal movement particularly in and from Europe, was blighted by the "white plague" (tuberculosis), an indiscriminate killer – irrespective of class, wealth, national boundaries, and unstoppable, a foreshadowing of AIDS: a heroine in the throes of consumption, a last hemoptysis, death – stuff of opera. Into this hopelessness strides the surgeon to deal with pulmonary cavities, septic foci, decayed and destroyed lung, bleeding points, and copious, poisonous secretions that were more than capable of drowning the patient. Surgical repertoire after the Sauerbruch revelation was the artificial pneumothorax, empyema drainage, plombage (insertion of inert material into the thoracic cavity to promote lung collapse as therapy for tuberculosis), phrenic nerve crush, the thoracoplasty, and some tentative steps at resection – ordeals staged over days and weeks but with an accrual of lifesaving consequences for countless (Fig. 1.3).

With no mechanisms of control of secretions and an ever-present danger of respiratory failure, standards for anesthesiology were sedation with opiates, topical, regional, and field blockade with local anesthetics to preserve self-ventilation so that cough and the ability to clear the airway were not lost.

Operating position became important. That of Trendelenburg was most effective to ensure that secretions, blood, and lung detritus drained gravitationally and not into

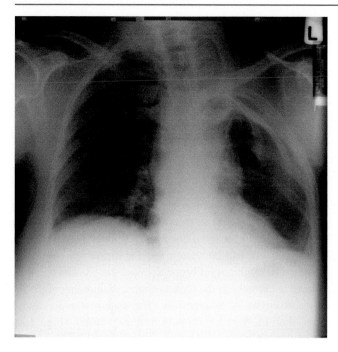

Fig. 1.3 Chest X-ray of a left-sided thoracoplasty, the ribs of the upper left hemithorax have been resected to promote left upper lobe collapse for tuberculosis therapy

the nonoperated lung. But, in the cachectic and septic sufferer of pulmonary tuberculosis or bronchiectasis, adoption of such steep head-down postures could prove fatal. The prone and semiprone positions were gentler and less compromising. Surgeons got used to operating and approaching the lung and its constituents through a posterior thoracotomy. This spawned the posterolateral thoracotomy, once tracheal intubation techniques enabled alternative, nongravitational ways of dealing with the secretion problem. The lung, esophagus, and heart became grist to the thoracic surgical mill.

As the era closed, the anesthesiologist (and the dawn of the specialist was at hand) had an experience of nitrous oxide and several volatile agents other than ether, notably chloroform and cyclopropane. Insufflation techniques, tracheal intubation, and rudimentary bronchial blocking techniques, which required a skill in rigid bronchoscopy, were tools of the expert. Several were using assisted ventilation before the advent of muscle relaxants. Prototype endobronchial tubes, bronchial blockers, and early positive-pressure ventilation techniques were in position for a new age – ushered in with curare.

There is no greater symbol of the transition than the pneumonectomy of the British King, *George VI (1895–1952)*. Operated on in 1951 – for lung cancer – by a surgeon (*C. Price Thomas (1893–1973)*) who was credited with his own operation (sleeve resection) for tuberculosis, the anesthesiologist (*Dr R. Machray*) had devised his own tracheal tube (but on the occasion used a Thompson bronchus blocker) and wielded measured doses of diamorphine and pethidine,

nitrous oxide, and the new agent, curare. And in the wings, spurred by intraoperative problems with ventilation, a trainee anesthesiologist (*William Pallister (1926–2008)*) was inspired to invent a new endobronchial tube specifically for the surgeon and his operation to avoid such critical incidents in the future. The surgeon later developed lung cancer for which he was operated on! The cigarette was yet to be seen as the cause and that this particular blight was largely man-made.

Surgery for Lung Cancer

Pulmonary resection for lung cancer came to dominate operating lists as the tuberculosis hazard receded to a point of rarity in developed countries with advances in public health that followed the Second World War. The favored method was general anesthesia with volatiles such as the new agent halothane, lung separation – commonly with double-lumen tubes – muscle relaxants, and, after the polio epidemics of the 1950s, positive-pressure ventilation with increasingly sophisticated ventilators. The Academic of the day, having acquired scientific tools, was beginning to recognize and investigate the subtle pathophysiological changes wrought by one-lung anesthesia.

In general, advances were defined by greater understanding of pulmonary physiology, limits and limitations of surgery particularly degree of resectability, and the fitness of patients to withstand ordeals of process, and more regard for quality of postresection existence. The crude practice of inserting a blocker through a rigid bronchoscope under topical anesthesia applied with Krause's Forceps, to test for the potential to survive a pulmonary resection, could be abandoned! Besides safeguarding the technological skills of an earlier era, the anesthesiologist needed to acquire a bedside expertise of the potential for respiratory failure to develop in a particular patient, based on simple pulmonary function tests (wet spirometry). In this era predating a foundation or philosophy for prolonged recovery with ventilator support and postoperative care resource, forecasting was on the basis that fatalities were theoretically due to carbon dioxide retention or right heart failure if excess lung was resected in reaching for a cure for a cancer: in practice sepsis and renal failure usually proved terminal.

The ending of this work pattern followed advances of plastics technology on equipment, fiber optics on diagnostics and operating instruments, and computers on monitoring and performance. Surgery was moving into an age that had a patient demand to push operability beyond limits established for cancer. This desire was to be met with larger resource for intensive levels of postoperative care.

Although advances were truly innovative, these were fraught with risk. For a perspective on this, recall that pulse oximeters were experimental not universal and end-tidal carbon dioxide measurement nonexistent: operational decisions depended on blood gas monitoring with unsophisticated and slow automated systems and the occasional use outside the laboratory of Swan-Ganz type pulmonary flotation catheters.

Surgery for Respiratory Failure

Defining elements include transplantation but also revisits to treatment of emphysema (which had with chronic bronchitis reached significant proportions in developed countries) and technological and material advances for trachea-bronchial disease which heretofore were off limits to all but a few establishments with special expertise and cardiopulmonary bypass technology.

Orthotopic lung transplantation had been attempted in extremis (1963), but success in terms of long-term viability was not to be achieved for another two decades (1986). A new immunosuppressant therapeutic era was to enable further, and this time, successful efforts. Much of the credit goes to the Toronto group, under Dr. Joel Cooper, whose selection and management templates resolved problems previously encountered by attempting to treat paraquat poisoning, routine use of corticosteroids for airway disease, tracheobronchial dehiscence, and reimplantation. Matching of lung preservation techniques to those for cardiac donors was a final step from experimental to mainstream and to the current healthy state of a thoracic organ transplant discipline.

Chronologically, not far behind, is lung volume reduction surgery, driven by many of the same innovators. Historically, this was just a revisitation of old ideas and not a monumental surgical advance; but the lessons learnt were in particular for anesthesiology. In learning to deal with emphysema lung pathophysiology, a "downside" of positive-pressure ventilation was encountered with great frequency. The prevention and treatment of dynamic hyperinflation scenarios ("breath stacking") is now, after a century, as big a challenge as that of "pendelluft" breathing was in its day.

Lung Separators

Three systems have evolved to facilitate one-lung ventilation: bronchus blocker, endobronchial tube, and double-lumen tube. The first two were of concept and had prototypes about the same time. Gale and Waters in 1931 have the credit for intubation of the contralateral bronchus prior to pneumonectomy: Craford and Magill as firsts for bronchial blocking. The double-lumen tube is a later development and as concept was taken from catheters, most notably the Carlens,

devised for bronchospirometric research, assessment, and investigation.

Devices were manufactured out of red rubber, and over the years many adaptations were made: right- and left-sided versions, carinal hooks, right upper lobe slots, and extra-inflatable cuffs, cuffs of red rubber and of latex rubber, net-covered – to mention but a few.

The Blocker Story

It is to the particular genius of *Ivan Magill (1888–1986)* that the bronchus blocker is owed. With minor modifications it became a dominant technique for practitioners, use of which, as mentioned, had become a test for fitness for operation. Inserted through a rigid bronchoscope, the blocker could be placed accurately in the most complex of anatomical distortions wrought by tuberculosis. The state-of-the-art device was that of *Vernon Thompson (1905–1995)* (Fig. 1.4). However, endobronchial tube availability and the versatility of double-lumen tubes meant that by the latter part of the twentieth century, there were few but a dedicated band of practitioners with the skill to place and use blockers effectively and first choice status was lost. Plastics and fiber optics led to reinvention for the twenty-first century. "Univent," Arndt, and Cohen systems follow in quick succession as the concept was revitalized.

The Endobronchial Tube Story

These very obvious adaptations of tracheal tubes gave anesthesiologists a range of devices that served purpose for half a century. That of Machray was a long, single-cuffed tracheal tube and was placed in the left main bronchus under direct vision using an intubating bronchoscope as introducer

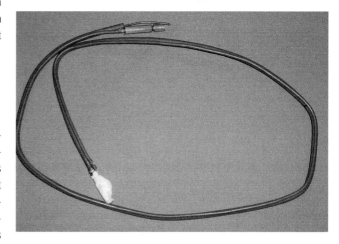

Fig. 1.4 Vernon Thompson bronchus blocker (circa 1943)

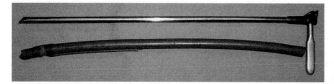

Fig. 1.5 Machray endobronchial tube and intubating bronchoscope

(Fig. 1.5). Being able to mount these devices on a rigid scope, again a Magill credited idea, defined these tubes. The characteristic facilitated placement in the most distorted of airways and allowed for ventilation through a wide-bore tube, bettered only by using a bronchus blocker outside and beside an endotracheal tube. Left-sided Macintosh-Leatherdale and Brompton-Pallister and the right-sided Gordon-Green were to prove the most enduring.

The Double-Lumen Tube Story

Unlike the other types of lung separators, the double-lumen tube was adapted and adopted rather than invented for the purpose of one-lung anesthesia and ventilation. The prototypes, notably that of *Eric Carlens (1908–1990)*, were for physiological investigation. Models with the ventilation lumens positioned coaxially and anterior-posterior were tried but that of *Frank Robertshaw (1918–1991)* with its side-by-side lumens, anatomical shape, range of size, and low resistance characteristic dominated, to be later reproduced as plastic and disposable materials (e.g., Sheridan, Broncho-Cath) that replaced the increasingly unsuitable and anachronistic red rubber. The right-sided version was actually invented from a Gordon-Green endobronchial tube, the slot of which has remained the most effective device to ventilate the right upper lobe – an efficacy dependent on properties of red rubber (Fig. 1.6).

Plastic and practice penetration by fiberoptic bronchoscopes of decreasing size and increasing sophistication and practicality led to much contemporary discussion about the "blind" placement of lung separators that replaced the tradition of rigid bronchoscopy as an aid to lung separation and bronchial cannulation. Though modern protocols are more fail-safe than reliance on clinical and observational skills, the modern didactic of medicolegality has trumped debate and stifled argument.

Origins of Thoracic Endoscopy

The ancient entertainment of sword swallowing had long demonstrated the feasibility of inserting rigid instruments into the esophagus. In 1895 a scope was first passed through a tracheotomy opening to be quickly followed by

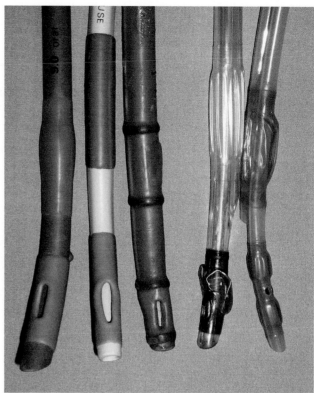

Fig. 1.6 Tubes with right upper lobe ventilation slots. From left to right: Gordon-Green endobronchial, Robertshaw double lumen, Carlens (White model) double lumen, "Broncho-Cath" double lumen, and "Portex" prototype double lumen

endoral attempts but at the limits of proximal lighting systems. *Chevalier Jackson (1865–1958)* was not the originator, but he certainly was a pioneer and the first master of distal lighting systems, with a record on removal of foreign bodies that stands unsurpassed to this day (Fig. 1.7). To him are owed the rules that made the dangerous art of sword swallowing into a scientific tool for therapy and diagnosis both in the esophagus and in the tracheobronchial tree and the subtleties of neck positioning that ensure either the esophagus or trachea is cannulated: a whole philosophy of skill that has been negated by the flexible nature of modern tools.

Now the only indications for rigid bronchoscopy are foreign body removal and occasional stent insertion, but there was a time when rigid bronchoscopy was indispensible for operative assessment, bronchography, diagnostics, insertion of lung separators, postoperative lung toilet, and treatment of bronchopleural fistula. Under careful local anesthetic application, topical, regional, and cricothyroid puncture, the technique could be conducted with such skill that no less an illustrious patient than *Geoffrey Organe (1908–1989)*, the Professor of Anaesthesia, Westminster Hospital, London, was able to declare the experience as "more pleasant than going to the dentist."

Fig. 1.7 A series of safety pins removed from the airway by rigid bronchoscopy. (From Jackson C. Foreign bodies in air and food passages. Charted experience in cases from no. 631 to no. 1155 at the Bronchoscopic Clinic; 1923)

Fbdy. 768 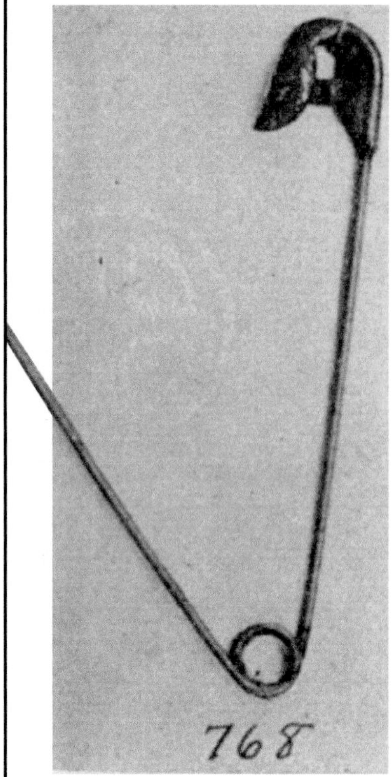	15 yrs.	Safety-pin open	Right main bron-chus, 3 weeks
Fbdy. 786 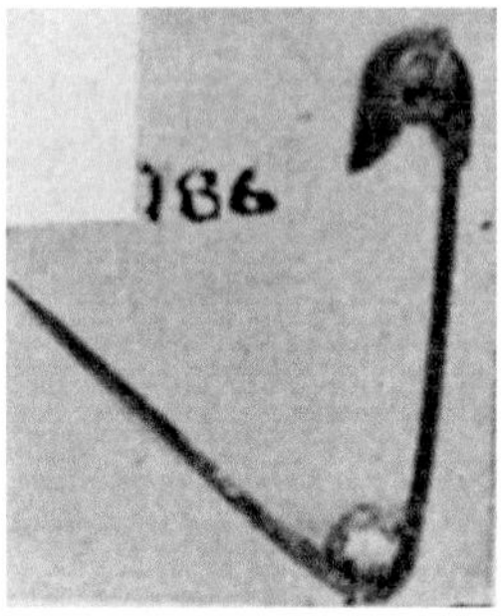	4 yrs.	Safety-pin open	Larynx, point up, 3 days
Fbdy. 794 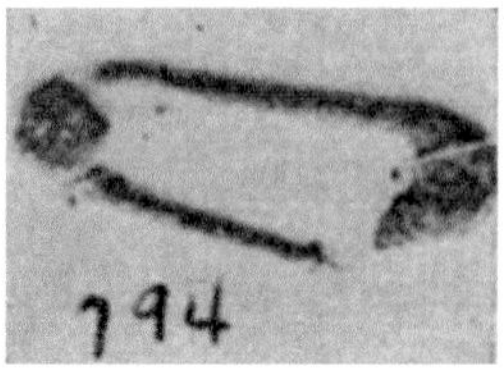	18 yrs.	Safety-pin open	Right lower lobe bronchus. Point up. 1 yr. 10 mos.

Trying to produce an artificial pneumothorax frequently failed because of adhesions. In 1913, a Swedish surgeon, Hans Christian Jacobaeus, reported on the use of a modified cystoscope to look into the chest and used a second port for instruments, such as probes and cautery, to deal with recalcitrant adhesions. It is not hard to see how this concept has evolved.

Tracheobronchial Stenosis

As technological advance is on the brink of tracheal reconstruction using biological methods, it is important not to forget that this state has been reached by a long and hard struggle to overcome the challenge for surgery and healing inherent in innately poor mammalian vascular supply of the tracheobronchial tree. The era of tracheal resection and repair was to be dominated by *Hermes Grillo (1923–2006)*, the Chief of Thoracic Surgery at the Massachusetts General Hospital. There was a brief period of tracheoplasty and silicon replacements, all of which were major anesthesiological undertakings, but developments in stents, largely modeled on similar devices for esophageal stricture, had become prevalent at the end of the twentieth century. Solid-state devices of silicon were replaced by a range of self-expanding ones made of nonreactive and malleable materials such as nitinol which have resulted in less challenging anesthesia scenarios.

Esophageal Surgery

Originally, surgery on the esophagus was very much a development of chest surgery. Several medical cultures retained a linkage late into the twentieth century, but this was largely a technical connection because of commonality of anesthesiological requirements like lung isolation. Most countries have now broken the connection, and the esophagus is largely seen as outside the hegemony of thoracic practice. Cancer, achalasia, and hiatus hernia, once part of the tougher end of the surgical diet, are now treated less traumatically and invasively.

As with pulmonary resection, early developments were based on totemic patients by small teams, whose successes and tribulations sustained knowledge that relief by surgical means ultimately was going to be of benefit to many more. A single case survivor of 13 years after transpleural esophagectomy by *Franz Torek (1861–1938)* in New York in 1913 was a beacon for three decades. The anesthetist was *Carl Eggers (1879–1957)* who administered ether through a woven silk tracheal tube to a self-ventilating patient. In 1941, the world experience of the technique was 17 survivors of 58 patients.

Pain Relief

Modern analgesics can be traced to the coca leaf, opium poppy, and willow bark, but administration other than by ingestion or inhalation needed the hypodermic needle. Spinal injection (1898), intercostal nerve blockade (1906), paravertebral injection (1906), and extradural (1921) are the historical sequence for local anesthetic procedures of context.

Survivors of thoracoplasty operations tell of hearing their ribs being cracked as, in the later stages of the operation, the thoracic cage was rearranged: few attendants were prepared to risk general anesthesia. A specimen technique of Magill's for this operation, first performed in the UK by *Hugh Morriston Davies (1879–1965)* in 1912, included premedication with opiates, supraclavicular brachial plexus block, intercostal nerve block, dermal infiltration of skin incision site and towel clip points as well as subscapular infiltration and much titration of dilutions of adrenalin (epinephrine). *J Alfred Lee (1906–1989)* (author of the classic *A Synopsis of Anaesthesia*, first produced in 1947) states advantages of local as opposed to general anesthesia: reduced risk of spread of disease, better elimination of secretions as cough reflex is not abolished, quicker convalescence because patient is less upset by drugs and needs less nursing care, and abolition of explosion risk.

Paravertebral blockade, first credited to Sellheim, went on to be used for operative pain relief, postthoracotomy neuralgia, and even angina and thoracic pain of unknown etiology. Subarachnoid block enjoyed a period in thoracic surgery, but the "high" nature meant that it was a hazardous technique because of uncontrolled hypotension and suppression of respiration. Epidural anesthesia was limited by the toxicity of agents, hazard of hemodynamic collapse, the short-lived nature of single-shot procedures, and logistics and feasibility of process in the context of hospital environment. Continuous analgesia perioperatively was only realistic with small-bore tubing and got impetus from the link to improved postoperative respiratory function.

Correlation of pain relief and reversal of some of the negative effects of surgery led to recognition that pain relief objectives could be broadened from humanitarian and reactive. A new philosophy has arisen: it is a proactive one to capitalize on observations that pain relief techniques contribute to the healing process by promoting a sense of well-being, preserving gastrointestinal function, improving anastomotic blood flow, and facilitating management of comorbidity.

Conclusion

The impetus for surgical development and advance are all in context, and in none more than thoracic practice is this true: phases, even paradigm shifts, defined by disease, sociology and advances in knowledge, and therapeutics and, in the case of anesthesiology, by drugs, materials, and technology. As historical evolution, much of current practice is recognizable.

A modern age is already characterized by a circumspect use of volatile agents, but predictable forces of surgery are the demand for minimal access and the use of once-only disposable materials that have already seen the demise of much of local infrastructure to process sterile equipment and surgical hygiene. Hospital-acquired infection morbidity is a given, as are epidemics of asbestosis-related pleural-pulmonary disease as this ubiquitous "pathogen" escapes from the twentieth-century confines. A new epidemic, obesity, will gain momentum. Lung cancer treatment options show little sign of being bettered by other than surgical methods. Tuberculosis has a new drug-resistant guise. Could history repeat itself? Many countries, notably in Africa and those previously part of the USSR, have endemic populations harboring and, sadly, nurturing drug-resistant tuberculosis. Some are now contemplating revisiting and revising early surgical techniques (e.g., thoracoplasty) to add

to future projects to tackle what has to be one of the most predictable and threatening of microbial conditions with a future to impact on thoracic anesthesiology and on all health-care systems.

Further Reading

1. Ellis H. The pneumonectomy of George VI. In: Operations that made history. London: Greenwich Medical Media; 1996. p. 123–30.
2. Hurt R. The history of cardiothoracic surgery from early times. New York: Parthenon; 1996.
3. Jackson C. Foreign bodies in the air and food passages. Trans Am Laryngol Rhinol Otol Soc. 1923;
4. Jackson C, Jackson CL. Bronchoesophagology. Philadelphia: WB Saunders; 1950.
5. Lee JA. Anaesthesia for thoracic surgery. In: A synopsis of anaesthesia. 3rd ed. Bristol: John Wright; 1955. p. 386–402.
6. Maltby JR, editor. Notable names in anaesthesia. London: Royal Society of Medicine; 1998.
7. Mushin WW, editor. Thoracic anaesthesia. Philadelphia: FA Davis; 1963.
8. Mushin WW, Rendell-Baker L, editors. The principles of thoracic anaesthesia: past and present. Oxford: Blackwell Scientific; 1953.
9. Sellors TH. Surgery of the thorax. London: Constable; 1933.

Part II

Preoperative Evaluation

Preanesthetic Assessment for Thoracic Surgery

2

Peter Slinger and Gail Darling

Key Points

- All patients having pulmonary resections should have a preoperative assessment of their respiratory function in three areas: Lung mechanical function, pulmonary parenchymal function, and cardiopulmonary reserve (the "three-legged stool" of respiratory assessment).
- Following pulmonary resection surgery, it is usually possible to wean and extubate patients with adequate predicted postoperative respiratory function in the operating room provided they are "AWaC" (alert, warm, and comfortable).
- Preoperative investigation and therapy of patients with coronary artery disease for noncardiac thoracic surgery are becoming a complex issue. An individualized strategy in consultation with the surgeon, cardiologist, and patient is required. Myocardial perfusion imaging and stress echocardiography are used increasingly in these patients.
- Geriatric patients are at a high risk for cardiac complications, particularly arrhythmias, following large pulmonary resections. Preoperative exercise capacity is the best predictor of post-thoracotomy outcome in the elderly.
- In the assessment of patients with malignancies, the "four M's" associated with cancer must be considered: Mass effects, metabolic effects, metastases, and medications.
- Perioperative interventions which have been shown to decrease the incidence of respiratory complications in high-risk patients undergoing thoracic surgery include cessation of smoking, physiotherapy, and thoracic epidural analgesia.

Introduction

Thoracic anesthesia encompasses a wide variety of diagnostic and therapeutic procedures involving the lungs, airways, and other intrathoracic structures. As the patient population presenting for noncardiac thoracic surgery has changed, so have the anesthetic techniques required to manage these patients. Thoracic surgery at the beginning of the last century was primarily for infectious indications (lung abscess, bronchiectasis, empyema, etc.). Although these cases still present for surgery in the post-antibiotic era, now the commonest indications are related to malignancies (pulmonary, esophageal, and mediastinal). In addition, the last two decades have seen the beginnings of surgical therapy for end-stage lung diseases with procedures such as lung transplantation and lung-volume reduction.

Recent advances in anesthetic management, surgical techniques, and perioperative care have expanded the envelope of patients now considered to be operable [1]. This chapter will focus primarily on preanesthetic assessment for pulmonary resection surgery in cancer patients. However, the basic principles described apply to diagnostic procedures, other types of nonmalignant pulmonary resections, and other chest surgeries. The major difference is that in patients with malignancy, the risk/benefit ratio of canceling or delaying surgery pending other investigation/therapy is always complicated by the risk of further spread of cancer

P. Slinger (✉)
Department of Anesthesia, Toronto General Hospital, Toronto, ON, Canada
e-mail: peter.slinger@uhn.ca

G. Darling
Department of Surgery, Division of Thoracic Surgery, Toronto General Hospital, University Health Network, Toronto, ON, Canada

© Springer Nature Switzerland AG 2019
P. Slinger (ed.), *Principles and Practice of Anesthesia for Thoracic Surgery*, https://doi.org/10.1007/978-3-030-00859-8_2

during any extended interval prior to resection. Cancer surgery is never completely "elective" surgery.

A patient with a "resectable" lung cancer has a disease that is still local or local-regional in scope and can be encompassed in a plausible surgical procedure. An "operable" patient is someone who can tolerate the proposed resection with acceptable risk. Anesthesiologists are not gatekeepers. Normally, it is not the anesthesiologist's function to assess these patients to decide who is or is not an operative candidate. In the majority of situations, the anesthesiologist will be seeing the patient at the end of a referral chain from chest or family physician to surgeon. At each stage there should have been a discussion of the risks and benefits of operation. It is the anesthesiologist's responsibility to use the preoperative assessment to identify those patients at elevated risk and then to use that risk assessment to stratify perioperative management and focus resources on the high-risk patients to improve their outcome (Fig. 2.1). This is the primary function of the preanesthetic assessment. However, there are occasions when the anesthesiologist is asked to contribute his/her opinion whether a specific high-risk patient will tolerate a specific surgical procedure. This may occur preoperatively but also occurs intraoperatively when the surgical findings suggest that a planned procedure, such as a lobectomy, may require a larger resection such as

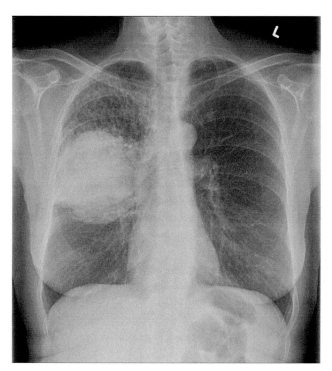

Fig. 2.1 Chest X-ray of a patient with a carcinoma of the right upper lobe scheduled for possible lobectomy or pneumonectomy. The purpose of the preoperative anesthetic assessment of this patient is to stratify the patient's risk and to identify factors which can be managed to improve the perioperative outcome

a pneumonectomy. For these reasons, it is imperative that the anesthesiologist have a complete preoperative knowledge of the patient's medical status and also an appreciation of the pathophysiology of lung resection surgery. There has been a comparatively small volume of research on the short-term (<6 weeks) outcome of these patients. However, this research area is currently very active, and there are several studies which can be used to guide anesthetic management in the perioperative period where it has an influence on outcome.

Thoracic surgeons are now being trained to perform "lung-sparing" resections such as sleeve lobectomies or segmentectomies and to perform resections with minimally invasive techniques such as video-assisted thoracoscopic surgery (VATS) and robotic surgery. The postoperative preservation of respiratory function has been shown to be proportional to the amount of the functioning lung parenchyma preserved. To assess patients with limited pulmonary function, the anesthesiologist must appreciate these newer surgical options in addition to the conventional open lobectomy or pneumonectomy.

Pre-thoracotomy assessment naturally involves all of the factors of a complete anesthetic assessment: past history, allergies, medications, upper airway, etc. This chapter will concentrate on the additional information, beyond a standard anesthetic assessment, that the anesthesiologist needs to manage a thoracic surgical patient. Practice patterns in anesthesia have evolved such that a patient is commonly assessed initially in an outpatient clinic and often not by the member of the anesthesia staff who will actually administer the anesthesia. The actual contact with the responsible anesthesiologist may be only 10–15 min prior to induction. It is necessary to organize and standardize the approach to preoperative evaluation for these patients into two temporally disjoint phases: the initial (clinic) assessment and the final (day-of-admission) assessment. There are elements vital to each assessment which will be described.

Assessment of Respiratory Function

The major cause of perioperative morbidity and mortality in the thoracic surgical population is respiratory complications. Major respiratory complications such as atelectasis, pneumonia, and respiratory failure occur in 15–20% of patients and account for the majority of the expected 3–4% mortality [2]. Cardiac complications such as arrhythmia, ischemia, etc. occur in 10–15% of the thoracic population. Postoperative outcomes after lobectomy are listed in Table 2.1 [3]. The primary focus for the anesthesiologist is to assess the risk of postoperative pulmonary complications.

Table 2.1 Post-lobectomy complications

	Thoracoscopy	Thoracotomy	p value
n	10,173	30,886	
Mortality	1.6%	2.3%	0.06
Length of stay	5 (3–8)	7 (5–9)	<0.001
Any complication	46.5%	50.4%	0.003
Pneumonia	7.3%	8.2%	0.17
Empyema	0.8%	1.4%	0.007
Supraventricular arrhythmia	13.7%	17.9%	<0.0001
Pulmonary embolus	0.6%	1.0%	0.018
Myocardial infarction	0.3%	0.7%	0.01

Based on data from the Nationwide Inpatient Sample Database, Paul et al. [3]

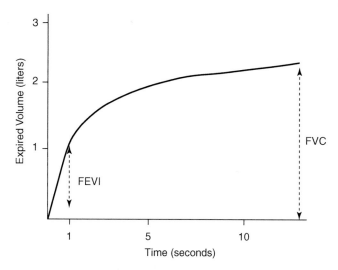

Fig. 2.2 Spirometry should be performed in all pulmonary resection patients to assess the forced expiratory volume in 1 second (FEV1) which can then be corrected for the patient's age, sex, and height to give a percentage of the normal predicted value (FEV1%)

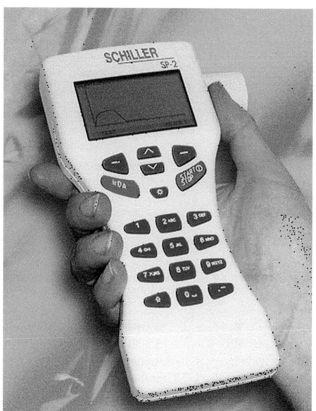

Fig. 2.3 An example of a portable handheld spirometer which can be easily used in the preoperative assessment clinic or at the bedside to measure forced expiratory flows and volumes

The best assessment of respiratory function comes from a detailed history of the patient's quality of life. All pulmonary resection patients should have baseline simple spirometry preoperatively to measure forced expiratory volume in 1 second (FEV1) and forced vital capacity (FVC) (Fig. 2.2) [4]. Simple portable spirometers are available that can be used easily in the clinic or at the bedside to make these measurements (Fig. 2.3). Objective measures of pulmonary function are required to guide anesthetic management and to have this information in a format that can be easily transmitted between members of the healthcare team. Much effort has been spent to try and find a single test of respiratory function that has sufficient sensitivity and specificity to predict outcome for all pulmonary resection patients. It is now clear that no single test will ever accomplish this. It is useful to assess each patient's respiratory function in three related but largely independent areas: respiratory mechanics, pulmonary parenchymal function, and cardiorespiratory interaction.

These can be remembered as the basic functional units of extracellular respiration, which are to get atmospheric oxygen (1) into the alveoli, (2) into the blood, and (3) to the tissues (the process is reversed for carbon dioxide removal).

Lung Mechanical Function

Many tests of respiratory mechanics and volumes show correlation with post-thoracotomy outcome: forced expiratory volume in 1 second (FEV1), forced vital capacity (FVC), maximal voluntary ventilation (MVV), and residual volume/total lung capacity (RV/TLC) ratio. For preoperative assessment, these values should always be expressed as a percent of predicted volumes corrected for age, sex, and height (e.g., FEV1%). Of these the most valid single test for post-thoracotomy respiratory complications is the predicted postoperative FEV1 (ppoFEV1%) [5] which is calculated as:

$$ppoFEV1\% = preoperative\,FEV1\%\times$$
$$\left(1-\%functional\,lung\,tissue\,removed\,/100\right)$$

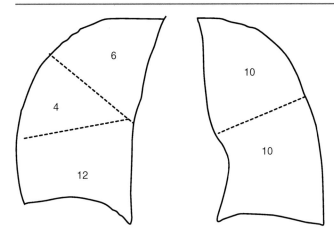

Fig. 2.4 The number of subsegments of each lobe is used to calculate the predicted postoperative (ppo) pulmonary function. For example, following a right lower lobectomy, a patient with a preoperative FEV1 (or DLCO) 70% of normal would be expected to have a ppoFEV1 = 70% × (1−29/100) = 50%

One method of estimating the percent of functional lung tissue is based on a calculation of the number of functioning subsegments of the lung removed (Fig. 2.4). Nakahara et al. [4] found that patients with a ppoFEV1 > 40% had no or minor post-resection respiratory complications. Major respiratory complications were only seen in the subgroup with ppoFEV1 < 40% (although not all patients in this subgroup developed respiratory complications), and 10/10 patients with $ppoFEV_1$ < 30% required postoperative mechanical ventilatory support. These key threshold ppoFEV1 values 40% and 30% are extremely useful to remember when managing these patients. The schema of Fig. 2.4 may be overly complicated, and it can be useful just to simply consider the right upper and middle lobes combined as being approximately equivalent to each of the other three lobes with the right lung 10% larger than the left. These data of Nakahara are from work done in the 1980s, and recent advances, such as improved postoperative analgesia, have decreased the incidence of complications in the high-risk (ppoFEV1 < 30%) group [6]. The use of minimally invasive thoracic surgery has also allowed safe pulmonary resection to be performed in individuals traditionally considered to have increased risk [7].

However, a ppoFEV1 value of ≤40% remains useful as a reference point for the anesthesiologist to identify the patient at increased risk. The ppoFEV1 is the most significant independent predictor of complications among a variety of historical, physical, and laboratory tests for these patients. In the 30 years since the original publication by Nakahara, repeated trials in different populations have consistently supported the use of ppoFEV1 < 40% as a

threshold for increased risk and ppoFEV1 < 30% as the threshold for high risk [8].

Patients with ppoFEV1 values <40% can be operated on with acceptable morbidity and mortality in certain circumstances. Linden et al. [9] reported on a series of 100 patients with ppoFEV1 < 35% who had lung resections for cancer with only 1 mortality and with a 36% complication rate. Whenever possible, these patients had VATS procedures and thoracic epidural analgesia. The authors propose an absolute lower limit of acceptability for resection as a ppoFEV1 < 20%. It should be appreciated that this report is from a center with a very high volume of thoracic surgery and surgical outcomes for lung cancer are correlated to the volume of surgery. High-volume hospitals had complication and mortality rates (20% and 3%, respectively) that were approximately one-half of low-volume hospitals (44% and 6%) [10]. However, the majority of institutions currently perform VATS procedures without thoracic epidural analgesia.

The actual measured postoperative FEV1 will not be the same as the ppoFEV1 for several reasons. First, it is impossible to predict the actual intraoperative surgical trauma to the chest wall and residual lung segments. Most patients will have FEV1 values immediately postoperatively that are less than the ppoFEV1, and these will improve over a period of 6 months [11]. Second, emphysematous patients will tend to have a lung-volume reduction effect on the residual lobe(s) and may exceed their ppoFEV1 if a hyperinflated lobe is resected. The actual postoperative FEV1 has been shown to be a better predictor of outcome than the ppoFEV1; however, the actual postoperative FEV1 is not available preoperatively.

Absolute predicted postoperative values for FEV1 were used in the past to assess patients. Absolute limits for ppoFEV1 such as 0.8 L were suggested as the lower limits of acceptability for resection. However, absolute values for pulmonary function tests do not take into consideration the wide variation in the size of patients who present for thoracic surgery. An absolute FEV1 result of 1 L for an 80-year-old male 5 ft. (152 cm) in height is normal (100% of predicted), but an FEV1 of 1 L for a 6 ft. (183 cm) 50-year-old male is severely abnormal (24% predicted). It is important always to consider patients' spirometry results as a percentage of their predicted normal.

Patients at increased risk of respiratory complications (ppoFEV1 < 40%) should have complete pulmonary function testing in a pulmonary function laboratory which will include an assessment of lung volumes and airway resistance (Fig. 2.5). These are more sensitive than an examination of the FEV1/FVC ratio to distinguish between obstructive and restrictive lung pathologies and will confirm the clinical

Lung volumes and capacities

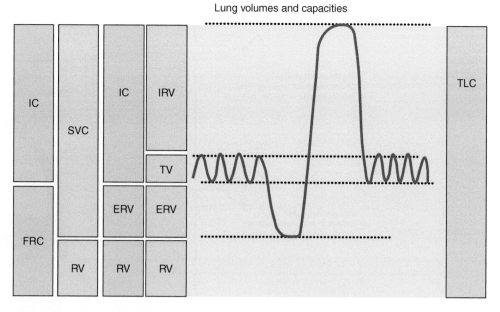

Fig. 2.5 Complete pulmonary function testing will provide data on lung volumes and capacities to differentiate obstructive from restrictive diseases. FRC = functional residual capacity; IC = inspiratory capacity; RV = residual volume; SVC = slow vital capacity; ERV = expiratory reserve volume; TV = tidal volume; IRV = inspiratory reserve volume; TLC = total lung capacity. Measuring closing volume and closing capacity requires insoluble gas washout techniques and is not included in routine pulmonary function testing. However, an appreciation of the variable relationship between closing capacity and FRC and the effects of anesthesia on FRC is essential for the anesthesiologist to understand the changes in gas exchange that occur during anesthesia (the reader is referred to Lumb AB, Nunn's Applied Respiratory Physiology, 7th ed., p. 58, Churchill Livingston Elsevier, Philadelphia, 2010, for a detailed explanation)

diagnosis of the underlying lung disease. Also this permits for optimization of intraoperative management during both two-lung and one-lung ventilation by individualization of settings for mechanical ventilation depending on the lung pathology [12]. There are two basic methods of measurement of lung volumes: insoluble gas dilution and plethysmography (Fig. 2.6). Plethysmography is the common method used in pulmonary function laboratories to measure lung volumes and has largely replaced insoluble gas dilution techniques. The difference (plethysmography-dilution) in measured lung volumes between the two techniques can be used to estimate the volume of bullae in the lung. Previously, maximal breathing capacity was also used to assess patients for pulmonary resection. This simple test was used in the era of pulmonary resection for tuberculosis and has been replaced by modern spirometry.

Pulmonary Parenchymal Function

As important to the process of respiration as the mechanical delivery of air to the distal airways is the subsequent ability of the lung to exchange oxygen and carbon dioxide between the pulmonary vascular bed and the alveoli. Traditionally arterial blood gas data such as $PaO_2 < 60$ mmHg or $PaCO_2 > 45$ mmHg have been used as cutoff values for pulmonary resection. Cancer resections have now been successfully done or even combined with volume reduction in patients who do not meet these criteria, although they remain useful as warning indicators of increased risk. The most useful test of the gas exchange capacity of the lung is the diffusing capacity for carbon monoxide (DLCO). The DLCO is a reflection of the total functioning surface area of alveolar-capillary interface. This simple noninvasive test which is included with spirometry and plethysmography by most pulmonary function laboratories is a useful predictor of perioperative morbidity and mortality [13]. The corrected DLCO can be used to calculate a post-resection (ppo) value using the same calculation as for the FEV1 (Fig. 2.7). A ppoDLCO <40% predicted correlates with both increased respiratory and cardiac complications and is, to a large degree, independent of the FEV1. The National Emphysema Treatment Trial has shown that patients with a preoperative FEV_1 or DLCO <20% had an unacceptably high perioperative mortality rate [14]. These can be considered as the absolute minimal values compatible with successful outcome. Complete pulmonary function testing, as performed in a pulmonary function laboratory, generates a report with

Fig. 2.6 Measurement of lung volumes is commonly performed with whole-body plethysmography with the patient seated in an airtight box. Lung volumes can be calculated from changes in the airway and box pressure since the volume of the box is known

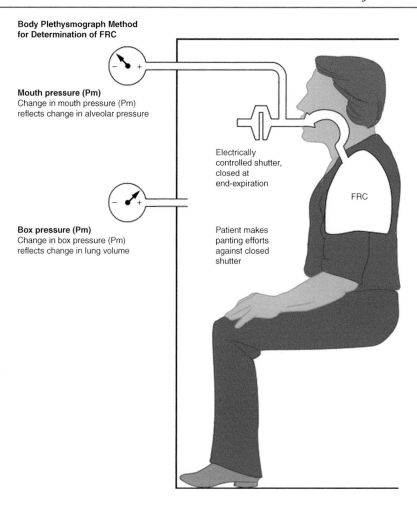

Body Plethysmograph Method for Determination of FRC

Mouth pressure (Pm)
Change in mouth pressure (Pm) reflects change in alveolar pressure

Electrically controlled shutter, closed at end-expiration

FRC

Box pressure (Pm)
Change in box pressure (Pm) reflects change in lung volume

Patient makes panting efforts against closed shutter

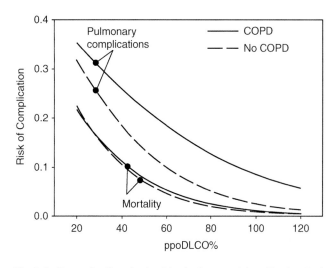

Fig. 2.7 Regression lines for the risk of pulmonary (upper lines) or fatal (lower lines) complications vs. predicted postoperative diffusing capacity for carbon monoxide (ppoDLCO%) following lung resection in patients with (solid lines) and without (dashed lines) chronic obstructive pulmonary disease (COPD). Note that both morbidity and mortality increase sharply when the ppoDLCO falls below a threshold value of 40%. (Reprinted from Ferguson and Vigneswaran [12] with permission)

often >12 test results (Fig. 2.8). Of these results, the two most valid tests for the anesthesiologist to use to assess perioperative risk are the % predicted FEV1 and DLCO. In evaluating a patient for pulmonary resection, the lower of the two values (ppoFEV1 or ppoDLCO) should be used as the guide for risk evaluation [15].

Cardiopulmonary Interaction

The final and perhaps most important assessment of respiratory function is an assessment of the cardiopulmonary interaction. Formal laboratory exercise testing is currently the "gold standard" for assessment of cardiopulmonary function [16], and the maximal oxygen consumption (VO$_2$ max) is the most useful predictor of post-thoracotomy outcome. The test is performed on a bicycle ergometer or treadmill. Resting measurements are made for 3–5 min. Three minutes of unloaded cycling is performed as a warm-up period. The workload is incremented at a rate designed to allow reaching maximum work capacity in 8–12 min. The test continues to

Test Performed		Pred.val	Pre BD		Post BD	
			Obs.	%Pred.val.	Obs.	%Pred.val.
Total Lung Capacity	(TLC), L	4.2	7.4	175	----	----
Functional Residual Capacity	(FRC), L	2.6	6.2	239	----	----
Inspiratory Capacity	(IC), L	1.6	1.2	74	----	----
Vital Capacity	(VC), L	2.4	1.5	63	----	----
Residual Volume	(RV), L	1.8	5.9	322	----	----
RV/TLC Ratio	(RV/TLC), %	43	80	184	----	----
Forced Vital Capacity	(FVC), L	2.4	1.5	62	----	----
Forced Exp. Volume In 1 sec.	(FEV1), L	1.7	0.6	34	----	----
FEV1/FVC Ratio	(FEV1/FVC), %	71	39	55	----	----
Max. Exp. Flow @ 50% VC	(V50), L/sec	2.4	0.17	7	----	----
Max. Exp. Flow @ 25% VC	(V25), L/sec	1.2	0.07	6	----	----
Mid Expiratory Flow 25-75%	(FEF 25–75), L/sec	2.0	0.2	12	----	----
Airway Resistance	(Raw), cmH2O/L/sec	0.7	2.5	387		
Max. Voluntary Ventilation	(MVV), L/min	50	----	----		
Lung Diffusion Capacity	(DLco), ml/min/mmHg	12.6	7.5	59	Normal limits: 75–125%	
VA @ BTPS from DLco	(VA@BTPS), L	4.2	2.5	60		

NOTE: %Pred. values are BOLD when outside of normal limits. (All except Raw & DLco values.)

Fig. 2.8 A copy of the pulmonary function laboratory test report for a patient with severe emphysema. Of the 15 different results in this report, the 2 results highlighted are the % predicted FEV1 and DLCO, which are the most useful tests for the anesthesiologist assessing a patient for possible pulmonary resection. This patient had taken a bronchodilator immediately before the test so the usual post-bronchodilator (Post BD) test was not repeated. Pred. val. = predicted value corrected for the patient's age, sex, and height. Obs. = patient's measured result. VA = the single-breath dilutional estimate of TLC from the DLCO

a point of symptom limitation (e.g., severe dyspnea) or discontinuation by medical staff (e.g., significant ECG abnormalities) or achievement of maximum predicted heart rate. Estimated VO_2 max is based on the patient's age, sex, and height. For sedentary males, estimated VO_2 max (ml/min) = (height [cm] – age [y]) × 20, i.e., for a 50-year-old male, height 170 cm, and weight 70 kg, the predicted VO_2 max = [(170–50) × 20]/70 = 34 ml/kg/min. For a sedentary woman, age 50, 160 cm, and 60 kg, estimated VO_2 max = [(160–50) × 14]/60 = 26 ml/kg/min (for comparison: the highest VO_2 max recorded in an exercise laboratory is 85 ml/kg/min by the American cyclist Lance Armstrong in 2005 [17]).

The risk of morbidity and mortality is unacceptably high if the preoperative VO_2 max is <15 ml/kg/min [18]. Few patients with a VO_2 max >20 ml/kg/min have respiratory complications. Exercise testing is particularly useful to differentiate between patients who have poor exercise tolerance due to respiratory and cardiac etiologies (Fig. 2.9). The anaerobic threshold measured during exercise testing has also been suggested as a predictor of postoperative complications [19]. The anaerobic threshold is the exercise level at which lactate begins to accumulate in the blood and anaerobic metabolism begins. The anaerobic threshold is approximately 55% of VO_2 max in untrained individuals but rises to >80% in trained athletes. The anaerobic threshold can be documented by repeated blood lactate analysis during exercise or by a threshold increase in CO_2 production above the initial respiratory quotient (ratio of CO_2 production to O_2 consumption, commonly approximately 0.8). A threshold value for AT of <11 ml/kg/min has been suggested as a marker for increased risk, but this has not been well validated [20]. Like FEV1 and DLCO, the VO_2 can be corrected for predicted values. A VO_2 max <60% predicted has been suggested as a threshold for increased risk; however, the % predicted VO_2 max has not been shown to be more useful than the absolute value of VO_2 max as a predictor postoperative of outcomes [21].

Complete laboratory exercise testing is time-consuming and thus expensive. It is generally not cost-effective to use as

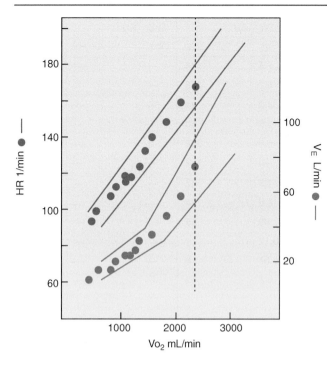

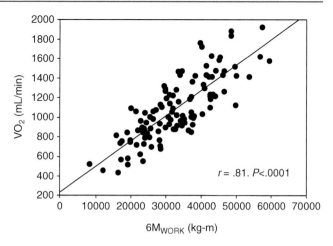

Fig. 2.10 The maximal oxygen consumption VO_2 (ml/min) shows a strong correlation with work ($6M_{WORK}$) for patients with moderate or severe COPD during a 6 min walk test. Work = distance traveled × weight (kg.m). A 70 kg patient who walks 450 m does 31,500 kg.m of work which correlates with an estimated VO_2 max of 1100 ml/min (or 16 ml/kg/min). A simple estimate of the VO_2 max can be made by diving the 6 min walk distance by 30 (i.e., 450 m/30 = 15 ml/kg/min). (Reprinted with permission from Carter et al. [21])

Fig. 2.9 A normal cardiopulmonary exercise test result. As the patient exercises, the increase in oxygen consumption (horizontal axis) is plotted against the heart rate (green dots, left vertical axis) and the minute ventilation (V_E, orange dots, right vertical axis). Normal responses for heart rate and ventilation lie within the green and orange lines. The vertical dashed line is the predicted upper limit of normal based on age. Patients with primarily cardiac causes for exercise limitation will show an excessive increase in heart rate with exercise. Patients with primarily respiratory limitation will show a disproportionate increase in ventilation. Patients with pulmonary vascular disease will have both abnormal heart rate and ventilation responses. (Reprinted with permission from Pearson GF, Thoracic Surgery 3rd. Ed. 2008, Elsevier, Philadelphia, PA)

a routine part of the preoperative assessment for all pulmonary resection patients. Several alternatives have been demonstrated to be valid surrogate tests for pre-thoracotomy assessment. The distance that a patient can walk during a 6-minute walk test (6MWT) shows an excellent correlation with VO_2 max and requires little or no laboratory equipment (Fig. 2.10). For patients with moderate or severe COPD, the 6MWT distance can be used to estimate the VO_2 max by dividing by a figure of 30 (i.e., 600-m distance is equivalent to a VO_2 max of 600/30 = 20 ml/kg/min) [22].

The 6MWT has become the most valid low-tech assessment of exercise capacity [23]. In a series of lobectomy patients, those with a preoperative 6MWT <500 m (approximate VO_2 max = 17 ml/kg) had a significantly higher rate of postoperative complications (61% vs. 37%) compared to those with a 6MWT >500 m [24].

Some centers also assess the fall in oximetry (SpO_2) during exercise. Patients with a decrease of SpO_2 > 4% during exercise (stair climbing 2 or 3 flights or equivalent) [25] are at increased risk of morbidity and mortality. Post-resection exer-

cise capacity can also be estimated based on the amount of functioning lung tissue removed (see Fig. 2.4). An estimated $ppoVO_2$ max <10 ml/kg/min can be considered a contraindication to pulmonary resection. In a small series [26], mortality was 100% (3/3) patients with a $ppoVO_2$ max <10 ml/kg/min.

The traditional, and still useful, test in ambulatory patients is stair climbing [27]. Stair climbing is done at the patient's own pace but without stopping and is usually documented as a certain number of flights. There is no exact definition for a "flight," but 20 steps at 6 in./step is a frequent value. The ability to climb five flights correlates with a VO_2 max >20 ml/kg/min, and climbing two flights corresponds to a maximal oxygen consumption (VO_2 max) of 12 ml/kg/min. A patient unable to climb two flights is extremely high risk [28].

After pulmonary resection, there is a degree of right ventricular dysfunction that seems to be in proportion to the amount of functioning pulmonary vascular bed removed. The exact etiology and duration of this dysfunction remain unknown. Clinical evidence of this hemodynamic problem is minimal when the patient is at rest but is dramatic when the patient exercises leading to elevation of pulmonary vascular pressures, limitation of cardiac output, and absence of the normal decrease in pulmonary vascular resistance usually seen with exertion [29].

Regional Lung Function

Prediction of post-resection pulmonary function can be further refined by assessment of the preoperative contribution of the lung or lobe to be resected by imaging of regional lung function [30]. If the lung region to be resected is nonfunctioning or minimally functioning, the prediction of postoperative function can be modified accordingly. This is particularly useful in pneumonectomy patients [31], and regional lung function imaging should be ordered for any potential pneumonectomy patient who has a preoperative FEV1 and/or DLCO <80% (i.e., if ppo values <40% predicted). Regional lung function imaging can be performed by three techniques: radionuclide ventilation/perfusion (V/Q) lung scanning, pulmonary quantitative CT scanning, or three-dimensional dynamic perfusion magnetic resonance imaging (MRI).

Ventilation/perfusion lung scanning is the gold standard. Regional ventilation is assessed by scanning after inhalation of a radiolabeled insoluble gas (commonly xenon-133). Regional lung perfusion is assessed by scanning after intravenous injection of radiolabeled particles that are trapped in the pulmonary capillaries (commonly technetium-99 m macroaggregated albumin) (Fig. 2.11). Actual postoperative lung function has shown a high correlation with predicted values based on preoperative V/Q scanning for FEV1 ($r = 0.92$), DLCO ($r = 0.90$), and VO$_2$ max ($r = 0.85$). Prediction is more accurate for post-pneumonectomy vs. post-lobectomy values. If there is a discrepancy between the ventilation and perfusion scan results, it is preferable to use the result which attributes the larger proportion of ventilation or perfusion to the diseased lung to estimate the post-resection pulmonary function.

Quantitative CT lung scans can be used to estimate post-resection values [32]. Each CT slice is quantified for areas of normal parenchyma, emphysema, and atelectasis. The contribution of each lobe or lung can be estimated based on the volume of normal parenchyma and then used to predict postoperative lung function. Quantitative CT primarily focuses on areas of ventilation and is more accurate for post-lobectomy vs. post-pneumonectomy values. Predicted postoperative values for FEV1 and DLCO were comparable to those derived from V/Q scans but less accurate for VO$_2$ max. This is a newer technique than V/Q scanning and requires specific imaging expertise. However, due to the routine preoperative CT scanning of most pulmonary resection patients, it may become more available.

Dynamic MRI uses estimates of regional pulmonary blood volume to assess regional blood flow [33]. This is the newest of the three techniques and is not widely used. It has shown a high level of correlation between predicted and actual values for postoperative FEV1. It has not been assessed for predicting DLCO or VO$_2$ max.

Split-Lung Function Studies

A variety of methods have been described to try and simulate the postoperative respiratory situation by preoperative unilateral exclusion of a lung or lobe with a double-lumen tube or bronchial blocker and/or by pulmonary artery balloon occlusion of a lung or lobe artery [34]. These tests have not shown sufficient predictive validity for universal adoption in lung resection patients. Lewis et al. [35] have shown that in a group of patients with COPD (ppoFEV1 < 40%) undergoing pneumonectomy, there were no significant changes in the pulmonary vascular pressures intraoperatively when the pulmonary artery was clamped but the right ventricular ejection fraction and cardiac output decreased. Echocardiography may offer more useful information than vascular pressure monitoring in these patients [36]. Split-lung function studies have been replaced in most centers by a combined assessment involving spirometry, DLCO, exercise tolerance, and imaging of regional lung function.

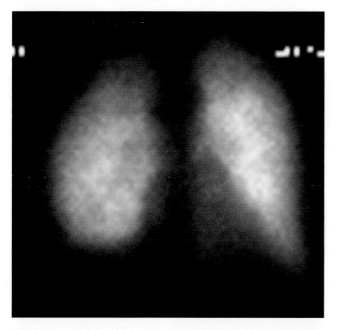

Fig. 2.11 Perfusion scan of a patient with a right lung tumor being assessed for possible pneumonectomy. The perfusion of the right lung (seen on the left in the image) was 37% and the left 63%. Preoperative FEV1 = 74% predicted and DLCO = 70%. Based on the anatomic number of subsegments to be excised, the predicted postoperative (ppo) FEV1 = 74 × 22/42 = 39% and the ppoDLCO = 70 × 22/42 = 37%. Using the regional lung imaging to predict postoperative values, the ppoFEV1 = 74 × 0.63 = 47% and the ppoDLCO = 70 × 0.63 = 44%, which are above the threshold values for increased perioperative risk

Combination of Tests

No single test of respiratory function has shown adequate validity as a sole preoperative assessment. Prior to surgery, an estimate of respiratory function in all three areas, lung mechanics, parenchymal function, and cardiopulmonary interaction, should be made for each patient. These three aspects of pulmonary function form the "three-legged stool" which is the foundation of pre-thoracotomy respiratory testing (Fig. 2.12). The three-legged stool can also be used to guide intra- and postoperative management (Fig. 2.13) and also to alter these plans when intraoperative surgical factors necessitate that a resection becomes more extensive than foreseen. If a patient has a ppoFEV1 > 40%, it should be possible for that patient to be extubated in the operating room at the conclusion of surgery assuming the patient is alert, warm, and comfortable ("AWaC"). Patients with a ppoFEV1 < 40% will usually comprise about one-fourth of an average thoracic surgical population. If the ppoFEV1 is >30% and exercise tolerance and lung parenchymal function exceed the increased risk thresholds, then extubation in the operating room should be possible depending on the status of associated medical

conditions. Those patients in this subgroup who do not meet the minimal criteria for cardiopulmonary and parenchymal function should be considered for staged weaning from mechanical ventilation postoperatively so that the effect of the increased oxygen consumption of spontaneous ventilation can be assessed. Patients with a ppoFEV1 20–30% and favorable predicted cardiorespiratory and parenchymal function can be considered for early extubation if thoracic epidural analgesia is used or if the resection is performed with VATS. Otherwise, these patients should have a postoperative staged weaning from mechanical ventilation. In the borderline group (ppoFEV1 30–40%), the presence of several associated factors and diseases which should be documented during the preoperative assessment will enter into the considerations for postoperative management (see below).

Jordan and Evans have outlined a protocol for planned elective admission of pulmonary resection patients to the intensive care unit postoperatively [37]. In their scheme, patients age ≥ 70 years or with fibrotic lung disease or with positive cardiovascular risk assessment or with an elevated ASA score or poor lung function (preoperative FEV <47%) would be admitted to ICU. Others would go to the recovery unit and then a monitored ward bed.

Concomitant Medical Conditions

Cardiac Disease

Cardiac complications are the second most common cause of perioperative morbidity and mortality in the thoracic surgical population. The commonest major cardiac complications are myocardial ischemia/infarction, arrhythmias, and heart failure. Several schemes have been developed to predict overall perioperative cardiac risk (see Table 2.2). The revised cardiac risk score [38] was developed for all major noncardiac sur-

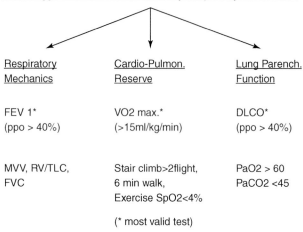

The "3-legged" Stool of Pre-thoracotomy Respiratory Assessment

Respiratory Mechanics	Cardio-Pulmon. Reserve	Lung Parench. Function
FEV 1* (ppo > 40%)	VO2 max.* (>15ml/kg/min)	DLCO* (ppo > 40%)
MVV, RV/TLC, FVC	Stair climb>2flight, 6 min walk, Exercise SpO2<4%	PaO2 > 60 PaCO2 <45
	(* most valid test)	

Fig. 2.12 The "three-legged stool" of pre-thoracotomy respiratory assessment involves evaluation of lung mechanical function, pulmonary parenchymal function, and cardiopulmonary interaction for each patient. The most valid test in each area is denoted by *. The threshold values below which risk increases are in parentheses. Ppo = predicted postoperative value as a % of the patient's normal value

Fig. 2.13 Anesthetic management guided by preoperative assessment and the amount of functioning lung tissue removed during surgery

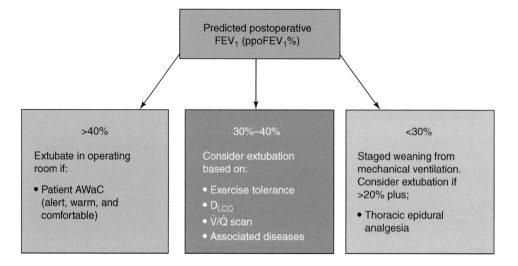

gery, and the thoracic revised cardiac risk score was developed specifically for thoracic surgery patients [39]. However, the predictive ability of these two scores in prospective studies has not always been high [40]. There is always a delay of several years between the time of development of these risk indices and actual prospective clinical studies. Their lack of accuracy in prospective studies may be due in part to the evolving underlying characteristics of the population with cardiac disease and also due to the rapid progress in preventing and treat-

ing major cardiovascular complications. Patients being treated with angiotensin-converting enzyme inhibitors or angiotensin II receptor blockers preoperatively are at an increased risk of postoperative cardiovascular complications if these medications are continued in the 24-h period before surgery [41].

Ischemia

Because the majority of pulmonary resection patients have a smoking history, they already have one risk factor for coronary artery disease (other factors include male sex, heredity, diabetes, obesity, high blood pressure, and elevated cholesterol). Elective pulmonary resection surgery is regarded as an "intermediate-risk" procedure in terms of perioperative cardiac ischemia [42]. The overall documented incidence of post-thoracotomy ischemia is 5% and peaks on days 2–3 postoperatively [43]. Beyond the standard history, physical, and electrocardiogram, further routine testing for cardiac disease does not appear to be cost-effective for all pre-thoracotomy patients.

The American College of Cardiology and American Heart Association have developed algorithms for preoperative cardiac investigations [44]. These guidelines are inclusive for all patients and not specific to thoracic surgery patients. A simplified algorithm, based on these recommendations, is presented in Fig. 2.14. Patients with intermediate clinical predictors of

Table 2.2 A comparison of the preoperative revised cardiac risk index and the thoracic revised cardiac risk index

Revised cardiac risk index (RCRI)	Points	Thoracic RCRI	Points
High-risk surgery (all major thoracic surgery)	1	Pneumonectomy	1.5
Coronary artery disease	1	Coronary artery disease	1.5
Congestive heart failure	1		
Cerebrovascular disease	1	Cerebrovascular disease	1.5
Diabetes on insulin	1		
Serum creatinine >2 mg/ml (>177 umol/L)	1	Serum creatinine >2 mg/ml (>177 umol/L)	1

Based on Licker et al. [95]

RCRI: 0–1 point = low-risk mortality (0.8%); 2 points = moderate risk (2.4%); >2 points = high risk (5.4%)

Thoracic RCRI: 0 points = low risk (<5%); 1–1.5 points = moderate risk (5–10%); ≥2 points = high risk (11–20%)

Fig. 2.14 An algorithm for cardiac risk assessment prior to noncardiac thoracic surgery. (Based on Fleisher et al. [43]). OR = operating room (i.e., proceed with surgery without further cardiac investigation). Cath. = coronary catheterization. Once a patient is found to have an abnormal result on noninvasive testing of myocardial perfusion, choosing the optimal pathway becomes complicated and requires a combined consultation with the surgeon, cardiologist, and patient

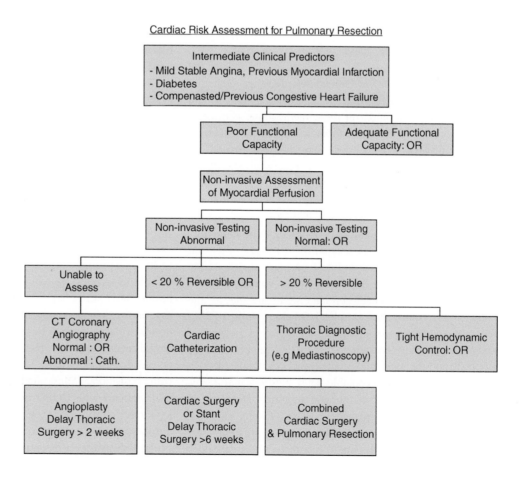

Cardiac Risk Assessment for Pulmonary Resection

increased cardiac risk (stable angina, diabetes, etc.) who have adequate functional capacity do not need further cardiac investigation prior to pulmonary surgery. Patients with these intermediate predictors and poor functional capacity should have noninvasive testing of myocardial perfusion at rest and during stress. The estimate of myocardial perfusion can be performed by nuclear medicine (technetium sestamibi or thallium injection) or transthoracic echocardiography at rest and during stress. The stress can be either with exercise or by injection of a coronary vasodilator (dipyridamole) or an inotrope (dobutamine). Based on the results from studies in vascular surgery [45], it can be extrapolated that patients with normal perfusion or who have areas of reversibility in <20% of myocardial segments can proceed to surgery without further cardiac investigation.

For patients who have major reversibility on a myocardial perfusion test, the diagnostic and therapeutic pathway is less clear. The standard recommendation is to proceed to cardiac catheterization. However, in individual circumstances, it could be an option to proceed with a minor diagnostic procedure (such as an endobronchial ultrasound or mediastinoscopy) first if there is a reasonable possibility that the patient may not have a resectable cancer. Or, it may be considered to proceed with the pulmonary resection with very tight perioperative hemodynamic control since it is not clear that coronary intervention improves perioperative outcome in patients who are not clear candidates for intervention outside the perioperative period [46]. The wisdom of elective perioperative β-blockade in these patients is debatable [47]. β-blockade may decrease the perioperative cardiac risk but increase the risk of stroke. Patients who have an indication for β-blockade apart from the perioperative context should be started and continued on these medications perioperatively, appreciating that many thoracic surgical patients have reactive airways disease that may be exacerbated by β-blockade. The use of β-blockers otherwise should be guided by specific hemodynamic indications.

For patients who require coronary catheterization, the results may necessitate angioplasty with or without stenting or coronary artery bypass surgery before or at the same time as pulmonary surgery (see Chap. 40). It is very important that the interventional cardiologist be made aware of the patient's diagnosis and the perioperative context prior to angiography. If bare metal coronary stents are placed, the patient will require dual antiplatelet therapy with a $P2Y_{12}$ receptor antagonist (clopidogrel, prasugrel, or ticagrelor) and aspirin for 4–6 weeks before the $P2Y_{12}$ inhibitor can be stopped (and the aspirin continued) preoperatively [48]. In some cases this is an acceptable delay before a major pulmonary resection or other thoracic surgeries. However, if drug-eluting stents are placed, the risk of stent stenosis, which is often fatal, is unacceptable if dual antiplatelet therapy is discontinued in the first 6 months. This is generally not an acceptable delay for cancer surgery.

Timing of lung resection surgery following a myocardial infarction is always a difficult decision. Limiting the delay to 4–6 weeks in a medically stable and fully investigated and optimized patient seems acceptable after myocardial infarction. The anesthesiologist needs to appreciate that the preoperative assessment and the therapeutic options for patients with significant coronary artery disease presenting for lung surgery are becoming very complicated and no single algorithm can be applied given the complexities of each individual case and the local availability of diagnostic equipment and personnel. Each of these patients needs to be managed by a team consultation that includes the thoracic surgeon, the cardiologist, the anesthesiologist, and the patient and family. The management of a patient who is discovered to have an incidental lung lesion during preoperative assessment for coronary artery or cardiac valvular surgery is discussed in Chap. 40.

Arrhythmias

The management of post-thoracotomy arrhythmias is discussed in Chap. 56. Arrhythmias are a common complication of pulmonary resection surgery, and the incidence is 30–50% of patients in the first week postoperatively when Holter monitoring is used [49]. Of these arrhythmias, 60–70% are atrial fibrillation. Several factors correlate with an increased incidence of arrhythmias; these include extent of lung resection (pneumonectomy 60% vs. lobectomy 40% vs. non-resection thoracotomy 30%), intrapericardial dissection, intraoperative blood loss, and age of the patient. Extrapleural pneumonectomy patients are a particularly high-risk group [50].

Two factors in the early post-thoracotomy period interact to produce atrial arrhythmias.

1. Increased flow resistance through the pulmonary vascular bed due to permanent (lung resection) or transient (atelectasis, hypoxemia) causes, with attendant strain on the right side of the heart.
2. Increased sympathetic stimuli and oxygen requirements, maximal on the second postoperative day as patients begin to mobilize.

In some pneumonectomy patients, the right heart may not be able to increase its output adequately to meet the usual postoperative stress. Transthoracic echocardiographic studies have shown that pneumonectomy patients develop an increase in right ventricular systolic pressure as measured by the tricuspid regurgitation jet (TRJ) on postoperative day 2 but not on day 1. An increase in TRJ velocity has been associated with post-thoracotomy supraventricular tachyarrhythmias [36]. Patients with COPD are more resistant to pharmacologic rate control when they develop post-thoracotomy atrial fibrillation and often require multiple drugs [51].

A wide variety of antiarrhythmics have been tried to decrease the incidence of atrial arrhythmias after lung surgery. The best known of these are digoxin preparations. It has been demonstrated that digoxin does not prevent arrhythmias after pneumonectomy or other intrathoracic procedures. Other agents which have been tried to prevent post-thoracotomy arrhythmias include β-blockers, verapamil, and amiodarone. All of these agents decrease arrhythmias in thoracic patients. At present the consensus statement of the American Association for Thoracic Surgery [52] recommends continuing β-blockers for patients who are already on them and intravenous magnesium for any patient who may have low or depleted serum and/or body stores of magnesium. In patients at high risk of postoperative supraventricular arrhythmias (lobectomy, pneumonectomy, esophagectomy, etc.), consideration of prophylactic therapy with diltiazem or amiodarone should be considered.

In one study [53] patients who subsequently developed atrial tachyarrhythmias could be identified in the early postoperative period by their right ventricular response to the withdrawal of supplemental oxygen. On the first postoperative day, a decrease of FiO_2 from 0.35 to 0.21 caused a significant rise of right ventricular end-diastolic pressure (RVEDP) in the patients who subsequently developed arrhythmias. Thoracic epidural analgesia (TEA) with local anesthetics may decrease the incidence and severity of arrhythmias. This effect is thought to be due to increasing myocardial refractory period, decreasing ventricular diastolic pressures, and improving endocardial/epicardial blood flow ratios [54].

Age

Perioperative management of the geriatric patient for thoracic surgery is discussed in Chap. 32. There is no maximum age that is a cutoff for pulmonary resection surgery. In one series, the operative mortality in a group of patients 80–92 years of age was 3%, a very respectable figure [55]. However, the rate of respiratory complications (40%) was double than expected in a younger population, and the rate of cardiac complications (40%), particularly arrhythmias, was nearly triple than which would be seen in younger patients. Naturally, the long-term (5-year) postoperative survival is decreased in the geriatric population [56].

In the elderly, thoracotomy should be considered a high-risk procedure for cardiac complications, and cardiopulmonary function is the most important part of the preoperative assessment. An algorithm for the cardiac assessment of the geriatric patient for thoracic surgery is presented in Fig. 2.15. Exercise tolerance seems to be the primary determinant of outcome in the elderly [57]. The ACC/AHA guidelines [43] suggest that with adequate functional capacity, patients with "intermediate" predictors of coronary artery disease do not need further cardiac assessment. However, this recommendation should not be extrapolated to elderly patients. The ACC/AHA guidelines define "adequate functional capacity"

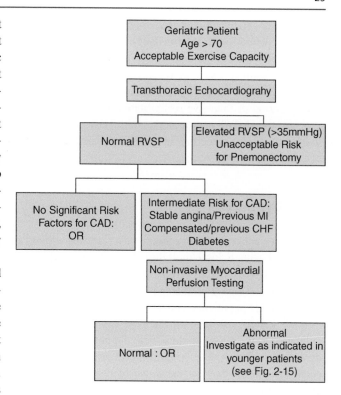

Fig. 2.15 An algorithm for preoperative cardiac investigation in a geriatric patient prior to pulmonary resection surgery. RVSP = right ventricular systolic pressure estimated by echocardiography. CAD = coronary artery disease. OR = operating room (i.e., proceed with surgery without further cardiac investigation)

Table 2.3 Energy consumption in metabolic equivalents (METS) of various activities

Activity	METS
Sitting quietly	1
Walking 1 block	2
Playing the accordion	2
Climbing 1 flight stairs	4
Sexual intercourse[a]	6
Bowling[a]	8
Ice hockey	8
Running 6 mph	10
Cross-country ski racing	14

MET = basal oxygen consumption = 3.5 ml/kg/min. Based on data from Hlatky MA, et al. Am J Cardiol 1989; 64: 651–654; Fleisher et al. [42]
[a]Bowling and sexual intercourse are given fewer METS in some classifications: Ainsworth BA, et al. Med Sci Sports Exerc 1992; 25: 71–80

as four metabolic equivalents (METS). One MET is the basal resting energy output which is commonly equated to an oxygen consumption of 3.5 ml/kg/min. Four METS are the equivalent of climbing one flight of stairs (Table 2.3) which does not represent an adequate level of exercise capacity for a geriatric patient for major pulmonary resection. The elderly should have, as a minimum cardiac investigation, a transthoracic echocardiogram, to rule out pulmonary hypertension. Although the mortality resulting from lobectomy among the elderly is acceptable, the mortality from pneumonectomy, particularly right pneumonectomy, is excessive [58]. Geriatric patients with intermediate-risk indicators of coronary artery disease should also have noninvasive myocardial perfusion testing. The elderly may benefit from efforts to increase exercise capacity preoperatively. Even a short, 7-day, period of intensive rehabilitation has been shown to increase the 6MWT and decrease pulmonary complications and length of stay in a group of geriatric patients having lung cancer surgery [59].

Renal Dysfunction

Renal dysfunction following pulmonary resection surgery is associated with a high mortality. In 1994, Golledge and Goldstraw [60] reported an incidence of renal impairment after thoracic surgery of 24% with a perioperative mortality of 19% (6/31) in patients who developed a significant elevation of serum creatinine in the post-thoracotomy period, compared to 0% (0/99) in those who did not show any renal dysfunction. Fortunately, a more recent study by Ishikawa et al. has shown that the incidence of postoperative renal injury in thoracic surgery (as defined by the acute kidney injury score) has decreased to 6% and there was no increase in mortality associated with acute kidney injury [61]. Factors associated with an elevated risk of renal impairment were identified in a multivariate analysis by Ahn et al. [62]. (see Table 2.4). Of note, in this study, there was no correlation between intraoperative fluid restriction and postoperative renal dysfunction. Nonsteroidal anti-inflammatory agents (NSAIDs) were not associated with renal impairment in this series but are clearly a concern in any thoracotomy patient with an increased risk of renal dysfunction. The high mortality in pneumonectomy patients from either renal failure or postoperative pulmonary edema emphasizes the importance of fluid management in these patients [63] and the need for close and intensive perioperative monitoring, particularly in those patients on diuretics or with a history of renal dysfunction. The importance of renal dysfunction, either preoperative dialysis or a serum creatinine value >2 mg/dL (>175 umol/L), as a predictor for prolonged length of stay after lobectomy was reconfirmed in an analysis of the Society of Thoracic Surgeons database for the period 2002–2006 [4].

Table 2.4 Factors associated with an increased risk of post-thoracotomy renal impairment

1. Decreased renal function + intraoperative hydroxyethyl starch
2. Preoperative angiotensin-converting enzyme inhibitor/angiotensin receptor blocker therapy
3. Pneumonectomy/esophagectomy
4. Diabetes mellitus
5. Cerebrovascular disease
6. Low serum albumin level

Chronic Obstructive Pulmonary Disease

The most common concurrent illness in the thoracic surgical population is chronic obstructive pulmonary disease (COPD) which incorporates three disorders: emphysema, peripheral airways disease, and chronic bronchitis. Any individual patient may have one or all of these conditions, but the dominant clinical feature is impairment of expiratory airflow [64]. Assessment of the severity of COPD has traditionally been on the basis of the FEV1% of predicted values. The American Thoracic Society categorizes stage I > 50% predicted FEV1% (this category previously included both "mild" and "moderate" COPD), stage II 35–50%, and stage III <35%. Life expectancy may be less than 3 years in stage III patients >60 years of age. Stage I patients should not have significant dyspnea, hypoxemia, or hypercarbia, and other causes should be considered if these are present. A complete discussion of perioperative management of patients with COPD is presented in Chap. 31. Of specific importance in the preoperative assessment of the patient with COPD prior to pulmonary resection is to assess for chronic carbon dioxide retention and to initiate therapy for any potentially treatable complications of COPD.

Carbon Dioxide Retention

Many stage II or III COPD patients have an elevated $PaCO_2$ at rest. It is not possible to differentiate these "CO_2 retainers" from non-retainers on the basis of history, physical examination, or spirometric pulmonary function testing [65]. This CO_2 retention seems to be more related to an inability to maintain the increased work of respiration (W_{resp}) required to keep the $PaCO_2$ normal in patients with mechanically inefficient pulmonary function and not primarily due to an alteration of respiratory control mechanisms. The $PaCO_2$ rises in these patients when a high FiO_2 is administered due to a relative decrease in alveolar ventilation [66] and an increase in alveolar dead space and shunt by the redistribution of perfusion away from lung areas of relatively normal V/Q matching to areas of very low V/Q ratio because regional hypoxic pulmonary vasoconstriction (HPV) is decreased [67] and also due to the Haldane effect [68]. However, supplemental oxygen must be administered to these patients postoperatively to prevent the hypoxemia associated with the unavoidable fall in functional residual capacity (FRC). The attendant rise in $PaCO_2$ should be anticipated and monitored. To identify these patients preoperatively, all stage II or III COPD patients need an arterial blood gas. Also, it is important to know the patient's baseline preoperative $PaCO_2$ to guide weaning if mechanical ventilation becomes necessary in the postoperative period.

Preoperative Therapy of COPD

There are four treatable complications of COPD that must be actively sought and therapy begun at the time of the initial pre-thoracotomy assessment. These are atelectasis, broncho-

Table 2.5 Concurrent problems that should be treated prior to anesthesia in COPD patients

Problem	Method of diagnosis
Bronchospasm	Auscultation
Atelectasis	Chest X-ray
Infection	History, sputum analysis
Pulmonary edema	Auscultation, chest X-ray

spasm, respiratory tract infections, and pulmonary edema (see Table 2.5). Atelectasis impairs local lung lymphocyte and macrophage function predisposing to infection [69]. Pulmonary edema can be very difficult to diagnose by auscultation in the presence of COPD and may present very abnormal radiological distributions (unilateral, upper lobes, etc.) [70]. Bronchial hyper-reactivity may be a symptom of congestive failure [71] or may represent an exacerbation of reversible airway obstruction. All COPD patients should receive maximal bronchodilator therapy as guided by their symptoms. Only 20–25% of COPD patients will respond to corticosteroids. In a patient who is poorly controlled on sympathomimetic and anticholinergic bronchodilators, a trial of corticosteroids may be beneficial [72]. It is not clear if corticosteroids are as beneficial in COPD as they are in asthma; pharmacotherapy for reactive airway diseases is discussed in Chap. 8.

Physiotherapy

Patients with COPD have fewer postoperative pulmonary complications when a perioperative program of intensive chest physiotherapy is initiated preoperatively [73]. Among COPD patients, those with excessive sputum benefit the most from chest physiotherapy. Among the different modalities available (cough and deep breathing, incentive spirometry, PEEP, CPAP, etc.), there is no clearly proven superior method. The important variable is the quantity of time spent with the patient and devoted to chest physiotherapy. Family members or non-physiotherapy hospital staff can easily be trained to perform effective preoperative chest physiotherapy, and this should be arranged at the time of the initial preoperative assessment. Even in the most severe COPD patient, it is possible to improve exercise tolerance with a physiotherapy program. Little improvement is seen before 1 month. In one small study, eight patients who had been refused pulmonary resection on the basis of poor pulmonary function were enrolled in a 4-week program of pulmonary rehabilitation. After the program, the mean 6-min walk test distance for the group increased 29%, and the mean FEV1 increased 5%. All eight patients then had lobectomies without any perioperative mortality [74].

Comprehensive 8–12-week programs of pulmonary rehabilitation involving physiotherapy, exercise, nutrition, and education have been clearly shown to improve functional capacity for patients with severe COPD [75]. These longer programs are generally not an option in resections for malignancy although for nonmalignant resections in severe COPD patients, rehabilitation should be considered. The concept of trying to increase a patient's exercise capacity preoperatively has recently been suggested. In a small randomized controlled trial, Morano et al. [76]. compared standard preoperative chest physiotherapy with pulmonary rehabilitation for a 4-week period before lung resection for cancer in patients with borderline pulmonary function (mean preoperative FEV1 50% predicted). Pulmonary rehabilitation involved 1-h sessions 5 days/week and included periods of interval training to 80% maximal capacity. The 6MWT distance increased significantly in the rehabilitation group (mean 425 to 475 m, $p < 0.05$) vs. no change in the control group, and there was a significant decrease in postoperative morbidity and length of stay (7.8 vs. 12.2 days, $p = 0.04$).

Restrictive Lung Diseases

Restrictive lung physiology is characterized on pulmonary function testing by decreased lung volumes but preserved forced expiratory volume in 1 second to forced vital capacity (FEV1/FVC) ratio. This pattern can be caused by diseases of the lung parenchyma (e.g., interstitial lung diseases), extrinsic problems affecting the pleura or chest wall (e.g., pleural effusions, scoliosis, severe obesity), or disorders causing weakness of the muscles of breathing (e.g., myasthenia gravis, Guillain-Barré syndrome).

Interstitial lung diseases (ILDs) are a heterogeneous group of disorders characterized by inflammation and fibrosis of the lung parenchyma affecting the alveolar-capillary unit. They are usually discerned from other restrictive lung diseases by an impaired diffusion capacity of the lungs for carbon monoxide (DLCO). The most common identifiable causes are related to exposure to occupational or environmental agents (e.g., silica, asbestos), drug-related toxicity (e.g., bleomycin, amiodarone), or radiation-induced lung injury. However, for a significant proportion of patients, a specific cause is never identified. These patients are broadly grouped into the diagnostic category of idiopathic interstitial pneumonia (IIP). There are multiple subcategories of IIP, and unfortunately the terminology has been confusing and overlapping in the literature. Preoperative risk assessment for pulmonary resection in patients with restrictive lung disease should proceed as outlined above with evaluation of ppoFEV1, ppoDLCO, and exercise capacity.

Among the subtypes of IIP, the one which is particularly relevant to the anesthesiologist is idiopathic pulmonary fibrosis (IPF) which is also called usual interstitial pneumonia (UIP). Differentiation of IPF from the other types of IIP is based on a combination of clinical and radiologic findings and may require histologic confirmation [77]. One study of pulmonary resections for non-small cell lung cancer in patients with IIP found significant differences in short- and long-term morbidity and mortality between an IPF group ($n = 46$) and non-IPF ($n = 57$) patients. Although other pre- and intraoperative risk factors were equal, the IPF patients tended to have a lower FRC with a preservation of the FEV1/FRC ratio. IPF patients had a higher 30-day mortality (7%) than non-IPF patients (0%) and a lower 5-year survival: 22% vs. 53%. Patients with IPF seem to be particularly at risk for perioperative lung injury during pulmonary resection [78].

Pulmonary Hypertension

A detailed discussion of the management of the patient with pulmonary hypertension for thoracic surgery is presented in Chap. 34. In one series, 19/279 patients having a lobectomy for cancer had pulmonary hypertension (right ventricular systolic pressure >36 mmHg on preoperative transthoracic echocardiography). Although there were trends toward increased morbidity and mortality in the pulmonary hypertension group, they did not reach statistical significance in this small sample. Pulmonary hypertension is not an automatic contraindication to thoracic surgery.

Smoking

Pulmonary complications are decreased in thoracic surgical patients who cease smoking for >4 weeks before surgery [79]. Carboxyhemoglobin concentrations decrease if smoking is stopped >12 h [80]. It is extremely important for patients to avoid smoking postoperatively. Smoking leads to a prolonged period of tissue hypoxemia. Wound tissue oxygen tension correlates with wound healing and resistance to infection. Wound healing is improved in patients who stop smoking >4 weeks preoperatively [81]. There is no rebound increase in pulmonary complications if patients stop for shorter (<8 weeks) periods before surgery [82]. The balance of evidence suggests that thoracic surgical patients should be counseled to stop smoking and advised that the longer the period of cessation, the greater the risk reduction for postoperative pulmonary complications [83]. Levels of successful cessation of smoking can exceed 50% at 1 year with a program of counseling and nicotine replacement [84].

Type of Surgical Procedure

It is important for the anesthesiologist to have an appreciation of the implications of the proposed type and extent of surgical resection. Pneumonectomy is the classic pulmonary resection operation for lung cancer. Prediction of postoperative pulmonary function and risks with a combination of pulmonary function tests and ventilation/perfusion scans, as outlined earlier, is accurate in pneumonectomy patients.

Even in geriatric patients, short-term morbidity and mortality are acceptable using these pre-resection prediction criteria [85]. It has been suggested that a preoperative VO$_2$ max of 20 ml/kg/min should be used as the lower limit for acceptability in pneumonectomy patients [86]. However, it is now appreciated that many patients do not have an acceptable quality of life after a pneumonectomy [87]. Because of this, surgeons are more likely to use lung-sparing procedures such as a bi-lobectomy or bronchial-sleeve lobectomy whenever possible to avoid a pneumonectomy. The frequency of pneumonectomies as a percentage of all lung cancer operations has decreased in the past 20 years from approximately 20% to 5% [88].

A bi-lobectomy is a useful alternative procedure to a right pneumonectomy when surgically possible. The complication rate following bi-lobectomies is intermediate between that for lobectomies and pneumonectomies and lower for upper bi-lobectomies than lower bi-lobectomies [89]. A nonanatomic wedge resection of a lung cancer is also a possibility in high-risk cases. Although the cure rate is less than an anatomical resection, there is a lower short-term morbidity and mortality in high-risk cases [90].

Minimally invasive video-assisted thoracoscopic surgery (VATS) or robotic surgeries are rapidly becoming the commonest approaches for a majority of pulmonary resections. There is a general consensus that patients have fewer complications and less postoperative pain when comparable resections are performed by VATS than by open thoracotomy [91]. Increased-risk patients with a ppoFEV1 or ppoDLCO <40% seem to have a significantly lower morbidity and mortality after lobectomy via VATS vs. thoracotomy [92]. A non-randomized comparison of matched patients having lobectomies via thoracotomy ($n = 167$) or VATS ($n = 173$) suggested that the threshold for increased risk could be shifted down from a ppoFEV1 of 40% in the thoracotomy patients to 30% in the VATS patients (see Fig. 2.16) [93]. It was not possible to identify a lower threshold of ppoDLCO for complications after VATS lobectomy (see Fig. 2.17); however, there were very few patients with a ppoDLCO <40% in this population.

Combined Strategies for Preoperative Assessment

Several multisystemic schemes to assess perioperative risk and guide preoperative evaluation have been developed. The American College of Surgeons has developed an online risk calculator based on the National Surgical Quality Improvement Program (NSQIP) database [94] (http://risk-calculator.facs.org/RiskCalculator). This calculator includes 21 preoperative factors (demographics, comorbidities, and procedure). It allows for individualized estimation of risks of

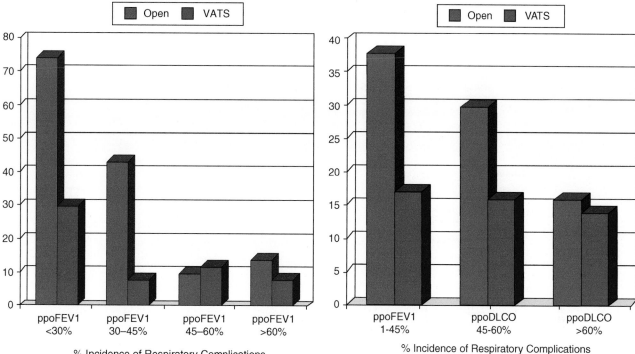

Fig. 2.16 A comparison of the incidence of postoperative respiratory complications after open (thoracotomy) vs. VATS lobectomies for lung cancer. ppo = predicted postoperative value. FEV1 = forced expiratory volume in 1 second. This was a non-randomized retrospective study. It appears that the threshold for increased risk may have decreased from <40% ppoFEV1 in the open group to <30% in the VATS group. (Based on data from Berry et al. [93])

Fig. 2.17 A comparison of the incidence of postoperative respiratory complications after open (thoracotomy) vs. VATS lobectomies for lung cancer. ppo = predicted postoperative value. DLCO = diffusing capacity for carbon monoxide. This was a non-randomized retrospective study. It appears there is a threshold for increased risk in open procedures under 60% ppoDLCO. A threshold for VATS procedures could not be identified; however, there were very few patients with a ppoDLCO <40% in this study. (Based on data from Berry [93])

mortality and specific major complications (see Fig. 2.18). Although this tool is very useful to explain to patients and families the perioperative risks from a specific operation, it does not allow for a stratified approach to preoperative evaluation for an individual patient. A combined cardiorespiratory algorithm specific to patients having lung cancer surgery is presented in Fig. 2.19 [95].

Perioperative Considerations in Thoracic Malignancies

The majority of patients presenting for major pulmonary surgery will have some type of malignancy. Because the different types of thoracic malignancies have varying implications for both surgery and anesthesia, it is important for the anesthesiologist to have some knowledge of the presentation and biology of these cancers. By far the most common tumor is lung cancer. It is estimated that at present rates over 210,000 new cases of lung cancer occur in the United States annually. Of these only 26% will be resectable. However, this represents >55,000 patients/year who can be offered potentially curative surgery [96]. Lung cancer is currently the leading cause of cancer deaths in both sexes in North America

subsequent to the peak incidence of smoking in the period 1940–1970 (Fig. 2.20) [97]. The mortality rate from lung cancer has shown a slight decrease in the last decade for men related to decreased smoking rates and appears to have plateaued in women.

Lung cancer is broadly divided into small-cell lung cancer (SCLC) and non-small cell lung cancer (NSCLC), with about 75–80% of these tumors being NSCLC. Other less common and less aggressive tumors of the lung include the carcinoid tumors (typical and atypical) and adenoid cystic carcinoma. In comparison with lung cancer, primary pleural tumors are rare. They include the solitary fibrous tumors of the pleura (previously referred to as benign mesotheliomas) and malignant pleural mesothelioma (MPM). Asbestos exposure is implicated as a causative effect in up to 80% of MPM. A dose-response relationship is not always apparent, and even brief exposures can lead to the disease. An exposure history is often difficult to obtain because the latent period before clinical manifestation of the tumor may be as long as 40–50 years.

Tobacco smoke (both primary and secondhand) is responsible for approximately 90% of all lung cancers, and

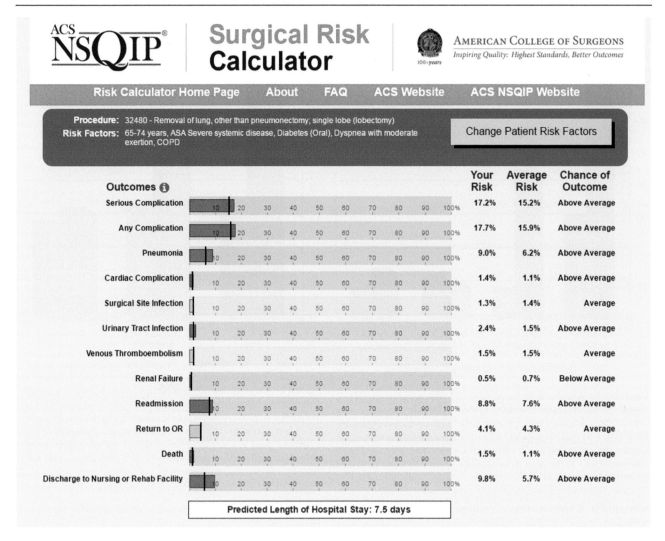

Fig. 2.18 A calculation of perioperative risks for a theoretical 70-year-old, nonobese, male with COPD and non-insulin-dependent diabetes scheduled for a pulmonary lobectomy using the NSQIP web-based cal- culator (http://riskcalculator.facs.org/RiskCalculator) (Note there is no quantification of the severity of COPD using this calculator)

the epidemiology of lung cancer follows the epidemiology of cigarette smoking with approximately a three-decade lag time [98]. Other environmental causes include asbestos and radon gas (a decay product of naturally occurring uranium) which act as cocarcinogens with tobacco smoke. For a pack-a-day cigarette smoker, the lifetime risk of lung cancer is approximately 1 in 14. Smoking cessation reduces the risk of lung cancer but never to that for never smokers. Assuming current mortality patterns continue, cancer will pass heart disease as the leading cause of death in North America in this decade.

Prior to pulmonary resection, lung cancer patients will undergo staging tests to determine the extent of their cancer. These will include radiographic tests such as CT scan, positron emission tomography (PET), and in some cases brain magnetic resonance imaging. Additionally, many patients will have invasive mediastinal staging to determine histo- logically whether or not the cancer has spread to the mediastinal lymph nodes. In general, if mediastinal lymph nodes contain cancer, primary surgical resection is not recommended. Cervical mediastinoscopy which is performed under general anesthesia has been the gold standard for invasive mediastinal staging. More recently, endobronchial ultrasound with transbronchial needle aspiration (EBUS-TBNA) and endoscopic ultrasound mediastinal node biopsy have become popular. These procedures may be done under topical anesthesia with intravenous sedation and are less invasive than mediastinoscopy. Regardless of the technique, the indication for invasive mediastinal staging is the same. Any patient with enlarged mediastinal nodes on CT or FDG-avid ("hot") nodes on PET scan should have invasive staging. Additional indications include T3 or T4 tumors, central tumors, and those with suspicion of hilar lymph node involvement [99].

Fig. 2.19 A flow diagram for preoperative evaluation for lung cancer patients. RCRI = Revised Cardiac Risk Index (see Table 2.2). MET = basal oxygen consumption (3.5 ml/kg/min). Ascent = height in meters nonstop stair climbing (Reproduced with permission from Licker et al. [95])

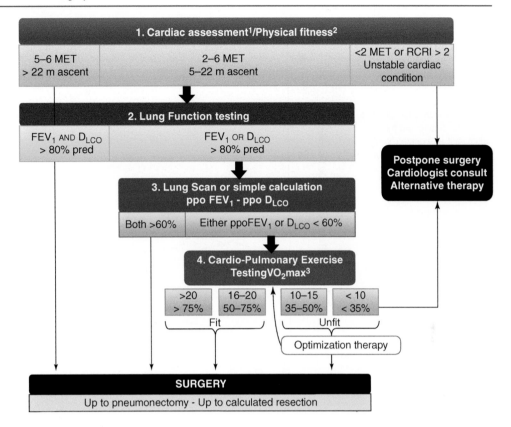

Non-Small Cell Lung Cancer (NSCLC)

This pathologically heterogeneous group of tumors includes squamous cell, adenocarcinoma, and large-cell carcinoma with several subtypes and combined tumors (Table 2.6). This represents the largest grouping of lung cancers and the vast majority of those that present for surgery. They are grouped together because the surgical therapy, and by inference the anesthetic implications, is similar and depends on the stage of the cancer at diagnosis (Tables 2.6, 2.7, and 2.8). Survival can approach 80% for stage I lesions. Unfortunately, 70–80% patients present with advanced disease (stage III or IV). Overall 5-year survival with surgery for NSCLC approaches 40%. This seemingly low figure must be viewed in the light of an estimated 5-year survival without surgery of <10%.

Although it is not always possible to be certain of the pathology of a given lung tumor preoperatively, many patients will have a known tissue diagnosis at the time of preanesthetic assessment on the basis of prior cytology, bronchoscopy, mediastinoscopy, or transthoracic needle aspiration. This is useful information for the anesthesiologist to obtain preoperatively. Specific anesthetic implications of the different types of lung cancer are listed in Table 2.9.

Adenocarcinoma

Adenocarcinoma is currently the most common NSCLC in both sexes. These tumors tend to be peripheral. Tumors identified by CT screening are most often in the adenocarcinoma spectrum. This is partly due to their increased frequency in general but also the slower growth rate of these tumors. Adenocarcinomas have been reclassified to include a broad spectrum of tumors including those previously classified as bronchoalveolar carcinoma (BAC). This spectrum of disease ranges from noninvasive carcinoma in situ to invasive adenocarcinomas. The biologic behavior can be very indolent such as in lepidic predominant (the former BAC) to aggressive with a high propensity for recurrence and metastases (e.g., papillary and micropapillary). With improved CT techniques, it is now recognized that these tumors may be multifocal such that multiple lesions actually represent multiple primary tumors rather than metastases. One variant of adenocarcinoma warrants further discussion: the pneumonic type lepidic variant which mimics pneumonia radiographically and is often associated with bronchorrhea. Because of its low potential to spread outside of the lungs, multifocal BAC may be treated by lung transplantation in selected cases [100].

Adenocarcinoma may invade extrapulmonary structures, including the chest wall, diaphragm, and pericardium. The majority of Pancoast tumors (see Chap. 37) are now due to adenocarcinomas. A variety of paraneoplastic metabolic factors can be secreted by adenocarcinomas such as growth hormone and corticotropin. Hypertrophic pulmonary osteoarthropathy (HPOA) is particularly associated with adenocarcinoma.

Fig. 2.20 Age-adjusted
mortality rates for women (**a**)
and men (**b**) in the United
States 1930–2008.
Respiratory malignancies
remain the leading cause of
cancer deaths in both sexes,
but the incidence has begun to
decrease in men and has
plateaued in women (National
Health Statistics of the United
States 2016. www.cancer.org)

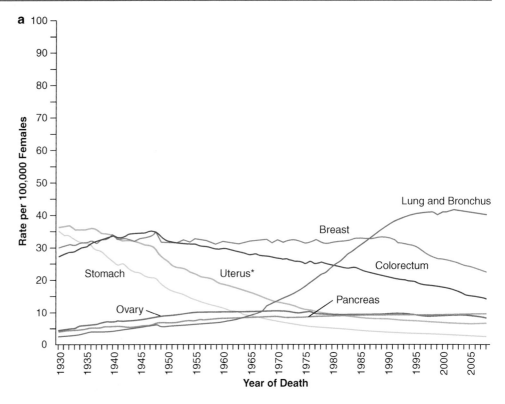

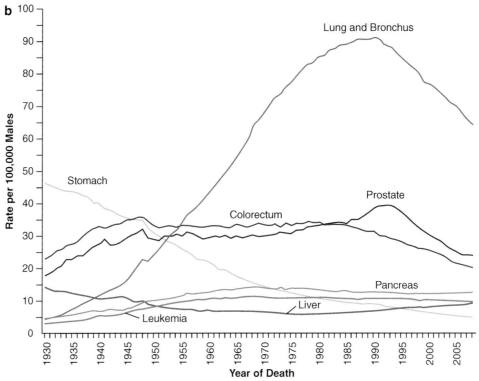

Table 2.6 Frequency of cell types of primary lung cancers

Histologic type	Proportion (%)
Adenocarcinoma	40
Squamous cell	27
Small cell	19
Large cell	8
Bronchoalveolar cell	4
Mixed adeno/squamous	2
Carcinoid	1

Based on Ref. [98]

Table 2.7 Proposed revised non-small cell lung cancer staging

Stage IA	T1a, b	N0	M0
Stage IB	T2a	N0	M0
Stage IIA	T1a, b	N1	M0
	T2a	N1	M0
	T2b	N0	M0
Stage IIB	T2b	N1	M0
	T3	N0	M0
Stage IIIA	T1, T2	N2	M0
	T3	N1, N2	M0
	T4	N0, N1	M0
Stage IIIB	T4	N2	M0
	Any T	N3	M0
Stage IV	Any T any N	M1a, b	

T1a: ≤ 2 cm; T1b: >2, ≤3 cm

T2a: >3 cm, ≤5 cm; T2b: >5–7 cm

T3: >7 cm

T3: Invasion of the chest wall, diaphragm, mediastinal pleura, phrenic nerve, parietal pericardium, tumor in the main bronchus <2 cm from the carina

T3: Separate tumor nodule in the same lobe (satellite)

T4: Invades the mediastinum, heart, great vessels, trachea, recurrent laryngeal nerve, esophagus, vertebral body, carina

N0

N1: Metastasis in ipsilateral peribronchial, hilar, or intrapulmonary nodes

N2: Metastasis in ipsilateral mediastinal nodes or subcarinal nodes

N3: Metastasis in contralateral mediastinal nodes or ipsilateral or contralateral supraclavicular/scalene nodes

M1a: Malignant pleural effusion, malignant pericardial effusion, separate tumor nodule in the contralateral lung

M1b: Distant metastases

[a]Goldstraw P, Crowley J, Chansky K, Girous DJ, Groome PA, Rami-Porta R, Postmus PE, Rusch V, Sobin L on behalf of the IASLC International Staging Committee. J Thorac Oncol 2007; 2:706–14

Squamous Cell Carcinoma

This is the subgroup of NSCLC most strongly linked to cigarette smoking. The tumors tend to grow to a large size, are often central, and metastasize later than others. They tend to cause symptoms related to local effects of a large tumor mass with a dominant endobronchial component, such as cavitation, hemoptysis, obstructive pneumonia, superior vena cava syndrome, and involvement of the

Table 2.8 Indications for surgery in non-small cell lung cancer

Stage I a and b	Primary resection, no postoperative chemo–/radiotherapy
Stage II	Primary resection, adjuvant postoperative chemotherapy
Stage IIIa, N2	Definitive chemoradiotherapy
In select patients induction chemoradiotherapy followed by resection in patients with stable or responding disease	
(For patients with N2 disease identified at thoracotomy: Postoperative chemotherapy, possibly radiation)	
Stage IIIb	Surgery rarely indicated. Chemoradiotherapy
Resection of select T4, N0–1, M0 tumors	
Stage IV	Palliative therapy. Possible exception: Selected patients with a resected isolated cerebral metastasis

Table 2.9 Anesthetic considerations for different types of lung cancer

Type	Considerations
Squamous cell	Central lesions (predominantly)
	Mass effects: obstruction, cavitation
	Hypercalcemia
	Hypertrophic pulmonary osteoarthropathy
Adenocarcinoma	Peripheral lesions
	Metastases (distant)
	Growth hormone, corticotropin
Small cell	Central lesions (predominantly)
	Few surgically treatable
	Paraneoplastic syndromes
	Lambert-Eaton syndrome
	Fast growth rate
	Early metastases
Carcinoid	Proximal, intrabronchial
	Predominantly benign
	No association with smoking
	5-year survival >90%
	Carcinoid syndrome (rarely)
Mesothelioma	Intraoperative hemorrhage
	Direct extension to the diaphragm, pericardium, etc.

mainstem bronchus, trachea, carina, and main pulmonary arteries. Hypercalcemia is specifically associated with this cell type due to elaboration of a parathyroid-like factor and not due to bone metastases.

Large Cell Undifferentiated Carcinoma

This is the least common of the NSCLCs. They tend to present as large, often cavitating, peripheral tumors. Their rapid growth rate may lead to widespread metastases, similar to adenocarcinoma.

Small-Cell Lung Cancer

This tumor of neuroendocrine origin is considered metastatic on presentation and is usually regarded as a medical, not a surgical disease [101]. Previously, the staging system for small-cell lung cancer was divided simply into limited stage and extensive stage; however, it is now staged according to the TNM system used for NSCLC. Limited disease is defined as disease confined to one hemithorax that may be encompassed by one radiotherapy field. Treatment of limited-stage SCLC with combination chemotherapy (etoposide/cisplatin or cyclophosphamide/doxorubicin/vincristine) gives objective response rates in over 80% of patients. In addition, these patients typically receive radical radiotherapy to the primary lung tumor and prophylactic cranial irradiation. Despite this initial response, the tumor invariably recurs and is quite resistant to further treatment. The overall survival rate is no better than 10%. Extensive-stage disease is treated with chemotherapy and palliative radiation as needed.

There are three situations in which surgery for SCLC might be considered. In the rare instance in which a solitary pulmonary nodule is diagnosed as SCLC (very limited stage or stage I), treatment should be surgical resection followed by chemotherapy. Salvage resection of a residual mass following chemotherapy for limited-stage disease may offer some long-term survival in selected cases. Many of these patients will have mixed SCLC/NSCLC in which the small-cell component has responded to chemotherapy and the non-small cell component is then resected. The third situation wherein patients with treated small-cell lung cancer should be considered for surgery is the finding of a new lung tumor. Patients with treated small cell have an increased rate of second primary lung cancers, which are usually non-small cell.

SCLC is known to cause a variety of paraneoplastic syndromes due to the production of peptide hormones and antibodies. The commonest of these is hyponatremia usually due to an inappropriate production of antidiuretic hormone (SIADH). Cushing's syndrome and hypercortisolism through ectopic production of adrenocorticotropic hormone (ACTH) are also commonly seen.

A well-known but rare neurologic paraneoplastic syndrome associated with small-cell lung tumors is the Lambert-Eaton myasthenic syndrome due to impaired release of acetylcholine from nerve terminals. This typically presents as proximal lower limb weakness and fatigability that may temporarily improve with exercise. The diagnosis is confirmed by electromyography (EMG) showing increasing amplitude of unusual action potentials with high-frequency stimulation and by serum antibodies. Similar to true myasthenia gravis patients (see Chap. 15), myasthenic syndrome patients are extremely sensitive to non-depolarizing muscle

relaxants. However, unlike true myasthenics, they respond poorly to anticholinesterase reversal agents [102]. Clinical differences between myasthenia and the myasthenic syndrome are discussed in Chap. 15 [103]. Diaminopyridine has been reported to be useful both as a maintenance medication and to reverse residual postoperative neuromuscular blockade in these patients [104]. Other treatments of the Lambert-Eaton syndrome include plasmapheresis, immunoglobulin, and guanidine. It is important to realize that there may be subclinical involvement of the diaphragm and muscles of respiration. Thoracic epidural analgesia has been used following thoracotomy in these patients without complication. These patients' neuromuscular function may improve following resection of the lung cancer. A patient with a lung cancer and unusual symptoms of weakness should be referred to neurology to rule out myasthenic syndrome. Non-depolarizing muscle relaxants should be avoided, if possible, during anesthesia in these patients.

Carcinoid Tumors

Carcinoid tumors are low-grade neuroendocrine malignancies and may be typical or atypical. Typical carcinoid tumors are most commonly found in the central airways and may present with obstructive symptoms or hemoptysis. Bronchoscopic biopsy or resection may cause significant bleeding. Five-year survival following resection for typical carcinoid exceeds 90%. Metastases to lymph nodes or distant sites are rare. Similarly, the carcinoid syndrome, which is caused by the ectopic synthesis of vasoactive mediators, is rare in pulmonary carcinoid unless the tumor is very large. Carcinoid syndrome is usually seen with carcinoid tumors of gut origin that have metastasized to the liver. Atypical carcinoid tumors are more often peripheral and are more aggressive and have a reduced survival rate. They often metastasize both regionally and systemically.

Perioperative management of intrathoracic atypical carcinoid tumors is discussed in Chap. 15. These tumors can precipitate an intraoperative hemodynamic crisis or coronary artery spasm even during bronchoscopic resection [105]. The anesthesiologist should be prepared to deal with severe hypotension that may not respond to the usual vasoconstrictors and will require the use of the specific antagonists octreotide or somatostatin [106].

Pleural Tumors

Solitary fibrous tumors of the pleura are usually large, space-occupying masses that are usually attached to the visceral pleura. They can be either benign or malignant, but most are easily resected with good results.

Malignant pleural mesotheliomas are strongly associated with exposure to asbestos fibers. Their incidence in Canada has almost doubled in the past 15 years. With the phasing out of asbestos-containing products and the long latent period between exposure and diagnosis, the peak incidence is not predicted for another 10–20 years. The tumor initially proliferates within the visceral and parietal pleura, typically forming a bloody effusion. Patients present with shortness of breath or dyspnea on exertion, dry cough, or pain. Thoracentesis often relieves the symptoms but rarely provides a diagnosis. Pleural biopsy by video-assisted thoracoscopy is most efficient way to secure a diagnosis, and talc poudrage is performed under the same anesthetic to treat the effusion.

Malignant pleural mesotheliomas respond poorly to therapy, and the median survival is less than 1 year. In patients with very early disease, extrapleural pneumonectomy may be considered, but it is difficult to know whether survival is improved. Alternatively, pleurectomy-decortication has been increasingly used. Although by definition a palliative procedure, it is much less morbid than EPP and offers potential for more durable palliation. Recently, several groups have reported improved results with combinations of radiation, chemotherapy, and surgery. Extrapleural pneumonectomy is an extensive procedure that is rife with potential complications, both intra- and postoperative [107]. Blood loss from the denuded chest wall or major vascular structures is always a risk. Complications related to resection of diaphragm and pericardium are additional risks to that of pneumonectomy. Perioperative management for extrapleural pneumonectomy is discussed in Chap. 36.

Preoperative Assessment of the Patient with Lung Cancer

At the time of initial assessment, cancer patients should be assessed for the "four M's" associated with malignancy (Table 2.10): mass effects, metabolic abnormalities, metastases, and medications. The prior use of medications which can exacerbate oxygen-induced pulmonary toxicity such as

Table 2.10 Anesthetic considerations in lung cancer patients (the "four M's")

1. Mass effects: Obstructive pneumonia, lung abscess, SVC syndrome, tracheobronchial distortion, Pancoast's syndrome, recurrent laryngeal nerve or phrenic nerve paresis, chest wall or mediastinal extension
2. Metabolic effects: Lambert-Eaton syndrome, hypercalcemia, hyponatremia, Cushing's syndrome
3. Metastases: Particularly to the brain, bone, liver, and adrenal
4. Medications: Chemotherapy agents, pulmonary toxicity (bleomycin, mitomycin), cardiac toxicity (doxorubicin), renal toxicity (cisplatin)

bleomycin should be considered [108]. Bleomycin is not used to treat primary lung cancers, but patients presenting for excision of lung metastases from germ-cell tumors will often have received prior bleomycin therapy. Although the association between previous bleomycin therapy and pulmonary toxicity from high inspired oxygen concentrations is well documented, none of the details of the association are understood (i.e., safe doses of oxygen or safe period after bleomycin exposure). The safest anesthetic management is to use the lowest FiO2 consistent with patient safety and to closely monitor oximetry in any patient who has received bleomycin. We have seen lung cancer patients who received preoperative chemotherapy with cisplatin, which is mildly nephrotoxic, and then developed an elevation of serum creatinine when they received nonsteroidal anti-inflammatory analgesics (NSAIDs) postoperatively. For this reason, we do not routinely administer NSAIDs to patients who have been treated recently with cisplatin.

Postoperative Analgesia

The strategy for postoperative analgesia should be developed and discussed with the patient during the initial preoperative assessment; full discussion of postoperative analgesia is presented in Chap. 46. Many techniques have been shown to be superior to the use of on-demand parenteral (intramuscular or intravenous) opioids alone in terms of pain control [109]. These include the addition of neuraxial blockade, intercostal/paravertebral blocks, interpleural local anesthetics, NSAIDs, etc. to narcotic-based analgesia. Only epidural techniques have been shown to consistently have the capability to decrease post-thoracotomy respiratory complications [110, 111]. It is becoming more evident that thoracic epidural analgesia is superior to lumbar epidural analgesia. This seems to be due to the synergy which local anesthetics have with opioids in producing neuraxial analgesia. Studies suggest that epidural local anesthetics increase segmental bioavailability of opioids in the cerebrospinal fluid [112] and also that they increase the binding of opioids by spinal cord receptors [113]. Although lumbar epidural opioids can produce similar levels of post-thoracotomy pain control at rest, only the segmental effects of thoracic epidural local anesthetic and opioid combinations can reliably produce increased analgesia with movement and increased respiratory function following a chest incision [114, 115]. In patients with coronary artery disease, thoracic epidural local anesthetics seem to reduce myocardial oxygen demand and supply in proportion [116].

It is at the time of initial preanesthetic assessment that the risks and benefits of the various forms of post-thoracotomy analgesia should be explained to the patient. Potential contraindications to specific methods of analgesia should be determined such as coagulation problems, sepsis, or neurologic disorders. When it is not possible to place a thoracic epidural due to problems with patient consent or other contraindications, a reasonable second choice for analgesia is a paravertebral infusion of local anesthetic via a catheter placed intraoperatively in the open hemithorax by the surgeon [117]. This is combined with intravenous patient-controlled opioid analgesia and NSAIDS whenever possible.

If the patient is to receive prophylactic anticoagulants and it is elected to use epidural analgesia, appropriate timing of anticoagulant administration and neuraxial catheter placement need to be arranged. ASRA guidelines suggest an interval of 2–4 h before or 1 h after catheter placement for prophylactic heparin administration [118]. Low molecular weight heparin (LMWH) precautions are less clear, and an interval of 12–24 h before and 24 h after catheter placement is recommended.

Premedication

Premedication should be discussed and ordered at the time of the initial preoperative visit. The most important aspect of preoperative medication is to avoid inadvertent withdrawal of those drugs which are taken for concurrent medical conditions (bronchodilators, antihypertensives, beta-blockers, etc.). For some types of thoracic surgery, such as esophageal reflux surgery, oral antacid and H_2 blockers or proton pump inhibitors are routinely ordered preoperatively. We do not routinely order preoperative sedation or analgesia for pulmonary resection patients. Mild sedation such as an intravenous short-acting benzodiazepine is often given immediately prior to placement of invasive monitoring lines and catheters. In patients with copious secretions, an antisilalgogue (such as glycopyrrolate) is useful to facilitate fiber-optic bronchoscopy for positioning of a double-lumen tube or bronchial blocker. To avoid an intramuscular injection, this can be given orally or intravenously immediately after placement of the intravenous catheter. It is a common practice to use short-term intravenous antibacterial prophylaxis such as a cephalosporin in thoracic surgical patients. If it is the local practice to administer these drugs prior to admission to the operating room, they will have to be ordered preoperatively. Consideration for those patients allergic to cephalosporins or penicillin will have to be made at the time of the initial preoperative visit.

Summary of The Initial Preoperative Assessment

The anesthetic considerations which should be addressed at the time of the initial preoperative assessment are summarized in Table 2.11. Patients need to be specifically assessed for risk factors associated with respiratory complications, which are the major cause of morbidity and mortality following thoracic surgery. Risk factors which can be modified preoperatively are listed in Table 2.12 [119].

Final Preoperative Assessment.

The final preoperative anesthetic assessment for the majority of thoracic surgical patients is carried out immediately prior to admission of the patient to the operating room. At this time it is important to review the data from the initial prethoracotomy assessment and the results of tests ordered at that time. In addition, two other specific areas affecting thoracic anesthesia need to be assessed: the potential for difficult lung isolation and the risk of desaturation during one-lung ventilation (Table 2.13).

Table 2.11 Initial preanesthetic assessment for thoracic surgery

1. For all patients: Assess exercise tolerance, simple spirometry; estimate ppoFEV1%; discuss postoperative analgesia, smoking cessation
2. Patients with ppoFEV1 < 40%: Full pulmonary function testing to include DLCO, ventilation/perfusion lung scan if possible pneumonectomy, exercise testing
3. Cancer patients: Consider the "four M's," mass effects, metabolic effects, metastases, medications
4. COPD patients: Physiotherapy, bronchodilators, arterial blood gas if moderate or severe COPD
5. Increased renal risk: Measure creatinine

Table 2.12 Probability for preoperative interventions to reduce the risk of pulmonary complications

Risk factor	Intervention	Probability
Smoking	Cessation >8 weeks	++++
	Cessation <8 weeks	+
Exacerbation of COPD or asthma	Steroids, bronchodilators and delay elective surgery	++++
		+++
	Antibiotics indicated by sputum	
Stable COPD or asthma	Physiotherapy	++++
	Bronchodilators	+++
	Rehabilitation	++
Obesity	Physiotherapy	++++
	Weight loss	++
Malnutrition	Oral nutrition program	++

From data in Ref. [91]

++++ = Multiple studies confirming

+++ = Both some data and physiologic rationale supporting

++ = Either some data or good physiologic rationale

+ = Limited data or physiologic rationale

Table 2.13 Final preanesthetic assessment for thoracic surgery

1. Review initial assessment and test results
2. Assess difficulty of lung isolation: examine preoperative chest imaging
3. Assess risk of hypoxemia during one-lung ventilation

Difficult Endobronchial Intubation

Anesthesiologists are familiar with the clinical assessment of the upper airway for ease of endotracheal intubation. In a similar fashion, each thoracic surgical patient must be assessed for the ease of endobronchial intubation. At the time of the preoperative visit, there may be historical factors or physical findings which lead to suspicion of difficult endobronchial intubation (previous radiotherapy, infection, prior pulmonary, or airway surgery). In addition, there may be a written bronchoscopy report with a detailed description of anatomical features. The most useful predictor of difficult endobronchial intubation is the plain chest X-ray (Fig. 2.21).

The anesthesiologist should view the chest imaging himself/herself prior to induction of anesthesia since neither the radiologist's nor the surgeon's report of the X-ray is made with the specific consideration of lung isolation in mind. A large portion of thoracic surgical patients will also have had a chest CT scan done preoperatively. As anesthesiologists have learned to assess X-rays for potential lung-isolation difficulties, it is also worthwhile to learn to examine the CT scan. Distal airway problems not detectable on the plain chest film can sometimes be visualized on the CT scan: a side-to-side compression of the distal trachea, the so called "saber-sheath" trachea, can cause obstruction of the tracheal lumen of a left-sided double-lumen tube during ventilation of the dependent lung for a left thoracotomy [120]. Similarly, extrinsic compression or intraluminal obstruction of a mainstem bronchus which can interfere with endobronchial tube placement may only be evident on the CT scan. The major factors in successful lower airway management are anticipation and preparation based on the preoperative assessment. Management of lung isolation in patients with difficult upper and lower airways is discussed in Chap. 18.

Prediction of Desaturation During One-Lung Ventilation

In the vast majority of cases, it is possible to identify preoperatively those patients which are most at risk of desaturation during one-lung ventilation (OLV) for thoracic surgery. The factors which correlate with desaturation during OLV are listed in Table 2.14. In patients at high risk of desaturation, prophylactic measures can be used during OLV to decrease this risk. The most useful prophylactic measures are the use of continuous positive airway pressure (CPAP) 2–5 cm H_2O of oxygen to the non-ventilated lung and/or positive end-expiratory pressure (PEEP) to the dependent lung.

The most important predictor of PaO_2 during OLV is the PaO_2 during two-lung ventilation, specifically the intraoperative PaO_2 during two-lung ventilation in the lateral position prior to OLV [121]. The proportion of perfusion or ventilation to the non-operated lung on preoperative V/Q scans also correlates with the PaO_2 during OLV [122]. If the operative lung has little perfusion preoperatively due to unilateral disease, the patient is unlikely to desaturate during OLV. The side of the thoracotomy has an effect on PaO_2 during OLV. The left lung being 10% smaller than the right, there is less shunt when the left lung is collapsed. In a series of patients, the mean PaO_2 during left thoracotomy was approximately 70 mmHg higher than during right thoracotomy [123]. Finally, the degree of obstructive lung disease correlates in an inverse fashion with PaO_2 during OLV. Other factors being equal, patients with more severe airflow limitation on preoperative spirometry will tend to have a better PaO_2 during OLV than patients with normal spirometry (see Chap. 6) [124].

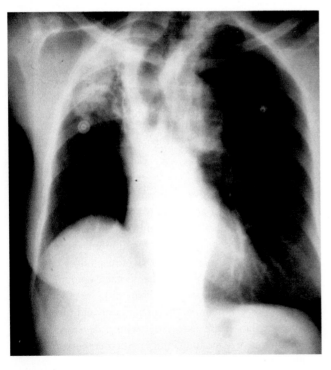

Fig. 2.21 Preoperative chest X-ray of a patient with a history of previous tuberculosis, right upper lobectomy, and recent hemoptysis presenting for right thoracotomy and possible completion pneumonectomy. The potential problems positioning a left-sided double-lumen tube in this patient are easily appreciated by viewing the X-ray but are not mentioned in the radiologist's report. The anesthesiologist must examine the chest imaging himself/herself preoperatively to anticipate problems in lung isolation (From Slinger and Johnston [126] with permission)

Table 2.14 Factors which correlate with an increased risk of desaturation during one-lung ventilation

High percentage of ventilation or perfusion to the operative lung on preoperative V/Q scan
Poor PaO_2 during two-lung ventilation, particularly in the lateral position intraoperatively
Right-sided thoracotomy
Normal preoperative spirometry (FEV1 or FVC) or restrictive lung disease
Supine position during one-lung ventilation

Assessment for Repeat Thoracic Surgery

Patients who survive lung cancer surgery form a high-risk cohort to have a recurrence of the original tumor or to develop a second primary. The incidence of developing a second primary lung tumor is estimated at 2%/year. The use of routine postoperative follow-up screening with low-dose spiral CT scans will probably increase the rate of early detection of recurrent or repeat primary tumors [125]. Patients who present for repeat thoracotomy should be assessed using the same framework as those who present for surgery the first time. Predicted values for postoperative respiratory function based on the preoperative lung mechanics, parenchymal function, exercise tolerance, and the amount of functioning lung tissue resected should be calculated and used to identify patients at increased risk.

Clinical Case Discussion

Case A 65-year-old male presents for anesthesia preoperative assessment (Fig. 2.22). He is scheduled for a bronchoscopy/mediastinoscopy and right pneumonectomy. He is a smoker who presented to his family doctor 2 weeks ago after minor hemoptysis. He has no significant known comorbidities and past history is otherwise unremarkable. A fine needle biopsy has confirmed the diagnosis of non-small cell lung cancer. The anesthesia team will need to decide if the patient will tolerate the proposed procedure and, if so, then what management strategies can be used to improve the perioperative outcome.

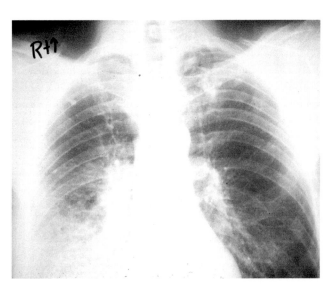

Fig. 2.22 Chest X-ray of a 65-year-old male with carcinoma involving the right middle and lower lobes, being assessed for possible right pneumonectomy

Questions

Apart from routine preoperative assessment for major surgery:

- What pulmonary function tests are indicated?
- What cardiac investigations are indicated?
- What specific anesthetic considerations are related to the patient's lung cancer?
- What other system function should be documented?

Focused Preoperative History, Physical and Investigations:

- Pulmonary function evaluation: lung mechanical function (spirometry: FEV1), pulmonary parenchymal function (DLCO), exercise capacity, and ventilation/perfusion scan (see Assessment of Respiratory Function)
- Cardiac evaluation: ECG (echocardiography and stress testing not indicated) (see Cardiovascular Disease)
- Tumor mass effects, metabolic (paraneoplastic) effects, metastases, and adjuvant medications
Other systems: renal function

Will the patient tolerate the procedure?

- Results of investigations: FEV1 65%, DLCO 70%, exercise tolerance: the patient can climb four flights of stairs without stopping. V/Q scan R/L 40/60 for both V and Q. Other investigations are all within normal limits.
- Predicted postoperative (ppo) FEV1 and DLCO will be in the range of 30–35% and adjusted for the V/Q scan possibly higher. These indicate increased risk but acceptable survival given the patient's age < 70. A bi-lobectomy could be considered for elderly or high-risk patients (see Age).

What management strategies will improve the patient's outcome?

- Smoking cessation
- Pre- and postoperative chest physiotherapy
- Thoracic epidural analgesia has not been clearly proven to improve outcomes in patients with normal pulmonary function but does improve function in moderate and severe COPD. This patient's risk of respiratory complications may be improved by either thoracic epidural or paravertebral analgesia (see also Chap. 59).
- Moderate perioperative fluid restriction and lung-protective ventilation are associated with a decreased risk of postoperative acute lung injury particularly after pneumonectomy (see also Chap. 10 and 21).
- Calcium channel blockers may be associated with a decreased risk of postoperative atrial fibrillation (see also Chap. 56).
- Preoperative ß-blockade, statins, or α-2 blockers are not proven to decrease cardiac ischemic risks in this patient at low risk of perioperative ischemia.

References

1. Taylor MD, LaPar D, Isbell J, et al. Marginal pulmonary function should not preclude lobectomy in selected patients with non-small cell lung cancer. J Thorac Cardiovasc Surg. 2014;147:738–46.

2. Licker M, Widikker I, Robert J, et al. Operative mortality and respiratory complications after lung resection for cancer: impact of chronic obstructive pulmonary disease and time trends. Ann Thorac Surg. 2006;81:1830–8.

3. Paul S, Sedrakyan A, Ya-lin C, et al. Outcomes after lobectomy using thoracoscopy vs thoracotomy. Eur J Cardiothorac Surg. 2013;43:813–7.

4. Brunelli A, Kim A, Berger K, et al. Physiological evaluation of the patient with lung cancer being considered for resectional surgery. Chest. 2013;143:e166s–90s.

5. British Thoracic Society. Guidelines on the selection of patients with lung cancer for surgery. Thorax. 2001;56:89–108.

6. Cerfolio RJ, Allen MS, Trastak VF, et al. Lung resection in patients with compromised pulmonary function. Ann Thorac Surg. 1996;62:348–51.

7. Donahoe LL, de Valence M, Atenafu EG, et al. High risk for thoracotomy but not thoracoscopic lobectomy. Ann Thorac Surg. 2017;103(6):1730–5.

8. Choi H, Mazzone P. Preoperative evaluation of the patient with lung cancer being considered for lung resection. Curr Opin Anesthesiol. 2015;28:18–25.

9. Linden PA, Bueno R, Colson YL, et al. Lung resection in patients with FEV1 < 35% predicted. Chest. 2005;127:1984–90.

10. Bach PB, Cramer LD, Schrag D. The influence of hospital volume on survival after resection for lung Cancer. N Eng J Med. 2001;345:181–8.

11. Brunelli A, Rocco G. Spirometry: predicting outcome and risk. Thorac Surg Clin. 2008;18:1–8.

12. Slinger PD, Kruger M, McRae K, Winton T. The relation of the static compliance curve and positive end-expiratory pressure to oxygenation during one-lung ventilation. Anesthesiology. 2001;95:1096–102.

13. Ferguson MK, Vigneswaran WT. Diffusing capacity predicts morbidity after lung resection in patients without obstructive lung disease. Ann Thorac Surg. 2008;85:1158–65.

14. National Emphysema Treatment Trial Research Group. A randomized trial comparing lung-volume-reduction surgery with medical therapy for severe emphysema. N Engl J Med. 2003;348:2059.

15. Lim E, Baldwin D, Beckles M, et al. Guidelines on the radical management of patients with lung cancer. Thorax. 2010;65:iii1–iii27.

16. Weisman IM. Cardiopulmonary exercise testing in the preoperative assessment for lung resection surgery. Semin Thorac Cardiovasc Surg. 2001;13:116–22.

17. Coyle EF. Improved muscular efficiency as Tour de France champion matures. J Appl Physiol. 2005;98:2191–6.

18. Walsh GL, Morice RC, Putnam JB, et al. Resection of lung cancer is justified in high risk patients selected by oxygen consumption. Ann Thorac Surg. 1994;58:704–10.

19. Nagamatsu Y, Shima I, Hayashi A, et al. Preoperative spirometry versus expired gas analysis during exercise testing as predictors of cardiopulmonary complications after lung resections. Surg Today. 2004;34:107–10.

20. Forshaw MJ, Strauss DC, Davies AR, et al. Is cardiopulmonary exercise testing a useful test before esophagectomy? Ann Thorac Surg. 2008;85:294–9.

21. Brunelli A, Pompili C, Salati M, et al. Preoperative maximum oxygen consumption is associated with prognosis after pulmonary resection in stage I non-small cell lung cancer. Ann Thorac Surg. 2014;98:238–42.

22. Carter R, Holiday DB, Stocks J, et al. Predicting oxygen uptake for men and women with moderate to severe chronic obstructive pulmonary disease. Arch Phys Med Rehabil. 2003;84:1158–64.

23. Lee L, Schwartzman K, Carli F, et al. The association of the distance walked in 6 min with preoperative peak oxygen consumption and complications 1 month after colorectal resection. Anaesthesia. 2013;68:811–6.

24. Marjanski T, Wnuk D, Bosakowski D. Patients who do not reach a distance 6of 500 m during the 6-min walk test have an increased risk of postoperative complications and prolonged hospital stay after lobectomy. Eur J Cardiothorac Surg. 2015;47:e213–9.

25. Ninan M, Sommers KE, Landranau RJ, et al. Standardized exercise oximetry predicts post-pneumonectomy outcome. Ann Thorac Surg. 1997;64:328–33.

26. Bolliger CT, Wyser C, Roser H, et al. Lung scanning and exercise testing for the prediction of postoperative performance in lung resection candidates at increased risk for complications. Chest. 1995;108:341–8.

27. Olsen GN, Bolton JWR, Weiman DS, Horning CA. Stair climbing as an exercise test to predict postoperative complications of lung resection. Chest. 1991;99:587–90.

28. Kinasewitz GT, Welsh MH. A simple method to assess postoperative risk. Chest. 2001;120:1057–8.

29. Heerdt PM. Post-thoracotomy cardiovascular adaptations and complications. In: Kaplan J, Slinger P, editors. Thoracic anesthesia. 3rd ed. Philadelphia: Churchill Livingston; 2003. p. 423–35.

30. Koegelenberg CFN, Bollinger CT. Assessing regional lung function. Thorac Surg Clin. 2008;18:19–29.

31. Win T, Larouche CM, Groves AM, et al. Use of quantitative lung scintigraphy to predict pulmonary function in lung cancer patients undergoing lobectomy. Ann Thorac Surg. 2004;78:1215–9.

32. Wu MT, Pan HB, Chiang AA, et al. Predicting postoperative lung function in patients with lung cancer. Am J Radiol. 2002;178:667–72.

33. Ohno Y, Koyama H, Nogami M, et al. Post-operative lung function in lung cancer patients: comparative analysis of predictive capacity of MRI, CT, SPECT. Am J Radiol. 2007;189:400–8.

34. Tisi GM. Preoperative evaluation of pulmonary function. Am Rev Resp Dis. 1979;119:293–301.

35. Lewis JW Jr, Bastanfar M, Gabriel F, Mascha E. Right heart function and prediction of respiratory morbidity in patients undergoing pneumonectomy with moderately severe cardiopulmonary dysfunction. J Thorac Cardiovasc Surg. 1994;108:169–75.

36. Amar D, Burt M, Roistacher N, Reinsel RA, Ginsberg RJ, Wilson R. Value of perioperative echocardiography in patients undergoing major lung resection. Ann Thorac Surg. 1996;61:516–22.

37. Jordan S, Evans TW. Predicting the need for intensive care following lung resection. Thorac Surg Clin. 2008;18:61–9.

38. Ford MK, Beattie WS. Systematic review: prediction of perioperative cardiac complications and mortality by the revised cardiac risk index. Ann Int Med. 2010;152:26–35.

39. Ferguson MK, Saha-Chaudhuri P, Mitchell JD, et al. Prediction of major cardiovascular events after lung resection using a modified scoring system. Ann Thorac Surg. 2014;97:1135–41.

40. Wotton R, Marshall A, Kerr A, et al. Does the revised cardiac risk index predict cardiac complications following elective lung resection? J Cardiothorac Surg. 2013;8:220–7.

41. Roshanov P, Rochwerg B, Patel A, et al. Withholding versus continuing angiotensin-converting enzyme inhibitors or angiotensin II receptor blockers before noncardiac surgery. Anesthesiology. 2017;126:16–27.

42. Fleisher LA, Beckman JA, Brown KA, et al. ACC/AHA 2007 guidelines on perioperative cardiovascular evaluation and care for noncardiac surgery. JACC. 2007;50:1707–32.

43. von Knorring J, Lepäntalo M, Lindgren L, Lindfors O. Cardiac arrhythmias and myocardial ischemia after thoracotomy for lung cancer. Ann Thorac Surg. 1992;53:642–7.

44. Fleisher LA, Fleishmann KE, Auerbach AD, et al. ACC/AHA guideline on perioperative cardiovascular evaluation and management of patients undergoing non-cardiac surgery. Circulation. 2014;130:2215–45.

45. Etchells E, Meade M, Tomlinson G, et al. Semiquantitative dipyridamole myocardial stress perfusion imaging before noncardiac vascular surgery: a metaanalysis. J Vasc Surg. 2002;36:534–40.

46. Brett AS. Are the current perioperative risk management strategies flawed? Circulation. 2008;117:3145–51.

47. Yang H, Beattie WS. POISE results and perioperative β-blockade. Can J Anesth. 2008;55:727–34.

48. 2016 ACC/AHA guideline focused update on duration of dual antiplatelet therapy in patients with coronary artery disease. J Thorac Cardiovasc Surg. 2016;152:1243–75.

49. Ritchie AJ, Bowe P, Gibbons JRP. Prophylactic digitalisation for thoracotomy: a reassessment. Ann Thorac Surg. 1990;50:86–8.

50. de Perrot M, McRae K, Anraku M, et al. Risk factors for major complications after extra-pleural pneumonectomy for malignant pleural mesothelioma. Ann Thorac Surg. 2008;85:1206–10.

51. Sekine Y, Kesler KA, Behnia M, et al. COPD may increase the incidence of refractory supraventricular arrhythmias following pulmonary resection for non-small cell lung cancer. Chest. 2001;120:1783–90.

52. Frendyl G, Sodickson AC, Chung MK, et al. 2014 AATS guidelines for the prevention and management of perioperative atrial fibrillation and flutter for thoracic surgical procedures. J Thorac Cardiovasc Surg. 2014;148:772–91.

53. Lindgren L, Lepantalo M, Von Knorring J, et al. Effect of verapamil on right ventricular pressure and atrial tachyarrhythmia after thoracotomy. Br J Anaesth. 1991;66:205–11.

54. Oka T, Ozawa Y, Ohkubo Y. Thoracic epidural bupivacaine attenuates supraventricular tachyarrhythmias after pulmonary resection. Anesth Analg. 2001;93:253–9.

55. Osaki T, Shirakusa T, Kodate M, et al. Surgical treatment of lung cancer in the octogenarian. Ann Thorac Surg. 1994;57:188–92.

56. Brunelli A, Salati M, Refai M, et al. Development of a patient-centered aggregate score to predict survival after lung resection for non-small cell lung cancer. J Thorac Cardiovasc Surg. 2013;146:385–90.

57. Brunelli A, Monteverde M, Al Refai M. Stair climbing as a predictor of cardiopulmonary complications after pulmonary lobectomy in the elderly. Ann Thorac Surg. 2004;77:266–70.

58. Pricopi C, Mordant O, Rivera C, et al. Postoperative morbidity and mortality after pneumonectomy. Interact Cardiovasc Thorac Surg. 2015;20:316–21.

59. Lai Y, Huang J, Yang M, et al. Seven-day preoperative rehabilitation for elderly patients with lung cancer. J Surg Res. 2017;209:30–6.

60. Golledge J, Goldstraw P. Renal impairment after thoracotomy: incidence, risk factors and significance. Ann Thorac Surg. 1994;58:524–8.

61. Ishikawa S, Greisdale D, Lohser J. Acute kidney injury after lung resection surgery. Anesth Analg. 2012;114:1256–62.

62. Ahn HJ, Kim JA, Lee AR, et al. The risk of acute kidney injury from fluid restriction and hydroxyethyl starch in thoracic surgery. Anesth Analg. 2016;122:186–93.

63. Slinger PD. Postpneumonectony pulmonary edema: good news, bad news. Anesthesiology. 2006;105:2–5.

64. American Thoracic Society. Standards for the diagnosis and care of patients with chronic obstructive pulmonary disease. Am J Resp Critic Care Med. 1995;152:s77–s121.

65. Parot S, Saunier C, Gauthier H, Milic-Emile J, Sadoul P. Breathing pattern and hypercapnia in patients with obstructive pulmonary disease. Am Rev Resp Dis. 1980;121:985–91.

66. Aubier M, Murciano D, Milic-Emili j.et al.. Effects of the administration of O2 on ventilation and blood gases in patients with chronic obstructive pulmonary disease during acute respiratory failure. American Rev Resp Dis. 1980;122:747–54.

67. Simpson SQ. Oxygen-induced acute hypercapnia in chronic obstructive pulmonary disease: what's the problem? Critic Care Med. 2002;30:258–9.

68. Hanson CW III, Marshall BE, Frasch HF, Marshall C. Causes of hypercarbia in patients with chronic obstructive pulmonary disease. Critic Care Med. 1996;24:23–8.

69. Nguyen DM, Mulder DS, Shennib H. Altered cellular immune function in atelectatic lung. Ann Thorac Surg. 1991;51:76–80.

70. Hublitz UF, Shapiro JH. Atypical pulmonary patterns of congestive failure in chronic lung disease. Radiology. 1969;93:995–1006.

71. Sasaki F, Ishizaki T, Mifune J, et al. Bronchial hyperresponsiveness in patients with chronic congestive heart failure. Chest. 1990;97:534–8.

72. Nisar M, Earis JE, Pearson MG, Calverly PMA. Acute bronchodilator trials in chronic obstructive pulmonary disease. Am Rev Resp Dis. 1992;146:555–9.

73. Warner DO. Preventing postoperative pulmonary complications. Anesthesiology. 2000;92:1467–72.

74. Cesario A, Ferri L, Cardaci V, et al. Pre-operative pulmonary rehabilitation and surgery for lung cancer. Lung Cancer. 2007;57:118–9.

75. Nici L. Preoperative and postoperative pulmonary rehabilitation in lung cancer patients. Thorac Surg Clin. 2008;18:39–43.

76. Morano M, Araujo A, Nascimento F, et al. Preoperative pulmonary rehabilitation vs. chest physical therapy in patients undergoing lung cancer resection. Arch Phys Med Rehab. 2013;94:53–8.

77. American Thoracic Society/European Respiratory Society international multidisciplinary consensus classification of the idiopathic interstitial pneumonias. Am J Resp Crit Care Med. 2002;165:277–304.

78. Kumar P, Goldstraw P, Yamada K. Pulmonary fibrosis and lung cancer: risk and benefit analysis of pulmonary resection. J Thorac Cardiovasc Surg. 2003;125:1321–7.

79. Vaporciyan AA, Merriman KW, Ece F, et al. Incidence of major pulmonary complications after pneumonectomy; association with timing of smoking cessation. Ann Thorac Surg. 2002;73:420–5.

80. Akrawi W, Benumof JL. A pathophysiological basis for informed preoperative smoking cessation counseling. J Cardiothorac Vasc Anesth. 1997;11:629–40.

81. Moller A, Tonnesen H. Risk reduction: perioperative smoking intervention. Best Pract Res Clin Anaesthesiol. 2006;20:237–48.

82. Barrera R, Shi W, Amar D, et al. Smoking and timing of cessation. Impact on pulmonary complications after thoracotomy. Chest. 2005;127:1977–83.

83. Warner DO. Feasibility of tobacco interventions in anesthesiology practices: a pilot study. Anesthesiology. 2009;110:1223–8.

84. Thomsen T, Tonnesen H, Moller AM. Effect of preoperative smoking cessation interventions on postoperative complications and smoking cessation. Br J Surg. 2009;96:451–61.

85. Rodriguez M, Gomez Hernandez M, Novoa N, et al. Morbidity and mortality in octogenarians with lung cancer undergoing pneumonectomy. Arch Bronconeumol. 2015;51:211–2.

86. Puente-Maestu L, Villar F, Gonzalez-Causurran G, et al. Early and long term validation of an algorithm assessing fitness for surgery in patients with postoperative FEV1 and diffusing capacity for carbon monoxide <40%. Chest. 2011;139:1430–8.

87. Schulte T, Schniewind B, Dohrmann P, et al. The extent of lung parenchymal resection significantly affects long-term quality of life in patients with non-small cell lung cancer. Chest. 2009;135:322–9.

88. Tang S, Redmond K, Griffiths M, et al. The mortality from acute respiratory distress syndrome after pulmonary resection

is decreasing: a 10-year single institutional experience. Eur J Cardiothorac Surg. 2009;34:898–902.

89. Thomas P, Falcoz P, Bernard A, et al. Bilobectomy for lung cancer: contemporary national early morbidity and mortality outcomes. Eur J Cardiothorac Surg. 2016;49:e38–43.

90. Linden P, D'Amico T, Perry Y, et al. Quantifying the safety benefits of wedge resection: a society of thoracic surgery database propensity-matched analysis. Ann Thorac Surg. 2014;98:1705–11.

91. Larsen L, Petersen R, Hansen H, et al. Video-assisted thoracoscopic surgery lobectomy for lung cancer is associated with a lower 30-day morbidity compared with lobectomy by thoracotomy. Eur J Cardiothorac Surg. 2016;49:870–5.

92. Burt B, Kosinski A, Shrager J, et al. Thoracoscopic lobectomy is associated with acceptable morbidity and mortality in patients with predicted postoperative forced expiratory volume in 1 second or diffusing capacity for carbon monoxide less than 40% of normal. J Thorac Cardiovasc Surg. 2014;148:19–28.

93. Berry M, Villamizar-Ortiz N, Tong B, et al. Pulmonary function tests do not predict pulmonary complications after thoracoscopic lobectomy. Ann Thorac Surg. 2010;89:1044–52.

94. Bilimoria K, liu Y, Paruch J, et al. Development and evaluation of the universal ACS NSQIP surgical risk calculator. J Am Coll Surg. 2013;217:833–42.

95. Licker M, Triponez F, Diaper J, et al. Preoperative evaluation of lung cancer patients. Curr Anesthesiol Rep. 2014;4:124–34.

96. Farjah F, Wood DE, Yanez D III, et al. Temporal trends in the management of potentially resectable lung cancer. Ann Thorac Surg. 2008;85:1850–6.

97. National Health Statistics of the United States 2007. www.cancer.org.

98. Feinstein MB, Bach PB. Epidemiology of lung cancer in lung cancer: past, present and future. Ginsberg RJ, Ruckdeschel JC eds. Chest Surg Clin. 2000;10:653–61.

99. Darling GE, Dickie AJ, et al. Invasive mediastinal staging of non-small-cell lung cancer: a clinical practice guideline. Curr Oncol. 2011;18(6):e304–10.

100. de Perrot M, Cherenko S, Waddell T, et al. Role of lung transplantation in the treatment of bronchogenic carcinomas for patients with end-stage pulmonary disease. J Clin Oncol. 2004;22:4351–6.

101. Johnson BE. Management of small cell lung cancer. Clin in Chest Med. 1993;14:173–87.

102. Levin KH. Paraneoplastic neuromuscular syndromes. Neurol Clin. 1997;15:597–614.

103. Petty R. Lambert-Eaton Myasthenic syndrome. Pract Neurol. 2007;7:265–7.

104. Telford RJ, Holloway TE. The myasthenic syndrome: anesthesia in a patient treated with 3-4 diaminopyridine. Br J Anaest. 1990;64:363–6.

105. Mehta AC, Rafanan AL, Bulkley R, et al. Coronary spasm and cardiac arrest from carcinoid syndrome during laser bronchoscopy. Chest. 1999;115:598–600.

106. Vaughan DJ, Brunner MD. Anesthesia for patients with the carcinoid syndrome. Int Anesthesiol Clin. 1997;35:129–42.

107. Hartigan PM, Ng JM. Anesthetic strategies for patients undergoing extrapleural pneumonectomy. Thorac Surg Clin. 2004;14:575–83.

108. Sleijfer S. Bleomycin-induced pneumonitis. Chest. 2001;120:617–24.

109. Kavanagh BP, Katz J, Sandler AN. Pain control after thoracic surgery: a review of current techniques. Anesthesiology. 1994;81:737–59.

110. Licker M, de Perrot M, Hohn L, et al. Perioperative mortality and major cardio-pulmonary complications after lung surgery for non-small call carcinoma. Eur J Cardiothorac Surg. 1999;15:314–9.

111. Rigg JRA, Jamrozik K, Myles PS. Epidural anaesthesia and analgesia and outcome of major surgery: a randomized trial. Lancet. 2005;359:1276–82.

112. Hansdottir V, Woestenborghs R, Nordberg G. The pharmacokinetics of continuous epidural sufentanil and bupivacaine infusion after thoracotomy. Anesth Analg. 1996;83:401–6.

113. Tejwani GA, Rattan AK, McDonald JS. Role of spinal opioid receptors in the antinociceptive interactions between intrathecal morphine and bupivacaine. Anesth Analg. 1992;74:726–34.

114. Hansdottir V, Bake B, Nordberg G. The analgesic efficiency and adverse effects of continuous epidural sufentanil and bupivacaine infusion after thoracotomy. Anesth Analg. 1996;83:394–400.

115. Bauer C, Hentz J-G, Ducrocq X, et al. Lung function after lobectomy: a randomized trial comparing thoracic epidural ropivacaine/sufentanil and intra-venous morphine for patient-controlled analgesia. Anesth Analg. 2007;105:238–44.

116. Saada M, Catoire P, Bonnet F, et al. Effect of thoracic epidural anesthesia combined with general anesthesia on segmental wall motion assessed by transesophageal echocardiography. Anesth Analg. 1992;75:329–35.

117. Karmakar MK. Thoracic paravertebral block. Anesthesiology. 2001;95:771–80.

118. Liu SS, Mulroy MF. Neuraxial anesthesia and analgesia in the presence of standard heparin. Reg Anesth Pain Med. 1998;23(6 Suppl 2):157–63.

119. Kempainen RR, Benditt JO. Evaluation and management of patients with pulmonary disease before thoracic and cardiovascular surgery. Semin Thorac Cardiovasc Surg. 2001;13:105–15.

120. Bayes J, Slater EM, Hadberg PS, Lawson D. Obstruction of a double-lumen tube by a saber-sheath trachea. Anesth Analg. 1994;79:186–8.

121. Slinger P, Suissa S, Triolet W. Predicting arterial oxygenation during one-lung anaesthesia. Can J Anaesth. 1992;39:1030–5.

122. Hurford WE, Kolker AC, Strauss HW. The use of ventilation/perfusion lung scans to predict oxygenation during one-lung anesthesia. Anesthesiology. 1987;67:841–4.

123. Lewis JW, Serwin JP, Gabriel FS, Bastaufar M, Jacobsen G. The utility of a double-lumen tube for one-lung ventilation in a variety of non-cardiac thoracic surgical procedures. J Cardiothorac Vasc Anesth. 1992;6:705–10.

124. Katz JA, Lavern RG, Fairley HB, et al. Pulmonary oxygen exchange during endobronchial anesthesia, effect of tidal volume and PEEP. Anesthesiology. 1982;56:164–71.

125. Naunheim KS, Virgo KS. Postoperative surveillance following lung cancer resection. Chest Surg Clin. 2001;11:213–25.

126. Slinger PD, Johnston M. Preoperative assessment: an anesthesiologist's perspective. Thorac Surg Clin. 2005;15:11–5.

Thoracic Imaging

Javier Campos and Kalpaj R. Parekh

Key Points

- Radiological images play an important role during the evaluation of patients undergoing thoracic surgery.
- Radiological studies must be reviewed, including a posterior–anterior chest radiograph and computed tomography scan of the chest.
- Special emphasis should be given to mediastinal mass with compromise to the airway or great vessels by reviewing the computed tomography scan of the chest.
- Multidetector computed tomography (CT) scan and tracheobronchial reconstruction are more specific studies in the thoracic surgical patient and allow measurements of the airway.
- Magnetic resonance imaging (MRI) provides greater contrast resolution than CT scans and offers the potential for tissue characterization. An MRI is indicated in selected cases, i.e., mediastinal mass with invasion of the superior vena cava.

Introduction

Radiological images play an important role in the preoperative, intraoperative, and postoperative evaluation and diagnosis of patients undergoing thoracic surgery. During the preoperative visit evaluation of the thoracic surgical patient, the clinician must have an understanding of the disease and also become familiar with radiological studies to be able to identify abnormal airway anatomy or compromises to the airway or to use caliper measurements in the tracheobronchial tree if necessary when selecting lung isolation devices. Another important component to a successful preoperative evaluation is an understanding of normal tracheobronchial anatomy. This chapter will be focused on reviewing normal tracheobronchial anatomy and radiological images, with special interest for anesthesiologists involved in the care of the thoracic surgical patient.

Normal Tracheobronchial Anatomy

The trachea is a cartilaginous and fibromuscular structure that extends from the inferior aspect of the cricoid cartilage to the level of the carina [1]. The adult trachea is, on average, 15 cm long. The trachea is composed of 16–22 C-shaped cartilages. The cartilages compose the anterior and lateral walls of the trachea and are connected posteriorly by the membranous wall of the trachea, which lacks cartilage and is supported by the trachealis muscle.

The average diameter in a normal trachea is 22 mm in men and 19 mm in women. In men, the coronal diameter ranges from 13 to 22 mm, and the sagittal diameter ranges from 13 to 27 mm. In women, the average coronal diameter is 10–21 mm and the sagittal is 10–23 mm [2]. The tracheal wall is about 3 mm in thickness in both men and women, with a tracheal lumen that is often ovoid in shape.

The trachea is located in the midline position but often can be deviated to the right at the level of the aortic arch, with a greater degree of displacement in the setting of an atherosclerotic aorta and advanced age or in the presence of severe chronic obstructive pulmonary disease (COPD). With COPD or aging, the lateral diameter of the trachea may decrease with a corresponding increase in the antero-

J. Campos (✉)
Department of Anesthesia, University of Iowa Health Care, Roy and Lucille Carver College of Medicine, Iowa City, IA, USA
e-mail: javier-campos@uiowa.edu

K. R. Parekh
Department of Cardiothoracic Surgery, University of Iowa Hospitals and Clinics, Iowa City, IA, USA

© Springer Nature Switzerland AG 2019
P. Slinger (ed.), *Principles and Practice of Anesthesia for Thoracic Surgery*, https://doi.org/10.1007/978-3-030-00859-8_3

posterior diameter. Conversely, COPD may also lead to softening of the tracheal rings with a decrease in the anteroposterior diameter of the trachea [3]. The cricoid cartilage is the narrowest part of the trachea with an average diameter of 17 mm in men and 13 mm in women.

The trachea bifurcates at the carina into the right and left mainstem bronchus. An important fact is that the tracheal lumen narrows slightly as it progresses toward the carina. The tracheal bifurcation is located at the level of the sternal angle anteriorly and the fifth thoracic vertebra posteriorly. The right mainstem bronchus continues as the bronchus intermedius after the takeoff of the right upper lobe bronchus. In men, the average distance from the tracheal carina to the takeoff of the right upper lobe bronchus is 2.0 cm, whereas it is approximately 1.5 cm in women. One in every 250 individuals from the general population may have an abnormal takeoff of the right upper lobe bronchus emerging from above the tracheal carina on the right side [4]. The diameter of the right mainstem bronchus is an average of 17.5 mm in men and 14.0 mm in women. The trifurcation of the right upper lobe bronchus consists of the apical, anterior, and posterior divisions. The average distance from the tracheal carina to the bifurcation of the left upper and left lower lobe is approximately 5.0 cm in men and 4.5 cm in women. The left mainstem bronchus is longer than the right mainstem bronchus, and it divides into the left upper and the left lower lobe bronchus. The left upper lobe bronchus has a superior and inferior division [5].

Chest Radiographs

The most common study in the patient undergoing thoracic, esophageal, or cardiac surgery is the chest X-radiograph (X-ray). The standard routine chest radiography consists of an erect radiograph made in the posterior–anterior (PA) projection and a left lateral radiograph, both obtained at full inspiration. The normal chest cavity contains four radiographic densities that are easily identified: air, fat, water, and calcium and other metals including bones, granulomas, and vascular calcification. The lungs, which are mostly air and contain some water, blood vessels, bronchi, nerves, lymphatics, alveolar walls, and interstitial tissues, provide the natural contrast that is the basis of chest radiology. When evaluating a chest X-ray, the changes in these densities, which provide natural contrast, are what are observed.

Radiologists in general refer to two regions: the silhouette sign and summation. Depending on the part or parts of the lungs that are involved, the result of this change in the absorption of X-rays is seen by the effect on the normal surface of a hemidiaphragm, for example, or if the descending aorta cannot be seen, then this is an indication that an unusual amount of aerated lung no longer touches the anatomic part. This occurs in part because the alveolar spaces are wholly or partially filled with fluid usually blood, pus, or water or in part because the lung has collapsed and decreased the normal ratio of air and soft tissue. The end result in the latter case would be an increase in opacity which is what the X-ray beam reveals. The heart border and the diaphragm are normally seen because of their interface with aerated lung. When the contiguous lung is not aerated, the opaque tissue of the affected lung blends visually with the soft tissue opacity of the heart, and the heart border is no longer visible. This is what is termed the silhouette sign. Summation by definition is the result of superimposition of many layers of lung tissue, so that the final visual effect is that of a greater amount of tissue in the path of a particular part of the X-ray beam. This is observed when the opacity of fluid in the pleural space, interstitial space, or even lung parenchyma is added on the normal structure of the lung [6]. The most important skill for evaluating a chest X-ray is the knowledge of normal anatomic variants, the specific patterns with pathological changes, and the common signs of abnormal states. Lateral decubitus radiographs are commonly employed to determine the presence or mobility of pleural effusions. These views can also be obtained to detect small pneumothoraces, particularly in patients who are confined to bed and unable to sit or stand erect. A new generation of digital X-ray systems based on flat panel detections is now emerging, and these provide good image quality and very rapid direct access to digital images.

Chest Radiographs and Pulmonary Disease

The basic underlying change in the chest film that allows the detection and diagnosis of abnormalities is usually due to an alteration in lung opacity. This can be caused by technical factors, physiologic variation, or pathologic mechanisms [7]. Diseases that affect the chest can usually be thought of as either those that make the film lighter (increase opacity) or those that make it darker (increase lucency).

For chest disease with increased opacity on radiographs, the conditions that are marked by focal or global increase in the opacity of the film are first examined. These conditions include atelectasis, pulmonary edema, acute respiratory distress syndrome, etc.

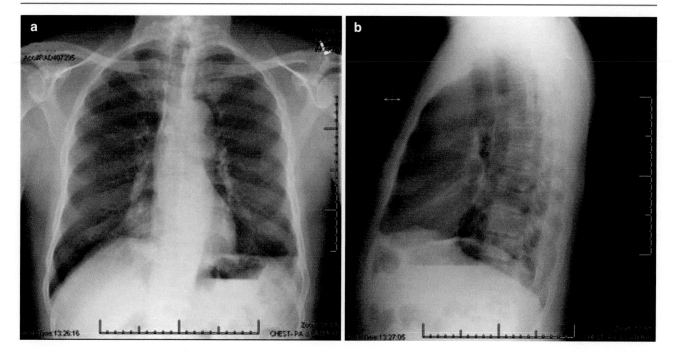

Fig. 3.1 (**a**) Shows a posteroanterior chest radiograph on a 68-year-old male with a lung neoplasm on the right lower lobe. The mass is clearly visible between the 8th and 9th rib on the right hemithorax. (**b**) Shows a lateral chest radiograph showing a round mass on the right hemithorax

Lung Mass and Chest X-Rays

Pulmonary neoplasia presents as opacities on films although usually as a more focal area with varying contours. However, smaller lesions may be very difficult to visualize, particularly when there are overlying bones or other soft tissue. Figure 3.1a shows a posteroanterior chest radiograph on a 68-year-old male with a lung neoplasm on the right lower lobe. The mass is clearly visible between the eighth and ninth rib on the right hemithorax. Figure 3.1b shows a lateral chest radiograph showing a round mass on the right hemithorax.

Mediastinal Mass and Chest X-Rays

In order to understand mediastinal masses and radiological images, it is important to be familiar with the anatomy of the mediastinum. The mediastinum is situated between the two pleural cavities. It extends superiorly from the root of the neck and the thoracic inlet to the hemidiaphragm inferiorly. It is divided into the superior and inferior mediastinum by the transverse thoracic plane, which is an imaginary plane extending horizontally from the sternal angle anteriorly to the border of the fourth thoracic vertebra posteriorly.

The inferior mediastinum is subdivided into anterior, middle, and posterior compartments. The anterior mediastinum contains the thymus, trachea, esophagus, vessels, and arteries as well as lymph nodes; any abnormal growth in this region will affect the adjacent area. A mass in this area may compress the tracheobronchial tree and/or major vessels (superior vena cava and pulmonary vessels). The middle mediastinum is the space occupied by the heart and pericardium [8, 9]. Figure 3.2a shows a schematic representation of mediastinal anatomy and Fig. 3.2b a lateral normal radiograph of the chest showing the potential location of mediastinal mass. A variety of neoplasms and other lesions present with anterior mediastinal involvement. Thymoma is the most common primary neoplasm of the anterior mediastinum [10].

Regarding radiological studies in patients with a suspected anterior mediastinal mass, the initial study generally is a standard biplane chest radiography, which will identify up to 97% of mediastinal tumors. The chest X-ray also provides important information regarding the size and the location of the mass [11].

In addition, in this patient group in particular, special attention must be paid to the lateral radiography of the chest to determine the overall extent of the mass and potential involvement of adjacent structures. A barium contrast

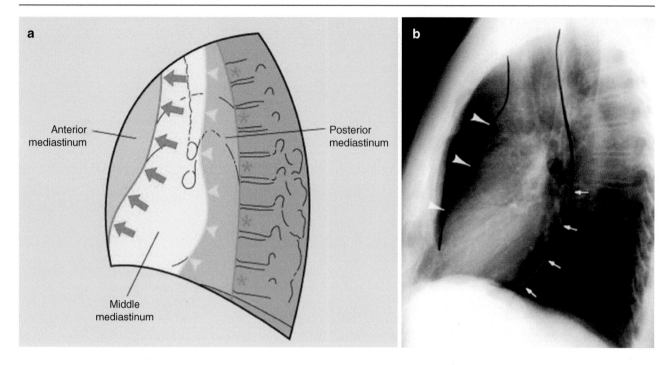

Fig. 3.2 (**a**) Shows a schematic representation of mediastinal anatomy and (**b**) a lateral normal radiograph of the chest showing the potential location of mediastinal mass. (With permission Ref. [10])

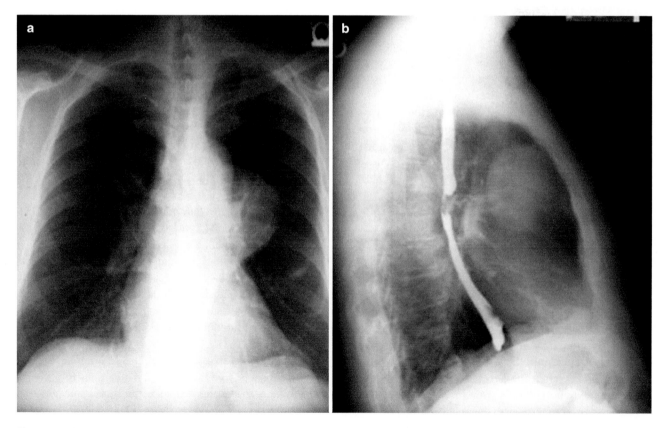

Fig. 3.3 (**a**) Shows an anterior mediastinal mass in the left hemithorax of the posteroanterior chest radiograph. (**b**) Shows a lateral radiograph with esophageal contrast where there is a mediastinal mass without compromise to the tracheobronchial tree

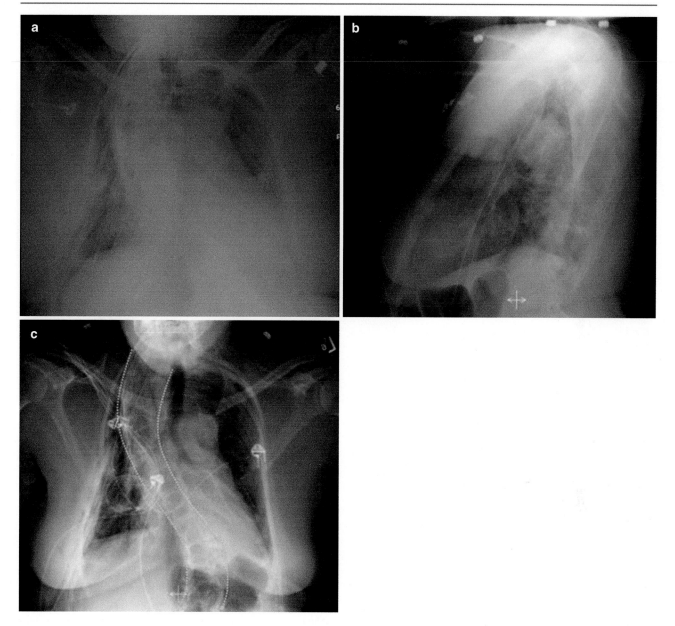

Fig. 3.4 Shows (**a**) a posterior mediastinal mass in the right hemithorax of the posterior–anterior chest radiograph in a female with severe kyphoscoliosis (**b**) a lateral radiograph showing the posterior mediastinal mass, (**c**) a portable posterior–anterior chest radiograph in the post-operative acute care unit after the resection of the posterior mediastinal mass. The yellow dots are showing the contour of the thoracic column showing severe kyphoscoliosis

esophagogram may help to determine whether there is esophageal or tracheobronchial involvement. Figure 3.3a shows an anterior mediastinal mass in the left hemithorax of the posteroanterior chest radiograph. Figure 3.3b shows a lateral radiograph with esophageal contrast where there is a mediastinal mass without compromise to the tracheobronchial tree (Fig. 3.4).

Bullae

Emphysema is characterized by a permanent increase in air spaces distal to the terminal bronchiole beyond the normal size. There is destruction of tissue, leading to a loss of alveolar surface available to participate in air exchange and, sometimes, severe displacement of the adjacent normal lung.

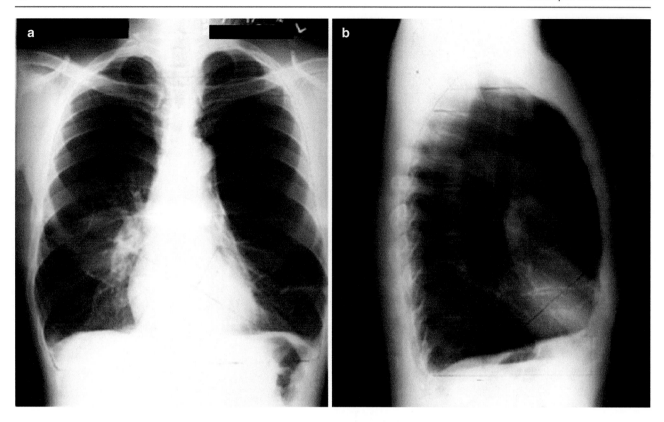

Fig. 3.5 (a) Shows a patient with emphysema. There is a marked hyperinflation with an increase in the anterior–posterior diameter of the chest. Also, there are flattening of the diaphragm bilaterally and gener- alized increase in the blackness of the film. (b) Shows the same patient a lateral chest X-ray

Many of the cases of emphysema seen in adult patients are strongly associated with cigarette smoking. The most strik- ing image in a patient with advanced emphysema is a marked hyperinflation with an increase in the anteroposterior diam- eter of the chest, flattening of the diaphragmatic surfaces, and a generalized increase in the blackness of the film. Also there is a change in the vascular pattern, with attenuated ves- sels thinned and spread apart.

Often bullous areas are noted as large thin-walled air cysts, especially the apices. A bulla is defined as an air- filled space 1 cm or greater in diameter within the lung parenchyma that forms as a result of this destructive pro- cess. Rarely, one or more bullae enlarge to such a degree that they occupy more than one-third of the hemithorax. The term giant bullae is then applied. These easily disten- sible reservoirs are preferentially filled during inspiration, causing the collapse of adjacent, more normal lung paren- chyma [12, 13]. Figure 3.5a shows a patient with emphy- sema, and Fig. 3.5b shows a lateral chest radiograph of the same patient. Figure 3.6 shows a PA chest X-ray and lateral radiograph of a patient with bullae. Figure 3.7 displays the chest X-ray showing a giant bulla occupying more than two-thirds of the right hemithorax and compressing the underlying lung.

Pneumothorax

Pneumothorax is the presence of air in the pleural space that is between the lung and the chest wall. Primary pneu- mothoraces arise in otherwise healthy people without any lung disease. Secondary pneumothoraces arise in subjects with underlying lung disease. Despite the absence of under- lying pulmonary disease in patients with primary pneumo- thorax, subpleural blebs and bullae are likely to play a role in the pathogenesis. It is frequently the result of trauma, although sometimes the source of air leak cannot be readily detected.

The radiographic diagnosis of pneumothorax is usually straightforward. A visceral pleural line is seen without distal lung markings. On standard lateral views, a visceral pleural line may be seen in the retrosternal position or overlying the vertebrae, parallel to the chest wall [14, 15].

Pneumothoraces present as appearances on lateral chest radiographs; although the value of expiratory views is controversial, many clinicians still find them useful in the detection of small pneumothoraces when clinical suspicion is high and an inspiratory radiograph appears normal. The British Thoracic Society guidelines divide pneumothoraces into small and large based on the distance from visceral

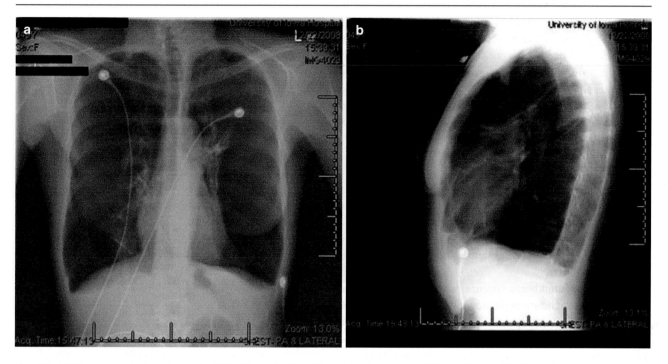

Fig. 3.6 (**a**) Shows a posterior–anterior chest X-radiograph of a patient with a bullae on the left hemithorax. (**b**) Shows the same patient on the lateral radiograph

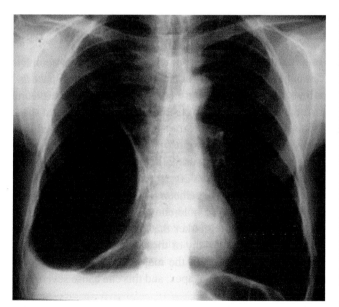

Fig. 3.7 Displays the chest X-ray showing a giant bullae occupying more than two-thirds of the right hemithorax and compressing the underlying lung

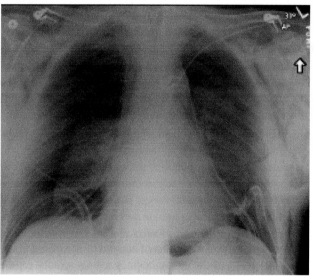

Fig. 3.8 Shows the chest radiograph of a patient with right-sided pneumothorax and bilateral chest tubes

pleural surface (lung edge) to chest wall, with less than 2 cm being small and more than 2 cm large [16]. A small rim of air around the lung actually translates into a relatively large loss of lung volume, with a 2-cm-deep pneumothorax occupying about 50% of the hemithorax.

In the supine position, air in the pleural space will usually be most readily visible at the lung bases in the cardiophrenic recess and may enlarge the costophrenic angle. Figure 3.8 shows the chest radiograph of a patient with right-sided pneumothorax.

Several well-known artifactual appearances can mimic the presence of a pneumothorax and should always be remembered during evaluation of chest radiography. The medial border of the scapula can imitate a lung edge but once considered can be traced in continuity with the rest of the bone, revealing its true nature. Skinfolds overlying

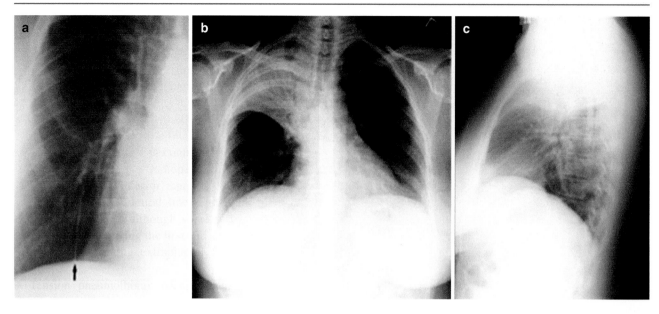

Fig. 3.12 (**a**) Shows a patient who had a right upper lobectomy showing a thin juxtaphrenic peak pointed with an arrow. (**b**) Shows a right upper lobectomy without the juxtaphrenic line. (**c**) Shows the same patient with the lateral chest radiograph

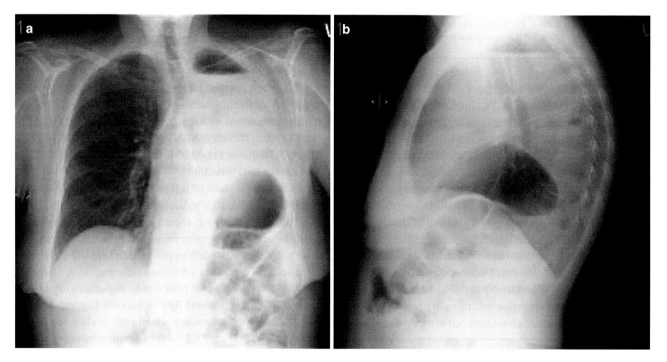

Fig. 3.13 (**a, b**) Shows a chest radiograph in anterior–posterior and lateral position in a patient with a left-sided pneumonectomy. On the left hemithorax, the white image corresponds to fluid in the hemithorax

margins of the heart and diaphragm. After pneumonectomy, air in the operated hemithorax is gradually reabsorbed and replaced by fluid with a net volume loss. As a result, the trachea and mediastinum gradually shift toward the surgical side. In the immediate postoperative period, a mediastinal shift away from the surgical side indicates atelectasis of the contralateral lung or an abnormal accumulation of air or fluid on the surgical side [23]. A rapid mediastinal shift can signify the presence of an air leak with a "ball valve" effect leading to a tension pneumothorax. There are usually some elevation of the hemidiaphragm and a shift of the heart and other midline structures toward the operated side as the remaining lung expands to take some of the space. Gradually the hemithorax fills with fluid, showing a distinct air fluid level if the patient is upright, or a more subtle increase in opacity if the patient is in the supine position. Figure 3.13

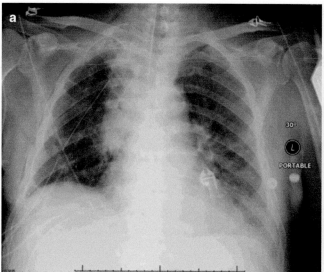 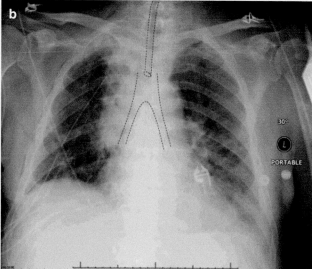

Fig. 3.14 (**a**) Shows a male patient who underwent a right upper lobectomy and remained intubated in the postoperative period with a single-lumen endotracheal tube. (**b**) Shows the same patient with a reconstruction of the single-lumen endotracheal tube. Notice that the tip of the single-lumen endotracheal tube should be placed 3 cm above the tracheal carina

shows a chest radiograph in anterior, posterior, and lateral position in a patient with a left-sided pneumonectomy.

After a thoracic surgical procedure, a chest radiograph film is required in order to assess lung expansion and chest tube placement, and if the patient remains intubated, the proper placement of the endotracheal tube must be assessed. The proper position of a single-lumen endotracheal tube as seen in the chest radiograph is that the distal tip of the tube is located approximately 3 cm above the tracheal carina. All endotracheal tubes have opaque markers that can be clearly identified in the radiographs. Figure 3.14a shows a male patient that underwent a right upper lobectomy and remained intubated in the postoperative period with a single-lumen endotracheal tube. Figure 3.14b shows the same patient with a reconstruction of the single-lumen endotracheal tube.

Double-Lumen Endotracheal Tubes

With any thoracic surgical procedure involving lung isolation devices, the anesthesiologist must review the tracheobronchial anatomy in the preoperative visit to determine whether or not abnormal anatomy exists. A view of the posteroanterior chest radiograph will allow assessment of the shadow of the tracheobronchial anatomy along with the bronchial bifurcation. It is estimated that in 75% of the films, the left mainstem bronchus shadow is seen. In addition, the chest radiograph can be useful to determine the proper size of a left-sided DLT. Brodsky et al. [24] reported that measurement of the tracheal diameter at the level of the clavicle on the preoperative posteroanterior chest

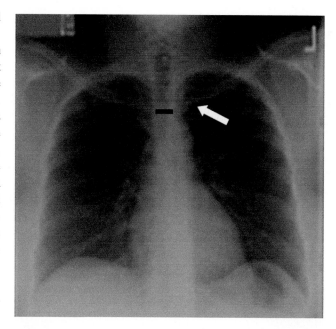

Fig. 3.15 Shows the measurement of the tracheal width at the level of the clavicles to estimate the proper size of the left-sided DLT from a chest radiograph

radiograph can be used to determine proper left-sided DLT size (refer to Chap. 16). Figure 3.15 shows the measurement of the tracheal width at the level of the clavicles to estimate the proper size of the left-sided DLT from a chest radiograph. In addition, the chest radiograph will allow the visualization of the already placed DLT. The tip of each lumen is identified with a radiopaque marker. Figure 3.16a shows the chest radiograph of a patient with a left-sided

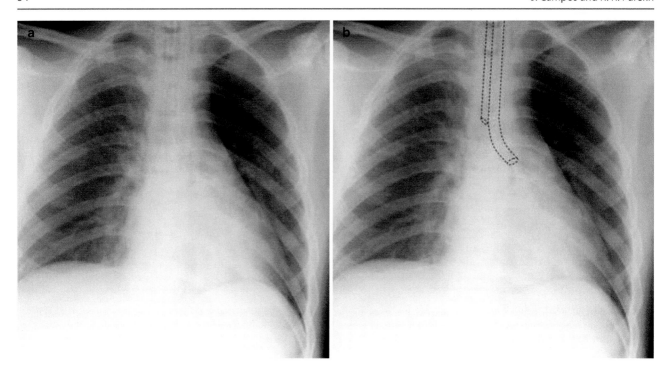

Fig. 3.16 (**a**) Shows the chest radiograph of a patient with a left-sided DLT in place. Notice the endobronchial lumen is approximately 2 cm below the tracheal carina into the left mainstem bronchus. (**b**) Shows a reconstruction of the DLT which is marked in the chest radiograph

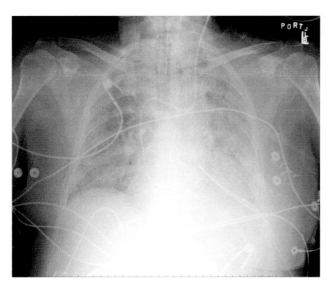

Fig. 3.17 Shows a patient with an acute lung injury (ALI) 72 h after the interstitial edema has progressed in the chest X-radiograph. There is a single-lumen endotracheal tube in place; also a pulmonary artery catheter introduced via the left internal jugular vein is seen. The chest radiograph also shows bilateral diffuse fluffy opacities typical of interstitial pulmonary edema postlobectomy

DLT in place. Notice the endobronchial lumen is approximately 2 cm below the tracheal carina into the left mainstem bronchus. Figure 3.16b shows a reconstruction of the DLT which is marked in the chest radiograph.

Postoperative Acute Lung Injury

Acute lung injury (ALI) may complicate thoracic surgery and is a major contributor to postoperative mortality. The incidence of ALI after thoracic surgery is estimated to be 4.2% [25, 26]. In a study by Licker et al. [25], they found a biphasic distribution pattern of ALI after lung resection. The primary form developed within the first 3 days after surgery and a secondary form triggered the onset of ALI after the third postoperative day.

The clinical presentation is a severe respiratory insufficiency with a progressive hypoxemia that does not respond to a conventional treatment including O_2 therapy. The chest radiograph of a patient with an ALI appears as patchy, unilateral or bilateral infiltrates, dependent pulmonary edema. In addition, atelectatic zones can be seen in the chest radiograph. Figure 3.17 shows a 60-year-old female following a left lower lobectomy who developed ALI in the immediate postoperative period; on the chest radiograph taken after 72 h, the interstitial edema has progressed. There is a single-lumen endotracheal tube in place; also a pulmonary artery catheter introduced via the left internal jugular vein can be seen. The chest radiograph also shows bilateral diffuse fluffy opacities typical of interstitial pulmonary edema postlobectomy after ALI.

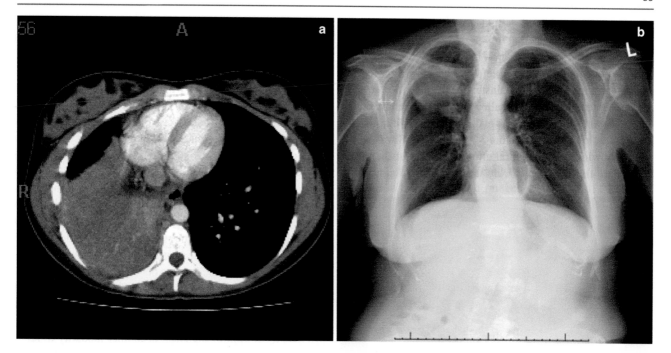

Fig. 3.18 (**a**) Shows a computed tomography (CT) scan of the chest. Diagnosis of pseudotumor of the lung. (**b**) Shows the chest radiograph showing the lung mass in the right upper lobe in the same patient. Diagnosis of right upper lobe adenocarcinoma

Computed Tomography Scan and Pulmonary Disease

CT scan of the chest is used as a diagnostic study; this is usually done after abnormal findings on a standard chest radiograph [27]. Common indications of CT include staging of lung cancer, solitary pulmonary nodule, mass or opacity, diffuse infiltrative lung disease, widened mediastinum, mediastinal mass, or other abnormalities of the mediastinum pleural abnormities, chest wall lesions, trauma, etc. Also, CT provides valuable information for the clinician with regard to the airway compression at any level of the tracheobronchial tree, as well as vascular compression diagnosis [28–31].

CT scans are performed in deep inspiration and at total lung capacity. For a routine helical CT of the chest, 2.5–5 mm sections are usually recommended. Thinner (1–2.5 mm) sections can be used to study fine details of the lung parenchyma. On routine studies, the field of view is adjusted to the size of the thorax, but small fields of view may be selected for smaller anatomic parts that require study. In addition, a contrast CT scan is useful in suspected vascular abnormalities such as pulmonary embolism. Recent improvements in scanner technology have led to the introduction of spiral or helical volumetric CT.

Computed Tomography Scan and Lung Mass, Mediastinal Mass, Pleural Effusion, and Pericardial Effusion

CT scan of the chest will confirm the presence of a mass in the chest and in many instances the specific location. Figure 3.18a shows a CT scan of the chest. There is the presence of a lung mass on the right lung. Figure 3.18b shows the chest radiograph showing the lung mass in the right upper lobe in a female patient. In addition, the CT scan of the chest will define the precise size and location of the mediastinal mass, any involvement with adjacent structures, as well as the degree of compression of the airway (trachea and/or bronchi). It is important during the assessment of the CT scan to identify the location of the mass, define its relationship to adjacent structures, assess the extent and degree of tracheal and/or vascular compression, and assess the patency of the airway at the tracheal and bronchial level. The CT scan also will permit accurate measurement of the airway diameter and will determine the precise level and extent of compression of the trachea. As mentioned previously, the average cross-sectional diameter of the trachea in a 70-kg, 170-cm tall person is approximately 18–23 mm. A tracheal diameter narrowing of 10 mm on CT corresponds to a 50% reduction in the tracheal cross-sectional area at

Fig. 3.23 Shows a tracheal stent in a patient with mediastinal mass. (**a**) Metallic expandable stent, (**b**) CT scan showing a mediastinal mass compressing the trachea, (**c**) airway stent in place seen by CT scan, (**d**) a chest X-ray showing the stent in place. (With permission Ref. [37])

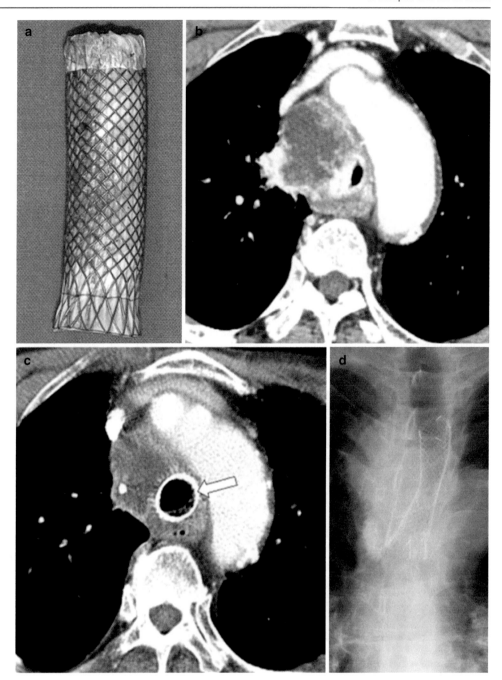

just in axial sections. Direct sagittal and coronal images enable the radiologist to evaluate involvement of lung parenchyma [41], mediastinal structure, and the chest wall with greater clarity than with a CT scan. In addition, MRI is an adjunct to CT scan evaluation reserved for patients in whom CT scans did not resolve the anatomic issues or for whom additional information about the mediastinal and its relationship to other vital organs are required including invasion to heart or great vessels [30, 42, 43]. Figure 3.25 shows MRI of the chest in a patient with a mediastinal mass.

Fig. 3.24 Shows a multidetector computed tomography scan of the chest on a male patient

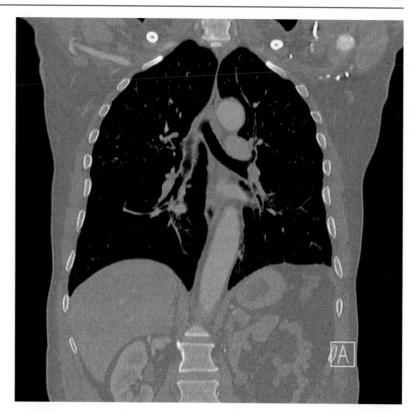

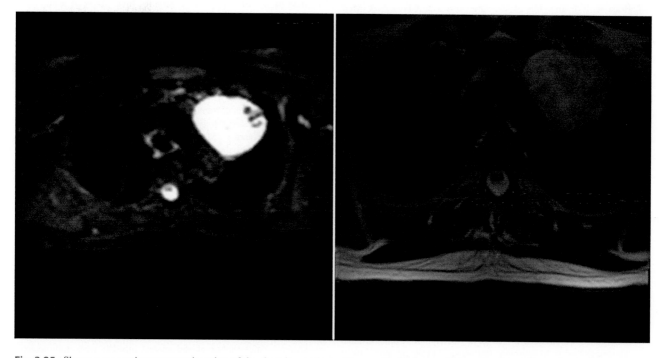

Fig. 3.25 Shows a magnetic resonance imaging of the chest in a patient with a mediastinal mass. This patient has a diagnosis of schwannoma

Summary

Radiological studies play an important role in the diagnosis and treatment of the thoracic surgical patient in the preoperative, intraoperative, and postoperative period. Chest radiographs allow us to identify distorted tracheobronchial anatomy, presence of lung masses, lung collapse, chest tube placement, endotracheal tube placement, and lung expansion or shifting of mediastinum in cases of tension pneumothorax. CT scans of the chest permit an identification and precise location of lung masses and mediastinal masses or the presence of fluid and compromise to adjacent structures; in addition it allows to identify the precise location of airway stents [44].

Multidetector computed tomography scan and 3D reconstruction allow identification of tracheobronchial anatomy in a more precise form. All radiological studies must be reviewed in the preoperative evaluation of thoracic surgical patients. In cases where the diagnosis or anatomy is unclear, these studies must be reviewed in conjunction with a thoracic surgeon or a radiologist.

References

1. Boiselle PM. Imaging of the large airways. Clin Chest Med. 2008;29:181–93.
2. Seymour AH. The relationship between the diameters of the adult cricoid ring and main tracheobronchial tree: a cadaver study to investigate the basis for double-lumen tube selection. J Cardiothorac Vasc Anesth. 2003;17:299–301.
3. Minnich DJ, Mathisen DJ. Anatomy of the trachea, carina and bronchi. Thorac Surg Clin. 2007;17:571–85.
4. Stene R, Rose M, Weigner MB, et al. Bronchial trifurcation at the carina complicating use of a double-lumen tracheal tube. Anesthesiology. 1994;80:162–1164.
5. Campos JH. Update on tracheobronchial anatomy and flexible fiberoptic bronchoscopy in thoracic anesthesia. Curr Opin Anaesthesiol. 2009;22:4–10.
6. Goldwin RL, Reed JC. Chapter 2: Radiology of the chest. In: Kaplan J, Slinger P, editors. Thoracic anesthesia. 3rd ed. New York: Churchill Livingstone; 2003. p. 24–56.
7. Fraser RS, Pare JA, Fraser RG, et al. Synopsis of diseases of the chest. 2nd ed. Philadelphia: WB Saunders; 1994.
8. Datt V, Tempe DK. Airway management in patients with mediastinal masses. Indian J Anaesth. 2005;49:344–52.
9. Ahmed-Nusrath A, Swanevelder J. Anesthesia for mediastinoscopy. Contin Educ Anaesth Crit Care Pain. 2007;7:6–9.
10. Campos JH. Chapter 11: Managing the patient with an anterior mediastinal mass In: Cohen NH, editor. Medically challenging patients undergoing cardiothoracic surgery, Society of Cardiovascular Anesthesiologists Monograph. Baltimore: Lippincott Williams & Wilkins; 2009. p. 285–302.
11. Harris GJ, Harman PK, Trinkle JK, et al. Standard biplane roentgenography is highly sensitive in documenting mediastinal masses. Ann Thorac Surg. 1987;44:238–41.
12. Morgan MDL, Edward CW, Morris J, et al. Origin and behavior of emphysematous bullae. Thorax. 1989;44:533–8.
13. Schipper PH, Meyers BF, Battafarano RJ, et al. Outcomes after resection of giant emphysematous bullae. Ann Thorac Surg. 2004;78:976–82.
14. O'Connor AR, Morgan WE. Radiological review of pneumothorax. BMJ. 2005;330:1493–7.
15. Glazer H, Anderson DJ, Wilson BS, et al. Pneumothorax: appearances on lateral chest radiographs. Radiology. 1989;173:707–11.
16. Henry M, Arnold T, Harvey J. BTS guidelines for the management of spontaneous pneumothorax. Thorax. 2003;58(Suppl 2):ii39–52.
17. Light RW. Tension pneumothorax. Intensive Care Med. 1994;20:468–9.
18. Baumann MH, Sahn SA. Tension pneumothorax: diagnostic and therapeutic pitfalls. Crit Care Med. 1994;22:896.
19. Symbas PN. Chest drainage tubes. Surg Clin North Am. 1989;69:41–6.
20. Baldt MM, Bankier AA, Germann PS, et al. Complications after emergency tube thoracostomy: assessment with CT. Radiology. 1995;195:539–43.
21. Maunder RJ, Pierson DJ, Hudson LD. Subcutaneous and mediastinal emphysema. Pathophysiology, diagnosis, and management. Arch Intern Med. 1984;144:1447–53.
22. Konen E, Rozenman J, Simansky DA, et al. Prevalence of the juxtaphrenic peak after upper lobectomy. Am J Roentgenol. 2001;177:869–73.
23. Wechsler RJ, Goodman LR. Mediastinal position and air-fluid height after pneumonectomy: the effect of the respiratory cycle. Am J Roentgenol. 1985;145:1173–6.
24. Brodsky JB, Macario A, Mark JB. Tracheal diameter predicts double-lumen tube size: a method for selecting left double-lumen tubes. Anesth Analg. 1996;82:861–4.
25. Licker M, de Perrot M, Spiliopoulos A, et al. Risk factors for acute lung injury after thoracic surgery for lung cancer. Anesth Analg. 2003;97:1558–65.
26. Hayes JP, Williams EA, Goldstraw P, et al. Lung injury in patients following thoracotomy. Thorax. 1995;50:990–1.
27. McLoud T. Chapter 36: Imaging the lungs. In: Patterson C, Deslauriers L, Luketich R, editors. Pearson's thoracic surgery. 3rd ed. New York: Churchill Livingstone; 2008. p. 415–28.
28. Harte BH, Jaklitsch MT, McKenna SS, et al. Use of a modified single-lumen endobronchial tube in severe tracheobronchial compression. Anesthesiology. 2002;96:510–1.
29. Slinger P, Karsli C. Management of the patient with a large anterior mediastinal mass: recurring myths. Curr Opin Anaesthesiol. 2007;20:1–3.
30. Chiles C, Woodard PK, Gutierrez FR, et al. Metastatic involvement of the heart and pericardium: CT and MR imaging. Radiographics. 2001;21:439–49.
31. Shepard JA, Grillo HC, McLoud TC, et al. Right-pneumonectomy syndrome: radiologic findings and CT correlation. Radiology. 1986;161:661–4.
32. Le Guen M, Beigelman C, Bouhemad B, et al. Chest computed tomography with multiplanar reformatted images for diagnosing traumatic bronchial rupture: a case report. Crit Care. 2007;11:1–8.
33. Rubin GD, Beaulieu CF, Argiro V, et al. Perspective volume rendering of CT and MR images: applications for endoscopic imaging. Radiology. 1996;199:321–30.
34. Boiselle PM, Reynolds KF, Ernst A. Multiplanar and three-dimensional imaging of the central airways with multidetector CT. Am J Roentgenol. 2002;179:301–8.
35. Higgins WE, Ramaswamy K, Swift RD, et al. Virtual bronchoscopy for three-dimensional pulmonary image assessment: state of the art and future needs. Radiographics. 1998;18:761–78.
36. Laroia AT, Thompson BH, Laroia ST, et al. Modern imaging of the tracheo-bronchial tree. World J Radiol. 2010;2:237–48.

37. Shin JH, Song HY, Ko GY, et al. Treatment of tracheobronchial obstruction with a polytetrafluoroethylene-covered retrievable expandable nitinol stent. J Vasc Interv Radiol. 2006;17: 657–63.

38. Higgins WE, Helferty JP, Lu K, et al. 3D CT-video fusion for image-guided bronchoscopy. Comput Med Imaging Graph. 2008;32:159–73.

39. Moore EH, Webb WR, Muller N, et al. MRI of pulmonary airspace disease: experimental model and preliminary clinical results. Am J Roentgenol. 1986;146:1123–8.

40. Bader TR, Semelka RC, Pedro MS, et al. Magnetic resonance imaging of pulmonary parenchymal disease using a modified breath-hold 3D gradient-echo technique: initial observations. J Magn Reson Imaging. 2002;15:31–8.

41. Bergin CJ, Glover GH, Pauly JM. Lung parenchyma: magnetic susceptibility in MR imaging. Radiology. 1991;180:845–8.

42. Bremerich J, Roberts TP, Wendland MF, et al. Three-dimensional MR imaging of pulmonary vessels and parenchyma with NC100150 injection (Clariscan). J Magn Reson Imaging. 2000;11:622–8.

43. Bittner RC, Felix R. Magnetic resonance (RM) imaging of the chest: state-of-the-art. Eur Respir J. 1998;11:1392–404.

44. Marchese R, Poidomani G, Paglino G, et al. Fully covered self-expandable metal stent in tracheobronchial disorders: clinical experience. Respiration. 2015;89:49–56.

Part III

Thoracic Anatomy, Physiology, and Pharmacology

Essential Anatomy and Physiology of the Respiratory System and the Pulmonary Circulation

4

J. Michael Jaeger, Brian J. Titus, and Randal S. Blank

Key Points

- Knowledge of the clinical anatomy and function of the respiratory system is essential for the safe, efficient, and appropriate perioperative management of intubation, mechanical ventilation, and anesthesia for the thoracic surgical patient.
- The lung has ten (third-generation airway) bronchopulmonary segments on the right and eight segments on the left that are readily identifiable by fiberoptic bronchoscopy (two segmental bronchi on the left are considered "fused").
- The anesthetic employed, both general and regional, will impact the control of respiration, reactivity of the airways, and the patient's ability to maintain their airway, take a deep breath, and cough.
- Dynamic influences of ventilatory pattern, posture, body habitus, agitation or pain, and inflammation can cause "air trapping" and drastically reduce alveolar ventilation.
- The compliance and resistance of the respiratory system will change during the course of surgery, especially those procedures requiring one-lung ventilation, and may necessitate frequent adjustments of the ventilator to optimize gas exchange and reduce lung injury.
- Many drugs employed during cardiothoracic surgery will impact the lung's intrinsic mechanisms to match ventilation to perfusion matching either directly on hypoxic pulmonary vasoconstriction (HPV) or indirectly by altering cardiac output or vascular resistance.

Introduction

Appropriate perioperative management of the thoracic surgical patient requires an appreciation of the uniqueness and complexity of the anatomy and function of the respiratory system. It is particularly suited to perform a wealth of tasks including gas exchange between the lungs and blood, speech, protection from airborne environmental insults and pathogens, and a host of metabolic functions (repair, growth). While some of these functions have little importance to the anesthesiologist during the course of a surgical procedure, optimizing gas exchange, controlling pulmonary arterial pressure, and maintaining blood flow require constant attention. Furthermore, the dynamic interaction between the cardiovascular system and the respiratory system can be altered by changes in position, medications and anesthetics, mechanical ventilation, surgical interventions, disease processes, etc. The impact of these alterations cannot be underestimated. The entire cardiac output passes from the right side of the heart to the left side with each heartbeat; therefore what affects the pulmonary circulation ultimately impacts the systemic circulation. While an in-depth discussion of the physiology and anatomy of the entire respiratory system is beyond the scope of this chapter, the essentials will be discussed with the goal of providing insights into the clinical relevance and application of this knowledge by the thoracic anesthesiologist.

Functional Anatomy

Upper Airway Anatomy

Oropharynx and Nasopharynx

The collection of air passages extending from the nares and lips through the labyrinthine nasopharynx and oropharynx extending through the larynx to the cricoid cartilage can be

J. Michael Jaeger (✉) · B. J. Titus · R. S. Blank
Department of Anesthesiology, University of Virginia Health System, Charlottesville, VA, USA
e-mail: jmj4w@virginia.edu

© Springer Nature Switzerland AG 2019

P. Slinger (ed.), *Principles and Practice of Anesthesia for Thoracic Surgery*, https://doi.org/10.1007/978-3-030-00859-8_4

defined as the functional upper airway. This airway complex serves a host of functions: warming and humidifying the passage of air, filtering particulate matter, and preventing aspiration during deglutition.

In normal quiet breathing, air enters the nose, a complex chamber separated medially its entire length by a cartilaginous and bony septum (vomer). It is bounded laterally by the inferior, middle, and superior turbinates overlying the sinus ostia and inferiorly by the hard and soft palates before emptying into the nasopharynx. The mucosa covering these structures is highly vascular and innervated which must be appreciated when performing nasopharyngeal intubation with endotracheal tubes and passage of nasogastric sumps, feeding tubes, or fiberoptic bronchoscopes. Furthermore the nasal passages represent a significant resistance to airflow, normally double that found in mouth-breathing. Airflow resistance increases dramatically when nasal polyps are present, the mucosa is inflamed and edematous, or when high air flows must be achieved as in heavy exercise.

The adult pharynx is 12–15 cm long and is divided into the nasopharynx (from the soft palate to the tip of the uvula), the oropharynx (from the anterior pillars of the tonsillar fossa to the epiglottis) that includes the pharyngeal portion of the genioglossus muscle, and finally the laryngopharynx lying posterior to the larynx. Supination, sleep, and general anesthesia may promote obstruction of the oropharynx by the tongue, hard palate, and pharyngeal musculature as their tone decreases [1, 2]. Hyperextension or hyperflexion of the cervical spine generally increases upper airway resistance [3]. During inspiration, a non-sedated, spontaneously breathing patient dilates the oropharyngeal pharynx by contracting the genioglossus muscle and elevating the tongue off the pharyngeal wall in a coordinated reflex possibly involving thoracic muscle activity [2, 3].

Larynx

The larynx is a complex structure overlying the fourth to the sixth cervical vertebra and consists of several muscles, their ligaments and cartilaginous anchors, and significant innervation (Fig. 4.1). The inlet of the larynx is defined by the epiglottis, aryepiglottic folds, and the arytenoids. The larynx itself bulges into the pharynx posteriorly creating a deep pharyngeal recess anterolaterally on either side, the pyriform fossa. The bilateral pyriform fossae or recesses are clinically relevant because of their tendency to trap food or foreign objects (and tubes or probes) in the pharynx and as potential sites for the application of topical anesthesia to block the internal branch of the superior laryngeal nerve. The larynx serves as the organ of phonation, plays an important role in coughing, and in protection of the airway during deglutition [4].

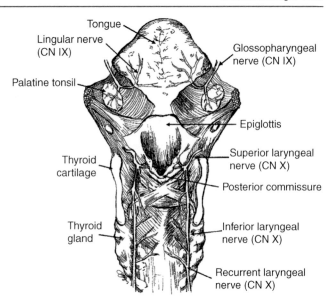

Fig. 4.1 Diagram of the larynx from the base of the tongue to below the thyroid cartilage as viewed from its posterior aspect. Note the relationship of the superior laryngeal, inferior laryngeal, and recurrent laryngeal nerves and the posterior aspect of the larynx, thyroid, and trachea. Tracheal and thyroid surgery places these nerves at risk

The primary structure of the larynx is the thyroid cartilage that forms the point of articulation of the paired arytenoid cartilages with the vocal ligaments and their controlling musculature. However other essential structures include the hyoid bone and its attachments, the epiglottis, the cricoid cartilage, and the corniculate cartilages. The hyoid bone is a U-shaped bone that is attached to the mandible and tongue by the hyoglossus, the mylohyoid, geniohyoid, and digastric muscles, to the stylohyoid ligament and muscle, and to the pharynx by the middle pharyngeal constrictor muscle. Beneath the hyoid bone is slung the remainder of the larynx by its attachment, the thyrohyoid membrane and muscle. While its function other than as a flexible anchor is unclear, it is possible to bisect its mandibular attachments ("suprahyoid release") and mobilize the larynx in order to facilitate its caudal displacement in tracheal resection procedures. The epiglottis is the midline "leaf-shaped" elastic cartilage found inferior to the base of the tongue. It is anchored anteriorly to the hyoid bone and inferiorly to the inside of the anterior portion of the thyroid cartilage immediately above the vocal cords. Bilateral folds of the epiglottis curve posteriorly to form a mucosal ridge attaching to the arytenoid cartilages sitting on top of the posterior lamina of the cricoid, the aryepiglottic folds. The epiglottis, aryepiglottic folds, and the corniculate tubercles form the readily recognizable inlet into the glottis below. The large thyroid cartilage defines the larynx with its paired lamina fused anteriorly at the laryngeal prominence and extending posteriorly to terminate in superior and inferior horns or cornu. The thyroid cartilage serves

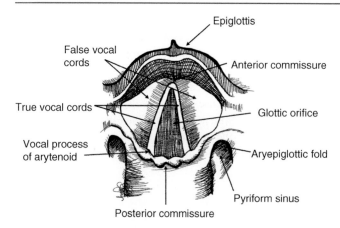

Fig. 4.2 Diagram of the glottis as seen from above using a laryngoscope or fiberoptic bronchoscope. Note the triangular shaped glottic introitus with its narrowest aspect at the anterior commissure. Passage of bronchoscopes, endotracheal tubes, and especially double-lumen tubes should be directed posteriorly where the vocal cords will spread the widest. Note that the vocal process of the arytenoid cartilage pivots on a small point and can be traumatized and displaced with rough handling

as a stable point of attachment for numerous small muscles and ligaments that manipulate the small arytenoids, corniculates, and vocal cords. The thyroid cartilage also attaches to the cricoid ring in ways that afford it some degree of mobility. One key ligament deserves special attention, the vocal ligament or true vocal cord. The paired vocal cords attach posteriorly to the vocal process of each arytenoid and stretch anteriorly to meet at the junction of the thyroepiglottic ligament of the anterior thyroid cartilage. The triangular opening formed by the vocal ligaments is the glottis with its apex anterior (Fig. 4.2). The mean length of the relaxed open glottis is approximately 23 mm in males and 17 mm in females. The glottis at its widest (posterior) point is 6–9 mm but can be "stretched" to 12 mm [5]. It should be noted that the vocal cords are covered by only a thin, adherent mucosa, producing the pearly white appearance. The absence of any submucosa implies that the vocal cords are unlikely to "swell" significantly as there is minimal space to accumulate edema fluid. The folds of mucosa and fibrous tissue lying parallel to the true vocal cords and just superior within the glottis, known as the vestibular folds or "false vocal cords," can become edematous. The intrinsic laryngeal musculature function to open the glottis in inspiration, close the glottis and constrict the superior structures in deglutition, and finely control abduction, adduction, and tension of the true vocal cords in phonation.

Pharyngeal Innervation

Innervation of the pharynx is distributed among several sensory and motor branches of the glossopharyngeal and vagus (external and internal branches of the superior laryngeal nerves, recurrent laryngeal nerves). The nasopharynx sensory innervation is derived from the maxillary division of the trigeminal nerve, while the oropharynx is diffusely innervated by sensory branches from the glossopharyngeal nerve. The internal branch of the superior laryngeal nerve pierces the lateral aspect of the thyrohyoid membrane along with the superior laryngeal artery and vein to provide sensation for the base of the tongue, vallecula, epiglottis, aryepiglottic folds, pyriform recesses, and the superior aspect of the true vocal cords. The external branch of the superior laryngeal nerve provides motor to the cricothyroid muscle, a tensor of the true vocal cords. The recurrent laryngeal nerves supply sensation to the vocal cords and tracheobronchial tree as well as motor to the remaining intrinsic musculature of the larynx. The right recurrent laryngeal nerve originates at the level of the right subclavian artery but the left originates at the level of the aortic arch and loops around the ligamentum arteriosum before both ascend cephalad along the tracheoesophageal groove. This relationship must be appreciated during esophageal surgery and during both cervical and anterior mediastinoscopy, as these structures can be at risk. The larynx receives its blood supply from the superior and inferior laryngeal arterial branches of the superior and inferior thyroid arteries, respectively [6]. These arteries follow the course of the superior and recurrent laryngeal nerves.

Upper Airway Function

Homeostatic Mechanisms

The most obvious function of the upper airways is to provide a durable protective conduit for the initial inhalation and then exhalation of gases to and from the lung while simultaneously performing multiple other functions, e.g., eating, drinking, speaking, etc. With respect to inhalation, the nasopharynx and posterior pharynx warm the inspired gas close to body temperature and humidify it to a water vapor pressure of 47 mmHg at 37 °C. This aids in maintaining core temperature and protects the more delicate epithelia lining the lower airways from desiccation. Glandular cells within the airway epithelium secrete mucus which coats the airway surface and maintains tissue hydration and also serves to trap particulate matter, bacteria, and viruses. Mucus also contains a number of enzymes with antioxidant, antiprotease, and antibacterial properties [7].

Another important role of the airways and its mucus coat is the filtering of inhaled particulate matter by an elaborate defense system that takes advantage of the airflow characteristics of the upper and lower airways and their associated epithelium. There are three mechanisms at work to produce mechanical filtering. The first, inertial impaction, is capable of trapping particulates larger than 10 μm by virtue of the turbulent flow, mucus lining the passageways, and complex structure. It accomplishes this task in minutes with mucus and saliva eventually swallowed. The bifurcating and branching tracheobronchial tree slows the gas flow until it becomes more laminar. Particulates impact the airway wall according to particle size (sedimentation). Normally the particles, bacteria, etc. trapped in the mucus at this level are transported cephalad by the constant motion of the cilia, an apical feature of the respiratory epithelium, at a rate of approximately 2.5 mm/min in the bronchi but over 5 mm/min in the trachea [8]. Lower airway mucus is usually cleared in about 24 hours although this can be drastically retarded in disease states such as cystic fibrosis or chronic bronchitis or conditions altering ciliary function or growth, e.g., smoking [9]. The filtering processes appear effective down to particles approximately 0.01 μm in diameter.

The Cough Reflex

An essential protective function of the respiratory system for expelling secretions and foreign bodies from the respiratory tract is the cough. The cough is a complex maneuver that is either voluntary or triggered by stimulation of airway irritant mechanoreceptors diffusely distributed throughout the larynx, trachea, and bronchi, especially the carina. Irritant chemoreceptors are distributed more diffusely in the distal central airways and at airway junctions, where noxious vapor particles are more likely to rain out on the epithelium. The vagus nerve serves as the primary afferent limb of the cough reflex, but the efferent limb encompasses the motor input to the phrenic, intercostal, other spinal motor neurons to the accessory respiratory muscles and the vagus nerve branches to the larynx and pharynx.

There are several acts involved in generating an explosive flow of air and material out of the airways. The first is an exaggerated inspiration through a widely abducted glottis to achieve a high lung volume, which may be as high as 50% of vital capacity. By enlarging the intrathoracic volume, this produces a lengthening in the expiratory muscles and improves their length-tension relationship allowing greater force generation. The second compressive phase begins with rapid adduction of the glottis simultaneous with the onset of expiratory muscle contraction. Glottic closure is accentuated by the tight adduction of the supraglottic ventricular folds. This phase lasts only hundredths of a second but is sufficient to produce a coordinated compression of the alveolar gas and increase in the intrathoracic pressure, briefly as high as 300 cm H_2O [4]. Abrupt initiation of the final expiration phase occurs with glottic

release of this pressure producing nearly a subatmospheric drop in central airway pressures accentuating the pressure gradient from the continually rising alveolar and pleural pressures as a consequence of expiratory muscle contraction. An additional effect is dynamic compression of the airways which increases airflow velocity in relation to the volume of air expired per second. The total effect is a shearing force across the surface of the mucus-covered airway epithelia and mucus expulsion.

Clinical Issues

Airway Obstruction

Patients with tracheal or laryngeal mass lesions and those with vocal cord dysfunction can have significant flow resistance during inspiration and/or expiration depending on the intrathoracic vice extrathoracic location of lesions. High airflow rates through the site of the restrictive lesion can accentuate the increase in airway resistance. Less obvious is the effort-dependent dynamic compression that can occur in those portions of the airway that lie on either side of the lesion during the period of high flow [10]. Attempts to generate high flows create the greatest Bernoulli effect (acceleration-induced negative pressure) on the surrounding structures and can result in airway narrowing. This has clinical importance in managing patients pre- and post-procedure for laryngeal or tracheobronchial resections. Slow, easy breathing is more efficacious than rapid, forced breaths; therefore judicious use of a sedative in addition to good postoperative pain management may improve gas exchange. This scenario is in contrast to that of patients with primary muscle weakness of the upper airway musculature either from residual neuromuscular blockade, general anesthesia, myasthenia, or extrapyramidal disorders [11]. These conditions require mechanical support until strength can be recovered or optimized.

Nebulized Medications

The features of the upper airway also impact the design and utility of multidose inhalers and medication nebulizers. Typically less than 30% of aerosolized drug delivered with the standard nebulizer or inhaler reaches the small airways [12]. Most drug particles in current inhalers range in size from 1.5 to 4.0 μm [13, 14]. Consequently, these particles frequently fail to reach the distal small airways sufficiently such that even with new particle manufacturing technologies, only about 50% of the drug penetrates to the intended target [13, 14]. Even aerosolizing chambers attached to endotracheal tubes or ventilator circuits provide only a marginal improvement in efficiency at delivering drug to the distal airways.

Tracheobronchial and Respiratory Anatomy

Tracheal and Bronchial Structure

The trachea originates at the cricoid cartilage (opposite vertebra C6) and extends approximately 12 cm (females) to 14 cm (males) to terminate in a bifurcation (carina) at the T4/5 vertebral level (second intercostal space, the angle of Louis). It is about 22 ± 1.5 mm (males) to 19 ± 1.5 mm (females) in diameter and consists of 16–20 U-shaped cartilaginous "rings" that are closed posteriorly by fibrous tissue and a longitudinal smooth muscle band or trachealis muscle.

The right main bronchus is wider (14–17.5 mm), shorter (1.4–1.8 cm), and more vertical than the left. The right main bronchus gives off the upper lobar bronchus then continues on as the bronchus intermedius giving off the right middle lobar bronchus and right lower lobar bronchus at the hilum of the lung at T5. The azygos vein arches over it from behind to reach the superior vena cava. The right pulmonary artery lies first inferiorly and then anterior to the bronchus intermedius. The left main bronchus ranges an average of 4.4–4.9 cm in length and 13–16.5 mm in diameter. It passes inferiorly and laterally below the aortic arch, anterior to the esophagus and descending thoracic aorta to reach the hilum of the lung opposite T6. At this point, it first lies behind and then slightly below the left pulmonary artery in its course. These dimensions can be quite variable among individuals, and chest pathology can drastically change the anticipated relationships. We recommend always consulting available computed tomograms of the chest prior to any thoracic procedure to provide the anesthesiologist with more appropriate dimensions and structural relationships in their patient.

The lobar bronchi (right upper, right middle, right lower and the left upper, left lower) diverge into their segmental bronchi that can be readily visualized during flexible bronchoscopy (Table 4.1). The right upper lobar bronchus gives off three segmental bronchi (apical, anterior, posterior), the right middle lobar bronchus splits into two segmental bronchi (lateral, medial), and the right lower lobar bronchus diverges into the superior segment with the basal segmental bronchus immediately diverging into four additional segments (medial basal, anterior basal, lateral basal, posterior basal) for a total of ten segmental branches on the right. The left upper lobar bronchus splits into the superior division with "three" segments (a "fused" apical-posterior, anterior) and the inferior division or lingual with two segments (superior lingular, inferior lingular). The left lower lobar bronchus branches into four lower segmental branches (superior, another "fused" anteromedial basal, lateral basal, posterior basal) for a total of "ten" segments on the left. Note that segmental nomenclature can vary in the literature [15].

Table 4.1 Bronchopulmonary segments

	Right lung			Left lung
		Upper lobe		
Apical	1		*Superior division*	
Anterior	2		Apical + posterior	1 + 3
Posterior	3		Anterior	2
			Inferior division – lingula	
			Superior lingular	4
			Inferior lingular	5
		Middle lobe		
Lateral	4			
Medial	5			
		Lower lobe		
Superior	6		Superior	6
Medial basal	7		Anteromedial basal	7 + 8
Anterior basal	8		Lateral basal	9
Lateral basal	9		Posterior basal	10
Posterior basal	10			

Tracheobronchial Circulation and Lymphatic System

The trachea and bronchi derive their blood supply from branches of several sources, and the variation can be substantial. The common pattern is as follows. The cervical trachea derives its blood supply from branches of the inferior thyroid artery. The carina and distal trachea receive their blood supply from the bronchial arteries (superior, middle, and inferior) coming off of the internal thoracic artery, branches from the innominate artery, and the descending aorta [6]. The segmental branches off the three bronchial arteries then form a longitudinal network over the length of the tracheal lateral wall. These arteries subsequently branch into an anterior and posterior intercartilagenous arteries. The anterior vessels enter the tracheal wall bilaterally, join within the wall at the midline, and then form a diverse submucosal vascular net that supplies their respective segment of trachea. The posterior intercartilagenous branches join with branches from esophageal segmental arteries to provide the blood supply to the membranous portion of the trachea.

There is great variation in the bronchial blood supply as well. In general though, the left mainstem bronchus is perfused by the inferior bronchial artery derived from two left-sided aortic sources. The right mainstem bronchus is most often supplied by a single branch from a right-sided aortic source [6]. The bronchial arteries frequently originate from the descending aorta between the level of the 5th and 6th thoracic vertebral level, but contributions can come from branches off of the arch or subclavian arteries [16]. The bronchial arteries originate from the anterolateral aspect of the descending aorta in a somewhat "tight" group of usually four ostia approximately 18 mm apart. This becomes relevant in lung transplantation as this "aortic patch of bronchial arteries" could be harvested *in toto* for bronchial revascularization.

Lymphatic drainage of the lung parenchyma occurs through a network of lymph capillaries located in the connective tissue surrounding the airways and their accompanying vascular structures. The lymphatic vessels are located between the alveolar walls and the assorted interlobular, peribronchial, and perivascular structures. However, they do not reside in any of the alveolar septae specialized for gas exchange nor are they within the interalveolar septum [16]. Lymphatic capillaries also course over the surface of the lung where they become confluent and join at the hilum with the peribronchial vessels. Smooth muscle and unidirectional valves within the lymphatic vessel walls ensure antegrade flow of the fluid. Of course lymph nodes are abundant within the lung and mediastinum belying their proximity to the airways exposed to the environment. Ultimately the lymphatic system drains into the venous system either via the internal jugulosubclavian venous confluence or via the thoracic duct after joining [17].

Respiratory Airways and Alveolar Histology

The airways continue to diverge into smaller and smaller diameter conduits until one arrives at the bronchioles with diameters less than 0.8 mm. At this level the airways lose all remnants of cartilage and begin the transformation from purely conducting airways to those described as respiratory bronchioles. Respiratory bronchioles eventually diverge into the final four generations of alveolar ducts that consist primarily of openings into the terminal alveolar sacs. In the descriptive model of E.R. Weibel, the trachea branches into 23 generations of pulmonary airways. The first 15 generations serve as conducting airways, and the subsequent 8 generations become sufficiently thin-walled to allow some degree of gas exchange and bear the moniker, acinar airways. One clinical aspect of this geometric progression of increasingly narrower airways (and blood vessels) by divergence and multiplication is that the overall cross-sectional area and therefore resistance to gas flow (or blood flow) becomes markedly less compared to the resistance of the individual airway (or blood vessel). This has an important impact on distribution of gas and blood flow, flow velocity, and, hence, transit time through key areas of gas exchange.

The trachea interior is lined with ciliated columnar epithelium, Goblet cells responsible for mucus production, and with interspersed specialized chemical and tactile afferent nerve receptors. This transitions from pseudostratified columnar epithelia in the larger bronchi to a thinner cuboidal ciliated variety in the small bronchi. The airway epithelium and submucosa also contain lymphocytes, mast cells, and a variety of neuroendocrine cell types. The next layer consists of circumferential bands of smooth muscle cells and a connective tissue layer containing submucosal glands and plates of cartilage (replacing the solid cartilage rings in the very large airways). The outermost layer is a loose adventitial shell with lymphatic vessels, sympathetic and parasympathetic nerves, and nourishing blood vessels.

The respiratory bronchioles empty into a pulmonary acinus, which has the appearance of a cluster of grapes on a network of stems. Each pulmonary acinus may contain multiple alveolar ducts communicating with 2000 alveoli arranged in a ring-like, honeycomb network. The alveolus is considered the primary site of gas exchange between the blood and gas in the lung. The alveolar septa are about 5–8 μm thick and are opposed by an alveolar surface on either side with the alveolar capillary bed sandwiched inside. The walls of the alveoli are extremely thin, between 0.1 and 0.2 μm, a feature that promotes rapid equilibration of gas by diffusion with the pulmonary capillary blood. In addition, gas can exchange between alveoli through pores of Kohn. There are approximately 300 million alveoli in the human lung that provide an extraordinary surface area for gas exchange (70 m²).

There are three major cell types found in the alveolus: Alveolar Type I, Alveolar Type II, and alveolar macrophages. However, there are others found under certain conditions in the lung, e.g., inflammation. Alveolar Type I cells are a squamous epithelium class that cover an estimated 95–97% of the total alveolar surface [18]. These nucleated cells have few cytoplasmic organelles and a sparse cytoplasm splayed out in sheets over the alveolar surface forming a thin barrier between the air space and the pulmonary capillary endothelium. While their role in gas exchange is obvious, new information suggests a more diversified role than previously thought. New protein analysis of the Type I cells suggests that they may play an important role in regulation of cell proliferation, ion transport and water flow, peptide metabolism, and signaling events in the peripheral lung [19]. Alveolar Type II cells are fewer in number, somewhat spherical, and coated on their apical surface with microvilli. In contrast to Type I cells, Alveolar Type II cells possess many organelles including multilayered granular structures called lamellar bodies. These lamellar bodies are considered the source of pulmonary surfactant, a lipoprotein coating the interior surface of the alveolus, and capable of significantly reducing the surface tension of the alveolus air-surface interface. Surface tension reduction is considered an important physical mechanism to reduce any tendency for alveolar collapse at very low lung volumes.

The immune defenses of the lung are extremely important because of its relative exposure to the environment via the airways. There are a number of excellent reviews of the immune function of the lung, but it is important to realize that there are many questions unanswered about how the lung responds to invasion and inflammation [20]. From a clinical standpoint, the pulmonary inflammatory response will greatly influence the perioperative management of the thoracic surgical patient. A few major defensive cell types residing in the alveolar air spaces and interstitium are worth mentioning. Alveolar macrophages are derived from bone marrow monoblast precursor cells and migrate to the lung parenchyma [21]. Alveolar macrophages are free to move over the surface of the alveolus and phagocytize foreign material that enters the alveolus including bacteria and particulates. Macrophages are cleared either through the lymphatics or are carried up and expelled via the airways. Lymphocytes, largely T-lymphocytes, are widely distributed in the normal lung within paratracheal and hilar lymph nodes, in the interstitium of the bronchial tree as nodules or individual cells, in the alveolar walls, and on the surface of the alveolus [22]. They play a critical role in the lung's primary immune response to inhaled antigens. Under some pathologic conditions in the lung, it is becoming apparent that an exaggerated inflammatory response and the activity of these cells and others may be harmful to the lung; the acute respiratory distress syndrome (ARDS) and emphysema are examples. Recent investigations have revealed another key cell in the lung's immune response to foreign material. Dendritic cells are potent antigen-presenting cells in the respiratory tract and elsewhere that possess dendrites that project to the airway luminal surface between the epithelial cells [23]. Dendritic cells are capable of sampling luminal contents, binding to foreign peptides, and then migrating to regional lymph nodes where they present these peptides to antigen-specific T-cells. In addition, they are sensitive to environmental signals from microbes, allergens, pollutants, or the products of tissue damage [23].

Innervation

The hilum of each lung serves as the entry point of the bronchi, pulmonary vessels, bronchial vessels, lymph vessels, and nerves. The lungs receive their innervation from the autonomic nervous system with branches from the vagus nerves and upper thoracic sympathetic ganglia (primarily second, third, and fourth). The vagal and thoracic sympathetic ganglia form anterior and posterior pulmonary plexuses at the hilum. From there, two main neural networks develop; one accompanies the bronchi, the peribronchial plexus, and the other associates with the pulmonary vasculature, the periarterial plexus. Virtually all afferent nerve fibers entering the CNS from the airways travel through the vagus nerve [24].

Neural Control of Respiration

Respiratory Centers

It is generally accepted that the medulla contains the respiratory centers within the brain that are responsible for coordinating numerous voluntary and involuntary inputs that generate the appropriate respiratory pattern to fulfill the body's requirements. The classical view described a dorsal respiratory group of neurons receiving modulatory input and controlling the timing of inspiration. A ventral respiratory group of dispersed nuclei was responsible for both inspiratory and expiratory respiration [25].

New evidence has led to the concept of a three-phase respiratory pattern in normal or "eupneic" breathing controlled by a complex architectural network of nuclei from the pons to the medulla that is highly conserved phylogenetically in mammals [26]. The three phases are inspiration, post-inspiration (post-I), and active expiration (E-2) [26, 27]. Inspiration begins with a synchronized neuronal discharge that increases to a maximal intensity then abruptly terminates. Subsequently, a secondary declining neuronal burst termed "post-inspiratory (post-I) afterdischarge" represents the active phase of the "passive" exhalation (E-2) from the lungs that is controlled by the upper airway adductor muscles [25–28].

The critical nucleus for inspiratory rhythm generation is widely accepted as centered in the pre-Bötzinger complex (pre-BötC) located in the ventral medulla respiratory column (Fig. 4.3). The pre-BötC neurons in turn project to numerous other neuron groups, e.g., rostral to the adjacent Bötzinger complex (BötC), which modifies and refines the post-inspiratory and expiratory phases [28]. BötC and pre-BötC are influenced by convergent inputs including the retrotrapezoid nucleus/parafacial respiratory group (RTN/pFRG) that are thought to provide a rhythmic expiratory drive. It is this region with its chemosensitive neurons in conjunction with input from the dorsal group of respiratory neurons in the nuclei of the solitary tract (NTS) that is poised to modify respiratory drive to match metabolic needs [29]. The NTS receives tonic activation from peripheral arterial chemoreceptors and from rhythmically activated lung stretch receptor afferent inputs. The NTS responds by influencing inspiratory termination after lung inflation [28]. Of note, there is debate whether lung stretch receptor reflexes actually play a significant role in humans as they clearly do in lower mammals [25]. One final important respiratory control center resides in the rostral pons. Here the Köllicker-Fuse (KF) and parabrachial nuclei are essentially relay nuclei for a large array of inputs from reflex afferents and higher CNS input controlling breathing. In particular, the KF area may regulate the inspiratory-expiratory phase transition and the dynamic control of upper air-

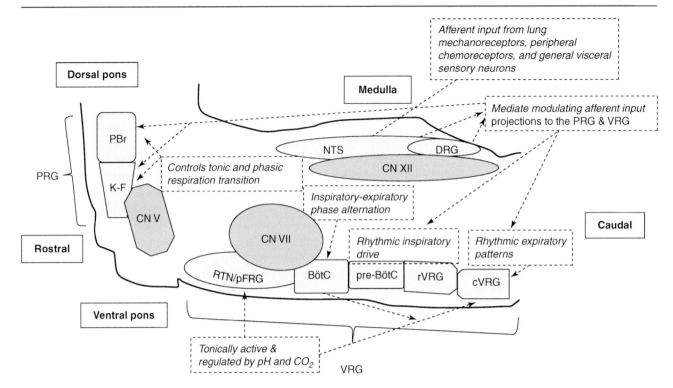

Fig. 4.3 Diagram of brainstem respiratory centers demonstrating the locations and relationships between key control centers, both ventral and dorsal respiratory groups. Rostral pons includes the pontine respiratory group (PRG) containing the Kölliker-Fuse (K-F) and parabrachial nuclei (PBr) important in phase transition from inspiration to expiration. These centers receive modulating input from the caudal nucleus tractus solitaries (NTS) and dorsal respiratory group (DRG). Located caudally in ventral respiratory group (VRG) are the tonically active retrotrapezoid nucleus (RTN)/parafacial respiratory group (pRFG) which generate rhythmic patterns and receive input from the central chemoreceptors. More caudal still lie the pre-Bötzinger complex (normal rhythmic inspiratory phase) and the Bötzinger complex (control inspiratory-expiratory phase transitions). Both of these areas receive modulating input from other sites and integrate the signals to produce the desired breathing pattern. The NTS and associated afferent nuclei of the DRG are sites of chemoreception and integration of afferent input from peripheral sensory neurons. This sensory integration modifies depth and rate of respiration and the states of arousal and airway patency to maintain homeostasis. (From data in Refs. [26–29])

way during the respiratory cycle and receives input from visceral sensory afferents via the vagus and glossopharyngeal nerves [25, 27, 28, 30].

Chemoreception and Respiratory Control

A fundamental concept in the regulation of breathing rate and depth is maintenance of an appropriate arterial PCO_2 and PO_2 as important components of acid-base regulation in a bicarbonate-based buffer system and of oxygen delivery, respectively [31]. The system must be able to adapt to a wide variety of conditions: awake at rest, during exercise, asleep, pregnancy, high-altitude exposure, or during illness, for example. Ventilation is far more sensitive to alterations in arterial PCO_2 within a fairly restricted range when compared to arterial PO_2. Determining the transduction mechanisms and location of the chemoreceptors as well as their relative contribution to control rate and depth of breathing has been difficult [32]. The experimental process may confound the results especially those studies performed on anesthetized subjects since many anesthetics have the ability to blunt respiratory drive via effects on reflex pathways and directly on chemoreception as a consequence of inducing acidosis in plasma and cerebrospinal fluid [33]. Nonetheless it is clear that there are central chemoreceptor areas and specific peripheral chemoreceptor structures that are capable of measuring arterial CO_2, hydrogen ions, and arterial O_2 and then generate a graded signal response transmitted to the central respiratory centers. There is also good evidence for the modulation of the inputs from these chemoreceptor sites by their interaction. Subsequent elegant studies performed in awake animals in the 1960s established the view that the respiratory centers were primarily sensitive to CO_2 and hydrogen ion concentration measured by central chemoreceptors located in the ventrolateral medulla [34, 35]. They found that a decrease of 0.05 pH unit can double alveolar ventilation, and inhalation of 5.6% CO_2 increases alveolar ventilation by 300% [34]. Further refinement of these studies and the addition of multiple new, sophisticated techniques revealed a more complicated picture involving multiple central and peripheral sites integrated to coordinate the response to acidemia, alkalemia, hypercarbia, and hypoxemia. It is estimated that approximately two-thirds of the ventilator response to CO_2 or hydrogen ions is contributed by the central chemoreceptors, while the remaining third is contributed by peripheral chemoreceptors, mainly the carotid body [33].

The molecular mechanism involved in the transduction of CO_2 or hydrogen ions into a graded signal relayed to the respiratory control centers remains a matter of debate [36]. The molecular details are beyond the scope of this chapter (for excellent review, see reference [37]). However, it has become clearer that it involves several different potassium ion channels (leading candidates are in the Kir and K_{2P} subfamilies) that either respond directly to pH changes or indirectly as effectors responding to an unidentified, possible G-protein coupled, proton-sensitive membrane receptor [37, 39]. It is well established that inhibition of one or more of these potassium channels results in depolarization of afferent neurons in the retrotrapezoid nucleus (RTN), locus coeruleus (LC), nucleus tractus solitarius (NTS), and medullary raphe, all in superficial locations readily exposed to CSF and the generously vascular areas within the ventrolateral and caudodorsal medulla [36–39].

The ventilator response to hypoxia is primarily initiated by the carotid bodies with O_2 sensors in the aortic bodies secondary. The carotid bodies are located bilaterally in the carotid bifurcations close to the carotid sinus. For their small size, they are complex organs that are richly innervated and possess a dense network of capillaries. The latter enable a relatively high degree of blood flow delivery with small diffusion distances between cells. The carotid bodies sensitivity to arterial PO_2 is a primary response, but they also have been shown to respond to pressure, hypercapnia, acidosis, hyperkalemia, hypoosmolality, certain hormones, hyperthermia, and hypoglycemia [40]. Two unique types of cells are present. Type I glomus cells similar to sensory neurons and a Type II glial-like "supportive" cells. The role of the latter remains unclear and will not be discussed further.

Carotid body Type I cells appear to contain the O_2-sensing apparatus that, when appropriately stimulated, release excitatory neurotransmitters, perhaps ATP, dopamine, or acetylcholine (ACh), which act on adjacent afferent nerve endings of the carotid sinus nerve. The carotid sinus (and carotid body) nerve is a component of the glossopharyngeal nerve and transmits a corresponding intensity of nerve impulses to the NTS [41]. Sensory discharge under normal conditions (arterial PO_2 of approximately 100 mmHg) elicits a low rate of neuronal discharge but increases exponentially beginning with only modest degree of hypoxemia (arterial PO_2 of approximately 60 mmHg). It appears to plateau at an arterial PO_2 of about 30–40 mmHg, but the gain can be modulated depending on local pH [42, 43]. As with the central chemo-

receptor cells, the actual mechanism of O_2 sensing is debatable. Many hypotheses have been put forth but most incorporate some pathway that ultimately inhibits potassium ion channels (TASK family) or activates voltage-dependent calcium ion channels resulting in membrane depolarization of the Type I glomus cell and the release of vesicles containing neurotransmitter [44, 45]. The exact mechanism varies. One hypothesis suggests that Type I cell mitochondria possess a unique cytochrome oxidase with an especially low affinity for O_2 such that electron transport system and ATP production are affected far sooner than in other mitochondria [45]. Others have suggested that reactive oxygen species or a number of "gasotransmitters" such as nitric oxide, carbon monoxide, or hydrogen sulfide might modulate carotid body chemotransduction by virtue of their production by heme-containing proteins and a requirement for molecular O2 as found in mitochondria [46, 47]. Obviously further work needs to be done and the mechanism substantiated in humans. For an extensive review of O_2-sensing mechanisms in the carotid body, see reference [48].

Finally, it is well established that there is considerable cross talk between the peripheral chemoreceptors and the central chemoreceptors in all mammals including humans [49]. While stimulation of central chemoreceptors likely does not impact the output of the peripheral chemoreceptors, there is considerable evidence that the gain of the central chemoreceptors to CO_2 and hydrogen ion concentration can be critically dependent upon activity in the carotid body afferent nerve output [50–52]. These relationships must be appreciated when managing patients intraoperatively under anesthesia and postoperatively where residual sedation, opioid analgesia, and a degree of metabolic disarray may exist. In addition, all of the aforementioned respiratory control processes are altered or dysfunctional in common conditions such as aging or immaturity, congenital central hypoventilation syndrome, obstructive sleep apnea, or central sleep apnea secondary to congestive heart failure [25].

Neural Control of the Airways

Neural control of the airway smooth muscle is important in determining airway caliber, and pharmacologic modulation of this input is clinically relevant. The main neurotransmitters identified are acetylcholine (ACh) that acts on several muscarinic subtypes, epinephrine and norepinephrine acting on both α- and β-adrenergic receptors, and a variety of purported non-adrenergic, non-cholinergic neurotransmitters such as vasoactive intestinal peptide (VIP), nitric oxide (NO), substance P, and neurokinin A acting via second messenger cascades to elicit a variety of responses. See Barnes for a detailed discussion [53]. Although some of these neurotransmitters can have non-pulmonary sources, it is now clear that airway parasympathetic and sympathetic nerves can release more than one class of neurotransmitter. The end terminals of parasympathetic nerves can release ACh, VIP, NO, and others that have inhibitory and excitatory properties on either the primary target end-organ or the presynaptic terminus to modify release of the primary neurotransmitter. Similarly, sympathetic nerves release norepinephrine but also may secrete substance P, neurokinin A, VIP, calcitonin gene-related peptide, cholecystokinin octapeptide, etc. [54]. The effects of many of these substances on the airway diameter, mucus secretion, and blood flow are still to be defined.

Cholinergic nerve influence on the human respiratory system is mediated via a family of muscarinic receptors on airway smooth muscle. Five muscarinic subtypes have been cloned, but only four have been identified in the lungs. These are M_1, M_2, M_3, and M_4 receptors, although only M_3 appears to be responsible for the contractile response on human airway smooth muscle [55]. M_2 receptors on the airway smooth muscle cells act through an inhibitory G-protein to block adenyl cyclase activity and lower cyclic AMP concentrations. Its role is yet to be determined, perhaps opposing the effects of β_2 agonists. However, M_2 receptors are also found on the human cholinergic presynaptic nerve terminal and likely functional as feedback inhibition to the further release of ACh. Alterations in the sensitivity or function of these receptor subtypes have been implicated in several disease states, especially influenza, asthma, and emphysema.

Adrenergic innervation of the human airways is present but despite the fact that airway smooth muscle possesses both α- and β-adrenergic receptors, direct adrenergic bronchodilator activity has not been demonstrated in contrast to observations in many animal models [56]. It appears that the more dominant role of adrenergic nerve stimulation is in presynaptic modulation of ACh release from airway cholinergic nerves via pre-junctional β_2-adrenergic receptors. Of note, β-blockers can have a profound negative impact on asthma exacerbations and yet have minimal effect on the bronchial tone of normal individuals. The mechanism behind this clinical observation is not known but may reflect expression of the asthmatic disease genotype. The absence of α-adrenergic receptors on human airway smooth muscle suggests that neuronal and adrenal catecholamines act directly only on arterial smooth muscle in the lung.

Respiratory Muscles

Bulk movement of air into and out of the lungs occurs as a result of changes in intrathoracic pressure created by rhythmic changes in the volume of the thorax. Expansion of the chest cavity occurs when three distinct respiratory muscle groups work in concert. The diaphragm, intercostal muscles, and the accessory muscles (sternocleidomastoids, sca-

lenes) are controlled by the respiratory centers of the brain to contract in a rhythmic pattern designed to carefully match ventilation to gas exchange requirements. The abdominal musculature (rectus abdominis, external oblique, internal oblique, and transversus abdominis) can be recruited when more force is required for exhalation, although abdominal muscle tone may stabilize the rib cage during inspiration as well.

Inspiration

The diaphragm is unique in that its muscle fibers radiate from a central tendinous structure to insert peripherally on the ventrolateral aspect of the first three lumbar vertebrae and on the aponeurotic arcuate ligaments, and the costal portion inserts on the xiphoid process and the upper margins of the lower six ribs. Its motor innervation is solely from the right and left phrenic nerves that originate from the third, fourth, and fifth cervical nerve roots. In the relaxed state, it forms a pronounced "dome" that closely apposes the chest wall for some distance before arching across the midline. Contraction of the diaphragm causes a large caudal displacement of the central tendon resulting in a longitudinal expansion of the chest cavity. Simultaneously, its insertions on the costal margins cause the lower ribs to rise and the chest to widen. This diaphragmatic motion is responsible for the majority of quiet respiration. Note that as the dome of the diaphragm descends, it displaces the abdominal contents caudally. The fall in pleural pressure and accompanying lung expansion produce an increase in abdominal pressure and some outward movement of the abdominal wall. The supine and Trendelenburg positions or surgical retractors can significantly impact this abdominal motion especially in the morbidly obese necessitating controlled ventilation under anesthesia.

The intercostal muscles are thin sheet-like muscles with origins and insertions between the ribs. The internal intercostal muscles have their fibers oriented obliquely caudad and dorsally from the rib above to the rib below. The external intercostal muscles have their fibers oriented obliquely caudad and ventrally from the rib above to the rib below. All intercostals are innervated by the intercostal nerves running in the neurovascular bundle within a groove on the inferior aspect of each rib. Contraction of the external intercostals produces an inspiratory action by elevating the upper ribs to increase the anteroposterior dimensions of the chest in a "well pump-handle" motion. The lower ribs are also elevated by virtue of the force applied and their point of rotation to increase the transverse diameter of the thorax. The internal intercostals apply their force in such a direction as to rotate the ribs downward, decreasing the thoracic anteroposterior dimension to aid in active expiration. In general, the intercostal muscle activity is minimal in quiet respiration but increases in conditions requiring a high minute ventilation like exercise.

The principal accessory respiratory muscles are the sternocleidomastoid and scalenes. The scalene muscles originate from the transverse processes of the fourth through the eighth cervical vertebrae and slope caudally to insert on the first two ribs. Their contraction during periods of high ventilatory demand elevates and fixes the cephalad rib cage during inspiration. Similarly, the sternocleidomastoid elevates the sternum and increases the longitudinal dimensions of the thorax.

Expiration

Expiration is a passive process in quiet breathing. It is a response to relaxation of the inspiratory muscles and the balance of forces generated by the elastic recoil of the lungs and chest wall. When high levels of ventilation are required as in exercise or if airway resistance increases as in exacerbations of asthma, the expiratory phase becomes an active process with forceful contraction of the rectus abdominis, the transverse abdominis, and the internal and external oblique muscles. The contraction of the abdominal musculature retracts the abdominal wall and pulls the lower ribs downward which increases intra-abdominal pressure and accelerates the cephalad displacement of the diaphragm during exhalation. The internal intercostal muscles depress the rib cage and provide a minor contribution to forced expiration. Innervation of the abdominal musculature is from thoracic nerves 7 through 12 and the first lumbar nerve. These nerves are commonly affected by epidural anesthesia and thus can impact cough and other forced expiratory maneuvers.

Like most skeletal muscles, the diaphragm and intercostal muscles are a heterogeneous mix of fiber types, containing between 40% and 60% slow oxidative (Type I) fibers. The human diaphragm probably has between 49% and 55% Type I fibers, the remainder a mix of the "faster-high activity" Type IIA and IIB fibers [57]. The types of skeletal muscle fibers seem to be distributed fairly evenly throughout the diaphragm. Of note, the respiratory muscles, especially the diaphragm, retain the ability to adapt to stress and training [58]. Not all adaptation is favorable. Mechanical ventilation (>18 hours) rapidly produces atrophy and dysfunction in the human diaphragm [59]. Diaphragm muscle fibers show increased proteolysis, reduced protein synthesis, possible mitochondrial oxidative stress (mitochondrial DNA deletions), and sarcoplasmic lipid accumulation [60, 61]. Lung pathology can produce maladaptive responses as well. Emphysema is a good example. The diaphragm undergoes changes at the sarcomere level, physically "losing or altering" key sarcomere proteins (slow heavy myosin, titin) and changes in the proportion of Type I to Type II fibers [62–64]. These changes result in an easily fatigued diaphragm and intercostal muscles causing the characteristic increased thoracic dimensions and "flattening" of the diaphragm, thus contributing to the limited exercise capacity in these patients [62].

The Respiratory "System"

The Pleural Pressure

The lungs and chest wall move together as a system. This is made possible by the enclosed, airtight thoracic cavity where the outer surface of the lungs and its visceral pleura are in close proximity to the parietal pleura covering the chest wall and mediastinal structures. Changes in the intrathoracic volume are only possible because the inside of the lung is in continuity with the ambient atmosphere outside the thorax via the trachea and pharynx. The intimate contact between the layers of pleura are maintained by a negative intrapleural pressure generated in part by the intermolecular forces of the pleural fluid excluding gas from this space. This lubricating fluid allows freedom of the pleural layers to slide over one another but highly resists separation of the layers much like two panes of glass with a thin layer of water between them. Deforming forces are thereby directly and reliably transmitted between the chest wall and lung and allow for a unified motion.

Normally the intrapleural pressure is about -5 cm H_2O when the respiratory system is in a "resting configuration or equilibrium state," but it can vary significantly. Recoil of the chest wall either outward or inward as with active exhalation and changes in elastic recoil of the expanded or contracted lung, diaphragm position, and body position (gravitational effects) will summate to define the magnitude of the intrapleural pressure (Fig. 4.4). Pathologic conditions like the introduction of air or blood into the intrapleural space can rapidly disrupt this relationship leading to a compromise in respiratory function but also interfere with cardiovascular function. Examples of disruption of the intrapleural space would be a pneumothorax, a large empyema or pleural effusions, or a tension pneumothorax.

Lung Volumes

Clinical pulmonary physiology is based in part upon a common nomenclature of the measured lung volumes during a variety of respiratory maneuvers. Mastering this language facilitates effective communication across all disciplines within medicine and surgery. First, most lung volumes and

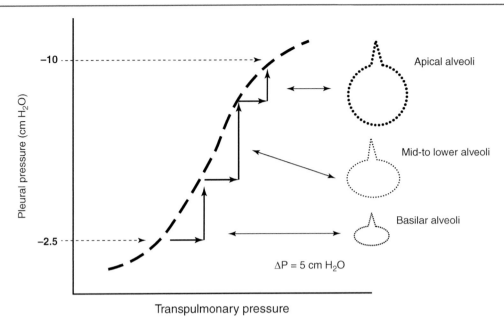

Fig. 4.4 The static relationship between the transpulmonary pressure (alveolar pressure – pleural pressure) and the pressure in the pleural space. Pleural pressure is normally negative relative to atmospheric pressure. The gradient is small at the base of the lung (P_{pl} least negative) but larger at the apex (P_{pl} most negative) because of the recoil pressure of the elastic lung tissue. This disparity results in larger alveoli at the apex then the dependent alveoli at the base. When atelectasis develops the alveoli are collapsed, a condition frequently seen in patients post-thoracotomy even when sitting upright. As a result a given change in transpulmonary pressure produces the largest change in volume (and pleural pressure) where the alveoli sit on the steepest portion of this curve

capacities are measured by a device referred to as a spirometer. Spirometry and other associated measurement techniques have combined to define four major subdivisions of *lung volume*: (1) residual volume (RV), (2) tidal volume (TV), (3) expiratory reserve volume (ERV), and (4) inspiratory reserve volume (IRV). These four lung volumes then can be combined to define the clinically useful four *lung capacities*: (1) total lung capacity (TLC), (2) vital capacity, (3) inspiratory capacity (IC), and (4) functional residual capacity (FRC). These terms and relationships are defined in Table 4.2. Details of their measurement are described in Chap. 2.

Differences in individual lung volumes are related to a large extent by body habitus, in particular, height. However, since TLC is influenced by lung and chest wall elastic recoil properties, inspiratory muscle strength, and body position, many conditions can alter its measurement. As an example, a "standard young adult male of average height" would likely have a TLC of about 6.5 L, of which 1.56 L is residual volume. Therefore his vital capacity would be about 5 L. However the magnitude of the residual volume, RV, is a balance between expiratory muscle strength and the outward recoil of the chest wall at complete active exhalation. Although these predominantly static measurements are made without any confounding flow resistance factors, "dynamic compression" of the airways from either extreme expiratory effort or loss of structural integrity with aging does occur and will increase lung residual volume. The lung

Table 4.2 Lung volumes and capacities

	Definition
Lung volumes	
Tidal volume (V_T)	Air volume inspired and expired during a relaxed breathing cycle
Residual volume (RV)	Volume remaining in the lung after a maximal expiratory effort
Expiratory reserve volume (ERV)	The volume of air that can be forcibly exhaled between the resting end-expiratory volume and RV
Inspiratory reserve volume (IRV)	The volume of air that can be inspired with maximal effort above the normal resting end-expiratory position of a V_T
Lung capacities	
Vital capacity (VC)	The amount of air that can be exhaled from the point of maximal inspiration to the point of maximal expiration [IRV+ERV]
Total lung capacity (TLC)	Total volume of air in the lungs after a maximal inspiration [IRV+ERV+RV]
Functional residual capacity (FRC)	Amount of air in the lung at the end of a quiet exhalation [ERV+RV]

volume at the end of a spontaneous exhalation during quiet breathing, the functional residual capacity or FRC, marks a passive balance between the opposing elastic forces of the lung and the chest wall, i.e., the resting volume of the respiratory system. At this lung volume, airway pressure is zero (or equal to ambient atmospheric pressure), i.e., no pressure gradient exists between the inside of the alveoli and the mouth and therefore no air flow.

Dynamic Mechanical Aspects of the Respiratory System

The Pressure-Volume Relationship

Both the chest wall and lungs are elastic structures, and each has unique physical properties that define this elasticity. As elastic structures, the lungs and chest wall will return to their original configuration when deforming forces are removed. The equilibrium positions or volumes are not the same for the lung and chest wall. In fact, it is possible to define the relationship between volume of the lung or chest wall (thoracic cavity) and a deforming pressure independently under experimental conditions. The static pressure-volume curve for an isolated lung is compared to that of a chest wall in Fig. 4.5. Note that the equilibrium position of the lung is at or near residual volume, RV. To sustain any lung volume above, this point requires the application of a distending force. The lung will recoil with an equal and opposing force. At all volumes above RV, the lung tends to recoil inwards as indicated by the positive pressure or distending force required (x-axis). On the other hand, the equilibrium position of the chest wall is at a relatively large volume, estimated at approximately 60% of the total lung capacity. To attain any "chest wall volume" above, this point requires

active inspiratory muscle force, and likewise to decrease the volume below, this point requires a significant input of expiratory muscle force. The thick solid line shows a summation of the two individual curves to define the static volume-pressure relationship for the total respiratory system. The recoil pressure of the respiratory system (P_{rs}) is defined as the algebraic sum of the individual recoil pressures of the lung (P_L) and the chest wall (P_{cw}).

$$P_{rs} = P_L + P_{cw}$$

The volume at which the P_{rs} is zero is the relaxation volume (V_{rx}) of the respiratory system. In the normal healthy individual during quiet breathing, the volume of the lung at end of expiration (FRC) approximates the V_{rx}. However, under different circumstances, FRC may deviate from V_{rx} significantly. Numerous static factors such as posture, respiratory muscle tone, body habitus, and other external forces may reduce end-expiratory lung volume, while dynamic mechanisms such as dynamic airway compression or asthma may increase it.

Postural influences on the pressure-volume relationship of the respiratory system are primarily related to gravitational forces on the abdominal contents. In the erect posture, the downward pull of gravity displaces the abdominal contents and tends to exert an inspiratory action on the

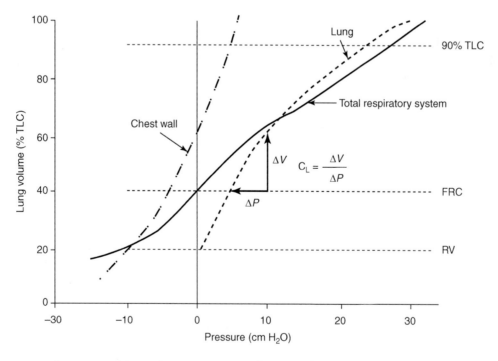

Fig. 4.5 Static pressure-volume curves of the respiratory system. The isolated chest wall pressure (P_{cw}) – thoracic cavity volume curve (large dash-dot line) crosses the zero pressure or equilibrium point at approximately 60% of TLC. The isolated lung pressure (P_L) – volume curve (small dash-dot line) approaches its equilibrium point at about 20% TLC or RV. Note that P_{cw} can be positive (force provided by contraction of the inspiratory muscles to achieve TLC) or negative (even greater

force exerted by expiratory muscles to collapse the chest wall to reach RV). The algebraic summation of the chest wall and lung compliance ($\Delta V/\Delta P$) curves defines the static pressure-volume relationship of the total respiratory system (solid line). Note that in the totally relaxed state, the balance between outward recoil of the chest wall and the inward recoil of the lung is at a lung volume (V_{rx}) that usually approximates FRC

diaphragm. In contrast, the upright posture affects the rib cage in a manner more like expiration, with gravity pulling the rib cage inward and downward. In the supine position, gravity exerts a small expiratory action on the rib cage but a more pronounced expiratory action on the abdominal contents and diaphragm. The pressure-volume curve for the chest wall is shifted to the right (i.e., produces less opposition to the inward recoil of the lung) and results in a shift in the V_{rx} and, hence, FRC to smaller volumes (in normal individuals about 10% or more). The Trendelenburg position can emphasize this decrease in FRC by an additional 10% of TLC. This fact should be kept in mind when a patient is emerging from anesthesia following surgery in the supine or Trendelenburg position.

Lung Compliance, Lung Volume, and Dynamic Modifiers

Healthy adults with relatively stiff chest walls or low chest wall compliance (C_{cw}) tend to breathe near their relaxation volumes or FRC because the respiratory system is most efficient when under these conditions. In other words, the necessary pressure gradient (ΔP) that must be generated to produce an adequate resting tidal volume (V_T or ΔV) is optimized on the steeper slope of this pressure-volume relationship to require the least amount of work of breathing (WOB). The slope of the pressure-volume relationship defines the respiratory system compliance (C_{rs}). For the sake of brevity, we will only discuss static (vs dynamic) compliance. The compliance of the respiratory system is calculated in a similar fashion to P_{rs}. Since the pressure (at a given volume) is inversely proportional to compliance, the total compliance of the respiratory system (C_{rs}) is the algebraic sum of the reciprocals of the compliance of the lung (C_L) and the chest wall (C_{cw}). Therefore, the equation of respiratory system recoil pressure can be rewritten as follows:

$$\frac{1}{C_{rs}} = \frac{1}{C_L} + \frac{1}{C_{cw}}$$

By definition, compliance, C_{rs}, equals $\Delta V_{rs}/\Delta P_{rs}$ and is normally in the range 50–80 mL/cm H_2O. To estimate the lung compliance and potential stress to the lung parenchyma would require a substitution of the transpulmonary pressure gradient. The traditional definition of transpulmonary pressure is the pressure difference between the airway opening (mouth) and the pleural space as estimated by esophageal manometry; both measured with respect to atmospheric pressure. Caution should be exercised in its interpretation [65]. Examples of pathologic conditions that alter respiratory system compliance are pulmonary fibrosis (a decrease in lung compliance) and scoliosis (a decrease in chest wall

compliance) through its effect on the spine and rib cage. To sustain the respiratory system at high lung volumes is disadvantageous from a mechanical standpoint and requires a considerable increase in work of breathing to balance the increased elastic chest wall and lung components. A secondary factor establishing the FRC is the interplay of dynamic factors [66]. During quiet breathing, there is sufficient time for passive emptying of the lungs. However at high rates of ventilation during exercise or when emptying is delayed because of obstruction to flow, end-expiratory volumes may be determined more by dynamic factors rather than a static equilibrium. In obstructive lung diseases, despite the general increase in C_L by destruction of the alveolar architecture and decline in elastic recoil, the increase in V_{rx} (FRC) is as much a reflection of effort-dependent dynamic airway compression and expiratory flow limitation. Therefore, dynamic factors can play an important role in setting the equilibrium point for the volume of the respiratory system and FRC.

The notion that dynamic factors can impact FRC is an important one that influences not only normal physiology but thoracic pathology and artificial conditions such as general anesthesia and mechanical ventilation. Dynamic FRC is determined by the balance between two major factors: the time available for expiration (t_E) and the rate of lung emptying or flow. The expiratory time (t_E) is highly influenced by the expiratory time constant (τ), which in its simplest form is the product of airway resistance to flow (R_{aw}) and compliance (C_{rs}). As an example, neonates have an increased R_{aw} because of the small diameter of their airways and have a highly compliant chest wall (increased C_{rs}) due to their underdeveloped rib cage and musculature. Thus τ, which equals ($R_{aw} \times C_{rs}$), is relatively prolonged. If the ratio t_E/τ is less than 3, dynamic FRC exceeds V_{rx}, and airway pressure at end-expiration does not reach zero. Therefore, there is incomplete expiration down to V_{rx}, and retention of gas occurs. This phenomenon continues to about 1 year of age whereupon sufficient maturity of the respiratory system produces a reduction in τ and increases in t_E to favor the normal adult pattern [67].

The same "air trapping" process can occur in adult individuals with prolonged expiratory times as a result of airway obstruction from COPD, asthma, or external airway compression from masses, for example. Incomplete expiration may occur during either spontaneous or mechanical ventilation. When describing a mechanically ventilated patient, the condition is referred to as "dynamic hyperinflation" and reflects a measurable increase in airway pressure above the normal zero pressure at end-expiration. In the literature, this has often been referred to as "intrinsic PEEP" and reflects the pulmonary end-expiratory pressure produced by the elastic recoil of the respiratory system at the higher lung volume.

Distribution of Ventilation

Ventilation is not homogeneous in the lung due to a number of factors, some of which still remain controversial. The most frequent explanation for this nonuniformity is the effect of gravity and the balance of all of the previously mentioned forces acting on the lung and chest wall. In the upright posture, the lung attains its greatest vertical height. Because the lung consists of a honeycomb of interconnected thin-walled sacs and airways and holds a considerable volume of blood within the blood vessels interspersed within its structure, it has mass that is acted upon by gravitational forces. Gravity will tend to favor blood flow to the dependent portions of the lung, and therefore, its weight will add to the weight of the lung tissue. This has multiple effects. First since the elastic lung septae are all interconnected, they distribute this force throughout the lung. The tendency for the lung to retract away from the chest wall at its apex creates a more negative (subatmospheric) pleural pressure than the pleural pressure at the lower dependent portions of the lung where its weight reduces the magnitude of the negative pleural pressure [68]. The gradient of pleural pressure from the lung apex to its base has been estimated at 0.4 cm H_2O per each centimeter of vertical height. Second, the increased stretch on the alveoli at the apex of the upright lung creates regions of larger, more inflated alveoli that become progressively smaller as one moves closer to the dependent lung base (Fig. 4.4). A consequence of this apical alveolar enlargement is to decrease compliance and create an inhomogeneous distribution of air within the lung during a breath at FRC, greater distribution of the breath to the base as opposed to the apex [68, 69]. Obviously, one might expect less of a transpulmonary pressure gradient from nondependent to dependent portions of the lung when supine or prone as compared to the upright position. In addition, the bronchi are supported by the radial traction of the surrounding lung parenchyma. Airway caliber will increase as the lung expands and contract when the lung shrinks significantly impacting airway resistance. At very low lung volumes, the small airways may close completely, a condition frequently seen at the very base of the lung where it is less well expanded. Also, the rate of inspiration directly impacts the homogeneity of gas distribution. At high inspiratory rates, air is distributed more evenly throughout the lung than at very slow rates [70].

In summary, numerous studies using a variety of tracer gases (e.g., N_2, He, ^{133}Xe) to measure alveolar gas washout have demonstrated that inspired gas distribution is inhomogeneous [69]. In the ideal, upright individual, during a spontaneous breath, inspired gas will tend to preferentially enter those open alveoli near the base of the lung which are the most compliant. As the breath continues, the gas will enter the more apical, less compliant alveoli and any previously atelectatic basilar alveoli as they become recruited by the traction exerted by the remainder of the expanding lung. In other words, although the nondependent lung areas are more distended at FRC, a given transpulmonary pressure gradient generated during a normal breath produces a greater volume change and therefore ventilation, to the dependent areas. Review Figs. 4.4 and 4.5. Numerous factors are responsible for the distribution of ventilation, and their potential impact in the thoracic surgical patient must be anticipated as body position, anesthetic gases, intravenous fluid shifts, surgical trauma, one-lung ventilation with positive pressure, and any broncho- or vasoactive drugs are introduced. These regional differences in ventilation are important in matching ventilation to perfusion for optimal gas exchange.

The Physiology of the Pulmonary Circulation

Anatomical Considerations

The lung circulation is comprised of two sources of blood flow: the pulmonary circulation from the main pulmonary artery and the smaller, bronchial circulation arising from the aorta [6]. The pulmonary circulation dominates, by volume, and serves to deliver the mixed venous blood to the alveolar capillaries to facilitate gas exchange and to act as a large, low resistance reservoir for the entire cardiac output from the right ventricle. The bronchial circulation serves to provide nutritional support to the airways and their associated pulmonary blood vessels [71]. The bronchial circulation also provides a constant source of heat and moisture for warming and humidification of the inspired air. Of note, not all of the bronchial circulation drains into the systemic venous system. A small portion of the bronchial venous drainage mixes with the pulmonary venous drainage and contributes a small physiological shunt.

Pulmonary Hemodynamics

Despite receiving all of the cardiac output from the right ventricle, the pulmonary vasculature maintains a relatively low pulmonary blood pressure. The normal adult mean pulmonary artery pressure (P_{PA}) is between 9 and 16 mmHg with systolic P_{PA} between 18 and 25 mmHg. Several features enable the pulmonary circulation to maintain this high flow at such low pressures. First, the pulmonary vasculature is extremely thin-walled with far less arterial vascular smooth muscle than its systemic counterparts. The result is a highly compliant reservoir capable of accommodating an average 3.2 L/min/m² blood flow at rest or six to eight times that flow during exercise. Second, the total pulmonary vascular resistance (PVR) is quite low, on the order of less than 250 dynes/s/cm⁵. This minimizes the pressure work faced by the less robust right ventricle while still enabling the right ventricle to match the output of the left ventricle. Pulmonary vascular resistance can change as a result of numerous factors, hypoxia, acidosis, mitral valve stenosis or regurgitation, left ventricular failure, primary pulmonary hypertension, or pulmonary emboli, to name just a few. Pulmonary vascular resistance can be calculated using data from a pulmonary artery catheter as:

$$PVR = \left[\frac{(P_{PA} - PAOP)}{CO} \right] \times 79.9$$

where PAOP is the pulmonary artery catheter occlusion pressure which is assumed to reflect the left atrial pressure, CO is cardiac output (L/min), and the factor, 79.9, converts from mmHg/L/min to units of absolute resistance, dynes.s/cm^{-5}.

Cardiopulmonary Interactions

Factors Affecting Right Ventricular Performance

Cardiopulmonary interactions can be described based on the effects of both changes in intrathoracic pressure and tidal volumes on venous return and left ventricular (LV) cardiac output and the energy required to create these changes. During spontaneous ventilation (normal breathing), venous return (right atrial filling) increases congruently with negative deflections in intrathoracic pressure, which, in turn, increases right ventricular (RV) volume and causes leftward deviation of the intraventricular septum. This, in turn, causes a spontaneous inspiration-associated decrease in left ventricular end-diastolic volume and decreased left ventricular diastolic compliance. The resultant attenuated left ventricular preload causes an immediate decrease in left ventricular stroke volume and pulse pressure which is referred to as *pulsus paradoxus* – its degree directly related to the magnitude of the resultant negative intrathoracic pressure [72, 73].

Both spontaneous and positive-pressure ventilation can significantly alter cardiopulmonary physiology through numerous complex interactions involving myocardial reserve, ventricular pump function, intravascular volume, autonomic vascular tone, lung volume, and intrathoracic pressure [72]. During spontaneous inspiration, intrathoracic pressure *decreases* (as described previously). During positive-pressure lung inflation, intrathoracic pressure *increases* (as a result of passive lung inflation and increasing airway pressure) [74].

As the right atrium is located within the thorax, spontaneous inspiration leads to a decrease in right atrial pressure relative to atmospheric pressure. Right atrial pressure is effectively the resistance to systemic venous return, which should result in augmentation of the pressure gradient of systemic venous return and thereby accelerate blood flow toward the right heart and increase preload [73, 75].

In healthy humans, ventilation typically requires less than 5% of total oxygen consumption. However in critically ill patients and those with pulmonary disease, the metabolic consequences of increased respiratory work of breathing may demand up to 25% of the total oxygen delivery [76, 77]. It therefore follows that if cardiac output is also reduced, through preexisting heart failure or other structural pathology (e.g., aortic stenosis, mitral regurgitation), blood flow and – more specifically – oxygen delivery to end organs can be significantly compromised [74]. Use of mechanical ventilation is known to decrease intrinsic work of breathing. In fact, even noninvasive modalities such as BiPAP and CPAP have been demonstrated to improve both cardiac output and oxygen delivery [78].

The process of lung inflation, either through normal spontaneous breathing or through positive-pressure mechanical ventilation, results in various and specific effects on a number of cardiopulmonary parameters. Chief among them are changes in autonomic tone, cyclical alterations in intrathoracic pressure, changes in systemic venous return, variation in both right and left ventricular output and afterload, and perturbations of intraventricular interdependence.

Increases in lung volume have immediate and significant effects on autonomic tone. Lung inflation provokes immediate changes in autonomic output [79], resulting in increases in heart rate – otherwise referred to as *respiratory sinus arrhythmia* [80], which occurs in humans with intact (normal) autonomic responsiveness [81]. Lung hyperinflation (>15 mL/kg PBW) results in relative bradycardia (which may be profound) through vagal responses and withdrawal of sympathetic tone. Additionally, several studies have demonstrated a reflex arterial vasodilation caused by lung overinflation through pathways involving inducible nitric oxide production [82].

Pulmonary Vascular Resistance

Increases in lung volume have a significant influence on cardiac performance through its effects on altering right ventricular preload and afterload [83]. Additionally, ventilatory changes can have a profound effect on RV afterload through hypoxic pulmonary vasoconstriction, which typically becomes clinically relevant when regional alveolar PO_2 falls below 60 mmHg: pulmonary vasoconstriction occurs, reducing local blood flow [84]. Patients with acute hypoxemic (Type I) respiratory failure typically have small lung volumes [85]. Decreases in end-expiratory lung volumes promote alveolar collapse that will increase PVR to a degree that may trigger acute RV failure. Restoration of normal lung volumes through standard recruitment maneuvers and the addition of extrinsic PEEP typically reverses this reduction in PVR. However, lung hyperinflation also results in the compression of alveolar vessels that serves to increase PVR [85]. Significant increases in pulmonary hypertension can cause acute RV failure or cor pulmonale [86] and RV ischemia [87]. PEEP then will have differential effects on pulmonary hypertension depending on the clinical context: it may serve to decrease PVR and RV afterload if it reduces hypoxic pulmonary vasoconstriction (see section on HPV below) [88], or it has potential to increase PVR if the end result is lung overinflation [89].

Changes in Intrathoracic Pressure

As the heart is a pressure-producing chamber that functions within a pressure chamber, it follows that changes in intrathoracic pressure (ITP) will affect the pressure gradients for both systemic venous blood return to the RV and systemic blood outflow from the LV (independent of intrinsic myocardial function). Interventions which cause an *increase* in intrathoracic pressure (e.g. positive-pressure ventilation) will cause an increase in right atrial pressure and a decreased transmural LV systolic pressure, reducing the pressure gradients for venous return and LV ejection and decreasing intrathoracic blood volume. *Decreases* in intrathoracic pressure will augment venous return, impede LV ejection, and increase intrathoracic blood volume.

Systemic Venous Return

Right atrial pressure (RAP) is essentially resistance to systemic venous return [90] which is comprised of low pressure, low resistance venous circuits. RAP is known to change rapidly throughout the ventilatory cycle due to simultaneous changes in ITP [91]. As mentioned previously, positive-pressure ventilation increases ITP and RAP decreasing the pressure gradient for venous blood return, resulting in decreased RV stroke volume and ultimately cardiac output [92]. However, decreases in venous return in the setting of increased ITP are offset to some extent by the resulting increase in intra-abdominal pressure caused by the caudal movement of the diaphragm and contraction of abdominal wall muscles [93]. Van den berg demonstrated that increasing CPAP up to 20 cm H_2O does not seem to have clinically relevant effects on cardiac output, provided that intra-abdominal pressures also increased similarly [94].

Factors Affecting Left Ventricular Performance

LV Preload and Ventricular Interdependence

Changes in venous return (and therefore RV output) necessarily influence LV preload and systemic cardiac output (where changes are typically observed after two to three beats, as observed with a standard Valsalva maneuver) [95]. This inherent phase delay between RV output and LV output is exaggerated in two clinical situations: hypovolemia and high tidal volumes [96].

Ventricular interdependence can be modified by a number of clinically relevant conditions. Increasing RV volume shifts the intraventricular septum into the LV throughout the cardiac cycle and simultaneously decreases LV diastolic compliance. During positive-pressure ventilation, RV volumes are typically decreased, minimizing ventricular interdependence [96, 97]. Positive-pressure ventilation-induced increases in lung volume compress the two ventricles into each other, decreasing biventricular volumes [98]. Restoring LV end-diastolic volume with fluids returns cardiac output during PEEP therapy without LV diastolic compliance changes [99]. However, during spontaneous inspiration, as RV volumes transiently increase, septal shift into the LV lumen is the rule [100], decreasing LV diastolic compliance and end-diastolic volume [88, 97]. This interdependence is the primary cause of inspiration-associated decreases in arterial pulse pressure, otherwise known as *pulsus paradoxus* [73].

LV Afterload

Maximal LV wall tension, or afterload, normally occurs at the end of isovolumic contraction. LV afterload normally decreases during ejection because LV volume decreases markedly despite the small increase in ejection pressure. With LV dilation, however, as in congestive heart failure, maximal LV wall stress occurs during LV ejection, making the heart more sensitive to changes in ejection pressure. Since arterial pressure with respect to atmosphere is kept constant by baroreceptor feedback [101], if arterial pressure were to remain constant as ITP increases, then LV ejection pressure must decrease [102]. Similarly, decreases in ITP with a constant arterial pressure will increase LV ejection pressure [102, 103]. As such, any process associated with significant decreases in ITP must also be associated with increased LV afterload and myocardial oxygen consumption; consider weaning-induced cardiac stress.

Rapid increases in ITP, as in coughing, will increase arterial pressure but not alter LV ejection pressure [73, 104] or aortic blood flow [105]; however, sustained increases in ITP, as seen with a Valsalva maneuver, will eventually decrease aortic blood flow and arterial pressure because venous return decreases [73].

The cardiovascular benefits of positive airway pressure can be achieved by withdrawing negative swings in ITP (which attenuate preload and augment LV afterload). Increasing levels of CPAP improve cardiac function in patients with heart failure but only once the negative swings in ITP are abolished [106]. Interestingly, prolonged nighttime nasal CPAP can selectively improve respiratory muscle strength, as well as LV contractile function if the patient had preexisting heart failure [107].

Hyperinflation, as can occur in obstructive airway diseases, for example, will compress the heart, increase PVR, and impede RV filling. Intrinsic PEEP (hyperinflation) alters hemodynamic function similar to extrinsic PEEP; thus, matching intrinsic PEEP with ventilator-derived PEEP does not alter hemodynamics [108]. There is little hemodynamic difference between increasing airway pressure to generate a breath and decreasing extrathoracic pressure (iron lung-negative pressure ventilation) [109].

Impact of Weaning from Mechanical Ventilation

The process of weaning from mechanical ventilator support is a significant cardiovascular stressor [74]. It is therefore not surprising that various studies have demonstrated ECG and thallium perfusion evidence of myocardial ischemia [110, 111]. Likewise, initiation of mechanical respiratory support in patients with heart failure can attenuate some of the signs of ischemia [112]. Ventilator-dependent patients who fail a weaning trial may show signs of heart failure only during the weaning process; transitioning from positive pressure to spontaneous breathing can induce pulmonary edema [113], tachycardia [110], mesenteric ischemia [114], and myocardial ischemia [115]. Jubran and colleagues showed that all subjects increased their cardiac output during the transition from positive pressure to spontaneous breathing as a result of increased metabolic demand [115]. Those patients who subsequently failed to wean showed an increase in their S_vO_2. Of note, some patients who fail a T-tube trial actually pass an extubation trial, likely reflecting increased work of breathing to overcome increased flow resistance through the endotracheal tube and not inherent respiratory dysfunction [116].

Distribution of Lung Perfusion

Gravity and Pulmonary Blood Flow

Blood flow within the normal lung is distributed in a non-homogeneous fashion. Many studies have demonstrated this behavior although explanations vary [117–119]. The earliest studies used radioactive tracers injected into the bloodstream and measured the radioactive emissions by sandwiching the subject between two external arrays of scintillation counters. The most common tracer employed was xenon-133 which has an extremely low solubility in the blood so most of it rapidly moves into the alveoli during the first pass, i.e., little recirculation. The time to achieve a steady state in the lung after injection was estimated at 3–4 s. Data acquisition of a 30 cm scan of the chest could be completed in about 30 s enabling single breath-hold studies at different static lung volumes. The data were limited to a

two-dimensional representation of the lung and failed to account for the very apex and base of the lung for technical reasons. Nonetheless the studies clearly showed a gradient of perfusion from the apex and increasing toward the base in the upright lung, presumably reflecting the effects of gravity [159]. However more refined techniques using radioactive microspheres and advanced computerized three-dimensional imaging techniques have revealed that blood flow distribution is highly variable even in those portions of the lung at a uniform vertical height [120, 121]. Indeed it appears that there are "high-flow" and "low-flow" regions of the lung whose perfusion is only minimally altered by changes in body position. Several studies performed under zero gravity [122, 123] and microgravity [124] support the notion that the whole-lung gravitational and postural changes seen in blood flow distribution are primarily determined by shifts in the lung parenchymal density which are augmented by smaller gravitational contributions to individual alveolar flow within the dependent regions of the lung.

Architecture and Pulmonary Blood Flow

If gravitational influences fail to completely explain the heterogeneity of lung perfusion, then other factors must be present. One popular concept is the role played by the branching pattern of the blood vessels. At each pulmonary vascular branch point, that proportion of the pulmonary blood flow that continues down each subsequent arterial branch is dependent upon its downstream resistance to flow. The progressive branching pattern of the blood vessels is assumed to be similar in geometry within each generation. However the number of generations will be influenced by the size of lung region. This "fractal geometry" theory has been employed in a number of biological systems to analyze flow [125]. However, its use as a foundation to explain heterogeneity in the distribution of gas and blood through generations of branching airways and vasculature has proven particularly useful [126, 127].

When ^{133}Xe blood flow studies are performed at different lung volumes in the same individual, a marked variation in the distribution occurs [128]. The greatest changes occur at the apex and base of the lung. Going from TLC to RV results in large drop in the percentage of blood flow to the base, while a modest increase in the flow to the apex occurs at RV compared to TLC. One explanation for this pattern of regional blood flow is that, similar to the effects on airway resistance, traction exerted on the small arteries within the lung parenchyma decreases their resistance. The greater the traction, e.g., at high lung volumes, the lower the arterial resistance. However to explain the improvement in apical blood flow at RV requires that we suppose that large lung volumes compress the alveolar capillaries and increase their resistance to flow. Therefore there must be a balance between alveolar pressure effects on the alveolar capillaries and the interstitial traction effects on the extra-alveolar pulmonary arterioles. Figure 4.5 illustrates this concept of lung volume and vascular resistance of intra-alveolar and extra-alveolar blood vessels.

Regional "Zones of Blood Flow"

A common conceptualization of the effects of posture and hemodynamics on the distribution of blood flow within the whole lung, the "Zones of West" model, has been useful clinically. First described in 1964 by J. B. West and colleagues, the model describes the dependence of pulmonary perfusion upon the interaction between three basic pressures: alveolar pressure, pulmonary arterial, and venous pressures [129, 159]. The notion of three (or four) "lung zones" dictated the blood flow through the acinus (see Table 4.3). In Zone 1 the alveolar pressure (P_A) is considered to be greater than both the arteriole (P_a) and venule (P_v) pressures thus creating a decreased transmural pressure favoring compression of the alveolar capillary and impeding blood flow (Fig. 4.6). Zone 1 (most nondependent region of the lung) is considered to be fairly small in the spontaneously breathing individual but can enlarge during positive-pressure ventilation. Zone 2 (a transition region between the most nondependent and dependent regions) is where the arteriole pressure (P_a) is greater than alveolar pressure (P_A) but venule pressure (P_v) remains less than the other two pressures throughout most of the respiratory cycle. The net effect is a resistance to blood flow governed by the difference between P_a and P_A. The transition is likely a gradual one and will vary throughout the respiratory cycle, especially when mechanical ventilation is employed. The size of Zone 2 will be subject to a wide variety of clinical conditions. The bulk of the normal lung is likely described by Zone 3 (dependent region of the lung) where both arteriole and venule pressures are greater than alveolar pressure during all phases of the respiratory cycle such that blood flow is

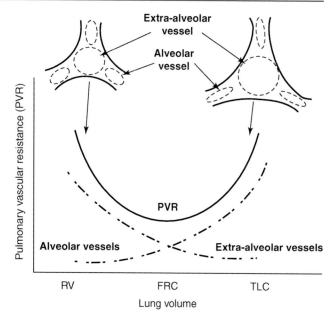

Fig. 4.6 Pulmonary vascular resistance changes with lung volume. Small pulmonary blood vessels are affected by lung volume as a result of their location with relation to alveolar sac. Alveolar capillaries are most compressed between alveoli at high lung volumes, while extra-alveolar vessels are stretched by the radial traction of the lung elastic recoil. The relationship is just the opposite at low lung volumes. As a result total pulmonary vascular resistance is highest at both extremes of lung volume and has its nadir at FRC

unimpeded and, presumably, gas exchange continues unabated. Finally, Zone 4 has been proposed. It is that region where atelectasis or severe pulmonary interstitial edema has developed and results in blood flow determined by the difference between P_a and the pulmonary interstitial fluid pressure (P_{isf}).

The pulmonary vasculature can best be viewed as a large branching tree with two components defining the distribution of blood flow within it. One component is the fixed structure that is the primary determinant of regional perfusion. However superimposed on this fixed component is a highly variable component that is influenced by numerous local factors. While fractal geometry can explain properties of the fixed component, the variable component is less predictable and subject to both passive and active regional factors. Some examples of regional factors are recruitment and distension due to changing cardiac output and blood pressure, lung distension, or vasomotion in response to hypoxic pulmonary vasoconstriction, shearing stresses, or pharmacologic interventions. The importance of all of these influences on ventilation and perfusion in the lung cannot be overstated. To optimize gas exchange requires the best possible "match" between alveolar ventilation and the delivery by the blood of CO_2 to the alveolus for removal and the absorption of O_2 for delivery to the body to sustain metabolism.

Table 4.3 Regional flow zones of the lung

Zone	Pressure relationships	Blood vessels	Determinants of blood flow
1	$P_{alv} > P_{pa} > P_v$	Collapsed	Minimal flow
2	$P_{pa} > P_{alv} > P_v$	Intermittent patency	$P_{pa} - P_{alv}$
3	$P_{pa} > P_v > P_{alv}$	Distended	$P_{pa} - P_v$
4	$P_{pa} > P_{isf} > P_v > P_{alv}$	Restriction	$P_{pa} - P_{isf}$

P_{alv} alveolar pressure, P_{pa} pulmonary artery pressure, P_v pulmonary venous pressure, P_{isf} interstitial fluid pressure

Ventilation to Perfusion Matching (The V_A/Q Ratio)

In a perfect world, the ventilation perfectly matches the perfusion in the lung. Therefore with a typical resting value of alveolar ventilation of 4 L/min and 5.1 L/min for pulmonary blood flow, we could calculate a global ventilation to perfusion ratio (V_A/Q) of 0.8. However as we have already discussed, the lung does not enjoy a homogeneous distribution of either ventilation or perfusion. A gradation exists between alveoli that are underventilated to those that are grossly underperfused. As expected, the V_A/Q ratios will vary from zero where an alveolus is perfused but not ventilated to a V_A/Q ratio of infinity where there is no alveolar blood flow but the alveolus remains ventilated. Useful physiologic descriptors of these two extremes are "physiological shunt" for a V_A/Q ratio nearing zero and "physiological dead space" when the V_A/Q ratio approaches infinity. The prefix "physiological" connotes that physiologic events can be superimposed to create these conditions in contrast to fixed anatomical arterial-venous shunts or the non-respiratory airways, i.e., anatomical dead space.

In the healthy conscious individual, the expected shunt or venous admixture is only about 1–2% of the cardiac output. This degree of venous admixture is likely to produce an alveolar to arterial PO_2 gradient of about 7 mmHg or less in someone breathing ambient air. However, the degree of venous admixture has been shown to increase with age. Administration of 100% inspired oxygen can achieve acceptable PaO_2 in the face of venous admixture up to about 30%. During most general anesthetics, an inspired FiO_2 of 40% is sufficient unless moderately severe shunting is present. Shunting developing during general anesthesia likely has two sources, atelectasis and redistribution of ventilation to regions of high V_A/Q ratio. The former can be corrected or significantly reduced by the application of PEEP. The latter may actually be worsened by PEEP. The end result will depend on the condition predominantly causing the increased venous admixture.

These conditions have significant consequences for metabolic homeostasis because of its impact on gas exchange. Alveoli with no ventilation will have a P_AO_2 and P_ACO_2 identical to that of mixed venous blood because the trapped alveolar gas will equilibrate with the CO_2 and O_2 levels in the mixed venous blood. Likewise for those alveoli ventilated but not perfused, the P_ACO_2 and P_AO_2 will be identical to the inspired gas since there is no blood to either add CO_2 or remove O_2 from the alveolus. Therefore for all alveoli with ratios in-between these extremes, their alveolar gas partial pressures will reflect the degree of both ventilation and perfusion. V_A/Q ratios have been measured under a variety of conditions and modeled to show a basic pattern in the normal upright lung under spontaneous respiration (see Fig. 4.7).

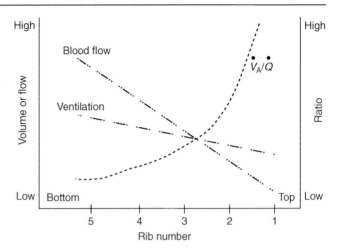

Fig. 4.7 General distribution of blood flow and ventilation and the ventilation-to-perfusion ratio as a function of distance from the base of the upright lung to its apex. Both ventilation and blood flow are significantly greater at the base of the lung than its apex. However the relation is much steeper for blood flow than for ventilation. Therefore the ventilation-perfusion ratio (V_A/Q) is greater at the apex or nondependent regions of the lung than the base or dependent regions of the lung

Note that perfusion changes relatively more than ventilation as you progress from the lung base to its apex resulting in V_A/Q ratios ranging from 0.6 to 3.3 [129]. Even these ratios may not represent the extreme values in the upright lung since the apex and base of the lung do not lend themselves to accurate assessment for technical reasons.

One method that has been used extensively in the laboratory to detect and quantify the disparity between ventilation and perfusion in normal and diseased human lungs is the multiple inert gas elimination technique (MIGET) [130]. Multiple tracer gases dissolved in a physiologic medium are infused intravenously for 30 min. The original mix included SF6, ethane, cyclopropane, halothane, ether, and acetone that are nonreactive with hemoglobin and possess a wide range of solubilities. After 30 min, mixed venous, arterial and mixed expired samples are taken and analyzed by gas chromatography for the arterial retention and alveolar excretion of each gas. Cardiac output and minute ventilation are measured. Each tracer gas has a linear dissociation curve and a single blood-gas solubility coefficient. Plots of ventilation and blood flow versus calculated V_A/Q ratio are derived for each gas. The composite V_A/Q distribution is fitted to 48 discrete compartments plus 1 for shunt ($V_A/Q = 0$) and 1 for alveolar dead space ($V_A/Q = \infty$). Note the characteristic plots in Fig. 4.8. Figure 4.8a shows a normal subject characterized by a near-perfect match between the blood flow curve and the ventilation curve. You should note that both distributions are bell-shaped curves supporting the notion of heterogeneity of both ventilation and perfusion in the normal lung. In comparison, Fig. 4.8b demonstrates a characteristic graph with a large degree of mismatch produced, in this case, by multiple pulmonary emboli. Note the significant physiologic

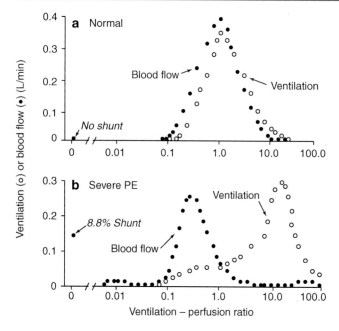

Fig. 4.8 Ventilation (open circles) or pulmonary blood flow (closed circles) as a function of computed ventilation-perfusion ratio (V_A/Q) using the multiple inert gas elimination technique (MIGET). See text for details of the experimental method. (**a**) Normal distribution of ventilation, blood flow and calculated V_A/Q ratios demonstrating a good match between alveolar blood flow and alveolar ventilation. (**b**) A characteristic plot in the presence of multiple pulmonary emboli. Note the dispersion of blood flow to regions of the lung with low V_A/Q ratios and the ventilation distributed to areas of high V_A/Q ratios. Ventilation is wasted presumably because of the obstruction of the pulmonary blood flow to many regions by emboli. The high calculated shunt of 8.8% likely reflects pulmonary edema and possibly the increased blood flow through anatomic arterial-venous shunts as a result of pulmonary hypertension. (Based on data from Wagner et al. [181])

dead space indicated by considerable ventilation to underperfused regions. In addition, there are large regions of perfusion to areas that are relatively underventilated producing areas in the lung of physiologic shunt. Finally, note the calculated shunt fraction of 8.8%, likely the result of pulmonary edema. It is also possible that under this pathologic condition, a portion of the cardiac output is passing through the lung through anatomic a-v shunts as well. These paths may become recruited when pulmonary vascular resistance increases as a compensatory mechanism to limit the increase in PVR or to accommodate gross increases in pulmonary blood volume as in congestive heart failure.

Hypoxic Pulmonary Vasoconstriction

Hypoxic pulmonary vasoconstriction (HPV) is an adaptive vasomotor response to alveolar hypoxia, which redistributes blood to optimally ventilated lung segments by an active process of vasoconstriction, thereby improving ventilation-perfusion matching. This is the major intrinsic mechanism of

the lung to divert blood flow from pulmonary acini served by occluded or partially ventilated bronchioles to neighboring well-ventilated pulmonary acini. Such conditions can transiently develop under a number of conditions, microatelectasis, mucus plugging, edema or inflammation, for example. HPV provides for a rapid and reversible response to changing conditions in the local environment. The mechanism is most efficient when the adjustments are restricted to small distances between adjacent pulmonary acini or at most, bronchiole segments. It tends to be less effective when the involved areas become large such as whole-lung segments or lobes. When global hypoxia is present as in the fetus in utero, HPV mechanisms lead to very high pulmonary arterial pressures that divert blood through the foramen ovale and ductus arteriosus, a useful adaptation to life with a placenta. However when alveolar hypoxia is global as upon ascent to high altitude, acute respiratory distress syndrome, hypoventilation syndromes, severe cystic fibrosis, or emphysema, HPV responses can be maladaptive and lead to pulmonary hypertension and potentially right heart failure.

The molecular and subcellular mechanisms subserving HPV are a contemporary polemic. However several aspects are well documented and are important to the clinician. We will focus on these in our discussion. Bradford and Dean were credited with the first modern observation of HPV as a result of asphyxia in 1894 and noted the dichotomy between the vasodilatory response of systemic arteries and the vasoconstriction of pulmonary arteries by the same stimulus [131]. Recognition of HPV as an important adaptive mechanism for ventilation-perfusion matching is attributed to Von Euler and Liljestrand in 1946 [132]. They noted the vasoconstriction of small intrapulmonary arteries in response to hypoxia without hypercapnia, a response limited to the pulmonary circulation. Later it was shown that the predominant stimulus was an inspired hypoxic gas mixture and not hypoxemia per se. Initial animal experiments showed that if the normal alveolar O_2 partial pressure was maintained in the face of a hypoxic blood perfusate to the lung, minimal HPV occurred [133, 134]. However, subsequent studies have clearly demonstrated that a low mixed venous PO_2 and therefore low pulmonary artery P_aO_2 will augment the HPV response to a hypoxic F_iO_2 but low pulmonary venous PO_2 has no effect [135, 136]. Indeed, as the size of the hypoxic lung increases, pulmonary vascular resistance increases, mixed venous oxygen tensions begin to fall, and the ability of HPV to shunt blood to the remaining well-ventilated lung becomes compromised. In fact if mixed venous PO_2 drops significantly, P_AO_2 in the ventilated alveoli drops sufficiently that the pulmonary perfusion pressure of those segments increases as well [135, 137]. Others have demonstrated that HPV remains intact despite chemical sympathectomy, bilateral vagotomy, and denervation of the carotid and aortic chemoreceptors [138, 139]. Finally bilateral lung transplants in man retain their hypoxic pulmonary vasoconstrictive responses [140]. HPV is augmented by conditions and chemicals which globally enhance pulmonary vascular resistance such as acidemia, hypercapnia, histamine, serotonin, and angiotensin II to name a few.

The actual cellular oxygen sensor has yet to be determined. Current research appears to implicate the mitochondria and regulatory processes of intracellular calcium within the pulmonary vascular smooth muscle cell as the primary site [141–143]. Numerous biochemical studies have indicated that selective interruption of the mitochondrial electron transport chain complexes can impair HPV. Some favor a hypoxia-induced change in the level of oxygen free radicals and hydrogen peroxide in the smooth muscle cell [144]. These changes affect the release of calcium from the sarcoplasmic reticulum and the voltage-dependent membrane conductance to potassium resulting in depolarization and contraction of the smooth muscle, hence vasoconstriction [141, 142, 145]. There appears to be a two-step response to hypoxia with an immediate increase in PVR and pulmonary perfusion pressure occurring within minutes followed by gradual increase to a maximum that occurs over hours and can be sustained [146–148]. The response can be enhanced by hypercapnia and may involve decreased production of nitric oxide by the pulmonary epithelium and endothelium [146].

Clinical Applications

Anesthesia and Atelectasis

J.F. Nunn was one of the first to show that during anesthesia and spontaneous ventilation, gas exchange was altered by shunt and inhomogeneous V/Q ratios [149]. He concluded from his observations that a normal range of P_aO_2 could be maintained if the alveolar PO_2 (P_AO_2) was at least 200 mmHg which would require an F_iO_2 of at least 35%. Many have speculated that induction of general anesthesia led to the decline in oxygenation as a result of alveolar collapse (atelectasis), but it was an important observation by Brismar and colleagues in 1985 that demonstrated the regional collapse of the lung. They were able to demonstrate using computed tomography that within 5 min of the induction of anesthesia, dependent edges of the lung developed an increase in density consistent with atelectasis [150]. It is now accepted that this occurs in dependent lung regions in approximately 90% of patients who undergo general anesthesia using a wide variety of agents [151]. Epidural anesthesia may be the one modality that appears to cause very little atelectasis and no change in V_A/Q matching or oxygenation [152, 153].

Three basic mechanisms are currently implicated in the cause of atelectasis under general anesthesia. See the excellent review of the topic by Magnusson and Spahn [154]. The near universal finding of rapid lung collapse upon induction of anesthesia and the rapid reappearance after discontinuation of PEEP has led to the conclusion that atelectasis was due to compression of lung tissue rather than alveolar gas absorption behind occluded airways [150]. The fluoroscopic study by Froese and Bryan of the diaphragmatic motion of spontaneously breathing volunteers demonstrated that in the supine position, the dependent portion of the diaphragm had the greatest caudad displacement. Initiation of paralysis with neuromuscular blocking agents and positive-pressure ventilation created a reversal of this motion with the nondependent or superior aspect of the diaphragm which underwent the greatest displacement with each ventilated breath [155]. Others have confirmed and extended these observations using CT scans [156, 157]. It is now apparent that the geometry of the chest and diaphragm is altered under general anesthesia with greater relaxation of the chest wall and a marked cephalad displacement of the most dorsal portion of the diaphragm in end-expiration.

Absorption atelectasis can occur when the rate of gas uptake into the blood exceeds the rate of ventilation of the alveolus. The extreme condition is total occlusion of an airway that isolates the alveolar gas in the distal alveolar and respiratory airways. The gas pressure within this compartment initially is nearly at atmospheric pressure. However given that mixed venous blood continues to perfuse this area, and the fact that the sum of the gas partial pressures within mixed venous blood is subatmospheric, gas uptake from the occluded compartment by blood continues and the alveoli collapses [158]. Computer modeling has demonstrated that the rate of gas absorption from unventilated areas is dependent upon the initial F_iO_2 [159]. However in many clinical situations, the airways are not completely occluded, but rather ventilation to an area becomes severely reduced. If the inspired V_A/Q ratio of a respiratory unit is reduced, a point is reached where the rate at which inspired gas enters the alveolus is exactly balanced by the gas uptake into the blood. If V_A/Q ratio drops below this critical equilibrium point, the volume of the alveolus declines and collapse ensues. Again this process is augmented by the presence of a high P_AO_2 and a rapid rate of gas uptake [160, 161].

Finally, loss of alveolar surfactant may play a role in alveolar instability at low alveolar volumes and collapse. The rapidity of alveolar collapse following alveolar recruitment maneuvers and discontinuation of PEEP has suggested that atelectasis per se may interfere with surfactant production. Therefore, atelectatic regions of the lung may be predisposed to recurrence of collapse because of reduced levels of surfactant, increased alveolar surface tension, and the aforementioned mechanisms, all contributing to reduced alveolar volumes.

Anesthesia and V_A/Q Matching

Of great interest to anesthesiologists is the impact of their anesthetic or pharmacologic interventions on the pulmonary homeostatic mechanisms. A wide variety of drugs have been investigated with their respect to hypoxic pulmonary vasoconstriction and V_A/Q matching. See review by Lumb and Slinger [162]. In general volatile anesthetics do not have a large impact on HPV. However volatile anesthetics could have a significant clinical effect in those patients with diseased lungs or poor cardiac function. Isoflurane can decrease cardiac output and is a potent vasodilator. As such it has been possible to demonstrate a concentration-dependent reduction of regional HPV by isoflurane during one-lung ventilation in experimental animals [163]. Domino and colleagues calculated that this increased the degree of shunt flow by approximately 4%. It is likely that this effect on blood flow and V_A/Q mismatch would be amplified in a thoracotomy patient with diffuse lung disease and with a significant preoperative fraction of cardiac output going to the nondependent lung. The newer volatile anesthetics cause less vasodilation but still produce some, albeit small, degree of shunt possibly through their general effects on cardiac output [164–166]. Studies in animals indicate that 70% nitrous oxide moderately diminishes the HPV response [167]. The general impression is that all volatile anesthetics can affect the HPV mechanism to some degree, but rather it is their impact on the patient's general physiology that may warrant greater consideration in their selection. When volatile anesthetics are compared with propofol or propofol and narcotic infusions, there appear to be only slight differences, none reaching statistical significance [166, 168, 169]. Intravenous drugs of most classes used in anesthesia such as barbiturates, opioids, benzodiazepines, and ketamine do not appear to have a measurable effect on the HPV response. However these drugs can still influence hemodynamics in other ways that can impact blood flow through the lung. Therefore except for possible changes in emergence pharmacokinetics or pharmacodynamics, there are no known significant advantages of using total intravenous anesthesia over volatile anesthetics with regard to HPV in the thoracotomy patient.

The effects of thoracic epidural anesthesia or analgesia on hypoxic pulmonary vasoconstriction have not been as extensively studied. However those animal studies examining the effects of thoracic epidural local anesthetics have not seen a significant blunting of HPV and any changes in shunt fraction are more likely to represent changes in global hemodynamics [170].

Non-anesthetic Drugs and HPV

In addition to volatile anesthetics, there are numerous drug classes that influence pulmonary vascular resistance, and several have been shown to modify HPV directly. A partial list of common drugs that can affect the pulmonary vasculature is compiled in Table 4.4. Unfortunately detailed pharmacodynamic studies are missing for many of these drugs that are commonly being used in patients. So it is quite difficult to extrapolate experimental findings to the clinical setting. Nonetheless the thoracic anesthesiologist must be aware of the potential effects of using vasoactive drugs in a perioperative setting where undesirable effects on HPV may be manifest.

Interventions to modify blood pressure or improve inotropic state can have direct effects on the pulmonary vasculature. Sodium nitroprusside, nitroglycerin, and hydralazine are potent vasodilators that can worsen P_aO_2 rapidly by reducing HPV, although preexisting vascular tone can influence the response [171, 172]. Attempts to improve the inotropic state of the heart, especially the right ventricle, with milrinone will concurrently vasodilate the pulmonary vasculature [173]. The improvement in cardiac output can enhance systemic O_2 delivery and mixed venous PO_2 so that the net effect on V_A/Q matching could be beneficial. Perioperative administration of inhaled nitric oxide (NO), inhaled PGI_2, and sildenafil to control pulmonary hypertension and improve the right ventricular afterload will also modulate HPV [174, 175]. Fortunately inhaled pulmonary vasodilators are more selective and theoretically are distributed to those better-ventilated lung regions to enhance pulmonary blood flow [176]. The intention is to amplify the response of HPV in the poorly ventilated regions. Newer pharmacologic approaches to treating coronary artery disease and chronic heart failure including those with chronic pulmonary hypertension have salient effects on the remodeling of both the heart and pulmonary vasculature. However new findings also suggest that angiotensin II receptor blockers and angiotensin-

Table 4.4 Drug Effects on Pulmonary Vascular Resistance

Decrease PVR	Increase PVR
Angiotensin II receptor blockers	α_1-Adrenergic receptor agonists
ACE inhibitors	Almitrine
β_2-Adrenergic receptor agonists	Angiotensin II
Calcium channel blockers	β-Adrenergic receptor blockers
Inhaled nitric oxide	Cyclooxygenase inhibitors
Milrinone	Histamine (H_1)
Nitroglycerin	Serotonin
Sildenafil	
Sodium nitroprusside	
Theophylline	
PGE_1 and PGI_2	

converting enzyme inhibitors may attenuate HPV response in acute hypoxia [177, 178].

Finally, future research will need to sort out the effects of acute hypoxia from chronic hypoxemia. It is apparent that a condition of chronic hypoxemia such as can be found in chronic pulmonary disease can slowly alter the normal acute response to a drop in inspired FiO_2 [179]. A downregulation of the HPV mechanisms might occur in the face of chronic hypoxia such that interventions such as inhaled NO may prove less efficacious [180].

In summary, the etiology of abnormal gas exchange in the patient undergoing thoracic surgery is complex, highly variable, and in a state of flux throughout the course of surgery. While certain aspects of the effect of pulmonary mechanics and control of pulmonary blood flow distribution are known, the subtle interaction between the inflammatory response to surgical trauma, mechanical ventilation (especially one-lung ventilation), and the poorly understood impact of both acute and chronic pharmacologic interventions have yet to be satisfactorily defined. Until more is known, it will be extremely difficult to predict with any certainty the consequences of our anesthetic management.

References

1. Hudgel DW, Hendricks C. Palate and hypopharynx – sites of inspiratory narrowing of the upper airway during sleep. Am Rev Respir Dis. 1988;138:1542–7.
2. Wheatley JR, Kelly WT, Tully A, Engel LA. Pressure-diameter relationships of the upper airway in awake supine subjects. J Appl Physiol. 1991;70(5):2242–51.
3. Spann RW, Hyatt RE. Factors affecting upper airway resistance in conscious man. J Appl Physiol. 1971;31(5):708–12.
4. Bartlett D. Respiratory function of the larynx. Physiol Rev. 1989;69:33–57.
5. Gal TJ. Anatomy and physiology of the respiratory system and the pulmonary circulation. In: Kaplan JA, Slinger PD, editors. Thoracic anesthesia. 3rd ed. Philadelphia: Churchill Livingstone; 2003. p. 57–70.
6. Minnich DJ, Mathisen DJ. Anatomy of the trachea, carina, and bronchi. Thorac Surg Clin. 2007;17:571–85.
7. Voynow JA, Rubin BK. Mucins, mucus, and sputum. Chest. 2009;135:505–12.
8. Foster WM, Langenback E, Bergofsky EH. Measurement of tracheal and bronchial mucus velocities in man: relation to clearance. J Appl Physiol Respirat Environ Exercise Physiol. 1980;48(6):965–71.
9. Gonda I. Particle deposition in the human respiratory tract. In: Crystal RG, West JB, Weibel ER, Barnes PJ, editors. The lung: scientific foundations. 2nd ed. Philadelphia: Lipincott-Raven; 1997. p. 2289–308.
10. Gibson GJ, Pride NB, Empey DW. The role of inspiratory dynamic compression in upper airway obstruction. Am Rev Respir Dis. 1973;108:1352–60.
11. Vincken WG, Gauthier SG, Dollfuss RE, Hanson RE, Darauay CM, Cosio MG. Involvement of upper-airway muscles in extrapyramidal disorders. N Engl J Med. 1984;311:438–42.
12. Phipps PR, Gonda I, Bailey DC, Borham P, Bautovich G, Anderson SD. Comparison of planar and tomographic gamma scintigraphy to measure the penetrating index of inhaled aerosols. Amer Rev Resp Dis. 1989;139:1516–23.
13. Lavorini F, Pederson S, Usmani OS. Dilemmas, confusion, and misconceptions related to small airways directed therapy. Chest. 2017;151(6):1345–55.
14. Usmanni OS. Small-airway disease in asthma: pharmacological considerations. Curr Opin Pulm Med. 2015;21:55–67.
15. Sealy WC, Connally SR, Dalton ML. Naming the bronchopulmonary segments and the development of pulmonary surgery. Ann Thorac Surg. 1993;55:184–8.
16. Riquet M. Bronchial arteries and lymphatics of the lung. Thorac Surg Clin. 2007;17:619–38.
17. Riquet M, Le Pimpec Barthes F, Souilamas R, et al. Thoracic duct tributaries from intrathoracic organs. Ann Thorac Surg. 2002;73:892–9.
18. Crapo JD, Barry BE, Gehr P, Bachoen M, Weibel ER. Cell numbers and cell characteristics in the normal lung. Am Rev Respir Dis. 1982;126(3):332–7.
19. Williams MC. Alveolar type I cells: molecular phenotype and development. Ann Rev Physiol. 2003;65:669–95.
20. Crapo JD, Harmsen AG, Sherman MP, et al. Pulmonary immunobiology and inflammation in pulmonary diseases. Am J Respir Crit Care Med. 2000;162:1983–6.
21. Johnston RB. Monocytes and macrophages. N Engl J Med. 1988;318:747–52.
22. Bienenstock J. Bronchus-associated lymphoid tissue. Int Arch Allergy Appl Immunol. 1985;76:62–9.
23. Upham JW, Xi Y. Dendritic cells in human lung disease, recent advances. Chest. 2017;151(3):668–73.
24. Richardson JB, Ferguson CC. Neuromuscular structure and function in the airways. Fed Proc. 1979;38:292–308.
25. Chowdhuri S, Badr MS. Control of ventilation in health and disease. Chest. 2017;151(4):917–29.
26. Smith JC, Abdala APL, Borgmann A, et al. Brainstem respiratory networks: building blocks and microcircuits. Trends in Neurosci. 2013;36(3):152–62.
27. Abdala APL, Rybak IA, Smith JC, et al. Multiple pontomedullary mechanisms of respiratory rhythmogenesis. Respir Physiol Neurobiol. 2009;168:19–25.
28. Richter DW Smith JC. Respiratory rhythm generation in vivo. Physiology (Bethesda). 2014;29(1):58–71.
29. Guyenet PG. The 2008 Carl Ludwig Lecture: retrotrapezoid nucleus, CO_2 homeostasis, and breathing automaticity. J Apply Physiol. 2008;105:404–16.
30. Morschel M, Deutschmann M. Pontine respiratory activity involved in inspiratory/expiratory phase transition. Phil Trans R Soc B. 2009;364:2517–26.
31. Dean JB, Nattie EE. Central CO_2 chemoreception in cardiorespiratory control. J Appl Physiol. 2010;108:976–8.
32. Bruce EN, Cherniack NS. Central chemoreceptors. J Appl Physiol. 1987;62(2):389–402.
33. Forster HV, Smith CA. Contributions of central and peripheral chemoreceptors to the ventilator response to CO_2/H^+. J Appl Physiol. 2010;108:989–94.
34. Pappenheimer JR, Fencl V, Heisey SR, et al. Role of cerebral fluids in control of respiration as studied in unanesthetized goats. Am J Physiol. 1965;208(3):436–50.
35. Fencl V, Miller TB, Pappenheimer JR. Studies on the respiratory response to disturbances of acid-base balance, with deductions concerning the ionic composition of cerebral interstitial fluid. Am J Physiol. 1966;210(3):459–72.
36. Nattie E, Comroe JH Jr. Distinguished Lecture: Central chemoreception: then …and now. J Appl Physiol. 2011;110:1–8.

37. Sepulveda FV, Cid LP, Teulon J, et al. Molecular aspects of structure, gating, and physiology of pH-sensitive background K_{2P} and Kir K^+-transport channels. Physiol Rev. 2015;95:179–217.

38. Nattie E, Li A. Central chemoreceptor: locations and functions. Compr Physiol. 2012;2(1):221–54.

39. Guyenet PG, Bayliss DA, Stornetta RL, et al. Proton detection and breathing regulation by the retrotrapezoid nucleus. J Physiol. 2016;594(6):1529–51.

40. Kumar P, Bin-Jaliah I. Adequate stimuli of the carotid body: more than an oxygen sensor? Respir Physiol Neurobiol. 2007;157:12–21.

41. Teppema LJ, Dahan A. The ventilator response to hypoxia in mammals: mechanisms, measurement, and analysis. Physiol Rev. 2010;90:675–754.

42. Hornbein TF, Griffo ZJ, Roos A. Quantitation of chemoreceptor activity: interrelation of hypoxia and hypercapnia. J Neurophysiol. 1961;24:561–8.

43. Hornbein TF, Roos A. Specificity of H ion concentration as a carotid chemoreceptor stimulus. J Appl Physiol. 1963;18(3):580–4.

44. Rocher A, Geijo-Barrientos E, Caceres AI, et al. Role of voltage-dependent calcium channels in stimulus-secretion coupling in rabbit carotid body chemoreceptor cells. J Physiol. 2005;562(2):407–20.

45. Turner PJ, Buckler KJ. Oxygen and mitochondrial inhibitors modulate both monomeric and heteromeric TASK-1 and TASK-3 channels in mouse carotid body type-1 cells. J Physiol. 2013;591(23):5977–98.

46. Gonzalez C, Sanz-Alfayate G, Agapito MT, et al. Significance of ROS in oxygen sensing in cell systems with sensitivity to physiological hypoxia. Respir Physiol Neurobiol. 2002;132:17–41.

47. Prabhakar NR, Peers C. Gasotransmitter regulation of ion channels: a key step in O_2 sensing by the carotid body. Physiology. 2014;29:49–57.

48. Lahiri S, Roy A, Baby SM, et al. Oxygen sensing in the body. Prog Biophys Mol Biol. 2006;91:249–86.

49. Robbins PA. Evidence for interaction between the contributions to ventilation from the central and peripheral chemoreceptors in man. J Physiol. 1988;401:503–18.

50. Clement ID, Pandit JJ, Bascom DA, et al. An assessment of central-peripheral ventilator chemoreflex interaction using acid and bicarbonate infusions in humans. J Physiol. 1995;485(2):561–70.

51. Blain GM, Smith CA, Henderson KS, et al. Peripheral chemoreceptors determine the respiratory sensitivity of central chemoreceptors to CO_2. J Physiol. 2010;588(13):2455–71.

52. Smith CA, Blain GM, Henderson KS, et al. Peripheral chemoreceptors determine the respiratory sensitivity of central chemoreceptors to CO2; role of carotid body CO2. J Physiol. 2015;593(18):4225–43.

53. Barnes PJ. Neural control of airway smooth muscle. Chapter 91. In: Crystal RG, West JB, Barnes PJ, Weibel ER, editors. The lung: scientific foundations. 2nd ed. Philadelphia: Lippincott-Raven Publishers; 1997. p. 1269–85.

54. Belvisi MG. Overview of the innervation of the lung. Curr Opin Pharmacol. 2002;2:211–5.

55. Caulfield MP. Muscarinic receptors, characterization, coupling and function. Pharmacol Ther. 1993;58:319–79.

56. Barnes PJ. Modulation of neurotransmission in airways. Physiol Rev. 1992;72:699–729.

57. McKenzie DK, Gandevia SC. Skeletal muscle properties: diaphragm and chest wall. In: Crystal RG, West JB, Weibel ER, Barnes PJ, editors. The lung: scientific foundations. 2nd ed. Philadelphia: Lipincott-Raven; 1997. p. 981–91.

58. Coirault C, Chemla D, Lecarpentier Y. Relaxation of the diaphragm. J Appl Physiol. 1999;87(4):1243–52.

59. Levine S, Nguyen T, Taylor N, et al. Rapid disuse atrophy of diaphragm fibers in mechanically ventilated humans. N Engl J Med. 2008;358(13):1327–35.

60. Powers SK, Kavazis AN, Levine S. Prolonged mechanical ventilation alters diaphragmatic structure and function. Crit Care Med. 2009;37(Suppl):S347–53.

61. Picard M, Jung B, Liang F, et al. Mitochondrial dysfunction and lipid accumulation in the human diaphragm during mechanical ventilation. Am J Respir Crit Care Med. 2012;186(11):1140–9.

62. Levine S, Kaiser L, Leferovich J, et al. Cellular adaptations in the diaphragm in chronic obstructive pulmonary disease. N Engl J Med. 1997;337(25):1799–806.

63. Levine S, Nguyen T, Kaiser LR, et al. Human diaphragm remodeling associated with chronic obstructive pulmonary disease. Clinical implications. Am J Respir Crit Care Med. 2003;168:706–13.

64. Ottenheijm CAC, Heunks LMA, Hafmans T, et al. Titin and diaphragm dysfunction in chronic obstructive pulmonary disease. Am J Respir Crit Care Med. 2006;173:527–34.

65. Loring SH, Topulos GP, Hubmayr RD. Transpulmonary pressure: the importance of precise definitions and limiting assumptions. Am J Respir Crit Care Med. 2016;194(12):1452–7.

66. Leith DE, Mead J. Mechanisms determining residual volume of the lungs in normal subjects. J Appl Physiol. 1967;23:221–7.

67. Colin AA, Wohl MEB, Mead J, et al. Transition from dynamically maintained to relaxed end-expiratory volume in human infants. J Appl Physiol. 1989;67:2107–11.

68. Milic-Emili J, Henderson JAM, Dolovich MB, et al. Regional distribution of inspired gas in the lung. J Appl Physiol. 1966;21:749–59.

69. West JB, Dollery CT. Distribution of blood flow and ventilation-perfusion ratio in the lung, measured with radioactive carbon dioxide. J Appl Physiol. 1960;15:405–10.

70. Bake B, Wood L, Murphy B, et al. Effect of inspiratory flow rate on regional distribution of inspired gas. J Appl Physiol. 1974;37:8–17.

71. Widdicombe J. Anatomy and physiology of the airway circulation. Am Rev Respir Dis. 1992;146:S3–7.

72. Pinsky MR. Heart-lung interactions. Curr Opin Crit Care. 2007;13:528–31.

73. Hamzaoui O, Monnet X, Teboul JL. Pulsus paradoxus. Euro Respir J. 2013;42(6):1696–705.

74. Pinsky MR. Cardiovascular issues in respiratory care. Chest. 2005;128:592S–7S.

75. Wise RA, Robotham JL, Summer WR. Effects of spontaneous ventilation on the circulation. Lung. 1981;159:175–86.

76. Roussos C, Macklem PT. The respiratory muscles. N Engl J Med. 1982;307:786–97.

77. Aubier M, Viires N, Syllie G, et al. Respiratory muscle contribution to lactic acidosis in low cardiac output. Am Rev Respir Dis. 1982;126:648–52.

78. Baratz DM, Westbrook PR, Shah PK, et al. Effect of nasal continuous positive airway pressure on cardiac output and oxygen delivery in patients with congestive heart failure. Chest. 1992;102:1397–401.

79. Glick G, Wechsler AS, Epstein SE. Reflex cardiovascular depression produced by stimulation of pulmonary stretch receptors in the dog. J Clin Invest. 1969;48:467–73.

80. Anrep GV, Pascual W, Rossler R. Respiratory variations of the heart rate: I. The reflex mechanism of the respiratory arrhythmia. Proc R Soc Lond B Biol Sci. 1936;119:191–217.

81. Taha BH, Simon PM, Dempsey JA, et al. Respiratory sinus arrhythmia in humans: an obligatory role for vagal feedback from the lungs. J Appl Physiol. 1995;78:638–45.

82. Persson MG, Lonnqvist PA, Gustafsson LE. Positive end expiratory pressure ventilation elicits increases in endogenously formed

nitric oxide as detected in air exhaled by rabbits. Anesthesiology. 1995;82:969–74.

83. Luce JM. The cardiovascular effects of mechanical ventilation and positive end-expiratory pressure. JAMA. 1984;252:807–11.

84. Madden JA, Dawson CA, Harder DR. Hypoxia-induced activation in small isolated pulmonary arteries from the cat. J Appl Physiol. 1985;59:113–8.

85. Hakim TS, Michel RP, Chang HK. Effect of lung inflation on pulmonary vascular resistance by arterial and venous occlusion. J Appl Physiol. 1982;53:1110–5.

86. Block AJ, Boysen PG, Wynne JW. The origins of cor pulmonale: a hypothesis. Chest. 1979;75:109–10.

87. Johnston WE, Vinten-Johansen J, Shugart HE, et al. Positive end-expiratory pressure potentiates the severity of canine right ventricular ischemia-reperfusion injury. Am J Physiol. 1992;262:H168–76.

88. Canada E, Benumof JL, Tousdale FR. Pulmonary vascular resistance correlates in intact normal and abnormal canine lungs. Crit Care Med. 1982;10:719–23.

89. Vieillard-Baron A, Loubieres Y, Schmitt JM, et al. Cyclic changes in right ventricular output impedance during mechanical ventilation. J Appl Physiol. 1999;87:1644–50.

90. Guyton AC, Lindsey AW, Abernathy B, et al. Venous return at various right atrial pressures and the normal venous return curve. Am J Physiol. 1957;189:609–15.

91. Pinsky MR. Instantaneous venous return curves in an intact canine preparation. J Appl Physiol. 1984;56:765–71.

92. Pinsky MR. Determinants of pulmonary arterial flow variation during respiration. J Appl Physiol. 1984;56:1237–45.

93. Fessler HE, Brower RG, Wise RA, et al. Effects of positive end-expiratory pressure on the canine venous return curve. Am Rev Respir Dis. 1992;146:4–10.

94. van den Berg PCM, Jansen JR, Pinsky MR. Effect of positive pressure on venous return in volume-loaded cardiac surgical patients. J Appl Physiol. 2002;92:1223–31.

95. Buda AJ, Pinsky MR, Ingels NB Jr, et al. Effect of intrathoracic pressure on left ventricular performance. N Engl J Med. 1979;301:453–9.

96. Jardin F, Farcot JC, Gueret P, et al. Echocardiographic evaluation of ventricles during continuous positive airway pressure breathing. J Appl Physiol. 1984;56:619–27.

97. Olsen CO, Tyson GS, Maier GW, et al. Dynamic ventricular interaction in the conscious dog. Circ Res. 1983;52:85–104.

98. Bell RC, Robotham JL, Badke FR, et al. Left ventricular geometry during intermittent positive pressure ventilation in dogs. J Crit Care. 1987;2:230–44.

99. Qvist J, Pontoppidan H, Wilson RS, et al. Hemodynamic responses to mechanical ventilation with PEEP: the effect of hypervolemia. Anesthesiology. 1975;42:45–55.

100. Brinker JA, Weiss JL, Lappe DL, et al. Leftward septal displacement during right ventricular loading in man. Circulation. 1980;61:626–33.

101. Vatner SF, Rutherford JD. Control of the myocardial contractile state by carotid chemo- and baroreceptor and pulmonary inflation reflexes in conscious dogs. J Clin Invest. 1978;61:1593–601.

102. Beyar R, Goldstein Y. Model studies of the effects of the thoracic pressure on the circulation. Ann Biomed Eng. 1987;15:373–83.

103. Pinsky MR, Summer WR, Wise RA, et al. Augmentation of cardiac function by elevation of intrathoracic pressure. J Appl Physiol. 1983;54:950–5.

104. Denault AY, Gorcsan J III, Pinsky MR. Dynamic effects of positive-pressure ventilation on canine left ventricular pressure-volume relations. J Appl Physiol. 2001;91:298–308.

105. Butler J. The heart is in good hands. Circulation. 1983;67:1163–8.

106. Naughton MT, Rahman MA, Hara K, et al. Effect of continuous positive airway pressure on intrathoracic and left ventricular transmural pressures in patients with congestive heart failure. Circulation. 1995;91:1725–31.

107. Kaneko Y, Floras JS, Usui K, et al. Cardiovascular effects of continuous positive airway pressure in patients with heart failure and obstructive sleep apnea. N Engl J Med. 2003;348:1233–41.

108. Ranieri VM, Giuliani R, Mascia L, et al. Patient-ventilator interaction during acute hypercapnia: pressure-support vs. proportional-assist ventilation. J Appl Physiol. 1996;81:426–36.

109. Ambrosino N, Cobelli F, Torbicki A, et al. Hemodynamic effects of negative-pressure ventilation in patients with COPD. Chest. 1990;97:850–6.

110. Hurford WE, Lynch KE, Strauss HW, et al. Myocardial perfusion as assessed by thallium-201 scintigraphy during the discontinuation of mechanical ventilation in ventilator-dependent patients. Anesthesiology. 1991;74:1007–16.

111. Srivastava S, Chatila W, Amoateng-Adjepong Y, et al. Myocardial ischemia and weaning failure in patients with coronary artery disease: an update. Crit Care Med. 1999;27:2109–12.

112. Rasanen J, Vaisanen IT, Heikkila J, et al. Acute myocardial infarction complicated by left ventricular dysfunction and respiratory failure: the effects of continuous positive airway pressure. Chest. 1985;87:158–62.

113. Lemaire F, Teboul JL, Cinotti L, et al. Acute left ventricular dysfunction during unsuccessful weaning from mechanical ventilation. Anesthesiology. 1988;69:171–9.

114. Mohsenifar Z, Hay A, Hay J, et al. Gastric intramural pH as a predictor of success or failure in weaning patients from mechanical ventilation. Ann Intern Med. 1993;119:794–8.

115. Jubran A, Mathru M, Dries D, et al. Continuous recordings of mixed venous oxygen saturation during weaning from mechanical ventilation and the ramifications thereof. Am J Respir Crit Care Med. 1998;158:1763–9.

116. Straus C, Louis B, Isabey D, et al. Contribution of the endotracheal tube and the upper airway to breathing workload. Am J Respir Crit Care Med. 1998;157:23–30.

117. Galvin I, Drummond GB, Nirmalan M. Distribution of blood flow and ventilation in the lung: gravity is not the only factor. Brit J Anaesth. 2007;98:420–8.

118. Hughes M, Point WJB. Gravity is the major factor determining the distribution of blood flow in the human lung. J Appl Physiol. 2008;104:1531–3.

119. Glenny RW. Counterpoint: Gravity is not the major factor determining the distribution of blood flow in the healthy human lung. J Appl Physiol. 2008;104:1533–5.

120. Glenny RW, Bernard S, Robertson HT. Gravity is an important but secondary determinant of regional pulmonary blood flow in upright primates. J Appl Physiol. 1999;86:623–32.

121. Robertson HT, Hlastala MP. Microsphere maps of regional blood flow and regional ventilation. J Appl Physiol. 2007;102:1265–72.

122. Prisk GK, Guy HJB, Elliott AR, et al. Inhomogeneity of pulmonary perfusion during sustained microgravity on SLS-1. J Appl Physiol. 1994;76:1730–8.

123. Prisk GK, Guy HJB, Elliott AR, et al. Ventilatory inhomogeneity determined from multiple-breath washouts during sustained microgravity on Spacelab SLS-1. J Appl Physiol. 1995;78:597–607.

124. Glenny RW, Lamm WJ, Bernard SL, et al. Selected contribution: redistribution of pulmonary perfusion during weightlessness and increased gravity. J Appl Physiol. 2000;89:1239–48.

125. Weibel ER. Fractal geometry: a design principle for living organisms. Am J Physiol Lung Cell Mol Physiol. 1991;261:L361–9.

126. Glenny RW. Blood flow distribution in the lung. Chest. 1998;114:8S–16S.

127. Altemeier WA, McKinney S, Glenny RW. Fractal nature of regional ventilation distribution. J Appl Physiol. 2000;88:1551–7.

128. Hughes JMB, Glazier JB, Maloney JE, et al. Effect of lung volume on the distribution of pulmonary blood flow in man. Respir Physiol. 1968;4:58–72.

129. West JB. Regional differences in gas exchange in the lung of erect man. J Appl Physiol. 1962;17:893–8.

130. Wagner PD, Dantzker DR, Dueck R, et al. Ventilation-perfusion inequality in chronic obstructive pulmonary disease. J Clin Invest. 1977;59:203–6.

131. Bradford J, Dean H. The pulmonary circulation. J Physiol. 1894;16:34–96.

132. Von Euler U, Liljestrand G. Observations on the pulmonary arterial pressure in the cat. Acta Physiol Scand. 1946;12:301–20.

133. Duke HN. Pulmonary vasomotor responses of isolated perfused cat lungs to anoxia and hypercapnia. Q J Exper Physiol. 1951;36:75–88.

134. Bergofsky EH, Haas F, Porcelli R. Determination of the sensitive vascular sites from which hypoxia and hypercapnia elicit rises in pulmonary arterial pressure. Fed Proc. 1968;27:1420–5.

135. Domino KB, Wetstein L, Glasser SA, et al. Influence of mixed venous oxygen tension (PvO₂) on blood flow to atelectatic lung. Anesthesiology. 1983;59:428–34.

136. Marshall C, Marshall BE. Influence of perfusate PO₂ on hypoxic pulmonary vasoconstriction in rats. Circ Res. 1983;52:691–6.

137. Marshall BE, Marshall C, Benumof J, et al. Hypoxic pulmonary vasoconstriction in dogs: effects of lung segment size and oxygen tension. J Appl Physiol Respirat Environ Exercise Physiol. 1981;51:1543–51.

138. Naeije R, Lejeune P, Leeman M, et al. Pulmonary vascular responses to surgical chemodenervation and chemical sympathectomy in dogs. J Appl Physiol. 1989;66:42–50.

139. Lejeune P, Vachiaery JL, Leeman M, et al. Absence of parasympathetic control of pulmonary vascular pressure-flow plots in hyperoxic and hypoxic dogs. Respir Physiol. 1989;78:123–33.

140. Robins ED, Theodore J, Burke CM, et al. Hypoxic vasoconstriction persists in the human transplanted lung. Clin Sci. 1987;72:283–7.

141. Aaronson PI, Robertson TP, Knock GA, et al. Hypoxic pulmonary vasoconstriction: mechanisms and controversies. J Physiol. 2006;570:53–8.

142. Evans AM. The role of intracellular ion channels in regulating cytoplasmic calcium in pulmonary arterial smooth muscle: which store and where? Adv Exp Biol Med. 2010;661:57–76.

143. Sylvester JT, Shimoda LA, Aaronson PI, Ward JPT. Hypoxic pulmonary vasoconstriction. Physiol Rev. 2012;92:367–520.

144. Waypa GB, Chandel NS, Schumacker PT. Model for hypoxic pulmonary vasoconstriction involving mitochondrial oxygen sensing. Circ Res. 2001;88:1259–66.

145. Evans AM, Dipp M. Hypoxic pulmonary vasoconstriction: cyclic adenosine diphosphate-ribose, smooth muscle Ca2+ stores and the endothelium. Respir Physiol Neurobiol. 2002;132:3–15.

146. Yamamoto Y, Nakano H, Ide H, et al. Role of airway nitric oxide on the regulation of pulmonary circulation by carbon dioxide. J Appl Physiol. 2001;91:1121–30.

147. Talbot NP, Balanos GM, Dorrington KL, et al. Two temporal components within the human pulmonary vascular response to ~2 h of isocapnic hypoxia. J Appl Physiol. 2005;98:1125–39.

148. Weissmann N, Zeller S, Schafer RU, et al. Impact of mitochondria and NADPH oxidases on acute and sustained hypoxic pulmonary vasoconstriction. Am J Respir Cell Mol Biol. 2006;34:505–13.

149. Nunn JF. Factors influencing the arterial oxygen tension during halothane anaesthesia with spontaneous respiration. Br J Anaesth. 1964;36:327–4.

150. Brismar B, Hedenstierna G, Lundquist H, et al. Pulmonary densities during anesthesia with muscular relaxation – a proposal of atelectasis. Anesthesiology. 1985;62:422–8.

151. Lundquuist H, Hedenstierna G, Strandberg A, et al. CT-assessment of dependent lung densities in man during general anesthesia. Acta Radiol. 1995;36:626–32.

152. Reber A, Bein T, Hogman M, et al. Lung aeration and pulmonary gas exchange during lumbar epidural anaesthesia and in the lithotomy position in elderly patients. Anaesthesia. 1998;53:854–61.

153. Tenling A, Joachimsson PO, Tyden H, et al. Thoracic epidural anesthesia as an adjunct to general anesthesia for cardiac surgery: effects on ventilation-perfusion relationships. Anesthesiology. 1987;66:157–67.

154. Magnusson L, Spahn DR. New concepts of atelectasis during general anaesthesia. Br J Anaesth. 2003;91:61–72.

155. Froese AB, Bryan AC. Effects of anesthesia and paralysis on diaphragmatic mechanics in man. Anesthesiology. 1974;41:242–55.

156. Warner DO, Warner MA, Ritman EL. Atelectasis and chest wall shape during halothane anesthesia. Anesthesiology. 1996;85:49–59.

157. Reber A, Nylund U, Hedenstierna G. Position and shape of the diaphragm: implications for atelectasis formation. Anaesthesia. 1998;53:1054–61.

158. Loring SH, Butler JP. Gas exchange in body cavities. In: Farhi LE, Tenney SM, editors. Handbook of physiology. Section 3. The respiratory system, Gas exchange, vol. 4. Bethesda: American Physiological Society; 1987. p. 283–95.

159. Joyce CJ, Baker AB, Kennedy RR. Gas uptake from an unventilated area of the lung: computer model of absorption atelectasis. J Appl Physiol. 1993;74:1107–16.

160. Joyce CJ, Williams AB. Kinetics of absorption atelectasis during anesthesia: a mathematical model. J Appl Physiol. 1999;86:1116–25.

161. Rothen HU, Sporre B, Engberg G, et al. Influence of gas composition on recurrence of atelectasis after a re-expansion maneuver during general anesthesia. Anesthesiology. 1995;82:832–42.

162. Lumb AB, Slinger P. Hypoxic pulmonary vasoconstriction. Physiology and anesthetic implications. Anesthesiology. 2015;122(4):932–46.

163. Domino KB, Borowec L, Alexander CM, et al. Influence of isoflurane on hypoxic pulmonary vasoconstriction in dogs. Anesthesiology. 1986;64:423–9.

164. Abe K, Mashimo T, Yoshiya I. Arterial oxygenation and shunt fraction during one-lung ventilation: a comparison of isoflurane and sevoflurane. Anesth Analg. 1998;86:1266–70.

165. Pagel PS, Fu JL, Damask MC, et al. Desflurane and isoflurane produce similar alterations in systemic and pulmonary hemodynamics and arterial oxygenation in patients undergoing one-lung ventilation during thoracotomy. Anesth Analg. 1998;87:800–7.

166. Schwarzkopf K, Schreiber T, Preussler N-P, et al. Lung perfusion, shunt fraction, and oxygenation during one-lung ventilation in pigs: the effects of desflurane, isoflurane, and propofol. J Cardiothorac Vasc Anesth. 2003;17:73–5.

167. Benumof JL, Wahrenbrock EA. Local effects of anesthetics on regional hypoxic pulmonary vasoconstriction. Anesthesiology. 1975;43:525–32.

168. Reid CW, Slinger PD, Lenis S. A comparison of the effects of propofol-alfentanil versus isoflurane anesthesia on arterial oxygenation during one-lung ventilation. J Cardiothorac Vasc Anesth. 1996;10:860–3.

169. Beck DH, Doepfmer UR, Sinemus C, et al. Effects of sevoflurane and propofol on pulmonary shunt fraction during one-lung ventilation for thoracic surgery. Br J Anaesth. 2001;86:38–43.

170. Ishibe Y, Shiokawa Y, Umeda T, et al. The effect of thoracic epidural anesthesia on hypoxic pulmonary vasoconstriction in dogs: an analysis of the pressure-flow curve. Anesth Analg. 1996;82:1049–55.

171. Parsons GH, Leventhal JP, Hansen MM, et al. Effect of sodium nitroprusside on hypoxic vasoconstriction in the dog. J Appl Physiol Respirat Environ Exercise Physiol. 1981;51: 288–92.

172. Casthely PA, Lear S, Cottrell JE, et al. Intrapulmonary shunting during induced hypotension. Anesth Analg. 1982;61: 231–5.

173. Kato R, Sato J, Hishino T. Milrinone decreases both pulmonary arterial and venous resistances in the hypoxic dog. Br J Anaesth. 1998;81:920–4.

174. Weissmann N, Gerigk B, Kocer O, et al. Hypoxi-induced pulmonary hypertension: different impact of iloprost, sildenafil, and nitric oxide. Respir Med. 2007;101:2125–32.

175. Reichenberger F, Kohstall MG, Seeger T, et al. Effect of sildenafil on hypoxia-induced changes in pulmonary circulation and right ventricular function. Respir Physiol Neurobiol. 2007;159:196–201.

176. Fesler P, Pagnamenta A, Rondelet B, et al. Effects of sildenafil on hypoxic pulmonary vascular function in dogs. J Appl Physiol. 2006;101:1085–90.

177. Kiely DG, Cargill RI, Lipworth BJ. Angiotensin II receptor blockade and effects on pulmonary hemodynamics and hypoxic pulmonary vasoconstriction in humans. Chest. 1996;110:698–703.

178. Cargill RI, Lipworth BJ. Lisinopril attenuates acute hypoxic pulmonary vasoconstriction in humans. Chest. 1996;109:424–9.

179. McMurty IF, Petrun MD, Reeves JT. Lungs from chronically hypoxic rats have decreased pressor response to acute hypoxia. Am J Physiol. 1978;235:H104–9.

180. Weissmann N, Nollen M, Gerigk B, et al. Down-regulation of hypoxic vasoconstriction by chronic hypoxia in rabbits: effects of nitric oxide. Am J Physiol. 2003;284:H931–8.

181. Wagner PD, Laravuso RB, Goldzimmer E, et al. Distribution of ventilation-perfusion ratios in dogs with normal and abnormal lungs. J Appl Physiol. 1975;38(6):1099–109.

Physiology of the Lateral Decubitus Position, Open Chest, and One-Lung Ventilation

5

Sean R. McLean and Jens Lohser

Key Points
- Ventilation and perfusion matching is optimized for gas exchange.
- Induction of anesthesia, one-lung ventilation (OLV), and opening of the chest progressively uncouple ventilation–perfusion (V/Q) homeostasis.
- Hypoxic pulmonary vasoconstriction (HPV) improves V/Q matching during OLV but can be impaired by anesthetic interventions.

Introduction

Early attempts at intrathoracic surgery in nonventilated patients were fraught with rapidly developing respiratory distress and a fast moving operative field. The difficulty with performing a thoracotomy in a spontaneously breathing patient, for both the patient and the surgeon, is explained by two phenomena: *pendel-luft* and *mediastinal shift* (Fig. 5.1) [1]. Both phenomena occur due to the fact that the pleural interface has been disrupted in the open hemithorax, which means that no negative intrathoracic pressure is being created in response to a spontaneous inspiratory effort and chest-wall expansion. In the closed hemithorax, on the other hand, chest-wall expansion and the resulting negative intrathoracic pressure will produce gas flow into the lung via the mainstem bronchus. However, inspiratory gas flow will not only come from the trachea but also from the operative lung, which is free to collapse due to the surgical pneumothorax. Inspiration therefore results in nonoperative lung expansion and operative lung retraction. The reverse process occurs during expiration, where bulk expiratory gas flow, from the nonoperative lung, not only escapes via the mainstem bronchus into the trachea but also back into the operative lung causing it to re-expand. This process results in the "pendular" motion of the lung with inspiration and expiration. Mediastinal shift occurs due to a similar process. The negative inspiratory pressure in the closed hemithorax is equally applied to the mediastinum, which is secondarily pulled away from the open thorax during inspiration. The reverse is true during expiration, where positive intrathoracic pressure pushes the mediastinum across into the open thorax. When combined, these two mechanisms explain the difficulty encountered by the operating surgeon in terms of a fast moving operating field and the potential for rapidly developing respiratory distress in the patient secondary to inefficient to-and-fro ventilation with limited CO_2 elimination and fresh gas entrainment (Fig. 5.1).

Selective ventilation of one lung was first described in 1931 and quickly resulted in increasingly complex lung resection surgery [3]. While infinitely better tolerated than spontaneous respiration, hypoxia was a frequent occurrence during the early years of OLV. Extensive research over the ensuing decades has clarified the basic physiology governing pulmonary perfusion (Q) and ventilation (V), as well as the disturbances that are caused by anesthetic and surgical interventions. Knowledge of the basic physiology is necessary to appreciate ventilation/perfusion (V/Q) disturbances during OLV.

Perfusion

Pulmonary blood flow is essential for multiple processes. Pulmonary arterial blood carries carbon dioxide to the alveoli for removal and exhalation. Pulmonary venous blood provides filling and oxygen to the left heart to support systemic perfusion and metabolic oxygen demand, respectively. Because of the closed nature of the circulatory system, the entire cardiac output (CO) has to pass through the pulmonary circulation. Pulmonary perfusion pressures are significantly

S. R. McLean · J. Lohser (✉)
Department of Anesthesiology, Pharmacology, and Therapeutics, University of British Columbia, Vancouver General Hospital, Vancouver, BC, Canada
e-mail: jens.lohser@vch.ca

© Springer Nature Switzerland AG 2019
P. Slinger (ed.), *Principles and Practice of Anesthesia for Thoracic Surgery*, https://doi.org/10.1007/978-3-030-00859-8_5

Fig. 5.1 Pendel-luft and mediastinal shift in an awake subject in the lateral decubitus with a surgical pneumothorax. During expiration, air moves out (blue arrows) from the dependent lung (DL) since alveolar pressure (P_{alv}) becomes higher than atmospheric pressure (P_{atm}). Part of the exhaled gases inflate (red arrow) the nondependent lung (NDL), in which Palv equalizes (P_{atm}). During inspiration, atmospheric air inflates the DL in which Palv becomes subatmospheric, whereas the NDL deflates, contributing (red arrow) to the ventilation of the DL. (Modified from Pompeo, 2012 with permission [2])

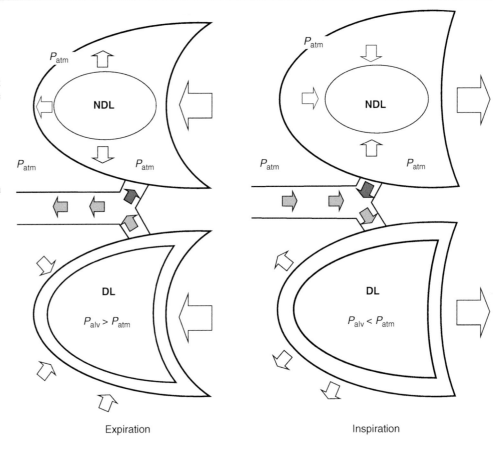

Expiration   Inspiration

lower than systemic perfusion pressures and become further reduced by 1 cm H_2O for each centimeter of elevation that blood flow has to travel above the level of the heart. Perfusion is therefore not uniform across the lung, as pulmonary arterial (P_{pa}) and venous (P_{pv}) pressures are dependent on the relative elevation above the heart, whereas the extrinsic compressive force of the alveolar distending pressure (P_A) is relatively constant. The interplay of pressures across the lung results in distinct territories of lung perfusion, which are known as the West zones (Fig. 5.2a) [4, 5]. Zone 1 exists in the most superior aspect of the lung and is characterized by alveolar pressures that exceed intravascular pressures ($P_A > P_{pa} > P_{pv}$). This results in capillary collapse and secondary complete obstruction of blood flow. Zone 1 therefore represents alveolar "dead space." While Zone 1 is minimal under normal circumstances, it may increase in the presence of increased P_A (positive-pressure ventilation) or decreased P_{pa} (decreased CO). Moving inferiorly in the lung, P_{pa} values increase due to the lesser elevation above the heart and begin to exceed P_A. This characterizes Zone 2 ($P_{pa} > P_A > P_{pv}$), where P_{pa} exceeds P_A resulting in capillary blood flow. As P_A continues to exceed P_{pv}, capillary blood flow remains dependent on the differential between P_{pa} and P_A. This relationship has been likened to a waterfall, as the amount of flow is dependent on the upstream "water level" (P_{pa}), relative to the height of the dam (P_A), but independent of the downstream

"water level" (P_{pv}). Zone 3 ($P_{pa} > P_{pv} > P_A$) is reached when P_{pv} begins to exceed P_A, resulting in pulmonary perfusion independent of P_A and only determined by difference between P_{pa} and P_{pv}. Zone 4 ($P_{pa} > P_{is} > P_{pv} > P_A$) is that portion of the lung where interstitial pressure P_{is} is higher than venous pressure P_{pv}, resulting in a reduction in blood flow relative to the pressure differential between P_{pa} and P_{is}. This is analogous to the patient with increased intracranial pressure (ICP), where the "interstitial" pressure (analogous to ICP) exceeds the venous outflow pressure (CVP) and therefore reduces the cerebral perfusion pressure. Zone 4 can exist in the most inferior portions of the lung or may alternatively be created by exhalation to low lung volumes or increased interstitial pressures such as in volume overload [5]. One should keep in mind that the West zones are an oversimplified static picture of a dynamic, cyclical system, as lung regions may move through various zones depending on the stage of the cardiac and respiratory cycle that they are in. For example, a given Zone 2 lung region may become Zone 1 during diastole (low P_{pa}) and positive-pressure inspiration (high P_A) or may become Zone 3 in systole (high P_{pa}) and mechanical expiration (low P_A). The gravitational model of the West zones helps to illustrate the basis of V/Q mismatch in the lungs but only partially reflects human physiology. In vivo perfusion scanning has demonstrated a combination of gravitational distribution and an "onion-like" layering, with

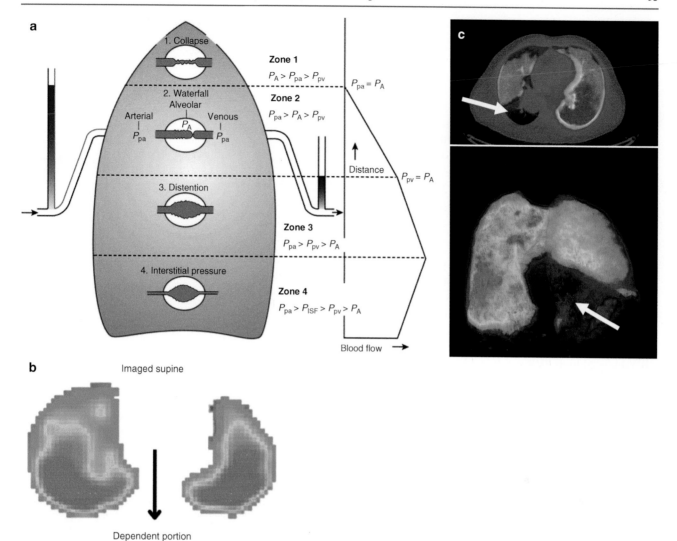

Fig. 5.2 Classic West zones of blood flow distribution in the upright position. Pulmonary blood flow distribution as it relates to the alveolar pressure (P_A), the pulmonary arterial pressure (P_{pa}), the pulmonary venous pressure (P_{pv}), and the interstitial pressure (P_{is}) at various gravitational levels (**a**). In vivo perfusion scanning illustrating central-to-peripheral, in addition to gravitational blood flow distribution, in the upright position (**b**). Single-photon emission computed tomography (SPECT) images of perfusion in a transverse section of the lung. Coloring is according to a relative scale of perfusion with red representing maximal and green representing minimal perfusion (**c**). Positron emission tomography/computed tomography (PET/CT) demonstrates both a gravity-dependent distribution and an onion-layered type perfusion distribution. The arrow indicates a perfusion defect secondary to cancer. (Modified from (**a**) West [4], (**b**) Petersson [6], and (**c**) Siva [7] with permission)

reduced flow at the periphery of the lung and higher flow toward the hilum (Fig. 5.2b, c) [6, 7]. It has also been shown that the perfusion of the left lung, in the dependent left lateral decubitus position, is lower than would be expected based simply on gravity redistribution. Compression and/or distortion elicited by the heart and mediastinum is the likely cause for this reduction [8].

The pulmonary vascular bed is a low-resistance conduit and possesses significant recruitable territory, which helps to offset any increases in pressure. Initial increases in P_{pa} or flow cause progressive recruitment of previously nonperfused vasculature. Once recruitment is complete, further increases in P_{pa} distend the pulmonary vessels, which mitigates increases in blood flow and helps to minimize increases in right ventricular afterload. These modifications allow pulmonary pressures to stay low, even when CO is increased to levels as high as 30 L/min during exercise [9]. At extreme levels of P_{pa}, distention of blood vessels will fail to decrease intravascular pressures resulting in transudation of fluid into the interstitium via mechanotransduction of the endothelial surface layer [10, 11]. Vascular resistance within the pulmonary circulation is also influenced by the degree of lung inflation. Overall pulmonary blood volume changes more than two-fold throughout the respiratory cycle, from a peak at end expiration (i.e., residual volume) to a nadir at total lung capacity. There are two populations of pulmonary vessels that exhibit opposing responses to lung inflation. Alveolar capillaries are exposed to intra-alveolar pressures and therefore experience increasing resistance to flow, or may actually collapse, as lung volumes increase. Intraparenchymal, extra-alveolar vessels, on the other hand, experience outward radial traction with lung expansion, which progressively decreases their resistance. The cumulative effect is a parabolic resistance curve, with minimal pulmonary vascular resistance (PVR) at functional residual capacity (FRC) and progressive increases in resistance at extremes of lung volume.

Hypoxic Pulmonary Vasoconstriction (HPV)

Oxygen-sensing mechanisms in the human body, including HPV of the pulmonary arterial bed, have been well studied and reviewed extensively [12, 13]. In the fetus HPV-induced high PVR results in diversion of blood flow across the foramen ovale and ductus arteriosus. HPV remains important ex utero, as it allows V/Q matching by reducing perfusion to poorly oxygenated lung tissue. HPV is active in the physiologic range (P_AO_2 40–100 mmHg in the adult) and proportional to not only the severity of the hypoxia but also the amount of hypoxic lung. HPV is maximal if between 30% and 70% of the lung is hypoxic. Low partial pressure of oxygen results in inhibition of potassium currents, which leads to membrane depolarization and calcium entry through L-type calcium channels. Extracellular calcium entry, plus calcium release from the sarcoplasmic reticulum, culminates in smooth muscle contraction, primarily in low-resistance pulmonary arteries with a diameter less than 500 μm [12]. The primary stimulus for HPV appears to be the alveolar partial pressure of oxygen (P_AO_2); however, the pulmonary venous partial pressure of oxygen (P_vO_2) is also involved. HPV is maximal at normal P_vO_2 levels but is inhibited at high or low levels. Low P_vO_2, for example in low CO states, results in a decrease in P_aO_2 and therefore generalized, competing vasoconstriction. Conversely, high P_vO_2 in the setting of sepsis will decrease the vasoconstrictor response in hypoxic areas due to the generalized increase in P_aO_2. Vasoconstriction occurs in a biphasic temporal fashion. The early response occurs within seconds and reaches an initial plateau at 15 min, followed by a late response result-

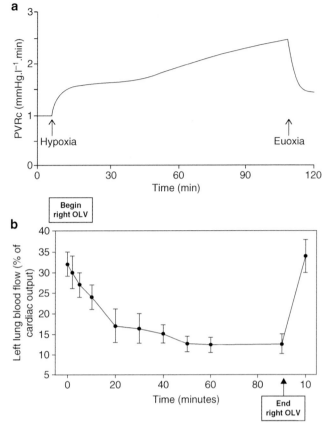

Fig. 5.3 (**a**) The biphasic nature of hypoxic pulmonary vasoconstriction (HPV) in hypoxic healthy subjects (end-tidal PO2 of 50 mmHg). Phase 1 of the response is complete within minutes, with a second phase occurring approximately 40 min later. Note the incomplete release of HPV after restitution of normoxemia. *PO2* partial pressure of oxygen, *PVRc* pulmonary vascular resistance corrected for cardiac output. (Reproduced from Lumb and Slinger with permission [13]). (**b**) The time course for redistribution of pulmonary blood flow to the non-ventilated left lung of anesthetized dogs over a 90-min interval of right-lung ventilation. (Reproduced from Heerdt with permission [20])

ing in maximal vasoconstriction at 4 h [14–17] (Fig. 5.3a). There is animal data demonstrating that this HPV response persists for at least 90 min after the restoration of normoxemia (Fig. 5.3a) [18]. HPV reduces the shunt flow through the operative lung by roughly 40%, facilitating the safe conduct of OLV (Fig. 5.4), although some have questioned its true clinical importance [19].

Extremes of HPV may cause harm. Overactivity, particularly during exercise at high altitudes, may result in high-altitude pulmonary edema [15]. The opposite is true in thoracic anesthesia where inhibition of HPV may result in intraoperative hypoxemia. Many studies have attempted to

$\dot{V}/\dot{Q}$ mismatch without HPV

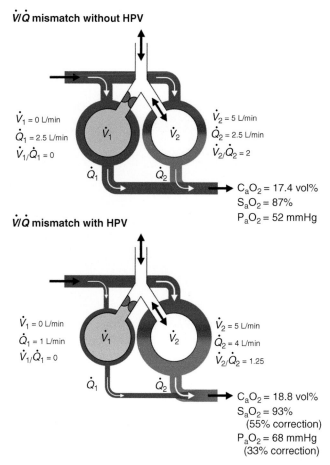

$\dot{V}/\dot{Q}$ mismatch with HPV

Fig. 5.4 Effects of ventilation–perfusion ($\dot{V}/\dot{Q}$) relationships on oxygen exchange in a 2-compartment lung during $\dot{V}/\dot{Q}$ mismatch without hypoxic pulmonary vasoconstriction (HPV) (top) and $\dot{V}/\dot{Q}$ mismatch with HPV (bottom). Values for total ventilation ($\dot{V}$), inspired O2 tension (PIO2), total cardiac output ($\dot{Q}$), and mixed venous O2 concentration (CmvO2), tension (PmvO2), and hemoglobin saturation (SmvO2) shown are the same for all conditions. Compartmental ventilation ($\dot{V}$ 1, $\dot{V}$ 2), perfusion ($\dot{Q}$ 1, $\dot{Q}$ 2), ventilation–perfusion ratio ($\dot{V}$ 1/$\dot{Q}$ 1, $\dot{V}$ 2/$\dot{Q}$ 2), the resulting systemic arterial O2 concentration (CaO2, calculated as the perfusion-weighted mean of the O2 concentrations in blood flowing from each compartment), and corresponding systemic arterial oxyhemoglobin saturation (SaO2) and O2 tension (PaO2) are also indicated for each condition. For simplicity, O2 concentrations were calculated as the product of hemoglobin concentration (15 g/dl), hemoglobin O2 binding capacity (1.34 vol% per g/dl), and oxyhemoglobin saturation, and ignore the concentration of O2 physically dissolved in plasma, which would be small at these O2 tensions. Vol% indicates ml O2/100 ml blood. (Reproduced from Sylvester with permission [21])

identify agents or interventions that potentiate or inhibit the pulmonary vasoconstrictor response to hypoxia. Most research has been performed on animals, as interventions are more easily standardized. Perioperative HPV modifiers are summarized in Table 5.1.

Anesthetic Modifiers

Inhibition of HPV by inhalational anesthesia has long been recognized. Ether, halothane, and nitrous oxide inhibit HPV in a dose-dependent fashion, and the underlying intracellular mechanisms have been described for halothane [71]. The effect of the newer inhalation anesthetics such as isoflurane, desflurane, and sevoflurane is less certain. All three of these agents appear to be equally neutral toward HPV or at least not cause significant depression at clinically relevant doses. Intravenous anesthesia with propofol has been proposed as a means of avoiding HPV modulation, but the improvement in oxygenation is clinically insignificant, except in marginal patients. Results on the influence of thoracic epidural anesthesia (TEA) on oxygenation have been conflicting. Garutti et al. showed an increase in pulmonary venous admixture and secondary worse oxygenation, which may have been due to a drop in CO [72]. Multiple other studies failed to demonstrate an effect of TEA on oxygenation during OLV, when hemodynamic variables were maintained [38–40]. Traditional thoracic teaching has emphasized to keep patients warm and dry, which is supported by the fact that hypothermia and both, hemodilution and increased left atrial pressure, inhibit HPV. Although altering HPV to improve oxygenation during OLV would be an appealing premise, studies have failed to elucidate an HPV modifying agent for routine use. Amiltrine, which is not available in North America, augments the HPV response, increases pulmonary vascular resistance on OLV, but fails to improve oxygenation [73]. Endogenous NO causes vasodilation and thereby inhibits HPV; if given by the inhalational route to the ventilated lung during OLV, exogenous NO causes localized vasodilation and thereby decreases shunt fraction. However, it has been demonstrated that, in the absence of arterial hypoxemia or pulmonary hypertension, inhaled NO does not improve oxygenation during OLV [74]. Therefore European consensus guidelines do not recommend the routine use of NO or amiltrine for desaturation during OLV [75]. Initial studies of other HPV augmenting agents, such as phenylephrine [76] and intravenous iron [77], have demonstrated improvements

Table 5.1 Perioperative modifiers of hypoxic pulmonary vasoconstriction

	Effect	References
Patient factors		
COPD	−	[22]
Cirrhosis	−	[23]
Sepsis	−	[24][a]
Pregnancy	−	[25][a]
Female sex	−	[26][a]
Exercise	−	[27][a]
Systemic HTN	+	[28]
EtOH	+	[29][a]
Physiologic changes		
Metabolic acidosis	+	[30][a]
Respiratory acidosis	0	[30][a]
Metabolic alkalosis	−	[30][a]
Respiratory alkalosis	−	[30][a]
Hypercapnea	+	[14]
Hypocapnea	−	[14]
Hyperthermia	+	[31][a]
Hypothermia	−	[31][a]
Increased LAP	−	[32][a]
Increased P_vO_2	−	[33][a]
Decreased P_vO_2	+	[33][a]
Perioperative interventions		
Trendelenburg	−	[34]
Lateral decubitus	+	[35]
Supine position	0	[35]
Surgical lung retraction	+	[36]
Hemodilution	−	[37]
Epidural anesthesia	0	[38–41]
Inhaled NO	0	[41]
Pharmacologic agents		
Inhalational anesthetics		
Nitrous oxide	−	[42]
Halothane	−	[43]
Enflurane	0	[44]
Isoflurane	0/−	[45]
Desflurane	0	[46]
Sevoflurane	0	[47]
Intravenous anesthetics		
Propofol	0/+	[47, 48][a]
Dexmedetomidine	0/+	[49]
Ketamine	0	[48][a]
Opioids	0	[50][a]
Calcium channel blockers		
Verapamil	−	[43]
Diltiazem	0	[51]
Adrenergic blockers		
Propranolol	+	[52][a]
Phenoxybenzamine	−	[52][a]
Phentolamine	−	[53]
Clonidine	+	[54][a]
Vasodilators		
Hydralazine	−	[53]
Nitroglycerin	−	[55][a]
Nitroprusside	−	[56]
Sildenafil	−	[57]

Table 5.1 (continued)

	Effect	References
Vasoactive agents		
Dopamine	?	[58][a]
Isoproterenol	−	[59][a]
Norepinephrine	−	[59][a]
Phenylephrine	+	[60]
Vasopressin	0	[61][a]
Other		
Losartan (ARB)	−	[62]
Lisinopril (ACE-I)	−	[63]
Methylprednisolone	0	[64]
Indomethacin	+	[55][a]
ASA	+	[55][a]
Prostacyclin	−	[65]
PGE_1	−	[66][a]
Salbutamol	+	[67]
Atrovent	+	[67]
Lidocaine	+	[42][a]
Iron	+	[68]
Desferoxamine	−	[68]
Ascorbate (vitamin C)	0	[69]

Modified from Lohser [70] with permission

[a]Animal data

in oxygenation, although further studies for use in OLV are warranted. Although clearly efficacious, the focus on HPV manipulation with potentially dangerous agents such as almitrine has been called a distraction from more common reasons for desaturation, such as hypoventilation of the dependent lung [19].

Other Modifiers of HPV

Surgical retraction can assist HPV by increasing PVR in the operative lung [36]; however, the release of vasoactive substances secondary to the manipulation may conversely result in an inhibition of HPV [78]. Ligation of pulmonary vessels during lung resection results in the permanent exclusion of vascular territory and thereby a reduction in shunt flow [78]. The side of surgery influences the extent of shunt flow, as the larger right lung receives a 10% higher proportion of CO than the left lung. Positioning is important as the lateral decubitus position allows for a gravity-induced reduction in shunt flow to the nondependent lung. Procedures that call for supine positioning, on the other hand, are hampered by higher shunt flow to the nondependent lung and may have higher rates of intraoperative desaturations [35]. Similarly, addition of a head-down tilt to the left lateral position has been shown to worsen oxygenation during OLV, likely due to dependent lung compression by abdominal contents [34].

Cardiac Output and Arterial Oxygenation

Arterial oxygen content (CaO_2) is influenced by end-capillary oxygen content (CcO_2), oxygen consumption (VO_2), CO (Q_t), and shunt flow (Q_s). CaO_2 can be calculated using Eq. (5.1):

$$CaO_2 = CcO_2 - (VO_2 / Q_t) \times \left(\frac{Q_s / Q_t}{10 \times (1 - Q_s / Q_t)} \right) \quad (5.1)$$

The influence of CO on arterial oxygenation during OLV has been studied repeatedly. Slinger and Scott showed a direct correlation between increasing CO and improving oxygenation in patients during OLV [79]. Similarly, CO augmented by a small dose of dobutamine (5 µg/kg/min) has been shown to improve arterial oxygenation and decrease shunt fraction [80, 81]. However, larger doses of dobutamine have been shown to adversely affect arterial oxygenation in a porcine model of OLV. Russell and James increased CO to supranormal levels (two to three times normal) with dopamine, dobutamine, adrenaline, or isoproterenol [82, 83]. They demonstrated that while high CO increases mixed venous oxygenation, this benefit is overridden by an increase in shunt fraction, resulting in impaired arterial oxygenation. The shunt fraction is likely increased due to weakened HPV in the face of increases in pulmonary arterial pressure and increased P_vO_2 [32, 84]. Animal studies have similarly shown that high doses (20–25 µg/kg/min) of dopamine and dobutamine inhibit HPV response in dogs with left lower lobe hypoxia [85] and one-lung atelectasis [58]. At low CO, oxygenation will therefore be impaired secondary to a low mixed venous oxygen saturation, despite a relatively low shunt fraction. At supranormal CO, on the other hand, oxygenation will be impaired due to an increased shunt fraction, despite the high mixed venous saturation (Fig. 5.5). This interplay bears some resemblance to the opposing effects of alveolar and parenchymal vascular resistance on PVR. Maintenance or restoration of "normal" CO is therefore important for oxygenation during OLV. The availability of noninvasive monitoring devices makes CO data more readily available and allows for appropriate titration of inotropes when required.

Ventilation

Similar to pulmonary perfusion, gravitational forces also affect the distribution of ventilation throughout the lung. The negative pressure of the visceral–parietal pleural interface forces the lung to maintain the shape of the hemitho-

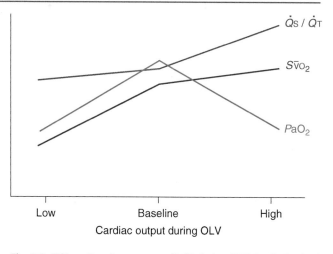

Fig. 5.5 Effect of cardiac output on PaO2 during OLV (on the basis of the data from Slinger and Scott [79] and Russell and James [82]. (Reproduced from Lumb [13] with permission)

rax. Disruption of that interface (as in a pneumothorax) results in recoil deflation of the lung, which, analogous to a fluid-filled balloon, will take on a more globular shape. The same forces are active even with an intact pleural interface and affect the cumulative transpulmonary pressure. The inherent tendency of the lung to want to collapse away from the upper chest wall adds to the negative pleural pressure at the top of the lung, while the tendency of the dependent lung to want to push outward reduces negative pleural pressure at the bottom of the lung. The resulting vertical pressure gradient accounts for a change of 0.25 cm H_2O per centimeter of vertical distance along the lung. On the basis of a height of 30 cm of the upright lung, this corresponds to a change in transpulmonary pressure (P_{pl}) of $30 \times 0.25 = 7.5$ cm H_2O between the top and the bottom of the lung [86]. The distending force (P_A) is the same for all alveoli; however, P_{pl} becomes less negative toward the bottom of the lung. The net effect is that the transpulmonary pressure ($P_A - P_{pl}$) is higher at the top of the lung, resulting in a larger alveolar volume compared to the bottom of the lung. In fact, this difference in size can be as much as fourfold. While the dependent alveoli are relatively small and compressed, they fall on the steep (compliant) portion of the volume–compliance curve and receive a disproportionately larger amount of the alveolar ventilation. The larger alveoli of the upper lung fall on the flat (noncompliant) portion of the volume–compliance curve and therefore change little during tidal respiration [87]. While this model of ventilation distribution is applicable to the healthy lung, recent advances in the imaging of dynamic changes in the distribution of ventilation during tidal breathing have confirmed that ventilation in the diseased lung (e.g., COPD) is much more heterogeneous [88].

Ventilation–Perfusion Matching

Efficient gas exchange hinges on matching of perfusion and ventilation. Both ventilation and perfusion increase progressively from nondependent to dependent areas, but the change in perfusion is more extreme and ranges from zero flow to high flows. As a result, nondependent areas tend to be relatively underperfused ($V/Q \gg 1$), whereas the dependent areas are relatively overperfused ($V/Q \ll 1$). Postcapillary blood from the underventilated, dependent lung zones ($V/Q \ll 1$), therefore, tends to be relatively hypoxemic and slightly hypercapnic. Nondependent lung zones, which are relatively overventilated ($V/Q \gg 1$), are able to compensate by removing excess CO_2, but due to the flat O_2-hemoglobin curve, they are less capable of increasing oxygen uptake. High V/Q areas therefore compensate for carbon dioxide, but not for oxygen, exchange. As a result, the alveolar–arterial (A–a) gradient, in the setting of significant V/Q mismatch, is large for oxygen and relatively small for carbon dioxide [89].

OLV provides a significant challenge to V/Q matching. Once lung isolation has been established, residual oxygen is gradually absorbed from the nonventilated lung until complete absorption atelectasis has occurred. At that point, pulmonary blood flow to the operative lung is entirely wasted perfusion. The resulting right-to-left shunt through the nonventilated lung is in addition to the normal 5% of shunt in the ventilated lung. As blood flow to each lung is roughly equal (right lung 55% of CO, left lung 45% of CO), this mathematically results in a shunt fraction upwards of 50%, at which point even high oxygen administration would be incapable of ensuring normoxemia (Fig. 5.6). Observed shunt fractions are fortunately much lower as illustrated above (Fig. 5.4).

Both passive and active mechanisms decrease the blood flow through the operative lung. Surgical manipulation and, in the lateral position, gravity passively reduce the blood flow to the nonventilated lung. In addition, HPV actively increases vascular resistance in the nonventilated lung, resulting in a gradual decrease in shunt fraction.

V/Q Matching in the Lateral Position

Awake

The distribution of alveoli on the compliance curve is maintained when an awake, spontaneously breathing patient assumes the lateral position. Dependent alveoli remain small and compliant, whereas nondependent alveoli stay large and noncompliant. Because of the position change, however, different areas of the lung are now dependent and nondependent. While caudal regions are small and compliant in the upright position, in the lateral position, it is the dependent (down) lung, which receives most of the ventilation. Additionally, the cephalad displacement of the dependent diaphragm by abdominal contents results in more effective diaphragmatic muscle contraction. The net result is preferential ventilation of the dependent lung in the lateral position relative to the nondependent lung [16, 91].

Perfusion is similarly altered by assuming the lateral decubitus position. The gravity-dependent distribution of flow is maintained, with a roughly 10% shift of CO to the dependent lung. A dependent right lung will therefore receive 65% of CO, compared to the 55% it receives in the upright or supine position. For a dependent left lung, this will result in an increase from the normal 45% of CO toward 55% of CO [92]. When combined, the lateral position favors the dependent lung in ventilation and perfusion, and V/Q matching is maintained similar to the upright position.

Anesthetized

Induction of anesthesia decreases diaphragmatic and inspiratory muscle tone, which results in a 15–20% drop in FRC in both lungs [93]. The change in lung volume alters the relative position of each lung on the compliance curve. The dependent lung drops from the steep portion of the volume–pressure curve, to the flat, noncompliant position. The nondependent lung on the other hand drops from the shallow position of the curve into the steeper portion previously occupied by the dependent lung. As a result, the nondependent lung is now more compliant than the dependent lung and becomes preferentially ventilated [91, 94, 95]. The distribution of perfusion, on the other hand, is not affected by the induction of anesthesia. The reduction in

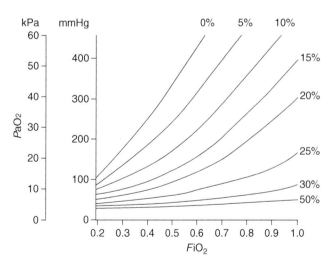

Fig. 5.6 Isoshunt diagram. Theoretical relationship between arterial oxygen (PaO2) and inspired oxygen concentration (FiO2) for different values of shunt at stable levels of hemoglobin, arterial carbon dioxide, and Alveolar–arterial gradient. (Modified from Benatar with permission [90])

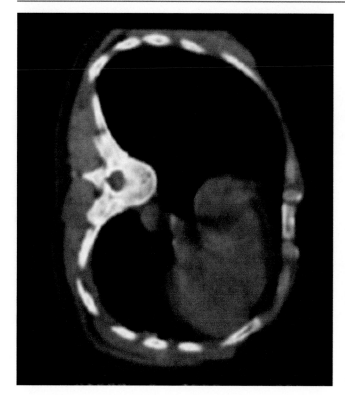

Fig. 5.7 Computed tomography image of a patient in the lateral decubitus position during mechanical two-lung ventilation and paralysis, demonstrating gravity-dependent mediastinal shift (**a**). Ventilation/perfusion diagrams in the same patient scenario indicating uncoupling of ventilation and perfusion (**b**). (Modified from Klingstedt with permission [97])

ventilation of the dependent lung disrupts V/Q matching beyond what was seen for the anesthetized, spontaneously breathing patient [91].

Paralyzed/Ventilated

Muscle relaxation, which entirely removes diaphragmatic and inspiratory muscle tone, further alters the distribution of ventilation. Diaphragmatic contraction played a more dominant role due to the favorable, higher resting position in the lateral decubitus position. Once paralyzed, static displacement of the relaxed diaphragm by abdominal contents and the gravitational force of the mediastinum further compromise the compliance of the lower lung and result in a 35% decrease in lower lung FRC [96] (Fig. 5.7). Coupled with the institution of positive-pressure ventilation, this further favors nondependent lung ventilation. Pulmonary perfusion is unaffected by muscle relaxation. However, the increase of P_A due to the institution of positive-pressure ventilation will increase Zone 1 ($P_A > P_{pa}$) and Zone 2 territory ($P_A > P_{pv}$). Consequently, ventilation and perfusion have become uncoupled with the nondependent lung receiving the bulk of ventilation (but little perfusion) and the dependent lung receiving the majority of perfusion (but little ventilation) [16, 91].

Open Chest

Establishment of the surgical pneumothorax with its loss of negative intrapleural pressure releases the mediastinal weight onto the dependent lung, further compromising its compliance. The nondependent lung on the other hand is now free to move independent of chest-wall constraints, solely based on parenchymal compliance. Consequently, the lung will collapse, if lung isolation has been applied, or will be able to herniate through the thoracotomy incision if still ventilated. The distribution of pulmonary blood flow will not be affected by opening the chest unless there is distortion of the mediastinal structures. V/Q matching will depend on whether lung isolation is being employed. During TLV, opening of the chest will result in a deterioration of V/Q matching, due to increase in Zone 1 ventilation with nondependent lung herniation through the thoracotomy incision. Application of lung isolation, however, will divert all ventilation to the dependent lung, which already receives most of the perfusion and therefore dramatically improves V/Q matching.

Most thoracic procedures are accomplished in the anesthetized, paralyzed, and mechanically ventilated patient. As we have seen in the preceding sections, induction of anesthesia, lateral decubitus positioning, paralysis, and mechanical ventilation result in progressive disruption of the close V/Q matching that is part of normal physiology. Pulmonary perfusion has remained rather undisturbed, with preferential perfusion of dependent areas. Conversely, ventilation has become progressively diverted to the nondependent lung, as the dependent lung experiences extrinsic compression by mediastinum and abdominal contents. The application of lung isolation forces ventilation back into the dependent lung and reestablishes relative V/Q matching in the dependent lung, at the expense of true shunt in the nondependent lung [16, 91].

Positions Other Than Lateral

Supine

Although not routine for thoracic surgery, a certain number of OLV cases are being performed in the supine position (e.g., chest-wall resections, sympathectomy, minimally invasive cardiac procedures). Lung compliance changes occur with induction of anesthesia, paralysis, and mechanical ventilation, as previously described, however, unlike the lateral decubitus position, now affect both lungs equally. Abdominal, and to some degree mediastinal, compression affects each lung. Pulmonary perfusion gradients are maintained in the supine position with preferential perfusion of dependent areas. As gravity affects both lungs equally, the percentage of CO perfusing each lung is unaffected. V/Q matching is disturbed, with dependent areas receiving more perfusion but less ventilation. Because of the minimal vertical distance from anterior to posterior compared to the lateral position, this disruption is relatively minimal in the supine position. However, initiation of OLV in the supine position is less well tolerated than in the lateral position. Because of the lack of gravity redistribution of blood flow, the shunt through the nonventilated lung is substantially larger than in the lateral decubitus position, resulting in worse oxygenation [35].

Prone

OLV in the prone position is rare; however, isolated reports of lung resection and minimally invasive esophagectomy in the prone position have been published [98–100]. In fact, prone positioning for minimally invasive esophagectomy may obviate the need for lung isolation due to the gravity displacement of the lung from the surgical field even during TLV [99]. The effects of prone positioning during TLV have been extensively investigated [101]. In contrast to the supine position, V/Q matching and FRC are better maintained, with secondary marked improvement in P_aO_2 values. Lung compliance is improved, in part due to the lack of compression of lung tissue by mediastinal structures [102]. The prone position lacks gravity redistribution of pulmonary blood flow similar to the supine position. The shunt fraction and oxygenation during OLV should therefore be comparable or better than the supine position but worse than the lateral position.

Alternative Approaches

Capnothorax

Intrathoracic CO_2 insufflation has been used routinely to facilitate thoracoscopic surgery when lung isolation is difficult or impossible to achieve, particularly in the neonatal and pediatric setting [103]. In the adult setting, CO_2 insufflation may be required to improve surgical exposure during OLV, particularly during mediastinal or cardiac procedures [104, 105]. Even reasonably low insufflation pressures of 10 mmHg result in decreases in cardiac index during minimally invasive cardiac procedures [104]. Insufflation pressures above 10 mmHg should likely be avoided as they are associated with increases in HR, CVP, PAP, and peak inspiratory pressures with concomitant decreases in cardiac index, arterial O_2 tension, and mixed venous oxyen saturation [105, 106].

Awake Non-intubated Lung Surgery

Minimally invasive techniques are associated with accelerated postoperative recovery and have enabled lung surgery in progressively older and sicker patients, a trend that is likely to continue. There is renewed interest in non-intubated lung surgery, given that thoracoscopic surgery, which avoids opening of the hemithorax, minimizes the degree of pendelluft and mediastinal shift [107]. The combination of video-assisted thoracoscopic surgery (VATS) in a non-intubated patient (known as NIVATS), which can be performed under regional anesthesia with sedation, has been touted as a further reduction in invasiveness to facilitate surgery in high-risk candidates [108–110]. Current support for this approach beyond minor pleural-based procedures to actual anatomic resections is restricted to a limited number of institutions [2].

Summary

OLV is a well-established anesthetic technique that is routinely used to improve surgical exposure for a myriad of pulmonary and nonpulmonary intrathoracic procedures. Although well tolerated in the majority of patients, lung compliance and oxygenation are significantly impaired and may complicate the care of some patients. A thorough knowledge of pulmonary physiology explains the majority of the intraoperative trespasses that one encounters during OLV and enables appropriate interventions.

References

1. Maloney JV, Schmutzer KJ, Raschke E. Paradoxical respiration and "pendelluft". J Thorac Cardiovasc Surg. 1961;41:291–8.
2. Pompeo E. Awake thoracic surgery – is it worth the trouble? Semin Thorac Cardiovasc Surg. 2012;24(2):106–14.
3. Brodsky JB, Lemmens HJ. The history of anesthesia for thoracic surgery. Minerva Anestesiol. 2007;73(10):513–24.
4. West JB, Dollery CT, Naimark A. Distribution of blood flow in isolated lung; relation to vascular and alveolar pressures. J Appl Physiol. 1964;19(4):713–24.
5. West JB, Dollery CT, Heard BE. Increased pulmonary vascular resistance in the dependent zone of the isolated dog lung caused by perivascular edema. Circ Res. 1965;17:191–206.
6. Petersson J, Rohdin M, Sánchez-Crespo A, Nyrén S, Jacobsson H, Larsson SA, et al. Posture primarily affects lung tissue distribution with minor effect on blood flow and ventilation. Respir Physiol Neurobiol. 2007;156(3):293–303.
7. Siva S, Callahan J, Kron T, Martin OA, MacManus MP, Ball DL, et al. A prospective observational study of gallium-68 ventilation and perfusion PET/CT during and after radiotherapy in patients with non-small cell lung cancer. BMC Cancer. 2014;14:740.
8. Chang H, Lai-Fook SJ, Domino KB, Schimmel C, Hildebrandt J, Robertson HT, et al. Spatial distribution of ventilation and perfusion in anesthetized dogs in lateral postures. J Appl Physiol. 2002;92(2):745–62.
9. Groves BM, Reeves JT, Sutton JR, Wagner PD, Cymerman A, Malconian MK, et al. Operation everest II: elevated high-altitude pulmonary resistance unresponsive to oxygen. J Appl Physiol (1985). 1987;63(2):521–30.
10. Maseri A, Caldini P, Harward P, Joshi RC, Permutt S, Zierler KL. Determinants of pulmonary vascular volume: recruitment versus distensibility. Circ Res. 1972;31(2):218–28.
11. Dull RO, Cluff M, Kingston J, Hill D, Chen H, Hoehne S, et al. Lung heparan sulfates modulate K(fc) during increased vascular pressure: evidence for glycocalyx-mediated mechanotransduction. Am J Physiol Lung Cell Mol Physiol. 2012;302(9):L816–28.
12. Weir EK, López-Barneo J, Buckler KJ, Archer SL. Acute oxygen-sensing mechanisms. N Engl J Med. 2005;353(19):2042–55.
13. Lumb AB, Slinger P. Hypoxic pulmonary vasoconstriction: physiology and anesthetic implications. Anesthesiology. 2015;122(4):932–46.
14. Balanos GM, Talbot NP, Dorrington KL, Robbins PA. Human pulmonary vascular response to 4 h of hypercapnia and hypocapnia measured using doppler echocardiography. J Appl Physiol (1985). 2003;94(4):1543–51.
15. Nagendran J, Stewart K, Hoskinson M, Archer SL. An anesthesiologist's guide to hypoxic pulmonary vasoconstriction: implications for managing single-lung anesthesia and atelectasis. Curr Opin Anaesthesiol. 2006;19(1):34–43.
16. Grichnik KP, Clark JA. Pathophysiology and management of one-lung ventilation. Thorac Surg Clin. 2005;15(1):85–103.
17. Talbot NP, Balanos GM, Dorrington KL, Robbins PA. Two temporal components within the human pulmonary vascular response to approximately 2 h of isocapnic hypoxia. J Appl Physiol (1985). 2005;98(3):1125–39.
18. Dorrington KL, Clar C, Young JD, Jonas M, Tansley JG, Robbins PA. Time course of the human pulmonary vascular response to 8 hours of isocapnic hypoxia. Am J Phys. 1997;273(3 Pt 2):H1126–34.
19. Conacher ID. 2000—time to apply Occam's razor to failure of hypoxic pulmonary vasoconstriction during one lung ventilation. Br J Anaesth. 2000;84(4):434–6.
20. Heerdt PM, Stowe DF. Single-lung ventilation and oxidative stress: a different perspective on a common practice. Curr Opin Anaesthesiol. 2017;30(1):42–9.
21. Sylvester JT, Shimoda LA, Aaronson PI, Ward JPT. Hypoxic pulmonary vasoconstriction. Physiol Rev. 2012;92(1):367–520.
22. Peinado VI, Santos S, Ramírez J, Roca J, Rodriguez-Roisin R, Barberà JA. Response to hypoxia of pulmonary arteries in chronic obstructive pulmonary disease: an in vitro study. Eur Respir J. 2002;20(2):332–8.
23. Nakos G, Evrenoglou D, Vassilakis N, Lampropoulos S. Haemodynamics and gas exchange in liver cirrhosis: the effect of orally administered almitrine bismesylate. Respir Med. 1993;87(2):93–8.
24. Reeves JT, Grover RF. Blockade of acute hypoxic pulmonary hypertension by endotoxin. J Appl Physiol. 1974;36(3):328–32.
25. Moore LG, Reeves JT. Pregnancy blunts pulmonary vascular reactivity in dogs. Am J Phys. 1980;239(3):H297–301.
26. Wetzel RC, Zacur HA, Sylvester JT. Effect of puberty and estradiol on hypoxic vasomotor response in isolated sheep lungs. J Appl Physiol Respir Environ Exerc Physiol. 1984;56(5):1199–203.
27. Favret F, Henderson KK, Allen J, Richalet JP, Gonzalez NC. Exercise training improves lung gas exchange and attenuates acute hypoxic pulmonary hypertension but does not prevent pulmonary hypertension of prolonged hypoxia. J Appl Physiol (1985). 2006;100(1):20–5.
28. Guazzi MD, Berti M, Doria E, Fiorentini C, Galli C, Pepi M, Tamborini G. Enhancement of the pulmonary vasoconstriction reaction to alveolar hypoxia in systemic high blood pressure. Clin Sci (Lond). 1991;80(4):403.
29. Doekel RC, Weir EK, Looga R, Grover RF, Reeves JT. Potentiation of hypoxic pulmonary vasoconstriction by ethyl alcohol in dogs. J Appl Physiol Respir Environ Exerc Physiol. 1978;44(1):76–80.
30. Brimioulle S, Lejeune P, Vachiery JL, Leeman M, Melot C, Naeije R. Effects of acidosis and alkalosis on hypoxic pulmonary vasoconstriction in dogs. Am J Phys. 1990;258(2 Pt 2):H347–53.
31. Benumof JL, Wahrenbrock EA. Dependency of hypoxic pulmonary vasoconstriction on temperature. J Appl Physiol Respir Environ Exerc Physiol. 1977;42(1):56–8.
32. Benumof JL, Wahrenbrock EA. Blunted hypoxic pulmonary vasoconstriction by increased lung vascular pressures. J Appl Physiol. 1975;38(5):846–50.
33. Marshall C, Marshall B. Site and sensitivity for stimulation of hypoxic pulmonary vasoconstriction. J Appl Physiol Respir Environ Exerc Physiol. 1983;55(3):711–6.
34. Choi YS, Bang SO, Shim JK, Chung KY, Kwak YL, Hong YW. Effects of head-down tilt on intrapulmonary shunt fraction and oxygenation during one-lung ventilation in the lateral decubitus position. J Thorac Cardiovasc Surg. 2007;134(3):613–8.
35. Bardoczky GI, Szegedi LL, dHollander AA, Moures JM, de Francquen P, Yernault JC. Two-lung and one-lung ventilation in patients with chronic obstructive pulmonary disease: the effects of position and fio2. Anesth Analg. 2000;90(1):35.
36. Ishikawa S, Nakazawa K, Makita K. Progressive changes in arterial oxygenation during one-lung anaesthesia are related to the response to compression of the non-dependent lung. Br J Anaesth. 2003;90(1):21–6.
37. Szegedi LL, Van der Linden P, Ducart A, Cosaert P, Poelaert J, Vermassen F, et al. The effects of acute isovolemic hemodilution on oxygenation during one-lung ventilation. Anesth Analg. 2005;100(1):15–20.
38. Von Dossow V, Welte M, Zaune U, Martin E, Walter M, Rückert J, et al. Thoracic epidural anesthesia combined with general anesthesia: the preferred anesthetic technique for thoracic surgery. Anesth Analg. 2001;92(4):848–54.
39. Casati A, Mascotto G, Iemi K, Nzepa-Batonga J, De Luca M. Epidural block does not worsen oxygenation during one-lung ventilation for lung resections under isoflurane/nitrous oxide anesthesia. Eur J Anaesthesiol. 2005;22(5):363–8.

40. Ozcan PE, Sentürk M, Sungur Ulke Z, Toker A, Dilege S, Ozden E, Camci E. Effects of thoracic epidural anaesthesia on pulmonary venous admixture and oxygenation during one-lung ventilation. Acta Anaesthesiol Scand. 2007;51(8):1117–22.

41. Moutafis M, Liu N, Dalibon N, Kuhlman G, Ducros L, Castelain MH, Fischler M. The effects of inhaled nitric oxide and its combination with intravenous almitrine on pao2 during one-lung ventilation in patients undergoing thoracoscopic procedures. Anesth Analg. 1997;85(5):1130–5.

42. Bindslev L, Cannon D, Sykes MK. Effect of lignocaine and nitrous oxide on hypoxic pulmonary vasoconstriction in the dog constant-flow perfused left lower lobe preparation. Br J Anaesth. 1986;58(3):315–20.

43. Kjaeve J, Bjertnaes LJ. Interaction of verapamil and halogenated inhalation anesthetics on hypoxic pulmonary vasoconstriction. Acta Anaesthesiol Scand. 1989;33(3):193–8.

44. Carlsson AJ, Hedenstierna G, Bindslev L. Hypoxia-induced vasoconstriction in human lung exposed to enflurane anaesthesia. Acta Anaesthesiol Scand. 1987;31(1):57–62.

45. Carlsson AJ, Bindslev L, Hedenstierna G. Hypoxia-induced pulmonary vasoconstriction in the human lung. The effect of isoflurane anesthesia. Anesthesiology. 1987;66(3):312–6.

46. Kerbaul F, Guidon C, Stephanazzi J, Bellezza M, Le Dantec P, Longeon T, Aubert M. Sub-MAC concentrations of desflurane do not inhibit hypoxic pulmonary vasoconstriction in anesthetized piglets. Can J Anesth. 2001;48(8):760–7.

47. Pruszkowski O, Dalibon N, Moutafis M, Jugan E, Law-Koune JD, Laloë PA, Fischler M. Effects of propofol vs sevoflurane on arterial oxygenation during one-lung ventilation. Br J Anaesth. 2007;98(4):539–44.

48. Nakayama M, Murray PA. Ketamine preserves and propofol potentiates hypoxic pulmonary vasoconstriction compared with the conscious state in chronically instrumented dogs. Anesthesiology. 1999;91(3):760–71.

49. Xia R, Xu J, Yin H, Wu H, Xia Z, Zhou D, et al. Intravenous infusion of dexmedetomidine combined isoflurane inhalation reduces oxidative stress and potentiates hypoxia pulmonary vasoconstriction during one-lung ventilation in patients. Mediat Inflamm. 2015;2015:238041.

50. Bjertnaes L, Hauge A, Kriz M. Hypoxia-induced pulmonary vasoconstriction: effects of fentanyl following different routes of administration. Acta Anaesthesiol Scand. 1980;24(1):53–7.

51. Clozel JP, Delorme N, Battistella P, Breda JL, Polu JM. Hemodynamic effects of intravenous diltiazem in hypoxic pulmonary hypertension. Chest. 1987;91(2):171–5.

52. Thilenius OG, Candiolo BM, Beug JL. Effect of adrenergic blockade on hypoxia-induced pulmonary vasoconstriction in awake dogs. Am J Phys. 1967;213(4):990–8.

53. Hackett PH, Roach RC, Hartig GS, Greene ER, Levine BD. The effect of vasodilators on pulmonary hemodynamics in high altitude pulmonary edema: a comparison. Int J Sports Med. 1992;13(S 1):S68–71.

54. Lübbe N, Bornscheuer A, Kirchner E. The effect of clonidine on the intrapulmonary right-to-left shunt in one-lung ventilation in the dog. Anaesthesist. 1991;40(7):391–6.

55. Hales CA, Westphal D. Hypoxemia following the administration of sublingual nitroglycerin. Am J Med. 1978;65(6):911–8.

56. Parsons GH, Leventhal JP, Hansen MM, Goldstein JD. Effect of sodium nitroprusside on hypoxic pulmonary vasoconstriction in the dog. J Appl Physiol. 1981;51(2):288–92.

57. Zhao L, Mason NA, Morrell NW, Kojonazarov B, Sadykov A, Maripov A, et al. Sildenafil inhibits hypoxia-induced pulmonary hypertension. Circulation. 2001;104(4):424–8.

58. Marin JL, Orchard C, Chakrabarti MK, Sykes MK. Depression of hypoxic pulmonary vasoconstriction in the dog by dopamine and isoprenaline. Br J Anaesth. 1979;51(4):303–12.

59. Silove ED, Grover RF. Effects of alpha adrenergic blockade and tissue catecholamine depletion on pulmonary vascular response to hypoxia. J Clin Invest. 1968;47(2):274–85.

60. Doering EB, Hanson CW, Reily DJ, Marshall C, Marshall BE. Improvement in oxygenation by phenylephrine and nitric oxide in patients with adult respiratory distress syndrome. Anesthesiology. 1997;87(1):18–25.

61. Hüter L, Schwarzkopf K, Preussler NP, Gaser E, Bauer R, Schubert H, Schreiber T. Effects of arginine vasopressin on oxygenation and haemodynamics during one-lung ventilation in an animal model. Anaesth Intensive Care. 2008;36(2):162–6.

62. Kiely DG, Cargill RI, Lipworth BJ. Acute hypoxic pulmonary vasoconstriction in man is attenuated by type I angiotensin II receptor blockade. Cardiovasc Res. 1995;30(6):875–80.

63. Cargill RI, Lipworth BJ. Lisinopril attenuates acute hypoxic pulmonary vasoconstriction in humans. Chest. 1996;109(2):424–9.

64. Leeman M, Lejeune P, Mélot C, Deloof T, Naeije R. Pulmonary artery pressure: flow relationships in hyperoxic and in hypoxic dogs. Effects of methylprednisolone. Acta Anaesthesiol Scand. 1988;32(2):147–51.

65. Lorente JA, Landin L, de Pablo R, Renes E. The effects of prostacyclin on oxygen transport in adult respiratory distress syndrome. Medicina Clinica. 1992;98(17):641–5.

66. Weir EK, Reeves JT, Grover RF. Prostaglandin E1 inhibits the pulmonary vascular pressor response to hypoxia and prostaglandin f2alpha. Prostaglandins. 1975;10(4):623–31.

67. Pillet O, Manier G, Castaing Y. Anticholinergic versus beta 2-agonist on gas exchange in COPD: A comparative study in 15 patients. Monaldi Arch Chest Dis. 1998;53(1):3–8.

68. Smith TG, Balanos GM, Croft QP, Talbot NP, Dorrington KL, Ratcliffe PJ, Robbins PA. The increase in pulmonary arterial pressure caused by hypoxia depends on iron status. J Physiol. 2008;586(24):5999–6005.

69. Smith TG, Talbot NP, Dorrington KL, Robbins PA. Intravenous iron and pulmonary hypertension in intensive care. Intensive Care Med. 2011;37:1720.

70. Lohser J. Evidence-based management of one-lung ventilation. Anesthesiol Clin. 2008;26(2):241–72, v.

71. Gurney AM, Osipenko ON, MacMillan D, McFarlane KM, Tate RJ, Kempsill FE. Two-pore domain K channel, TASK-1, in pulmonary artery smooth muscle cells. Circ Res. 2003;93(10):957–64.

72. Garutti I, Quintana B, Olmedilla L, Cruz A, Barranco M, Garcia de Lucas E. Arterial oxygenation during one-lung ventilation: combined versus general anesthesia. Anesth Analg. 1999;88(3):494–9.

73. Bermejo S, Gallart L, Silva-Costa-Gomes T, Vallès J, Aguiló R, Puig MM. Almitrine fails to improve oxygenation during one-lung ventilation with sevoflurane anesthesia. YJCAN. 2014;28(4):919–24.

74. Rocca GD, Passariello M, Coccia C, Costa MG, di Marco P, Venuta F, et al. Inhaled nitric oxide administration during one-lung ventilation in patients undergoing thoracic surgery. J Cardiothorac Vasc Anesth. 2001;15(2):218–23.

75. Germann P, Braschi A, Della Rocca G, Dinh-Xuan AT, Falke K, Frostell C, et al. Inhaled nitric oxide therapy in adults: European expert recommendations. Intensive Care Med. 2005;31(8):1029–41.

76. Schloss B, Martin D, Beebe A, Klamar J, Tobias JD. Phenylephrine to treat hypoxemia during one-lung ventilation in a pediatric patient. Thorac Cardiovasc Surg Rep. 2013;2(1):16–8.

77. Talbot NP, Croft QP, Curtis MK, Turner BE, Dorrington KL, Robbins PA, Smith TG. Contrasting effects of ascorbate and iron on the pulmonary vascular response to hypoxia in humans. Physiol Rep. 2014;2(12):e12220.

78. Szegedi LL. Pathophysiology of one-lung ventilation. Anesthesiol Clin North Am. 2001;19(3):435–53.

79. Slinger P, Scott WA. Arterial oxygenation during one-lung ventilation. A comparison of enflurane and isoflurane. Anesthesiology. 1995;82(4):940–6.

80. Nomoto Y, Kawamura M. Pulmonary gas exchange effects by nitroglycerin, dopamine and dobutamine during one-lung ventilation in man. Can J Anaesth. 1989;36(3 Pt 1):273–7.

81. Mathru M, Dries DJ, Kanuri D, Blakeman B, Rao T. Effect of cardiac output on gas exchange in one-lung atelectasis. Chest. 1990;97(5):1121–4.

82. Russell WJ, James MF. The effects on arterial haemoglobin oxygen saturation and on shunt of increasing cardiac output with dopamine or dobutamine during one-lung ventilation. Anaesth Intensive Care. 2004;32(5):644–8.

83. Russell W, James M. The effects on increasing cardiac output with adrenaline or isoprenaline on arterial haemoglobin oxygen saturation and shunt during one-lung ventilation. Anaesth Intensive Care. 2004;32:644–8.

84. Malmkvist G, Fletcher R, Nordström L, Werner O. Effects of lung surgery and one-lung ventilation on pulmonary arterial pressure, venous admixture and immediate postoperative lung function. Br J Anaesth. 1989;63(6):696–701.

85. McFarlane PA, Mortimer AJ, Ryder WA, Madgwick RG, Gardaz JP, Harrison BJ, Sykes MK. Effects of dopamine and dobutamine on the distribution of pulmonary blood flow during lobar ventilation hypoxia and lobar collapse in dogs. Eur J Clin Investig. 1985;15(2):53–9.

86. Hoppin FG, Green ID, Mead J. Distribution of pleural surface pressure in dogs. J Appl Physiol. 1969;27(6):863–73.

87. Milic-Emili J, Henderson JAM, Dolovich MB, Trop D, Kaneko K. Regional distribution of inspired gas in the lung. J Appl Physiol. 1966;21(3):749–59.

88. Hamedani H, Clapp JT, Kadlecek SJ, Emami K, Ishii M, Gefter WB, et al. Regional fractional ventilation by using multibreath wash-in (3)he MR imaging. Radiology. 2016;279(3):917–24.

89. West JB. Regional differences in gas exchange in the lung of erect man. J Appl Physiol (1985). 1962;17(6):893.

90. Benatar SR, Hewlett AM, Nunn JF. The use of iso-shunt lines for control of oxygen therapy. Br J Anaesth. 1973;45(7):711–8.

91. Benumof JL. Anesthesia for thoracic surgery. London: WB Saunders; 2005. p. 2005r.

92. Wulff KE, Aulin I. The regional lung function in the lateral decubitus position during anesthesia and operation. Acta Anaesthesiol Scand. 1972;16(4):195–205.

93. Wahba RW. Perioperative functional residual capacity. Can J Anaesth. 1991;38(3):384–400.

94. Rehder K, Hatch DJ, Sessler AD, Fowler WS. The function of each lung of anesthetized and paralyzed man during mechanical ventilation. Anesthesiology. 1972;37(1):16.

95. Rehder K, Wenthe FM, Sessler AD. Function of each lung during mechanical ventilation with ZEEP and with PEEP in man anesthetized with thiopental-meperidine. Anesthesiology. 1973;39(6):597–606.

96. Chang H, Lai-Fook SJ, Domino KB, Hildebrandt J, Robertson HT, Glenny RW, et al. Ventilation and perfusion distribution during altered PEEP in the left lung in the left lateral decubitus posture with unchanged tidal volume in dogs. Chin J Physiol. 2006;49(2):74–82.

97. Klingstedt C, Hedenstierna G, Baehrendtz S, Lundqvist H, Strandberg A, Tokics L, Brismar B. Ventilation-perfusion relationships and atelectasis formation in the supine and lateral positions during conventional mechanical and differential ventilation. Acta Anaesthesiol Scand. 1990;34(6):421–9.

98. Conlan AA, Moyes DG, Schutz J, Scoccianti M, Abramor E, Levy H. Pulmonary resection in the prone position for suppurative lung disease in children. J Thorac Cardiovasc Surg. 1986;92(5):890–3.

99. Fabian T, Martin J, Katigbak M, McKelvey AA, Federico JA. Thoracoscopic esophageal mobilization during minimally invasive esophagectomy: a head-to-head comparison of prone versus decubitus positions. Surg Endosc. 2008;22(11):2485–91.

100. Turner MWH, Buchanan CCR, Brown SW. Paediatric one lung ventilation in the prone position. Pediatr Anesth. 1997;7(5):427–9.

101. Albert RK. Prone ventilation. Clin Chest Med. 2000;21(3):511–7.

102. Pelosi P, Croci M, Calappi E, Cerisara M, Mulazzi D, Vicardi P, Gattinoni L. The prone positioning during general anesthesia minimally affects respiratory mechanics while improving functional residual capacity and increasing oxygen tension. Anesth Analg. 1995;80(5):955–60.

103. Hammer GB, Fitzmaurice BG, Brodsky JB. Methods for single-lung ventilation in pediatric patients. Anesth Analg. 1999;89(6):1426–9.

104. Brock H, Rieger R, Gabriel C, Pölz W, Moosbauer W, Necek S. Haemodynamic changes during thoracoscopic surgery the effects of one-lung ventilation compared with carbon dioxide insufflation. Anaesthesia. 2000;55(1):10–6.

105. Deshpande SP, Lehr E, Odonkor P, Bonatti JO, Kalangie M, Zimrin DA, Grigore AM. Anesthetic management of robotically assisted totally endoscopic coronary artery bypass surgery (TECAB). J Cardiothorac Vasc Anesth. 2013;27(3):586–99.

106. Reinius H, Borges JB, Fredén F, Jideus L, Camargo ED, Amato MB, et al. Real-time ventilation and perfusion distributions by electrical impedance tomography during one-lung ventilation with capnothorax. Acta Anaesthesiol Scand. 2015;59(3):354–68.

107. Tacconi F, Pompeo E, Forcella D, Marino M, Varvaras D, Mineo TC. Lung volume reduction reoperations. Ann Thorac Surg. 2008;85(4):1171–7.

108. Gonzalez-Rivas D, Bonome C, Fieira E, Aymerich H, Fernandez R, Delgado M, et al. Non-intubated video-assisted thoracoscopic lung resections: the future of thoracic surgery? Eur J Cardio-thorac Surg Off J Eur Assoc Cardio-thorac Surg. 2016;49(3):721–31.

109. Pompeo E, Sorge R, Akopov A, Congregado M, Grodzki T, Group EN-ITSW. Non-intubated thoracic surgery-a survey from the European society of thoracic surgeons. Ann Transl Med. 2015;3(3):37.

110. Gonzalez-Rivas D, Fernandez R, de la Torre M, Bonome C. Uniportal video-assisted thoracoscopic left upper lobectomy under spontaneous ventilation. J Thorac Dis. 2015;7(3):494–5.

Clinical Management of One-Lung Ventilation

6

Travis Schisler and Jens Lohser

Key Points
- OLV needs to be individualized for the underlying lung pathology, BMI, and ventilatory mechanical characteristics.
- OLV is a modifiable risk factor for acute lung injury.
- Protective OLV is a combination of small tidal volumes, low peak and plateau pressures, routine PEEP (adequate PEEP to facilitate open lung ventilation), and permissive hypercapnia.
- Hypoxemia during one-lung ventilation is rare and often secondary to alveolar de-recruitment in the face of hypoventilation.
- Management of hypoxemia requires a structured treatment algorithm.

Introduction

The development of thoracic surgery as a subspecialty only occurred after lung isolation and OLV had been reported. Prior to the description of endotracheal intubation and the cuffed endotracheal tube, only short intrathoracic procedures had been feasible [1]. Rapid lung movement and quickly developing respiratory distress due to the surgical pneumothorax made all but minimal procedures impossible. Selective ventilation of one lung was first described in 1931 by Gale and Waters and quickly led to increasingly complex lung resection surgery, with the first published pneumonectomy for cancer in 1933 [1]. Much has since been learned about the physiology of OLV, particularly the issue of ventilation/perfusion matching (see Chap. 5). Hypoxemia used to be the primary concern during OLV. However, hypoxemia has become less frequent due to more effective lung isolation techniques with routine use of fiber-optic bronchoscopy and the use of anesthetic agents with little or no detrimental effects on hypoxic pulmonary vasoconstriction (HPV). Acute lung injury (ALI) has replaced hypoxemia as the chief concern associated with OLV [2]. Data has emerged in the past 10 years from both critical care and the operating room that has better elucidated the causative biomechanical and ventilatory factors involved in ventilator-induced lung injury (VILI). Translation of this data has yielded significant progress in harm reduction strategies in the routine application of mechanical ventilation.

Acute Lung Injury

Lung injury after lung resection was first recognized in the form of post-pneumonectomy pulmonary edema [3], which is now referred to as post-thoracotomy ALI [4]. Pneumonectomy carries a particularly high risk of lung injury, but lesser lung resections and even non-pulmonary intrathoracic procedures, which employ OLV, can create the same pathology [5]. Post-thoracotomy ALI is part of a spectrum of disease, which in its most severe form is recognized as acute respiratory distress syndrome (ARDS). Diagnosis is based on the oxygenation index of PaO_2/FiO_2 (P/F). Critical care consensus guidelines define ALI as a P/F ratio < 300 and ARDS as a P/F ratio < 200 [6]. The criteria have recently been made more stringent by requiring that a minimum of 5 cmH$_2$O of PEEP or CPAP be applied at the time of the P/F ratio determination [7]. ALI after lung resection is fortunately infrequent, occurring in 2.5–3.1% of all lung resections combined; however, the incidence can be as high as 7.9–10.1% after pneumonectomies. Although infrequent, ALI after lung resection may be associated with significant morbidity (prolonged intubation and hospitalization)

T. Schisler · J. Lohser (✉)
Department of Anesthesiology, Pharmacology, and Therapeutics, University of British Columbia, Vancouver General Hospital, Vancouver, BC, Canada
e-mail: jens.lohser@vch.ca

© Springer Nature Switzerland AG 2019
P. Slinger (ed.), *Principles and Practice of Anesthesia for Thoracic Surgery*, https://doi.org/10.1007/978-3-030-00859-8_6

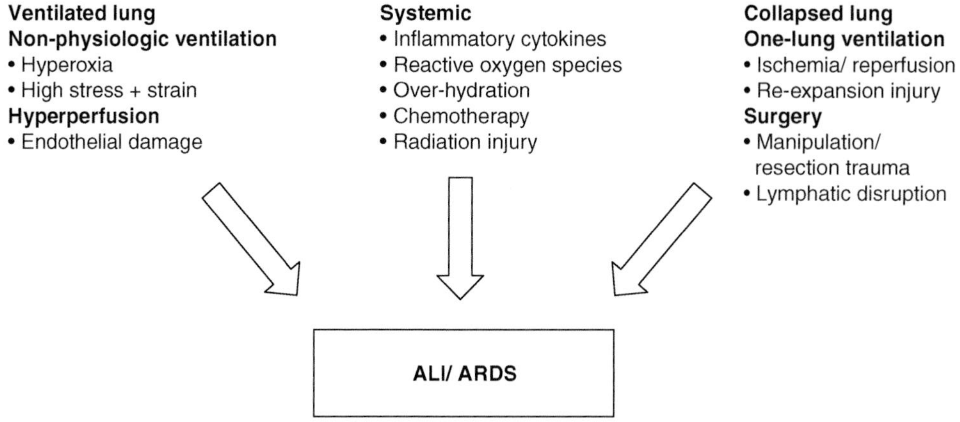

Fig. 6.1 Proposed mechanisms for ALI and ARDS after lung resection surgery

| **Ventilated lung** **Non-physiologic ventilation** • Hyperoxia • High stress + strain **Hyperperfusion** • Endothelial damage | **Systemic** • Inflammatory cytokines • Reactive oxygen species • Over-hydration • Chemotherapy • Radiation injury | **Collapsed lung** **One-lung ventilation** • Ischemia/ reperfusion • Re-expansion injury **Surgery** • Manipulation/ resection trauma • Lymphatic disruption |

ALI/ ARDS

and mortality [5]. Mortality, which was reported to be as high as 37–64% among patients with ALI [8–10], appears to be on the decline, as more recent reports indicated a mortality rate of 25–40% [11]. Similarly, Tang et al. reported a decrease in both the ARDS incidence of (3.2–1.6%) and mortality (72–45%) after pulmonary resection in a single institution cohort over a 10-year period. Their data have to be interpreted with caution, however, as the number of pneumonectomies was drastically higher in the historical cohort (17.4 versus 6.4%), which may explain the higher morbidity and mortality [12].

The etiology of lung injury is complex and likely multifactorial (Fig. 6.1). Historically, risk factors were felt to be right-sided surgery and large perioperative fluid loads. However, impaired lymphatic drainage, surgical technique, mechanical ventilation, transfusion, aspiration, infection, oxidative stress, and ischemia-reperfusion have all since been implicated (Table 6.1) [13]. The fact that ventilation may have detrimental effects in the critically ill patients in the form of ventilator-induced lung injury has long been recognized. Early animal studies demonstrated that high tidal volumes (45 mL/kg) are particularly injurious to the lung, irrespective of the applied pressure. This has led to the term "volutrauma" and the realization that end-inspiratory stretch plays a dominant role in lung injury [14]. In ARDS patients, application of protective lung ventilation (PLV) with smaller tidal volumes and high positive end-expiratory pressure (PEEP) improved survival [15]. Additionally, protective ventilation was shown to inhibit progression of lung injury compared to high tidal volume ventilation [14] and to inhibit the development of lung injury in ICU patients [16–19]. It is now generally accepted that mechanical ventilation by itself may induce lung injury even in the patient with healthy lungs [20]. In patients undergoing either non-thoracic or thoracic surgery, mechanical ventilation with high tidal volumes and low PEEP is associated with lung injury, increased postoperative morbidity (including prolonged hospital and critical care length of stay), and most importantly increased mortality [21]. The first large-scale multi-

Table 6.1 Risk factors for ALI after OLV

Patient
Poor postoperative predicted lung function
Preexisting lung injury
Trauma
Infection
Chemotherapy
EtOH abuse
Female gender
Procedure
Prolonged OLV (>100 min)
Lung transplantation
Larger resections (pneumonectomy > lobectomy)
Esophagectomy
Transfusion
Large perioperative fluid load

center randomized controlled trial to investigate this principle occurred in 2013 in high-risk patients undergoing major abdominal surgery. Patients were randomized to a protective two-lung ventilation (TLV) strategy characterized by tidal volumes of 6–8 mL/kg, PEEP 6 to 8 cmH$_2$O, and frequent recruitment maneuvers or to a conventional strategy with tidal volumes of 10 mL/kg, no PEEP, and no recruitment maneuvers. Postoperative pulmonary complications occurred in 27% of the conventional ventilation group and in only 10% of the protective ventilation group [22]. Several studies have substantiated this report, and meta-analyses support the use of low tidal volumes (< 8 mL/kg during TLV) and some PEEP (greater than 3 cmH$_2$O) [23, 24]. It should be pointed out that low tidal volumes without adequate PEEP are harmful as evidenced by a greater incidence of hypoxemia, postoperative complications, and mortality [25]. Sufficient PEEP in addition to low tidal volumes is equally important in thoracic surgery and supported by an ever-increasing body of literature. In patients undergoing lobectomy, protective ventilation led to fewer postoperative pulmonary complications [26]. A retrospective analysis of over a thousand patients undergoing one-lung ventilation found that low tidal volume ventilation was protective but only when accompanied with adequate PEEP [27]. During minimally invasive three-hole esophagectomy, a protective strategy reduced postoperative pulmonary complications [28]. Tidal volume reduction to 4–6 mL/kg for all patients undergoing one-lung ventilation with PEEP titrated to at least 5–10 cmH$_2$O should now be considered routine practice [29].

OLV predisposes the patient to ALI. Radiologic density changes in patients with ALI after thoracic surgery are more pronounced in the nonoperative, ventilated lung [30]. An increased duration of OLV was found to be an independent predictor of ALI in a retrospective analysis [8]. In animal models, OLV causes histological changes compatible with lung injury, including vascular congestion, diffuse alveolar wall thickening and damage, as well as a decrease in nitric oxide in the ventilated lung [31, 32]. Re-expansion of lung tissue after short-term OLV incites pro-inflammatory cytokine release in animals [33]. Similar cytokine elevations are found in patients undergoing thoracic surgery [34, 35]. Much of the early attention focused on the use of high tidal volumes during OLV. The analogy to ARDS has been drawn, as both involve ventilation of a so-called "baby lung" with reduced lung capacities [36]. Analogous to ARDS, high tidal volumes were therefore hypothesized to cause excessive end-inspiratory stretch during OLV.

Beyond ventilatory management, even anesthetic agents themselves appear to have the potential to modify the inflammatory response to OLV and surgery. De Conno et al. allocated adult patients undergoing lung resection surgery to propofol or sevoflurane anesthesia and found that the increase in inflammatory mediators during OLV was significantly less pronounced in the sevoflurane group. Composite adverse events were significantly higher in the propofol group, but the groups differed in OLV duration and the need for surgical re-exploration [37]. The possible benefit of inhalational anesthesia is not without merit, as volatile anesthetics have been shown to confer attenuating effects in a model of alveolar epithelial injury [38]. Inhalational anesthesia has been shown to minimize ischemia-reperfusion injury [39] and secondary glycocalyx breakdown [40, 41]. Significantly elevated levels of pro-inflammatory cytokine levels have been demonstrated in the alveolus of patients undergoing thoracic surgery under propofol anesthesia, when compared to patients done using inhalational anesthesia with sevoflurane or desflurane [42, 43], although no difference was demonstrated in circulating cytokine levels [43]. These studies indicate that anesthetic agents themselves may influence the pro-inflammatory response to OLV, but the true clinical relevance of that decrease remains to be established. This however illustrates the fact that the true answer to lung injury avoidance is more complex than simple tidal volume reduction.

Individual Ventilator Settings

Tidal Volume

Tidal volumes used during TLV (10–12 mL/kg) used to be maintained into the period of OLV [44, 45]. Large tidal volumes were recommended because they had been found to improve oxygenation and decrease shunt fraction, during both TLV [46] and OLV, irrespective of the level of PEEP applied [47]. Large tidal volumes were shown to provide end-inspiratory alveolar recruitment (Fig. 6.2), resulting in improved oxygenation in the setting of zero end-expiratory pressure (ZEEP). Excessive tidal volumes (e.g., 15 mL/kg), on the other hand, were shown to worsen oxygenation, secondary to elevations in pulmonary vascular resistance (PVR) resulting in increased shunt flow [48]. However, computed tomography images demonstrate gross overexpansion of the dependent lung during OLV in pigs when using tidal volumes of 10 ml/kg as compared to 5 ml/kg (Fig. 6.2). Based on the recent literature on patients with both healthy and injured lungs, it is clear that large tidal volumes during OLV expose the patient to undue risk of postoperative respiratory complications.

Two retrospective case series by Van de Werff and Licker identified multiple risk factors among more than 1000 patients undergoing lung resection surgery. Both studies demonstrated a significant association between high ventilating pressures and ALI but failed to provide a link to intraoperative tidal volumes [8, 50]. Fernández-Pérez et al., on the other hand, showed a significant association between larger intraoperative tidal volumes (8.3 vs. 6.7 mL/kg) and the development of postoperative respiratory failure in a single institution review of 170 pneumonectomies [51]. The study was criticized for the fact that ventilatory pressures were not analyzed; tidal volumes referred to the largest volume charted on the anesthetic record, with the assumption that they had been carried over to OLV; and patients that developed respiratory failure received a median of 2.2 liters of fluid intraoperatively [52]. However, the results were essentially duplicated in another single-institution review of 146 pneumonectomy patients. In that study, larger tidal volumes were independently associated with the development of ALI/ARDS (8.2 vs. 7.7 mL/kg) with an odds ratio (OR) of 3.37 per one mL/kg increase in tidal volume per predicted body weight (95% confidence interval 1.65–6.86). Peak airway pressure was an additional independent risk factor with an OR 2.32 per cmH$_2$O increase (95% confidence interval 1.46–3.67) [53].

One of the earliest trials of tidal volume reduction during OLV was an animal study published in 2003 [54]. Isolated rabbit lungs were subjected to OLV with either 8 mL/kg ZEEP or the "protective" 4 mL/kg – average PEEP 2.1 cmH$_2$O (based on the dynamic pressure-time curve). OLV was

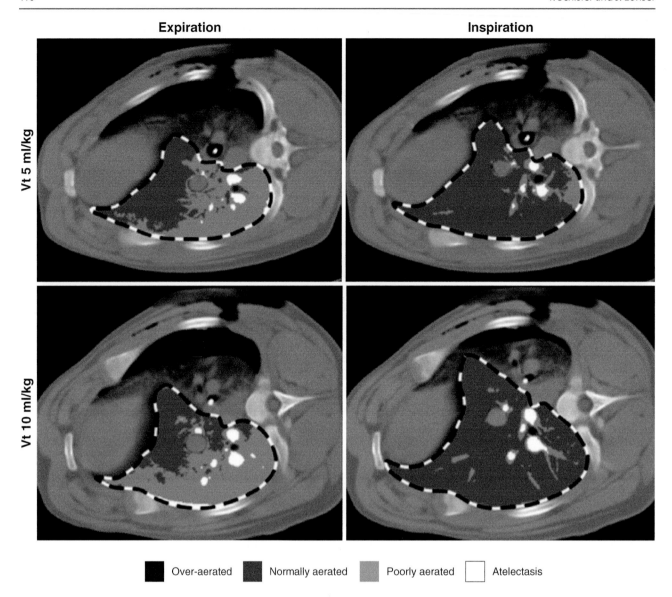

Fig. 6.2 Juxtadiaphragmatic lung computed tomographic scans of pigs during one-lung ventilation (OLV) with a tidal volume of 5 or 10 ml/kg. In each image, the region of interest includes the following (Hounsfield units in parentheses): over-aerated (from −1000 to −900), normally aerated (from −900 to −500), poorly aerated (from −500 to −100), and atelectatic (from −100 to 100) lung areas. The regions are coded by gray scale. The dependent lung border is outlined by the dashed line. Note the marked lung heterogeneity at end-expiration and the marked hyperinflation at end-inspiration with 10 ml/kg tidal volume. (Reprinted from Kozian et al. [49] with permission)

associated with increases in multiple surrogate markers of lung injury (pulmonary artery pressure [PAP], lung weight gain [LWG], and TXB_2 cytokine levels), which occurred to a lesser degree in the protective ventilation group. The protective ventilation group, however, only received half the minute ventilation of the control group, as no compensatory increase in respiratory rate was used in the low tidal volume group. Based on the study design, it was therefore not possible to state whether the outcome benefit was due to any one, or all, of minute ventilation reduction, tidal volume reduction, and/ or application of external PEEP [54]. Kuzkov et al. showed that when comparing equal minute ventilation in anesthetized sheep undergoing pneumonectomies, protective ventilation

with 6 mL/kg PEEP 2 cmH_2O lowered extravascular lung water (EVLW, a surrogate for lung injury), compared to 12 mL/kg ZEEP [55]. This finding has recently been refined in a trial demonstrating increases in EVLW when using tidal volumes of 6 or 8 ml/kg during OLV, while EVLW actually decreased when using tidal volumes of 4 ml/kg (Fig. 6.3) [56]. Tidal volume reduction by itself, however, is unlikely to be sufficient to improve outcomes. This point was best illustrated by an animal study comparing low versus high tidal volume ventilation with or without PEEP in ALI. While animals with high tidal volume ventilation and ZEEP clearly had significant cytokine elevations, all animals exposed to low tidal volumes and ZEEP died during the experiment [57].

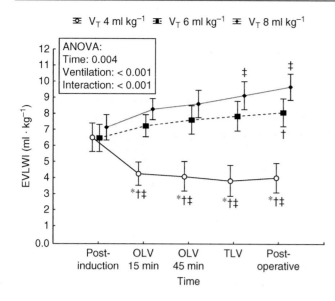

Fig. 6.3 Perioperative changes in the extravascular lung water index. Data are presented as mean (95% CI). ANOVA analysis of variance, EVLWI extravascular lung water index, OLV one-lung ventilation, TLV two-lung ventilation, VT tidal volume. $P < 0.05$ compared with *6 ml/kg, †8ml/kg and ‡postinduction values. (Reproduced from Qutub [56] with permission)

Due to the infrequent occurrence of lung injury, prospective clinical studies have focused on cytokine levels as a surrogate marker for potentially harmful ventilation. Cytokine elevations are part of the disease process, as levels of IL-6, IL-8, sICAM-1, and vWF are elevated even prior to intubation in patients with ALI [58] and baseline plasma levels of IL-6, IL-8, and IL-10 are associated with an increased risk of death in patients with ARDS [59]. Wrigge et al. failed to demonstrate a difference in tracheal cytokine levels between patients ventilated with 12–15 mL/kg ZEEP or 6 mL/kg PEEP 10 cmH₂O during TLV and OLV for laparotomy or thoracotomy. Cytokine levels before, during, and after OLV were no different between the groups [60]. However, tracheal aspirates may not be sensitive enough to detect early alveolar damage. Michelet randomized 52 patients with normal lung functions undergoing esophagectomy to OLV 9 mL/kg ZEEP or 5 mL/kg PEEP 5 cmH₂O. In this study, serum cytokine levels (IL-1, IL-6, IL-8) increased perioperatively, but to a lesser degree in the protective ventilation group [35]. The degree of lung injury and cytokine elevation may have been exaggerated by the fact that despite an average of 6 h of mechanical ventilation and 8 liters of fluid, only the low tidal volume group received PEEP during OLV, and no patient received PEEP during the remainder of the operation [35]. Esophageal surgery may also present a higher risk for lung injury as it is associated with cytokine elevations secondary to intestinal ischemia, potentially acting as a first hit [61]. The most compelling experimental evidence that tidal volumes per se are linked to the etiology of ALI after lung surgery comes from a

randomized trial, which investigated 32 patients scheduled for OLV and thoracotomy. Patients received OLV with 10 or 5 mL/kg, both without PEEP but identical minute ventilation. While OLV increased cytokine levels (TNF-α, sICAM-1) in both groups, levels were lower in the low tidal volume ventilation group [34].

More important than cytokine elevations, clinically significant outcomes of ALI, ICU admission, and hospital stay were shown to be reduced in a cohort analysis of patients who routinely received PLV (2003–2008), as compared to historical controls (1998–2003) [4]. While historical controls are fraught with limitations due to concomitant developments and improvements in medical care, this analysis by Licker et al. showed a dramatic reduction in adverse postoperative respiratory outcomes after the routine implementation of a PLV strategy. The ventilation strategy consisted of an open lung concept, with tidal volumes <8 mL/kg, routine PEEP, pressure-control ventilation (PCV), and frequent recruitment maneuvers. The statistically averaged ventilation parameters among the 558 patients in their protective ventilation group consisted of a tidal volume of 5.3 mL/kg (standard deviation [SD] 1.1), plateau pressure of 15 cmH₂O (SD 6), PEEP of 6.2 cmH₂O (SD 2.4), and respiratory rate of 15 bpm (SD 2). While the historical control already had a mean tidal volume of 7.1 mL/kg, only 24% of patients received tidal volumes less than 8 mL/kg, compared to the 92% compliance with low tidal volumes in the PLV cohort. As mentioned above, historical comparisons of ICU admission and length of hospitalization are difficult to interpret as criteria change, and moves toward fast-tracking of patients are established. However, the definition of ALI was consistent during the study period, and the authors were able to show a significant reduction in ALI from 3.8% to 0.9% [62].

While the benefits of protective ventilation for lung injury prevention are becoming clearer, its impact on oxygenation is uncertain. Two studies that investigated PLV (lower tidal volume and PEEP) during OLV reported improved oxygenation and shunt fraction as compared to traditional high tidal volume OLV [35, 55]. However, with inadequate or no PEEP, low tidal volume ventilation may be associated with worse shunt and oxygenation [34]. Recruitment studies performed during protective OLV have shown that despite a PEEP of 8 cmH₂O, patient ventilated with a tidal volume of 6 mL/kg showed significant recruitability of the ventilated lung, suggesting relative hypoventilation and atelectasis formation (see expiratory images in Fig. 6.2). Despite the presence of atelectatic lung prior to the recruitment maneuver, however, oxygenation was adequate in all patients [63]. Postoperative arterial oxygenation was not affected in a historical cohort analysis of patients undergoing lung cancer surgery with a PLV protocol incorporating lower tidal volumes [62].

Additional tools are emerging to support the clinician in the appropriate selection of tidal volume during one-lung ventilation. Hoftman and colleagues demonstrated that forced vital capacity (FVC) may be a better predictor of ideal tidal volume during thoracic surgery than predicted body weight. FVC below 3.5 liters was found to be a good predictor of reduced lung compliance, and adjustment for preoperative FVC (VT = FRC/8) allowed for more appropriate one-lung tidal volume selection [64].

PEEP

Positive-end expiratory pressure minimizes alveolar collapse and atelectasis formation by providing resistance to airway collapse during exhalation. Applied PEEP should therefore be routine for all ventilated patients during TLV [65]. Klingstedt et al. demonstrated that the mediastinal weight results in significant compression of the dependent lung in the lateral position during TLV, which can be resolved with the application of selective PEEP to the dependent lung [66]. Due to the relative position of the heart in the left hemithorax, mediastinal shift and dependent lung compression are more marked in the left lateral position than the right lateral position (Fig. 6.4) [67].

PEEP does attenuate lung injury, both in the setting of high and low tidal volumes [13]. Intrinsic or auto-PEEP occurs if expiratory time is too short to allow lung units to empty toward their resting volume. Lung areas with high compliance, characteristically found in patients with emphysema, are particularly prone due to their poor elastic recoil. Auto-PEEP is inhomogeneous throughout the lung and can therefore not be relied upon for effective avoidance of derecruitment [68]. The total PEEP after application of external

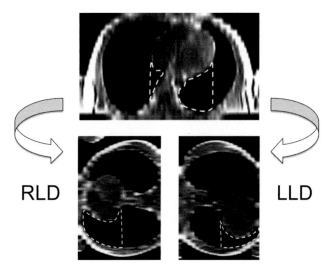

RLD   LLD

Fig. 6.4 Mediastinal shift as imaged with magnetic resonance images. Hashed areas indicate compressed areas of the lung. Note that while right lateral decubitus does expose more lung area to compression, the compression is more severe in left lateral decubitus. (Modified from an open access article by Mase et al. [67])

PEEP is also unpredictable, due to the heterogeneous nature of auto-PEEP [69].

Endotracheal intubation prevents glottic closure, resulting in complete absence of auto-PEEP in patients without obstructive lung disease on TLV. However, initiation of OLV with 10 mL/kg ZEEP has been shown to create auto-PEEP and air trapping. Measured auto-PEEP was minimal in patients without obstructive lung disease, but patients with severe COPD developed auto-PEEP levels up to 16 cmH_2O, which was associated with air trapping of 284 mL [68]. These values are unlikely to be reflective of the amount of auto-PEEP that develops with one-lung tidal volumes of 4–5 ml/kg. Patients with preexisting auto-PEEP have an unpredictable response to the application of extrinsic PEEP. In a study of ICU patients on TLV, application of PEEP changed total PEEP up, down, or not at all [70]. In a small study of patients during OLV, the additive effect of applied PEEP to auto-PEEP was inversely related to the preexisting auto-PEEP level. In other words, extrinsic PEEP contributed less to total PEEP in patients with already high auto-PEEP than patients with low auto-PEEP; however, the extent of the response was not predictable [69]. Excessive total PEEP and dynamic hyperinflation are clearly undesirable as they may cause cardiovascular depression and may require fluid loading and/or inotropic support [71].

Traditionally OLV has been performed with ZEEP, with selective application of PEEP to the nonoperative lung as part of a hypoxemia treatment algorithm. The effect of PEEP on oxygenation during OLV is variable. It is beneficial in patients whose intrinsic PEEP is well below the lower inflection point (LIP) of the compliance curve, more commonly the patient with normal lung function. In that scenario application of external PEEP will increase the total PEEP toward the LIP of the pressure-volume curve, resulting in more open (recruited) lung and improved oxygenation. Oxygenation is worse, however, if total PEEP is increased well above the LIP, likely due to alveolar overdistension, and increases in PVR resulting in an increased shunt fraction (Fig. 6.5) [72]. Neither intrinsic PEEP nor the compliance curve is routinely or easily acquired during thoracic surgery, which is why preoperative prediction of PEEP responders would be ideal. Valenza et al. showed that patients with relatively normal lung function ($FEV_1 > 72\%$) exhibited improved oxygenation on application of PEEP 10 cmH_2O during OLV [73].

Whether applied PEEP is able to decrease ALI after OLV is unclear, as it has not been studied in isolation. PEEP application as part of a "protective" ventilation regime has been shown to decrease surrogate markers of lung injury [35, 54, 55]. Additionally, routine PEEP in patients with or without COPD as part of a PLV strategy was shown to be associated with a significant decrease in the incidence of ALI and atelectasis after OLV [62].

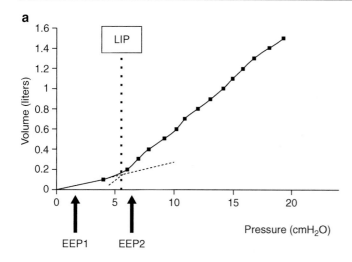

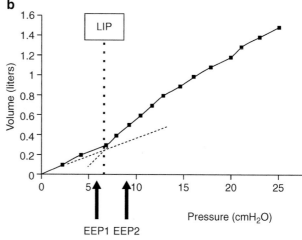

Fig. 6.5 Effect of applied PEEP on total PEEP and oxygenation during OLV. Static compliance curves of patients undergoing OLV. End-expiratory pressure before (EEP1) and after application of 5 cmH2O PEEP (EEP2) as well as lower inflection points (LIP) are indicated. Patients with normal pulmonary function and low EEP1 (**a**), in whom

EEP2 moved closer to LIP, were more likely to show oxygenation benefits after PEEP application than patients with poor lung function and intrinsic PEEP (**b**). See text for details. (Modified from Slinger et al. with permission [72])

Use of "protective" OLV with low tidal volumes but no PEEP does not appear sensible, as de-recruitment is harmful and auto-PEEP unreliable in terms of homogeneous lung recruitment. Additionally, due to the compression by abdominal contents and the mediastinal structures, marked de-recruitment and lung heterogeneity is present in the dependent lung at end-expiration (Fig. 6.2). Lack of PEEP in the setting of low tidal volume OLV has been shown to worsen oxygenation [34]. Low levels of PEEP are safe, likely beneficial for lung injury avoidance, and should be used in all patients. The only true contraindication to PEEP application would be the presence of a bronchopleural fistula. PEEP levels, however, need to be adjusted to the individual and their respiratory mechanics. Patients with normal lung function or restrictive lung disease should benefit from, and will tolerate, 5–10 cmH$_2$O PEEP or more. Patients with severe obstructive lung disease, as evidenced by preoperative hyperinflation (RV/TLC $>>$ 140%), exhibit significant air trapping during OLV, but as previously stated may not exhibit a significant increase in total PEEP with the application of external PEEP. Low levels of extrinsic PEEP 2–5 cmH$_2$O are likely well tolerated and should routinely be applied. Clearly dynamic hyperinflation must be considered in the differential for intraoperative hypotensive episodes in patients at risk. However, based on the static compliance analysis by Licker et al., who used routine PEEP in all patients as part of their PLV strategy, hyperinflation (and secondary decrease in static compliance) does not appear to be a significant concern, as the compliance actually increased in their cohort exposed to PLV with routine PEEP [62]. Early, routine application of PEEP helps to prevent atelectasis and shunt formation and thereby improves oxygenation during OLV [74].

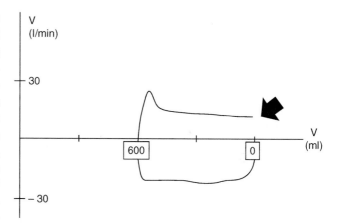

Fig. 6.6 Auto-PEEP detection by in-line spirometry. Flow-volume curve with expiration above and inspiration below the line. Expiratory flow normally returns to zero prior to inspiration. Interrupted airflow at end-expiration (arrow) indicates the presence of auto-PEEP. (Modified from Bardoczky et al. [75] with permission)

Clearly it would be best to measure total PEEP for each patient in order to rationally apply external PEEP [69]. This, however, is difficult or impossible in most intraoperative settings due to the inability of anesthetic ventilators to perform an end-expiratory hold maneuver. The simplest approximation of intrinsic PEEP can be derived from inline spirometry where interruptions of the end-expiratory flow curve indicate the presence of auto-PEEP (Fig. 6.6) [75]. Alternatively, compliance can be approximated by simple calculation (compliance = tidal volume/driving pressure), which may serve as an indicator of potential air-trapping, realizing that hyperinflation is only one of the possible explanations for a decrease in compliance.

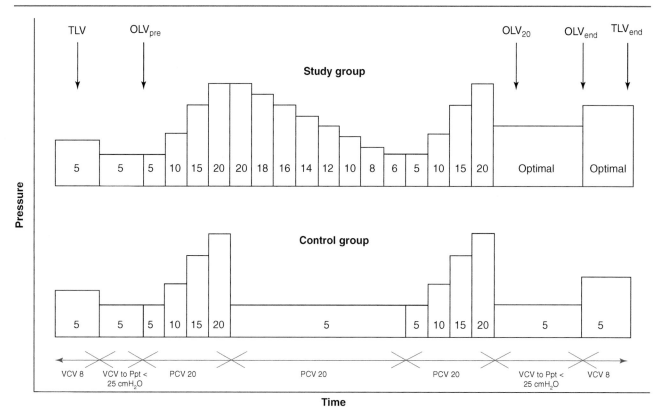

Fig. 6.7 PEEP titration during OLV after formal lung recruitment. In the study arm, optimal PEEP was determined by a stepwise decrement trial toward the point of optimal lung compliance. The control arm patients received a standard PEEP of 5 cmH2O. Individualized PEEP was higher than routinely used (10 ± 2 cmH2O) and resulted in better oxygenation both during and after OLV. (Reproduced from Ferrando et al. with permission [78])

It is possible to find the optimal level of PEEP for each individual patient during both one- and two-lung ventilation [76]. Static or dynamic lung compliance as calculated from the ventilator is influenced by FRC and the recruitable lung volume [76]. As the lung is recruited and FRC improves, so do PaO2, dead space, and lung compliance. Lung compliance is therefore a reliable surrogate of FRC during general anesthesia. A PEEP titration study utilizing a PEEP decrement trial whereby PEEP is titrated to the best compliance following a recruitment maneuver is a reliable method to determine adequate PEEP [77] and tends to result in higher levels of PEEP than traditionally selected (Fig. 6.7) [78].

FiO2

One hundred percent oxygen used to be a routine component of OLV, as hypoxemia was its most feared complication. However, with the decline in the incidence of hypoxemia and the realization that high FiO2 may be detrimental, even this practice has been questioned. Oxygen toxicity is a well-recognized consequence of prolonged exposure to high FiO2, characterized by histopathologic changes similar to ALI. Oxygen toxicity occurs during OLV and involves ischemia-reperfusion injury and oxidative stress [13]. Collapse of the operative lung and surgical manipulation results in relative organ ischemia, and reperfusion at the time of lung expansion leads to the production of radical oxygen species. Increasing durations of OLV and the presence of tumor result in increased markers of oxidative stress, which after 120 min are associated with significant increases in the rates of respiratory failure and death [79]. Lung re-expansion should likely occur at a lower FiO2, as hypoxemic reperfusion has been shown to attenuate the reperfusion syndrome [80]. This is of particular relevance after lung transplantation. Even short-term exposure to high FiO2 during the induction of anesthesia has been shown to cause significant absorption atelectasis [81]. Studies have shown that an FiO2 as low as 0.4 may provide adequate oxygenation for OLV in the lateral decubitus position [82]. Due to the potential for lung injury, particularly in the high-risk patient, after adjuvant therapy or undergoing lung transplantation, FiO2 should be titrated to effect. At the initiation of OLV, a FiO2 of 0.8 may be appropriate, but 15–20 min later, when the nadir of oxygenation has occurred, the FiO2 should be gradually decreased to the minimum that is required to maintain a stable saturation level above 90–92%. During lung resection surgery, further reductions in FiO2 are possible once the vasculature to the resected lobe or lung has been disrupted. Stapling of the vasculature effectively reduces, or, in the setting of a pneumonectomy, essentially eliminates the shunt flow.

The oxygen content and gas mixture are not only important for oxygenation but also for the speed of nonventilated lung collapse during OLV. This is of particular importance for surgical exposure during video-assisted thoracoscopic surgery (VATS). Ko et al. compared three different gas mixtures during TLV immediately prior to OLV (air/O_2, N_2O/O_2, O_2) and investigated which gas mixture would best collapse the operative lung while maintaining arterial oxygenation in patients undergoing lung resection surgery [83]. FiO_2 was 0.4 in the air/O_2 and N_2O/O_2 group and 1.0 in the O_2 group during TLV. All groups received 100% oxygen on initiation of OLV. Not surprisingly, lung deflation was worse if nitrogen (i.e., air) was administered prior to lung collapse, due to the poor solubility of nitrogen in blood. A nitrous oxide/O_2 mixture was superior to oxygen alone for lung collapse, but nitrous oxide is rarely used nowadays. Administering 100% oxygen pre-OLV temporarily improved OLV oxygenation but only until the nonventilated lung becomes atelectatic. Once the operative lung has collapsed at around 15 min of OLV, that oxygen reservoir and any benefit from it have disappeared [83].

While 100% oxygen facilitates collapse of the operative lung, it also facilitates the development of de-recruitment and atelectasis in the nonoperative lung, producing shunt and facilitating hypoxemia. The greater the FiO_2 following endotracheal intubation, the larger the degree of atelectasis is seen on computed tomography [84]. While no prospective studies have evaluated the impact of lower than 100% oxygen prior to lung collapse, the individual practitioner should weigh the risks and benefits of lower FiO_2 and consider using the lowest inspired oxygen necessary to maintain acceptable arterial oxygenation.

Minute Ventilation/Permissive Hypercapnia

Permissive hypercapnia has been a key component of the critical care management for ALI/ARDS. Reduction of the minute ventilation allows for a decrease in tidal volumes and ventilatory pressures, thereby minimizing mechanical stress and secondary volu- or barotrauma. Beyond the reduction in minute ventilation and mechanical trauma, the actual elevated CO_2 level itself may be beneficial [85], as hypercapnia appears to attenuate the cytokine response [86].

Permissive hypercapnia has been investigated in the OLV setting. In the previously mentioned study by Gama de Abreu et al., isolated rabbit lungs were exposed to OLV with 8 mL/kg ZEEP or 4 mL/kg PEEP 2.1 cmH$_2$O (based on the dynamic pressure-time curve), without respiratory rate compensation. The protective ventilation group, which received half the minute ventilation, exhibited a reduction in surrogate markers for lung injury (PAP, LWG, cytokine levels) [54]. Similar ventilatory parameters were studied during OLV in thoracotomy patients. Sticher et al. ventilated patients with 7 mL/kg PEEP 2 cmH$_2$O or 3.5 mL/kg PEEP 2 cmH$_2$O, again without respiratory rate compensation, effectively halving minute ventilation similar to Gama de Abreu. $PaCO_2$ values rose from 42 to 64 mmHg, which was associated with a 42% increase in PVR, but no change in oxygenation. Hypercapnia was well tolerated; however, higher-risk patients with pulmonary hypertension or major cardiac rhythm disturbances were excluded [87]. In a case series of 24 patients undergoing volume reduction surgery for advanced emphysema, permissive hypercapnia was used electively as part of a barotrauma avoidance strategy. The mean $PaCO_2$ value was 56 mmHg with a peak of 86 mmHg, resulting in pH values between 7.11 and 7.41 (mean 7.29). The authors state that hypercapnia was well tolerated; however, inotropic support was required in over 50% of patients [88]. Even higher $PaCO_2$ levels have been described in a small series of ten patients with severe emphysema that were again managed with elective hypoventilation for barotrauma avoidance. $PaCO_2$ values rose to peak levels of 70–135 mmHg, resulting in pH values as low as 7.03 (despite bicarbonate administration). Hypercapnia was poorly tolerated at these high levels. All patients required inotropic support during anesthesia. Four patients developed ventricular dysrhythmias and three patients required tracheal gas insufflation for treatment of hypoxemia [89]. Significant hypercapnia can cause increased intracranial pressure, pulmonary hypertension, decreased myocardial contractility, decreased renal blood flow, and release of endogenous catecholamines. At extremely high levels, CO_2 can be lethal due to excessive sympathetic stimulation, cardiac rhythm disturbances, and/or cardiac collapse [71, 89]. Moderate hypercapnia potentiates the HPV response and is therefore unlikely to adversely affect oxygenation [90]; however, the same may not hold true for extreme CO_2 elevations [89]. A protective ventilation strategy including permissive hypercapnia has been shown to reduce the incidence of ALI in a cohort analysis by Licker et al. [62]. While not explicitly discussed in the manuscript, permissive hypercapnia clearly was part of their strategy. The PLV group had significantly lower tidal volumes with only marginal rate compensation. Based on the manuscript, the minute ventilation of the historical cohort was 92 vs. 80 mL/kg/min in the PLV group. The PLV group therefore had smaller minute ventilation and increased anatomic dead space ventilation (increased respiratory rate), resulting in decreased CO_2 elimination [62]. Permissive hypercapnia should be considered a routine component of a PLV strategy for OLV. Assuming a reasonable cardiovascular reserve, and in particular right ventricular function, $PaCO_2$ levels

<70 mmHg are well tolerated in the short term and clearly beneficial in terms of lung injury avoidance and attenuation. Higher levels should be avoided in the majority of patients due to the risk of hemodynamic instability.

I:E Ratio and Respiratory Rate

Each ventilatory cycle consists of time spent in inspiration and expiration. The appropriate ratio of inspiratory to expiratory (I:E) time depends on underlying lung mechanics. Restrictive lung disease is characterized by poorly compliant lungs, which resist passive lung expansion but rapidly recoil to FRC. Increasing the I:E ratio to 1:1 (or using inverse ratio ventilation) maximizes the time spent in inspiration, thereby reducing peak and plateau ventilatory pressures. For illustration, at a respiratory rate of 15 bpm and an I:E ratio of 1:1, each respiratory cycle lasts 4 s, with 2 s spent in each of inspiration and expiration, respectively. Obstructive lung disease, on the other hand, is characterized by lungs, which have difficulty to empty toward FRC, due to poor elastic recoil and conducting airway collapse. Decreasing the I:E ratio toward 1:4 allows for more expiratory time and helps to minimize the risk of auto-PEEP and dynamic hyperinflation. For illustration, at a respiratory rate of 15 bpm, now with the I:E ratio to 1:4, each respiratory cycle is still 4 s; however, expiration now takes up 3.2 s of the entire cycle.

Respiratory rate modification may be equally necessary depending on the underlying lung mechanics. Extreme airflow obstruction may require very long expiratory times. After reducing the I:E ratio to the minimum of 1:4, this can only be achieved by increasing the overall cycle length, i.e., reducing the respiratory rate. Clinical examples, such as the patient with severe cystic fibrosis requiring a respiratory rate of 4–6 to allow for complete exhalation have been reported [91]. In restrictive lung disease, on the other hand, dividing a given minute volume by a higher respiratory frequency may be beneficial in reducing peak and plateau ventilatory pressures. It has to be realized, however, that as anatomic dead space remains unchanged, dividing the minute volume by a higher respiratory rate results in reduced CO_2 elimination as the unchanged size of the anatomic dead space makes up a larger component of the tidal volume [92]. For illustration, a patient ventilated at 20 bpm of 400 ml receives the same minute ventilation as a patient ventilated at 10 bpm of 800 ml. However, dead space ventilation, which occupies about 150 mL of each breath, has doubled from 1500 mL at 10 bpm to 3000 mL at 20 bpm. Alveolar ventilation has therefore been reduced from 6500 mL (8000–1500) to 5000 mL (8000–3000). Additionally, OLV with small tidal volume and rapid respiratory rate results in statistically higher auto-PEEP [65]. While auto-PEEP elevations in this study were unlikely to be clinically significant, they serve as a reminder that rapid, shallow ventilation has the potential to increase dynamic hyperinflation.

Peak/Plateau Pressure

The peak inspiratory pressure is a reflection of the dynamic compliance of the respiratory system and airway resistance. It depends on tidal volume, inspiratory time, endotracheal size, and airway tone (bronchospasm). Plateau pressure, on the other hand, relates to the static compliance of the respiratory system, i.e., chest wall and lung compliance. Double-lumen endobronchial tubes have small internal diameters resulting in increased resistance to air flow [93]. Application of the full TLV minute volume to a single lumen of the double lumen tube (DLT) results in a 55% increase in peak inspiratory pressure and 42% increase in plateau pressure [92]. While plateau pressure reflects alveolar pressure, peak pressure is unlikely to be fully applied to the alveolus. A retrospective study of 197 pneumonectomy patients did, however, show that peak ventilation pressures above 40 cmH_2O were associated with the development of PPPE [50]. Recently, Fernández-Pérez et al. reviewed 4420 consecutive patients without preexisting lung injury undergoing high-risk elective surgeries for postoperative pulmonary complications and demonstrated that mean first hour airway pressure (OR 1.07; 95% CI 1.02–1.15 cmH_2O) but not tidal volume, PEEP, or FiO_2 were associated with ALI after adjusting for nonventilatory parameters [94]. Similarly, patients exposed to a plateau pressure of 29 cmH_2O were at significantly higher risk of developing ALI after lung resection surgery than those with a plateau pressure of 14 cmH_2O [7]. Based on the critical care literature, there does not appear to be a critical plateau pressure level above which injury occurs, but rather any elevation in plateau pressure increases the relative risk of lung injury. With the implementation of permissive hypoventilation, peak pressure levels less than 35 cmH_2O and plateau pressures less than 25 cmH_2O should therefore be achievable in the majority of patients during OLV. This was confirmed in the cohort study by Licker et al. who showed that implementation of a PLV strategy for OLV resulted in mean plateau pressures of 15 cmH_2O [62].

Driving Pressure

One of the primary mechanisms driving ventilator-induced lung injury (VILI) is excessive stress and strain on lung parenchyma during inspiration. Transpulmonary pressure is calculated as plateau pressure minus pleural pressure and is a surrogate of both lung stress and strain [95]. Calculating transpulmonary pressure requires a plateau pressure measurement. Plateau pressure can be measured on most present-day anesthetic machines by simply setting an inspiratory hold of at least 40% of the delivery time during a square wave flow delivery (volume control ventilation) [96]. Driving pressure is calculated as the plateau pressure minus the PEEP and frequently and closely approximates transpulmonary pressure when PEEP equals pleural pressure [95]. Driving pressure is a surrogate of lung stress and strain and should be kept as low as possible and ideally below 13 cmH$_2$O [97] as higher levels are associated with excessive lung stress [95]. Driving pressure is now considered an important independent predictor of mortality in ARDS and more influential than tidal volume or plateau pressure. In fact, any ventilator maneuver (PEEP titration, tidal volume titration) that reduces driving pressure also reduces mortality in patients with ARDS [97]. Driving pressure is also an important marker of postoperative pulmonary complications in patients with healthy lungs in the operating room. An analysis of individual patient data from several randomized controlled trials demonstrated that an increase in driving pressure resulted in a greater incidence of postoperative pulmonary complications [98]. Importantly, any change in PEEP (increase or decrease) that resulted in a lower driving pressure translated to a lower incidence of postoperative pulmonary complications. To date, a similar analysis has not been reported in patients undergoing one-lung ventilation; however Blank and colleagues found an association between driving pressure and postoperative pulmonary complications in their retrospective analysis [27].

Ventilatory Mode

Volume-control ventilation (VCV) has been the predominant ventilatory mode both in the intensive care and operating room. VCV uses a constant inspired flow (square wave), creating a progressive increase in airway pressure toward the peak inspiratory pressure, which is reached as the full tidal volume has been delivered. Inspiratory pressure during VCV depends on the set tidal volume and PEEP, gas flow rates and resistance, as well as respiratory system compliance. The set tidal volume will be delivered unless the inspiratory pressure exceeds the pressure limit, in which case the flow ceases. With the realization that ventilatory pressures may be one of the inciting factors of lung injury, other ventilatory modes have been explored.

Pressure-control ventilation (PCV) uses a decelerating flow pattern, with maximal flow at the beginning of inspiration until the set pressure is reached, after which flow rapidly decreases balancing the decreasing compliance of the expanding lung. This resembles the spontaneous mammalian breath, which also follows a decelerating pattern, as negative intrathoracic pressure induced by contracting diaphragm and intercostal muscles cause a high initial airflow [65]. Tidal volumes can be highly variable during PCV and may fall precipitously with changes in lung compliance, particularly with surgical manipulation. As the majority of the tidal volume is delivered in the early part of the inspiration, mean airway and alveolar pressure tend to be higher during PCV. The decelerating flow pattern results in a more homogeneous distribution of the tidal volume, improving static and dynamic lung compliance due to recruitment of poorly ventilated lung regions and improving oxygenation and dead space ventilation [99]. Whether PCV during OLV improves oxygenation is controversial. Tuğrul et al. studied 48 patients undergoing thoracotomy and lung resection. Patients received VCV or PCV during OLV, both delivering 10 mL/kg ZEEP 100% O$_2$, in a crossover fashion. PCV was associated with statistically significant decreases in peak and plateau airway pressures, as well as improved oxygenation and shunt fraction. Oxygenation improved more in patients with poor preoperative lung function, which may relate to the more homogeneous distribution of ventilation achieved with the pressure-control breath [100]. The same group investigated the benefit of adding PEEP 4 cmH$_2$O to OLV with PCV and showed that it provided an additional significant improvement in oxygenation and shunt fraction in their patients [101]. Other groups, however, have failed to reproduce the oxygenation benefit in PCV studies during OLV [102–104].

The effect of intraoperative ventilatory mode on postoperative oxygenation is equally controversial. Although a better postoperative oxygenation was shown in the PCV group compared with VCV in a trial of patients undergoing MIDCAB surgery [105], no significant difference was demonstrated in a study of patients after thoracic surgery [106]. Despite the lack of a clear oxygenation benefit, PCV is likely preferable over VCV due to the potential to decrease ventilatory pressures and the ability to recruit lung units.

High-frequency jet ventilation (HFJV) is another ventilatory mode that has been successfully used in thoracic surgery [107]. HFJV, when applied to the operative lung during prolonged OLV in aortic surgery, is more effective than continuous positive airway pressure (CPAP) in improving PaO$_2$ [108]. This may be particularly relevant in the poor operative candidate after prior contralateral lung resection [109, 110]. Misiolek et al. evaluated the value of two-lung HFJV via a standard endotracheal tube for thoracic surgery. Sixty patients were randomized to HFJV (1 atm pressure, rate 200/min, 100% O$_2$) or standard OLV (10 mL/kg, 100% O$_2$, ZEEP). HFJV was associated with lower ventilating pressures, improved oxygenation, and shunt fraction and importantly no detriment in surgical exposure or intraoperative hemodynamic variables [111]. Buise et al. reported that HFJV was associated with a lower mean blood loss and less crystalloids administration during esophagectomy, compared with the OLV group. They speculated that higher ventilatory pressures in the OLV group resulted in higher intrathoracic pressure and central venous pressure, and thus splanchnic congestion, which increased blood loss relative to the HFJV group [112]. Difficulties in monitoring ventilatory pressures, tidal volumes, and end-tidal CO_2 concentrations, in addition to the inherent risks of barotrauma associated with this technique, continue to limit its widespread adoption [107].

Another ventilatory mode, which has only been used as a CPAP equivalent at this point, is high-frequency percussive ventilation (HFPV). It is a ventilatory technique providing convective and diffusive ventilation that can reduce the physiologic right-to-left shunt and improve arterial oxygenation [113–115]. Lucangelo et al. assessed the effects of HFPV (FiO_2 1.0, 500 cycles/min, mean pressure 5 cmH_2O, with pressures oscillating between 2 and 8 cmH_2O) applied to the nondependent lung compared to standard CPAP in patients undergoing elective lung resection. HFPV patients showed higher PaO_2 during OLV than CPAP and exhibited better clearance of secretions and shortened hospital stays [116].

Recruitment/Re-expansion

Atelectasis has long been known to occur in dependent lung areas of anesthetized patients. The primary reasons for alveolar collapse during anesthesia are extrinsic compression and gas resorption. Studies have shown that atelectatic alveoli are not simply airless, but may also be fluid- or foam-filled. Beyond simple lung collapse, atelectasis is therefore now considered both a potential cause and a manifestation of ALI [81]. Interestingly, re-expansion of collapsed alveoli causes injury not only to the alveoli that are being recruited but also to remote nonatelectatic alveoli [81]. This may be in part due to the early realization by Mead that expansion of a gas-free alveolus with a transpulmonary pressure of 30 cmH_2O creates a shear force of 140 cmH_2O to adjacent alveoli [14, 117]. PEEP has been shown to prevent lung injury associated with both high and low tidal volumes, by stabilizing alveoli and preventing their collapse [81]. In animal models of ARDS, it has been shown that atelectasis is associated with vascular leak, right ventricular failure, and eventual death in 31% of rats and is easily avoided with PEEP [118].

Atelectasis formation in the nonoperative lung is highly undesirable during OLV as it worsens the already high shunt fraction, increasing the potential for hypoxemia. Among the risk factors that predispose to lung de-recruitment during OLV are high FiO_2, traditional lack of PEEP, and extrinsic compression by abdominal contents, the heart and mediastinum. The best evidence for the presence of atelectasis during

OLV comes from a lung recruitment study, which investigated an aggressive alveolar recruitment maneuver (ARM) with increasing pressure breaths over a 4-min period up to a peak pressure of 40 cmH_2O and a PEEP level of 20 cmH_2O (Fig. 6.7). Recruitment increased PaO_2 on OLV from a mean of 144 mmHg to a mean of 244 mmHg (Fig. 6.8) [63].

However, it is not only for oxygenation purposes that lung recruitment is important. Establishment (and retention) of open lung optimizes lung compliance and optimizes ventilation by reducing dead space ventilation to its lowest level (Fig. 6.9). It is an often overlooked benefit of lung recruitment that it optimizes the amount of CO_2 clearance and therefore may in fact allow for a reduction in minute ventilation with secondary further decreases in lung stress and strain.

Cinnella et al. demonstrated that the alveolar recruitment achieved by a formal ARM resulted in a significant decrease in static elastance of the dependent lung [120]. Hemodynamic instability is a well-recognized risk of such an aggressive ARM as the sustained intrathoracic pressure increases right ventricular afterload, resulting in impaired venous return and left heart preload [35, 121]. A recent study showed that stroke volume variation (an indicator of preload responsiveness) increases dramatically after an ARM, while both

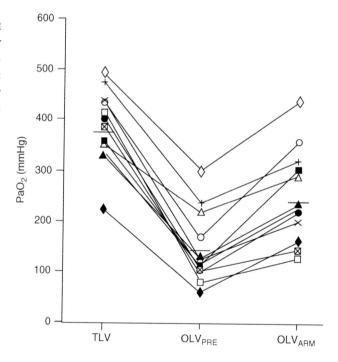

Fig. 6.8 Lung recruitment improves oxygenation during OLV. PaO2 (mmHg) in all patients during two-lung ventilation (TLV) and during one-lung ventilation before (OLVPRE) and after (OLVARM) the alveolar recruitment maneuver consisting of stepwise increases in PEEP from 5 to 20 cmH2O with a stable pressure-control driving pressure. Each symbol represents one patient in every point of the study. Horizontal bars represent mean values at each point. (Reprinted from Tusman et al. [63] with permission)

Fig. 6.9 Dynamic changes in dead space during thoracic surgery in one representative patient. All the measurements were performed in the right lateral position. The PEEP at the bottom is used as a marker of the RM and PEEP titration. The sequences of different representative periods of ventilation with two-lung (TLV, VT 8 ml/kg) or one-lung (OLV, VT 6 ml/kg) before and after RM are depicted. Rectangle: the time scale of the RM and PEEP titrations was magnified to highlight the interventions and their effects. The arrows indicate the closing pressure, thus the level of PEEP needed to maintain the lungs open after the RM, as identified by the highest dynamic compliance (Cdyn), which coincides with the lowest physiological (VD/VT) and alveolar (VDalv/VTalv) dead space values. PEEP, positive end-expiratory pressure; RM, recruitment maneuver. (Modified from Tusman et al. with permission [119])

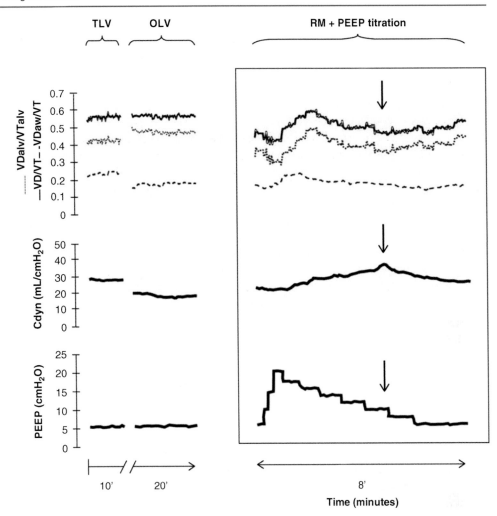

cardiac index and venous oxygen saturation decrease. These changes, however, were transient and completely recovered within 3 min [122].

Caution is required with the implementation of PLV, as low tidal volumes and plateau pressures may promote atelectasis formation and increase FiO_2 and PEEP requirements [71]. Frequent de-recruitment and therefore need for repeated recruitment maneuvers, as may be the case with low tidal volume ventilation with insufficient PEEP, are potentially deleterious. In animal models of lung injury, repeated de-recruitment and recruitment maneuvers are associated with histological evidence of lung injury [123, 124]. Even a single recruitment maneuver of 40 cmH_2O for 40 s has been shown to elevate biomarkers of lung injury in the rat model without preexisting lung injury [125]. The same may potentially be true in humans, although this aspect has only been studied in critically ill patients. Halbertsma et al. demonstrated that a single ARM could increase translocation of pro-inflammatory cytokines from the alveolar space into the systemic circulation in ventilated critically ill children. Fifteen minutes after the ARM, an increase was observed in plasma TNFα, IL-6, and IL-1β [93]. Another critical care study found that 4 out

of 28 patients with ALI/ARDS developed barotrauma necessitating intervention following an ARM [126]. This does create a curious dilemma as the increased use of PLV, with low tidal volumes, may promote atelectasis formation and therefore increase the need for recruitment maneuvers [71]. The best ventilatory strategy is therefore one that follows the "open lung" concept and maintains lung recruitment with appropriate levels of PEEP.

Atelectasis formation in the operative lung is routine and occurs gradually over a 10–20-min period as residual oxygen is being absorbed, which parallels the gradual decline in PaO_2 on OLV. Ko et al. compared three different gas mixtures during TLV immediately prior to OLV (air/O_2, N_2O/O_2, O_2) and investigated which gas mixture would best collapse the operative lung while maintaining arterial oxygenation in patients undergoing lung resection surgery. FiO_2 was 0.4 in the air/O_2 and N_2O/O_2 group and 1.0 in the O_2 group during TLV. All groups received 100% oxygen on initiation of OLV. Not surprisingly, lung deflation was worse if nitrogen (i.e., air) was administered prior to lung collapse, due to the poor solubility of nitrogen in blood. A nitrous oxide/O_2 mixture was superior to oxygen alone for lung collapse, but nitrous oxide is contraindicated in many thoracic patients. Administering 100% oxygen pre-OLV temporarily improved OLV oxygenation but only until the nonventilated lung becomes atelectatic. Once the operative lung has collapsed at around 15 min of OLV, that oxygen reservoir and any benefit from it have disappeared [83].

Atelectasis is complete, unless CPAP is applied to the operative lung. CPAP, or its variant HFJV, if applied to the at least partially recruited operative lung, effectively improves *V/Q* matching and hypoxemia [108]. Gradual re-expansion of the operative lung at the conclusion of OLV is achieved with a continuous pressure hold of 20–30 cmH_2O, which is lower than standard recruitment regimens, in order to prevent disruption of staple lines. As discussed, re-expansion of lung tissue may be harmful. Re-expansion injury after prolonged lung collapse consists of alveolar-capillary membrane edema and increase in lymphocyte and neutrophil infiltration [127]. Re-expansion of isolated rabbit lungs after 55 min of lung collapse showed significant elevations in myeloperoxidase (MPO) levels, as well as IL-1β and TNF-α mRNA, when compared to an open lung control [33]. Intermittent lung re-expansion may mitigate these effects, as intermittent recruitment of the operative lung during OLV has been shown to decrease pro-inflammatory mediators during esophagectomy [128]. Lung recruitment with continuous high-pressure hold may result in significant hypotension if applied to both lungs. However, even in the setting of hypovolemia, recruitment is well tolerated, if it is selectively applied to one lung at a time, with the other lung open to the atmosphere [129]. Re-expansion pulmonary edema is fortunately rare if a gradual, gentle recruitment technique is applied and is more likely after sudden recruitment of long-standing lung collapse [130]. Low oxygen tensions should likely be used for re-expansion, as recruitment of the operative lung is associated with substantial oxidative stress, particularly after prolonged OLV [79, 80].

OLV Duration

Mechanical stress due to OLV can be minimized by optimization of ventilatory parameters. However, even minimal stress using "protective" parameters becomes significant if exposure is prolonged. Retrospective case series have shown that OLV lasting more than 100 min is associated with an increased risk for postoperative lung injury [8]. Part of the damage may be due to oxidative stress. A recent animal study exposed rats to increasing durations of OLV from 1 to 3 h. At the conclusion of the experiment, animals were sacrificed and analyzed for biochemical indicators of oxidative stress and histologic changes in lung tissue. Increasing the duration of OLV from 1 to 3 h resulted in significant elevations of malondialdehyde (MDA) activity and increased the amount

of tissue damage on histological analysis [131]. A prospective analysis of patients undergoing lobectomy for non-small cell cancer with either TLV or OLV lasting more than 60, 90, or 120 min compared MDA plasma levels at lung re-expansion. Again, MDA levels increased significantly with increasing OLV duration, indicating cumulative oxidative stress [79]. Anesthesiologists have limited control over the duration of OLV as it is mostly determined by the surgical procedure. However, initiation of OLV should occur as close to pleural opening as possible (except for thoracoscopic procedures), and TLV should resume as early as possible. With the increasing use of OLV outside the thoracic theater, it is essential to ensure that the nonthoracic surgeon appreciates the need to minimize the length of OLV.

Combined Ventilator Strategy

The cumulative evidence is overwhelmingly in favor of adopting a protective lung ventilatory strategy for OLV, which has been shown to decrease surrogate markers of lung injury as well as the incidence of ALI itself. Protective ventilation is not synonymous with low tidal volume ventilation but also must include all of routine PEEP (set above the closing pressure and lower inflection point), lower FiO_2 (sufficient to maintain adequate arterial oxygenation), and particularly lower ventilatory pressures (driving pressure primarily) through the use of PCV and permissive hypercapnia. This strategy follows the "open lung" concept that has been widely adopted for the critical care management of ARDS patients but has since been expanded to include patients in the ICU without ARDS and to high-risk patients in the operating room or those undergoing major surgery. As part of the open lung concept, frequent recruitment of the lung has to be considered as another component of a PLV strategy. Recruitment should occur at a minimum following endotracheal intubation, at the beginning of OLV and on resumption of TLV. In addition, lung recruitment should be considered whenever oxygenation and lung compliance deteriorate. Lung de-recruitment may potentially be more prevalent with low tidal volumes due to the loss of end-inspiratory stretch in the setting of high FiO_2. Appropriate levels of external PEEP minimize de-recruitment in the setting of low tidal volume ventilation. PEEP titration is possible in the operating room with the use of spirometry and real-time measurement of pulmonary compliance. When PEEP is titrated to the best pulmonary compliance following maximal recruitment, FRC is maximized, atelectasis and dead space are reduced, oxygenation is improved, and atelectrauma is lessened [70]. Titrating PEEP to compliance individualizes the ventilator strategy to each patient's unique respiratory pathophysiology. As driving pressure is equal to tidal volume divided by pulmonary compliance, a reduction in driving pressure is achieved through an improvement in compliance. Titrating PEEP allows one to also avoid overdistension which may produce pulmonary blood flow diversion to the operative lung and worsen hypoxemia and, as mentioned above, increases pulmonary complications [98]. There is no one-size-fits-all solution to PEEP selection as has become evident in recent RCTs [23]. Meta-analyses in both the ICU and the operating room have clearly demonstrated that PEEP titration toward lower driving pressure (due to improved compliance) improves patient outcomes [97, 98]. Once PEEP has been titrated to an optimal setting, the provider should then turn their attention to tidal volume. Excessive tidal volumes are often unintentionally provided in females, in the morbidly obese, and in patients of shorter stature, a fact that is avoidable by calculating ideal or predicted body weight [132]. Using driving pressure to optimize tidal volume is an important area that requires further investigation keeping in mind that driving pressure greater than 13 cmH_2O is an independent risk factor for postoperative pulmonary complications. One should consider decreasing tidal volume if this driving pressure threshold has been reached until more definitive data emerges.

Other than the ICU, where as long as cardiac output is maintained, PEEP can be increased to maintain "open lung"; in the OLV setting, excessive PEEP will cause pulmonary blood flow diversion to the operative lung and worsens oxygenation. As such, low tidal volume ventilation has the potential to worsen oxygenation, either due to lung de-recruitment with inadequate PEEP or due to pulmonary blood flow diversion with excessive PEEP. Low tidal volume ventilation increases dead space and CO_2 elimination is therefore consistently worse with this technique. This should not present a problem in the majority of patients, unless CO_2 elimination is already compromised by severe obstructive lung disease (e.g., cystic fibrosis). In cases of severe respiratory acidosis, marked pulmonary hypertension, or right ventricular dysfunction, "protective" low-tidal volume – high rate ventilation – may need to be aborted in favor of higher tidal volume ventilation at a lower respiratory rate (to maximize CO_2 elimination), as the imminent risk of hemodynamic dysfunction trumps the potential risk of ALI. Dynamic hyperinflation is common during OLV and is increased with the application of PEEP and the use of higher respiratory rates. The risk of hyperinflation may be increased with a PLV strategy, which has to be considered, particularly in patients with severe emphysema and during periods of hemodynamic instability. Providing adequate expiratory time and use of permissive hypoventilation should minimize the risk of significant hyperinflation in all but the patients with the most severe form of obstructive lung disease.

While PLV should be the norm for all patients, it is particularly important in patients with risk factors for ALI and during procedures that trigger a higher inflammatory response, such as pneumonectomy, esophageal surgery, or lung transplantation. Respiratory mechanics vary widely between restrictive and obstructive lung disease so that any ventilatory strategy needs to be individualized for the particular patient (Table 6.2).

Table 6.2 Summary of ventilatory strategies

Tidal volume: protective, 3–5 mL/kg; hypoxemia or severe hypercapnia (consider 6–8 mL/kg (with decreased RR))
PEEP (approximate): normal lungs, 10 cmH_2O; obstructive, 2–5 cmH_2O (minimize intrinsic PEEP); restrictive, 10+ cmH_2O
RR: protective, 12–15 bpm; severe hypercapnia, 6–8 bpm (with increased VT)
FiO_2: transplant: 21%+, routine 50–80%, hypoxemia 100%
I:E ratio: restrictive, 1:1 or inverse ratio; normal, 1:1–1:2; obstructive, 1:3–4 (reduced RR)
Pressures: driving <15 cmH_2O, plateau <20 cmH_2O, peak <35 cmH_2O
Minute volume: $PaCO_2$ 40–60 mmHg (rarely higher: severe obstruction, lung transplantation)
Ventilator mode: PCV

Hypoxemia

Prediction

Hypoxemia used to be the major concern during OLV. Early reports indicated that 40–50% of patients suffered hypoxemia during OLV [133]. Predictors for possible desaturation have been identified (Table 6.3). Hurford et al. examined the intraoperative oxygenation of patients who had undergone preoperative V/Q scanning [133]. They found that the amount of preoperative perfusion (and ventilation) to the operative lung inversely correlated with PaO_2 after 10 min of OLV. As HPV is only able to halve blood flow through the operative lung during OLV, the authors concluded that the extent of preoperative blood flow helped to predict the amount of intraoperative shunt. Slinger et al. showed that PaO_2 during OLV relates to multiple factors. Poor oxygenation during TLV was predictive of continued oxygenation difficulties as were right-sided operations (due to the increased perfusion to that side). Good preoperative pulmonary function (FEV_1) was found to be predictive of poor OLV oxygenation, which is felt to be due to the lack of auto-PEEP and secondary de-recruitment in normal lungs [134]. Two recent studies correlated the risk of hypoxemia to the end-tidal CO_2 gradients. One study showed that the difference of end-tidal CO_2 between the lungs in the lateral position significantly correlates with the P/F ratio at 15 min of OLV [135]. The other study demonstrated that there was a significant negative correlation between the lowest PaO_2 recorded during the first 45 min of OLV and the end-tidal CO_2 difference between TLV and the early phase of OLV

Table 6.3 Predictors of hypoxemia during one-lung ventilation

Preferential perfusion of the operative lung
Right-sided surgery
Prior contralateral resection
Supine position
Normal FEV_1
Poor oxygenation on TLV
High $A–a$ gradient for CO_2

Table 6.4 Approach to hypoxemia during one-lung ventilation

Mild hypoxemia (90–95%)
Confirm position of lung isolation device
Recruit ventilated lung
Ensure adequate cardiac output
Increase FiO_2 toward 1.0
Optimize PEEP to nonoperative lung (up or down, toward lower inflection point)
CPAP/HFJV/O_2 insufflation to operative lung (IPAP, FOB)
Consider reduction in vapor anesthetic and/or total intravenous anesthesia
Ensure adequate oxygen carrying capacity (hemoglobin)
Severe (<<90%) or refractory hypoxemia
Resume TLV with 100% O_2
If not possible, consider
Pulmonary artery clamp on operative side during pneumonectomy, transplant
Inhaled NO and/or infusions of almitrine/phenylephrine
Extracorporeal support (ECMO, CPB)

[136]. Both studies postulated that elevated CO_2 gradients were indicative of V/Q mismatching and therefore explained the risk of hypoxemia.

Over the years the incidence of hypoxemia has been declining. Improvements in anesthetic technique including improved lung isolation, confirmation of lung isolation with fiber-optic bronchoscopy, and use of anesthetic agents with less effects on HPV are being credited for the reduction of oxygenation difficulties. In 1993 the incidence of hypoxemia (SpO_2 < 90%) occurring during OLV was quoted at 9% [133]. By 2003 the published incidence of hypoxemia was down to 1% of OLV cases in some hands [137]. However, another more recent study again showed a 10% incidence of hypoxemia <90% in a single institution between 2003 and 2004. The discrepancy could be due to variations in clinical management. Alternatively, it may indicate the difference between manual and electronic charting, as the latter study consisted of automatic recording of saturation every 30 s [138]. Although rare, significant hypoxemia may still occur, at times without warning [139].

Treatment

For a rational approach to hypoxemia during OLV, it has to be appreciated that CPAP and TLV are uniformly effective (Table 6.4). CPAP always decreases shunt flow and TLV essentially eliminates shunt flow. Aside from procedures such as pneumonectomy and lung transplantation where these techniques are not available, patients should therefore not have to suffer prolonged hypoxemia. Assuming that the lung isolation device is properly positioned, these two maneuvers are the most effective treatments for hypoxemia. They are not chosen as first-line interventions, however, because they will impair surgical access to the lung, particularly during thoracoscopic procedures. CPAP is easily applied via one of the commercially available units that connect to the open lumen of the DLT, or the suction port of the bronchial blocker via the CPAP adaptor. Alternatively, a standard AMBU bag with a PEEP valve can be used if no CPAP unit is available. CPAP does require some degree of lung recruitment, which is not always feasible (lung lavage, bronchopleural fistula) and will impact surgical exposure. Recently, Russell et al.

described an intermittent positive airway pressure (IPAP) technique, which does not elicit lung inflation and therefore should not impact surgical exposure. While the technique does not call for lung recruitment, it is unlikely to be of benefit in the setting of complete lung collapse. It is based on intermittent delivery of short bursts of low-flow oxygen (2 LPM) to the nonventilated lung to treat hypoxemia, circumventing significant lung movement in the surgical field. Placing a standard bacteriostatic filter on the open lumen of the DLT, with oxygen connected to the CO_2 sampling port, manual occlusion of open filter end allows for "jet insufflation" of oxygen into the collapsed lung. A 2-second burst of flow will deliver 66 mL of oxygen to the nonventilated lung. In their study, all patients with relative hypoxemia (SpO_2 < 95%) were successfully treated with repeated 2-second bursts of oxygen, followed by 10-second exhalations, while no impairment in surgical exposure was noted [140]. Apneic oxygen insufflation via an endotracheal suction catheter at 3 LPM is another successful method that has been shown to reduce the incidence of hypoxemia while on OLV. This technique should result in fewer interruptions to surgery during a VATS procedure [141].

Hypoxemia during OLV for VATS presents a particular problem, as TLV and CPAP techniques are generally considered to be contraindicated. Ku et al. presented a novel method, which may be of benefit in select cases. They described the treatment of refractory hypoxemia during left-sided VATS for lung volume reduction surgery. A 4-mm fiber-optic bronchoscope was inserted into the basilar segment of the left lower lobe bronchus, and 5 L/min of oxygen was insufflated for approximately 20 s via the suction port (Fig.6.10). Oxygenation successfully recovered within 2 min without impairing the surgical field and remained adequate for 20 min. There are two important considerations to this technique. First, it can only be applied if the insufflation

Fig. 6.10 Schematic illustration of oxygen supplementation during thoracoscopic surgery via bronchoscopy suction channel. See text for details. (Reprinted from Ku et al. [142] with permission)

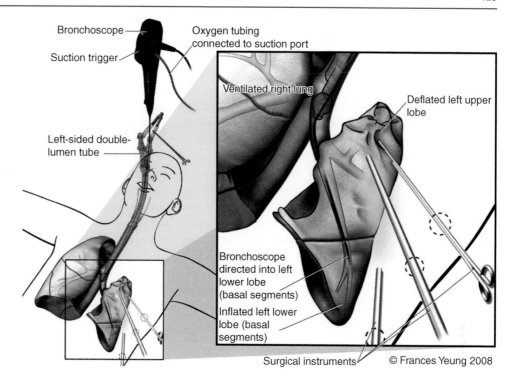

Bronchoscope

Suction trigger

Oxygen tubing connected to suction port

Ventilated right lung

Deflated left upper lobe

Left-sided double-lumen tube

Bronchoscope directed into left lower lobe (basal segments)

Inflated left lower lobe (basal segments)

Surgical instruments

© Frances Yeung 2008

occurs in a lung territory that is remote to the surgical site and is therefore unlikely to be successful in case of a central lesion. In this case report, oxygen was insufflated into basilar segments while lung resection occurred at the apex. Second, insufflation of relatively high-flow oxygen has the potential to cause lung overdistension or barotrauma if the bronchoscope tip is allowed to wedge in the airway. The authors guarded against this by having the surgeon visualize the basilar lung segments throughout the period of insufflation [142]. Distal oxygen insufflation, particularly at relatively high flow rates as described in this report, should never be applied blindly. As another option, HFJV has been successfully employed during VATS procedures [143]. In order for this technique to succeed, the lung has to be allowed to collapse away from the chest wall prior to the institution of HFJV, and driving pressures have to be low enough to only cause partial lung inflation. As previously stated, however, with proper attention to adequate lung isolation, "open lung" ventilation, and maintenance of a normal cardiac output, these interventions should rarely be necessary.

Lung de-recruitment in the ventilated lung is common, easily reversed with recruitment maneuvers and preventable with appropriate PEEP levels. Low mixed venous oxygen saturation secondary to low cardiac output is another frequent and easily treatable cause of desaturation. Pharmacological modulation with vasoconstrictors (almitrine, phenylephrine) to strengthen HPV in the operative lung and vasodilators (inhaled NO) to improve pulmonary vascular capacitance in the ventilated lung may be helpful in extreme cases.

Systemic Effects

Even though hypoxemia has become less of an anesthetic issue during OLV, relative hypoxemia may have a significant impact on vital nonpulmonary organ function given the ever-increasing rate of comorbid conditions in thoracic patients. In addition to hypoxemia, release of inflammatory cytokines and reactive oxygen metabolites may have yet unknown effects on organ function.

A recent study by Mierdl et al. analyzed the impact of hypoxemia during OLV on myocardial metabolism in patients with severe multivessel coronary artery disease. Patients underwent minimally invasive coronary artery bypass grafting via small lateral thoracotomy. In their study measurements of arterial and coronary sinus PO_2, pH and lactate did not show any evidence of anaerobic metabolism, despite arterial PaO_2 values between 50 and 70 mmHg during OLV. Additionally, no patient exhibited myocardial ischemia, which led the authors to conclude that OLV may be used in patients with multivessel coronary artery disease with an acceptable low risk of inducing anaerobic myocardial metabolism [144].

Neurocognitive dysfunction is a well-known complication of cardiac surgery and has been shown to be associated with intraoperative episodes of cerebral oxygen desaturation. Standard pulse oximetry is insufficient to detect these events. Monitoring for and treating cerebral desaturation events may decrease the incidence of postoperative neurocognitive dysfunction [145, 146]. Tobias et al. investigated the incidence and risk factors for cerebral desaturation by monitoring cerebral oxygenation (rSO_2) using near-infrared spectroscopy in patients who required OLV for thoracic surgery [147]. In 8 of 40 patients, prolonged decreases in rSO_2 to less than 75% of the baseline value were recorded during OLV. These eight patients were older, weighed more, and were more likely to be ASA III than the remainder of the patients. Since there was no significant difference in patient background or other monitoring values, the authors concluded that rSO_2 monitoring might be useful to detect cerebral desaturation and allow for early intervention in patients during OLV. Jugular bulb venous oxygen saturations during OLV were assessed in a study comparing sevoflurane- and propofol-based anesthesia in patients undergoing lung surgery [148]. The SjO_2 values were significantly higher in the sevoflurane group than in the propofol group, despite identical SaO_2 values. The lower SjO_2 values observed with propofol anesthesia may be explained by the fact that propofol reduces cerebral blood flow more than cerebral metabolic rate [149, 150].

Interestingly, cerebral oxygen desaturation also appears to be predictive of noncerebral postoperative complications. In a trial of 50 patients undergoing major thoracotomy with OLV, a minimal absolute regional cerebral oxygen saturation of less than 65% was found to be predictive of postoperative organ dysfunction based on the Sequential Organ Failure Assessment (SOFA) scoring system with an OR of 2.37 (95% CI 1.18–4.39, $P = 0.043$) [151]. Cerebral tissue oxygenation depends on arterial oxygen content, oxygen delivery (cardiac output), and metabolic consumption and may therefore be a superior monitor to simple pulse oximetry.

Reactive oxygen metabolites are known to occur after re-expansion of the nonventilated lung. These metabolites may have deleterious effects on cellular function. Yuluğ et al. investigated the effects of OLV and re-expansion on the tissue damage of the liver and ileum in rats [152]. Plasma aspartate aminotransferase (AST), alanine aminotransferase (ALT), tissue MDA, and MPO activities in both tissues were significantly increased associated with OLV and re-expansion. Tissue damage and apoptotic index increased in rats with longer OLV duration, suggesting that OLV may cause tissue damage in the liver and ileum. These are some of the early indicators that OLV may indeed have effects beyond lung tissue; future research will help to delineate the significance of these findings.

Alternatives to One-Lung Ventilation

With the uncommon yet legitimate concern about acute lung injury following one-lung ventilation, clinicians have sought alternatives to general anesthesia and positive pressure ventilation for patients undergoing thoracic surgery. One approach which has reemerged is the avoidance of endotra-

cheal intubation and mechanical ventilation for thoracic surgery [153]. This has also been termed NIVATS, which stands for non-intubated video-assisted thoracic surgery. The goal of NIVATS is to avoid the risks associated with endotracheal intubation, general anesthesia, and positive pressure ventilation including mechanical airway injury, ventilator-induced lung injury, hypoxemia, cardiac arrhythmias, cognitive dysfunction, and other organ injury [154]. NIVATS has been used for a range of thoracic procedures from simple pneumothorax, effusions and empyema, wedge resection, mediastinal biopsy, bullectomy to more invasive procedures including lobectomy, pneumonectomy, thymectomy, and even carinal and tracheal resection. NIVATS is often facilitated with varying degrees of conscious sedation combined with regional anesthesia via an epidural, paravertebral, intercostal, or serratus anterior block with the maintenance of spontaneous ventilation in the lateral position, which favors ventilation perfusion matching. Complications associated with NIVATS include hypercapnia, coughing, disruption of the surgical field from mediastinal and diaphragm motion, and patient intolerance, which may require conversion to general anesthesia [155]. In a recent survey to members of the European Society of Thoracic Surgeons, 62 out of 105 respondents claimed an experience with NIVATS. The most common approach included intercostal blocks with minimal sedation followed by laryngeal mask with sedation and thoracic epidural blockade with sedation. The most common procedures in which NIVATS was utilized included the management of pleural effusion and lung or mediastinal biopsy [157]. So far data on outcomes using NIVATS compared to general anesthesia (GAVATS) is sparse but points to shorter hospital length of stay and less postoperative morbidity in high-risk individuals [154]. NIVATS offers a promising alternative to general anesthesia and endotracheal intubation in high-risk individuals for primarily simple thoracic procedures when the thoracic surgeon and anesthesiologist are comfortable using this modality and are prepared to convert to general anesthesia if the need arises. There is insufficient evidence to recommend this approach in more involved lung resections.

Conclusion

The last two decades have seen a shift in OLV research from studies investigating hypoxemia to various aspects of lung injury pathophysiology and prevention. Much has been learned about ventilation strategies that minimize lung injury. Evidence to date supports PLV based on reduction of surrogate markers but more importantly now also indicates reduction of adverse outcomes. Ventilatory parameters have to be individualized for each patient's unique pulmonary mechanics but should focus on an "open lung" strategy.

Performing a PEEP titration study and routinely monitoring and limiting driving pressure are two recent developments in the literature that deserve special attention and further investigation. Hypoxemia is infrequent and should lead to a re-evaluation of ventilatory parameters. Routine algorithms for treatment of hypoxemia, as well as advanced management techniques, are available, such that prolonged hypoxemia should be exceedingly rare. There are early indicators that OLV may impact systemic organ function, but future research is needed to address end-organ effects.

References

1. Brodsky JB. The evolution of thoracic anesthesia. Thorac Surg Clin. 2005;15(1):1–10.
2. Lohser J. Evidence-based management of one-lung ventilation. Anesthesiol Clin. 2008;26(2):241–72. v
3. Zeldin RA, Normandin D, Landtwing D, Peters RM. Postpneumonectomy pulmonary edema. J Thorac Cardiovasc Surg. 1984;87(3):359–65.
4. Licker M, Fauconnet P, Villiger Y, Tschopp JM. Acute lung injury and outcomes after thoracic surgery. Curr Opin Anaesthesiol. 2009;22(1):61–7.
5. Dulu A, Pastores SM, Park B, Riedel E, Rusch V, Halpern NA. Prevalence and mortality of acute lung injury and ARDS after lung resection. Chest. 2006;130(1):73–8.
6. Bernard GR, Artigas A, Brigham KL, Carlet J, Falke K, Hudson L, et al. The American-European Consensus Conference on ARDS. Definitions, mechanisms, relevant outcomes, and clinical trial coordination. Am J Respir Crit Care Med. 1994;149(3):818–24.
7. Ferguson ND, Fan E, Camporota L, Antonelli M, Anzueto A, Beale R, et al. The berlin definition of ARDS: an expanded rationale, justification, and supplementary material. Intensive Care Med. 2012;38(10):1573–82.
8. Licker M, de Perrot M, Spiliopoulos A, Robert J, Diaper J, Chevalley C, Tschopp J-M. Risk factors for acute lung injury after thoracic surgery for lung cancer. Anesth Analg. 2003;97(6):1558–65.
9. Ruffini E, Parola A, Papalia E, Filosso PL, Mancuso M, Oliaro A, et al. Frequency and mortality of acute lung injury and acute respiratory distress syndrome after pulmonary resection for bronchogenic carcinoma. Eur J Cardiothorac Surg. 2001;20(1):30–6. discussion 36-7
10. Kutlu CA, Williams EA, Evans TW, Pastorino U, Goldstraw P. Acute lung injury and acute respiratory distress syndrome after pulmonary resection. Ann Thorac Surg. 2000;69(2):376–80.
11. Della Rocca G, Coccia C. Acute lung injury in thoracic surgery. Curr Opin Anaesthesiol. 2013;26(1):40–6.
12. Tang SS, Redmond K, Griffiths M, Ladas G, Goldstraw P, Dusmet M. The mortality from acute respiratory distress syndrome after pulmonary resection is reducing: a 10-year single institutional experience. Eur J Cardiothorac Surg. 2008;34(4):898–902.
13. Jordan S, Mitchell JA, Quinlan GJ, Goldstraw P, Evans TW. The pathogenesis of lung injury following pulmonary resection. Eur Respir J. 2000;15(4):790–9.
14. Tremblay LN, Slutsky AS. Ventilator-induced lung injury: from the bench to the bedside. Intensive Care Med. 2006;32(1):24–33.
15. Amato MB, Barbas CS, Medeiros DM, Magaldi RB, Schettino GP, Lorenzi-Filho G, et al. Effect of a protective-ventilation strategy on mortality in the acute respiratory distress syndrome. N Engl J Med. 1998;338(6):347–54.
16. Determann RM, Royakkers A, Wolthuis EK, Vlaar AP, Choi G, Paulus F, et al. Ventilation with lower tidal volumes as compared with conventional tidal volumes for patients without acute lung injury: a preventive randomized controlled trial. Crit Care. 2010;14(1):R1.
17. Gajic O, Frutos-Vivar F, Esteban A, Hubmayr RD, Anzueto A. Ventilator settings as a risk factor for acute respiratory distress syndrome in mechanically ventilated patients. Intensive Care Med. 2005;31(7):922–6.
18. Gajic O, Dara SI, Mendez JL, Adesanya AO, Festic E, Caples SM, et al. Ventilator-associated lung injury in patients without acute lung injury at the onset of mechanical ventilation. Crit Care Med. 2004;32(9):1817–24.
19. Neto AS, Simonis FD, Barbas CS, Biehl M, Determann RM, Elmer J, et al. Lung-protective ventilation with low tidal volumes and the occurrence of pulmonary complications in patients without acute respiratory distress syndrome: a systematic review and individual patient data analysis. Crit Care Med. 2015;43(10):2155–63.
20. Silva PL, Negrini D, Macêdo Rocco PR. Mechanisms of ventilator-induced lung injury in healthy lungs. Best Pract Res Clin Anaesthesiol. 2015;29(3):301–13.
21. Serpa Neto A, Hemmes SN, Barbas CS, Beiderlinden M, Fernandez-Bustamante A, Futier E, et al. Incidence of mortality and morbidity related to postoperative lung injury in patients who have undergone abdominal or thoracic surgery: a systematic review and meta-analysis. Lancet Respir Med. 2014;2(12):1007–15.
22. Futier E, Constantin JM, Paugam-Burtz C, Pascal J, Eurin M, Neuschwander A, et al. A trial of intraoperative low-tidal-volume ventilation in abdominal surgery. N Engl J Med. 2013;369(5):428–37.
23. Hemmes SN, Serpa Neto A, Schultz MJ. Intraoperative ventilatory strategies to prevent postoperative pulmonary complications: a meta-analysis. Curr Opin Anaesthesiol. 2013;26(2):126–33.
24. Serpa Neto A, Hemmes SNT, Barbas CSV, Beiderlinden M, Biehl M, Binnekade JM, et al. Protective versus conventional ventilation for surgery. Anesthesiology. 2015;123(1):66–78.
25. Levin MA, McCormick PJ, Lin HM, Hosseinian L, Fischer GW. Low intraoperative tidal volume ventilation with minimal PEEP is associated with increased mortality. Br J Anaesth. 2014;113(1):97–108.
26. Yang M, Ahn HJ, Kim K, Kim JA, Yi CA, Kim MJ, Kim HJ. Does a protective ventilation strategy reduce the risk of pulmonary complications after lung cancer surgery?: a randomized controlled trial. Chest. 2011;139(3):530–7.
27. Blank RS, Colquhoun DA, Durieux ME, Kozower BD, McMurry TL, Bender SP, Naik BI. Management of one-lung ventilation: impact of tidal volume on complications after thoracic surgery. Anesthesiology. 2016;124(6):1286–95.
28. Shen B. Low tidal volume ventilation in the operating room—where are we now? Anesthesia Patient Safety Foundation Newsletter. 2016:1–4.
29. Lohser J, Slinger P. Lung injury after one-lung ventilation: a review of the pathophysiologic mechanisms affecting the ventilated and the collapsed lung. Anesth Analg. 2015;121(2):302–18.
30. Padley SP, Jordan SJ, Goldstraw P, Wells AU, Hansell DM. Asymmetric ARDS following pulmonary resection: CT findings initial observations. Radiology. 2002;223(2):468–73.
31. Yin K, Gribbin E, Emanuel S, Orndorff R, Walker J, Weese J, Fallahnejad M. Histochemical alterations in one lung ventilation. J Surg Res. 2007;137(1):16–20.
32. Kozian A, Schilling T, Fredén F, Maripuu E, Röcken C, Strang C, et al. One-lung ventilation induces hyperperfusion and alveolar damage in the ventilated lung: an experimental study. Br J Anaesth. 2008;100(4):549–59.
33. Funakoshi T, Ishibe Y, Okazaki N, Miura K, Liu R, Nagai S, Minami Y. Effect of re-expansion after short-period lung collapse

on pulmonary capillary permeability and pro-inflammatory cytokine gene expression in isolated rabbit lungs. Br J Anaesth. 2004;92(4):558–63.

34. Schilling T, Kozian A, Huth C, Bühling F, Kretzschmar M, Welte T, Hachenberg T. The pulmonary immune effects of mechanical ventilation in patients undergoing thoracic surgery. Anesth Analg. 2005;101(4):957–65. table of contents

35. Michelet P, D'Journo XB, Roch A, Doddoli C, Marin V, Papazian L, et al. Protective ventilation influences systemic inflammation after esophagectomy: a randomized controlled study. Anesthesiology. 2006;105(5):911–9.

36. Sentürk M. New concepts of the management of one-lung ventilation. Curr Opin Anaesthesiol. 2006;19(1):1–4.

37. De Conno E, Steurer MP, Wittlinger M, Zalunardo MP, Weder W, Schneiter D, et al. Anesthetic-induced improvement of the inflammatory response to one-lung ventilation. Anesthesiology. 2009;110(6):1316–26.

38. Giraud O, Molliex S, Rolland C, Leçon-Malas V, Desmonts JM, Aubier M, Dehoux M. Halogenated anesthetics reduce interleukin-1beta-induced cytokine secretion by rat alveolar type II cells in primary culture. Anesthesiology. 2003;98(1):74–81.

39. Erturk E, Topaloglu S, Dohman D, Kutanis D, Beşir A, Demirci Y, et al. The comparison of the effects of sevoflurane inhalation anesthesia and intravenous propofol anesthesia on oxidative stress in one lung ventilation. Biomed Res Int. 2014;2014:360936.

40. Chappell D, Heindl B, Jacob M, Annecke T, Chen C, Rehm M, et al. Sevoflurane reduces leukocyte and platelet adhesion after ischemia-reperfusion by protecting the endothelial glycocalyx. Anesthesiology. 2011;115(3):483–91.

41. Casanova J, Simon C, Vara E, Sanchez G, Rancan L, Abubakra S, et al. Sevoflurane anesthetic preconditioning protects the lung endothelial glycocalyx from ischemia reperfusion injury in an experimental lung autotransplant model. J Anesth. 2016;30(5):755–62.

42. Schilling T, Kozian A, Kretzschmar M, Huth C, Welte T, Bühling F, et al. Effects of propofol and desflurane anaesthesia on the alveolar inflammatory response to one-lung ventilation. Br J Anaesth. 2007;99(3):368–75.

43. Schilling T, Kozian A, Senturk M, Huth C, Reinhold A, Hedenstierna G, Hachenberg T. Effects of volatile and intravenous anesthesia on the alveolar and systemic inflammatory response in thoracic surgical patients. Anesthesiology. 2011;115(1):65–74.

44. Cohen E. Management of one-lung ventilation. Anesthesiol Clin North Am. 2001;19(3):475–95. vi

45. Brodsky JB, Fitzmaurice B. Modern anesthetic techniques for thoracic operations. World J Surg. 2001;25(2):162–6.

46. BENDIXEN HH, HEDLEY-WHYTE J, LAVER MB. Impaired oxygenation in surgical patients during general anesthesia with controlled ventilation. A concept of atelectasis. N Engl J Med. 1963;269:991–6.

47. Katz JA, Laverne RG, Fairley HB, Thomas AN. Pulmonary oxygen exchange during endobronchial anesthesia: effect of tidal volume and PEEP. Anesthesiology. 1982;56(3):164–71.

48. Flacke JW, Thompson DS, Read RC. Influence of tidal volume and pulmonary artery occlusion on arterial oxygenation during endobronchial anesthesia. South Med J. 1976;69(5):619–26.

49. Kozian A, Schilling T, Schütze H, Senturk M, Hachenberg T, Hedenstierna G. Ventilatory protective strategies during thoracic surgery: effects of alveolar recruitment maneuver and low-tidal volume ventilation on lung density distribution. Anesthesiology. 2011;114(5):1025–35.

50. van der Werff YD, van der Houwen HK, Heijmans PJ, Duurkens VA, Leusink HA, van Heeswijk HP, de Boer A. Postpneumonectomy pulmonary edema. A retrospective analysis of incidence and possible risk factors. Chest. 1997;111(5):1278–84.

51. Fernández-Pérez ER, Keegan MT, Brown DR, Hubmayr RD, Gajic O. Intraoperative tidal volume as a risk factor for respiratory failure after pneumonectomy. Anesthesiology. 2006;105(1):14–8.

52. Neustein S. Association of high tidal volume with postpneumonectomy failure. Anesthesiology. 2007;106(4):875–6.

53. Jeon K, Yoon JW, Suh GY, Kim J, Kim K, Yang M, et al. Risk factors for post-pneumonectomy acute lung injury/acute respiratory distress syndrome in primary lung cancer patients. Anaesth Intensive Care. 2009;37(1):14–9.

54. Gama de Abreu M, Heintz M, Heller A, Széchényi R, Albrecht DM, Koch T. One-lung ventilation with high tidal volumes and zero positive end-expiratory pressure is injurious in the isolated rabbit lung model. Anesth Analg. 2003;96(1):220–8. table of contents.

55. Kuzkov VV, Suborov EV, Kirov MY, Kuklin VN, Sobhkhez M, Johnsen S, et al. Extravascular lung water after pneumonectomy and one-lung ventilation in sheep. Crit Care Med. 2007;35(6):1550–9.

56. Qutub H, El-Tahan MR, Mowafi HA, El Ghoneimy YF, Regal MA, Al Saflan AA. Effect of tidal volume on extravascular lung water content during one-lung ventilation for video-assisted thoracoscopic surgery: a randomised, controlled trial. Eur J Anaesthesiol. 2014;31:466.

57. Chiumello D, Pristine G, Slutsky AS. Mechanical ventilation affects local and systemic cytokines in an animal model of acute respiratory distress syndrome. Am J Respir Crit Care Med. 1999;160(1):109–16.

58. Cepkova M, Brady S, Sapru A, Matthay MA, Church G. Biological markers of lung injury before and after the institution of positive pressure ventilation in patients with acute lung injury. Crit Care. 2006;10(5):R126.

59. Parsons PE, Eisner MD, Thompson BT, Matthay MA, Ancukiewicz M, Bernard GR, et al. Lower tidal volume ventilation and plasma cytokine markers of inflammation in patients with acute lung injury. Crit Care Med. 2005;33(1):1–6. discussion 230-2

60. Wrigge H, Uhlig U, Zinserling J, Behrends-Callsen E, Ottersbach G, Fischer M, et al. The effects of different ventilatory settings on pulmonary and systemic inflammatory responses during major surgery. Anesth Analg. 2004;98(3):775–81.

61. Boyle NH, Pearce A, Hunter D, Owen WJ, Mason RC. Intraoperative scanning laser doppler flowmetry in the assessment of gastric tube perfusion during esophageal resection. J Am Coll Surg. 1999;188(5):498–502.

62. Licker M, Diaper J, Villiger Y, Spiliopoulos A, Licker V, Robert J, Tschopp JM. Impact of intraoperative lung-protective interventions in patients undergoing lung cancer surgery. Crit Care. 2009;13(2):R41.

63. Tusman G, Böhm SH, Sipmann FS, Maisch S. Lung recruitment improves the efficiency of ventilation and gas exchange during one-lung ventilation anesthesia. Anesth Analg. 2004;98(6):1604–9. table of contents

64. Hoftman N, Eikermann E, Shin J, Buckley J, Navab K, Abtin F, et al. Utilizing forced vital capacity to predict low lung compliance and select intraoperative tidal volume during thoracic surgery. Anesth Analg. 2017;125:1922.

65. Schultz MJ, Haitsma JJ, Slutsky AS, Gajic O. What tidal volumes should be used in patients without acute lung injury? Anesthesiology. 2007;106(6):1226–31.

66. Klingstedt C, Hedenstierna G, Baehrendtz S, Lundqvist H, Strandberg A, Tokics L, Brismar B. Ventilation-perfusion relationships and atelectasis formation in the supine and lateral positions during conventional mechanical and differential ventilation. Acta Anaesthesiol Scand. 1990;34(6):421–9.

67. Mase K, Noguchi T, Tagami M, Imura S, Tomita K, Monma M, et al. Compression of the lungs by the heart in supine, side-lying, semi-prone positions. J Phys Ther Sci. 2016;28(9):2470–3.

68. Ducros L, Moutafis M, Castelain MH, Liu N, Fischler M. Pulmonary air trapping during two-lung and one-lung ventilation. J Cardiothorac Vasc Anesth. 1999;13(1):35–9.

69. Slinger PD, Hickey DR. The interaction between applied PEEP and auto-peep during one-lung ventilation. J Cardiothorac Vasc Anesth. 1998;12(2):133–6.

70. Caramez MP, Borges JB, Tucci MR, Okamoto VN, Carvalho CR, Kacmarek RM, et al. Paradoxical responses to positive end-expiratory pressure in patients with airway obstruction during controlled ventilation. Crit Care Med. 2005;33(7):1519–28.

71. Putensen C, Wrigge H. Tidal volumes in patients with normal lungs: one for all or the less, the better? Anesthesiology. 2007;106(6):1085–7.

72. Slinger PD, Kruger M, McRae K, Winton T. Relation of the static compliance curve and positive end-expiratory pressure to oxygenation during one-lung ventilation. Anesthesiology. 2001;95(5):1096–102.

73. Valenza F, Ronzoni G, Perrone L, Valsecchi M, Sibilla S, Nosotti M, et al. Positive end-expiratory pressure applied to the dependent lung during one-lung ventilation improves oxygenation and respiratory mechanics in patients with high FEV1. Eur J Anaesthesiol. 2004;21(12):938–43.

74. Ren Y, Peng ZL, Xue QS, Yu BW. The effect of timing of application of positive end-expiratory pressure on oxygenation during one-lung ventilation. Anaesth Intensive Care. 2008;36(4):544–8.

75. Bardoczky GI, d'Hollander AA, Cappello M, Yernault JC. Interrupted expiratory flow on automatically constructed flow-volume curves may determine the presence of intrinsic positive end-expiratory pressure during one-lung ventilation. Anesth Analg. 1998;86(4):880–4.

76. Henderson WR, Chen L, Amato MB, Brochard LJ. Fifty years of research in ARDS. Respiratory mechanics in acute respiratory distress syndrome. Am J Respir Crit Care Med. 2017;196:822.

77. Tusman G, Böhm SH. Prevention and reversal of lung collapse during the intra-operative period. Best Pract Res Clin Anaesthesiol. 2010;24(2):183–97.

78. Ferrando C, Mugarra A, Gutierrez A, Carbonell JA, García M, Soro M, et al. Setting individualized positive end-expiratory pressure level with a positive end-expiratory pressure decrement trial after a recruitment maneuver improves oxygenation and lung mechanics during one-lung ventilation. Anesth Analg. 2014;118(3):657–65.

79. Misthos P, Katsaragakis S, Theodorou D, Milingos N, Skottis I. The degree of oxidative stress is associated with major adverse effects after lung resection: a prospective study. Eur J Cardiothorac Surg. 2006;29(4):591–5.

80. Douzinas EE, Kollias S, Tiniakos D, Evangelou E, Papalois A, Rapidis AD, et al. Hypoxemic reperfusion after 120 mins of intestinal ischemia attenuates the histopathologic and inflammatory response. Crit Care Med. 2004;32(11):2279–83.

81. Duggan M, Kavanagh BP. Atelectasis in the perioperative patient. Curr Opin Anaesthesiol. 2007;20(1):37–42.

82. Bardoczky GI, Szegedi LL, dHollander AA, Moures JM, de Francquen P, Yernault JC. Two-lung and one-lung ventilation in patients with chronic obstructive pulmonary disease: the effects of position and fio2. Anesth Analg. 2000;90(1):35.

83. Ko R, McRae K, Darling G, Waddell TK, McGlade D, Cheung K, et al. The use of air in the inspired gas mixture during two-lung ventilation delays lung collapse during one-lung ventilation. Anesth Analg. 2009;108(4):1092–6.

84. Edmark L, Kostova-Aherdan K, Enlund M, Hedenstierna G. Optimal oxygen concentration during induction of general anesthesia. Anesthesiology. 2003;98(1):28–33.

85. Kregenow DA, Rubenfeld GD, Hudson LD, Swenson ER. Hypercapnic acidosis and mortality in acute lung injury. Crit Care Med. 2006;34(1):1–7.

86. Lang CJ, Barnett EK, Doyle IR. Stretch and CO2 modulate the inflammatory response of alveolar macrophages through independent changes in metabolic activity. Cytokine. 2006;33(6):346–51.

87. Sticher J, Müller M, Scholz S, Schindler E, Hempelmann G. Controlled hypercapnia during one-lung ventilation in patients undergoing pulmonary resection. Acta Anaesthesiol Scand. 2001;45(7):842–7.

88. Zollinger A, Zaugg M, Weder W, Russi EW, Blumenthal S, Zalunardo MP, et al. Video-assisted thoracoscopic volume reduction surgery in patients with diffuse pulmonary emphysema: gas exchange and anesthesiological management. Anesth Analg. 1997;84(4):845–51.

89. Morisaki H, Serita R, Innami Y, Kotake Y, Takeda J. Permissive hypercapnia during thoracic anaesthesia. Acta Anaesthesiol Scand. 1999;43(8):845–9.

90. Balanos GM, Talbot NP, Dorrington KL, Robbins PA. Human pulmonary vascular response to 4 h of hypercapnia and hypocapnia measured using Doppler echocardiography. J Appl Physiol (1985). 2003;94(4):1543–51.

91. Robinson RJ, Shennib H, Noirclerc M. Slow-rate, high-pressure ventilation: a method of management of difficult transplant recipients during sequential double lung transplantation for cystic fibrosis. J Heart Lung Transplant. 1994;13(5):779–84.

92. Szegedi LL, Barvais L, Sokolow Y, Yernault JC, d'Hollander AA. Intrinsic positive end-expiratory pressure during one-lung ventilation of patients with pulmonary hyperinflation. Influence of low respiratory rate with unchanged minute volume. Br J Anaesth. 2002;88(1):56–60.

93. Slinger PD, Lesiuk L. Flow resistances of disposable double-lumen, single-lumen, and univent tubes. J Cardiothorac Vasc Anesth. 1998;12(2):142–4.

94. Fernández-Pérez ER, Sprung J, Afessa B, Warner DO, Vachon CM, Schroeder DR, et al. Intraoperative ventilator settings and acute lung injury after elective surgery: a nested case control study. Thorax. 2009;64(2):121–7.

95. Chiumello D, Carlesso E, Brioni M, Cressoni M. Airway driving pressure and lung stress in ARDS patients. Crit Care. 2016;20:276.

96. Helwani MA, Saied NN. Intraoperative plateau pressure measurement using modern anesthesia machine ventilators. Can J Anaesth. 2013;60(4):404–6.

97. Amato MB, Meade MO, Slutsky AS, Brochard L, Costa EL, Schoenfeld DA, et al. Driving pressure and survival in the acute respiratory distress syndrome. N Engl J Med. 2015;372(8):747–55.

98. Neto AS, Hemmes SNT, Barbas CSV, Beiderlinden M, Fernandez-Bustamante A, Futier E, et al. Association between driving pressure and development of postoperative pulmonary complications in patients undergoing mechanical ventilation for general anaesthesia: a meta-analysis of individual patient data. Lancet Respir Med. 2016;4(4):272–80.

99. Nichols D, Haranath S. Pressure control ventilation. Crit Care Clin. 2007;23(2):183–99. viii-ix

100. Tuğrul M, Camci E, Karadeniz H, Sentürk M, Pembeci K, Akpir K. Comparison of volume controlled with pressure controlled ventilation during one-lung anaesthesia. Br J Anaesth. 1997;79(3):306–10.

101. Sentürk NM, Dilek A, Camci E, Sentürk E, Orhan M, Tuğrul M, Pembeci K. Effects of positive end-expiratory pressure on ventilatory and oxygenation parameters during pressure-controlled one-lung ventilation. J Cardiothorac Vasc Anesth. 2005;19(1):71–5.

102. Unzueta MC, Casas JI, Moral MV. Pressure-controlled versus volume-controlled ventilation during one-lung ventilation for thoracic surgery. Anesth Analg. 2007;104(5):1029–33. tables of contents

103. Leong LM, Chatterjee S, Gao F. The effect of positive end expiratory pressure on the respiratory profile during one-lung ventilation for thoracotomy. Anaesthesia. 2007;62(1):23–6.

104. Choi YS, Shim JK, Na S, Hong SB, Hong YW, Oh YJ. Pressure-controlled versus volume-controlled ventilation during one-lung ventilation in the prone position for robot-assisted esophagectomy. Surg Endosc. 2009;23(10):2286–91.

105. Heimberg C, Winterhalter M, Strüber M, Piepenbrock S, Bund M. Pressure-controlled versus volume-controlled one-lung ventilation for MIDCAB. Thorac Cardiovasc Surg. 2006;54(8):516–20.

106. Pardos PC, Garutti I, Piñeiro P, Olmedilla L, de la Gala F. Effects of ventilatory mode during one-lung ventilation on intraoperative and postoperative arterial oxygenation in thoracic surgery. J Cardiothorac Vasc Anesth. 2009;23(6):770–4.

107. Ihra G, Gockner G, Kashanipour A, Aloy A. High-frequency jet ventilation in european and north american institutions: developments and clinical practice. Eur J Anaesthesiol. 2000;17(7):418–30.

108. Abe K, Oka J, Takahashi H, Funatsu T, Fukuda H, Miyamoto Y. Effect of high-frequency jet ventilation on oxygenation during one-lung ventilation in patients undergoing thoracic aneurysm surgery. J Anesth. 2006;20(1):1–5.

109. Knüttgen D, Zeidler D, Vorweg M, Doehn M. Unilateral high-frequency jet ventilation supporting one-lung ventilation during thoracic surgical procedures. Anaesthesist. 2001;50(8):585–9.

110. Durkin C, Lohser J. Oxygenation and ventilation strategies for patients undergoing lung resection surgery after prior lobectomy or pneumonectomy. Curr Anesthesiol Rep. 2016;6(2):135–41.

111. Misiolek H, Knapik P, Swaneveldder J, Wyatt R, Misiolek M. Comparison of double-lung jet ventilation and one-lung ventilation for thoracotomy. Eur J Anaesthesiol. 2008;25(1):15–21.

112. Buise M, van Bommel J, van Genderen M, Tilanus H, van Zundert A, Gommers D. Two-lung high-frequency jet ventilation as an alternative ventilation technique during transthoracic esophagectomy. J Cardiothorac Vasc Anesth. 2009;23(4):509–12.

113. Lentz CW, Peterson HD. Smoke inhalation is a multilevel insult to the pulmonary system. Curr Opin Pulm Med. 1997;3(3):221–6.

114. Reper P, Dankaert R, van Hille F, van Laeke P, Duinslaeger L, Vanderkelen A. The usefulness of combined high-frequency percussive ventilation during acute respiratory failure after smoke inhalation. Burns. 1998;24(1):34–8.

115. Velmahos GC, Chan LS, Tatevossian R, Cornwell EE, Dougherty WR, Escudero J, Demetriades D. High-frequency percussive ventilation improves oxygenation in patients with ARDS. Chest. 1999;116(2):440–6.

116. Lucangelo U, Antonaglia V, Zin WA, Confalonieri M, Borelli M, Columban M, et al. High-frequency percussive ventilation improves perioperatively clinical evolution in pulmonary resection. Crit Care Med. 2009;37(5):1663–9.

117. Mead J, Takishima T, Leith D. Stress distribution in lungs: a model of pulmonary elasticity. J Appl Physiol. 1970;28(5):596–608.

118. Duggan M, McCaul CL, McNamara PJ, Engelberts D, Ackerley C, Kavanagh BP. Atelectasis causes vascular leak and lethal right ventricular failure in uninjured rat lungs. Am J Respir Crit Care Med. 2003;167(12):1633–40.

119. Tusman G, Böhm SH, Suarez-Sipmann F. Dead space during one-lung ventilation. Curr Opin Anesthesiol. 2015;28(1):10–7.

120. Cinnella G, Grasso S, Natale C, Sollitto F, Cacciapaglia M, Angiolillo M, et al. Physiological effects of a lung-recruiting strategy applied during one-lung ventilation. Acta Anaesthesiol Scand. 2008;52(6):766–75.

121. Vieillard-Baron A, Charron C, Jardin F. Lung recruitment or lung overinflation maneuvers? Intensive Care Med. 2006;32(1):177–8.

122. Garutti I, Martinez G, Cruz P, Piñeiro P, Olmedilla L, de la Gala F. The impact of lung recruitment on hemodynamics during one-lung ventilation. J Cardiothorac Vasc Anesth. 2009;23(4):506–8.

123. Koh WJ, Suh GY, Han J, Lee SH, Kang EH, Chung MP, et al. Recruitment maneuvers attenuate repeated derecruitment-associated lung injury. Crit Care Med. 2005;33(5):1070–6.

124. Suh GY, Koh Y, Chung MP, An CH, Kim H, Jang WY, et al. Repeated derecruitments accentuate lung injury during mechanical ventilation. Crit Care Med. 2002;30(8):1848–53.

125. Farias LL, Faffe DS, Xisto DG, Santana MC, Lassance R, Prota LF, et al. Positive end-expiratory pressure prevents lung mechanical stress caused by recruitment/derecruitment. J Appl Physiol (1985). 2005;98(1):53–61.

126. Meade MO, Cook DJ, Griffith LE, Hand LE, Lapinsky SE, Stewart TE, et al. A study of the physiologic responses to a lung recruitment maneuver in acute lung injury and acute respiratory distress syndrome. Respir Care. 2008;53(11):1441–9.

127. Sivrikoz MC, Tunçözgür B, Cekmen M, Bakir K, Meram I, Koçer E, et al. The role of tissue reperfusion in the reexpansion injury of the lungs. Eur J Cardiothorac Surg. 2002;22(5):721–7.

128. Ojima H, Kuwano H, Kato H, Miyazaki T, Nakajima M, Sohda M, Tsukada K. Relationship between cytokine response and temporary ventilation during one-lung ventilation in esophagectomy. Hepato-Gastroenterology. 2007;54(73):111–5.

129. Hansen LK, Koefoed-Nielsen J, Nielsen J, Larsson A. Are selective lung recruitment maneuvers hemodynamically safe in severe hypovolemia? An experimental study in hypovolemic pigs with lobar collapse. Anesth Analg. 2007;105(3):729–34.

130. Mahfood S, Hix WR, Aaron BL, Blaes P, Watson DC. Reexpansion pulmonary edema. Ann Thorac Surg. 1988;45(3):340–5.

131. Tekinbas C, Ulusoy H, Yulug E, Erol MM, Alver A, Yenilmez E, et al. One-lung ventilation: for how long? J Thorac Cardiovasc Surg. 2007;134(2):405–10.

132. Fernandez-Bustamante A, Wood CL, Tran ZV, Moine P. Intraoperative ventilation: incidence and risk factors for receiving large tidal volumes during general anesthesia. BMC Anesthesiol. 2011;11:22.

133. Hurford WE, Kolker AC, Strauss HW. The use of ventilation/perfusion lung scans to predict oxygenation during one-lung anesthesia. Anesth. 1987;67(5):841–3.

134. Slinger P, Suissa S, Adam J, Triolet W. Predicting arterial oxygenation during one-lung ventilation with continuous positive airway pressure to the nonventilated lung. J Cardiothorac Anesth. 1990;4(4):436–40.

135. Yamamoto Y, Watanabe S, Kano T. Gradient of bronchial end-tidal CO_2 during two-lung ventilation in lateral decubitus position is predictive of oxygenation disorder during subsequent one-lung ventilation. J Anesth. 2009;23(2):192–7.

136. Fukuoka N, Iida H, Akamatsu S, Nagase K, Iwata H, Dohi S. The association between the initial end-tidal carbon dioxide difference and the lowest arterial oxygen tension value obtained during one-lung anesthesia with propofol or sevoflurane. J Cardiothorac Vasc Anesth. 2009;23(6):775–9.

137. Brodsky JB, Lemmens HJ. Left double-lumen tubes: clinical experience with 1,170 patients. J Cardiothorac Vasc Anesth. 2003;17(3):289–98.

138. Ehrenfeld JM, Walsh JL, Sandberg WS. Right- and left-sided mallinckrodt double-lumen tubes have identical clinical performance. Anesth Analg. 2008;106(6):1847–52.

139. Baraka AS, Taha SK, Yaacoub CI. Alarming hypoxemia during one-lung ventilation in a patient with respiratory bronchiolitis-associated interstitial lung disease. Can J Anesth. 2003;50(4):411–4.

140. Russell WJ. Intermittent positive airway pressure to manage hypoxia during one-lung anaesthesia. Anaesth Intensive Care. 2009;37(3):432–4.

141. Jung DM, Ahn HJ, Jung SH, Yang M, Kim JA, Shin SM, Jeon S. Apneic oxygen insufflation decreases the incidence of hypoxemia during one-lung ventilation in open and thoracoscopic pulmonary lobectomy: a randomized controlled trial. J Thorac Cardiovasc Surg. 2017;154:360.

142. Ku CM, Slinger P, Waddell TK. A novel method of treating hypoxemia during one-lung ventilation for thoracoscopic surgery. J Cardiothorac Vasc Anesth. 2009;23(6):850–2.

143. Lohser J, McLean SR. Thoracoscopic wedge resection of the lung using high-frequency jet ventilation in a postpneumonectomy patient. A&A Case Reports. 2013;1:39–41.

144. Mierdl S, Meininger D, Dogan S, Wimmer-Greinecker G, Westphal K, Bremerich DH, Byhahn C. Does poor oxygenation during one-lung ventilation impair aerobic myocardial metabolism in patients with symptomatic coronary artery disease? Interact Cardiovasc Thorac Surg. 2007;6(2):209–13.

145. Casati A, Fanelli G, Pietropaoli P, Proietti R, Tufano R, Danelli G, et al. Continuous monitoring of cerebral oxygen saturation in elderly patients undergoing major abdominal surgery minimizes brain exposure to potential hypoxia. Anesth Analg. 2005;101(3):740–7.

146. Murkin JM, Adams SJ, Novick RJ, Quantz M, Bainbridge D, Iglesias I, et al. Monitoring brain oxygen saturation during coronary bypass surgery: a randomized, prospective study. Anesth Analg. 2007;104(1):51–8.

147. Tobias JD, Johnson GA, Rehman S, Fisher R, Caron N. Cerebral oxygenation monitoring using near infrared spectroscopy during one-lung ventilation in adults. J Minim Access Surg. 2008;4(4):104.

148. Iwata M, Inoue S, Kawaguchi M, Takahama M, Tojo T, Taniguchi S, Furuya H. Jugular bulb venous oxygen saturation during one-lung ventilation under sevoflurane- or propofol-based anesthesia for lung surgery. J Cardiothorac Vasc Anesth. 2008;22(1):71–6.

149. Van Hemelrijck J, Fitch W, Mattheussen M, Van Aken H, Plets C, Lauwers T. Effect of propofol on cerebral circulation and autoregulation in the baboon. Anesth Analg. 1990;71(1):49–54.

150. Vandesteene A, Trempont V, Engelman E, Deloof T, Focroul M, Schoutens A, Rood M. Effect of propofol on cerebral blood flow and metabolism in man. Anaesthesia. 1988;43(s1):42–3.

151. Kazan R, Bracco D, Hemmerling TM. Reduced cerebral oxygen saturation measured by absolute cerebral oximetry during thoracic surgery correlates with postoperative complications. Br J Anaesth. 2009;103(6):811–6.

152. Yuluğ E, Tekinbas C, Ulusoy H, Alver A, Yenilmez E, Aydin S, et al. The effects of oxidative stress on the liver and ileum in rats caused by one-lung ventilation. J Surg Res. 2007;139(2):253–60.

153. Pompeo E. State of the art and perspectives in non-intubated thoracic surgery. Ann Transl Med. 2014;2(11):106.

154. Tacconi F, Pompeo E. Non-intubated video-assisted thoracic surgery: where does evidence stand? J Thorac Dis. 2016;8(Suppl 4):S364–75.

155. Al-Abdullatief M, Wahood A, Al-Shirawi N, Arabi Y, Wahba M, Al-Jumah M, et al. Awake anaesthesia for major thoracic surgical procedures: an observational study. Eur J Cardiothorac Surg. 2007;32(2):346–50.

156. Pompeo E, Sorge R, Akopov A, Congregado M, Grodzki T, ESTS Non-intubated Thoracic Surgery Working Group. Non-intubated thoracic surgery-a survey from the european society of thoracic surgeons. Ann Transl Med. 2015;3(3):37.

Nonrespiratory Functions of the Lung

7

Amanda M. Kleiman and Keith E. Littlewood

Key Points

- Pulmonary endothelial cells metabolize endogenous substances and xenobiotics via ectoenzymes on their luminal surface and caveolae as well as enzyme systems within their cytosol.
- Pulmonary metabolism results in the activation of several endogenous substances and medications of importance to the anesthesiologist.
- Pulmonary uptake is often not associated with metabolism, but still markedly affects pharmacokinetics by initially attenuating peak concentrations and then returning unchanged substance to the circulation.
- The lung's ability to serve as a vascular reservoir is directly related to the capacitance of the pulmonary vessels.
- The lung serves as a physical filter, but this function may be compromised with high cardiac output and in several disease states.
- The respiratory epithelium's functions include humidification and trapping of particles and pathogens.
- The airway surface film has antimicrobial capacity beyond its mechanical removal of debris from the airway.

Introduction

For nearly two millennia of Western medicine, the lungs were thought to primarily protect the heart from overheating by exhaling warm air and from direct injury both by their position and cushioning structure. These views are ascribed to the teachings of Galen and, to some extent, Aristotle [1, 2]. Traditional Chinese medicine emphasized the interconnectedness of the organ groupings of the five phases, but within this construct, the lung was seen as a minister to the emperor heart and in partnership with the bowel to have the responsibility of maintaining the boundary of the body and outside world. In the thirteenth century, Ibn-an-Nafis of Cairo described the purification of blood by mixing with air in the lungs in one of the earliest known descriptions of gas exchange [3].

Over the last sever-al centuries, however, the biochemistry and physiology of respiration have become essentially synonymous with the lungs. From the work of pioneers such as Boyle, Lower, Priestly, Haldane, and others, most clinicians now think of the lung first and foremost as an organ of gas exchange. In more recent years, other important roles of the lung have emerged, roles that are largely in keeping with the concepts of our medical heritages.

In this sense, we now return to historic views of the lung as protector and modulator. Specifically, nonrespiratory functions of the lung including its metabolic processes, endocrine role, mechanical filtration of venous blood, warming of inspired gasses, and protection against inhaled pathogens and toxins are discussed. Focused aspects of organ structure and cellular function are reviewed as required by this discussion.

Uptake and Metabolism Within the Lung

The lungs are particularly suited for critical metabolic activities. They continuously receive essentially the entire cardiac output, and their vascular area, depending upon the

A. M. Kleiman (✉) · K. E. Littlewood
Department of Anesthesiology, University of Virginia Health System, Charlottesville, VA, USA
e-mail: ak8zg@hscmail.mcc.virginia.edu

© Springer Nature Switzerland AG 2019
P. Slinger (ed.), *Principles and Practice of Anesthesia for Thoracic Surgery*, https://doi.org/10.1007/978-3-030-00859-8_7

degree of recruitment, is an enormous 70–100 m^2. Further, the lungs contain nearly half of the body's endothelium [4] and have an extraordinarily high perfusion of 14 mL/min/g tissue (as opposed to the next-highest renal perfusion of 4 mL/min/g tissue). Thus, there is ample blood–endothelial interface for surface enzyme activity as well as uptake and secretion. The largest population of cells involved in pulmonary metabolism of blood-borne substances is, as might be expected, the pulmonary endothelium. Consistent with high metabolic activity, endothelial cells have both extensive cytoplasmic vesicles and prominent caveolae. The caveolae are tiny membrane invaginations and near-membrane vesicles similar to those found elsewhere in the body, measuring 50–100 nm, associated with caveolin proteins, and derived from lipid rafts within the membrane. The predominant activities of these caveolae, thought to include endocytosis [5] and signal transduction, have not been fully delineated and may be pleiotropic [6]. The endothelial cells structurally have large luminal projections and invaginations, providing an even greater interface area at the microscopic level.

Metabolism by the endothelial cell occurs either on the surface of the cell via enzymes associated with the membrane ("ectoenzymes") or by cytosolic processing after the substances are taken up by the cell. Some surface enzymes are distributed along the luminal membrane [7], while others are associated exclusively with the caveolae [8]. Figure 7.1 schematically depicts these processes with example substances and pathways. Metabolism may be further divided

into exogenous vs. endogenous substances as well as deactivated vs. activated products. Regardless of these considerations, it should be remembered that intensive investigation of pulmonary metabolism has developed only over the last several decades [9]. Much remains to be discovered, and conflicting data exist for drugs as central to clinical anesthesiology as propofol [10, 11].

The literature's terminology of pulmonary metabolism can be confusing and sometimes inconsistent. The careful reader must sometimes deduce the actual processes described and investigated through context. In general, "pulmonary uptake" or "extraction" is simply used to describe transfer from blood to the lung and does not indicate whether the substance of interest is subsequently metabolized or returned back into the blood with or without alteration. "First-pass" uptake is used to describe the amount of substance removed from the blood on the first cycle through the lungs, although data from techniques such as tissue slices have been used to infer this behavior. "Extraction" is also sometimes used synonymously with first-pass uptake. "Clearance" may be used to describe a substance undergoing actual elimination, either in terms similar to renal clearance as volume of blood from which the substance would be completely removed (mL/min or mL/kg min) or as a comparison of pulmonary arterial concentration vs. systemic arterial concentration. Terms used for isolated lung studies include "accumulation," the percentage of substance retained in the lungs after equilibrium, and "persistence," percentage of substance retained after washout.

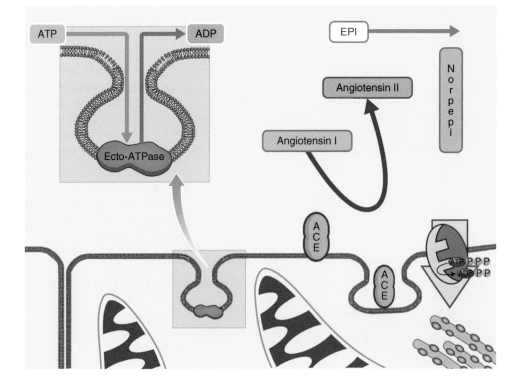

Fig. 7.1 Schematic examples of pulmonary endothelial metabolism. Surface enzymes may be restricted to the caveolae (Ecto-ATPase in the inset above is an example) or present on both the luminal surface and caveola (e.g., angiotensin-converting enzyme [ACE]). Another characteristic of pulmonary endothelium is selective uptake, here exemplified by the ATP-dependent uptake of norepinehrine (NOREPI), while epinephrine (EPI) is not taken up. See text for details

It is beyond the scope of this discussion to fully detail the experimental methods used in the investigation of pulmonary metabolism, but the challenges of investigation and data interpretation merit at least mention. As implied above, lung metabolism has been investigated in vitro and in vivo. In vitro techniques include the use of cellular fractionates, tissue homogenates, and tissue slices. Recent advances in uniform preparation and cryoprotection have made tissue slices an attractive, cost-efficient option [12] despite concerns regarding the impact of processing on enzyme behavior. Tissue slices have a particular advantage in lung research because they include all cell types. The isolated and perfused animal lung model represents the next level of fidelity. The lung can remain within the animal or be explanted, and the uses of various perfusion managements (e.g., nonpulsatile vs. pulsatile, blood vs. crystalloid, and one-pass vs. recirculation) have been described with little standardization. Further, various investigators commonly subject the lung to no inflation, constant airway pressure, or positive pressure ventilation. The impact of these differences in ventilation on resultant data is unknown. In the next level of modeling, in intact animals and human subjects, the pulmonary uptake is assessed by measurements of the difference between pulmonary arterial and pulmonary venous (animals) or systemic arterial (human) concentrations of the substance in question, typically after a controlled bolus and/or infusion when possible. These invasive requirements do not lend themselves to large volunteer studies. In fact, most human subjects are critically ill and/or undergoing complex procedures. This variation in disease and treatment may produce data that in turn has great variance [13]. Conversely, inclusion criteria rigorous enough to provide consistent results produce a patient population in which the results are of limited general applicability [14]. A variation of the method just described is the double-indicator dilution technique [15]. In this technique, the substance of interest and a substance with no (or no known) pulmonary uptake are injected, typically into the right atrium. Samples are then taken from a systemic artery, with the known substance serving as the control to which the investigated substance's concentration curve is compared. This technique is more practical in terms of decreased frequency of sampling and somewhat decreased invasiveness.

It is important to reemphasize that the lung has a profound impact on the blood concentration of substances even when it does not ultimately metabolize or secrete them. This is because of the simple uptake and retention of substances, often followed by release back into the blood. This "capacitor effect" [16] of the lungs in which any rapid rise or fall in concentration is attenuated will be revisited in the discussion below as it pertains to local anesthetic toxicity.

With these limitations in mind, we shall first review the current understanding of drug metabolism with focus on medications of particular interest to the anesthesiologist, and

Table 7.1 The lung and medications of interest to anesthesiologists

Drug class	Impact of passage through the pulmonary circulation	
	Minimal or none	First-pass uptake and/or metabolism
Hypnotics		Thiopental +
		Ketamine ++
		Propofol ++
Benzodiazepines		Diazepam ++
Nondepolarizing muscle relaxants	Rocuronium	
	Vecuronium	
	Rapacuronium	
	d-tubocurarine	
Opiates	Morphine	Fentanyl ++
		Sufentanil +
		Alfentanil ±
Catecholamines	Dopamine	Norepinephrine +
	Epinephrine	
	Isoproterenol	
Local anesthetics		Bupivacaine +
		Lidocaine ++

then look at metabolism of endogenous substances. Even though they are also administered therapeutically and duplicated in the summary of medications, endogenously produced substances such as catecholamines will be included in the latter discussion (Table 7.1).

Drugs

The cytochrome P-450 monooxygenase enzyme systems are the most studied metabolic pathways for medications. The lungs have substantial concentrations of P-450 isoenzymes, particularly within type II pneumocytes, Clara cells, and endothelial cells [17]. This implies that the lung has the capacity for drug metabolism via P-450 systems. While P-450 and other enzyme systems have long been known to exist in the human lung (Table 7.2), the actual activity of lung enzymes ranges from negligible to 33% of that of the liver [19]. The difference between organ enzyme activity of different species is large (lung to liver activity varying from a few percent to 111%) and mandates caution when interpreting animal data [20].

Opioids

Fentanyl has been shown to have a markedly variable first-pass uptake of up to 90% in humans [21]. The same investigators found that significant amounts of fentanyl are returned from the lungs into the blood with a biphasic pattern, equilibrating after about a minute in the fast phase and nearly 25 min for the slow phase. The uptake of fentanyl is higher than expected even for this basic and lipophilic drug. In fact,

Table 7.2 Enzyme systems of the lung [18]

Cytochrome P-450 oxygenase
Sulfotransferase
Nitroreductase
N-Methyltransferase
Glutathione-S-epoxide transferase
Glutathione-S-aryl transferase
Glucuronyl transferase
Epoxide hydrolase
Amine oxidase

active uptake of fentanyl has been demonstrated in human lung endothelial cells [22].

The study of alfentanil has led to widely variant first-pass uptake data. Uptakes of 67% have been reported [21], although more commonly uptakes of approximately 10% are reported [23]. Of note, these studies included other medications (sufentanil and morphine in one study and fentanyl in the other) that were found to behave similarly to accepted data for those drugs. This makes the discrepancy for alfentanil behavior particularly hard to interpret.

Sufentanil demonstrates uptake that is a little more than half that of fentanyl. A study in which patients had received alfentanil for induction followed by a sufentanil infusion of 50 μg/min for 10 min showed sufentanil first-pass uptake of about 50% with a 20-min retention of about 20% [24]. The investigators incidentally noted that smokers had a statistically higher retention of the infused dose.

Early work with morphine in the perfused rabbit lung model showed about 30% first-pass uptake [25]. Interestingly, subsequent work in intact animals and in humans has found much lower uptake of about 10% [23, 26], including postoperative bolus and infusion [27]. Metabolism has generally been found to be negligible.

Muscle Relaxants

There is a paucity of data on pulmonary pharmacokinetics of muscle relaxants. This may be because the agents studied, including vecuronium, rocuronium, d-tubocurarine, rapacuronium, and Org 7617, demonstrated no first-pass uptake or metabolism in the intact porcine model [28]. This would appear to have generated little enthusiasm for further investigation of this class of drugs.

Local Anesthetics

Lidocaine has a long history of investigation in terms of pulmonary uptake and metabolism. The general consistencies across species include a first-pass uptake of approximately 50% with significant retention at 10 min [29–31]. The uptake of lidocaine has also been examined in a variety of physiological circumstances. Under extremes of metabolic acidosis and alkalosis [30], lidocaine demonstrates increased uptake with higher blood pH. It is postulated that this finding is the consequence of increased drug lipophilicity, since, in a less acidic environment, more of the drug is in its nonionized form. Under extremes of FiO_2 in in vivo isolated lobes of dogs under nitrous oxide and halothane anesthesia, there were no differences demonstrated in lidocaine uptake [32]. Of interest, the prolonged retention in all groups was less than that commonly reported in other studies, raising the issue of the effects of this particular model on uptake.

Bupivacaine has been investigated less extensively than lidocaine with less consistent results. In most animal species, peak extraction has been reported as high with variable first-pass retention between species and methodology [33–35]. In humans, however, the effective first-pass extraction appears to be lower when studied by epidural dosing [36, 37]. As in the case of lidocaine, the pulmonary pharmacokinetics of bupivacaine have also been investigated in acidosis. In a rabbit model, animals with a pH of 7.0–7.1 demonstrated decreased maximum pulmonary extraction as a group [38] with resultant higher peak systemic concentrations of drugs.

Two recent areas of interest in the practice of clinical anesthesia are intimately linked with the pulmonary uptake of local anesthetics. The first is the relative safety of levobupivacaine and ropivacaine in comparison to bupivacaine. These drugs have, in fact, been the subject of several investigations. Early animal studies suggested decreased toxicity of these newer preparations [39, 40]. The discussion continues, however, with more recent work regarding the pulmonary uptake of these drugs. In rabbits, for example, the uptake of levobupivacaine is higher than ropivacaine with resultant lower systemic blood concentrations of levobupivicaine [41]. The authors thus caution that the lower absolute toxicity of ropivacaine may be tempered by the lung's greater attenuation of peak levobupivacaine levels in inadvertent intravenous injections. A recent review of the pharmacodynamics and pharmacokinetics of local anesthetics [42] focuses on the challenges of comparing toxicities in clinical practice [43–45]. Animal models, with the limitations already discussed among many more [46], must be utilized since clinical toxicity is an uncontrolled, rare, and dangerous event [47]. Other questions are raised by the relative central nervous system and cardiovascular toxicity between drugs and study variation in drug administration and measurement. The inconsistencies in the data of pulmonary uptake are thus one of many challenges in understanding the clinical toxicities of local anesthetics.

A second, related, area of great contemporary interest is the treatment of local anesthetic toxicity with lipid emulsion [48, 49]. A recent case report, in particular, is germane to the discussion of pulmonary uptake [50]. Briefly, a patient undergoing brachial plexus block with bupivacaine demonstrated evidence of toxicity by progressive symptomatology, seizures, widening QRS tachycardia, and asystole. Successful emulsified lipid "rescue" was followed nearly an hour later by recurrence of episodic ventricular tachycardia. The authors believe that this represented the first reported recurrence of toxic bupivacaine levels after lipid treatment. Several possible causes were postulated for this phenomenon, including postresuscitation hepatic dysfunction, reversal of generalized peripheral ion trapping of bupivacaine, and, appropriately, release of bupivacaine from the pulmonary vasculature. Thus, it seems that the issue of pulmonary uptake and release of local anesthetics must be considered in the treatment of suspected local anesthetic toxicity with emulsified lipid.

Hypnotics

There are limited, and sometimes dated, data regarding the pulmonary metabolism of intravenous induction agents. Thiopental has been found to have nearly 15% first-pass uptake in humans [51] with little or no metabolism. Ketamine shows marked species variation in its metabolism. In rabbit homogenate, the eventual complete disappearance of ketamine with only half being metabolized to norketamine implies the production of other metabolite(s) [52]. Lung tissue homogenate was more quickly saturated than liver tissue. As previously mentioned, the applicability of this homogenate data to intact animals, and certainly to humans, is unknown. In dogs under halothane anesthesia, the pulmonary uptake of ketamine was found to be slightly less than 10% without subsequent metabolism [53]. Human data are lacking.

The clarification of propofol uptake and metabolism by the lungs has taken many turns. One of the earliest studies in sheep with propofol administered as the sole medication demonstrated an apparent steady-state pulmonary clearance of 1.21 L/min [54] with negligible drug accumulation in the lung tissue, while a later study in sheep demonstrated a similar 1.14 L/min pulmonary clearance [55]. Other early works found that propofol uptake in cats was nearly 60%, but this uptake was particularly decreased in the presence of halothane or fentanyl [56]. Microsomal fractions from rat, rabbit, and human lung showed no glucuronidation of propofol [57]. Turning to data from human clinical studies, most recent work shows about 30% first-pass uptake and negligible metabolism of propofol by the lungs [11, 58]. It is interesting that a recently developed model of propofol pharmacodynamics and pharmacokinetics [59] has produced a very good fit with data from human studies [60, 61]. In this work, the lung is modeled as three tanks in series with the full cardiac output sequentially flowing to each, a model previously proven effective [62] in simulating the behavior of markers indocyanine green and antipyrine as well as the narcotic alfentanil.

Inhaled Medications

A number of medications include inhaled formulations. The inhaled route offers multiple benefits for drug delivery including a large absorptive surface area, high epithelial permeability, increased vascularity, avoidance of first-pass metabolism, and fast onset [63]. The majority of inhaled medications are used to treat the lungs directly, offering localized, targeted delivery and avoidance of systemic absorption. However, several drugs to treat illnesses from migraine headaches to diabetes are currently under development [63].

The handling of aerosolized drugs occurs via four processes including deposition, dissolution, absorption, and clearance. The site of deposition in the respiratory tract determines the treatment of most inhaled medications and is determined by the size of the particle. Chronic lung diseases including asthma, chronic bronchitis, and emphysema affect the deposition of aerosolized particles by narrowing the smaller airways resulting in deposition in larger airways [64]. The epithelial lining fluid has direct contact with the aerosolized particles, and the thickness and composition of the layer vary according to the site of deposition. Dissolution of particles into the fluid layer is controlled by the hydrophilicity of the particle. Water-soluble particles (e.g., albuterol, insulin) dissolve into the fluid and are freely absorbed [65]. In poorly water-soluble drugs (e.g., budesonide, fluticasone), the dose exceeds the aqueous solubility and the absorption is determined by dissolution-controlled kinetics [65]. Once dissolved, the speed of absorption depends on the size of the particle with smaller drugs quickly absorbed within minutes. The absorption of larger proteins is more complex but typically slower with more variable bioavailability [66]. Absorption occurs via several mechanisms. Passive diffusion occurs primarily via intercellular junction pores for hydrophilic compounds and transcellular diffusion for hydrophobic compounds. Drugs with low passive permeability utilize drug carrier transporters for uptake and transfer across cell membranes [67]. Like deposition, absorption may be impacted by chronic pulmonary disease due to deposition in the diseased upper airways, thickened mucous, and reduced surface area of diseased lungs. This may be beneficial in the treatment of chronic pulmonary diseases by preventing systemic absorption and increasing local drug effects. Hydrophilic substances may have increased absorption in the presence of chronic inflammation due to decreased epithelial barrier function and tight junction dysregulation with

full response to pulmonary embolism [88]. The infusion of a serotonin antagonist in animals was found to attenuate the increase in pulmonary pressures associated with pulmonary embolism [89], supporting the role of 5-HT in this response.

Histamine, in contrast to 5-HT, has almost no uptake in the pulmonary circulation. Lung homogenates are capable of histamine metabolism [90], but the intact lung appears to lack an uptake mechanism for histamine.

Just as the lung has the enzymes to metabolize both histamine and serotonin but the ability to take up only serotonin, its uptake of catecholamines also demonstrates marked selectivity. Norepinephrine demonstrates a 35–50% first-pass uptake with subsequent metabolism by catechol-O-methyltransferase (COMT), MAO, aldehyde reductase, and aldehyde dehydrogenase [91]. Dopamine and epinephrine, however, have essentially no uptake although they would be susceptible to the cytosolic enzymes, as again proven by cell homogenates. The synthetic catecholamine isoproterenol also has no appreciable uptake by the lung.

Arachidonic Acid Metabolites

Extensive production and metabolism of arachidonic acid derivatives occur in the lung. The term eicosanoids refers to the 20-carbon carboxylic acids derived from the metabolism of the lipid membrane component icosatetraenoic acid, more commonly known as arachidonic acid. The action of phospholipase A_2 converts the esterified form, as found in the membrane, and releases arachidonic acid from structural glycerol. Once free, arachidonic acid may follow three main metabolic pathways in the lung. The lipoxygenase pathway produces leukotrienes, lipoxins, and some of the hydroxyeicosatetraenoic acids (HETEs). The cyclooxygenase (COX) pathway produces prostaglandins, thromboxane, and prostacyclin. The cytochrome P-450 monooxygenase system produces cis-epoxyeicosatrienoic acids and HETEs that are different than the products of the lipoxygenase pathway.

The lipoxygenase pathways produce leukotrienes and lipoxins. The formation of all leukotrienes starts from a common precursor. 5-Lipoxygenase, located in the perinuclear cytosol, responds to increased calcium in concert with its activating protein to generate 5-hydroperoxyeicosatetraenoic acids (5-HPETE) from arachidonic acid. A dehydrase then yields the relatively unstable leukotriene A_4 (LTA$_4$), which may undergo transformation by epoxide hydrolase (LTA$_4$ hydrolase) to LTB$_4$ which leaves the cell via a transport protein. The alternative pathway for LTA$_4$ is via LTC$_4$ synthase to form LTC$_4$, which is converted by nonspecific interstitial peptidases to the leukotrienes LTD$_4$ and LTE$_4$ (commonly referred to as slow-reacting substance of anaphylaxis). Whereas closely related prostanoids (see below) demonstrate opposing biological actions, the leukotrienes uniformly promote inflammatory responses in the lung. They are responsible for bronchoconstriction and increased pulmonary vascular permeability, are chemotactic and chemokinetic for neutrophils, and facilitate eosinophil degranulation [92–94]. They are produced by activated inflammatory cells within the lung as well as those arriving in response to inflammation. It should be no surprise that leukotrienes have been the subject of investigation in processes ranging from hypoxic pulmonary vasoconstriction in normal as well as damaged lungs [95, 96] to the pathogenesis of adult respiratory distress syndrome (ARDS) [97–99] and asthma [100]. This work has been especially fruitful in the case of asthma, for which leukotriene modifiers are a mainstay of treatment [101–103].

There appears to be little specialized pulmonary uptake or metabolism of the leukotrienes beyond the inactivation of LTB$_4$ and LTC$_4$ by neutrophils in the lung. Nonspecific hydroxylation and carboxylation of leukotrienes also occur in the interstitium, similar to that of other tissues [104].

The lipoxins have been identified as critical factors in the resolution of inflammation throughout the body, now seen more as an active process than the simple "burnout" of pro-inflammatory processes [105, 106]. There are three main synthetic routes of lipoxin formation, involving interactions of products from 5-lipoxygenase, 15-lipoxygenase, and/or 12-lipoxygenase, with the eventual formation of the two lipoxins, the positional isomers lipoxin A_4 (LxA$_4$) and B$_4$ (LxB$_4$). The lipoxins have a variety of antiinflammatory effects. They inhibit eosinophil and neutrophil chemotaxis and adhesion, as well as natural killer cell activation [107–110]. They are endothelium-dependent vasodilators of both pulmonary and systemic vasculature [111]. The lipoxins have been investigated extensively for their role in lung physiology and disease. Asthma, in particular, has received a great deal of attention [112]. Work thus far indicates that lipoxins are decreased in the sputum [113] and blood [114] of patients with severe asthma. The balance between leukotriene and lipoxin activity, in particular, has been found related to disease severity [115], raising the possibility of inducing lipoxin activity [116] as an adjunct to leukotriene modifiers. The role of lipoxins has also been considered in the active resolution of acute lung injury [117].

The lipoxins are predominately taken up by circulating monocytes with subsequent dehydrogenation [118]. No specific pulmonary uptake or metabolism of lipoxins has been described.

As implied by its name, COX catalyzes the cyclization and oxygenation of arachidonic acid, producing prostaglandin PGG$_2$, which is converted by nonspecific peroxidase(s) to the unstable precursor PGH$_2$. There are subtypes of COX, most notably COX-1 and COX-2. There has been great interest in COX-2 since its discovery in the 1990s because its inhibition was hoped to be more specific in controlling pain and inflammation without injury to the gastroduodenal mucosa [119,

120]. Although effective, the emergence of a small but real increase in cardiovascular risk of COX-2 inhibitors [121] has tempered their use. Complicating this issue further is that many of the "traditional" COX inhibitors such as acetaminophen, salicylates, and the nonsteroidal antiinflammatory agents ibuprofen and naproxen show only slightly less COX-2 avidity than some of the newer COX-2 inhibitors.

Following the production of PGH_2, the metabolic pathway divides into branches producing the various bioactive prostanoids; the enzymes of particular interest here are PGD synthase, PGE synthase, prostacyclin synthase, and thromboxane synthase. The final products of these pathways typically have oppositional or balancing effects locally and regionally. Prostaglandin E_2 (PGE_2) and PGI_2 are bronchodilators, for example, while $PGF_{2\alpha}$, PGD_2, and thromboxane A_2 (TXA_2) cause bronchoconstriction. Similarly, PGD_2, PGE_2, $PGF_{2\alpha}$, and TXA_2 are potent vasoconstrictors, while PGE_1 and PGF_2 are vasodilators.

Pulmonary endothelial cell cultures demonstrate virtually all COX pathway products to some extent, but the level of in vivo production is less clear. PGI_2 appears to be continuously produced, with modulation by vascular flow [122]. PGD_2, PGE_1, PGE_2, PGI_2, $PGF_{2\alpha}$, and TXB_2 have all been found to be produced by human lungs, although under varying circumstances [123, 124].

The discussion of the pulmonary metabolism of COX products includes the now familiar theme of a broad range of intracellular enzymes (by cell culture and cellular homogenate investigation) but selective uptake. In this way, at least 80–90% of PGD_1, PGE_2, and $PGF_{2\alpha}$ are taken up and metabolized in a first-pass through intact pulmonary circulation; but PGA_1, PGA_2, and PGI_2 demonstrate essentially no uptake [24, 125, 126]. TXA_2, a relatively unstable compound, presents a special case in the discussion of pulmonary uptake. TXA_2 undergoes hydrolysis in the blood, forming TXB_2. It is TXB_2 that is taken up by a carrier for cytosolic metabolism and is often utilized as an investigative marker of TXA_2 activity [127].

The P-450 monooxygenase system provides three pathways of arachidonic acid metabolism which results in epoxyeicosatetraenoic acids (EETs), HETEs, or dihydroxyeicosatetraenoic acids (dHETEs). These pathways are not unique to the endothelium, epithelium, and smooth muscle of the lung, being found in several other organs including the gastrointestinal tract, liver, and kidney [128]. Subfamilies of cytochrome P-450 systems have been identified within the lung. The CYPA4 family produces 20-HETE, while the CYP2J family is found in epithelial, bronchial, and vascular smooth muscle cells, as well as endothelial and alveolar macrophages [129].

The HETEs and EETs have been shown experimentally to affect pulmonary vascular and bronchomotor tone. 20 HETE and 5, 6, 11, and 12-EETs all have relaxing effects on both the lung vasculature and airways [130, 131]. They are further known to have general antiinflammatory effects, to modulate

reperfusion injury, and to inhibit platelet aggregation. Within the lung, 15-HETE and 20-HETE may both modify hypoxic vasoconstriction [132].

Natriuretic Peptides

The natriuretic peptides currently consist of, in order of their discovery during the 1980s, atrial natriuretic peptide (ANP), brain natriuretic peptide, and C-type natriuretic peptide. ANP has received the most attention in terms of pulmonary pharmacokinetics. It is a pulmonary artery (and to a lesser extent, venous) vasodilator whose action is independent of endothelial function. ANP is known to interact with the renin–angiotensin–aldosterone system at several points. Best described are suppression of renin release, decrease in angiotensin-converting enzyme activity, and blocking of aldosterone release. These actions promote natriuresis and diuresis. ANP is mainly produced in the cardiac atria, but both ANP and its prohormone have been found in the human fetal lung [133] and adult pulmonary veins [134]. Lung production is suppressed by hypovolemia and increased with hypoxemia, hypervolemia, and in the presence of glucocorticoids. In terms of elimination, the rabbit lung demonstrates a 25% first-pass uptake of ANP [135].

Other Endogenous Substances

The number of substances handled by the lung and the intricacies of their metabolism precludes full discussion here. For the interested reader, several historically and/or clinically important substances are listed in Table 7.3, and references

Table 7.3 Lung effects on endogenous substances relevant to the anesthesiologist

Group	Impact of passage through the pulmonary circulation		
	Activated	Minimal or none	First-pass uptake and/or metabolism
Peptides	Angiotensin I	Angiotensin II	Endothelins
		Vasopressin	Bradykinin
		Oxytocin	
		Atrial natriuretic peptide	
Steroids	Cortisone		Beclomethasone
			Progesterone
Purine family			Adenosine phosphates (AMP, ADP, ATP)
Arachidonic acid family		PGA_2	PGD_2
		Prostacyclin (PGI_2)	PGE_2
			PGF_2
			Leukotrienes
Biogenic amines		Dopamine	5-HT
		Epinephrine	Norepinephrine
		Histamine	

are provided for the activation of cortisone to cortisol in health [136, 137] and disease [138], the behavior of endothelin in several clinical circumstances [76, 139, 140], and new perspectives on purine metabolism by endothelial ectoenzymes [138].

The Lung as Vascular Reservoir and Filter

The volume of blood within the lungs under various conditions has been a subject of investigation for over 80 years [141]. What is known is that the pulmonary vasculature in health has remarkable capacitance, allowing it to accept wide ranges of right ventricular output with minimal change in pressure. This ability to load and offload volume allows the lungs to serve as a vascular reservoir to meet the preload needs of the left heart as they change due to factors such as posture, exercise, changes in intrathoracic pressure (e.g., Valsalva maneuver), and daily volume shifts [142]. The role of pulmonary vascular capacitance is also emerging in our understanding of disease processes relevant to clinical anesthesiology. Models of heart failure, for example, now incorporate the role of vascular compliance in general and the pulmonary vasculature capacitance and permeability specifically [143]. Also of interest to anesthesiologists, researchers have found that following the release of the tourniquet in total knee arthroplasty, there is an actual decrease in pulmonary vascular resistance. A clue to the mechanism of this finding was metabolic evidence of increased endothelial recruitment with this obligatory microembolism [144].

The unique anatomical position of the lungs as they receive the entire right heart output allows them to serve as physical filters, in much the same way that they metabolically play a pivotal role in the uptake of endogenous substances and xenobiotics. Particles normally filtered by the lung before reaching the systemic circulation include small blood clots, fat droplets, agglutinated white blood cells, and amniotic fluid in the case of pregnancy. The literature commonly alludes to the ability of 350 and even 500 μm glass beads to pass through the pulmonary vasculature in animal models. Given that normal pulmonary capillaries have a diameter of 7–10 μm, this implies other arteriovenous communications under normal conditions. Recent work in isolated, but normally ventilated, animal and human lungs and, especially, exercised human subjects implies a more complicated picture. It now appears that, indeed, arteriovenous passage of particles larger than 50 μm occurs in isolated lungs, although more than 99% of such glass microspheres are trapped by the lungs [145]. In human volunteers, aggregated albumin tagged with technetium-99 and with diameters of 7–25 μm was found to have about 0.7% transpulmonary passage at rest. This rose to 3%

passage with exercise, as demonstrated by aggregate trapping in systemic capillaries. This implies the recruitment of intrapulmonary arteriovenous pathways with exercise which presumably allow decreased resistance to flow but also compromise the lung's competence as a mechanical filter [146]. The lung's protection of systemic circulation from embolus can also, of course, be completely subverted by anatomic variants and pathological states. The latter is exemplified by the hepatopulmonary syndrome's intrapulmonary vascular dilatations, which have been associated with patient injury from embolism [147]. The patent foramen ovale and its potential for catastrophic embolic phenomena in the perioperative period [18, 146, 148] have long been appreciated and feared by anesthesiologists as the classic anatomic variant which bypasses the protective filtration of the pulmonary vasculature.

The Respiratory Epithelium

The lung defends the body not only by mechanical filtration and metabolism of substances from the blood but also from airborne agents. In this way, the constantly renewing airway epithelium is responsible for helping to maintain normal gas exchange from the trachea to the terminal alveoli. The respiratory epithelium represents a huge surface area that is a gateway from the outside world to the exquisitely delicate alveoli, a path taken by both life-sustaining oxygen and potentially damaging particles and gasses. This defensive challenge is especially impressive when considering both the wide range of conditions to which the modern human is exposed and the simple fact that even a somewhat sedentary adult can be expected to inhale well over 10,000 L of gas from his/her environment in a day. The discussion below will briefly review the structure and function of this system and then the way in which it provides protection through the mucociliary apparatus, trapping of particles, and response to particles and pathogens.

The Cells of the Respiratory Epithelium

While some 50 distinct cell types have been identified in the human airway [149], our discussion will focus on those most important to the lung's nonrespiratory functions.

Ciliated Columnar Cells

These cells are the most common of the respiratory epithelium. Their most obvious defining feature is several hundred cilia moving at a rate of about 12 cycles per second, always toward the trachea. As might be expected, this

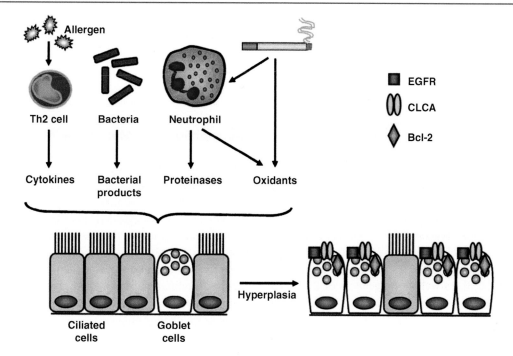

Fig. 7.3 Airway goblet cell hyperplasia. Simplified schematic outlining selected pathways generating increased epithelial mucin production. Cytokines (e.g., interleukin-4, interleukin-9 and interleukin-13), bacterial products (e.g., lipopolysaccharide and lipoteichoic acid), proteinases (e.g., elastase and cathepsin G), and oxidants from T helper-2 (Th2) lymphocytes, bacteria, neutrophils, and cigarette smoke upregulate mucin production and/or induce goblet cell hyperplasia with asso-

ciated increases in expression of epidermal growth factor receptors (EGFR), calcium-activated chloride channels (CLCA), and the anti-apoptotic factor Bcl-2. Note: not all stimuli have yet been shown to induce expression of each of EGFR, CLCA, and Bcl-2. In addition, production of new goblet cells appears to involve differentiation of non-granulated epithelial cells rather than goblet cell division. (Reproduced with permission. Rogers [150]. Copyright Elsevier)

process requires large energy expenditures, and, in fact, the cells have extensive populations of mitochondria for energy production. The cellular architecture and shape change according to position in the respiratory tract. In the nose, pharynx, and large airways, the columnar cells are pseudostratified, layered over the basal cells which are thought to be the stem cells for both ciliated and goblet cells. Moving down the bronchi, they gradually thin to a single layer. Further still, in the bronchioles, the columnar cells transition to a layer of cuboidal cells and then, approaching the terminal airways, they mix with type I alveolar cells.

Goblet Cells

These specialized columnar epithelial cells can rapidly secrete mucins (high molecular weight mucous glycoproteins) which provide a protective layer over the epithelium when it combines with other lipid, glycoconjugate, and protein components [150]. Mucin is released by exocytosis in response to a variety of stimuli such as dust, microorganisms, fumes, and debris within the airway. Hyperplasia in response to chronic stimulation is a

hallmark of the goblet cell population (Fig. 7.3) and typical of disease processes such as asthma, bronchitis, and cystic fibrosis [151].

Submucosal Secretory Cells

There are actually two types of submucosal secretory cells. Both are associated with the submucosal glands of the trachea and large bronchi. These glands are innervated by cholinergic fibers from the vagus [152] and are located in the submucosa between the smooth muscle and cartilage plate. The serous-type cells account for more than half of the submucosal gland in health and contain multiple secretory granules. Proteoglycans, lysozyme, lactoferrin, IgA receptor complex, peroxidase, and antiproteases are among the contents of these granules. The mucous-type cells are columnar cells with a high density of cell granules containing mucin. It is thought that serous cells transdifferentiate to mucous cells in response to injury from inhaled agents and the resulting predominance of mucous cells plays a role in the change of the character of mucus in response to injury. While it is accepted that both the submucosal secretory cells and goblet cells contribute to airway mucus, there is apparent variability in the relative contribution of these cells on the basis of airway level, experimental model, and species [153–156].

Clara Cells

Clara cells (nonciliated bronchial secretory cells) are normally found predominately in the terminal bronchioles (Fig. 7.4). Their granules secrete Clara cell secretory protein (CCSP), the function of which is poorly defined. In an animal model, antigenic challenge results in proliferation of tracheobronchial Clara cells that secret not only CCSP but also demonstrate secretion of mucin [156]. Conversely, in normal humans, bronchiolar goblet cells have been found to secrete CCSP, leading to speculation that Clara cells may be goblet cell precursors [158], as well as progenitors of the epithelium [157].

Mast Cells

Mast cells are located throughout the lung, from typical locations under the airway epithelium and in the alveolar septum to those freely positioned in the airway. They have traditionally been associated with acquired immunity, but

recent evidence indicates that mast cells also have important roles in innate immunity and inflammatory regulation [159]. Specifically, their role as sentinel for innate immunity seems to bridge the classic with the more recently appreciated roles [160].

Macrophages and Monocytes

Macrophages and monocytes can be categorized as (1) airway and alveolar macrophages, (2) interstitial macrophages, and (3) pulmonary vascular monocytes. This scheme does not include the monocyte derivative dendritic cells. There are limited data regarding the sparse interstitial macrophage population, mostly from animal preparations. There is no evidence that the intravascular monocytes of the lung are particularly different from monocytes throughout the body's vascular system, transforming into macrophages within the tissue to which they migrate.

The alveolar macrophages must routinely phagocytize a dizzying array of invaders of the airspace. These include dust and particulates as well as bacteria, yeasts, and other organic and inorganic debris. Phagosomes initially envelope the ingested target and then are merged with lysosomes. The latter contain hydrolytic enzymes, which efficiently destroy the majority of bacteria, yeasts, and debris encountered. For some

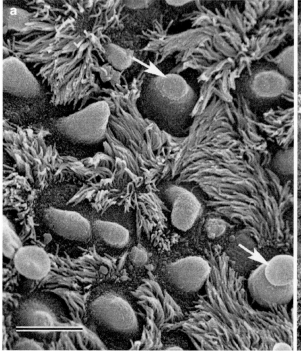
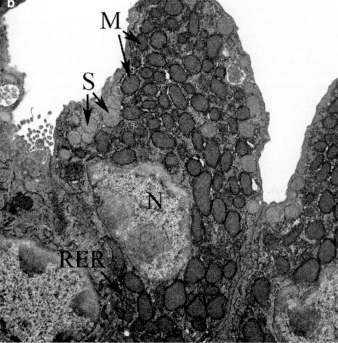

Fig. 7.4 (**a**) Scanning electron micrograph of the lining of the proximal bronchiole of a rat showing Clara cells, some of which are undergoing apocrine secretion (*arrows*), surrounded by ciliated cells (bar = 10 μm). (**b**) Transmission electron micrograph of a terminal bron- chiolar Clara cell. Numerous mitochondria (M), secretory granules (S), rough endoplasmic reticulum (RER), and the basal nucleus (N) are indicated. (Reproduced with permission. Reynolds and Malkinson [157]. Copyright Elsevier)

microorganisms (e.g., mycobacteria and many gram-negative bacteria) and materials, the lysosomal system is not effective. In this case, secondary lysosomes are now used essentially as storage areas, where the material is isolated for the life of the macrophage. The fate of these laden cells is not uniform. It appears that some are swept away by the mucociliary apparatus for mechanical elimination and others remain in the lung for as long as months before dying and releasing their sequestered contents for uptake by successor macrophages. There has been recent attention to the translocation of particles from the lung to lymph nodes and other organs [161, 162], presumably in conjunction with alveolar macrophage activity.

Alveolar Epithelial Cells

Alveolar epithelial type I and type II cells (also referred to as type I and II pneumocytes) line the terminal alveoli. Type I cells are thin sheets lining the alveoli with each covering several capillaries. Type I cells cover approximately 90% of lung surface area and are responsible for maintaining lung fluid homeostasis. The tight junctions between cells are well described and thought to provide only a 1-μm gap under normal circumstances. Historically thought to serve as a barrier to the movement of solutes and water into the alveoli, more recent work with sodium and chloride transporters has found evidence of active epithelial mechanisms for fluid transport in both health and diseased states [163, 164]. Additionally, the presence of caveolae and intracellular vacuoles suggests that type I cells may also have endocytic function and participate in metabolic activities [165]. Type II alveolar epithelial cells tend to be clustered at alveolar junction points. They are cuboidal cells with lamellar bodies in the cytoplasm and numerous mitochondria. The lamellar bodies are inclusions of variable size and composed of stacked layers of membrane-like material. It is this material which is processed and released as surfactant by the type II cell [166]. Four types of surfactant proteins A, B, C, and D (SP-A through SP-D) have been identified. SP-A and SP-D modulate surfactant release, while SP-B and SP-C stabilize the surfactant monolayer discussed below [167]. SP-B is the protein absolutely required for survival, but important contributions have been discovered for the other SP proteins. SP-A and SP-D, for example, play immune roles by direct antimicrobial activity and enhancement of macrophage recognition of microorganisms.

Functions of the Respiratory Epithelium

The functions of the respiratory epithelium that will be reviewed here include maintenance of the complex liquid film of the airway, humidification, removal of inhaled materials, and response to inhaled pathogens.

Airway Surface Film

The surface liquid of the airway, in health, is about 10 μm thick. It consists of two layers, namely, the periciliary sol underneath a second layer of mucus gel. The sol is a low-viscosity watery liquid that surrounds the cilia. The mucus, as discussed previously, is produced by the submucosal glands and goblet cells in response to a variety of irritants. The complex gel-aqueous becomes progressively thinner from the trachea (100 μm) to the bronchi (8 μm) and then to terminal bronchioles (3 μm) [168]. The cilia are too tightly arranged for the mucus gel to find its way between cilia, thus the gel layer contacts only the ciliary tips along its bottom edge. The cilia, then, are free to move in their well-characterized rhythmic pattern with relatively less resistance from the minimally viscous sol. In this manner, the cilia propel the mucous layer toward the trachea at a rate of 3–4 mm/min [169]. The thickness of the layers of this system, especially the sol, must be maintained within very narrow tolerances for mechanical efficiency. This is achieved in large extent by simple osmotic gradient and probably accounts for much of the adjustment that occurs as larger amounts of mucus converge in the larger airways. Adjustments of sol osmolarity to effect this mechanism occur through the activity of the amiloride-sensitive chloride channel, more commonly referred to as the cystic fibrosis transmembrane conductance regulator (CFTR) protein. Indeed, the ravages of cystic fibrosis are now thought to start at least in part because of the relative depletion of the sol, emphasizing the delicate nature of the system just described [170]. The antimicrobial capabilities of the mucociliary apparatus will be discussed below.

Humidification

The respiratory system has enormous capacity to humidify inspired gas. At rest, air is completely saturated with water vapor as it passes through the nose and upper airway, before it reaches the trachea. As minute ventilation (MV) increases, smaller and smaller airways are required to contribute to humidification, such that at a MV of 50 L min^{-1}, airways of only a few millimeters in diameter receive incompletely humidified gas [171]. The airways do reclaim some of the heat and moisture imparted on the inhaled gas during its exhalation. Thus, bypassing of the nasopharyngeal passages and upper trachea by devices such as endotracheal tubes not only decreases humidification of the gasses delivered to the distal airways but also cheats the opportunity to recoup heat and moisture on exhalation.

Removal of Inhaled Particles

The regions of the respiratory tract in which particles are deposited depend upon respiratory pattern, environmental conditions, and the nature of the particles themselves. Accepting these variations, it is possible to generalize particle behavior under normal circumstances. Particles larger than 10 μm (e.g., dust and particulates from low-grade petroleum combustion) are often trapped at the level of the nose or pharynx. Those that enter the airway of the lung, and particles of 3–10 μm, are caught on the liquid film layer and transported out of the lung for swallowing or expectoration as previously described. They tend to be deposited in higher concentration in areas of high turbulence such as airway bifurcations. Particles smaller than 3 μm may reach the alveoli. They will either be subsequently exhaled or settle in the alveolus, where they will be subject to the activity of macrophages as discussed in a previous section. There are, of course, particular substances that instigate a detrimental response from the body, for example, asbestos with resultant pulmonary fibrosis.

Response to Inhaled Organisms

There are several mechanisms with which the airway defends the body against inhaled microorganisms. The first is simple impact and capture by the nasal and pharyngeal mucosa with subsequent swallowing and destruction in the hostile gastrointestinal tract or expectoration. Those organisms that enter the lung may be similarly trapped on the surface film and moved out of the lung by ciliary action. The surface film is more than a simple transport mechanism, having a variety of antimicrobial mechanisms. These capabilities make teleological sense, because the potentially damaging agents are not immediately removed.

Surfactants, consisting of 80% phospholipids, 5–10% proteins, and 5–10% other lipids, are best known for their ability to reduce surface tension and thus equalize pressures within airspaces of differing sizes [168]. Less appreciated is the fact that SP-A and SP-D (following terminology introduced in the discussion of type II alveolar cells) are members of the collectin protein family. Collectins have an N-terminal collagen-type region and a C-terminal lectin region that bind carbohydrates. The C-terminal's preferential binding site is nonhost oligosaccharides, giving them the ability to opsonize bacterial and viral pathogens and to facilitate macrophage phagocytosis [172]. SP-A and SP-D are also known to be directly antimicrobial, without immune cells, against a variety of pathogens [173, 174].

The surface films of the large bronchi (and the mucosa of the nasopharynx) have generous amounts of IgA, which acts as an opsonin and has a role in complement induction. In smaller airways and alveoli, IgG becomes the predominant surface antibody in normal circumstances.

The airway epithelium also acts as an immune barrier via interactions between Fas receptors (CD95/Apo-1) and Fas ligand (FasL, CD95L, CD178), found on airway epithelium, in response to immune reactions and infection [175, 176]. The interaction between Fas and FasL activates intracellular caspases leading to apoptosis of infiltrating immune cells, protecting against tissue injury [177, 178]. FasL appears to be cleaved and made inactive in asthma, contributing to the chronic inflammation and damage to the epithelium seen in chronic lung diseases [179]. Toll-like receptors are also found in airway epithelial cells, upregulating the production of cytokines, chemokines, and other antimicrobial peptides in response to bacteria and viruses [180, 181]. Epithelial cells also secrete antimicrobial peptides including ß-defensins and LL-37, preventing the growth of inhaled microorganisms prior to clearance or phagocytosis [181].

Lung epithelial cells can release soluble factors including IL-1ß and IL-8, while alveolar macrophages release TNF-α and IL-6 resulting in the release of neutrophils from bone marrow as well as neutrophil chemotaxis in response to pollutants, including cigarette smoke, and pathogens [182, 183]. Once present at the source of infection, neutrophils secrete granules containing lactoferrin, lysozymes, defensins, and other proteolytic enzymes as well as generate oxygen free radicals to destroy pathogens [184]. Stimulated bronchial epithelial cells can also secrete and/or facilitate adhesion molecules, growth factors, and collagen. Epithelial cells produce high levels of nitric oxide (NO), and production is increased in the presence of respiratory viruses acting to inhibit viral replication [185]. The absence of upregulation of nitric oxide synthase-2 in cystic fibrosis is implicated in increased viral susceptibility in these patients [186].

Summary

Historically, practitioners of the medical arts from around the globe viewed the lung as a defender of the body from a hostile outside world and as a trusted modulator of its internal processes. More recently, respiratory function became the focus of attention with advances that have been central to the development of anesthesiology and upon which modern clinicians base much of our practice in cardiopulmonary medicine. The purpose of this discussion, which returns to the concepts of lung as protector and minister, has been to highlight important nonrespiratory lung functions in terms of both current areas of discovery and clinical implications. It is hoped that the reader will agree that familiarity with these aspects of pulmonary function is pivotal to a complete understanding of the lung and to the advancement of clinical practice.

References

1. Major R. A history of medicine. Springfield: Thomas; 1954.
2. Lumb AB. The history of respiratory physiology. In: Lumb AB, editor. Nunn's applied respiratory physiology. 6th ed. Oxford: Buttterworth-Heinemann; 2005.
3. Shoja MM, Tubbs RS. The history of anatomy in Persia. J Anat. 2007;210(4):359–78.
4. Simionescu M. Lung endothelium: structure-function correlates. In: Crystal RG, editor. Lung: scientific foundations. New York: Raven Press; 1991. p. 301–21.
5. Klein IK, Predescu DN, Sharma T, Knezevic I, Malik AB, Predescu S. Intersectin-2L regulates caveola endocytosis secondary to Cdc42-mediated actin polymerization. J Biol Chem. 2009;284(38):25953–61.
6. Parat M, Kwang WJ. The biology of caveolae: achievements and perspectives. In: International review of cell and molecular biology, vol. 273. Amsterdam: Academic; 2009. p. 117–62.
7. Ryan US, Ryan JW. Relevance of endothelial surface structure to the activity of vasoactive substances. Chest. 1985;88(4 Suppl):203S–7.
8. Ryan JW, Smith U. Metabolism of adenosine 5′-monophosphate during circulation through the lungs. Trans Assoc Am Phys. 1971;84:297–306.
9. Vane JR. The release and fate of vaso-active hormones in the circulation. Br J Pharmacol. 1969;35(2):209–42.
10. Dawidowicz ALP, Fornal EPD, Mardarowicz MPD, Fijalkowska APD. The role of human lungs in the biotransformation of propofol. Anesthesiology. 2000;93(4):992–7.
11. Hiraoka H, Yamamoto K, Miyoshi S, et al. Kidneys contribute to the extrahepatic clearance of propofol in humans, but not lungs and brain. Br J Clin Pharmacol. 2005;60(2):176–82.
12. de Graaf IAM, Koster HJ. Cryopreservation of precision-cut tissue slices for application in drug metabolism research. Toxicol In Vitro. 2003;17(1):1–17.
13. Klem C, Dasta JF, Reilley TE, Flancbaum LJ. Pulmonary extraction of dobutamine in critically ill surgical patients. Anesth Analg. 1995;81(2):287–91.
14. Hayashi Y, Sumikawa K, Yamatodani A, Kamibayashi T, Mammoto T, Kuro M. Quantitative analysis of pulmonary clearance of exogenous dopamine after cardiopulmonary bypass in humans. Anesth Analg. 1993;76(1):107–12.
15. Matot I, Pizov R. Pulmonary extraction and accumulation of lipid formulations of amphotericin B. Crit Care Med. 2000;28(7):2528–32.
16. Upton RN, Doolette DJ. Kinetic aspects of drug disposition in the lungs. Clin Exp Pharmacol Physiol. 1999;26(5–6):381–91.
17. Serabjit-Singh CJ, Nishio SJ, Philpot RM, Plopper CG. The distribution of cytochrome P-450 monooxygenase in cells of the rabbit lung: an ultrastructural immunocytochemical characterization. Mol Pharmacol. 1988;33(3):279–89.
18. Mizuguchi KA, Fox AA, Burch TM, Cohn LH, Fox JA. Tricuspid and mitral valve carcinoid disease in the setting of a patent foramen ovale. Anesth Analg. 2008;107(6):1819–21.
19. Pacifici GM, Franchi M, Bencini C, Repetti F, Di Lascio N, Muraro GB. Tissue distribution of drug-metabolizing enzymes in humans. Xenobiotica. 1988;18(7):849–56.
20. Litterst CL, Mimnaugh EG, Reagan RL, Gram TE. Comparison of in vitro drug metabolism by lung, liver, and kidney of several common laboratory species. Drug Metab Dispos. 1975;3(4):259–65.
21. Taeger K, Weninger E, Schmelzer F, Adt M, Franke N, Peter K. Pulmonary kinetics of fentanyl and alfentanil in surgical patients. Br J Anaesth. 1988;61(4):425–34.
22. Waters CM, Krejcie TC, Avram MJ. Facilitated uptake of fentanyl, but not alfentanil, by human pulmonary endothelial cells. Anesthesiology. 2000;93(3):825–31.
23. Boer F, Bovill JG, Burm AG, Mooren RA. Uptake of sufentanil, alfentanil and morphine in the lungs of patients about to undergo coronary artery surgery. Br J Anaesth. 1992;68(4):370–5.
24. Boer F, Olofsen E, Bovill JG, et al. Pulmonary uptake of sufentanil during and after constant rate infusion. Br J Anaesth. 1996;76(2):203–8.
25. Davis ME, Mehendale HM. Absence of metabolism of morphine during accumulation by isolated perfused rabbit lung. Drug Metab Dispos. 1979;7(6):425–8.
26. Roerig DL, Kotrly KJ, Vucins EJ, Ahlf SB, Dawson CA, Kampine JP. First pass uptake of fentanyl, meperidine, and morphine in the human lung. Anesthesiology. 1987;67(4):466–72.
27. Persson MP, Wiklund L, Hartvig P, Paalzow L. Potential pulmonary uptake and clearance of morphine in postoperative patients. Eur J Clin Pharmacol. 1986;30(5):567–74.
28. Beaufort TM, Proost JH, Houwertjes MC, Roggeveld J, Wierda JM. The pulmonary first-pass uptake of five nondepolarizing muscle relaxants in the pig. Anesthesiology. 1999;90(2):477–83.
29. Bertler A, Lewis DH, Lofstrom JB, Post C. In vivo lung uptake of lidocaine in pigs. Acta Anaesthesiol Scand. 1978;22(5):530–6.
30. Post C, Eriksdotter-Behm K. Dependence of lung uptake of lidocaine in vivo on blood pH. Acta Pharmacol Toxicol (Copenh). 1982;51(2):136–40.
31. Krejcie TC, Avram MJ, Gentry WB, Niemann CU, Janowski MP, Henthorn TK. A recirculatory model of the pulmonary uptake and pharmacokinetics of lidocaine based on analysis of arterial and mixed venous data from dogs. J Pharmacokinet Biopharm. 1997;25(2):169–90.
32. Hasegawa K, Yukioka H, Hayashi M, Tatekawa S, Fujimori M. Lung uptake of lidocaine during hyperoxia and hypoxia in the dog. Acta Anaesthesiol Scand. 1996;40(4):489–95.
33. Sjostrand U, Widman B. Distribution of bupivacaine in the rabbit under normal and acidotic conditions. Acta Anaesthesiol Scand Suppl. 1973;50:1–24.
34. Irestedt L, Andreen M, Belfrage P, Fagerstrom T. The elimination of bupivacaine (Marcain) after short intravenous infusion in the dog: with special reference to the role played by the liver and lungs. Acta Anaesthesiol Scand. 1978;22(4):413–22.
35. Rothstein P, Cole JS, Pitt BR. Pulmonary extraction of [3H] bupivacaine: modification by dose, propranolol and interaction with [14C]5-hydroxytryptamine. J Pharmacol Exp Ther. 1987;240(2):410–4.
36. Kietzmann D, Foth H, Geng WP, Rathgeber J, GundertRemy U, Kettler D. Transpulmonary disposition of prilocaine, mepivacaine, and bupivacaine in humans in the course of epidural anaesthesia. Acta Anaesthesiol Scand. 1995;39(7):885–90.
37. Sharrock NE, Mather LE, Go G, Sculco TP. Arterial and pulmonary arterial concentrations of the enantiomers of bupivacaine after epidural injection in elderly patients. Anesth Analg. 1998;86(4):812–7.
38. Palazzo MG, Kalso EA, Argiras E, Madgwick R, Sear JW. First pass lung uptake of bupivacaine: effect of acidosis in an intact rabbit lung model. Br J Anaesth. 1991;67(6):759–63.
39. Chang DH, Ladd LA, Wilson KA, Gelgor L, Mather LE. Tolerability of large-dose intravenous levobupivacaine in sheep. Anesth Analg. 2000;91(3):671–9.
40. Ohmura S, Kawada M, Ohta T, Yamamoto K, Kobayashi T. Systemic toxicity and resuscitation in bupivacaine-, levobupivacaine-, or ropivacaine-infused rats.[see comment]. Anesth Analg. 2001;93(3):743–8.
41. Ohmura S, Sugano A, Kawada M, Yamamoto K. Pulmonary uptake of ropivacaine and levobupivacaine in rabbits. Anesth Analg. 2003;97(3):893–7.

42. Mather LE, Copeland SE, Ladd LA. Acute toxicity of local anesthetics: underlying pharmacokinetic and pharmacodynamic concepts [see comment]. Reg Anesth Pain Med. 2005;30(6):553–66.

43. Heavner JE. Let's abandon blanket maximum recommended doses of local anesthetics [comment]. Reg Anesth Pain Med. 2004;29(6):524.

44. Rosenberg PH, Veering BT, Urmey WF. Maximum recommended doses of local anesthetics: a multifactorial concept [see comment]. Reg Anesth Pain Med. 2004;29(6):564–75; discussion 524.

45. Reynolds F. Maximum recommended doses of local anesthetics: a constant cause of confusion [comment]. Reg Anesth Pain Med. 2005;30(3):314–6.

46. Groban L. Central nervous system and cardiac effects from long-acting amide local anesthetic toxicity in the intact animal model. Reg Anesth Pain Med. 2003;28(1):3–11.

47. Mulroy MF. Systemic toxicity and cardiotoxicity from local anesthetics: incidence and preventive measures. Reg Anesth Pain Med. 2002;27(6):556–61.

48. Rosenblatt MA, Abel M, Fischer GW, Itzkovich CJ, Eisenkraft JB. Successful use of a 20% lipid emulsion to resuscitate a patient after a presumed bupivacaine-related cardiac arrest [see comment]. Anesthesiology. 2006;105(1):217–8.

49. Felice K, Schumann H. Intravenous lipid emulsion for local anesthetic toxicity: a review of the literature. J Med Toxicol. 2008;4(3):184–91.

50. Marwick PC, Levin AI, Coetzee AR. Recurrence of cardiotoxicity after lipid rescue from bupivacaine-induced cardiac arrest [see comment]. Anesth Analg. 2009;108(4):1344–6.

51. Roerig DL, Kotrly KJ, Dawson CA, Ahlf SB, Gualtieri JF, Kampine JP. First-pass uptake of verapamil, diazepam, and thiopental in the human lung. Anesth Analg. 1989;69(4):461–6.

52. Pedraz JL, Lanao JM, Hernandez JM, Dominguez-Gil A. The biotransformation kinetics of ketamine "in vitro" in rabbit liver and lung microsome fractions. Eur J Drug Metab Pharmacokinet. 1986;11(1):9–16.

53. Henthorn TK, Krejcie TC, Niemann CU, Enders-Klein C, Shanks CA, Avram MJ. Ketamine distribution described by a recirculatory pharmacokinetic model is not stereoselective. Anesthesiology. 1999;91(6):1733–43.

54. Mather LE, Selby DG, Runciman WB, McLean CF. Propofol: assay and regional mass balance in the sheep. Xenobiotica. 1989;19(11):1337–47.

55. Kuipers JA, Boer F, Olieman W, Burm AG, Bovill JG. First-pass lung uptake and pulmonary clearance of propofol: assessment with a recirculatory indocyanine green pharmacokinetic model. Anesthesiology. 1999;91(6):1780–7.

56. Matot I, Neely CF, Katz RY, Neufeld GR. Pulmonary uptake of propofol in cats. Effect of fentanyl and halothane. Anesthesiology. 1993;78(6):1157–65.

57. Le Guellec C, Lacarelle B, Villard PH, Point H, Catalin J, Durand A. Glucuronidation of propofol in microsomal fractions from various tissues and species including humans: effect of different drugs. Anesth Analg. 1995;81(4):855–61.

58. Bulger EM, Maier RV. Lipid mediators in the pathophysiology of critical illness. Crit Care Med. 2000;28(4 Suppl):N27–36.

59. Upton RN, Ludbrook G. A physiologically based, recirculatory model of the kinetics and dynamics of propofol in man. Anesthesiology. 2005;103(2):344–52.

60. Kazama T, Ikeda K, Morita K, Ikeda T, Kikura M, Sato S. Relation between initial blood distribution volume and propofol induction dose requirement [see comment]. Anesthesiology. 2001;94(2):205–10.

61. Kazama T, Morita K, Ikeda T, Kurita T, Sato S. Comparison of predicted induction dose with predetermined physiologic characteristics of patients and with pharmacokinetic models incorporating those characteristics as covariates. Anesthesiology. 2003;98(2):299–305.

62. Krejcie TC, Jacquez JA, Avram MJ, Niemann CU, Shanks CA, Henthorn TK. Use of parallel Erlang density functions to analyze first-pass pulmonary uptake of multiple indicators in dogs. J Pharmacokinet Biopharm. 1996;24(6):569–88.

63. Wang WB, Watts AB, Peters JI, Williams RO III. The impact of pulmonary disease on the fate of inhaled medicines- a review. Int J Phram. 2014;461:112–28.

64. Sweeney TD, Skornik WA, Brain JD, Hatch V, Godleski JJ. Chronic bronchitis alters the pattern of aerosol deposition in the lung. Am J Respir Crit Care Med. 1995;151:482–8.

65. Patton JS, Brain JD, Davies LA, et al. The particle has landed-characterizing the fate of inhaled pharmaceuticals. J Aerosol Med Pulm Drug Deliv. 2010;23(Suppl 2):S71–87.

66. Patton JS, Fishburn CS, Weers JG. The lungs as a portal of entry for systemic drug delivery. Proc Am Thorac Soc. 2004;1:338–44.

67. Olsson B, Bodesson E, Borgstom L. Pulmonary drug metabolism, clearance, and absorption. In: Smyth HDC, Hickey AJ, editors. Controlled pulmonary drug delivery. 1st ed. New York: Springer; 2011.

68. Ryan JW. Processing of endogenous polypeptides by the lungs. Annu Rev Physiol. 1982;44:241–55.

69. Orfanos SE, Langleben D, Khoury J, et al. Pulmonary capillary endothelium-bound angiotensin-converting enzyme activity in humans. Circulation. 1999;99(12):1593–9.

70. Skidgel RA. Bradykinin-degrading enzymes: structure, function, distribution, and potential roles in cardiovascular pharmacology. J Cardiovasc Pharmacol. 1992;20(Suppl 9):S4–9.

71. Chand N, Altura BM. Acetylcholine and bradykinin relax intrapulmonary arteries by acting on endothelial cells: role in lung vascular diseases. Science. 1981;213(4514):1376–9.

72. Skidgel RA, Erdos EG. Angiotensin converting enzyme (ACE) and neprilysin hydrolyze neuropeptides: a brief history, the beginning and follow-ups to early studies. Peptides. 2004;25(3):521–5.

73. Simke J, Graeme ML, Sigg EB. Bradykinin induced bronchoconstriction in guinea pigs and its modification by various agents. Arch Int Pharmacodyn Ther. 1967;165(2):291–301.

74. Collier HO. Humoral factors in bronchoconstriction. Sci Basis Med Annu Rev. 1968:308–35.

75. Suguikawa TR, Garcia CA, Martinez EZ, Vianna EO. Cough and dyspnea during bronchoconstriction: comparison of different stimuli. Cough. 2009;5:6.

76. Enseleit F, Hurlimann D, Luscher TF. Vascular protective effects of angiotensin converting enzyme inhibitors and their relation to clinical events. J Cardiovasc Pharmacol. 2001;37(Suppl 1):S21–30.

77. Muntner P, Krousel-Wood M, Hyre AD, et al. Antihypertensive prescriptions for newly treated patients before and after the main antihypertensive and lipid-lowering treatment to prevent heart attack trial results and seventh report of the joint national committee on prevention, detection, evaluation, and treatment of high blood pressure guidelines [see comment]. Hypertension. 2009;53(4):617–23.

78. Alabaster VA, Bakhle YS. Removal of 5-hydroxytryptamine in the pulmonary circulation of rat isolated lungs. Br J Pharmacol. 1970;40(3):468–82.

79. Gonmori K, Rao KS, Mehendale HM. Pulmonary synthesis of 5-hydroxytryptamine in isolated perfused rabbit and rat lung preparations. Exp Lung Res. 1986;11(4):295–305.

80. Cook DR, Brandom BW. Enflurane, halothane, and isoflurane inhibit removal of 5-hydroxytryptamine from the pulmonary circulation. Anesth Analg. 1982;61(8):671–5.

81. Junod AF. Uptake, metabolism and efflux of 14 C-5-hydroxytryptamine in isolated perfused rat lungs. J Pharmacol Exp Ther. 1972;183(2):341–55.

82. Righi L, Volante M, Rapa I, Scagliotti GV, Papotti M. Neuro-endocrine tumours of the lung. A review of relevant pathological and molecular data. Virchows Arch. 2007;451(Suppl 1):S51–9.

83. Shah PM, Raney AA. Tricuspid valve disease. Curr Probl Cardiol. 2008;33(2):47–84.

84. Sandmann H, Pakkal M, Steeds R. Cardiovascular magnetic resonance imaging in the assessment of carcinoid heart disease. Clin Radiol. 2009;64(8):761–6.

85. Bernheim AM, Connolly HM, Pellikka PA. Carcinoid heart disease. Curr Treat Options Cardiovasc Med. 2007;9(6):482–9.

86. Droogmans S, Cosyns B, D'Haenen H, et al. Possible association between 3, 4-methylenedioxymethamphetamine abuse and valvular heart disease. Am J Cardiol. 2007;100(9):1442–5.

87. Utsunomiya T, Krausz MM, Shepro D, Hechtman HB. Prostaglandin control of plasma and platelet 5-hydroxytryptamine in normal and embolized animals. Am J Phys. 1981;241(5):H766–71.

88. Stratmann G, Gregory GA. Neurogenic and humoral vasoconstriction in acute pulmonary thromboembolism [see comment]. Anesth Analg. 2003;97(2):341–54.

89. Huval WV, Mathieson MA, Stemp LI, et al. Therapeutic benefits of 5-hydroxytryptamine inhibition following pulmonary embolism. Ann Surg. 1983;197(2):220–5.

90. Said SI. Metabolic functions of the pulmonary circulation. Circ Res. 1982;50(3):325–33.

91. Philpot RM, Andersson TB, Eling TE. Uptake, accumulation, and metabolism of chemicals by the lung. In: Bakhle YS, Vane JR, editors. Metabolic functions of the lung. New York: Marcel Dekker; 1977. p. 123–71.

92. Garcia JG, Noonan TC, Jubiz W, Malik AB. Leukotrienes and the pulmonary microcirculation. Am Rev Respir Dis. 1987;136(1):161–9.

93. Samuelsson B, Dahlen SE, Lindgren JA, Rouzer CA, Serhan CN. Leukotrienes and lipoxins: structures, biosynthesis, and biological effects. Science. 1987;237(4819):1171–6.

94. Haeggstrom JZ, Kull F, Rudberg PC, Tholander F, Thunnissen MMGM. Leukotriene A4 hydrolase. Prostaglandins Other Lipid Mediat. 2002;68–69:495–510.

95. Yang G, Chen G, Wang D. Effects of prostaglandins and leukotrienes on hypoxic pulmonary vasoconstriction in rats. J Tongji Med Univ. 2000;20(3):197–9.

96. Caironi P, Ichinose F, Liu R, Jones RC, Bloch KD, Zapol WM. 5-lipoxygenase deficiency prevents respiratory failure during ventilator-induced lung injury [see comment]. Am J Respir Crit Care Med. 2005;172(3):334–43.

97. Leitch AG. The role of leukotrienes in asthma. Ann Acad Med Singap. 1985;14(3):503–7.

98. Sprague RS, Stephenson AH, Dahms TE, Lonigro AJ. Proposed role for leukotrienes in the pathophysiology of multiple systems organ failure. Crit Care Clin. 1989;5(2):315–29.

99. Orfanos SE, Mavrommati I, Korovesi I, Roussos C. Pulmonary endothelium in acute lung injury: from basic science to the critically ill. Intensive Care Med. 2004;30(9):1702–14.

100. Huang SK, Peters-Golden M. Eicosanoid lipid mediators in fibrotic lung diseases: ready for prime time? Chest. 2008;133(6):1442–50.

101. Del Giudice MM, Pezzulo A, Capristo C, et al. Leukotriene modifiers in the treatment of asthma in children. Ther Adv Respir Dis. 2009;3(5):245–51.

102. O'Byrne PM, Gauvreau GM, Murphy DM. Efficacy of leukotriene receptor antagonists and synthesis inhibitors in asthma. J Allergy Clin Immunol. 2009;124(3):397–403.

103. Tantisira KG, Drazen JM. Genetics and pharmacogenetics of the leukotriene pathway. J Allergy Clin Immunol. 2009;124(3):422–7.

104. Murphy RC, Gijon MA. Biosynthesis and metabolism of leukotrienes [erratum appears in Biochem J. 2007 Sep 15;406(3):527]. Biochem J. 2007;405(3):379–95.

105. Romano M. Lipid mediators: lipoxin and aspirin-triggered 15-epi-lipoxins. Inflamm Allergy Drug Targets. 2006;5(2):81–90.

106. Romano M, Recchia I, Recchiuti A. Lipoxin receptors. Sci World J. 2007;7:1393–412.

107. Soyombo O, Spur BW, Lee TH. Effects of lipoxin A4 on chemotaxis and degranulation of human eosinophils stimulated by platelet-activating factor and N-formyl-L-methionyl-L-leucyl-L-phenylalanine. Allergy. 1994;49(4):230–4.

108. Raud J, Palmertz U, Dahlen SE, Hedqvist P. Lipoxins inhibit microvascular inflammatory actions of leukotriene B4. Adv Exp Med Biol. 1991;314:185–92.

109. Le Y, Li B, Gong W, et al. Novel pathophysiological role of classical chemotactic peptide receptors and their communications with chemokine receptors. Immunol Rev. 2000;177:185–94.

110. Colgan SP, Serhan CN, Parkos CA, Delp-Archer C, Madara JL. Lipoxin A4 modulates transmigration of human neutrophils across intestinal epithelial monolayers. J Clin Invest. 1993;92(1):75–82.

111. Brezinski ME, Gimbrone MA Jr, Nicolaou KC, Serhan CN. Lipoxins stimulate prostacyclin generation by human endothelial cells. FEBS Lett. 1989;245(1–2):167–72.

112. Wenzel SE, Busse WW, The National Heart, Lung, Blood Institute's Severe Asthma Research Program. Severe asthma: lessons from the Severe Asthma Research Program. J Allergy Clin Immunol. 2007;119(1):14–21; quiz 22–13.

113. Vachier I, Bonnans C, Chavis C, et al. Severe asthma is associated with a loss of LX4, an endogenous anti-inflammatory compound. J Allergy Clin Immunol. 2005;115(1):55–60.

114. Levy BD, Bonnans C, Silverman ES, et al. Diminished lipoxin biosynthesis in severe asthma. Am J Respir Crit Care Med. 2005;172(7):824–30.

115. Kupczyk M, Antczak A, Kuprys-Lipinska I, Kuna P. Lipoxin A4 generation is decreased in aspirin-sensitive patients in lysine-aspirin nasal challenge in vivo model. Allergy. 2009;64(12):1746–52.

116. Van Hove CL, Maes T, Joos GF, Tournoy KG. Chronic inflammation in asthma: a contest of persistence vs. resolution. Allergy. 2008;63(9):1095–109.

117. Bonnans C, Levy BD. Lipid mediators as agonists for the resolution of acute lung inflammation and injury. Am J Respir Cell Mol Biol. 2007;36(2):201–5.

118. Serhan CN. Lipoxins and novel aspirin-triggered 15-epi-lipoxins (ATL): a jungle of cell-cell interactions or a therapeutic opportunity? Prostaglandins. 1997;53(2):107–37.

119. Ramalho TC, Rocha MVJ, da Cunha EFF, Freitas MP. The search for new COX-2 inhibitors: a review of 2002–2008 patents. Expert Opin Ther Pat. 2009;19(9):1193–228.

120. Grosser T. Variability in the response to cyclooxygenase inhibitors: toward the individualization of nonsteroidal anti-inflammatory drug therapy. J Investig Med. 2009;57(6):709–16.

121. Funk CD, FitzGerald GA. COX-2 inhibitors and cardiovascular risk. J Cardiovasc Pharmacol. 2007;50(5):470–9.

122. Frangos JA, Eskin SG, McIntire LV, Ives CL. Flow effects on prostacyclin production by cultured human endothelial cells. Science. 1985;227(4693):1477–9.

123. Eling TE, Ally AI. Pulmonary biosynthesis and metabolism of prostaglandins and related substances. Environ Health Perspect. 1984;55:159–68.

124. Robinson C, Hardy CC, Holgate ST. Pulmonary synthesis, release and metabolism of prostaglandins. J Allergy Clin Immunol. 1985;76(2 Pt 2):265–71.

125. McGiff JC, Terragno NA, Strand JC, Lee JB, Lonigro AJ, Ng KK. Selective passage of prostaglandins across the lung. Nature. 1969;223(5207):742–5.

126. Dusting GJ, Moncada S, Vane JR. Recirculation of prostacyclin (PGI2) in the dog. Br J Pharmacol. 1978;64(2):315–20.

127. Gardiner PJ. Eicosanoids and airway smooth muscle. Pharmacol Ther. 1989;44(1):1–62.

128. Regner KR, Connolly HM, Schaff HV, Albright RC. Acute renal failure after cardiac surgery for carcinoid heart disease: incidence, risk factors, and prognosis. Am J Kidney Dis. 2005;45(5):826–32.

129. Zeldin DC, Foley J, Ma J, et al. CYP2J subfamily P450s in the lung: expression, localization, and potential functional significance. Mol Pharmacol. 1996;50(5):1111–7.

130. Salvail D, Dumoulin M, Rousseau E. Direct modulation of tracheal cl – channel activity by 5, 6- and 11, 12-EET. Am J Phys. 1998;275(3 Pt 1):L432–41.

131. Birks EK, Bousamra M, Presberg K, Marsh JA, Effros RM, Jacobs ER. Human pulmonary arteries dilate to 20-HETE, an endogenous eicosanoid of lung tissue. Am J Phys. 1997;272(5 Pt 1):L823–9.

132. Jacobs ER, Zeldin DC. The lung HETEs (and EETs) up. Am J Physiol Heart Circ Physiol. 2001;280(1):H1–10.

133. Sirois P, Gutkowska J. Atrial natriuretic factor immunoreactivity in human fetal lung tissue and perfusates. Hypertension. 1988;11(2 Pt 2):I62–5.

134. Di Nardo P, Peruzzi G. Physiology and pathophysiology of atrial natriuretic factor in lungs. Can J Cardiol. 1992;8(5):503–8.

135. Turrin M, Gillis CN. Removal of atrial natriuretic peptide by perfused rabbit lungs in situ. Biochem Biophys Res Commun. 1986;140(3):868–73.

136. Tomlinson JW, Walker EA, Bujalska IJ, et al. 11beta-hydroxysteroid dehydrogenase type 1: a tissue-specific regulator of glucocorticoid response. Endocr Rev. 2004;25(5):831–66.

137. Garbrecht MR, Klein JM, Schmidt TJ, Snyder JM. Glucocorticoid metabolism in the human fetal lung: implications for lung development and the pulmonary surfactant system. Biol Neonate. 2006;89(2):109–19.

138. Baker RW, Walker BR, Shaw RJ, et al. Increased cortisol: cortisone ratio in acute pulmonary tuberculosis. Am J Respir Crit Care Med. 2000;162(5):1641–7.

139. Huang CH, Huang HH, Chen TL, Wang MJ. Perioperative changes of plasma endothelin-1 concentrations in patients undergoing cardiac valve surgery. Anaesth Intensive Care. 1996;24(3):342–7.

140. Dupuis J, Cernacek P, Tardif JC, et al. Reduced pulmonary clearance of endothelin-1 in pulmonary hypertension. Am Heart J. 1998;135(4):614–20.

141. Drinker CK, Churchill ED, Ferry RM. The volume of blood in the heart and lungs. Am J Phys. 1926;77(3):590–622.

142. Campbell I, Waterhouse J. Fluid balance and non-respiratory functions of the lung. Anaesth Intensive Care Med. 2005;6(11):370–1.

143. Cotter G, Metra M, Milo-Cotter O, Dittrich HC, Gheorghiade M. Fluid overload in acute heart failure – re-distribution and other mechanisms beyond fluid accumulation. Eur J Heart Fail. 2008;10(2):165–9.

144. Jules-Elysee K, Blanck TJJ, Catravas JD, et al. Angiotensin-converting enzyme activity: a novel way of assessing pulmonary changes during total knee arthroplasty. Anesth Analg. 2004;99(4):1018–23.

145. Lovering AT, Stickland MK, Kelso AJ, Eldridge MW. Direct demonstration of 25- and 50-microm arteriovenous pathways in healthy human and baboon lungs. Am J Physiol Heart Circ Physiol. 2007;292(4):H1777–81.

146. Lovering AT, Haverkamp HC, Romer LM, Hokanson JS, Eldridge MW. Transpulmonary passage of 99mTc macroaggregated albumin in healthy humans at rest and during maximal exercise. J Appl Physiol. 2009;106(6):1986–92.

147. Abrams GA, Rose K, Fallon MB, et al. Hepatopulmonary syndrome and venous emboli causing intracerebral hemorrhages after liver transplantation: a case report. Transplantation. 1999;68(11):1809–11.

148. Colohan AR, Perkins NA, Bedford RF, Jane JA. Intravenous fluid loading as prophylaxis for paradoxical air embolism. J Neurosurg. 1985;62(6):839–42.

149. Breeze RG, Wheeldon EB. The cells of the pulmonary airways. Am Rev Respir Dis. 1977;116(4):705–77.

150. Rogers DF. The airway goblet cell. Int J Biochem Cell Biol. 2003;35(1):1–6.

151. Huffmyer JL, Littlewood KE, Nemergut EC. Perioperative management of the adult with cystic fibrosis. Anesth Analg. 2009;109(6):1949–61.

152. Nadel JA. Neural control of airway submucosal gland secretion. Eur J Respir Dis Suppl. 1983;128(Pt 1):322–6.

153. Reid L. Measurement of the bronchial mucous gland layer: a diagnostic yardstick in chronic bronchitis. Thorax. 1960;15:132–41.

154. Gallagher JT, Kent PW, Passatore M, Phipps RJ, Richardson PS. The composition of tracheal mucus and the nervous control of its secretion in the cat. Proc R Soc Lond B Biol Sci. 1975;192(1106):49–76.

155. Heidsiek JG, Hyde DM, Plopper CG, St George JA. Quantitative histochemistry of mucosubstance in tracheal epithelium of the macaque monkey. J Histochem Cytochem. 1987;35(4):435–42.

156. Evans CM, Williams OW, Tuvim MJ, et al. Mucin is produced by clara cells in the proximal airways of antigen-challenged mice. Am J Respir Cell Mol Biol. 2004;31(4):382–94.

157. Reynolds SD, Malkinson AM. Clara cell: progenitor for the bronchiolar epithelium. Int J Biochem Cell Biol. 2009;42(1):1–4.

158. Boers JE, Ambergen AW, Thunnissen FB. Number and proliferation of clara cells in normal human airway epithelium. Am J Respir Crit Care Med. 1999;159(5 Pt 1):1585–91.

159. Krishnaswamy G, Ajitawi O, Chi DS. The human mast cell: an overview. Methods Mol Biol. 2006;315:13–34.

160. Taube C, Stassen M. Mast cells and mast cell-derived factors in the regulation of allergic sensitization. Chem Immunol Allergy. 2008;94:58–66.

161. Peters A, Veronesi B, Calderon-Garciduenas L, et al. Translocation and potential neurological effects of fine and ultrafine particles a critical update. Part Fibre Toxicol [Electronic Resource]. 2006;3:13.

162. Jakubzick C, Tacke F, Llodra J, van Rooijen N, Randolph GJ. Modulation of dendritic cell trafficking to and from the airways. J Immunol. 2006;176(6):3578–84.

163. Matthay MA, Folkesson HG, Clerici C. Lung epithelial fluid transport and the resolution of pulmonary edema. Physiol Rev. 2002;82(3):569–600.

164. Matthay MA, Clerici C, Saumon G. Invited review: active fluid clearance from the distal air spaces of the lung. J Appl Physiol. 2002;93(4):1533–41.

165. Dobbs LG, Johnson MD. Alveolar epithelial transport in the adult lung. Respir Physiol Neurobiol. 2007;159:283–300.

166. Andreeva AV, Kutuzov MA, Voyno-Yasenetskaya TA. Regulation of surfactant secretion in alveolar type II cells. Am J Physiol Lung Cell Mol Physiol. 2007;293(2):L259–71.

167. Weaver TE, Conkright JJ. Function of surfactant proteins B and C. Annu Rev Physiol. 2001;63:555–78.

168. Ungaro F, d'Angelo I, Miro A, La Rotonda MI, Quaglia F. Engineered PLGA nano- and micro-carriers for pulmonary delivery: challenges and promises. J Pharm Pharmacol. 2012;64:1217–35.

169. Wanner A, Salathe M, O'Riordan TG. Mucociliary clearance in the airways. Am J Respir Crit Care Med. 1996;154(6 Pt 1):1868–902.

170. Boucher RC. Evidence for airway surface dehydration as the initiating event in CF airway disease. J Intern Med. 2007;261(1):5–16.

171. McFadden ER Jr. Heat and water exchange in human airways. Am Rev Respir Dis. 1992;146(5 Pt 2):S8–10.

172. Crouch E, Wright JR. Surfactant proteins a and d and pulmonary host defense. Annu Rev Physiol. 2001;63:521–54.

173. Wu H, Kuzmenko A, Wan S, et al. Surfactant proteins a and D inhibit the growth of gram-negative bacteria by increasing membrane permeability [see comment]. J Clin Invest. 2003;111(10):1589–602.

174. Wright JR. Pulmonary surfactant: a front line of lung host defense [comment]. J Clin Invest. 2003;111(10):1453–5.

175. Hamann KJ, Dorscheid DR, Ko FD, et al. Expression of Fas (CD95) and FasL (CD95L) in human airway epithelium. Am J Respir Cell Mol Biol. 1998;19:537–42.

176. Fine A, Anderson NL, Rothstein TL, Williams MC, Gochuico BR. Fas expression in pulmonary alveolar type II cells. Am J Phys. 1997;273:L64_L71.

177. Muzio M, Salvesen GS, Dixit VM. FLICE induced apoptosis in a cell-free system. Cleavage of caspase zymogens. J Biol Chem. 1997;272:2952–6.

178. Griffith TS, Brunner T, Fletcher SM, Green DR, Ferguson TA. Fas ligand-induced apoptosis as a mechanism of immune privilege. Science. 1995;270:1189–92.

179. Wadsworth SJ, Atsuta R, McIntyre JO, Hackett TL, Singhera GK, Dorscheid DR. IL-13 and T(H)2 cytokine exposure triggers matrix metalloproteinase 7-mediated Fas ligand cleavage from bronchial epithelial cells. J Allergy Clin Immunol. 2011;126(2):366–74, 374 e1–8.

180. Kaisho T, Akira S. Toll-like receptor function and signaling. J Allergy Clin Immunol. 2006;117:979–87.

181. Bals R, Hiemstra PS. Innate immunity in the lung: how epithelial cells fight against respiratory pathogens. Eur Respir J. 2004;23:327–33.

182. Mio T, Romberger DJ, Thompson AB, Robbins RA, Heires A, Rennard SI. Cigarette smoke induces interleukin-8 release from human bronchial epithelial cells. Am J Respir Crit Care Med. 1997;155:1770–6.

183. Chung KF. Cytokines in chronic obstructive pulmonary disease. Eur Respir J. 2001;34(Suppl):50s–9s.

184. Russo RG, Liotta LA, Thorgeirsson U, Brundage R, Schiffmann E. Polymorphonuclear leukocyte migration through human amnion membrane. J Cell Biol. 1981;91:459–67.

185. Kao YJ, Piedra PA, Larsen GL, Colasurdo GN. Induction and regulation of nitric oxide synthase in airway epithelial cells by respiratory syncytial virus. Am J Respir Crit Care Med. 2001;163:532–9.

186. Zheng S, De SBP, Choudhary S, et al. Impaired innate host defense causes susceptibility to respiratory virus infections in cystic fibrosis. Immunity. 2003;18:619–30.

Pharmacology of the Airways

8

Cassandra Bailey, Paul J. Wojciechowski,
and William E. Hurford

Key Points

- Short-acting beta-2 adrenergic agonists are administered for the acute relief of bronchospasm, wheezing, and airflow obstruction. Long-acting beta-2 adrenergic agonists are for long-term control of symptoms.
- Inhaled anticholinergics are first-line therapy in COPD. They are useful for both maintenance therapy and in acute exacerbations.
- Inhaled corticosteroids are used to control inflammation in asthma and COPD. In asthma, they can be used as monotherapy. In COPD, they are used in conjunction with long-acting beta-adrenergic agonists.
- Systemic corticosteroids are used for the reduction of inflammation in asthma and COPD exacerbations and are not typically prescribed as maintenance therapy.
- Phosphodiesterase 4 inhibitors can be used in patients with severe COPD, chronic bronchitis, and a history of exacerbations.
- Leukotriene modifiers, mast cell stabilizers, and methylxanthines are alternative therapies used in asthma when symptoms are not well-controlled on first-line therapy.

- Volatile and intravenous anesthetics provide a degree of bronchodilation that may be useful in treating intraoperative bronchoconstriction.
- Helium/oxygen mixtures, antihistamines, and magnesium sulfate are alternative therapies used when bronchospasm does not respond to conventional therapies.

Introduction

This chapter reviews the pharmacology of agents commonly encountered in anesthetic practice that are either administered to treat pulmonary diseases or administered into the airway for action at end organs other than the lung but have effects on the airway. Drugs that modify the state of the autonomic nervous system (ANS) and the airway will be reviewed along with medications that modify or suppress inflammation of the airway. Lastly, the action of anesthetic agents on the airway will be reviewed along with the actions of several adjunctive agents.

Pharmacologic agents administered via the lungs take advantage of the unique interface between air and blood allowing for rapid uptake of drugs into the bloodstream or immediate utilization by cells that populate the airway. The delivery of medications to the lungs can have systemic effects, direct effects on the airway, or both. For example, inhaled anesthetics are delivered via the lungs to act in the brain and have bronchodilatory effects. Conversely, beta-adrenergic agonists delivered via aerosol exert direct effects on bronchial smooth muscle with few systemic effects. Drugs administered directly to the airway are ideal for treating pulmonary parenchymal diseases such as asthma and chronic obstructive pulmonary disease (COPD).

C. Bailey (✉) · P. J. Wojciechowski · W. E. Hurford
Department of Anesthesiology, University of Cincinnati,
Cincinnati, OH, USA
e-mail: barryca@ucmail.uc.edu

© Springer Nature Switzerland AG 2019
P. Slinger (ed.), *Principles and Practice of Anesthesia for Thoracic Surgery*, https://doi.org/10.1007/978-3-030-00859-8_8

Influence of the Autonomic Nervous System on the Airway and Modulation of the Response

Traditionally, the ANS has been divided into two major parts, the parasympathetic and sympathetic nervous systems. The parasympathetic nervous system regulates airway caliber, airway glandular activity, and airway microvasculature [1–4]. The vagus nerve provides the preganglionic fibers which synapse with postganglionic fibers in airway parasympathetic ganglia [1–4]. Acetylcholine activates the muscarinic (M3) receptor of postganglionic fibers of the parasympathetic nervous system to produce bronchoconstriction [5]. Anticholinergics can provide bronchodilation even in the resting state since the parasympathetic nervous system produces a basal level of resting bronchomotor tone [3, 4, 6]. Activated eosinophils may play a role in airway hyperresponsiveness through release of major basic protein that prevents acetylcholine from binding the M2 receptors, leading to inhibition of negative feedback control and increasing release of acetylcholine [7].

Although the sympathetic nervous system plays no direct role in control of airway muscle tone, beta-2 adrenergic receptors are present on airway smooth muscle cells and cause bronchodilation via G-protein and secondary messenger mechanisms [1–5]. The abundance of these receptors in the airway allows for pharmacologic manipulation of airway tone [8].

The ANS also influences bronchomotor tone through the nonadrenergic noncholinergic (NANC) system [2, 4, 9, 10]. The exact role of NANC in humans is not well defined; it has excitatory and inhibitory neuropeptides that influence inflammation and smooth muscle tone, respectively [2, 9]. Vasoactive intestinal peptide (VIP) and nitric oxide (NO) are the main inhibitory transmitters thought to be responsible for airway smooth muscle relaxation [2, 9]. Substance P (SP) and neurokinin A (NKA) are the main excitatory transmitters and have been shown to cause neurogenic inflammation, including bronchoconstriction [2, 9]. The precise role of NANC in healthy and diseased human lung is unclear. Further study is needed to fully elucidate the role that this group of neuropeptides has in the regulation of bronchial smooth muscle responsiveness.

Inhaled Adrenergic Agonists

The mainstay of therapy for bronchospasm, wheezing, and airflow obstruction is beta-adrenergic agonists. Beta-adrenergic agonists used in clinical practice are typically delivered via inhalers or nebulizers, are beta-2 selective, and are divided into short- and long-acting therapies [11]. Short-acting beta-2 agonist therapy is effective for the rapid relief of wheezing, bronchospasm, and airflow obstruction [11]. Longer-acting beta-2 agonists are used as maintenance ther-

Table 8.1 Pharmacologic influence on the autonomic nervous system

Systemic adrenergic agonists	Inhaled adrenergic agonists	Inhaled cholinergic antagonists	Systemic cholinergic antagonists
	Short-acting	Short-acting	
Terbutaline	Albuterol	Ipratropium	Atropine
Epinephrine	Levalbuterol		Scopolamine
Albuterol	Metaproterenol		Glycopyrrolate
	Pirbuterol		
	Long-acting	Long-acting	
	Salmeterol	Tiotropium	
	Formoterol		
	Arformoterol		

Adapted from Fanta et al. [11]

apy providing improvement in lung function and reduction in symptoms and exacerbations [11]. Please refer to Table 8.1 for a selection of beta-2 selective agonists that play a role in the management of airway diseases and symptoms both in and out of the operating room.

Mechanism of Action

Short-acting beta-2 agonists bind to the beta-2 adrenergic receptor located on the plasma membrane of smooth muscle cells, epithelial, endothelial, and many other types of airway cells [8, 12]. Figure 8.1 demonstrates how a ligand binding to the receptor causes a G-stimulatory protein to activate adenylate cyclase-converting adenosine triphosphate (ATP) into cyclic adenosine monophosphate (cAMP) [8, 12]. It is unknown precisely how cAMP causes smooth muscle relaxation; however, decreases in calcium release and alterations in membrane potential are the most likely mechanisms [8]. Longer-acting beta-2 agonists have the same mechanism of action as short-acting beta-2 agonists; however, they have unique properties that allow for a longer duration of action. For example, salmeterol has a longer duration of action because a side chain binds to the beta-2 receptor and prolongs the activation of the receptor [12, 13]. The lipophilic side chain of formoterol allows for interaction with the lipid bilayer of the plasma membrane and a slow, steady release prolonging its duration of action [12].

Clinical Applications

Beta-2 agonists have a central role in the management of obstructive airway diseases allowing for control of symptoms and improvement in lung function. Short-acting beta-2 agonists such as albuterol, levalbuterol, metaproterenol, and pirbuterol are prescribed for the rapid relief of wheezing, bronchospasm, and airflow obstruction [11]. Clinical effect is seen in a matter of minutes and lasts up to 4–6 h [12]. Scheduled, daily use of short-acting beta-2 agonists has

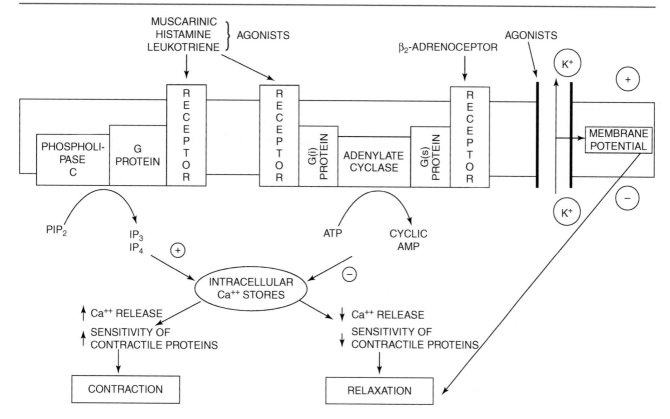

Fig. 8.1 Effects of agonists at the beta-2 receptor and at the muscarinic receptor. Stimulation of the beta-2 receptor will cause a decrease in calcium release and relaxation of smooth muscle. Blockade of the muscarinic receptor will prevent the release of calcium and smooth muscle contraction. ATP, adenosine triphosphate; AMP, adenosine monophos- phate; IP, inositol phosphate; PIP2, phosphoinositide bisphosphate. (Reprinted with permission of the Thoracic Society. Copyright© American Thoracic Society. Johnson [8]. Official Journal of the American Thoracic Society)

fallen out of favor, and they are now used primarily as rescue therapy [14–16]. Long-acting beta-2 agonists can be prescribed for control of symptoms when rescue therapies (i.e., short-acting beta-2 agonists) are used frequently within a week [11, 17]. In asthma, combination therapy including a long-acting beta-2 agonist and an inhaled corticosteroid (IC) are effective in reducing symptoms, reducing the risk of exacerbation, and improving lung function while minimizing the dose of IC [11, 18]. In COPD, combination therapy composed of inhaled long-acting beta-2 agonists, IC, and long-acting muscarinic antagonists can improve lung function and reported patient outcomes; however more studies are needed before triple therapy can be fully recommended [19].

Side Effects

Systemic absorption of inhaled beta-2 agonists is responsible for a myriad of side effects, most of which are not serious. Most commonly, beta-2 agonist therapy leads to tremors and tachycardia secondary to direct stimulation of the beta-2 adrenergic receptor in skeletal muscle or vasculature, respectively [11, 12, 20, 21]. In severe asthma, beta-2 agonists may cause a temporary reduction in arterial oxygen tension of

5 mmHg or more secondary to beta-2-mediated vasodilation in poorly ventilated lung regions [12, 22]. Hyperglycemia, hypokalemia, and hypomagnesemia also can occur with beta-2 agonist therapy, but the severity of these side effects tends to diminish with regular use [12]. Tolerance to beta-2 agonists can occur with regular use over a period of weeks and, while not affecting peak bronchodilation, can be evidenced by a decrease in the duration of bronchodilation and the magnitude of side effects (tremor, tachycardia, etc.) [12, 23, 24]. Tolerance likely reflects beta-2 adrenergic receptor downregulation [12]. Last, beta-2 agonist therapy withdrawal after regular use can produce transient bronchial hyperresponsiveness [12].

Safety Concerns

Evidence has associated the use of long-acting beta-2 agonist therapy without concomitant use of a steroid inhaler with fatal and near-fatal asthma attacks [11, 25]. In light of this evidence, it seems prudent to save long-acting beta-2 agonists for asthmatic patients that are poorly controlled on inhaled steroids alone or for those patients with symptoms sufficiently challenging to warrant the potential extra risk associated with use of the agents [11, 25].

Systemic Adrenergic Agonists

Systemic administration of adrenergic agonists for asthma was used more frequently in the past. Oral, intravenous, or subcutaneous administration of beta-specific or nonspecific adrenergic agonists is now reserved for rescue therapy.

Mechanism of Action

The mechanism of action of systemically administered adrenergic agonists is the same as it is for inhaled agents. Binding of the drug to the beta-2 adrenergic receptor on smooth muscle cells in the airway is responsible for the bronchodilatory effects [8]. Specifically, beta-2 receptor stimulation induces a G-stimulatory protein to convert ATP to cAMP and in turn reduces intracellular calcium release and alters membrane potential [8, 12].

Clinical Applications

Terbutaline can be given orally, subcutaneously, or intravenously (IV), albuterol (salbutamol) can be given intravenously, and epinephrine is usually given subcutaneously or intravenously. Regardless of the route of administration, all three will produce bronchodilation. Comparison of intravenous and inhaled formulations of terbutaline failed to demonstrate any difference in bronchodilation, and, with the propensity for IV formulations to cause side effects, inhaled therapy should be considered the first-line treatment [26, 27]. This principle not only applies to terbutaline but also to all beta-adrenergic agonists that are available in IV and inhaled forms [17]. If inhaled therapy is not readily available or if inhaled therapy is maximized and symptoms persist, then subcutaneous epinephrine or terbutaline can be administered with improvement in symptoms and spirometry values [28]. In summary, subcutaneous or IV beta agonists should be reserved only for rescue therapy.

Side Effects

The side-effect profile of systemic adrenergic agonists is similar to that for inhalational adrenergic agonists. The most common side effects are tremor and tachycardia [11, 12]. Arterial oxygen tension can be transiently decreased, and hyperglycemia, hypokalemia, and hypomagnesemia can also be present [11, 12]. Escalating oral, subcutaneous, or IV doses can be associated with a greater incidence of side effects for the same degree of bronchodilation compared to inhaled beta-adrenergic agonists [11, 12].

Inhaled Cholinergic Antagonists

The use of anticholinergics (antimuscarinics) for maintenance therapy and treatment of acute exacerbations in obstructive airway diseases is common. The parasympathetic nervous system is primarily responsible for bronchomotor tone, and inhaled anticholinergics act on muscarinic receptors in the airway to reduce tone [2]. The parasympathetic nervous system plays a role in determining resting heart rate, and suppression of the parasympathetic nervous system can cause tachyarrhythmias. The use of inhaled anticholinergics (see Table 8.1) in COPD as maintenance and rescue therapy is considered first-line, standard treatment [29]. Anticholinergics are not used for first-line maintenance therapy in asthma and are only recommended for use in acute exacerbations or as therapy steps up [11, 17, 29, 30].

Mechanism of Action

The targets of therapy for anticholinergics are the muscarinic receptors located in the airway. There are three subtypes of muscarinic receptors found in the human airway [31]. Muscarinic 2 (M2) is present on postganglionic cells and is responsible for limiting production of acetylcholine and protects against bronchoconstriction [31]. M2 is not the target of inhaled anticholinergics but is antagonized by them [31]. Muscarinic 1 (M1) and muscarinic 3 (M3) receptors are responsible for bronchoconstriction and mucus production and are the targets of inhaled anticholinergic therapy [31]. Acetylcholine binds to the M3 and M1 receptors and causes smooth muscle contraction (see Fig. 8.1) via increases in cyclic guanosine monophosphate (cGMP) or by activation of a G-protein (Gq) [5, 6, 31]. Gq activates phospholipase C to produce inositol triphosphate (IP3), which causes release of calcium from intracellular stores and activation of myosin light-chain kinase causing smooth muscle contraction [5, 6, 31]. Anticholinergics inhibit this cascade and reduce smooth muscle tone by decreasing release of calcium from intracellular stores [5, 6].

Clinical Applications

Inhaled antimuscarinics are approved for the treatment of obstructive airway diseases. Ipratropium is classified as a short-acting anticholinergic and is commonly used as maintenance therapy for COPD and as rescue therapy for both COPD and asthmatic exacerbations [29, 31]. It is not indicated for the routine management of asthma [11, 17, 29, 30]. Patients treated with ipratropium experience an increase in exercise tolerance, decrease in dyspnea, and improved gas exchange [31]. Tiotropium is an example of inhaled long-acting antimuscarinic available for COPD maintenance therapy. Tiotropium has been shown to reduce COPD exacerbations, respiratory failure, and all-cause mortality [32]. Combination bronchodilators with both LABA and LAMA are available and improve symptoms and reduce exacerbations greater than with a single bronchodilator. Tiotropium also improves the effectiveness of pulmonary rehabilitation [19]. The newer long-acting muscarinic antagonist, inhaled glycopyrronium, has a faster onset of bronchodilation on the first day when compared to tiotropium. A randomized controlled trial showed comparable improvements in lung function and health status when combination glycopyrronium with LABA and ICs was compared to tiotropium with LABA and ICs. This study also demonstrated benefits of triple therapy compared to combination LABA/ICs [33]. In asthmatics who are poorly controlled on ICs and LABA, the addition of tiotropium reduces severe exacerbations [34].

Side Effects

Inhaled anticholinergics are poorly absorbed and therefore serious side effects are uncommon. Most commonly, patients experience dry mouth and urinary retention and can experience pupillary dilation and blurred vision if the eyes are inadvertently exposed to the drug [31]. Inhaled anticholinergic medications have been shown to increase the risk of serious cardiovascular events including cardiovascular mortality [35]. Tachyarrhythmias and atrial tachycardias are side effects, and inhaled anticholinergics should be used with caution in patients with known concomitant cardiovascular disease.

Systemic Cholinergic Antagonists

The systemically administered anticholinergics atropine and glycopyrrolate act via the same mechanisms as inhaled anticholinergics. While these anticholinergics can be administered by IV or inhalation, significant systemic absorption occurs, and their use is generally limited by side effects. Atropine, in particular, is limited in use because of its tertiary ammonium structure [29]. It has a tendency to cause tachy-

cardia, gastrointestinal upset, blurred vision, dry mouth, and central nervous system effects secondary to its ability to cross the blood–brain barrier [29]. Glycopyrrolate has a quaternary ammonium structure and is insoluble in lipids, similar to ipratropium and tiotropium, and has fewer systemic side effects than atropine [29, 31]. Intravenous glycopyrrolate is also clinically limited in use secondary to side effects [36]. Glycopyrrolate has been studied as inhaled therapy, however, and is an effective bronchodilator with an intermediate duration of action [37–40]. Clinically, it has never been popular as a mainstay of therapy for obstructive airway diseases. Atropine and glycopyrrolate are both used clinically to reduce secretions.

Influence of Inflammation on the Airway and Modulation of the Response

Asthma and COPD, the most common obstructive airway diseases, have a component of inflammation as part of their pathogenesis. Although inflammation is a common pathogenesis, the characteristics and prominent cellular elements involved in the inflammatory process for each disease are distinct [41]. In COPD, neutrophils, macrophages, CD8+ T lymphocytes, and eosinophils are more prominent in the inflammatory composition [41]. In asthma, eosinophils play a more prominent role followed by mast cells, CD 4+ T lymphocytes, and macrophages in the inflammatory composition [41]. Inflammatory cell types present in sputum, biopsy specimens, and bronchoalveolar lavage fluid can help predict the response to anti-inflammatory therapy [41]. For example, eosinophilia in induced sputum of a patient presenting with a COPD exacerbation predicts an increase in steroid responsiveness [41–43]. Treatment aimed at reducing eosinophilia in COPD patients has been shown to reduce exacerbations and hospitalization [44, 45]. Patients presenting to the operating room with obstructive airway diseases have a high likelihood of being prescribed and taking or being exposed to one of the anti-inflammatory therapies in Table 8.2 for control of their disease.

Table 8.2 Pharmacologic influence on inflammation

Inhaled corticosteroids	Leukotriene modifiers	Mast cell stabilizers	Methylxanthines
Monotherapy	Antagonists		
Beclomethasone	Montelukast	Cromolyn sodium	Theophylline
Budesonide	Zafirlukast	Nedocromil	Aminophylline
Ciclesonide	Pranlukast (not in the United States)		
Flunisolide			
Fluticasone	Inhibitors		
Mometasone	Zileuton		
Triamcinolone			
Combination therapy			
Budesonide/formoterol			
Fluticasone/salmeterol			

Adapted from Fanta et al. [11]

Inhaled Corticosteroids

In the treatment of asthma, the use of ICs reduces the inflammatory changes associated with the disease, thereby improving lung function and reducing exacerbations that result in hospitalization and death [11, 46–48]. On the contrary, the use of ICs as monotherapy in COPD is discouraged [31]. In COPD, ICs are used as a part of combination therapy along with long-acting beta-adrenergic agonists (LABA) and possibly long-acting antimuscarinic antagonists [19]. The combination of drugs acts synergistically and is useful for reducing inflammation [31]. Currently, combination therapy of ICs and LABA is recommended for use in severe to very severe COPD [31, 49]. Triple therapy with ICs, LABA, and LAMA improves lung function and reduces exacerbations more than ICs combined with only LABA [19].

Mechanism of Action

The glucocorticoid receptor alpha (GRα) located in the cytoplasm of airway epithelial cells is the primary target of ICs [50, 51]. Passive diffusion of steroids into the cell allows for binding of the steroid ligand to GRα, dissociation of heat shock proteins, and subsequent translocation to the nucleus [51]. Figure 8.2 shows how the steroid–receptor complex can have a multitude of actions when it enters the nucleus [51]. The complex can bind to promoter regions of DNA sequences and either induce or suppress gene expression [51]. Additionally, the steroid–receptor complex can interact with

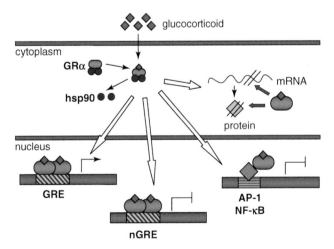

Fig. 8.2 Action of glucocorticoids. Glucocorticoids can bind to promoter regions inducing or repressing gene expression, act on promoters with transcription factors in place, or influence the structure of chromatin. GRα, glucocorticoid receptor alpha; hsp90, heat shock proteins; mRNA, messenger ribonucleic acid; GRE, glucocorticoid responsive elements; nGRe, negative glucocorticoid responsive elements; NF-KB, nuclear factor kappa beta; AP-1, activator protein-1. (Reprinted from Pujols et al. [51] with permission)

transcription factors already in place, such as the ones responsible for proinflammatory mediators, without binding to DNA and repressing expression of those genes [50, 51]. Corticosteroids may inhibit the transcription of proinflammatory mediators and upregulate production of anti-inflammatory proteins [52]. The steroid–receptor complex also can affect chromatin structure by association with transcription factors that influence the winding of DNA around histones, reducing access of RNA polymerase and other transcription factors, and thus reducing expression of inflammatory gene products [50, 51]. Corticosteroids are able to modulate B2-adrenoreceptor and their function by protecting against desensitization and development of tolerance, increasing the efficiency of receptor coupling, and mitigating the risk of inflammation-induced receptor downregulation and uncoupling [52].

Clinical Applications

ICs are used in asthma as part of a multimodal treatment regimen and are added to a therapeutic regimen when there is an increase in severity or frequency of asthma exacerbations [11]. There is good evidence to show that ICs can reduce both hospitalizations and death in asthma [47, 48]. The use of ICs in COPD is limited to use in severe to very severe COPD and in combination with LABA [19, 31]. Although no improvement in mortality has been consistently demonstrated with combination therapy (ICs/LABA), an ICs combined with LABA is more effective than the individual components in improving lung function and health status and reducing exacerbations [19]. Triple therapy with the addition of LAMA is more effective in reducing exacerbations. In COPD, the benefits of corticosteroids have been shown to be greater in patients with eosinophilic airway inflammation [19]. Research is ongoing looking at the use of eosinophil counts as potential biomarkers to direct treatment decisions. Further investigation is needed, but the use of eosinophil counts may lead to an improved risk–benefit ratio for inhaled corticosteroid treatment in severe COPD [53].

Side Effects and Safety Concerns

Side effects have been reported with the use of ICs in asthma and COPD. A recent meta-analysis reported an increase in pneumonia and serious pneumonia but not pneumonia-related deaths when ICs was used in the treatment of COPD [54]. Patients at higher risk of pneumonia are smokers, age 55 years or older, BMI less than 25 kg/m², or have a history of prior pneumonia or exacerbations [55]. Other reported side effects in COPD and asthma include oropharyngeal candidiasis, pharyngitis, hoarseness, easy bruising, osteoporosis, cataracts, elevated intraocular pressure, dysphonia, cough, and growth retardation in children [11, 31, 49]. As with any pharmacotherapy, the risks and benefits of therapy must be weighed, and the patient must be carefully monitored for adverse effects. This is especially true with the use of ICs in obstructive lung diseases.

Systemic Corticosteroids

Systemic corticosteroids given in intravenous or oral form are used for treatment of asthma and COPD exacerbations. The mechanism of action is the same as it is for ICs, activation or suppression of gene products at a transcriptional level and alteration of chromatin structure [50, 51]. Patients that are hospitalized with a COPD exacerbation will typically receive corticosteroids to suppress any inflammatory component that may be contributing to the flare-up. Therapy with oral prednisolone is equally as effective as IV administration [56]. A study done at the Veterans Affairs medical centers in the United States published in 1999 reported that corticosteroid therapy shortened hospital length of stay and improved forced expiratory volume in 1 second vs. placebo. The study also compared a 2-week regimen vs. an 8-week regimen of corticosteroids and found no difference [57]. The REDUCE randomized clinical trial compared 5 days to 14 days of therapy with 40 mg prednisone daily for treatment of COPD exacerbations. The trial showed that 5-day treatment was noninferior [58]. Current guidelines state that duration of therapy for systemic corticosteroids should not be more than 5–7 days [19]. In asthma, corticosteroids are recommended for exacerbations that are either severe, with a peak expiratory flow of less than 40% of baseline, or a mild to moderate exacerbation with no immediate response to short-acting beta-adrenergic agonists [17]. The recommended duration of therapy is 3–10 days without tapering [17]. Alternatively, some patients with asthma and COPD will be receiving long-term oral corticosteroid therapy because their disease is difficult to manage. Side effects of systemic corticosteroids are well described and numerous. Hypertension, hyperglycemia, adrenal suppression, increased infections, cataracts, dermal thinning, psychosis, and peptic ulcers are reported complications of corticosteroid therapy [59].

Leukotriene Modifiers

Leukotriene modifiers can be used for the treatment of asthma. They are prescribed primarily for long-term control in addition to short-acting beta-adrenergic agonists or in conjunction with ICs and short-acting beta agonists. Leukotriene modifiers are taken by mouth, produce bronchodilatation in hours, and have maximal effect within days of administration [11]. Their role in the management of COPD is not defined. Future investigations will need to focus on the role these medications can play in the outpatient management of COPD [60].

Mechanism of Action

Arachidonic acid is converted to leukotrienes via the 5-lipoxygenase pathway [61]. Leukotrienes C_4, D_4, and E_4 are the end products of the pathway and cause bronchoconstriction, tissue edema, migration of eosinophils, and increased airway secretions [61]. Leukotriene modifiers come in two different varieties, leukotriene receptor antagonists and leukotriene inhibitors [11]. Figure 8.3 shows how the binding of leukotrienes C_4, D_4, and E_4 at the type 1 cysteinyl leukotriene receptor is blocked by the leukotriene receptor antagonists montelukast, zafirlukast, and pranlukast (not available in the United States) [11, 61]. The leukotriene inhibitor zileuton antagonizes 5-lipoxygenase (Fig. 8.3), inhibiting the production of cysteinyl leukotrienes [11, 61].

Clinical Applications

Leukotriene modifiers improve lung function, reduce exacerbations, and are used as long-term asthma therapy [11, 17, 62, 63]. Clinical trials have reported that ICs are superior to leukotriene modifiers for long-term control and should be the first-line choice [17, 64, 65]. Leukotriene modifiers provide an additional pharmacologic option for the control of asthma. Addition of leukotriene modifiers to ICs will improve control of symptoms of asthma as opposed to ICs alone [66].

Side Effects

Overall, leukotriene antagonists are well-tolerated without significant side effects. Links between Churg-Strauss syndrome and the use of leukotriene antagonists have been reported, but it is not clear whether these reports reflect unmasking of a pre-existing condition or whether there is a direct link between the two [11, 61]. Zileuton is known to cause a reversible hepatitis in 2–4% of patients [11]. Liver function tests should be checked frequently at first and periodically thereafter to monitor for hepatocellular damage [11, 61].

Mast Cell Stabilizers

Cromolyn sodium and nedocromil are the two prototypical agents in this category that are used in the treatment of asthma. These agents are delivered by powder inhaler and are not first-line therapy for asthma. They do provide an alternative treatment when the control of asthma is not optimal on other conventional therapies [17].

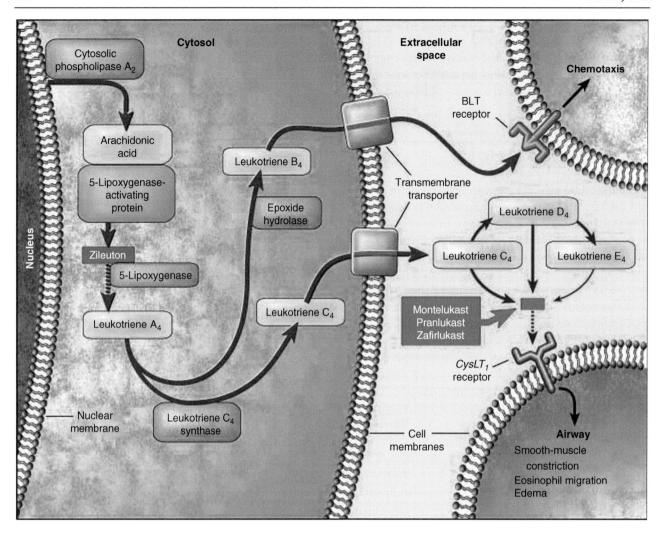

Fig. 8.3 Generation of leukotrienes and action of leukotriene-modifying drugs. Leukotriene antagonists block the action of leukotrienes at the cysteinyl leukotriene receptor (CysLT1), and leukotriene inhibitors block the conversion of arachidonic acid to leukotriene A4.

BLT leukotriene receptor B. (Reprinted from Drazen et al. [61] with permission, © 1999 Massachusetts Medical Society. All Rights Reserved)

Mechanism of Action

Cromolyn sodium and nedocromil stabilize submucosal and intraluminal mast cells [17, 67]. These drugs interfere with the antigen-dependent release of mediators, such as histamine and slow-reacting substance of anaphylaxis, that cause bronchoconstriction, mucosal edema, and increased mucus secretion [67].

Clinical Applications

Large systematic reviews of the available literature and consensus statements favor the use of ICs over cromolyn sodium or nedocromil as first-line agents to control symptoms of asthma [17, 68]. Alternatively, cromolyn sodium and nedocromil may be used as preventative treatment before exercise or known allergen exposure causing symptoms of asthma [17].

Side Effects

There are no major side effects reported with the use of cromolyn sodium and nedocromil. The most commonly reported side effects are gastrointestinal upset and coughing or irritation of the throat [67].

Methylxanthines

The role of theophylline, a prototypical methylxanthine, has changed since the introduction of ICs and LABA. Theophylline was a common choice for the control of asthma and COPD because of its bronchodilatory and anti-inflammatory effects [69]. Currently, theophylline is recommended only as an alternative therapy and is not a first-line choice for asthma or COPD [17, 70, 71].

Mechanism of Action

Theophylline is thought to act via multiple pathways causing improvement in symptoms in obstructive lung diseases. Theophylline is a nonselective inhibitor of phosphodiesterase and increases levels of cyclic AMP and GMP causing smooth muscle relaxation [69]. Antagonism of the A_1 and A_2 adenosine receptors also causes smooth muscle relaxation via inhibition of the release of histamine and leukotrienes from mast cells, another reported action of theophylline [69]. In asthma, theophylline reduces the number of eosinophils in bronchial specimens and, in COPD, reduces the number of neutrophils in sputum, having an anti-inflammatory effect in both conditions [69]. In addition, theophylline activates histone deacetylase and reduces the expression of inflammatory genes [69]. Theophylline and aminophylline are reported to improve diaphragmatic function; however data have not demonstrated this effect consistently [69, 72].

Clinical Applications

Theophylline has been relegated to an alternative therapy in both asthma and COPD. This has occurred largely because of its significant side-effect profile and the subsequent need for monitoring of blood levels [17, 69–71]. Patients that are already on an ICs and a LABA and still have symptoms may benefit from the addition of theophylline, especially if leukotriene modifiers and other alternatives are not tolerated [17, 70, 71]. Theophylline is not recommended for use in COPD exacerbations due to significant toxicity.

Side Effects

Theophylline can cause significant and life-threatening side effects if not dosed carefully and monitored appropriately. Toxicity is dose related, and side effects tend to be more prominent when blood levels exceed 20 mg/L [69]. The most common side effects include headache, nausea, vomiting, restlessness, abdominal discomfort, gastroesophageal reflux, and diuresis [69]. The most significant side effects include seizures, cardiac arrhythmias, and death [69]. Adverse effects from theophylline may be avoided if the clinician follows the patient carefully, monitors blood levels regularly, and educates the patient on the signs and symptoms of overdose.

Phosphodiesterase 4 Inhibitors

Mechanism of Action

Phosphodiesterase 4 (PDE4) is an enzyme that breaks down cyclic AMP. The enzyme is present in inflammatory and immune cells such as eosinophils, macrophages, and T lymphocytes. Inhibition of PDE4 has anti-inflammatory effects. Roflumilast, a PDE4 inhibitor, has been shown to decrease the expression of T cell adhesion molecules and decrease release of inflammatory mediators and cytokines [73].

Clinical Applications

Roflumilast is available for management in COPD in patients whose disease is not adequately controlled with long-acting bronchodilators. It is recommended for patients with severe airflow limitation, symptoms of chronic bronchitis, and history of exacerbations [74].

Side Effects

PDE4 inhibitors have a significant side-effect profile, which has limited their use. The main side effects are nausea, weight loss, and diarrhea. Less frequent side effects include insomnia, anxiety, and depression. In clinical trials, the side effects appeared to be dose dependent. Other PDE4 inhibitors are being studied for use in asthma and COPD [73, 74].

Influence of Anesthetics on the Airway

Volatile Anesthetics

Volatile anesthetics have a host of effects on the respiratory system. Volatile anesthetics reduce bronchomotor tone. All commonly used volatile anesthetics (see Table 8.3), except desflurane, produce a degree of bronchodilatation that may be helpful in patients with obstructive lung disease or in patients that experience any degree of bronchoconstriction [75, 77]. Rooke and colleagues in 1997 reported that sevoflurane produced a greater reduction in respiratory system resistance than isoflurane or halothane 10 min after the induction of anesthesia [75].

Mechanism of Action

The precise mechanisms by which volatile anesthetics induce bronchodilatation are not completely clear. Animal studies

Table 8.3 Anesthetics with a favorable influence on bronchomotor tone

Volatile anesthetics[a]	Intravenous anesthetics[b]
Isoflurane	Propofol
Sevoflurane	Ketamine
Halothane	Midazolam

[a]Adapted from Rooke et al. [75]
[b]Adapted from Cheng et al. [76]

suggest that volatile anesthetics inhibit tracheal smooth muscle contraction by decreasing intracellular calcium, mediated by an increase in intracellular cAMP and by suppression of protein kinase C which, in the absence of volatile anesthetics, sensitizes contractile elements to calcium and inhibits myosin light-chain phosphatase [78]. The effect is seen to a greater degree in distal airway smooth muscle secondary to the T-type voltage-dependent calcium channel, which is sensitive to volatile anesthetics [79].

Clinical Applications

Volatile anesthetics are administered to provide amnesia and blunt the response to surgical stimulation but can be of use in patients who have obstructive airway diseases or experience bronchoconstriction in the operating room. Multiple case reports provide examples of how volatile agents were used solely for the treatment of status asthmaticus [80–83].

Side Effects

The main concern with the use of volatile anesthetics is the rare occurrence of malignant hyperthermia. Hypotension can also be a concern with volatile anesthetics; however the blood pressure is usually easily restored with small amounts of IV fluids or vasopressors. Nausea and vomiting is a known side effect of volatile anesthetics, and prophylactic antiemetics should be considered based on patient risk factors. Deep levels of anesthesia associated with high concentrations of volatile anesthetics may be undesirable, and prolonged administration outside the operating room is problematic.

Intravenous Anesthetics

Intravenous anesthetics can have positive effects on bronchomotor tone when used for induction or intravenous anesthesia in the operating room. Ketamine, propofol, and midazolam (see Table 8.3) have relaxant effects on airway smooth muscle [76]. Etomidate and thiobarbiturates do not affect bronchomotor tone to the same extent [84]. The choice of intravenous anesthetics for induction and maintenance of anesthesia may be important for a patient with hard to manage bronchospasm or reactive airway disease.

Mechanism of Action

The precise mechanism of reduction of bronchomotor tone for the intravenous anesthetics is largely unknown. Ketamine is thought to have a direct relaxant effect on smooth muscle

[85]. Propofol is thought to reduce vagal tone and have a direct effect on muscarinic receptors by interfering with cellular signaling and inhibiting calcium mobilization [86, 87]. The preservative metabisulfite in propofol prevents the inhibition of vagal-mediated bronchoconstriction [88].

Clinical Applications

Choosing an agent such as propofol or ketamine can be beneficial in patients with bronchospasm or obstructive airway disease [76, 84]. The use of these intravenous agents for induction or maintenance of anesthesia over other agents can be useful in minimizing the intraoperative effects of bronchospasm.

Side Effects

Although each of the intravenous anesthetics carries a unique side-effect profile, the major effects are not related to the airway. The use of ketamine is associated with increased salivation, and coadministration of a small dose of anticholinergic can attenuate secretion production. Propofol is associated with hypotension that usually is easily corrected with IV fluids and vasopressors.

Local Anesthetics

Local anesthetics are primarily used to suppress coughing and blunt the hemodynamic response to tracheal intubation [89, 90]. Although animal models have demonstrated some ability of local anesthetics to relax bronchial smooth, in clinical practice the use of local anesthetics as pure bronchodilators is limited by toxicity and the ready availability of more potent bronchodilators such as short-acting beta-adrenergic agonists [85].

Influence of Adjunctive Agents on the Airway

Heliox

Helium (administered as a mixture of helium and oxygen [heliox]) has the advantage of having a low Reynolds' number and less resistance during turbulent airflow especially in large airways [6]. Helium and oxygen mixtures are recommended as alternative therapies in asthma to support patients when traditional therapies have initially failed to make improvements [17, 70]. A recent trial in patients with COPD exacerbations failed to demonstrate a statistically significant reduction in the necessity for endotracheal intubation in patients treated with noninvasive ventilation and helium/

oxygen mixtures [91]. The use of helium–oxygen mixtures is limited by a progressive reduction in efficacy at higher inspired oxygen concentrations.

Antihistamines

Histamine release from mast cells and basophils is responsible for airway inflammation and bronchoconstriction in asthma [92]. Antihistamines are not standard therapy for asthma, but the use of antihistamines and leukotriene modifiers for allergen-induced bronchoconstriction has shown promise for diminishing the early and late responses to allergens [92, 93]. Patients that have allergen-induced asthma or patients that experience an allergic reaction in the operating room may benefit from antihistamines to attenuate the role that histamine plays in bronchoconstriction.

Magnesium Sulfate

Magnesium sulfate is not a standard therapy for asthma exacerbations. Magnesium sulfate is thought to produce additional bronchodilation when given in conjunction with standard therapy for asthma exacerbations. Currently, intravenous magnesium therapy is reserved as an alternative therapy when the patient has not responded to standard therapy [17, 70, 94]. The combination of nebulized magnesium sulfate and beta-adrenergic agonists has also been studied and shows potential benefit in asthma exacerbations [95]. Overall, magnesium sulfate, IV or nebulized, is not a first-line therapy for asthma exacerbations and should be reserved for situations when the patient is not responding to conventional therapy [17, 70].

Summary

Patients with obstructive lung diseases presenting to the operating room for thoracic surgical procedures usually will be receiving pharmacotherapy to modify their symptoms or disease process. Understanding the role of pharmacotherapy in obstructive lung disease is essential to proper preoperative evaluation, perioperative risk reduction, and intraoperative management.

Clinical Case

A 65-year-old-man with COPD who quit smoking 2 years ago now presents to the preoperative clinic for evaluation before a right upper lobe lobectomy for a lung nodule. The patient has no other medical history and a recent cardiac stress test is normal.

Questions

Preoperative evaluation:

- How often does he need rescue inhalers? Has the frequency increased recently?
- When was the last time he was in the hospital with a COPD exacerbation?
- What medications for the treatment of COPD is the patient receiving?
- When was the last time he needed systemic corticosteroids for an exacerbation?
- Has there been any recent change in sputum or use of antibiotics?

Intraoperative Management:

- What medications will provide quickest relief of wheezing?
- Are prophylactic systemic corticosteroids indicated?
- What role do helium/oxygen mixtures and magnesium sulfate play in the management of wheezing?

Answers

Preoperative evaluation:

- Asking patients about the use of rescue inhalers gives some indication of how well their symptoms are controlled at baseline. Any increase in frequency of inhaler use may indicate disease progression or potential acute exacerbation.
- Inquiring about previous hospitalizations and the extent of illness (i.e., intubation, ICU admission) is important in determining the severity of disease.
- This patient will likely present on an IC and long-acting beta-adrenergic agonist combination along with an antimuscarinic such as ipratropium.
- The most recent use of systemic corticosteroids not only provides information as to how well the disease is being controlled but also gives the evaluator an idea if the patient is prone to adrenal suppression during surgical stress.
- Discussing the use of antibiotics and changes in sputum allows the evaluator to know if the patient is experiencing an exacerbation or if the patient is at risk for infection with multidrug-resistant bacteria.

Intraoperative management:

- Intraoperative wheezing can be due to endotracheal intubation, light anesthesia, or allergic reaction. Short-acting beta-2 adrenergic agonists, followed by inhaled anticholinergics, will give the most prompt relief. The additional use of intravenous and inhaled anesthetics may also be an effective treatment of bronchoconstriction. Epinephrine may be used for severe bronchoconstriction.

- Prophylactic IV corticosteroids are not indicated. Steroids should be given if the patient has recently received steroids and stress doses are needed or the patient experiences an allergic reaction and steroids are administered to reduce the inflammatory response associated with the exposure.

- Helium/oxygen mixtures and magnesium sulfate are only indicated when the patient fails to adequately respond to maximum conventional therapy.

References

1. Jordan D. Central nervous pathways and control of the airways. Respir Physiol. 2001;125(1–2):67–81.
2. Lewis MJ, Short AL, Lewis KE. Autonomic nervous system control of the cardiovascular and respiratory systems in asthma. Respir Med. 2006;100(10):1688–705.
3. Burwell DR, Jones JG. The airways and anaesthesia – I. Anatomy, physiology and fluid mechanics. Anaesthesia. 1996;51(9):849–57.
4. Canning BJ, Fischer A. Neural regulation of airway smooth muscle tone. Respir Physiol. 2001;125(1–2):113–27.
5. Barnes PJ. Pharmacology of airway smooth muscle. Am J Respir Crit Care Med. 1998;158(5):S123–32.
6. Lumb AB, Nunn JF. Nunn's applied respiratory physiology. 6th ed. Edinburgh: Elsevier Butterworth Heinemann; 2005.
7. Jartti T. Asthma, asthma medication and autonomic nervous system dysfunction. Clin Physiol. 2001;21:260–9.
8. Johnson M. The beta-adrenoceptor. Am J Respir Crit Care Med. 1998;158(5 Pt 3):S146–53.
9. Widdicombe JG. Autonomic regulation. i-NANC/e-NANC. Am J Respir Crit Care Med. 1998;158(5 Pt 3):S171–5.
10. Drazen JM, Gaston B, Shore SA. Chemical regulation of pulmonary airway tone. Annu Rev Physiol. 1995;57:151–70.
11. Fanta CH. Asthma. N Engl J Med. 2009;360(10):1002–14.
12. Nelson HS. Beta-adrenergic bronchodilators. N Engl J Med. 1995;333(8):499–506.
13. Johnson M, Butchers PR, Coleman RA, et al. The pharmacology of salmeterol. Life Sci. 1993;52(26):2131–43.
14. Drazen JM, Israel E, Boushey HA, et al. Comparison of regularly scheduled with as-needed use of albuterol in mild asthma. Asthma Clinical Research Network. N Engl J Med. 1996;335(12):841–7.
15. Israel E, Chinchilli VM, Ford JG, et al. Use of regularly scheduled albuterol treatment in asthma: genotype-stratified, randomised, placebo-controlled cross-over trial. Lancet. 2004;364(9444):1505–12.
16. Israel E, Drazen JM, Liggett SB, et al. The effect of polymorphisms of the beta(2)-adrenergic receptor on the response to regular use of albuterol in asthma. Am J Respir Crit Care Med. 2000;162(1):75–80.
17. Expert panel report 3 (EPR-3): guidelines for the diagnosis and management of asthma – summary report 2007. 2009. http://www.nhlbi.nih.gov/health/pubs/pub_prof.htm#asthma. Accessed 29 Dec 2009.
18. Gibson PG, Powell H, Ducharme FM. Differential effects of maintenance long-acting beta-agonist and inhaled corticosteroid on asthma control and asthma exacerbations. J Allergy Clin Immunol. 2007;119(2):344–50.
19. Global strategy for the diagnosis, management, and prevention of chronic obstructive lung disease 2017 report. GOLD executive summary. www.goldcopd.org. Accessed on 30 June 2017.
20. Bengtsson B. Plasma concentration and side-effects of terbutaline. Eur J Respir Dis Suppl. 1984;134:231–5.
21. Teule GJ, Majid PA. Haemodynamic effects of terbutaline in chronic obstructive airways disease. Thorax. 1980;35(7):536–42.
22. Wagner PD, Dantzker DR, Iacovoni VE, Tomlin WC, West JB. Ventilation-perfusion inequality in asymptomatic asthma. Am Rev Respir Dis. 1978;118(3):511–24.
23. Repsher LH, Anderson JA, Bush RK, et al. Assessment of tachyphylaxis following prolonged therapy of asthma with inhaled albuterol aerosol. Chest. 1984;85(1):34–8.
24. Georgopoulos D, Wong D, Anthonisen NR. Tolerance to beta 2-agonists in patients with chronic obstructive pulmonary disease. Chest. 1990;97(2):280–4.
25. Nelson HS, Weiss ST, Bleecker ER, Yancey SW, Dorinsky PM. The Salmeterol Multicenter Asthma Research Trial: a comparison of usual pharmacotherapy for asthma or usual pharmacotherapy plus salmeterol. Chest. 2006;129(1):15–26.
26. Williams SJ, Winner SJ, Clark TJ. Comparison of inhaled and intravenous terbutaline in acute severe asthma. Thorax. 1981;36(8):629–31.
27. Pierce RJ, Payne CR, Williams SJ, Denison DM, Clark TJ. Comparison of intravenous and inhaled terbutaline in the treatment of asthma. Chest. 1981;79(5):506–11.
28. Spiteri MA, Millar AB, Pavia D, Clarke SW. Subcutaneous adrenaline versus terbutaline in the treatment of acute severe asthma. Thorax. 1988;43(1):19–23.
29. Flynn RA, Glynn DA, Kennedy MP. Anticholinergic treatment in airways diseases. Adv Ther. 2009;26(10):908–19.
30. Karpel JP, Schacter EN, Fanta C, et al. A comparison of ipratropium and albuterol vs albuterol alone for the treatment of acute asthma. Chest. 1996;110(3):611–6.
31. Restrepo RD. A stepwise approach to management of stable COPD with inhaled pharmacotherapy: a review. Respir Care. 2009;54(8):1058–81.
32. Tashkin DP, Celli B, Senn S, et al. A 4-year trial of tiotropium in chronic obstructive pulmonary disease. N Engl J Med. 2008;359(15):1543–54.
33. Frith PA, Thompson PJ, Ratnavadivel R, et al. Glycopyrronium once-daily significantly improves lung function and health status when combined with Salmeterol/fluticasone in patients with COPD: the GLISTEN study – a randomized controlled trial. Thorax. 2015;70:519–27.
34. Kerstjens HA, Engel M, Dahl R, et al. Tiotropium in asthma poorly controlled with standard combination therapy. NEJM. 2012;367:1198–207.
35. Singh S, Loke Y, Enright P, Furberg CD. Pro-arrhythmic and pro ischaemic effects of inhaled anticholinergic medications. Thorax. 2013;68:114–6.
36. Gal TJ, Suratt PM. Atropine and glycopyrrolate effects on lung mechanics in normal man. Anesth Analg. 1981;60(2):85–90.
37. Gal TJ, Suratt PM, Lu JY. Glycopyrrolate and atropine inhalation: comparative effects on normal airway function. Am Rev Respir Dis. 1984;129(5):871–3.
38. Villetti G, Bergamaschi M, Bassani F, et al. Pharmacological assessment of the duration of action of glycopyrrolate vs tiotropium and ipratropium in guinea-pig and human airways. Br J Pharmacol. 2006;148(3):291–8.
39. Haddad EB, Patel H, Keeling JE, Yacoub MH, Barnes PJ, Belvisi MG. Pharmacological characterization of the muscarinic receptor

antagonist, glycopyrrolate, in human and guinea-pig airways. Br J Pharmacol. 1999;127(2):413–20.

40. Tzelepis G, Komanapolli S, Tyler D, Vega D, Fulambarker A. Comparison of nebulized glycopyrrolate and metaproterenol in chronic obstructive pulmonary disease. Eur Respir J. 1996;9(1):100–3.

41. Sutherland ER, Martin RJ. Airway inflammation in chronic obstructive pulmonary disease: comparisons with asthma. J Allergy Clin Immunol. 2003;112(5):819–27; quiz 828.

42. Fujimoto K, Kubo K, Yamamoto H, Yamaguchi S, Matsuzawa Y. Eosinophilic inflammation in the airway is related to glucocorticoid reversibility in patients with pulmonary emphysema. Chest. 1999;115(3):697–702.

43. Pizzichini E, Pizzichini MM, Gibson P, et al. Sputum eosinophilia predicts benefit from prednisone in smokers with chronic obstructive bronchitis. Am J Respir Crit Care Med. 1998;158(5 Pt 1):1511–7.

44. Postma DS, Rabe KF. The asthma-COPD overlap syndrome. NEJM. 2015;373:1241–9.

45. Postma DS, Reddel HK, ten Hacken NHT, van den Berge M. Asthma and chronic obstructive pulmonary disease: similarities and differences. Clin Chest Med. 2014;35:143–56.

46. Chanez P, Bourdin A, Vachier I, Godard P, Bousquet J, Vignola AM. Effects of inhaled corticosteroids on pathology in asthma and chronic obstructive pulmonary disease. Proc Am Thorac Soc. 2004;1(3):184–90.

47. Suissa S, Ernst P, Benayoun S, Baltzan M, Cai B. Low-dose inhaled corticosteroids and the prevention of death from asthma. N Engl J Med. 2000;343(5):332–6.

48. Donahue JG, Weiss ST, Livingston JM, Goetsch MA, Greineder DK, Platt R. Inhaled steroids and the risk of hospitalization for asthma. JAMA. 1997;277(11):887–91.

49. Calverley PM, Anderson JA, Celli B, et al. Salmeterol and fluticasone propionate and survival in chronic obstructive pulmonary disease. N Engl J Med. 2007;356(8):775–89.

50. Barnes PJ. Molecular mechanisms of corticosteroids in allergic diseases. Allergy. 2001;56(10):928–36.

51. Pujols L, Mullol J, Torrego A, Picado C. Glucocorticoid receptors in human airways. Allergy. 2004;59(10):1042–52.

52. Glaab T, Taube C. Effects of inhaled corticosteroids in stable chronic obstructive pulmonary disease. Pulm Pharmacol Ther. 2011;24:15–22.

53. Pascoe S, Locantore N, Dransfield M, Barnes N, Pavord ID. Blood eosinophil counts, exacerbations, and response to the addition of inhaled fluticasone furoate to vilanterol in patients with chronic obstructive pulmonary disease: a secondary analysis of data from two parallel randomized controlled trials. Lancet. 2015;3:435–42.

54. Singh S, Amin AV, Loke YK. Long-term use of inhaled corticosteroids and the risk of pneumonia in chronic obstructive pulmonary disease: a meta-analysis. Arch Intern Med. 2009;169(3):219–29.

55. Crim C, Dransfield MT, Bourbeau J, Jones PW, Hanania NA, Mahler DA, Vestbo J, Wachtel A, Martinez FJ, Barnhart F, et al. Pneumonia risk with inhaled fluticasone furoate and vilanterol compared with vilanterol alone in patients with COPD. Ann Am Thorac Soc. 2015;12:27–34.

56. deJong YP, Uil SM, Grotjohan HP, Postma DS, Kerstjens HA, van den Berg JW. Oral or IV prednisolone in the treatment of COPD exacerbations: a randomized controlled, double-blind study. Chest. 2007;132:1741–7.

57. Niewoehner DE, Erbland ML, Deupree RH, et al. Effect of systemic glucocorticoids on exacerbations of chronic obstructive pulmonary disease. Department of Veterans Affairs Cooperative Study Group. N Engl J Med. 1999;340(25):1941–7.

58. Leuppi JD, et al. Short-term vs conventional glucocorticoid therapy in acute exacerbations of chronic obstructive pulmonary disease. The REDUCE randomized clinical trial. JAMA. 2013;309:2223–31.

59. McEvoy CE, Niewoehner DE. Adverse effects of corticosteroid therapy for COPD. A critical review. Chest. 1997;111(3):732–43.

60. Usery JB, Self TH, Muthiah MP, Finch CK. Potential role of leukotriene modifiers in the treatment of chronic obstructive pulmonary disease. Pharmacotherapy. 2008;28(9):1183–7.

61. Drazen JM, Israel E, O'Byrne PM. Drug therapy: treatment of asthma with drugs modifying the leukotriene pathway. N Engl J Med. 1999;340(3):197–206.

62. Reiss TF, Chervinsky P, Dockhorn RJ, Shingo S, Seidenberg B, Edwards TB. Montelukast, a once-daily leukotriene receptor antagonist, in the treatment of chronic asthma: a multicenter, randomized, double-blind trial. Montelukast Clinical Research Study Group. Arch Intern Med. 1998;158(11):1213–20.

63. Israel E, Rubin P, Kemp JP, et al. The effect of inhibition of 5-lipoxygenase by zileuton in mild-to-moderate asthma. Ann Intern Med. 1993;119(11):1059–66.

64. Brabson JH, Clifford D, Kerwin E, et al. Efficacy and safety of low-dose fluticasone propionate compared with zafirlukast in patients with persistent asthma. Am J Med. 2002;113(1):15–21.

65. Malmstrom K, Rodriguez-Gomez G, Guerra J, et al. Oral montelukast, inhaled beclomethasone, and placebo for chronic asthma. A randomized, controlled trial. Montelukast/Beclomethasone Study Group. Ann Intern Med. 1999;130(6):487–95.

66. Price DB, Hernandez D, Magyar P, et al. Randomised controlled trial of montelukast plus inhaled budesonide versus double dose inhaled budesonide in adult patients with asthma. Thorax. 2003;58(3):211–6.

67. Bernstein IL. Cromolyn sodium. Chest. 1985;87(1 Suppl):68S–73.

68. Guevara JP, Ducharme FM, Keren R, Nihtianova S, Zorc J. Inhaled corticosteroids versus sodium cromoglycate in children and adults with asthma. Cochrane Database Syst Rev. 2006;(2):CD003558.

69. Barnes PJ. Theophylline: new perspectives for an old drug. Am J Respir Crit Care Med. 2003;167(6):813–8.

70. Global Intiative for Asthma. http://www.ginasthma.com. 2009. Accessed 5 Jan 2010.

71. Global Initiative for Chronic Obstructive Lung Disease. http://www.goldcopd.com. 2009. Accessed 7 Jan 2010.

72. Aubier M, De Troyer A, Sampson M, Macklem PT, Roussos C. Aminophylline improves diaphragmatic contractility. N Engl J Med. 1981;305(5):249–52.

73. Hatzelmann A, Morcillo EJ, Lungarello G, Adnot S, Sanjar S, Beume R, Schudt C, Tenor H. The preclinical pharmacology of roflumilast – a selective, oral phosphodiesterase inhibitor in development for chronic obstructive pulmonary disease. Pulm Pharmacol Ther. 2010;23:235–56.

74. Beghe B, Rabe KF, Fabbri LM. Phosphodiesterase-4 inhibitor therapy for lung diseases. Am J Respir Crit Care Med. 2013;188:271–8.

75. Rooke GA, Choi JH, Bishop MJ. The effect of isoflurane, halothane, sevoflurane, and thiopental/nitrous oxide on respiratory system resistance after tracheal intubation. Anesthesiology. 1997;86(6):1294–9.

76. Cheng EY, Mazzeo AJ, Bosnjak ZJ, Coon RL, Kampine JP. Direct relaxant effects of intravenous anesthetics on airway smooth muscle. Anesth Analg. 1996;83(1):162–8.

77. Goff MJ, Arain SR, Ficke DJ, Uhrich TD, Ebert TJ. Absence of bronchodilation during desflurane anesthesia: a comparison to sevoflurane and thiopental. Anesthesiology. 2000;93(2):404–8.

78. Yamakage M. Direct inhibitory mechanisms of halothane on canine tracheal smooth muscle contraction. Anesthesiology. 1992;77(3):546–53.

79. Yamakage M, Chen X, Tsujiguchi N, Kamada Y, Namiki A. Different inhibitory effects of volatile anesthetics on T- and L-type voltage-dependent Ca^{2+} channels in porcine tracheal and bronchial smooth muscles. Anesthesiology. 2001;94(4):683–93.

80. Gold MI, Helrich M. Pulmonary mechanics during general anesthesia: V. Status asthmaticus. Anesthesiology. 1970;32(5):422–8.

81. Parnass SM, Feld JM, Chamberlin WH, Segil LJ. Status asthmaticus treated with isoflurane and enflurane. Anesth Analg. 1987;66(2):193–5.

82. Johnston RG, Noseworthy TW, Friesen EG, Yule HA, Shustack A. Isoflurane therapy for status asthmaticus in children and adults. Chest. 1990;97(3):698–701.

83. Schwartz SH. Treatment of status asthmaticus with halothane. JAMA. 1984;251(20):2688–9.

84. Eames WO, Rooke GA, Wu RS, Bishop MJ. Comparison of the effects of etomidate, propofol, and thiopental on respiratory resistance after tracheal intubation. Anesthesiology. 1996;84(6):1307–11.

85. Wanna HT, Gergis SD. Procaine, lidocaine, and ketamine inhibit histamine-induced contracture of guinea pig tracheal muscle in vitro. Anesth Analg. 1978;57(1):25–7.

86. Lin CC, Shyr MH, Tan PP, et al. Mechanisms underlying the inhibitory effect of propofol on the contraction of canine airway smooth muscle. Anesthesiology. 1999;91(3):750–9.

87. Brown RH, Wagner EM. Mechanisms of bronchoprotection by anesthetic induction agents: propofol versus ketamine. Anesthesiology. 1999;90(3):822–8.

88. Brown RH, Greenberg RS, Wagner EM. Efficacy of propofol to prevent bronchoconstriction: effects of preservative. Anesthesiology. 2001;94(5):851–5; discussion 856A.

89. Yukioka H, Hayashi M, Terai T, Fujimori M. Intravenous lidocaine as a suppressant of coughing during tracheal intubation in elderly patients. Anesth Analg. 1993;77(2):309–12.

90. Hamill JF, Bedford RF, Weaver DC, Colohan AR. Lidocaine before endotracheal intubation: intravenous or laryngotracheal? Anesthesiology. 1981;55(5):578–81.

91. Maggiore SM, Richard JC, Abroug F, et al. A multicenter, randomized trial of noninvasive ventilation with helium-oxygen mixture in exacerbations of chronic obstructive lung disease. Crit Care Med. 2010;38(1):145–51.

92. Lordan JL, Holgate ST. H1-antihistamines in asthma. Clin Allergy Immunol. 2002;17:221–48.

93. Richter K, Gronke L, Janicki S, Maus J, Jorres RA, Magnussen H. Effect of azelastine, montelukast, and their combination on allergen-induced bronchoconstriction in asthma. Pulm Pharmacol Ther. 2008;21(1):61–6.

94. Rowe BH, Bretzlaff JA, Bourdon C, Bota GW, Camargo CA Jr. Magnesium sulfate for treating exacerbations of acute asthma in the emergency department. Cochrane Database Syst Rev. 2000;(2):CD001490.

95. Blitz M, Blitz S, Hughes R, et al. Aerosolized magnesium sulfate for acute asthma: a systematic review. Chest. 2005;128(1):337–44.

Pharmacology of the Pulmonary Circulation

9

Cara Reimer and John Granton

Abbreviations

(m)PAP	(mean) Pulmonary artery pressure
CI	Confidence interval
CO	Cardiac output
LAP	Left atrial pressure
PHTN	Pulmonary hypertension
PVB	Paravertebral block
PVR(I)	Pulmonary vascular resistance (index)
SVR(I)	Systemic vascular resistance (index)
TEA	Thoracic epidural analgesia

> **Key Points**
> - The pulmonary vasculature is a complex system, and studies of the effects of anesthetic drugs on this system are often contradictory.
> - A balanced anesthetic technique with adherence to the hemodynamic goals of maintenance of right ventricular preload and right coronary perfusion is the safest choice for patients with PHTN.
> - There are no absolute contraindications to most anesthetic drugs in patients with pulmonary hypertension.
> - Inhaled pulmonary vasodilators can be used to optimize hemodynamic variables perioperatively, although effects on gas exchange are variable.

C. Reimer (✉)
Department of Anesthesiology and Perioperative Medicine, Kingston Health Sciences Centre, Kingston, ON, Canada
e-mail: cara.reimer@kingstonhsc.ca

J. Granton
Division of Respirology, Department of Medicine, University of Toronto and University Health Network, Mount Sinai Hospital, Women's College Hospital, Toronto, ON, Canada

Introduction

Drugs affecting the pulmonary vascular bed are routinely administered perioperatively in thoracic anesthesia, and their effects are of particular interest in patients with pulmonary hypertension (PHTN). In addition, the increase in right ventricular (RV) afterload afforded by positive pressure ventilation may have adverse effects on patients with more advanced PHTN and reduced RV function.

Pulmonary hypertension is defined as a mean pulmonary arterial pressure ≥ 25 mmHg at rest. PHTN is classified according to the recent international guidelines into five groups: pulmonary arterial hypertension (PAH; group 1), PHTN secondary to left-sided heart or valvular disease (group 2), PHTN secondary to parenchymal or hypoxic/hypercapnic respiratory disease (group 3), chronic thrombo-embolic pulmonary hypertension (CTEPH; group 4), and miscellaneous causes of PHTN (group 5) [1, 2]. Group 1 PHTN embraces idiopathic, heritable, congenital cardiac, connective tissue disease, HIV, portal hypertension, and schistosomiasis-related pulmonary arterial hypertension. The rational for differentiation of PAH from other forms of PHTN relates to the distinctive arteriopathy that characterizes this condition as well as response to pulmonary vasodilator therapies. Irrespective of the etiology, patients with PHTN are high-risk candidates for cardiothoracic and non-cardiothoracic surgery. Although defined as an increase on pulmonary pressure, the consequence and severity of PHTN are likely best judged by the degree of right ventricular function [3]. Although the studies to date have not systematically evaluated the degree of RV function and outcome in patients with PHTN undergoing surgery, data from mixed populations of patients undergoing cardiac surgery supports the notion that RV function is associated with short- and longer-term outcomes [4]. Owing to the influence of afterload on the thinner walled RV, these patients have poor cardiorespiratory reserve and are at risk of having perioperative complications including pulmonary hypertensive crises with resultant heart failure, respiratory failure, and dysrhythmias [5, 6]. In patients undergoing valve repair or coronary artery bypass surgery, the presence of preoperative PHTN is associated with worse perioperative and long-term outcomes [7–9]. Management of these patients should not focus on pulmonary arterial pressure rather the goals should be centered on improving RV function and oxygen delivery [10]. Owing to the limited reserve of the RV, however, anesthetic management of these patients can be complex and challenging.

Drugs can interact with the pulmonary vascular bed both directly, through receptor binding, and indirectly, by changes in cardiac output. The effects of anesthetic, vasopressor, and vasodilator drugs on the pulmonary vessels will be reviewed in this chapter, with a special emphasis on perioperative drug choices in patients with pulmonary hypertension.

Anesthetic Drugs

Introduction

Evaluating the effects of anesthetic drugs on the pulmonary vasculature is challenging. In clinical practice, these drugs are rarely administered in isolation. Their administration can lead to concurrent changes in non-pulmonary hemodynamic parameters such as cardiac output (CO) that ultimately affect pulmonary artery pressure (PAP). An increase in PAP may be the result of increased PVR, increased CO, or an increase in LAP (PAP = (PVR × CO) + LAP). In addition, general anesthesia involves manipulation of variables that affect PVR, including FiO_2, carbon dioxide (CO_2), and positive pressure ventilation (PPV). Issues that arise in interpreting studies and making useful conclusions include reliance on and extrapolation from animal data, small study sample sizes, the questionable application of results in normal patients to patients with PHTN, children to adults and vice versa, and a vast supply of contradictory results. It is with acknowledgment of these limitations that we will review the effects of routinely administered anesthetic drugs on the pulmonary system.

Ketamine

Ketamine has occupied a controversial position in anesthesia for patients with PHTN [11]. Despite its current widespread use in these challenging patients, it has been classically taught that ketamine causes pulmonary vasoconstriction and should be used with extreme caution in this group.

The mechanism of action of ketamine is complex and not fully elucidated. It is an N-methyl-D-aspartic acid (NMDA) receptor antagonist and also binds to opioid receptors and muscarinic receptors [12]. It appears to stimulate release [13] as well as inhibit neuronal uptake of catecholamines [14]

which may account for its cardiostimulatory and bronchodilatory effects. Some animal studies have shown an endothelium-independent vasodilatory response to ketamine in the pulmonary bed [15, 16]. NMDA receptor subunits have been demonstrated in human pulmonary vascular cells, and antagonism of NMDA receptors prevents glutamate-mediated lung injury and reverses pulmonary hypertension in rats [17].

The effects of ketamine on the human pulmonary vasculature appear to be complex, and, indeed, review of the clinical literature reveals heterogeneity in regard to results. Factors known to affect pulmonary vasoreactivity such as FiO_2, CO_2, presence of PHTN, and presence of premedicants are not reported or acknowledged in many studies. The hemodynamic effects of a bolus of ketamine can be attenuated or abolished with premedicants like droperidol [18], dexmedetomidine [19], or benzodiazepines [20].

Early study of the drug's hemodynamic profile in adult patients showed increases of PAP and PVR in the range of 40–50% [21, 22]. This, combined with increases in variables contributing to myocardial oxygen consumption, raised concern about the use of ketamine in patients with CAD and PHTN. In the pediatric literature, Williams et al. [23] showed no change in PVR or mPAP after ketamine administration in spontaneously breathing children with severe pulmonary hypertension undergoing cardiac catheterization. In another pediatric study, ketamine maintained pulmonary to systemic blood flow and did not affect pulmonary pressure or resistance in children with intracardiac shunt undergoing cardiac catheterization [24]. Propofol, on the other hand, decreased SVR leading to increased right to left shunting in this study. More recently, a bolus of ketamine (2 mg/kg) has been shown to increase mPAP by a negligible amount clinically (mean 2 mmHg [95% CI 0.2, 3.7]) in pediatric patients with pulmonary hypertension with no change in PVRI or SVRI [25]. As part of a balanced anesthetic induction for open lung biopsy, ketamine has been used in Eisenmenger syndrome with good results [26]. In adult patients undergoing OLV for lung resection, ketamine did not significantly increase PAP or PVR compared to enflurane [27]. Other case reports highlight the value of the cardiostability of the drug in patients with minimal cardiorespiratory reserve [28–30]. Many clinicians, including those at our institutions, incorporate this drug into their routine inductions for patients with severe pulmonary hypertension. The advantages, in particular maintenance of stable hemodynamics and coronary artery perfusion pressure, seem to outweigh the potential disadvantages.

Propofol

Propofol is ubiquitously used in anesthesia, including for patients with pulmonary hypertension. It is frequently used to maintain anesthesia during and after lung transplantation.

The effects of propofol are thought to be primarily mediated by GABA receptors [31]. GABA inhibits peripheral sympathetic neurotransmission, and chronic treatment with GABA has been shown to decrease extent of pulmonary artery medial thickening and decrease right ventricular hypertrophy in mice with induced pulmonary hypertension [32].

As mentioned in the discussion on ketamine, the concerning hemodynamic effect of propofol in the context of pulmonary hypertension is a decrease in SVR, which can not only have effects on intracardiac shunting if present, but can lead to decreased coronary artery perfusion of the right ventricle and resultant right ventricular dysfunction. In regard to direct effects on the pulmonary vasculature, animal studies have shown that during increased tone conditions in the pulmonary vasculature, propofol may act as a pulmonary vasoconstrictor [33, 34]. Propofol has also been shown to interfere with acetylcholine-induced pulmonary vasodilation in dogs [35]. On the other hand, in isolated pulmonary arteries from human and chronically hypoxic rats, etomidate and (to a lesser extent) propofol showed vessel relaxation [36]. The clinical significance of these contradictory results is unknown. It has been suggested that to avoid hypotension, a vasopressor should be used at the time of anesthetic induction with propofol, etomidate, or volatile gas in patients with Eisenmenger syndrome [37].

Etomidate

Etomidate is an imidazole that mediates its clinical actions primarily at GABA A receptors. As mentioned above, it appears to have vasorelaxant properties in isolated pulmonary arteries [36]. Its major attribute as an induction agent is its stable hemodynamic profile. In patients with cardiac disease, an induction dose of etomidate increased MAP, decreased SVR, and decreased PAP [38]. In pediatric patients without pulmonary hypertension presenting for cardiac catheterization, there were no significant changes in any hemodynamic parameters, including PAP, after a bolus dose of etomidate (0.3 mg/kg) [39].

The drug has successfully been used in patients with pulmonary hypertension in obstetrics [40] and other procedures requiring general anesthesia or sedation [37].

Dexemedetomidine

An $\alpha 2$ adrenergic agonist, dexmedetomidine acts at preganglionic sites in the central nervous system and the autonomic nervous system to inhibit norepinephrine release, in addition to acting on postsynaptic receptors to cause vasoconstriction and vasodilation [41, 42]. Whereas the sympathetic nerve fibers of the human pulmonary artery possess

presynaptic $\alpha 2$ receptors [43], there is minimal evidence for postsynaptic $\alpha 2$ receptors in the arterial system of the lung [44]. However, this data is from canine pulmonary arteries which may have a different $\alpha 2$ receptor distribution than humans [45].

The drug has been shown to cause transient increases in MAP and a dose-dependent persistent decrease in noninvasively measured CO and increase in SVR at higher bolus doses (>1 mcg/kg over 2 min) in healthy volunteers [45]. These higher bolus doses caused small increases (~5 mmHg) in CO_2 and decrease in minute ventilation by approximately 30% [46]. Dose-dependent increases in dexmedetomidine cause increases in PAP, PVRI, and SVRI in healthy volunteers with pulmonary artery catheters [47]. While a bolus dose of 0.5–1 mcg/kg dexmedetomidine over 10 min caused an increase in MAP and SVRI, there were minimal changes in PAP and PVRI in children with pulmonary hypertension undergoing cardiac catheterization [48]. The increase in SVRI was theorized to take place via stimulation of postsynaptic $\alpha 1$ receptors in the peripheral vessels. A 1 mcg/kg bolus followed by 0.4 mcg/kg/h infusion prior to surgical incision in patients with pulmonary hypertension undergoing mitral valve replacement surgery caused significant decreases in HR, MAP, CI, and mPAP with no significant increases in PVRI or SVRI. The decrease in heart rate seen with dexmedetomidine is thought to occur via decreased inhibition of cardiac vagal neurons [49]. It would appear that (as with most drugs used in patients with pulmonary hypertension) titrated lower bolus doses of dexmedetomidine (<1 mcg/kg) with subsequent infusion titration would be appropriate for patients with pulmonary hypertension given the widespread hemodynamic effects of the drug. Dexmedetomidine used during one-lung ventilation decreased volatile and opioid requirements and increased phenylephrine requirements in a randomized trial [50].

Opioids

Mu, delta, and kappa opioid receptors have been shown to exist in the pulmonary artery of rats [51]. The number of kappa opioid receptors in rat pulmonary artery is increased under hypoxic conditions [52]. Kappa receptor agonism attenuates proliferation of pulmonary artery smooth muscle cells and lowers mean pulmonary artery pressure in these animals [53].

In anesthetized cats, administration of histamine, morphine, fentanyl, remifentanil, and sufentanil causes a vasodilatory response under elevated tone conditions in isolated lobar artery [54]. The mechanism seems to involve histamine- and opioid-mediated receptor pathways. Morphine causes a prostanoid-dependent vasodilation in isolated dog pulmonary arteries and veins [55].

The presence of opioid receptors and their significance in human pulmonary arteries are unknown as per the author's literature search. Clinical experience would echo the cardiostability of judicious opioid administration in hemodynamically fragile patients.

Neuromuscular Blockers

Pancuronium increases PAP in dogs with lung injury [56]. It is theorized to do so indirectly by increases in cardiac output and directly by increasing PVR, possibly by its antagonist actions at muscarinic receptors in the pulmonary vasculature. The drug has been shown to be an antagonist at acetylcholine M3 receptors in transfected hamster cells [57]. Rocuronium and succinylcholine also were antagonists at M3 receptors in this study, but not at clinically relevant concentrations. In human pulmonary arteries, M3 receptors present on endothelial cells are involved in vasodilation, and M3 receptors on smooth muscle cells mediate vasoconstriction [58].

In humans, rocuronium, cisatracurium, and vecuronium have little to no effect on most cardiac indices in patients undergoing CABG [59, 60].

Vasopressors and Inotropes

Vasopressors and inotropes are commonly required in thoracic anesthesia to counteract the effects of cardiodepressant and vasodilating drugs. Treatment of hypotension in these patients can be difficult to manage given the typical cautious fluid administration in this patient population. Neurotransmitter receptors in this system include those from the adrenergic, cholinergic, and dopaminergic families as well as histamine, serotonin, adenosine, purines, and peptides [61]. The pulmonary vasculature's response to sympathetic activation will generally result in an increase in PVR [62]. In human pulmonary artery, administration of acetylcholine induces pulmonary relaxation at the endothelial level [58, 63].

The response of the pulmonary system to exogenous vasoinopressor administration is dependent on the clinical situation. Consequently, results of studies are heterogeneous. In anesthetized dogs without pulmonary hypertension, dopamine, epinephrine, norepinephrine, and phenylephrine all increase PAP to varying degrees by varying mechanisms but with no drug is there a significant increase in PVR [64]. Dopamine does not increase PVR after lung transplantation in pigs [65]. In anesthetized patients with chronic secondary pulmonary hypertension undergoing cardiac surgery, both norepinephrine and phenylephrine increase PAP and PVRI with minimal change in CI [66]. Within the clinically relevant MAP target in this study, norepinephrine decreased the mPAP to MAP ratio, but phenylephrine did not, suggesting it (norepi-

nephrine) may be a better choice in this patient cohort. In a dog model of acute pulmonary hypertension, however, phenylephrine restored perfusion to the ischemic right ventricle and therefore increased CO [67]. This is a relevant observation, as it illustrates the importance of coronary artery perfusion in the setting of right ventricular strain and that maintenance of systemic pressure by whatever method may be the most important guiding principle in this subset of patients.

Vasopressin has also been studied. In a chronic hypoxic rat model, vasopressin administration resulted in a V1 receptor-mediated pulmonary vasodilation [68]. In an acute PHTN model in dogs, vasopressin increased PVR and resulted in a substantial decrease in right ventricular contractility [69]. Human studies of the effects of vasopressin on the pulmonary vasculature are limited. Vasopressin has been used successfully after cardiac surgery in patients with pulmonary hypertension and resistant hypotension [70]. The use of vasopressin to treat acute right ventricular failure in patients with IPPH has been described in obstetric anesthesia [71]. In isolated human pulmonary arteries, both norepinephrine and phenylephrine cause vasoconstriction, whereas vasopressin does not [72]. In dogs, phenylephrine and vasopressin have been shown to increase pulmonary artery pressure "passively" by increasing pulmonary blood volume. This is associated with minimal increases in PVR, increases in left atrial pressure, and SVR and is worse during left ventricular dysfunction [73].

Magnesium

Magnesium is a vasodilator in both the systemic and pulmonary circulations. The mechanism of action of magnesium's effects on vasodilation is likely through its effects on membrane channels involved in calcium flux and through its action in the synthesis of cyclic AMP [74]. It would appear to be an important cofactor for endothelial-dependent pulmonary vasodilation [75]. It has been used successfully to wean nitric oxide in pulmonary hypertension [76]. Increasing doses of magnesium in piglets with acute embolic pulmonary hypertension decreased mean PAP, increased CO, and decreased PVR [77]. Magnesium has been used to treat persistent pulmonary hypertension of the newborn, but controversy surrounds its use here, and a systematic review concluded that there is a lack of evidence to support its use in this population [78].

Volatile Anesthetics

At clinically relevant concentrations, modern volatile anesthetics likely have little to no direct vasodilating effect on the pulmonary vasculature. At MAC levels of 1.5, neither sevoflurane nor desflurane had an effect on the relationship between the pulmonary artery pressure-left atrial pressure gradient and pulmonary blood flow in healthy dogs [79]. In a dog model (without PHTN), isoflurane decreased right ventricular function more than left ventricular function with no effect on PVR [80]. Likewise in pigs, sevoflurane administration depressed right ventricular function with no change in PVR [81]. This suggests that the decreases in PAP observed with volatile anesthetics [82] may partially occur secondary to the decreases in cardiac output seen with these agents. Nitrous oxide is typically avoided in patients with pulmonary hypertension as it is believed to cause pulmonary vasoconstriction, perhaps via release of catecholamines from sympathetic nerves supplying the pulmonary vasculature [83]. In patients with mitral stenosis and pulmonary hypertension presenting for cardiac surgery, administration of nitrous oxide after fentanyl anesthesia (7.5–10 mcg/kg) increased PVR, PAP, and CI [84]. However, a subsequent study showed that in the presence of high-dose fentanyl (50–75 mcg/kg), 70% nitrous oxide actually was associated with a decrease in PAP and CO in patients with secondary PHTN, with no echocardiographic changes in right ventricular function [85]. Interestingly, in univariate analysis in one retrospective cohort study, *not* using nitrous oxide was associated with postoperative mortality and increased length of stay in patients with PHTN presenting for non-cardiac surgery [5]. The ENIGMA-II international randomized trial demonstrated the safety of nitrous oxide use in a large group of patients with coronary artery disease undergoing non-cardiac surgery [86]. The incidence of pulmonary hypertension in this cohort of patients was not indicated, but thoracic procedures were excluded given the usual requirement for higher FiO2 in these patients. Death and cardiovascular complications occurred with equal frequencies in both intervention and control groups. In addition, the risk of postoperative nausea was only slightly increased in the nitrous oxide group (15% vs 11%). Similarly at 1-year follow-up, nitrous oxide did not increase the risk of death or complications [87].

Perioperative Analgesia

Pain can increase PVR [88]. Perioperative thoracic epidural analgesia (TEA) and paravertebral blockade (PVB) are used routinely in thoracic surgery. TEA may decrease PAP through decreases in CO or via attenuation of the pulmonary sympathetic outflow [89]. In humans without pulmonary hypertension, TEA during one-lung ventilation depresses right ventricular contractility but maintains cardiac output by increases in right diastolic function and a decrease in pulmonary artery elastance [90]. In this study, right ventricular contractility increased in response to pulmonary artery clamping. Unilateral thoracic paravertebral block with lidocaine has been shown to decrease myocardial contractility up to 30% and significantly decrease systemic pressure, an effect that may be attenuated by epinephrine [91]. In general, the potential benefits of regional anesthesia in thoracic surgery probably outweigh the risks of hypotension and right ventricular dysfunction. As with most anesthetic interventions in patients with PHTN, careful titration and monitoring are paramount. Indeed, case reports illustrate successful use of epidural analgesia in this patient population [92–94].

Conclusion

In general, no anesthetic drug is contraindicated in patients with PHTN. The aim of any anesthetic intervention in these patients is hemodynamic neutrality, which can be accomplished by a variety of agents and techniques. An awareness of the potential advantages and disadvantages of drugs is key to proper decision-making. In the PHTN population, the general principles remain the same: adequate anesthesia and analgesia, maintenance of gas exchange to the best extent possible, and support of the right ventricle. In reality, most clinicians who deal with these patients regularly use a wide variety of medications with success.

Support of the Right Ventricle

RV failure can occur acutely when the right ventricular afterload suddenly increases. Unlike the left ventricle, the naïve right ventricle is not capable of generating flow against a high afterload. In the setting of chronic pulmonary hypertension, RV failure can occur following arrhythmias, sepsis, pulmonary embolism, pregnancy, surgery/anesthesia, or progression of their primary disease [95]. The mainstay to supporting the right ventricle includes ensuring an adequate systemic blood pressure (to preserve coronary perfusion), optimizing RV volumes (to reduce RV wall tension and myocardial work and improve RV–LV interaction), and reducing RV afterload [10, 96]. Inotropes may not be effective in acute RV failure owing to the relatively small muscle mass of the right ventricle or the presence of RV ischemia. Additionally, inotropes may lead to an increase in heart rate and a reduction in RV and LV filling time. In addition to avoiding agents that may have a direct adverse effect on cardiac function or those that may adversely increase RV afterload, agents that can reduce RV afterload can be used acutely. Although not systematically studied in the context of acute RV failure, the anesthetist should have an understanding of the agents used to treat chronic pulmonary arterial hypertension and how to manage these agents in the perioperative setting.

Pulmonary Vasodilators (PO/IV/Inhaled)

Pulmonary vascular resistance (PVR) is commonly considered clinically as reflective of the degree of right ventricular afterload. However, afterload to the right ventricle also includes pulmonary vascular compliance and impedance as well as RV wall tension [97, 98]. The naïve and decompensated RV is exquisitely sensitive to increases in its afterload. Consequently, even small changes in RV afterload may have profound effects on RV function. There are three main pathways that have been exploited acutely and more commonly chronically to reduce right ventricular afterload and increase cardiac output and oxygen delivery to metabolically active tissues. The various agents, pathway, and route of administration are provided in Table 9.1. Therapies directed toward the nitric oxide/guanylate cyclase pathway, the endothelin pathway, and the prostanoid/adenylate cyclase pathway have been the subject of several randomized controlled trials in patients with WHO group I pulmonary hypertension (pulmonary arterial hypertension – PAH). The use of these agents in the acute setting however is based more on biological plausibility and often small case series. In the acute setting, the ideal pulmonary vasodilator would have a rapid onset, short half-life, and selectivity for the pulmonary (as opposed to systemic) vasculature. In general, the only way to confer pulmonary vascular selectivity is by delivering the drug by inhalation. However, many agents administered by inhalation may be absorbed and "spill over" producing systemic effects. Systemic agents are also limited by possible increase in ventilation perfusion mismatching (shunt) owing to dilation of blood vessels to alveolar units that are not effectively participating in gas exchange.

Table 9.1 Comparison of currently available pulmonary vasodilators used to treat pulmonary hypertension and RV failure

Pathway	Agent/therapy	Route
Prostanoids		
Prostaglandin analogues	Epoprostenol sodium	IV, Inhaled
	Treprostinil	IV, SC, Inhaled
	Beraprost sodium	Oral
Prostaglandin receptor agonist	Selexipag	Oral
Endothelin		
Endothelin receptor blockers	Bosentan, ambrisentan, macitentan	Oral
Nitric oxide/cGMP		
	Nitric oxide	Inhaled
Inhibition of phosphodiesterase	Sildenafil	Oral, IV
	Tadalafil	Oral
Guanylate cyclase agonist	Riociguat	Oral

Nitric Oxide/Cyclic-GMP Pathway

Nitric oxide (NO) exerts its vasodilatory effects, in part, by binding to soluble guanylate cyclase (sGC) leading to the production of cyclic GMP (cGMP) that in turn activates protein kinase G [99–101]. The ensuing reduction in cytosolic calcium causes smooth muscle dilation by inhibition of phosphorylation and subsequent cross-linking of myosin or through activation of myosin light chain phosphatases that dephosphorylate myosin light chains. Direct activation of calcium-dependent potassium channels is another mechanism and leads to hyperpolarization of cells/reduced contraction [100].

Nitric Oxide

Inhaled nitric oxide (iNO) leads to an improvement in perfusion to alveoli that can participate in gas exchange. This "selective effect" leads to a decrease in intrapulmonary shunt [102, 103]. Nitric oxide may be administered either noninvasively or through a ventilator circuit using a device that can regulate the concentration of NO and monitor levels of nitrogen dioxide – a byproduct of NO when it combines with oxygen. Although there is controversy about a dose response relationship for NO and pulmonary vasodilation, the typical dose ranges from 10 to 40 ppm [104, 105]. The effect of NO on gas exchange and hemodynamics may be increased when used in combination with phosphodiesterase inhibitors [106–108]. Methemoglobin levels need to be monitored when NO is administered for more than 24 h. At present iNO is only approved for infants with respiratory distress syndrome. This approval stems from two large prospective placebo controlled studies demonstrating that NO reduced the need for ECMO and reduced the requirement for oxygen therapy following ICU discharge [109, 110]. However, iNO is still used for patients with refractory hypoxemia, acute pulmonary hypertension and RV failure, primary graft dysfunction, and acute RV failure following heart transplant [111, 112]. The acute right ventricular failure complicating heart transplantation may be attenuated with the use of a pulmonary vasodilator. Although several studies suggest that NO may be useful preoperatively in risk stratifying patients scheduled for cardiac transplant, only case series support the use of inhaled NO to reverse the right ventricular dysfunction following cardiac transplant [111, 113]. However, based on clinical experience, inhaled NO has become a standard of care in many transplant centers for the management of primary graft dysfunction (PGD). The beneficial immune-modulating effects of inhaled NO in addition to its vasodilating properties were felt to be responsible for preliminary studies of using inhaled NO to prevent PGD after lung transplantation [114, 115]. Although a randomized clinical trial failed to show benefit in preventing PGD, it is commonly used to treat the hypoxemia and pulmonary hypertension seen in established, severe PGD [116]. Owing to the inherent cost of using inhaled NO, other pulmonary vasodilators have been evaluated.

In non-transplant thoracic surgery, NO has been studied as a potential treatment for the gas exchange abnormalities associated with OLV. Its effects are controversial, but it would appear that it exerts its maximal benefits in patients with elevated PVRI and the poorest gas exchange before administration [117–120]. There is no evidence for the routine use of this expensive drug in otherwise normal patients undergoing routine thoracic surgery.

cGMP/cAMP Pathway

Phosphodiesterase (PDE) inhibitors prevent the degradation of cyclic guanosine monophosphate (cGMP) and adenosine monophosphate (cAMP). Owing to the relatively higher expression of PDE_5 in the pulmonary circulation relative to the systemic circulation, PDE_5 inhibitors have a relative selective effect on PVR as opposed to SVR [121, 122]. In addition to their relatively selective pulmonary vasodilatory effects, their effects on smooth muscle proliferation and cellular apoptosis [123, 124] may be responsible for benefit of these agents when administered chronically in patients with idiopathic PAH [125, 126]. A direct inotropic effect of sildenafil on the right ventricle has been postulated; however, the clinical relevance of this finding is uncertain [127].

Although the benefits of sildenafil and tadalafil in chronic PAH have been evaluated in prospective controlled trials, most of the acute applications for these agents have been described in case reports or small cohort studies and as such have not been approved for these indications. In the acute setting, sildenafil has been demonstrated to enhance the effects of inhaled NO and may also be useful in blunting the rebound in pulmonary pressures that occurs during weaning of inhaled NO [106, 121, 128]. The benefits of sildenafil in acute pulmonary embolism and cardiac transplantation and in patients with pulmonary hypertension being considered for pulmonary thromboendarterectomy have also been described [107, 108, 129–131]. Although pulmonary vasodilators can improve hemodynamics in patients with CTEPH [132], the merits of attempting to optimize RV function in patients with pulmonary hypertension and planned pulmonary thromboendarterectomy were recently challenged in a retrospective analysis of chronic thromboembolic pulmonary hypertension patients referred to a single center during 2005–2007 [133]. There was minimal benefit of treatment with medication on pre-PTE mean pulmonary artery pressure, but its use was associated with a significant delay in time to referral for PTE. Importantly

the two groups did not differ significantly in any post-PTE outcome. Although this study did not specifically evaluate the use of sildenafil for this purpose, it suggests at the very least that planned, potentially curative surgery should not be delayed while exploring theoretic benefits of this agent on RV function. Whether it can modify surgical risk in patients with very high PVR or who have evidence of shock remains speculative [134]. Although some reports have demonstrated acute beneficial effects of sildenafil in patients with pulmonary hypertension in the context of systolic and diastolic dysfunction [135–138], and in patients undergoing valve surgery [139], the negative results of a study evaluating continuous intravenous epoprostenol for the same purpose supports the notion that a controlled trial be conducted before these agents are routinely used for this purpose [140, 141].

The activity of soluble guanylate cyclase (sGC) may also be directly influenced by sGC activators and stimulators [142]. Riociguat (sGC stimulator) has a dual mechanism of action on sGC by increasing both the sensitivity of sGC to endogenous NO and via a direct (NO independent) stimulation of sGC [143]. Unlike other agents mentioned thus far, riociguat must be up-titrated gradually over several weeks to ensure that the medication is tolerated. The efficacy of riociguat has been demonstrated in chronic pulmonary hypertension. In patients with PAH and in inoperable or persistent chronic thromboembolic disease post-endarterectomy [144, 145], riociguat improved exercise capacity (assessed by 6-min walk distance), symptoms of dyspnea, quality of life, and hemodynamics. The main relevant limitation to riociguat is twofold. First hemoptysis and pulmonary hemorrhage have been reported within the confines of the acute and long-term trials (generally less than 3% of the study cohort). Second, riociguat can cause systemic hypotension. Particularly noteworthy is the adverse interaction between this agent and the PDE_5 inhibitor class of agents and a theoretic adverse interaction between this agent and NO donors, in causing systemic hypotension [146]. The effects of endogenous/inhaled NO in combination with riociguat have not been systematically evaluated.

Endothelin Antagonists

Endothelin-1 (ET-1) is a peptide produced primarily by endothelial cells. It acts on ET-A and ET-B receptors, both of which are located on pulmonary vascular smooth muscle cells. The ET-B receptor is also located on endothelial cells. Abnormally high concentration of ET-1 in PAH is the result of increased production and decreased clearance of the peptide [147, 148]. Both circulating and pulmonary concentrations of ET-1 have been correlated with disease severity and prognosis in PAH [149].

Bosentan, ambrisentan, and macitentan are approved as treatment for patients with PAH. Both ambrisentan and bosentan have been shown to improve symptom severity, hemodynamics, and exercise capacity (quantified by improvements in the standardized 6-min walk test – 6MWT) [150]. The SERAPHIN trial (macitentan 3 mg vs 10 mg vs placebo) was the first endpoint-driven trial and demonstrated an improvement in time to clinical worsening (hospitalizations, escalation in treatments, death, or transplantation) [151]. This composite primary endpoint was primarily driven by a reduction in hospitalizations or escalation in medical treatments for PAH.

The tolerability as a class is most commonly limited by hepatotoxicity, followed by several less frequent hematologic, neurologic, cardiovascular, respiratory, and gastrointestinal adverse effects. The newer agents, ambrisentan and macitentan, have the lowest incidence of hepatotoxicity and fewer drug-drug interactions than bosentan [152]. However, interactions with agents undergoing CYP metabolism remain a potential concern for this class. The effect on cyclosporine metabolism is particularly relevant. Although effective in the chronic setting, these agents have not been utilized for acute RV failure or acute pulmonary hypertensive crisis.

In the chronic setting, medical therapies are often combined to capitalize on the different therapeutic pathways. Indeed, recent data from a randomized controlled trial suggests that upfront combination therapy (ambrisentan and tadalafil) is associated with improved outcomes compared to monotherapy with either agent [153]. In the acute setting, combination therapy (e.g., with iNO and a PDE$_5$ inhibitor) may also be of benefit.

Milrinone is an adenosine-3′, 5′-cyclic monophosphate (cAMP)-selective phosphodiesterase enzyme (PDE) inhibitor. When nebulized it has been shown to lead to a relative reduction in PVR compared to SVR [154–156]. Haraldsson et al. evaluated a cohort of post cardiac surgery patients and reported upon the hemodynamic effects of the combination inhaled milrinone and inhaled prostacyclins [157]. The inhalation of milrinone selectively dilated the pulmonary vasculature without systemic effects. When milrinone is combined with inhaled prostacyclin, there appears to be a potentiation and prolongation of the pulmonary vasodilatory effect [157, 158].

Prostaglandins

Prostanoids induce relaxation of vascular smooth muscle, inhibit growth of smooth muscle cells, and are powerful inhibitors of platelet aggregation [159]. Inhaled prostanoids involve an aerosol delivery system that uses a nebulizer attached to the ventilator circuit. Treatment may be limited by inefficiencies in aerosolization. Owing to the short half-life of epoprostenol, the drug must also be continuously nebulized. As a result, changes of dose delivery with alterations in ventilator volumes, FiO$_2$, airway pressures, and solvent evaporation may be challenging [160]. The synthetic prostanoids, treprostinil and iloprost, hold promise as inhaled vasodilators as they may only require intermitted administration. Studies of prostanoids in chronic PAH demonstrated that they were effective in improving symptoms and exercise tolerance [161, 162]. When nebulized, prostanoids can lead to similar improvements in oxygenation and pulmonary pressures as compared to inhaled NO [163–167]. Indeed, several cohort studies have failed to demonstrate a benefit of iNO over inhaled prostanoids in treating acute pulmonary hypertension [168, 169]. Similarly in critically ill patients with refractory hypoxemia, inhaled epoprostenol ($n = 52$) and iNO ($n = 53$) had similar acute effects on gas exchange. The effects on pulmonary pressures or RV function were not assessed [170]. Similar to iNO, the effects of inhaled prostanoids on gas exchange and hemodynamics may be increased with the co-administration of PDE$_5$ inhibitors [171].

Use of intravenous prostaglandins during OLV results in a decrease in both systemic and pulmonary pressures and either no change or a decrease in PaO$_2$ [172, 173]. Selective infusion of prostaglandin into the pulmonary artery of the ventilated lung in a dog model during OLV resulted in stable systemic pressure and a reduction in PVR and increase in PaO$_2$ [174]. However, this route of administration is not practical in routine thoracic anesthesia practice. Inhaled prostacyclin decreases PVRI and PAP with maintenance of favorable systemic pressures but does not change PaO$_2$ during OLV [173].

Both inhaled nitric oxide and prostaglandins have been shown to affect platelet function [175, 176]. This could theoretically contribute to perioperative bleeding during large surgeries such as lung transplantation and a consideration in regard to the risks of neuraxial analgesia. It is important to emphasize however that the clinical relevance of platelet inhibition with these inhaled agents has not been systematically evaluated. Indeed, in cardiac surgery patients, laboratory confirmation of platelet dysfunction with inhaled prostacyclin did not correlate with chest tube losses [175]. Also, in an obstetrical patient with pulmonary hypertension on intravenous prostacyclin, conversion to inhaled prostacyclin allowed for a successful labor epidural placement with no complications [177].

Until recently an efficacious oral prostanoid has remained elusive. Selexipag is an oral selective IP receptor agonist that was shown to reduce clinical events (time to clinical worsening endpoints such as hospitalization and escalation of PAH treatments) compared to placebo in patients with group I PH. Although of benefit when administered chronically, it is unlikely that this oral agent will have clinical utility in the acute setting as it shares the same limitations as other parenteral prostanoids for the management of acute RV failure/pulmonary hypertension.

Pulmonary Vasodilators in Thoracic Surgery

Unsurprisingly, the bulk of research studying pulmonary vasodilators in thoracic surgery is in lung transplantation. Preoperatively transplant patients may be on oral, intravenous, or inhaled drugs for pulmonary hypertension. These must be continued perioperatively. Intraoperatively, inhaled pulmonary vasodilators such as nitric oxide (NO) and prostaglandins are commonly employed in attempts to decrease right ventricular afterload and optimize gas exchange. Addition of inhaled prostacyclin to inhaled NO after implantation of the first lung during bilateral sequential transplantation decreases pulmonary shunt, $PaCO_2$, and PAP while increasing PaO_2/FiO_2 with no effect on systemic hemodynamics [119]. Posttransplant, these drugs have been shown to improve the gas exchange abnormalities and increased pulmonary pressures associated with reperfusion injury [163] [114, 178]. Initial excitement over the potential ability of prophylactic NO to prevent acute graft rejection after lung transplantation [179] was tempered when a randomized trial did not show a statistically significant difference between placebo and NO for preventing reperfusion injury or changing postoperative outcome when administered 10 min after reperfusion in the operating room [116].

In non-transplant thoracic surgery, NO has been studied as a potential treatment for the gas exchange abnormalities associated with OLV. Its effects are controversial, but it would appear that it exerts its maximal benefits in patients with elevated PVRI and the poorest gas exchange before administration [117, 118, 120]. There is no evidence for the routine use of this expensive drug in otherwise normal patients undergoing routine thoracic surgery.

Inhaled prostacyclin decreases PVRI and PAP with maintenance of favorable systemic pressures but does not change PaO_2 during OLV [173].

Use of intravenous prostaglandins during OLV results in a decrease in both systemic and pulmonary pressures and either no change or a decrease in PaO_2 [172]. Selective infusion of prostaglandin into the pulmonary artery of the ventilated lung in a dog model during OLV resulted in stable systemic pressure and a reduction in PVR and increase in PaO_2 [174]. However, this route of administration is not practical in routine thoracic anesthesia practice.

Both inhaled nitric oxide and prostaglandins have been shown to affect platelet function [175, 176]. This could theoretically contribute to perioperative bleeding during large surgeries such as lung transplantation and is a concern in regard to neuraxial analgesia. The clinical relevance of platelet inhibition with these inhaled agents is unknown. Indeed, in cardiac surgery patients, laboratory confirmation of platelet dysfunction with inhaled prostacyclin did not correlate with chest tube losses [175]. Also, in an obstetrical patient with pulmonary hypertension on intravenous prostacyclin, conversion to inhaled prostacyclin allowed for a successful labor epidural placement with no complications [177].

To date there are few systematic concealed trials of pulmonary vasodilators on the acute management of intraoperative/perioperative pulmonary hypertension or RV failure. A recent systematic review of inhaled pulmonary vasodilators in cardiac surgery identified ten studies of inhaled pulmonary vasodilators (vs intravenous route or placebo) [180]. The authors concluded that while these agents seemed to be acutely better than systemic agents in improving RV function, there was no clear benefit of these agents when compared to placebo on clinical outcomes. Given the costs associated with these agents, a systematic study of their benefit to patient-relevant outcomes is needed.

Clinical Case Study

A 46-year-old woman with interstitial lung disease (ILD) presents to the pre-anesthetic clinic before an open lung biopsy.

What are the Anesthetic Considerations for This Case?

Considerations include those of ILD and the proposed case itself. In regard to the ILD, its etiology and severity (including associated connective tissue disorders and multisystem involvement), and associated right heart dysfunction should be delineated. In regard to the biopsy, the usual considerations of lung separation, analgesic options, invasive monitoring and, in this patient, the potential requirement for perioperative inhaled vasodilator therapy are present.

Besides the Usual Anesthetic History and Physical, What Would You Want to Elicit on History and Look for on Physical Exam in This Case?

On history, a careful assessment of functional status and current symptoms, personal and family history of connective tissue diseases should be undertaken.

On physical exam, vital signs including respiratory rate, potential clubbing, crackles on lung auscultation, and signs of right heart dysfunction (including increased JVP, hepatomegaly, lower extremity edema, increased P2 on heart auscultation and right ventricular heave on palpation) should be assessed.

The patient has been experiencing progressive worsening of shortness of breath for approximately 2 years. Her ability to exercise has declined markedly, to the point where she cannot climb a flight of stairs. She had a recent admission to hospital where she was started on home oxygen therapy and referred to a respirologist. An echocardiogram done at that time revealed an RVSP of 89 with mild right ventricular dilation and hypokinesis. ECG shows sinus tachycardia at 105. The respirologist suggests a biopsy to shed light on the etiology.

Physical exam reveals a thin woman with a respiratory rate of 18 wearing oxygen via nasal prongs at 4 L/min. Her oxygen saturation is 95%, her heart rate is 95, and her blood pressure is 100/60. Airway exam is reassuring. She has coarse crackles bilaterally. JVP is normal, but P2 is increased on cardiac auscultation. There is no hepatomegaly or pedal edema.

What Can be Done to Optimize These Patients' Perioperative Course?

After communicating with the patient's respirologist, a decision is made to bring the patient to the hospital the day before the planned operation to perform a right heart catheterization and assess the patient's response to inhaled prostacyclin. A pulmonary artery catheter is inserted under local anesthesia in the intensive care unit. PAP is 75/40. Systemic blood pressure is 90/60. After institution of inhaled prostacyclin, the PAP decreases to 60/30 with no change in systemic pressure.

What is the Anesthetic Plan?

TEE is arranged to be available for the case. After an appropriate fasting interval, the patient is transferred to the operating room with inhaled prostacyclin (10 ng/kg/min) and oxygen. A baseline ABG is drawn and shows pH of 7.38, $PaCO_2$ 44, PaO_2 65, and HCO_3 28. Baseline vital signs are sinus tachycardia 103, PAP 65/37, BP 98/62, and 96% on FiO_2 40%. An epidural is placed and tested at T5/6. An epidural infusion of bupivacaine and hydromorphone is started. Preoxygenation continues without interruption of the inhaled prostacyclin, and norepinephrine is started at 0.05 mcg/kg/min. After ensuring the surgeons are in the room, induction medications are titrated to effect and include midazolam 2 mg, fentanyl 250 mcg, and ketamine 50 mg. Rocuronium 50 mg is given to facilitate endotracheal intubation. A 37F left-sided double-lumen tube is placed without difficulty, and anesthesia is maintained with sevoflurane and 100% oxygen. Inhaled prostacyclin is continued via the anesthetic circuit. Vital signs are stable with assumption of positive pressure ventilation. The patient is turned to the lateral position and surgery is started. After commencement of OLV, the patient's PAP climbs to 80/45, BP decreases to 78/40, and ST depression occurs in lead II on ECG. Oxygen saturation drops to 87% on 100%. Pre-existing right ventricular hypokinesis and dilation are seen to worsen on TEE. A temporizing bolus of phenylephrine 200 mcg is given, while the norepinephrine is titrated up to 0.1 mcg/kg/min. A bolus of 250 cc of normal saline is administered, keeping in mind the delicate balance between overloading a failing right ventricle and maintenance of adequate preload to ensure systemic cardiac output. Inhaled prostacyclin is titrated up to 30 ng/kg/min. Vital signs move back toward baseline. The surgery is completed,

the patient is extubated, awake, and comfortable. Norepinephrine is titrated off in recovery, and the prostacyclin is titrated down to baseline. The patient returns back to intensive care for close observation.

References

1. Galiè N, Simonneau G. The fifth world symposium on pulmonary hypertension. J Am Coll Cardiol. 2013;62(25 Suppl):D1–3.
2. Galiè N, Humbert M, Vachiéry J-L, et al. 2015 ESC/ERS Guidelines for the diagnosis and treatment of pulmonary hypertension: The Joint Task Force for the Diagnosis and Treatment of Pulmonary Hypertension of the European Society of Cardiology (ESC) and the European Respiratory Society (ERS): endorsed by: Association for European Paediatric and Congenital Cardiology (AEPC), International Society for Heart and Lung Transplantation (ISHLT). Eur Heart J. 2016;37(1):67–119.
3. Hemnes AR, Kawut SM. The right ventricle in pulmonary hypertension: from dogma to data. Am J Respir Crit Care Med. 2010;182(5):586–8.
4. Bootsma IT, de Lange F, Koopmans M, et al. Right ventricular function after cardiac surgery is a strong independent predictor for long-term mortality. J Cardiothorac Vasc Anesth. 2017;31(5):1656–62.
5. Ramakrishna G, Sprung J, Ravi BS, Chandrasekaran K, McGoon MD. Impact of pulmonary hypertension on the outcomes of noncardiac surgery: predictors of perioperative morbidity and mortality. J Am Coll Cardiol. 2005;45(10):1691–9.
6. Lai HC, Wang KY, Lee WL, Ting CT, Liu TJ. Severe pulmonary hypertension complicates postoperative outcome of non-cardiac surgery. Br J Anaesth. 2007;99(2):184–90.
7. Yang B, DeBenedictus C, Watt T, et al. The impact of concomitant pulmonary hypertension on early and late outcomes following surgery for mitral stenosis. J Thorac Cardiovasc Surg. 2016;152(2):394–400.e391.
8. Patel HJ, Likosky DS, Pruitt AL, Murphy ET, Theurer PF, Prager RL. Aortic valve replacement in the moderately elevated risk patient: a population-based analysis of outcomes. Ann Thorac Surg. 2016;102(5):1466–72.
9. Mentias A, Patel K, Patel H, et al. Effect of pulmonary vascular pressures on long-term outcome in patients with primary mitral regurgitation. J Am Coll Cardiol. 2016;67(25):2952–61.
10. Hoeper MM, Granton J. Intensive care unit management of patients with severe pulmonary hypertension and right heart failure. Am J Respir Crit Care Med. 2011;184(10):1114–24.
11. Maxwell BG, Jackson E. Role of ketamine in the management of pulmonary hypertension and right ventricular failure. J Cardiothorac Vasc Anesth. 2012;26(3):e24–5; author reply e25–26.
12. Hirota K, Lambert DG. Ketamine: its mechanism(s) of action and unusual clinical uses. Br J Anaesth. 1996;77(4):441–4.
13. Baraka A, Harrison T, Kachachi T. Catecholamine levels after ketamine anesthesia in man. Anesth Analg. 1973;52(2):198–200.
14. Lundy PM, Lockwood PA, Thompson G, Frew R. Differential effects of ketamine isomers on neuronal and extraneuronal catecholamine uptake mechanisms. Anesthesiology. 1986;64(3):359–63.
15. Maruyama K, Maruyama J, Yokochi A, Muneyuki M, Miyasaka K. Vasodilatory effects of ketamine on pulmonary arteries in rats with chronic hypoxic pulmonary hypertension. Anesth Analg. 1995;80(4):786–92.
16. Lee TS, Hou X. Vasoactive effects of ketamine on isolated rabbit pulmonary arteries. Chest. 1995;107(4):1152–5.

17. Dumas SJPF, Bru-Mercier G, Ranchoux B, Rücker-Martin C, Gouadon E, Vocelle M, Dorfmüller P, Fadel E, Humbert M, Cohen-Kaminsky S. Role of NMDA receptors in vascular remodelling associated to pulmonary hypertension. Eur Respir J. 2014;44(Supp 58):314.

18. Balfors E, Haggmark S, Nyhman H, Rydvall A, Reiz S. Droperidol inhibits the effects of intravenous ketamine on central hemodynamics and myocardial oxygen consumption in patients with generalized atherosclerotic disease. Anesth Analg. 1983;62(2):193–7.

19. Levanen J, Makela ML, Scheinin H. Dexmedetomidine premedication attenuates ketamine-induced cardiostimulatory effects and postanesthetic delirium. Anesthesiology. 1995;82(5):1117–25.

20. Reich DL, Silvay G. Ketamine: an update on the first twenty-five years of clinical experience. Can J Anaesth. 1989;36(2):186–97.

21. Tweed WA, Minuck M, Mymin D. Circulatory responses to ketamine anesthesia. Anesthesiology. 1972;37(6):613–9.

22. Gooding JM, Dimick AR, Tavakoli M, Corssen G. A physiologic analysis of cardiopulmonary responses to ketamine anesthesia in noncardiac patients. Anesth Analg. 1977;56(6):813–6.

23. Williams GD, Philip BM, Chu LF, et al. Ketamine does not increase pulmonary vascular resistance in children with pulmonary hypertension undergoing sevoflurane anesthesia and spontaneous ventilation. Anesth Analg. 2007;105(6):1578–84, table of contents.

24. Oklu E, Bulutcu FS, Yalcin Y, Ozbek U, Cakali E, Bayindir O. Which anesthetic agent alters the hemodynamic status during pediatric catheterization? Comparison of propofol versus ketamine. J Cardiothorac Vasc Anesth. 2003;17(6):686–90.

25. Friesen RH, Twite MD, Nichols CS, et al. Hemodynamic response to ketamine in children with pulmonary hypertension. Paediatr Anaesth. 2016;26(1):102–8.

26. Heller AR, Litz RJ, Koch T. A fine balance – one-lung ventilation in a patient with Eisenmenger syndrome. Br J Anaesth. 2004;92(4):587–90.

27. Rees DI, Gaines GY 3rd. One-lung anesthesia – a comparison of pulmonary gas exchange during anesthesia with ketamine or enflurane. Anesth Analg. 1984;63(5):521–5.

28. Aye T, Milne B. Ketamine anesthesia for pericardial window in a patient with pericardial tamponade and severe COPD. Can J Anaesth. 2002;49(3):283–6.

29. Kopka A, McMenemin IM, Serpell MG, Quasim I. Anaesthesia for cholecystectomy in two non-parturients with Eisenmenger's syndrome. Acta Anaesthesiol Scand. 2004;48(6):782–6.

30. Burbridge MA, Brodt J, Jaffe RA. Ventriculoperitoneal shunt insertion under monitored anesthesia care in a patient with severe pulmonary hypertension. A A Case Rep. 2016;7(2):27–9.

31. Trapani G, Altomare C, Liso G, Sanna E, Biggio G. Propofol in anesthesia. Mechanism of action, structure-activity relationships, and drug delivery. Curr Med Chem. 2000;7(2):249–71.

32. Suzuki R, Maehara R, Kobuchi S, Tanaka R, Ohkita M, Matsumura Y. Beneficial effects of gamma-aminobutyric acid on right ventricular pressure and pulmonary vascular remodeling in experimental pulmonary hypertension. Life Sci. 2012;91(13–14):693–8.

33. Kondo U, Kim SO, Nakayama M, Murray PA. Pulmonary vascular effects of propofol at baseline, during elevated vasomotor tone, and in response to sympathetic alpha- and beta-adrenoreceptor activation. Anesthesiology. 2001;94(5):815–23.

34. Edanaga M, Nakayama M, Kanaya N, Tohse N, Namiki A. Propofol increases pulmonary vascular resistance during alpha-adrenoreceptor activation in normal and monocrotaline-induced pulmonary hypertensive rats. Anesth Analg. 2007;104(1):112–8.

35. Kondo U, Kim SO, Murray PA. Propofol selectively attenuates endothelium-dependent pulmonary vasodilation in chronically instrumented dogs. Anesthesiology. 2000;93(2):437–46.

36. Ouedraogo N, Mounkaila B, Crevel H, Marthan R, Roux E. Effect of propofol and etomidate on normoxic and chronically hypoxic pulmonary artery. BMC Anesthesiol. 2006;6:2.

37. Bennett JM, Ehrenfeld JM, Markham L, Eagle SS. Anesthetic management and outcomes for patients with pulmonary hypertension and intracardiac shunts and Eisenmenger syndrome: a review of institutional experience. J Clin Anesth. 2014;26(4):286–93.

38. Colvin MP, Savege TM, Newland PE, et al. Cardiorespiratory changes following induction of anaesthesia with etomidate in patients with cardiac disease. Br J Anaesth. 1979;51(6):551–6.

39. Sarkar M, Laussen PC, Zurakowski D, Shukla A, Kussman B, Odegard KC. Hemodynamic responses to etomidate on induction of anesthesia in pediatric patients. Anesth Analg. 2005;101(3):645–50, table of contents.

40. Coskun D, Mahli A, Korkmaz S, et al. Anaesthesia for caesarean section in the presence of multivalvular heart disease and severe pulmonary hypertension: a case report. Cases J. 2009;2:9383.

41. Lazol JP, Lichtenstein SE, Jooste EH, et al. Effect of dexmedetomidine on pulmonary artery pressure after congenital cardiac surgery: a pilot study. Pediatr Crit Care Med. 2010;11(5):589–92.

42. Kaur M, Singh PM. Current role of dexmedetomidine in clinical anesthesia and intensive care. Anesth Essays Res. 2011;5(2):128–33.

43. Hentrich F, Gothert M, Greschuchna D. Noradrenaline release in the human pulmonary artery is modulated by presynaptic alpha 2-adrenoceptors. J Cardiovasc Pharmacol. 1986;8(3):539–44.

44. De Mey J, Vanhoutte PM. Uneven distribution of postjunctional alpha 1-and alpha 2-like adrenoceptors in canine arterial and venous smooth muscle. Circ Res. 1981;48(6 Pt 1):875–84.

45. Bloor BC, Ward DS, Belleville JP, Maze M. Effects of intravenous dexmedetomidine in humans. II. Hemodynamic changes. Anesthesiology. 1992;77(6):1134–42.

46. Belleville JP, Ward DS, Bloor BC, Maze M. Effects of intravenous dexmedetomidine in humans. I. Sedation, ventilation, and metabolic rate. Anesthesiology. 1992;77(6):1125–33.

47. Ebert TJ, Hall JE, Barney JA, Uhrich TD, Colinco MD. The effects of increasing plasma concentrations of dexmedetomidine in humans. Anesthesiology. 2000;93(2):382–94.

48. Friesen RH, Nichols CS, Twite MD, et al. The hemodynamic response to dexmedetomidine loading dose in children with and without pulmonary hypertension. Anesth Analg. 2013;117(4):953–9.

49. Sharp DB, Wang X, Mendelowitz D. Dexmedetomidine decreases inhibitory but not excitatory neurotransmission to cardiac vagal neurons in the nucleus ambiguus. Brain Res. 2014;1574:1–5.

50. Kernan S, Rehman S, Meyer T, Bourbeau J, Caron N, Tobias JD. Effects of dexmedetomidine on oxygenation during one-lung ventilation for thoracic surgery in adults. J Minim Access Surg. 2011;7(4):227–31.

51. Bhargava HN, Villar VM, Cortijo J, Morcillo EJ. Binding of [3H][D-Ala2, MePhe4, Gly-ol5] enkephalin, [3H][D-Pen2, D-Pen5] enkephalin, and [3H]U-69,593 to airway and pulmonary tissues of normal and sensitized rats. Peptides. 1997;18(10):1603–8.

52. Peng P, Huang LY, Li J, et al. Distribution of kappa-opioid receptor in the pulmonary artery and its changes during hypoxia. Anat Rec (Hoboken). 2009;292(7):1062–7.

53. Zhang L, Li J, Shi Q, et al. Role of kappa-opioid receptor in hypoxic pulmonary artery hypertension and its underlying mechanism. Am J Ther. 2013;20(4):329–36.

54. Kaye AD, Hoover JM, Kaye AJ, et al. Morphine, opioids, and the feline pulmonary vascular bed. Acta Anaesthesiol Scand. 2008;52(7):931–7.

55. Greenberg S, McGowan C, Xie J, Summer WR. Selective pulmonary and venous smooth muscle relaxation by furosemide: a comparison with morphine. J Pharmacol Exp Ther. 1994;270(3):1077–85.

56. Du H, Orii R, Yamada Y, et al. Pancuronium increases pulmonary arterial pressure in lung injury. Br J Anaesth. 1996;77(4):526–9.

57. Hou VY, Hirshman CA, Emala CW. Neuromuscular relaxants as antagonists for M2 and M3 muscarinic receptors. Anesthesiology. 1998;88(3):744–50.

58. Norel X, Walch L, Costantino M, et al. M1 and M3 muscarinic receptors in human pulmonary arteries. Br J Pharmacol. 1996;119(1):149–57.

59. McCoy EP, Maddineni VR, Elliott P, Mirakhur RK, Carson IW, Cooper RA. Haemodynamic effects of rocuronium during fentanyl anaesthesia: comparison with vecuronium. Can J Anaesth. 1993;40(8):703–8.

60. Searle NR, Thomson I, Dupont C, et al. A two-center study evaluating the hemodynamic and pharmacodynamic effects of cisatracurium and vecuronium in patients undergoing coronary artery bypass surgery. J Cardiothorac Vasc Anesth. 1999;13(1):20–5.

61. Kobayashi Y, Amenta F. Neurotransmitter receptors in the pulmonary circulation with particular emphasis on pulmonary endothelium. J Auton Pharmacol. 1994;14(2):137–64.

62. Barnes PJ, Liu SF. Regulation of pulmonary vascular tone. Pharmacol Rev. 1995;47(1):87–131.

63. Greenberg B, Rhoden K, Barnes PJ. Endothelium-dependent relaxation of human pulmonary arteries. Am J Phys. 1987;252(2 Pt 2):H434–8.

64. Pearl RG, Maze M, Rosenthal MH. Pulmonary and systemic hemodynamic effects of central venous and left atrial sympathomimetic drug administration in the dog. J Cardiothorac Anesth. 1987;1(1):29–35.

65. Roscher R, Ingemansson R, Algotsson L, Sjoberg T, Steen S. Effects of dopamine in lung-transplanted pigs at 32 degrees C. Acta Anaesthesiol Scand. 1999;43(7):715–21.

66. Kwak YL, Lee CS, Park YH, Hong YW. The effect of phenylephrine and norepinephrine in patients with chronic pulmonary hypertension*. Anaesthesia. 2002;57(1):9–14.

67. Vlahakes GJ, Turley K, Hoffman JI. The pathophysiology of failure in acute right ventricular hypertension: hemodynamic and biochemical correlations. Circulation. 1981;63(1):87–95.

68. Jin HK, Yang RH, Chen YF, Thornton RM, Jackson RM, Oparil S. Hemodynamic effects of arginine vasopressin in rats adapted to chronic hypoxia. J Appl Physiol. 1989;66(1):151–60.

69. Leather HA, Segers P, Berends N, Vandermeersch E, Wouters PF. Effects of vasopressin on right ventricular function in an experimental model of acute pulmonary hypertension. Crit Care Med. 2002;30(11):2548–52.

70. Tayama E, Ueda T, Shojima T, et al. Arginine vasopressin is an ideal drug after cardiac surgery for the management of low systemic vascular resistant hypotension concomitant with pulmonary hypertension. Interact Cardiovasc Thorac Surg. 2007;6(6):715–9.

71. Price LC, Forrest P, Sodhi V, et al. Use of vasopressin after Caesarean section in idiopathic pulmonary arterial hypertension. Br J Anaesth. 2007;99(4):552–5.

72. Currigan DA, Hughes RJ, Wright CE, Angus JA, Soeding PF. Vasoconstrictor responses to vasopressor agents in human pulmonary and radial arteries: an in vitro study. Anesthesiology. 2014;121(5):930–6.

73. Jiang C, Qian H, Luo S, et al. Vasopressors induce passive pulmonary hypertension by blood redistribution from systemic to pulmonary circulation. Basic Res Cardiol. 2017;112(3):21.

74. Dube L, Granry JC. The therapeutic use of magnesium in anesthesiology, intensive care and emergency medicine: a review. Can J Anaesth. 2003;50(7):732–46.

75. Fullerton DA, Hahn AR, Agrafojo J, Sheridan BC, McIntyre RC Jr. Magnesium is essential in mechanisms of pulmonary vasomotor control. J Surg Res. 1996;63(1):93–7.

76. al-Halees Z, Afrane B, el-Barbary M. Magnesium sulfate to facilitate weaning of nitric oxide in pulmonary hypertension. Ann Thorac Surg. 1997;63(1):298–9.

77. Haas NA, Kemke J, Schulze-Neick I, Lange PE. Effect of increasing doses of magnesium in experimental pulmonary hypertension after acute pulmonary embolism. Intensive Care Med. 2004;30(11):2102–9.

78. Ho JJ, Rasa G. Magnesium sulfate for persistent pulmonary hypertension of the newborn. Cochrane Database Syst Rev. 2007;3:CD005588.

79. Nakayama M, Kondo U, Murray PA. Pulmonary vasodilator response to adenosine triphosphate-sensitive potassium channel activation is attenuated during desflurane but preserved during sevoflurane anesthesia compared with the conscious state. Anesthesiology. 1998;88(4):1023–35.

80. Priebe HJ. Differential effects of isoflurane on regional right and left ventricular performances, and on coronary, systemic, and pulmonary hemodynamics in the dog. Anesthesiology. 1987;66(3):262–72.

81. Kerbaul F, Bellezza M, Mekkaoui C, et al. Sevoflurane alters right ventricular performance but not pulmonary vascular resistance in acutely instrumented anesthetized pigs. J Cardiothorac Vasc Anesth. 2006;20(2):209–16.

82. Cheng DC, Edelist G. Isoflurane and primary pulmonary hypertension. Anaesthesia. 1988;43(1):22–4.

83. Rorie DK, Tyce GM, Sill JC. Increased norepinephrine release from dog pulmonary artery caused by nitrous oxide. Anesth Analg. 1986;65(6):560–4.

84. Schulte-Sasse U, Hess W, Tarnow J. Pulmonary vascular responses to nitrous oxide in patients with normal and high pulmonary vascular resistance. Anesthesiology. 1982;57(1):9–13.

85. Konstadt SN, Reich DL, Thys DM. Nitrous oxide does not exacerbate pulmonary hypertension or ventricular dysfunction in patients with mitral valvular disease. Can J Anaesth. 1990;37(6):613–7.

86. Myles PS, Leslie K, Chan MT, et al. The safety of addition of nitrous oxide to general anaesthesia in at-risk patients having major non-cardiac surgery (ENIGMA-II): a randomised, single-blind trial. Lancet. 2014;384(9952):1446–54.

87. Leslie K, Myles PS, Kasza J, et al. Nitrous oxide and serious long-term morbidity and mortality in the evaluation of nitrous oxide in the gas mixture for anaesthesia (ENIGMA)-II trial. Anesthesiology. 2015;123(6):1267–80.

88. Houfflin Debarge V, Sicot B, Jaillard S, et al. The mechanisms of pain-induced pulmonary vasoconstriction: an experimental study in fetal lambs. Anesth Analg. 2007;104(4):799–806.

89. Veering BT, Cousins MJ. Cardiovascular and pulmonary effects of epidural anaesthesia. Anaesth Intensive Care. 2000;28(6):620–35.

90. Wink J, de Wilde RB, Wouters PF, et al. Thoracic epidural anesthesia reduces right ventricular systolic function with maintained ventricular-pulmonary coupling. Circulation. 2016;134(16):1163–75.

91. Garutti I, Olmedilla L, Cruz P, Pineiro P, De la Gala F, Cirujano A. Comparison of the hemodynamic effects of a single 5 mg/kg dose of lidocaine with or without epinephrine for thoracic paravertebral block. Reg Anesth Pain Med. 2008;33(1):57–63.

92. Armstrong P. Thoracic epidural anaesthesia and primary pulmonary hypertension. Anaesthesia. 1992;47(6):496–9.

93. Mallampati SR. Low thoracic epidural anaesthesia for elective cholecystectomy in a patient with congenital heart disease and pulmonary hypertension. Can Anaesth Soc J. 1983;30(1):72–6.

94. Swamy MC, Mukherjee A, Rao LL, Pandith S. Anaesthetic management of a patient with severe pulmonary arterial hypertension for renal transplantation. Indian J Anaesth. 2017;61(2):167–9.

95. Sztrymf B, Souza R, Bertoletti L, et al. Prognostic factors of acute heart failure in patients with pulmonary arterial hypertension. Eur Respir J. 2010;35(6):1286–93.

96. Fox DL, Stream AR, Bull T. Perioperative management of the patient with pulmonary hypertension. Semin Cardiothorac Vasc Anesth. 2014;18(4):310–8.

97. Vonk-Noordegraaf A, Haddad F, Chin KM, et al. Right heart adaptation to pulmonary arterial hypertension: physiology and pathobiology. J Am Coll Cardiol. 2013;62(S):D22–33.

98. Haddad F, Hunt SA, Rosenthal DN, Murphy DJ. Right ventricular function in cardiovascular disease, part I: anatomy, physiology, aging, and functional assessment of the right ventricle. Circulation. 2008;117(11):1436–48.

99. Moncada S, Higgs A. The L-arginine-nitric oxide pathway. N Engl J Med. 1993;329(27):2002–12.

100. Bolotina VM, Najibi S, Palacino JJ, Pagano PJ, Cohen RA. Nitric oxide directly activates calcium-dependent potassium channels in vascular smooth muscle. Nature. 1994;368(6474):850–3.

101. Lundberg JO, Weitzberg E, Gladwin MT. The nitrate-nitrite-nitric oxide pathway in physiology and therapeutics. Nat Rev Drug Discov. 2008;7(2):156–67.

102. Troncy E, Collet JP, Shapiro S, et al. Inhaled nitric oxide in acute respiratory distress syndrome: a pilot randomized controlled study. Am J Respir Crit Care Med. 1998;157(5 Pt 1):1483–8.

103. Michael JR, Barton RG, Saffle JR, et al. Inhaled nitric oxide versus conventional therapy: effect on oxygenation in ARDS. Am J Respir Crit Care Med. 1998;157(5 Pt 1):1372–80.

104. Solina AR, Ginsberg SH, Papp D, et al. Response to nitric oxide during adult cardiac surgery. J Investig Surg. 2002;15(1):5–14.

105. Solina AR, Ginsberg SH, Papp D, et al. Dose response to nitric oxide in adult cardiac surgery patients. J Clin Anesth. 2001;13(4):281–6.

106. Bigatello LM, Hess D, Dennehy KC, Medoff BD, Hurford WE. Sildenafil can increase the response to inhaled nitric oxide. Anesthesiology. 2000;92(6):1827–9.

107. Dias-Junior CA, Montenegro MF, Florencio BC, Tanus-Santos JE. Sildenafil improves the beneficial haemodynamic effects of intravenous nitrite infusion during acute pulmonary embolism. Basic Clin Pharmacol Toxicol. 2008;103(4):374–9.

108. Suntharalingam J, Hughes RJ, Goldsmith K, et al. Acute haemodynamic responses to inhaled nitric oxide and intravenous sildenafil in distal chronic thromboembolic pulmonary hypertension (CTEPH). Vasc Pharmacol. 2007;46(6):449–55.

109. Roberts JD Jr, Fineman JR, Morin FC 3rd, et al. Inhaled nitric oxide and persistent pulmonary hypertension of the newborn. The Inhaled Nitric Oxide Study Group. N Engl J Med. 1997;336(9):605–10.

110. Inhaled nitric oxide and hypoxic respiratory failure in infants with congenital diaphragmatic hernia. The Neonatal Inhaled Nitric Oxide Study Group (NINOS). Pediatrics. 1997;99(6):838–45.

111. Ardehali A, Hughes K, Sadeghi A, et al. Inhaled nitric oxide for pulmonary hypertension after heart transplantation. Transplantation. 2001;72(4):638–41.

112. Adhikari N, Granton JT. Inhaled nitric oxide for acute lung injury: no place for NO? JAMA. 2004;291(13):1629–31.

113. Paniagua MJ, Crespo-Leiro MG, Rodriguez JA, et al. Usefulness of nitric oxide inhalation for management of right ventricular failure after heart transplantation in patients with pretransplant pulmonary hypertension. Transplant Proc. 1999;31(6):2505–6.

114. Date H, Triantafillou AN, Trulock EP, Pohl MS, Cooper JD, Patterson GA. Inhaled nitric oxide reduces human lung allograft dysfunction. J Thorac Cardiovasc Surg. 1996;111(5):913–9.

115. Yamashita H, Akamine S, Sumida Y, et al. Inhaled nitric oxide attenuates apoptosis in ischemia-reperfusion injury of the rabbit lung. Ann Thorac Surg. 2004;78(1):292–7.

116. Meade MO, Granton JT, Matte-Martyn A, et al. A randomized trial of inhaled nitric oxide to prevent ischemia-reperfusion injury after lung transplantation. Am J Respir Crit Care Med. 2003;167(11):1483–9.

117. Wilson WC, Kapelanski DP, Benumof JL, Newhart JW 2nd, Johnson FW, Channick RN. Inhaled nitric oxide (40 ppm) during one-lung ventilation, in the lateral decubitus position, does not decrease pulmonary vascular resistance or improve oxygenation in normal patients. J Cardiothorac Vasc Anesth. 1997;11(2):172–6.

118. Ismail-Zade IA, Vuylsteke A, Ghosh S, Latimer RD. Inhaled nitric oxide and one-lung ventilation in the lateral decubitus position. J Cardiothorac Vasc Anesth. 1997;11(7):926–7.

119. Rocca GD, Coccia C, Pompei L, et al. Hemodynamic and oxygenation changes of combined therapy with inhaled nitric oxide and inhaled aerosolized prostacyclin. J Cardiothorac Vasc Anesth. 2001;15(2):224–7.

120. Rocca GD, Passariello M, Coccia C, et al. Inhaled nitric oxide administration during one-lung ventilation in patients undergoing thoracic surgery. J Cardiothorac Vasc Anesth. 2001;15(2):218–23.

121. Ghofrani HA, Voswinckel R, Reichenberger F, et al. Differences in hemodynamic and oxygenation responses to three different phosphodiesterase-5 inhibitors in patients with pulmonary arterial hypertension: a randomized prospective study. J Am Coll Cardiol. 2004;44(7):1488–96.

122. Michelakis E, Tymchak W, Lien D, Webster L, Hashimoto K, Archer S. Oral sildenafil is an effective and specific pulmonary vasodilator in patients with pulmonary arterial hypertension: comparison with inhaled nitric oxide. Circulation. 2002;105(20):2398–403.

123. Archer SL, Michelakis ED. Phosphodiesterase type 5 inhibitors for pulmonary arterial hypertension. N Engl J Med. 2009;361(19):1864–71.

124. Wharton J, Strange JW, Moller GM, et al. Antiproliferative effects of phosphodiesterase type 5 inhibition in human pulmonary artery cells. Am J Respir Crit Care Med. 2005;172(1):105–13.

125. Galie N, Brundage BH, Ghofrani HA, et al. Tadalafil therapy for pulmonary arterial hypertension. Circulation. 2009;119(22):2894–903.

126. Galie N, Ghofrani HA, Torbicki A, et al. Sildenafil citrate therapy for pulmonary arterial hypertension. N Engl J Med. 2005;353(20):2148–57.

127. Nagendran J, Archer SL, Soliman D, et al. Phosphodiesterase type 5 is highly expressed in the hypertrophied human right ventricle, and acute inhibition of phosphodiesterase type 5 improves contractility. Circulation. 2007;116(3):238–48.

128. Atz AM, Wessel DL. Sildenafil ameliorates effects of inhaled nitric oxide withdrawal. Anesthesiology. 1999;91(1):307–10.

129. Boffini M, Sansone F, Ceresa F, et al. Role of oral sildenafil in the treatment of right ventricular dysfunction after heart transplantation. Transplant Proc. 2009;41(4):1353–6.

130. De Santo LS, Mastroianni C, Romano G, et al. Role of sildenafil in acute posttransplant right ventricular dysfunction: successful experience in 13 consecutive patients. Transplant Proc. 2008;40(6):2015–8.

131. Ghofrani HA, Schermuly RT, Rose F, et al. Sildenafil for long-term treatment of nonoperable chronic thromboembolic pulmonary hypertension. Am J Respir Crit Care Med. 2003;167(8):1139–41.

132. Nagaya N, Sasaki N, Ando M, et al. Prostacyclin therapy before pulmonary thromboendarterectomy in patients with chronic thromboembolic pulmonary hypertension. Chest. 2003;123(2):338–43.

133. Jensen KW, Kerr KM, Fedullo PF, et al. Pulmonary hypertensive medical therapy in chronic thromboembolic pulmonary hypertension before pulmonary thromboendarterectomy. Circulation. 2009;120(13):1248–54.

134. Delcroix M, Lang I, Pepke-Zaba J, et al. Long-term outcome of patients with chronic thromboembolic pulmonary hypertension: results from an international prospective registry. Circulation. 2016;133(9):859–71.

135. Lewis GD, Shah R, Shahzad K, et al. Sildenafil improves exercise capacity and quality of life in patients with systolic heart failure and secondary pulmonary hypertension. Circulation. 2007;116(14):1555–62.

136. Andersen MJ, Ersbøll M, Axelsson A, et al. Sildenafil and diastolic dysfunction after acute myocardial infarction in patients

Perioperative Lung Injury

Peter Slinger

Key Points

- Traditional patterns of mechanical ventilation with large (e.g., 10–12 mL/kg) tidal volumes and without PEEP cause a subclinical injury in healthy lungs in proportion to the duration of ventilation.
- Perioperative acute lung injury becomes clinically important when injurious ventilation patterns are used in patients who have other concomitant lung injuries such as large pulmonary resection, cardiopulmonary bypass, or transfusion-related lung injury.
- One-lung ventilation causes a lung injury in both the ventilated and non-ventilated lungs.
- This lung injury is usually subclinical and increases with the duration of one-lung ventilation.
- Lung-protective patterns of mechanical ventilation, using more physiologic tidal volumes and appropriate PEEP, appear to reduce the severity of this lung injury.
- At present, there is no convincing evidence that the use of lung-protective strategies has improved patient outcomes in thoracic surgery.
- The majority of the recent decrease in the incidence of lung injury after pulmonary resections is primarily due to a decrease in the frequency of pneumonectomy.

Introduction

Perioperative lung injury is defined as pneumonitis or acute respiratory distress syndrome (ARDS) occurring in the immediate postoperative period during the initial hospitalization. ARDS definitions include a PaO_2/FiO_2 ratio (mild <300, moderate <200, and severe <100) and radiographic infiltrates characteristic of pulmonary edema in accordance with the European Society of Intensive Care Medicine definition [1]. Lung injury following thoracic surgery has been described by a number of terms over the past 30 years including post-pneumonectomy pulmonary edema, permeability pulmonary edema, and postoperative lung injury. While other causes of postoperative morbidity and mortality in thoracic surgery such as atelectasis, pneumonia, and bronchopleural fistula have declined dramatically in the past 30 years [2], lung injury remains a major problem and now has become the leading cause of death after pulmonary surgery [3].

Acute Lung Injury in Patients with Healthy Lungs

Traditionally, anesthesiologists have been taught to ventilate patients in the operative and postoperative periods with relatively large tidal volumes. Volumes as large as 15 mL/kg ideal body weight have been suggested to avoid intraoperative atelectasis [4]. This far exceeds the normal spontaneous tidal volumes (6 mL/kg) common to most mammals [5]. The use of nonphysiologic large tidal volumes for one-lung anesthesia evolved in the 1960–70s because it was discovered that very large tidal volumes improved PaO_2 during thoracic surgery [6]. However, the incidence of serious oxygen desaturation during one-lung ventilation has decreased from approximately 20–25% of cases in the 1970s to <5% currently [7]. This decrease is primarily due to the development of anesthetic agents that cause less inhibition of hypoxic pulmonary vasoconstriction (see Chaps. 6 and 26) and improved

P. Slinger (✉)
Department of Anesthesia, Toronto General Hospital, Toronto, ON, Canada
e-mail: peter.slinger@uhn.ca

© Springer Nature Switzerland AG 2019
P. Slinger (ed.), *Principles and Practice of Anesthesia for Thoracic Surgery*, https://doi.org/10.1007/978-3-030-00859-8_10

lung isolation techniques (see Chaps. 16 and 17). Thus, it is no longer necessary to use large tidal volumes during one-lung anesthesia.

Recently, it has become obvious that these nonphysiologic large tidal volumes can cause a degree of subclinical injury in healthy lungs. Gajic et al. [8] reported that 25% of patients without lung injury ventilated in an ICU setting for 2 days or longer developed acute lung injury (ALI) or acute respiratory distress syndrome (ARDS). The main risk factors associated with the development of lung injury were the use of large tidal volumes, restrictive lung disease, and transfusion of blood products. In a prospective study, the same group have found that tidal volumes >700 mL and peak airway pressures >30 cm H_2O were independently associated with the development of ARDS [9]. In an intraoperative study of patients having esophageal surgery, Michelet et al. [10] compared the use of tidal volumes of 9 mL/kg without positive end-expiratory pressure (PEEP) during two- and one-lung ventilation vs. 9 mL/kg during two-lung ventilation and 5 mL/kg during one-lung ventilation with PEEP 5 cm H_2O throughout. They found significantly lower serum makers of inflammation (cytokines IL-1ß, IL-6ß, and IL-8ß) in the lower tidal volume plus PEEP group (see Fig. 10.1). This study did not find any major difference in postoperative outcome between the two groups; however, it was not powered to do this. The study did demonstrate better oxygenation in the lower tidal volume group during and immediately after one-lung ventilation (see Fig. 10.2) but not after 18 h. In a study of major abdominal surgery patients ventilated for >5 h, Choi et al. [11] compared the use of 12 mL/kg tidal volumes without PEEP vs. 6 mL/kg plus PEEP 10 cm

H_2O. Bronchiolar lavages were performed before and after 5 h of mechanical ventilation. Lavage fluid from the high tidal volume group showed a pattern of leakage of plasma into the alveoli with increased levels of thrombin-antithrombin complexes (see Fig. 10.3), soluble tissue factor, and factor VIIa. This is the hallmark of alveolar lung injury. A clear pattern seems to be appearing from the clinical research that, even in patients with no lung disease, the use of nonphysiologic patterns of ventilation with large tidal volumes and without PEEP causes a degree of systemic inflammation and lung injury. The severity of this injury seems to be directly related to the duration of mechanical ventilation.

Atelectasis is a frequent postoperative complication of surgical procedures. Atelectasis occurs intraoperatively as part of essentially any general anesthetic [12]. Anesthesiologists are aware of this, and techniques to avoid it with air-oxygen mixtures, PEEP, and recruitment maneuvers are used frequently

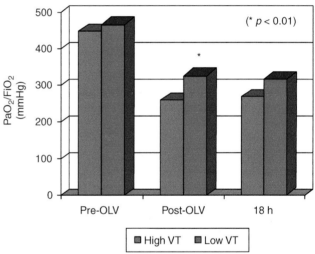

Fig. 10.2 Ratio of arterial oxygen tension to inspired oxygen concentration (PaO_2/FiO_2) in patients ventilated with either a large tidal volume (9 mL/kg) or a small tidal volume (5 mL/kg) plus PEEP (5 cm H_2O) during OLV. (Based on data from Ref. [10])

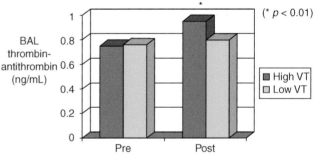

Fig. 10.3 Bronchoalveolar lavage (BAL) levels of thrombin-antithrombin complexes as a marker of lung epithelial injury in patients ventilated for >5 h during abdominal surgery with either a large tidal volume (12 mL/kg) without PEEP vs. a small tidal volume (6 mL/kg) with PEEP (10 cm H_2O). (Based on data from Ref. [11])

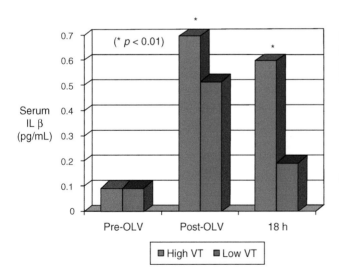

Fig. 10.1 Serum levels of inflammatory cytokine IL-1ß before and after periods of one-lung ventilation (OLV) in patients having esophagectomies. Patients' lungs were ventilated with either a large tidal volume (9 mL/kg) or a small tidal volume (5 mL/kg) plus PEEP (5 cm H_2O) during OLV. (Based on data from Ref. [10])

[13]. However, anesthesiologists are often not aware that atel-ectasis is a pathological state and, if it persists in the post-operative period, leads to an increased capillary permeability and an inflammatory response with subsequent lung injury. Atelectasis injures the lung while it is atelectatic due to local release of inflammatory mediators, and it injures the lung if the lung is repeatedly subjected to collapse and recruitment [14]. Atelectasis also contributes to injury in the non-atelec-tatic lung regions which develop a volutrauma injury due to excessive distribution of inspiration to these remaining, ven-tilated, lung regions [15]. Both retrospective [16] and pro-spective [17] studies have consistently shown that appropriate thoracic epidural analgesia reduces the incidence of respira-tory complications (atelectasis, pneumonia, and respiratory failure) after major abdominal and thoracic surgery. The ben-efits of epidural analgesia seem to be in direct proportion to the severity of the patients underlying lung disease. Patients with COPD seem to derive the most benefit from epidural analgesia. It has also been recently demonstrated that aggres-sive physiotherapy with CPAP in the postoperative period in patients who develop early desaturation after major abdomi-nal surgery leads to lower rates of major respiratory compli-cations [18].

Pulmonary Resection

There are some situations when the anesthesiologist appreci-ates that a patient presenting for surgery may have a lung injury (trauma/ARDS, lung transplantation, etc.). However, there are many more cases where the lung injury is subclini-cal and underappreciated in the perioperative period (cardio-pulmonary bypass, large pulmonary resections [19]). Acute lung injury following pulmonary resection has been described since the beginning of one-lung ventilation (OLV) for thoracic surgery. One-lung ventilation is injurious to both the ventilated and non-ventilated lung. This injury seems to be more serious in the ventilated lung (see Fig. 10.4), and this injury increases with the duration of one-lung ventilation [20].The most publicized report is a compilation of ten cases of pulmonary edema following pneumonectomy published in 1984 [21] which focused on the role of intravenous over-hydration as a cause of post-pneumonectomy pulmonary edema. Subsequently there have been several reviews of this topic identifying a variety of other potentially causative fac-tors for lung injury such as the administration of fresh frozen plasma, mediastinal lymphatic damage, inflammation, and oxygen toxicity [22]. The most thorough study to date [23] is a retrospective survey of 806 pneumonectomies which found 21 cases (2.5%) of post-pneumonectomy pulmonary edema, one of the lowest incidences reported of this complication. There were no differences in perioperative fluid balance between post-pneumonectomy pulmonary edema cases (positive fluid balance at 24 h, 10 mL/kg) and matched pneu-monectomy controls (13 mL/kg). These authors used rigor-ous fluid restriction compared to other reports [24] (e.g., 24 h positive balance, 21 ± 9 mL/kg) suggesting that limiting intraoperative fluids might decrease but not eliminate post-pneumonectomy pulmonary edema. Subsequent reports demonstrate improved survival from post-pneumonectomy pulmonary edema due to improved postoperative manage-ment of established cases [25].

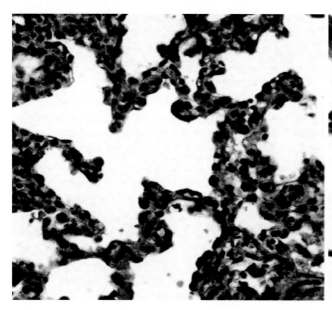
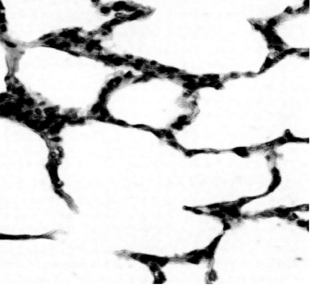

Fig. 10.4 Histologic specimens from the ventilated lung (left) and the non-ventilated lung (right) show evidence of lung injury with neutro-phil infiltration in the alveolar septa after 90 min of one-lung ventilation in a pig model. The injury is more severe in the ventilated lung. (Reproduced with permission from Lohser and Slinger [20])

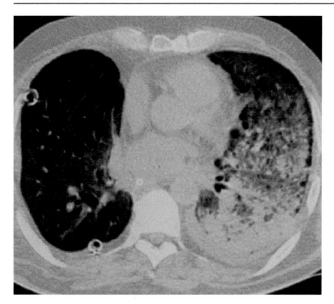

Fig. 10.5 Axial CT scan image of a patient who developed acute lung injury of the left lung (on the right in the image) after a right-sided lobectomy. The majority of lung injury after lobectomy presents in the ventilated (anesthesiologist's) lung, not the non-ventilated (surgeon's) lung

Post-pneumonectomy lung injury [26] has been found to have a bimodal distribution of onset. Late cases (10/37, 27%) presented 3–10 days postoperatively and were secondary to obvious causes such as bronchopneumonia, aspiration, etc. "Primary" lung injury (27/37, 73% of cases) presented on postoperative days 0–3. Four factors were independently significant predictors of primary lung injury: high intraoperative ventilation pressures, excessive intravenous volume replacement, pneumonectomy, and preoperative alcohol abuse. The known facts about lung injury following lung surgery include an incidence of 2–4% following pneumonectomy, greater frequency in right vs. left pneumonectomies, symptomatic onset 1–3 days after surgery, high associated mortality (25–50%), and resistance to standard therapies. While lung injury occurs following lesser pulmonary resections such as lobectomy, it has a much lower mortality rate. Of interest, in 8/9 cases who developed unilateral lung injury following lobectomy, the injury was in the nonoperated (i.e., the ventilated) lung (see Fig. 10.5) [27].

While there is some association between postoperative lung injuries with fluid overload, the finding of low/normal pulmonary artery wedge pressures and high-protein edema fluid in affected patients suggests a role of endothelial damage (low-pressure pulmonary edema). Postoperative increases in lung capillary permeability of the nonoperated lung occur after pneumonectomy but not lobectomy [28]. This capillary-leak injury may be due to an inflammatory cascade affecting even the nonoperative lung that is triggered by lung resection and is proportional to the amount of lung tissue resected (Table 10.1) [29, 30]. Free oxygen radical

Table 10.1 Factors associated with acute lung injury following pulmonary resection

Large pulmonary resections (right pneumonectomy, extrapleural pneumonectomy)
Large tidal volumes during OLV (>9 mL/kg ideal body weight)
Excessive intravenous fluids (>20 mL/kg positive fluid balance first 24 h)
Decreased lung function (low predicted postoperative DLCO or FEV1)
Duration of OLV
Preoperative chemotherapy
Restrictive lung disease
Administration of fresh frozen plasma and other blood products
Age
Preoperative alcohol abuse

DLCO diffusing capacity of the lung for carbon monoxide; *FEV1* forced expiratory volume in 1 s

Table 10.2 Causes of post-resection lung injury

Probable	Possible
Endothelial injury	Inflammatory response
Epithelial injury (large tidal volumes)	Right ventricular dysfunction (raised CVP)
Increased pulmonary capillary pressure	Oxygen toxicity
Fluid overload	
Lung lymphatic injury	

generation in lung cancer patients is related to the duration of OLV [31]. Nonetheless, there is no single mechanism that can fully explain acute lung injury after lung resection, and its etiology is likely multifactorial (Table 10.2). A unifying hypothesis is that post-pneumonectomy pulmonary edema is one end of a spectrum of lung injury that occurs during all lung resections. The more extensive the resection, the more likely there is to be a postoperative injury (see Fig. 10.6). The increased dissection and trauma associated with extrapleural pneumonectomy place these patients at high risk to develop postoperative ALI [32].

Understanding that lung endothelial injury occurs after lung resection supports management strategies similar to other conditions associated with ARDS. As a general principle, it seems that the lung is least injured when a pattern of ventilation as close as possible to normal spontaneous ventilation can be followed: FiO_2 as low as acceptable, variable tidal volumes [33], beginning inspiration at FRC, and avoiding atelectasis with frequent recruitment maneuvers [34]. Studies in ARDS demonstrate that lung injury is exacerbated by the use of large tidal volumes and that lung-protective ventilation strategies with low tidal volumes and PEEP are less injurious. The most important factor in the etiology of ventilator-induced lung injury seems to be the end-inspiratory lung volume [35]. Many patients, particularly those with emphysema, develop auto-PEEP during one-lung ventilation [36], thus beginning inspiration at a lung volume above functional

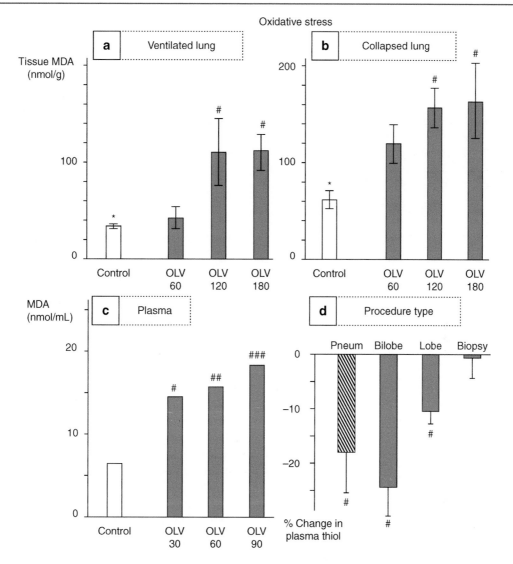

Fig. 10.6 Oxidative stress rises with increasing OLV duration and is more pronounced in the collapsed lung. Panel (**a/b**): bronchoalveolar MDA levels are higher during OLV than TLV controls at all time points (*; $p < 0.01$). The increase is time-dependent, with levels at 120 and 180 min significantly higher than after 60 min (#; $p < 0.005$). Higher levels are achieved in the collapsed lung (**b**) than the ventilated lung (**a**). Panel (**c**): plasma MDA levels increase dramatically after re-ventilation of the collapsed lung. Each increase in OLV duration of 30 min was associated with a significant increase in MDA levels over shorter OLV durations (#/##/###; $p < 0.001$). Panel (**d**): changes in plasma thiol concentration associated with OLV comparing levels from post-induction and postemergence. Major lung resections cause significant decreases in antioxidant activity from baseline values (#; $p < 0.05$), as opposed to lung biopsy or wedge resections. Bx, lung biopsy; lobe, lobectomy; 2-lobe, bilobectomy; MDA, malondialdehyde; OLV, one-lung ventilation; pneum, pneumonectomy. (Reproduced with permission from Lohser and Slinger [20])

residual capacity. It is conceivable that routine use of a large tidal volume (10–12 mL/kg) during OLV in such patients produces end-inspiratory lung volumes close to levels that contribute to lung injury.

Changes in respiratory function during OLV in the lateral position with an open nondependent hemithorax are complex. Initial studies of the application of PEEP during OLV suggested that it led to a deterioration of arterial oxygenation [37]. It is now appreciated that the effects of applied PEEP during OLV depend on the lung mechanics of the individual patient. Most patients with COPD develop auto-PEEP during OLV, and thus adding external PEEP leads to hyperinflation and increased shunt [38] (see Fig. 10.7). However, patients with normal lung parenchyma or those with restrictive lung diseases tend to fall below their FRC at end-expiration during OLV (see Fig. 10.8) and benefit from applied external PEEP [39]. Intraoperative atelectasis may contribute to injury in the dependent lung. It is now appreciated that atelectasis is a pre-inflammatory state predisposing to injury both in the atelectatic portion of the lung and in ventilated regions in the same lung which become hyperinflated [40].

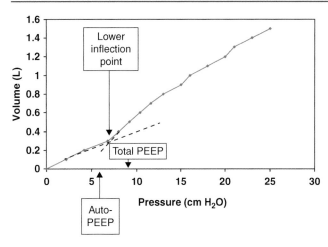

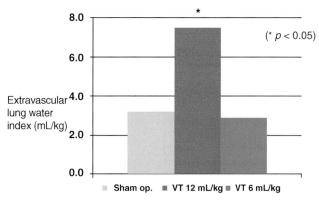

Fig. 10.9 Postmortem extravascular lung water index measured by gravimetry after 4 h of mechanical ventilation in sheep. Sham op. = control thoracotomy group, no lung resection, tidal volume two-lung ventilation 12 mL/kg. VT 12 mL/kg = pneumonectomy group ventilated with tidal volume 12 mL/kg no added PEEP. VT 6 mL/kg = pneumonectomy group ventilated with tidal volume 6 mL/kg + PEEP 5 cm H_2O. (Based on data from Ref. [44])

Fig. 10.7 The inspiratory compliance curve (lung volume vs. airway pressure) during one-lung ventilation as the lung is slowly inflated by 100 mL increments in a patient with COPD. The lower inflection point of the curve (thought to represent functional residual capacity (FRC)) is at 7 cm H_2O. During OLV this patient developed an intrinsic PEEP (measured by end-expiratory airway occlusion plateau pressure "auto-PEEP") of 6 cm H_2O. The addition of 5 cm PEEP through the ventilator resulted in a total PEEP in the circuit of 9 cm. The addition of PEEP in this patient raised the end-expiratory lung volume above FRC, thus raising pulmonary vascular resistance in the ventilated lung and caused a deterioration in oxygenation. (Based on data from Ref. [36])

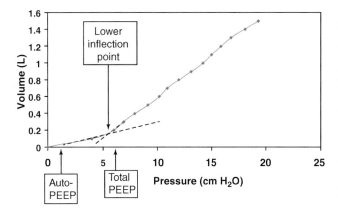

Fig. 10.8 The inspiratory compliance curve during OLV in a patient with normal pulmonary function. The lower inflection point of the curve is at 6 cm H_2O. During OLV this patient developed an intrinsic PEEP of 2 cm H_2O. The addition of 5 cm PEEP through the ventilator resulted in a total PEEP in the circuit of 7 cm. The addition of PEEP in this patient raised the end-expiratory lung volume to FRC, thus decreasing pulmonary vascular resistance in the ventilated lung and caused an improvement in oxygenation. (Based on data from Ref. [36])

There is evidence that when an element of lung injury is added to large tidal volume ventilation during OLV, this contributes to lung injury. In a rabbit model of OLV during isolated perfusion, large tidal volume (8 mL/kg) ventilation produced a picture of lung injury absent in animals randomized to a lung-protective ventilation pattern (4 mL/kg plus PEEP). Another consideration is the management of patients who have received preoperative chemotherapy with agents

such as cis-platinum and gemcitabine that may affect respiratory function and may increase the risk of postoperative respiratory complications including lung injury in some patients [41]. Large pulmonary resections (pneumonectomy or bilobectomy) should be considered to be associated with some degree of lung injury. Acute lung injury, diagnosed radiographically, was reported in 42% of pneumonectomy patients who had been ventilated with peak airway pressures >40 cm H_2O [42]. A small retrospective study found that post-pneumonectomy respiratory failure was associated with the use of higher intraoperative tidal volumes (8.3 vs. 6.7 mL/kg in pneumonectomy patients who did not develop respiratory failure) [43]. In a sheep model, Kuzkov et al. demonstrated that the use of large tidal volume ventilation without PEEP for 4 h following a pneumonectomy resulted in an increase of extravascular lung model more than double compared to a control (sham operation) group or a pneumonectomy group ventilated with 6 mL/kg tidal volume plus PEEP 5 cm H_2O (see Fig. 10.9) [44].

Since it is not always possible to predict which patient scheduled for a lobectomy may require a pneumonectomy for complete tumor resection, the routine use of several lung-protective strategies during OLV seems logical. Overinflation of the nonoperated lung should be avoided using lung-protective ventilation (5–6 mL/kg) adding PEEP to those patients without auto-PEEP and limiting plateau and peak inspiratory pressures to <25 cm H_2O and <35 cm H_2O, respectively. Minimizing pulmonary capillary pressures by avoiding overhydration for patients undergoing pneumonectomy is reasonable while acknowledging that not all increases in pulmonary artery pressures perioperatively are due to intravascular volume replacement. Other factors such as hypercarbia, hypoxemia, and pain can all increase pulmonary pressures and must be treated. Finally, it must be appreciated that not all hyperinflation of the residual lung occurs in the operating room. Overexpansion of the remaining lung after a pneumonectomy may occur postoperatively either with or without a chest drain in place. The use of a balanced chest drainage system to keep the mediastinum in a neutral position and avoid hyperinflation of the residual lung following a pneumonectomy has been suggested to contribute to a marked decline in this complication in some centers [45].

Cardiopulmonary bypass causes a subclinical lung injury that can be aggravated by injurious ventilation patterns. Zupancich et al. [46] compared the use of non-protective high tidal volumes (10–12 mL/kg) plus low PEEP (2–3 cm H_2O) vs. lung-protective low tidal volumes (8 mL/kg) plus high PEEP (10 cm H_2O) in patients ventilated for 6 h following cardiopulmonary bypass for coronary artery bypass surgery. Serum and bronchiolar lavage levels of the inflammatory cytokines IL-6 and IL-8 were significantly increased at 6 h only in the non-protective ventilation group.

The Role of the Glycocalyx in Lung Injury

The glycocalyx is a dynamic, fragile, and complex layer of membrane-bound macromolecules that forms an intravascular carpet on the luminal surface of the vascular endothelium [47]. The composition and thickness of the glycocalyx change constantly, as it is continually sheared by plasma flow and replaced. Its components have a net negative charge and therefore repel negatively charged molecules and blood cells. A primary function of the endothelial glycocalyx is to regulate and influence vascular permeability [48]. Together with circulating substances, it forms a barrier that prevents circulating cells and macromolecules from entering the interstitium. In contrast to the original Starling model, which explained the regulation of fluid balance occurring across the entire endothelial cell, a revised model has been proposed whereby the hydrostatic and osmotic forces act only across the glycocalyx surface layer on the luminal aspect of the endothelium. These forces reach equilibrium very quickly, resulting in a much lower fluid flux than predicted by the traditional Starling equation.

The glycocalyx has other functions. It regulates blood cell-endothelial interaction by its negative charge and via specific adhesion molecules for leukocytes and platelets. These are normally hidden deep within the glycocalyx structure but become exposed following damage to the glycocalyx. It also protects the vascular endothelium from shear stress and oxidative damage via nitric oxide-induced vasodilation and scavenging of oxygen free radicals.

The glycocalyx may be injured by inflammatory cytokines, surgical trauma, and ischemia-reperfusion (see Fig. 10.10). Hypervolemia damages the glycocalyx, both by dilution of plasma proteins and via release of atrial natriuretic peptide, which strips the glycocalyx. Loss of the intact glycocalyx causes increased vascular permeability and fluid extravasation. Loss of plasma proteins further compounds this. Leukocyte adhesion molecules are exposed, promoting cellular adhesion,

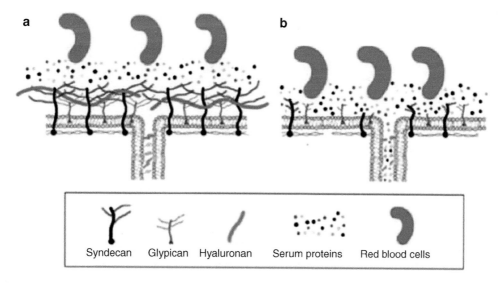

Fig. 10.10 The glycocalyx is a complex layer of proteoglycans, glycosaminoglycans, and glycolipids on the endothelial surface. (**a**) An intact glycocalyx limits water and protein flux into the cell-cell junction by forming a molecular filter over the junctional orifice. The glycocalyx also creates scaffolding on which serum proteins accumulate and form the immobile plasma layer directly adjacent to the vessel wall. Collectively the glycocalyx and the protein layer create the red blood cell exclusion zone used to determine the functional thickness of the glycocalyx. (**b**) During inflammation, proteases degrade the glycocalyx, and endothelial cells shed constituents through cell-associated sheddases. Loss of the glycocalyx scaffolding eliminates the immobile plasma layer. Breakdown of the glycocalyx is associated with increased vascular permeability due to loss of the junctional barrier and opening of the intracellular junction, as evidenced by increased water and protein flux through the junction. Note the protein-free space under the glycocalyx (left panel) that may significantly affect Starling forces across the cell-cell junction. (Reproduced form Ref. [48] with permission)

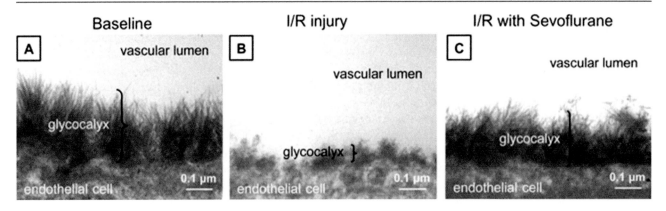

Fig. 10.11 (**a**) Electron micrograph of an intact endothelial glycocalyx from a guinea pig heart. (**b**) The glycocalyx from an animal exposed to ischemia-reperfusion (I/R) injury. (**c**) The glycocalyx from an animal exposed to I/R after pretreatment with sevoflurane. (Reproduced from Ref. [20] with permission)

migration, and further inflammation. This vicious cycle of increased permeability, extravasation, and inflammation leads to pulmonary edema, as is observed in ALI.

Several empiric strategies, based on animal experiments, have been proposed to protect the glycocalyx, including avoiding hypervolemia, albumin infusion, corticosteroids, antithrombin III, and direct inhibitors of inflammatory cytokines. Volatile anesthetic agents have been associated with less injury to the alveolar-capillary tight junction [49], less local release of inflammatory mediators, and less glycocalyx destruction (see Fig. 10.11) [20].

Transfusion-Related Acute Lung Injury (TRALI)

Over the past 30 years, acute lung injury secondary to transfusion of blood products has become recognized as a distinct clinical entity. It crosses the boundaries between patients with and without lung injury because it can cause injury to healthy lungs or it can exacerbate incipient lung injury [50]. The etiology of TRALI is primarily due to anti-white blood cell antibodies in the transfused serum. These antibodies can be either human leukocyte antigens (HLAs) or human neutrophil antigens (HNAs). HNA antibodies can bind to and trigger neutrophils and leukocytes in the recipient. HLAs are more widespread, and these antibodies can react with white blood cells and/or the pulmonary endothelium of the recipient. Neutrophils normally are flexible and are deformed as they pass through the lung, since the diameter of 50% of the pulmonary capillaries is smaller than the neutrophils. Priming of the neutrophils by sepsis, inflammation, or immune triggering (as in the case of TRALI) stiffens the neutrophils which then become sequestered in the pulmonary capillary bed. This process can be aggravated by any physical injury to the endothelium which causes the release of intercellular adhesion molecules which then cause trans-endothelial migration of the sequestered neutrophils into the interstitium of the lung parenchyma, beginning the process of injury. The process seems to be a two-hit phenomenon usu-

ally requiring both a degree of lung injury and priming of the circulating neutrophils. Although TRALI can occur unrelated to surgery, a disproportionate number of cases occur in the perioperative period [51]. Since its first identification 30 years ago, the incidence of TRALI has decreased primarily due to donor management strategies for plasma-containing products that have been adopted by blood bankers. These strategies include some or all of donor deferral based on antibody screening, donor deferral based on a history of pregnancy or transfusion, and deferral of all female donors [52]. However the major burden of prevention falls on the anesthesiologist to avoid unnecessary transfusion of blood products and to decrease the potential for perioperative mechanical lung injury.

Prevention and Therapy for Acute Lung Injury

Much of the research on lung injury due to ARDS has focused on high volume overdistention of distal lung units (volutrauma). However, there is another facet to lung injury in ARDS that involves repeated tidal opening and collapse of alveolar units at low lung volumes [53]. This repeated opening is referred to by several names such as atelectrauma and repeated alveolar collapse and expansion (RACE). Although the histological lung injury may be similar between atelectrauma and volutrauma, the inflammatory response appears to be less with atelectrauma [54]. However, the inflammatory response to atelectrauma appears to be more severe than that due to atelectasis [55]. As can be seen from Fig. 6.2, it appears that between 1/2 and 2/3 of the ventilated lung is repeatedly opening and closing every breath during one-lung ventilation. Thus, a degree of ventilator-induced lung injury to the ventilated lung seems almost unavoidable with our present techniques of anesthetic management.

Apart from mechanical ventilation strategies, a number of other therapies have been suggested to prevent or treat acute lung injury. Early reports comparing the use of volatile vs. intravenous anesthetics [56] have shown mixed results with respect to the ability of anesthetic agents to affect immune

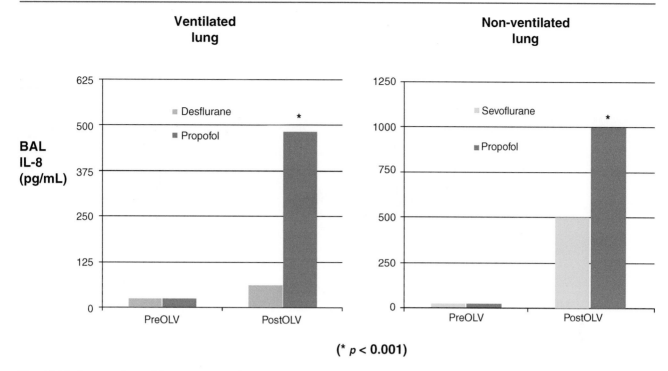

(* p < 0.001)

Fig. 10.12 A comparison of intravenous anesthesia (propofol) vs. volatile anesthesia on the inflammatory cytokine IL-8 obtained by bronchoalveolar lavage (BAL) from the ventilated lung (left) and the non-ventilated lung (right) before (preOLV) and after (postOLV) one-lung ventilation for thoracic surgery. The increase in inflammatory markers was significantly attenuated in both lungs by volatile anesthesia. (Based on data from Refs. [62, 63])

responses and lung endothelial injury [57]. Randomized placebo-controlled trials of several different therapies including surfactant, prone positioning, inhaled nitric oxide, and anti-inflammatories have not shown significant clinical benefits in patients with established acute lung injury [58]. ß-Agonists increase the rate of alveolar fluid clearance by increasing cellular cyclic adenosine monophosphate (cAMP) in the epithelium [59], and ß-agonists have anti-inflammatory properties. In a randomized placebo-controlled study in 40 patients with acute lung injury, Perkins et al. [60] found that the use of intravenous salbutamol decreased lung water and plateau airway pressure, although there were no significant differences in outcome. A randomized study of inhaled salmeterol has shown that it can reduce the incidence of high-altitude pulmonary edema in subjects at risk [61].

The use of volatile vs. intravenous anesthetics for one-lung ventilation has been shown to decrease the local inflammatory response of both the ventilated [62] and non-ventilated lung [63] (see Fig. 10.12). Also, volatile anesthetics have been shown to decrease ischemia-reperfusion injury in an animal model of lung transplantation (see Fig. 10.13) [64].

Outcomes

There have been no convincing data that demonstrate that the lung-protective strategies outlined above actually improve patient outcomes. In a retrospective study of over 1000 thoracic surgery cases involving OLV, tidal volumes of

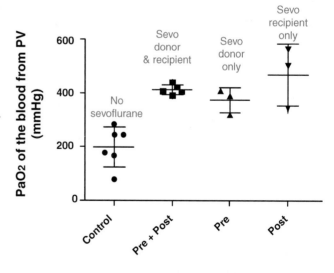

Blood gas 2 h after reperfusion

Rat Single-Lung Transplants

Fig. 10.13 The PaO_2 of the blood from the pulmonary vein (PV) of the donor's lung 2 h after single-lung transplantation. One MAC sevoflurane was associated with significantly improved oxygenation when administered to the donor (pre) and/or the recipient (post). (Based on data form Ref. [64])

5–8 mL/kg ideal body weight were recorded during OLV [65]. There was an inverse relationship between OLV tidal volume and respiratory complication and postoperative morbidity (i.e., low tidal volumes tended to be associated with poorer

Modifiers of inflammation

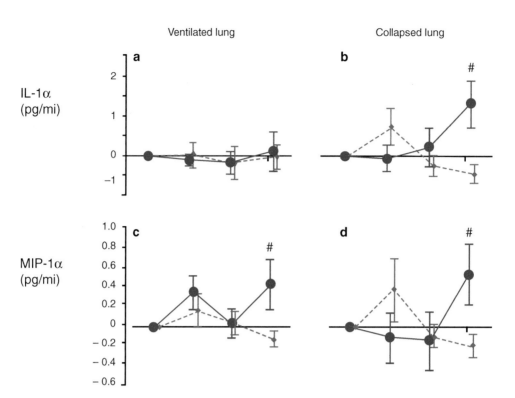

Fig. 10.14 The inflammatory cytokine response to OLV can be modulated with continuous CPAP to the non-ventilated lung. Bronchoalveolar lavage cytokine levels in the ventilated and collapsed (non-ventilated) lung during and after OLV in patients undergoing transthoracic esophagectomy. Panel (**a**): the application of CPAP (green dashed line) to the collapsed lung does not significantly decrease cytokine IL-1α levels in the ventilated lung vs. control (blue solid line) but (panel **b**) does in the collapsed lung itself (#; $p < 0.03$). Panels (**c**) and (**d**): the application of CPAP abolishes the postoperative increase in MIP-1α in both the ventilated and collapsed lungs. Time points: preoperative, 2 h after collapse, 2 h after re-insufflation, postoperative. CPAP, continuous positive airway pressure; IL-1α, interleukin 1 alpha; MIP-1α, macrophage inflammatory protein 1α; OLV, one-lung ventilation. (Based on data from Ref. [67])

outcomes). There was a positive association between ventilator driving pressure (plateau airway pressure, PEEP) and complications. The use of PEEP and recruitment maneuvers could not be analyzed from the data in this study.

A randomized controlled study [66] of >400 patients having lung surgery and OLV compared volatile anesthesia with desflurane vs. intravenous anesthesia with propofol. The incidence of major complications within 6 months of surgery (propofol 40.4%, desflurane 39.6%) was not different between the groups. At present, the reasons why logical strategies for lung protection have not been shown to improve outcome in thoracic surgery remain unclear. This may be because simple strategies to avoid lung injury, such as small tidal volumes, PEEP, and volatile anesthetics, have a small effect compared to the large proportion of the ventilated lung that is exposed to cyclic atelectrauma during OLV.

Avoiding One-Lung Ventilation

Since there seems to be some subclinical lung injury associated with the use of one-lung ventilation, it seems reasonable to limit periods of one-lung ventilation to those clinical situations where it is necessary or to avoid one-lung ventilation whenever possible. Several strategies to modify or avoid one-lung ventilation have been described.

The use of continuous positive airway pressure (CPAP) to the non-ventilated lung whenever possible will improve oxygenation and may decrease the inflammatory response to OLV in both the ventilated and non-ventilated lungs (see Fig. 10.14) [67]. Although the use of CPAP can impede surgery during VATS lung procedures, for many other intrathoracic operations such as open thoracotomies, esophagectomies, vascular surgery, and minimally invasive cardiac

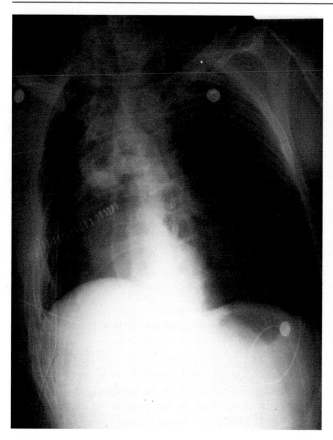

Fig. 10.15 Immediate postoperative chest X-ray of a 68-year-old male following a right pneumonectomy. This is normal post-pneumonectomy film

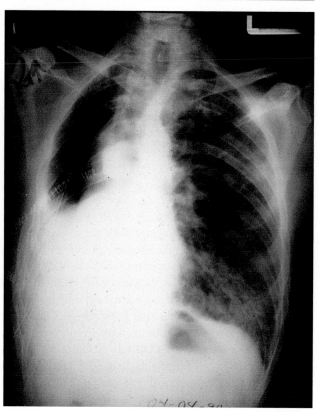

Fig. 10.16 Chest X-ray on postoperative day 3 of the same patient in Fig. 10.15. The patient has gradually become more dyspneic and has significant arterial oxygen desaturation breathing air. Chest X-ray shows signs of increased lung interstitial markings suggestive of pulmonary edema

procedures, the use of CPAP should be considered if a prolonged period of OLV is foreseen.

In some clinical situations, it may be possible to avoid OLV by maintaining spontaneous two-lung ventilation during thoracic procedures [68]. There has been an increase in the reports of case series of non-intubated VATS procedures (see Chap. 25). To date, the numbers are too small to be certain if the outcomes are improved compared to more traditional anesthetic techniques.

Clinical Case Discussion

A 68-year-old 70 kg male presents with bronchogenic carcinoma of the right middle and lower lobes. The patient is a smoker (30 pack-year) with good exercise tolerance. Preoperative FEV1 is 80% predicted and DLCO is 70% predicted. V/Q scan shows 50% ventilation and perfusion to the right lung. The patient has an uncomplicated 3 h right pneumonectomy. During the procedure, he receives 1.5 L of crys-

talloid and is ventilated with a tidal volume of 700 mL, FiO_2 1.0, during both two- and one-LV. Postoperatively, the patient is stable in the recovery room (see Fig. 10.15) with thoracic epidural analgesia and is discharged to the thoracic surgical floor.

On postoperative day 3, the patient complains of increasing dyspnea. The patient's oximetry saturation is 85% on air and 93% with FiO_2 0.4 mask. His pulse is sinus rhythm at 104 and blood pressure 130/80. A repeat chest X-ray is taken (see Fig. 10.16).

- What is the differential diagnosis?
- How can the diagnosis be confirmed?

The differential diagnosis should include postthoracotomy ARDS, pulmonary embolus, congestive heart failure and/or myocardial ischemia, aspiration, and pneumonia. ARDS in this setting is a diagnosis of exclusion. A perfusion lung scan should be obtained to rule out emboli and an electrocardiogram to rule out subclinical ischemia, which is unlikely in the absence of a prior history of coronary heart disease or diabetes. A transthoracic echocardiogram should be performed to rule out myocardial dysfunction. Major aspiration is unlikely without a history of a decreased level of consciousness. Pneumonia is a possibility, but unlikely without signs of sepsis or an elevated white blood cell count, sputum for culture and sensitivity should be obtained. If other common possibilities of postoperative respiratory failure are ruled out, the provisional diagnosis is ARDS.

- What therapy is indicated?

The patient should be transferred to an intensive care unit. All therapy is basically palliative with the aim to support respiratory function and minimize any exacerbation of the lung injury pending spontaneous resolution. Initially respiratory support should begin with noninvasive ventilation and minimizing the FiO_2 to maintain normal physiologic oxygen saturations. Attempts to reduce the pulmonary vascular pressures with inhaled nitric oxide or prostacyclin are logical although not proven and are unlikely to cause harm. The same applies to inhaled β-adrenergic agents. The benefit of corticosteroids is uncertain. If gas exchange deteriorates, then mechanical ventilation using the principles of lung protection will need to be added. In severe ARDS, unresponsive to conventional therapy, the use of extracorporeal lung support should be considered (see also Chap. 55).

References

1. ARDS Definition Task Force. Acute respiratory distress syndrome, the Berlin Definition. JAMA. 2012;307:2526–33.
2. Licker M, Widikker I, Robert J, et al. Operative mortality and respiratory complications after lung resection for cancer: impact of chronic obstructive pulmonary disease and time trends. Ann Thorac Surg. 2006;81:1830–8.
3. Alam N, Park BM, Wilton A, et al. Incidence and risk factors for lung injury after lung cancer resection. Ann Thorac Surg. 2007;84:1085–91.
4. Bendixen HH, Hedley-White J, Laver MB. Impaired oxygenation in surgical patients during general anesthesia with controlled ventilation: a concept of atelectasis. N Engl J Med. 1963;96:156–66.
5. Tenny SM, Remmers JE. Comparative quantitative morphology of the mammalian lung: diffusing area. Nature. 1963;197:54–6.
6. Katz JA, Laverne RG, Fairley HB, Thomas AN. Pulmonary oxygen exchange during endobronchial anesthesia: effect of tidal volume and PEEP. Anesthesiology. 1982;56:164–71.
7. Karzai W, Schwarzkopf K. Hypoxemia during one-lung ventilation. Anesthesiology. 2009;110:1402–11.
8. Gajic O, Dara SI, Mendez JL, et al. Ventilator associated lung injury in patients without acute lung injury at the onset of mechanical ventilation. Crit Care Med. 2004;32:1817–24.
9. Gajic O, Frutos-Vivar F, Esteban A, et al. Ventilator settings as a risk factor for acute respiratory distress syndrome in mechanically ventilated patients. Intens Care Med. 2005;31:922–6.
10. Michelet P, D'Journo X-B, Roch A, et al. Protective ventilation influences systemic inflammation after esophagectomy. Anesthesiology. 2006;105:911–9.
11. Choi G, Wolthuis EK, Bresser P, et al. Mechanical ventilation with lower tidal volumes and positive end-expiratory pressure prevents alveolar coagulation in patients without lung injury. Anesthesiology. 2006;105:689–95.
12. Lindberg P, Gunnarsson L, Tokics L, et al. Atelectasis and lung function in the postoperative period. Acta Anaesthesiol Scand. 1992;36:546–53.
13. Tusman G, Bohm SH, Suarez-Sipmann F. Alveolar recruitment improves ventilatory efficiency of the lungs during anesthesia. Can J Anesth. 2004;51:723–7.
14. Duggan M, Kavanagh B. Pulmonary Atelectasis a pathological perioperative entity. Anesthesiology. 2005;102:838–54.
15. Tsuchida S, Engelberts D, Peltekova V, et al. Atelectasis causes alveolar injury in nonatelectatic lung regions. Am J Respir Crit Care Med. 2006;174:279–89.
16. Ballantyne JC, Carr DB, deFerranti S. The comparative effects of postoperative analgesic therapies on pulmonary outcome: cumulative meta-analysis of randomized, controlled trials. Anesth Analg. 1998;86:598–612.
17. Rigg J, Jamrozik K, Myles P, et al. Epidural anaesthesia and analgesia and outcome of major surgery: a randomized trial. Lancet. 2002;359:1276–82.
18. Squadrone V, Coha M, Cerutti E, et al. Continuous positive airway pressure for treatment of postoperative hypoxemia. JAMA. 2005;293:589–95.
19. Grichnik KP, D'Amico TA. Acute lung injury and acute respiratory distress syndrome after pulmonary resection. Sem Cardiothorac Vasc Anesth. 2004;8:317–34.
20. Lohser J, Slinger P. Lung injury after one-lung ventilation: a review of the pathophysiologic mechanisms affecting the ventilated and collapsed lung. Anesth Analg. 2015;121:302–18.
21. Zeldin RA, Normadin D, Landtwing BS, Peters RM. Postpneumonectomy pulmonary edema. J Thorac Cardiovasc Surg. 1984;87:359–65.
22. Slinger P. Post-pneumonectomy pulmonary edema: is anesthesia to blame? Curr Opin Anesthesiol. 1999;12:49–54.
23. Turnage WS, Lunn JL. Postpneumonectomy pulmonary edema. A retrospective analysis of associated variables. Chest. 1993;103:1646–50.
24. Waller DA, Gebitekin C, Saundres NR, Walker DR. Noncardiogenic pulmonary edema complicating lung resection. Ann Thorac Surg. 1993;55:140–3.
25. Keegan MT, Harrison BA, De Ruyter ML, Deschamps C. Postpneumonectomy pulmonary edema are we making progress? Anesthesiology. 2004;101:A431.
26. Licker M, De Perrot M, Spiliopoulos A, et al. Risk factors for acute lung injury after thoracic surgery for lung cancer. Anesth Analg. 2003;97:1558–65.
27. Padley SPG, Jordan SJ, Goldstraw P, et al. Asymmetric ARDS following pulmonary resection. Radiology. 2002;223:468–73.
28. Waller DA, Keavey P, Woodfine L, Dark JH. Pulmonary endothelial permeability changes after major resection. Ann Thorac Surg. 1996;61:1435–40.
29. Williams EA, Quinlan GJ, Goldstraw P, et al. Postoperative lung injury and oxidative damage in patients undergoing pulmonary resection. Eur Respir J. 1998;11:1028–34.
30. Tayama K, Takamori S, Mitsuoka M, et al. Natriuretic peptides after pulmonary resection. Ann Thorac Surg. 2002;73:1582–6.
31. Misthos P, Katsaragikis A, Milingos N, et al. Postresectional pulmonary oxidative stress in lung cancer patients. The role of one-lung ventilation. Eur J Cardiothorac Surg. 2005;27:379–83.
32. Stewart DJ, Martin-Uncar AE, Edwards JG, et al. Extra-pleural pneumonectomy for malignant mesothelioma: the risks of induction chemotherapy, right-sided procedures and prolonged operations. Eur J Cardiothorac Surg. 2005;27:373–8.
33. Boker A, Haberman C, Girling L, et al. Variable ventilation improves perioperative lung function in patients undergoing abdominal aortic aneurysmectomy. Anesthesiology. 2004;100:608–16.

34. Mols G, Priebe H-J, Guttmann. Alveolar recruitment in acute lung injury. Br J Anaesth 2006, 96: 156–166

35. Dreyfuss D, Soler P, Basset G, et al. High inflation pressure pulmonary edema. Am Rev Respir Dis. 1988;137:1159–64.

36. Slinger P, Hickey DR. The interaction between applied PEEP and auto-PEEP during one-lung ventilation. J Cardiothorac Vasc Anesth. 1998;12:133–6.

37. Capan LM, Turndorf H, Patel C, et al. Optimization of arterial oxygenation during one-lung anesthesia. Anesth Analg. 1980;59:847–51.

38. Slinger P, Kruger M, McRae K, Winton T. Relation of the static compliance curve and positive end-expiratory pressure to oxygenation during one-lung. Anesthesiology. 2001;95:1096–102.

39. Fujiwara M, Abe K, Mashimo T. The effect of positive end-expiratory pressure and continuous positive airway pressure on the oxygenation and shunt fraction during one-lung ventilation with propofol anesthesia. J Clin Anesth. 2001;13:473–7.

40. Tsuchida S, Engleberts D, Peltekova V, et al. Atelectasis causes alveolar injury in nonatelectatic lung regions. AJRCCM. 2006;174:279–89.

41. Leo F, Solli P, Spaggiari L, et al. Respiratory function changes after chemotherapy: an additional risk for post-operative respiratory complications? Ann Thorac Surg. 2004;77:260–5.

42. Van der Werff YD, van der Houwen HK, Heilmans PJM, et al. Postpneumonectomy pulmonary edema. A retrospective analysis of incidence and possible risk factors. Chest. 1997;111:1278–84.

43. Fernandez-Perez E, Keegan M, Brown DR. Intraoperative tidal volume as a risk factor for respiratory failure after pneumonectomy. Anesthesiology. 2006;105:14–8.

44. Kuzkov V, Subarov E, Kirov M. Extravascular lung water after pneumonectomy and one-lung ventilation in sheep. Crit Care Med. 2007;35:1550–9.

45. Alvarez JM, Panda RK, Newman MAJ, et al. Postpneumonectomy pulmonary edema. J Cardiothorac Vasc Anesth. 2003;17:388–95.

46. Zupancich E. Mechanical ventilation affects inflammatory mediators in patients undergoing cardiopulmonary bypass for cardiac surgery: a randomized controlled trial. J Thorac Cardiovasc Surg. 2005;130:378–83.

47. Ashes C, Slinger P. Volume management and resuscitation in thoracic surgery. Curr Anesthesiol Rep. 2014;4:386–96.

48. Collins SR, Blank RS, Deatherage LS, et al. The endothelial glycocalyx: emerging concepts in pulmonary edema and acute lung injury. Anesth Analg. 2013;117:664–74.

49. Englebert J, Macias A, Amador-Munoz D, et al. Isoflurane ameliorates acute lung injury by preserving epithelial tight junction integrity. Anesthesiology. 2015;123:377–88.

50. Bux J, Sachs UJH. The pathogenesis of transfusion related lung injury (TRALI). Br J Haem. 2007;136:788–99.

51. Popovsky MA, Moore SB. Diagnostic and pathogenic considerations in transfusion-related acute lung injury. Transfusion. 1985;25:573–7.

52. Muller MC, van Stein D, Binnekade JM, et al. Low-risk transfusion-related acute lung injury donor strategies and the impact on the onset of transfusion-related lung injury: a meta-analysis. Transfusion. 2015;55:164–075.

53. Dreyfuss D, Ricard J, Gaudry S. Did studies on HFOV fail to improve ARDS survival because they did not decrease VILI? On the potential validity of a physiological concept enounced several decades ago? Intensive Care Med. 2015;41:2210–2.

54. Guldner A, Braune A, Ball L, et al. Comparative effects of volutrauma and atelectrauma on lung inflammation in experimental acute respiratory distress syndrome. Crit Care Med. 2016;44:e854–65.

55. Chu E, Whitehead T, Slutsky A. Effects of cyclic opening and closing at low- and high-volume ventilation on bronchoalveolar lavage cytokines. Crit Care Med. 2004;32:168–74.

56. Schilling T, Kozian A, Kretzschmar M, et al. Effects of desflurane or propofol on pulmonary and systemic immune response s to one-lung ventilation. Br J Anaesth. 2007;99:368–75.

57. Balyasnikova I, Vistinine D, Gunnerson H, et al. Propofol attenuates lung endothelial injury induced by ischemia-reperfusion and oxidative stress. Anesth Analg. 2005;100:929–36.

58. Bernard GR. Acute respiratory distress syndrome. Am J Respir Crit Care Med. 2005;171:1125–8.

59. Matthay M. ß-Adrenergic agonist therapy as a potential treatment for acute lung injury. Am J Respir Crit Care Med. 2006;173:254–5.

60. Perkins GD, McAuley DF, Thickett DR, et al. The ß-agonist lung injury trial. Am J Respir Crit Care Med. 2006;173:281–7.

61. Sartori C, Allemann Y, Duplain H, et al. Salmeterol for the prevention of high altitude pulmonary edema. New Engl J Med. 2002;346:1631–6.

62. Schilling T, Kozian A, Kretzschmar M, et al. Effects of propofol and desflurane anaesthesia on the alveolar inflammatory response to one-lung ventilation. Br J Anaesth. 2007;99:368–75.

63. De Conno E, Steurer MP, Wittlinger M, et al. Anesthetic-induced improvement of the inflammatory response to one-lung ventilation. Anesthesiology. 2009;110:1316–26.

64. Oshumi A, Marseu K, Slinger P, et al. Sevoflurane attenuates ischemia-reperfusion injury in a rat lung transplantation model. Ann Thorac Surg. 2017;103:1578–158.

65. Blank R, Colquhoun D, Durieux M, et al. Management of one lung ventilation, impact of tidal volume on complications after thoracic surgery. Anesthesiology. 2016;124:1286–95.

66. Beck-Schimmer B, Bonvini JM, Braun J, et al. Which anesthesia regimen is best to reduce morbidity and mortality in lung surgery? A multicenter randomized controlled trial. Anesthesiology. 2016;125:313–21.

67. Verhage R, Boone J, Rijkers G, et al. Reduced local immune response with continuous positive airway pressure during one-lung ventilation for oesophagectomy. Br J Anaesth. 2014;112:920–8.

68. Gonzalez-Rivas D, Bonome C, Fieira E, et al. Non-intubated video-assisted thoracoscopic lung resections: the future of thoracic surgery? Eur J Cardiothorac Surg. 2016;49:721–31.

Bronchoscopic Procedures

Gordon N. Finlayson, Tawimas Shaipanich,
and Chris Durkin

Key Points
- Diagnostic flexible bronchoscopy is safely performed outside of the operating room with light to moderate sedation and topical anesthesia.
- Rigid bronchoscopy is typically performed in patients with central airway obstruction and major comorbidities. Primary concerns include the risk of complete airway obstruction and inability to ventilate or dynamic hyperventilation with hemodynamic compromise.
- A fluid transition between ventilation strategies is often required for these procedures.
- Extracorporeal membrane oxygenation may be utilized in high-risk cases.
- Multimodal techniques employed by interventional bronchoscopists to acutely re-establish patency of obstructed central airways include stenting, laser, endobronchial electrosurgery, cryotherapy, argon plasma coagulation, and balloon bronchoplasty.
- Major intraoperative complications associated with these techniques include hemorrhage, airway trauma, perforation, fire, systemic gas embolism, and dissemination of postobstructive pneumonia.
- Alternative indications for these procedures include treatment of low-grade malignancies and carcinoma in situ. These lesions may also respond to brachytherapy, cryotherapy, or photodynamic therapy.
- Interventional bronchoscopy is an evolving field with expanding applications. Future indications may include endobronchial valve insertion for persistent air leaks and COPD as well as bronchial thermoplasty for treatment-resistant asthma.

Introduction

Routine diagnostic flexible bronchoscopy is a well-established, safe procedure that rarely demands the presence of an anesthesiologist. Interventional bronchoscopy is an evolving, specialized discipline that has a pivotal role in the strategic relief of central airway obstruction and the anastomotic complications of lung transplantation. Many of these procedures require general anesthesia and provide significant challenges in establishing a patent airway and maintaining adequate ventilation. There are a number of newer interventions adopted by bronchoscopists for the detection and management of precancerous lesions and early-stage malignancies. With improvements in lung cancer screening, the frequency of these procedures is expected to increase substantially in the coming years. Emerging roles for interventional pulmonologists include minimally invasive lung volume reduction with placement of endobronchial valves and bronchial thermoplasty for severe asthma.

G. N. Finlayson (✉)
Department of Anesthesiology, Division of Critical Care,
Vancouver General Hospital, University of British Columbia,
Vancouver, BC, Canada
e-mail: Gordon.Finlayson@vch.ca

T. Shaipanich
Interventional Pulmonology, Respiratory Medicine, and Integrative
Oncology, St Paul's Hospital, BC Cancer Agency and University
of British Columbia, Vancouver, BC, Canada

C. Durkin
Department of Anesthesiology, Pharmacology and Therapeutics,
University of British Columbia; Vancouver General Hospital,
Vancouver, BC, Canada

© Springer Nature Switzerland AG 2019
P. Slinger (ed.), *Principles and Practice of Anesthesia for Thoracic Surgery*, https://doi.org/10.1007/978-3-030-00859-8_11

Anesthetic Considerations

Therapeutic bronchoscopic interventions have historically been aimed at the relief of airway obstruction using a rigid endoscope. The first reported use of bronchoscopy by Gustav Killian in 1897 was for the removal of a right mainstem foreign body. Soon thereafter, attempts were aimed at resection of tumor, dilation of infectious strictures, and drainage of obstructive secretions [1].

Rigid bronchoscopy involves the placement of a non-cuffed, straight metal endoscope directly into the trachea, precluding the placement of an endotracheal tube. This is a key distinction when compared to flexible bronchoscopy which can be performed on an intubated patient with a secured airway. Rigid rather than flexible bronchoscopy is most commonly used for interventional procedures, as it allows for the passage of large instruments and removal of bulky objects while simultaneously providing a patent airway for provision of positive pressure ventilation (Table 11.1).

During rigid bronchoscopy gas exchange is most commonly maintained by jet ventilation as the open-circuit design renders conventional positive pressure ventilation prone to gas leak. Using a handheld injector or high-frequency jet ventilator, high-flow oxygen at variable concentrations can be delivered to the lungs. The precise fraction of inspired oxygen achieved is somewhat less than that selected on the injector because entrainment of room air ultimately dilutes the delivered oxygen content. Similarly, the use of volatile agents is unreliable because its delivery and measurement cannot be guaranteed. Since the breathing circuit is not sealed, leakage of anesthetic gas also contaminates the operating room. Jet injection of a blended oxygen/air mixture is typically delivered through high-pressure tubing connected either directly to an intraluminal port incorporated in the bronchoscope or to a catheter placed within the airway.

Various other ventilation strategies are also available during rigid bronchoscopy though these may be more challenging to perform effectively. Spontaneous breathing is an option [2]; however many bronchoscopists insist on paralysis as unanticipated coughing or straining may lead to increased technical challenges and complications. Placement of a rigid bronchoscope requires considerable neck extension and extensive manipulation of the airway such that most patients are intolerant without inducing apnea. There are ventilating bronchoscopes available that are designed to allow the use of an anesthetic breathing circuit; however these mandate closely matching the size of the bronchoscope with the trachea, to prevent gas leakage [3]. Theoretically it is possible to provide conventional ventilation in this circumstance, but any significant leak would reduce the efficacy of this technique. Finally, with judicious preoxygenation and passive insufflation of oxygen, short periods of apnea are generally well tolerated in select patients. For procedures requiring extended airway manipulation, this strategy may be interrupted intermittently to provide positive pressure ventilation.

Anesthetic considerations for interventional bronchoscopy include the operative indication, patient comorbidities, and appreciation of procedure-specific complications. Airway obstruction remains the most common indication requiring bronchoscopic intervention, and these procedures are typically performed urgently or emergently on physiologically distressed patients [4]. Ultimately, this may lead to conflicting anesthetic goals including balancing a full stomach with an unsecured airway, high oxygen requirements with the risk of fire ignition, and jet ventilation through obstructing stenoses with the risk of air trapping and barotrauma (Table 11.2).

Total intravenous anesthesia (TIVA) avoids operating room contamination with inhalational agents during

Table 11.1 Comparison of flexible and rigid bronchoscopy

Flexible bronchoscopy	Rigid bronchoscopy
Minimal sedation	Requires general anesthesia
May be used through endotracheal tube	Difficult with endotracheal tube in situ
No absolute contraindications	Cervical spine pathology contraindicated
Minimal risk of trauma	Significant risk of trauma
Inability to ventilate through scope (?Excluding HFJV)	Provides airway for ventilation
Requires small instruments	May use larger instruments
May need to remove scope when extracting specimen	Able to remove large objects through scope
Can access distal airways	Limited to central airways
Technically straightforward	Specialized training required

Table 11.2 Anesthetic considerations of rigid bronchoscopy

1. *Stimulating*
   Likely require general anesthesia
   ± Neuromuscular blockade
2. *Unprotected airway*
   Aspiration risk
   Potentially challenging ventilation
   Potential for loss of airway access
3. *Considerations of jet ventilation*
   Potential for barotrauma
4. *Technical considerations*
   Shared airway with bronchoscopist
   Open circuit: room contamination with volatile anesthetic
   Need for total intravenous anesthesia
5. *Potential for procedure-specific complications*
   Airway fire
   Hemorrhage
   Gas embolism
   Traumatic injuries

interventional bronchoscopy [5] (see Chap. 12). Another advantage of intravenous agents is avoiding the dependence of anesthetic delivery on ventilation – an important consideration when novel ventilation strategies are anticipated. Standard monitors recommended by the American Society of Anesthesiologists are mandatory for interventional procedures. Arterial cannulation or transcutaneous pCO_2 monitoring is useful for assessing the adequacy of gas exchange because of the frequent interruption to end-tidal carbon dioxide sampling. Patients receiving TIVA and muscle relaxants are at higher risk for awareness; therefore extended monitoring (e.g., BIS) and the addition of benzodiazepines may be considered. As the presence of an intratracheal instrument is a strong stimulator of cough, patients almost invariably require paralysis. Including a potent, short-acting opioid (e.g., remifentanil) in the TIVA regimen can help suppress this powerful and disruptive reflex. Given the unique and potentially unanticipated technical challenges presented by these cases, an extended procedural duration may require ongoing neuromuscular blockade with close monitoring of depth of paralysis.

Complications of rigid bronchoscopy including dental, vocal cord, and airway trauma usually occur during placement of the scope. The potential for difficulties in tracheal intubation must be kept in mind as this may result in a catastrophic inability to ventilate the patient, specifically in those with difficult anatomy or supraglottic distortion. Often these procedures are performed in nonoperative settings; these unfamiliar surroundings have been shown to be a factor in increasing the risk of adverse events [6]. Emergency equipment should include alternatives to direct laryngoscopy and possibly setup for surgical airway access. Other complications associated with specific interventional bronchoscopic procedures include airway fire, air embolism, and severe hemorrhage; these are discussed in more detail in the remainder of the chapter.

Central Airway Obstruction

Central airway obstruction may originate from intrinsic, extrinsic, or mixed lesions (Fig. 11.1) [7]. These lesions are further characterized by location (intrathoracic vs. extrathoracic), etiology (malignant vs. nonmalignant) (Table 11.3), and presence of fixed or dynamic airflow obstruction [8]. Specific interventional strategies for alleviating an obstruction are dictated by these features and considered within the context of the patient's appropriate level of care. Generally speaking, the comorbidities of these patients reflect the predisposing risks of the underlying malignancy, extrapulmonary features of an associated systemic inflammatory disease, or posttransplant status. Because central airway obstructions often progress insidiously, symptoms of dyspnea, wheeze, or stridor only manifest with advanced (5–8 mm) airway narrowing [9]. Still, lesions that rapidly encroach upon the airway or involve long segments may prove symptomatic with lesser degrees of obstruction.

Owing to its relative infancy, the perioperative risks of therapeutic bronchoscopy for the relief of central airway obstruction are not clearly defined. Although interventional bronchoscopy may efficiently re-establish patency of an obstructed airway, data from high-volume centers underscore the vigilance demanded in caring for these patients. Approximately 20% of patients will experience perioperative complications with an overall 30 day mortality of 7.8% (primarily attributed to underlying disease progression) [4].

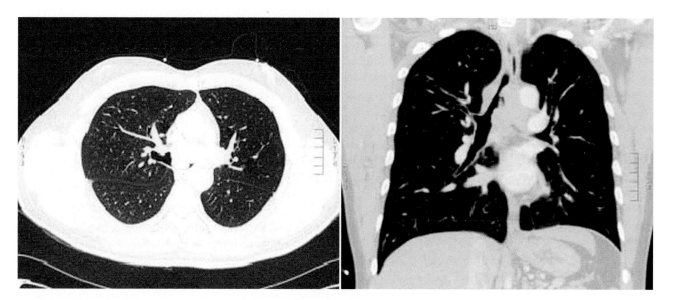

Fig. 11.1 CT demonstrating severe intrinsic central airway obstruction involving the tracheal carina and left main bronchus

Table 11.3 Causes of central airway obstruction

Benign
Traumatic: Post intubation; blunt, penetrating, or inhalational injury
Inflammatory: Wegener's; amyloidosis; SLE
Infectious: Papillomas; tuberculosis; rhinoscleroma; viral tracheobronchitis; bacterial tracheitis; diphtheria
Vascular: Rings; aneurysms; postpneumonectomy syndrome; anomalies (e.g., right innominate artery; double aortic arch)
Neoplastic: Neurofibroma, chondroma, chondroblastoma, hemangioma, pleomorphic adenoma
Anastomotic: Lung transplant; sleeve resection
Other: Tracheomalacia; relapsing polychondritis; sarcoidosis; foreign body
Malignant
Primary malignancy intraluminal
Adenoid cystic
Carcinoid
Mucoepidermoid
Bronchogenic
Primary malignancy extraluminal
Esophageal
Mediastinal (thymus, thyroid, germ cell)
Lymphoma
Sarcoma
Metastatic malignancy
Bronchogenic
Renal cell
Breast
Thyroid
Melanoma
Colon

Reprinted from Finlayson and Brodsky [39]. With permission

Evaluation of patients with central airway obstruction is largely determined by clinical status and degree of physiologic compromise. Excluding those with impending respiratory arrest, the nature and extent of obstruction must be clearly defined [10]. Traditionally, evaluation with flow volume loops has been advocated. While considered crucial in the assessment of patients suspected of central airway obstruction, their value in preoperative planning is limited [11]. Furthermore, performance of spirometry may provoke respiratory failure in advanced obstructions [12]. Reconstructed, multislice CT scans of the airway convey crucial information regarding location, extent, dynamic collapse, and invasion of adjacent structures that is paramount for safe preoperative planning [13–16]. If demanded by the patient's symptoms, CT scanning may be performed in the prone position.

Owing to the clinical urgency of these cases, the opportunity for optimization of medical comorbidities is limited. Depending upon the indication for intervention, several comorbidities including tobacco use, hypertension, moderate to severe COPD, and diabetes have been associated with increasing the likelihood of complications including bleeding and hypoxemia [4]. Although yet unproven to influence

perioperative outcomes for these types of cases, attentive management of coexisting illnesses seems prudent. Preoperatively, selective use of antisialogogues [17] is beneficial for facilitating airway topicalization and fiber-optic examination. Steroids are advocated when repeated instrumentation of the airway threatens postoperative glottic edema [18]. In patients with respiratory distress, heliox (gas mixtures of helium and oxygen, usually with an FiO_2 approximately 30%) can temporarily reduce work of breathing and improve gas exchange when the obstruction causes turbulent airflow [19].

Of foremost concern in managing patients with central airway lesions is the threat of precipitating complete obstruction with routine induction of general anesthesia. Critical central obstructions may also contribute to dynamic hyperinflation and cardiovascular compromise [17]. Because there is a paucity of literature to guide critical decisions in these challenging patients, strategies for the provision of safe anesthesia depend heavily on experience and judgment.

Traditional teaching advocates anesthetic techniques that maintain spontaneous ventilation during acute obstruction in order to avoid airway collapse after paralysis of respiratory musculature [20]. However, experienced centers have documented successful management with intravenous induction and neuromuscular blockade in patients with stridor at rest [21]. Similarly, case series attest to the safe application of innovative ventilation strategies during interventional bronchoscopy [22]. Effective ventilation may be maintained with intermittent, assisted, positive pressure delivered through the side-arm adapter of a rigid bronchoscope. The Sanders technique of manual jet ventilation also provides uninterrupted ventilation delivered through the rigid bronchoscope [8]. High-frequency jet ventilation demonstrates reliable gas exchange and operative conditions without relying on the presence of a rigid bronchoscope [22]. Finally, for those patients with reversible illnesses and critically obstructive lesions, selected use of extracorporeal membrane oxygenation may be justified [23, 24]. Unfortunately, there are limited data comparing the effectiveness and safety of these ventilation techniques during therapeutic endoscopy [25]. Whichever technique is employed, attention should be dedicated to reassessing the adequacy of ventilation and presence of dynamic hyperinflation throughout the procedure. Oftentimes these cases demand dynamic decision-making and flexible transition between various modes of ventilation – preparation is crucial.

The fundamental components to the safe relief of a central airway obstruction include a wide selection of rigid bronchoscopes and a veteran endoscopist to immediately access the airway. Although few general respirologists maintain competency in rigid bronchoscopy [26], many interventional pulmonologists are highly qualified [27]. If there is an anticipated potential for an emergent thoracotomy, the presence of a thoracic surgeon is mandatory. Blind tracheal intubation in patients with central airway lesions should be avoided as it risks precipitating hemorrhage or airway obstruction from unnecessary trauma. Routine use of flexible bronchoscopy will help minimize these complications.

Within the past decade, worldwide utilization of veno-veno (VV) extracorporeal membrane oxygenation (ECMO) has increased. While reported applications for managing central airway obstruction continue to evolve, high-volume centers have developed clinical maturity in managing patients on ECMO for alternate indications [28]. Veno-veno ECMO can replace gas exchange when native pulmonary function is impaired or absent; venoarterial (VA) ECMO can be utilized when cardiac function is inadequate. While a comprehensive discussion of the considerations of ECMO is beyond the scope of this chapter, there are some important practicalities to highlight when relying on this technology for patients with central airway obstruction not treatable by conventional approaches. First and foremost, ECMO is best instituted by an experienced team with flexibility in approaches to cannulation and its various configurations. Cannulation is usually performed with transient anticoagulation (typically 5000 units unfractioned heparin), but is not imperative. Fluoroscopy and/or echocardiography is needed to ensure safe and appropriate cannula positioning. Maintenance anticoagulation can be withheld for patients requiring VV ECMO, if heparinization is deemed prohibitive and bleeding risk is excessive. Experienced operators can successfully cannulate within ~20 min, but additional time is required for mobilization of equipment and human resources. These time limitations must be recognized if ECMO is employed to manage a critically obstructed airway at risk of cardiac/respiratory arrest. Initiation of ECMO can be performed in awake (or lightly sedated) patients, but is more challenging if there is no capacity to lie supine (Fig. 11.2).

Finally, if the indication for ECMO is to entirely replace native gas exchange, cannula size and circuit configuration should establish sufficient flow to match a patient's intrinsic cardiac output. Recent case reports and case series emphasize the utility of ECMO in managing impending airway obstruction – either in lieu of establishing a secured airway or to facilitate bronchoscopic or surgical intervention [29–34].

Successful bronchoscopic management of central airway lesions often mandates multimodal techniques. The following sections will highlight these techniques and specific anesthetic considerations.

Airway Stents

Montgomery pioneered the application of airway stents for the management of subglottic stenosis in the 1960s [35]. In 1990, Dumon introduced a silicone stent positioned com-

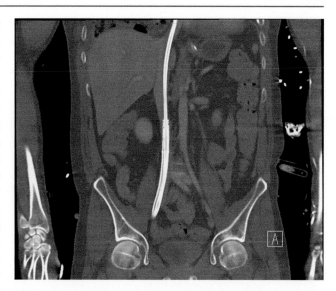

Fig. 11.2 VV ECMO can be employed by cannulating only the femoral vessels if dictated by the clinical circumstance. This CT image depicts a dual lumen femoral venous cannulae with access ports in the distal IVC and the returning orifice in the right atrium

pletely within the tracheal lumen [36]. Today, the armamentarium of interventional bronchoscopists includes a wide selection of stents aimed at restoring the patency of obstructed airways. Generally speaking, modern stents are composed of silicone, metal, or combination thereof. Ideally, an airway stent should demonstrate easy insertion and removal, stability within the airway limiting the tendency for migration, durability to compressive forces and sufficient elasticity to conform to the airway, resistance to granuloma formation and infection, and preservation of mucociliary transport [18, 37].

Currently there are no manufactured stents that satisfy these demanding design properties, though innovations in stent technology continue to progress [38]. Silicone stents are suitable for benign diseases of the central airways because of their ease of removal. Limitations of silicone stents include migration, obstruction with secretions, flammability, and reduced inner diameter [39]. Both bare metal stents and covered metal stents are available (Fig. 11.3) (Table 11.4). Advantages of metal stents include preservation of mucociliary transport, large inner diameter, and relatively easier placement. The Achilles heel of metal stents remains their tendency toward granuloma formation. Additionally, bare metal stents can transmit laser energy and injury surrounding tissue, while covered versions may pose a fire risk during laser procedures [40, 41]. Because of concerns surrounding in-stent obstruction and complicated removal, experts suggest that metal stent insertion should be reserved for malignant or palliative situations [42, 43]. Despite this consideration, other authors report successful management of benign

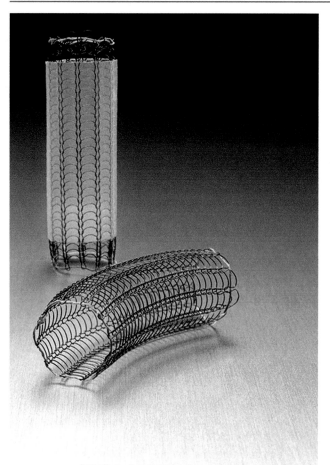

Fig. 11.3 Example of covered and uncovered varieties of expandable metal stents. (Image courtesy of Boston Scientific)

Table 11.4 Stent properties

Metal
Advantages
Large inner to outer diameter ratio
Resistant to migration
Preserved mucociliary clearance
May be placed under local anesthesia
Disadvantages
Prone to granulation and restenosis
Transmission of laser energy
Flammable when covered
Risk of long-term airway perforation
Difficult removal (*considered permanent*)
Silicone
Advantages
Easily repositioned and extracted
Disadvantages
Requires rigid bronchoscopy
Reduced inner to outer diameter ratio
Prone to migration
Inhibition of mucociliary clearance
Secretion impaction
Flammable

Reprinted from Finlayson and Brodsky [39]. With permission

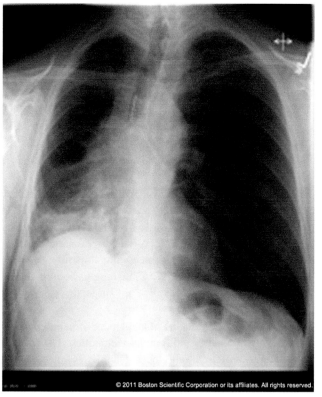

Fig. 11.4 CXR of Boston scientific dynamic y stent placed under fluoroscopy and rigid bronchoscopy. (Images courtesy of Boston Scientific)

conditions with application of metal stents, though thoughtful patient selection is crucial [44, 45].

Deployment of silicone stents requires the use of rigid bronchoscopy. Metal stents can be positioned in the airway using flexible bronchoscopy or fluoroscopy (Fig. 11.4). Primary anesthetic considerations for airway stenting overlap with the guiding principles of managing central airway lesions. During stent placement, maintenance of an immobile surgical field is preferred. Strategies to avoid coughing, including judicious airway topicalization, are advocated to minimize the risk of stent dislodgment. Specific intraoperative complications include airway hemorrhage, obstruction, and perforation with resultant pneumothorax or pneumomediastinum. When relieving a chronic airway obstruction, positioning maneuvers to minimize dissemination of a postobstructive pneumonia are recommended [13, 46]. Major chronic complications of airway stents include fistula formation to adjacent structures, which may lead to massive hemoptysis as a result of a bronchovascular fistula or aspiration pneumonia due to an esophagorespiratory fistula [47].

In instances where patients have had remote airway stenting, preoperative evaluation should consider the possibility of stent migration or obstruction from secretions, granuloma formation, or tumor invasion. Generally speaking, airway instrumentation should be avoided in these patients, with preference given to regional anesthesia if feasible. For general anesthesia, use of a laryngeal mask avoids stent disruption [48]. When tracheal intubation is indicated, fiber-optic inspection of the airway should guide tube placement proximal to (preferred) or within the stent lumen and should be repeated upon extubation [36, 49].

Other Modalities

Since the advent of flexible bronchoscopy as a diagnostic tool in the 1960s, there has been a push to use this versatile instrument for therapeutic purposes as well. Contemporary indications for therapeutic bronchoscopy extend beyond providing relief of acute central airway obstruction. The innovative techniques of interventional bronchoscopists have facilitated new opportunities for palliation of intraluminal obstructing lesions and curative resection of early-staged cancers. Often these bronchoscopic interventions are used in concert with external beam radiation or chemotherapy to facilitate surgical debulking (Fig. 11.5).

Laser

Laser technology involves the focused synchronization of light at a specific wavelength to induce thermal changes leading first to photocoagulation and ultimately to vaporization of tissue [50]. The term is an acronym for light amplification by stimulated emission of radiation. At shorter wavelengths, the beam coagulates vascular structures and prevents bleeding. At longer wavelengths, the energy delivered can be used to resect tissue as it induces vaporization. The application of laser can be accomplished by contact or noncontact probes (usually <1 cm). There are a variety of lasers available; however for medical purposes, the Nd:YAG (neodymium/yttrium aluminum garnet, wavelength 1064 nm) and CO_2 (wavelength 10 µm) types are most widely used [51]. The former is preferred by bronchoscopists as it offers a better coagulation profile and can be used through either a flexible or rigid bronchoscope, though incisions are less precise. CO_2 laser equipment is cumbersome, and its articulated arm cannot deliver the beam around corners, beyond the trachea. As such, its use is better suited for otolaryngologists working above the carina and around the larynx.

Surgical laser can be applied by interventionalists through flexible or rigid bronchoscopes. Experienced practitioners prefer rigid bronchoscopy because of the improved airway access and control [52]. In addition to isolated laser vaporization of the tumor, an alternate strategy is to devascularize and core out the bulk of the mass in combination with physical resection using forceps or a scalpel [53]. Beyond the general anesthetic considerations of bronchoscopy, the use of laser confers the rare but catastrophic risk of airway fire. For this reason, it is prudent to minimize the inspired oxygen concentration (<40% FiO_2) as tolerated. Should an endotracheal tube be required during fiber-optic laser use, specialized tubes or reflective wrap may be utilized to minimize the risk of plastic combustion with the CO_2 laser [54]. However, no material used in an airway device, except metal, is completely safe from combustion if struck by a Nd:YAG laser.

Overall, complication rates are low with laser (~1%) [55] and include the aforementioned risk of endobronchial burns, hemorrhage, airway perforation, hypoxemia, arrhythmia, and even stroke. The remote possibility of cerebral air embolism is caused by the use of air for coaxial cooling of the laser and is greatly reduced by substituting CO_2 for this purpose [56]. Extra care must be taken when using laser on highly vascular posterior structures for this reason. Also, Nd:YAG laser light can lead to retinal damage in the case of inadvertent exposure; protective eyewear is recommended for all operating room occupants. Similarly, smoke evacuation systems have been advocated in response to reports that viral particles are present in laser plume [57]. In fact, transmission of HPV to physicians during laser vaporization of papillomas has been documented [58], though others have shown that HIV particles isolated from laser exhaust are not viable in vitro [59].

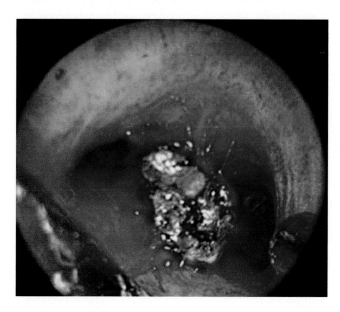

Fig. 11.5 Example of tumor debulking. (Image courtesy of Dr. Tawimas Shaipanich BC Cancer Agency)

Endobronchial Electrosurgery

Endobronchial electrosurgery (EBES) refers to therapeutic interventions using the direct application of electric current to tissue in a patient who is electrically grounded with an adhesive grounding pad. The delivery of thermal energy by this method will either induce coagulation or incision ("cut") depending on the precise levels of amperage and voltage [60]. Practitioners can blend these two parameters to induce the type of tissue changes they are seeking (e.g., arrest of bleeding or resection of tissue). Using a wire loop, pedunculated lesions can be cleanly excised by circumferential cutting of the supporting stalk, while sessile lesions can be debulked with dissecting probes. Essentially, the technology can be employed in virtually the same scenarios as those where laser is applied [61]. The main difference between the two is that EBES is much less expensive and requires less sophisticated equipment and technical expertise to perform [62]. Complications are also largely the same as those for laser with a significant risk of airway fire during cauterization of tissue. Electromagnetic interference during EBES may lead to malfunction of implanted electrical devices including pacemakers and AICDs [63].

Argon Plasma Cautery

Argon plasma cautery (APC) also uses electrical current to induce thermal destruction of endobronchial tissues for resection and coagulation. However, rather than using direct contact with an electrically grounded patient to conduct current, ionized argon gas released from the tip of the probe acts as the conductor allowing for a noncontact technique [64]. The nature of the gas flow allows for energy to be directed in multiple planes from the probe tip and for targeting lesions that would otherwise be inaccessible by other modalities [65].

The depth of penetration using APC is less than that of laser or EBES, so it is most useful for superficial lesions (e.g., hemorrhagic foci) and may be used more safely near endobronchial stents [66]. Along with the usual complications of interventional bronchoscopy, APC confers both the risk of electromagnetic interference and air embolus (thought to be related to entrainment of argon gas) [67].

Balloon Bronchoplasty

Balloon bronchoplasty involves navigating a silicone balloon into a stenotic region using fiber-optic or rigid bronchoscopy alone or in combination with fluoroscopy and then applying incremental, pressurized inflation. Oftentimes the airway patency achieved with isolated balloon bronchoplasty is not sustained, and either demands repeated attempts or combined intervention (e.g., stenting). Malignant strictures are at notable risk for rapid restenosis. Although mucosal damage associated with balloon bronchoplasty is limited when compared with laser photoresection or bougie dilation, airway rupture and hemorrhage remain a risk. Other reported complications with this technique include bronchospasm, tracheitis, fever, atelectasis, and pneumomediastinum [68].

Delayed Resection Techniques

A major advantage of laser, EBES, APC, and balloon bronchoplasty is the immediate effective relief of airway obstruction and return of airway patency. There are a number of other techniques (Table 11.5) whose mode of action is delayed including photodynamic therapy, cryotherapy, and brachytherapy. They are most often employed for nonsurgical candidates with nonobstructing lesions, for palliation of advanced malignancy, and for potential cure of early-stage cancer, such as carcinoma in situ [69]. They can all be performed via fiber-optic bronchoscopy and therefore rarely require the service of an anesthesiologist (except cryoadhesion and spray cryotherapy; see below). Acute decompensation due to procedural complications with these techniques is less frequent than with the more invasive techniques described above.

Of the delayed resection techniques, cryotherapy is the most commonly applied therapy (Fig. 11.6). Utilizing the cytotoxic effects of rapid freezing and thawing cycles, it can destroy (cryoablation), adhere (cryoadhesion), or biopsy (cryobiopsy) tissue. Destruction of biologic material is influenced by the cooling and thawing rates as well as the lowest temperature delivered. Exploitation of the Joule-Thomson effect (rapid cooling of a gas as it expands from a high-pressure delivery system to the atmosphere) enables this process, with nitrous oxide being the favored agent. Monitoring of tissue freezing remains a problem, relying on operator experience although a usual freeze cycle is approximately 30 s and repeated two or three times. Tissues with high cellular water content (tumor cells, skin, mucous membranes, granulation tissue) are more sensitive than those without (fat, cartilage, connective tissue). Delivery requires a cryoprobe, bronchoscope, and cooling agent. Initially only available as a rigid probe which demanded a rigid bronchoscope, the advent of flexible devices with delivery via the working

Table 11.5 Nonoperative tumor resection techniques

Modality	Description	Complications
Photodynamic therapy	Injection of photosensitive agent (dihemato-porphyrin ester) which is activated by direct exposure to light	Prolonged susceptibility to burn from sunlight
		Requires bronchial lavage due to pronounced tissue sloughing
Cryotherapy	Tissue destruction by rapid freezing using decompressed gas	Requires bronchial lavage due to pronounced tissue sloughing
		Transient fever
Brachytherapy	Radioactive beads (iridium 192) placed directly in tumor	Hemorrhage
		Fistula formation
		Bronchial stenosis
		Radiation exposure

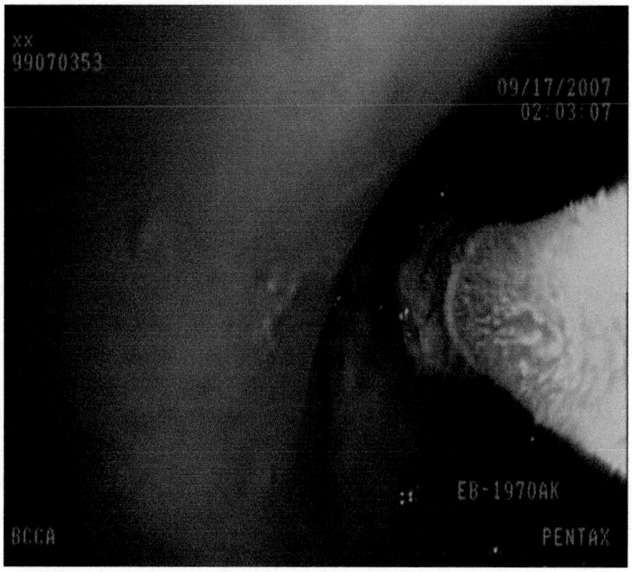

Fig. 11.6 Cryotherapy of a left upper lobe tumor; picture shows ice crystal formation at the catheter

channel of a flexible bronchoscope has expanded the diagnostic and therapeutic utility.

The primary role of cryotherapy remains palliative or adjunctive therapy for inoperable malignant central airway obstruction where supportive literature (primarily observational) suggests symptomatic relief in over 90% of patients [70, 71]. Minimal complications, relative ease of use, and economical superiority are advantages as compared to other modalities [71]. Occasionally, it is used in nonmalignant central airway obstruction (granulation tissue, blood clots, and mucus plug) but should be avoided in fibrotic processes as these are cryoresistant and may be exacerbated. Tissue sloughing continuing for days afterward is the main limitation and necessitates repeat bronchoscopy 5–10 days following the index procedure. Depth of penetration is low (3 mm) allowing for a reduced risk of airway perforation, and the lack of spark eliminates any concern of airway fire.

Cryoadhesion is a relatively new technique that facilitates tissue removal (tumor debulking) faster than standard cryoablation by allowing the frozen probe tip to "stick" to the tissue of interest with rapid removal prior to the thaw cycle. Extraction of large samples can be achieved although bleeding refractory to conservative measures that requires APC or electrocautery remains a concern (~4%) [72]. This technique mandates general anesthesia with a laryngeal mask or endotracheal tube to allow frequent, repeated removal of specimen. The same principle has been applied to allow for intraluminal tissue biopsy (cryobiopsy) with a high diagnostic yield as well as transbronchial biopsy of peripheral lung lesions using fluoroscopic guidance, although this is currently used for investigation purposes only.

Recently, a special catheter (cryospray) was released allowing for the treatment of large areas rapidly and uniformly without the requirement of direct contact [73]. Instead of nitrous oxide, liquid nitrogen (LN_2) is used which brings a unique set of anesthetic considerations centered around barotrauma from rapid gas expansion and hypoxemia as LN_2 displaces inspired oxygen [74]. Additionally, delivery over 5–10 s requires apnea. This constellation of issues requires general anesthesia with an open ventilation circuit (deflate endotracheal cuff if intubated). Newer units reducing the flow of LN_2 are mitigating these risks. Delayed treatment effect with an inflammatory response is similar to standard cryotherapy.

Foreign Body Extraction and Emerging Techniques

In the absence of history, the diagnosis of foreign body aspiration may be allusive. The classic "penetration syndrome" of choke, cough, and wheeze is present only in a fraction of patients. Patients at extremes of ages are at greatest risk for aspiration owing to immature or blunted airway and swallowing reflexes [75]. In adults, the foreign body tends to impact in the distal airway, whereas in children, the material often settles in the mainstem bronchi (R > L).

The host response and complications of foreign body aspiration are primarily dependent upon the physical properties of the aspirated object (organic vs. inorganic; sharp vs. dull), location, and duration of involvement. Organic material elicits a robust local inflammatory response culminating in tissue granulation. Prolonged impaction may cause atelectasis, postobstructive pneumonia, bronchiectasis, and bronchial stenosis. Perforation or erosion of the airway may be associated with pneumothorax, pneumomediastinum, or hemoptysis [75].

Traditionally, the rigid bronchoscope has been the instrument of choice for foreign body extraction. Contemporary strategies for managing foreign body aspiration in adults primarily employ flexible bronchoscopy [76]. Diagnostic imaging (e.g., CXR and CT scan) has a limited role in evaluating foreign body aspiration; flexible bronchoscopy remains the gold standard for diagnosis. Further, the armamentarium of devices deployed through the working channel of a flexible bronchoscope typically obviates the need for rigid bronchoscopy. These tools include a selection of grasping forceps, balloon catheters, baskets, snares, magnets, as well as laser and cryotherapy probes (cryoadhesion).

Extraction in adults is often performed with airway topicalization, light sedation, and spontaneous ventilation. If clinical status permits, an appropriate period of fasting should be respected to minimize the risk of aspiration. Tracheal intubation and mechanical ventilation may be required in the subset of patients with respiratory distress preoperatively or in those at high risk of aspiration. In either case, experts advocate strategies to avoid distal dislodgement of the foreign body during the procedure. Assuming a low risk of airway perforation or laceration, this typically will involve placement of a balloon catheter beyond the object and pulling it proximal to the tracheal carina. Once in the trachea, the foreign body can then be secured with a grasping device that is then removed from the patient's airway in tandem with the bronchoscope. For ventilated patients, temporary tracheal extubation during the final stage of removal may avoid the need to navigate the object through an endotracheal tube and the attendant risk of dislodgement or airway obstruction.

Pediatric foreign body removal is typically performed in the operating room under general anesthesia with rigid bronchoscopy. Owing to the reduced airway diameter, there is a greater perceived risk of obstruction and asphyxiation as well as air trapping from a ball valve mechanism. Gas exchange is supported with either spontaneous ventilation or intermittent positive pressure ventilation. Theoretical advantages of a spontaneous breathing technique include fewer interruptions to ventilation, as well as a reduced risk of distal dislodgement and dynamic hyperinflation. Advocates of positive pressure ventilation cite a quiet operative field as advantageous. Evidence supporting the superiority of either technique is lacking [77].

Endobronchial Valves

Newly defined roles for interventional bronchoscopists continue to emerge. Specifically, innovative interventional techniques are evolving in the management of severe emphysema and asthma. Unlike interventional strategies designed to relieve acute central airway obstruction, the role of bronchoscopy in these areas is suited for evaluation in well-designed clinical trials.

Lung volume reduction surgery (LVRS) improves pulmonary function, exercise capacity, and quality of life in selected patients at the expense of high perioperative morbidity [78]. Patients with a heterogeneous pattern of emphysema most predictably benefit from LVRS. Bronchoscopic lung volume reduction surgery (bLVRS) arose in response to the excessive morbidity associated with LVRS (see Chap. 36) and may target a wider population to include those with homogenous emphysema [79].

Bronchoscopic management of severe heterogeneous emphysema involves insertion of one-way endobronchial valves (Fig. 11.7) in segmental or subsegmental bronchi thereby restricting flow during inspiration and allowing passive exhalation and secretion clearance. Ultimately, the physiologic intent is to minimize dynamic hyperinflation through atelectasis (Fig. 11.8). Radiographic documentation of atelectasis in targeted lung segments is infrequently achieved, though clinical improvement often persists [80]. Improvement in cardiac function, diaphragm and inspiratory muscle performance, as well as recruitment of compressed alveoli may account for the clinical response [80]. A multicenter randomized controlled trial (VENT) in this population demonstrated improved exercise tolerance and modest improvement in quality of life but was hampered by a significant incidence of complications [81]. A more recent trial selecting for patients with a low probability of collateral ventilation, cited as the mechanism for failure to achieve the intended atelectasis, similarly demonstrated improved pulmonary function and exercise tolerance, but the frequent occurrence of serious adverse events has reduced enthusiasm for this technique [82]. Endobronchial valve technology continues to be limited to clinical trials until an improved safety profile can be achieved. Recently, a number of studies have considered the utility of bronchoscopic deployment of coils into subsegmental airways to allow for collapse of emphysematous tissue but have shown variable improvement and encountered similar limitations to endobronchial valves [83, 84].

Insertion may be performed under local or general anesthesia using flexible bronchoscopy. Relatively common complications include bronchospasm, COPD exacerbation, and pneumothorax (~20%) [82]. Valve migration and obstructing pneumonia are less frequent (~5%); fortunately, device extraction is easily performed [78]. Interestingly, compassionate use of endobronchial valves has aided in the successful management of persistent postoperative air leaks (Fig. 11.9) [85]. In all likelihood this will materialize as a new indication for device insertion.

Bronchoscopic lung volume reduction may benefit patients with homogenous emphysema where hyperinflation occurs from closure of small airways. An airway bypass system that establishes a shunt between a central airway and targeted region of hyperinflated lung theoretically allows for more efficient lung emptying. This technique involves endobronchial ultrasound for vascular mapping, followed by targeted radiofrequency ablation and drug-eluting stent insertion [86]. Although preliminary literature was promising, a multicenter randomized trial (EASE) failed to show benefit of this modality and has halted further evaluation [87].

Bronchial Thermoplasty

Difficult-to-control asthma has also received attention from bronchoscopists. Bronchial thermoplasty is a technique of applying radiofrequency energy to the airway wall, generating a tissue temperature of ~65 °C. This thermal injury reduces smooth muscle mass but avoids tissue destruction and scarring [88]. Reduction in smooth muscle mass should

Fig. 11.7 (**a**) Olympus endobronchial valve and (**b**) schematic representation of device deployment. (Images courtesy of Olympus)

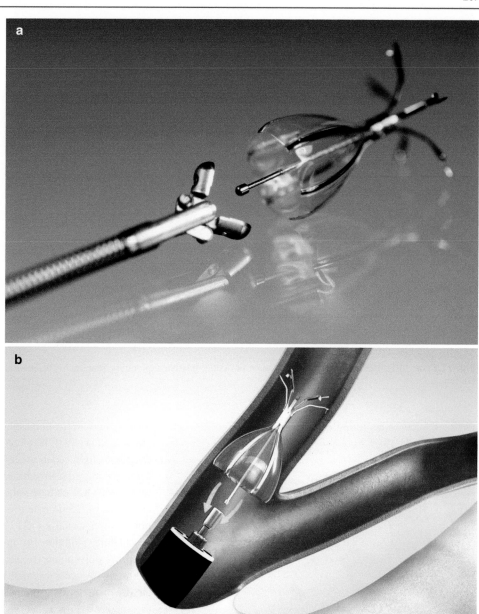

theoretically improve airflow in asthmatics with airway hyperresponsiveness [89]. Further randomized studies are required in this area to elucidate the safety profile and ideal candidates.

Diagnostic Bronchoscopy

Diagnostic bronchoscopy is almost exclusively practiced in nonoperative settings, using a flexible bronchoscope with topicalized local anesthesia and intravenous sedation. The presence of an anesthesiologist is generally reserved for patients who have tenuous cardiopulmonary reserve, impending airway compromise, or for procedures which are likely to require rigid bronchoscopy or immediately before or after other thoracic surgical procedures. Flexible bronchoscopy can be supplemented by a variety of modalities to aid in the diagnosis and staging of lung cancer, as well as a host of other pulmonary diseases. Aside from endobronchial assessment of the large airways via direct visualization, the addition of bronchial brushing, lavage, and sampling expands the diagnostic yield significantly [90]. Sampling submucosal and peribronchial lesions, which cannot be directly visualized, is aided with autofluorescence bronchoscopy, optical coherence tomography (OCT), CT, fluoroscopy, or endobronchial ultrasound imaging to improve diagnostic yield and limit complications. Complications attributable to these procedures are reported as less than 0.3% and include hypoxemia and cardiac arrhythmias, which are generally transient and rarely life-threatening [91].

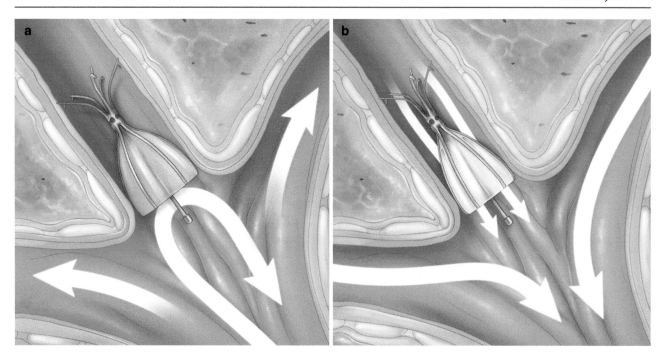

Fig. 11.8 (**a, b**) Endobronchial valve mechanism of action: passive exploratory flow and restriction of inspiring flow. (Images courtesy of Olympus)

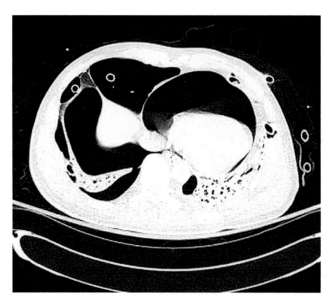

Fig. 11.9 Endobronchial valve placement was considered in this young patient with a massive air leak associated with tumor necrosis following induction chemotherapy for lymphoma

Optical coherence tomography (Fig. 11.10a) is a new imaging modality in pulmonary medicine. It enables higher-resolution (at least an order of magnitude) imaging as compared to conventional white-light bronchoscopy, facilitating subluminal airway examination and early lung cancer detection. Ex vivo studies have shown that OCT can visualize structural features associated with pulmonary nodules that precisely correlate with those on histopathology [92] and trained readers can identify nodules from normal lung tissue with good sensitivity and specificity [93]. It can be performed via flexible bronchoscopy with light sedation although deep sedation can improve exam accuracy due to reduced respiratory motion. Miniaturized fiber-optic OCT catheters allow endoscopic imaging of peripheral airways, while extensions of OCT such as Doppler and polarization-sensitive OCT can be used to examine pulmonary vasculature. Additionally, in benign airway stenosis such as relapsing polychondritis and granulomatosis with polyangiitis (formerly Wegener's granulomatosis), OCT has been used in airway diameter measurement to improve accuracy and assist therapeutic balloon dilation.

Noninvasive Techniques

Bronchial washing involves the use of small amounts (10–15 mL) of fluid instilled in the bronchial tree to be suctioned through the bronchoscope and then sent for culture, stain, and cytology. Bronchoalveolar lavage (BAL) is the same process using larger volumes of fluid (100–200 mL) which may have greater sensitivity for the diagnosis of *Pneumocystis jirovecii* (formerly *P. carinii*), legionella, tuberculosis, and respiratory viruses such as influenza and respiratory syncytial virus. Additionally, BAL may establish a diagnosis for other noninfectious pulmonary pathologies including malignancies, alveolar proteinosis (where it can also be used therapeutically), and histiocytosis, for example [94].

Complications encountered during these procedures are generally the same as those for fiber-optic bronchoscopy,

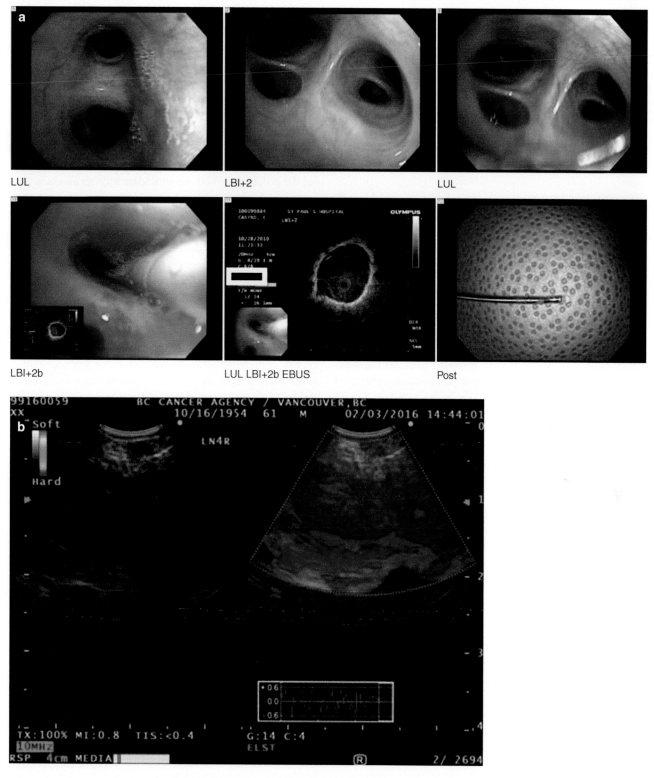

Fig. 11.10 (**a**) OCT examination of the tracheal stenosis with detailed airway measurement. (**b**) Linear EBUS examination of a paratracheal lymph node with elastography study (blue area indicates hard texture of the lymph node comparing to adjacent tissue)

though hypoxemia may be more profound depending on the amount of fluid administered and the number of lung segments involved [95]. It seems that temperature of the lavage fluid can also have an impact on respiratory mechanics – room temperature fluids have been shown to lead to impaired TLC, FEF 25–75, and increased RV [96]. These changes do not occur with fluids at body temperature. Lavage can precipitate bronchospasm in patients with reactive airways, and thus pretreatment with beta-agonists and steroids, as well as the use of warmed fluid, has been advocated [97]. The release of cytokines resulting from inflamed tissues may lead to transient fevers and chills. Hemorrhage is rare and self-limiting, occurring mainly in patients with bleeding dyscrasias or uremia. Alveolar infiltrates may remain present on chest X-ray for up to 24 h [98].

Invasive Techniques

Bronchoscopic lung biopsy (BLB) and transbronchial needle aspiration (TBNA) are nonsurgical approaches for the procurement of tissue samples required for diagnosing and staging lung pathology. The main issue with these techniques is the difficulty in delineating the location of pathologic tissue and avoiding important intrathoracic and mediastinal structures. This is problematic for two reasons: firstly, diagnostic yields are low using a blind technique, and secondly, the opportunity for iatrogenic misadventure resulting in hemorrhage or air leak is heightened. The use of high-resolution CT and real-time fluoroscopy goes a long way to resolving these issues; however, these strategies are cumbersome and require a higher level of technical skill and resources. Due to the increased risk of serious complications, these approaches have fallen out of favor with many bronchoscopists and surgeons [99].

In recent years, the advent of endobronchial ultrasound (EBUS) has led to a resurgence in the interest in transbronchial tissue sampling [100]. There are two main types of EBUS technology. An EBUS radial probe is a small ultrasound catheter that can be inserted via the working channel of a regular bronchoscope to assist with locating peripheral lung lesions that can then be biopsied using a guided sheath system. Linear EBUS (as opposed to radial) uses a small ultrasound probe on the end of a larger fiber-optic bronchoscope to identify mediastinal and hilar lymph nodes. Transbronchial needle aspiration can then be performed via the linear EBUS scope under direct and real-time visualization. Doppler ultrasound can be used to identify adjacent vascular structures that need to be avoided. Moreover, elastography is an additional feature of the EBUS which can examine density of the lymph nodes and help select site of biopsy within the targeted lymph node in order to increase sensitivity and specificity of the biopsy (Fig. 11.10b).

Accurate sampling with EBUS is cited to exceed 90% [101, 102]. The same technology has been applied to esophagoscopy (EUS); the combination of the two approaches allows for a complete assessment of the mediastinum including all nodes accessible via traditional mediastinoscopy [103]. Both EBUS and EUS can be done under local anesthetic with sedation; however, in some centers they are conducted in the operating room under general anesthesia in conjunction with other surgical procedures.

Serious complications associated with endobronchial tissue sampling result primarily from bleeding or pneumothorax [104]. Rarer issues include transient fever, purulent pericarditis, or hemomediastinum [105]. Overall, complication rates for BLB are the highest among these techniques with as many as 3% of cases reported to have an adverse event of some kind and associated mortality of up to 0.1% [106]. Contraindications to BLB include coagulopathy, extensive bullous disease, vascular malformations, severe asthma, uncontrollable cough, or inability to cooperate during the procedure. Work-up should include an assessment of coagulation profile, including platelet count and kidney function. Pretreatment may include the use of DDAVP, cough suppressant, and bronchodilators. Cessation of antiplatelet agents for 5–7 days before the procedure reduces the incidence of bleeding significantly [107].

Mechanical ventilation is not a contraindication to BLB; however, the risk of pneumothorax is three times higher in this population than in spontaneously breathing patients [108]. Reduction of PEEP below 5 cmH$_2$O, adequate sedation, and prophylactic neuromuscular blockade may reduce the risk of pneumothorax. In anticipation of potential cardiopulmonary collapse due to tension pneumothorax, the availability of thoracostomy tube and personnel facile in rapid insertion are recommended [109].

Airway bleeding can usually be efficiently handled by the interventionalist using equipment available in the bronchoscopy suite. Standard techniques include wedging the bronchoscope into the involved segment to tamponade bleeding or instilling 10–15 mL of iced saline (with or without epinephrine) to induce vasoconstriction [90]. Should bleeding prove more severe and unresponsive to these simple interventions, isolation of the affected lung with either a double-lumen endobronchial tube or bronchial blocker may be required to prevent widespread aspiration of blood. Ultimately, urgent embolization of bronchial arteries or even surgical resection may be necessary in severe cases.

Awake Fiber-Optic Intubation

Fiber-optic bronchoscopy is often employed by anesthesiologists to facilitate safe tracheal intubation in situations where conventional laryngoscopy is difficult or contraindicated. Difficult laryngoscopy may be encountered in patients with distorted anatomy or limited neck or soft tissue mobility that impedes the direct visualization of the larynx. Mask ventilation may also be a challenge in these patients, culminating in a potentially catastrophic "can't intubate, can't ventilate" scenario if spontaneous ventilation is compromised. Relative contraindications to direct laryngoscopy include situations where manipulation of the cervical spine may be harmful, as with ligamentous instability or unstable fractures.

The advantage of a fiber-optic bronchoscopic intubation (FOBI) is that excessive movement of the patient's neck or mouth is not required to enable visualization of the upper airway and trachea. The bronchoscope can be guided through relatively small openings (either orally or nasally), and its maneuverability allows the operator to achieve excellent visualization without necessitating the same anatomic alignment required with direct laryngoscopy. Once the bronchoscope has been positioned beyond the vocal cords into the trachea, it can serve as a guide over which an endotracheal tube can be passed. Some advocate approaching FOBI through the nose, as the natural curvature of the nasopharynx often results in the bronchoscope being aligned directly at the laryngeal inlet. However, nasal intubation may be less tolerated by patients, demands the use of a smaller tube, and can precipitate epistaxis. The decision as to which approach is used depends on the circumstances of the individual case.

When access to the larynx is likely to be difficult, maintenance of spontaneous ventilation during intubation is the safest method of securing the airway. Often described as an awake intubation, the technique is best performed with an appropriately sedated (ideally cooperative) and reasonably comfortable patient. The type of sedation used is preferably short acting or quickly reversible, to allow for rapid return of spontaneous ventilation should the patient become apneic. Used judiciously, short-acting opioids such as fentanyl or remifentanil provide excellent sedation though they can easily lead to apnea if overdosed. Midazolam is a rapid onset intravenous benzodiazepine with amnestic properties that has a higher threshold for suppressing respiration. It should be kept in mind that the combined use of sedatives may have synergistic effects resulting in an unconscious or apneic patient at lower than anticipated doses. Reversal agents including naloxone and flumazenil should be available in case of accidental overdose. In recent years dexmedetomidine, a short-acting highly selective alpha-2-adrenoceptor agonist, has gained popularity due to its favorable sedative and anxiolytic effects combined with a minimal impact on respiratory drive. The ability to induce a level of sedation similar to sleep while the patient remains easily rousable and cooperative makes it an appealing agent for awake intubation. Other adjuvant medications to consider include antisialogogues to reduce airway secretions. Anticholinergic agents used for this purpose include atropine, glycopyrrolate, and scopolamine, each of which has a characteristic side-effect profile, including tachycardia (atropine > glycopyrrolate) and sedation (scopolamine > atropine) [110, 111].

As previously described, awake patients often poorly tolerate the placement of a bronchoscope and endotracheal tube in the oropharynx and trachea. Even with effective sedation, the cough and gag reflexes are difficult to suppress and remain disruptive to the bronchoscopist. These powerful reflexes are key defenses in protecting the lungs from aspiration and are rudimentary indicators of intact brainstem function. An understanding of the basic innervation of the pharynx and larynx allows one to interrupt the afferent and efferent neural limbs to facilitate instrumentation of the airway. Basically, there are three nerves responsible for sensation in the airway: the trigeminal nerve supplies the nasopharynx, the glossopharyngeal supplies the oropharynx, and the vagus supplies the larynx and the trachea [112]. In the upper airway, the gag response includes afferent input from the glossopharyngeal and an efferent motor arc from branches of the vagus nerve. In the lower airway, innervation above the vocal cords is primarily provided by the supralaryngeal nerve (SNL) and below the cords by the recurrent laryngeal and external SNL, all of which are vagal branches. As such the SNL controls the glottic closure reflex (which leads to laryngospasm if hyper stimulated), while the remaining vagal inputs control the cough reflex.

The application of topical anesthetic to the mucosal surfaces of the airway is the simplest way to minimize sensory stimulation and thus interrupt the afferent arm of the airway reflexes before attempting an awake intubation [113]. These can be administered either by inhalation of a nebulized liquid (via face mask), direct application using an atomized spray (either blindly or through the bronchoscope itself), placement of gauze soaked in local anesthetic solution (intranasally or at the tonsillar bases), or gargling [114]. The ideal agent for topicalization is one that is quick in onset and has a few side effects, with limited risk of toxicity. Absorption of these drugs through the mucous membranes of the oropharynx and lungs is unpredictable; it is possible to achieve toxic plasma levels with excessive topicalization [115]. Table 11.6 outlines the most commonly used topical agents.

Through effective topicalization, practitioners are able to achieve excellent conditions for awake intubation. Despite this, some advocate the use of nerve blocks to enhance the blunting of airway reflexes by selectively targeting the three nerves described above. These blocks are useful in clinical scenarios when local infection, blood, or secretions hinder effective

Table 11.6 Topical airway anesthetic agents

Agent	Speed of onset	Duration (min)	Maximum dose	Toxicity
Cocaine	Slow	30–60	1.5 mg/kg	Hypertension, myocardial ischemia
Lidocaine	Moderate	30–60	3 mg/kg (7 mg/kg with epinephrine)	Tinnitus, seizures, arrhythmia
Benzocaine	Fast	5–10	200 mg	Methemoglobinemia

Table 11.7 Airway nerve blocks

Nerve	Approach	Considerations
Glossopharyngeal	Intraoral: Injection at base of posterior tonsillar pillar	Requires adequate mouth opening Risk of carotid injection
	Peri-styloid: Injection between the mastoid process and angle of jaw	Requires palpable landmarks Risk of carotid injection
Superior laryngeal	Injection between the greater cornu of hyoid bone and superior cornu of thyroid cartilage	Requires palpable landmarks and neck extension Risk of intravascular injection
Vagus (infraglottic and upper tracheal)	Intratracheal injection through cricothyroid membrane	Requires palpable landmarks Risk of airway compromise from bleeding or trauma

topicalization. Lidocaine is usually the agent of choice for airway blocks. If nerve blocks are used in addition to topical agents, be wary of exceeding toxic levels. Obviously, these techniques involve a higher level of skill and risk the complications of intravascular injection, hematoma, and nerve injury. Further, as they require insertion of needles in the patient's neck, the performance of these blocks may themselves add to an already anxiety provoking procedure. Table 11.7 outlines the main approaches to airway nerve blocks.

Clinical Case Discussion

A 65-year-old woman with a remote transhiatal esophagectomy for cancer presented with 2 days of increasing dyspnea. She remains hypoxemic following intubation for respiratory failure in the emergency department, despite maximal conventional ventilation. CT imaging demonstrates near-complete obstruction of the left main bronchus and significant obstruction of the right main bronchus (Fig. 11.11). The Interventional Pulmonologist intends to perform balloon dilatation, tumor resection, and stent insertion in the left main bronchus via rigid bronchoscopy.

Questions

Outline the considerations of providing anesthesia for patients with central airway obstruction:

- Risk of complete airway obstruction and impossible ventilation

- Potential for dynamic hyperinflation resulting in hemodynamic compromise or barotrauma
- Considerations and complications of rigid and interventional bronchoscopy

Describe the ventilation techniques applied during rigid bronchoscopy:

- Spontaneous
- Assisted
- Sanders jet ventilation
- HFJV

Describe the acute complications of balloon bronchoplasty, airway stenting, and electrocautery:

- Tracheitis
- Fever
- Atelectasis
- Bronchospasm
- Airway disruption
- Dissemination of obstructing pneumonia
- Hemorrhage
- Airway fire
- Electromagnetic interference

Authors' Management

General anesthesia was maintained by TIVA and neuromuscular blockade. Fiber-optic inspection of the tracheobronchial tree was expeditiously performed to further evaluate the tumor and characterize the anatomy of the obstruction. Given the degree of hypoxemia, an exchange catheter was inserted adjacent to the endotracheal tube, to allow for temporary oxygenation during the transition between tracheal extubation and access with the rigid bronchoscope. Ventilation following tracheal placement of the rigid bronchoscope was supported with a Sanders jet injector. Left mainstem patency was re-established using a combination of balloon dilation, electrocautery, and stent placement. Following restoration of normal gas exchange, balloon dilation of the right mainstem was employed, the trachea was extubated, and a laryngeal mask was inserted. Once the patient recovered from intravenous anesthesia, neuromuscular blockade was reversed, adequate spontaneous ventilation was established, and the patient was observed in the operating room until fully awake (Fig. 11.11).

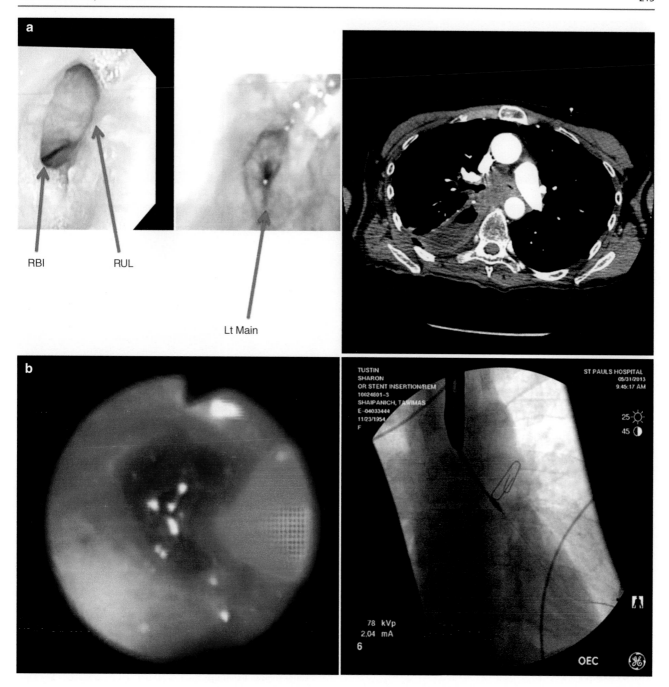

Fig. 11.11 (**a**) Bronchoscopic picture of the right bronchus intermediate (RBI) stenosis and left main bronchial stenosis (Lt main); CT scan of the chest demonstrates near occlusion of the left main airway by tumor. (**b**) Balloon dilation of the left main bronchus (left). Fluoroscopy image shows stent insertion via rigid bronchoscopy (right) (**c**) Bronchoscopic examination shows left main airway stent and patent right main airway post balloon dilation and stent placement

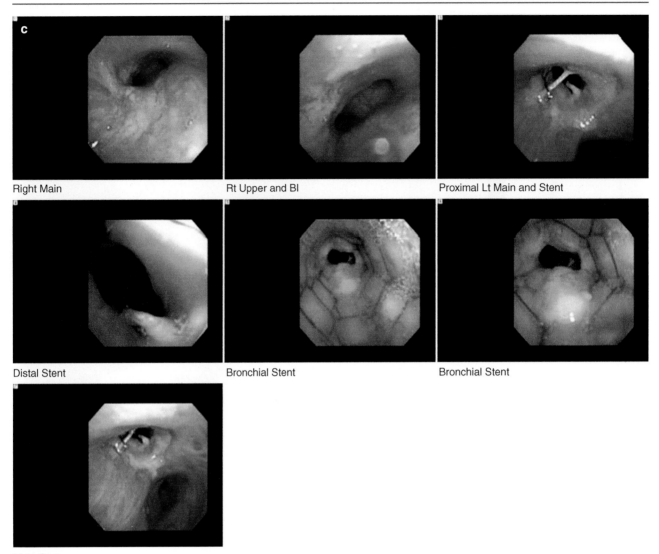

Right Main

Rt Upper and Bl

Proximal Lt Main and Stent

Distal Stent

Bronchial Stent

Bronchial Stent

Main Carina

Fig. 11.11 (continued)

References

1. Limper AH, Prakash UB. Tracheobronchial foreign bodies in adults. Ann Intern Med. 1990;112(8):604–9.
2. Conacher ID, Curran E. Local anaesthesia and sedation for rigid bronchoscopy for emergency relief of central airway obstruction. Anaesthesia. 2004;59(3):290–2.
3. Chadha M, Kulshrestha M, Biyani A. Anaesthesia for bronchoscopy. Indian J Anaesth. 2015;59(9):565–73.
4. Ernst A, Simoff M, Ost D, Goldman Y, Herth FJ. Prospective risk-adjusted morbidity and mortality outcome analysis after therapeutic bronchoscopic procedures: results of a multi-institutional outcomes database. Chest. 2008;134(3):514–9.
5. Perrin G, Colt HG, Martin C, Mak MA, Dumon JF, Gouin F. Safety of interventional rigid bronchoscopy using intravenous anesthesia and spontaneous assisted ventilation. A prospective study. Chest. 1992;102(5):1526–30.
6. Metzner J, Posner KL, Domino KB. The risk and safety of anesthesia at remote locations: the US closed claims analysis. Curr Opin Anaesthesiol. 2009;22(4):502–8.
7. Folch E, Mehta AC. Airway interventions in the tracheobronchial tree. Semin Respir Crit Care Med. 2008;29(4):441–52.
8. Brodsky JB. Bronchoscopic procedures for central airway obstruction. J Cardiothorac Vasc Anesth. 2003;17(5):638–46.
9. Pinsonneault C, Fortier J, Donati F. Tracheal resection and reconstruction. Can J Anaesth. 1999;46(5):439–55.
10. Mason RA, Fielder CP. The obstructed airway in head and neck surgery. Anaesthesia. 1999;120(4):1152–6.
11. Hnatiuk OW, Corcoran PC, Sierra A. Spirometry in surgery for anterior mediastinal masses. Chest. 2001;120(4):1152–6.
12. Ernst A, Feller-Kopman D, Becker HD, Mehta AC. Central airway obstruction. Am J Respir Crit Care Med. 2004;169(12): 1278–97.
13. Walser EM. Stent placement for tracheobronchial disease. Eur J Radiol. 2005;55(3):321–30.

14. Lee KS, Lunn W, Feller-Kopman D, Ernst A, Hatabu H, Boiselle PM. Multislice CT evaluation of airway stents. J Thorac Imaging. 2005;20(2):81–8.

15. Burke AJ, Vining DJ, McGuirt WF, Postma G, Browne JD. Evaluation of airway obstruction using virtual endoscopy. Laryngoscope. 2000;110(1):23–9.

16. Baroni RH, Ashiku S, Boiselle PM. Dynamic CT evaluation of the central airways in patients undergoing tracheoplasty for tracheobronchomalacia. Am J Roentgenol. 2005;184(5):1444–9.

17. Conacher ID. Anaesthesia and tracheobronchial stenting for central airway obstruction in adults. Br J Anaesth. 2003;90(3):367–74.

18. Wood D. Airway stenting. Chest Surg Clin N Am. 2003;13(2):211–29.

19. Ho AM, Dion PW, Karmakar MK, Chung DC, Tay BA. Use of heliox in critical upper airway obstruction. Physical and physiologic considerations in choosing the optimal helium:Oxygen mix. Resuscitation. 2002;52(3):297–300.

20. Stephens KE, Wood DE. Bronchoscopic management of central airway obstruction. J Thorac Cardiovasc Surg. 2000;119(2):289–96.

21. Vonk-Noordegraaf A, Postmus PE, Sutedja TG. Tracheobronchial stenting in the terminal care of cancer patients with central airways obstruction. Chest. 2001;120(6):1811–4.

22. Hautmann H, Gamarra F, Henke M, Diehm S, Huber RM. High frequency jet ventilation in interventional fiberoptic bronchoscopy. Anesth Analg. 2000;90(6):1436–40.

23. Smith IJ, Sidebotham DA, McGeorge AD, Dorman EB, Wilsher ML, Kolbe J. Use of extracorporeal membrane oxygenation during resection of tracheal papillomatosis. Anesthesiology. 2009;110(2):427–9.

24. Zhou YF, Zhu SJ, Zhu SM, An XX. Anesthetic management of emergent critical tracheal stenosis. J Zhejiang Univ Sci B. 2007;8(7):522–5.

25. Vourc'h G, Fischler M, Michon F, Melchior JC, Seigneur F. Manual jet ventilation v. high frequency jet ventilation during laser resection of tracheo-bronchial stenosis. Br J Anaesth. 1983;55(10):973–5.

26. Vaitkeviciute I, Ehrenwerth J. Con: bronchial stenting and laser airway surgery should not take place outside the operating room. J Cardiothorac Vasc Anesth. 2005;19(1):121–2.

27. Wahidi MM, Herth FJ, Ernst A. State of the art: interventional pulmonology. Chest. 2007;131(1):261–74.

28. Barbaro RP, Odetola FO, Kidwell KM, Paden ML, Bartlett RH, Davis MM, Annich GM. Association of hospital-level volume of extracorporeal membrane oxygenation cases and mortality. Analysis of the extracorporeal life support organization registry. Am J Respir Crit Care Med. 2015;191(8):894–901.

29. Kim CW, Kim DH, Son BS, Cho JS, Kim YD, Hoseok I, Ahn HY. The feasibility of extracorporeal membrane oxygenation in the variant airway problems. Ann Thorac Cardiovasc Surg. 2015;21(6):517–22.

30. McLenon M, Bittle GJ, Jones K, Menaker J, Pham SM, Iacono AT, et al. Extracorporeal lung support as a bridge to airway stenting and radiotherapy for airway-obstructing pancoast tumor. Ann Thorac Surg. 2016;102(1):e7–9.

31. Willms DC, Mendez R, Norman V, Chammas JH. Emergency bedside extracorporeal membrane oxygenation for rescue of acute tracheal obstruction. Respir Care. 2012;57(4):646–9.

32. Ko M, dos Santos PR, Machuca TN, Marseu K, Waddell TK, Keshavjee S, Cypel M. Use of single-cannula venous-venous extracorporeal life support in the management of life-threatening airway obstruction. Ann Thorac Surg. 2015;99(3):e63–5.

33. Natt B, Knepler J Jr, Kazui T, Mosier JM. The use of extracorporeal membrane oxygenation in the bronchoscopic management of critical upper airway obstruction. J Bronchol Interv Pulmonol. 2017;24(1):e12–4.

34. Hong Y, Jo KW, Lyu J, Huh JW, Hong SB, Jung SH, et al. Use of venovenous extracorporeal membrane oxygenation in central airway obstruction to facilitate interventions leading to definitive airway security. J Crit Care. 2013;28(5):669–74.

35. Guha A, Mostafa SM, Kendall JB. The montgomery t-tube: Anaesthetic problems and solutions. Br J Anaesth. 2001;87(5):787–90.

36. Dumon JF. A dedicated tracheobronchial stent. Chest. 1990;97(2):328–32.

37. Saito Y. Endobronchial stents: past, present, and future. Semin Respir Crit Care Med. 2004;25(4):375–80.

38. Stehlik L, Hytych V, Letackova J, Kubena P, Vasakova M. Biodegradable polydioxanone stents in the treatment of adult patients with tracheal narrowing. BMC Pulm Med. 2015;15:164.

39. Finlayson GN, Brodsky JB. Anesthetic considerations for airway stenting in adult patients. Anesthesiol Clin. 2008;26(2):281–91.

40. Zakaluzny SA, Lane JD, Mair EA. Complications of tracheobronchial airway stents. Otolaryngol Head Neck Surg. 2003;128(4):478–88.

41. Bolliger CT, Sutedja TG, Strausz J, Freitag L. Therapeutic bronchoscopy with immediate effect: laser, electrocautery, argon plasma coagulation and stents. Eur Respir J. 2006;27(6):1258–71.

42. Grillo HC. Stents and sense. Ann Thorac Surg. 2000;70(4):1142.

43. Grewe PH, Müller KM, Lindstaedt M, Germing A, Müller A, Mügge A, Deneke T. Reaction patterns of the tracheobronchial wall to implanted noncovered metal stents. Chest. 2005;128(2):986–90.

44. Thornton RH, Gordon RL, Kerlan RK, LaBerge JM, Wilson MW, Wolanske KA, et al. Outcomes of tracheobronchial stent placement for benign disease 1. Radiology. 2006;240(1):273–82.

45. Eller RL, Livingston WJ, Morgan CE, Peters GE, Sillers MJ, Magnuson JS, Rosenthal EL. Expandable tracheal stenting for benign disease: worth the complications? Ann Otol Rhinol Laryngol. 2006;115(4):247–52.

46. Makris D, Marquette CH. Tracheobronchial stenting and central airway replacement. Curr Opin Pulm Med. 2007;13(4):278–83.

47. Urschel JD. Delayed massive hemoptysis after expandable bronchial stent placement. J Laparoendosc Adv Surg Tech A. 1999;9(2):155–8.

48. Hung WT, Liao SM, Su JM. Laryngeal mask airway in patients with tracheal stents who are undergoing non-airway related interventions: report of three cases. J Clin Anesth. 2004;16(3):214–6.

49. Davis N, Madden BP, Sheth A, Crerar-Gilbert AJ. Airway management of patients with tracheobronchial stents. Br J Anaesth. 2006;96(1):132–5.

50. Yan Y, Olszewski AE, Hoffman MR, Zhuang P, Ford CN, Dailey SH, Jiang JJ. Use of lasers in laryngeal surgery. J Voice. 2010;24(1):102–9.

51. Van Der Spek AF, Spargo PM, Norton ML. The physics of lasers and implications for their use during airway surgery. Br J Anaesth. 1988;60(6):709–29.

52. Cortese DA. Rigid versus flexible bronchoscope in laser bronchoscopy pro rigid bronchoscopic laser application. J Bronchol Interv Pulmonol. 1994;1(1):72–5.

53. Moghissi K, Dixon K, Hudson E, Stringer M, Brown S. Endoscopic laser therapy in malignant tracheobronchial obstruction using sequential nd YAG laser and photodynamic therapy. Thorax. 1997;52(3):281–3.

54. Geffin B, Shapshay SM, Bellack GS, Hobin K, Setzer SE. Flammability of endotracheal tubes during nd-yag laser application in the airway. Anesthesiology. 1986;65(5):511–5.

55. Lee P, Kupeli E, Mehta AC. Therapeutic bronchoscopy in lung cancer. Laser therapy, electrocautery, brachytherapy, stents, and photodynamic therapy. Clin Chest Med. 2002;23(1):241–56.

56. Tellides G, Ugurlu BS, Kim RW, Hammond GL. Pathogenesis of systemic air embolism during bronchoscopic nd:YAG laser operations. Ann Thorac Surg. 1998;65(4):930–4.

57. Lobraico RV, Schifano MJ, Brader KR. A retrospective study on the hazards of the carbon dioxide laser plume. J Laser Appl. 1988;1(1):6–8.

58. Garden JM, O'Banion MK, Shelnitz LS, Pinski KS, Bakus AD, Reichmann ME, Sundberg JP. Papillomavirus in the vapor of carbon dioxide laser-treated verrucae. JAMA. 1988;259(8):1199–202.

59. Baggish MS, Poiesz BJ, Joret D, Williamson P, Refai A. Presence of human immunodeficiency virus DNA in laser smoke. Lasers Surg Med. 1991;11(3):197–203.

60. Barlow DE. Endoscopic applications of electrosurgery: a review of basic principles. Gastrointest Endosc. 1982;28(2):73–6.

61. Coulter TD, Mehta AC. The heat is on: impact of endobronchial electrosurgery on the need for nd-yag laser photoresection. Chest. 2000;118(2):516–21.

62. Boxem TV, Muller M, Venmans B, Postmus P, Sutedja T. Nd-YAG laser vs bronchoscopic electrocautery for palliation of symptomatic airway obstruction: a cost-effectiveness study. Chest. 1999;116(4):1108–12.

63. Ernst A, Silvestri GA, Johnstone D. Interventional pulmonary procedures: guidelines from the american college of chest physicians. Chest J. 2003;123(5):1693–717.

64. Grund KE, Storek D, Farin G. Endoscopic argon plasma coagulation (APC) first clinical experiences in flexible endoscopy. Endosc Surg Allied Technol. 1994;2(1):42–6.

65. Sheski FD, Mathur PN. Endobronchial electrosurgery: argon plasma coagulation and electrocautery. Semin Respir Crit Care Med. 2004;25(4):367–74.

66. Morice RC, Ece T, Ece F, Keus L. Endobronchial argon plasma coagulation for treatment of hemoptysis and neoplastic airway obstruction. Chest. 2001;119(3):781–7.

67. Reddy C, Majid A, Michaud G, Feller-Kopman D, Eberhardt R, Herth F, Ernst A. Gas embolism following bronchoscopic argon plasma coagulation: a case series. Chest. 2008;134(5):1066–9.

68. McArdle JR, Gildea TR, Mehta AC. Balloon bronchoplasty: its indications, benefits, and complications. J Bronchol Interv Pulmonol. 2005;12(2):123–7.

69. Vergnon JM, Huber RM, Moghissi K. Place of cryotherapy, brachytherapy and photodynamic therapy in therapeutic bronchoscopy of lung cancers. Eur Respir J. 2006;28(1):200–18.

70. Schumann C, Hetzel M, Babiak AJ, Hetzel J, Merk T, Wibmer T, et al. Endobronchial tumor debulking with a flexible cryoprobe for immediate treatment of malignant stenosis. J Thorac Cardiovasc Surg. 2010;139(4):997–1000.

71. Mohamed AS, El-Din MAA. Fiberoptic bronchoscopic cryoablation of central bronchial lung cancer. Egypt J Chest Dis Tuberc. 2016;65(2):527–30.

72. Inaty H, Folch E, Berger R, Fernandez-Bussy S, Chatterji S, Alape D, Majid A. Unimodality and multimodality cryodebridement for airway obstruction. A single-center experience with safety and efficacy. Ann Am Thorac Soc. 2016;13(6):856–61.

73. Browning R, Parrish S, Sarkar S, Turner JF. First report of a novel liquid nitrogen adjustable flow spray cryotherapy (SCT) device in the bronchoscopic treatment of disease of the central tracheobronchial airways. J Thorac Dis. 2013;5(3):E103–6.

74. Browning R, Turner JF, Parrish S. Spray cryotherapy (SCT): institutional evolution of techniques and clinical practice from early experience in the treatment of malignant airway disease. J Thorac Dis. 2015;7(Suppl 4):S405–14.

75. Rafanan AL, Mehta AC. Adult airway foreign body removal. What's new? Clin Chest Med. 2001;22(2):319–30.

76. Swanson KL. Airway foreign bodies: What's new? Semin Respir Crit Care Med. 2004;25(4):405–11.

77. Zur KB, Litman RS. Pediatric airway foreign body retrieval: surgical and anesthetic perspectives. Paediatr Anaesth. 2009;19(Suppl 1):109–17.

78. McKenna RJ. Endobronchial valves for the treatment of emphysema. Semin Thorac Cardiovasc Surg. 2008;20(4):285–9.

79. Valipour A, Slebos DJ, Herth F, Darwiche K, Wagner M, Ficker JH, et al. Endobronchial valve therapy in patients with homogeneous emphysema. Results from the IMPACT study. Am J Respir Crit Care Med. 2016;194(9):1073–82.

80. Hopkinson NS. Bronchoscopic lung volume reduction: indications, effects and prospects. Curr Opin Pulm Med. 2007, Mar;13(2):125–30.

81. Sciurba FC, Ernst A, Herth FJ, Strange C, Criner GJ, Marquette CH, et al. A randomized study of endobronchial valves for advanced emphysema. N Engl J Med. 2010, Sep 23;363(13):1233–44.

82. Klooster K, ten Hacken NH, Hartman JE, Kerstjens HA, van Rikxoort EM, Slebos D-J. Endobronchial valves for emphysema without interlobar collateral ventilation. N Engl J Med. 2015;373(24):2325–35.

83. Sciurba FC, Criner GJ, Strange C, Shah PL, Michaud G, Connolly TA, et al. Effect of endobronchial coils vs usual care on exercise tolerance in patients with severe emphysema: the RENEW randomized clinical trial. JAMA. 2016;315(20):2178–89.

84. Deslée G, Mal H, Dutau H, Bourdin A, Vergnon JM, Pison C, et al. Lung volume reduction coil treatment vs usual care in patients with severe emphysema: the REVOLENS randomized clinical trial. JAMA. 2016;315(2):175–84.

85. Travaline JM, McKenna RJ, De Giacomo T, Venuta F, Hazelrigg SR, Boomer M, et al. Treatment of persistent pulmonary air leaks using endobronchial valves. Chest. 2009;136(2):355–60.

86. Ingenito EP, Wood DE, Utz JP. Bronchoscopic lung volume reduction in severe emphysema. Proc Am Thorac Soc. 2008;5(4):454–60.

87. Shah PL, Slebos DJ, Cardoso PF, Cetti E, Voelker K, Levine B, et al. Bronchoscopic lung-volume reduction with exhale airway stents for emphysema (EASE trial): randomised, sham-controlled, multicentre trial. Lancet. 2011;378(9795):997–1005.

88. Bel EH. "Hot Stuff" bronchial thermoplasty for asthma. Am J Respir Crit Care Med. 2006;173:941–2.

89. Cox G. New interventions in asthma including bronchial thermoplasty. Curr Opin Pulm Med. 2008;14(1):77–81.

90. Lee P, Mehta AC, Mathur PN. Management of complications from diagnostic and interventional bronchoscopy. Respirology. 2009;14(7):940–53.

91. Burns DM, Shure D, Francoz R, Kalafer M, Harrell J, Witztum K, Moser KM. The physiologic consequences of saline lobar lavage in healthy human adults. Am Rev Respir Dis. 1983;127(6):695–701.

92. Hariri LP, Applegate MB, Mino-Kenudson M, Mark EJ, Bouma BE, Tearney GJ, Suter MJ. Optical frequency domain imaging of ex vivo pulmonary resection specimens: obtaining one to one image to histopathology correlation. J Vis Exp. 2013;71:e3855.

93. Hariri LP, Mino-Kenudson M, Applegate MB, Mark EJ, Tearney GJ, Lanuti M, et al. Toward the guidance of transbronchial biopsy: identifying pulmonary nodules with optical coherence tomography. Chest. 2013;144(4):1261–8.

94. Strumpf IJ, Feld MK, Cornelius MJ, Keogh BA, Crystal RG. Safety of fiberoptic bronchoalveolar lavage in evaluation of interstitial lung disease. Chest. 1981;80(3):268–71.

95. Pingleton SK, Harrison GF, Stechschulte DJ, Wesselius LJ, Kerby GR, Ruth WE. Effect of location, ph, and temperature of instillate in bronchoalveolar lavage in normal volunteers. Am Rev Respir Dis. 1983;128(6):1035–7.

96. Wardlaw AJ, Collins JV, Kay AB. Mechanisms in asthma using the technique of bronchoalveolar lavage. Int Arch Allergy Appl Immunol. 1987;82(3–4):518–25.

97. Klech H, Pohl W. Technical recommendations and guidelines for bronchoalveolar lavage (BAL). Eur Respir J. 1989;2(6):561–85.

98. Schreiber G, McCrory DC. Performance characteristics of different modalities for diagnosis of suspected lung cancer: summary of published evidence. Chest. 2003;123:115S–28S.

99. Colt HG, Prakash UB, Offord KP. Bronchoscopy in north america: survey by the american association for bronchology, 1999. J Bronchol Interv Pulmonol. 2000;7(1):8–25.

100. Sheski FD, Mathur PN. Endobronchial ultrasound. Chest. 2008;133(1):264–70.
101. Krasnik M, Vilmann P, Larsen SS, Jacobsen GK. Preliminary experience with a new method of endoscopic transbronchial real time ultrasound guided biopsy for diagnosis of mediastinal and hilar lesions. Thorax. 2003;58(12):1083–6.
102. Herth FJ, Lunn W, Eberhardt R, Becker HD, Ernst A. Transbronchial versus transesophageal ultrasound-guided aspiration of enlarged mediastinal lymph nodes. Am J Respir Crit Care Med. 2005;171(10):1164–7.
103. Kennedy MP, Jimenez CA, Morice RC, Eapen GA. Ultrasound-guided endobronchial, endoscopic, and transthoracic biopsy. Semin Respir Crit Care Med. 2008;29(4):453–64.
104. Kucera F, Wolfe GK, Perry ME. Hemomediastinum after transbronchial needle aspiration. Chest. 1990;3:466.
105. Epstein SK, Winslow CJ, Brecher SM, Faling LJ. Polymicrobial bacterial pericarditis after transbronchial needle aspiration. Case report with an investigation on the risk of bacterial contamination during fiberoptic bronchoscopy. Am Rev Respir Dis. 1992;146(2):523–5.
106. Simpson FG, Arnold AG, Purvis A, Belfield PW, Muers MF, Cooke NJ. Postal survey of bronchoscopic practice by physicians in the United Kingdom. Thorax. 1986;41(4):311–7.
107. Ernst A, Eberhardt R, Wahidi M, Becker HD, Herth FJ. Effect of routine clopidogrel use on bleeding complications after transbronchial biopsy in humans. Chest. 2006;129(3):734–7.
108. Papin TA, Grum CM, Weg JG. Transbronchial biopsy during mechanical ventilation. Chest. 1986;89(2):168–70.
109. O'Brien JD, Ettinger NA, Shevlin D, Kollef MH. Safety and yield of transbronchial biopsy in mechanically ventilated patients. Crit Care Med. 1997;25(3):440–6.
110. Rose DD. Review of anticholinergic drugs: their use and safe omittance in preoperative medications. AANA J. 1984.
111. Corallo CE, Whitfield A, Wu A. Anticholinergic syndrome following an unintentional overdose of scopolamine. Ther Clin Risk Manag. 2009;5(5):719–23.
112. Simmons ST, Schleich AR. Airway regional anesthesia for awake fiberoptic intubation. Reg Anesth Pain Med. 2002;27(2):180–92.
113. Kundra P, Kutralam S, Ravishankar M. Local anaesthesia for awake fibreoptic nasotracheal intubation. Acta Anaesthesiol Scand. 2000;44(5):511–6.
114. Mostafa SM, Murthy BVS, Hodgson CA, Beese E. Nebulized 10% lignocaine for awake fibreoptic intubation. Anaesth Intensive Care. 1998;26(2):222.
115. Chung DC, Mainland PA, Kong AS. Anesthesia of the airway by aspiration of lidocaine. Can J Anaesth. 1999;46(3):215–9.

Intravenous Anesthesia for Thoracic Procedures

12

Javier D. Lasala and Ron V. Purugganan

Introduction

Over the last century and a half, thoracic surgery has evolved from hurried operations with high mortality to relatively safe and controlled procedures with a good chance of survival. In early procedures, anesthetic agents and their delivery were crude, resulting in suboptimal surgical conditions in which anesthetic depth was questionable, hemodynamics were unstable, and ventilation/oxygenation is subpar. The development of endotracheal intubation, lung isolation techniques, and modern anesthetic drugs was instrumental in the evolution of thoracic surgery. Modern anesthetics can reliably render a patient unconscious and immobile while maintaining hemodynamic and respiratory stability. Through these improvements of surgical conditions, more complex and time-consuming operations became possible. Furthermore, the continued evolution of intravenous anesthetic agents has made it possible for thoracic anesthesiologists to better adapt their techniques to suit specific surgical scenarios. This chapter reviews the rationale for using intravenous anesthesia for thoracic operations, the drugs and equipment required, and the methodology involved.

Rationale for Total Intravenous Anesthesia

Traditional inhalational anesthetics have been associated (at least in animal studies) with a direct inhibition of hypoxic pulmonary vasoconstriction (HPV), the reflex arteriolar constriction that diverts blood from hypoxic segments of the lung to normal areas of the lung, thereby decreasing shunt fraction. In

Key Points

- Total intravenous anesthesia (TIVA) is indicated for procedures in which inhalational anesthetics may not be safely or effectively delivered, including endobronchial procedures using flexible or rigid bronchoscopy and proximal airway-disrupting surgeries. TIVA may also be beneficial in lung volume reduction surgery, lung transplantation, and thymectomy.
- TIVA is safer and more practical for thoracic procedures performed outside of the operating room, such as off-site locations, military field, or impoverished areas of the world.
- Target-controlled infusion (TCI) is a delivery system for TIVA that is based on pharmacokinetic models to optimize intravenous anesthetic delivery. TCI has many advantages over conventional calculator pumps but is not currently available in the United States.
- Because well-established MAC-type systems for intravenous anesthetics are not available, anesthetic depth monitors are useful in monitoring patients undergoing TIVA.
- Propofol, dexmedetomidine, ketamine, lidocaine, and remifentanil may be used in combination with anesthetic depth monitoring to execute an effective TIVA regimen.
- This chapter reviews the balanced TIVA technique currently used at the University of Texas MD Anderson Cancer Center, which encompasses enhanced recovery after surgery principles.

J. D. Lasala (✉)
Department of Anesthesiology and Perioperative Medicine,
The University of Texas MD Anderson Cancer Center,
Houston, TX, USA
e-mail: jlasala@mdanderson.org

R. V. Purugganan
Department of Anesthesiology and Perioperative Medicine,
The University of Texas MD Anderson Cancer Center,
Cardiothoracic Anesthesia Group, Unit 409, Faculty Center,
Houston, TX, USA
e-mail: rpurugga@mdanderson.org

© Springer Nature Switzerland AG 2019
P. Slinger (ed.), *Principles and Practice of Anesthesia for Thoracic Surgery*, https://doi.org/10.1007/978-3-030-00859-8_12

thoracic procedures, this inhibition of HPV may be detrimental to patient oxygenation levels during one-lung ventilation. In contrast, intravenous anesthetics do not appear to directly inhibit HPV, in vitro or in patients. Consequently, interest has focused on whether total intravenous anesthesia (TIVA) might provide better oxygenation and lesser shunt fraction than inhaled anesthetics in thoracic procedures. As little work has been done to answer this question more recently, research published in the last decade is summarized here.

Several studies have shown an advantage to using TIVA. Abe and colleagues studied patients receiving either isoflurane or sevoflurane followed by TIVA (propofol). PaO_2 increased significantly, and shunt fraction decreased significantly after the initiation of TIVA [1]. In another study, PaO_2 was also significantly higher in patients who received TIVA for pulmonary resection than in those who received volatile anesthetics [2]. Özcan and colleagues compared oxygenation and shunt fraction in 100 patients undergoing one of four anesthesia techniques during one-lung ventilation: TIVA with or without thoracic epidural anesthesia (TEA) and isoflurane with or without TEA. Patient oxygenation was significantly higher, and shunt was significantly lower in the two groups receiving TIVA; the addition of TEA in either study group had no significant effect [3]. A retrospective study examined changes in saturation in patients receiving propofol and fentanyl intravenous anesthesia compared to inhalation anesthesia. In this study they showed patients in the TIVA group to have an 8% chance of developing hypoxemia compared to literature, which suggests hypoxemia ranging from 13% to 40% in patients receiving inhalation anesthesia, hence demonstrating TIVA as a suitable anesthetic to maintain saturation during one-lung ventilation [4]. A study conducted on the effect of remifentanil on arterial oxygenation during one-lung ventilation revealed that an infusion can be successful with propofol during one-lung ventilation without significant changes in PaO_2 [5].

Alternatively, a few studies fail to support any advantage of TIVA. Beck and colleagues studied 40 patients who received either propofol or sevoflurane during one-lung ventilation for thoracic surgery. They found no significant difference in shunt fraction between the two groups. Hemodynamic variables known to influence HPV (cardiac index, mixed venous oxygen tension, and arterial carbon dioxide partial pressure) were also similar between the two groups [6]. Pruszkowski and colleagues compared oxygenation levels in patients undergoing lung lobectomy. The patients received a thoracic epidural and either sevoflurane or propofol at levels required to maintain a bispectral index (BIS) between 40 and 60. The authors found no difference in PaO_2 levels between the sevoflurane and propofol groups. They suggest that the titration of anesthetics to appropriate BIS levels (which distinguished their study) could avoid potential negative effects of inhalational anesthetics on hemodynamics that affect the shunt [7]. Yondov and col-

leagues in a comparative study of the effect of halothane, isoflurane, and propofol on partial arterial oxygen pressure during one-lung ventilation concluded that TIVA with propofol/fentanyl can be applied as an alternative of general anesthesia with halogenated volatile anesthetics, as there was no significant difference in the PaO_2 between the three groups during ventilation [8]. Lastly, Von Dossow and colleagues divided 50 patients undergoing pulmonary surgery into two groups—isoflurane with TEA or TIVA (propofol)—and measured shunt fraction, PaO_2, and cardiac output. They found that the decrease in PaO_2 level following the conversion from two-lung to one-lung ventilation was less in the isoflurane group. Shunt fraction remained the same in both groups. Cardiac output was greater in the TIVA group, which may have contributed to the effect on PaO_2 [9].

Most likely, even though inhalational anesthetics suppress HPV, other factors such as surgical manipulation, cardiac output, mixed venous oxygen tension, and positive end-expiratory pressure may have a greater influence on shunt fraction than the influence of inhalational agents on HPV. Therefore, further studies are required to define the clinical significance of inhaled anesthetics on HPV in thoracic surgery.

Immunomodulatory effects of inhaled vs. TIVA techniques on the lung are another area of ongoing investigation. Animal studies have shown that propofol may have a protective effect on the lungs, especially in acute lung injury resulting from endotoxin exposure [10]. In patients undergoing cardiopulmonary bypass, propofol has been shown to regulate the pulmonary inflammatory response [11]. However, studies of thoracic surgery patients undergoing one-lung ventilation may favor the use of volatile anesthetics to decrease the inflammatory response to lung isolation [12–14]. Resuming two-lung ventilation from one-lung induces oxidative stress; this attributed to superoxide release. Huang and colleagues looked to see if there was any difference between inhalational anesthesia with isoflurane and propofol infusion. They measured reactive oxygen species and total antioxidant status before one-lung ventilation, before resuming two-lung ventilation, and at intervals of 5 and 20 min after resuming two-lung ventilation. They revealed that propofol infusion, compared with isoflurane, attenuates reactive oxygen species production and limits it for 20 min after resuming two-lung ventilation [15]. In another investigators looked to see the effects of sevoflurane inhalation anesthesia only versus propofol total intravenous anesthesia on perioperative cytokine balance in lung cancer patients. Venous blood samples were obtained before one-lung ventilation, before the conclusion of one-lung ventilation, after closed chest surgery, and after 24 h; they measured the serum concentrations of IL-6, IL-8, and IL-10 by ELISA. It was shown that propofol causes less inflammatory mediator release and can also modulate the balance of cytokines. In the authors' opinion, they advocate that propofol is a better anesthetic for lung cancer than sevoflurane [16]. Wakabayashi and colleagues study the effects of anesthesia with sevoflurane and propofol on the cytokine/chemokine production at the airway epithelium during esophagectomy; the levels of inflammatory cytokines and chemokine in the epithelial lining were obtained from the ventilated dependent lung and collapsed non-dependent lung by bronchoscopic microsampling method, and these were measured before and after one-lung ventilation. The results of the study suggest that propofol anesthesia more potently suppresses the surgical stress-induced inflammatory perturbation at the local milieu of the airway during esophagectomy compared with sevoflurane anesthesia [17]. Wigmore and colleagues looked at overall long-term survival for patients undergoing volatile versus IV anesthesia for all cancer surgical procedures. In this retrospective analysis, the authors compared mortality after cancer surgery in more than 7000 patients given volatile general anesthesia or total IV anesthesia. This retrospective analysis demonstrates an association between the type of anesthetic delivered and survival; mortality was approximately 50% greater with volatile than IV anesthesia, with an adjusted hazard ratio of 1.46 (1.29–1.66) [18]. Alternatively, one study comparing pulmonary morbidity using sevoflurane or propofol-remifentanil anesthesia in an Ivor Lewis operation showed different results in regard to IL-6 levels. In this study sevoflurane anesthesia attenuated an increase in blood IL-6 at the end of surgery but did not provide any advantages over propofol-remifentanil in terms of postoperative pulmonary complications [19]. These studies are promising in that they show not only a significant reduction in measured inflammatory response but also an improvement in clinical outcome. Further studies are warranted.

Although neither TIVA nor inhaled anesthetic agents provide a clear *physiologic* advantage over the other for thoracic surgery, there is solid rationale for the use of TIVA in certain circumstances (Table 12.1):

- When the delivery of inhaled anesthetics is impossible or disadvantageous, due to the nature of the operation
- In scenarios where traditional anesthetic delivery systems may be unavailable or impractical

Table 12.1 Situations in which TIVA may be indicated

Special surgical conditions
Tracheal/carinal surgery
Lung volume reduction surgery
Lung transplantation
Endobronchial procedures
Thymectomy
Non-ideal environments
Off-site locations requiring anesthesia
Austere environments (military, developing countries)

TIVA in Special Thoracic Surgical Conditions

Procedures or trauma that disrupts the trachea and carina complicate the delivery of inhaled anesthesia. When the proximal airways are breached, volatile agents may escape, and the quantity of anesthesia reaching the patient is uncertain. Also, the operating room is at risk of pollution from the escaped anesthetics, posing a hazard to personnel. This situation is most likely during cross-field ventilation, a technique in which the distal airways (main bronchi) are directly intubated in the surgical field to facilitate ventilation and oxygenation. Intubation and extubation are often repeated, and airway seals are frequently compromised. Also, certain cases may require high-frequency jet ventilation or other specialized modes of ventilation incompatible with the delivery of inhalational anesthetics [20].

Patients undergoing lung volume reduction surgery (LVRS) also benefit from a TIVA approach. Because these patients suffer from chronic obstructive pulmonary disease (COPD) and have increased dead space, end-tidal volatile anesthetic concentration is inaccurate and anesthetic levels questionable [21]. Also, air trapping is common, and the elimination of volatile anesthetic may be hindered, delaying awakening and extubation.

In the case of lung transplantation, volatile anesthetics have several drawbacks. During lung transplantation, the right ventricle is subject to increased afterload and potential failure, and the cardiodepressant effects of volatile anesthetics could be detrimental. In addition, significant intrapulmonary shunt and dead space in the transplanted lung interfere with the accuracy of end-tidal anesthetic measurements. Consequently, narcotic-based anesthetic regimens are usually administered for lung transplantation surgery. However, this is not always an ideal solution, because narcotic levels may decline unpredictably during the procedure. This decline has several possible causes: (1) narcotics may be sequestered in the CPB circuit in cases using cardiopulmonary bypass (CPB); (2) narcotics tend to accumulate in lung tissue during first pass, and a considerable amount of drug might be removed when the diseased, native lung is resected; and (3) when the donor lung is transplanted, first-pass uptake is repeated, and systemic narcotic levels may again drop [22]. When narcotic levels drop, more volatile anesthetics and/or narcotics must be given—but with older anesthetics, overaccumulation and delayed awakening may occur. Newer, rapidly metabolized intravenous anesthetics, on the other hand, are able to rapidly counter changes in anesthetic depth without significant risk of overaccumulation. Furthermore, in pulmonary transplant surgery requiring CPB (i.e., double-lung or heart-lung transplant), TIVA allows an uninterrupted transition to the CPB phase and back to native circulation.

Endobronchial procedures that use flexible or rigid bronchoscopy (e.g., stent placement, dilatation, biopsy, and laser procedures) also benefit from a TIVA approach. These procedures are frequently complicated by periods of apnea, the need for special ventilatory techniques such as high-frequency jet ventilation, and compromised airway seals. Thus, the delivery of volatile anesthetics may be problematical. Furthermore, these procedures frequently involve repeated alternating periods of high and low stimulation, and intravenous anesthetics can be more rapidly titrated to meet fluctuating demands. Lastly, accurate measurements of volatile anesthetics by standard mass spectrometry are hindered in procedures where helium/oxygen will be used [23].

Lastly, patients with myasthenia gravis undergoing thymectomy may benefit from a TIVA approach. Myasthenia gravis (MG) is associated with autoimmune damage to the acetylcholine (ACH) receptors; therefore, patients exhibit baseline muscle weakness. The thymus gland is implicated in the autoimmune response against the ACH receptors; in a select population of those with MG, symptoms improve post-thymectomy. MG patients are exquisitely sensitive to neuromuscular blocking agents and volatile anesthetics, which may cause prolonged paralysis or residual muscle weakness [24]. The ideal anesthetic for such patients would avoid neuromuscular blocking agents and volatile anesthetics. Successful thymectomies have been performed without neuromuscular blocking agents using TIVA +/− high thoracic epidurals. Conditions for intubation and surgery were excellent [25, 26].

Scenarios that Benefit from TIVA

TIVA is the anesthetic administration system of choice in scenarios where the logistics of having fully functional anesthesia machines may be impractical or impossible. For example, off-site anesthesia has recently become more commonplace. Many minimally invasive thoracic procedures are being carried out in nonoperating room "procedure suites." In these circumstances, TIVA is more versatile because (1) its administration does not require a full anesthesia machine setup, and (2) it can provide different levels of anesthesia (from MAC/sedation to general).

TIVA also offers several advantages in austere environments such as battlefields, disaster zones, and developing nations. For example, volatile anesthetics are considered hazardous materials—they are difficult to store and transport, and they generate waste gases that must be properly scavenged. In addition volatile anesthetics are known emitters of greenhouse gases. Sherman and colleagues looked at the greenhouse gas emissions of anesthetic drugs and their environmental impact, and the entire life cycle of five anesthetic drugs were examined: sevoflurane, desflurane, isoflurane, nitrous oxide, and propofol. Data from their study reveals and reiterates previous data regarding the greenhouse gases emitted by volatile anesthetics. From the results techniques that can substitute volatile anesthetics, such as total intravenous anesthesia and neuraxial or peripheral nerve blocks, would be the least harmful to the environment [27]. In contrast, TIVA agents are more easily stored, transported, and disposed. A second advantage is the reduced logistical footprint—basic TIVA equipment (infusion pump and ventilator) eliminates the traditional anesthesia machine. Additionally, TIVA equipment is more robust than traditional anesthesia machines and is more likely to perform reliably in less-than-ideal conditions. Although specialized anesthesia machines developed for military applications are available, they are more costly and complex than a simple ventilator and infusion pump setup. In fact, in its most basic form, TIVA can be administered with only a syringe and ambu-bag, which is even simpler than a basic draw-over (volatile) system. Hospitals in developed countries are routinely set up for inhalational anesthetics; thus, TIVA is usually more costly, due to the price of the agents. In developing nations, however, the cost of hardware and its maintenance usually outweighs the cost of drug, making TIVA a more economical option.

Intravenous Anesthetic Agents

Several intravenous anesthetic agents may be used in combination to execute an effective TIVA regimen. Propofol, the model drug for TIVA, and useful adjuncts for TIVA—dexmedetomidine, remifentanil, ketamine, and lidocaine—are reviewed below.

Propofol

Propofol remains the mainstay drug for TIVA. In addition to its favorable pharmacodynamics and pharmacokinetic profile, propofol offers distinct benefits over inhaled anesthetics. In studies comparing propofol with inhaled anesthetics in thoracic procedures, propofol reduced the postoperative decline of lung function after lung resection [28] and inhibited the catecholamine surge and adrenocorticotropic hormone (ACTH) response during lung lobectomy [29]. Studies of propofol in non-thoracic operations have also shown advantages that may apply to thoracic procedures; propofol reduced coughing during emergence from anesthesia [30] and the depression in bronchial mucus transport velocity associated with general anesthesia [31]. In addition, the stress hormone response [32] and the expression of pro-inflammatory cytokines in alveolar macrophages [33] were lower in patients receiving propofol than in those receiving inhaled anesthetics. When looking at the effects of propofol versus isoflurane on liver function after open thoracotomy, both have a comparable minor effect on liver function after an elective thoracotomy [34]. Given that thoracotomy is one of the most painful surgical incisions, another study focused on the incidence of post-thoracotomy pain, comparing total intravenous anesthesia and inhalational anesthesia. A prospective randomized trial looked at two groups' propofol and remifentanil versus sevoflurane anesthesia. The incidence of chronic post-thoracotomy pain syndrome was compared at 3- and 6-month intervals. Results demonstrated total intravenous anesthesia may reduce the incidence of chronic post-thoracotomy pain syndrome at 3 and 6 months [35].

Dexmedetomidine

Dexmedetomidine is an alpha-2 agonist sedative-analgesic that inhibits endogenous norepinephrine release. Dexmedetomidine is eight times more selective for the alpha-2 receptor than clonidine, with an alpha-2/alpha-1 receptor ratio of 1600:1 [36]. Evidence suggests that its main effector sites are the locus coeruleus for sedative action and the spinal cord for analgesic action. Interestingly, sedation with dexmedetomidine has been observed to mimic natural sleep in that hypercapnic arousal phenomenon upon exposure to a CO_2 challenge is preserved [37]. In addition to its direct sedative-analgesic properties, dexmedetomidine also reduces opioid requirements [38–45] and minimum alveolar concentration levels for inhalational anesthetics [46–48].

In thoracic surgery, dexmedetomidine may offer several physiologic benefits. It reduces perioperative oxygen consumption [49] and the sympathetic response to surgical stimulus [38, 50, 51], which may confer cardioprotective benefits. In studies of thoracic surgery patients, the use of dexmedetomidine as an adjunct to epidural analgesia reduced the need for epidural fentanyl [45] and resulted in postoperative diuresis and favorable indices of glomerular filtration, suggesting enhanced renal function [52]. In patients with pulmonary hypertension undergoing mitral valve replacement, dexmedetomidine lessened the rise in systemic and pulmonary vascular resistance post-sternotomy and decreased mean arterial, mean pulmonary artery, and pulmonary capillary wedge pressures [53]. Lastly, patients recovering from thoracic surgery may benefit from the reduced occurrence of respiratory depression [54–56], improved pain control [57–59], and postoperative shivering [60, 61] associated with dexmedetomidine. Of note the use of intraoperative dexmedetomidine is not associated with a reduction in acute kidney injury after lung cancer surgery [62]. Dexmedetomidine is clearly an important adjuvant for total intravenous anesthesia for the thoracotomy patient.

Remifentanil

Remifentanil is an ultrashort-acting fentanyl derivative that is particularly suited to thoracic procedures. Remifentanil's rapid onset time (1 min) and short duration of action (3–10 min) [63] are ideal for managing the fluctuating periods of high and low surgical stimulations that characterize most thoracic procedures. Because thoracic epidural anesthesia is the main modality for pain relief in most thoracic surgeries, there is little need for long-acting IV narcotics that may prolong extubation and cause postoperative respiratory depression. Some situations, however (e.g., multiple surgical sites), require supplemental longer-acting narcotics for adequate postoperative analgesia. In these cases, remifentanil may be co-administered with longer-acting narcotics to provide intraoperative analgesia for periods of high surgical stimuli without risk of overaccumulation of the accompanying narcotics.

Ketamine

Ketamine is an N-methyl-o-aspartate receptor antagonist that induces a "dissociative state" in which sensory input (sight, hearing, touch) normally perceived by the patient is blocked from reaching consciousness. Because of its profound analgesic, sedative, and amnestic properties, it is occasionally used as an adjunct to propofol in TIVA regimens. Ketamine is particularly valuable for thoracic surgery because it (1) has bronchodilating properties; (2) does not depress respiration; (3) may reduce pain for up to 3 months postoperatively when used in conjunction with TEA for thoracotomy [64]; (4) reduces narcotic requirement; and (5) exerts sympathomimetic effects, which may be beneficial in thoracic trauma and in situations where perfusion pressure must be maintained in the presence of volume restriction. In thoracotomies preemptive administration of ketamine may be an effective adjuvant; a study by Fiorelli and colleagues showed patients in a ketamine group compared to a placebo to have better satisfaction of pain relief, significant reduction in inflammatory response, and decreased morphine consumption [65]. There is still ongoing research needed in relation to post-thoracotomy pain syndrome. Moyse and colleagues reviewed evidence for the efficacy of intravenous and epidural administration of ketamine in acute post-thoracotomy pain management and its effectiveness. They concluded that the majority of randomized controlled trials presently show no role for ketamine in attenuating or preventing post-thoracotomy pain syndrome although there is clear benefit for acute post-thoracotomy pain [66]. There is potential for ketamine to have benefits in reducing chronic postoperative pain, but the optimum treatment duration and dose for different operations have yet to be identified [67].

Lidocaine

Intravenous lidocaine has also been described as an adjuvant in total intravenous anesthetics. It has been described as having analgesic, antihyperalgesic, and anti-inflammatory properties. The mechanism of action and mechanism of analgesia of intravenous lidocaine reveal its potential advantages in a total intravenous anesthetic technique. Intravenous lidocaine infusion in the perioperative period is safe and has clear advantages, such as decreased intraoperative anesthetic requirements, lower pain scores, reduced postoperative analgesic requirements, as well as faster return of bowel function and decreased length of hospital stay [68–75]. The final analgesic action of intravenous lidocaine is a reflection of its multifactorial action. It has been suggested that its central sensitization is secondary to a peripheral antihyperalgesic action on somatic pain and central on neuropathic pain, which result in the blockade of central hyperexcitability. The intravenous dose should not exceed the toxic plasma concentration of 5 microg mL (−1); doses smaller than 5 mg kg (−1), administered slowly (30 min), under monitoring, are considered safe [76]. Its use in thoracic surgery still requires more studies to find its true benefit in this specific population, but the evidence for its use as an adjuvant and part of a total intravenous anesthetic is compelling.

Infusion Systems

Delivery of TIVA is more complicated than that of volatile anesthetics via the lung. While concentrations of volatile anesthetics may be approximated intraoperatively by MAC, the "MAC equivalent" for IV agents, Cp50—the plasma concentration that will prevent a response to a given stimulus in 50% of patients—has not been fully developed for the wide range of IV anesthetics and specific clinical conditions in which they are used.

Traditionally, TIVA has been administered through calculator pumps that deliver a preset dose per unit of time. Dosages are based on recommended minimum infusion rates determined by the drug's manufacturer and titrated to clinical effect through measurement of hemodynamics and subjective patient assessment. However, intravenous agents have a narrow therapeutic window that may be difficult to target and maintain [77]. Additionally, calculator pumps are not capable of adjusting infusion rates in response to the dynamic real-time changes in pharmacodynamics and pharmacokinetics, which can lead to under- or overdosage of the anesthetic. Therefore, computer-controlled IV drug delivery systems, or target-controlled infusion (TCI) systems, have been developed to address the shortcomings of traditional calculator pumps and mimic the convenience, advantages, and familiarity of vaporizers [78].

TCI systems (Fig. 12.1) administer intravenous anesthesia based on real-time pharmacokinetic models, derived from population studies specific for each intravenous agent. These studies consider multiple factors—demographics, altered physiology, or comorbidities—that may influence drug pharmacokinetics. Appropriate administration is accomplished by incorporating a computer program coded with pharmacokinetic models of the selected agent to drive its rate of delivery—a more sensitive and accurate method of controlling concentrations than the constant rate of infusions provided by calculator pumps to achieve steady state. In other words, the practitioner focuses on target concentration, not infusion rate. The computer adjusts infusion rate constantly based on pharmacokinetic simulation of the current serum concentration of anesthetic agent in a particular patient. TCI systems reduce the subjective estimation of TIVA delivery, may deliver more consistent levels of anesthesia, and can automatically tailor the dose of anesthetic to specific phases of the surgery.

While pharmacokinetic models serve as the computational basis for TCI drug delivery, the regimen is based on the method of bolus-elimination-transfer (BET) [79, 80]. The system delivers a bolus (B) to achieve target concentration, compensates for elimination (E) by continuous infusion, and corrects for transfer (T) to peripheral tissues with an exponentially decreasing infusion. The software allows the fine-tuning of anesthetic delivery to target the steep slope of the concentration-effect curve, in which small changes in anesthetic concentration have a relatively large effect. This tuning is accomplished through three approaches: pharmacodynamics, pharmacokinetic, and pharmaceutical [81].

The pharmacodynamic approach examines the response of the body to the anesthetic agent and adjusts delivery as needed to achieve the desired effect. This approach is usually linked with some sort of monitoring device. In contrast, the pharmacokinetic approach focuses on achieving absolute target concentrations, based on known therapeutic windows appropriate for specific anesthetic applications. Drug effect in this approach is not considered. Lastly, the pharmaceutical approach is tied to the short action (favorable pharmacokinetics) of the newer anesthetic agents. Because these agents are short-acting, it is easier to maintain a patient in the steep slope of the concentration-effect curve. If the patient is over-anesthetized, a rapid titration down of anesthetic agent results in a quick correction; if under-anesthetized, a rapid titration up is better controlled, and the patient is unlikely to experience the adverse effects of "overshooting" for a prolonged period.

Because TCI systems work by *estimating* drug concentration in the bloodstream, concerns arise over the accuracy of this estimation and overall performance of TCI. Evaluation of TCI performance depends on four parameters [82]:

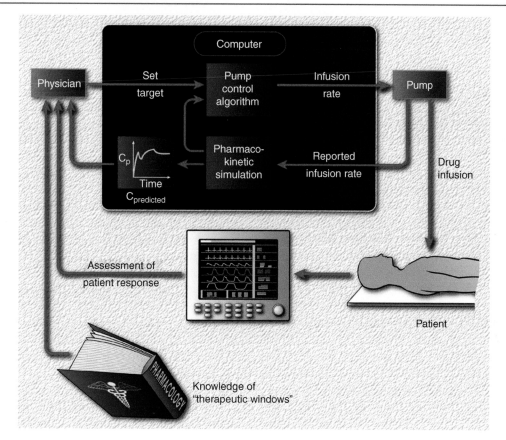

Fig. 12.1 Delivery of intravenous anesthetic agents via target controlled infusion (TCI) The practitioner sets a target for anesthetic concentration based on three pieces of information: knowledge of therapeutic windows for a particular drug, assessment of patient response, and predicted current concentration in the bloodstream (Cpredicted). The TCI computer calculates an infusion rate based on the input target concentration and pharmacokinetic models for the drug. The pump delivers the anesthetic at the calculated rate and reports this rate back to the computer, which uses pharmacokinetic simulation to update Cpredicted. (Adapted from [78], used with permission; adapted from Ron V Purugganan, in the journal *Current Opinion in Anaesthesiology*, published by Wolters Kluwer Health/Lippincott Williams & Wilkins, 2008, Vol. 21, pp 1–7 Reprinted with permission)

- Median absolute performance error (MDAPE): a measure of the accuracy of the TCI system—the median value for how close each estimate is to actual concentration
- Median prediction error (MDPE): a measure of the direction of error of the estimates—whether the system tends to over-administer or under-administer
- Divergence: fluctuation in the difference between estimated and actual concentrations (accuracy) over time
- Wobble: failure to maintain a stable plasma concentration over time.

Typical MDAPE for TCI systems ranges from about 15–30%, while typical MDPE ranges from 3% to 20% (reviewed in [78]). MDPE has been called "clinically acceptable" in the 10–20% range [83].

Research and development for TCI currently focuses on several areas. Among the greatest of these is the fact that TCI targets plasma (not effect-site) concentration. To address this discrepancy, research is focused on further modifying and refining the pharmacokinetic models to take into account effect-site concentration instead of plasma concentration and achieving effect-site control via closed loop systems (e.g., anesthetic depth monitoring) [77, 84]. In the pain management of post-thoracotomy patients, newly developed pharmacokinetic models for TCI patient-controlled analgesia may be an alternative to the standard method of postoperative pain management—thoracic epidural—when it is contraindicated or not feasible [85]. In fact, the greater control offered by TCI may be advantageous in these patients, who are more susceptible to the adverse effects of inadequate or excessive narcotic dosing. Another area of investigation is the use of simulation of drug delivery to compare context-sensitive half-times (CSHTs)—that is, the time required to reduce by half the drug concentration after terminating an infusion at steady state [86].

Although TCI systems are widely available throughout the world, in at least 96 countries, they have yet to be introduced commercially in the United States, the use only for propofol and opioids if using research software in IRB-approved research studies. Because TCI systems inherently fuse drug and device, the US Food and Drug Administration is uncertain whether to regulate TCI as a drug or a device and has stalled TCI system approval; this regulatory roadblock has, unfortunately, hindered commercial interest in furthering TCI technology for the US market [78, 87, 88].

Anesthetic Depth Monitors

Anesthetic depth monitors analyze and process a patient's spontaneous electroencephalogram (EEG) and/or mid-latency auditory evoked potentials (MLAEP) to gauge hypnotic depth [89]. To date, however, studies have failed to show that anesthetic depth monitors are consistently capable of either detecting intraoperative awareness or distinguishing between consciousness states [90], although anecdotal reports are encouraging. This may be of concern to anesthesia providers who consider TIVA more difficult to administer and worry that the risk of intraoperative awareness may be increased. Many of these providers are less familiar with TIVA administration than volatile anesthetic administration; for instance, they may be less familiar with the concept of Cp50 than with the analogous minimum alveolar concentration for volatile anesthetics. And even with advanced delivery systems such as TCI, direct control of effect-site concentrations is currently not available.

However, an increased risk of intraoperative recall in TIVA has never been documented using the Brice interview [91] (the primary diagnostic structured interview for the assessment of intraoperative recall). Furthermore, the anesthetic depth monitor is more properly used as part of a larger overall clinical assessment scheme. Certainly, in combination with other clinical signs of inadequate hypnosis (themselves nonspecific), anesthetic depth monitors may help in the titration of intravenous anesthesia. This may be particularly important for unstable patients susceptible to the cardiovascular depressant effects associated with moderate to high doses of anesthetic agents [92]. In fact, in a study of non-cardiac surgery patients, mortality was correlated with cumulative deep hypnotic time as measured by bispectral index (BIS) <45 [93].

Methodology

At the University of Texas MD Anderson Cancer Center, our TIVA technique for special thoracic procedures is a balanced technique, which allows for reduced dosages of medications and opioid sparing/reduction. Our regimen consists of midazolam for amnesia, propofol and dexmedetomidine for hypnosis, and ketamine and lidocaine as adjuvants if clinically applicable, and TEA or posterior intercostal block by the surgeon for analgesia, and muscle relaxants for immobiliza-

tion. Anesthetic depth monitors are used routinely. Our protocol is detailed below; drug dosages are typical (and may be adjusted according to patient variability). Currently, we practice using principles of enhanced recovery after thoracic surgery, which can be found more in depth in the corresponding chapter dedicated to this modality of care.

Premedication and Thoracic Epidural Placement

In the holding area, supplemental oxygen and IV midazolam (0.5–2 mg) are administered. Immediately prior to transport to the operating room by the anesthesia team, a dexmedetomidine infusion (0.2–0.4 mcg/kg/h) is begun. A small bolus of dexmedetomidine (0.1–0.2 mcg/kg) is administered rather than the manufacturer's recommended bolus-loading dose (1 mcg/kg) to minimize the adverse effects associated with dexmedetomidine loading—hypo-/hypertension, bradycardia, and atrial fibrillation [94]. During transport, pulse oximetry and constant communication are used to monitor the patient.

In the operating room, additional monitors (BP cuff and ECG) are applied, and the patient is positioned for thoracic epidural placement. Upon completion of the epidural placement, anesthetic depth monitoring is initiated, and a smooth transition to induction is accomplished by adding a propofol infusion (20–50 mcg/kg/min) and gradually increasing the infusions of dexmedetomidine (to 0.5–0.7 mcg/kg/h). If no epidural is placed, another technique utilized is the posterior intercostal block by the surgery team using liposomal bupivacaine [95].

Induction

Infusions are continued through induction. Hemodynamics, anesthetic depth monitoring, and subjective assessment guide the induction dosing of propofol (10–30 mg) and muscle relaxant to achieve adequate conditions for intubation.

Once the airway is secured, preoperative fiber-optic bronchoscopy is performed to assess airway anatomy. This potentially stimulating time for the patient may be remedied with small boluses of propofol (20–40 mg). In addition, laryngotracheal anesthesia (2% lidocaine) administered prior to bronchoscopy may lessen this response.

Invasive monitors and additional IV access may be placed pre- or post-induction as needed. A dedicated infusion line(s) ensures proper titration of IV anesthetics and prevents incompatibility issues that may arise between different medications.

Upon completion of the initial bronchoscopy, lung isolation devices are placed (if necessary), and the patient is positioned and prepped for surgery. Epidural narcotics if applicable are administered prior to skin incision, and dexmedetomidine, propofol, and remifentanil/narcotic infusions are adjusted to reflect changes in anesthetic depth monitoring and/or hemodynamics.

Maintenance

Anesthesia is maintained with propofol and dexmedetomidine titrated according to anesthetic depth monitoring and hemodynamics; as stated above ketamine and lidocaine infusions are used as adjuvants if indicated. Muscle relaxants are used if spontaneous ventilation is not required; they are administered by infusion to keep a train-of-four ratio of 0.4–0.5. If necessary, IV antihypertensive (rather than more anesthesia) may be used in situations where sympathetic stimulation is high, yet a sufficient amount of anesthesia is being administered, and anesthetic depth monitoring shows an adequate depth of hypnosis. Administration of local anesthesia via the epidural if in place is usually withheld or administered in dilute concentrations to avoid sympathectomy in patients where strict volume restriction will be followed.

Emergence

In preparation for emergence, a bolus of local anesthesia followed by a constant infusion is administered via the thoracic epidural. At the start of skin closure, propofol is discontinued, and muscle relaxant reversal is administered. The patient is maintained on dexmedetomidine (0.1–0.2 mcg/kg/h) until extubation in order to impart the cardioprotective benefits of alpha-2 agonism: stable hemodynamics and rapid awakening/extubation.

Clinical Case Discussion: TIVA for Thoracic Procedures (Fig. 12.2)

Case A 52-year-old male smoker diagnosed with advanced pulmonary squamous cell carcinoma (stage IV) presents with progressive shortness of breath and orthopnea. Bronchoscopy reveals a distal tracheal mass causing moderate to severe airway obstruction. He is scheduled for rigid bronchoscopy with stent placement to lessen tracheal obstruction. This procedure will be performed in the pulmonary procedure suite.

Questions

1. What are the disadvantages of using volatile anesthetics in this operation?

    For discussion, see section "TIVA in special thoracic surgical conditions" and "Scenarios that benefit from TIVA."

2. What are the advantages of using (1) propofol, (2) dexmedetomidine, (3) remifentinil in this patient?

    For discussion, see section "Intravenous anesthetic agents."

3. What is the basic concept of target controlled infusion, and how is it advantageous over manually controlled infusion?

    For discussion, see section "Infusion systems."

Fig. 12.2 Left: rigid bronchoscopy view of an intratracheal mass obstructing the airway. Right: trachea after stent placement

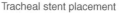

Tracheal stent placement

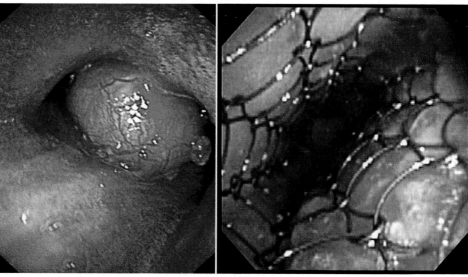

pain control: a meta-analysis of randomized controlled trials. Can J Anaesth. 2011;58(1):22–37.

74. Wu CT, Borel CO, Lee MS, Yu JC, Liou HS, Yi HD, et al. The interaction effect of perioperative cotreatment with dextromethorphan and intravenous lidocaine on pain relief and recovery of bowel function after laparoscopic cholecystectomy. Anesth Analg. 2005;100(2):448–53.

75. Bakan M, Umutoglu T, Topuz U, Uysal H, Bayram M, Kadioglu H, et al. Opioid-free total intravenous anesthesia with propofol, dexmedetomidine and lidocaine infusions for laparoscopic cholecystectomy: a prospective, randomized, double-blinded study. Braz J Anesthesiol. 2015;65(3):191–9.

76. Lauretti GR. Mechanisms of analgesia of intravenous lidocaine. Rev Bras Anestesiol. 2008;58(3):280–6.

77. Viviand X, Leone M. Induction and maintenance of intravenous anaesthesia using target-controlled infusion systems. Best Pract Res Clin Anaesthesiol. 2001;15(1):19–33.

78. Egan TD. Target-controlled drug delivery: progress toward an intravenous "vaporizer" and automated anesthetic administration. Anesthesiology. 2003;99(5):1214–9.

79. Kruger-Thiemer E. Continuous intravenous infusion and multicompartment accumulation. Eur J Pharmacol. 1968;4(3):317–24.

80. Schwilden H. A general method for calculating the dosage scheme in linear pharmacokinetics. Eur J Clin Pharmacol. 1981;20(5):379–86.

81. Egan TD. Advances in the clinical pharmacology of intravenous anesthetics: pharmacokinetic, pharmacodynamic, pharmaceutical, and technological considerations. ASA Refresher Courses Anesthesiol. 2004;32(1):71–83.

82. Varvel JR, Donoho DL, Shafer SL. Measuring the predictive performance of computer-controlled infusion pumps. J Pharmacokinet Biopharm. 1992;20(1):63–94.

83. Glass PJ, Jacobs JR, Reeves JG. Intravenous drug delivery. In: Milder RD, editor. Anesthesia. 3rd ed. New York: Churchill Livingstone; 1990. p. 367–88.

84. Van Poucke GE, Bravo LJ, Shafer SL. Target controlled infusions: targeting the effect site while limiting peak plasma concentration. IEEE Trans Biomed Eng. 2004;51(11):1869–75.

85. Van den Nieuwenhuyzen MC, Engbers FH, Burm AG, Vletter AA, Van Kleef JW, Bovill JG. Target-controlled infusion of alfentanil for postoperative analgesia: a feasibility study and pharmacodynamic evaluation in the early postoperative period. Br J Anaesth. 1997;78(1):17–23.

86. Hughes MA, Glass PS, Jacobs JR. Context-sensitive half-time in multicompartment pharmacokinetic models for intravenous anesthetic drugs. Anesthesiology. 1992;76(3):334–41.

87. Dryden PE. Target-controlled infusions: paths to approval. Anesth Analg. 2016;122(1):86–9.

88. Absalom AR, Glen JI, Zwart GJ, Schnider TW, Struys MM. Target-controlled infusion: a mature technology. Anesth Analg. 2016;122(1):70–8.

89. Bruhn J, Myles PS, Sneyd R, Struys MM. Depth of anaesthesia monitoring: what's available, what's validated and what's next? Br J Anaesth. 2006;97(1):85–94.

90. Schneider G, Gelb AW, Schmeller B, Tschakert R, Kochs E. Detection of awareness in surgical patients with EEG-based indices--bispectral index and patient state index. Br J Anaesth. 2003;91(3):329–35.

91. Nordstrom O, Engstrom AM, Persson S, Sandin R. Incidence of awareness in total i.v. anaesthesia based on propofol, alfentanil and neuromuscular blockade. Acta Anaesthesiol Scand. 1997;41(8):978–84.

92. Leonard IE, Myles PS. Target-controlled intravenous anaesthesia with bispectral index monitoring for thoracotomy in a patient with severely impaired left ventricular function. Anaesth Intensive Care. 2000;28(3):318–21.

93. Monk TG, Saini V, Weldon BC, Sigl JC. Anesthetic management and one-year mortality after noncardiac surgery. Anesth Analg. 2005;100(1):4–10.

94. Ickeringill M, Shehabi Y, Adamson H, Ruettimann U. Dexmedetomidine infusion without loading dose in surgical patients requiring mechanical ventilation: haemodynamic effects and efficacy. Anaesth Intensive Care. 2004;32(6):741–5.

95. Rice DC, Cata JP, Mena GE, Rodriguez-Restrepo A, Correa AM, Mehran RJ. Posterior intercostal nerve block with liposomal bupivacaine: an alternative to thoracic epidural analgesia. Ann Thorac Surg. 2015;99(6):1953–60.

Tracheal Resection and Reconstruction

Karen McRae

Key Points
- The tracheal imaging (CT scan and/or MRI) must be examined by the anesthesiologist to plan the anesthetic management.
- Patients with tracheal stenosis may not become symptomatic until the tracheal diameter is narrowed to <50% of normal.
- Initial surgical management for tracheal stenosis will commonly involve rigid bronchoscopy and dilation.
- The two major methods of distal airway management for resection of tracheal stenosis are cross-field ventilation with an endotracheal tube or jet ventilation with a tracheal catheter.
- Maintenance of anesthesia during the period of tracheal resection is commonly managed with intravenous anesthesia techniques.

Historical Note

Surgery of the conducting airway requires diagnostic and therapeutic manipulation of the respiratory tree despite ongoing ventilation. From the very beginning of tracheal surgery, the greatest challenge facing the anesthesiologist has been how to ventilate the patient adequately before and during airway resection. Close collaboration between anesthesia and surgical colleagues was required. Early reports of tracheal tumor resection by Belsey [1] described reconstruction of the mid-trachea after the intratracheal tube was advanced by the surgeon beyond the tracheal defect. A wire coil was constructed over the cuff of the intratracheal tube, a free graft of fascia covered the wire skeleton, and the intratracheal tube was withdrawn. In 1957 Barclay [2] reported the resection of the carina for a low tracheal tumor with deliberate endobronchial intubation of the left side by the surgeon across the surgical field. The right main stem bronchus was sutured to the remaining trachea, while the left lung was ventilated. Ventilation was then resumed via the orotracheal tube, and the left bronchial was sutured to the right bronchus intermedius during intermittent periods of apnea. In 1963 Grillo and Bendixen [3] described the performance of a similar procedure under critical circumstances, in a patient whose tracheal obstruction had progressed to severe dyspnea and pulmonary hyperinflation. During cross-field ventilation of the left lung, the right pulmonary artery was lightly clamped so that the unventilated lung was not perfused (Fig. 13.1). Elimination of shunt maintained "the best possible tissue oxygenation" permitting an unhurried reconstruction. "The operative requirement for complete anesthetic control during all phases of tracheal surgery is met by the technic of transitory physiologic pneumonectomy." The same group in 1969 reported the anesthetic management of 31 patients who underwent tracheal resection and reconstruction [4]. The problems of anesthetic induction and control of the airway were fully described in a paper first presented at the International Anesthesia Research Society in March 1969. The upper and lower airway management strategies used during a pivotal period of the development of tracheal resection and reconstruction at the Massachusetts General Hospital were elegantly presented. The discussion of the paper at the meeting reveals the increasing appreciation of the etiology of postintubation stenoses and the clinical dilemmas these injuries presented.

Prolonged incision and complex reconstruction of the airway in patients with compromised pulmonary function have demanded further innovation on the part of anesthesiologists and surgeons. A spectrum of ventilation strategies has been used, not only to maintaining ventilation but to optimize

K. McRae (✉)
Department of Anesthesia and Pain Management,
The Toronto General Hospital, University Health Network,
Toronto, ON, Canada
e-mail: karen.mcrae@uhn.ca

© Springer Nature Switzerland AG 2019
P. Slinger (ed.), *Principles and Practice of Anesthesia for Thoracic Surgery*, https://doi.org/10.1007/978-3-030-00859-8_13

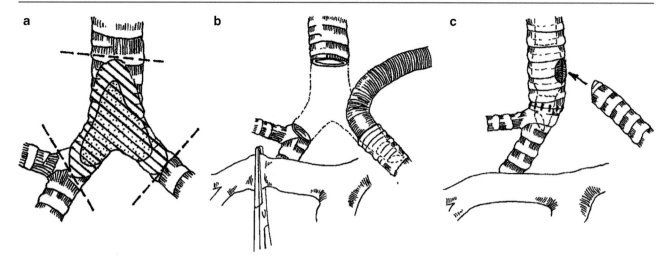

Fig. 13.1 Cross-field ventilation for carinal resection. (**a**) The tumor is at the carina; the patient is intubated with an orotracheal tube (not shown). (**b**) A sterile endobronchial tube is placed across the surgical field after the left main stem bronchus is incised. (**c**) After anastomosis of the right main stem bronchus to the remaining trachea, the cross-field endobronchial tube is removed; the orotracheal tube is advanced into a right endobronchial position, during anastomosis of the left main stem bronchus to the trachea. Early descriptions of this technique included snaring of the right pulmonary artery during (**b**) to minimize shunt during one-lung ventilation (as shown here); this was later deemed unnecessary in most cases. (Adapted from Ref. [3])

operating conditions. Evidence of the success of this evolving collaboration lies in the large series of successful procedures reported.

Etiology of Tracheal Lesions

The trachea, carina, and major bronchi may be affected by a variety of conditions that are amenable to surgical resection and reconstruction. Airway lesions can be a result of benign or malignant etiologies (Table 13.1) and may or may not result in significant stenosis. Congenital stenosis is typically resected during infancy, after presentation in the first few months of life. In adults many cases of subglottic stenosis are idiopathic; frequently patients have increasing respiratory symptoms for many years, often incorrectly attributed to asthma. Post-intubation injury is the most common cause of benign tracheal stenosis despite the widespread use of high-volume, low-pressure cuffs. Posterior glottic stenosis and circumferential subglottic stenosis are the result of direct trauma from the tube and the cuff, respectively. This results in mucosal ulceration; subsequently the exposed tracheal cartilage is devitalized and disappears, followed by replacement of the tracheal wall with scar tissue [5]. Mucosal injury leading to ulceration has been observed after as little as 2–3 h of intubation with a high-volume low-pressure cuff in a subgroup of patients who received standard anesthesia care [6]. After extubation most lesions heal as a fibrous scar; however some lesions develop malacic components. Post-intubation strictures typically show concentric narrowing, whereas post-tracheotomy stomal strictures tend to result in more side-to-side rather than

Table 13.1 Etiology of tracheal lesions amenable to resection and reconstruction

Benign lesions
Congenital
Tracheal atresia
Congenital stenosis
Congenital chondromalacia
Vascular rings
Idiopathic
Post-intubation or post-tracheotomy injury
Posterior glottic stenosis
Subglottic stenosis (including cuff injuries)
Tracheoinnominate artery fistula (anterior trachea)
Tracheoesophageal fistula (posterior trachea)
Stomal stenosis (from tracheotomy)
Trauma
Inflammatory
Wegener's granulomatosis
Postinfection (after treatment)
Tuberculosis
Syphilis
Diphtheria
Typhoid
Malignant lesions
Primary malignancies
Squamous cell carcinoma
Adenoid cystic carcinoma (cylindroma)
Mucoepidermoid carcinoma
Carcinoid adenoma
Sarcoma
Mesenchymal tumors
Secondary malignancies
Bronchogenic carcinoma
Thyroid carcinoma
Laryngeal carcinoma
Esophageal carcinoma

anteroposterior narrowing. Penetrating or blunt trauma may cause life-threatening tracheal disruption or, if less severe and unrecognized, may present later as stenosis [7]. A variety of inflammatory diseases can cause airway stenosis; however due to widespread involvement of the airway, few are considered suitable for surgical resection. Most inflammatory lesions are therefore treated with chronic tracheostomy, intermittent dilation, or stenting. A notable exception is Wegener's granulomatosis, which can produce focal stenosis amenable to resection. Postinfectious stenotic lesions may be resected after treatment of the underlying infection. Tracheal resection is performed for primary malignancies unless metastases preclude curative surgery; secondary neoplasms invading the trachea typically arise from the adjacent structures and are less often amenable to surgical resection. When curative resection is not possible, many patients are treated with palliative endoscopic debridement. Similarly, endoluminal metastases which are the result of hematogenous spread from distant malignancies (including breast, colon and renal cell carcinomas, and melanoma) are typically debrided or stented.

Planning Tracheal Surgery

Planning is essential in these challenging and varied procedures and should be clearly outlined in the preoperative interdisciplinary checklist (Table 13.2). A number of elements are required, starting with a clear understanding of the patient's tracheal anatomy and the resection proposed. A detailed plan for ventilation throughout induction, during the period of open airway and on emergence, must be clear to the anesthesia and surgical teams. Appropriate airway equipment should be assembled and tested to ensure that it is in good working order including rigid bronchoscopes of a variety of diameters and a way of ventilation through a bronchoscope. A supraglottic airway device usually a laryngeal mask airway (LMA) should be available, as well as endotracheal tubes in a range of sizes to be placed orotracheally or into the distal airway by the surgeon. If cross-field intubation is anticipated, sterile endotracheal tubes and a sterile breathing circuit are needed.

Fundamental questions in planning a case include whether there is airway stenosis, where it lies within the airway, and how small is the residual airway. Glottic and subglottic lesions almost always require dilation by the surgeon at the beginning of the procedure usually with rigid bronchoscopes of increased diameter, although some centers use smooth round dilators. An endotracheal tube may be then be placed, although often of a smaller size than would usually be used. If the lesion is in the mid-trachea or lower, and the lumen is adequate, an endotracheal tube may be placed above the lesion, without prior dilatation. The anesthetic technique has influenced the chosen mode of ventilation. Anesthetic agents with rapid onset and short duration permit a deep plane of general anesthesia with prompt recovery and resumption of spontaneous ventilation necessary to successful extubation of patients with compromised airway anatomy. A crucial decision is when it is appropriate to suppress the patient's spontaneous breathing and conversion to controlled techniques. In some centers it is preferred to secure the airway each time with an inhalational induction, maintenance of spontaneous ventilation, and avoidance of muscle relaxants until the initial airway is established. Most airway resections are performed in centers with experienced surgical and anesthesia teams. In many circumstances it is suitable to induce general anesthesia with intravenous agents and give muscle relaxant prior to rigid bronchoscopy, dilation, or laser resection of the airway in preparation for definitive resection. This is particularly true of patients who have had a recent, uneventful rigid bronchoscopy as part of their preoperative care.

Many experienced clinical groups recommend a staged approach which starts with cautious fiberoptic bronchoscopy, after airway topicalization in the awake, spontaneously breathing patient. This permits evaluation of vocal cord function and for any malacic segments. This is often followed by rigid bronchoscopy under general anesthesia to dilate stenosis or debride obstructing tumor from the airway. The rigid bronchoscope is also the best tool to measure the position and length of the lesion in the trachea. The following measurements are made relative to the patient's upper incisors: the carina, the distal and proximal ends of the lesion, and the vocal cords. This permits an estimate of both the length of the lesion and the remaining trachea available for reconstruction. The airway can be temporarily improved in the vast majority of patients allowing patient optimization for the definitive resection, to ensure that any bronchospasm and pulmonary infections are reversed, and weaning of steroids if needed.

Excellent analgesia is required to optimize the chances of prompt extubation and is planned according to the incision required by the resection. Postoperative positive pressure ventilation is undesirable as pressure on new anastomoses increase the risk of airway dehiscence.

Table 13.2 Planning for tracheal surgery

Tracheal anatomy, resection proposed
Incision required and patient position
Preoperative assessment
Patient monitoring
Ventilation
Transition from spontaneous to controlled ventilation
Apparatus required for ventilation
Mode of ventilation
Anesthetic drug regimen
Analgesia
Emergence, airway configuration at the end of the case

Tracheal Anatomy and Surgical Management

The position of the lesion within the trachea will determine the site of incision and the extent of trachea requiring resection. This is often described by the number of tracheal rings removed. Using cadaver studies, Grillo investigated how much of the trachea could be removed with end-to-end reconstruction without causing undue tension or compromise of the blood supply. He determined that a median length of 4.5 cm was achievable, equivalent to seven rings [8]. The blood supply to the upper trachea is predominantly from the inferior thyroid artery, whereas the lower trachea and carina are supplied by the bronchial arteries [9]. The blood supply enters the walls of the trachea laterally in a segmental fashion; therefore the trachea is best mobilized with anterior and posterior dissection to prevent devascularization.

Knowledge of the location of the tracheal lesion and the proposed extent of airway resection are essential for planning the induction of anesthesia and the maintenance of oxygenation and ventilation. Additionally, the position of the lesion will determine the incision required and the patient position.

The Subglottis and Upper Trachea

Resection of the subglottis and upper third of the trachea may be accomplished via a collar (cervical) incision with the neck fully extended and a bolster placed behind the scapulae. The subglottic airway extends from just below the vocal cords to the lower border of the cricoid cartilage. Post-intubation stenosis is the most common cause of subglottic stenosis. Complete transection of the subglottic airway will divide the recurrent laryngeal nerves; resection is therefore modified to preserve the posterior shell of the cricoid cartilage in order to protect the entry point of these nerves [10]. Most post-intubation strictures involve relatively short segments, between 1 and 4 cm, and can be managed by segmental resection and reconstruction with a primary anastomosis. Malignancies may require more extensive resection including concomitant laryngectomy.

Prolonged trans-laryngeal intubation frequently results in synchronous laryngotracheal injury. The most common glottic injury is a posterior inter-arytenoid stenosis, which restricts vocal cord movement. These combined injuries require simultaneous high tracheal resection and laryngofissure, with excision of the inter-arytenoid scar. When the subglottic anastomosis lies within a few millimeters of the vocal cords, there is significant risk of glottic edema. A Montgomery T-tube (Fig. 13.2) is placed to support the airway and left in place several months to minimize restenosis. The T-tube is a cylindrical silicone stent with a perpendicular limb which is positioned in a small tracheostomy which makes it unlikely to become dislodged or migrate [11]. Following laryngotracheoplasty the upper limb of the silicone stent lies 0.5–1.0 cm above the cords. In cases of stenotic or malacic segments of the cervical trachea without laryngeal injury, a T-tube may be left in place with the upper limb of the T-tube that is positioned below the cords, allowing for voice preservation.

Head flexion during primary anastomosis delivers the cervical trachea into the mediastinum to facilitate re-approximation of the edges of the trachea, and if the anastomosis appears to be at risk of being under tension, a guardian stitch is placed after skin closure, between the skin of the chin and the anterior chest and maintained for approximately a week (Fig. 13.2).

Mid-Trachea

A cervico-mediastinal incision is used for tumors of the mid-trachea (Fig. 13.3) and most benign lesions throughout the trachea. The upper trachea is explored through a cervical incision, which is extended via a partial sternotomy to just below the sternal angle, and separated with a pediatric chest spreader. Through this incision the anterior carina and the right and left tracheobronchial angles can be exposed without sacrifice of the innominate vein, artery, or other great vessels. The trachea is then mobilized and incised and distal ventilation is secured. Many surgeons will request for the patient's neck to temporarily be flexed to test the ease with which the tracheal ends will come together. The length of trachea that can be safely incised is influenced by the patient's age, body habitus, pathology, and prior treatment. If it is clear that the anastomosis will be under excessive tension, or a long segment of trachea requires resection, a release maneuver is performed, most often a suprahyoid release. Muscle attachments to superior surface of the hyoid bone and the hyoid bone itself are divided allowing the larynx to drop, adding between 1 and 2 cm of additional mobility to the trachea [12].

The resection of long segments of trachea which cannot be repaired with a primary anastomosis presents a formidable problem and underscores the fact that the trachea is not simply a tube but is an armored structure capable of sustaining cyclical intrathoracic pressures. Historically, prosthetic grafts fail in the long term due to the formation of granulation tissue and fistulas, and while devascularized aortic grafts have been used, they tend to develop malacic components. More promising reconstructive techniques include fasciocutaneous forearm flaps stiffened with C-shaped segments of rib cartilage [13]. Reports of decellularized tracheal allograft repopulated with the recipient's own chondrocytes and airway epithelial cells were recently used to replace the trachea in a small number of patients, by a single lead surgeon [14].

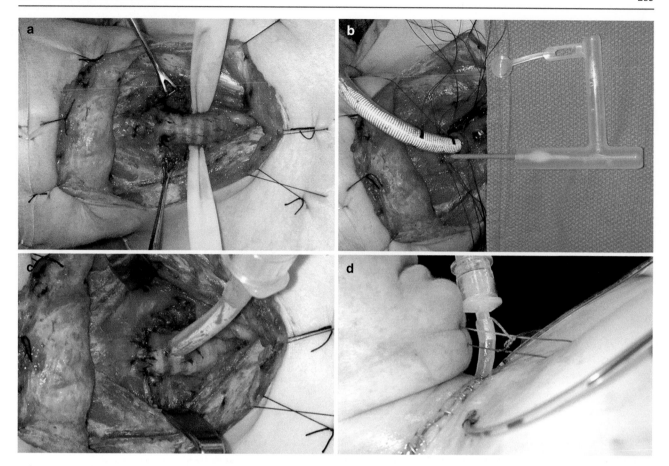

Fig. 13.2 Airway management for high tracheal resection. (**a**) Mobilization of the trachea, the patient's head is to the left of the photograph. (**b**) A sterile cross-field endotracheal tube has been placed in the distal trachea. A Montgomery T-tube will be placed; the balloon of a Fogarty catheter will be inflated to obstruct the proximal limb, to allow ventilation via the distal limb. The Fogarty catheter is passed retrograde through the patient's mouth. (**c**) Ventilation via the Montgomery T-tube external limb during closure of the incision. A standard endotracheal tube connector has been inserted into the external limb of the T-tube. (**d**) Head flexion and the guardian ("chin") stitch. The Fogarty catheter is deflated and removed when spontaneous ventilation is reestablished. The guardian stitch is removed after a week. (Photos courtesy of Dr. Andrew Pierre, Division of Thoracic Surgery, Department of Surgery, Toronto General Hospital)

This clinical experience that has been recently heavily criticized for incomplete reporting of poor long-term outcomes must be considered experimental at this time.

Carinal Resection

The incision depends on the type of carinal resection. Carinal resection without pulmonary parenchymal resection is approached through a full sternotomy. The pericardium is opened anteriorly, and the exposure is facilitated by mobilization of the aorta and both main pulmonary arteries (Fig. 13.4). Tracheal resection is usually limited to less than 4 cm at the carinal level. When there is anastomotic tension, a hilar release is performed with a U-shaped incision of the pericardium, which allows hilar structures to advance by about 2 cm. Laryngeal release is not deemed helpful for carinal resection and a chin stitch is not routinely used. Resection of the carina may be combined with a right or left pneumo-

nectomy or right upper lobe bronchial sleeve resection. Left carinal pneumonectomy may be performed via a sternotomy, a left posterolateral thoracotomy, or clamshell incisions. When all or part of the right lung requires resection, a right posterolateral approach is used. Careful patient selection and optimization are essential to the success of these technically demanding and high-risk surgeries [15].

Patient Characteristics

Idiopathic tracheal stenosis is a diagnosis almost exclusively in females often presenting for resection in their fifth decade of life; many have had progressive symptoms for up to 10 years. At least one third report clinically significant reflux, and at least as many are obese which may be due to their exercise limitation. Patients with post-intubation and post-tracheotomy stenoses have a mean age in their 40s at the time of presentation and not infrequently have diabetes

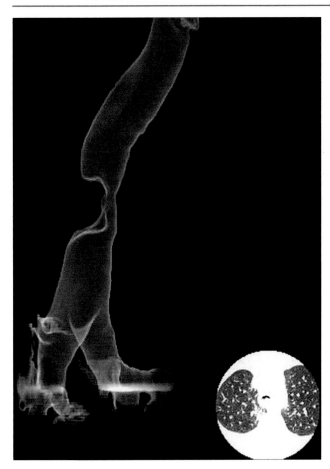

Fig. 13.3 A three-dimensional CT reconstruction of a mid-tracheal tumor. This patient was managed with rigid bronchoscopy and debridement prior to tracheal resection

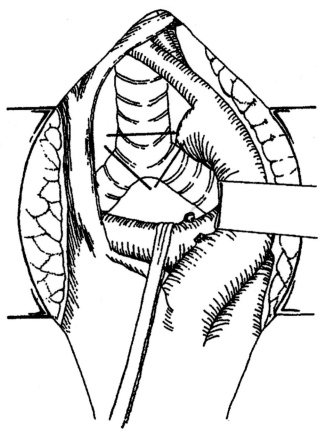

Fig. 13.4 Exposure of the carina via a sternotomy

mellitus, cardiovascular disease, asthma, or chronic obstructive pulmonary disease, all conditions that may have required prior intubation. These comorbidities increase the likelihood of perioperative complications. Patients with tracheal tumors tend to be a decade older, tend less to be diabetic or obese, and are more likely to smoke, with the associated risk of vascular disease. It must be noted that some primary tracheal tumors are not associated with smoking and can present at any age [16].

Most patients are symptomatic, the most common being dyspnea on exertion, but a careful history may reveal orthopnea, a brassy cough, difficulty clearing secretions, and wheezing. Malignant tumors may produce hemoptysis. Patients should be examined for evidence of airway obstruction and the use of accessory muscles or stridor. In adults narrowing of the lumen to less than 50% of its normal cross section results in dyspnea with significant exertion, and narrowing to less than 25% of its normal cross section will usually produce dyspnea and stridor at rest. Stridor is a sign of significant airway obstruction; likely the tracheal diameter is 6 mm or less [17]. These patients are at risk of acute airway

obstruction with a mucus plug. Stridor is classically more pronounced in inspiration when stenosis is extra-thoracic; if the lesion is intrathoracic, the stridor may be predominant in expiration, particularly if there is significant malacia. In addition to auscultation of the lungs and trachea, patient's neck mobility should be evaluated.

Preoperative Assessment

The anesthesiologist should review all available information delineating the patient's airway pathology. The chest X-ray may be deceptively normal. A CT scan of the neck and thorax will have typically been performed, with thin cuts along the entire airway. Increasingly three-dimensional images are being constructed from helical CT data. This imaging is helpful in defining the relationship of the lesion to the vocal cords and carina and, as a complement to prior endoscopy, helps in planning airway management.

Pulmonary function tests, including spirometry and flow-volume loops, are usually performed unless the patient is at risk of imminent airway obstruction. Fixed airway stenoses cause limitation of both inspiratory and expiratory flow at similar flowrates. A variable extra-thoracic airway obstruction limits inspiration much more than exhalation. Conversely, with a variable intrathoracic lesion, the patient is able to inhale reasonably well, but expiratory flow limitation is produced. It should be noted that the quality of flow-volume loops is very much dependent on patient effort. The characteristic findings of expiratory flow limitation may be obscured by small airways disease such as asthma or COPD [18]. The absence of classic spirometric patterns does not predict the absence of pathology, and the presence of findings does not reliably indicate the degree of obstruction. Imaging of the airway is far more useful in planning surgery.

Manipulation of airway and mediastinal structures intraoperatively may provoke a significant sympathoadrenal stress response [19]. Increases in heart rate and both systemic and pulmonary artery pressures are seen and may be prolonged. Myocardial oxygen consumption rises and dysrhythmias may occur. The incidence of myocardial ischemia in older smokers during and after rigid bronchoscopy alone may be as high as 10–15% of patients [20]. Preoperative ECG should be obtained in all patients to assess cardiac rhythm. Patients over 40 with symptoms or significant risk factors for coronary artery disease should be investigated with echocardiography, Persantine-thallium stress testing, and coronary angiography if indicated. Risk stratification is then possible, with appropriate institution of treatment. Cardiac assessment is recommended when carinal resection is required especially when combined with pneumonectomy. If significant coronary artery lesions are identified, the decision to proceed with definitive surgery rather than palliation should be decided on a case-by-case basis. Quantitative ventilation and perfusion scans may be warranted when the resection of considerable lung parenchymal is anticipated [21]. In all patients considered for tracheal resection, the identification and treatment of reversible pulmonary disease are important. Repeated airway dilation or stenting may permit a period of medical optimization of the patient [22]. Smoking cessation is vital, particularly as patients who have undergone airway resection often struggle to mobilize secretions. Postoperative mechanical ventilation is undesirable: the presence of an endotracheal tube may predispose new suture lines to necrosis and dehiscence. Severe respiratory compromise due to parenchymal lung disease or neuromuscular disorder is a serious concern and may preclude tracheal resection [23].

Patient Monitoring

In addition to secure peripheral intravenous access and standard anesthetic monitors, an arterial catheter is placed for continuous blood pressure measurement. When an intrathoracic approach to the trachea is used, many anesthesiologists choose the left side for the radial arterial line; the innominate artery lies anterior to the trachea, and compression or division of this vessel will render inaccurate arterial measurement in the right arm. Arterial cannulation also provides immediate access to blood gas analysis essential during interrupted ventilation, during ventilation with techniques that preclude capnography, and in the event of postoperative respiratory distress. Central venous cannulation may be used if indicated by the proposed surgery (i.e., including a major pulmonary resection) and cardiopulmonary status of the patient. Avoidance of the area of incision must be considered in catheter placement; jugular, subclavian, or antecubital approach may be used. A urinary catheter is placed, even if a simple resection is accomplished quickly; the patient's mobility is often reduced for several days due to postoperative neck flexion. The patient's temperature is monitored and normothermia should be maintained. In the rare instance of cervical exenteration, where elective division of the innominate artery is contemplated, placement of EEG monitoring has been recommended [7].

Ventilation Strategies

Surgical intervention in the airway presents unique ventilation difficulties. Clinicians have devised creative solutions for these challenges, and there has been a proliferation of ventilation techniques applied to the open airway (Table 13.3). Overarching consideration includes adequate gas exchange while minimizing airway occupancy, movement and the spraying of blood, and secretions.

Distal Tracheal Intubation, Intermittent Positive Pressure Ventilation (IPPV)

Early reports of tracheal tumor resection described reconstruction of the trachea after an intratracheal tube was advanced by the surgeon beyond the tracheal defect [1]. Advancement of a full-sized orotracheal tube across the surgical field into the distal trachea or bronchus is an option currently seldom used, as the large diameter obstructs access to the surgical field. Endobronchial tubes are long tubes of reduced diameter, with a small volume and shorter cuff positioned close to the tip. They are favored by some clinicians for certain tracheal resections. They can be positioned in the trachea beyond the lesion under bronchoscopic guidance past a mid-tracheal lesion or placed in the contralateral bronchus when a thoracotomy is required for carinal resection or carinal pneumonectomy. The endobronchial tube's slender profile allows much of the surgery to be accomplished while the tube remains within the tracheal lumen, and distal ventilation is maintained. Alternatively, these tubes can be withdrawn when the airway is opened and distal ventilation

Table 13.3 Characteristics of modes of ventilation during airway surgery

	Able to ventilate open airway	Immobility of operative field	Specialized equipment required	Airway pressure – pressure/monitoring	Potential for barotrauma	Gas entrainment	Airway gas composition
IPPV	No	No	No	Pressure is dependent on ventilator settings/reliable	Minor	No	Stable, accurate monitoring
LFJV	Yes	No	No	Intermittently high/difficult	Yes, high	Yes	Variable, difficult to monitor
HFJV	Yes	Yes	Yes	Can be high, gas trapping common/difficult, especially around jet nozzle	Yes	Yes	Variable, difficult to monitor
HFPPV	Yes	Yes	Yes	Low peak and mean transpulmonary pressure/difficult	Yes	Minor	Stable, accurate monitoring

IPPV intermediate positive pressure ventilation, *LFJV* low-frequency jet ventilation, *HFJV* high-frequency jet ventilation, *HFPPV* high-frequency positive pressure ventilation

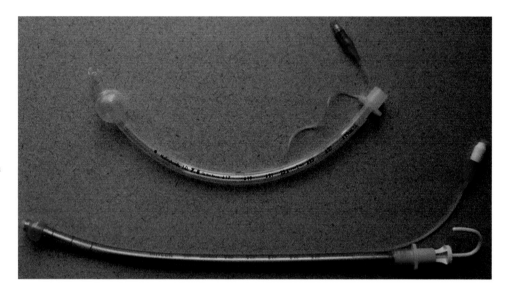

Fig. 13.5 A 7.5 mm ID Phycon endobronchial tube (lower tube) (Fuji Systems, Tokyo, Japan) as compared to a 7.5 mm ID standard endotracheal tube (above). The standard tube is 32 cm long; the armored endobronchial tube is 40 cm and is also available in 5.5 and 6.5 mm ID sizes. Note the small endobronchial cuff size, the lack of both bevel and Murphy eye on the distal end of the endobronchial tube

provided on the surgical field. Drawbacks of these tubes include the frequent air leak that occurs when an endobronchial tube is positioned in the trachea, as the balloon has a relatively small volume.

The cuffs are prone to being ruptured when the trachea is being repaired around its circumference, requiring replacement [24]. A variety of endobronchial cuffs have been described although many are no longer available [25]. In our institution, the Phycon endobronchial tube (Fuji Systems, Tokyo, Japan) is used (Fig. 13.5). The ideal endotracheal tube for tracheal reconstruction has been described as a long, flexible, reinforced tube with a short, low-pressure, high-volume cuff and a short segment beyond the cuff, to allow the ventilation of both lungs through a short tracheal stump without encroachment on the operative site; unfortunately no such endotracheal tube is currently manufactured [26].

The use of cross-field intubation and ventilation of the distal airway was first described for the resection of a low tracheal tumor; the left bronchus was cannulated on the field by the surgeon, while the right main stem bronchus was sutured to the remaining trachea. Ventilation was then resumed via the endotracheal tube and left bronchial anastomosis was performed [2]. Geffin fully described the variations of cross-field ventilation to be used for high and low tracheal lesions [4]. An orotracheal tube is placed, above the lesion. As the airway is divided, the surgeon advances a second, sterile endotracheal tube across the field into the distal trachea (Fig. 13.6). In our institution, when subglottic resection is performed, a sterile reinforced endotracheal tube is inserted in the distal trachea, and the proximal end of the tube is passed by the patient's cheek, under the sterile drapes to be connected to the anesthetic circuit. Resection of the mid- or lower trachea necessitates the use of a second, sterile anesthetic circuit originating from the surgical field, passed over the drapes. Typically, a relatively small endotracheal tube is placed in the distal airway to permit the placement of posterior sutures, while the tube remains in the distal airway, held anterior by the surgeons. After reanastomosis of the posterior trachea, the distal tube is withdrawn; the orotracheal tube is readvanced and is used

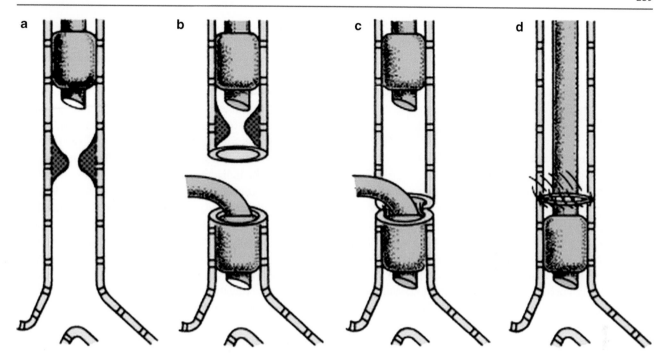

Fig. 13.6 Airway management for resection of a high tracheal lesion. (**a**) Orotracheal intubation above the lesion. (**b**) With tracheal incision, a sterile cross-field endotracheal tube is placed distal to the lesion. (**c**) The posterior wall of the anastomosis is sutured. (**d**) The cross-field endotracheal tube is removed, the orotracheal tube is advanced across the anastomosis, and the anterior anastomosis is completed. (With permission from the Society for Thoracic Surgeons, previously published in [84])

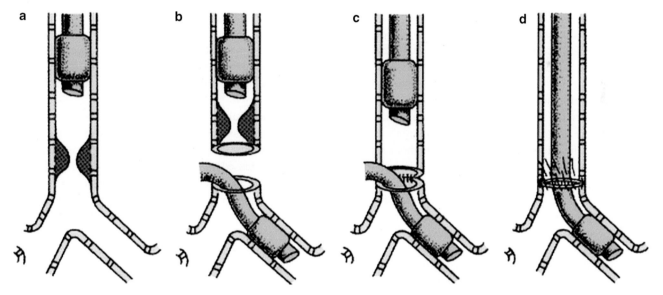

Fig. 13.7 Airway management for resection of a low tracheal lesion. (**a**) Orotracheal intubation above the lesion. (**b**) A sterile cross-field endotracheal tube is placed in the left main stem bronchus. (**c**) The posterior wall of the anastomosis is sutured. (**d**) The cross-field endotracheal tube is removed, the orotracheal tube is advanced across the anastomosis into an endobronchial position, and the anterior anastomosis is completed. (With permission of the Society for Thoracic Surgeons, previously published in [84])

for ventilation. Lower tracheal and carinal resection requires some modification of the technique (Fig. 13.7). The distal tube is advanced into the left main stem bronchus below the lesion. The resected trachea and the right main stem bronchus are anastomosed, the orotracheal tube is advanced through the suture line, and one-lung ventila-

tion to the right side is accomplished, while the left main stem bronchus is anastomosed to the side of the trachea. The orotracheal tube is withdrawn above both suture lines until extubation. This technique necessitates intermittent periods of apnea as surgeons withdraw the distal tracheal tube for better exposure and placement of sutures. Increased oxygen concentration is used when ventilating (>70%) in order to delay desaturation. Periods of moderate hypercapnia are inevitable but are usually well tolerated. Independent distal cannulation of both bronchi has been described; a variety of endotracheal tubes of different sizes should be available for distal cannulation [27].

Low-Frequency Jet Ventilation (LFJV)

Jet ventilation releases high gas flow through a small orifice, permitting ventilation via laryngoscopes, bronchoscopes, and the open airway with minimal obstruction of the surgical field. Low-frequency jet ventilation (LFJV) is accomplished by the release of gas under high-pressure (50–60 psi) through an orifice (~1 mm) as described by Sanders [28]. A pressure regulator is required to maintain constant flow, and a handheld on-off valve is released intermittently; jet pulses are delivered at a rate of 10–20/min. A distinct advantage of this approach is its simplicity and lack of specialized equipment. The use of lengthy catheters of small caliber, advanced through the orotracheal tube, permits ventilation of distal airways. Physiologic tidal volumes are generated and chest or lung movement is clearly visible.

LFJV with intermittent apnea was first described in tracheal resection in the 1970s [29, 30], and a variation of this technique is still favored by some groups [31]. The use of a narrow lengthy catheter permits ventilation of the distal airway using a device well away from the surgical field; their diameter is unlikely to obstruct surgical access to the airway. The ultimate catheter position varies with the procedure performed. A high tracheal stenosis may not admit a regular size endotracheal tube; jet ventilation via a long small orotracheal tube has been used throughout resection [32]. More often an orotracheal tube is placed above the tracheal lesion, and the narrow ventilation catheter is advanced into the distal airway after incision of the trachea. The use of independent, simultaneous catheter ventilation of each bronchus has been described in carinal resection [33]. Unpredictable tidal volumes are generated using LFJV; they are however sufficiently large to cause disruption of the surgical field, and intermittent apnea is usually required. When high driving pressure (50–60 psi) is used through a narrow catheter, a high flow jet is produced (up to 100 l/min) entraining air, blood, and debris from the field into the distal airway. Blood may spray from the surgical field. When larger ventilation catheters are used, high flows can be maintained with lower driving pressure; air entrainment is reduced, permitting less dilution of the oxygen jet as demonstrated by the high arterial oxygen tensions that can be achieved; longer periods of apnea are therefore possible [30].

High-Frequency Jet Ventilation

High-frequency jet ventilation (HFJV) resembles its low-frequency counterpart in that gas is delivered from a high-pressure gas source via a stiff, small-bore catheter positioned in the airway. Rather than a handheld switch, the jet stream is cut by a high-frequency pneumatic or electronically controlled flow interrupter. As the high-velocity gas jet enters the airway, additional gas is entrained at the jet nozzle, contributing to the delivered tidal volumes which remain small compared to conventional ventilation considerably less than airways dead space [34]. Variables that can be regulated during HFJV include driving pressure, frequency, and inspiratory time, usually set at 20–30% of the cycle. Ventilation rates span 100–400 breaths/min; tidal volumes delivered are 2–5 ml/kg. The mechanical effects of the use of high frequencies are crucial to the understanding of gas transfer in high-frequency ventilation. Increasing the respiratory rate decreases the emptying time of the lung, moderate gas trapping occurs, and the lung is held in a distended state. Peripheral airway pressures have been shown to be continuously positive using all high-frequency techniques with low mean and peak pressures maintained [34–37]. An obvious advantage when ventilating the open airway is that lower peak pressures are generated as compared to conventional ventilation optimizing lung recruitment with much less air leak. The use of low tidal volumes at high respiratory rates produces minimal movement of the operative field, and interruption of ventilation is not required during many procedures. The slender catheters used minimally obstruct the surgical field.

HFJV has been studied in experimental tracheal airway disruption; the gas driving pressure and size of the jet nozzle were shown to be crucial. When a constant driving pressure was used, increased nozzle size was required to maintain gas exchange with increasing air leak; however a larger nozzle used with a smaller air leak resulted in lung overdistension and systemic hypotension [38]. Clinically, increased driving pressure and inspiratory time can result in impedance in expiratory gas flow, gas trapping, development of auto-PEEP, and impaired CO_2 elimination [39].

When HFJV is used in the intensive care unit, the ventilating catheter is advanced through an orotracheal tube; however the optimum position of the catheter tip is the subject of considerable debate [40]. During airway surgery, the ventilating catheter is advanced across a stenosis or surgically created defect; catheter position is therefore dictated by the nature of the procedure. The use of HFJV via a catheter placed through an LMA has been described for the resection of a high tracheal stenosis either with [41] or without addition cross-field IPPV [32]. Catheters may be advanced through an orotracheal tube into the mid- or distal trachea for

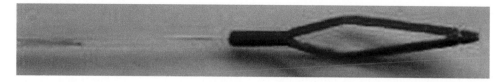

Fig. 13.8 The basket tip of the Hunsaker MonJet ventilation catheter. The collapsible basket is designed to center the catheter in the airway and to reduce catheter-whip injuries to the walls of the airway during jet ventilation. The catheter had a second lumen for monitoring distal airway pressure and presence of CO_2

resection of tracheal segments [42, 43], into the distal bronchus for carinal or sleeve resection [42], and bilateral bronchial catheters have been reported in carinal resection in a patient with limited respiratory reserve, when desaturation occurred during HFJV of one lung [44]. These reports emphasize that ventilator frequency and driving pressure must be adjusted to the patient's respiratory compliance and the proportion of lung segments being ventilated at the time.

"Whip motion" of the distal catheter tip possibly causing tracheal laceration and pneumothorax is a concern with all jet catheter ventilation techniques. The Hunsaker jet ventilation catheter (MonJet, Medtronic Xomed, Jacksonville FL) has a distal, collapsible basket-like support to maintain the jet port tip in the center of the airway and reduce whip injuries. It has been used extensively for endoscopic laryngeal surgery and has been used in some centers for airway resection [32] (see Fig. 13.8). A recent review describes commercially available high-frequency ventilators and catheters [45].

High-Frequency Positive Pressure Ventilation (HFPPV)

High-frequency positive pressure ventilation (HFPPV) of small tidal volumes (3–5 ml/kg breaths at 60 breaths/min) may be delivered using a conventional ventilator of low internal volume and negligible internal compliance; known volumes and gas mixtures are delivered. External PEEP may be added and there is little hemodynamic derangement described. HFPPV is applied via an insufflation catheter placed at the tip of an endotracheal tube. An injection catheter with multiple side holes is recommended to both increase turbulence, thereby reducing airway injury from the jet of gas, and to minimize gas entrainment [36]. Eriksson [46] first described tracheal resection using HFPPV with gas delivery via a rigid bronchoscope during examination of the lesion and via a 5 mm diameter insufflation catheter threaded into the distal trachea during resection and anastomosis. El-Baz [47] described the use of HFPPV during complex tracheal reconstruction using a 2 mm insufflation catheter via a Montgomery T-tube. The same type of catheter inserted down the endotracheal tube and across the resected airway for HFPPV during sleeve resection and carinal resection was further reported

[48, 49]. Excellent surgical conditions with minimal motion of the field and uninterrupted access to the circumference of the anastomosis were described; continuous outflow of gas through the open bronchus was felt to minimize soiling with blood. Placement of a sterile ventilation catheter in the distal airway across the surgical field has also been used to deliver HFPPV [17]. It should be noted that the use of the high-frequency oscillation ventilation, which is used in intensive care units to treat hypoxia, is not useful for airway surgery due to excessive movement of the airways produced by this modality [37].

Disadvantages of the use of high-frequency techniques include requirement for specialized ventilator equipment and technical difficulty in monitoring ventilation parameters. The variable positioning of ventilation catheters during airway surgery precludes the use of optimal sites for airway pressure monitoring. Peripheral airway pressures may be markedly different from those in the large airways due to gas trapping inherent to the use of high respiratory rates, short expiratory times, and expiratory flow limitation. Delivered breath volumes are nearly impossible to quantify with an open airway; therefore serial blood gas analysis is essential to detect hypoventilation. Provision for humidification of gases must be made for longer procedures to avoid drying of the airway mucosa and desiccation of secretions; this is a particular problem when jet techniques are used. All modes of high-frequency ventilation require that the delivery circuit have minimal compliance. Review of the HFV literature is notable for the variation in devices used in different clinical reports. Many ventilators and breathing circuits are institution specific, having been built in a hospital laboratory. A description of operating conditions is often lacking. Many devices are in fact hybrids, superimposing a high-frequency mode on conventional IPPV or displaying features of two forms of high-frequency ventilation [40]. Similarly, many catheters used for the delivery of high-frequency jet ventilation are either institution specific or intended for other purposes such as urethral catheters or airway suction catheters, for example. There is inherent risk in the use of high flow, high-pressure gas pulses in the airway, even more so when delivered at rapid rates. Catheter position and alignment within the tracheobronchial tree must be known at all times and are made more difficult by manipulation of the airway during surgery. Free egress of expired gas and adequate expiratory time must be maintained in order to avoid inadvertent hyperinflation and barotrauma. Whereas continuous positive airway pressure is expected in HFV and is beneficial in maintaining lung recruitment, the use of higher ventilation rates and higher volumes may result in occult PEEP [35]. The resulting lung hyperinflation can lead to impedance of venous return and hemodynamic compromise, particularly if the chest is closed. Barotrauma and volutrauma in the form of pneumothorax, pneumomediastinum, and subcutaneous emphysema have been reported with all forms of high-frequency ventilation and with LFJV. The use of not only distal airway pressure monitoring but automatic shutoff mechanisms to prevent further gas flow into the lungs in the event of high airway pressure is recommended [40].

While there are many reports of the adaptation of volatile agent vaporizers for use with high-frequency ventilation [46, 50], this is unnecessary as current practice offers ideal total intravenous anesthetic regimens. The use of short-acting volatile agent using the high flows required of HFV would be wasteful and difficult to scavenge.

Extraordinary Ventilation Strategies

Cardiopulmonary Bypass (CPB) and Extracorporeal Oxygenation (ECMO)

Cardiopulmonary bypass without circulatory arrest was first used for resection of a carinal tumor in 1959 followed by reports of small series in both adults and children [51]. Then as now, systemic anticoagulation required for CPB may introduce formidable problems, notably intrapulmonary hemorrhage [4]. Currently, CPB is considered only under specific circumstances: tracheoplasty of long segments in small children in whom small airway caliber precludes other options [52], combined cardiac and pulmonary procedures for malignant disease in adults [53], the repair of complex tracheobronchial injuries [54], or when tracheal occlusion is imminent from a lesion unlikely to be bypassed by tracheotomy or rigid bronchoscopy [55]. Recently, reports of tracheal reconstruction in pediatric [56] and adult patients [56, 57] using extracorporeal membrane oxygenation (ECMO) have emphasized that this form of lung assist is amenable to peripheral rather than central vascular cannulation and reduced levels of anticoagulation (see also Chap. 27). The practice of performing particularly complex tracheal reconstruction only in centers where extracorporeal support is available can be justified.

Spontaneous Ventilation

A departure from the use of neuromuscular relaxants and positive pressure ventilation are case reports of a small number of patients allowed to breathe spontaneously throughout tracheal resection [58] and tracheoesophageal fistula repair [59]. Total intravenous anesthesia was provided with endotracheal oxygen insufflation. Some aspiration of blood and debris from the surgical field was noted. The reported patients were well oxygenated and stable despite moderate respiratory acidosis; however it is unlikely that patients with significant limitation of pulmonary reserve would tolerate this approach. A pilot study in 20 patients of the feasibility performing upper tracheal resection awake using cervical epidural anesthesia and remifentanil sedation reported that surgical conditions were facilitated by the absence of any tube or catheters within the airway and the opportunity to assess vocal cord motion. The authors did not discuss what they would have done if a patient has suffered complete airway obstruction [60]. Since that time there have been single cases described of upper tracheal resection under cervical plexus block, and VATS assisted mid-tracheal and carinal resection under thoracic epidural block supplemented by vagus nerve block to suppress coughing. All patients received intravenous anesthesia (propofol, remifentanil +/− dexmedetomidine) and had an LMA placed to secure the supraglottic airway, spontaneous breathing oxygen-enriched air. Anesthetic infusions were titrated to electroencephalogram bispectral index. These cases were reported by a multidisciplinary group with an interest and expertise in non-intubated thoracic surgery; they suggest that their approach leads to accelerated recovery. They have developed exclusion criteria for patients unsuitable for the technique. Contingency plans for rescue tracheal intubation were described but not required [61, 62, 63].

Hyperbaric Oxygenation

The use of hyperbaric oxygenation has been reported to supplement differential lung ventilation by conventional and HFV modes when these methods failed in the repair of a large tracheal tear [64]. Hyperbaric conditions enhance oxygen delivery via increased oxygen dissolved in the plasma. This approach requires the performance of surgery within a hyperbaric chamber with compression of the entire surgical team and must be considered experimental.

Anesthesia Induction and Maintenance

Careful questioning of the patient will reveal position-dependent increase in airway obstruction, particularly intolerance to lying supine. Anesthetic induction may be performed in a sitting or semi-sitting position. Any difficulty encountered at previous intubation or bronchoscopy should be known to the team. All team members should be present. A clear, coordinated plan is required and ongoing communication is essential. All equipment anticipated for airway management should be ready and confirmed to be working.

When there is little or no tracheal obstruction, the induction of anesthesia, neuromuscular relaxation, and intubation is performed as per the anesthesiologist's usual practice. In the presence of significant airway obstruction or stenosis, induction is followed by rigid bronchoscopy, dilation of tracheal stenosis, or debridement of tumor prior to placement of an orotracheal tube. A variety of anesthetic strategies have been described including airway topicalization and awake intubation, inhalational induction with volatile anesthetics, and intravenous induction agents with and without the use of neuromuscular relaxants [23]. Awake intubation is of questionable value in this circumstance; in patients with high stenosis, endotracheal tube placement is not possible, and in those with lower lesions, the tube must shortly be removed for rigid bronchoscopy after the induction of general anesthesia. When an inhalation induction is chosen, currently sevoflurane is most often used. Complete preoxygenation/denitrogenation will take more than the usual time, often more than 5 min, due to restriction of tidal volumes. In the setting of airway compromise, inhalation induction with a slowly increasing concentration of a volatile anesthetic in 100% oxygen will also take increased time. Patients often require some ongoing continuous positive airway pressure via the anesthetic circuit to maintain even modest tidal volumes. When a deep plane of anesthesia is achieved, a local anesthetic (often lidocaine) is applied to the vocal cords and upper airway prior to instrumentation. While this approach attempts to maintain the ability to turn off the anesthetic and to wake up the patient if difficulties are encountered, it is not without drawbacks. The decision to attempt airway dilation without the use of relaxant may make placement of the rigid bronchoscope considerably more difficult. Coughing can result in profound desaturation. If the patient forcefully breathes against a nearly obstructed airway as a very small bronchoscope fills the remaining lumen, the patient is put at risk of negative-pressure pulmonary edema. Another option after inhalation induction is to use a rapid-acting muscle relaxant (such as succinylcholine) to facilitate the introduction of the bronchoscope. Intravenous induction of anesthesia, with the use of short- or intermediate-acting muscle relaxant to facilitate rigid bronchoscopy, is described in many reports and is particularly appropriate when prior rigid bronchoscopy has been uneventful. This is the approach most often used in the author's center. Spirometric studies before and after the induction of anesthesia in patients undergoing upper tracheal reconstruction surgery showed that intravenous induction of anesthesia with muscle relaxation, placement of a LMA, and initiation of IPPV resulted in improvement in airflow across even severe intraluminal, extra-thoracic stenosis as compared to the patients' awake spontaneous efforts [65]. However it is clear that the decision of what induction agent to use and when to give muscle relaxant and control the patient's ventilation must be made by the anesthesiologist and surgeon based on their assessment of the patient and their level of experience.

The sympathetic response to airway instrumentation may be reduced by the use of intravenous lidocaine (1–1.5 mg/kg) bolus prior to induction. The intravenous induction may be with propofol or a combination of propofol and an opioid; fentanyl or remifentanil infusion is frequently used. Another choice of induction agent is ketamine, an N-methyl-D-aspartate receptor antagonist that produces dissociative anesthesia. Ketamine depresses ventilation less than many other sedative or general anesthetic drugs. It has the additional advantage of having bronchodilator and sympathomimetic effects and may contribute to the prevention of post-incisional pain. After induction patient may be mask ventilated until the introduction of the rigid bronchoscope, or a laryngeal mask airway may be placed. When the tracheal obstruction is relieved, the trachea is intubated and positive pressure ventilation usually instituted, a dose of an intermediate-acting muscle relaxant is usually given, and provision is made for ventilation during the period of open airway.

Anesthesia may be maintained with an inhalational agent while the trachea is intact, but during cross-field ventilation, where there are frequent periods where the endotracheal tube is out of the airway and the inhaled anesthetic is not delivered to the patient. Many anesthesiologists will convert to a total intravenous technique with propofol and an opioid, often a remifentanil infusion. Similarly, intravenous anesthesia is used when high-frequency jet ventilation techniques are required. The α-2 adrenergic agonist dexmedetomidine has several desirable properties for sedation while securing a critically compromised airway including anxiolysis, analgesia, and amnesia with minimal respiratory depression [66]. It is likely the sole intravenous agent that can replace inhalational induction when a spontaneous breathing technique is chosen for airway manipulation and may prove to be particularly useful in obese patients [67]. Dexmedetomidine may facilitate controlled emergence and has been used as a prolonged infusion for patients requiring a few days of mechanical support following tracheal reconstruction [68].

Reconstruction of the Airway

When the airway is open, the surgeon is able to manipulate the endotracheal tube within the trachea. During distal cross-field ventilation, in order to easily retrieve the distal tip of the orotracheal tube, the surgeon may affix a suture to the Murphy eye which remains in the surgical field and can be used to reposition the orotracheal tube. If the orotracheal tube is damaged, specifically if the cuff is ruptured, it may be replaced if the trachea is still open. After removal of the connector of the new tube, the surgeon can insert the pilot balloon within the lumen tube and pass the tube retrograde up the trachea into the oropharynx where it is retrieved by the anesthesiologist. During airway reconstruction, the use of uncut endotracheal tubes is recommended, as positioning distal to surgical anastomoses is frequently required. When the airway is closed, conventional positive pressure ventilation through the orotracheal tube is resumed.

When a Montgomery T-tube is left in the trachea, there are several ways to maintain ventilation. An inflated Fogarty catheter can remain in the proximal limb, while positive pressure ventilation is provided by the tracheotomy limb. This can be facilitated by the use of a multiport ventilation of the type used for insertion of a bronchial blocker. The multiport adaptor is connected to the tracheal limb of the T-tube via an endotracheal tube connector (from a 5.0 or 6.0 endotracheal tube), and the Fogarty catheter is placed in the proximal limb of the Montgomery T-tube via the side port [69]. Alternately, the surgeon will fit a small (usually 6.0 mm) endotracheal tube into the proximal limb. This press fit permits positive pressure ventilation via the proximal limb with the tracheotomy limb corked. With spontaneous ventilation reestablished, the endotracheal tube is removed by steady traction while the surgeon maintains the position of the T-tube with a clamp.

In upper and mid-tracheal resections, the head is flexed as the anastomosis is created to reduce anastomotic tension. The guardian stitch is placed after skin closure, between the skin of the chin and the anterior chest (Fig. 13.2d). Patients should be warned of this positioning that their head will be flexed at the time of emergence, and all efforts should be made to maintain the flexed position during the postoperative period to avoid traction on the new repair.

Emergence After Airway Surgery

The resumption of sustained spontaneous ventilation is highly desirable. Prompt extubation is a priority after airway reconstruction to avoid positive pressure or endotracheal tube cuff trauma to the new anastomosis, which might predispose to dehiscence. Most patients breathe more comfortably in a sitting position, removing the weight of abdominal contents from the diaphragm and increasing the patient's functional lung capacity. The oropharynx is thoroughly suctioned, neuromuscular blockade is fully reversed, and the patient is extubated when awake, able to maintain patency of their upper airway and to mobilize secretions. Intravenous anesthesia by infusion for the final stages of the procedure is useful, which permits rapid emergence to a wakeful state without agitation in most cases. It is important to avoid abrupt neck extension with possible traction injury to the anastomosis. The patient should be warned in advance of the need to maintain head flexion and the presence of the guardian stitch. Alternatively, the tracheal may be extubated when

the patient is still anesthetized, breathing spontaneously, and a laryngeal mask placed. This permits fiber-optic bronchoscopy and assessment of both the anastomosis and vocal cord function. Emergence with the LMA in place provokes minimal airway irritation and coughing; the patient will often atraumatically remove the device themselves. A drawback of this approach is that the laryngeal mask is not always easily seated in the supraglottis; this technique is best reserved for patients who were easy to bag-mask ventilate.

Maintenance of normothermia is important; shivering increases oxygen consumption, which is particularly problematic if the patient's airway is compromised. Humidification of inhaled gases minimizes the inspissated airway secretions.

Re-intubation after tracheal reconstruction may be difficult. After subglottic resection the patient's neck may be positioned in extreme flexion, the airway may be edematous and bloody, and there is potential for mechanical injury to new anastomosis. If required, endotracheal tube repositioning is best accomplished under direct vision with a fiberoptic bronchoscope. When an airway stent is left in place, the trachea should not be blindly intubated from above. Telescoping of a small endotracheal tube into the stent may be possible using a bronchoscope. This technique should be applied with great care when a self-expanding metal stent has been placed for airway stenosis; the stents require several hours to completely expand. Insertion of an endotracheal tube may distort or dislodge the stent, especially if the balloon cuff becomes snagged. An LMA may be positioned above the stented airway, particularly if a short period of ventilatory assistance is required, to facilitate emergence from anesthesia. The airway with a Montgomery T-tube can be ventilated in several ways. The side arm protruding via a tracheal stoma will accommodate an endotracheal tube connector (from a 5.0 to 6.0 mm ETT), permitting connection to standard ventilation circuits. If positive pressure is required, the open upper limb must be obstructed to prevent loss of ventilating gas. The patient's mouth and nose may be manually held shut, packing may be placed in the pharynx, or a bronchial blocker or an embolectomy catheter (Fogarty #14) may be directed into to upper limb via the side arm of the stent and the balloon inflated [70]. Low-frequency jet ventilation may also be initiated via the side arm [71].

Immediate Postoperative Complications Specific to Airway Surgery

In all surgical patients, residual anesthetics, analgesics, and neuromuscular blockade may contribute to hypoventilation, atelectasis, and poor mobilization of secretions, leading to postoperative respiratory compromise. Additional pulmonary complications may be a direct result of surgery to the airway. Airway obstruction should be suspected if the patient is in respiratory distress particularly if stridor is evident. Prior to emergence the tracheobronchial tree should be examined and any residual blood in the airway should be carefully removed; despite this, bleeding may be ongoing, or old clot may be mobilized from the lung periphery. Airway caliber may be further compromised by edema. Diuresis and steroids are used empirically; however controlled studies of their use in airway surgery are entirely lacking. Dexamethasone is frequently chosen for its long duration of action; however several hours may be required after dosing (4–10 mg intravenously) for edema to subside. For many years, nebulized racemic epinephrine has been recommended for treatment of post-intubation edema. The racemic form which is an equal mixture of the dextro- and levo-isomers of epinephrine is increasingly unavailable. The more commonly available 1% levo-epinephrine is proposed to be equally effective. In our institution, 5 ml of 1:1000 epinephrine is administered by nebulizer unless limited by tachycardia. Helium and oxygen mixtures provided by non-rebreathing facemask may permit increased ventilation in patients with narrowed conducting airway and are useful as a supportive measure while definitive therapy is pursued. Breathing with airway obstruction may be viewed as breathing through an orifice, which creates turbulent flow. Under turbulent conditions, gas flow varies with inverse square root of density. The low density of helium permits a 1.5 fold increase in relative flow of the commercially available heliox (70% helium/30% oxygen) over air and oxygen mixtures [72]. The high helium fraction required to significantly reduce the work of breathing precludes a high delivered oxygen concentrations which may be undesirable if the patient has low oxygen saturation. When airway compromise is refractory to medical therapy, reintubation may be required.

Pulmonary parenchymal injury may occur. In a review of cases of pulmonary edema associated with airway obstruction after surgery, more than 20% of cases were in adults that were being treated for airway tumor [73]. Spontaneous inspiratory efforts against an obstructed upper airway result in marked negative intrapleural and transpulmonary pressures, causing edema formation, usually within minutes. Laryngospasm is a frequent precursor. Bronchoscopic findings include pink frothy secretions and punctate hemorrhagic lesions throughout tracheobronchial tree [74]. Treatment is supportive and includes re-establishment of airway patency, oxygen supplementation, and diuresis; 85% of patients require reintubation, usually of short duration [73].

Pulmonary aspiration of acidic stomach contents is a particular concern during and after airway surgery where the trachea is not consistently protected by an endotracheal tube. Aspiration may occur at the time of airway manipulation or after completion of the airway procedure. Patients with newly placed T-tubes may have difficulty closing their glot-

tis. Laryngeal dysfunction can occur after suprahyoid release but is less common than after previously used thyrohyoid release procedures [74]. Swallowing dysfunction usually improves after a few days. Recurrent laryngeal nerve paralysis is possible after tracheal surgery [16]. Chemoprophylaxis with antacids, H2 blockers, and gastric propulsants remains unproven in the prevention of the secondary lung injury of acid aspiration. Once aspiration has occured treatment is supportive: bronchoscopy for removal of particulate matter and ventilation with positive end-expiratory pressure if indicated.

Tracheal Procedures with Specific Considerations

Two clinical scenarios present the challenge of a pre-existing defect in the trachea prior to the induction of anesthesia: traumatic injury to the airway and tracheoesophageal fistula.

Airway Trauma

Iatrogenic airway injury may occur during airway instrumentation, most often the posterior membranous portion of the trachea. This may occur during intubation with a single-lumen endotracheal tube or advancement of a bougie, bronchoscope, or other inflexible devices. Injury during placement of a double-lumen tube is most frequently located in the membranous trachea near the carina. If not noted intraoperatively, most injuries become apparent immediately after extubation. While small tears may be managed conservatively, urgent repair is required when significant clinical manifestations hemoptysis, dyspnea, or pneumomediastinum or if bronchoscopic examination reveals gaping of the edges of the tear during respiratory flow. Repair of injuries in the upper trachea may be possible via an extended cervicotomy, whereas thoracotomy is required for tears that extend lower in the airway [75]. Preoperative assessment is limited by the urgency of the procedure. Pulmonary function testing with spirometry is contraindicated as positive airway pressure will increase subcutaneous emphysema. Intubation of the patient for surgery is best accomplished under bronchoscopic guidance while the patient is breathing spontaneously, either awake with upper airway topicalization or after inhalation induction, until the lesion is bypassed. When a transtracheal approach is used, the surgeon will make an anterior tracheotomy and pass a small endotracheal tube distally to be used intermittently for ventilation. The repair is performed during periods of apnea when the cross-field tube is withdrawn. Repairs via thoracotomy may be repaired with a small diameter single-lumen endobronchial tube guided under direct vision to the side contralateral to the tear.

A double-lumen tube may be used but has a larger diameter which may make placement more difficult and may impede the surgical repair.

Injury to the conducting airways may be a result of blunt or penetrating trauma; often other injuries are present. Respiratory distress and subcutaneous emphysema are the most common physical findings [76]. Approximately 6% of penetrating neck injuries involve tracheal trauma as compared to less than 1% of patients with penetrating chest injuries. Most patients with blunt trauma severe enough to cause a tracheal tear do not survive long enough to present to the hospital. But in those who do, cervical spine injury is common and must be considered in securing the airway. The disruption of the trachea is most likely to occur within 2 cm of the carina. Airway control beyond the injury is required, and intubation with the aid of fiber-optic bronchoscopy in the spontaneously ventilating awake patient is recommended both to inspect the injury and to secure ventilation. When lower airway injury is identified, endobronchial intubation of side contralateral to the injury may be desirable. Trauma cases are particularly fraught with technical difficulties, patient agitation, and competing medical concerns. If the initial plan for securing the airway fails, an alternate plan should be identified. A surgical tracheostomy is useful in injuries of the cervical trachea, but if the tear is intrathoracic, then it is of no value. Cardiopulmonary bypass via femoral cannula has been described to provide lifesaving oxygenation and ventilation in such scenarios but is certainly not available in all trauma centers and has the significant drawback of the requirement for full anticoagulation of a polytrauma patient [77]. ECMO has been described for multiday support for both conservative treatment of airway trauma and for surgical repair [78] (see also Chap. 27).

Tracheoesophageal Fistula

Congenital TE fistula is recognized in the neonatal period; adults may acquire such a lesion from trauma, neoplasia, or radiotherapy of the trachea. In cases of TE fistula, contamination of the airway with gastric contents and pre-existing pulmonary injury likely will have occurred, resulting in preoperative pneumonitis. Positive pressure ventilation is avoided prior to securing the airway as gastric insufflation may result in increased intrathoracic pressure, difficult ventilation, and impaired venous return [79]. Placement of an endotracheal tube beyond the fistula while maintaining spontaneous ventilation is recommended. A novel variation of this strategy was described in an adult who presented for resection of a large carinal tracheoesophageal fistula. To independently isolate each lung, two 5.0 mm microlaryngoscopy endotracheal tubes were place sequentially in each bronchus following inhalation induction of anesthesia using sevoflurane. Conventional IPPV was then initiated [80].

Pediatrics

Congenital tracheal stenosis in infants and children typically occur in the presence of complete tracheal rings and may involve significant lengths of the trachea. Not infrequently these lesions are associated with cardiovascular anomalies which also require repair, most often a pulmonary artery sling. Surgical reconstruction of long-segment tracheal stenoses has been described with a number of techniques including simple resection, incision and patching with pericardium, rib cartilage or tracheal autograft, and slide tracheoplasty all performed via median sternotomy [81, 82]. Slide tracheoplasty is performed by dividing the stenotic trachea at midpoint, incising the proximal and distal narrowed segments vertically on opposite anterior and posterior surfaces and sliding these together. The advantage of this approach is that only fully vascularized, cartilage-supported tissue is used which permits early extubation of many patients. There remains some debate among surgeons which procedure should be performed, whether CPB is always required when only airway reconstruction is performed and if cardiovascular repair is required if the procedures should be staged or performed as a single operation. These surgeries are performed in highly specialized centers, and early referral is recommended to avoid complications associated with lengthy preoperative periods of mechanical ventilation (see also Chap. 50).

Management of the Patient with a T-Tube

A T-tube may be placed for a finite period of time to allow an upper airway prone to malacia or scarring to heal and stabilize or in some cases becomes essentially permanent airway support. Patients with T-tubes may require airway examination, replacement, or adjustment of their T-tube or surgery unrelated to their airway. They present a significant challenge to the anesthesiologist. When a patient with a T-tube in situ required a general anesthetic, the risk of aspiration should be considered. If the procedure is elective, the upper airway can be controlled by a laryngeal mask airway either with spontaneous or controlled ventilation, in which the tracheostomy limb is capped. Alternately the use of a well-seated LMA which is then capped to block the escape from the proximal tracheal limb while ventilating the patient via the tracheostomy limb has been described [11]. Other methods of ventilation through the T-tube offer only partial airway protection from aspiration such as the placement of a Fogarty catheter through the tracheotomy limb into the proximal limb to block egress of gas into the upper airway, with simultaneous ventilation through the tracheotomy limb. Awake fiber-optic telescoping of a small endotracheal tube into the proximal tracheal limb of the T-tube has been described, but aspiration around the T-tube is still possible. One report of airway management of a patient with a full stomach described awake fiber-optic placement of a 5mm microlaryngoscopy tube through both the proximal and distal limbs of the T-tube with the inflation of the cuff in the trachea [83]. Adult T-tube sizes vary from 8 to 16 mm external diameter. This approach may only be possible with the larger sizes. Finally, the T-tube can be removed, ideally with the help of the patient's surgeon, and replaced by a tracheotomy tube. If the tracheotomy is left for any length of time, the patient could suffer a recurrence of their airway compromise. They would require another general anesthetic for replacement of a T-tube.

References

1. Belsey R. Resection and reconstruction of the intrathoracic trachea. Br J Surg. 1950;38:200.
2. Barclay RS, McSwan N, Welsh TH. Tracheal reconstruction without the use of grafts. Thorax. 1957;12:177.
3. Grillo HC, Bendixen HH, Gephart T. Resection of the carina and lower trachea. Ann Surg. 1963;158:889.
4. Geffin B, Bland J, Grillo HC. Anesthetic management of tracheal resection and reconstruction. Anesth Analg. 1969;48:884.
5. Cooper JD, Grillo HC. The evolution of tracheal injury due to ventilator assistance through cuffed tubes: a pathological study. Ann Surg. 1969;169:334–48.
6. Liu J, Zhang X, Gong W, et al. Correlations between controlled endotracheal tube cuff pressure and post procedural complications: a multicenter study. Anesth Analg. 2010;111:1133–7.
7. Grillo HC, Mathisen DJ. Cervical exenteration. Ann Thorac Surg. 1990;49:401.
8. Miura T, Grillo HC. The contribution of the inferior thyroid artery to the blood supply of the human trachea. Surg Gynecol Obstet. 1966;123:99–102.
9. Minnich DJ, Mathisen DJ. Anatomy of the trachea, carina, and bronchi. Thorac Surg Clin. 2007;17:571–85.
10. Pearson FG, Cooper JD, Nelems JM, et al. Primary tracheal anastomosis after resection of the cricoid cartilage with preservation of recurrent laryngeal nerves. J Thorac Cardiovasc Surg. 1975;70:806–16.
11. Agrawal S, Payal YS, Sharma JP, et al. Montgomery T-tube: anesthetic management. J Clin Anesth. 2007;19:135–7.
12. Merritt RE, Mathisen DJ. Tracheal resection. In: Patterson GA, Cooper JD, Deslauriers J, et al., editors. Pearson's thoracic and esophageal surgery. 3rd ed. Philadelphia: Churchill Livingston; 2008. p. 377–82.
13. Fabre D, Fadel E, Mussot S, et al. Autologous tracheal replacement for cancer. Chin Clin Oncol. 2015;4(4):46.
14. Macchiarini P, Jungebluth P, Go T, et al. Clinical transplantation of a tissue-engineered airway. Lancet. 2008;372:2023–30.
15. De Perrot M, Fadel E, Dartevelle P. Carinal resection. In: Patterson GA, Cooper JD, Deslauriers J, et al., editors. Pearson's thoracic and esophageal surgery. 3rd ed. Philadelphia: Churchill Livingstone; 2008. p. 383–92.
16. Wright C, Grillo H, Wain JC, et al. Anastomotic complications after tracheal resection: prognostic factors and management. J Thorac Cardiovasc Surg. 2004;128:731–9.
17. Young-Beyer P, Wilson RS. Anesthetic management for tracheal resection and reconstruction. J Cardiothorac Anesth. 1988;2:821–35.
18. Pellegrino R, Viegi G, Brusasco V, et al. Interpretative strategies for lung function tests. Eur Respir J. 2005;26:948–68.
19. Tomori Z, Widdicombe JG. Muscular, bronchomotor and cardiovascular reflexes elicited by mechanical stimulation of the respiratory tract. J Physiol. 1969;200:25.
20. Hill AJ, Feneck RO, Underwood SM, et al. The haemodynamic effects of bronchoscopy, comparison of propofol and thiopentone with and without alfentanil pretreatment. Anaesthesia. 1991;46:266–70.
21. De Perrot M, Fadel E, Mercier O, et al. Long term results after carinal resection for carcinoma. J Thorac Cardiovasc Surg. 2006;131:81–9.
22. Licker M, Schweizer A, Nicolet G, et al. Anesthesia of a patient with an obstructing tracheal mass: a new way to manage the airway. Acta Anaesthesiol Scand. 1997;41:34.
23. Pinsonneault C, Fortier J, Donati F. Tracheal resection and reconstruction. Can J Anaesth. 1999;46:439.
24. Fischler M, Troche G, Guerin Y, et al. Evolution des techniques d'anesthesie pour resection-anastamose de trachee. Ann Fr Anesth Reanim. 1988;7:125–7.
25. Conacher ID, Velasquez H, Morrice DJ. Endobronchial tubes – a case for re-evaluation. Anaesthesia. 2006;61:587.
26. Hannallah MS. The optimal breathing tube for tracheal resection and reconstruction. Anesthesiology. 1995;83:419.
27. Theman TE, Kerr JH, Nelems JM, et al. Carinal resection, a report of two cases and a description of the anesthetic technique. J Thorac Cardiovasc Surg. 1976;71:314.
28. Sanders RD. Two ventilating attachments for bronchoscopes. Del Med J. 1967;39:170–3.
29. Lee P, English ICW. Management of anesthesia during tracheal resection. Anaesthesia. 1974;29:305.
30. Ellis RH, Hinds CJ, Gadd LT. Management of anaesthesia during tracheal resection. Anaesthesia. 1976;31:1076.
31. McClish A, Deslauriers J, Beaulieu M, et al. High-flow catheter ventilation during major tracheobroncheal reconstruction. J Thorac Cardiovasc Surg. 1985;89:508.
32. Baraka A. Oxygen-jet ventilation during tracheal reconstruction in patients with tracheal stenosis. Anesth Analg. 1977;56:429.
33. Clarkson WB, Davies JR. Anaesthesia for carinal resection. Anaesthesia. 1978;33:815.
34. Carlon GC, Kahn RC, Howland WS, et al. Clinical experience with high frequency ventilation. Crit Care Med. 1981;9:1.
35. Howland WS, Carlon GC, Goldiner PL, et al. High-frequency jet ventilation during thoracic surgical procedures. Anesthesiology. 1987;67:1009.
36. Sjostrand U. High-frequency positive-pressure ventilation: a review. Crit Care Med. 1980;8:345.
37. Glenski JA, Crawford M, Rehder K. High-frequency, small volume ventilation during thoracic surgery. Anesthesiology. 1980;59:577.
38. Carlon GC, Griffin J, Ray C Jr. High-frequency jet ventilation in experimental airway disruption. Crit Care Med. 1983;11:353–5.
39. Beamer WC, Prough DS, Royster RL, et al. High-frequency jet ventilation produces auto-PEEP. Crit Care Med. 1984;12:734.
40. Froese AS, Bryan AC. High frequency ventilation. Am Rev Respir Dis. 1987;135:1363.
41. Adelsmayr E, Keller C, Erd G, et al. The laryngeal mask and high-frequency jet ventilation for resection of high tracheal stenosis. Anesth Analg. 1998;86:907.
42. Watanabe Y, Murakami S, Iwa T, et al. The clinical value of high-frequency jet ventilation in major airway reconstructive surgery. Scand J Thorac Cardiovasc Surg. 1988;22:227.
43. Magnusson L, Lang FJW, Monnier P, et al. Anaesthesia for tracheal resection: report of 17 cases. Can J Anaesth. 1997;44:1282.
44. Perera ER, Vidic DM, Zivot J. Carinal resection with two high-frequency jet ventilation delivery systems. Can J Anaesth. 1993;40:59.

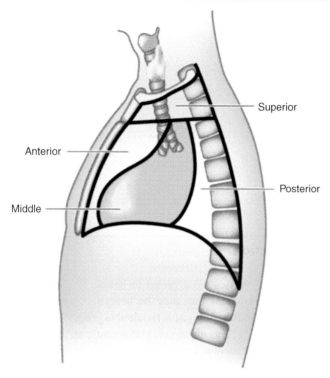

Fig. 14.1 Anatomic location of the four compartments of the mediastinum. (Reprinted from Warren [10] with permission)

Table 14.1 Masses in the mediastinal compartments

	Adult	Children
Superior mediastinum	*Benign* Thymoma Retrosternal thyroid Zenker's diverticulum Aortic aneurysm *Malignant* Lymphoma Metastatic carcinoma Parathyroid tumors	Lymphoma Thymoma Retrosternal thyroid Parathyroid tumors
Anterior mediastinum	*Benign* Thymoma Thymic cyst Thymic hyperplasia Thyroid (goiter, ectopic thyroid tissue) Parathyroid adenoma *Malignant* Thymic carcinoma Thyroid carcinoma Seminoma Germ cell tumors (seminoma, teratoma, non-seminoma) Lymphoma	Lymphoma Teratoma Cystic hygroma Thymoma Pericardial cysts Diaphragmatic hernia (Morgagni)
Middle mediastinum	*Benign* Benign lymphadenopathy Cysts Esophageal masses Hiatus hernia Cardiac/vascular structures (pericardial cysts, aneurysm) *Malignant* Lymphoma Metastases Esophageal cancer Thyroid cancer	
Posterior mediastinum	*Benign* Neurofibroma Schwannoma Chemodectoma Hiatus hernia *Malignant* Neuroblastoma	

Anatomy and Pathophysiology

The mediastinum is bound by the sternum anteriorly and the vertebral bodies posteriorly and extends from the thoracic inlet to the diaphragm (Fig. 14.1) [11]. It is divided into superior and inferior regions, which is further subdivided into the anterior, middle, and posterior mediastinum. Table 14.1 shows the typical masses in the various mediastinal compartments [11, 12].

Because of the proximity to other airway and cardiovascular structures, mediastinal masses can lead to complications under anesthetic due to compression or encroachment of these structures. Although the majority of complications are described for masses in the anterior mediastinum, masses in the middle mediastinum [13] and posterior mediastinum [14] have also been associated with hemodynamic and respiratory collapse with general anesthesia (GA).

During normal spontaneous ventilation, there is preferential perfusion to dependent areas of the lung and distribution of ventilation controlled mainly by lung compliance [15]. Most studies evaluating ventilation changes under anesthesia have shown a decrease in functional reserve capacity (FRC) [15]. With muscle paralysis and supine positioning, there is cephalad shift of the diaphragm that further contributes to impaired gas exchange under anesthesia. Neuman stated three reasons for the dangers of general anesthesia: (1) the reduction of lung volume by as much as 500–1500 ml under

GA, (2) relaxation of bronchial smooth muscle leading to greater compressibility, and (3) loss of spontaneous diaphragmatic movement with paralysis, which reduces the normal transpleural pressure gradient that helps dilate the airways [16]. These normal changes that occur under general anesthesia are especially pronounced in patients with mediastinal masses who may have limited reserve or further alteration of ventilation-perfusion matching due to extrinsic airway compression.

Induction of general anesthesia is a sequence of events, and complications can occur at any of these stages, including (1) changing patient position from upright to supine, (2) transitioning from awake to anesthetized state, (3) moving from spontaneous negative pressure ventilation to positive pressure ventilation, and (4) changing of muscle tone from unparalyzed to paralyzed state. Furthermore, complications do not occur solely at the time of induction and intubation but can extend into the maintenance phase, at extubation, or even into the postoperative period [17].

Numerous case studies documenting airway collapse [3, 6, 18] and cardiovascular collapse [5, 7, 18, 19] under anesthesia have been described. Most anesthetic deaths have been described in the pediatric population, possibly due to increased compressibility of pediatric airways or the lack of awareness of the extent of airway involvement [3–5], as well as the intolerance of any cardiovascular insult.

Hemodynamic decompensation may occur if there is compression of the heart or great vessels such as the pulmonary artery (PA) and superior vena cava (SVC). If the PA is compressed, decreased pulmonary perfusion can lead to hypoxemia, acute right ventricular dysfunction, and even cardiac arrest [17]. Compression of SVC leads predominantly to a reduction in venous return and the subsequent reduction in cardiac output [20]. Direct compression of the heart is rare but can lead to arrhythmias, pericardial effusion, or reduction in preload from mechanical compression [17].

Preanesthetic Assessment

Clinical Signs and Symptoms

Common symptoms include dyspnea, cough, hoarseness, new-onset wheezing, syncope, chest pain, night sweats, weight loss, dysphagia, and superior vena cava (SVC) obstruction [1, 17]. These symptoms are especially worrisome if it worsens in the supine position.

SVC syndrome can present with edema of the upper body (face, neck, larynx, upper limbs), plethora, dilation of veins (neck and thorax), and development of collateral veins if slowly evolving [11, 17, 20]. Patients can also present with CNS symptoms including headache, visual distortion, or altered mentation [11]. Respiratory symptoms can accompany SVC obstruction due to concurrent compression of the airway by tumor or engorged veins [7].

Clinical signs may include tachypnea, stridor, rhonchi, or decreased breath sounds. Severity of respiratory symptoms may not correlate with degree of airway obstruction, especially in the pediatric population [6, 21, 22].

Coexisting systemic syndromes such as myasthenia gravis or thyroid dysfunction may be present, and their concurrent optimization needs to be considered, but the specific management of these conditions will not be discussed here.

Mediastinal masses may also be asymptomatic and found incidentally through work-up being performed for other indications. Occasionally these masses come to light due to perioperative complications for an unrelated surgical procedure, and patients are subsequently found to have a mediastinal mass [8, 9].

Investigations

Following chest radiography, computed tomography (CT) is often the next choice of imaging modality as it can provide exact anatomical detail of the mass, including size and relation to adjacent structures [1, 23]. CT can provide useful information regarding the location and extent of airway compression, as well as cardiovascular involvement [17]. Unfortunately, CT scans are static images that only assess one time-point and do not provide information about dynamic compression or position-related changes [16]. MRI may provide more details regarding soft tissue but is not routinely performed. However, it may be useful for neurogenic and vascular lesions, especially when the use of contrast is contraindicated [24].

Azizkhan examined a series of 50 children with anterior mediastinal mass and found that the severity of pulmonary symptoms is not a reliable indicator of the degree of compression in children [25]. Rather, those who had decreases in cross-sectional area of the trachea of at least 50% had the highest association of complications under general anesthetic. Retrospective analysis by Shamberger confirmed the absence of major complications in pediatric patients with a tracheal diameter greater than 50% predicted who underwent general anesthesia [26]. A follow-up prospective study confirmed that GA was well tolerated in children with tracheal area and peak expired flow rate (PEFR) greater than 50% predicted. It was, however, unable to conclude whether impaired pulmonary function as measured by PEFR would be predictive of respiratory collapse during GA as the highest-risk patients were all operated on under local anesthesia [27].

Neuman et al. first advocated for pulmonary function testing and flow-volume loops in 1984, and it soon became widespread recommendation as part of the preoperative work-up of anterior mediastinal masses despite being based on anecdotal recommendations [16, 28]. Subsequent studies have failed to correlate degree of changes in spirometry with perioperative airway complication rates [29]. Hnatiuk et al. assessed upright and supine spirometry and showed no correlation between abnormal spirometry results and respiratory symptoms, abnormal CT results, and anesthetic complications [30]. Spirometry and flow-volume loops do not predict intraoperative morbidity and mortality beyond the information obtained on imaging studies [1, 28].

Transthoracic echocardiography (TTE) and transesophageal echocardiography (TEE) are indicated if clinical or CT information suggests cardiac or great vessel involvement.

They provide additional information about encroachment or compression of cardiac structures [23]. These exams can also be performed in recumbent and lateral positions to determine any positional changes in tumor compression effects [17]. As some masses can enlarge and progress rapidly, imaging should be performed as close to the time of surgery as possible.

Other modalities that are sometimes employed include fluorodeoxyglucose positron emission tomography (FDG-PET), which may provide additional information for staging, diagnosis, and prognosis, as it evaluates the metabolic activity of the tumor to predict its response to neoadjuvant therapy [23].

An awake fiber-optic bronchoscopic exam assessing any dynamic airway compression, especially with positional changes, is a useful adjunct to preoperative evaluation and planning.

Anesthetic Risks

Risk Stratification (Fig. 14.2)

Risk assessment in this patient population depends on clinical signs and symptoms (with emphasis on presence of supine symptoms), radiologic studies (CXR and CT chest), and possibly echocardiography (if cardiac or vascular compression is suspected). Table 14.2 outlines several high-risk criteria that are useful for risk stratification of these patients.

Neuman et al. presented a flowchart of suggested management of anterior mediastinal masses [16]. Since then, there have been modifications on this flowchart with continued emphasis on maintaining spontaneous ventilation and avoidance of muscle relaxation if possible.

Knowledge and documentation of "position of comfort" for patient in terms of respiration and circulation may be useful [17].

Risk of complications in the pediatric population has been reported to be 7–20% [4, 25, 31, 32]. Bechard examined 105 anesthetics in the adult population and had an incidence of airway obstruction of 0% during the intraoperative period. However, some patients with the most worrisome features received preoperative chemotherapy or had their tissue biopsy obtained by other means [33]. The overall intraoperative cardiorespiratory complication rate was 3.8%, and postoperative respiratory complication rate was 10.5% [33]. This study found a correlation between the presence of cardiorespiratory symptoms and perioperative complications, with no perioperative complications seen in asymptomatic patients. Although an abnormal pulmonary function test (PEFR <40% predicted) did not predict intraoperative complications, it was associated with a tenfold increase in postoperative complications. Also, a combination of obstruction/restrictive pattern was also associated with a higher rate of postoperative complications [33].

Preoperative Treatment

Preoperative chemotherapy, steroids, or radiation therapy may reduce the size of the tumor and reduce intraoperative risk but may distort histological diagnosis. However, the recommendation of preoperative radiation may be warranted in cases of SVC syndrome as massive hemorrhage, respiratory obstruction, or fatal exacerbation of the SVC obstruction can occur with induction of general anesthesia [7].

Piro recommended preoperative radiation based on their series of 139 patients, where all 5 acute life-threatening complications were encountered in patients with untreated AMM [4]. This recommendation is echoed by other authors [3, 18], while others [12, 31] feel that in the absence of tissue diagnosis, empiric treatment with radiation therapy may delay diagnosis or lead to inappropriate treatment of the mediastinal mass.

Tracheobronchial stenting can also be performed either via flexible or rigid bronchoscopy. This may provide a bridge to chemotherapy or radiation, used to maintain adequate airway prior to excision of mediastinal mass, or for palliation [12]. Spontaneous ventilation maintained with the use of an LMA has been successfully described for placement of a self-expanding metallic stent [34]. There is however a small chance that airway stenting may worsen patient hemodynamics by displacing the mass into adjacent cardiovascular structures.

Anesthetic Management

The choice of anesthetic is based on preoperative risk stratification. For those with high-risk criteria (Table 14.2), the avoidance of general anesthesia and utilization of local or regional anesthesia is advocated if feasible, but this is less practical in the pediatric population.

The ability to rapidly change patient's position should be considered prior to the initiation of anesthesia or surgery.

Sedation

Judicious use (or avoidance) of sedation in the highest-risk population is recommended as respiratory depression, upper airway obstruction, and any amount of muscle relaxation may worsen compressive symptoms exerted by the mediastinal mass [17].

Dexmedetomidine has been used successfully in this population as a sole anesthetic without the use of muscle relaxant, with the ability to maintain spontaneous respirations with minimal respiratory depression [35].

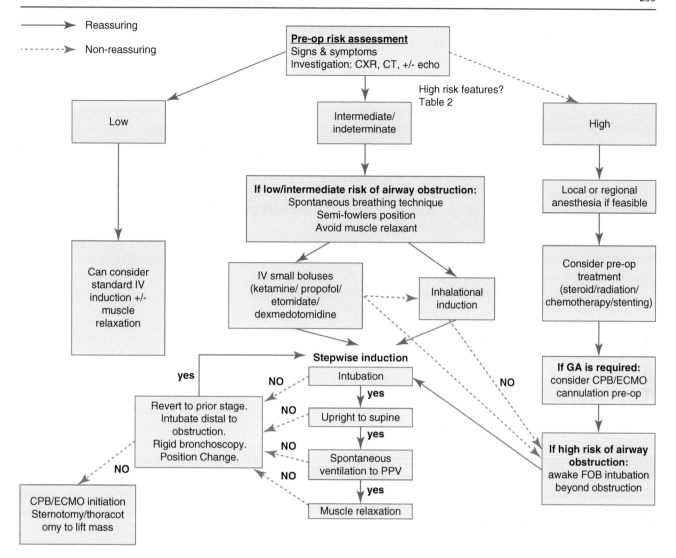

Fig. 14.2 Flowchart of potential management strategies of patients with anterior mediastinal mass based on preoperative risk stratification

Table 14.2 Preoperative high-risk criteria

High-risk criteria
Dyspnea when supine (orthopnea)
Increased cough when supine
Syncope
SVC syndrome
Pericardial effusion
Tracheal compression to <50% of predicted cross-sectional area (pediatric)

Induction and Intubation

This should be performed in a stepwise approach, with verification of adequate ventilation and circulation at each step prior to proceeding [1, 17]. The use of short-acting medications allows for the resumption of the previously tolerated state (e.g., spontaneous ventilation).

Options for induction include:

1. No induction (local vs. regional, with or without sedation).
2. Awake fiber-optic intubation with placement of ETT beyond area of compression or stenosis; then proceed with induction.
3. Maintenance of spontaneous ventilation using small boluses of IV anesthetic (e.g., Ketamine [36], propofol, or etomidate) or inhalational induction.
4. Standard IV induction (with or without muscle relaxation).

Maintenance of spontaneous ventilation has been advocated. However, cases of airway collapse have also been documented despite maintenance of spontaneous respirations [37].

Prior to induction of anesthesia, alternative airway management and rescue for hemodynamic complications should be laid out. This may include long endotracheal tubes of varying diameters (e.g., endobronchial tubes, microlaryngeal tubes [MLT]), double-lumen tubes or bronchial blockers, flexible fiber-optic bronchoscope, rigid bronchoscope, (and an experienced bronchoscopist), and potential equipment and personnel to initiate extracorporeal circulation (ECC) if cannulation is planned prior to induction. Glycopyrrolate is useful in this population to reduce airway secretions prior to awake bronchoscopic airway assessments, as well as lessening any vagal responses to airway manipulation.

Muscle relaxation should be avoided whenever possible. If muscle relaxation is required for surgical reasons, a small dose of short-acting muscle relaxant such as succinylcholine should be given and mechanical ventilation attempted. If mechanical ventilation can proceed without any significant increase in airway pressure or hemodynamic compromise, subsequent doses of muscle relaxant can be considered [17].

The use of ECC including full cardiopulmonary bypass (CPB) and extracorporeal membrane oxygenation (ECMO) in high-risk patients may be considered. This will be discussed in more detail below.

Maintenance of Anesthesia and Intraoperative Monitoring

Intraoperative transesophageal echocardiography (TEE) may play an increasing role during tumor resection, as it is an invaluable tool in the monitoring and diagnosis of hemodynamically unstable patients [28]. It provides real-time imaging of the heart and nearby structures and can help establish anatomical and functional involvement of the tumor during resection [37–40]. TEE can also provide information regarding contractility, degree of right ventricular outflow tract (RVOT) obstruction or compression [14], volume status, and presence of pericardial effusion [39, 41]. The American Society of Anesthesiologist and Society of Cardiovascular Anesthesiologists Task Force on Transesophageal Echocardiography supports the use of TEE in noncardiac surgical patients with known or suspected cardiovascular pathology that might result in hemodynamic, pulmonary, or neurologic compromise [42]. Furthermore, its use should be considered in those with unexplained persistent hypotension as well as unexplained hypoxemia [42].

Emergence and Postoperative Care

Complications related to mediastinal masses have been reported in the postoperative periods; therefore increased vigilance must continue during this time. Transitioning from the anesthetized state to the awake state can pose an issue if pain, anxiety, or coughing leads to increased airflow and turbulence through a compromised airway [31]. Tracheomalacia

can occur with prolonged compression of airway by enlarging masses. Furthermore, upper airway obstruction and decreased muscle tone will further aggravate airway collapse during high inspiratory pressure exerted against a closed glottis. Patients with SVC obstruction may encounter postextubation breathing issues due to airway edema [43].

Most of these patients will require intensive postoperative monitoring especially after diagnostic procedures where the cause of obstruction has not been addressed [17, 43].

Complications

Mediastinal mass syndrome (MMS) is a term describing the clinical picture caused by mediastinal mass in anesthetized patients, encompassing acute respiratory and hemodynamic decompensation [17].

Airway Compression

Respiratory decompensation is caused by mechanical compression of the trachea, main bronchi, or both [17]. Table 14.3 outlines rescue options for acute airway obstruction.

Even asymptomatic patients can develop life-threatening obstruction at induction and maintenance of anesthetic [24, 37, 44]. Preoperative chest CT can provide accurate measurement of airway diameter, and it is important to determine the precise level and extension of compression [25, 44]. Any indication of tracheal or bronchial compression may be associated with airway complications under anesthetic.

Azizkhan et al. examined 50 consecutive cases of children with anterior mediastinal mass and found that all 5 cases of life-threatening complications occurred in those with tracheal compression >50% [25].

Spontaneous ventilation with the avoidance of muscle relaxant has often been advocated for this patient population, but this is not a failsafe option as airway collapse has been described in a case of anterior mediastinal mass despite spontaneous ventilation and avoidance of muscle relaxation [37].

Alternative airway management may include wire-reinforced endotracheal tubes, long endotracheal tubes, flexible

Table 14.3 Rescue options for airway obstruction

Rescue options for airway obstruction
Double-lumen tube or long endotracheal tube advanced beyond obstruction or compression [24]
Reposition patient to position of comfort (if known), lateral or prone (to decrease the weight of tumor on airway)
Resumption of previous tolerated state (e.g., upright position, spontaneous ventilation, awaken from anesthetic)
Rigid bronchoscopy beyond stenosis
Initiation of cardiopulmonary bypass or ECMO

Table 14.4 Management of SVC syndrome

Management of SVC syndrome
Augmentation of preload
Positioning to minimize compression of heart or major vessels (e.g., lateral position)
Lower extremity IV access
Spontaneous ventilation to augment venous return
Sternotomy and lifting of mass to relieve compression

fiber-optic bronchoscope, and rigid bronchoscope. Lee describes a case of airway obstruction on induction that was relieved with rigid bronchoscopy and subsequent placement of a double-lumen tube to act as an endobronchial stent [24].

Aggressive ventilation through a partially obstructed airway may lead to dynamic hyperinflation and worsened hemodynamics. These patients may benefit from transient disconnection from airway circuit or utilization of zero end-expiratory pressure (ZEEP).

Cardiovascular Compression

SVC compression and obstruction can lead to excessive bleeding, insufficient drug delivery, and possible airway swelling. These patients may require postoperative ventilation as airway edema can extend into the postoperative period. If worsening of SVC syndrome is suspected, optimization of preload and attempt to relieve compression from the mediastinal mass should be made (Table 14.4).

Compression of the pulmonary trunk or main pulmonary artery (PA) can also occur [19]. Unlike the SVC, PA is relatively protected by the aortic arch, making it less vulnerable to external compression. If cyanosis does occur; the possibility of RVOT obstruction and subsequent hypoxemia, hypotension, or cardiac arrest should be considered [11, 19].

Extracorporeal Circulation (ECC)

Preinduction femoral cannulation for CPB can be considered in extremely high-risk patients as the use of CPB as an emergency rescue can take 10–20 min to initiate and can lead to anoxic brain injury [14, 28, 37]. Patient positioning, inadequate access to femoral vessels, and near-arrest conditions may further complicate vessel cannulation once the surgical procedure has commenced [45].

Femoral-femoral cardiopulmonary bypass (CPB) initiated in an awake patient under local anesthesia has been utilized in patients at high risk of airway or hemodynamic collapse with general anesthesia in which awake fiber-optic intubation may not always be feasible or successful [46–49].

Increasingly, extracorporeal membrane oxygenation (ECMO) is being initiated prior to intubation as part of the airway plan in patients with mediastinal tumors with evidence of airway compromise [50, 51].

On the other hand, preinduction initiation of CPB carries with it the risks of anticoagulation and potentially unnecessary access to vessels. Occasionally, the patient may not tolerate attempts at awake cannulation, as they cannot endure supine positioning [52]. Some authors have advocated for the placement of wires in femoral vessels without full commencement of CPB as a compromise [28].

Anesthesia for Mediastinoscopy

Mediastinoscopy can be performed for staging of lung cancer, for evaluation of mediastinal lymph nodes, or for obtaining tissues biopsy samples for diagnosis of mediastinal masses [53]. The more common procedure is the cervical mediastinoscopy, where the mediastinoscope is inserted toward the carina through a small transverse incision in the suprasternal notch [53] and requires general anesthesia. The less commonly performed anterior mediastinoscopy is performed through the interchondral space along the second rib. This procedure can be performed under local anesthesia or general anesthesia while maintaining spontaneous respiration [54, 55], but coughing or movement can lead to catastrophic surgical complications.

Monitoring of the pulse in the right arm is recommended (either through pulse oximeter or arterial line in the right arm) as compression of the innominate artery by the mediastinoscope can occur and lead to decreased cerebral perfusion and ischemia [53] (Fig. 14.3). Noninvasive blood pressure monitoring in the left arm will provide information regarding systemic perfusion pressures.

The most significant immediate complication of mediastinoscopy is major hemorrhage. Adequate IV access in a lower extremity and availability of blood products should be considered. In a retrospective review of over 300 mediastinoscopies, Park et al. had a major hemorrhage rate of 0.4% [56]. Ninety-three percent of the patients had control of hemorrhage through packing, and only one patient required emergency sternotomy. Once local tamponade was in place, all patients eventually underwent surgical exploration and management of bleeding. The most commonly injured vessels were the azygos vein and the innominate and pulmonary arteries [56]. Lower limb IV access may be required if SVC injury is suspected. Principles of massive transfusion should be utilized until control of hemorrhage has occurred.

Pneumothorax is an uncommon complication but can lead to increased airway pressures, tracheal shift, hypotension, and cyanosis [53]. Other rare complications include injury to

Fig. 14.3 Diagram of a mediastinoscope in the pretracheal fascia along with relevant surrounding structures. Note the innominate artery immediately anterior to the mediastinoscope. The azygos vein drains into the superior vena cava, which has been omitted from the drawing because it would cover the location of the mediastinoscope. (Reprinted from Slinger and Campos [53] with permission)

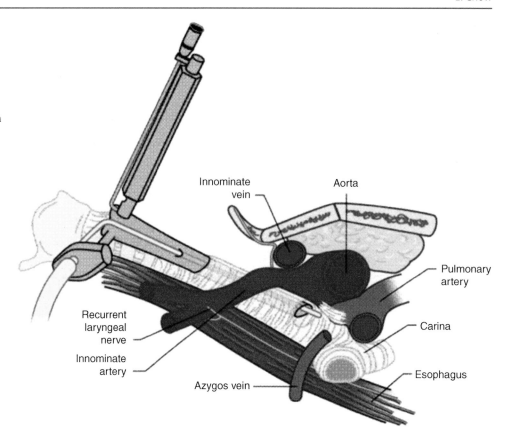

the recurrent laryngeal nerve, which can cause vocal cord dysfunction, vagus nerve, and thoracic duct and compression of the aorta, which may lead to reflex bradycardia [56].

Summary

Improved understanding of the pathophysiology of mediastinal masses has improved the perioperative morbidity, and mortality has been reduced in this patient population. Careful preoperative assessment and knowledge of the location of the mass and its relationship to adjacent structures are paramount for anesthesia planning. Diagnostic procedures should be performed under local or regional anesthesia whenever possible. Close communication with the surgical team thorough risk assessment and devising a plan for intraoperative airway or hemodynamic complications all contribute to the successful management of these cases.

Clinical Case Discussion

A 24-year-old female presented with a 1-week history of progression of dry cough and increased facial and neck swelling (especially in the morning on awakening). She also

notes increasing shortness of breath, especially when lying flat. Chest X-ray (Fig. 14.4 a, b) demonstrates a large anterior mediastinal mass as well as a right pleural effusion. CT scan demonstrates a 6.3 x 8.7 x 8.0 cm soft tissues mediastinal mass that is encasing the superior vena cava, both brachiocephalic veins, and the right pulmonary artery (Fig. 14.5 a–d). The trachea and mainstem bronchi are compressed. Percutaneous CT-guided biopsy was nondiagnostic (Fig. 14.6 a–c).

Question 1

Anterior mediastinoscopy is planned to obtain tissue biopsy samples. What are your options for induction of anesthesia?

Answer

This patient has several high-risk features (increased shortness of breath and cough when supine as well as SVC syndrome). Options include local anesthesia (if feasible), awake fiber-optic intubation, and inhalational induction with avoidance of muscle relaxation. Discussion with the surgical team should also include the possibility of preinduction CPB or

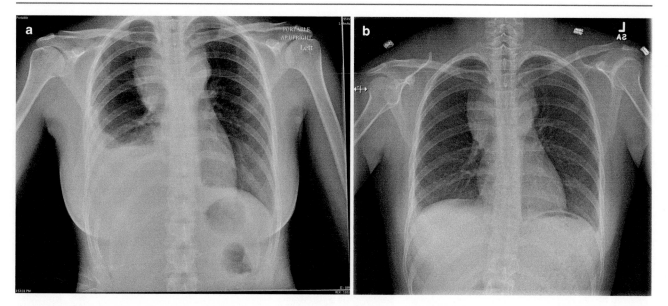

Fig. 14.4 Chest X-ray of a 24-year-old female patient with a large anterior mediastinal mass presenting for biopsy of the mass under GA. (**a**) CXR shows presence of a right-sided pleural effusion. (**b**) Repeat CXR after pleural effusion was drained. Recent percutaneous CT-guided biopsies were nondiagnostic. She presented with symptoms of SVC obstruction. The trachea appears midline and patent on CXR

ECMO with the encasement of SVC. If local anesthesia is not feasible, awake fiber-optic assessment of the airway, followed by passage of endotracheal tube distal to obstruction, may be the safest technique. This also allows for assessment of any dynamic airway obstruction during spontaneous ventilation, association with any positional changes, and identification of the least obstructed bronchus.

SVC compression will lead to decreased venous return and subsequent reduction in cardiac output. The cessation of spontaneous ventilation will also augment the decrease in venous return. Profound hypotension will lead to insufficient pulmonary perfusion and hypoxemia.

Cyanosis and hypoxemia can also occur with RVOT obstruction and should be considered in this patient.

Question 2

You successfully performed an awake fiber-optic intubation of this patient. There is moderate mid-tracheal compression and mild compression of bilateral bronchi on examination. A long endotracheal tube (ETT) is placed beyond the area of tracheal compression. Soon after administration of a muscle relaxant, ventilation becomes more difficult, and patient begins to desaturate. BP is 60/42. What do you suspect?

Answer

The differential diagnosis includes acute airway obstruction as well as potential compression of major cardiovascular structures.

Increase in airway pressure may suggest obstruction distal to the ETT. A quick check with the bronchoscopy may help verify this, and the ETT can be advanced beyond the obstruction (endobronchial intubation may be required).

Question 3

The patient begins to desaturate despite attempts at bronchoscopic adjustment of the endotracheal tube and adjustment of patient position from supine to upright. The surgeons are scrubbing. What should you do?

Answer

Immediately alert the surgeon. The plan may be to proceed immediately to sternotomy to lift the mediastinal mass to relieve its compressive effects. CPB and ECMO may be considered but may not be achieved quickly enough if preinduction cannulation of vessels was not performed.

The surgeons quickly perform a sternotomy, and upon lifting the mass off the trachea and right pulmonary artery, the airway pressure, saturation, and blood pressure improved dramatically.

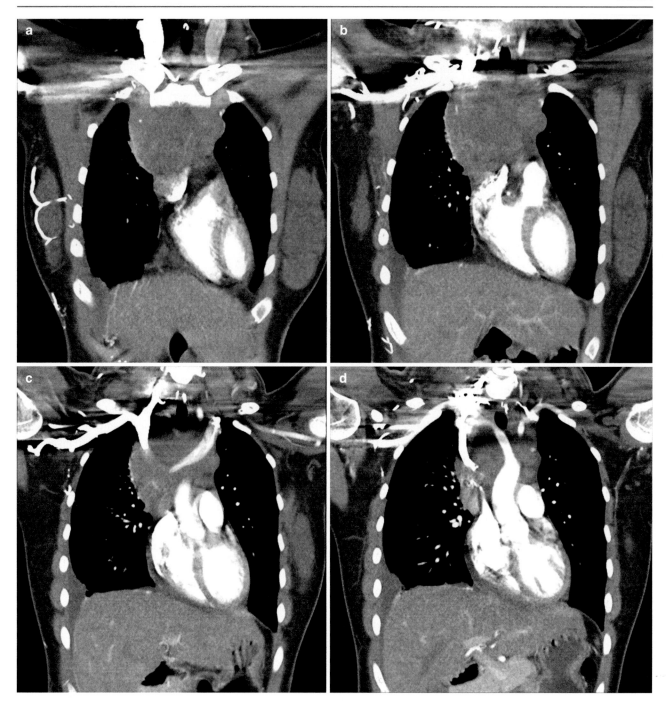

Fig. 14.5 (**a–d**) CT scan (sagittal views) of the same patient shows a large anterior mediastinal mass measuring 6.3 × 8.7 × 8.0 cm. There is encasement and compression of the SVC, both brachiocephalic veins, and the right pulmonary artery

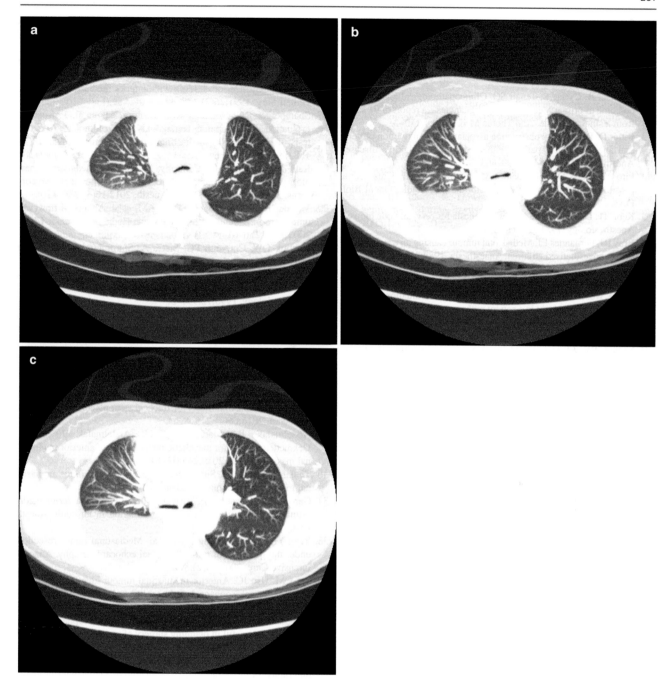

Fig. 14.6 (**a–c**) CT scan (coronal views) of the same patient shows tracheal and bilateral mainstem bronchi compression by anterior mediastinal mass to almost a slit. The patient was intubated awake beyond the area of maximal tracheal compression

Thymic Surgery and Paraendocrine Syndromes

15

Daniel Sellers and Karen McRae

Abbreviations

ACTH	Adrenocorticotrophic hormone
CRH	Corticotrophin-releasing hormone
CT	Computed tomography
CVP	Central venous pressure
ECG	Electrocardiogram
GHRH	Growth-hormone-releasing hormone
IVIG	Intravenous immunoglobulin
LES	Lambert-Eaton syndrome
LRP-4	Lipoprotein receptor-related protein 4
MEN	Multiple endocrine neoplasia
MG	Myasthenia gravis
MGFA	Myasthenia Gravis Foundation of America
MuSK	Muscle-specific kinase
NDMR	Nondepolarizing muscle relaxants
NMJ	Neuromuscular junction
SCLC	Small cell lung cancer
SIADH	Syndrome of inappropriate release of antidiuretic hormone
TEA	Thoracic epidural anesthesia
TIVA	Total intravenous anesthesia
TSH	Thyroid-stimulating hormone
VATS	Video-assisted thoracic surgery

Key Points

- Indications for thymic surgery typically include thymic mass or nonthymomatous myasthenia gravis (MG).
- Considerations for a patient with a thymic mass include potential for invasion or compression of cardiopulmonary structures causing life-threatening compromise particularly at induction of general anesthesia.
- Thymectomy for MG is never an emergency procedure and should not proceed without preoperative optimization by a multidisciplinary team specializing in the care of myasthenic patients.
- Anesthetic considerations for a patient with MG focus on preventing an exacerbation and minimizing the effect of surgical pain and residual anesthetics on postoperative respiratory function.
- Muscle relaxants and their reversal agents should be avoided in patients with MG whenever possible. Other principles include the use of short-acting agents, use of regional anesthesia for opioid-sparing effects, and proper perioperative management of anticholinesterases.
- Despite repeated efforts to determine what clinical features predict the need for postoperative ventilation, no criteria have been proven to be universally applicable in the myasthenic population.
- Many thoracic malignancies have commonly associated paraneoplastic syndromes with important implications for the anesthesiologist.
- The most common extraintestinal location of carcinoid tumors is the lungs; however, unlike their gastrointestinal counterparts, bronchial carcinoids are rarely secretory.

D. Sellers · K. McRae (✉)
Department of Anesthesia and Pain Management, Toronto General Hospital, University Health Network, Toronto, ON, Canada
e-mail: karen.mcrae@uhn.ca

© Springer Nature Switzerland AG 2019
P. Slinger (ed.), *Principles and Practice of Anesthesia for Thoracic Surgery*, https://doi.org/10.1007/978-3-030-00859-8_15

- Carcinoid syndrome must be optimized with at least 24 h of preoperative octreotide to minimize the life-threatening cardiopulmonary instability that can occur during a carcinoid crisis.
- Advanced carcinoid disease is associated with fibrosis which can lead to pulmonary hypertension or significant valvulopathy with progressive, severe, right-sided heart failure. For these reasons, patients presenting with carcinoid syndrome must have a preoperative echocardiogram.

Introduction

The thymus gland is situated in the anterior mediastinum; protected by the sternum and ribcage, it is nestled amid vital cardiopulmonary structures. Its function is primarily as a site for maturation of T cells from hemopoietic progenitors and as such is a critical part of the development of the adaptive immune system. It is largest in childhood, becomes quiescent in early adolescence, and after puberty is increasingly replaced by fat. Its autoimmune function gives rise to pathology with which the thoracic anesthesiologist must be familiar, myasthenia gravis (MG) in particular. The implications of acquired myasthenia are essential material for the anesthesiologist, and therefore, much of this chapter is devoted to this important neuromuscular condition. Other paraneoplastic and paraendocrine syndromes with important perioperative implications include Lambert-Eaton syndrome (LES) and other endocrine derangements commonly associated with malignancies. The final part of this chapter deals with this.

Thymic Surgery

Common indications for thymectomy include MG and the presence of thymic masses. Thymectomy for MG is covered in the following section. Here, the common masses of the thymus are briefly reviewed along with general anesthetic considerations. As an anterior mediastinal structure, the reader is also referred to Chap. 14 which addresses anterior mediastinal masses and the potential for compressive effects.

The most common tumor of the thymus and the anterior mediastinum is thymoma. Thymoma may be invasive or noninvasive, and 40% have associated paraneoplastic syndromes [1]. The most commonly associated paraneoplastic syndrome is MG (30%), but systemic lupus erythematosus, Cushing's syndrome, syndrome of inappropriate antidiuretic hormone secretion, and pure red cell aplasia may be associated [2].

Thymic carcinomas are much more rare than thymoma, and in contrast, they are always invasive and often present with symptoms reflective of their aggressive nature [3]. Paraneoplastic syndromes are possible but are much less common [4].

Thymic carcinoid is the most common member of the rare group of thymic neuroendocrine neoplasms. It is a potentially secretory tumor, commonly manifesting as Cushing's syndrome rather than the typical carcinoid syndrome [5]. At least 15% of thymic carcinoids present as part of multiple endocrine neoplasia (MEN-1) syndrome [1]. Surgery plays an important role in the management of thymic masses. Removal of all thymic tissue and perithymic fat is the current standard of care [6, 7] for malignant masses for optimal oncological clearance. The anesthesia considerations for non-myasthenia thymic surgery are similar to those for any anterior mediastinal mass. The anesthetist must maintain suspicion of compression of the major cardiopulmonary structures [8–10]. A history of cough, chest discomfort, dyspnea, palpitations, and syncope should be sought including any change associated with assuming the supine position. Symptoms may also occur due to paraneoplastic and paraendocrine syndromes, as detailed later in this chapter. Clinicians should screen for MG by inquiring about blurring vision, difficulty swallowing, or difficulty with speech. Invasive thymoma and thymic carcinoma tend to invade surrounding structure including major airways, pericardium, and great vessels; therefore imaging should be reviewed and resection of major structures discussed with the surgeon preoperatively [11]. A history of any preceding treatment should also be sought. Radiation to the chest can result in pulmonary fibrosis, coronary artery disease, valvular heart disease, and pericarditis [12]. Many chemotherapeutic agents have known implications for perioperative management, particularly cisplatin (a potential nephrotoxin) which is one of the most common chemotherapeutic drugs used in the treatment of thymoma; doxorubicin (with potential for decreased left ventricular function), vincristine (which causes neuropathy), and others may also be used [13, 14].

Myasthenia Gravis

First described in the seventeenth century, MG did not become a recognized entity until over 200 years later when Dr Friedrich Jolly titled the syndrome "myasthenia gravis pseudoparalytica" [15, 16]. At that time, MG almost uniformly caused death by respiratory failure within 1–2 years of illness. With a prevalence of 1:17,000 [17] and an established role for surgery in its management, the anesthesiologist must know how to optimize and safely manage these patients perioperatively.

Pathophysiology

MG is an autoimmune disease due to antibody-mediated destruction of nicotinic acetylcholine receptors [18] or other related proteins such as muscle-specific kinase (MuSK) or lipoprotein receptor-related protein 4 (LRP-4). As a result, the neuromuscular junctions (NMJs) of all muscles, even clinically unaffected muscles, have a reduced number of acetylcholine receptors [19, 20]. In addition to a reduced number of acetylcholine receptors, other abnormalities of the NMJ include reduced number and depth of the junctional folds in the postsynaptic membrane [21]. Autoantibodies are detectable in most cases, and the 10–20% of patients once considered "sero-negative" actually have AChR antibodies which are detectable through more advanced laboratory techniques or antibodies to MuSK or LRP-4.

Patients present with fluctuating skeletal muscle weakness which is made worse by activity and improves with rest. The reduction in postsynaptic acetylcholine receptors results in generation of fewer motor end-plate potentials; therefore fewer muscle fibers contract. With repeated or continued stimulation, even less motor end-plate potentials reach threshold, and weakness becomes more pronounced.

The cause of the immune reaction leading to MG is unknown. A very strong link exists between MG and thymic pathology. Most patients with MG exhibit thymic abnormalities which can range from hyperplasia (70–80%) to the presence of thymoma (10–15%), and 15% of patients with thymoma have MG. Furthermore, removal of the thymus results in clinical improvement in the majority of cases of MG [20, 22, 23].

MG is often associated with other conditions which share an underlying autoimmune tendency [17]. Diabetes and thyroid disorders (hyperthyroid or hypothyroid) are present in 5–6%, and 1–2% have rheumatoid arthritis. Systemic lupus erythematosus, leukemia, scleroderma, and polymyositis have also been found in higher numbers in the myasthenic population than in the general population [24].

Presentation

The majority of patients initially present due to diplopia (leading to blurring vision) or ptosis. Other presentations include difficulty swallowing or speaking due to bulbar dysfunction, dyspnea due to respiratory muscle compromise, or weakness of the neck or limbs. Symptoms always worsen with the use of the affected muscles, and strength returns after rest [16, 17]. The muscle groups affected can vary according to the serological profile: patients with AChR antibodies tend to have ocular involvement which progresses through limb weakness to bulbar symptoms, whereas MuSK antibodies tend to be ocular-sparing, and LRP-4 antibodies cause very mild generalized disease [25].

Acetylcholine receptor antibodies in MG are specific to the neuromuscular junction, so MG does not cause hemodynamic instability directly; however cardiac antibodies (such as anti-$\beta_1\beta_2$, ryanodine, and Kv1.4) are commonly also found, which can cause palpitations, dyspnea, mild hypertension, first-degree atrioventricular block, atrial fibrillation, and myocarditis. Diastolic dysfunction has also been noted [26–31].

Diagnosis

Since 1952, the first-line diagnostic test for MG has been the "Tensilon test" [32]. As an anticholinesterase of rapid onset (30 s) and offset (5 min), edrophonium (Tensilon™) is ideal for diagnostic testing. The inhibition of acetylcholine breakdown allows acetylcholine to accumulate and stimulate the reduced number of postjunctional receptors. Intravenous edrophonium is administered, and muscle performance is assessed within 30–90s. Clear improvement in the affected muscles, as measured qualitatively and quantitatively, is found in of MG [20, 24]. However, this test has a significant false-positive rate, and current guidelines [33–35] advise AChR antibody assay, with MuSK antibody assay if negative, in conjunction with thyroid function tests and CT of the chest as first-line investigations. In cases of diagnostic dilemma, referral for formal neurophysiological testing, including Tensilon test, as well as MRI brain is made.

Classification

In 1971, Dr. Osserman based a classification scheme on the observation of over 1200 patients at the Myasthenia Gravis Clinic in New York [24]. In its modified form, this continues to be of use today (see Table 15.1). Patients are placed into a grade based on their weakest muscle group. More recently, a task force put together by the Myasthenia Gravis Foundation of America (MGFA) developed a clinical classification scheme to facilitate standardization of reporting (see Table 15.2).

Medical Management

Pyridostigmine is the anticholinesterase of choice for management of MG. Others are available for oral use; however, the effectiveness, kinetics, and tolerability of pyridostigmine are the most favorable [38]. Side effects, usually uncommon or mild, include diarrhea, bronchorrhea, and abdominal cramping.

After an oral dose of pyridostigmine, an effect may be seen as early as 30 min later, and the peak effect is reached

Table 15.1 Modified Osserman grades

Type I	Disease localized to ocular muscles Tends not to progress if remains confined to ocular muscles for first 2 years
Type IIA	Mild generalized myasthenia Slowly progressive often from ocular muscles to skeletal and bulbar muscles, however spares muscles of respiration Good response to drug therapy and low mortality
Type IIB	Moderate generalized myasthenia Gradual onset, usually ocular, progressing to more generalized bulbar and skeletal muscle involvement Respiratory muscles are not involved More bulbar symptoms than IIA Less responsive to medical therapy than IIA
Type III	Severe disease Progression may be gradual or sudden deterioration Poor response to drug therapy High mortality
Type IV	Myasthenic crisis with respiratory failure Require intubation

Based on data from Refs. [24, 36]

Table 15.2 MGFA clinical classification

Class	Description	Subclassification (where applicable)
I	Isolated ocular weakness	–
II	Mild weakness of extraocular muscles	(a) Predominantly affecting limb, axial muscles, or both
III	Moderate weakness of extraocular muscles	(b) Predominantly affecting oropharyngeal, respiratory muscles, or both
IV	Severe weakness of extraocular muscles	(a) Swallowing unaffected (b) Requiring feeding tube without intubation
V	Intubation	

Adapted from Ref. [37]

1 to 2 h later. The duration of action is usually between 3 and 6 h. The nonsustained release formulation can be crushed and given via nasogastric tube. If required, pyridostigmine can also be given intravenously with an oral to intravenous conversion ratio of 30:1.

There is great interindividual variability in the kinetics of oral pyridostigmine; therefore the dose and frequency are titrated to reach optimum effect for each individual [38, 39]. The symptomatic control provided by anticholinesterases is often incomplete, so most patients find themselves on additional medication in the form of immunosuppression.

Corticosteroids are commonly used to treat MG; however, the considerable side effect profile (see Table 15.3) of long-term corticosteroids makes them undesirable as an immunosuppressant. Once a patient has achieved remission, corticosteroids are usually tapered to their lowest effective dose. Frequently, corticosteroids are helpful to gain more control of the disease process, while other immunosuppressants are being initiated [40].

Table 15.3 Adverse effects of corticosteroids

Gastrointestinal	Dyspepsia Peptic ulcers
Body habitus	Truncal obesity
Skin and musculoskeletal	Acne Easy bruising Delayed wound healing Aseptic necrosis of the femoral head Osteoporosis
Metabolic, fluid, and electrolyte	Hypertension Peripheral edema Hypokalemia Hyperglycemia/glucose intolerance Adrenal suppression
Muscle	Myopathy
Behavior	Anxiety Psychosis

Azathioprine is one such alternative immunosuppressant which may take months to have an effect. A maximal benefit may take up to 24 months; however its use allows corticosteroids to be minimized [38]. Adverse effects include bone marrow suppression, hepatotoxicity (usually mild and reversible), and gastrointestinal upset.

Cyclosporine is a potent immunosuppressant agent with onset much sooner than azathioprine. Greater risks of toxicity limit its use. Common and severe adverse side effects include hypertension, nephrotoxicity, hepatotoxicity, and bone marrow suppression. Levels must be monitored regularly [38, 40].

First reported in 1976 [41], the role of plasmapheresis for the treatment of MG has grown substantially. Treatments occur over 1–2 weeks and consist of three to five exchanges of plasma via a temporarily placed dialysis catheter. Each treatment removes 1–3 L. There is a reduction in acetylcholine receptor antibody titers in patients who have measurable antibodies. Benefits are usually seen after one or two exchanges, and, once a course is completed, the improvement can last for 2 weeks to 2 months. Indications for treatment include bulbar symptoms, myasthenic crisis, or preoperative optimization in patients who are at high risk of postoperative respiratory failure [42].

Intravenous immunoglobulin (IVIG) represents a similar immune-mediating therapy for MG. Its role is not as extensively studied as plasmapheresis, and a Cochrane review based on six randomized controlled trials found limited evidence for its use in chronic MG [42]. However, it is recommended as a first-line treatment in patients with acute relapse requiring hospital admission, in particular requiring intensive care [33]. IVIG is preferred to plasmapheresis as its efficacy is similar and it is more easily applied [43]. As a blood product pooled from a large volume of donor plasma, it carries with it risks inherent to any blood product. The dose is given intravenously over 2–5 days, and adverse reactions are mild and tolerable (fever, nausea, headache). Benefit is seen within 4 days and peaks by 2 weeks; it may last 40–100 days. The mechanism of action remains unknown.

Surgical Management

In 1939, the first thymectomy was performed by Dr. Blalock and resulted in remission of MG [44]. Dr Blalock followed this success with a series of thymectomies with similarly positive results [45, 46]. Today, thymectomy remains an important part of the management of MG although there remains controversy regarding its indications, timing, and preferred surgical approach [47–52]. Despite the first thymectomy for MG being reported in 1939, a randomized trial demonstrating effectiveness has only just been completed, which demonstrated that patients who received thymectomy in addition to immunosuppression required lower prednisolone doses (44 vs 60 mg, $P < 0.001$), were less likely to need supplemental immunosuppression with azathioprine (17 vs 48%, $P < 0.001$), and were less likely to be hospitalized for exacerbations (9 vs 37%, $P < 0.001$) [53]. Thymectomy for MG, while already established in clinical practice, is now backed by high-quality evidence. Remission does not immediately follow removal of the thymus gland. It may take months to years for remission or significant improvement in the disease to occur. By 5 years, 34–46% of patients have complete remission, and another 33–40% are significantly improved [38]. The other indication for thymectomy is the presence of a thymoma or thymic carcinoma, for relief or mass effect and oncological clearance [38, 39].

The preferred surgical approach for removal of thymoma remains median sternotomy, as this provides optimal surgical access to facilitate a full oncological clearance.

However, a wide range of minimally invasive approaches are practiced for nonthymomatous MG, including transcervical, subxiphoid, ministernotomy, and both right and left VATS [54]. The rarity of MG makes performing randomized controlled trials of these surgical approaches difficult, but published case series demonstrate similar long-term outcomes in terms of reduction of MG symptoms [48, 55]. The anesthesiologist may encounter any combination of different approaches, depending on surgical and institutional preference.

Myasthenic vs Cholinergic Crisis

A myasthenic crisis refers to rapidly deteriorating strength which threatens the life of the patient. The most common causes of crisis are infection, surgery, and drugs (see Table 15.4); however, in many cases no underlying precipitant can be found.

Table 15.4 Precipitants of myasthenic crisis

Stress
Surgery
Infection
Drugs
Aminoglycosides
Quinolones
Macrolides
Beta-blockers
Calcium channel blockers
Magnesium salts
Iodinated contrast agents
Phenytoin
Procainamide

Based on data from Ref. [56]

Table 15.5 Manifestations of cholinergic crisis

Motor: fasciculations, weakness
Cardiac: bradycardia
Respiratory: bronchorrhea
Ocular: miosis
Gastrointestinal: salivation, nausea, vomiting, colic, diarrhea
General: pallor, diaphoresis

Patients with myasthenic crisis will be in respiratory failure due to weakness of the diaphragm and other muscles of respiration. Management requires intubation and admission to and intensive care unit for respiratory care [57]. Correctable causes should be sought and treated, high-dose prednisolone reinstituted, and IVIG given as first-line treatment. Patients who have not recovered at 5 days may require second dose of IVIG or plasmapheresis.

In contrast to myasthenic crisis, a cholinergic crisis is caused by too much acetylcholine at the cholinergic receptors. It is most often caused by a relative overdose of anticholinesterase. This syndrome has become uncommon with present-day management because the use of immunosuppressants has meant that smaller doses of anticholinesterases are used [56]. The high levels of acetylcholine at all cholinergic receptors have multi-system effects. At the NMJ, it creates an endogenous depolarization type of phenomenon causing fasciculations and muscle weakness [58]. The respiratory distress due to muscle weakness may be further compounded by bronchorrhea. Other manifestations are attributable to muscarinic stimulation (Table 15.5).

Differentiating a cholinergic vs myasthenic crisis can be difficult as both can present with weakness and respiratory distress. In addition to a history of recent events, pupil size, muscarinic signs, and Tensilon test may be helpful, but should be applied with caution in acutely ill patients, as it may precipitate complete respiratory failure. The pupils are constricted in a cholinergic crisis and dilated in a myasthenic crisis (due to sympathetic activation). Treatment includes intubation, antimuscarinics, and supportive care.

Anesthetic Considerations

The anesthesiologist will be confronted with myasthenic patients coming for thymectomy as well as those coming for surgery unrelated to their disease. Whenever possible, surgery should never be undertaken without preoperative stabilization and optimization of MG.

Anesthetic considerations include minimizing the risk of a myasthenic crisis and facilitating sustained extubation at the end of a general anesthetic. If a thymectomy is planned, then considerations of thymoma and anterior mediastinal mass may also apply (see earlier).

Preoperatively, it is important to ask about the duration of disease and its severity, particularly with respect to ocular, bulbar, respiratory, and generalized symptoms. Many attempts have been made to delineate preoperative characteristics which predict the need for postoperative ventilation. The Leventhal criteria are often cited for this purpose [59] and are based on a retrospective review of 24 patients who underwent transsternal thymectomy (see Table 15.6). The criteria have been evaluated in other settings and have been found inaccurate in predicting the need for postoperative ventilation in patients undergoing other types of thymectomy as well as nonthymectomy surgery [60, 61]. Despite continued attempts to develop a model predictive of the need for postoperative ventilation, no such model has been consistently reliable. Anesthesiologists may use a series of preoperative factors examined in the literature which have been suggested to be predictive in various settings (see Table 15.7)

Patients should be questioned for any cardiac symptoms of palpitations, syncope, dyspnea, and any manifestations of congestive heart failure. A history of associated autoimmune conditions, particularly thyroid dysfunction, should be sought. In order to plan perioperative medical management, detailed history of current medications should be noted on the chart. Use of corticosteroids is usually tapered or discontinued preoperatively where possible, but ongoing use may necessitate a stress dose of steroids preoperatively. Use of other immunosuppressants should also prompt a search for signs of toxicity or adverse effects. Table 15.8 lists suggested preoperative investigations

Preoperative optimization should be undertaken in cooperation with a neurologist familiar with the care of myasthenia. Plasmapheresis or IVIG may be arranged to reduce the chances of perioperative respiratory failure. As these treatments are not without adverse effects, their routine use may

expose patients to unnecessary risk [64]. In general, patients with advanced disease, bulbar symptoms, or poor pulmonary function receive these immune-modulating therapies [28, 65]. It should be noted that preoperative plasmapheresis depletes plasma cholinesterase, so the duration of some neuromuscular-blocking drugs (e.g., succinylcholine, mivacurium, and remifentanil) will be prolonged [36].

There are different approaches to perioperative dosing of anticholinesterases. Some advocate the complete omission of anticholinesterase medications on the day of surgery in order to reduce the need for muscle relaxants [66]. Anticholinesterases may be given intraoperatively near the end of the procedure to facilitate extubation with this approach. See Table 15.9 for useful conversion factors of

Table 15.6 Leventhal criteria

| Disease duration >6 years |
| Pyridostigmine dose >750 mg/day |
| Preoperative vital capacity <2.9 L |
| Presence of other respiratory disease |

Based on data from Ref. [59]

Table 15.7 Prediction of myasthenia gravis patients at high risk of prolonged postoperative ventilator support

| Advanced disease |
| Myasthenia Gravis Foundation class II or higher |
| Myasthenia gravis for >6 years |
| History of steroid requirement for myasthenia gravis |
| History of myasthenia gravis-induced respiratory insufficiency |
| Vital capacity <2.9 L |
| Pyridostigmine dose >750 mg/day |
| Maximum respiratory force <40–50 cmH20 |

Based on data from Refs. [28, 59, 60, 62, 63]

Table 15.8 Suggested preoperative investigations for the patient with myasthenia gravis

Complete blood count	May have pernicious anemia, red cell aplasia, bone marrow suppression from immunosuppressants
Electrolytes, creatinine, liver function	As required depending on immunosuppressants
TSH	Commonly have thyroid dysfunction
Chest X-ray	Rule out thymoma/mediastinal mass, pneumonia (particularly aspiration if bulbar symptoms)
ECG	Arrhythmias, atrial fibrillation
Echo	If signs or symptoms of cardiac involvement
Pulmonary function tests	Useful to compare to previous for baseline

Table 15.9 Conversion between anticholinesterases for management of myasthenia gravis

Drug and formulation	Dose equivalent	Onset	Time to maximum response	Duration of action
Pyridostigmine oral	60 mg	40 min	1 h	4 h
Neostigmine oral	15 mg	1 h	1.5 h	30 min
Neostigmine IM	1.5 mg	30 min	1 h	30 min
Neostigmine IV	0.5 mg	5–10 min	20 min	30 min

Reprinted with permission from Ropper and Samuels [67]. McGraw-Hill companies. Copyright 2009

anticholinesterase drugs. Another approach is to give half the usual morning dose for patients with grade I or II disease and the full dose for more severe cases [68]. Still others advocate giving patients their full dose at their usual schedule [69].

The approach followed at our institution, as well as others, is to give patients their usual dose of pyridostigmine preoperatively. Ideally, the patient delays their morning dose until immediately preoperatively when it is given with a sip of water. Patients are scheduled as early in the day as possible to facilitate this approach. The goal is optimal strength at the time of extubation. While myasthenics have intact respiratory drive in response to arterial CO_2 and are not at greater risk of respiratory depression caused by opioids or benzodiazepines, it is conceivable that preoperative sedation may act synergistically with respiratory muscle weakness to cause respiratory compromise, so these drugs should be used cautiously if at all. Monitors and invasive lines are dictated by the individual patient and the planned surgery; however, regardless of whether neuromuscular-blocking drugs are used, the use of nerve monitoring is essential.

Myasthenic patients are exquisitely sensitive to all nondepolarizing muscle relaxants (NDMR) [70–72]. The underlying muscle weakness due to the disease combined with the muscle-relaxing properties of intravenous and volatile anesthetics often makes the use of muscle relaxants unnecessary. The use of remifentanil can reduce the response to airway manipulation and allow intubation without NMDRs; however Fujita et al. report a rate of postoperative respiratory failure of 28% with this technique [73], so it cannot be regarded as fail-safe.

Circumstances may rise when paralysis becomes necessary. For intermediate-acting neuromuscular-blocking agents, a dose reduction to one-fifth the usual is recommended. Long-acting neuromuscular blockade should be avoided [74, 75]. Patients who have received their pyridostigmine preoperatively may have a prolonged action of mivacurium due to the interaction with plasma cholinesterase [76].

The reversal of neuromuscular blockade is another area of controversy. The safest recommendation is to choose a minimal dose of short-acting NDMR and ensure that the effect has completely terminated spontaneously [69]. Sugammadex, a cyclodextrin which rapidly and completely terminates the action of rocuronium and vecuronium, is a very attractive option for NMDR reversal in MG. There are a number of case reports [77, 78] and case series [79, 80] which support this as a strategy. However, it may not always be successful [81], as other intraoperative factors and drugs can affect the NMJ (see Table 15.4). In addition, if a patient appears weak and in respiratory distress postoperatively, differentiating between insufficient reversal and cholinergic crisis is very difficult. If such a situation is encountered, supportive care with appropriate ventilation is recommended until the diagnosis becomes clear, and appropriate anticholinesterase levels are re-established.

In contrast to the response to NDMR, myasthenic patients show resistance to succinylcholine due to the loss of nicotinic receptors [82, 83]. Eisenkraft et al. have demonstrated that the ED50 is twice normal and recommend using a dose of 1.5–2 mg/kg if rapid sequence induction conditions are required [82]. The onset of the depolarizing block may take longer than expected [69]. Myasthenics are also more likely to develop a phase II block, particularly with repeated doses [84], and the duration of action may be prolonged if cholinesterase inhibitors have been taken that day.

Volatile anesthetics (halothane and particularly sevoflurane and isoflurane) have potent muscle relaxation effects in normal patients and have been shown to reduce neuromuscular transmission by close to 50% [85–87]. The dose of volatile required to achieve this depth may lead to hemodynamic instability. To minimize inhalational agents, they have been combined with regional anesthesia [88] or remifentanil infusion. Desflurane's lower blood-gas partition coefficient has a theoretical advantage and has been used with good results [89, 90].

The use of total intravenous anesthesia (TIVA) for patients with MG has grown, particularly with the widespread use of remifentanil [89, 91, 92]. Propofol, etomidate, and ketamine have also been used uneventfully, and effects on neuromuscular transmission are minimal [93]. Opioids should be minimized because of the central respiratory depression as described earlier. For pain management perioperatively, consideration should be given to opioid-sparing techniques such as regional anesthesia or multimodal analgesia plans.

The use of regional anesthesia for myasthenics has many advantages; however, possible drug interactions must be kept in mind [94]. Local anesthetics (ester and amide) have some inhibitory effect on neuromuscular transmission, and this can be potentiated further in the presence of NDMR [95]. If regional anesthesia is used, it is recommended to reduce the maximum dose of local anesthetic [39, 74]. However, modern ultrasound-guided regional anesthesia practice allows much lower volumes of local anesthetic to be used, much reducing the risk of this rare interaction.

The place of thoracic epidural anesthesia (TEA) in the perioperative management of MG has changed dramatically. Traditionally, concern over blockade of intercostal muscles causing respiratory distress precluded the use of TEA [69]. Many examples now exist of the successful use of TEA intraoperatively as well as postoperatively [92, 96–98]. The benefits of excellent analgesia, muscle relaxation, and opioid sparing have translated into earlier extubation and a reduced need for postoperative ventilator support [92, 97]. Intrathecal opioids have similarly proven beneficial in terms of analgesia and optimizing respiratory function postoperatively [99, 100].

The perioperative management of patients with MG coming for surgery requires a team of experts in neurology, surgery, and anesthesia. No anesthetic technique has been shown to be superior in MG. The individualization of a perioperative plan encompassing the principles presented here is suggested.

Paraendocrine and Paraneoplastic Syndromes

Paraendocrine and paraneoplastic syndromes must be kept in mind when patients present with malignancy. Table 15.10 contains the most common paraneoplastic syndromes that may be encountered. The remainder of this chapter will be devoted to the discussion of the carcinoid syndrome (a paraendocrine syndrome) and LES (a paraneoplastic syndrome). Although not common, both have important implications for the anesthesiologist.

Carcinoid Tumors

Carcinoid tumors are most commonly found in the gastrointestinal tract where they often present due to bowel obstruction or are discovered due to symptoms of carcinoid syndrome. Primary carcinoids outside of the GI tract have originated in the ovary [102], liver [103, 104], and thymus [105, 106], but the most common extraintestinal location is the lung [107].

Bronchial carcinoids account for 2–5% of primary lung tumors; however, this makes up 20–30% of all carcinoids [107]. Seventy-five percent of bronchial carcinoids are centrally located therefore present with symptoms of postobstructive pneumonia, hemoptysis, and dyspnea [108]. The remaining one-quarter occur peripherally in the lung, are asymptomatic, and are usually detected on routine chest radiography [108].

It is estimated that 15–20% of all carcinoids give rise to paraendocrine syndromes, most notable the "carcinoid syn-

drome" [107]. Carcinoid tumors may secrete well over a dozen compounds, including serotonin, histamine, catecholamines (norepinephrine and dopamine), bradykinins, ACTH, GHRH, and others [109]. The secretory behavior of the tumor as well as the exposure to the systemic circulation determines whether a paraendocrine syndrome will develop. Enzymes capable of metabolizing the secretory products are present in the liver and lung. Tumor products secreted from gastrointestinal carcinoids travel to the liver via the portal circulation and are inactivated before a paraendocrine syndrome can be manifested. If metastases to the liver occur, secretory products may enter the systemic circulation via the hepatic vein and exert their systemic effects.

The carcinoid syndrome is classically described as the triad of flushing, diarrhea, and bronchospasm. In addition, patients complain of sweating, tachycardia, and dyspnea. Diarrhea can be particularly troublesome, occurring up to 30 times per day and causing fluid and electrolyte disturbances as well as weight loss [110]. The limerick below aptly describes the classic patient with carcinoid syndrome:

> *This man was addicted to moanin'*
> *Confusion, edema and groanin'*
> *Intestinal rushes*
> *Great tricolored blushes*
> *And died from too much serotonin*
> Samuel A. Wells [111]

Carcinoid crises are life-threatening, severe episodes of profound flushing, hypertension or hypotension, arrhythmia, bronchoconstriction, and alteration of mental status [110, 112]. Crisis may be triggered by emotional stress, heat, cold, ingestion of certain foods (such as alcohol, chocolate), straining, as well as physical manipulation of the tumor (abdominal palpation or biopsy) [109, 113].

A significant proportion of carcinoid syndromes occur in the bronchus and, less commonly, in the thymus [106] and therefore will be encountered by the thoracic anesthesiologist. In contrast to gastrointestinal carcinoids, bronchial and thymic carcinoids are seldom secretory. Less than 5% of

Table 15.10 Common paraneoplastic syndromes

	Humoral hypercalcemia	SIADH	Cushing's syndrome
Associated malignancy	Squamous cell cancers of the lung, esophagus, head, and neck. Breast cancer, more rarely ovarian cancer	Small cell lung cancer and squamous cell cancer of the head and neck	Small cell lung cancer bronchial carcinoid, medullary thyroid cancer, pancreatic islet cell tumors, pheochromocytoma
Presentation	Muscle weakness, cardiac arrhythmias, nausea and vomiting, renal failure	Hyponatremia, decreased serum osmolarity, inappropriately increased urine osmolarity, euvolemia, normal thyroid, and adrenal function	Hypokalemia, alkalosis, hypertension, psychosis
Etiology	Increased release of parathyroid-related peptides and other cytokines	Production of arginine vasopressin by tumor	Abnormally high secretion of ACTH or CRH
Management	Treat malignancy, hydrate, diuresis, calcitonin, steroids, bisphosphonates	Treat malignancy, fluid restriction, demeclocycline	Dexamethasone suppression (for some tumors), bromocriptine, ketoconazole

Based on data from Ref. [101]
ACTH adrenocorticotrophic hormone, *CRH* corticotrophin-releasing hormone

bronchial carcinoids exhibit paraendocrine syndromes [108]. When the rare secretory bronchial carcinoid is encountered, the symptoms described above may be unusually severe and prolonged. In addition to the classical carcinoid syndrome, bronchial and thymic carcinoids may secrete exclusively ACTH (causing Cushing's syndrome) or even GHRH (causing acromegaly) [114–118]. In fact, bronchial and thymic carcinoids are the most common causes of ectopic ACTH outside the pituitary and adrenal glands [105]. Therefore, although the lung is the most common location of extraintestinal carcinoids, secretion of metabolically active compounds is rare. Although often nonsecretory, the vascularity of these tumors should be kept in mind in the cases of bronchoscopy and particularly biopsy. Severe hemorrhage can result and may require emergency thoracotomy [119].

Advanced carcinoid disease is associated with fibrosis which is attributed to the mitogenic effect of serotonin on smooth muscle and connective tissue. In the abdomen, this may present as retroperitoneal or omental fibrosis, but in the cardiopulmonary system, this can lead to pulmonary hypertension and carcinoid heart disease [109, 120].

Carcinoid heart disease manifests as right-sided valvulopathy, most notably with severe tricuspid regurgitation with progressive volume overload of the right-sided heart chambers. Its onset is usually preceded by a history of carcinoid syndrome indicating passage of secretory products into the systemic circulation and therefore into the chambers of the right heart [121]. Although most often attributed to serotonin, the reduction of serotonin levels by medical management does not alter progression of heart disease indicating that other secretory products are involved in the pathophysiology [122]. The left-sided cardiac chambers are considered to be "protected" by the pulmonary circulation which metabolizes carcinoid products; however, in the presence of a secretory bronchial carcinoid or a right to left shunt, left-sided carcinoid heart disease is seen and manifests as regurgitant mitral and aortic valve lesions [122]. With time, the right ventricle becomes hypokinetic, and right-sided heart failure develops with severe dyspnea, ascites, and peripheral edema. Management options are limited. Medical therapies used for left-sided heart failure often have limited effect or may even worsen right-sided heart failure [121, 122]. Surgical management is the only option and carries a 35% mortality rate [119].

Medical management of carcinoid syndrome was revolutionized by the discovery that the tumor cells often possess somatostatin receptors. Somatostatin, or its longer-acting analog octreotide, is able to suppress tumor secretion and alleviate the symptoms of carcinoid syndrome in most patients [123]. Prior to the introduction of octreotide, management of the carcinoid syndrome involved a variety of antihistamine and antiserotonergic drugs with limited efficacy. Despite the ability to control symptoms of carcinoid

disease, octreotide has no effect on tumor growth. Use of chemotherapeutic agents has had limited success in carcinoid tumors making surgical resection the definitive therapy.

Preoperative assessment of patients with carcinoid tumors is influenced by whether the tumor is secretory or not. This is determined by history or by urinary levels of 5-HIAA (a serotonin metabolite) in the case of asymptomatic patients. A nonsecretory tumor has less significance for the anesthesiologist. In the case of carcinoid syndrome, the history should ascertain the severity of symptoms as well as how well they are controlled with medical therapy. The severity of symptoms does not predict the intraoperative course; however, it is helpful to know that the tumor is responsive to octreotide [124]. Physical examination should look for signs of right-sided valvulopathy and heart failure. Preoperative investigations should include complete blood count, electrolytes, liver function tests, and creatinine as well as measurement of blood glucose. All patients should have an electrocardiogram and chest X-ray to screen for cardiac disease; however, an echocardiogram is the definitive test for carcinoid heart disease.

Perioperative care of the patient with carcinoid syndrome involves avoidance of triggers and preparation to manage crisis, particularly at times of tumor manipulation.

Preoperative optimization should correct hypovolemia and electrolyte imbalances. Preoperative sedation with benzodiazepine (lorazepam sublingual 2 mg, 90 min preoperatively) is highly recommended, and consideration may be given to use of cyproheptadine (4 mg; antihistamine and antiserotonergic) as well. Patients should receive octreotide 50–100 mcg sc BID for at least 24 h prior to induction with an additional 100mcg sc 1 h preoperatively [119, 121, 124].

Intraoperatively, monitors should be placed while the patient is awake. In addition to standard monitors, invasive blood pressure monitoring is required, and central access is indicated for CVP monitoring, rapid administration of drugs, fluids, and blood if required. Temperature monitoring and body warmers should be used as hypothermia is a trigger of crises. In the presence of cardiac disease, transesophageal echocardiography should be readily available. Octreotide infusion at 100–250mcg/h is recommended [112, 119] and may be started once in the operating room. A smooth induction and blunting of airway reflexes for intubation are ideal. Nonhistamine-releasing opioids such as fentanyl or remifentanil may be used with good results [125]. The use of NDMR is safe provided histamine release is avoided. Succinylcholine use is controversial. Some practitioners strictly avoid it due to concern over histamine release and concern over precipitating a crisis secondary to fasciculations [112, 119]. In a review of 21 patients with carcinoid syndrome, Veall et al. [126] used succinylcholine in half of patients uneventfully. Therefore, in optimized patients, the use of succinylcholine should not be considered contraindicated when airway or other concerns make it the best choice of muscle relaxant.

Intraoperatively, electrolytes and glucose should be monitored, and hyperglycemia may require insulin infusion. Octreotide, diluted to 10–50 mcg/mL, should be readily available for emergency use in doses of 50–100mcg iv titrated to response.

Carcinoid crisis may manifest as profound hypertension or hypotension accompanied by bronchospasm. Hypertension may be treated by increasing anesthetic depth, administering a bolus of short-acting opioid [126], using β-blockade (metoprolol or esmolol) [124], or administering octreotide. Kataserin, a selective serotonin antagonist with α-1 blocking effects, has also been described as useful (dose 5–10 mg) but has Vaughn-Williams class I and III antiarrhythmic effects and may prolong QT interval [121, 124]. Cyproheptadine (1 mg) and methotrimeprazine (2.5 mg) are serotonin antagonists which have also been described for the management of hypertensive carcinoid crisis.

Profound hypotension is a more common manifestation of crisis intraoperatively and may be severe. The treatment of choice is octreotide boluses as described above. Intravenous octreotide reaches peak effect after 4 min; there are no significant side effects, and doses may need to be escalated until a response is seen [126]. Vasopressin or phenylephrine has also been described as an additional therapy if hypotension is refractory [124, 127]. Additional management of hypotension includes fluid resuscitation, reduction of anesthetic depth, and cessation of surgical manipulation. Catecholamines are usually avoided in the treatment of hypotension as they may precipitate further crisis; however recent data suggest they may be used in patients who have been optimized with somatostatin analogs [122]. If necessary, small boluses should be administered and the response observed carefully. In addition to the above, calcium, angiotensin, and milrinone are also considered safe [112, 126].

The management of bronchospasm with salbutamol is another area of controversy. Noncatecholamine bronchodilators (ipratropium bromide), steroids, antihistamines, and octreotide have been suggested as effective for crisis-associated bronchospasm [124]. Others describe the safe and effective use of salbutamol and advocate its use despite sympathomimetic activity [102, 126]. While noncatecholamine bronchodilators should be considered first, salbutamol is not contraindicated particularly in the optimized patient with bronchospasm.

Neuraxial anesthesia is controversial in a patient population at risk for acute hemodynamic instability; however both epidural [125, 128] and spinal anesthesias [129] have been described even in the presence of severe carcinoid heart disease. Keys to this approach noted by all authors included fluid loading, and minimization of hemodynamic changes with careful drug selection.

Postoperatively, delayed awakening has been described and attributed to the high serotonin levels. Patients require an intensive care environment where hemodynamic monitoring and continuation of drug infusions are possible. Manifestations of carcinoid syndrome may continue due to residual tumor or unresected metastases. Octreotide infusions should be continued or weaned slowly while monitoring for manifestations of secretory activity. Postoperative analgesia is imperative to avoid triggering crisis, and for this reason, the benefits of a carefully titrated epidural infusion may outweigh the risks.

Lambert-Eaton Myasthenic Syndrome (LEMS)

LEMS is a common paraneoplastic neurological syndrome associated with lung cancer [130]. Fifty to sixty percent of patients with LEMS will subsequently be diagnosed with a malignancy, most commonly small cell lung cancer (SCLC), within 2 years [131].

LEMS bears a striking resemblance to MG at first glance, but there are many important differences (Table 15.11). While MG is a disease affecting the postsynaptic membrane, LEMS is due to a reduction in acetylcholine release from the presynaptic nerve terminal [132–134]. An autoimmune attack directed against the voltage-gated calcium channels of the presynaptic nerve terminal reduces calcium entry into the presynaptic nerve terminal. As a result of reduced calcium influx, there is markedly reduced acetylcholine release leading to symptoms of LEMS.

The most common symptom of LEMS is proximal lower extremity weakness. Many also experience autonomic symptoms such as dry mouth, impotence, constipation, and orthostatic hypotension. Ocular and bulbar muscle involvement may be present, but it is often mild and usually not the presenting feature. Respiratory muscle weakness can occur but usually as a late complication [135].

Table 15.11 Myasthenia gravis vs. Lambert-Eaton syndrome

Feature	Myasthenia gravis	Lambert-Eaton syndrome
Most common malignancy	Thymoma (40%)	Small cell lung cancer (1–3%)
Antibody target	Post synaptic acetylcholine, MuSK, LRP-4 receptors	Presynaptic voltage-gated calcium channels
Common presenting feature	Ocular progressing to limb and then bulbar weakness	Limb weakness, ocular and bulbar sparing
Autonomic dysfunction	Rare	Common
Deep tendon reflexes	Normal	Reduced
Exercise effect	Weakness exacerbated	Weakness reduced

Management of LEMS is usually medical as patients with SCLC are often not operative candidates for resection of their malignancy. 3,4-Diaminopyridine is a potassium channel-blocking drug which causes the depolarization of the presynaptic nerve terminal to be prolonged. This allows time for increased calcium influx which results in increased acetylcholine release and greater clinical strength [131]. There may also be a role for IVIG and plasmapheresis in some cases [102].

Patients with LEMS presenting for anesthesia are very sensitive to both succinylcholine and NDMR [131]. Therapy with 3,4-diaminopyridine should be continued up to the time of surgery. The use of paralytics should be minimized and, if necessary, should be titrated in very small doses and monitored closely. Reversal of neuromuscular blockade by usual means is seldom effective. The administration of 3,4-diaminopyridine concomitantly with reversal agents has met with some success [136, 137]. Additional consideration should be given to the potential for autonomic disturbances, and provision should be made preoperatively for postoperative ventilation if required.

Case Discussion

Case A 32-year-old female presents for preoperative assessment. She is booked for a transcervical thymectomy for MG. In addition to the usual preoperative assessment, consider:

- What additional information, specific to this patient, should be gathered at the preoperative anesthesia consultation?
- Appropriate investigations
- How will you optimize her for her upcoming surgery?
- What premedication will she require including dosing of her current medication?
- Appropriate preoperative disposition
- Your anesthetic technique of choice including acute postoperative pain management

What Additional Information, Specific to This Patient, Should Be Gathered at the Preoperative Anesthesia Consultation?

In addition to the usual elements of a preoperative consultation, the preoperative visit should serve to characterize the severity of MG in this patient as well as determine if there are any mediastinal compressive symptoms. A history of associated autoimmune disorders should also be sought.

Determine when the patient was diagnosed with MG and how the disease has progressed. Determine if the symptoms have been purely ocular or if they have involved bulbar muscles (putting the patient at risk for dysphagia and aspiration), axial or limb muscles, or if the patient has had any episodes of respiratory failure requiring ventilator support. Determine the management history, particularly the dose and frequency of pyridostigmine and what consequences are of delaying a dose. Is there a history of steroid requirements or the use of any other immunosuppressant drugs?

A history of palpitations, chest pain, or dyspnea on exertion as well as findings consistent with heart failure should be sought due to the possibility of cardiac involvement. The association with thyroid dysfunction, rheumatoid arthritis, and lupus should prompt screening questions which may or may not require additional medical consultation and optimization.

To screen for a thymoma with mass effect, a history of orthopnea, supine dyspnea, or cough should be sought. Changes in voice (dysphonia, hoarseness), palpitations, syncope, edema of the face or tongue, and dysphagia are other signs of mediastinal compression; however, dysphagia and dysphonia may also be due to MG.

This patient has been diagnosed with MG for 5 years. She initially presented with oculobulbar symptoms which were well controlled with pyridostigmine. Over the last few years, increasing doses have been required eventually prompting referral for surgical treatment. She does not have any associated autoimmune disorders and denies all symptoms of mass compression. To her knowledge, there is no thymoma present. She takes 80 mg of pyridostigmine every 4 h and feels weakness if she is more than an hour later with her dose. Her usual first dose is around 6 o'clock in the morning.

Appropriate Investigations

Bloodwork: CBC (pernicious anemia) and crossmatch are mandatory. Strongly consider electrolytes and creatinine, coagulation profile, and TSH as well.

Imaging must be reviewed, CXR and chest CT for the presence of thymoma. Bloodwork in this patient is all within normal limits. Her TSH is normal. The radiologist's reports do not mention any sign of aspiration pneumonia nor any thymoma causing compression of cardiopulmonary structures.

How Will You Optimize Her for Her Upcoming Surgery?

Confirm that the patient's neurologist is aware of the upcoming surgery and discuss possible plasmapheresis or IVIG to optimize the patient's muscle strength and minimize the chances of postoperative respiratory failure and the need for postoperative ventilation. Pyridostigmine should be continued up to the day of surgery, and the surgery should be scheduled first thing in the morning. The patient should be instructed to take their morning dose of pyridostigmine as close to the time of surgery as possible. If surgery takes longer than expected, an intravenous supplemental anticholinesterase may be given or an additional dose of oral pyridostigmine may be given via nasogastric tube. No premedication with sedating effects should be ordered.

What Is the Anesthetic Technique of Choice Including Postoperative Pain Management?

General anesthesia with endotracheal intubation is the technique of choice under these circumstances. Induction with propofol and remifentanil is recommended (no neuromuscular blockade). Maintenance may be achieved with a volatile such as desflurane or with a propofol infusion. Remifentanil may be used as an analgesic infusion. Pre- or intraoperative acetaminophen and nonsteroidal anti-inflammatory (such as Naprosyn or ketorolac) should also be used and continued postoperatively. The surgeon should also be asked to infiltrate the wound with local anesthetic solution at closure.

What Is the Most Appropriate Postoperative Disposition?

Patients undergoing transcervical thymectomy for nonthymomatous MG have significantly less pain and respiratory dysfunction than patients undergoing transsternal thymectomy. Provided that the patient can be optimized preoperatively with plasmapheresis or equivalent, an overnight stay in a regular ward is appropriate. Pain is likely to be manageable with oral opioids, and multimodal analgesia with acetaminophen and anti-inflammatories will be beneficial. Based on the history, optimization, and low analgesic requirements, the risk of postoperative respiratory failure is low. Pyridostigmine dosing must be continued, and ongoing collaboration with neurology and the postoperative care team is important.

References

1. Souza C, Muller N. Imaging of the mediastinum. In: Patterson G, Cooper J, Deslauriers J, Lerut A, Luketich J, Rice T, editors. Pearson's thoracic and esophageal surgery. 3rd ed. Philadelphia: Churchill Livingstone; 2008. p. 1477–505.
2. Souadjian JV, Enriquez P, Silverstein MN, Pépin JM. The spectrum of diseases associated with thymoma. Coincidence or syndrome? Arch Intern Med. 1974;134(2):374–9.
3. Maggi G, Casadio C, Cavallo A, Cianci R, Molinatti M, Ruffini E. Thymoma: results of 241 operated cases. Ann Thorac Surg. 1991;51(1):152–6.
4. Blumberg D, Burt ME, Bains MS, Downey RJ, Martini N, Rusch V, et al. Thymic carcinoma: current staging does not predict prognosis. J Thorac Cardiovasc Surg. 1998;115(2):303–9.
5. Miller BS, Rusinko RY, Fowler L. Synchronous thymoma and thymic carcinoid in a woman with multiple endocrine neoplasia type 1: case report and review. Endocr Pract. 2008;14(6):713–6.
6. Falkson CB, Bezjak A, Darling G, Gregg R, Malthaner R, Maziak DE, et al. The management of thymoma: a systematic review and practice guideline. J Thorac Oncol. 2009;4(7):911–9.
7. Tomaszek S, Wigle DA, Keshavjee S, Fischer S, Cowen D, Richaud P, et al. Thymomas: review of current clinical practice. Ann Thorac Surg. 2009;87(6):1973–80.
8. Lerro A, De Luca G. Giant Thymolipoma causing cardiocompressive syndrome with chronic heart failure. Ann Thorac Surg. 2009;87(2):644.
9. Jiang X, Fang Y, Wang G. Giant thymolipoma involving both chest cavities. Ann Thorac Surg. 2009;87(6):1960.
10. Ceran S, Tulek B, Sunam G, Suerdem M. Respiratory failure caused by giant thymolipoma. Ann Thorac Surg. 2008;86(2):661–3.
11. Johnson SB, Eng TY, Giaccone G, Thomas CR. Thymoma: update for the new millennium. Oncologist. 2001;6(3):239–46.
12. Korst RJ, Kansler AL, Christos PJ, Mandal S. Adjuvant radiotherapy for thymic epithelial tumors: a systematic review and meta-analysis. Ann Thorac Surg. 2009;87(5):1641–7.
13. Girard N, Mornex F, Van Houtte P, Cordier J-F, van Schil P. Thymoma: a focus on current therapeutic management. J Thorac Oncol. 2009;4(1):119–26.
14. Venuta F, Rendina EA, Coloni GF. Multimodality treatment of thymic tumors. Thorac Surg Clin. 2009;19(1):71–81.
15. Pascuzzi RM. The history of myasthenia gravis. Neurol Clin. 1994;12(12):231–42.
16. Jolly F. Uber myasthenia gravis pseudoparalytica. Berliner Klin Wochenshur. 1895;32:1.
17. Grob D, Brunner N, Namba T, Pagala M. Lifetime course of myasthenia gravis. Muscle Nerve. 2008;37(2):141–9.
18. Engel AG, Lambert EH, Howard FM. Immune complexes (IgG and C3) at the motor end-plate in myasthenia gravis: ultrastructural and light microscopic localization and electrophysiologic correlations. Mayo Clin Proc. 1977;52(5):267–80.
19. Pestronk A, Drachman DB, Self SG. Measurement of junctional acetylcholine receptors in myasthenia gravis: clinical correlates. Muscle Nerve. 1985;8(3):245–51.
20. Drachman DB. Myasthenia gravis. N Engl J Med. 1994;330(25):1797–810.
21. Engel AG, Tsujihata M, Lindstrom JM, Lennon VA. The motor end plate in myasthenia gravis and in experimental autoimmune myasthenia gravis. A quantitative ultrastructural study. Ann N Y Acad Sci. 1976;274:60–79.
22. Thomas CR, Wright CD, Loehrer PJ. Thymoma: state of the art. J Clin Oncol. 1999;17:2280–9.
23. Castleman B. The pathology of the thymus gland in myasthenia gravis. Ann N Y Acad Sci. 1966;135(1):496–503.
24. Osserman KE, Genkins G. Studies in myasthenia gravis: review of a twenty-year experience in over 1200 patients. Mt Sinai J Med. 1971;38(6):497–537.
25. Gilhus NE, Verschuuren JJ. Myasthenia gravis: subgroup classification and therapeutic strategies. Lancet Neurol. 2015;14:1023–36.
26. Gibson TC. The heart in myasthenia gravis. Am Heart J. 1975;90(3):389–96.
27. Johannessen KA, Mygland A, Gilhus NE, Aarli J, Vik-Mo H. Left ventricular function in myasthenia gravis. Am J Cardiol. 1992;69(1):129–32.
28. Hofstad H, Ohm OJ, Mørk SJ, Aarli JA. Heart disease in myasthenia gravis. Acta Neurol Scand. 1984;70(3):176–84.
29. Shivamurthy P, Matthew W, Parker A. Cardiac manifestation of myasthenia gravis: a systematic review. IJC Metab Endocr. 2014;5:3–6.
30. Suzuki S, Baba A, Kaida K, Utsugisawa K, Kita Y, Tsugawa J, et al. Cardiac involvements in myasthenia gravis associated with anti-Kv1.4 antibodies. Eur J Neurol. 2014;21(2):223–30.
31. Suzuki S, Utsugisawa K, Yoshikawa H, Motomura M, Matsubara S, Yokoyama K, et al. Autoimmune targets of heart and skeletal muscles in myasthenia gravis. Arch Neurol. 2009;66(11): 1334–8.
32. Daroff RB. The office Tensilon test for ocular myasthenia gravis. Arch Neurol. 1986;43(8):843–4.
33. Sussman J, Farrugia ME, Maddison P, Hill M, Leite MI, Hilton-Jones D. Myasthenia gravis: Association of British Neurologists' management guidelines. Pract Neurol. 2015;15(3):199–206.
34. Sanders DB, Wolfe GI, Benatar M, Evoli A, Gilhus NE, Illa I, et al. International consensus guidance for management of myasthenia gravis. Neurology. 2016;87(4):419–25.
35. Skeie GO, Apostolski S, Evoli A, Gilhus NE, Illa I, Harms L, et al. Guidelines for treatment of autoimmune neuromuscular transmission disorders. Eur J Neurol. 2010;17(7):893–902.

36. Osserman KE. Myasthenia gravis. New York: Grune & Stratton; 1958.

37. Jaretzki A, Barohn RJ, Ernstoff RM, Kaminski HJ, Keesey JC, Penn AS, et al. Myasthenia gravis: recommendations for clinical research standards. Task Force of the Medical Scientific Advisory Board of the Myasthenia Gravis Foundation of America. Ann Thorac Surg. 2000;70(1):327–34.

38. Nicolle MW. Myasthenia gravis. Neurologist. 2002;8(1):2–21.

39. Baraka A. Anaesthesia and myasthenia gravis. Reply Can J Anaesth. 1992;39(5):1002–3.

40. Sathasivam S. Steroids and immunosuppressant drugs in myasthenia gravis. Nat Clin Pract Neurol. 2008;4(6):317–27.

41. Pinching AJ, Peters DK, Newsom DJ. Remission of myasthenia gravis following plasma exchange. Lancet. 1976;308(8000):1373–6.

42. Gajdos P, Chevret S, Toyka K. Intravenous immunoglobulin for myasthenia gravis. Gajdos P, editor. Cochrane Database Syst Rev. 2008;(1):CD002277.

43. Arsura E. Experience with intravenous immunoglobulin in myasthenia gravis. Clin Immunol Immunopathol. 1989;53(2):S170–9.

44. Blalock A, Mason MF, Morgan HJ, Riven SS. Myasthenia gravis and tumors of the thymic region: report of a case where the tumor was removed. Ann Surg. 1939;110(4):544–61.

45. Blalock A, Harvey A, Ford F. The treatment of myasthenia gravis by removal of the thymus gland. JAMA. 1941;117:1529–33.

46. Blalock A. Thymectomy for the treatment of myasthenia gravis. Report of twenty cases. J Thorac Surg. 1944;13:316–39.

47. Mulder DG, Graves M, Herrmann C. Thymectomy for myasthenia gravis: recent observations and comparisons with past experience. Ann Thorac Surg. 1989;48(4):551–5.

48. de Perrot M, Bril V, McRae K, Keshavjee S. Impact of minimally invasive trans-cervical thymectomy on outcome in patients with myasthenia gravis. Eur J Cardiothorac Surg. 2003;24(5):677–83.

49. Bachmann K, Burkhardt D, Schreiter I, Kaifi J, Busch C, Thayssen G, et al. Long-term outcome and quality of life after open and thoracoscopic thymectomy for myasthenia gravis: analysis of 131 patients. Surg Endosc Other Interv Tech. 2008;22(11):2470–7.

50. Prokakis C, Koletsis E, Salakou S, Apostolakis E, Baltayiannis N, Chatzimichalis A, et al. Modified maximal thymectomy for myasthenia gravis: effect of maximal resection on late neurologic outcome and predictors of disease remission. Ann Thorac Surg. 2009;88(5):1638–45.

51. Pompeo E, Tacconi F, Massa R, Mineo D, Nahmias S, Mineo TC. Long-term outcome of thoracoscopic extended thymectomy for nonthymomatous myasthenia gravis. Eur J Cardio Thorac Surg. 2009;36(1):164–9.

52. Gronseth GS, Barohn RJ. Practice parameter: thymectomy for autoimmune myasthenia gravis (an evidence-based review): report of the Quality Standards Subcommittee of the American Academy of Neurology. Neurology. 2000;55:7–15.

53. Wolfe GI, Kaminski HJ, Aban IB, Minisman G, Kuo H-C, Marx A, et al. Randomized trial of thymectomy in myasthenia gravis. N Engl J Med. 2016;375(6):511–22.

54. Lucchi M, Van Schil P, Schmid R, Rea F, Melfi F, Athanassiadi K, et al. Thymectomy for thymoma and myasthenia gravis. A survey of current surgical practice in thymic disease amongst EACTS members. Interact Cardiovasc Thorac Surg. 2012;14:765–70.

55. Calhoun RF, Ritter JH, Guthrie TJ, Pestronk A, Meyers BF, Patterson GA, et al. Results of transcervical thymectomy for myasthenia gravis in 100 consecutive patients. Ann Surg. 1999;230(4):555–559–561.

56. Howard J. Physician issues. In: Howard J, editor. Myasthenia gravis a manual for the healthcare provider. St Paul: Myasthenia Gravis Foundation of America; 2008. p. 8–30.

57. Gracey DR, Divertie MB, Howard FM. Mechanical ventilation for respiratory failure in myasthenia gravis. Two-year experience with 22 patients. Mayo Clin Proc. 1983;58(9):597–602.

58. Fernando M, Paterson HS, Byth K, Robinson BM, Wolfenden H, Gracey D, et al. Outcomes of cardiac surgery in chronic kidney disease. J Thorac Cardiovasc Surg. 2014;148(5):2167–73.

59. Leventhal SR, Orkin FK, Hirsh RA. Prediction of the need for postoperative mechanical ventilation in myasthenia gravis. Anesthesiology. 1980;53(1):26–30.

60. Eisenkraft JB, Papatestas AE, Kahn CH, Mora CT, Fagerstrom R, Genkins G. Predicting the need for postoperative mechanical ventilation in myasthenia gravis. Anesthesiology. 1986;65(1):79–82.

61. Grant RP, Jenkins LC. Prediction of the need for postoperative mechanical ventilation in myasthenia gravis: thymectomy compared to other surgical procedures. Can Anaesth Soc J. 1982;29(2):112–6.

62. Gracey DR, Divertie MB, Howard FM, Payne WS. Postoperative respiratory care after transsternal thymectomy in myasthenia gravis. A 3-year experience in 53 patients. Chest. 1984;86(1):67–71.

63. Younger DS, Braun NM, Jaretzki A, Penn AS, Lovelace RE. Myasthenia gravis: determinants for independent ventilation after transsternal thymectomy. Neurology. 1984;34(3):336–40.

64. El-Bawab H, Hajjar W, Rafay M, Bamousa A, Khalil A, Al-Kattan K. Plasmapheresis before thymectomy in myasthenia gravis: routine versus selective protocols. Eur J Cardio Thorac Surg. 2009;35(3):392–7.

65. Spence PA, Morin JE, Katz M. Role of plasmapheresis in preparing myasthenic patients for thymectomy: initial results. Can J Surg. 1984;27(3):303–5.

66. Baraka A, Taha S, Yazbeck V, Rizkallah P. Vecuronium block in the myasthenic patient: influence of anticholinesterase therapy. Anaesthesia. 1993;48(7):588–90.

67. Ropper A, Samuels M. Myasthenia gravis and related disorders of the neuromuscular junction. In: Adams and Victor's principles of neurology. 9th ed. New York: McGraw-Hill; 2009. p. 1405–21.

68. Girnar DS, Weinreich AI. Anesthesia for transcervical thymectomy in myasthenia gravis. Anesth Analg. 1976;55(1):13–7.

69. Krucylak PE, Naunheim KS. Preoperative preparation and anesthetic management of patients with myasthenia gravis. Semin Thorac Cardiovasc Surg. 1999;11(1):47–53.

70. Kim JM, Mangold J. Sensitivity to both vecuronium and neostigmine in a sero-negative myasthenic patient. Br J Anaesth. 1989;63(4):497–500.

71. Lumb AB, Calder I. "Cured" myasthenia gravis and neuromuscular blockade. Anaesthesia. 1989;44(10):828–30.

72. Azar I. The response of patients with neuromuscular disorders to muscle relaxants: a review. Anesthesiology. 1984;61(2):173–87.

73. Fujita Y, Moriyama S, Aoki S, Yoshizawa S, Tomita M, Kojima T, et al. Estimation of the success rate of anesthetic management for thymectomy in patients with myasthenia gravis treated without muscle relaxants: a retrospective observational cohort study. J Anesth [Internet]. 2015 [cited 2016 Dec 20];29(5):794–7. Available from: http://www.ncbi.nlm.nih.gov/pubmed/25796520

74. Postevka E. Anesthetic implications of myasthenia gravis: a case report. AANA J. 2013;81(5):386–8.

75. Blitt CD, Wright WA, Peat J. Pancuronium and the patient with myasthenia gravis. Anesthesiology. 1975;42(5):624–6.

76. Book W, Abel M, Eisenkraft J. Anesthesia and neuromuscular diseases. Anesthesiol Clin North Am. 1996;14:515–42.

77. Petrun AM, Mekiš D, Kamenik M. Successful use of rocuronium and sugammadex in a patient with myasthenia. Eur J Anaesthesiol. 2010;27(10):917–8.

78. Unterbuchner C, Fink H, Blobner M. The use of sugammadex in a patient with myasthenia gravis. Anaesthesia. 2010;65(3):302–5.

79. de Boer HD, Shields MO, Booij LHDJ. Reversal of neuromuscular blockade with sugammadex in patients with myasthenia gravis: a case series of 21 patients and review of the literature. Eur J Anaesthesiol [Internet]. 2014 [cited 2016 Aug 24];31(12):715–21. Available from: http://www.ncbi.nlm.nih.gov/pubmed/25192270

80. Ulke ZS, Yavru A, Camci E, Ozkan B, Toker A, Senturk M. Rocuronium and sugammadex in patients with myasthenia gravis undergoing thymectomy. Acta Anaesthesiol Scand. 2013;57(6):745–8.

81. Ortiz-Gó Mez JR, Palacio-Abizanda FJ, Fornet-Ruiz I. Failure of sugammadex to reverse rocuronium-induced neuromuscular blockade a case report. Eur J Anaesthesiol. 2014;31:708–9.

82. Eisenkraft JB, Book WJ, Mann SM, Papatestas AE, Hubbard M. Resistance to succinylcholine in myasthenia gravis: a dose-response study. Anesthesiology. 1988;69(5):760–3.

83. Juste BJ, Ibañez C. Bats of the Gulf of Guinea islands: faunal composition and origins. Biodivers Conserv. 1994;3(9):837–50.

84. Baraka A, Baroody M, Yazbeck V. Repeated doses of suxamethonium in the myasthenic patient. Anaesthesia. 1993;48(9):782–4.

85. Nilsson E, Muller K. Neuromuscular effects of isoflurane in patients with myasthenia gravis. Acta Anaesthesiol Scand. 1990;34(2):126–31.

86. Kiran U, Choudhury M, Saxena N, Kapoor P. Sevoflurane as a sole anaesthetic for thymectomy in myasthenia gravis. Acta Anaesthesiol Scand. 2000;44(3):351–3.

87. Nishi M, Nakagawa H, Komatsu R, Natsuyama T, Tanaka Y. Neuromuscular effects of sevoflurane in a patient with myasthenia gravis. J Anesth. 1993;7(2):237–9.

88. Madi-Jebara S, Yazigi A, Hayek G, Haddad F, Antakly MC. Sevoflurane anesthesia and intrathecal sufentanil-morphine for thymectomy in myasthenia gravis. J Clin Anesth. 2002;14:558–9.

89. Gritti P, Carrara B, Khotcholava M, Bortolotti G, Giardini D, Lanterna LA, et al. The use of desflurane or propofol in combination with remifentanil in myasthenic patients undergoing a video-assisted thoracoscopic-extended thymectomy. Acta Anaesthesiol Scand. 2009;53(3):380–9.

90. Hübler M, Litz RJ, Albrecht DM. Combination of balanced and regional anaesthesia for minimally invasive surgery in a patient with myasthenia gravis. Eur J Anaesthesiol. 2000;17(5):325–8.

91. Sener M, Bilen A, Bozdogan N, Kilic D, Arslan G. Laryngeal Mask Airway insertion with total intravenous anesthesia for transsternal thymectomy in patients with myasthenia gravis: report of 5 cases. J Clin Anesth. 2008;20(3):206–9.

92. Mekis D, Kamenik M. Remifentanil and high thoracic epidural anaesthesia: a successful combination for patients with myasthenia gravis undergoing transsternal thymectomy. Eur J Anaesthesiol. 2005;22(5):397–9.

93. Bouaggad A, Bouderka MA, Abassi O. Total intravenous anaesthesia with propofol for myasthenic patients. Eur J Anaesthesiol. 2005;22(5):393–4.

94. de José Maria B, Carrero E, Sala X. Myasthenia gravis and regional anaesthesia. Can J Anaesth. 1995;42(2):178–9.

95. Matsuo S, Rao DB, Chaudry I, Foldes FF. Interaction of muscle relaxants and local anesthetics at the neuromuscular junction. Anesth Analg. 1978;57(5):580–7.

96. Burgess FW, Wilcosky B. Thoracic epidural anesthesia for transsternal thymectomy in myasthenia gravis. Anesth Analg. 1989;69(4):529–31.

97. Chevalley C, Spiliopoulos A, de Perrot M, Tschopp JM, Licker M. Perioperative medical management and outcome following thymectomy for myasthenia gravis. Can J Anaesth. 2001;48(5):446–51.

98. Akpolat N, Tilgen H, Gürsoy F, Saydam S, Gürel A. Thoracic epidural anaesthesia and analgesia with bupivacaine for transsternal thymectomy for myasthenia gravis. Eur J Anaesthesiol. 1997;14(2):220–3.

99. Kirsch JR, Diringer MN, Borel CO, Hanley DF, Merritt WT, Bulkley GB. Preoperative lumbar epidural morphine improves postoperative analgesia and ventilatory function after transsternal thymectomy in patients with myasthenia gravis. Crit Care Med. 1991;19(12):1474–9.

100. Nilsson E, Perttunen K, Kalso E. Intrathecal morphine for post-sternotomy pain in patients with myasthenia gravis: effects on respiratory function. Acta Anaesthesiol Scand. 1997;41(5):549–56.

101. Pierce ST. Paraendocrine syndromes. Curr Opin Oncol. 1993;5(4):639–45.

102. Toothaker TB, Rubin M. Paraneoplastic neurological syndromes. Neurologist. 2009;15(1):21–33.

103. Tohyama T, Matsui K, Kitagawa K. Primary hepatic carcinoid tumor with carcinoid syndrome and carcinoid heart disease: a case report of a patient on long-term follow-up. Intern Med. 2005;44(9):958–62.

104. Zhang A, Xiang J, Zhang M, Zheng S. Primary hepatic carcinoid tumours: clinical features with an emphasis on carcinoid syndrome and recurrence. J Int Med Res. 2008;36(4):848–59.

105. Claret C, Chillarón JJ, Flores JA, Benaiges D, Aguiló R, García M, et al. Carcinoid tumor of the thymus associated with Cushing's syndrome and dysgeusia: case report and review of the literature. Endocrine. 2010;37(1):1–5.

106. De Perrot M, Spiliopoulos A, Fischer S, Totsch M, Keshavjee S. Neuroendocrine carcinoma (carcinoid) of the thymus associated with Cushing's syndrome. Ann Thorac Surg. 2002;73:675–81.

107. Modlin IM, Lye KD, Kidd M. A 5-decade analysis of 13,715 carcinoid tumors. Cancer. 2003;97(4):934–59.

108. Gustafsson BI, Kidd M, Chan A, Malfertheiner MV, Modlin IM. Bronchopulmonary neuroendocrine tumors. Cancer. 2008;113:5–21.

109. Lips CJM, Lentjes EGWM, Höppener JWM, Hoppener JW. The spectrum of carcinoid tumours and carcinoid syndromes. Ann Clin Biochem. 2003;40(Pt 6):612–27.

110. Ghevariya V, Malieckal A, Ghevariya N, Mazumder M, Anand S. Carcinoid tumors of the gastrointestinal tract. South Med J. 2009;102(10):1032–40.

111. Wells SA. Foreword. Curr Probl Surg. 2009;46(3):189.

112. Dierdorf SF. Carcinoid tumor and carcinoid syndrome. Curr Opin Anaesthesiol. 2003;16(3):343–7.

113. Bendelow J, Apps E, Jones LE, Poston GJ. Carcinoid syndrome. Eur J Surg Oncol. 2008;34(3):289–96.

114. Athanassiadi K, Exarchos D, Tsagarakis S, Bellenis I. Acromegaly caused by ectopic growth hormone-releasing hormone secretion by a carcinoid bronchial tumor: a rare entity. J Thorac Cardiovasc Surg. 2004;128(4):631–2.

115. Scheithauer BW, Carpenter PC, Bloch B, Brazeau P. Ectopic secretion of a growth hormone-releasing factor. Report of a case of acromegaly with bronchial carcinoid tumor. Am J Med. 1984;76(4):605–16.

116. Shrager JB, Wright CD, Wain JC, Torchiana DF, Grillo HC, Mathisen DJ. Bronchopulmonary carcinoid tumors associated with Cushing's syndrome: a more aggressive variant of typical carcinoid. J Thorac Cardiovasc Surg. 1997;114(3):367–75.

117. Malchoff CD, Orth DN, Abboud C, Carney JA, Pairolero PC, Carey RM. Ectopic ACTH syndrome caused by a bronchial carcinoid tumor responsive to dexamethasone, metyrapone, and corticotropin-releasing factor. Am J Med. 1988;84(4):760–4.

118. Scanagatta P, Montresor E, Pergher S, Mainente M, Bonadiman C, Benato C, et al. Cushing's syndrome induced by bronchopulmonary carcinoid tumours: a review of 98 cases and our experience of two cases. Chir Ital. 2004;56(1):63–70.

119. Fischer S, Kruger M, McRae K, Merchant N, Tsao MS, Keshavjee S. Giant bronchial carcinoid tumors: a multidisciplinary approach. Ann Thorac Surg. 2001;71(1):386–93.

120. Modlin IM, Shapiro MD, Kidd M. Carcinoid tumors and fibrosis: an association with no explanation. Am J Gastroenterol. 2004;99:2466–78.

121. Anderson AS, Krauss D, Lang R. Cardiovascular complications of malignant carcinoid disease. Am Heart J. 1997;134(4):693–702.

122. Zuetenhorst JM, Bonfrer JMGM, Korse CM, Bakker R, van Tinteren H, Taal BG. Carcinoid heart disease. Cancer. 2003;97(7):1609–15.

123. Kvols LK, Moertel CG, O'Connell MJ, Schutt AJ, Rubin J, Hahn RG. Treatment of the malignant carcinoid syndrome. Evaluation of a long-acting somatostatin analogue. N Engl J Med. 1986;315(11):663–6.

124. Vaughan DJ, Brunner MD. Anesthesia for patients with carcinoid syndrome. Int Anesthesiol Clin. 1997;35(4):129–42.

125. Farling PA, Durairaju AK. Remifentanil and anaesthesia for carcinoid syndrome. Br J Anaesth. 2004;92:893–5.

126. Veall GRQ, Peacock JE, Bax NDS, Reilly CS. Review of the anaesthetic management of 21 patients undergoing laparotomy for carcinoid syndrome. Br J Anaesth. 1994;72:335–41.

127. Cortinez FLI. Refractory hypotension during carcinoid resection surgery. Anaesthesia. 2000;55(5):505–6.

128. Monteith K, Roaseg OP. Epidural anaesthesia for transurethral resection of the prostate in a patient with carcinoid syndrome. Can J Anaesth. 1990;37(3):349–52.

129. Orbach-Zinger S, Lombroso R, Eidelman LA. Uneventful spinal anesthesia for a patient with carcinoid syndrome managed with long-acting octreotide. Can J Anaesth. 2002;49(7):678–81.

130. Darnell RB, Posner JB. Paraneoplastic syndromes affecting the nervous system. Semin Oncol. 2006;33(3):270–98.

131. O'Neill GN. Acquired disorders of the neuromuscular junction. Int Anesthesiol Clin. 2006;44(2):107–21.

132. Lambert EH, Elmqvist D. Quantal components of end-plate potentials in myasthenic syndrome. Ann NY Acad Sci. 1971;183(1):183–99.

133. Elmqvist D, Lambert EH. Detailed analysis of neuromuscular transmission in a patient with the myasthenic syndrome sometimes associated with bronchogenic carcinoma. Mayo Clin Proc. 1968;43(10):689–713.

134. Molenaar PC, Newsom-Davis J, Polak RL, Vincent A. Eaton-Lambert syndrome: acetylcholine and choline acetyltransferase in skeletal muscle. Neurology. 1982;32(9):1061–5.

135. O'Neill JH, Murray NM, Newsom-Davis J. The Lambert-Eaton myasthenic syndrome. A review of 50 cases. Brain. 1988;111(Pt 3):577–96.

136. Telford RJ, Hollway TE, Telford RJ, Hollway TE. The myasthenic syndrome: anaesthesia in a patient treated with 3.4 diaminopyridine. Br J Anaesth. 1990;64(3):363–6.

137. Small S, Ali HH, Lennon VA, Brown RH, Carr DB, de Armendi A. Anesthesia for an unsuspected Lambert-Eaton myasthenic syndrome with autoantibodies and occult small cell lung carcinoma. Anesthesiology. 1992;76(1):142–5.

Lung Isolation

16

Javier Campos

Key Points
- During the preoperative period, review of the posteroanterior chest radiograph is necessary to measure the tracheal width and also appreciate the pattern of the tracheobronchial anatomy to determine what device and size to use.
- The left-sided DLT is the most common device used for lung isolation because of its greater margin of safety.
- The use of bronchial blockers is indicated in patients who present with difficult airways and require lung isolation.
- Patients with a tracheostomy in place requiring lung isolation are best managed with the use of an independent bronchial blocker and flexible fiberoptic bronchoscopy.
- Flexible fiberoptic bronchoscopy is the recommended method to achieve optimal position of lung isolation devices, first in supine position, later in lateral decubitus, or whenever a malposition occurs.

Introduction

Lung separation techniques are used to provide one-lung ventilation (OLV) in patients undergoing thoracic, mediastinal, cardiac, vascular, or esophageal procedures [1, 2]. Lung separation can be achieved with two different techniques. The first involves a device made of disposable polyvinylchloride material, the double-lumen endotracheal tube (DLT) [3]. The DLT is a bifurcated tube with both an endotracheal and an endobronchial lumen and can be used to achieve isolation of either the right or left lung. In addition the newly designed VivaSight® DLT has an integrated camera, allowing continuous visualization of its position within the trachea [4]. The second technique involves blockade of a mainstem bronchus to allow lung collapse distal to the occlusion [5]. Currently, there are different bronchial blockers available to facilitate lung separation collapse; these devices are either attached to a single-lumen endotracheal tube with an enclosed bronchial blocker (Torque Control Blocker Univent) (Vitaid, Lewiston, NY) [6] or are used independently over a standard single-lumen endotracheal tube, as with the wire-guided endobronchial blocker (Arndt® blocker) [7] (Cook Critical Care, Bloomington, IN), the Cohen tip-deflecting endobronchial blocker [8] (Cook Critical Care, Bloomington, IN), the Fuji Uniblocker® [9] (Fuji Corp, Tokyo, Japan], or the EZ-blocker® [10] (Teleflex Medical, Morrisville, NC). There are a number of recognized indications for OLV. In practice, the most common indications for lung separation are (1) for surgical exposure, (2) for prevention of contamination to the contralateral lung from bleeding pus material or saline lavage (abscess, hemoptysis, bronchiectasis, and lung lavage), and (3) during differential lung ventilation or for continuity of the airway gas exchange such as with bronchopleural fistula. Table 16.1 describes common indications for lung isolation with a DLT or a bronchial blocker.

Double-Lumen Endotracheal Tubes

Currently, all DLTs are based on a design suggested by Carlens and Björk [11]. There are two versions of DLTs, left-sided and a right-sided, which are designed to accommodate the unique anatomy of each mainstem bronchus [12]. DLTs are available from different manufacturers: Mallinckrodt Broncho-Cath (St. Louis, MO) is the most common brand name in North America; there are also the Sheridan Sher-I-Bronch (Argyle, NY) and DLTs from

J. Campos (✉)
Department of Anesthesia, University of Iowa Health Care, Roy and Lucille Carver College of Medicine, Iowa City, IA, USA
e-mail: javier-campos@uiowa.edu

Table 16.1 Indications for lung isolation with a double-lumen endotracheal tube (DLT) or a bronchial blocker

A. *Indications for lung isolation with the use of a DLT*
   Protection of one lung from a contralateral contamination
      Lung abscess
      Lung cyst
      Pulmonary hemorrhage
   Bronchopulmonary lavage
      Pulmonary alveolar proteinosis
   Control and continuity of the airway gas exchange
      Bronchopleural fistula
      Bronchial disruption (i.e., laceration with a knife)
      Pneumonectomy

B. *Indication for lung isolation with the use of a DLT or a bronchial blocker*
   Any operation that requires surgical exposure through the chest cavity with lung collapse
      Video-assisted thoracoscopic surgery
      Lobectomy and bilobectomy
      Mediastinal mass resection through the chest (selective cases)
      Esophageal surgery
      Orthopedic procedures (spine surgery involving chest)
      Minimally invasive cardiac surgery

C. *Specific indications for bronchial blockers*
   Difficult airways
      Limited mouth opening
         Nasotracheal intubation
      Awake orotracheal intubation
   Already intubated patient requiring lung isolation
   Tracheostomy patient requiring lung isolation
   Selective lobar blockade
   Potential for mechanical ventilation in the postoperative period

Table 16.2 Displays the external and internal diameters of the different sizes of DLTs and the size of the flexible fiberoptic bronchoscope recommended

DLT French size (F)				
F size	OD (mm)	Bronchial ID (mm)	Trachea ID (mm)	FOB size OD (mm)
26	8.7	3.5	3.5	2.2
28	9.3	3.2	3.1	2.2
32	10.7	3.4	3.5	2.2
35	11.7	4.3	4.5	3.5 or 4.2
37	12.3	4.5	4.7	3.5 or 4.2
39	13.0	4.9	4.9	3.5 or 4.2
41	13.7	5.4	5.4	3.5 or 4.2

OD outer diameter; *ID* internal diameter; *FOB* fiberoptic bronchoscope

Rüsch (Duluth, GA) and Portex (Keene, NH) and the VivaSight® DLT from Teleflex (St. Louis, MO). The sizes of the DLTs vary among manufacturers; the smallest available is 26 French (F) followed by 28, 32, 35, 37, 39, and 41 F. Table 16.2 displays the external and internal diameters of the different sizes of DLTs and the size of the flexible fiberoptic bronchoscope recommended (of note, the size of the DLTs varies among manufacturers). The ones described in this table are Mallinckrodt Broncho-Cath, Sher-I-Bronch, and Rüsch.

Size Selection

Regarding selection of the proper size of a DLT, all studies have focused on the left-sided DLT in part because the right-sided DLT is used infrequently. A common problem with the left-sided DLT is the lack of objective guidelines to properly choose the correct or approximate size of DLT.

A left-sided DLT that is too small requires a large endobronchial cuff volume, which might increase the incidence of malposition. In addition, a small DLT does not readily allow fiberoptic bronchoscope placement and can make suction difficult. A properly sized DLT is one in which the main body of the tube passes without resistance through the glottis and advances easily within the trachea and in which the bronchial component passes into the intended bronchus without difficulty. In a study performed in adult cadavers, it was shown that the cricoid ring diameter never exceeds the diameter of the glottis. If a DLT encounters resistance when passing the glottis, it is likely that the DLT would encounter resistance while passing the cricoid ring [13].

There are reports of complications related to the use of an undersized DLT. A tension pneumothorax and pneumomediastinum occurred after the endobronchial tip of an undersized DLT had migrated too far into the left lower bronchus, and the entire tidal volume was delivered into a single lobe [14]. Also, smaller DLTs might present with more resistance to gas flow and more intrinsic auto-positive end-expiratory pressure compared with the wider lumen of larger DLTs [15]. Airway-related complications have been reported with undersized left-sided DLTs. A rupture of the left mainstem bronchus by tracheal portion of a DLT has been reported [16]. A longitudinal laceration of the left mainstem bronchus occurred. The cause of this complication was believed to be an undersized DLT, which allowed the endotracheal portion of the DLT to enter the left mainstem bronchus. In addition, an oversized DLT also can be associated with bronchial rupture in a small adult patient [17].

Brodsky et al. [18] reported that measurement of tracheal diameter at the level of the clavicle on the preoperative posteroanterior chest radiograph can be used to determine proper left-sided DLT size. These methods lead to a 90% increase in the use of larger left-sided DLTs (i.e., 41 F DLT in men and 39 F and 41 F DLT in women). However, a study involving Asian patients by Chow et al. [19], using the methodology of Brodsky et al. [18], found this approach less reliable. In the Chow et al. [19] study, the overall positive predictive value for the proper left size of a left-sided DLT was 77% for men and 45% for women. This method seems to have limited use in patients of smaller stature, such as women and people of Asian descent, and an alternative method should be sought, including placement of a different lung isolation device such as an independent bronchial blocker through a single-lumen endotracheal tube. Figure 16.1 shows the guidelines to pre-

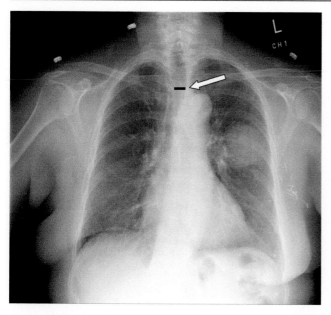

Measured Tracheal Width (mm)	Predicted Left Bronchus Width (mm)	Recommended DLT size (F)
≥18	≥12.2	41
≥16	≥10.9	39
≥15	≥10.2	37
≥14	≥9.5	35

Fig. 16.1 Left Broncho-Cath double-lumen endotracheal tubes guideline. (Modified from Brodsky et al. [16])

dict the proper left-sided DLT based upon measurements of the tracheal width from the chest X-ray according to Brodsky et al. [18].

A study involving thoracic anesthesiologists by Amar et al. [20] has shown that the use of a smaller DLT (i.e., 35 or 37 F left-sided DLT) rather than a conventionally large-sized DLT (i.e., 39 or 41 F) was not associated with any difference in clinical intraoperative outcomes, regardless of patient size or gender in 300 patients undergoing thoracic surgery requiring lung isolation. However, in their study, only 51 (35%) of the patients who received a 35 F DLT were males, and 92 (65%) were females. In practice, women usually receive a 35 F DLT; therefore, the question of whether or not a 35 F for all patients is favorable remains unclear.

Another alternative that has been suggested in order to predict the proper size of a right-sided or left-sided DLT is a three-dimensional image reconstruction of tracheobronchial anatomy generated from spiral computed tomography (CT) scans combined with superimposed transparencies of DLTs [21]. Taken together, these studies suggest that chest radiographs and CT scans are valuable tools for selection of proper DLT size, in addition to their proven value in assessment of any abnormal tracheobronchial anatomy. These images should be reviewed before placement of a DLT. Particular emphasis should be made in viewing a pos-

teroanterior chest radiograph in order to assess the shadow of tracheobronchial anatomy along with bronchial bifurcation. It is estimated that in 75% of the films, the left mainstem bronchus shadow is seen. The trachea is located in the midline position, but often can be deviated to the right at the level of the aortic arch, with a greater degree of displacement in the setting of an atherosclerotic aorta, advanced age, or in the presence of severe chronic obstructive pulmonary disease (COPD). With COPD or aging, the lateral diameter of the trachea may decrease with an increase in the anteroposterior diameter. Conversely, COPD may also lead to softening of the tracheal rings with a decrease in the anteroposterior diameter of the trachea. The cricoid cartilage is the narrowest part of the trachea with an average diameter of 17 mm in men and 13 mm in women.

Figure 16.2a shows a multidetector three-dimensional CT scan of the chest displaying the trachea and bronchial anatomy in a 25-year-old healthy volunteer; Fig. 16.2b shows the changes that occur in a 60-year-old man with severe COPD, which shows a deviated trachea and narrow bronchus. Points of importance include the recognition of any distorted anatomy identified in the films prior to placement of DLTs.

Methods of Insertion

Two techniques are used most commonly by anesthesiologists when inserting and placing a DLT. The first is the blind technique, that is, when the DLT is passed with direct laryngoscopy, then it is turned to the left (for a left-sided DLT) or right (for a right-sided DLT) after the endobronchial cuff has passed beyond the vocal cords. The DLT then is advanced until the depth of insertion at the teeth is approximately 29 cm for both men and women if the patient's height is at least 170 cm [23].

The second technique employs fiberoptic bronchoscopy guidance, where the tip of the endobronchial lumen is guided after the DLT passes the vocal cords; direction is sought with the aid of a flexible fiberoptic bronchoscope. A study by Boucek et al. [24] comparing the blind technique versus the fiberoptic bronchoscopy-guided technique showed that of the 32 patients who underwent the blind technique approach, primary success occurred in 30 patients. In contrast, in the 27 patients receiving the bronchoscopy-guided technique, primary success was achieved only in 21 patients and eventual success in 25 patients. This study also showed that the time spent placing a DLT was an average of 88 s for the blind technique and 181 s for the directed bronchoscopic approach. Although both methods resulted in successful left mainstem bronchus placement in most patients, more time was required when the fiberoptic bronchoscopy guidance technique was used. In addition, two patients in each group required an alternative method for tube placement. Either method may

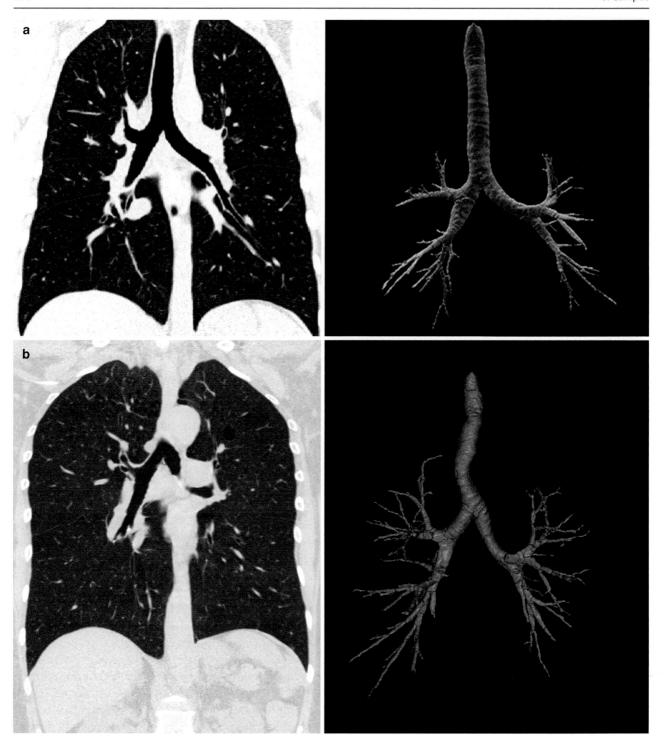

Fig. 16.2 (**a**) Male tracheobronchial tree via multidetector three-dimensional computer tomography scan in a healthy 25-year-old. (**b**) Male tracheobronchial tree via multidetector three-dimensional com- puter tomography scan in a 60-year-old with chronic obstructive pulmonary disease (COPD) [22]

fail when used alone. Figure 16.3 shows the blind method technique and Fig. 16.4 shows a fiberoptic bronchoscopy guidance technique for placement of a left-sided DLT.

In recent years video laryngoscopy has been introduced as an important tool in the management of patients with expected or unexpected difficult airways. Clinical studies have shown that video laryngoscopes improve visualization of laryngeal structures and facilitate insertion of a single-lumen endotracheal tube [26]. The use of the C-MAC video laryngoscope has been compared with the Macintosh blade (most common

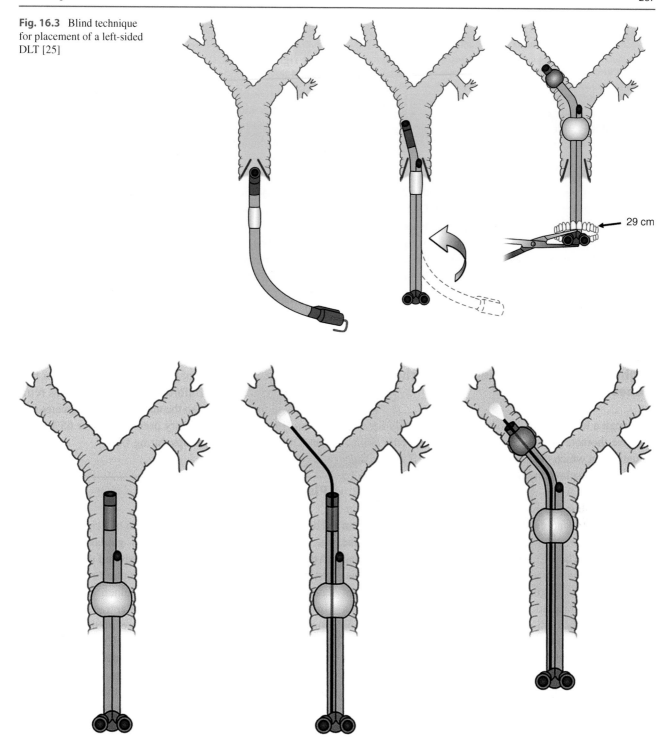

Fig. 16.3 Blind technique for placement of a left-sided DLT [25]

29 cm

Fig. 16.4 A fiberoptic bronchoscopy guidance technique for placing a left-sided DLT [25]

device used during laryngoscopy while using a DLT) and the Miller blade during DLT intubation in patients with normal airways. The authors of this retrospective study [27] showed that video laryngoscopy was similar to the views obtained with a Miller blade while passing a DLT. In contrast the group that used a Macintosh blade had reported higher difficult intubations with the DLTs. Another study [28], comparing the GlideScope® and the Macintosh laryngoscope for a DLT intubation, showed that the overall rate of successful endobronchial intubation was easier with the Macintosh blade compared with the GlideScope; also voice changes were less common in the Macintosh group. Therefore the authors do not recommend the routine use of the GlideScope in patients who have normal airways while using a DLT.

left side of the chest (left hemithorax). If none of these maneuvers are successful, or confusion ensues with breath sounds and the location of the DLT, a fiberoptic bronchoscopy exam takes precedent. In a study involving 200 patients who were intubated by the blind technique in whom confirmation of placement of DLTs was done first with auscultation and clamping, one of the ports of the connector of the DLT and with a second anesthesiologist with expertise in fiberoptic bronchoscopy reconfirming the placement of the DLT showed that 35% of the tubes placed were malpositioned when auscultation was used alone. All detected malpositions were eventually corrected [42]. A study by Brodsky and Lemmens [30] reported their clinical experience with the use of left-sided DLTs. Using auscultation and clinical signs, they reported 98% efficacy in lung collapse, yet in only 58 instances they used fiberoptic bronchoscopy to attempt to place the DLTs correctly. In this study, there were 71 patients (6.2%) in whom the DLT was found not to be in a satisfactory position, requiring readjustment after initial placement. What is important from the Brodsky study [30] is the fact that in 56 patients the DLT was considered too deep into the left bronchus, and indirectly this was a cause of hypoxemia in 21 of 56 patients who had a malpositioned tube. Anesthesiologists should be able to avoid this complication with the use of fiberoptic bronchoscope. In a report related to the national confidential inquiry into perioperative deaths in Great Britain [43], which detailed the management of patients undergoing esophagogastrectomy, it was shown that 30% of deaths reported were associated with malposition of DLTs. The problems ranged from use of multiple DLTs to prolonged periods of hypoxia and hypoventilation. The anesthesiologists did not use a fiberoptic bronchoscope to confirm DLT position before surgery, during surgery, or when the DLT was placed incorrectly [44].

In another report from Great Britain, Seymour [45] reported a survey among anesthesiologists in a single institution, in which they participated in 506 placements of left- or right-sided DLTs; in their report, only 56% of the cases managed used fiberoptic bronchoscopy to confirm the proper placement of the DLTs. In more than 10% of their cases, hypoxemia was present in the intraoperative period. An editorial by Slinger [46] pointed out the importance of using fiberoptic bronchoscopy to confirm placement of DLTs.

A study involving nonthoracic anesthesiologists with very limited experience in lung separation techniques showed that when placing lung isolation devices (DLTs or bronchial blockers), there was a 38% incidence in unrecognized malpositions when these devices were placed with the fiberoptic bronchoscope. The possible causes were lack of skill with fiberoptic bronchoscopy and lack of recognition of the tracheobronchial anatomy [47]. It is the author's opinion that fiberoptic bronchoscopy is essential and mandatory to achieve 100% success in placement and positioning of DLTs as long as the anesthesiologist is able to recognize proper tracheobronchial anatomy and has skills with flexible fiberoptic bronchoscopy. Table 16.4 displays the findings and outcomes when auscultation, clamping maneuvers, and or fiberoptic bronchoscopy were used to position and achieve optimal position of the DLTs.

In another study involving thoracic anesthesiologist [48], 104 patients were intubated with a left-sided DLT, and auscultation and clamping maneuver technique were used to confirm the optimal position of the DLT. An endoscopist with experience in flexible fiberoptic bronchoscopy was asked to confirm the optimal and proper position after auscultation, and it showed that in 37% of the patients, there were unrecognized malpositions while placing the DLT and all malpositions were easily corrected with the use of flexible fiberoptic bronchoscopy. This study clearly demonstrates that even experienced thoracic anesthesiologists can't rely on the optimal position of the DLT with just auscultation; therefore flexible fiberoptic bronchoscopy must be used to obtain optimal position.

Table 16.4 Role of auscultation, fiberoptic bronchoscopy, and/or both during lung isolation

References	Number of patients	Method	Outcome
Brodsky and Lemmens [30]	1170 DLTs (retrospective study)	Clinical experience over 8-year period (1993–2001)	Successful lung isolation 98%
		Auscultation and clinical signs	56 DLT too deep in the left bronchus (n = 21 hypoxemia)
			Fiberoptic bronchoscopy was used n = 58
Klein et al. [42]	200 L-R DLTs (prospective study)	Auscultation/clamping/followed by a fiberoptic bronchoscopy with a second anesthesiologist	35% malpositions
			Optimal position achieved with the use of fiberoptic bronchoscopy in all cases
Seymour et al. [45]	506 L-R DLTs (survey)	Audit of DLT	56% used fiberoptic bronchoscopy
		Auscultation/clamping maneuvers or fiberoptic bronchoscopy	>10% hypoxemia (SpO$_2$ < 88%)
Bellis, et al. [48]	104 L- DLTs (prospective study)	Auscultation/clamping maneuvers or fiberoptic bronchoscopy	37% unrecognized malposition when auscultation was used all malpositions were corrected with fiberoptic bronchoscopy

DLT double-lumen endotracheal tube; *R* right; *L* left

New Technology with Double-Lumen Endotracheal Tubes

Fuji Systems in Tokyo, Japan, has introduced the Silbroncho DLT, which is made of silicone. The unique characteristic of this device relies on the wire-reinforced endobronchial tip. Also, the short bronchial tip and reduced bronchial cuff should increase the margin of safety when compared with a Broncho-Cath left-sided DLT. At the present time, only a left-sided Silbroncho DLT is available on the market [49]. Its effectiveness has not been reported.

Also, there is a newly designed right-sided DLT, the Cliny® (Create Medic Co., Ltd., Yokohama, Japan). This device has a long oblique bronchial cuff and two ventilation slots for the right upper lobe. The proximal part of the bronchial cuff is located immediately opposite the tracheal orifice. This device can be useful in patients with a very short right mainstem bronchus [50]. Figure 16.9 (a) displays the Silbroncho left-sided DLT and (b) displays the Cliny® right-sided DLT (c) VivaSight DLT® left-sided.

Another newly designed DLT has been designed to enable rapid and reliable lung isolation using a bronchial blocker. The Papworth BiVent Tube [51, 52] is a DLT with two D-shaped lumens arranged in a side-by-side configuration, separated by a central position. The tube characteristics include a preformed single posterior concavity and a single inflatable, low-volume, high-pressure tracheal cuff. At the distal end, there are two pliable crescent-shaped flanges arising from the central position to form a forked tip. The purpose of the forked tip is to seat at the tracheal carina. A bronchial blocker can be advanced blindly through either lumen and is guided into a bronchus. The size available for the Papworth BiVent tube at the present time is 43 F. According to the developers, the Papworth BiVent tube

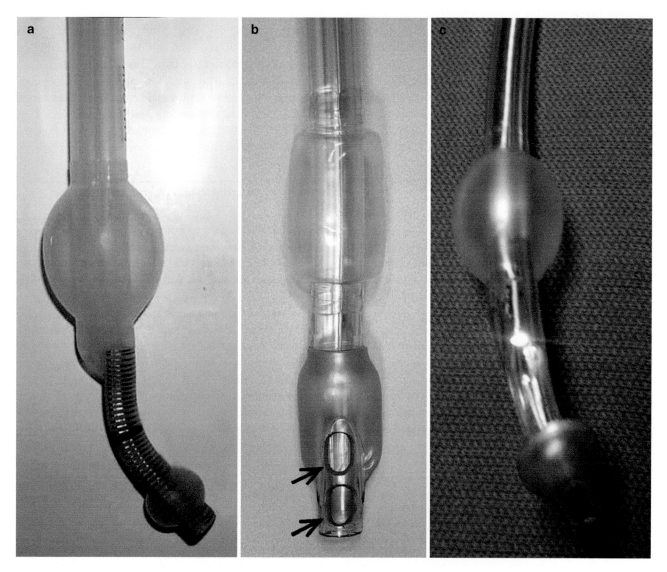

Fig. 16.9 (**a**) Silbroncho left-sided DLT. (**b**) Cliny® right-sided DLT. (**c**) VivaSight DLT® left-sided

can be used without the requirement for endoscopic guidance. Unfortunately, at the present time, there are no studies in humans to confirm its clinical use during lung separation.

A new DLT called the VivaSight DL® has an integrated high-resolution camera. The camera is embedded at the right end of the endotracheal lumen; when connected through a cable, the camera allows continuous visualization of the tracheal carina and blue cuff of the endobronchial lumen of the DLT [37]. The advantage of this device is the real-time image of the position of the DLT.

Complications Associated with Double-Lumen Endotracheal Tube Placement

The most common problems and complications from the use of DLTs are malpositions and airway trauma. A malpositioned DLT fails to allow collapse of the lung, causing gas trapping during positive pressure ventilation, or it may partially collapse the ventilated or dependant lung, producing hypoxemia. A common cause of malposition is dislodgement of the endobronchial cuff because of overinflation, surgical manipulation of the bronchus, or extension of the head and neck during or after patient positioning [53].

Airway trauma and rupture of the membranous part of the trachea or the bronchus continue to be infrequent problems with the use of DLTs [15, 17]. These complications can occur during insertion and placement, while the case is in progress, or during extubation [54–56]. Another problem that has been reported is the development of bilateral pneumothoraces or a tension pneumothorax in the dependent, ventilated lung [57, 58]. A 25-year review of the literature by Fitzmaurice and Brodsky [59] found that most airway injuries were associated with undersized DLTs, particularly in women who received a 35 or 37 F disposable DLT. It is likely that airway damage occurs when an undersized DLT migrates distally into the bronchus and the main tracheal body of the DLT advances into the bronchus, producing lacerations or rupture of the airway. Airway damage during the use of DLTs can present as unexpected air leaks, subcutaneous emphysema, massive bleeding into the lumen of the DLT, or protrusion of the endotracheal or endobronchial cuff into the surgical field, with visualization of this by the surgeon. If any of the aforementioned problems occur, a bronchoscopic examination should be performed and surgical repair performed.

Benign complications with the use of the DLT have been reported by Knoll et al. [60]. In their comparative study between the DLT and the endobronchial blocker, the development of postoperative hoarseness occurred significantly more commonly in the DLT group when compared to the endobronchial blocker group; however, the incidence of bronchial injuries was comparable between groups. A meta-analysis of a randomized controlled trial comparing the efficiency and adverse effects of DLT when compared with bronchial blockers showed that the DLTs were associated

with more patients having a sore throat and hoarseness and more minor airway injuries [61].

Also, a recent review on lung isolation for thoracic surgery reiterated that DLTs are quicker and more reliable to place but are associated with a higher incidence of airway injuries when compared to bronchial blocker [62]. A prospective randomized study [63] has shown that the use of dexamethasone 0.1 or 0.2 mg·kg is beneficial prior to the use of the DLT in order to reduce the incidence of sore throat and hoarseness up to 24 h.

Bronchial Blockers

An alternative method to achieve lung separation involves blockade of a mainstem bronchus to allow lung collapse distal to the occlusion [5]. Bronchial blockers also can be used selectively to achieve lobar collapse, if needed [64–70]. Currently, there are different bronchial blockers available to facilitate lung separation collapse; these devices either are attached to a single-lumen endotracheal tube with an enclosed bronchial blocker (Torque Control Blocker Univent) [5] or are used independently through or alongside a conventional single-lumen endotracheal tube, such as the wire-guided endobronchial blocker Arndt® blocker [6], the Cohen tip-deflecting endobronchial blocker [8], the Fuji Uniblocker® [9, 71], or the EZ-blocker® (Teleflex Medical, Morrisville, NC) [72, 73]. See Fig. 16.10.

Torque Control Blocker Univent

The Univent® tube consists of a single-lumen endotracheal tube with an enclosed and movable bronchial blocker made of flexible, nonlatex material, and it includes a flexible shaft that is easier to guide into a bronchus [6]. The bronchial balloon has a high-pressure, low-volume cuff that requires approximately 2 mL of air to produce an airtight seal if selective lobar blockade is used or 4–8 mL of air if the total blockade of the bronchus is desired. The bronchial blocker has a 2-mm-diameter lumen that can be used for suctioning or for oxygen administration and it should be closed before insertion. One of the advantages of the Univent® blocker is its utility in patients in whom the airway is considered difficult for direct laryngoscopy and during unanticipated difficult endotracheal intubation [74–80].

Placement of the Univent® blocker is straightforward. First the bronchial blocker is lubricated to facilitate passage. The enclosed bronchial blocker is fully retracted into the lumen of the tube. Conventional endotracheal tube placement is performed via direct laryngoscopy, and then a fiberoptic bronchoscope is passed through a Portex swivel adaptor into the endotracheal tube. Under direct vision, the enclosed bronchial blocker is advanced into the targeted bronchus. All bronchial blockers must be directed into the bronchus of the surgical side, where the lung collapse is to occur.

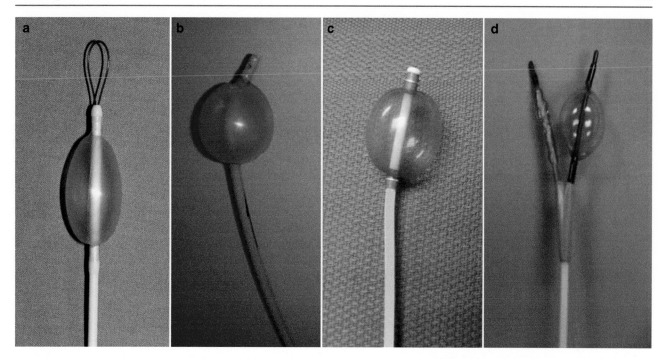

Fig. 16.10 Four independent bronchial blockers currently available in North America (see Table 16.6 for details). (**a**) The Arndt wire-guided endobronchial blocker (Arndt® Cook Critical Care), (**b**) the Cohen® tip-deflecting endobronchial blocker 9F (Cook Critical Care, Bloomington, IN), (**c**) the Fuji Uniblocker®, 9F (Fuji Corp., Tokyo, Japan), (**d**) EZ-blocker (Teleflex Medical, Morrisville, NC)

Independent Bronchial Blockers During Lung Isolation

Another alternative to achieve lung separation is by using an independent blocker passed through an in situ single-lumen endotracheal tube. The various devices considered to be independent blockers include the wire-guided endobronchial blocker (Arndt® blocker), the Cohen tip-deflecting endobronchial blocker, the Fuji Uniblocker®, and the EZ-blocker [9, 71].

Arndt® Wire-Guided Endobronchial Blocker

The Arndt® blocker [7] is an independent blocker attached to a 5 F, 7 F, or 9 F catheter that is available in 65- and 78-cm lengths with an inner lumen that measures 1.4 mm in diameter. Near the distal end of the catheter, side holes are incorporated to facilitate lung deflation. These side holes are present only in the 9 F Arndt® block. The Arndt® blocker has a high-volume, low-pressure cuff with either an elliptical or spherical shape (see Fig. 16.11). A unique feature of the Arndt® blocker compared with other blockers is that the inner lumen contains a flexible nylon wire passing through the proximal end of the catheter and extending to the distal end, which exits as a small flexible wire loop. This blocker comes with a multiport connector. The wire loop of the Arndt® blocker is coupled with the fiberoptic bronchoscope and serves as a guide wire to introduce the blocker into the bronchus [25]. For the Arndt® blocker to function properly and allow manipulation with the adult fiberoptic broncho-

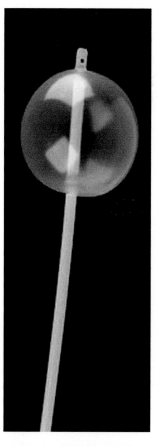

Fig. 16.11 The recently introduced Arndt® spherical bronchial blocker cuff (Cook Critical Care, Bloomington, IN). Some clinicians prefer to use this spherical cuff for right-sided surgery versus the original elliptical cuff because of the short length of the right mainstem bronchus

scope, the proper size endotracheal tube must be used. For a 7 F blocker which can be used for a 40-kg patient, a 7.5-mm internal diameter (ID) single-lumen endotracheal tube is used, and for the larger 9 F Arndt® blocker, at least an 8.0-mm ID single-lumen endotracheal tube is used. Figure 16.12a displays the placement of an Arndt® blocker through a single-lumen endotracheal tube with the fiberoptic bronchoscope advanced through the guide wire loop. Figure 16.12b displays the optimal position of the Arndt® blocker.

The advantages of the Arndt® blocker include its use in patients who are already tracheally intubated [81], who present a difficult airway and require an awake orotracheal or nasotracheal intubation [82], or who require OLV during acute trauma to the chest [83, 84]. In addition, an Arndt® blocker can be used as a selective lobar blocker in patients with previous pneumonectomy who require selective one-lobe ventilation [85] or as a selective blocker during severe pulmonary bleeding [86]. Figure 16.13a displays the use of a bronchial blocker for selective lobar blockade. Figure 16.13b displays the use of the Arndt® blocker in a patient with previous contralateral pneumonectomy and segmental lobar blockade.

Methods of Placement

The Arndt® blocker is an independent endobronchial blocker that is passed through an existing single-lumen endotracheal tube. To facilitate insertion through the endotracheal tube, the blocker and the fiberoptic bronchoscope are lubricated. For a right-sided mainstem bronchus intubation, the spherically shaped blocker is recommended; for the left mainstem bronchus intubation, the elliptical or the spherical blocker is used.

The placement of the Arndt® blocker involves placing the endobronchial blocker through the endotracheal tube and using the fiberoptic bronchoscope and wire-guided loop to direct the blocker into a mainstem bronchus. The fiberoptic bronchoscope has to be advanced distally enough so that the Arndt® blocker enters the bronchus while it is being advanced. When the deflated cuff is beyond the entrance of the bronchus, the fiberoptic bronchoscope is withdrawn, and the cuff is fully inflated with fiberoptic visualization with 4–8 mL of air to obtain total bronchial blockade.

For right mainstem bronchus blockade, the Arndt® blocker can be advanced independently of the wire loop by observing its entrance into the right mainstem bronchus under fiberoptic visualization. Before turning the patient into a lateral decubitus position, the cuff of the blocker should be deflated and then advanced 1 cm deeper to avoid proximal dislodgement while changing the patient's position; the placement again is confirmed in the lateral decubitus position. The wire loop can be withdrawn to convert the 1.4-mm channel into a suction port to expedite lung collapse. The newest version of the Arndt® blocker has a cone-shaped device that is attached

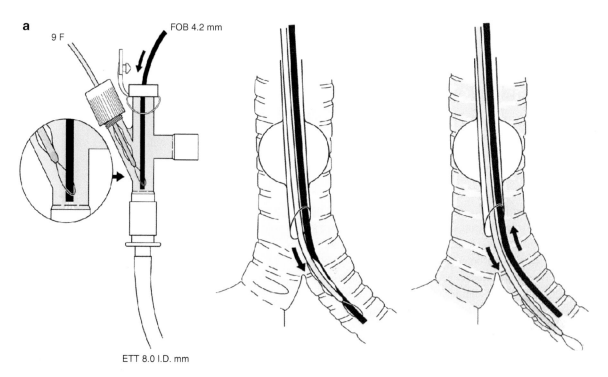

Fig. 16.12 (**a**) Placement of an Arndt® blocker through a single-lumen endotracheal tube with the fiberoptic bronchoscope advanced through the guide wire loop. (**b**) Optimal position of a bronchial blocker in the right or left mainstem bronchus as seen with a fiberoptic bronchoscope. (**A**) Right mainstem blocker; (**B**) Left mainstem blocker [25]

b

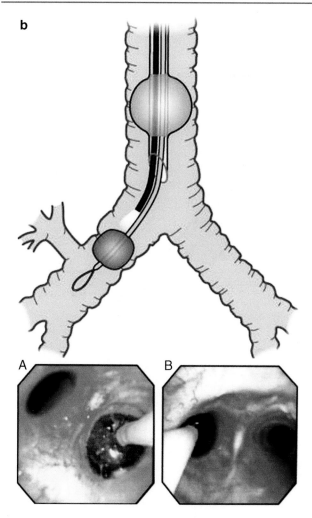

Fig. 16.12 (continued)

that allows deflection of the tip of the distal part of the blocker into the desired bronchus [2, 8, 73]. This device has been purposely preangled at the distal tip to facilitate insertion into a target bronchus. Also, there is a torque grip located at the 55-cm mark to allow rotating the blocker. In the distal tip above the balloon, there is an arrow that when seen with the fiberoptic bronchoscope indicates in which direction the tip deflects. This Cohen® blocker also comes with a multiport adaptor to facilitate an airtight seal when in place. The indications for use of the Cohen® blocker are the same as for the Arndt® blocker. Figure 16.14 displays the Cohen® blocker.

Methods of Placement

The Cohen® blocker is advanced through an 8.0-mm ID single-lumen endotracheal tube; before insertion, the blocker balloon is tested and then fully deflated. This blocker needs

to the center channel to connect and facilitate suction [87, 88]. It is important to remove the wire loop to avoid inclusion in the stapling line of the bronchus [89]. The optimal position of the Arndt® blocker in the left or in the right bronchus is achieved when the blocker balloon's outer surface is seen with the fiberoptic bronchoscope at least 5 mm below the tracheal carina on the targeted bronchus and the proper seal is obtained.

Cohen® Flexitip Endobronchial Blocker

The Cohen® blocker is an independent endobronchial blocker that is available only in size 9 F and 65-cm length with an inner lumen measuring 1.4 mm in diameter. This device comes with a spherically shaped balloon. Near the distal end of the catheter, there are side holes incorporated to facilitate lung deflation. This bronchial blocker has a high-volume, low-pressure cuff. The Cohen® blocker relies on a wheel-turning device located in the most proximal part of the unit

a

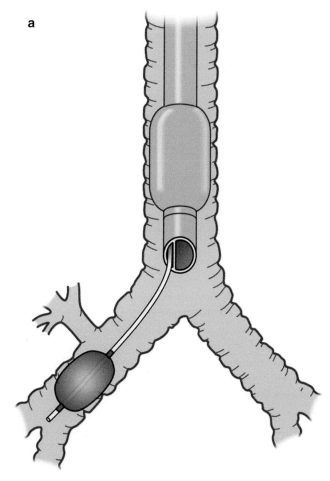

Fig. 16.13 (**a**) Selective lobar blockade where the blocker is sealing the right bronchus intermedius. (**b**) Patient with a previous right pneumonectomy where selective lobar blockade is used to occlude the left upper lobe. *R* stump of right mainstem bronchus; *C* main carina; *L* left mainstem bronchus; *LUL* left upper lobe; *LLL* left lower lobe [70]

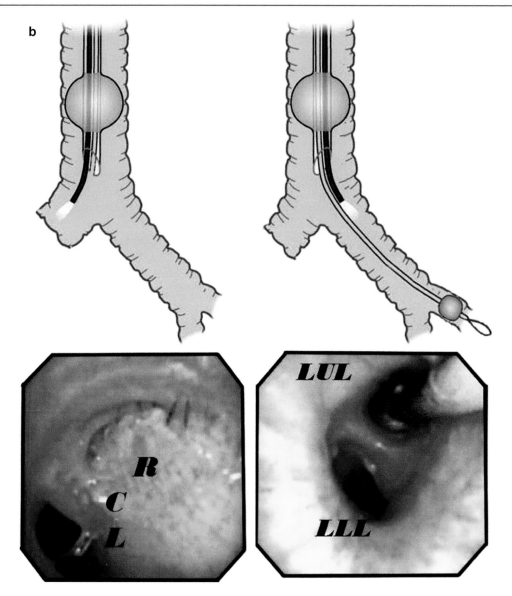

Fig. 16.13 (continued)

to be lubricated to facilitate insertion and passage through the single-lumen endotracheal tube.

The placement of the Cohen® blocker involves placing the endobronchial blocker through the endotracheal tube and using the fiberoptic bronchoscope to observe the direction of the blocker into a mainstem bronchus. For blocking the right mainstem bronchus, the optimal position is the one that provides a view of the outer surface of the fully inflated balloon (4–8 mL of air) with the fiberoptic bronchoscope at least 5 mm below the tracheal carina on the right mainstem bronchus.

Intubation of the left mainstem bronchus can be facilitated by allowing the tip of the single-lumen endotracheal tube to be near the entrance of the left bronchus and then twisting the Cohen® blocker to the left side. After the blocker is seen inside the left bronchus, the single-lumen endotracheal tube is withdrawn a few centimeters. A different alternative is to turn

the head toward the right allowing the left main bronchus to displace to the midline. This maneuver will facilitate the placement of a Cohen® blocker into the left mainstem bronchus. The optimal position in the left mainstem bronchus is achieved when the blocker balloon's outer surface is seen with the fiberoptic bronchoscope at least 5 mm below the trachea carina inside the left mainstem bronchus.

Fuji Uniblocker®

The Fuji Uniblocker® is an independent bronchial blocker that is available in 4.5 and 9 F size and is 65 cm in length that has a high-volume balloon made of silicone with a gas barrier property to reduce diffusion of gas into or out of the cuff. Also, with its maximal cuff inflation of 6 mL of air, this new bronchial blocker's transmitted pressure tested in vitro was

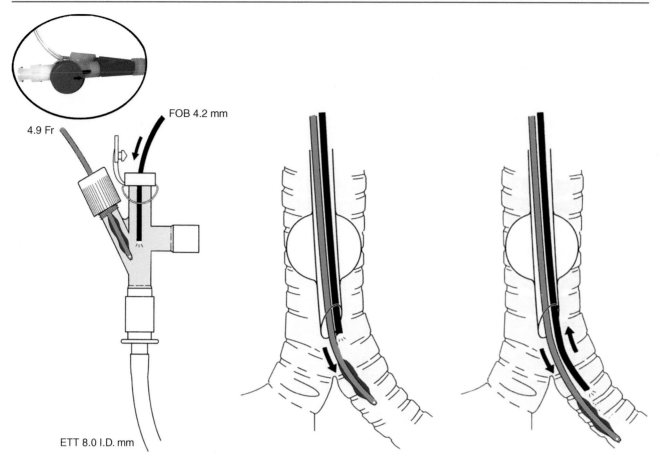

Fig. 16.14 The Cohen flexitip bronchial blocker with a multiport connector [90]

<30 mmHg, which does not exceed the recommended safety limit in relationship to bronchial mucosa [91]. In addition, the Fuji Uniblocker® is equipped with a swivel connector. The swivel connector allows easy insertion of the fiberoptic bronchoscope. The Fuji Uniblocker® has a torque control blocker with an incorporated shaft that allows the guidance through the desired bronchus. A recent study [9] involving the use of the Fuji Uniblocker® compared with the Arndt® and Cohen® blocker showed that surgical exposure was clinically equivalent to left-sided DLTs for thoracoscopic or open thoracotomies; however, the bronchial blockers including the Fuji Uniblocker® took a longer time to position and required more intraoperative repositioning when compared to left-sided DLTs. Another report [92], this one examining the use Fuji Uniblocker® in patients undergoing thoracoscopic surgery, showed a better quality of lung collapse with left-sided procedures than right-sided procedures. The indications for use of the Fuji Uniblocker® are the same as for the Arndt® blocker. Table 16.5 displays the characteristics of the Arndt® blocker, the Cohen® flexitip endobronchial blocker, the Fuji Uniblocker®, and the EZ-blocker. The Cohen® and Fuji® blockers can be easily placed through the glottis or tracheostomy external to an endotracheal tube, if required in small patients, and the blocker position confirmed with a FOB passed through the endotracheal tube.

Methods of Placement

The Fuji Uniblocker® size 9 F is advanced through an 8.0-mm ID single-lumen endotracheal tube; before insertion the blocker balloon is tested and then fully deflated. This blocker needs to be lubricated to facilitate insertion and passage through the single-lumen endotracheal tube.

The placement of the Fuji Uniblocker® involves placing the endobronchial blocker through the endotracheal tube and using the fiberoptic bronchoscope to observe the direction of the blocker into a mainstem bronchus. The torque control shaft with the blocker allows guidance into the desired target bronchus. For blocking the right mainstem bronchus, the optimal position is the one that provides a view of the outer surface of the fully inflated balloon (4–8 mL of air) with the fiberoptic bronchoscope at least 5 mm below the tracheal carina on the right mainstem bronchus. The optimal position in the left mainstem bronchus is achieved when the blocker balloon's outer surface is seen with the fiberoptic bronchoscope at least 5–10 mm below

Table 16.5 Characteristics of the Arndt® blocker, the Cohen® flexitip endobronchial blocker, the Fuji Uniblocker®, and the EZ-Blocker

	Cohen blocker	Arndt® blocker	Fuji Uniblocker®	EZ-blocker
Size	9 F	5 F, 7 F, and 9 F	4.5 F, 9 F	7 F
Balloon shape	Spherical	Spherical or elliptical	Spherical	Spherical Two balloons
Guidance mechanism	Wheel device to deflect the tip	Nylon wire loop that is coupled with the fiberoptic bronchoscope	None, preshaped tip	None
Smallest recommended *ETT for coaxial use	9 F (8.0 ETT)	5 F (4.5 ETT), 7 F (7.0 ETT), 9 F (8.0 ETT)	4.5 F (4.5 ETT) 9 F (8.0 ETT)	(7.5 or 8.0 ETT)
Murphy eye	Present	Present in 9F	Not present	Not present
Center channel	1.6-mm internal diameter	1.4-mm internal diameter	2.0-mm internal diameter	1.0-mm internal diameter

Reprinted and modified from Campos [71], with permission
ETT single endotracheal tube

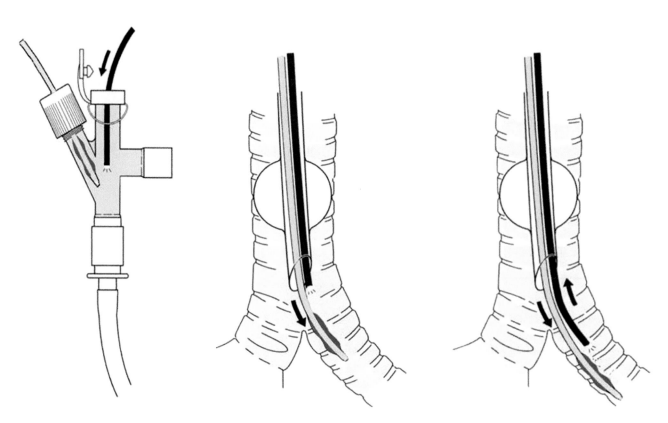

Fig. 16.15 Placement of the Fuji blocker

the trachea carina inside the left mainstem bronchus. Figure 16.15 displays the Fuji blocker and placement.

The EZ-Blocker

The EZ-blocker is an independent bronchial blocker that is available in a 7.0 F size and made of polyurethane material. The EZ-blocker is manufactured with a Y-shaped distal end. Both limbs of the distal end are fitted with an inflatable balloon and a central channel in each to allow suction. Also, each limb is color coded (yellow or blue) for easy

identification with the matching pilot balloon. The EZ-blocker is inserted through a port on the enclosed multiport adapter that is attached to a single-lumen endotracheal tube. The optimal size of the single-lumen endotracheal tube should be 7.5 or 8.0 mm internal diameter so it allows the blocker and the fiberoptic bronchoscope to navigate together.

The multiport adaptor of the EZ-blocker is designed to connect to a connector of the single-lumen endotracheal tube and it contains two additional ports, one to allow advancement of the blocker and the other port for passing the flexible fiberoptic bronchoscope.

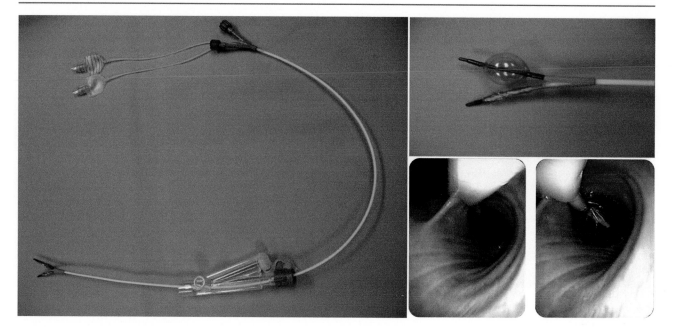

Fig. 16.16 Placement of the EZ-Blocker

Methods of Placement

The EZ-blocker is tested and lubricated prior to passing into the lumen of the single-lumen endotracheal tube and the multiport connector. After advancing the blocker, the Y-shaped end should be seated in the tracheal carina and each independent tip should be located in the entrance of right and left bronchus. Only the balloon where lung isolation occurs should be inflated under direct fiberoptic bronchoscopy. The pilot of the cuff is color coded to allow identification of the respective balloon (one is yellow and the other one is blue). After the tip of the deflated balloon is in the bronchus, inflation of the balloon should be performed with flexible fiberoptic bronchoscopy. Unfortunately the balloon of the EZ-blocker sometimes requires between 10 and 14 cc of air to block the left or right bronchus [72]. Proper and optimal position is when the outer surface of the balloon is seen 5–10 mm below the entrance of the bronchus. A common problem with the EZ blocker is that both limbs initially enter the right mainstem bronchus. This requires withdrawing the blocker above the carina and readvancement under direct vision with the bronchoscope. The distal end of the single-lumen ETT should be at least 4 cm above the carina to minimize this problem. The distal Y-junction of the two limbs of the blocker must be firmly seated on the carina to minimize displacement of the blocker during surgery. Figure 16.16 displays the optimal position of the EZ-blocker.

Complications with the Use of Bronchial Blockers

Although serious complications have been reported with the use of current bronchial blockers, these complications appear to be more benign than those involving DLTs. A structural complication has been reported in the torque control Univent blocker in which a fracture of the blocker cap connector occurred in 2 of the first 50 tubes used [93]. Failure to achieve lung separation because of abnormal anatomy, in which the entrance of the right upper lobe bronchus was located above the tracheal carina, or lack of seal within the bronchus also has been reported [94, 95]. Inclusion of the enclosed bronchial blocker into the stapling line has been reported during a right upper lobectomy [96]. Communication with the surgical team regarding the presence of a bronchial blocker in the surgical side is crucial. Another potential and dangerous complication with the bronchial cuff of the Univent has been reported: the cuff of the bronchial blocker was inflated mistakenly near the tracheal lumen, precluding all airflow and producing respiratory arrest [97].

Complications with the Arndt® blocker include a report of a sheared balloon of the Arndt® blocker that occurred when the blocker was removed through the multiport blocker side [98]. It is advised that when an independent bronchial blocker is not in use, it needs to be removed with the multiport connector in place rather than through the connector to prevent shredded material into the single-lumen endotracheal tube. Another near-fatal complication reported with the use of the

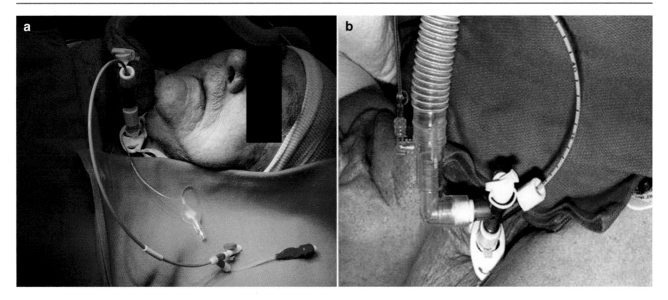

Fig. 16.17 (**a**) Cohen® blocker in a patient with a tracheostomy. (**b**) Use of an Arndt® blocker via a tracheostomy

Arndt® blocker occurred when the fully inflated balloon of the blocker dislodged into the patient's trachea, leading to a complete airway obstruction. Severe air trapping led to pulseless activity in the patient, who was undergoing a rupture descending thoracic aortic aneurysm. A prompt deflation of the bronchial blocker cuff resolved the problem [99].

Another complication reported with the Arndt® blocker involved inadvertent resection of the guide wire and part of the tip of the bronchial blocker during stapler resection of the left lower lobe; this complication required surgical reexploration after unsuccessful removal of the bronchial blocker after extubation [89].

In a retrospective review of 302 consecutive cases from a single institution, no major complications were found with the use of different bronchial blockers during lung isolation [100]. A recent report involving three cases where the balloon of the Fuji blocker failed to deflate at the conclusion of the surgery. In two of the cases, the already inflated bronchial blocker had to be removed along with the single-lumen endotracheal tube during extubation [101]. It is recommended to test the pilot and the balloon prior to use to ensure that the air that is injected is aspirated and the balloon completely deflates. When compared the complications the DLTs outnumber the reported complications with the bronchial blockers.

Lung Isolation in Patients with Tracheostomy in Place

OLV can be a challenge in patients with a tracheostomy in place because the airway has been shortened and the stoma can be small and restrictive. Although a shortened version of a DLT for tracheostomy patients has been used [102, 103], there is no shortened DLT available for tracheostomy patients

in the United States. An alternative to achieve successful lung separation through a tracheostomized patient involves the use of a bronchial blocker, either attached to a single-lumen endotracheal tube such as the Univent® blocker [104, 105], or passed independently through a Shiley 8.0-mm ID tracheostomy tube (Mallinckrodt, St. Louis, MO) with the Arndt® bronchial blocker [69], or placed independently through a single-lumen endotracheal tube [106]. An alternative way to manage these cases is with the Cohen® Blocker [8] or the Fuji Uniblocker® [9]; when passing a 9 F bronchial blocker through a tracheostomy tube, the recommended flexible fiberoptic bronchoscope should be 3.5-mm ID so the independent blocker and the fiberscope can navigate together to achieve optimal position of these devices into the designed bronchus. In some instances when using a Shiley tracheostomy tube, the multiport connector is attached to the ventilating port of the Shiley cannula to maintain the bronchial blocker in place. Optimal position is achieved with the fiberoptic bronchoscope. Figure 16.17 displays the use of an independent blocker through a tracheostomy stoma.

Lung Collapse During Lung Isolation

A challenge for every anesthesiologist is to properly position a lung isolation device and make it work by allowing the lung to collapse. In a study [6] comparing the Broncho-Cath left-sided DLT with the Univent® torque control blocker and the Arndt® wire-guided blocker, it was shown that the average time for lung collapse is 17 min for a DLT (spontaneous lung collapse without suction) versus 19–26 min for the Univent® or Arndt® bronchial blocker (assisted with suction). Once lung isolation was achieved, however, the overall clinical performance was similar for the three devices studied.

Another study [9] involving left-sided DLTs and comparing it with the Arndt®, the Cohen®, or the Fuji® blocker showed that the surgical exposure was equivalent among the devices studied. However, the bronchial blockers required longer time to position and were more prone to intraoperative reposition. It is important to emphasize that these two studies involved at least one senior thoracic anesthesiologist with broad experience with lung isolation devices.

A study [107] has shown that denitrogenation of the lung which is to be collapsed with a FiO$_2$ 1.0 is a useful strategy to improve surgical conditions during OLV; in contrast, the use of air in the inspired gas mixture during two-lung ventilation and prior to OLV delays lung collapse during OLV. A recent study involving the use of a bronchial blocker showed that the use of nitrous oxide in a mixture of N$_2$O/O$_2$ (FiO$_2$ = 0.5) facilitated lung collapse after opening the chest compared with a comparative group using 100% oxygen. Both groups also have a suction assisted in place during one-lung ventilation [108]. Another study involving morbidly obese patients undergoing one-lung ventilation where a left-sided DLT was compared with the Arndt wire-guided blocker reported that there was no overall advantage of one device over the other during intubation or the success of lung collapse both devices were very comparable [109].

A recent study comparing the Fuji blocker with a left-sided DLT in video-assisted thoracoscopic surgery reported that the bronchial blocker had a faster time to obtain lung collapse and overall superior quality of lung deflation when compared to a left-sided DLT [110].

Combining all studies my recommendation is that all anesthesiologists should be familiar with the use of bronchial blockers and DLTs during lung isolation techniques. Editorial reports, scientific evidence, and topic of debates support this recommendation [6, 111, 112].

Table 16.6 displays the advantages and disadvantages of DLTs and bronchial blockers.

Future Trends in Lung Isolation

With the advances in thoracic, cardiac, esophageal surgery, and minimally invasive surgery, it has led to an increased need for lung isolation techniques among anesthesiologists. A previous study [47] has shown that anesthesiologists with limited thoracic experience often fail to correctly place lung isolation devices. Increased clinical experience would likely reduce this failure rate, but greater experienced may not be possible, particularly for anesthesiologists working in centers that perform relatively few thoracic cases. Therefore, improved nonclinical training methods are needed.

Anesthesia simulators have been used to enhance learning and to improve performance [113–115], usually under

Table 16.6 Advantages and disadvantages of DLTs and bronchial blockers

Double-lumen endotracheal tubes	Bronchial blockers (Arndt®, Cohen®, Fuji®)
Advantages	
Large lumen facilitates suctioning	Easy recognition of anatomy if the tip of a single tube is above carina
Best device for absolute indications for lung separation, to protect the lung from soiling	Best device for patients with difficult airways
Conversion from two- to one-lung ventilation and back easy and reliable	Cuff damage during intubation rare
	No need to replace a tube if mechanical ventilation is needed
Disadvantages	
Difficulties in selecting proper size	Small channel for suctioning
More difficult to place during laryngoscopy	Conversion from one- to two- and then to one-lung ventilation problematic more complicated
Potential damage to tracheal cuff during intubation	High maintenance device (frequent dislodgement or loss of seal during surgery)
Rare major tracheobronchial injuries	

Modified from Campos [71]

the personal direction of an experienced clinician. Therefore, one educational approach to lung isolation techniques might involve training on an airway simulator mentored by an experienced thoracic anesthesiologist. An alternative is to train in a fiberoptic bronchoscopy simulator [116] on lung isolation techniques particularly for the occasional anesthesiologist who does not perform thoracic cases on a regular basis. In a study involving anesthesiologists with limited thoracic experience comparing the simulator intubation model versus computer didactic-based material in how to place a left-sided DLT, it showed that both teaching methods had similar outcomes when this group of anesthesiologists placed the DLTs after their training [117].

Another study involving high-fidelity simulation of lung isolation with double-lumen endotracheal tubes and bronchial blockers in anesthesiology residents showed that their performance to place lung isolation devices was very successful [118]. A similar model/study was performed involving senior medical students to teach basic lung isolation skills on a simulator, and it showed that video-didactic and simulation-based methods were very comparable and successful in training novices for lung isolation techniques [119]. This study also reported that the acquired skills particularly decreased without practice. Regardless of the method to teach lung isolation techniques, it should be used periodically in anesthesiologist with limited thoracic experience in order to retain their level of skills.

It is the author's personal opinion that every surgical center that performs lung isolation techniques must consider the

Fig. 16.18 Ideal teaching facility with a pulmonary work station for placement of lung isolation devices by trainees

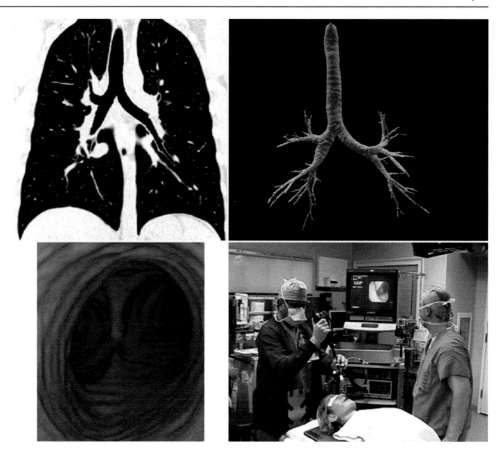

development of a pulmonary workstation along with simulator training facility to enhance teaching to residents, fellows, and staff anesthesiologists [117–119]. Figure 16.18 displays a pulmonary workstation including simulator. Also, a free online bronchoscopy simulator is available on the website www.thoracicanesthesia.com to teach anesthesiologists tracheobronchial anatomy (see Fig. 16.19).

Summary

The basic principle of successful lung separation requires (1) recognition of tracheobronchial anatomy with a posteroanterior chest radiograph in the preoperative evaluation and with flexible fiberoptic bronchoscopy in the perioperative period, (2) familiarity and skills with flexible fiberoptic bronchoscopy, and (3) familiarity and expertise with DLTs and bronchial blockers.

Because of its greater margin of safety, a left-sided DLT is the more common and easiest device used during lung separation. A right-sided DLT is recommended for a left-sided pneumonectomy or any contraindication to placement of a left-sided DLT. For patients with a difficult abnormal airway or a tracheostomy in place, the use of a bronchial blocker is indicated. Bronchial blockers require more time for placement and are more prone to intraoperative dislodgement. Lung collapse is facilitated with a denitrogenation technique using FiO_2 1.0 during two-lung ventilation prior to lung col-

lapse. Every lung isolation device placement requires auscultation and clamping maneuvers followed by a fiberoptic bronchoscopy to obtain 100% success during lung separation techniques. The optimal position of these devices (DLTs and bronchial blockers) is achieved best with the use of fiberoptic bronchoscopy techniques with the patient first in the supine and then in the lateral decubitus position or whenever repositioning of the device is needed.

Clinical Case Discussion

Case: A 60-year-old female, weight 61 kg and is 161 cm tall, has a left lower lobe mass and is scheduled for a left lower lobectomy (Fig. 16.17a, b). She is a former smoker and the predicted value of forced expiratory volume in 1 s (FEV_1) is 75% of the predicted value. She has no significant known comorbidities and past history otherwise unremarkable (see Fig. 16.20).

Questions

- What lung isolation device will be indicated?
- What side and size of lung isolation device will be indicated?
- What anatomical structures in the chest radiograph are relevant while planning the use of lung isolation devices?

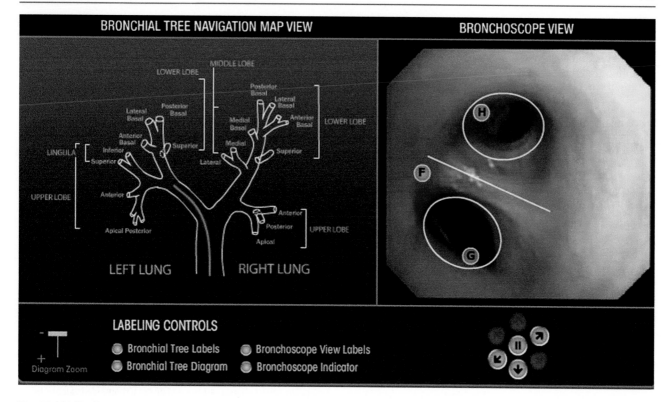

Fig. 16.19 The free online bronchoscopy simulator at www.thoracic-anesthesia.com. The user can navigate the tracheobronchial tree using real-time video by clicking on the lighted directional arrows under the "Bronchoscopic view" (right). Clicking on the labels on the "Bronchoscopic view" gives details of the anatomy seen. The process is aided by the "Bronchial Tree Navigational Map" (left), which shows the simultaneous location of the bronchoscope as the orange line in the airway

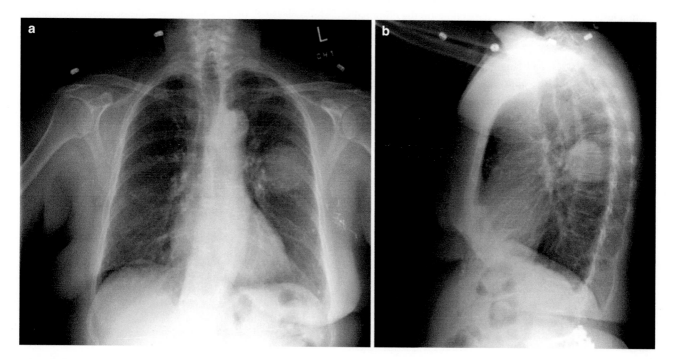

Fig. 16.20 (**a, b**) Chest X-ray of a female patient with a carcinoma of the left lower lobe undergoing a lobectomy

- What are the different alternatives for lung isolation devices?
- What technique should be used to achieve optimal position of lung isolation devices?
- What are the common problems in the intraoperative period with lung isolation devices?
- What are the complications associated with lung isolation devices?

Focus on the Patient's Gender, Size, Height, and Preoperative Chest Radiograph

- To determine the lung isolation device.
- Focus on the use of left-sided DLT for routine, uncomplicated cases or a right-sided DLT for selective cases.
- Focus on the indication of lung isolation.
- Knowledge of tracheobronchial anatomy and the use of flexible fiberoptic bronchoscopy to confirm device placement are essential for success on lung isolation.
- Alternative devices for lung isolation such as bronchial blockers should be considered in specific cases.

Choice of Lung Isolation Device

- If there is nothing in the patient's history or physical examination to suggest the possibility of difficult airway in a left- or right-sided DLT, depending on the clinician's preference, would be equivalent first choices to manage this case.
- The patient's sex and height suggest that either a 35 or 37 F DLT would be appropriate and the choice can be further refined by measuring the tracheal width on the PA chest X-ray (see Fig. 16.1).
- In the absence of a difficult airway, the problem of intraoperative displacement with bronchial blockers makes them a second choice for lung isolation in this patient.
- Correct positioning of the device for lung isolation should be confirmed with fiberoptic bronchoscopy.

Expected Intraoperative Problems During Lung Isolation

- Malpositions and the potential for tracheobronchial injuries

References

1. Campos JH. Current techniques for perioperative lung isolation in adults. Anesthesiology. 2002;97:1295–301.
2. Campos JH. Progress in lung separation. Thorac Surg Clin. 2005;15:71–83.
3. Lewis JW Jr, Serwin JP, Gabriel FS, Bastanfar M, Jacobsen G. The utility of a double-lumen tube for one-lung ventilation in a variety of noncardiac thoracic surgical procedures. J Cardiothorac Vasc Anesth. 1992;6:705–10.
4. Schuepbach R, Grande B, Camen G, et al. Intubation with VivaSight or conventional left-sided double-lumen tubes: a randomized trial. Can J Anaesth. 2015;62:762–9.
5. Campos JH. An update on bronchial blockers during lung separation techniques in adults. Anesth Analg. 2003;97:1266–74.
6. Campos JH, Kernstine KH. A comparison of a left-sided Broncho-Cath with the torque control blocker univent and the wire-guided blocker. Anesth Analg. 2003;96:283–9.
7. Arndt GA, Kranner PW, Rusy DA, Love R. Single-lung ventilation in a critically ill patient using a fiberoptically directed wire-guided endobronchial blocker. Anesthesiology. 1999;90:1484–6.
8. Cohen E. The Cohen flexitip endobronchial blocker: an alternative to a double lumen tube. Anesth Analg. 2005;101:1877–9.
9. Narayanaswamy M, McRae K, Slinger P, et al. Choosing a lung isolation device for thoracic surgery: a randomized trial of three bronchial blockers versus double-lumen tubes. Anesth Analg. 2009;108:1097–101.
10. Ruetzler K, Grubhofer G, Schmid W, et al. Randomized clinical trial comparing double-lumen tube and EZ-blocker for single-lung ventilation. Br J Anaesth. 2011;106:896–0.
11. Bjork VO, Carlens E. The prevention of spread during pulmonary resection by the use of a double-lumen catheter. J Thorac Surg. 1950;20:151–7.
12. Campos JH, Massa FC, Kernstine KH. The incidence of right upper-lobe collapse when comparing a right-sided double-lumen tube versus a modified left double-lumen tube for left-sided thoracic surgery. Anesth Analg. 2000;90:535–40.
13. Seymour AH, Prakash N. A cadaver study to measure the adult glottis and subglottis: defining a problem associated with the use of double-lumen tubes. J Cardiothorac Vasc Anesth. 2002;16:196–8.
14. Sivalingam P, Tio R. Tension pneumothorax, pneumomediastinum, pneumoperitoneum, and subcutaneous emphysema in a 15-year-old Chinese girl after a double-lumen tube intubation and one-lung ventilation. J Cardiothorac Vasc Anesth. 1999;13:312–5.
15. Bardoczky G, d'Hollander A, Yernault JC, et al. On-line expiratory flow-volume curves during thoracic surgery: occurrence of auto-PEEP. Br J Anaesth. 1994;72:25–8.
16. Sakuragi T, Kumano K, Yasumoto M, Dan K. Rupture of the left main-stem bronchus by the tracheal portion of a double-lumen endobronchial tube. Acta Anaesthesiol Scand. 1997;41:1218–20.
17. Hannallah M, Gomes M. Bronchial rupture associated with the use of a double-lumen tube in a small adult. Anesthesiology. 1989;71:457–8.
18. Brodsky JB, Macario A, Mark JB. Tracheal diameter predicts double-lumen tube size: a method for selecting left double-lumen tubes. Anesth Analg. 1996;82:861–4.
19. Chow MY, Liam BL, Lew TW, Chelliah RY, Ong BC. Predicting the size of a double-lumen endobronchial tube based on tracheal diameter. Anesth Analg. 1998;87:158–60.
20. Amar D, Desiderio DP, Heerdt PM, et al. Practice patterns in choice of left double-lumen tube size for thoracic surgery. Anesth Analg. 2008;106:379–83.
21. Eberle B, Weiler N, Vogel N, Kauczor HU, Heinrichs W. Computed tomography-based tracheobronchial image reconstruction allows selection of the individually appropriate double-lumen tube size. J Cardiothorac Vasc Anesth. 1999;13:532–7.
22. Campos JH. Update on tracheobronchial anatomy and flexible fiberoptic bronchoscopy in thoracic anesthesia. Curr Opin Anaesthesiol. 2009;22:4–10.
23. Brodsky JB, Benumof JL, Ehrenwerth J, Ozaki GT. Depth of placement of left double-lumen endobronchial tubes. Anesth Analg. 1991;73:570–2.

24. Boucek CD, Landreneau R, Freeman JA, Strollo D, Bircher NG. A comparison of techniques for placement of double-lumen endobronchial tubes. J Clin Anesth. 1998;10:557–60.

25. Campos JH. How to achieve successful lung separation. SAJAA. 2008;14:22–6.

26. Cavus E, Kieckhaefer J, Doerges V, et al. The C-MAC videolaryngoscope: first experiences with a new device for videolaryngoscopy-guided intubation. Anesth Analg. 2010 Feb;110:473–7.

27. Purugganan RV, Jackson TA, Heir JS, et al. Video laryngoscopy versus direct laryngoscopy for double-lumen endotracheal tube intubation: a retrospective analysis. J Cardiothorac Vasc Anesth. 2012;26:845–8.

28. Russell T, Slinger P, Roscoe A, et al. A randomised controlled trial comparing the GlideScope(®) and the Macintosh laryngoscope for double-lumen endobronchial intubation. Anaesthesia. 2013;68:1253–8.

29. Chastel B, Perrier V, Germain A, et al. Usefulness of the Airtraq DL™ videolaryngoscope for placing a double-lumen tube. Anaesth Crit Care Pain Med. 2015;34:89–93.

30. Brodsky JB, Lemmens HJ. Left double-lumen tubes: clinical experience with 1,170 patients. J Cardiothorac Vasc Anesth. 2003;17:289–98.

31. Benumof JL, Partridge BL, Salvatierra C, Keating J. Margin of safety in positioning modern double-lumen endotracheal tubes. Anesthesiology. 1987;67:729–38.

32. McKenna MJ, Wilson RS, Botelho RJ. Right upper lobe obstruction with right-sided double-lumen endobronchial tubes: a comparison of two tube types. J Cardiothorac Anesth. 1988;2:734–40.

33. Campos JH, Gomez MN. Pro: right-sided double-lumen endotracheal tubes should be routinely used in thoracic surgery. J Cardiothorac Vasc Anesth. 2002;16:246–8.

34. Bussières JS, Lacasse Y, Côté D, et al. Modified right-sided Broncho-Cath® double lumen tube improves endobronchial positioning: a randomized study. Can J Anaesth. 2007;54:276–82.

35. Stene R, Rose M, Weinger MB, Benumof JL, Harrell J. Bronchial trifurcation at the carina complicating use of a double-lumen tracheal tube. Anesthesiology. 1994;80:1162–3.

36. Ehrenfeld JM, Walsh JL, Sandberg WS. Right- and left-sided Mallinckrodt double-lumen tubes have identical clinical performance. Anesth Analg. 2008;106:1847–52.

37. Campos JH, Hanada S. DLT with incorporated fiberoptic bronchoscopy. Chapter 116. In: Rosenblatt WH, Popescu WM, editors. Master techniques in upper and lower airway management: Wolters Kluwer Health; 2015. p. 250–1.

38. Saracoglu A, Saracoglu KT. VivaSight: a new era in the evolution of tracheal tubes. J Clin Anesth. 2016;33:442–9.

39. Heir JS, Purugganan R, Jackson TA, et al. A retrospective evaluation of the use of video-capable double-lumen endotracheal tubes in thoracic surgery. J Cardiothorac Vasc Anesth. 2014;28:870–2.

40. Massot J, Dumand-Nizard V, Fischler M, et al. Evaluation of the double-lumen tube vivasight-DL (DLT-ETView): a prospective single-center study. J Cardiothorac Vasc Anesth. 2015;29:1544–9.

41. Levy-Faber D, Malyanker Y, Nir RR, et al. Comparison of VivaSight double-lumen tube with a conventional double-lumen tube in adult patients undergoing video-assisted thoracoscopic surgery. Anaesthesia. 2015;70:1259–63.

42. Klein U, Karzai W, Bloos F, et al. Role of fiberoptic bronchoscopy in conjunction with the use of double-lumen tubes for thoracic anesthesia: a prospective study. Anesthesiology. 1998;88:346–50.

43. Sherry K. Management of patients undergoing oesophagectomy. In: Gray AJG, Hoile RW, Ingram GS, Sherry K, editors. The report of the national confidential enquiry into perioperative deaths 1996/1997. London: NCEPOD; 1998. p. 57–61.

44. Pennefather SH, Russell GN. Placement of double lumen tubes – time to shed light on an old problem. Br J Anaesth. 2000;84:308–10.

45. Seymour AH, Prasad B, McKenzie RJ. Audit of double-lumen endobronchial intubation. Br J Anaesth. 2004;93:525–7.

46. Slinger P. A view of and through double-lumen tubes. J Cardiothorac Vasc Anesth. 2003;17:287–8.

47. Campos JH, Hallam EA, Van Natta T, Kernstine KH. Devices for lung isolation used by anesthesiologists with limited thoracic experience: comparison of double-lumen endotracheal tube, Univent torque control blocker, and Arndt wire-guided endobronchial blocker. Anesthesiology. 2006;104:261–6.

48. de Bellis M, Accardo R, Di Maio M, et al. Is flexible bronchoscopy necessary to confirm the position of double-lumen tubes before thoracic surgery? Eur J Cardiothorac Surg. 2011;40:912–6.

49. Lohser J, Brodsky JB. Silbronco double-lumen tube. J Cardiothorac Vasc Anesth. 2006;20:129–31.

50. Hagihira S, Takashina M, Mashimo T. Application of a newly designed right-sided, double-lumen endobronchial tube in patients with a very short right mainstem bronchus. Anesthesiology. 2008;109:565–8.

51. Ghosh S, Falter F, Goldsmith K, Arrowsmith JE. The Papworth BiVent tube: a new device for lung isolation. Anaesthesia. 2008;63:996–1000.

52. Ghosh S, Klein AA, Prabhu M, Falter F, et al. The Papworth BiVent tube: a feasibility study of a novel double-lumen endotracheal tube and bronchial blocker in human cadavers. Br J Anaesth. 2008;101:424–8.

53. Saito S, Dohi S, Naito H. Alteration of double-lumen endobronchial tube position by flexion and extension of the neck. Anesthesiology. 1985;62:696–7.

54. Yüceyar L, Kaynak K, Cantürk E, Aykaç B. Bronchial rupture with a left-sided polyvinylchloride double-lumen tube. Acta Anaesthesiol Scand. 2003;47:622–5.

55. Liu H, Jahr JS, Sullivan E, Waters PF. Tracheobronchial rupture after double-lumen endotracheal intubation. J Cardiothorac Vasc Anesth. 2004;18:228–33.

56. Benumof JL, Wu D. Tracheal tear caused by extubation of a double-lumen tube. Anesthesiology. 2002;97:1007–8.

57. Sucato DJ, Girgis M. Bilateral pneumothoraces, pneumomediastinum, pneumoperitoneum, pneumoretroperitoneum, and subcutaneous emphysema following intubation with a double-lumen endotracheal tube for thoracoscopic anterior spinal release and fusion in a patient with idiopathic scoliosis. J Spinal Disord Tech. 2002;15:133–8.

58. Weng W, DeCrosta DJ, Zhang H. Tension pneumothorax during one-lung ventilation: a case report. J Clin Anesth. 2002;14:529–31.

59. Fitzmaurice BG, Brodsky JB. Airway rupture from double-lumen tubes. J Cardiothorac Vasc Anesth. 1999;13:322–9.

60. Knoll H, Ziegeler S, Schreiber JU, et al. Airway injuries after one-lung ventilation: a comparison between double-lumen tube and endobronchial blocker: a randomized, prospective, controlled trial. Anesthesiology. 2006;105:471–7.

61. Clayton-Smith A, Bennett K, Alston RP, et al. A comparison of the efficacy and adverse effects of double-lumen endobronchial tubes and bronchial blockers in thoracic surgery: a systematic review and meta-analysis of randomized controlled trials. J Cardiothorac Vasc Anesth. 2015;29:955–66.

62. Falzon D, Alston RP, Coley E, et al. Lung isolation for thoracic surgery: from inception to evidence-based. J Cardiothorac Vasc Anesth. 2017;31:678–93.

63. Park SH, Han SH, Do SH, et al. Prophylactic dexamethasone decreases the incidence of sore throat and hoarseness after tracheal extubation with a double-lumen endobronchial tube. Anesth Analg. 2008;107:1814–8.

64. Campos JH. Effects of oxygenation during selective lobar versus total lung collapse with or without continuous positive airway pressure. Anesth Analg. 1997;85:583–6.

65. Campos JH, Ledet C, Moyers JR. Improvement of arterial oxygen saturation with selective lobar bronchial block during hemorrhage

in a patient with previous contralateral lobectomy. Anesth Analg. 1995;81:1095–6.

66. Amar D, Desiderio DP, Bains MS, Wilson RS. A novel method of one-lung isolation using a double endobronchial blocker technique. Anesthesiology. 2001;95:1528–30.

67. Espí C, García-Guasch R, Ibáñez C, Fernández E, Astudillo J. Selective lobar blockade using an Arndt endobronchial blocker in 2 patients with respiratory compromise who underwent lung resection. Arch Bronconeumol. 2007;43:346–8.

68. Ng JM, Hartigan PM. Selective lobar bronchial blockade following contralateral pneumonectomy. Anesthesiology. 2003;98:268–70.

69. Hagihira S, Maki N, Kawaguchi M, Slinger P. Selective bronchial blockade in patients with previous contralateral lung surgery. J Cardiothorac Vasc Anesth. 2002;16:638–42.

70. Campos JH. Update on selective lobar blockade during pulmonary resections. Curr Opin Anaesthesiol. 2009;22:18–22.

71. Campos JH. Which device should be considered the best for lung isolation: double-lumen endotracheal tube versus bronchial blockers. Curr Opin Anaesthesiol. 2007;20:27–31.

72. Mourisse J, Liesveld J, Verhagen A, et al. Efficiency, efficacy, and safety of EZ-blocker compared with left-sided double-lumen tube for one-lung ventilation. Anesthesiology. 2013;118:550–61.

73. Kus A, Hosten T, Gurkan Y, et al. A comparison of the EZ-blocker with a Cohen flex-tip blocker for one-lung ventilation. J Cardiothorac Vasc Anesth. 2014;28:896–9.

74. Hagihira S, Takashina M, Mori T, Yoshiya I. One-lung ventilation in patients with difficult airways. J Cardiothorac Vasc Anesth. 1998;12:186–8.

75. Baraka A. The univent tube can facilitate difficult intubation in a patient undergoing thoracoscopy. J Cardiothorac Vasc Anesth. 1996;10:693–4.

76. Ransom ES, Carter SL, Mund GD. Univent tube: a useful device in patients with difficult airways. J Cardiothorac Vasc Anesth. 1995;9:725–7.

77. Campos JH. Difficult airway and one-lung ventilation. Curr Rev Clin Anesth. 2002;22:197–208.

78. García-Aguado R, Mateo EM, Tommasi-Rosso M, et al. Thoracic surgery and difficult intubation: another application of univent tube for one-lung ventilation. J Cardiothorac Vasc Anesth. 1997;11:925–6.

79. García-Aguado R, Mateo EM, Onrubia VJ, Bolinches R. Use of the Univent System tube for difficult intubation and for achieving one-lung anaesthesia. Acta Anaesthesiol Scand. 1996;40:765–7.

80. Takenaka I, Aoyama K, Kadoya T. Use of the univent bronchial-blocker tube for unanticipated difficult endotracheal intubation. Anesthesiology. 2000;93:590–1.

81. Arndt GA, DeLessio ST, Kranner PW, et al. One-lung ventilation when intubation is difficult-presentation of a new endobronchial blocker. Acta Anaesthesiol Scand. 1999;43:356–8.

82. Arndt GA, Buchika S, Kranner PW, DeLessio ST. Wire-guided endobronchial blockade in a patient with a limited mouth opening. Can J Anaesth. 1999;46:87–9.

83. Grocott HP, Scales G, Schinderle D, King K. A new technique for lung isolation in acute thoracic trauma. J Trauma. 2000;49:940–2.

84. Byhahn C, Habler OP, Bingold TM, et al. The wire-guided endobronchial blocker: applications in trauma patients beyond mere single-lung ventilation. J Trauma. 2006;61:755–9.

85. Campos JH, Kernstine KH. Use of the wire-guided endobronchial blocker for one-lung anesthesia in patients with airway abnormalities. J Cardiothorac Vasc Anesth. 2003;17:352–4.

86. Kabon B, Waltl B, Leitgeb J, Kapral S, Zimpfer M. First experience with fiberoptically directed wire-guided endobronchial blockade in severe pulmonary bleeding in an emergency setting. Chest. 2001;120:1399–402.

87. Kazari W. Alternative method to deflate the operated lung when using wire-guided endobronchial blockade. Anesthesiology. 2003;99:239–40.

88. Campos JH. In response: an alternative method to deflate the operated lung when using wire guided endobronchial blockade. Anesthesiology. 2003;99:241.

89. Soto RG, Oleszak SP. Resection of the Arndt bronchial blocker during stapler resection of the left lower lobe. J Cardiothorac Vasc Anesth. 2006;20:131–2.

90. Campos J. Lung isolation. In: Slinger P, editor. Principles and practice of anesthesia for thoracic surgery. 1st ed. New York; London: Springer; 2011.

91. Roscoe A, Kanellakos GW, McRae K, Slinger P. Pressures exerted by endobronchial devices. Anesth Analg. 2007;104:655–8.

92. Lizuka T, Tanno M, Hamada Y, Shga T, Ohe Y. Uniblocker® bronchial blocker tube to facilitate one-lung ventilation during thoracoscopic surgery. Anesthesiology. 2007;108:A1815.

93. Campos JH, Kernstine KH. A structural complication in the torque control blocker Univent: fracture of the blocker cap connector. Anesth Analg. 2003;96:630–1.

94. Peragallo RA, Swenson JD. Congenital tracheal bronchus: the inability to isolate the right lung with a univent bronchial blocker tube. Anesth Analg. 2000;91:300–1.

95. Asai T. Failure of the Univent bronchial blocker in sealing the bronchus. Anaesthesia. 1999;54:97.

96. Thielmeier KA, Anwar M. Complication of the Univent tube. Anesthesiology. 1996;84:491.

97. Dougherty P, Hannallah M. A potentially serious complication that resulted from improper use of the Univent tube. Anesthesiology. 1992;77:835.

98. Prabhu MR, Smith JH. Use of the Arndt wire-guided endobronchial blocker. Anesthesiology. 2002;97:1325.

99. Sandberg WS. Endobronchial blocker dislodgement leading to pulseless electrical activity. Anesth Analg. 2005;100:1728–30.

100. Ueda K, Goetzinger C, Gauger EH, et al. Use of bronchial blockers: a retrospective review of 302 cases. J Anesth. 2012;26:115–7.

101. Honikman R, Rodriguez-Diaz CA, Cohen E. A ballooning crisis: three cases of bronchial blocker malfunction and a review. J Cardiothorac Vasc Anesth. 2017;31:1799–804.

102. Brodsky JB, Tobler HG, Mark JB. A double-lumen endobronchial tube for tracheostomies. Anesthesiology. 1991;74:387–8.

103. Saito T, Naruke T, Carney E, et al. New double intrabronchial tube (Naruke tube) for tracheostomized patients. Anesthesiology. 1998;89:1038–9.

104. Bellver J, García-Aguado R, De Andrés J, Valía JC, Bolinches R. Selective bronchial intubation with the univent system in patients with a tracheostomy. Anesthesiology. 1993;79:1453–4.

105. Dhamee MS. One-lung ventilation in a patient with a fresh tracheostomy using the tracheostomy tube and a Univent endobronchial blocker. J Cardiothorac Vasc Anesth. 1997;11:124–5.

106. Tobias JD. Variations on one-lung ventilation. J Clin Anesth. 2001;13:35–9.

107. Ko R, McRae K, Darling G, et al. The use of air in the inspired gas mixture during two-lung ventilation delays lung collapse during one-lung ventilation. Anesth Analg. 2009;108:1092–6.

108. Yoshimura T, Ueda K, Kakinuma A, et al. Bronchial blocker lung collapse technique: nitrous oxide for facilitating lung collapse during one-lung ventilation with a bronchial blocker. Anesth Analg. 2014;118:666–70.

109. Campos JH, Ueda K, Hallam EA. Lung isolation in the morbidly obese patient: a comparison of a left-sided double-lumen endotracheal tube with the Arndt® wire-guided blocker. Br J Anaesth. 2012;109:630–5.

110. Bussières JS, Somma J, Del Castillo JL, et al. Bronchial blocker versus left double-lumen endotracheal tube in video-assisted thoracoscopic surgery: a randomized-controlled trial examining time and quality of lung deflation. Can J Anaesth. 2016;63:818–27.

111. Neustein SM. Pro: bronchial blockers should be used routinely for providing one-lung ventilation. J Cardiothorac Vasc Anesth. 2015;29:234–6.

112. Cohen E. Strategies for lung isolation: to block or not to block? Can J Anaesth. 2016;63:797–801.

113. Hesselfeldt R, Kristensen MS, Rasmussen LS, et al. Evaluation of the airway of the SimMan® full-scale patient simulator. Acta Anaesthesiol Scand. 2005;49:1339–45.

114. Wong AK. Full scale computer simulators in anesthesia training and evaluation. Can J Anaesth. 2004;51:455–64.

115. Nyssen AS, Larbuisson R, Janssens M, et al. A comparison of the training value of two types of anesthesia simulators: computer screen-based and mannequin-based simulators. Anesth Analg. 2002;94:1560–5.

116. Duffy CH, Myles PS. Review: thoracic-anesthesia.com. J Cardiothorac Vasc Anesth. 2008;22:644.

117. Campos JH, Hallam EA, Ueda K. Training in placement of the left-sided double lumen tube among non-thoracic anesthesiologists: intubation model simulator versus computer-based DVD, a randomized control trial. Eur J Anaesthesiol. 2011;28:169–74.

118. Failor E, Bowdle A, Jelacic S, et al. High-fidelity simulation of lung isolation with double-lumen endotracheal tubes and bronchial blockers in anesthesiology resident training. J Cardiothorac Vasc Anesth. 2014;28:865–9.

119. Latif RK, VanHorne EM, Kandadai SK, et al. Teaching basic lung isolation skills on human anatomy simulator: attainment and retention of lung isolation skills. BMC Anesthesiol. 2016;20:16:1–7.

Fiberoptic Bronchoscopy for Positioning Double-Lumen Tubes and Bronchial Blockers

17

Javier Campos

Key Points
- Recognition of tracheobronchial anatomy structures is a key component during flexible fiberoptic bronchoscopy.
- Flexible fiberoptic bronchoscopy is the recommended method to achieve optimal position of lung isolation devices, first in supine position, later in lateral decubitus, or whenever a malposition occurs.
- The preferred technique for placement of a right-sided double-lumen endotracheal tube is with the fiberoptic bronchoscopy guidance technique.
- Any suspicion of airway trauma, unexpected air leaks, subcutaneous emphysema, massive bleeding, or protrusion of the cuff balloon into the surgical field, a flexible fiberoptic bronchoscopy examination should be performed followed by surgical repair if needed.
- The use of flexible fiberoptic bronchoscopy should be considered an art in thoracic anesthesia.

Introduction

Flexible fiberoptic bronchoscopy is a diagnostic and therapeutic procedure of great value in the clinical practice of thoracic anesthesia [1]. The most common method to perform flexible fiberoptic bronchoscopy is with the use of a single-lumen endotracheal tube. Once the tube is advanced beyond the vocal cords and inside the trachea, the tip of the endotracheal tube should come to rest 3–4 cm above the tracheal carina. A Portex fiberoptic bronchoscope (SSL American, Inc. Norcross, Georgia, USA) swivel adapter with a self-

J. Campos (✉)
Department of Anesthesia, University of Iowa Health Care, Roy and Lucille Carver College of Medicine, Iowa City, IA, USA
e-mail: javier-campos@uiowa.edu

sealing valve is used to facilitate ventilation and manipulation of the bronchoscope at the same time. When using a large single-lumen endotracheal tube, an adult fiberoptic bronchoscope should be used (i.e., 4.1 mm inner diameter). Another alternative to perform fiberoptic bronchoscopy is with the use of a laryngeal mask airway (LMA). This technique allows visualization of the vocal cords and subglottic structures with lower resistance than a single-lumen endotracheal tube when the bronchoscope is inserted.

A systematic and complete fiberoptic bronchoscopy examination (refer to Fig. 17.1) includes a clear view of the anterior wall (tracheal cartilage) and posterior wall (membranous portion) of the trachea below the vocal cords and of the tracheal carina. When advancing the bronchoscope through the right mainstem bronchus, a clear view of the bronchus intermedius should be seen, and at 3 o'clock the orifice of the right upper bronchus should also be seen. The distance from the tracheal carina to the takeoff of the right upper lobe is between 1.0 and 2.0 cm as the fiberscope is advanced inside the takeoff of the right upper bronchus; a clear view of three orifices is found in 98% of the population, and four orifices are found in less than 2%. These orifices are apical anterior and posterior segments. This is the only structure in the tracheobronchial tree that has three orifices. After withdrawing the bronchoscope from the right upper bronchus, it is advanced distally into the bronchus intermedius in order to identify the middle and lower right lobe bronchi. The right middle bronchus has the shape of a letter D. Infrequently seen is the takeoff of the right upper bronchus that emerges above the tracheal carina on the right side [2–4]. Once the complete examination has been performed on the right mainstem bronchus, the flexible bronchoscope is withdrawn until the tracheal carina is seen again, and then the bronchoscope is readvanced into the left mainstem bronchus in which the bifurcation into the left upper and lower lobe is visualized. The anatomical distance from the tracheal carina to the bifurcation on the left-sided bronchus is approximately 4–5 cm in length. Also in a very limited occurrences

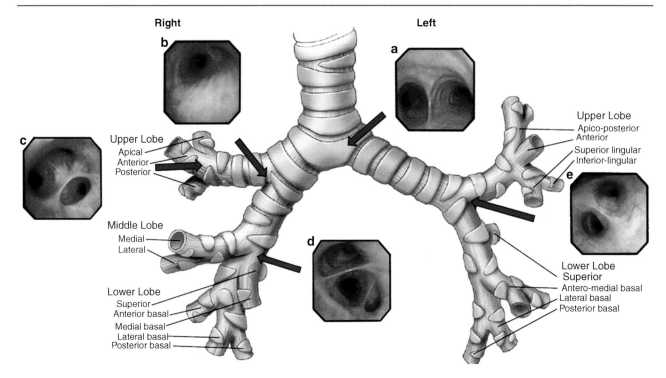

Fig. 17.1 Tracheobronchial anatomy and fiberoptic bronchoscopy exam with the view of the trachea and right and left bronchus. (**a**) shows a clear view of the tracheal carina with the flexible fiberoptic bronchoscope, (**b**) shows the takeoff of the right upper bronchus, (**c**) shows the apical upper (center) anterior toward the left and posterior segment toward the right of the right upper lobe bronchus, (**d**) shows the right middle (D shaped) and the right lower lobe bronchus (middle) and the superior segment of right lower lobe, and (**e**) shows a view of the left upper lobe and left lower lobe bronchus

an observant left upper or left lower bronchus can emerge above the tracheal carina [5]. Fig. 17.1 shows tracheobronchial anatomy [6] and fiberoptic bronchoscopy exam with the view of the trachea and right and left bronchus.

Flexible Fiberoptic Bronchoscopy and Double–Lumen Endotracheal Tube Placement

Placement and positioning of a left-sided DLT can be accomplished with the flexible fiberoptic bronchoscopy guidance technique, in which the endobronchial tip is passed beyond the vocal cords and guided through the trachea with the aid of the fiberoptic bronchoscope until the entrance of the left mainstem bronchus is identified and the tube is introduced into the left bronchus.

Optimal Position of the Left-Sided Double-Lumen Tube with Flexible Bronchoscopy

Flexible fiberoptic bronchoscopy is the recommended method to confirm the optimal position of the DLT [7–9]. Recognition of tracheobronchial anatomy and familiarity with the use of flexible fiberoptic bronchoscopy are mandatory in order to successfully achieve optimal position of the DLT. Previous studies [10, 11] involving non-thoracic anesthesiologist with very limited experience in lung separation techniques showed up to 38% incidence of unrecognized malpositions when DLTs were placed with fiberoptic bronchoscope.

The optimal position for a left-sided DLT as seen with the fiberoptic bronchoscope is completed in two steps: First the flexible fiberscope is advanced to the tracheal lumen, after the tracheal carina is identified the fiberscope is guided towards the entrance of the right mainstem bronchus, in a distance of approximately 1.0–2.0 cm to the takeoff of the right upper bronchus is seen at 3–4 o'clock on the lateral wall. Advancing the fiberoptic bronchoscope inside this orifice should provide a clear view of the apical, anterior, and posterior segments (the "cloverleaf" view). This is the only structure in the tracheobronchial tree that has tree orifices. In addition, in less than 2% of the population, a quadrivial pattern (four orifices) can be seen inside the right upper lobe bronchus [5]. Figure 17.2 shows a trifurcated and quadrivial view of the apical, anterior, and posterior segments.

After the right bronchus is identified, the endobronchial cuff of the DLT is fully inflated with no more than 3 ml of air. The blue edge of the endobronchial balloon should be positioned at least 1 cm below the trachea carina into the entrance of the left mainstem bronchus. During inspection with the fiberscope, the fully inflated balloon should not show air bubbles (leak).

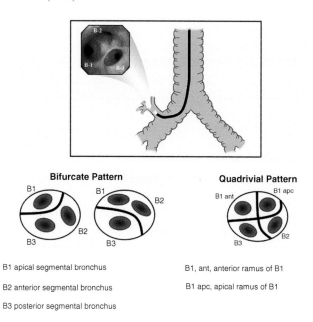

Bifurcate Pattern

Quadrivial Pattern

B1 apical segmental bronchus

B2 anterior segmental bronchus

B3 posterior segmental bronchus

B1, ant, anterior ramus of B1

B1 apc, apical ramus of B1

Fig. 17.2 A trifurcated and quadrivial view of the apical, anterior, and posterior segments

After the fiberoptic bronchoscopic inspection is completed from the tracheal lumen, the patient is ventilated, and then the next view is from the endobronchial lumen. Two observations are relevant: First the fiberoptic bronchoscope is advanced inside the endobronchial lumen, and the patency of the lumen is observed before advancing the bronchoscope through the blue inside portion of the tube; the second view is at the distal end of the endobronchial tip of the tube, where a clear and unobstructed view of the left upper and lower lobe bronchus entrance orifices is visualized distally. This view provides the margin of safety for a left-sided DLT [12]. Figure 17.3 shows the optimal position of a left-sided DLT seen with the flexible fiberoptic bronchoscope. This examination should be done in supine and after the patient is turned into lateral decubitus position.

A variation of the left-sided DLT is a newly designed DLT named VivaSight DLT that includes an integrated camera near to the tracheal lumen (distal) to allow a continuous view of the tracheal carina [13, 14]. A systematic review of randomized controlled trials comparing the VivaSight double-lumen tubes with a conventional double-lumen tubes showed that for optimal position of the VivaSight DLT, a flexible fiberoptic bronchoscopy is needed when this device is used [15]. Therefore, the optimal position of the VivaSight DLT is no different than placing a conventional left-sided DLT with the fiberoptic bronchoscope to achieve optimal position.

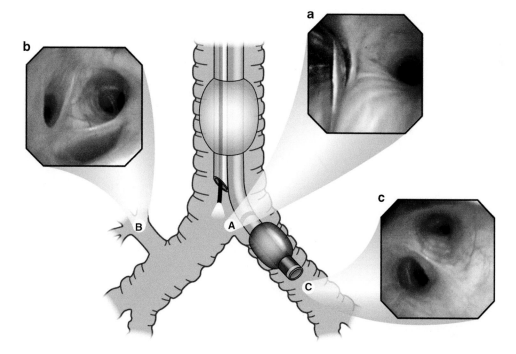

Fig. 17.3 The optimal position of a left-sided DLT seen with the flexible fiberoptic bronchoscope. This examination should be done in supine and after the patient is turned into lateral decubitus position. (**a**) shows an unobstructed view of the entrance of the right mainstem bronchus when the fiberscope is passed through the tracheal lumen and the edge of the fully inflated endobronchial cuff is below the tracheal carina in the left bronchus. (**b**) shows the takeoff of the right upper bronchus with the three segments (apical, anterior, and posterior); this is a landmark to reconfirm a right bronchus. (**c**) shows an unobstructed view of the left upper and left lower bronchus when the fiberoptic bronchoscope is advanced through the endobronchial lumen. (Campos [1])

Optimal Position of a Right-Sided Double-Lumen Tube with Flexible Bronchoscopy

The preferred technique for placement of a right-sided DLT is with the fiberoptic bronchoscopy guidance technique [16]. After the right-sided DLT is passed beyond the vocal cords under direct laryngoscopy, the fiberoptic bronchoscope is advanced through the endobronchial lumen. Before advancing the DLT, the tracheal carina, the entrance of the right mainstem bronchus, and the entrance of the right upper lobe bronchus are identified. Then the right-sided DLT is rotated toward the right and advanced with the aid of the fiberoptic bronchoscope. The optimal position of a right-sided DLT is one that provides good alignment between the opening slot of the endobronchial lumen in relationship to the entrance of the right upper lobe bronchus and, distally, a clear view of the bronchus intermedius and the right lower lobe bronchus seen from the endobronchial lumen. After the endobronchial inspection is completed and after ventilation is re-established, the next step is to inspect the DLT from the tracheal view; the optimal position for a right-sided DLT provides a view of the edge of the blue cuff just below the tracheal carina and a view of the entrance of the right mainstem bronchus. Figure 17.4 shows the optimal position of a right-sided DLT seen from the endobronchial or endotracheal view with a fiberoptic bronchoscope.

Flexible Fiberoptic Bronchoscopy and Bronchial Blockers

Another alternative to achieve lung separation is with the use of bronchial blockers passed through an in situ single-lumen endotracheal tube [17]. The various devices available at the present time include the wire-guided endobronchial blocker (Arndt® blocker), the Cohen tip-deflecting endobronchial blocker, the Fuji Uniblocker®, and the EZ-blocker [18, 19].

Placement of the Arndt® Blocker with Fiberoptic Bronchoscopy

The placement of the Arndt® blocker involves placing the endobronchial blocker through the endotracheal tube and using the fiberoptic bronchoscope and wire-guided loop to direct the blocker into a mainstem bronchus (Fig. 17.5). The fiberoptic bronchoscope has to be advanced distally enough so that the Arndt® blocker enters the bronchus while it is advanced. When the deflated cuff is beyond the entrance of the bronchus, the fiberoptic bronchoscope is withdrawn, and the cuff is fully inflated with fiberoptic visualization with 4–8 mL of air to obtain a total bronchial blockade. The optimal position of the Arndt® blocker in the left or in the right

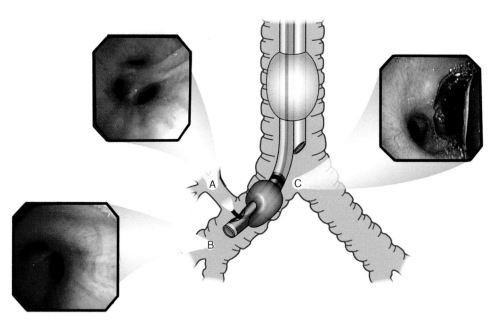

Fig. 17.4 The optimal position of a right-sided DLT seen from the endobronchial or endotracheal view with a fiberoptic bronchoscope. (**a**) shows the takeoff of the right upper bronchus with three segments (apical, anterior, and posterior) when the fiberoptic bronchoscope emerges from the opening slot located in the endobronchial lumen. (**b**) shows an unobstructed view of the entrance of the right middle and right lower lobe bronchus when the fiberscope is passed through the endobronchial lumen. (**c**) shows a view of the tracheal carina to the right edge of the blue balloon fully inflated, to the left unobstructed view of the entrance of the left mainstem bronchus when the fiberscope is advanced through the tracheal lumen. (Campos [1])

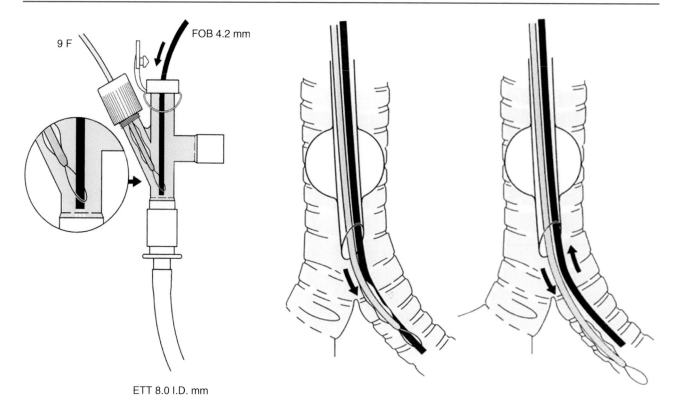

ETT 8.0 I.D. mm

Fig. 17.5 (**a**) The placement of an Arndt® blocker through a single-lumen endotracheal tube with the fiberoptic bronchoscope advanced through the guide-wire loop into the left mainstem bronchus.

Abbreviations: FOB fiberoptic bronchoscopy, ETT single-lumen endotracheal tube. (Campos [20])

bronchus is achieved when the blocker balloon's outer surface is seen with the fiberoptic bronchoscope at least 5–10 mm below the tracheal carina on the targeted bronchus and the proper real is obtained (Fig. 17.6).

Placement of the Cohen® Blocker with Fiberoptic Bronchoscopy

The Cohen® blocker relies on a wheel-turning device located in the most proximal part of the unit that allows deflection of the tip of the distal part of the blocker into the designated bronchus. This device has been purposely pre-angulated at the distal tip to facilitate insertion into a targeted bronchus. The Cohen® blocker is advanced through an 8.0 mmID single-lumen endotracheal tube. The placement of the Cohen® blocker involves placing the endobronchial blocker through the endotracheal tube and using the fiberoptic bronchoscope to observe the direction of the blocker into a mainstem bronchus. The advantage of the Cohen® blocker is that the tip of the blocker can be seen as it is advanced when the fiberoptic bronchoscope tip is placed a few centimeters from the tip of the blocker (Fig. 17.7).

The optimal position for the right of mainstem bronchus if the one that provides a view of the outer surface of the

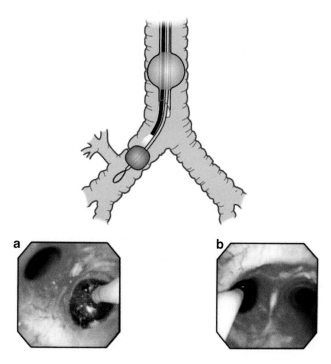

Fig. 17.6 The optimal position of a bronchial blocker in the right and left mainstem bronchus. The proximal edge of the fully inflated cuff is approximately 5–10 mm below the tracheal carina. (**a**) shows a bronchial blocker in the right mainstem bronchus, and (**b**) shows a bronchial blocker in the left mainstem bronchus. (Campos [20])

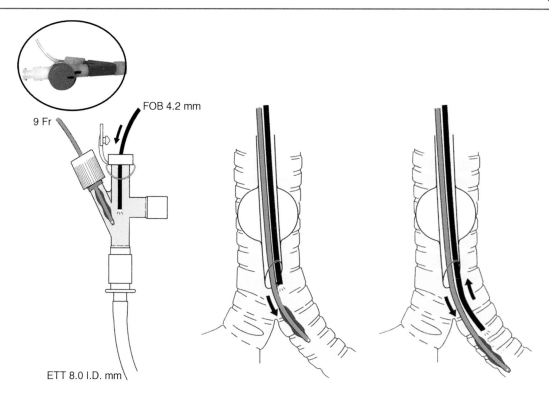

Fig. 17.7 The Cohen® blocker going into the left mainstem bronchus with the fiberoptic bronchoscope

fully inflated balloon (4–8 mL of air) with the fiberoptic bronchoscope at least 5–10 mm below the tracheal carina on the respective bronchus (Fig. 17.8).

Placement of the Fuji Uniblocker® with the Fiberoptic Bronchoscopy

The Fuji Uniblocker® is another independent bronchial blocker; the unique characteristic of this blocker is that the balloon is made of silicone with a gas barrier property to reduce diffusion of gas into or out of the cuff. The Fuji Uniblocker® size 9F (adult size) is advanced through an 8.0 mmID single-lumen endotracheal tube; before insertion, the blocker balloon is tested and then fully deflated. The tip of this blocker has a pre-angulated tip (hockey stick shape) to facilitate insertion into a targeted bronchus. The placement of the Fuji Uniblocker® involves placing the endobronchial blocker through the endotracheal tube and using the fiberoptic bronchoscope to observe the direction of the blocker into a mainstem bronchus. For blocking the right mainstem bronchus, the optimal position is the one that provides a view of the outer surface of the fully inflated

balloon (4–8 mL of air) with the fiberoptic bronchoscope at least 10 mm below the tracheal carina on the right mainstem bronchus (Fig. 17.9a, b). The optimal position in the left mainstem bronchus is achieved when the blocker balloon's outer surface is seen with the fiberoptic bronchoscope at least 10 mm below the trachea carina inside the left mainstem bronchus.

Placement of the EZ-Blocker with Fiberoptic Bronchoscopy

The EZ-blocker is an independent bronchial blocker that is available only in a 7.0F size (adult size) (Fig. 17.10a). The EZ-blocker is manufactured with a y-shaped distal end (Fig. 17.10b). Both limbs of the distal end are fitted with an inflatable balloon (Fig. 17.10c). Each limb is color-coded (yellow or blue) for easy identification with a matching pilot balloon. The optimal size of the single-lumen endotracheal tube should be 7.5 or 8.0 mmID so it allows the blocker and the fiberoptic bronchoscope to navigate together. The multiport adaptor of the EZ-blocker is designated to connect to the connector of the single-lumen

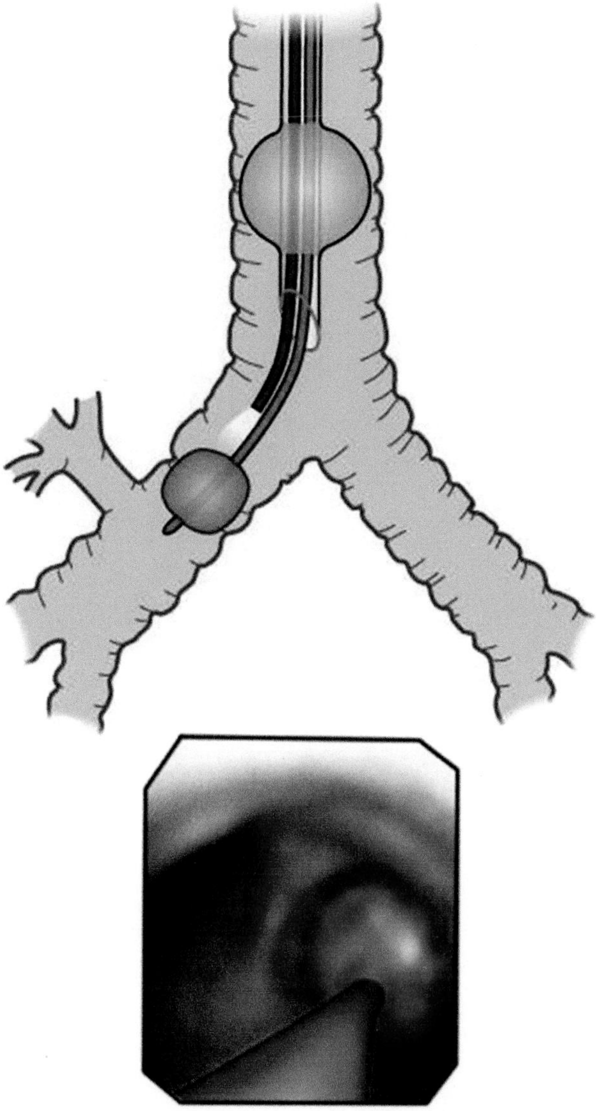

The pilot of the cuff is color-coded to allow identification of the respective balloon (one is yellow and the other one is blue). After the tip of the deflated balloon is in the bronchus, inflation of the balloon should be performed with flexible fiberoptic bronchoscopy. The balloon inflation requires between 8 and 14 mL of air to block a bronchus [21]. Proper and optimal position is when the outer surface of the balloon is seen at least 5–10 mm below the entrance of the bronchus. The distal end of the single-lumen endotracheal tube should be at least 4 cm above the carina to allow easy placement of the blocker into the bronchus. The distal y-junction of the two limbs of the blocker must be firmly seated on the carina to minimize displacement of the blocker during surgery. Optimal position with the fiberscope should be obtained in supine and lateral decubitus position.

Selective Lobar Blockade with Bronchial Blocker and Flexible Fiberoptic Bronchoscopy

Selective lobar blockade is a specific technique that allows one-lobe ventilation (OLV), while the operated lobe is collapsed during thoracic surgery in patients with previous pulmonary resection requiring subsequent resection or in patients with limited pulmonary reserve resulting from severe pulmonary disease [22–24]. During selective lobar blockade techniques, it is mandatory for the anesthesiologist to recognize the tracheobronchial anatomy with special emphasis on the previous bronchial resection. For instance, a patient who has previous right upper lobectomy lacks the right upper bronchus, which may contribute to difficulties in recognizing the right mainstem bronchus versus the left mainstem bronchus (Fig. 17.11). Owing to this loss of an anatomical landmark (right upper bronchus), the anesthesiologist may not be able to recognize the apical, anterior, and posterior segments seen inside the right upper bronchus with the fiberoptic bronchoscope.

Patients with previous lobectomy requiring another surgery in the contralateral lung may be at risk of developing hypoxemia during total lung collapse, barotrauma, or pulmonary hyperinflation of the remaining lung, which can lead to the development of acute lung injury. One alternative is to use a bronchial blocker to achieve selective lobar blockade to facilitate surgical exposure and improve oxygenation (Fig. 17.12).

Fig. 17.8 The optimal position of the Cohen® blocker in the right mainstem bronchus with the bronchial balloon fully inflated

endotracheal tube, and it contains two additional ports, one to allow advancement of the blocker and the other port for passing the flexible fiberoptic bronchoscope. The EZ-blocker is tested and lubricated prior to passing into the lumen of the single endotracheal tube and the multiport connector. After advancing the blocker, the y-shaped end should be seated in the tracheal carina, and each independent tip should be located in the entrance of the right or left bronchus. Only the balloon where lung isolation occurs should be inflated under direct fiberoptic bronchoscopy.

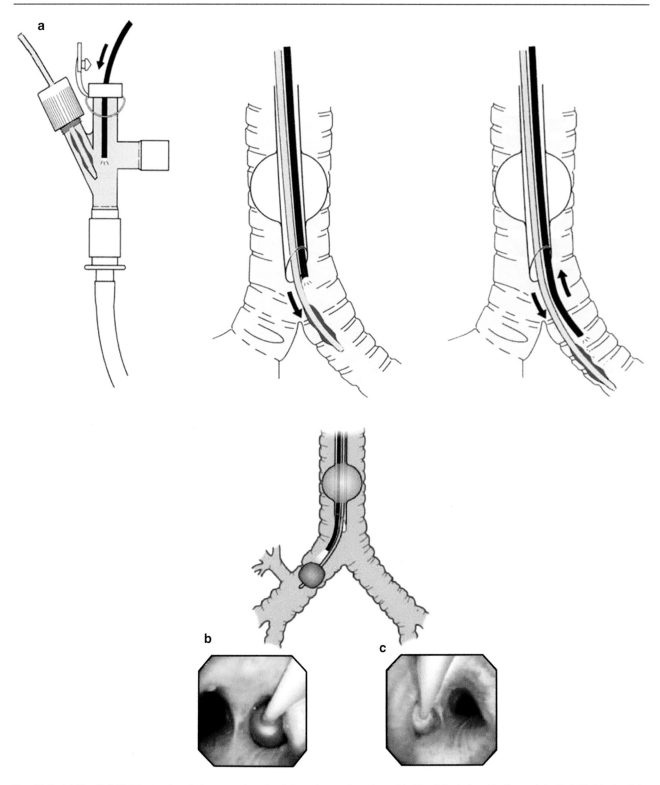

Fig. 17.9 (a) The Fuji Uniblocker® and placement into the right mainstem bronchus. (b). The fully inflated balloon of the Fuji Uniblocker® in the right mainstem bronchus and (c) the fully inflated balloon of the Fuji Uniblocker® in the left mainstem bronchus. (Campos [1])

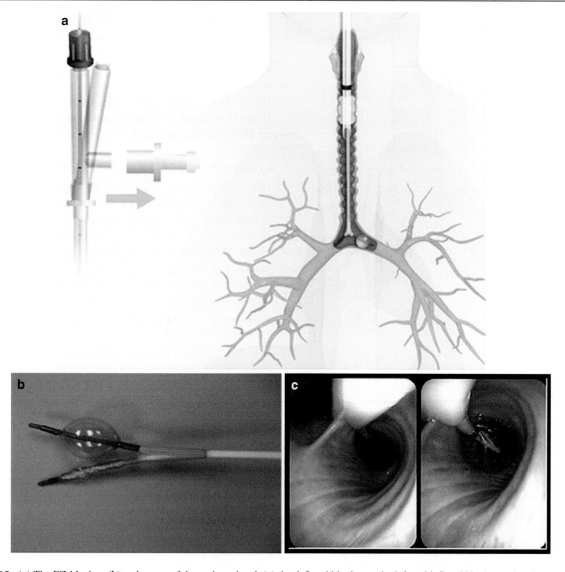

Fig. 17.10 (**a**) The EZ-blocker, (**b**) a close up of the y-shaped end, (**c**) the deflated blocker to the left and inflated blocker to the right

Fig. 17.11 The fiberoptic bronchoscopy view in a patient with previous right upper lobectomy

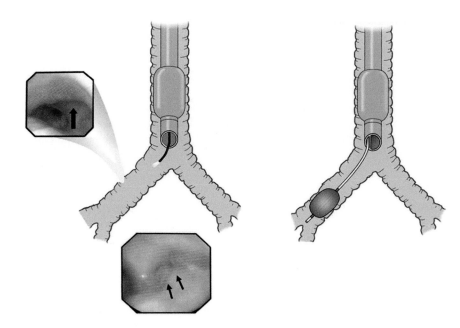

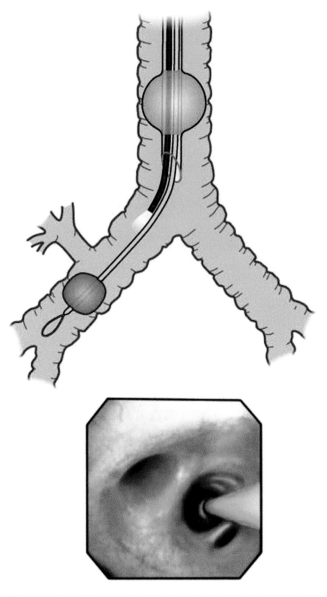

Fig. 17.12 A bronchial blocker placed in the bronchus intermedius. The fully inflated balloon is blocking the right middle and right lower lobe bronchus while the right upper lobe is being ventilated (selective lobar blockade). (Campos [24])

A bronchial blocker can be used through a single-lumen endotracheal tube. In order to achieve a bronchial blockade, it must be advanced and positioned with the aid of a fiberoptic bronchoscope into a selective bronchus (Fig. 17.13a). The

amount of air required to inflate a bronchial blocker balloon to achieve selective lobar blockage ranges between 2 and 4 mL (Fig. 17.13b).

Other Uses of Flexible Fiberoptic Bronchoscopy During Double-Lumen Tubes or Bronchial Blockers

Common problems and limited number of complications can occur with the use of DLTs and bronchial blockers, particularly malpositions and airway trauma. Therefore it is essential to keep the flexible fiberoptic bronchoscope during the entire case and remove it (after the patient leaves the operating room). Malpositions of lung isolation devices are easily corrected with the use of flexible fiberoptic bronchoscope. Airway trauma and rupture of the membranous part of the trachea or bronchus continue to be an infrequent problem with the use of DLTs, and this can occur during insertion, placement, while the case is in progress, or during extubation [25, 26]. Airway damage during the use of DLTs can present as unexpected air leaks, subcutaneous emphysema, massive bleeding, or protrusion of the cuff balloon into the surgical fields. If any of the aforementioned problems occur, a flexible fiberoptic bronchoscopic examination should be performed and surgical repair performed. Another use of flexible fiberoptic bronchoscopy is to inspect the airway after removal of a fully inflated blocker [27] after failure in the device to achieve deflation at the conclusion of surgery. Inspection with the fiberscope allows to identify any trauma to the airway.

Summary

The use of flexible fiberoptic bronchoscopy should be considered an art in thoracic anesthesia. To master this art, one must be able to recognize tracheobronchial anatomy and changes that occur with age, understand the anatomical distances of the airway, recognize the takeoff of the right upper lobe bronchus and its variants, and have familiarity and expertise with the use of the flexible fiberoptic bronchoscopy. This will lead to a successful placement of a right- or left-sided DLT as well as bronchial blocker during lung isolation techniques.

Fig. 17.13 (a) displays a fiberoptic bronchoscopy view of tracheal carina in a patient with a right-sided pneumonectomy. (b) displays an Arndt® blocker blocking the entrance of the left upper lobe in a patient that required left upper segmentectomy. (Campos [24])

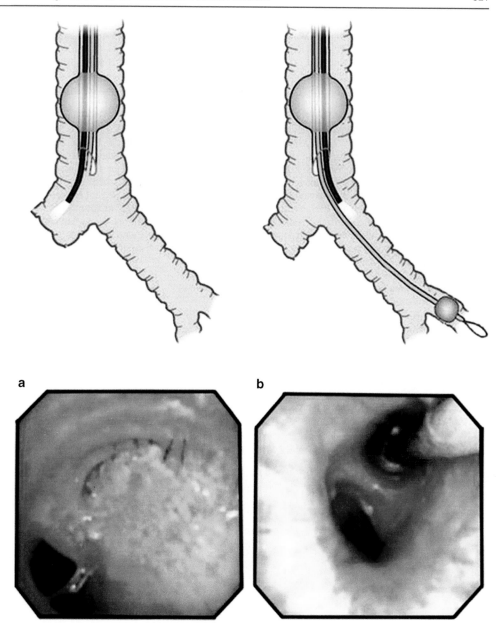

a

b

References

1. Campos JH. Update on tracheobronchial anatomy and flexible Fiberoptic bronchoscopy in thoracic anesthesia. Curr Opin Anaesthesiol. 2009;22:4–10.
2. Stene R, Rose M, Weinger MB, et al. Bronchial trifurcation at the carina complicating use of a double-lumen tracheal tube. Anesthesiology. 1994;80:1162–4.
3. Conacher ID. Implications of a tracheal bronchus for adult anaesthetic practice. Br J Anaesth. 2000;85:317–20.
4. Moon YJ, Kim SH, Park SW, et al. The implications of a tracheal bronchus on one-lung ventilation and fiberoptic bronchoscopy in a patient undergoing thoracic surgery: a case report. Can J Anaesth. 2015;62:399–402.
5. Gonlugur U, Efeoglu T, Kaptanoglu M, et al. Major anatomical variations of the tracheobronchial tree: bronchoscopic observation. Anat Sci Int. 2005;80:111–5.

6. Minnich DJ, Mathisen DJ. Anatomy of the trachea, carina, and bronchi. Thorac Surg Clin. 2007;17:571–85.

7. Klein U, Karzai W, Bloos F, et al. Role of fiberoptic bronchoscopy in conjunction with the use of double-lumen tubes for thoracic anesthesia: a prospective study. Anesthesiology. 1998;88:346–50.

8. Slinger PD. Fiberoptic bronchoscopic positioning of double-lumen tubes. J Cardiothorac Anesth. 1989;3:486–96.

9. Campos JH. Current techniques for perioperative lung isolation in adults. Anesthesiology. 2002;97:1295–301.

10. Campos JH, Hallam EA, Van Natta T, et al. Devices for lung isolation used by anesthesiologists with limited thoracic experience: comparison of double-lumen endotracheal tube, Univent torque control blocker, and Arndt wire-guided endobronchial blocker. Anesthesiology. 2006;104:261–6.

11. Campos JH, Hallam EA, Ueda K. Training in placement of the left-sided double lumen tube among non-thoracic anesthesiologists: intubation model simulator versus computer-based DVD, a randomized control trial. Eur J Anaesthesiol. 2011;28:169–74.

12. Benumof JL, Partridge BL, Salvatierra C, et al. Margin of safety in positioning modern double-lumen endotracheal tubes. Anesthesiology. 1987;67:729–38.

13. Koopman EM, Barak M, Weber E, et al. Evaluation of a new double-lumen endobronchial tube with an integrated camera (VivaSight-DL(™)): a prospective multicentre observational study. Anaesthesia. 2015;70:962–8.

14. Schuepbach R, Grande B, Camen G, et al. Intubation with VivaSight or conventional left-sided double-lumen tubes: a randomized trial. Can J Anaesth. 2015;62:762–9.

15. Saracoglu A, Saracoglu KT. VivaSight: a new era in the evolution of tracheal tubes. J Clin Anesth. 2016;33:442–9.

16. Campos JH, Massa CF, Kernstine KH. The incidence of right upper lobe collapse when comparing a right-sided double lumen tube versus modified left double lumen tube for left-sided thoracic surgery. Anesth Analg. 2000;90:535–40.

17. Campos JH. An update on bronchial blockers during lung separation techniques in adults. Anesth Analg. 2003;97:1266–74.

18. Narayanaswamy M, McRae K, Slinger P, et al. Choosing a lung isolation device for thoracic surgery: a randomized trial of three bronchial blockers versus double-lumen tubes. Anesth Analg. 2009;108:1097–101.

19. Kus A, Hosten T, Gurkan Y, et al. A comparison of the EZ-blocker with a Cohen flex-tip blocker for one-lung ventilation. J Cardiothorac Vasc Anesth. 2014;28:896–9.

20. Campos JH. How to achieve successful lung separation. SAJAA. 2008;14:22–6.

21. Mourisse J, Liesveld J, Verhagen A, et al. Efficiency, efficacy, and safety of EZ-blocker compared with left-sided double-lumen tube for one-lung ventilation. Anesthesiology. 2013;118:550–61.

22. Campos JH, Ledet CH, Moyers JR. Improvement of arterial oxygen saturation with selective lobar bronchial block during hemorrhage in a patient with previous contralateral lobectomy. Anesth Analg. 1995;81:1095–6.

23. Campos JH. Effects on oxygenation during selective lobar versus total lung collapse with or without continuous positive airway pressure. Anesth Analg. 1997;85:583–6.

24. Campos JH. Update on selective lobar blockade during pulmonary resections. Curr Opin Anaesthesiol. 2009;22:18–22.

25. Liu H, Jahr JS, Sullivan E, et al. Tracheobronchial rupture after double-lumen endotracheal intubation. J Cardiothorac Vasc Anesth. 2004;18:228–33.

26. Benumof JL, Wu D. Tracheal tear caused by extubation of a double-lumen tube. Anesthesiology. 2002;97:1007–8.

27. Honikman R, Rodriguez-Diaz CA, Cohen E. A ballooning crisis: three cases of bronchial blocker malfunction and a review. J Cardiothorac Vasc Anesth. 2017;31:1799–804.

Lung Isolation in Patients with Difficult Airways

18

Daniel Tran and Wanda M. Popescu

Key Points
- Recognition of a difficult airway prior to the use of lung isolation devices is essential.
- Securing the airway is the primary task in patients with difficult airways requiring lung isolation.
- The use of bronchial blocker is the first-line choice in patients with difficult airway who require lung isolation.
- In patients with difficult airways, the use of airway exchange catheters is recommended when changing single-lumen tubes to double-lumen tubes and vice versa.

Introduction

One-lung ventilation (OLV) in the thoracic surgical patient can be achieved with the use of a double-lumen endotracheal tube (DLT) or an independent bronchial blocker [1]. A number of patients requiring lung isolation may present as potentially difficult airways due to abnormalities of either the upper or lower airway [2]. In order to optimally manage these patients, it is important to understand the normal anatomy of the tracheobronchial tree, including the anatomical distances of the airway [3].

Patients with a potentially difficult airway who require OLV may be identified during the preoperative evaluation. However, others will present with airways that are unexpectedly difficult to intubate after induction of anesthesia. It is

estimated that between 5% and 8% of patients with primary lung carcinoma also have a carcinoma of the pharynx, usually in the epiglottic area [2]. Many of these patients may have had previous airway surgery or radiation therapy to the neck, making intubation and achievement of OLV difficult due to distorted upper airway anatomy. In addition, a patient who requires OLV might have distorted anatomy at or beyond the tracheal carina due to a descending thoracic aortic aneurysm compressing the entrance of the left mainstem bronchus or an extraluminal tumor compressing the tracheobronchial bifurcation, making the insertion of a left-sided DLT relatively difficult or impossible.

Preoperative Evaluation of the Difficult Airway and Lung Isolation Techniques

According to the ASA practice guideline for management of the difficult airway [4], an airway is termed difficult when conventional laryngoscopy reveals a grade III view (just the epiglottis is seen) or a grade IV view (just part of the soft palate is seen). However, in patients requiring OLV, the definition of a difficult airway is more comprehensive. It includes not only issues pertaining to the the upper airway, which could render a laryngoscopic grade III or IV view, but also problems with the lower airway (tracheobronchial tree). If the upper airway is recognized as being potentially difficult, a careful examination of the patient ensues. Previous anesthesia records should be examined for a history of airway management. Patients should be asked to open their mouths as widely as possible and extend their tongues. The mandibular opening should be assessed and the pharyngeal anatomy observed. The length of the submental space should also be noted. Patients should be evaluated from side to side to assess any degree of maxillary overbite and their ability to assume the sniffing position. Also, the patency of the nostrils must be assessed in patients who cannot open their mouths, as a nasotracheal approach might be considered. In patients

Electronic Supplementary Material The online version of this chapter (doi:10.1007/978-3-030-00859-8_18) contains supplementary material, which is available to authorized users.

D. Tran · W. M. Popescu (✉)
Department of Anesthesiology, Yale School of Medicine, New Haven, CT, USA
e-mail: daniel.tran@yale.edu; wanda.popescu@yale.edu

with previous radiation therapy to the neck, the external surface of the neck should be palpated to determine if the presence of very hard, rigid tissue could make intubation challenging. Similarly, patients with limited neck mobility can make laryngoscopy difficult. For patients who have a tracheostomy cannula in place and require OLV, it is important to determine if the cannula is cuffed or uncuffed and to assess the inlet of the stoma as well as the circumferential diameter in order to establish what type and size of lung isolation device can be used.

Another group of patients considered to have difficult airways during OLV are those who have distorted anatomy at the entrance of the mainstem bronchus. Such anomalies can be found by reviewing the chest radiographs and by reviewing the computer tomography scans of the chest regarding the mainstem bronchus diameter and anatomy, which can be distorted or compressed (see Fig. 18.1). Also, in specific patients, an examination with a flexible bronchoscope under local anesthesia and sedation prior to the selection of a specific OLV device could be useful to assess a distorted area of the airway. Table 18.1 displays the patients at risk of having a difficult intubation during OLV [5].

Difficult Airway and Lung Isolation: Securing the Airway First

In patients who require OLV and present with a difficult airway, the primary goal is to establish a secure airway. This task may be easier when using a single-lumen endotracheal tube placed orally. In selected patients who seem easy to ventilate, placing the endotracheal tube may be performed after induction of anesthesia with the use of a flexible bronchoscope or with a video laryngoscope [6–8]. Alternatively, a single-lumen endotracheal tube can be placed with flexible bronchoscopic guidance through a laryngeal mask airway.

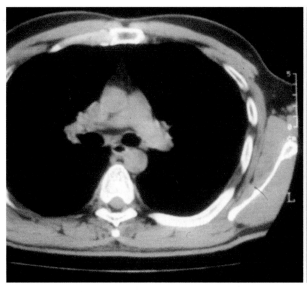 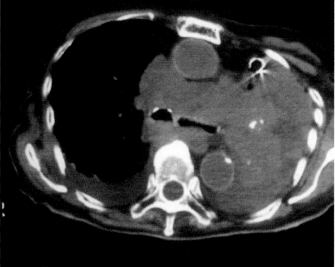

Fig. 18.1 Computed tomography (CT) scans from just below the level of the carinal bifurcation. *Left*: CT from a patient with no compression of the airway. *Right*: CT from patient scheduled for left lung biopsy. The patient has a left-sided lung tumor and effusion, which compresses the left mainstem bronchus. This bronchial compression was not evi- dent on the chest X-ray. It may be difficult to place a left-sided double-lumen endobronchial tube (DLT) in this patient. A right-sided DLT or a bronchial blocker would be the preferred method of lung isolation for this patient under flexible bronchoscopy guidance

Table 18.1 Characteristics of patients at risk of having a difficult intubation during one-lung ventilation

Upper airway	Lower airway
Short neck and increased neck circumference	Existing tracheostomy in place
Prominent upper incisors with a receding mandible	Distorted anatomy of the trachea or bronchus
Limited cervical mobility	Compression at the entrance of left mainstem bronchus by a tumor, descending thoracic aortic aneurysm, previous surgery, or radiation
Limited jaw opening	Previous lobectomy
Radiation therapy of the neck	Congenital abnormalities of the tracheobronchial tree (bronchus suis)
Hemiglossectomy/hemimandibulectomy Tumors (mouth, tongue, epiglottis)	Tracheoesophageal fistula

Use of a Flexible Bronchoscope During Awake Intubation

The administration of supplemental oxygen via nasal cannula as well as an antisialog medication such as glycopyrrolate is highly advisable during awake flexible bronchoscopic intubations. All local anesthetics used via spray or aerosolizer should be quantified to avoid overdose or complications, such as seizures or methemoglobinemia. A simple approach to anesthetize the posterior part of the tongue is to apply lidocaine 5% ointment to a tongue blade depressor and let the patient hold this in his or her mouth for about 5 min. After the tongue blade depressor is removed, the next step is to use a mucosal atomization device (MAD®) to spray the local anesthetic (lidocaine 4%, 10 mL) directly to the pharynx, larynx, and vocal cords. When the patient experiences a cough reflex, it is very likely that the anesthetic has entered the vocal cords. Before proceeding, all residual secretions accumulated in the airway should be suctioned. In order to test that the gag reflex is abolished, an intubating pharyngeal airway impregnated with lidocaine 5% ointment at the posterior tip can be advanced until it is completely inserted in the oral cavity. The oral intubating airway guides the bronchoscope toward the airway and prevents contact between the device and the patient's teeth.

The flexible bronchoscope is positioned in the midline such that the single-lumen endotracheal tube faces posteriorly during the intubation attempt. In some cases, retraction of the single-lumen endotracheal tube and 90° counterclockwise rotation will facilitate passage of the tube through the vocal cords. Sometimes it is necessary to complement the local anesthetic with an additional dose of lidocaine 4% (3 mL) through the suction channel of the bronchoscope to abolish the cough reflex during manipulation of the airway. The best indicator of proper placement of the bronchoscope and the endotracheal tube within the patient's trachea is the direct visualization of the tracheal rings and tracheal carina [9]. Once the patient is intubated with an endotracheal tube, then an independent bronchial blocker can be considered to achieve OLV.

Common independent bronchial blockers used through a single-lumen endotracheal tube include the following: a wire-guided endobronchial Arndt® blocker sizes 5.0, 7.0, and 9.0 F [10], the Cohen® Flex-Tip blocker size 9.0 F [11], and the Fuji Uniblocker® sizes 4.5 and 9.0 F [12, 13] (see Chap. 16).

The EZ-Blocker (IQ Medical Ventures BV, Rotterdam, Netherlands) is a new Y-shaped, symmetrical, bronchial blocker with two distal extensions, each with its own inflatable spherical cuff and central lumen. It is intended for use with a conventional endotracheal tube to provide lung isolation by inflation of either the left or right cuff while the distal extensions are located in the left and right mainstem bronchi. The design of the EZ-Blocker resembles the anatomic structure of the tracheobronchial tree which gives the device stability as it sits atop the carina, resulting in fewer dislodgements when compared to the Cohen Flex-Tip blocker [14]. The EZ-Blocker's polyurethane cuffs are "high pressure-low volume"; therefore the lowest required volumes should be used for inflation to avoid trauma to the bronchial mucosa. It is best to inflate the cuff of the bronchial blocker under direct visualization of the flexible bronchoscope in order to assure that the lowest amount of air is used while the entire bronchus is occluded. Limitations of the EZ-Blocker include the inability to perform selective lobar blockade, endobronchial suctioning, or lavage [15, 16].

If a patient cannot open his/her mouth and cannot be intubated orally, then an awake nasotracheal intubation can be performed. All precautions of a nasal intubation, including the application of a vasoconstrictor and a local anesthetic, should be taken. Once the airway is established with a nasal endotracheal tube, then an independent bronchial blocker can be advanced [17, 18]. Figure 18.2 shows a patient with previous hemimandibulectomy requiring nasotracheal intubation with an 8.0 mm internal diameter endotracheal tube and an Arndt® blocker passed through the multiport connector.

When a bronchial blocker is used, the smallest acceptable endotracheal tube size is 8.0-mm internal diameter to allow enough space between the bronchial blocker and the flexible bronchoscope. Once the endotracheal tube is secured in the patient's trachea, a bronchial blocker can be advanced with the aid of a flexible bronchoscope. An advantage of the Cohen® or the Fuji Uniblocker® over the Arndt® wire-guided endobronchial blocker is that while advancing it to a desired bronchus, the distal tip of the blocker can be seen while entering a bronchus. With the Arndt® blocker, the distal tip is looped into the fiberscope and cannot be seen until disengagement occurs. One of the advantages of bronchial

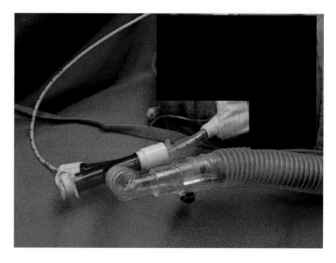

Fig. 18.2 A patient with previous hemimandibulectomy requiring nasotracheal intubation with an 8.0-mm internal diameter single-lumen endotracheal tube and an Arndt® blocker

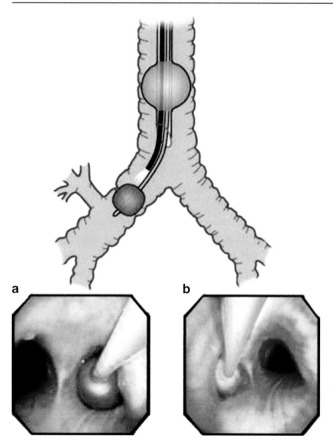

Fig. 18.3 The optimal position of an independent bronchial blocker through a single-lumen endotracheal tube. (**a**) The bronchial blocker balloon fully inflated into the right mainstem bronchus. (**b**) Fully inflated balloon in the entrance of the left mainstem bronchus [9]

blocker for lung isolation in a patient with a difficult airway is that at the end of the procedure, if postoperative ventilatory support is needed, the blocker is simply removed and the patient remains intubated with a single-lumen endotracheal tube [19].

In an adult the amount of air needed to achieve a complete seal within the bronchus varies significantly depending on the type of blocker utilized as well as on the size of the bronchi. The optimal position of a bronchial blocker is when the blocker balloon's outer surface is seen at least 10 mm below the tracheal carina inside the blocked bronchus and a proper seal is achieved. In order to identify an appropriate seal of the bronchus, the balloon should be inflated under bronchoscopic guidance. Figure 18.3 shows the optimal position of an independent bronchial blocker through a single-lumen endotracheal tube.

Special Consideration for Patients with High Aspiration Risk

Patients with difficult airways and high aspiration risk presenting for thoracic surgery require additional care given the

need to quickly and safely secure the airway. NPO guidelines should be strictly followed prior to surgery. The safest approach for securing the airway for this patient group is by performing an awake oral or nasal fiberoptic intubation with a single-lumen endotracheal tube, following proper airway topicalization. If lung isolation is required, an independent bronchial blocker is placed after the airway is safely secured. Alternatively, an awake DLT intubation can be done with the flexible bronchoscope inserted into the bronchial lumen of the DLT, then advanced into the correct mainstem bronchus under direct visualization. Awake DLT placement is more challenging due to the larger size of the tube which may not easily pass through the glottic opening. Intraoperatively, periodic suctioning of the oropharynx and gastric tubes before emergence and extubation is important to prevent reflux of contents from the esophagus. At the end of the procedure, patients should be extubated after being positioned with the head of the bed elevated and when fully awake [20].

Use of Laryngeal Mask Airway and a Bronchial Blocker During Difficult Airways

An alternative to achieve OLV in a patient with a difficult airway is with the use of a laryngeal mask airway in conjunction with the use of an independent bronchial blocker. A laryngeal mask airway can be modified by removing the aperture bar in order to facilitate the insertion of a flexible bronchoscope and bronchial blocker [21]. The ProSeal laryngeal mask airway has been used with a bronchial blocker in patients in whom the airway was deemed difficult and who required OLV during thoracoscopic surgery [22, 23].

Use of a Double-Lumen Endotracheal Tube in Patients with Difficult Airways

Intubation with a DLT can be more difficult than intubation with a single-lumen endotracheal tube. The larger size, the rigidity, and the shape of the DLT, without a bevel at the tip of the tube, can obscure the view of the glottis. In practice there are several different ways to place a DLT in patients with difficult airways. The first involves the use of airway topical anesthesia and awake bronchoscopy with passage of the flexible bronchoscope through the bronchial lumen of the DLT. The tube is advanced under bronchoscopic guidance while the patient is breathing spontaneously [24] (see Fig. 18.4). The second technique involves the use of ancillary lighted devices or video laryngoscopes that increase the visualization field of the epiglottis and vocal cords and aid the passage of the tube. The use of a malleable, lighted stylet

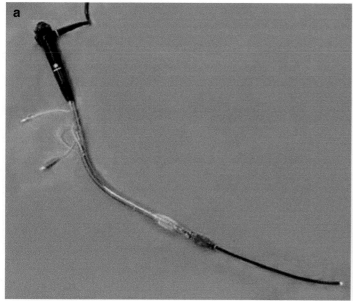

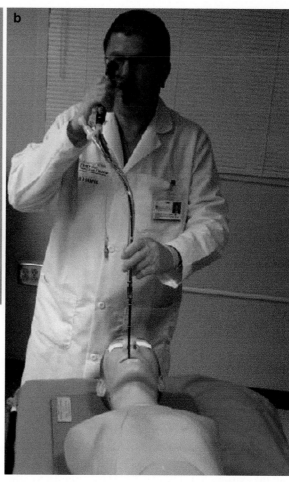

Fig. 18.4 (**a**) Pediatric fiberoptic bronchoscope passed through the endobronchial lumen of a double-lumen endotracheal tube (DLT) for fiberoptic intubation. Note that the actual working length of the DLT beyond the distal bronchial orifice is only approximately 20–25 cm. (**b**) Fiberoptic intubation of a mannequin with a left-sided DLT

(Mercury Medical, Clearwater, FL, USA) has been reported. The lighted stylet is placed via the endobronchial lumen of the DLT, where the tip of the bulb is positioned distally at the tip of the DLT [25]. Others have reported the use of a fiberoptic laryngoscope, the WuScope (Pentax Precision Instruments, Orangeburg, NJ, USA), during placement of a DLT in patients with abnormal airway anatomy [26]. One of the advantages of the fiberoptic laryngoscope is that it protects against rupture of the endotracheal cuff during laryngoscopy because the DLT is enclosed with the laryngoscope blade. A disadvantage of this device is the need for smaller-sized DLTs, such as 35–37 F.

Another option is the use of the VivaSight-DL. This is a new, single-use DLT with an integrated high-resolution camera embedded at the tip of the endotracheal lumen that allows for continuous visualization of the carina and position of the endobronchial balloon [27]. When used in a patient with a difficult airway, this device is placed in a similar manner as a standard DLT, with the advantage that the VivaSight-DL is connected to a screen monitor to provide a live view while the tube navigates the airway. In addition, after the VivaSight-DL is correctly positioned in the left mainstem bronchus, the continuous display of the carina and its position relative to the endobronchial balloon makes it easy to detect tube malposition in real time [28].

The Glidescope® video laryngoscope (Saturn Biomedical Systems, Burnaby, British Columbia, Canada) has been used in patients with a difficult airway during placement of a DLT [29]. Video-directed laryngoscopy may facilitate DLT intubation when direct laryngoscopy does not yield a clear view of the glottic opening for easy intubation. The Glidescope® technique offers several advantages including faster speed (in experienced hands), increased rate of first-pass success, and reduced risk of upper airway trauma. However, for patients with small oral apertures, the Glidescope® has limited utility.

The Glidescope® should be used with a dedicated semi-rigid intubating stylet (GlideRite DLT Stylet) while inserting a DLT, which maintains optimal curvature of the DLT and aligns the tip of the DLT with the tip of the Glidescope® blade

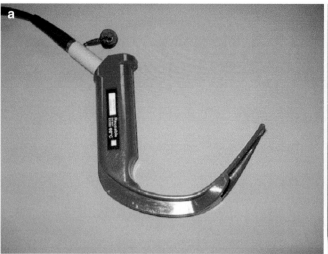
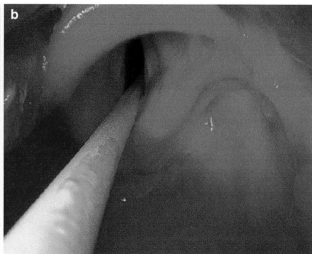

Fig. 18.5 (**a**) GlideScope® (Verathon Corp., Bothell, WA) video laryngoscope. Note the acute flexion of the laryngoscope blade. (**b**) View of the glottis from a GlideScope® during a tube exchange. A tube exchange catheter can be seen passing through the vocal cords. This clear view of the glottis facilitates manipulation of the airway device during replacement of a single-lumen endotracheal tube with a DLT or vice versa

[30]. Alternatively, the stylet of the DLT can be used; however, bending the tip of the DLT is recommended to facilitate insertion using the Glidescope®.

Another alternative is to intubate the patient's trachea with a single-lumen endotracheal tube during an awake or asleep flexible bronchoscopy. After induction of anesthesia, a DLT-specific Cook airway catheter can be used to exchange out the existing tube for a DLT [31] (see Fig. 18.5). The flexible beveled distal tip of the bronchial lumen of the Fuji Silbroncho doube-lumen tube is specifically designed for this purpose and facilitates this tube exchange [31] (see Fig. 18.6a–d).

The airway exchange catheter, single-lumen endotracheal tube, and the DLT combination should be tested in vitro before the exchange [32]. A sniffing position will facilitate tube exchange. After the airway exchange catheter is lubricated, it is advanced through a single-lumen endotracheal tube. The airway catheter should not be inserted deeper than 24 cm from the lips to avoid accidental rupture or laceration of the trachea, bronchi, or lung [33, 34]. After cuff deflation, the single-lumen endotracheal tube is withdrawn. The endobronchial lumen of the DLT is then advanced over the exchange catheter. It is optimal to use a video laryngoscope during the tube exchange to guide the DLT through the glottis under direct vision [35]. If a video laryngoscope is not available, then having an assistant per-

form a standard laryngoscopy during tube exchange partially straightens out the alignment of the oropharynx and glottis and facilitates the exchange. Proper final position of the DLT is then achieved with bronchoscopic examination. Replacement of a DLT for a single-lumen endotracheal tube can be done at the conclusion of surgery with the use of either a single or a double airway exchange catheter. One study using two airway exchange catheters to exchange a DLT for a single-lumen endotracheal tube showed that there was a reduction in the incidence of glottis impingement of the tracheal tube and that there was a higher success rate of passage of the single-lumen endotracheal tube when compared with the use of a single airway exchange catheter [36]. The use of a double airway exchange catheter involves the following techniques: two 11 F, 83-cm-long airway exchange catheters from Cook® Critical Care are used. One catheter is passed through the endobronchial lumen of the DLT, making sure that the tip of the airway exchanger does not protrude distally in the tip of the DLT. A second exchange catheter is passed through the tracheal lumen; both catheters provide easy placement of the new single-lumen endotracheal tube because of the increase rigidity with the two tube exchangers. For this technique to work, an 8.0-mm internal diameter single-lumen endotracheal tube must be used. Another variation of the tube exchanger technique is using a double-diameter coaxial airway exchange

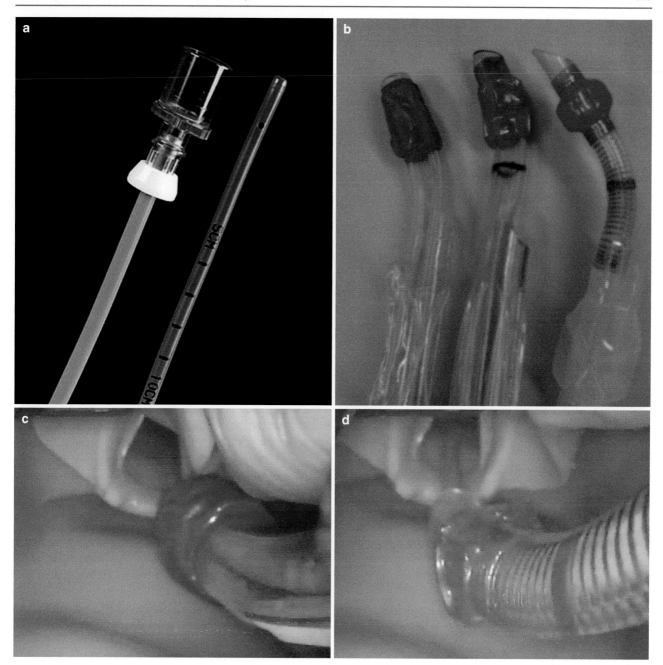

Fig. 18.6 (**a**) The Cook® airway catheter (Cook Critical Care, Bloomington, IN) for exchange between DLTs and a single-lumen endotracheal tube. This catheter has a soft distal (*purple*) tip to attempt to decrease the risk of distal airway injury during tube exchange (*right*). The proximal stiffer *green* end (*left*) has detachable connectors for emergency ventilation. Shown is the standard 15-mm outside diameter breathing circuit connector. The exchange catheter also comes with a jet ventilation connector (not shown). (**b**) Double-lumen tube manufacturers' designs of the distal tip of the bronchial lumen. From left to right: Rusch Brochopart, Teleflex, Research Triangle Park, NC; Mallinckrodt, Broncho-Cath, Covidien, Mansfield, MA; and Fuji, Silbroncho, Fuji Systems, Tokyo. (**c**) Single- to double-lumen tube exchange over a Cook catheter with a Rusch double-lumen tube seen via a video laryngoscope. The distal bronchial lumen of the tube is impacted on the right arytenoid. (**d**) Single- to double-lumen tube exchange over a Cook catheter with a Fuji double-lumen tube seen via a video laryngoscope. The bevel of the distal bronchial lumen of the tube facilitates entry into the glottis. (Figures reproduced from Ref. [31] with permission)

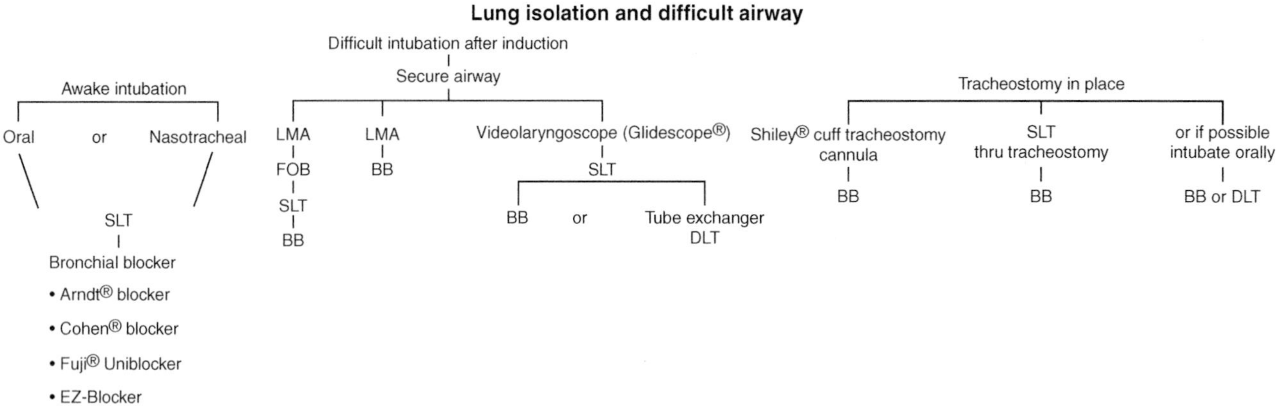

Lung isolation and difficult airway

Difficult intubation after induction
|
Secure airway

Awake intubation

Oral   or   Nasotracheal   LMA   LMA   Videolaryngoscope (Glidescope®)   Shiley® cuff tracheostomy   SLT   or if possible
                                             | | cannula   thru tracheostomy   intubate orally
                                            FOB   BB   SLT
                                             | | BB   BB   BB or DLT
                    SLT   SLT   BB   or   Tube exchanger
                     | | DLT
        Bronchial blocker   BB

        • Arndt® blocker

        • Cohen® blocker

        • Fuji® Uniblocker

        • EZ-Blocker

Tracheostomy in place

Fig. 18.7 Different alternatives to achieve lung isolation during difficult airways [6]. Abbreviations: LMA Laryngeal mask airway, FOB Fiberoptic bronchoscopy, SLT Single-lumen tube, BB Bronchial blocker, DLT Double-lumen tube

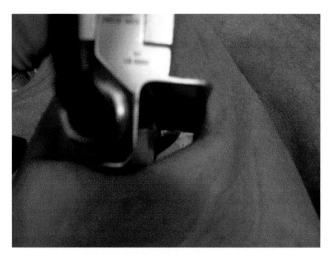

Fig. 18.8 Photograph of the Video MACINTOSH® System (Karl Storz, Culver City, CA) during intubation. Note the poor grade of view of the glottis seen with "line of sight". (Photo is courtesy of Dr. R. Purugganan)

catheter. This consists of a 4.0-mm outer diameter exchanger inside a 7.0-mm outer diameter exchanger. This device allows for a more rigid guide wire for replacing DLT with a single-lumen endotracheal tube. During tube exchanger techniques, it is recommended to use a video laryngoscope to visualize the proper exchange and move the tongue away from the tube. Figure 18.7 displays the different techniques to manage the patient who has a difficult airway and requires lung isolation. Several other manufacturers have introduced different designs of video laryngoscopes that are also useful for lung isolation with difficult airways (see Fig. 18.8).

Lung Isolation Techniques in Patients with Tracheostomies

Before placing any lung isolation devices through a tracheostomy stoma, it is important to consider whether it is a fresh stoma (i.e., few days old, when the airway can be lost immediately or decannulation can occur) versus an old tracheostomy. A standard DLT placed through a tracheostomy stoma can be prone to malposition because the upper airway has been shortened and a conventional DLT is too long.

When selecting a DLT as a replacement of the tracheostomy cannula, a specially designed short version of a DLT, such as the Naruke DLT, can be used. In a report involving six patients with permanent tracheostomies, the Naruke tube was used with satisfactory results in patients requiring thoracic surgery and OLV [37].

An alternative to achieve lung isolation in a tracheostomized patient includes the placement of a single-lumen endotracheal tube through the tracheostomy followed by insertion of a bronchial blocker [38] [see Video 18.1]. If possible the airway could be accessed orally for standard placement of a single-lumen endotracheal tube followed by a bronchial blocker. Another option is the use of a disposable cuff tracheostomy cannula with an independent bronchial blocker passed coaxially. In these cases, a small-size flexible bronchoscope (i.e., 3.5-mm outer diameter) is recommended. Figure 18.9 shows lung isolation in a patient with a small tracheal stoma. The tracheostomy device has been replaced; a small laryngeal mask airway LMA #3 has been used to ventilate the patient through the stoma. Also shown in the picture is a patient with a tracheostomy stoma where a 7.0-mm internal diameter single-lumen endotracheal tube has been advanced through the stoma followed by an Arndt® bronchial blocker.

Lower Airway Abnormalities and Lung Isolation

Patients with lower airway abnormalities, specifically distal tracheal or bronchial lesions, require special attention when OLV is required. A right-sided DLT is indicated when the lumen of the left mainstem bronchus is either constricted or compressed (e.g., by intraluminal tumor or descending thoracic aortic aneurysm), absent or stenosed due to previous

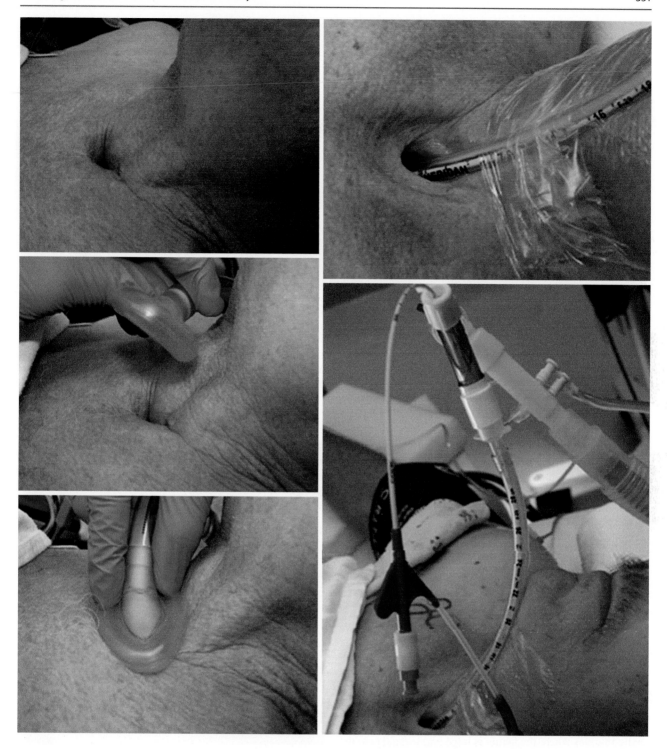

Fig. 18.9 Lung isolation in a patient with a small tracheal stoma. The tracheostomy device has been replaced; to the *left* a small laryngeal mask airway LMA #3 has been used to ventilate the patient through the stoma. To the *right* is shown a patient with a stoma where a 7.0-mm internal diameter single-lumen endotracheal tube has been advanced through the stoma followed by an Arndt® bronchial blocker

surgeries (e.g., pneumonectomy or lung transplantation), or when surgical repair involves the left mainstem bronchus [39]. Following endotracheal tube placement, flexible bronchoscopy should be used to verify the proper alignment between the right upper lobe bronchus and the ventilation slot of the right-sided DLT to avoid right upper lobe obstruction; also, the right lower and middle lobes should be unob-structed by the bronchial lumen. Studies have shown that there is no clinical ventilatory advantage between a left-sided and a right-sided DLT [40].

Patients who have undergone previous lobectomy surgery may present with distorted anatomy. Identifying the right and left bronchi may be difficult because of the loss of ana-tomical landmarks [41]. In order to properly identify the

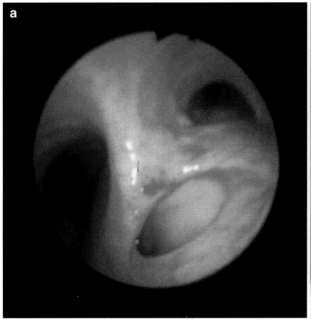

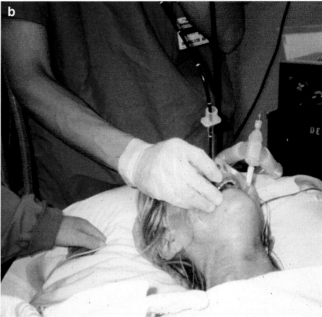

Fig. 18.10 (**a**) Flexible bronchoscopy view of a tracheoesophageal fistula caused by esophageal cancer. The fistula is seen posteriorly at the level of the carina at 5 o'clock. The left mainstem bronchus is at 9 o'clock, and the right mainstem bronchus is at 2 o'clock. (**b**)

Fiberoptic-guided placement of bilateral endobronchial tubes (5-mm internal diameter microlaryngoscopy tubes) for repair of tracheoesophageal fistula in the same patient. (Photos are courtesy of Dr. R Grant)

anatomy of the tracheobronchial tree, a complete broncho-scopic exam of the lower airway prior to placement of the lung isolation device is required.

Another lower airway abnormality to consider is the tracheoesophageal fistula (TEF). Improper positioning of the endotracheal tube in patients with TEF can lead to serious complications. Ultimately, the location and size of the fistula and surgical approach will dictate how the airway should be secured to facilitate lung isolation and exposure for repair. Generally, if a single-lumen endotracheal tube is employed, for instance, to facilitate the repair of a TEF that is located high in the trachea, it should be secured so that its tip is above the carina and its cuff is below the fistula in order to provide adequate ventilation while avoiding gastric insufflation which may lead to an unwanted aspiration event. Flexible bronchoscopy is an indispensable tool for TEF assessment prior to repair but also for quick confirmation of endotracheal tube migration and malposition, especially in cases where the fistula is large and located near the carina ("large and low-lying"). For TEF repair via a right thoracotomy incision, lung isolation with a left-sided DLT can be achieved effectively when the fistula is positioned above the cuff of the tracheal lumen. Alternatively, isolation of the right lung and fistula can be achieved simultaneously by inserting a single-lumen endotracheal tube down the left mainstem bronchus [42, 43]. Also, the use of two micro-laryngeal endotracheal tubes as endobronchial tubes placed under flexible bronchoscopy guidance can help secure the airway under these circumstances as shown in Fig. 18.10.

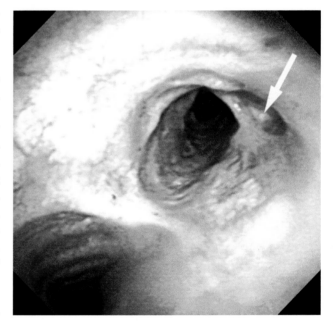

Fig. 18.11 Bronchoscopic view of the bronchus suis. White arrow indicates the supracarinal takeoff of the right upper lobe

Tracheal bronchus, also called bronchus suis or pig bronchus, is a congenital anatomical variant where the right upper lobe bronchus originates directly from the supracarinal trachea [see Fig. 18.11]. The incidence ranges from 0.1% to 5%, with the right tracheal bronchus being the more common presentation. Tracheal bronchi can be classified as supernumerary (the normal segmental bronchus is also present, in addition to the supernumerary bronchus) or displaced (the normal segmental bronchus is absent). Most patients with this condition are asymptomatic, but some may experience recurrent pneumonia, stridor, or chronic bronchitis due to retained secretions [44, 45].

Several challenges arise in the management of patients with tracheal bronchus undergoing surgery requiring lung isolation. Whether a single-lumen endotracheal tube or DLT is used, proper positioning of the endotracheal tube above the bronchial takeoff must be confirmed to ensure adequate ventilation of the anomalous bronchus. Additionally, care should be taken to avoid insertion of the endotracheal tube into the tracheal bronchus which could lead to injury from overventilation. Lung isolation for right-sided lung surgery in the setting of the tracheal bronchus can be achieved using a single-lumen endotracheal tube, DLT, and in certain situations a bronchial blocker. A left-sided DLT is the best option for tracheal bronchus with carinal takeoff. However, if the right upper lobe bronchus takeoff is supracarinal, then a single-lumen endotracheal tube (inserted into the left mainstem bronchus) or two bronchial blockers (one to isolate the normal and the other to isolate the anomalous bronchus) can be used. Close communication with the surgical team and a thorough bronchoscopic examination of the airway are recommended prior to formulating a complete anesthetic plan for patients with this congenital condition.

Lung Isolation in Patients with Cervical Spine Abnormalities

Injuries to the cervical spine occur in only 2–3% of all patients with blunt trauma but are significant because of their high level of associated mortality and morbidity [46, 47]. Some of these patients have experienced trauma to the chest with an injury to the descending thoracic aorta. In these trauma patients, the atlantoaxial region is the most common site of injury, and the sixth and seventh vertebrae are involved in over one third of all injuries [48]. In these patients, all precautions must be taken with regard to cervical spine injury [49].

Close communication with the surgical team is paramount in managing patients presenting after acute chest trauma with possible multiple injuries to intrathoracic structures. In a stable and cooperative patient, an approach which preserves spontaneous ventilation (e.g., awake flexible bronchoscopy-guided intubation) is ideal. In most cases, however, it is important to immediately and safely secure the airway to facilitate surgical treatment of injuries and for protection against aspiration of blood and gastric contents. Following thoracic trauma, a single-lumen endotracheal tube is recommended for rapidly securing an airway with ques-

tionable integrity. Videolaryngoscopy and flexible bronchoscopy approaches may be challenging due to the presence of blood in the airway. A bronchoscopic exam should immediately be performed after intubation to assess the extent of damage to the airway. After the integrity of the lower airway is confirmed, lung isolation can be achieved with a bronchial blocker [50].

Patients who present with cervical spine instability require additional care aimed at minimizing excessive force to the cervical spine which may lead to further injury. Manual in-line stabilization (MILS) is a standard practice performed during intubation with the goal of preventing cervical spine movement by the application of equal and opposite forces to those generated by the intubator. Rigid MILS, however, may cause problems during intubation by limiting the view for laryngoscopy and potentially increasing subluxation of unstable cervical segments. It is important to consider the application of additional intubating tools (e.g., stylet or bougie) for securing the airway [51]. If lung isolation is desired, a bronchial blocker can be placed under flexible bronchoscopic guidance only after the integrity of the lower airway has been established. A similar approach can be used in patients with cervical spine instability due to rheumatoid arthritis (see Fig. 18.12).

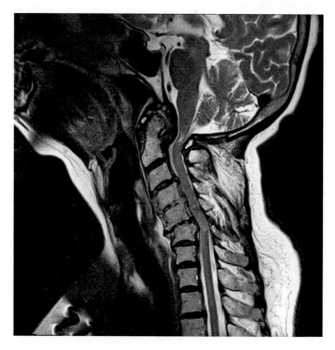

Fig. 18.12 This patient with rheumatoid arthritis has a retroflexed odontoid process and associated inflammatory mass (pseudogout) causing compression of the cervical spinal cord just inferior to the foramen magnum. The patient also had intervertebral subluxations and osteophytes from C3 to C5 that cause cord compression. The anesthetic plan included an awake fiberoptic intubation with a single-lumen endotracheal tube

Extubation or Mechanical Ventilation After Surgery

Extubation at the completion of surgery in a patient who has a difficult airway represents a challenge. Factors to consider prior to extubation include any mucosal edema, bleeding or lacerations to the airway during intubation, the length of surgery, and the amount of fluid administered during the intraoperative period. Continuous access to the airway should be maintained in case reintubation is needed. The single-lumen endotracheal tube or the DLT can be removed with an airway catheter exchanger left in place after extubation [52].

In some instances a patient with a difficult airway who has a DLT in place may require mechanical ventilation in the postoperative period. One option is to deflate both cuffs, withdraw the bronchial lumen above the carina, and then reinflate the tracheal cuff to effectively convert the DLT to a "single" lumen tube [53], particularly if the conversion to exchange a DLT for a single-lumen endotracheal tube is considered too risky.

An alternative technique is to exchange a DLT for a single-lumen endotracheal tube using an airway catheter exchanger under direct vision with a laryngoscope [54] or video laryngoscope [55–57].

Summary

In patients who require OLV, a key element during the preoperative assessment is the recognition and identification of the potentially difficult airway. The safest way to establish an airway is by securing the airway with a single-lumen endotracheal tube placed orally or nasotracheally with the aid of a flexible bronchoscope. Lung isolation in these patients is best achieved with the use of an independent bronchial blocker. An alternative can be the use of a DLT placed with an airway catheter exchange technique. For the patient who has a tracheostomy in place, the use of an independent bronchial blocker through a single-lumen endotracheal tube or through a tracheotomy cannula in place is recommended. For all these devices, a flexible bronchoscopic examination is recommended prior, during placement, and at the conclusion of the use of lung isolation devices.

Clinical Case Discussion

Case: A 61-year-old male with a right upper lobe lung mass is scheduled for a right upper lobectomy. He is 175 cm tall and weights 73 kg. Relevant history includes right manidibular mass resection and radiation therapy to the neck. He smoked two packs of cigarettes per day for 40 years.

Airway exam reveals the following: normal dentition, Mallampati score III, thyromental distance of two finger breadths, very limited neck range of motion, and scarring from previous surgery and radiation. Palpation of the anterior neck shows hard and rigid consistency of the tissue.

Questions

- What technique would you select to intubate this patient?
- What potential problems do you expect during an awake fiberoptic bronchoscopy in a patient with a previous neck resection and extensive surgery?
- What device and size would you use to provide lung isolation?
- What are the common problems in the intraoperative period with the use of bronchial blockers?
- What are the complications associated with the bronchial blocker?
- What are the advantages and disadvantages of using a bronchial blocker during a case with a difficult airway that requires lung isolation?

The Key Is to Focus on Patient's Anatomy in Order to Select the Lung Isolation Device

- Review the chest radiograph to appreciate the distorted tracheobronchial anatomy.
- Focus on lung isolation devices during difficult airways.
- Familiarity with the use of independent blockers is mandatory.
- Skills with flexible bronchoscopy during awake intubation, as well as during placement of bronchial blockers, are essential.

Expected Intraoperative Problems with the Use of Bronchial Blockers

- Possible malposition/dislodgement of bronchial blocker.
- The balloon of the bronchial blocker can occlude the trachea and impede ventilation.

Suggested Management

In patients requiring OLV who are identified during the preoperative evaluation to have difficult airway as in the case presented here, the main challenges include (1) to safely secure the airway and (2) to select the proper bronchial blocker to achieve lung isolation during OLV. Because of previous neck surgery with airway anatomy distortion, the main problem in this case is to safely establish an airway. An awake flexible bronchoscopy can be used. After nasal and oral airway topical anesthesia is achieved, a flexible bronchoscope is passed orally with an 8.5-mm internal diameter single-lumen endotracheal tube loaded on it.

The single-lumen endotracheal tube is advanced without difficulty. After the tube is secured, a complete flexible bronchoscopic exam is performed under general anesthesia. Successful lung isolation is achieved with a 9 F Fuji Uniblocker® that is passed under direct bronchoscopic view into the right mainstem bronchus. The bronchial blocker cuff is inflated under direct bronchoscopic view to confirm complete bronchial occlusion [see Video 18.2]. The optimal position is once again confirmed in the lateral decubitus position. After completion of the right upper lobectomy, two-lung ventilation is reestablished, the bronchial blocker is removed, and the patient can be extubated without any complications.

References

1. Campos JH. Progress in lung separation. Thorac Surg Clin. 2005;15:71–83.
2. Hagihira S, Takashina M, Mori T, Yoshiya I. One-lung ventilation in patients with difficult airways. J Cardiothorac Vasc Anesth. 1998;12:186–8.
3. Campos JH. Update on tracheobronchial anatomy and flexible fiberoptic bronchoscopy in thoracic anesthesia. Curr Opin Anaesthesiol. 2009;22:4–10.
4. American Society of Anesthesiologists Task Force on Management of the Difficult Airway. Practice guidelines for management ofthe difficult airway: an updated report by the American Society of Anesthesiologists Task Force on Management of the Difficult Airway. Anesthesiology. 2003;98:1269–77.
5. Campos JH. Difficult airway and one-lung ventilation. Curr Rev Clin Anesth. 2002;22:199–205.
6. Campos JH. Lung isolation techniques for patients with difficult airways. Curr Opin Anaesthesiol. 2010;23:12–7.
7. Poon KH, Liu EH. The airway scope for difficult double-lumen tube intubation. J Clin Anesth. 2008;20:319.
8. Davis L, Cook-Sather SD, Schreiner MS. Lighted stylet tracheal intubation: a review. Anesth Analg. 2000;90:745–6.
9. Campos JH. Fiberoptic bronchoscopy in anesthesia. Curr Rev Clin Anesth. 2008;29:61–72.
10. Arndt GA, Buchika S, Kranner PW, DeLessio ST. Wire-guided endobronchial blockade in a patient with a limited mouth opening. Can J Anaesth. 1999;46:87–9.
11. Cohen E. The Cohen flexitip endobronchial blocker: an alternative to a double lumen tube. Anesth Analg. 2005;101:1877–9.
12. Campos JH. Which device should be considered the best for lung isolation: double-lumen endotracheal tube versus bronchial blockers. Curr Opin Anaesthesiol. 2007;20:27–31.
13. Narayanaswamy M, McRae K, Slinger P, et al. Choosing a lung isolation device for thoracic surgery: a randomized trial of three bronchial blockers versus double-lumen tubes. Anesth Analg. 2009;108:1097–101.
14. Kus A, et al. A comparison of the EZ-Blocker with a Cohen Flex-Tip blocker for one-lung ventilation. J Cardiothorac Vasc Anesth. 2014 Aug;28(4):896–9.
15. Mourisse J, et al. Efficiency, efficacy, and safety of EZ-blocker compared with left-sided double-lumen tube for one-lung ventilation. Anesthesiology. 2013;118(3):550–61.
16. Ruetzler K, et al. Randomized clinical trial comparing double-lumen tube and EZ-Blocker for single-lung ventilation. Br J Anaesth. 2011;106(6):896–902.
17. Campos JH. Use of the wire-guided endobronchial blocker for one-lung anesthesia in patients with airway abnormalities. J Cardiothorac Vasc Anesth. 2003;17:352–4.
18. Angie Ho CY, Chen CY, Yang MW, Liu HP. Use of the Arndt wire-guided endobronchial blocker via nasal for one-lung ventilation in patient with anticipated restricted mouth opening for esophagectomy. Eur J Cardiothorac Surg. 2005;28:174–5.
19. Cohen E. Pro: the new bronchial blockers are preferable to double-lumen tubes for lung isolation. J Cardiothorac Vasc Anesth. 2008;22:920–4.
20. Carney A, Dickinson M. Anesthesia for esophagectomy. Anesthesiol Clin. 2015;33(1):143–63.
21. Robinson AR III, Gravenstein N, Alomar-Melero E, Peng YG. Lung isolation using a laryngeal mask airway and a bronchial blocker in a patient with a recent tracheostomy. J Cardiothorac Vasc Anesth. 2008;22:883–6.
22. Ozaki M, Murashima K, Fukutome T. One-lung ventilation using the ProSeal laryngeal mask airway. Anaesthesia. 2004;59:726.
23. Tsuchihashi T, Ide S, Nakagawa H, Hishinuma N, et al. Differential lung ventilation using laryngeal mask airway and a bronchial blocker tube for a patient with unanticipated difficult intubation. Masui. 2007;56:1075–7.
24. Patane PS, Sell BA, Mahla ME. Awake fiberoptic endobronchial intubation. J Cardiothorac Anesth. 1990;4:229–31.
25. O'Connor CJ, O'Connor TA. Use of lighted stylets to facilitate insertion of double-lumen endobronchial tubes in patients with difficult airway anatomy. J Clin Anesth. 2006;18:616–9.
26. Smith CE, Kareti M. Fiberoptic laryngoscopy (WuScope) for double-lumen endobronchial tube placement in two difficult intubation patients. Anesthesiology. 2000;93:906–7.
27. Huitink JM, et al. Tracheal intubation with a camera embedded in the tube tip (Vivasight™). Anaesthesia. 2013;68(1):74–8.
28. Koopman EM, et al. Evaluation of a new double-lumen endobronchial tube with an integrated camera (VivaSight-DL™): a prospective multicentre observational study. Anaesthesia. 2015;70(8):962–8.
29. Hernandez AA, Wong DH. Using a Glidescope for intubation with a double lumen endotracheal tube. Can J Anaesth. 2005;52:658–9.
30. Bussières JS. A customized stylet for GlideScope® insertion of double lumen tubes. Can J Anaesth. 2012;59(4):424–5.
31. Gamez R, Slinger P. A simulator study of tube exchange with 3 different designs of double-lumen tube. Anesth Analg. 2014;119:449–53.
32. Benumof JL. Difficult tubes and difficult airways. J Cardiothorac Vasc Anesth. 1998;12:131–2.
33. Thomas V, Neustein SM. Tracheal laceration after the use ofan airway exchange catheter for double-lumen tube placement. J Cardiothorac Vasc Anesth. 2007;21:718–9.
34. deLima LG, Bishop MJ. Lung laceration after tracheal extubation over a plastic tube changer. Anesth Analg. 1991;73:350–1.
35. Chen A, Lai HY, Lin PC, Chen TY, Shyr MH. GlideScope-assisted double-lumen endobronchial tube placement in a patient with an unanticipated difficult airway. J Cardiothorac Vasc Anesth. 2008;22:170–2.
36. Suzuki A, Uraoka M, Kimura K, Sato S. Effects of using two airway exchange catheters on laryngeal passage during change from a double-lumen tracheal tube to a single-lumen tracheal tube. Br J Anaesth. 2007;99:440–3.
37. Saito T, Naruke T, Carney E, et al. New double intrabronchial tube (Naruke tube) for tracheostomized patients. Anesthesiology. 1998;89:1038–9.
38. Tobias JD. Variations on one-lung ventilation. J Clin Anesth. 2001;13:35–9.

39. Campos JH, Ajax TJ, Knutson R, et al. Case conference 5–1990. A 76-year-old man undergoing an emergency descending thoracicaortic aneurysm repair has multiple intraoperative and postoperative complications. J Cardiothorac Anesth. 1990;4:631–45.

40. Ehrenfeld JM, et al. Performance comparison of right- and left-sided double-lumen tubes among infrequent users. J Cardiothorac Vasc Anesth. 2010;24:598–601.

41. Campos JH. Update on selective lobar blockade during pulmonary resections. Curr Opin Anaesthesiol. 2009;22:18–22.

42. Tercan E, Sungun MB, Boyaci A, Kucukaydin M. One lung ventilation of a preterm newborn during esophageal atresia and tracheoesophageal fistula repair. Acta Anaesthesiol Scand. 2002;46:332–3.

43. Taneja B, Saxenaet KN. Endotracheal intubation in a neonate with esophageal atresia and Trachea-Esophageal Fistula: pitfalls and techniques. J Neonatal Surg. 2014;3(2):18.

44. Ghaye B, Szapiro D, Fanchamps JM, Dondelinger RF. Congenital bronchial abnormalities revisited. Radiographics. 2001;21:105–19.

45. McLaughlin FJ, Strieder DJ, Harris GBC, et al. Tracheal bronchus: association with respiratory morbidity in childhood. J Pediatr. 1985;106:751–5.

46. Hoffman JR, Schriger DL, Mower WR, et al. Low-risk criteria for cervical-spine radiography in blunt trauma: a prospective study. Ann Emerg Med. 1992;21:1454–60.

47. Roberge RJ, Wears RC, Kelly M, et al. Selective application of cervical spine radiography in alert victims of blunt trauma: a prospective study. J Trauma. 1988;28:784–8.

48. Goldberg W, Mueller C, Panacek E, et al. Distribution and patterns of blunt traumatic cervical spine injury. Ann Emerg Med. 2001;38:17–21.

49. Crosby ET. Airway management in adults after cervical spine trauma. Anesthesiology. 2006;104:1293–318.

50. Surgical treatment of thoracic trauma: lung. In: DiSaverio S, Tugnoli G, Catena F, et al., editors. Trauma surgery, thoracic and abdominal trauma. Vol. 2. New York: Springer; 2014. p. 77–90.

51. Nolan JP, Wilson ME. Orotracheal intubation in patients with potential cervical spine injuries. An indication for the gum elastic bougie. Anaesthesia. 1993;48:630–3.

52. Mort TC. Continuous airway access for the difficult extubation:the efficacy of the airway exchange catheter. Anesth Analg. 2007;105:1357–62.

53. Merlone SC, Shulman MS, Allen MD, Mark JB. Prolonged intubation with a polyvinylchloride double-lumen endobronchial tube. J Cardiothorac Anesth. 1987;1:563–4.

54. Benumof JL. Airway exchange catheters: simple concept, potentially great danger. Anesthesiology. 1999;91:342–4.

55. Merli G, Guarino A, Della Rocca G, et al. Recommendations for airway control and difficult airway management in thoracic anesthesia and lung separation procedures. Minerva Anestesiol. 2009;75:59–78.

56. Pott LM, Murray WB. Review of video laryngoscopy and rigid fiberoptic laryngoscopy. Curr Opin Anaesthesiol. 2008;21:750–8.

57. Thong SY, Lim Y. Video and optic laryngoscopy assisted tracheal intubation–the new era. Anaesth Intensive Care. 2009;37:219–33.

Intraoperative Patient Positioning and Neurological Injuries

19

Cara Reimer and Peter Slinger

Key Points
- Thoracic cases usually involve repositioning the patient after induction of anesthesia. Vigilance is required to avoid major displacement of airway devices, lines, and monitors during and after position changes.
- Obtaining central venous access after changing to the lateral position is extremely difficult. If a central line may be needed, it should be placed at induction.
- Prevention of peripheral nerve injuries in the lateral position requires a survey of the patient from the head and sides of the operating table prior to draping.
- A large portion of the ipsilateral shoulder pain following thoracic surgery may be due to intraoperative positioning.
- Several centers now advocate minimally invasive esophagectomy surgery in the prone position to improve surgical access.
- Post-thoracotomy paraplegia is primarily a surgical complication.

The majority of thoracic procedures are performed in the lateral position, but depending on the surgical technique, a flexed-lateral (nephrectomy), supine, semi-supine, semi-prone lateral, or prone position may be used. These positions have specific implications for the anesthesiologist.

C. Reimer
Department of Anesthesiology and Perioperative Medicine, Kingston Health Sciences Centre, Kingston, ON, Canada

P. Slinger (✉)
Department of Anesthesia, Toronto General Hospital, Toronto, ON, Canada
e-mail: peter.slinger@uhn.ca

Position Change It is awkward to induce anesthesia in the lateral position. Thus, monitors will be placed, and anesthesia will usually be induced in the supine position, and the anesthetized patient will then be repositioned for surgery. Sometimes multiple repositionings are required during a single case. It is possible to induce anesthesia in the lateral position, and this may rarely be indicated with unilateral lung diseases such as bronchiectasis or hemoptysis until lung isolation can be achieved. However, even these patients will then have to be repositioned after induction and the diseased lung turned to the non-dependent position. The operating room team, led by the anesthesiologist, needs to follow a standardized protocol to avoid injury to the patient and displacement of lines, tubes, and monitors during each position change.

Due to the loss of venous vascular tone in the anesthetized patient, it is not uncommon to see hypotension when turning the patient to or from the lateral position. All lines and monitors will have to be secured during position change and their function reassessed after repositioning. The anesthesiologist should take personal responsibility for the head, neck, and airway during position change and must be in charge of the operating team to direct repositioning. It is useful to make an initial "head-to-toe" survey of the patient after induction and intubation checking oxygenation, ventilation, hemodynamics, lines, monitors, and potential nerve injuries. This survey then must be repeated and documented after repositioning (see Table 19.1). It is nearly impossible to avoid some movement of a double-lumen tube or bronchial blocker during repositioning [1]. The patient's head, neck, and endobronchial tube should be turned "en bloc" with the patient's thoracolumbar spine. However, the margin of error in positioning endobronchial tubes or blockers is often so narrow that even very small movements can have significant clinical implications [2]. The carina and mediastinum may shift independently with repositioning, and this can lead to proximal misplacement of a previously well-positioned tube.

Table 19.1 Neurovascular injuries specific to the lateral position routine "Head-to-Toe" survey

1) Dependent eye
2) Dependent ear pinna
3) Cervical spine in-line with thoracic spine
4) Dependent arm: (i) brachial plexus, (ii) circulation
5) Non-dependent arm[a]: (i) brachial plexus, (ii) circulation
6) Dependent and non-dependent suprascapular nerves
7) Non-dependent leg sciatic nerve
8) Dependent leg: (i) peroneal nerve, (ii) circulation

[a]Neurovascular injuries of the non-dependent arm are more likely to occur if the arm is suspended or held in an independently positioned armrest.

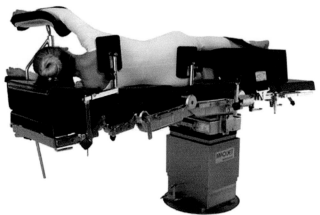

Fig. 19.2 Posterior view of a patient in the lateral view with a vacuum mat. It is very important to survey the patient from this perspective to ascertain that the cervicothoracic spine is in alignment prior to draping. After turning from the supine position, it is very easy to accidentally reposition the patient with a degree of lateral cervical flexion that is difficult to appreciate from the head of the table. Note the extra padding under the upper thorax below the axilla. Also note the gel ring preventing compression of the dependent ear pinna and the cushioning between the legs. (From Ref. [18])

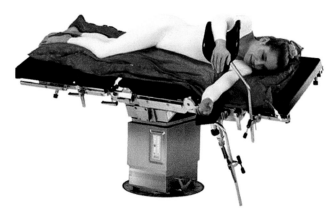

Fig. 19.1 Patient in the lateral position on a vacuum mat. Note both arms are supported on armrests which are fixed to the operating table. This position of the arms allows good access to the head for monitoring and airway management after surgical draping. The dependent leg is straight and the non-dependent leg flexed. (From Ref. [18])

Endobronchial tube/blocker position and the adequacy of ventilation must be rechecked by auscultation and fiber-optic bronchoscopy after patient repositioning.

The Lateral Position (also referred to as the lateral decubitus position) This is the commonest position for thoracic surgical procedures. The patient may be positioned on a vacuum mat (see Fig. 19.1) or on cushions (see Fig. 19.2). The operating table headrest and pillows must be adjusted so that the cervical spine remains in-line with the thoracic spine. It is very easy after repositioning the patient in the lateral position to cause excessive lateral flexion of the cervical spine because of improper positioning of the patient's head. This malpositioning, which exacerbates brachial plexus traction, can cause a "whiplash" syndrome and is difficult to appreciate from the head of the operating table, particularly after the surgical drapes have been placed. It is useful for the anesthesiologist to survey the patient from the side of the table immediately after turning to ensure that the entire vertebral column is aligned properly. Both eyes should be visible to the anesthesiologist throughout the procedure to avoid compression on the globes by pillows or lines. The dependent ear pinna may be positioned in the center of a gel ring.

The dependent arm is positioned on an armrest at 90° to the table, and the non-dependent arm is positioned on an armrest or pillows. The brachial plexus is the site of the majority of intraoperative nerve injuries related to the lateral position [3]. These are basically of two varieties: the majority are compression injuries of the brachial plexus of the dependent arm, but there is also significant risk of stretch injuries to the brachial plexus of the non-dependent arm. The brachial plexus is fixed at two points: proximally by the transverse processes of the cervical vertebrae and distally by the axillary fascia. This two-point fixation plus the extreme mobility of neighboring skeletal and muscular structures makes the brachial plexus extremely liable to injury (see Table 19.2). The patient should be positioned with padding under the dependent thorax (see Fig. 19.2) to keep the weight of the upper body off the dependent arm brachial plexus. Unfortunately this pad is called an "axillary pad" or "axillary roll" in some institutions. However, this padding will exacerbate the pressure on the brachial plexus if it migrates superiorly into the axilla.

The brachial plexus of the non-dependent arm is most at risk if it is suspended from an independently fixed arm support or "ether screen" (see Fig. 19.3). Traction on the brachial plexus in these situations is particularly likely to occur if the patient's trunk accidentally slips toward a semi-prone or semi-supine position after fixation of the non-dependent arm. Vascular compression of the non-dependent arm in this situation is also possible, and it is useful to monitor pulse oximetry in the non-dependent hand to observe for this. The arm should not be abducted beyond 90° and should not be extended posteriorly beyond the neutral position nor flexed

Table 19.2 Factors contributing to brachial plexus injury in the lateral position

a) Dependent arm (compression injuries):
1) Arm directly under thorax
2) Pressure on clavicle into retro-clavicular space
3) Cervical rib
4) Caudal migration of thorax padding into the axilla[a]
b) Non-dependent arm (stretch injuries):
1) Lateral flexion of cervical spine
2) Excessive abduction of arm (>90%)
3) Semi-prone or semi-supine repositioning after arm fixed to a support

[a]Unfortunately this padding under the thorax is misnamed an "axillary roll" in some institutions. This padding absolutely should NOT be placed in the axilla.

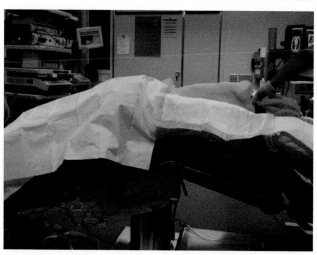

Fig. 19.4 Posterior view of the flexed-lateral position commonly used for thoracoscopic (VATS) surgery. The patient is on a vacuum mat, and a forced-air warmer has been applied to the lower body prior to draping. The flexed-lateral position is more likely to cause impairment of venous return and hypotension than the lateral position

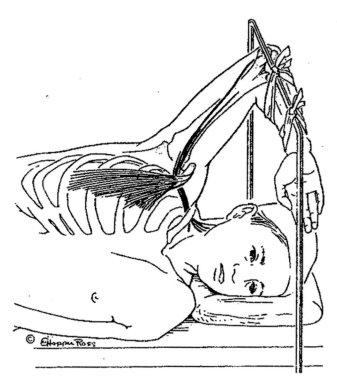

Fig. 19.3 Bilateral malpositioning of the arms in the lateral position. The non-dependent arm is hyperextended and fixed to the anesthetic screen. This causes traction of the brachial plexus as it passes under the clavicle and the tendon of the pectoralis minor muscle. This traction may increase if the patient's torso rotates during surgery, while the arm remains fixed. The dependent arm is directly under the thorax with the potential for vascular compression and/or injury to the brachial plexus. (From Ref. [3])

anteriorly greater than 90°. Fortunately, the majority of these nerve injuries resolve spontaneously over a period of months.

Anterior flexion of the non-dependent arm at the shoulder (circumduction) across the chest or lateral flexion of the neck toward the opposite side can cause a traction injury of the suprascapular nerve. Malpositioning can also cause a deep, musculoskeletal pain of the posterior and lateral

aspects of the shoulder and is responsible for a large proportion of cases of postoperative ipsilateral shoulder pain [4]. The anesthesiologist should question the patient before surgery about any shoulder problems, and, if there is any history, the intraoperative position should be tested preinduction to find a comfortable position for the non-dependent arm.

The dependent leg should be slightly flexed with padding under the knee to protect the peroneal nerve lateral to the proximal head of the fibula. The non-dependent leg is placed in a neutral extended position and padding placed between it and the dependent leg. The dependent leg must be observed for vascular compression. Excessively tight strapping at the hip level can compress the sciatic nerve of the non-dependent leg.

The Flexed-Lateral Position To lower the non-dependent iliac crest so that it does not interfere with surgical access, most patients for VATS surgery are placed in a flexed-lateral position (see Fig. 19.4) similar to the nephrectomy position with lateral flexion of the lower thoracolumbar spine, while the upper thoracic and cervical spine is maintained in a horizontal plane. Some surgeons also use this position for thoracotomies to try and open the intercostal spaces. After repositioning and stabilization, the hemodynamics of the lateral position are not significantly different from the supine position. However, the flexed-lateral position impairs venous return and is associated with significant reductions in blood pressure and cardiac index (3.0 vs. 2.4 l/min/m² in one study [5]). This can particularly be a problem in the elderly, who are more liable to have clinically important falls in blood pressure with decreases in pre-load.

Positive pressure ventilation during anesthesia in the lateral position is associated with significant increases in mismatching of ventilation and perfusion. These changes are discussed in Chap. 5.

Supine Position The standard supine position with arms abducted is used for a variety of thoracic surgical procedures such as sternotomies for mediastinal tumors or bilateral wedge resections. The arms are positioned prone with careful attention to padding the ulnar nerves at the elbow to prevent pressure. The supine position with the arms abducted may be used for bilateral trans-sternal thoracotomies (the "clamshell" incision) for bilateral lung transplantation or large anterior mediastinal mass resections or for bilateral thoracoscopic procedures (see Fig. 19.5). The arms are positioned supine and not abducted more than 90°. The arms should be padded with the joints slightly flexed, so that the wrist is higher than the elbow and the elbow higher than the shoulder.

Prone Position Recently, the use of the prone position for the intrathoracic portion of minimally invasive esophagectomy procedures has been adopted in several centers because the surgical access is felt to be improved vs. the lateral position [6] (see Chap. 38). This has implications for airway management since it may be difficult to accommodate a double-lumen tube in a standard prone head rest. Some centers use a bronchial blocker for lung isolation in these cases. It has been reported that esophagectomy in the prone position can be performed with a single-lumen tube with surgical capnothorax and without one-lung ventilation [7].

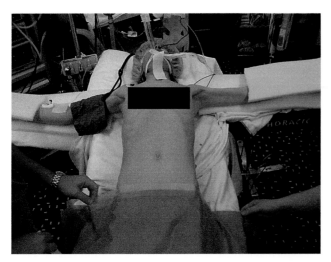

Fig. 19.5 The supine position with the arms abducted. This position is appropriate for bilateral thoracoscopic procedures or for bilateral lung transplantation

Central Neurological Injuries

Paraplegia With an estimated incidence of 0.08% [8], postthoracotomy paralysis (PTP) is a rare but devastating complication following thoracic surgery. PTP can occur as a result of spinal cord compression from an epidural hematoma or a foreign body or ligation of major arteries perfusing the vulnerable thoracic cord. Arterial embolus and perioperative hypotension have also been implicated.

Epidural hematoma (EH) is a rare but well-appreciated complication of neuraxial anesthesia. EH associated with epidural placement is estimated to occur with a frequency of 1:150000 [9]. Symptoms of EH vary but can include back pain, sensory and motor deficits, and incontinence. EH can present any time, including immediately postoperatively and after catheter removal. Prompt diagnosis, ideally with MRI scanning, can confirm the diagnosis. Immediate neurosurgical consultation should be obtained for decompression which has its best results within 12 h of onset of symptoms.

Surgical bleeding at or near the costovertebral junction with posterolateral thoracotomy incisions can be difficult to manage. There are multiple case reports [10] of oxidized cellulose polymer (Surgicel) positioned and left at or near the angle of the vertebral body to control bleeding. The material has subsequently swelled and compressed the ipsilateral nerve root or even migrated into the spinal canal, causing permanent paralysis [11]. The product monograph specifically contraindicates the use of the polymer in this situation. Neurologic deficit in this scenario presents within hours of surgery. Diagnosis is confirmed with imaging and treatment is removal.

Paralysis due to spinal cord ischemia is a commonly appreciated complication of vascular surgery, where its postoperative incidence can reach upward to 20% [12]. Nonvascular thoracic surgery can also lead to spinal cord ischemia. Anatomical considerations related to this have been reviewed [13]. The thoracic spinal cord has a less luxurious blood supply than its cervical and lumbar counterparts. The cord is supplied by the solitary anterior spinal artery (ASA) which provides blood supply to the anterior 2/3 of the cord and the paired posterior spinal (PSA) arteries which supply the posterior 1/3. In the thoracic region, the ASA receives important contributions from a few variable radicular arteries which are branches of the posterior intercostal arteries. Ligation of small but integral intercostal arteries during thoracic surgery, leading to hypoperfusion and ischemia of the spinal cord, has been implicated in PTP, both in lung resection and esophagectomy. The classic presentation of spinal cord ischemia from ASA supply interruption in the thoracic region is bilateral motor, pain, and temperature loss with maintenance of proprioception, the so-called anterior cord syndrome. There may be associated autonomic dysfunction.

Treatment of ischemia due to inadvertent surgical interruption of spinal cord blood supply is guided by interventions driven at optimizing supply and demand to the cord. Commonly used strategies include maintaining a normal to supranormal blood pressure with vaso-inopressors, an adequate hemoglobin, and a steroid administration. It should be noted that none of these interventions have been rigorously proven to improve neurologic outcome and some, in particular steroid administration, are controversial. Spinal drains are commonly placed electively in thoracic aneurysm repair to optimize spinal cord perfusion, but this treatment has not been utilized in the PTP literature.

To conclude, post-thoracotomy neurologic deficit is usually assumed to be an anesthetic complication related to epidural placement. Although anesthesiologists must always be vigilant and act quickly in these cases to image the spinal cord to rule out a hematoma, we must also remember the differential includes surgically related causes.

Blindness Postoperative visual loss (POVL) has been infrequently reported following surgery in the lateral position. Similar to the POVL more often reported after surgery in the prone position, the risk factors include prolonged surgery, hypotension, massive transfusion, diabetes, and obesity [14]. The etiology in non-cardiac surgery has been primarily due to posterior ischemic optic neuropathy. The perfusion pressure in the posterior portion of the optic nerve is directly related to mean arterial pressure and inversely related to venous drainage pressure. In one case report following spine surgery in the lateral position via VATS and open thoracotomy, the visual loss was complete in the dependent eye and partial in the non-dependent eye suggesting the potential impact of venous drainage pressure [15]. Of note, this patient also had marked facial edema after the end of the case. Since there is no monitor available to assess the perfusion pressure in the optic nerve, prevention involves avoiding the treatable associated factors (hypotension and anemia), regular intraoperative observation of the face to assure that there is no direct pressure on the eyes and careful neutral positioning of the cervical spine to avoid any compromise of venous drainage.

Ischemic optic neuropathy has been well described following orthopedic surgical procedures in the prone position. If the patient can be placed with a slight extension of the cervical spine (10° above neutral) while prone, this will decrease the intraocular pressure [16]. This may improve optic nerve perfusion but has not yet been demonstrated to have a beneficial effect on outcome. To date, there do not seem to have been any published reports of blindness following prone esophageal surgery.

Other Position-Related Injuries The lateral position has been reported to be associated with a variety of pressure-related injuries to the legs. These include myonecrosis, sciatic nerve palsy, and compartment syndromes [17]. The majority of these reports involve orthopedic procedures of long duration (>5 h). Increased vigilance for potential position-related injuries is required in long procedures.

Clinical Case Discussion

A 60-year-old woman presents for a left thoracotomy for left lower lobectomy for lung cancer. Past medical history includes a remote myocardial infarction with a preoperative ejection fraction of 40%, controlled hypertension, and diet-controlled diabetes mellitus. Regular medications are taken the morning of the OR, including metoprolol and aspirin 81 mg. A flexible epidural catheter with inner stainless steel coil wire is placed at T6/7 for postoperative analgesia. After an epidural test dose of 3 ml lidocaine 2%, an infusion of bupivacaine 0.1% plus hydromorphone 15ug/ml is started at 5 cc/h. A central line is placed after induction. The operation is remarkable for intraoperative hypotension requiring dopamine and norepinephrine and brisk bleeding near the costovertebral junction. Immediately postoperatively, blood pressure is in the patient's normal range with no support, there is no motor deficit, and pain is well-controlled. Six hours postoperatively, a nurse from the ward calls to report that the patient is complaining of bilateral lower extremity motor weakness.

1. What is the differential diagnosis?

At this point, the differential is wide and includes a motor block secondary to epidural local anesthetic solution, an intrathecal catheter, compression of the nerve roots or spinal cord from an epidural hematoma or a foreign body, arterial embolus to a radicular artery, or a hypoperfusion state.

2. What should be done immediately?

Vital signs should be taken and documented, the epidural solution should be stopped, and the catheter should be aspirated. A focused chart review should be undertaken with special note taken of any recently administered anticoagulants. The surgeon should be called and be advised of the problem. A complete neurological examination should be performed.

3. What does the initial assessment reveal?

The patient is awake and alert. Her blood pressure is 89/65 with a normal heart rate and oxygen saturation. No blood or CSF is aspirated through the catheter. She is unable to move her legs. She has loss of sensation to pain and temperature in both legs, but proprioception is intact. Thirty minutes after the epidural solution has been turned off, there is no change in her neurological status. The last documented INR is 1.29 5 h ago. The patient received subcutaneous heparin for DVT prophylaxis 1 h ago.

4. What should be done next? What bloodwork, imaging, and consults should be ordered?

Dopamine is started through the patient's central line to keep the blood pressure in her normal range (120/80) with continuous cardiac monitoring. "STAT" complete blood count and coagulation tests are drawn. There is hesitance to remove the epidural catheter in the context of a coagulation abnormality combined with recent heparin administration and aspirin. MRI is the preferred modality to diagnose an epidural hematoma. However, the in situ epidural catheter is not permitted in the scanner. After consultation with the radiologist, the epidural is left in place, and a CT is performed. The neurosurgeon and neurologist are called and made aware of the patient.

5. What is found on additional testing?

The CT shows no epidural hematoma or mass. The hemoglobin is 90 g/L. Platelets are normal. INR is 1.21. The patient is seen by the neurologist and given a provisional diagnosis of spinal cord ischemia causing an anterior cord syndrome.

6. What else can be done?

The patient is moved to a step-down unit with continuous monitoring. Neurologic vitals are done every 4 h. Dopamine is continued, and the patient is given 100 mg methylprednisolone IV q8h × 3 doses. Hemoglobin is maintained at 100 g/L. The epidural is removed 6 h after the last subcutaneous heparin dose. An MRI is then performed and is normal. Pain is controlled with hydromorphone intravenous PCA. Over the next 4 days, the patient gradually and completely recovers.

References

1. Desiderio DP, Burt M, Kolver AC, et al. The effects of endobronchial cuff inflation on double-lumen endobronchial tube movement after lateral positioning. J Cardiothorac Vasc Anesth. 1997;11:595–9.
2. Fortier G, Coté D, Bergeron C, et al. New landmarks improve the positioning of the left Broncho-Cath double-lumen tube: Comparison with the classic technique. Can J Anesth. 2001;48:790–5.
3. Britt BA, Gordon RA. Peripheral nerve injuries associated with anaesthesia. Can Anaesth Soc J. 1964;11(514):514–36
4. Blichfeldt-Eckhardt M, Andersen C, Ording H, et al. Shoulder pain after thoracic surgery; type and time course, a prospective study. J Cardiothorac Vasc Anesth. 2017;31:147–51.
5. Yokoyama M, Ueda W, Hirakawa M. Haemodynamic effects of the lateral decubitus position and the kidney rest lateral decubitus position during anaesthesia. Br J Anesth. 2000;84:753–7.
6. Shen Y, Feng M, Tan L, et al. Thoracoscopic esophagectomy in prone versus decubitus position; ergonometric evaluation from a randomized and controlled study. Ann Thorac Surg. 2014;98:1072–8.
7. Singh M, Uppal R, Chaudhary K, et al. Use of a single-lumen tube for minimally invasive and hybrid esophagectomies with prone thoracoscopic dissection: case series. J Clin Anesth. 2016;33:450–5.
8. Attar S. Paraplegia after thoracotomy: report of five cases and review of the literature. Ann Thorac Surg. 1995;59:1410–6.
9. Horlocker T. Regional anesthesia in the anticoagulated patient: defining the risks (the second ASRA consensus conference on neuraxial anesthesia and anticoagulation). Reg Anes Pain Med. 2003;28:172–97.
10. Kreppel D. Spinal hematoma: a literature survey with meta-analysis of 613 patients. Neurosurg Rev. 2003;26:1–49.
11. Short H. Paraplegia associated with the use of oxidized cellulose in posterolateral thoracotomy incisions. Ann Thorac Surg. 1990;50:288–90.
12. Greenberg R. Contemporary analysis of descending thoracic and thoracoabdominal aneurysm repair: a comparison of endovascular and open techniques. Circulation. 2008;118:808–17.
13. Shamji M. Circulation of the spinal cord: an important consideration for thoracic surgeons. Ann Thorac Surg. 2003;76:315–21.
14. Newman NJ. Perioperative visual loss after nonocular surgeries. Am J Opthalmol. 2008;145:604–10.
15. Heitz JW, Audu PB. Asymmetric postoperative visual loss after spine surgery in the lateral decubitus position. Br J Anaesth. 2008;101:380–2.
16. Emery S, Daffner S, France J, et al. Effect of head position on intraocular pressure during lumbar spine fusion; a randomized, prospective study. J Bone & Joint Surg. 2015;97:1817–23.
17. Cascio BM, Buchowski JM, Frassica FJ. Well-limb compartment syndrome after prolonged lateral decubitus positioning. J Bone Joint Surg. 2004;86:2038–40.
18. Kretteck C, Aschemann D. Positioning techniques in surgical applications. Hamburg: Springer; 2006.

Intraoperative Monitoring

Gabriel E. Mena, Karthik Raghunathan,
and William T. McGee

Key Points

- Continuous automated ST-segment analysis is especially important during thoracic surgery given the potential for cardiac ischemia, arrhythmias, pneumothorax, severe hypoxemia, and hemodynamic instability.
- Oxygenation during one-lung ventilation is determined by many factors including cardiac output, blood pressure, ventilation-perfusion matching, anesthetic effects on hypoxic pulmonary vasoconstriction, airway mechanics and reactivity, oxygen consumption, and preexisting pulmonary disease. Pulse oximetry with occasional intermittent arterial blood gas analysis provides warning of significant hypoxemia.
- The typical CO_2 vs. time waveform, displayed on most anesthesia monitors, has characteristic intervals that represent different physiologic events during ventilation.
- Continuous breath-by-breath spirometry (monitoring of inspiratory and expiratory volumes, pressures, and flows) enables the early detection of a malpositioned double-lumen tube and can reduce the potential for ventilatory-induced lung injury by guiding the optimization of ventilatory settings.
- Invasive arterial pressure monitoring is commonly used to assess beat-by-beat blood pressure and can also be used to derive functional hemodynamic information such as systolic pressure variation (SPV) and pulse pressure variation (PPV).
- SPV and PPV measure related aspects of cardiorespiratory interaction in the presence of adequate tidal volume. However, these variables do not predict the ability to increase cardiac output with fluid loading when tidal volumes are <8 cc/kg, as is typically the case with one-lung ventilation during thoracic surgery.
- Minimally invasive hemodynamic monitoring (arterial pressure waveform-based devices) coupled with certain maneuvers can identify whether inadequate tissue perfusion can be improved with intravenous fluid therapy.

Introduction

The general principles of intraoperative monitoring for thoracic surgery are similar to those for any major surgery. Monitoring guides the detection of problems and helps track the response to interventions. From a practical standpoint, this translates into the rather conservative approach of invasive monitoring from the outset, with the assumption that cardiac and pulmonary complications are more prone to occur (relative to other noncardiac procedures) and that access to the patient may be restricted (especially with the patient in the lateral decubitus position during lung isolation).

Monitoring techniques have rarely been subjected to the kind of scrutiny that pharmacologic and other therapeutic

G. E. Mena (✉)
Department of Anesthesiology and Perioperative Medicine,
The University of Texas MD Anderson Cancer Center,
Houston, TX, USA
e-mail: gmena@mdanderson.org

K. Raghunathan
Department of Anesthesiology, Duke University,
Durham, NC, USA
e-mail: karthik.raghunathan@duke.edu

W. T. McGee
Critical Care Division, Department of Medicine and Surgery,
University of Massachusetts Medical School,
Baystate Medical Center, Springfield, MA, USA
e-mail: William.mcgee@baystatehealth.org

© Springer Nature Switzerland AG 2019
P. Slinger (ed.), *Principles and Practice of Anesthesia for Thoracic Surgery*, https://doi.org/10.1007/978-3-030-00859-8_20

interventions are [1]. With improvements in monitoring technology and in our understanding of cardiorespiratory physiology, we hope to acquire and interpret data better, recognize errors, and generate and apply evidence-based goal-directed interventions to optimize outcomes in a cost-effective manner. Although this is self-evident, intraoperative monitoring, no matter how sophisticated, cannot *itself* improve outcomes. Monitoring coupled with physiologically derived protocol-driven care can improve outcomes by reducing unwarranted variation in practice while still allowing practitioners to use their clinical judgment [2]. For instance, protocol-driven goal-directed resuscitation in septic patients has been shown to reduce mortality [3], while invasive pulmonary artery catheter (PAC)-based monitoring during high-risk surgery has, in fact, been shown *not* to lead to better outcomes [4]. We will focus on intraoperative monitoring specifically relevant to thoracic surgical patients and will also emphasize minimally and noninvasive hemodynamic monitoring technologies.

ECG

Approximately 30% of patients exposed to anesthesia for surgical procedures in the United States have a known prior history of coronary artery disease (CAD) or coronary risk factors. Perioperative myocardial ischemia is more common in patients with poor cardiopulmonary reserve that typically present for thoracic surgery. Multivessel coronary disease is also more likely in the thoracic surgical population given their likelihood of being smokers and having related comorbidities [5]. An estimated 50,000 such patients per year, who receive noncardiac surgery, will experience a perioperative myocardial infarction, which carries a 40–70% mortality rate.

Continuous automated ST-segment analysis is fundamental during thoracic surgery due to the potential for cardiac ischemia as a result of arrhythmias, pneumothorax, the potential for severe hypoxemia from intrapulmonary shunting, and hemodynamic instability from the compression of large vessels with the potential for cardiac decompensation from pulmonary hypertension or hemorrhage [6]. The typical five-lead electrocardiographic system should be placed for thoracic surgical patients with suspected or known coronary disease undergoing thoracic surgery. Depending on the surgical site, careful positioning of leads is pivotal in order to both avoid errors in the ST-segment analysis and minimize interference with the sterile surgical field. Based on previous studies, lead II has a 90% sensitivity to detect arrhythmias, and the lateral lead V5 has 75% sensitivity to detect lateral wall ischemia. London M, et al. demonstrated that lead V4 was the second-most sensitive lead to detect intraoperative ischemia (61% sensitivity) and that the use of two lateral leads (V4 and V5) provided a combined sensitivity of 90% for the detection of lateral wall ischemia [7]. ST-segment trend analysis is pivotal

for the diagnosis of myocardial ischemia caused by and characteristic of multivessel coronary disease in patients with a significant history of smoking and with poor collateral circulation [8]. Specific coronary artery territories typically implicated in ischemia or infarction can be diagnosed based on the congruence of leads showing ST-segment changes (for instance, changes in leads II, III, and aVF typically represent RCA territory supply/demand mismatch). Although the diagnosis of acute MI in the presence of a left bundle branch block (LBBB) is difficult, criteria have been developed that may be applied for early detection and timely intervention [9].

ECG can also be used to monitor for various severe electrolyte disturbances (e.g., hyperkalemia, hypocalcemia, hypomagnesaemia) and the appropriate functioning of cardiac rhythm management devices. As a result of serious underlying cardiac rhythm disturbances or congestive heart failure, many patients undergoing thoracic surgery will have pacemakers or implantable cardiac defibrillators, and monitoring these devices during the surgical procedure is critical to ensuring appropriate responses. Atrial fibrillation is also more common with thoracic surgical procedures.

Pulse Oximetry

Pulse oximetry (SpO_2) is a continuous, noninvasive method of measuring the arterial oxygen saturation (SaO_2) from a processed infrared light signal transmitted through a pulsatile vascular bed (a practical application of the Beer-Lambert law). Plethysmography, the measurement of pulsatile volume changes that occur in tissue beds, can also be performed by most pulse oximeters and may have future applications in the noninvasive assessment of fluid responsiveness.

The main goal of pulse oximetry in thoracic surgery is to provide immediate warning of hypoxemia mainly during procedures at high risk for desaturation such as one-lung ventilation (OLV). This allows for prompt treatment to be initiated before irreversible metabolic derangements occur. During OLV, significant desaturation ($SpO_2 < 90\%$) can occur despite high-inspired oxygen concentration secondary to obligate shunt (nonventilated lung) and potentially treatable intrapulmonary shunting (ventilated lung). Oxygenation during OLV (and during other thoracic surgical procedures) is determined by many factors including cardiac output, blood pressure, blood flow through nonventilated lung, ventilation-perfusion matching in ventilated lung, anesthetic effects on hypoxic pulmonary vasoconstriction (HPV), airway mechanics and reactivity, oxygen consumption, and preexisting pulmonary disease. In the 1980s, a significant study by Brodsky J, et al. revealed (based on findings from 19 patients undergoing OLV with continuous pulse oximetry monitoring and simultaneous arterial blood gas analysis) that the pulse oximetry measurements were in good agreement with the arterial blood gas analysis [12]. The greatest discrepancy was about ±6%, and these authors concluded that the reliability of the pulse oximetry for the detection of changes in oxygenation was sufficient enough that frequent arterial blood gas analysis was not required. However, arterial blood gas analysis will always have a role in the determination of the safety margin before arterial desaturation in terms of the partial pressure of oxygen (PaO_2) measurement. Once the arterial oxygen saturation drops below 90%, the critical "steep portion" on the sigmoid oxy-hemoglobin dissociation curve, further desaturation might be drastic and need prompt evaluation and intervention. Since significant desaturation does not occur until the PaO_2 falls below 60 mmHg, the pulse oximeter (SpO_2) will not detect large changes in PaO_2. Interestingly enough, the maintenance of normocarbia is not problematic during OLV (described further in the section "Capnography"), while the inevitable intrapulmonary shunt during OLV makes desaturation likely. As most of the oxygen content in arterial blood is based largely on transportation by hemoglobin, when venous admixture occurs (with blood flow from nonventilated lung mixing with the blood flow from ventilated lung), the ability to compensate for this decrease in the oxygen content is limited. The lungs are unable to compensate for this decrease in the arterial oxygen content by increasing blood flow through ventilated lung.

During thoracotomy or thoracoscopy when the patient is placed in the lateral decubitus position, there is potential for rapid changes in SpO_2 from the compression of mediastinal great vessels in addition to intrapulmonary shunting (OLV). The manipulation of lung parenchyma and/or the mediastinum can lead to the development of cardiac arrhythmias that can affect the pulse oximetry readings as well. The use of electrocautery will also, occasionally, interfere with pulse oximetry.

Judicious perioperative fluid management is of crucial importance for thoracic surgical patients. Respiratory variations in invasive arterial pressure recordings (discussed later) such as systolic pressure variation (SPV) or pulse pressure variation (PPV) are sensitive and specific indicators of fluid responsiveness. There is growing interest in the use of variations in the pulse oximeter plethysmographic waveform amplitude as a noninvasive method of estimating fluid responsiveness. Such ventilatory variations in plethysmographic amplitude can be sensitive to changes in preload and can predict fluid responsiveness in mechanically ventilated patients [10]. The "Pleth Variability Index" (PVI, Masimo Corp., Irvine, CA) may be one such dynamic index automatically derived from pulse oximeter waveform analysis, with potential for clinical applications in the assessment of fluid responsiveness and in monitoring response to therapy. Studies showing that patients with significant dynamic plethysmographic variation will respond to a fluid bolus have

been published [8]. However, since different pulse oximeters use different nonstandardized proprietary signal processing plethysmographic algorithms, measurements obtained by one specific device or method may not be applicable to similar variables from other manufacturers [11]. There are several factors other than volume status that can affect plethysmography such as local temperature, site of measurement, influence of venous pressures, etc. [13]. The future application of this plethysmographic aspect of pulse oximetry is ripe for further investigation both during and after thoracic surgery.

Capnography

Monitoring the adequacy of ventilation via CO_2 waveform analysis is usually performed continuously during thoracic surgery by infrared dispersion spectrophotometry or mass spectrometry. Patients undergoing thoracic surgery usually have significant underlying lung disease and a chronic history of smoking, so it is extremely important to recognize the different phases of the time capnograph to recognize the underlying pulmonary pathology (such as obstructive patterns of expiration) as well as distinguish artifacts and errors. The typical CO_2 vs. time waveform (time capnography) is displayed on most anesthesia monitors and has characteristic intervals that represent different physiologic events during ventilation (see Fig. 20.1).

Phase I is the expiratory baseline and represents the exhalation of CO_2-free gas from anatomic dead space. Phase II is the expiratory upstroke or fast rise phase representing the mixing of dead space gas with alveolar gas containing CO_2. Phase III or the alveolar expiratory plateau phase represents the exhalation of CO_2-rich gas from the gas-exchanging alveoli. The angle between phases II and III has been referred to as the α angle and is an indirect indication of ventilation-perfusion (V/Q) matching. Finally, phase 0 is the inspiratory

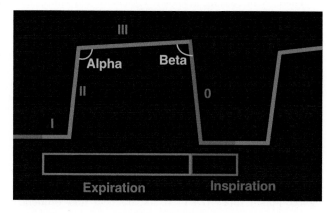

Fig. 20.1 Time capnograph. (From Bhavani Shankar Kodali MD. http://www.capnography.com Accessed 10 Feb 2010)

downslope during which time fresh gases are inhaled. The nearly 90° angle between phases III and 0 has been referred to as the β angle [14]. This β angle may increase during rebreathing. During thoracic surgery these phases are affected by cardiopulmonary conditions that need to be recognized by the anesthesiologist. A decrease in the slope of phase II may be seen in certain acute and chronic conditions that negatively impact expiratory flow (such as bronchospasm or COPD). This reduction in the slope is determined by the extent of mixing of parallel and series dead space gases with ideally well-mixed alveolar gas. An increase in the α angle appears as a prominent upsloping in phase III and signifies worsening V/Q matching. This may be due to changes in cardiac output, CO_2 production, airway resistance, and/or functional residual capacity.

In the lateral decubitus position, there are physiologic changes in ventilation and perfusion for both the dependent and nondependent lungs. Phase III of the capnograph has a characteristic biphasic appearance of the waveform. This is believed to occur because the nondependent lung will obtain significantly more ventilation relative to perfusion (high V/Q units) and will contain more alveolar dead space contributing to the earlier and lower part of an upsloping phase III. The dependent lung will receive more perfusion relative to ventilation (lower V/Q units) and less alveolar dead space consequently contributing to the later and higher part of the phase III plateau. During cross-field ventilation for procedures involving resection of main stem or tracheal masses that require jet ventilation or intermittent apnea, close monitoring and vigilance of the capnogram are pivotal because complete absence of a waveform implies no ventilation, no circulation, or a disconnected capnometer. The end-tidal CO_2 to arterial CO_2 gradient ($PaCO_2$–$PETCO_2$) is related to the extent of dead space ventilation and tends to increase during OLV. Despite occasionally significant oxygen desaturation, the maintenance of adequate ventilation or normocarbia during OLV is usually not problematic.

There is increasing acknowledgment of the similarities between adult respiratory distress syndrome (ARDS) and OLV [15]. Ventilation strategies originally developed for ARDS may have benefits during OLV. Permissive moderate hypercarbia is becoming a routine component of OLV management, and capnography (with intermittent arterial blood gas analysis) will aid in monitoring this approach to ventilation. Increasing minute ventilation to the dependent ventilated lung during OLV in the lateral position removes sufficient CO_2 to compensate for the higher CO_2 content of the pulmonary blood flow perfusing the nonventilated lung. Capnography also enables the detection of improperly placed double-lumen tubes (DLT) if the tracheal and bronchial lumens are separately and continuously monitored during tube positioning.

Intraoperative Spirometry

With the availability of real-time intraoperative spirometry in the current generation of anesthesia machines, it has become possible to continuously monitor inspiratory and expiratory volumes, pressures, and flows. During thoracic anesthesia, especially with OLV in the patient with preexisting pulmonary disease or at-risk for postoperative complications, breath-by-breath spirometry can guide the early detection of a malpositioned DLT and help minimize the potential for lung injury by guiding the optimization of ventilatory settings that are individualized to each patient [16].

With the loss of lung isolation, such as with cephalad migration of the DLT, the expired volume will, acutely, decrease significantly to well below the inspired volume (beyond the usual normal 20–30 mL/breath difference that results from the uptake of inspired oxygen) [16]. Similarly, unintentional caudad migration of the DLT can result in a readily apparent decrease in compliance as set tidal volume/pressure is delivered to a single lobe rather than the appropriate lung. The pressure-volume and flow-volume graphs can show characteristic changes. Additional uses for intraoperative spirometry include the identification of auto-PEEP (persistent end-expiratory flow) during OLV, which can be seen on the flow-volume loop. Intraoperative spirometry data (e.g., monitoring compliance and plateau pressures) can be combined with data from arterial blood gases, capnography, and oximetry to make adjustments to ventilatory parameters to optimize gas exchange [16]. The ability to accurately measure differences in inspiratory and expiratory tidal volumes can also be extremely useful to aid in the assessment and management of pulmonary air leaks during pulmonary resections.

Arterial Blood Pressure Monitoring

Given the potential for cardiovascular instability during intrathoracic procedures, the possible need for repeated blood gas analysis, and a patient population with significant underlying comorbidities, the use of invasive arterial blood pressure monitoring is common in current clinical thoracic anesthesia practice to assess beat-to-beat blood pressure and derived functional hemodynamics. Mean arterial pressure (MAP) is the most useful parameter to approximate organ perfusion pressure in noncardiac tissues provided venous or surrounding tissue pressures are not elevated [17].

Technical aspects of the invasive measurement of vascular pressures: the principles described here apply to the invasive measurement of vascular pressures (arterial blood pressure, central venous pressure (CVP), or PAC pressures). The monitoring system typically used in current clinical practice consists of a catheter connected via saline-filled, low-compliance tubing to an electronic transducer. Signal transduction, performed by these so-called dynamic pressure transducers, involves changing either electric resistance or capacitance in response to changes in pressure on a solid-state device (Wheatstone bridge system) [18]. Pressure waves recorded through intravascular catheters should be transmitted undistorted to the transducer, processed, and then displayed. Unfortunately, there are phenomena that can interfere with the accuracy of such systems. Distortion can result from either resonance or damping and produce errone-ous readings that need to be recognized. The "fast flush test" is a clinically useful method that allows for the detection of these errors. Readers are directed to comprehensive techni-cal reviews on this topic for further information [18, 19].

Digital numeric readouts of systolic and diastolic pres-sures that are displayed on the monitors are the running aver-age of values over a certain time interval. From a clinically relevant perspective, the transducer must be placed in the appropriate position relative to the patient. Correct position-ing of the pressure transducer is crucial and often most prone to error. Generally, pressures are referenced against ambient atmospheric pressure by exposing the pressure transducer system to air through an open stopcock and pressing the zero-pressure button on the monitor display. The transducer must be horizontally aligned with a specific position on the patient's body that represents the upper fluid level in the chamber or vessel from which pressure is to be measured [19]. Proper positioning of the pressure transducer is espe-cially critical for measurement of venous pressures (CVP, PAOP) because seemingly small errors in transducer height relative to the patient are amplified. Ideally, transducers should be positioned approximately 5 cm posterior to the left sternal border at the fourth intercostals space, since this point better represents the upper fluid level of the right atrium. This is especially relevant during thoracic surgery when patients are in a lateral position where errors in zeroing/ref-erencing can easily influence therapy. For instance, in the lateral decubitus position, invasive arterial pressure recorded directly from either the right or left radial arteries will remain unchanged relative to the supine position as long as the respective pressure transducers remain at heart level. However, noninvasively measured blood pressure will be higher in the dependent arm and lower in the nondependent arm. Such differences in noninvasive blood pressure mea-surement are determined by the positions of the arms above and below the level of the heart and are equal to the hydro-static pressure differences between the level of the heart and the respective arm. Blood pressure is directly related to the cardiac output (CO) and systemic vascular resistance (SVR). This is the hemodynamic corollary to Ohm's law where elec-tricity (flow or Q) is directly proportional to the voltage (driving pressure gradient across vascular beds or $MAP - CVP$) and is inversely proportional to resistance

(SVR). Adapted to circulation, this proportionality can be described as flow or $Q = (MAP - CVP)/SVR$. While a nor-mal blood pressure does not necessarily reflect hemody-namic stability, hypotension does represent a potential threat to adequate tissue perfusion.

As the arterial waveform is transmitted from the aortic root to the periphery, the actual pressure wave itself becomes distorted. Aging, hypertension, and atherosclerosis all rela-tively common in thoracic surgical patients can also influ-ence the displayed arterial waveform. In the peripheral arterial tree, the high-frequency components (such as the dicrotic notch) disappear, the diastolic trough decreases, the systolic peak increases, and there is a transmission delay because there is decreased arterial elastance. Thus, invasive pressure waveform morphology and actual pressure values depend on the site of pressure measurement. Pulse contour analysis-based devices are, therefore, susceptible to mechan-ical errors in arterial pressure measurement and to such distal pulse amplification. Consequently, clinical therapy is often better guided using mean arterial pressure than systolic or diastolic blood pressure measurements. The use of arterial pressure-derived variables such as SPV, PPV, deltaDown, etc. is discussed below under noninvasive hemodynamic monitoring.

Central Venous Pressure

Technical aspects of invasive pressure measurement are described in the previous section. CVP represents the back pressure to systemic venous return and is, in effect, an esti-mate of right ventricular filling pressure. An appropriately inserted central venous catheter is required for actual CVP measurement, and placing a catheter on the same side as the thoracic operation (internal jugular or subclavian) allows for an unintentional pneumothorax to be treated by the pleural drainage tube that is usually inserted for most thoracic surgi-cal procedures. Routine placement of central venous cathe-ters are not justified, but the risks may be worth taking if it is likely that infusions of vasoactive drugs will be used, if blood products may need to be rapidly administered, or when large-bore peripheral venous access is not obtainable.

CVP might be inaccurate after the establishment of a pneumothorax during thoracic surgery, during the resection of mediastinal masses compressing the right heart cham-bers, and also during lateral positioning or with an open chest. Tumors invading cardiac structures can also produce erroneous CVP values. The use of isolated CVP measures to guide fluid therapy during thoracic procedures is not desir-able given the evidence against the use of static hemody-namic measures. Changes in CVP over time are more clinically relevant than absolute numeric values. There are no clear CVP "cutoffs" that can reliably distinguish between

Table 20.1 Comparison of currently clinically useful minimally invasive hemodynamic monitoring devices

Noninvasive hemodynamic device	Calibration required	Arterial waveform high fidelity	Hemodynamic parameters calculated	Requires central line insertion
FloTrac and Vigileo	No	Yes	SVV, SV, CO, SVR	No
Esophageal Doppler monitoring (EDM)	No	No	SV, CO, and FTc (flow corrected time)	No
LiDCO (lithium dilution cardiac output)	Yes (lithium)	Yes	SVV, SV, CO, SVR, DO$_2$	Yes
LiDCO rapid	No	Yes	SVV, SV, CO, SVR	No
PiCCO (pulse intermittent continuous cardiac output)	Yes	Yes	SVV, SV, CO, SVR, EVLW, ITTV, CI	Yes
Cheetah BioReactance	No	Not applicable	SV, change in stroke volume with PLR	No

SVV stoke volume variation, *SV* stoke volume, *SVR* systemic vascular resistance, *CO/CI* cardiac output/index, *FTc* heart rate corrected flow time, *DO$_2$* oxygen delivery in cc/min, *EVLW* extravascular lung water, *ITTV* intrathoracic thermal volume, *PLR* passive leg raise

When compared with conventional intraoperative assessment (physical examination, fluid input and output measurements, etc.), fluid administration guided by flow monitoring can improve outcomes [28]. Furthermore, there is evidence that compared to catheter-based measurements (such as cardiac output by thermodilution or CVP), therapeutic management based on certain less invasive cardiac output monitors leads to fewer complications and shorter length of stay [26–28]. The dangers of inadequate cardiac output secondary to hypovolemia need to be balanced against the dangers of fluid overloading in these patients. Increasingly, dynamic indices of fluid responsiveness are being monitored to guide intraoperative fluid therapy [31, 32]. Functional hemodynamic monitoring is a term often used to describe the use of monitoring to evaluate treatment efficacy. The devices described below are minimally or noninvasive when compared with central venous catheters, PACs, and TEE. Table 20.1 provides a comparison of the different minimally invasive monitoring technologies.

Key functional hemodynamic questions applied to thoracic surgical patients include is flow (cardiac output) adequate to meet global tissue demands, will flow increase with fluid loading, and is hypotension a reflection of reduced flow or vascular tone or both. Therapies are consequently based on the identification of the potential for tissue hypoperfusion and the likelihood that fluid loading alone (preload responsiveness) and/or the use of inotropes or vasopressors will increase flow and mean arterial pressure. The stroke volume, systolic arterial pressure, and pulse pressure all vary in hypovolemic patients during positive-pressure ventilation with fixed tidal volumes [33, 34].

Stroke volume variation (SVV), SPV, and PPV measure different but related aspects of cardiorespiratory interaction. These variables have been shown to be superior to the conventional estimates for preload responsiveness such as CVP and PAOP. Figure 20.3 shows the receiver operating curve for SVV and PPV [26–28]. In other words, the ability to increase flow with volume loading is better predicted by the SVV, SPV, and/or PPV especially in patients undergoing sur-

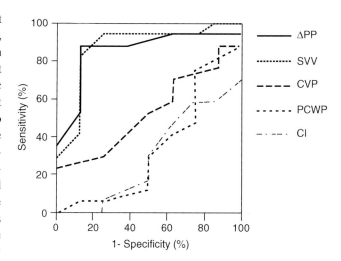

Fig. 20.3 Only the dynamic variables ΔPP (delta pulse pressure) and SVV (stroke volume variation) allow discrimination of responders from non-responders to a volume challenge, area under the ROC > 0.85. CVP central venous pressure, PCWP pulmonary capillary wedge pressure, CI cardiac input area under the ROC of 50% or less

gical procedures with an expected substantial blood loss or fluid-compartment shifts (compare with Fig. 20.2). These variables are directly measured from the arterial pressure tracing and its variation with ventilation. During controlled mechanical ventilation, there are respirophasic changes in venous return and consequently subtle changes in pulse pressure and systolic pressure with each respiratory cycle. Figures 20.4 and 20.5 graphically display the physiologic mechanisms underlying these observations.

Esophageal Doppler Monitoring

Esophageal Doppler monitoring (EDM) was first introduced in 1975. Since that time, it has been the most common minimally invasive hemodynamic monitor used and studied for

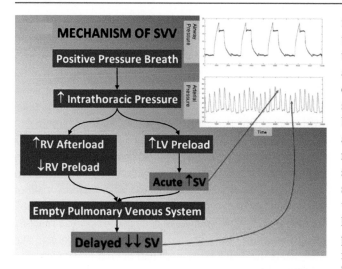

Fig. 20.4 Mechanism of stroke volume variation (SVV) from positive pressure ventilation. An acute increase in (left ventricular) LV stroke volume (SV) coincident with the inspiratory phase of positive pressure ventilation. Simultaneously displayed airway pressure and arterial pressure demonstrate that the increase in blood pressure and left ventricular stroke volume occurs during inspiration with positive pressure ventilation. This is the opposite of spontaneous breathing and is sometimes referred to as reverse pulsus paradoxus. RV right ventricular

individualized hemodynamic optimization and goal-directed therapy in thoracic surgery. Based on the Doppler principle, the probe which is inserted into the mid-esophagus transmits a continuous wave Doppler signal aligned with flow in the descending thoracic aorta at the tip of the device. The ultrasound beam is directed as parallel to the pathway of the red blood cells (traveling through the descending thoracic aorta) as possible. The constant motion of the red blood cells reflects a fraction of these ultrasound signals. The relative shift in the frequency of returned signals is called the Doppler shift, and this shift is proportional to the peak red blood cell velocity. The displayed velocity vs. time profile allows the hemodynamic calculation of stroke volume and cardiac output (based on certain assumptions). This device allows immediate real-time, comprehensive left ventricular flow-based assessment of the effects of changes in preload, afterload, contractility, and rhythm and on stroke volume. This device has been validated against the thermodilution PAC.

The caveat with this device is that it *estimates* the cross-sectional area of the descending thoracic aorta based on patients' demographics from a nomogram including age, height, and weight. Also, the angle between the direction of

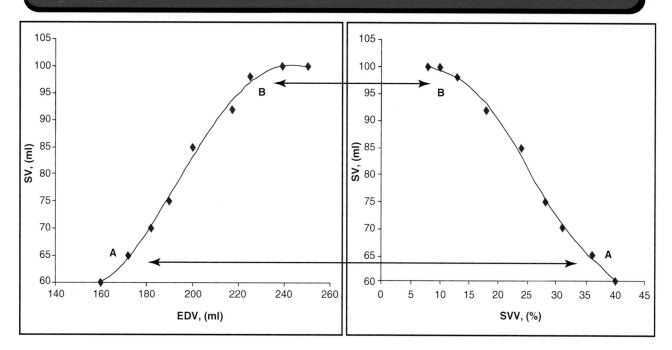

Fig. 20.5 Simultaneously developed Frank-Starling curve with the corresponding SV-SVV relationship in an individual patient undergoing volume resuscitation. The SV - SVV relationship mirrors the Frank Starling curve: as preload increases cardiac performance reaches a plateau, similarly declining SVV is associated with improved cardiac performance. SVV-SV pairs can provide information about cardiac performance similar to a Frank-Starling curve. *EDV* end diastolic volume

blood flow in the descending thoracic aorta and the Doppler signal sent by the esophageal probe is greater than the ideal 20° angle, so flow can be underestimated (although automated corrections are made for this difference). Furthermore, assumptions on the ratio of blood flow distribution to the upper vs. the lower body are also made. These correction factors can generate inaccuracies when exposed to interventions that affect blood flow distribution such as when using thoracic epidural analgesia. The esophageal Doppler device is very sensitive to positioning for the probe, leading to a need for frequent repositioning when trying to obtain accurate data. The use of electrocautery also interferes with data acquisition. The technology also allows for the calculation of flow time corrected for heart rate (FTc). This is the time that it takes for the left ventricle to eject the stroke volume or the systolic flow time in the descending thoracic aorta corrected for heart rate. The typical range for the FTc is 330–360 ms. The more volume loaded the ventricle is, the longer it takes to eject the stroke volume, conversely the more volume depleted the ventricle is, the lesser time it takes to eject the stroke volume. The FTc usually decreases to under 300 ms in volume-depleted patients. The FTc has been used in algorithms for goal-directed fluid therapy [35]; however, it remains a function of contractility, preload, and SVR, and as such, vascular impedance significantly affects this variable. In thoracic surgical patients, it has been demonstrated that this device can be used to detect and correct low-flow conditions and to guide hemodynamic support during the intraoperative period [35, 36].

Unfortunately, the EDM cannot be used during esophageal procedures where fluid management is pivotal to length of hospital stay and outcomes. The goals during these often lengthy procedures (such as esophagectomy for esophageal cancer) are to be more liberal with fluids during the abdominal portion of the surgery and more conservative during the thoracic portion of the procedure.

Continuous Pulse Contour Analysis (PiCCO)

This device estimates cardiac output using a combination of transpulmonary thermodilution and arterial contour waveform analysis. Both the thermal indicator and the pressure waveform must be measured simultaneously from a central line and an arterial line (either femoral or axillary) for calibration. This is impractical in the operating room setting, and consequently this technology is largely limited to use in Europe in the intensive care unit setting. Stroke volume is estimated from the portion of the arterial waveform that corresponds to systole. The pulsatile systolic pressure-time integral (multiplied by the heart rate to give an estimated cardiac output) is calibrated against the transpulmonary thermodilution technique of cardiac output measurement. The advan-

tage of calibration against transpulmonary thermodilution is its independence relative to the influence of ventilation and the respiratory cycle. PiCCO has also been validated against continuous cardiac output monitoring offered by the PAC. This technology relies on a high fidelity arterial waveform and is, therefore, sensitive to damping and resonance where errors in the estimation of the cardiac output may occur. Another limitation of the PiCCO system is that conditions that interfere with the calibration process or pulse contour waveform analysis such as intracardiac shunts, severe aortic valvular disease, and the use of intraaortic balloon pump devices introduce errors [37]. As of the time that this section was written, there have been no prospective randomized controlled outcome studies published in thoracic surgery using the PiCCO system as part of goal-directed therapy (GDT).

Lithium Dilution Cardiac Output

This technology is based on the physics of pulse power analysis, which is independent of the waveform morphology, and has a correction factor incorporated to account for impedance and arterial compliance. Based on an understanding that pulse pressure measured from the arterial trace is a combination of an incident pressure wave ejected from the aorta and a reflected wave from the periphery, stroke volume calculation requires that the two waves need to be separated. The algorithm takes into consideration the fact that the arterial pressure wave changes in size depending upon the proximity of the sampling site to the heart and also on patient's age. The use of an indicator dilution method for calibration (in this case lithium since it does not naturally occur in plasma and therefore can generate a high signal-to-noise ratio) allows the measurement of blood flow, with a lithium ion-selective electrode situated in an arterial line sensing the extent of dilution. These data are used to generate a concentration vs. time curve, and the cardiac output can then be calculated from the known amount of lithium and the area under the concentration-time curve (standard indicator-dilution technique for cardiac output estimation). Multiple studies have compared continuous cardiac output measurement via PACs with the lithium dilution cardiac output (LiDCO plus) system and have found acceptable correlation (defined as agreement of measured values within 15% of each other). There have been multiple studies confirming that lithium dilution is comparable to intrapulmonary thermodilution over a range of cardiac outputs. This is very important in thoracic surgical patients with poor ventricular function and in individual patients with a fluctuating cardiac output or with a hyperdynamic circulation [38].

This device has to be calibrated because the proprietary algorithm lacks the ability to independently assess the effects of constantly changing vascular tone on stroke volume measurement. Another limitation of this technology revolves around the use of lithium. Nondepolarizing muscle relaxants cross-react with the lithium sensor and can cause the sensor to drift. Calibration may also be unreliable in patients with severe hyponatremia. For intraoperative use, calibration needs to be performed either before induction or after the initial hemodynamic stress from airway management has had time to subside. The device can be onerous for the operating room, and it is currently mainly used in the ICU setting. The accuracy of the device is compromised in patients with severe peripheral vascular or aortic valve disease and in those requiring intraaortic balloon counter-pulsation therapy. A high fidelity arterial waveform is mandatory for accurate hemodynamic data.

The LiDCO Rapid is a recently introduced alternative designed for the operating room setting. This technology uses the same internal algorithm as the LiDCO plus but allows for the calculation of other hemodynamic parameters. The device analyzes the arterial pressure waveform and using the pulse power cardiac output algorithm converts pulse pressure into a nominal stroke volume and cardiac output. The device does not require calibration with lithium and uses a nomogram for calculation of arterial compliance. There are no published studies at the time of this review that examine the use of this technology during thoracic surgery.

Arterial Pressure Cardiac Output Device (APCO, FloTrac/Vigileo)

This technology is based on the physical principle of the relationship between pulse pressure and stroke volume. Arterial pulse pressure is directly proportional to left ventricular stroke volume and is inversely related to aortic compliance. Once stroke volume is determined by the internal algorithm, the pulse rate is counted, and cardiac output is estimated. The device does not require external calibration because the algorithm, in theory, corrects and compensates for dynamic changes in vascular tone. The device calculates cardiac output on a continuous basis (in a 20-s averaging cycle or a 5-min averaging cycle) [39–44]. With the FloTrac/Vigileo device, the arterial pressure waveform morphology is used to analyze the pulse rate and examine the variation (skewness, kurtosis, and standard deviation) of the waveform to determine changes in stroke volume. Finally, the device takes into account the multiple variables responsible for the changes in vasculature compliance (a so-called Ki factor). This constant is derived from the patient's specific vascular compliance based on biometric values (age, height, sex, and weight). The second-generation software tended to underestimate the cardiac output when the SVR was less than 800 dynes such as in sepsis and during liver transplants second-

ary to the hyperdynamic state typical of these situations. With the development of the third-generation software, the estimation of the cardiac output is more accurate, and newer data have demonstrated clinically acceptable precision in hyperdynamic states. Presumably, this will lead to further important studies in the near future in thoracic surgical patients. The accuracy of the device is compromised in patients with severe peripheral vascular or aortic valvular disease and in those requiring intraaortic balloon counter-pulsation therapy. A high fidelity arterial line waveform is mandatory for accurate hemodynamic data. The technology has been studied during cardiac surgery and in the postoperative cardiac surgical population. Precision and bias in the estimation of cardiac output (using Bland-Altman analyses) are acceptable relative to the gold standard thermodilution PAC measurement [41–44]. Data relevant to thoracic surgical patients are sparse.

In addition, central venous oximetry can be integrated into decision-making with this device. This technology allows for the measurement of the superior vena cava oxygen saturation ($SvcO_2$) via insertion of an 8 Fr fiber-optic double-lumen catheter into the jugular or subclavian veins (using the same physical principle of spectrophotometry used for pulse oximetry). The measured value is 5–7% higher than the true mixed venous oximetry since only the upper extremity, neck, and head venous effluent is captured. With PACs, mixed venous oximetry can be performed, and coronary sinus and lower extremity effluent causes the measured value to be lower (global mixed venous effluent saturation is measured rather than central venous saturation). Despite the fact that the difference in saturation is 5–7% higher with the $SvcO_2$ than with SvO_2, it is still a very good surrogate and may be used as a sensitive marker for GDT in high-risk surgical patients undergoing elective thoracic surgery.

BioReactance (Cheetah)

The principle underlying BioReactance is that ejection of blood from the left ventricle into the thoracic aorta creates changes in injected transthoracic electric signals, i.e., phasic changes in blood flow in the thoracic aorta are detectable as changes in the "phase" of a current that is injected into the body using electrodes placed on the chest. Data have demonstrated the feasibility of using "blood flow-related phase shifts" for noninvasive measurement of cardiac output [45]. The BioReactance system consists of four dual-electrode "stickers" (two on the right side and two on the left side of the chest) placed to establish electrical contact with the body. Within each sticker, one electrode is used to inject an oscillating high-frequency sine wave into the body (by a current generator), while the other is used as a receiver (voltage input amplifier). A "phase" shift is detected and is directly proportional to stroke volumes ejected from the left ventricle into the thoracic aorta. Stickers on a given side of the body are paired, so that the currents are passed between the outer electrodes of the pair and voltages are recorded from between the inner electrodes. Noninvasive cardiac output measurement signal is determined separately from each side of the body, and the final signal is obtained by averaging.

As with other noninvasive devices, rather than an absolute measurement of cardiac output, the utility of this device may lie in detection of relative changes when various maneuvers are instituted (passive leg raising or a fluid challenge). Volume responsiveness can be detected and fluid administered when clinically indicated. When compared with bioimpedance, which relies on measurement of changes in signal amplitude, thoracic bioreactance is based on analysis of relative phase shifts of oscillating currents. This is theoretically less impacted more by patient movement, variable environment, humidity, and sticker location (i.e., bioreactance is robust to interpatient body variance and electrode positioning) [46].

References

1. Wendon J. Cost effectiveness of monitoring techniques. In: Pinsky MR, Payen D, editors. Functional hemodynamic monitoring. 1st ed. New York: Springer; 2005.
2. Grocott MPW, Mythen MG, Gan TJ. Perioperative fluid management and clinical outcomes in adults. Anesth Analg. 2005;100:1093–106.
3. Rivers E, Nguyen B, Havstad S, et al. Early goal-directed therapy in the treatment of severe sepsis and septic shock. N Engl J Med. 2001;345:1368–77.
4. Sandham JD, Hull RD, Brant RF, et al. A randomized, controlled trial of the use of pulmonary-artery catheters in high-risk surgical patients. N Engl J Med. 2003;348:5–14.
5. Kaplan J, Slinger P, editors. Thoracic anesthesia. 3rd ed. Philadelphia: Churchill Livingstone; 2006.
6. Schroeder RA, Barbeito A, Bar-Yosef S, Mark JB. Cardiovascular monitoring. In: Miller R, Eriksson L, Fleisher L, Wiener-Kronish J, Young W, editors. Miller's anesthesia. 7th ed. Philadelphia: Churchill Livingstone; 2010. p. 1267–328.
7. Anesthesiology 1988 Aug;69(2):232-41. Intraoperative myocardial ischemia: localization by continuous 12-lead electrocardiography. London MJ1, Hollenberg M, Wong MG, Levenson L, Tubau JF, Browner W, Mangano DT.
8. Landesberg G, Mosseri M, Wolf Y, Vesselov Y, Weissman C. Perioperative myocardial ischemia and infarction. Identification by continuous 12-lead electrocardiogram with online ST-segment monitoring. Anesthesiology. 2002;96:264–70.
9. Sgarbossa EB, Pinski SL, Barbagelata A, et al. Electrocardiographic diagnosis of evolving acute myocardial infarction in the presence of left bundle-branch block. N Engl J Med. 1996;334:481–7.
10. Cannesson M, Delannoy B, Morand A, et al. Does the Pleth variability index indicate the respiratory-induced variation in the plethysmogram and arterial pressure waveforms? Anesth Analg. 2008;106(4):1189–94.
11. Natalini G, Rosano A, Taranto M, et al. Arterial versus plethysmographic dynamic indices to test responsiveness for testing fluid administration in hypotensive patients: a clinical trial. Anesth Analg. 2006;103(6):1478–84.
12. Brodsky JB, Shulman MS, Swan M, Mark JBD (1985) Pulse oximetry during onelung ventilation. Anesthesiology 63:212—214
13. Perel A. Automated assessment of fluid responsiveness in mechanically ventilated patients. Anesth Analg. 2008;106(4):1031–3.
14. Components of a time capnogram. http://www.capnography.com/new/index.php?option=com_content&view=article&id=72&Itemid=95. Accessed 10 Feb 2010.
15. Lohser J. Evidence-based management of one-lung ventilation. Anesthesiol Clin. 2008;26:241–72.
16. Van Limmen JGM, Szegedi LL. Peri-operative spirometry: tool or gadget? Acta Anaesthesiol Belg. 2008;59:273–82.
17. Pinsky MR, Payen D. Functional hemodynamic monitoring. Crit Care. 2005;9:566–72.
18. Barbeito A, Mark JB. Arterial and central venous pressure monitoring. Anesthesiol Clin. 2006;24:717–35.
19. Courtois M, Fattal PG, Kovacs SJ Jr, et al. Anatomically and physiologically based reference level for measurement of intracardiac pressures. Circulation. 1995;92(7):1994–2000.
20. Magder S, Georgiadis G, Cheong T. Respiratory variations in right atrial pressure predict the response to fluid challenge. J Crit Care. 1992;7:76–85.
21. Marik P, Baram M, Vahid B. Does central venous pressure predict fluid responsiveness? A systematic review of the literature and the tale of seven mares. Chest. 2008;134:172–8.
22. The National Heart, Lung, and Blood Institute Acute Respiratory Distress Syndrome (ARDS) Clinical Trials Network. Pulmonary-artery versus central venous catheter to guide treatment of acute lung injury. N Engl J Med. 2006;354:2213–24.
23. Caterino U, Dialetto G, Covino FE, et al. The usefulness of transesophageal echocardiography in the staging of locally advanced lung cancer. Monaldi Arch Chest Dis. 2007;67(1):39–42.
24. Arthur ME, Landolfo C, Wade M, Castresana MR. Inferior vena cava diameter (IVCD) measured with transesophageal echocardiography (TEE) can be used to derive the central venous pressure (CVP) in anesthetized mechanically ventilated patients. Echocardiography. 2009;26(2):140–9.
25. Michard F, Teboul JL. Predicting fluid responsiveness in ICU patients: a critical analysis of the evidence. Chest. 2002;121:2000–8.
26. Gan TJ, Soppitt A, Maroof M, et al. Goal-directed intraoperative fluid administration reduces length of hospital stay after major surgery. Anesthesiology. 2002;97(4):820–6.
27. Pearse R, Dawson D, Fawcett J, Rhodes A, Grounds M, Bennett D. Early goal-directed therapy after major surgery reduces complications and duration of hospital stay. A randomized, controlled trial. Crit Care. 2005;9:R687–93.
28. Donati A, Loggi S, Preiser J, Orsetti G, et al. Goal-directed intraoperative therapy reduces morbidity and length of hospital stay in high-risk surgical patients. Chest. 2007;132:1817–24.
29. Venn R, Steele A, Richardson P, et al. Randomized controlled trial to investigate influence of the fluid challenge on duration of hospital stay and perioperative morbidity in patients with hip fractures. Br J Anaesth. 2002;88:65–71.
30. Diaper J, Ellenberger C, Villiger Y, et al. Transoesophageal Doppler monitoring for fluid and hemodynamic treatment during lung surgery. J Clin Monit Comput. 2008;22(5):367–74.
31. Lobo S, Lobo F, Polachini C, Patini D, et al. Prospective, randomized trial comparing fluids and dobutamine optimization of oxygen delivery in high-risk surgical patients. Crit Care. 2006;10(R72):1–11.
32. Lobo S, Salgado P, Castillo V, Borim A, et al. Effects of maximizing oxygen delivery on morbidity and mortality in high-risk surgical patients. Crit Care Med. 2000;28(10):3396–404.

33. Michard F. Changes in arterial pressure during mechanical ventilation. Anesthesiology. 2005;103:419–28.

34. Michard F, Boussat S, Chemla D, et al. Relation between respiratory changes in arterial pulse pressure and fluid responsiveness in septic patients with acute circulatory failure. Am J Respir Crit Care Med. 2000;162:134–8.

35. Phan TD, Ismail H, Heriot AG, et al. Improving perioperative outcomes: fluid optimization with the esophageal Doppler monitor, a metaanalysis and review. J Am Coll Surg. 2008;207(6):935–41.

36. Slinger PD, Campos JH. Anesthesia for thoracic surgery. In: Miller RD, Eriksson LI, Fleisher LA, Wiener-Kronish JP, Young WL, editors. Miller's anesthesia. 7th ed. Philadelphia: Churchill Livingstone; 2009.

37. Morgan P, Al-Subaie N, Rhodes A. Minimally invasive cardiac output monitoring. Curr Opin Crit Care. 2008;14:322–6.

38. De Waal EC, Wappler F, Wolfgang F. Cardiac output monitoring. Curr Opin Anesthesiol. 2009;22:71–7.

39. Manecke GR, Auger WR. Cardiac output determination from the arterial pressure wave: clinical testing of a novel algorithm that does not require calibration. J Cardiothorac Vasc Anesth. 2007;21:3–7.

40. Breukers RM, Sepehrkhouy S, Spiegelenberg SR, et al. Cardiac output measured by a new arterial pressure waveform analysis method without calibration compared with thermodilution after cardiac surgery. J Cardiothorac Vasc Anesth. 2007;21:632–5.

41. Mayer J, Boldt J, Wolf MW, et al. Cardiac output derived from arterial pressure waveform analysis in patients undergoing cardiac surgery: validity of a second generation device. Anesth Analg. 2008;106:867–72.

42. Scheeren TW, Wiesenack C, Compton FD, et al. Performance of a minimally invasive cardiac output monitoring system (Flotrac/Vigileo). Br J Anaesth. 2008;101:279–80.

43. Mehta Y, Chand RK, Sawhney R, et al. Cardiac output monitoring: comparison of a new arterial pressure waveform analysis to the bolus thermodilution technique in patients undergoing off-pump coronary artery bypass surgery. J Cardiothorac Vasc Anesth. 2008;22:394–9.

44. McGee WT. A simple physiologic algorithm for managing hemodynamics using stroke volume and stroke volume variation. J Intensive Care Med. 2009;24(6):352–60.

45. Keren H, Burkhoff D, Squara P. Evaluation of a noninvasive continuous cardiac output monitoring system based on thoracic bioreactance. Am J Physiol Heart Circ Physiol. 2007 Jul;293(1):H583–9.

46. Fuller HD. The validity of cardiac output measurement by cardiothoracic impedance: a meta-analysis. Clin Invest Med. 1992;15:103–12.

Fluid Management in Thoracic Surgery

21

Rebecca Y. Klinger

Key Points

- Excess fluid administration in the perioperative period is associated with increased risk of postoperative pulmonary injury.
- The role of the endothelial surface layer (glycocalyx) is important to understand as it relates to intraoperative injury and resultant capillary leak.
- "Goal-directed" fluid therapy using dynamic indices has been helpful in non-cardiothoracic surgery but has many limitations in thoracic surgery.
- Although the risk of acute kidney injury remains a concern with restrictive fluid regimens, there is little evidence to support an association between fluid restriction and postoperative acute kidney injury after thoracic surgery.
- Thoracic surgical patients will benefit from smaller intraoperative crystalloid maintenance infusions, judicious colloid boluses to replace blood loss, the use of inotropes/vasopressors to combat anesthesia-/neuraxial-related relative hypovolemia, and a focus on limiting postoperative positive fluid balance.

Introduction

One of the most challenging aspects of the anesthetic management of patients undergoing thoracic surgery is achieving and maintaining optimal fluid balance. Too little fluid risks hypovolemia and organ dysfunction, while too much fluid risks edema, anastomotic leakage, and lung injury. Both scenarios can profoundly impact perioperative morbidity and mortality, so achieving the appropriate fluid balance is crucial.

The Fluid Problem

Intravenous fluid therapy is integral to the practice of anesthesia, but the optimal volume and composition of fluid therapy in the perioperative setting remain debated. Both too little, but more commonly too much, intravenous fluid administration has been associated with increased postoperative complications [1]. Fluid therapy is often the first-line approach for maintaining and/or restoring intraoperative hemodynamic stability. Anesthesia decreases the effective circulating blood volume, thus reducing perfusion pressure and potentially compromising adequate oxygen delivery to tissues. However, the effectiveness with which intravenous fluid administration will improve tissue oxygen delivery is highly dependent on global cardiovascular parameters [2]. In some settings, fluid administration is beneficial, while in other settings, it is deleterious.

In patients undergoing intraabdominal surgery, excessive intraoperative fluid administration appears to be associated with multiple postoperative complications, including ileus and delayed hospital discharge [3–5]. In thoracic surgery, the consequences of fluid overload, including pulmonary edema and lung injury, are arguably far graver.

Lung Injury After Thoracic Surgery

Incidence

Lung injury occurring after pulmonary resection is a significant contributor to postoperative morbidity and mortality [6]. What had formerly been known as "acute lung injury" (ALI)

R. Y. Klinger (✉)
Department of Anesthesiology, Duke University Medical Center, Durham, NC, USA
e-mail: rebecca.y.klinger@duke.edu

© Springer Nature Switzerland AG 2019
P. Slinger (ed.), *Principles and Practice of Anesthesia for Thoracic Surgery*, https://doi.org/10.1007/978-3-030-00859-8_21

Table 21.1 Criteria for acute respiratory distress syndrome (ARDS) per the Berlin criteria [7]

ARDS severity	PaO$_2$/F$_i$O$_2$	Associated mortality
Mild	200–300	27%
Moderate	100–200	32%
Severe	<100	45%

now falls under the definition of mild acute respiratory distress syndrome (ARDS) as of the 2012 publication of the Berlin criteria by the ARDS Definition Task Force [7]. Mild ARDS is characterized, as acute lung injury was, by a PaO$_2$/F$_i$O$_2$ of 200–300 occurring within 7 days of surgery. Worse degrees of hypoxemia are associated with moderate or severe classifications of ARDS (Table 21.1). Radiographic evidence of pulmonary edema, being most commonly unilateral in the case of pulmonary surgery, is also required for the diagnosis.

The overall incidence of ALI/mild ARDS after thoracic surgery consistently ranges from 2% to 7%, with an average of around 4% [8–11]. Lung injury is less common after smaller lung resections and increases with increasingly invasive pulmonary resection, peaking with pneumonectomy. In early studies, the overall mortality with ALI after thoracic surgery was up to 70%. While the overall mortality for postoperative lung injury has improved to closer to 26% [8], it remains higher after pneumonectomy at 40% [12]. Furthermore, ALI remains the leading cause of death after surgical lung resection [13].

Factors Contributing to Postoperative Lung Injury

While lung injury following extensive lung resection has long been known [14], it is important to recognize that this syndrome also occurs after lesser degrees of lung parenchyma removal and even after intrathoracic procedures requiring one-lung ventilation but without concomitant pulmonary resection [15, 16]. The etiology of lung injury after thoracic surgery is not fully elucidated and is most likely multifactorial in nature [17]. Radionucleotide lung scans have demonstrated an increase in the pulmonary vascular permeability in the remaining lung tissue after major pulmonary resections [18]. This altered permeability is thought to be due to several perioperative factors, including surgical trauma to the lung parenchyma, lymphatic disruption, lung hyperinflation during mechanical ventilation, and release of inflammatory mediators [19]. Furthermore, surgical factors, patient characteristics, and intraoperative management all play a role in modulating the risk of postoperative lung injury.

Surgical Risk Factors

The surgical approach and extent of resection both contribute to the risk of postoperative lung injury. A right pneumonectomy has been clearly linked to increased risk for the development of acute lung injury. Zeldin et al. [14], who were the first to identify postpneumonectomy pulmonary edema, noted in their case series that nine of the ten patients who developed pulmonary edema postoperatively had undergone right pneumonectomy. The reason right pneumonectomy carries a higher risk than left pneumonectomy is likely related to the fact that more lung tissue is resected with a right pneumonectomy, thereby forcing the entire cardiac output to flow through less residual lung and thus potentially injuring the pulmonary capillary endothelium. It is likely for similar reasons that more extensive pulmonary resections in general carry a greater risk of postoperative pulmonary injury than lesser resections. Further explanation for more extensive pulmonary edema with right pneumonectomy may relate to the fact that lymphatic drainage is not the same for the right and left lungs. Greater than 90% of the lymphatic drainage of the right lung is ipsilateral, while the left lung is drained partially on the left but more than 50% by right-sided lymphatics [20]. For this reason, a right pneumonectomy will compromise more than half of the lymphatic drainage of the remaining left lung, increasing the risk for pulmonary edema, while a left pneumonectomy will do little to compromise drainage of the remaining right lung [21].

Patient-Related Risk Factors

Fernandez-Perez et al. [22] described several patient-related risk factors that significantly contribute to acute lung injury after thoracic surgery. As may be expected, American Society of Anesthesiologists (ASA) physical status class is associated with increased risk [23]. Specific comorbidities associated with a higher risk of postoperative lung injury include diabetes, smoking, chronic obstructive pulmonary disease (COPD), and daily alcohol use (defined as >60 g alcohol consumed per day). Chronic alcohol abuse has also been noted as a risk factor by others [9]. This association was described in early studies of ARDS, which identified that the incidence of ARDS in patients with a history of alcohol abuse was 43% compared to only 22% in nonalcoholic patients [24]. Importantly, alcoholics who developed ARDS had a higher mortality (65%) than nonalcoholic patients (36%). The mechanism by which chronic alcohol ingestion increases the susceptibility to acute lung injury may be related to decreases in the levels of glutathione, which is known to serve as an important antioxidant at the alveolar membrane during periods of inflammatory stress.

Risk factors for developing postpneumonectomy pulmonary edema, specifically, have been described to include predicted postoperative lung perfusion ≤55% and predicted postoperative $FEV_1 < 45\%$ of preoperative values. History of chemotherapy or radiation therapy has also been linked to the risk for postoperative pulmonary edema [25], although this association was not observed in more recent studies [26–28]. Several other risk factors have also been identified, including advanced age, blood loss, reoperation, preoperative albumin level, pulmonary metastasis, altered mental status, shortness of breath, current or past history of smoking, and low body mass index [11, 26, 28–30].

Intraoperative Management

Multiple factors related to intraoperative anesthetic management have been identified to contribute to postoperative acute lung injury. These are discussed in detail in Chap. 10 (Perioperative Lung Injury). However, two key factors are mechanical ventilation strategy [22, 31] and intravenous fluid balance. In the remainder of this chapter, we focus on the contribution of perioperative fluid management to lung injury in the setting of thoracic surgery.

Perioperative Fluid Administration and Acute Lung Injury

Acute lung injury after thoracic surgery has been linked to the administration of excessive fluid in the perioperative period by several authors [14, 17, 25]. Zeldin and colleagues were the first to propose this connection based on data from a retrospective review of ten patients who developed postpneumonectomy pulmonary edema; those who developed pulmonary edema received 4.9 ± 1.2 L of fluid, while patients who did not develop pulmonary edema received 3.5 ± 1 L of fluid [14]. Concurrently the authors reported that excessive fluid administration led to postoperative pulmonary edema in a canine model. Dogs undergoing right pneumonectomy received either "liberal" (100 mL/kg rapid bolus followed by >100 mL/kg positive fluid balance) or a more "restrictive" (50 mL/kg rapid bolus followed by <100 mL/kg positive fluid balance) crystalloid administration in the first 48 hours after surgery. All dogs who received "liberal" fluid management developed pulmonary edema postoperatively, while no dogs receiving "restrictive" fluid management developed pulmonary edema. While Zeldin and colleagues lay much of the blame for postpneumonectomy pulmonary edema on fluid administration, Turnage and colleagues [21] found no correlation between postpneumonectomy pulmonary edema and 24-h fluid balance, although their standard fluid regimen

was comparatively restrictive to most. What these conflicting data do tell us is that while fluid balance clearly plays a role in pulmonary injury after surgery, it is not likely to be the only contributor.

The best human evidence to date addressing the issue of perioperative fluid management and ALI after thoracic surgery comes from a study by Licker and colleagues [8]. The authors evaluated 879 consecutive patients undergoing pulmonary resection via thoracotomy for non-small cell lung cancer. Within this cohort, only 4.2% developed lung injury (as defined by consensus guidelines); however, this acute lung injury was responsible for 43% of perioperative deaths (26–60%, depending on the etiology of the ALI). Licker et al. identified that excess fluid administration during surgery and within the first 24 h postoperatively was an independent risk factor (OR 2.9) for early acute lung injury after surgery. Those patients who developed acute lung injury received a mean cumulative intraoperative and postoperative fluid administration of 2.6 ± 1.2 mL/kg/h, while non-ALI patients received 2.0 ± 1.1 mL/kg/h ($p = 0.003$). This appeared to be driven primarily by intraoperative, rather than postoperative, fluid administration since fluid infusion in the first 24 h postoperatively did not differ between groups. Intraoperatively, patients who went on to develop ALI received a mean of 1.68 ± 0.60 L (9.1 ± 4.1 mL/kg/h) of crystalloid compared to 1.22 ± 0.72 L (7.2 mL/kg/h) in the non-ALI group. Interestingly, the difference in total fluid administration between ALI and non-ALI groups is rather narrow, making it difficult to define "liberal" compared to "restrictive" fluid strategies and suggesting a small margin of error in fluid administration before lung injury results.

Similar fluid volume cutoffs have been suggested by others. Parquin et al. [25] noted that intraoperative fluid administration >2 L is an independent risk factor for pulmonary edema after pneumonectomy [25]. Also in pneumonectomy patients, Blank et al. [32] found in univariate analysis that patients who suffered respiratory complications (inclusive of the need for initial mechanical ventilation for >48 h postoperatively, the need for reintubation due to respiratory insufficiency, ALI, ARDS, atelectasis requiring bronchoscopy, pneumonia, and bronchopleural fistula) received a median of 2.7 L of intravenous fluids compared to 1.8 L in patients without respiratory complications (p = 0.001). Importantly, this association was no longer seen in multivariate analysis.

The ARDS network conducted a randomized study aimed to identify the contribution of conservative vs. liberal fluid management strategies on outcomes in 1000 ALI patients in the intensive care unit (not necessarily operative patients) [33]. While this study did not address the contribution of fluid balance to the development of ALI, especially in the perioperative period, it did demonstrate a benefit to fluid restriction in patients with established ALI [34]. This benefit was primarily a significant increase in ventilator-free days at 28 days, with a trend toward a mortality benefit.

A similar study evaluated the role of fluid balance on outcomes in critically ill surgical patients. Barmparas and colleagues [35] prospectively followed 144 non-thoracic surgical patients admitted to the intensive care unit (ICU) and stratified them by positive or negative fluid balance achieved by ICU day 5 (or ICU discharge if before day 5). The positive fluid balance group had a significantly higher mean daily fluid intake than the negative fluid balance group (3728 ± 211 mL vs. 4579 ± 263 mL, p = 0.013), as would be expected. While there was no difference in the observed rate of ALI/ARDS, the negative fluid balance group had a 70% lower in-hospital mortality than the positive fluid balance group, after adjustment for potential confounders.

Several more recent studies have been performed in thoracic surgical patients, specifically, which add to the picture described early on by Zeldin and Licker. Arslantas and colleagues [36] evaluated data on perioperative fluid management in 139 patients undergoing multiple types of thoracic surgical procedures. Patients were divided into those suffering pulmonary complications (inclusive of ARDS, need for intubation, pneumonia, need for toilet bronchoscopy, atelectasis, air leak >7 days, and failure to expand the lung) compared to those without such pulmonary complications. Those thoracic surgical patients who developed postoperative pulmonary complications received significantly greater intraoperative crystalloids, blood products, and other fluids as well as a higher infusion rate of fluids in the first 48 hours after surgery. However, in multivariate logistic regression, only intraoperative crystalloid infusion rate (and smoking history) was significantly associated with pulmonary complications. Patients with pulmonary complications received a mean intraoperative fluid infusion rate of 6.58 ± 3.64 mL/kg/h compared to 4.61 ± 2.28 mL in those without pulmonary complications.

Fluid administration has also been implicated in ALI after esophagectomy by several groups. After multivariate analysis in 45 patients undergoing esophagectomy, Casado and colleagues [16] identified that intraoperative fluid administration plus 5-day fluid balance was the only factor in their analysis that was predictive of postoperative acute lung injury. Those who developed respiratory complications received a mean of 5410 ± 810 mL of fluid intraoperatively and had a 5-day positive fluid balance of 7873 ± 954 mL (compared with 4174 ± 1033 mL and 5928 ± 1047 mL, respectively, in the group without respiratory complications). Tandon and colleagues found that ARDS, developed in 14.5% of patients after esophagectomy, was associated with intraoperative fluid and transfusion requirements, and was associated with 50% mortality (compared to only 3.5% in esophagectomy patients who did not develop ARDS) [37].

Physiologic Basis of Fluid Overload

Intraoperative fluid administration has historically been targeted by anesthesiologists to replace perceived significant fluid deficits resulting from overnight fasting, insensible losses occurring through perspiration and exposure of organ surfaces during surgery, and third-space fluid shifts. We now know that these assumptions of fluid deficit requiring treatment with intravascular volume are grossly overestimated [38–40] and that this paradigm only leads to relative hypervolemia and perioperative fluid retention. Much of the fluid load given intravascularly during surgery shifts into the extracellular space, resulting in edema.

Shifting of administered fluid out of the intravascular compartment is well documented in the perioperative period. In the setting of major surgery, the difference between intravenous fluid input and measurable output (e.g., blood loss, urine output) reveals an approximate loss of 3–6 L from the vasculature [41–43]. While this shifting begins intraoperatively, it continues into the postoperative period, extending out to 72 h in certain cases [44]. Indeed, Lowell et al. described that 40% of patients admitted to a surgical intensive care unit were 10% over their preoperative weight, presumably due to fluid accumulation [45]. This additional fluid is also not rapidly cleared. Healthy volunteers require approximately 2 days to excrete an intravenous saline load of 22 mL/kg [46, 47], and postsurgical patients would conceivably require longer in the setting of tissue trauma and possible organ dysfunction.

What remains unclear is whether surgical trauma is the primary driver of fluid shifts from the intravascular space to the interstitium (that is then treated with aggressive intraoperative fluid administration) or if inappropriately high volumes of intravenous fluid administration lead to overload of the intravascular compartment and consequent interstitial edema. In a rabbit model, surgical manipulation and trauma are alone sufficient to increase interstitial fluid by 5–10% in the complete absence of intravenous fluid administration [48]. What is even more interesting is that the resultant postsurgical interstitial edema doubled in volume with the concomitant administration of intravenous crystalloid.

Role of the Glycocalyx

Tissue and pulmonary edema are produced by increased permeability of the capillary vasculature that then allows for the egress of protein-rich fluid from the vascular compartment into the interstitial compartment. Edema has long been understood in the context of the Starling principle; however, recent understanding of the role of the endothelial surface layer (ESL), which is comprised of the endothelial

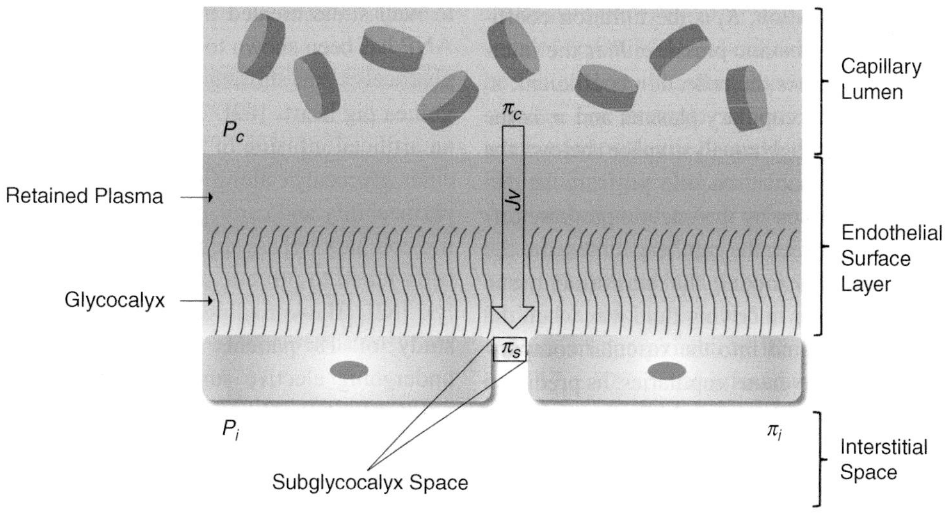

Fig. 21.1 The endothelial surface layer (ESL) is comprised of the endothelial glycocalyx and retained plasma proteins on the luminal surface of the capillary endothelium. The ESL acts as a sieve, allowing few plasma proteins to pass into the subglycocalyx space. These proteins are continuously cleared to the interstitial space; thus, the subglycocalyx space below the ESL has a very low oncotic pressure (π_s) compared to the capillary plasma oncotic pressure (π_c), creating an oncotic gradient favoring retention of fluid in the vascular lumen. The net flux of fluid across the endothelium (J_v) is driven by the balance between the capillary and interstitial hydrostatic pressures (P_c and P_i, respectively) and the oncotic gradient established between capillary lumen (π_c) and the subglyceal space (π_s). Compared to the traditional Starling principle, in this revised model, the oncotic pressure of the interstitium (π_i) does not contribute to fluid flux. (Adapted from [51, 57])

glycocalyx and bound plasma proteins, has expanded our understanding of fluid transit across the vasculature and called into question the classic Starling model.

The Starling principle [49] relies on a differential in hydrostatic and oncotic pressures between the intravascular and interstitial spaces to explain fluid transport across the capillary endothelium. However, several experiments have revealed that the calculations derived from the Startling equation are incorrect; specifically, the expected lymph flow based on calculations using the Starling principle far exceeds actual measured flow [50]. Adamson and colleagues demonstrated this phenomenon in rat mesentery. They measured trans-endothelial fluid in post-capillary venules while altering the interstitial oncotic pressure through albumin superfusion; this led to the finding that raising the interstitial oncotic pressure only increased fluid filtration by a small fraction of that predicted by the Starling model [51]. A similar study in frogs found that altering interstitial oncotic pressure had essentially no effect on fluid filtration [52].

Instead, the vascular endothelial glycocalyx appears to play a crucial role in modulating transvascular fluid flux. The glycocalyx is found on the luminal side of the vascular endothelium and is comprised of membrane-bound proteoglycans, glycoproteins, and glycolipids [53]. The glycocalyx adsorbs plasma proteins, primarily albumin, to form the ~1 μm-thick endothelial surface layer. The ESL is responsible for trapping approximately 700–1000 mL of plasma at the endothelial surface [54], thereby forming an inwardly directed oncotic force that retains plasma that would otherwise be hydrostatically forced into the interstitium

(Fig. 21.1). Furthermore, it appears to be the oncotic pressure of a small area below the glycocalyx (the subglycocalyx, or subglyceal, space) that is responsible for opposing vascular oncotic pressure rather than the interstitial tissue oncotic pressure; this again is based on experimental evidence that alterations of interstitial albumin concentration had no effect on fluid filtration. This subglycocalyx oncotic pressure is developed by diffusion of plasma albumin into this space under conditions of low transcapillary fluid filtration rates [55]. Proteins in the subglycocalyx space are rapidly cleared into the interstitium by protein transport, keeping the oncotic pressure in this space extremely low and favoring retention of fluid in the vascular compartment.

It has been proposed that the endothelial glycocalyx structure serves as a passive barrier to edema formation. Increases in vascular hydrostatic pressure (i.e., during exercise) will accelerate fluid filtration into the subglycocalyx space, thereby rapidly decreasing the subglycocalyx oncotic pressure and establishing a high trans-glycocalyx oncotic pressure gradient favoring retention of fluid in the vascular lumen [51]. Similarly, low vascular hydrostatic pressure and decreased fluid filtration rates would readjust the Starling forces across the capillary endothelium to allow for more fluid filtration into the interstitium. This "revised" Starling principle, reviewed in [56, 57], can be summarized by the following equation:

$$J_v = K_f \left[\left(P_c - P_i \right) - \sigma \left(\pi_c - \pi_s \right) \right],$$

thoracic surgery at 1.4%; notably this only reflects patients requiring renal replacement therapy [104]. The rate of renal failure after esophagectomy appears to be slightly higher at 2.0% [105]. Criteria have been devised to classify AKI, including the risk, injury, failure, loss, and end-stage disease (RIFLE) [106] and acute kidney injury network (AKIN) [107] criteria. Using these criteria, AKI after thoracic surgery appears to range around 6% and is associated with increased length of stay, morbidity, and mortality [108, 109].

In the study by Ishikawa and colleagues [108], AKI as defined by AKIN criteria occurred within the first 72 h of surgery in 5.9% of patients. Most of these cases were AKIN stage 1 (59/67), while a few were AKIN stage 2 (8/67). Using the RIFLE criteria, AKI was diagnosed in 2.3% in the same cohort of patients. As would be expected, the rate of AKI varied based on the invasiveness of the procedure, with pneumonectomy having the highest rate and wedge resection/bullectomy having the lowest rate. Several patient-related risk factors were identified in those who developed AKI. With regard to perioperative fluid management, only exposure to hydroxyethyl starch fluids was associated with AKI and in a dose-dependent manner, such that each 250 mL of hydroxyethyl starch increased the odds of AKI 1.5-fold. Rather than volume restriction, univariate analysis indicated that patients who developed AKI received *more* perioperative crystalloid than those without AKI; however, this association was not supported in multivariate analysis.

Licker and colleagues [109] identified a slightly higher rate of AKI (6.8%) after lung cancer surgery using RIFLE criteria. Again, risk was highest in patients undergoing more extensive surgery with longer operative and anesthesia times. Patients who developed AKI received higher volumes of colloids intraoperatively and had greater vasopressor requirements. However, logistic regression failed to identify any fluid-related risk factors; rather vasopressor requirement was one of the four identified independent predictors of AKI. While this observation has been noted by others in noncardiac surgical patients [110], it remains unclear whether the association between vasopressor use and AKI is reflective of arterial hypotension and uncompensated hypovolemia, as the authors suggest, or rather reflective of patient- or procedure-related comorbidity. The authors did note that AKI was more prevalent in patients who received chronic angiotensin receptor blocker therapy preoperatively. Furthermore, there was no difference in intravenous fluid administration between patients who developed AKI and those who did not.

In a more recent study, Ahn and colleagues [111] retrospectively evaluated the association between postoperative AKI, based on AKIN criteria, within 72 h after thoracic surgery in nearly 1500 patients. In their cohort, 5.1% of patients developed AKI with only 0.1% requiring renal replacement therapy. In this cohort, the highest risk of AKI was seen in esophagectomy patients (13%), followed by pneumonectomy (11%), lobectomy (5%), and finally wedge resection/segmentectomy (2%). Intraoperative crystalloid restriction was not associated with a higher incidence of AKI after thoracic surgery, even down to ≤2 mL/kg/h and in patients with preexisting abnormal renal function. However, and in support of the findings by Ishikawa et al., hydroxyethyl starch administration was associated with increased postoperative AKI, with each 500 mL increasing the odds for AKI 1.75-fold. Importantly, after multivariate adjustment, hydroxyethyl starch administration was only a risk factor for postoperative AKI in patients with preexisting abnormal renal function (odds ratio 7.6).

These findings are in line with the general surgical literature. A recent systematic review and meta-analysis evaluating a total of 1594 patients were unable to find an association between "restrictive" intraoperative fluid management and an increase in oliguria or AKI [112]. They also found no difference in AKI between studies that specifically targeted reversal of oliguria versus those that did not. In the pooled studies, intraoperative fluid administration was 1.9 L lower in the restrictive group versus the conventional fluid group when oliguria was not targeted and still 1.6 L lower in studies that targeted oliguria reversal. Similarly, the Fluids and Catheters Treatment Trial (FACCT) failed to demonstrate any difference in AKI-free days between restrictive and conventional fluid management approaches in patients with established ARDS [33].

In addition to the evidence that fluid restriction does not appear to increase the risk of AKI in thoracic surgery, there is also little support for generous hydration to improve perioperative renal function or urine output in thoracic surgical patients. In a study by Matot et al., urine output was the same (median, 300 mL) in 102 video-assisted thoracoscopic surgical patients, regardless of whether they received "high" (mean, 2131 ± 850 mL) or "low" (mean, 1035 ± 652 mL) intraoperative fluid. Serum creatinine levels decreased postoperatively from preoperative levels in both fluid groups to an equal extent, and there was no difference in postoperative creatinine between patients with urine output <1 mL/kg/h and those with urine output >1 mL/kg/h.

Based on the currently available evidence, it does not appear that intraoperative crystalloid fluid restriction is associated with an increased risk for postoperative renal injury.

Methods of Targeting Fluid Management

Maintaining dry lungs and relative normovolemia during the perioperative period has been espoused by many and appears to be a rational approach. However, the question remains as to how one can accomplish this goal without straying into either hypervolemia or hypovolemia. The general perioperative literature has proposed a conservative fluid management strategy referred to as the "zero-balance" approach, the goal of which is to minimize perioperative weight gain due to fluid administration and salt/water retention in response to surgical stress-induced antidiuretic hormone release [57] without inducing hypovolemia.

The so-called goal-directed fluid therapy has long been an objective in anesthesia practice. As might be expected, clinicians are not good at estimating the volume status of patients; only 50% of hemodynamically unstable patients will appropriately respond (increase their stroke volume by 10–15%) to fluid challenges administered based on clinical suspicion [113]. For a fluid bolus to cause an appropriate increase in stroke volume, the following must be true: the bolus must increase the mean circulatory filling pressure above the central venous pressure, thus driving venous return to the heart, and the heart must be on the ascending portion of the Frank-Starling curve [114]. Furthermore, volume loading of patients in the steep portion of the Frank-Starling curve (preload-insensitive patients) will only increase hydrostatic pressure and resultant edema with minimal gains in cardiac output (Fig. 21.2). The resultant tissue and pulmonary edema with inappropriate fluid loading is accentuated in patients with disease processes that increase endothelial permeability/glycocalyx damage, as described above. Increased extravascular lung water specifically is known to be strong predictor of morbidity and mortality in patients with critical illness [115, 116].

Initially, invasive monitors, including central venous pressure monitoring and pulmonary artery catheters, were utilized to help guide fluid therapy. However, central venous pressure was found to be inaccurate at assessing volume status or predicting response to a volume challenge [113, 117]. Pulmonary artery catheters are also poor predictors of fluid responsiveness [118, 119] and are associated with major morbidity [120]. The use of dynamic hemodynamic parameters to predict fluid responsiveness has been advocated, including variation (generally of >13%) in systolic pressure, stroke volume, or pulse pressure [121]. These indices are based on the principle that mechanical ventilation cyclically increases intrathoracic pressure, which then has variable effects on ventricular loading depending on the volume status of the patient. Thus, these indices can theoretically predict fluid responsiveness [122, 123] and are designed to offer the clinician an estimate of the position of the patient's cardiovascular system on the Frank-Starling curve. Unfortunately, there remains a "gray zone" (between 9% and 13% variation) in which fluid responsiveness cannot be reliably predicted in many patients [124].

Particularly problematic for adoption of these dynamic indices in thoracic surgery is the fact that their predictive value varies greatly with different delivered tidal volumes [125] and substantially decreases at tidal volumes less than 7 mL/kg [126]. Furthermore, the reliability of these dynamic indices under open-chest conditions has varied in different

studies, with some reporting loss of reliability [127–129] but others reporting no change [130]. Lee and colleagues interestingly reported the ability of pulse pressure variation to predict fluid responsiveness with protective one-lung ventilation (OLV) but not with non-protective OLV strategies in thoracotomy [131]. Patients were randomized to either protective strategies (OLV with tidal volumes of 6 mL/kg, FiO_2 of 0.5, and positive end-expiratory pressure [PEEP] of 5 cmH_2O) or "conventional" OLV (tidal volumes of 10 mL/kg and no PEEP). After the initiation of OLV, patients received volume loading with 7 mL/kg of 6% hydroxyethyl starch, and pulse pressure variation and cardiac index were measured. Pulse pressure variation was predictive of fluid responsiveness (cardiac index increase of at least 15%) only in the protective lung ventilation group and at a threshold of 5.8%. In contrast, a study in patients undergoing lobectomy identified that stroke volume variation was only able to predict fluid responsiveness during OLV if the tidal volume was at least 8 mL/kg [132]. Transesophageal echocardiography can be particularly useful in assessing volume responsiveness during open-chest procedures [133] but is unlikely to be used in the vast majority of thoracic surgical procedures. The various dynamic

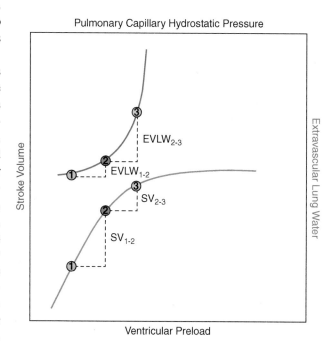

Fig. 21.2 Superimposition of the Frank-Starling curve (blue), which describes the relationship between left-ventricular preload and stroke volume/cardiac output, and the Marik-Phillips curve (red), which describes the relationship between pulmonary capillary hydrostatic pressure and extravascular lung water (EVLW). Movement from positions 1 to 2 on the curves produces a large increase in stroke volume (SV_{1-2}) with a relatively small increase in EVLW ($EVLW_{1-2}$); this describes a preload-dependent patient. In contrast, movement from positions 2 to 3 on the curves produces only a small gain in stroke volume (SV_{2-3}) but at the expense of a much larger increase in EVLW ($EVLW_{2-3}$); this describes a preload-independent patient. (Adapted from [114])

hemodynamic monitoring devices in clinical use today are reviewed elsewhere [134, 135].

While fluid challenges are known to predict fluid responsiveness [136], the actual hemodynamic response to fluid augmentation is generally fleeting and of unclear benefit. In a study of patients with shock, fluid responders experienced a 25% increase in their cardiac index following a fluid bolus; however, their cardiac index returned to baseline by 30 min after the completion of the bolus [137]. Similarly, in patients with sepsis, a fluid bolus increased the mean arterial pressure for only 1 h and did not augment urine output [138]. ARDS patients similarly experienced an augmentation of mean arterial pressure in response to a fluid bolus without any increase in urine production [139]. In the Fluid Expansion as Supportive Therapy (FEAST) trial in pediatric febrile patients, albumin and saline boluses both increased the rate of death due to cardiovascular collapse (not fluid overload) at 48 h compared to no fluid bolus, suggesting that bolus fluids may adversely impair normal neurohormonal compensatory mechanisms [140].

The currently employed paradigms for fluid administration are naturally only surrogates for the intended benefit, namely, optimizing tissue blood flow and oxygen delivery. The difficulty in monitoring the effects of fluid therapy at the intended site of action – the microcirculation – likely contributes to the ongoing controversy surrounding best practices for fluid administration. However, the use of the microcirculation as the end point of fluid resuscitation, via measures such as in vivo microscopy to identify the microvascular flow index or sublingual capnography to define the sublingual-systemic CO_2 gradient (reviewed in [141]), may bring us closer to defining optimal perioperative fluid management strategies in the future.

Approach to Fluid Management in Thoracic Surgery

Fluid management has become central to much of the literature surrounding enhanced recovery after surgery (ERAS) approaches. Careful and rational fluid management is also central to the perioperative management of thoracic surgical patients to mitigate postoperative morbidity. Borrowing from the broader ERAS literature, several recommendations may also make sense in the thoracic surgical population.

ERAS-Based Fluid Management

ERAS protocols have called into question the traditional thinking regarding *nil* per os (NPO) guidelines in the preoperative phase. Many centers and individuals still practice NPO after midnight, inclusive of any food and drink, except

for small amounts of clear liquids up to 2 h prior to surgery. However, there is sufficient evidence to support the notion that fasting of solid food for 6 h and oral fluid intake until 2 h prior to surgery is safe and may improve outcomes [142, 143]. Some protocols even encourage active carbohydrate drink consumption up to 2 h prior to surgery. While this strategy has not necessarily been shown to prevent fluid overload or acute lung injury and is derived largely from the abdominal surgery literature, there appears to be a signal toward reduced length of stay and attenuation of insulin resistance [144]. Whether carbohydrate drinks are superior to clear liquid consumption and whether these findings are applicable to thoracic surgical patients remain to be investigated. Furthermore, an exact target for volume of preoperative liquid consumption also remains unclear.

The second component of an ERAS-based fluid strategy is to restrict intraoperative fluid administration to avoid overt hypervolemia. While the correct amount of fluid needed to maintain normovolemia remains elusive and the definition of a "restrictive" approach is highly variable, some sort of protocol-driven fluid management appears to reduce the incidence of complications in major surgery [145–147]. In general, replacement of fluid losses into the "third space" has largely been discounted [57]. Based on the available evidence, ERAS advocates have argued for limiting intraoperative maintenance infusions designed to replace loss of fluid through the skin and airways, evaporation from the surgical field, and bodily secretions to 1–2 mL/kg/h [148]. Additional fluid should only be administered to account for blood loss. The results of many of the trials of goal-directed fluid therapy in a myriad of surgical procedure types are reviewed by the International Fluid Optimization Group [148]. It should be noted that goal-directed approaches are not synonymous with restrictive fluid administration approaches; in many trials, goal-directed patients received more fluids, in particular colloids, than control patients [148]. This may be particularly problematic for the translation of these approaches to thoracic surgical patients.

Managing Fluids in Lung Surgery

Thoracic patients are unique in their risk for postoperative lung injury; thus stricter fluid recommendations have been put forth [149]. In addition to protective lung ventilation strategies, a more restrictive fluid administration regimen targeted to maintaining normovolemia has been advocated in thoracic surgical patients. Assaad and colleagues suggested a protocol that maintained normal renal function without increasing extravascular lung water in a small prospective observational study [150]. Their preferred fluid regimen included the following: maintenance fluids administered as a balanced salt solution at 1.5 mL/kg/h and continued until oral intake resumed; repletion of fasting fluid deficit with a bolus equivalent to number of hours of fasting times the above maintenance rate; repletion of evaporative losses in open thoracotomy procedures at a rate of 1 mL/kg/h; and 1:1 repletion of blood loss with either a hetastarch solution or packed red blood cells if the hematocrit fell below 25%. They showed this protocol to maintain cardiac preload and tissue perfusion (as assessed by serum lactate and central venous oxygen saturation). There were no cases of ALI in this cohort, and their rate of postoperative AKI in the first 3 days was 7.5% (based on AKIN criteria). This study suffers from several limitations: the cohort size is very small, encompassing only 40 patients; arguably, the routine replacement of fasting fluid loses is outdated; and this study lacked an alternate fluid administration protocol group for comparison. Nevertheless, their results provide some guidelines as to fluid administration parameters that, in combination with lung-protective ventilation strategies, appear to be non-injurious.

Goal-directed approaches using dynamic indices have also been attempted in the thoracic surgical population with mixed results. A small study of 27 patients undergoing either lung surgery or esophagectomy by Haas and colleagues reported that a goal-directed fluid approach (an arguably aggressive maintenance crystalloid infusion of 9 mL/kg/h intraoperatively and 5 mL/kg starch colloid boluses for stroke volume variation >10%) did not result in an increase in extravascular lung water [151]. They did, however, report a decrease in the PaO_2/F_iO_2 ratio during surgery, although this value remained >300 mmHg outside of periods of OLV. A larger study of 60 patients undergoing thoracoscopic lobectomy randomized patients to receive either goal-directed fluid therapy or control therapy [152]. Control patients received a basal crystalloid infusion of 8 mL/kg/h and crystalloid or colloid boluses at the discretion of the anesthesiologist to maintain mean arterial pressure 65–90 mmHg, heart rate 60–100 beats/min, and urine output >0.5 mL/kg/h. Goal-directed patients received the same basal crystalloid infusion rate along with the following interventions: starch colloid boluses when stroke volume variation >11% to achieve stable stroke volume variation ≤9%; ephedrine boluses and continuous phenylephrine infusion of 2 mcg/min for mean arterial pressure <60 mmHg despite fluid resuscitation; and dobutamine infusion (2–5 mcg/kg/min) to maintain the cardiac index between 2.5–4 L/min/m². They demonstrated that the goal-directed group received significantly less colloids and overall less infused fluid volume than the control group and had fewer instances of nausea and vomiting. With regard to pulmonary outcomes, they report that the goal-directed group had a significantly higher PaO_2/F_iO_2 ratio before the end of OLV than the control group. Five of the 30 goal-directed patients required dobutamine infusions. The authors note in their discussion that stroke volume variation values became more difficult to treat and less predictably responsive to treatment in the lateral position, again highlighting that these dynamic indices may fall short given the complexities of thoracic surgery and one-lung ventilation.

In addition to focusing on the volume of fluid administered, the anesthesiologist must also remember that not all episodes of hypotension are due to hypovolemia and that hemodynamic optimization can and should include vasopressors and inotropes in addition to fluids. Several guidelines have encouraged the use of vasopressors in lieu of intravenous fluids to counteract anesthesia-induced vasodilation and accompanying relative hypovolemia. It is known from the sepsis literature that norepinephrine, for example, is quite effective in augmenting venous return to the heart, increasing stroke volume and cardiac output, and raising the mean arterial pressure; these effects should improve organ and tissue perfusion while minimizing the formation of edema [153, 154]. A randomized trial in radical cystectomy patients demonstrated that a so-called restrictive deferred hydration protocol (initial fluid therapy limited to 1 mL/kg/h with low-dose norepinephrine followed by a hydration phase at 3 mL/kg/h) resulted in a shorter hospital length of stay and lower transfusion rate compared to a liberal fluid regimen (6 mL/kg/h) without any difference in major complications [155, 156]. Finally, in a recent meta-analysis, perioperative hemodynamic optimization using a combination of fluids and inotropes was effective in reducing AKI after surgery [157].

Lastly, in addition to intraoperative fluid targets, attention should be paid to overall perioperative fluid balance and patient body weight in the early postoperative period. An excess positive fluid balance in the postoperative period should be avoided. Intravenous fluid administration should be terminated as soon as feasible, with the resumption of oral hydration and alimentation as soon after surgery as is safe.

Table 21.3 offers suggestions regarding perioperative fluid management for providers in thoracic anesthesia.

Managing Fluids in Esophagectomy

Esophagectomy deserves additional consideration, as this procedure has traditionally been approached with more aggressive fluid resuscitation. As noted above, lung injury after esophagectomy also occurs, but typically at a higher fluid threshold than for lung surgery. Regardless, excessive fluid administration should also be avoided in these patients. Both aggressive fluid resuscitation and the use of vasopressors have been feared to contribute to anastomotic complications after esophagectomy. While the data in esophagectomy is sparse, extrapolation of the abdominal surgery literature

Table 21.3 Suggestions for perioperative fluid management in thoracic surgical patients

Variable	Suggested value
Clear liquid consumption up to 2 h before surgery	Unrestricted
Fluid administration in first 24 h	≤2 mL/kg/h
Perioperative positive fluid balance	≤1.5 L
Vasopressors/inotropes	As needed for anesthesia-induced vasodilation or ongoing hypoperfusion
Mechanical ventilation	Lung-protective strategies

Based in part on Evans and Naidu [149]

suggests that avoiding excessive fluid administration may avoid anastomotic breakdown [158, 159].

A recent study evaluated the effects of goal-directed fluid therapy in 199 esophagectomy patients [160]. Control patients received crystalloids and colloids at the discretion of the anesthesiologist with the only goal to maintain mean arterial pressure >65 mmHg or <20% from baseline. Goal-directed patients received colloid boluses to reach and then maintain stroke volume within 10% below optimum. Phenylephrine, ephedrine, and norepinephrine were used in both groups to maintain mean arterial pressure. There were no differences in morbidity or mortality between the groups. The control group had a higher mean postoperative intensive care unit or post anesthesia care unit length of stay, but overall hospital length of stay did not differ. Goal-directed patients received overall less fluid intraoperatively, although they received more colloid than controls. Norepinephrine use was higher in the goal-directed group, but phenylephrine use was higher in controls. With regard to composite pulmonary complications, there was no difference between groups, although the goal-directed patients had a significantly lower incidence of pneumonia in secondary analyses. Important to esophagectomy patients, this study failed to demonstrate a benefit to goal-directed therapy in terms of anastomotic leakage.

Glatz and colleagues very recently published a retrospective study of 335 esophagectomy patients that identified an association between intra- and postoperative fluid overload and several complications, including both pulmonary (representing 53% of all complications) and anastomotic complications, along with in-hospital mortality [161]. Intraoperative fluid load (postoperative day zero fluid balance) along with ASA score were the only independent predictors of adverse outcomes (at least one complication) in multivariate analysis. The cutoff points for identifying liberal versus restrictive fluid strategies in terms of outcomes in this study were again quite large in comparison to those typically seen in lung surgery: a positive fluid balance on postoperative day zero (representative of intraoperative administration) of 6 L and on postoperative day 4 of 5.5 L. Anastomotic leakage occurred in 9% of the patients who received restrictive intraoperative fluids compared to 21% who received liberal management.

With respect to vasopressors use, earlier animal studies of esophagectomy indicated that treatment of hypotension with norepinephrine was associated with gastric conduit hypoperfusion [162]. However, small human studies have since indicated that treatment of epidural-induced hypotension during esophagectomy with epinephrine [163] or phenylephrine [164] were not detrimental and actually improved or restored compromised graft blood flow.

While larger fluid volumes appear to be tolerated in esophagectomy patients before complications occur, the available data suggests that the avoidance of an excessive (several liter) postoperative fluid balance is desirable and that the use of vasopressors and inotropes to improve intraoperative hemodynamics and offset anesthesia−/neuraxial-related hypotension is reasonable without risking overt anastomotic breakdown.

Conclusion

Lung injury after thoracic surgery remains a significant problem that is associated with postoperative morbidity and mortality. There is considerable evidence to associate postoperative lung injury with perioperative fluid administration, among other factors. While more research is required, the available evidence suggests that a more restrictive approach to fluid management along with the use of vasopressors and inotropes to offset anesthesia-related hypotension is likely beneficial to the thoracic surgical patient without significant risk of renal or other tissue injuries. Dynamic indices to guide fluid administration may be of benefit, although they are associated with many pitfalls in related to one-lung ventilation and open-chest approaches. Practitioners should pay attention to overall perioperative fluid balance in addition to limiting intraoperative fluid administration. Finally, the apparent synergism between volume status and mechanical ventilation strategies argues for the use of lung-protective ventilation along with judicious perioperative fluid management in the patient undergoing thoracic surgery.

References

1. Holte K, Sharrock NE, Kehlet H. Pathophysiology and clinical implications of perioperative fluid excess. Br J Anaesth. 2002;89(4):622–32.
2. Chawla LS, Ince C, Chappell D, Gan TJ, Kellum JA, Mythen M, et al. Vascular content, tone, integrity, and haemodynamics for guiding fluid therapy: a conceptual approach. Br J Anaesth. 2014;113(5):748–55.
3. Brandstrup B, Tonnesen H, Beier-Holgersen R, Hjortso E, Ording H, Lindorff-Larsen K, et al. Effects of intravenous fluid restriction on postoperative complications: comparison of two perioperative

fluid regimens: a randomized assessor-blinded multicenter trial. Ann Surg. 2003;238(5):641–8.

4. Lobo DN, Bostock KA, Neal KR, Perkins AC, Rowlands BJ, Allison SP. Effect of salt and water balance on recovery of gastro-intestinal function after elective colonic resection: a randomised controlled trial. Lancet. 2002;359(9320):1812–8.

5. Nisanevich V, Felsenstein I, Almogy G, Weissman C, Einav S, Matot I. Effect of intraoperative fluid management on outcome after intraabdominal surgery. Anesthesiology. 2005;103(1):25–32.

6. Alam N, Park BJ, Wilton A, Seshan VE, Bains MS, Downey RJ, et al. Incidence and risk factors for lung injury after lung cancer resection. Ann Thorac Surg. 2007;84(4):1085–91. discussion 91

7. Force ADT, Ranieri VM, Rubenfeld GD, Thompson BT, Ferguson ND, Caldwell E, et al. Acute respiratory distress syndrome: the Berlin definition. JAMA. 2012;307(23):2526–33.

8. Licker M, de Perrot M, Spiliopoulos A, Robert J, Diaper J, Chevalley C, et al. Risk factors for acute lung injury after thoracic surgery for lung cancer. Anesth Analg. 2003;97(6):1558–65.

9. Licker M, Fauconnet P, Villiger Y, Tschopp JM. Acute lung injury and outcomes after thoracic surgery. Curr Opin Anaesthesiol. 2009;22(1):61–7.

10. Ruffini E, Parola A, Papalia E, Filosso PL, Mancuso M, Oliaro A, et al. Frequency and mortality of acute lung injury and acute respiratory distress syndrome after pulmonary resection for bronchogenic carcinoma. Eur J Cardiothorac Surg. 2001;20(1):30–6. discussion 6–7

11. Kutlu CA, Williams EA, Evans TW, Pastorino U, Goldstraw P. Acute lung injury and acute respiratory distress syndrome after pulmonary resection. Ann Thorac Surg. 2000;69(2):376–80.

12. Park BJ. Respiratory failure following pulmonary resection. Semin Thorac Cardiovasc Surg. 2007;19(4):374–9.

13. Neto A, Hemmes S, Barbas C, Beiderlinden M, Fernandez-Bustamante A, Futier E, et al. Incidence of mortality and morbidity related to postoperative lung injury in patients who have undergone abdominal or thoracic surgery: a systematic review and meta-analysis. Lancet Respir Med. 2014;2(12):1007–15.

14. Zeldin RA, Normandin D, Landtwing D, Peters RM. Postpneumonectomy pulmonary edema. J Thorac Cardiovasc Surg. 1984;87(3):359–65.

15. Gothard J. Lung injury after thoracic surgery and one-lung ventilation. Curr Opin Anaesthesiol. 2006;19(1):5–10.

16. Casado D, Lopez F, Marti R. Perioperative fluid management and major respiratory complications in patients undergoing esophagectomy. Dis Esophagus. 2010;23(7):523–8.

17. Slinger PD. Acute lung injury after pulmonary resection: more pieces of the puzzle. Anesth Analg. 2003;97(6):1555–7.

18. Waller DA, Keavey P, Woodfine L, Dark JH. Pulmonary endothelial permeability changes after major lung resection. Ann Thorac Surg. 1996;61(5):1435–40.

19. Eichenbaum KD, Neustein SM. Acute lung injury after thoracic surgery. J Cardiothorac Vasc Anesth. 2010;24(4):681–90.

20. Nohl-Oser HC. An investigation of the anatomy of the lymphatic drainage of the lungs as shown by the lymphatic spread of bronchial carcinoma. Ann R Coll Surg Engl. 1972;51(3):157–76.

21. Turnage WS, Lunn JJ. Postpneumonectomy pulmonary edema. A retrospective analysis of associated variables. Chest. 1993;103(6):1646–50.

22. Fernandez-Perez ER, Sprung J, Afessa B, Warner DO, Vachon CM, Schroeder DR, et al. Intraoperative ventilator settings and acute lung injury after elective surgery: a nested case control study. Thorax. 2009;64(2):121–7.

23. Sen S, Sen S, Senturk E, Kuman NK. Postresectional lung injury in thoracic surgery pre and intraoperative risk factors: a retrospective clinical study of a hundred forty-three cases. J Cardiothorac Surg. 2010;5:62.

24. Moss M, Bucher B, Moore FA, Moore EE, Parsons PE. The role of chronic alcohol abuse in the development of acute respiratory distress syndrome in adults. JAMA. 1996;275(1):50–4.

25. Parquin F, Marchal M, Mehiri S, Herve P, Lescot B. Postpneumonectomy pulmonary edema: analysis and risk factors. Eur J Cardiothorac Surg. 1996;10(11):929–32. discussion 33

26. Dulu A, Pastores SM, Park B, Riedel E, Rusch V, Halpern NA. Prevalence and mortality of acute lung injury and ARDS after lung resection. Chest. 2006;130(1):73–8.

27. Perrot E, Guibert B, Mulsant P, Blandin S, Arnaud I, Roy P, et al. Preoperative chemotherapy does not increase complications after nonsmall cell lung cancer resection. Ann Thorac Surg. 2005;80(2):423–7.

28. Grichnik KP, D'Amico TA. Acute lung injury and acute respiratory distress syndrome after pulmonary resection. Semin Cardiothorac Vasc Anesth. 2004;8(4):317–34.

29. Harpole DH Jr, DeCamp MM Jr, Daley J, Hur K, Oprian CA, Henderson WG, et al. Prognostic models of thirty-day mortality and morbidity after major pulmonary resection. J Thorac Cardiovasc Surg. 1999;117(5):969–79.

30. Ely EW, Wheeler AP, Thompson BT, Ancukiewicz M, Steinberg KP, Bernard GR. Recovery rate and prognosis in older persons who develop acute lung injury and the acute respiratory distress syndrome. Ann Intern Med. 2002;136(1):25–36.

31. Fernandez-Perez ER, Keegan MT, Brown DR, Hubmayr RD, Gajic O. Intraoperative tidal volume as a risk factor for respiratory failure after pneumonectomy. Anesthesiology. 2006;105(1):14–8.

32. Blank RS, Hucklenbruch C, Gurka KK, Scalzo DC, Wang XQ, Jones DR, et al. Intraoperative factors and the risk of respiratory complications after pneumonectomy. Ann Thorac Surg. 2011;92(4):1188–94.

33. National Heart L, Blood Institute Acute Respiratory Distress Syndrome Clinical Trials N, Wiedemann HP, Wheeler AP, Bernard GR, Thompson BT, et al. Comparison of two fluid-management strategies in acute lung injury. N Engl J Med. 2006;354(24):2564–75.

34. Wiedemann HP. A perspective on the fluids and catheters treatment trial (FACTT). Fluid restriction is superior in acute lung injury and ARDS. Cleve Clin J Med. 2008;75(1):42–8.

35. Barmparas G, Liou D, Lee D, Fierro N, Bloom M, Ley E, et al. Impact of positive fluid balance on critically ill surgical patients: a prospective observational study. J Crit Care. 2014;29(6):936–41.

36. Arslantas MK, Kara HV, Tuncer BB, Yildizeli B, Yuksel M, Bostanci K, et al. Effect of the amount of intraoperative fluid administration on postoperative pulmonary complications following anatomic lung resections. J Thorac Cardiovasc Surg. 2015;149(1):314–20, 21 e1.

37. Tandon S, Batchelor A, Bullock R, Gascoigne A, Griffin M, Hayes N, et al. Peri-operative risk factors for acute lung injury after elective oesophagectomy. Br J Anaesth. 2001;86(5):633–8.

38. Jacob M, Chappell D, Conzen P, Finsterer U, Rehm M. Blood volume is normal after pre-operative overnight fasting. Acta Anaesthesiol Scand. 2008;52(4):522–9.

39. Lamke LO, Nilsson GE, Reithner HL. Water loss by evaporation from the abdominal cavity during surgery. Acta Chir Scand. 1977;143(5):279–84.

40. Jacob M, Chappell D, Rehm M. The 'third space'–fact or fiction? Best Pract Res Clin Anaesthesiol. 2009;23(2):145–57.

41. Rehm M, Haller M, Orth V, Kreimeier U, Jacob M, Dressel H, et al. Changes in blood volume and hematocrit during acute preoperative volume loading with 5% albumin or 6% hetastarch solutions in patients before radical hysterectomy. Anesthesiology. 2001;95(4):849–56.

42. Rehm M, Orth V, Kreimeier U, Thiel M, Haller M, Brechtelsbauer H, et al. Changes in intravascular volume during acute normovolemic hemodilution and intraoperative retransfusion in patients with radical hysterectomy. Anesthesiology. 2000;92(3):657–64.

43. Perko MJ, Jarnvig IL, Hojgaard-Rasmussen N, Eliasen K, Arendrup H. Electric impedance for evaluation of body fluid balance in cardiac surgical patients. J Cardiothorac Vasc Anesth. 2001;15(1):44–8.

44. Robarts WM. Nature of the disturbance in the body fluid compartments during and after surgical operations. Br J Surg. 1979;66(10):691–5.

45. Lowell JA, Schifferdecker C, Driscoll DF, Benotti PN, Bistrian BR. Postoperative fluid overload: not a benign problem. Crit Care Med. 1990;18(7):728–33.

46. Drummer C, Gerzer R, Heer M, Molz B, Bie P, Schlossberger M, et al. Effects of an acute saline infusion on fluid and electrolyte metabolism in humans. Am J Phys. 1992;262(5 Pt 2):F744–54.

47. Drummer C, Heer M, Baisch F, Blomqvist CG, Lang RE, Maass H, et al. Diuresis and natriuresis following isotonic saline infusion in healthy young volunteers before, during, and after HDT. Acta Physiol Scand Suppl. 1992;604:101–11.

48. Chan ST, Kapadia CR, Johnson AW, Radcliffe AG, Dudley HA. Extracellular fluid volume expansion and third space sequestration at the site of small bowel anastomoses. Br J Surg. 1983;70(1):36–9.

49. Starling EH. On the absorption of fluids from the connective tissue spaces. J Physiol. 1896;19(4):312–26.

50. Levick JR. Capillary filtration-absorption balance reconsidered in light of dynamic extravascular factors. Exp Physiol. 1991;76(6):825–57.

51. Adamson RH, Lenz JF, Zhang X, Adamson GN, Weinbaum S, Curry FE. Oncotic pressures opposing filtration across nonfenestrated rat microvessels. J Physiol. 2004;557(Pt 3):889–907.

52. Hu X, Adamson RH, Liu B, Curry FE, Weinbaum S. Starling forces that oppose filtration after tissue oncotic pressure is increased. Am J Physiol Heart Circ Physiol. 2000;279(4):H1724–36.

53. Becker BF, Chappell D, Jacob M. Endothelial glycocalyx and coronary vascular permeability: the fringe benefit. Basic Res Cardiol. 2010;105(6):687–701.

54. Pries AR, Secomb TW, Gaehtgens P. The endothelial surface layer. Pflugers Arch. 2000;440(5):653–66.

55. Curry FR. Microvascular solute and water transport. Microcirculation. 2005;12(1):17–31.

56. Chappell D, Jacob M. Role of the glycocalyx in fluid management: small things matter. Best Pract Res Clin Anaesthesiol. 2014;28(3):227–34.

57. Chappell D, Jacob M, Hofmann-Kiefer K, Conzen P, Rehm M. A rational approach to perioperative fluid management. Anesthesiology. 2008;109(4):723–40.

58. Woodcock TE, Woodcock TM. Revised Starling equation and the glycocalyx model of transvascular fluid exchange: an improved paradigm for prescribing intravenous fluid therapy. Br J Anaesth. 2012;108(3):384–94.

59. Rehm M, Bruegger D, Christ F, Conzen P, Thiel M, Jacob M, et al. Shedding of the endothelial glycocalyx in patients undergoing major vascular surgery with global and regional ischemia. Circulation. 2007;116(17):1896–906.

60. Nelson A, Berkestedt I, Schmidtchen A, Ljunggren L, Bodelsson M. Increased levels of glycosaminoglycans during septic shock: relation to mortality and the antibacterial actions of plasma. Shock. 2008;30(6):623–7.

61. Johansson PI, Stensballe J, Rasmussen LS, Ostrowski SR. A high admission syndecan-1 level, a marker of endothelial glycocalyx degradation, is associated with inflammation, protein C depletion, fibrinolysis, and increased mortality in trauma patients. Ann Surg. 2011;254(2):194–200.

62. Bruegger D, Schwartz L, Chappell D, Jacob M, Rehm M, Vogeser M, et al. Release of atrial natriuretic peptide precedes shedding of the endothelial glycocalyx equally in patients undergoing on- and off-pump coronary artery bypass surgery. Basic Res Cardiol. 2011;106(6):1111–21.

63. Chappell D, Bruegger D, Potzel J, Jacob M, Brettner F, Vogeser M, et al. Hypervolemia increases release of atrial natriuretic peptide and shedding of the endothelial glycocalyx. Crit Care. 2014;18(5):538.

64. Chappell D, Dorfler N, Jacob M, Rehm M, Welsch U, Conzen P, et al. Glycocalyx protection reduces leukocyte adhesion after ischemia/reperfusion. Shock. 2010;34(2):133–9.

65. Chappell D, Heindl B, Jacob M, Annecke T, Chen C, Rehm M, et al. Sevoflurane reduces leukocyte and platelet adhesion after ischemia-reperfusion by protecting the endothelial glycocalyx. Anesthesiology. 2011;115(3):483–91.

66. Schmidt EP, Yang Y, Janssen WJ, Gandjeva A, Perez MJ, Barthel L, et al. The pulmonary endothelial glycocalyx regulates neutrophil adhesion and lung injury during experimental sepsis. Nat Med. 2012;18(8):1217–23.

67. Parker JC. Hydraulic conductance of lung endothelial phenotypes and Starling safety factors against edema. Am J Physiol Lung Cell Mol Physiol. 2007;292(2):L378–80.

68. Parker JC, Stevens T, Randall J, Weber DS, King JA. Hydraulic conductance of pulmonary microvascular and macrovascular endothelial cell monolayers. Am J Physiol Lung Cell Mol Physiol. 2006;291(1):L30–7.

69. Stevens T, Phan S, Frid MG, Alvarez D, Herzog E, Stenmark KR. Lung vascular cell heterogeneity: endothelium, smooth muscle, and fibroblasts. Proc Am Thorac Soc. 2008;5(7):783–91.

70. Steppan J, Hofer S, Funke B, Brenner T, Henrich M, Martin E, et al. Sepsis and major abdominal surgery lead to flaking of the endothelial glycocalix. J Surg Res. 2011;165(1):136–41.

71. Nelson A, Berkestedt I, Bodelsson M. Circulating glycosaminoglycan species in septic shock. Acta Anaesthesiol Scand. 2014;58(1):36–43.

72. Nettelbladt O, Hallgren R. Hyaluronan (hyaluronic acid) in bronchoalveolar lavage fluid during the development of bleomycin-induced alveolitis in the rat. Am Rev Respir Dis. 1989;140(4):1028–32.

73. Nettelbladt O, Tengblad A, Hallgren R. Lung accumulation of hyaluronan parallels pulmonary edema in experimental alveolitis. Am J Phys. 1989;257(6 Pt 1):L379–84.

74. Constantinescu AA, Vink H, Spaan JA. Endothelial cell glycocalyx modulates immobilization of leukocytes at the endothelial surface. Arterioscler Thromb Vasc Biol. 2003;23(9):1541–7.

75. Vink H, Constantinescu AA, Spaan JA. Oxidized lipoproteins degrade the endothelial surface layer : implications for platelet-endothelial cell adhesion. Circulation. 2000;101(13):1500–2.

76. Huxley VH, Williams DA. Role of a glycocalyx on coronary arteriole permeability to proteins: evidence from enzyme treatments. Am J Physiol Heart Circ Physiol. 2000;278(4):H1177–85.

77. Dull RO, Cluff M, Kingston J, Hill D, Chen H, Hoehne S, et al. Lung heparan sulfates modulate K(fc) during increased vascular pressure: evidence for glycocalyx-mediated mechanotransduction. Am J Physiol Lung Cell Mol Physiol. 2012;302(9):L816–28.

78. Dull RO, Mecham I, McJames S. Heparan sulfates mediate pressure-induced increase in lung endothelial hydraulic conductivity via nitric oxide/reactive oxygen species. Am J Physiol Lung Cell Mol Physiol. 2007;292(6):L1452–8.

79. Curry FR. Atrial natriuretic peptide: an essential physiological regulator of transvascular fluid, protein transport, and plasma volume. J Clin Invest. 2005;115(6):1458–61.

80. Florian JA, Kosky JR, Ainslie K, Pang Z, Dull RO, Tarbell JM. Heparan sulfate proteoglycan is a mechanosensor on endothelial cells. Circ Res. 2003;93(10):e136–42.

81. Collins SR, Blank RS, Deatherage LS, Dull RO. Special article: the endothelial glycocalyx: emerging concepts in pulmonary edema and acute lung injury. Anesth Analg. 2013;117(3):664–74.

82. Dull RO, Jo H, Sill H, Hollis TM, Tarbell JM. The effect of varying albumin concentration and hydrostatic pressure on hydraulic

conductivity and albumin permeability of cultured endothelial monolayers. Microvasc Res. 1991;41(3):390–407.

83. McCluskey SA, Karkouti K, Wijeysundera D, Minkovich L, Tait G, Beattie WS. Hyperchloremia after noncardiac surgery is independently associated with increased morbidity and mortality: a propensity-matched cohort study. Anesth Analg. 2013;117(2):412–21.

84. Morgan TJ, Venkatesh B, Hall J. Crystalloid strong ion difference determines metabolic acid-base change during acute normovolaemic haemodilution. Intensive Care Med. 2004;30(7):1432–7.

85. Yunos NM, Bellomo R, Hegarty C, Story D, Ho L, Bailey M. Association between a chloride-liberal vs chloride-restrictive intravenous fluid administration strategy and kidney injury in critically ill adults. JAMA. 2012;308(15):1566–72.

86. Shaw AD, Bagshaw SM, Goldstein SL, Scherer LA, Duan M, Schermer CR, et al. Major complications, mortality, and resource utilization after open abdominal surgery: 0.9% saline compared to Plasma-Lyte. Ann Surg. 2012;255(5):821–9.

87. Myburgh JA, Mythen MG. Resuscitation fluids. N Engl J Med. 2013;369(25):2462–3.

88. Yunos NM, Bellomo R, Glassford N, Sutcliffe H, Lam Q, Bailey M. Chloride-liberal vs. chloride-restrictive intravenous fluid administration and acute kidney injury: an extended analysis. Intensive Care Med. 2015;41(2):257–64.

89. Haase N, Perner A, Hennings LI, Siegemund M, Lauridsen B, Wetterslev M, et al. Hydroxyethyl starch 130/0.38-0.45 versus crystalloid or albumin in patients with sepsis: systematic review with meta-analysis and trial sequential analysis. BMJ. 2013;346:f839.

90. Zarychanski R, Abou-Setta AM, Turgeon AF, Houston BL, McIntyre L, Marshall JC, et al. Association of hydroxyethyl starch administration with mortality and acute kidney injury in critically ill patients requiring volume resuscitation: a systematic review and meta-analysis. JAMA. 2013;309(7):678–88.

91. Perner A, Haase N, Guttormsen AB, Tenhunen J, Klemenzson G, Aneman A, et al. Hydroxyethyl starch 130/0.42 versus Ringer's acetate in severe sepsis. N Engl J Med. 2012;367(2):124–34.

92. Myburgh JA, Finfer S, Bellomo R, Billot L, Cass A, Gattas D, et al. Hydroxyethyl starch or saline for fluid resuscitation in intensive care. N Engl J Med. 2012;367(20):1901–11.

93. Meybohm P, Van Aken H, De Gasperi A, De Hert S, Della Rocca G, Girbes AR, et al. Re-evaluating currently available data and suggestions for planning randomised controlled studies regarding the use of hydroxyethyl starch in critically ill patients – a multidisciplinary statement. Crit Care. 2013;17(4):R166.

94. Mertes PM, Laxenaire MC, Alla F, Groupe d'Etudes des Reactions Anaphylactoides P. Anaphylactic and anaphylactoid reactions occurring during anesthesia in France in 1999–2000. Anesthesiology. 2003;99(3):536–45.

95. Barron ME, Wilkes MM, Navickis RJ. A systematic review of the comparative safety of colloids. Arch Surg. 2004;139(5):552–63.

96. Sirtl C, Laubenthal H, Zumtobel V, Kraft D, Jurecka W. Tissue deposits of hydroxyethyl starch (HES): dose-dependent and time-related. Br J Anaesth. 1999;82(4):510–5.

97. Van der Linden P, Ickx BE. The effects of colloid solutions on hemostasis. Can J Anaesth. 2006;53(6 Suppl):S30–9.

98. Jacob M, Chappell D, Hofmann-Kiefer K, Helfen T, Schuelke A, Jacob B, et al. The intravascular volume effect of Ringer's lactate is below 20%: a prospective study in humans. Crit Care. 2012;16(3):R86.

99. Jacob M, Rehm M, Orth V, Lotsch M, Brechtelsbauer H, Weninger E, et al. Exact measurement of the volume effect of 6% hydoxyethyl starch 130/0.4 (Voluven) during acute preoperative normovolemic hemodilution. Anaesthesist. 2003;52(10):896–904.

100. Perel P, Roberts I, Ker K. Colloids versus crystalloids for fluid resuscitation in critically ill patients. Cochrane Database Syst Rev. 2013;2:CD000567.

101. Verheij J, van Lingen A, Raijmakers PG, Rijnsburger ER, Veerman DP, Wisselink W, et al. Effect of fluid loading with saline or colloids on pulmonary permeability, oedema and lung injury score after cardiac and major vascular surgery. Br J Anaesth. 2006;96(1):21–30.

102. Huang CC, Kao KC, Hsu KH, Ko HW, Li LF, Hsieh MJ, et al. Effects of hydroxyethyl starch resuscitation on extravascular lung water and pulmonary permeability in sepsis-related acute respiratory distress syndrome. Crit Care Med. 2009;37(6):1948–55.

103. van der Heijden M, Verheij J, van Nieuw Amerongen GP, Groeneveld AB. Crystalloid or colloid fluid loading and pulmonary permeability, edema, and injury in septic and nonseptic critically ill patients with hypovolemia. Crit Care Med. 2009;37(4):1275–81.

104. Boffa DJ, Allen MS, Grab JD, Gaissert HA, Harpole DH, Wright CD. Data from the Society of Thoracic Surgeons General Thoracic Surgery database: the surgical management of primary lung tumors. J Thorac Cardiovasc Surg. 2008;135(2):247–54.

105. Raymond DP, Seder CW, Wright CD, Magee MJ, Kosinski AS, Cassivi SD, et al. Predictors of major morbidity or mortality after resection for esophageal cancer: a Society of Thoracic Surgeons General Thoracic Surgery database risk adjustment model. Ann Thorac Surg. 2016;102(1):207–14.

106. Bellomo R, Ronco C, Kellum JA, Mehta RL, Palevsky P, Acute dialysis quality Initiative w. Acute renal failure – definition, outcome measures, animal models, fluid therapy and information technology needs: the second international consensus conference of the Acute Dialysis Quality Initiative (ADQI) Group. Crit Care. 2004;8(4):R204–12.

107. Mehta RL, Kellum JA, Shah SV, Molitoris BA, Ronco C, Warnock DG, et al. Acute Kidney Injury Network: report of an initiative to improve outcomes in acute kidney injury. Crit Care. 2007;11(2):R31.

108. Ishikawa S, Griesdale DE, Lohser J. Acute kidney injury within 72 hours after lung transplantation: incidence and perioperative risk factors. J Cardiothorac Vasc Anesth. 2014;28(4):931–5.

109. Licker M, Cartier V, Robert J, Diaper J, Villiger Y, Tschopp JM, et al. Risk factors of acute kidney injury according to RIFLE criteria after lung cancer surgery. Ann Thorac Surg. 2011;91(3):844–50.

110. Kheterpal S, Tremper KK, Englesbe MJ, O'Reilly M, Shanks AM, Fetterman DM, et al. Predictors of postoperative acute renal failure after noncardiac surgery in patients with previously normal renal function. Anesthesiology. 2007;107(6):892–902.

111. Ahn HJ, Kim JA, Lee AR, Yang M, Jung HJ, Heo B. The risk of acute kidney injury from fluid restriction and hydroxyethyl starch in thoracic surgery. Anesth Analg. 2016;122(1):186–93.

112. Egal M, de Geus HR, van Bommel J, Groeneveld AB. Targeting oliguria reversal in perioperative restrictive fluid management does not influence the occurrence of renal dysfunction: a systematic review and meta-analysis. Eur J Anaesthesiol. 2016;33(6):425–35.

113. Marik PE, Cavallazzi R. Does the central venous pressure predict fluid responsiveness? An updated meta-analysis and a plea for some common sense. Crit Care Med. 2013;41(7):1774–81.

114. Marik PE. Fluid responsiveness and the six guiding principles of fluid resuscitation. Crit Care Med. 2016;44(10):1920–2.

115. Sakka SG, Klein M, Reinhart K, Meier-Hellmann A. Prognostic value of extravascular lung water in critically ill patients. Chest. 2002;122(6):2080–6.

116. Chung FT, Lin HC, Kuo CH, Yu CT, Chou CL, Lee KY, et al. Extravascular lung water correlates multiorgan dysfunction syndrome and mortality in sepsis. PLoS One. 2010;5(12):e15265.

117. Marik PE. Iatrogenic salt water drowning and the hazards of a high central venous pressure. Ann Intensive Care. 2014;4:21.

118. Michard F, Teboul JL. Predicting fluid responsiveness in ICU patients: a critical analysis of the evidence. Chest. 2002;121(6):2000–8.

119. Osman D, Ridel C, Ray P, Monnet X, Anguel N, Richard C, et al. Cardiac filling pressures are not appropriate to predict

hemodynamic response to volume challenge. Crit Care Med. 2007;35(1):64–8.

120. Hadian M, Pinsky MR. Evidence-based review of the use of the pulmonary artery catheter: impact data and complications. Crit Care. 2006;10(Suppl 3):S8.

121. Perel A, Habicher M, Sander M. Bench-to-bedside review: functional hemodynamics during surgery – should it be used for all high-risk cases? Crit Care. 2013;17(1):203.

122. Michard F, Boussat S, Chemla D, Anguel N, Mercat A, Lecarpentier Y, et al. Relation between respiratory changes in arterial pulse pressure and fluid responsiveness in septic patients with acute circulatory failure. Am J Respir Crit Care Med. 2000;162(1):134–8.

123. Feissel M, Michard F, Mangin I, Ruyer O, Faller JP, Teboul JL. Respiratory changes in aortic blood velocity as an indicator of fluid responsiveness in ventilated patients with septic shock. Chest. 2001;119(3):867–73.

124. Cannesson M, Le Manach Y, Hofer CK, Goarin JP, Lehot JJ, Vallet B, et al. Assessing the diagnostic accuracy of pulse pressure variations for the prediction of fluid responsiveness: a "gray zone" approach. Anesthesiology. 2011;115(2):231–41.

125. De Backer D, Heenen S, Piagnerelli M, Koch M, Vincent JL. Pulse pressure variations to predict fluid responsiveness: influence of tidal volume. Intensive Care Med. 2005;31(4):517–23.

126. Lansdorp B, Lemson J, van Putten MJ, de Keijzer A, van der Hoeven JG, Pickkers P. Dynamic indices do not predict volume responsiveness in routine clinical practice. Br J Anaesth. 2012;108(3):395–401.

127. Reuter DA, Goresch T, Goepfert MS, Wildhirt SM, Kilger E, Goetz AE. Effects of mid-line thoracotomy on the interaction between mechanical ventilation and cardiac filling during cardiac surgery. Br J Anaesth. 2004;92(6):808–13.

128. Rex S, Schalte G, Schroth S, de Waal EE, Metzelder S, Overbeck Y, et al. Limitations of arterial pulse pressure variation and left ventricular stroke volume variation in estimating cardiac pre-load during open heart surgery. Acta Anaesthesiol Scand. 2007;51(9):1258–67.

129. Wyffels PA, Sergeant P, Wouters PF. The value of pulse pressure and stroke volume variation as predictors of fluid responsiveness during open chest surgery. Anaesthesia. 2010;65(7):704–9.

130. Lorne E, Mahjoub Y, Zogheib E, Debec G, Ben Ammar A, Trojette F, et al. Influence of open chest conditions on pulse pressure variations. Ann Fr Anesth Reanim. 2011;30(2):117–21.

131. Lee JH, Jeon Y, Bahk JH, Gil NS, Hong DM, Kim JH, et al. Pulse pressure variation as a predictor of fluid responsiveness during one-lung ventilation for lung surgery using thoracotomy: randomised controlled study. Eur J Anaesthesiol. 2011;28(1):39–44.

132. Suehiro K, Okutani R. Influence of tidal volume for stroke volume variation to predict fluid responsiveness in patients undergoing one-lung ventilation. J Anesth. 2011;25(5):777–80.

133. de Waal EE, Rex S, Kruitwagen CL, Kalkman CJ, Buhre WF. Dynamic preload indicators fail to predict fluid responsiveness in open-chest conditions. Crit Care Med. 2009;37(2):510–5.

134. Naik BI, Durieux ME. Hemodynamic monitoring devices: putting it all together. Best Pract Res Clin Anaesthesiol. 2014;28(4):477–88.

135. Downs EA, Isbell JM. Impact of hemodynamic monitoring on clinical outcomes. Best Pract Res Clin Anaesthesiol. 2014;28(4):463–76.

136. Marik PE, Monnet X, Teboul JL. Hemodynamic parameters to guide fluid therapy. Ann Intensive Care. 2011;1(1):1.

137. Nunes TS, Ladeira RT, Bafi AT, de Azevedo LC, Machado FR, Freitas FG. Duration of hemodynamic effects of crystalloids in patients with circulatory shock after initial resuscitation. Ann Intensive Care. 2014;4:25.

138. Glassford NJ, Eastwood GM, Bellomo R. Physiological changes after fluid bolus therapy in sepsis: a systematic review of contemporary data. Crit Care. 2014;18(6):696.

139. Lammi MR, Aiello B, Burg GT, Rehman T, Douglas IS, Wheeler AP, et al. Response to fluid boluses in the fluid and catheter treatment trial. Chest. 2015;148(4):919–26.

140. Maitland K, George EC, Evans JA, Kiguli S, Olupot-Olupot P, Akech SO, et al. Exploring mechanisms of excess mortality with early fluid resuscitation: insights from the FEAST trial. BMC Med. 2013;11:68.

141. Veenstra G, Ince C, Boerma EC. Direct markers of organ perfusion to guide fluid therapy: when to start, when to stop. Best Pract Res Clin Anaesthesiol. 2014;28(3):217–26.

142. Brady M, Kinn S, Stuart P. Preoperative fasting for adults to prevent perioperative complications. Cochrane Database Syst Rev. 2003;4:CD004423.

143. Lobo DN, Macafee DA, Allison SP. How perioperative fluid balance influences postoperative outcomes. Best Pract Res Clin Anaesthesiol. 2006;20(3):439–55.

144. Awad S, Varadhan KK, Ljungqvist O, Lobo DN. A meta-analysis of randomised controlled trials on preoperative oral carbohydrate treatment in elective surgery. Clin Nutr. 2013;32(1):34–44.

145. Hamilton MA, Cecconi M, Rhodes A. A systematic review and meta-analysis on the use of preemptive hemodynamic intervention to improve postoperative outcomes in moderate and high-risk surgical patients. Anesth Analg. 2011;112(6):1392–402.

146. Lees N, Hamilton M, Rhodes A. Clinical review: goal-directed therapy in high risk surgical patients. Crit Care. 2009;13(5):231.

147. Gurgel ST, do Nascimento P Jr. Maintaining tissue perfusion in high-risk surgical patients: a systematic review of randomized clinical trials. Anesth Analg. 2011;112(6):1384–91.

148. Navarro LH, Bloomstone JA, Auler JO Jr, Cannesson M, Rocca GD, Gan TJ, et al. Perioperative fluid therapy: a statement from the international Fluid Optimization Group. Perioper Med (Lond). 2015;4:3.

149. Evans RG, Naidu B. Does a conservative fluid management strategy in the perioperative management of lung resection patients reduce the risk of acute lung injury? Interact Cardiovasc Thorac Surg. 2012;15(3):498–504.

150. Assaad S, Kyriakides T, Tellides G, Kim AW, Perkal M, Perrino A. Extravascular lung water and tissue perfusion biomarkers after lung resection surgery under a Normovolemic Fluid Protocol. J Cardiothorac Vasc Anesth. 2015;29(4):977–83.

151. Haas S, Eichhorn V, Hasbach T, Trepte C, Kutup A, Goetz AE, et al. Goal-directed fluid therapy using stroke volume variation does not result in pulmonary fluid overload in thoracic surgery requiring one-lung ventilation. Crit Care Res Pract. 2012;2012:687018.

152. Zhang J, Chen CQ, Lei XZ, Feng ZY, Zhu SM. Goal-directed fluid optimization based on stroke volume variation and cardiac index during one-lung ventilation in patients undergoing thoracoscopy lobectomy operations: a pilot study. Clinics (Sao Paulo). 2013;68(7):1065–70.

153. Georger JF, Hamzaoui O, Chaari A, Maizel J, Richard C, Teboul JL. Restoring arterial pressure with norepinephrine improves muscle tissue oxygenation assessed by near-infrared spectroscopy in severely hypotensive septic patients. Intensive Care Med. 2010;36(11):1882–9.

154. Hamzaoui O, Georger JF, Monnet X, Ksouri H, Maizel J, Richard C, et al. Early administration of norepinephrine increases cardiac preload and cardiac output in septic patients with life-threatening hypotension. Crit Care. 2010;14(4):R142.

155. Wuethrich PY, Burkhard FC, Thalmann GN, Stueber F, Studer UE. Restrictive deferred hydration combined with preemptive norepinephrine infusion during radical cystectomy reduces post-

operative complications and hospitalization time: a randomized clinical trial. Anesthesiology. 2014;120(2):365–77.

156. Wuethrich PY, Studer UE, Thalmann GN, Burkhard FC. Intraoperative continuous norepinephrine infusion combined with restrictive deferred hydration significantly reduces the need for blood transfusion in patients undergoing open radical cystectomy: results of a prospective randomised trial. Eur Urol. 2014;66(2):352–60.

157. Brienza N, Giglio MT, Marucci M, Fiore T. Does perioperative hemodynamic optimization protect renal function in surgical patients? A meta-analytic study. Crit Care Med. 2009;37(6):2079–90.

158. Marjanovic G, Villain C, Juettner E, zur Hausen A, Hoeppner J, Hopt UT, et al. Impact of different crystalloid volume regimes on intestinal anastomotic stability. Ann Surg. 2009;249(2):181–5.

159. Schnuriger B, Inaba K, Wu T, Eberle BM, Belzberg H, Demetriades D. Crystalloids after primary colon resection and anastomosis at initial trauma laparotomy: excessive volumes are associated with anastomotic leakage. J Trauma. 2011;70(3):603–10.

160. Veelo DP, van Berge Henegouwen MI, Ouwehand KS, Geerts BF, Anderegg MC, van Dieren S, et al. Effect of goal-directed therapy on outcome after esophageal surgery: a quality improvement study. PLoS One. 2017;12(3):e0172806.

161. Glatz T, Kulemann B, Marjanovic G, Bregenzer S, Makowiec F, Hoeppner J. Postoperative fluid overload is a risk factor for adverse surgical outcome in patients undergoing esophagectomy for esophageal cancer: a retrospective study in 335 patients. BMC Surg. 2017;17(1):6.

162. Theodorou D, Drimousis PG, Larentzakis A, Papalois A, Toutouzas KG, Katsaragakis S. The effects of vasopressors on perfusion of gastric graft after esophagectomy. An experimental study. J Gastrointest Surg. 2008;12(9):1497–501.

163. Al-Rawi OY, Pennefather SH, Page RD, Dave I, Russell GN. The effect of thoracic epidural bupivacaine and an intravenous adrenaline infusion on gastric tube blood flow during esophagectomy. Anesth Analg. 2008;106(3):884–7. table of contents

164. Pathak D, Pennefather SH, Russell GN, Al Rawi O, Dave IC, Gilby S, et al. Phenylephrine infusion improves blood flow to the stomach during oesophagectomy in the presence of a thoracic epidural analgesia. Eur J Cardiothorac Surg. 2013;44(1):130–3.

Intraoperative Ventilation Strategies for Thoracic Surgery

Jennifer A. Macpherson

Key Points

- Ventilatory strategies for one-lung ventilation (OLV) should take into account preventing intraoperative hypoxemia, intraoperative alveolar stress, and postoperative ventilator-induced lung injury (VILI).
- Based on available evidence, it seems appropriate to limit tidal volumes and inflation pressures during OLV, providing high breathing frequencies are not needed and mild to moderate hypercapnia is not contraindicated.
- A lung-protective strategy utilizing low tidal volumes, ≤6 mL/kg of predicted body weight and preferable 4–5 mL/kg, and limited plateau inspiratory pressures (<25 cm H_2O) is clearly indicated for patients at high risk for postoperative pulmonary complications.
- With appropriate use of pressure and tidal volume alarms, either pressure- or volume-controlled ventilation may be used to deliver the desired tidal volume and plateau pressure.
- Intrinsic positive end-expiratory pressure (PEEP) is common with OLV (utilizing a double-lumen endotracheal tube), and caution is warranted when high respiratory rates (short exhalation times) are utilized. The addition of external PEEP does not consistently greatly improve oxygenation and has not been shown to reduce the incidence of VILI.
- Any PEEP used should be titrated for the individual patient.
- A lung-opening procedure (LOP) utilizing several breaths of high inspiratory and expiratory pressures may improve oxygenation, but the hemodynamic consequences of the maneuver must be considered. The use of a LOP after the institution of OLV may be warranted.

Introduction

While not all thoracic surgery requires specialized intraoperative ventilation, techniques that ventilate only a single lung are the hallmarks of anesthesia for this type of surgery. One-lung ventilation (OLV), with the collapse of the contralateral lung, greatly facilitates surgery within the thorax. With the development of video-assisted thoracoscopic surgery, the collapse of the lung on the operative side has become a necessity. OLV during these operations must ensure adequate gas exchange (arterial oxygenation and venous carbon dioxide removal), full contralateral lung deflation, and reduction of the incidence of postoperative pulmonary complications (PPC) and acute lung injury (ALI). This last concern has grown more important as it has become clear that prevention of ventilator-induced lung injury (VILI) is important in intensive care unit treatment of acute respiratory distress syndrome (ARDS) and ALI [1] (see Chaps. 10 and 42 for a discussion of the definitions and treatment of ALI and ARDS). It may not always be possible to fully achieve these three goals, and anesthesiologists' skills are required to determine the best compromise for each individual patient.

Postthoracotomy ALI, while not common, has a high mortality rate [2]. Early studies indicated a correlation with high intraoperative fluid administration [3], but subsequent

Recognition of Denham S. Ward, MD, author of the first edition chapter and on whose work this edit is based.

J. A. Macpherson (✉)
Department of Anesthesiology and Perioperative Medicine, The University of Rochester Medical Center, Rochester, NY, USA
e-mail: jennifer_macpherson@urmc.rochester.edu

studies have not shown as strong a correlation [4]. Although the causes are multifactorial [5–7], including a possible genetic predisposition [8], recent studies have pointed to intraoperative mechanical ventilation with large tidal volumes as an important risk factor [2, 4, 9–15]. In an observational study, Licker et al. [9] used historical controls to compare outcomes from a lung-protective ventilation protocol. The protocol resulted in a decrease of ALI from 3.7% to 0.9% ($P < 0.01$) and an odds ratio of 0.34 (95% confidence interval of 0.23–0.75) adjusted for the other significant risk factors of chronic alcohol consumption, chemoradiation therapy, more advanced cancer stage, pneumonectomy, and increased fluid administration. For complications less severe than postoperative ALI, the data may not be as clear. Blank et al. [13] in a retrospective analysis of 1019 cases found, using multivariate logistic regression modeling, that higher tidal volumes were associated with a *decrease* in PPC but an increase in driving pressure was associated with an increase in complications. However, they noted that positive end-expiratory pressure (PEEP) of ≥ 5 cm H_2O was used in fewer than half of the patients and that 73.3% of the patients were ventilated with a tidal volume (V_T) > 5 mL/kg of predicted body weight. Liu et al. [11] performed a meta-analysis of 11 studies (657 patients) and found that a protective ventilatory strategy (tidal volume ≤ 6 mL/kg) decreases the incidence of postoperative pulmonary complications (OR 0.29 95% CI 0.15–0.57).

While the chosen ventilation strategy clearly has an immediate effect on oxygenation, the potential for opposing effects as well as many other important patient and surgical factors has made it difficult to determine the single best ventilation mode or even predict the best mode for an individual patient. Because there are so many options for ventilator parameters, e.g., tidal volume (V_T), pressure-controlled ventilation (PCV), volume-controlled ventilation (VCV), PEEP, and lung-opening procedures (LOP), few studies are directly comparable. The clinician needs a deep understanding of ventilation and gas exchange physiology and potential lung injury mechanisms [1] to place the clinical and animal studies into context and to be equipped for making appropriate clinical decisions.

Physiology of One-Lung Mechanical Ventilation (See Chap. 6 for a More Complete Discussion)

Although there is specific terminology describing certain "modes" of ventilation (e.g., pressure-controlled, volume-controlled, inverse I/E ratio, etc.), mechanical ventilation, in a fully paralyzed patient without any spontaneous ventilatory effort, fundamentally provides a time-varying pressure waveform at the interface between the lung and its external environment. For thoracic surgery, this is invariably at the proximal end of the ventilated lumen of the double-lumen endotracheal tube. The resulting movement of gas into and out of the lung depends on both this waveform and the resistance and compliance of the lung, chest wall, and endotracheal tube (the reader is referred to Chap. 7 of *Nunn's Applied Respiratory Physiology* [16] for a full discussion of the physiology). Even more germane, the flow of gas into and out of the individual gas-exchanging units depends on the relative airway resistance and alveolar compliance of each unit.

While this pressure waveform can be quite complex, obviously the key characteristic is a cyclic variation in pressure through a cycle of high (inspiration) to low (expiration). Several basic clinical measurements describe this waveform, including peak and plateau inspiratory pressure, inspiratory and expiratory times, inspiratory (tidal) volume, and end-expiratory pressure. This waveform not only determines the distribution of gas in the lung but, through changes in pulmonary vascular resistance and intrathoracic pressure, will influence regional perfusion and total cardiac output. The latter can become quite important during OLV, since the unventilated lung creates an obligate shunt and the oxygen level in the venous admixture directly determines arterial oxygenation.

While modern double-lumen endotracheal tubes and bronchial blockers, combined with the routine use of fiberoptic flexible bronchoscopy, have greatly reduced the incidence of hypoxemia during OLV [13–18], the selection of the mechanical ventilation mode clearly still plays a role. Hypoxemia during OLV is caused by venous admixture through shunts and areas of low ventilation/perfusion ratio (V/Q) gas-exchanging units. Thus, during OLV the collapsed lung is an obligate shunt, while the dependent lung also causes a venous admixture through shunt and areas of low V/Q. This is primarily through atelectatic areas of the lung seen with general anesthesia [19] and is perhaps increased with the lateral decubitus position through the weight of the mediastinum, abdominal organs, and low compliance of the chest wall in the dependent position [20, 21]. The ventilation strategy should therefore minimize perfusion to the collapsed lung and reduce areas of low V/Q in the ventilated lung. Since gas exchange not only involves providing adequate oxygenation but also adequate removal of CO_2, the total alveolar ventilation required is determined by the desired P_aCO_2. These considerations have resulted in the classic recommendation that tidal volume for OLV not be reduced (preventing atelectasis and maintaining elimination of CO_2) and the two-lung minute ventilation be maintained, often resulting in normocapnia to moderate hypocapnia with typical tidal volumes of 10 mL/kg. In this situation, the addition of PEEP causes a decrease in cardiac output and an increase in venous admixture, Fig. 22.1 [22].

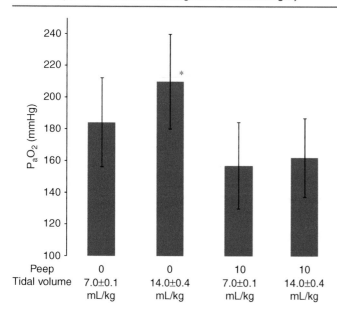

Fig. 22.1 Effect of 10 cm H_2O of positive end-expiratory pressure at tidal volumes of 8% and 16% of total lung capacity (approximately 7 and 17 mL/kg) during one-lung ventilation (OLV) (mean ± SEM, $n = 11$). Mean P_aCO_2 during all conditions was 35–38 mmHg. *$P < 0.05$ different from the other conditions by two-way ANOVA. P_aO_2 arterial oxygen partial pressure; FiO_2 fractional concentration of inspired oxygen; QT cardiac output; and QS/QT physiological shunt. (Based on data from Katz et al. [21])

Table 22.1 Effects of different ventilatory strategies on the determinants of arterial oxygenation

Determinants of arterial oxygen content	Effect of changes in ventilation
P_{50} of the hemoglobin dissociation curve	Increased ventilation will cause a respiratory alkalosis, left shifting the curve ($\downarrow P_{50}$). While this may increase arterial saturation, unloading of oxygen in the tissue may be impaired
	Decreased ventilation will cause a respiratory acidosis, right shifting the curve ($\uparrow P_{50}$). While this may decrease the arterial content when the P_aO_2 is low, this may be offset by the increased ease of unloading O_2 at the tissue (increased tissue PO_2)
Arterial carbon dioxide (P_aCO_2)	Hyperventilation lowers the P_aCO_2 and, for a given inspired oxygen tension (FiO_2), will increase the alveolar oxygen (P_AO_2), while hypercapnia will lower the P_AO_2. These are relatively small effects except at the extremes of P_aCO_2
Total cardiac output (Q_t)	Increased ventilation requires a higher mean alveolar pressure which can reduce the cardiac output via a decreased venous return and increased right ventricular afterload
Blood flow through the unventilated lung (Q_s)	Increased ventilation and/or increased PEEP to the dependent lung (higher mean alveolar pressure) may cause more blood to be diverted away from the ventilated lung and increase the blood flow to the unventilated lung
Blood flow through the unventilated (atelectatic or low V/Q) areas of the ventilated lung	Lower tidal volumes and/or ZEEP (zero end-expiratory pressure) may result in more atelectasis and shunt in the ventilated lung

Traditionally, the avoidance and treatment of arterial hypoxemia have been the essential concern of anesthesiologists during thoracic surgery with OLV [19]. Using the classic three-compartment model of gas exchange, the determinants of arterial oxygen content are hemoglobin concentration, hemoglobin dissociation curve (P_{50}), oxygen consumption, total cardiac output (Q_t) [23, 24], inspired oxygen fraction (FiO_2) and arterial carbon dioxide (P_aCO_2) (both of which determine the alveolar oxygen level, P_AO_2), blood flow through the unventilated lung, and unventilated (or low V/Q) areas of the ventilated lung [19, 24]. The latter two factors are often lumped together as shunt (Q_s) or shunt fraction (Q_s/Q_t) [25]; however, when considering the effects of ventilation on arterial oxygenation during OLV, it is often better to consider the blood flow through the unventilated lung ($V/Q = 0$) separately from the ventilation of the low V/Q areas of the ventilated lung, since ventilation strategy may have opposing effects on these causes of venous admixture. Changes in ventilation have both direct and indirect effects on these factors (Table 22.1). The first counter to hypoxemia during OLV is to utilize an FiO_2 of 100%, and many anesthesiologists use 100% FiO_2 routinely for OLV. The high-inspired oxygen concentration will reduce any residual hypoxic pulmonary vasoconstriction and increase P_AO_2 in the ventilated lung [26]. While concerns have been expressed about the absorption atelectasis caused by high FiO_2 and the possibility of oxidative damage to the lung, neither of these

factors have been explicitly studied as a possible contributor to postoperative ALI. Utilizing continuous positive airway pressure to the unventilated lung, while not possible in many procedures, e.g., video-assisted thoracotomy (VATS), this maneuver most often will ameliorate any significant hypoxemia [19, 27]. Since selection of the FiO_2 and the use of continuous positive airway pressure are not ventilatory strategies, they will not be discussed further in this chapter.

By not decreasing total V_T during OLV, the distension of the ventilated lung is essentially doubled. That is, if two-lung total ventilation is typically a V_T of 10 mL/kg (5 mL/kg/lung) with a rate of 8–12 breaths/minute, going to OLV would be the equivalent of increasing the total tidal volume to 20 mL/kg when still ventilating two lungs. With the increasing use of a lung-protective strategy of $V_T < 6$ mL/kg for two-lung ventilation, decreasing V_T by half for OLV may be unnecessary, as alveolar recruitment occurs without significant increase in plateau pressures [1, 12–14]. In addition, the distribution of ventilation is not uniform and is determined by regional airway resistance and alveolar; thus low-resistance, high-compliance alveoli may be greatly overdistended by

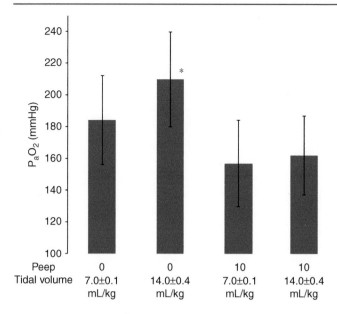

Fig. 22.1 Effect of 10 cm H_2O of positive end-expiratory pressure at tidal volumes of 8% and 16% of total lung capacity (approximately 7 and 17 mL/kg) during one-lung ventilation (OLV) (mean ± SEM, $n = 11$). Mean P_aCO_2 during all conditions was 35–38 mmHg. *$P < 0.05$ different from the other conditions by two-way ANOVA. P_aO_2 arterial oxygen partial pressure; FiO_2 fractional concentration of inspired oxygen; QT cardiac output; and QS/QT physiological shunt. (Based on data from Katz et al. [21])

Table 22.1 Effects of different ventilatory strategies on the determinants of arterial oxygenation

Determinants of arterial oxygen content	Effect of changes in ventilation
P_{50} of the hemoglobin dissociation curve	Increased ventilation will cause a respiratory alkalosis, left shifting the curve ($\downarrow P_{50}$). While this may increase arterial saturation, unloading of oxygen in the tissue may be impaired
	Decreased ventilation will cause a respiratory acidosis, right shifting the curve ($\uparrow P_{50}$). While this may decrease the arterial content when the P_aO_2 is low, this may be offset by the increased ease of unloading O_2 at the tissue (increased tissue PO_2)
Arterial carbon dioxide (P_aCO_2)	Hyperventilation lowers the P_aCO_2 and, for a given inspired oxygen tension (FiO_2), will increase the alveolar oxygen (P_AO_2), while hypercapnia will lower the P_AO_2. These are relatively small effects except at the extremes of P_aCO_2
Total cardiac output (Q_t)	Increased ventilation requires a higher mean alveolar pressure which can reduce the cardiac output via a decreased venous return and increased right ventricular afterload
Blood flow through the unventilated lung (Q_s)	Increased ventilation and/or increased PEEP to the dependent lung (higher mean alveolar pressure) may cause more blood to be diverted away from the ventilated lung and increase the blood flow to the unventilated lung
Blood flow through the unventilated (atelectatic or low V/Q) areas of the ventilated lung	Lower tidal volumes and/or ZEEP (zero end-expiratory pressure) may result in more atelectasis and shunt in the ventilated lung

Traditionally, the avoidance and treatment of arterial hypoxemia have been the essential concern of anesthesiologists during thoracic surgery with OLV [19]. Using the classic three-compartment model of gas exchange, the determinants of arterial oxygen content are hemoglobin concentration, hemoglobin dissociation curve (P_{50}), oxygen consumption, total cardiac output (Q_t) [23, 24], inspired oxygen fraction (FiO_2) and arterial carbon dioxide (P_aCO_2) (both of which determine the alveolar oxygen level, P_AO_2), blood flow through the unventilated lung, and unventilated (or low V/Q) areas of the ventilated lung [19, 24]. The latter two factors are often lumped together as shunt (Q_s) or shunt fraction (Q_s/Q_t) [25]; however, when considering the effects of ventilation on arterial oxygenation during OLV, it is often better to consider the blood flow through the unventilated lung ($V/Q = 0$) separately from the ventilation of the low V/Q areas of the ventilated lung, since ventilation strategy may have opposing effects on these causes of venous admixture. Changes in ventilation have both direct and indirect effects on these factors (Table 22.1). The first counter to hypoxemia during OLV is to utilize an FiO_2 of 100%, and many anesthesiologists use 100% FiO_2 routinely for OLV. The high-inspired oxygen concentration will reduce any residual hypoxic pulmonary vasoconstriction and increase P_AO_2 in the ventilated lung [26]. While concerns have been expressed about the absorption atelectasis caused by high FiO_2 and the possibility of oxidative damage to the lung, neither of these factors have been explicitly studied as a possible contributor to postoperative ALI. Utilizing continuous positive airway pressure to the unventilated lung, while not possible in many procedures, e.g., video-assisted thoracotomy (VATS), this maneuver most often will ameliorate any significant hypoxemia [19, 27]. Since selection of the FiO_2 and the use of continuous positive airway pressure are not ventilatory strategies, they will not be discussed further in this chapter.

By not decreasing total V_T during OLV, the distension of the ventilated lung is essentially doubled. That is, if two-lung total ventilation is typically a V_T of 10 mL/kg (5 mL/kg/lung) with a rate of 8–12 breaths/minute, going to OLV would be the equivalent of increasing the total tidal volume to 20 mL/kg when still ventilating two lungs. With the increasing use of a lung-protective strategy of $V_T < 6$ mL/kg for two-lung ventilation, decreasing V_T by half for OLV may be unnecessary, as alveolar recruitment occurs without significant increase in plateau pressures [1, 12–14]. In addition, the distribution of ventilation is not uniform and is determined by regional airway resistance and alveolar; thus low-resistance, high-compliance alveoli may be greatly overdistended by

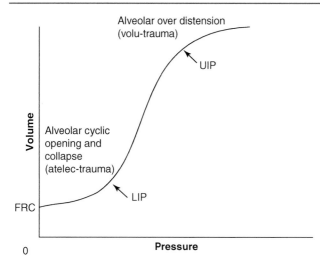

Fig. 22.2 Idealized lung pressure-volume curve. Under anesthesia, the functional residual capacity (FRC) falls too close to the residual volume, potentially causing a relatively noncompliant lung at low airway pressures as atelectatic regions of the lung are opened. At high airway pressures, the limits of distensibility may be reached. The lower inflection point (LIP) represents the pressure when the compliance increases as all atelectatic regions are opened; the upper inflection point (UIP) represents the pressure when alveoli are becoming less compliant due to overdistension

such high tidal volumes. The pressure-volume curve for the whole lung has an idealized sigmoid shape (Fig. 22.2). The relatively low compliance at low pressures represents the pressure needed to inflate the atelectatic collapsed portions of the lung, and the flatter, less compliant portion at high pressures represents the limits of elasticity. Tidal volumes at the lower end of the curve (no PEEP) may involve opening and closing atelectatic areas of the lung (atelectrauma); tidal volumes at the upper end (high PEEP) may cause barotrauma. However, Slinger et al. [27] actually measured the single-lung compliance curve, and while approximately a quarter of their patients did not have a lower inflection point, at volumes of 1500 mL or a maximum pressure of 30 cm H_2O, there was no decrease in compliance (no upper inflection point).

Modes of Mechanical Ventilation for OLV in the Operating Room

While modern operating room ventilators have a wide range of settings, a primary variation between ventilator types is the pressure waveform generated by a constant inspiratory *pressure* vs. a waveform generated by a constant inspiratory *flow*. These types are commonly referred to as pressure-controlled ventilators (PCV) and volume-controlled ventilators (VCV). The resulting V_T may be the same, but the pressure and flow waveforms are quite different, although when the constant flow ventilator is used with an

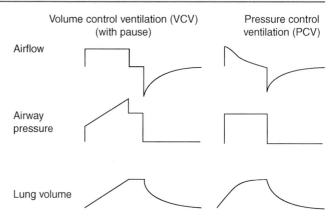

Fig. 22.3 Pressure, flow, and volume generated by constant flow or volume-controlled ventilation (VCV) (left) and constant pressure or pressure-controlled ventilation (PCV) (right). The constant flow ventilator incorporates an end-inspiratory pause, resulting in peak and plateau pressures, while the constant pressure ventilator only has a plateau pressure. With PCV, the airflow constantly declines from the initial maximum

end-inspiratory pause, the differences in the change in lung volume with time are not as pronounced (Fig. 22.3). There are three main areas of controversy in selecting the ventilation mode for OLV: (1) pressure vs. volume ventilation, (2) high vs. low tidal volume, and (3) use of PEEP. Until recently, most studies focused on which mode would most improve oxygenation. However, the use of modern double-lumen tubes (DLTs) or bronchial blockers correctly positioned with bronchoscopic confirmation has actually greatly reduced the incidence of clinically significant hypoxia [18]. Since the pulse oximeter permits continuous monitoring, saturations in the high 80s are frequently well tolerated (by both the patient and the anesthesiologist) during OLV. Current research has thus focused more on the ventilator mode, primarily high vs. low tidal volume, to prevent PPC and ALI.

Pressure- Versus Volume-Controlled Ventilation

The two primary modes of ventilation commonly used in the operating room are either PCV or VCV. Short-term effects of PCV or VCV on oxygenation during OLV as well as possible effects of VILI postoperatively are controversial. No definitive studies can conclusively provide specific recommendations. As can be seen from Fig. 22.3, the difference in the waveforms produced by the modes results from the decreasing airflow with PCV, when compared with the constant airflow with VCV. By adding an end-inspiratory pause to VCV, the volume trajectories of the two modes are not too dissimilar. Figure 22.4 illustrates the airway and average alveolar pressures that are generated by each of the two waveforms. The peak pressure generated by VCV for a given tidal volume

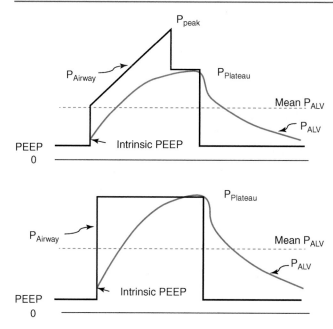

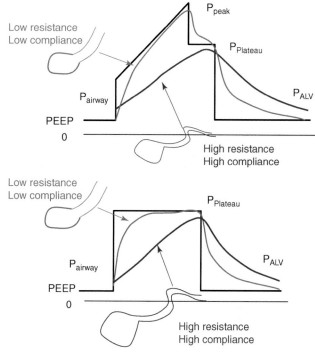

Fig. 22.4 Comparison of the airway (P_{airway}, black line) and alveolar (P_{ALV}, red line) pressures for VCV (top) and pressure-controlled ventilation (bottom). For VCV, both a peak (P_{peak}) and a plateau ($P_{Plateau}$) are observed. The difference between these pressures represents the resistance to gas flow. The PCV has only a plateau pressure

Fig. 22.5 The distribution of inspiratory pressure to different areas of the lung with different time constants for VCV (top) and PCV (bottom)

is due to both airway resistance and compliance, and the plateau pressure is due to the dynamic compliance (the difference between the peak and plateau pressure is determined by the airway resistance and flow). The plateau pressure for both modes is representative of the average maximum alveolar pressure and the resulting tidal volume. The mean airway pressure (the time-averaged pressure over the whole inspiratory-expiratory cycle) determines the average lung inflation.

Another way of looking at the two modes is that PCV has a high peak inspiratory flow, which is limited in VCV, while VCV has a high peak airway pressure that is limited in PCV. Although primarily based on animal studies, both high peak inspiratory flows [28] and high peak airway pressures [29] may contribute to VILI. By limiting the tidal volume and maintaining an adequate inspiratory time, both these factors can be minimized for either PCV or VCV. It is important to note that in acutely injured and inflamed lungs, the heterogeneity of the compliance, airflow resistance, and capillary blood flow of alveolar units result in a very uneven distribution of airflow, volume, and pressure throughout the respiratory cycle (Fig. 22.5). This may cause gross overinflation (volutrauma) of some units even though the airway pressure and total tidal volume are both limited. Both VCV with an end-inspiratory pause and PCV may permit a better distribution of the inspiration across alveolar-capillary units with

different airflow time constants because of the relatively longer time at full inspiration. However, this distribution fundamentally requires an adequately long total inspiratory time. This lengthened inspiratory time may be difficult during OLV because of the conflict between the need to increase the respiratory rate (to compensate for the lower tidal volumes now recommended) and the concern about development of intrinsic PEEP as the expiratory time becomes crowded out (see next sections of this chapter).

Prella et al. [30] found that in patients with ARDS, the use of PCV permits lower peak airway pressures when tidal volumes of 9 mL/kg are used. However, no differences in blood gas values were observed. Although not commonly available in the operating room, VCV with a decreasing inspiratory flow pattern (rather than the constant inspiratory flow pattern shown in Fig. 22.3) seems to provide all the advantages of PCV but limits the possible damaging effects of the initial high peak flow seen with PCV [31–33].

There have been a few direct comparisons of VCV and PCV in laparoscopic surgery [34, 35] and in thoracic surgery [36–39]. In general, these studies have shown either no or only small improvement in oxygenation with PCV over VCV. All studies for OLV used relatively large tidal volumes (9–10 mL/kg) with resulting normocapnia to mild hypocapnia. Among the four studies, only Tugrul et al. [38] showed a significant statistical improvement in P_aO_2, and that improvement was not clinically significant since the average S_aO_2 was above 98% with either mode. All studies used a 10% inspiratory pause during VCV. The addition of an end-inspiratory pause in this type of ventilation can help with distribution of the inspired gas and improve oxygenation, but, particularly in patients with chronic obstructive pulmonary disease undergoing OLV, a reduction in expiratory time to accommodate the end-inspiratory pause may increase intrinsic PEEP and reduce oxygenation [40]. No clinical studies have looked at PCV vs. VCV for prevention of post-thoracotomy lung injury. A meta-analysis of research about mechanical ventilation strategies during OLV published by Liu et al. [11] concluded that current data are insufficient to determine any decreased risk of postoperative lung injury when using PCV as opposed to VCV.

Monitoring for changes in airway pressure for VCV and in tidal volume for PCV can provide important early warning indicators of a malpositioned DLT. A possible advantage of PCV is that the tidal volume alarms can be set for increases or decreases from the current tidal volume. An increase in resistance or compliance (e.g., a left-sided DLT migrating into the left lower lobe during left lung ventilation) would cause a decrease in the delivered volume (for the set pressure) and would thereby sound the low-volume alarm. Alternately, a leak from the left side to right (e.g., from a leak around the bronchial cuff into the left lung when ventilating the right lung with a left DLT) would cause an increase in the delivered volume (but often a decrease in the returned volume, resulting in the bellows of the ventilator not completely filling if the fresh gas flow is low enough). For VCV, the airway pressure would increase if the left-sided DLT migrated into the left lower lobe orifice, but for a partial leak, only the loss of the full return volume would cause an alarm. Whichever mode is used, the anesthesiologist should carefully set the appropriate alarms close to the volume currently being delivered and understand the likely causes for any alarm activation. A timely response to an alarm, by repositioning the DLT under bronchoscopic guidance, can often prevent desaturation or unwanted inflation of the operative lung.

High Versus Low Tidal Volume

In a patient with ARDS, there is strong evidence that a lung-protective strategy improves outcomes [41–43] although Putensen et al. [43] have pointed out that there are still only a limited number of randomized controlled trials. This lung-protective strategy may include tidal volume of <6 mL/kg and plateau pressure below 25 cm H_2O, with the respiratory frequency adjusted to maintain CO_2 elimination (normocapnia to mild hypercapnia) and PEEP as needed to improve oxygenation without increasing the plateau pressure above

30 cm H_2O. This ventilation strategy is intended to prevent both the cyclic opening and closing of collapsed alveoli at the start of inspiration (atelectrauma) as well as the overdistension (barotrauma) of some alveoli at the end of inspiration (Fig. 22.5) [44–46]. The mild to moderate hypercapnia and respiratory acidosis induced by this strategy are not thought to be harmful [47, 48], and may even have some beneficial effects [49]. The basic mechanisms for low tidal volumes providing protection are not entirely known, but the prevention of the induction of a pulmonary and systemic inflammatory response seems to be the common pathway [30, 50–52]. Of interest, there is increasing evidence that a further reduction in tidal volume may be beneficial even when the P_{peak} is less than 30 cm H_2O [53] and a significant hypercapnia can be tolerated.

A low tidal volume protective strategy is not without drawbacks. In the PROVHILO trial [53], it was reported that the low tidal volumes in combination with high PEEP (12 cm H_2O) and LOPs led to an increased incidence of intraoperative hypotension and use of vasoactive medications without any decrease in PPC compared to low PEEP (2 cm H_2O). Although this study was not in thoracic patients, it might be expected that in OLV, with its obligate increased shunt, any decrease in cardiac output could cause significant hypoxemia. However, Ferrando and Belda [54] utilized a PEEP decrement trial to individualize PEEP (average of 10 cm H_2O) which did not decrease the cardiac index relative to the control group (fixed PEEP of 5 cm H_2O).

One point does need clarification, and that is whether the tidal volume is expressed as mL per actual or per PBW. Since lung volume is more closely related to height than body weight, using actual body weight may result in particularly large tidal volumes in short, obese individuals. It is better to set the tidal volume on the basis of PBW. PBW is calculated in males as PBW (kg) $= 50 + 2.3$ (height (in) -60) and in females as PBW (kg) $= 45.5 + 2.3$ (height (in) -60) [55]. The tidal volume recommendations in this chapter are based on PBW.

Although the anesthesiologist may be more concerned about acute intraoperative hypoxemia [19], the not infrequent rate of ARDS or ALI following thoracic surgery [4, 5, 10, 56, 57] has brought into focus the question of using a lung-protective strategy during OLV [58]. While the use of such a strategy during OLV has been controversial [59, 60], a recent large observational study [15] and other smaller clinical studies examining risk factors for ALI following OLV [3, 9] support the use of such a protective strategy. Fernández-Pérez et al. [4] found an odds ratio for postoperative respiratory failure after pneumonectomy of 1.56 (95% confidence interval of 1.12–2.23) per each mL/kg of PBW (Fig. 22.6).

However, the use of lower V_T during anesthesia has been implicated in the development of intraoperative atelectasis

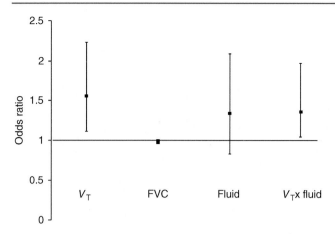

Fig. 22.6 Risk factors associated with postpneumonectomy acute lung injury. Odds ratio and 95% confidence interval from multivariate logistic regression analysis: V_T (tidal volume) is per each mL/kg predicted body weight; FVC (forced vital capacity) is for each percent decline; fluid is for each liter of fluid infused intraoperatively; and $V_T \times$ fluid is the cross product in the logistic regression model. (Based on data from Fernández-Pérez et al. [4])

which may contribute to both intraoperative hypoxemia and postoperative lung injury [60]. Levin et al. [61] in a large retrospective study found that a low tidal volume with minimal PEEP actually increased the 30-day mortality and suggested that a low tidal volume strategy is helpful only with used with PEEP.

The role of V_T in influencing the development of lung or systemic inflammatory markers in patients without ALI undergoing short-term mechanical ventilation has been investigated in several studies, with some finding a correlation [60, 62, 63] but others not finding that high tidal volumes had a pro-inflammatory effect [61]. In addition, other factors may also play a role in the development of inflammatory markers following OLV [63–66], including genetics [62, 66], the length of time of OLV [67, 68], and the patient's capacity to handle an oxidative stress [69].

The recommendations for low tidal volumes even in patients without ALI [70, 71] are based on the observed synergistic effects of high tidal volume with other lung injuries that might by themselves be subclinical ("two hit" hypothesis) [72]. This is clearest in situations where the second lung injury occurs during high tidal volume ventilation in previously healthy lungs or in a patient with developing ALI [70]. It is not as clear if the same synergism applies when the nonprotective ventilation occurs for a short period of time (intraoperative) and precedes rather than is concurrent with a second event that could cause lung injury.

Until there is a definite prospective clinical trial of sufficient size to decide the question, several factors must be considered when deciding the best strategy to use. First, as noted previously, OLV requires relatively high tidal volumes to a single lung to ensure even normocapnia to moderate

hypercapnia. The recommended lung-protective ventilation of 6 mL/kg is only 3 mL/kg/lung. Thus, with two-lung ventilation, 6 mL/kg may require a frequency of 12–16 breaths/min to maintain moderate hypercapnia (P_aCO_2 40–55 mmHg); initiating OLV and maintaining the 3 mL/kg/lung tidal volume may require a frequency of over 20 breaths/min and still may result in excessive hypercapnia. This rapid rate, together with the high-resistance DLT, may not permit adequate exhale time, and excessive intrinsic positive end-expiratory pressure (PEEPi) may occur [73]. The best current recommendation is to use a lower V_T, < 6 mL/kg (PBW) and preferably 4–5 mL/kg if moderate hypercapnia can be maintained without excessively rapid ventilatory rates.

Positive End-Expiratory Pressure

The use of PEEP is a mainstay for increasing oxygenation in patients with ARDS or ALI [74]. It can also be useful in preventing cyclic opening and closing of atelectatic areas of the lung (see Figs. 22.2 and 22.7), thus potentially reducing VILI in these patients. By increasing the functional residual capacity, PEEP can prevent the closure of alveoli at the end of expiration and accomplish both an increase in oxygenation and a reduction of VILI. However, the optimal level of PEEP for both objectives is still controversial [75]. The ARDS Clinical Trials Network investigators found no difference in outcomes in patients with ARDS with either low PEEP (8.3 ± 3.2 cm H_2O) or higher PEEP (13.2 ± 3.5 cm H_2O) adjusted to maintain oxygenation [75]; subsequent studies have confirmed this finding [76, 77]. However, there is still no clear means of determining the "optimal" PEEP in ARDS/ALI [67], and there may even be subgroups that would particularly benefit from a higher level of PEEP (while maintaining the peak airway pressure below 30 cm H_2O) [77, 78].

The factors considered for selecting PEEP for the ventilated lung in OLV differ from the factors determining PEEP in ARDS/ALI patients. First is the level of intrinsic PEEP (PEEPi) that is already present; second is the fact that the presence of the large shunt fraction in OLV is due to the blocked ventilation to the nondependent lung rather than to the heterogeneous lung injury in ARDS. Intrinsic PEEP results from incomplete emptying of the lung back to its passive recoil equilibrium by the start of the next inspiration (end exhale) and can result from factors related both to the patient (lung resistance and compliance) and to the mechanical ventilation (endotracheal tube expiratory resistance, tidal volume, and exhale time). Patients undergoing thoracic surgery with OLV are at risk for developing PEEPi (Fig. 22.8a) [80, 81]. However, the magnitude of PEEPi is not correlated with P_aO_2 during OLV (Fig. 22.8b) [79, 80]. It is important to remember that the magnitude of PEEPi is not indicated on the usual airway pressure manometer, but requires a special

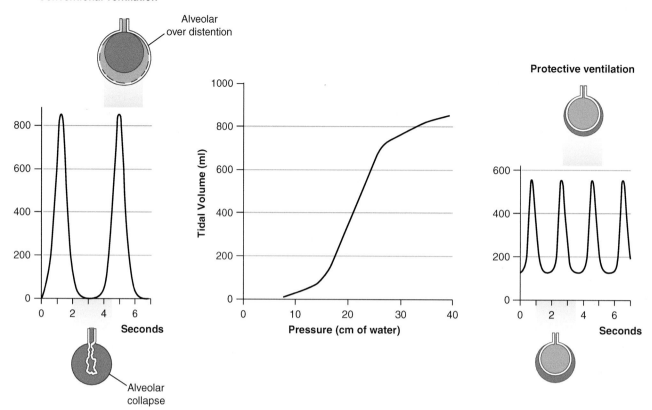

Fig. 22.7 The pressure-volume curve shown in the middle represents the compliance curve of a patient with acute respiratory distress syndrome. At low volumes, compliance is increased because of alveolar collapse, and at high volumes, it is decreased because of overdistension. In the illustration, these inflection points occur at 14 and 26 cm H_2O, respectively. With conventional high tidal volume (12 mL/kg) and no PEEP, alveoli collapse and are overdistended on every breath (left). With low tidal volumes (6 mL/kg) plus PEEP (LIP plus 2 cm H_2O), the tidal volume range stays in the nondistended, noncollapsed region (right). Note the increase in respiratory frequency with low tidal volume to maintain CO_2 elimination. (Reprinted with permission from Tobin [44]. © 2001 Massachusetts Medical Society. All rights reserved)

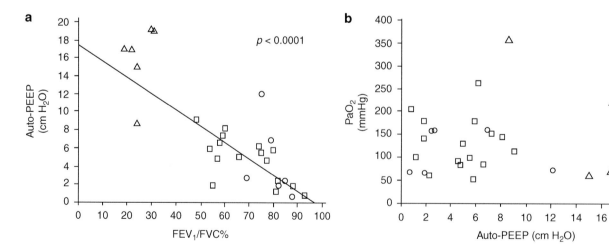

Fig. 22.8 The amount of intrinsic positive end-expiratory pressure (auto-PEEP) was measured in patients with moderate or no obstructive lung disease (open circle), severe emphysema (open triangle), or severe fibrotic lung disease (open square) during OLV with tidal volumes of 10 mL/kg and respiratory rates of 10–12. The amount of PEEPi was inversely related to FEV1/FVC% (**a**). PaO_2 was not correlated with PEEPi (**b**). (Reprinted from Ducros et al. [79]. © 1999 with permission from Elsevier)

maneuver to determine its presence [82, 83]. Additional factors to be considered include the relationship between PEEP and total cardiac output and relative blood flow between the ventilated and unventilated lungs. As PEEP is increased, the average alveolar pressure increases and causes compression of the pulmonary vasculature, increasing the pulmonary vascular resistance in the ventilated lung. This increased resistance may cause more blood to flow to the nonventilated lung, resulting in a greater venous admixture. In addition, the increased afterload on the right heart and increased intrathoracic pressure may decrease total cardiac output and reduce the mixed venous oxygen hemoglobin saturation, also resulting in an increased venous admixture. These negative effects of PEEP are countered by the improved oxygenation of the ventilated lung by assuring more open alveoli. It is not surprising that clinical studies of the effects of PEEP on arterial oxygenation during OLV have shown conflicting results [25, 79]. Current evidence does show that high tidal volume ventilation without PEEP causes injury, but low tidal volume ventilation without adequate PEEP may also [61].

Early studies of the best ventilatory pattern during OLV indicated that external PEEP tended to decrease P_aO_2; in these studies, the best ventilatory strategy was for relatively large tidal volumes and no PEEP to the ventilated lung (Fig. 22.1) [22] unless continuous positive airway pressure with oxygen was applied to the unventilated lung [27]. More recent studies have generally confirmed this finding [83, 84], although there may be subgroups in which PEEP will improve oxygenation [85–89].

Ferrando et al. [54] investigated individualizing PEEP compared to a standardized 5 cm H_2O. They utilized a LOP upon initiation of OLV with subsequent VCV adjusted to a plateau pressure of ≤25 cm H_2O in both groups. The individualized PEEP was selected by decrementing PEEP from 20 cm H_2O to determine the PEEP that yielded the maximum dynamic compliance. The resulting individualized PEEP was 10 ± 2. Oxygenation was high in the individualized PEEP group both during and after OLV without a difference in cardiac index. However, since 100% oxygen was used, no patient in either group was hypoxemic.

Since PEEPi is so common in OLV, it is important to understand the complex relationship between external PEEP and PEEPi: actual total PEEP is different from applied, measured PEEP, depending on preexisting PEEPi [80, 81]. The interaction between applied PEEP and PEEPi is not straightforward, although it is apparent from the study by Slinger and Hickey [73] that total PEEP does not increase greatly beyond PEEPi until the added PEEP approaches the value of PEEPi. It has been suggested that applying an external PEEP equal to PEEPi results in the best oxygenation [85], but PEEPi is not readily measurable in the operating room. Slinger et al. clarified the effects of PEEP on oxygenation in a study measuring the static lung compliance curve [27]. By

measuring the static compliance curve, the lower inflection point (Fig. 22.2) could be identified. Without the application of external PEEP, the lower inflection point was 4.5 ± 3.5 cm H_2O, but no lower inflection point could be identified in 24% of the 42 patients studied. The value of the lower inflection point was not significantly changed by the addition of 5 cm H_2O of external PEEP. When patients were ventilated with a tidal volume of 10 mL/kg at a rate of 10 breaths/min, the measured PEEPi was 4.2 ± 3.4 cm H_2O, and the total PEEP with 5 cm H_2O added externally was 6.8 ± 1.8 cm H_2O.

Overall, no significant improvement in oxygenation was observed with the addition of PEEP. However, improvements in oxygenation were seen when total PEEP was closest to the lower inflection point. Thus, external PEEP improved oxygenation depending on the relationship between the lower inflection point, intrinsic PEEP, and total PEEP at the time external PEEP was added. The minority of patients benefiting from external PEEP had a larger lower inflection point pressure and had good elastic recoil. Presumably this good recoil resulted in an end-expiratory lung volume in the dependent lung during OLV below the normal functional residual capacity with resulting atelectasis and increased vascular resistance.

Lung Opening Procedures

Atelectasis commonly occurs even in healthy lungs under general anesthesia, and the cyclic opening and closing of atelectatic areas of the lungs (Fig. 22.7) during mechanical ventilation may contribute to VILI (atelectrauma) [60]. Even with a lung-protective ventilation strategy, it may be necessary to periodically apply higher pressures, on both inspiration and end-expiration, to open atelectatic areas of the lung [90]. Such maneuvers are often called "alveolar recruitment" or "lung opening" maneuvers [91]. While such a strategy may improve oxygenation in the heterogeneously inflamed lung of ARDS, there may not be any decrease in mortality when combined with established low-tidal volume lung-protective ventilation [76, 92].

The use of an open-lung procedure during OLV has been proposed, not to reduce VILI by prevention of atelectrauma but rather to prevent or treat intraoperative hypoxemia. As with the use of PEEP, in OLV the open-lung procedure in a noninflamed lung is quite different from its use in ARDS or ALI. However, areas of atelectasis in the dependent lung may benefit from a lung-opening procedure. While the details of the procedure vary somewhat, in essence it consists of several breaths (often 6–10) at an inspiratory pressure of 40 cm H_2O and a PEEP of 20 cm H_2O. There is also a several-breath "ramp-up" to these high pressures. Tusman et al. [92] found that such a lung recruitment procedure, when combined with a tidal volume of 6 mL/kg (peak pressures less than 30 cm H_2O), respiratory rate of 15–18, and a PEEP of 8 cm H_2O, significantly increased P_aO_2 (see Chap. 6, Fig. 6.8). Subsequently, Cinnella et al. studied the physiological effects of a lung recruitment procedure during OLV with a tidal volume of 8 mL/kg and a respiratory rate of 12 and found a similar lasting increase in P_aO_2 [93]. They also noted a decrease in cardiac output and mean arterial pressure during the maneuver, but the hemodynamic variables returned to baseline following the maneuver.

Conclusion

Anesthesiologists have many options to consider in determining the intraoperative ventilation, and there is no definite evidence supporting a single strategy to prevent intraoperative hypoxemia, intraoperative alveolar injury, and postoperative ALI. Brassard et al. [14] has provided one "step-by-step" approach to the management of OLV. Current evidence supports a strategy to maintain endinspiratory plateau pressures no greater than 30 cm H_2O, preferably less than 25 cm H_2O. To do so, tidal volume should be reduced to a range of $\leq$6 mL/kg of PBW during OLV, and respiratory rate increased to maintain normocapnia to moderate hypercapnia (P_aCO_2 in a range of 40–50 mmHg). Using the measured P_aCO_2 (the $P_{ET}CO_2$ can be used as a guide, but there is often a significant gradient between the two) greatly facilitates the adjustment of the ventilator, but an initial ventilator setting should be based on ideal or PBW, since lung volume is more closely related to height than to actual weight. Caution is warranted if the respiratory rate must be increased above the mid-teens, since excessive PEEPi may develop, causing a reduced cardiac output and hypoxemia. The initial use of low to moderate PEEP (4–8 cm H_2O) is probably unnecessary to maintain adequate oxygenation, but the use of low to moderate PEEP is often used to prevent atelectrauma and may reduce PPC. The individualization of PEEP may be necessary to optimize oxygenation. However, the actual total PEEP may not change significantly with the addition of low external PEEP because of the probable existence of PEEPi during OLV. Either PCV or VCV can be used, as long as proper monitoring for changes in airway pressure and tidal volume is maintained. This ventilation strategy should prevent intraoperative hypoxemia in most patients and may even reduce the incidence of postoperative VILI, particularly in high-risk situations (e.g., pneumonectomy, patients with a history of alcohol abuse, large intraoperative fluid requirements, men over 60 years old, longer OLV, fresh frozen plasma administration, and/or preexisting ALI). If intraoperative hypoxemia develops, then careful adjustment of PEEP and a lung-opening procedure can be tried. Of course, correct positioning of the DLT or bronchial blocker must be verified whenever there is hypoxemia during OLV, and continuous positive airway pressure with oxygen to the unventilated lung may be successful if compatible with the surgical procedure.

Clinical Case Discussion

A 72-year-old woman, with weight = 98 kg, height = 168 cm (BMI = 34.7, PBW = 60.3 kg), and a 43 pack-year smoking history (stopped smoking 2 weeks ago), presents for left upper lobectomy for small cell carcinoma via a left VATS. Past medical history includes hypertension, type 2 DM, and obstructive sleep apnea (CPAP at 10 cm H_2O nightly).

Preoperative pulmonary function testing showed:

- FVC = 2.82 L (57% predicted).
- FEV_1 = 1.58 (42% predicted).
- FEV_1/FVC = 56%.
- DLCO = 23.9 mL/min/mmHg (79% predicted).

A left 37 French DLT was placed without difficulty, and its correct position was confirmed via fiber-optic bronchoscopy. Two-lung ventilation was initiated, while the patient was supine with VCV incorporating a 10% end-inspiratory pause with a tidal volume of 550 mL and a rate of 10 breaths/min. Peak airway pressures were 22 cm H_2O and the $P_{ET}CO_2$ was 45 mmHg. SpO_2 = 98% on 100% oxygen.

(a) What mode of ventilation and inspiratory gas concentration would you use for initiating OLV? What tidal volume would you use?
   - Either PCV or VCV would be acceptable. Initial tidal volume should be set based on the PBW, typically at 4–6 mL/kg. 6 mL/kg × 60.3 kg PBW = 361 mL, so initial tidal volume should be reduced and the OLV peak and plateau pressures noted.

(b) After setting the tidal volume to 361 mL with a rate of 14 and 0 end-expiratory pressure (ZEEP), the peak inspiratory pressure is 28 cm H_2O, and the $P_{ET}CO_2$ is 49 mmHg. Is any further adjustment of the ventilator required? Would other clinical measurements be useful?
   - With the peak inspiratory pressure less than 30 mmHg (presumable if VCV is being used, the plateau pressure, which is more reflective of the alveolar distending pressure, will be less than the peak) and the end-tidal CO_2 at an acceptable level, no further adjustments are needed. Initially observing the end-tidal CO_2 ($P_{ET}CO_2$) can guide the respiratory rate setting, but a blood gas would be helpful because the increased alveolar dead space associated with this patient's COPD may result in a significant arterial to end-tidal gradient.

(c) What would your recommendation for PEEP be after making these adjustments?

- At low tidal volumes and in patients with ALI, PEEP may help reduce the opening and closing of atelectatic regions of the lung, improving oxygenation and possibly prevent further lung injury. However, a high PEEP may also reduce oxygenation during OLV by forcing more blood flow to the unventilated lung. PEEP up to 5 cm H_2O may be used but higher levels should be instituted cautiously.

(d) Thirty minutes after the start of OLV, S_pO_2 falls to 88%. What maneuvers could be employed to stabilize the S_pO_2?

- Whenever there is an acute decrease in the S_pO_2, after increasing the FiO_2, the position of the DLT must be carefully checked with a fiber-optic bronchoscopy. In this case entry of the left bronchial lumen into the left lower lobe orifice could result in the tracheal opening of the DLT to abut the carina and result in a decrease in right lung ventilation.

A lung opening procedure (LOP) with a few breaths of high PEEP and inspiratory pressure may also be of benefit, but caution must be exercised if there is any indication of hemodynamic instability.

If hypoxemia still persists after optimal positioning of the DLT and a LOP, then CPAP to the unventilated lung is the most reliable way of decreasing the venous admixture; however, this is unlikely to provide acceptable operating conditions for a VATS. Switching to PCV or increasing the end-inspiratory pause with VCV may be useful. With a large DLT and a respiratory rate of only 14, significant intrinsic PEEP is unlikely, but a reduction in the inspiratory rate (with perhaps an increase in the tidal volume) can be tried.

A blood gas should be obtained and the surgeon notified that it may be necessary to return to two-lung ventilation intermittently if the saturation falls any lower. Since a low cardiac output will cause hypoxemia during OLV, interventions to increase the cardiac output may be of value.

References

1. Lohser J, Slinger P. Lung injury after one-lung ventilation: A review of the pathophysiologic mechanisms affecting the ventilated and collapsed lung. Anesth Analg. 2015;121:302–18.
2. Slinger PD. Postpneumonectomy pulmonary edema: good news, bad news. Anesthesiology. 2006;105:2–5.
3. Zeldin RA, Normandin D, Landtwing D, Peters RM. Postpneumonectomy pulmonary edema. J Thorac Cardiovasc Surg. 1984;87:359–65.
4. Fernández-Pérez ER, Keegan MT, Brown DR, Hubmayr RD, Gajic O. Intraoperative tidal volume as a risk factor for respiratory failure after pneumonectomy. Anesthesiology. 2006;105:14–8.
5. Gothard J. Lung injury after thoracic surgery and one-lung ventilation. Curr Opin Anaesthesiol. 2006;19:5–10.
6. Baudouin SV. Lung injury after thoracotomy. Br J Anaesth. 2003;91:132–42.
7. Williams EA, Evans TW, Goldstraw P. Acute lung injury following lung resection: is one lung anaesthesia to blame? Thorax. 1996;51:114–6.
8. Gao L, Barnes KC. Recent advances in genetic predisposition to clinical acute lung injury. Am J Physiol Lung Cell Mol Physiol. 2009;296:L713–25.
9. Licker M, de Perrot M, Spiliopoulos A, et al. Risk factors for acute lung injury after thoracic surgery for lung cancer. Anesth Analg. 2003;97:1558–65.
10. Jeon K, Yoon JW, Suh GY, et al. Risk factors for post-pneumonectomy acute lung injury/acute respiratory distress syndrome in primary lung cancer patients. Anaesth Intensive Care. 2009;37:14–9.
11. Liu Z, Liu X, Huang Y, Zhao J. Intraoperative mechanical ventilation strategies in patients undergoing one-lung ventilation: a meta-analysis. Springerplus. 2016;5:1251.
12. Gulder A, Kiss T, Serpa Neto T, Hemmes SN, Canet j SPM, Rocco PR, Schultz MJ, Pelosi P, Gama de Abreu M. Intraoperative protective mechanical ventilation for prevention of postoperative pulmonary complications: A comprehensive review of the role of tidal volume, positive end-expiratory pressure, and lung recruitment maneuvers. Anesthesiology. 2015;123(3):692–713.
13. Blank RS, Colquhoun DA, Durieux ME, Kozower BD, McMurray TL, Bender SP, Naik BI. Management of one-lung ventilation: impact of tidal volume on complications after thoracic surgery. Anesthesiology. 2016;124(6):1286–129.
14. Brassard CL, Lohser J, Donati F, Bussieres JS. Step by step clinical management of one-lung ventilation: continuing professional development. Can J Anaesth. 2014;61:1103–21.
15. Licker M, Diaper J, Villiger Y, et al. Impact of intraoperative lung-protective interventions in patients undergoing lung cancer surgery. Crit Care. 2009;13:R41.
16. Lumb AB. Nunn's applied respiratory physiology. 8th ed. Edinburgh, New York: Elsevier; 2017
17. Brodsky JB, Lemmens HJ. Left double-lumen tubes: clinical experience with 1,170 patients. J Cardiothorac Vasc Anesth. 2003;17:289–98.
18. Karzai W, Schwarzkopf K. Hypoxemia during one-lung ventilation: prediction, prevention, and treatment. Anesthesiology. 2009;110:1402–11.
19. Hedenstierna G, Tokics L, Strandberg A, Lundquist H, Brismar B. Correlation of gas exchange impairment to development of atelectasis during anaesthesia and muscle paralysis. Acta Anaesthesiol Scand. 1986;30:183–91.
20. Larsson A, Malmkvist G, Werner O. Variations in lung volume and compliance during pulmonary surgery. Br J Anaesth. 1987;59:585–91.
21. Katz JA, Laverne RG, Fairley HB, Thomas AN. Pulmonary oxygen exchange during endobronchial anesthesia: effect of tidal volume and PEEP. Anesthesiology. 1982;56:164–71.
22. Levin AI, Coetzee JF. Arterial oxygenation during one-lung anesthesia. Anesth Analg. 2005;100:12–4.
23. Levin AI, Coetzee JF, Coetzee A. Arterial oxygenation and one-lung anesthesia. Curr Opin Anaesthesiol. 2008;21:28–36.
24. Takala J. Hypoxemia due to increased venous admixture: influence of cardiac output on oxygenation. Intensive Care Med. 2007;33:908–11.
25. Nagendran J, Stewart K, Hoskinson M, Archer SL. An anesthesiologist's guide to hypoxic pulmonary vasoconstriction: implications for managing single-lung anesthesia and atelectasis. Curr Opin Anaesthesiol. 2006;19:34–43.
26. Capan LM, Turndorf H, Patel C, Ramanathan S, Acinapura A, Chalon J. Optimization of arterial oxygenation during one-lung anesthesia. Anesth Analg. 1980;59:847–51.

27. Slinger PD, Kruger M, McRae K, Winton T. Relation of the static compliance curve and positive end-expiratory pressure to oxygenation during one-lung ventilation. Anesthesiology. 2001;95:1096–102.

28. Maeda Y, Fujino Y, Uchiyama A, Matsuura N, Mashimo T, Nishimura M. Effects of peak inspiratory flow on development of ventilator-induced lung injury in rabbits. Anesthesiology. 2004;101:722–8.

29. Uhlig S. Ventilation-induced lung injury and mechanotransduction: stretching it too far? Am J Physiol Lung Cell Mol Physiol. 2002;282:L892–6.

30. Prella M, Feihl F, Domenighetti G. Effects of short-term pressure-controlled ventilation on gas exchange, airway pressures, and gas distribution in patients with acute lung injury/ARDS: comparison with volume-controlled ventilation. Chest. 2002;122:1382–8.

31. Davis K Jr, Branson RD, Campbell RS, Porembka DT. Comparison of volume control and pressure control ventilation: is flow waveform the difference? J Trauma. 1996;41:808–14.

32. Campbell RS, Davis BR. Pressure-controlled versus volume-controlled ventilation: does it matter? Respir Care. 2002;47:416–24.

33. Cadi P, Guenoun T, Journois D, Chevallier JM, Diehl JL, Safran D. Pressure-controlled ventilation improves oxygenation during laparoscopic obesity surgery compared with volume-controlled ventilation. Br J Anaesth. 2008;100:709–16.

34. Balick-Weber CC, Nicolas P, Hedreville-Montout M, Blanchet P, Stéphan F. Respiratory and haemodynamic effects of volume-controlled vs. pressure-controlled ventilation during laparoscopy: a cross-over study with echocardiographic assessment. Br J Anaesth. 2007;99:429–35.

35. Heimberg C, Winterhalter M, Strüber M, Piepenbrock S, Bund M. Pressure-controlled versus volume-controlled one-lung ventilation for MIDCAB. Thorac Cardiovasc Surg. 2006;54:516–20.

36. Unzueta MC, Casas JI, Moral MV. Pressure-controlled versus volume-controlled ventilation during one-lung ventilation for thoracic surgery. Anesth Analg. 2007;104:1029–33.

37. Choi YS, Shim JK, Na S, Hong SB, Hong YW, Oh YJ. Pressure-controlled versus volume-controlled ventilation during one-lung ventilation in the prone position for robot-assisted esophagectomy. Surg Endosc. 2009;23:2286–91.

38. Tugrul M, Çamci E, Karadeniz H, Sentürk M, Pembeci K, Akpir K. Comparison of volume controlled with pressure controlled ventilation during one-lung anaesthesia. Br J Anaesth. 1997;79:306–10.

39. Bardoczky GI, d'Hollander AA, Rocmans P, Estenne M, Yernault JC. Respiratory mechanics and gas exchange during one-lung ventilation for thoracic surgery: the effects of end-inspiratory pause in stable COPD patients. J Cardiothorac Vasc Anesth. 1998;12:137–41.

40. Malhotra A. Low-tidal-volume ventilation in the acute respiratory distress syndrome. N Engl J Med. 2007;357:1113–20.

41. Petrucci N, Iacovelli W. Lung protective ventilation strategy for the acute respiratory distress syndrome. Cochrane Database Syst Rev. 2007;(2):CD003844.

42. The Acute Respiratory Distress Syndrome Network. Ventilation with lower tidal volumes as compared with traditional tidal volumes for acute lung injury and the acute respiratory distress syndrome. N Engl J Med. 2000;342:1301–8.

43. Putensen C, Theuerkauf N, Zinserling J, Wrigge H, Pelosi P. Meta-analysis: ventilation strategies and outcomes of the acute respiratory distress syndrome and acute lung injury. Ann Intern Med. 2009;151:566–76.

44. Tobin MJ. Advances in mechanical ventilation. N Engl J Med. 2001;344:1986–96.

45. Mols G, Priebe HJ, Guttmann J. Alveolar recruitment in acute lung injury. Br J Anaesth. 2006;96:156–66.

46. Morisaki H, Serita R, Innami Y, Kotake Y, Takeda J. Permissive hypercapnia during thoracic anaesthesia. Acta Anaesthesiol Scand. 1999;43:845–9.

47. Sticher J, Müller M, Scholz S, Schindler E, Hempelmann G. Controlled hypercapnia during one-lung ventilation in patients undergoing pulmonary resection. Acta Anaesthesiol Scand. 2001;45:842–7.

48. Broccard AFM. Respiratory acidosis and acute respiratory distress syndrome: time to trade in a bull market? Crit Care Med. 2006;34:229–31.

49. Vaneker M, Heunks LM, Joosten LA, et al. Mechanical ventilation induces a toll/interleukin-1 receptor domain-containing adapter-inducing interferon beta-dependent inflammatory response in healthy mice. Anesthesiology. 2009;111:836–43.

50. Curley GF, Kevin LG, Laffey JG. Mechanical ventilation: taking its toll on the lung. Anesthesiology. 2009;111:701–3.

51. Dos Santos CC, Slutsky AS. Invited review: mechanisms of ventilator-induced lung injury: a perspective. J Appl Physiol. 2000;89:1645–55.

52. Hager DN, Krishnan JA, Hayden DL, Brower RG. Tidal volume reduction in patients with acute lung injury when plateau pressures are not high. Am J Respir Crit Care Med. 2005;172:1241–5.53.

53. Hemmes SN, Gamma de Abreu M, Pelosi P, Schultz MJ. High versus low positive end-expiratory pressure during general anesthesia for open abdominal surgery (PROVHILO trial): a multicenter randomized controlled trial. Lancet. 2014;384:495–503.

54. Ferrando C, Belda FJ. Personalized intraoperative positive end-expiratory pressure: a further step in protective ventilation. Minerva Anestesiol. 2018;84(2):147–9.

55. Predicted Body Weight Calculator. http://www.ardsnet.org/node/77460. Accessed 18 Dec 2009.

56. Tandon S, Batchelor A, Bullock R, et al. Peri-operative risk factors for acute lung injury after elective oesophagectomy. Br J Anaesth. 2001;86:633–8.

57. Kutlu CA, Williams EA, Evans TW, Pastorino U, Goldstraw P. Acute lung injury and acute respiratory distress syndrome after pulmonary resection. Ann Thorac Surg. 2000;69:376–80.

58. Lytle FT, Brown DR. Appropriate ventilatory settings for thoracic surgery: intraoperative and postoperative. Semin Cardiothorac Vasc Anesth. 2008;12:97–108.

59. Slinger P. Pro: low tidal volume is indicated during one-lung ventilation. Anesth Analg. 2006;103:268–70.

60. Gal TJ. Con: low tidal volumes are indicated during one-lung ventilation. Anesth Analg. 2006;103:271–3.

61. Levin MA, McCormick PJ, Lin HM, Hosseinian L, Fischer GW. Low intraoperative tidal volume ventilation with minimal PEEP is associated with increased mortality. Br J Anaesth. 2014;113(1):97–108.

62. Duggan M, Kavanagh BP. Pulmonary atelectasis: a pathogenic perioperative entity. Anesthesiology. 2005;102:838–54.

63. Michelet P, D'Journo XB, Roch A, et al. Protective ventilation influences systemic inflammation after esophagectomy: a randomized controlled study. Anesthesiology. 2006;105:911–9.

64. Schilling T, Kozian A, Huth C, et al. The pulmonary immune effects of mechanical ventilation in patients undergoing thoracic surgery. Anesth Analg. 2005;101:957–65.

65. Wrigge H, Uhlig U, Zinserling J, et al. The effects of different ventilatory settings on pulmonary and systemic inflammatory responses during major surgery. Anesth Analg. 2004;98:775–81.

66. Shaw AD, Vaporciyan AA, Wu X, et al. Inflammatory gene polymorphisms influence risk of postoperative morbidity after lung resection. Ann Thorac Surg. 2005;79:1704–10.

67. Tekinbas C, Ulusoy H, Yulug E, et al. One-lung ventilation: for how long? J Thorac Cardiovasc Surg. 2007;134:405–10.

68. Misthos P, Katsaragakis S, Milingos N, et al. Postresectional pulmonary oxidative stress in lung cancer patients. The role of one-lung ventilation. Eur J Cardiothorac Surg. 2005;27:379–82.

69. Cheng YJ, Chan KC, Chien CT, Sun WZ, Lin CJ. Oxidative stress during 1-lung ventilation. J Thorac Cardiovasc Surg. 2006;132:513–8.

70. Gajic O, Dara SI, Mendez JL, et al. Ventilator-associated lung injury in patients without acute lung injury at the onset of mechanical ventilation. Crit Care Med. 2004;32:1817–24.

71. Schultz MJ. Lung-protective mechanical ventilation with lower tidal volumes in patients not suffering from acute lung injury: a review of clinical studies. Med Sci Monit. 2008;14:RA22–6.

72. Bonetto C, Terragni P, Ranieri VM. Does high tidal volume generate ALI/ARDS in healthy lungs? Intensive Care Med. 2005;31:893–5.

73. Slinger PD, Hickey DR. The interaction between applied PEEP and auto-PEEP during one-lung ventilation. J Cardiothorac Vasc Anesth. 1998;12:133–6.

74. Levy MM. PEEP in ARDS – how much is enough? N Engl J Med. 2004;351:389–91.

75. Brower RG, Lanken PN, MacIntyre N, et al. Higher versus lower positive end-expiratory pressures in patients with the acute respiratory distress syndrome. N Engl J Med. 2004;351:327–36.

76. Meade MO, Cook DJ, Guyatt GH, et al. Ventilation strategy using low tidal volumes, recruitment maneuvers, and high positive end-expiratory pressure for acute lung injury and acute respiratory distress syndrome: a randomized controlled trial. JAMA. 2008;299:637–45.

77. Mercat A, Richard JC, Vielle B, et al. Positive end-expiratory pressure setting in adults with acute lung injury and acute respiratory distress syndrome: a randomized controlled trial. JAMA. 2008;299:646–55.

78. Gattinoni L, Caironi P. Refining ventilatory treatment for acute lung injury and acute respiratory distress syndrome. JAMA. 2008;299:691–3.

79. Ducros L, Moutafis M, Castelain MH, Liu N, Fischler M. Pulmonary air trapping during two-lung and one-lung ventilation. J Cardiothorac Vasc Anesth. 1999;13:35–9.

80. Yokota K, Toriumi T, Sari A, Endou S, Mihira M. Auto-positive end-expiratory pressure during one-lung ventilation using a double-lumen endobronchial tube. Anesth Analg. 1996;82:1007–10.

81. Bardoczky GI, Yernault JC, Engelman EE, Velghe CE, Cappello M, Hollander AA. Intrinsic positive end-expiratory pressure during one-lung ventilation for thoracic surgery. The influence of preoperative pulmonary function. Chest. 1996;110:180–4.

82. Blanch L, Bernabé F, Lucangelo U. Measurement of air trapping, intrinsic positive end-expiratory pressure, and dynamic hyperinflation in mechanically ventilated patients. Respir Care. 2005;50:110–23.

83. Bardoczky GI, d'Hollander AA, Cappello M, Yernault JC. Interrupted expiratory flow on automatically constructed flow-volume curves may determine the presence of intrinsic positive end-expiratory pressure during one-lung ventilation. Anesth Analg. 1998;86:880–4.

84. Benumof JL. One-lung ventilation: which lung should be PEEPed? Anesthesiology. 1982;56:161–3.

85. Mascotto G, Bizzarri M, Messina M, et al. Prospective, randomized, controlled evaluation of the preventive effects of positive end-expiratory pressure on patient oxygenation during one-lung ventilation. Eur J Anaesthesiol. 2003;20:704–10.

86. Leong LM, Chatterjee S, Gao F. The effect of positive end expiratory pressure on the respiratory profile during one-lung ventilation for thoracotomy. Anaesthesia. 2007;62:23–6.

87. Cohen E, Eisenkraft JB. Positive end-expiratory pressure during one-lung ventilation improves oxygenation in patients with low arterial oxygen tensions. J Cardiothorac Vasc Anesth. 1996;10:578–82.

88. Valenza F, Ronzoni G, Perrone L, et al. Positive end-expiratory pressure applied to the dependent lung during one-lung ventilation improves oxygenation and respiratory mechanics in patients with high FEV_1. Eur J Anaesthesiol. 2004;21:938–43.

89. Inomata S, Nishikawa T, Saito S, Kihara S. "Best" PEEP during one-lung ventilation. Br J Anaesth. 1997;78:754–6.

90. Lachmann B. Open up the lung and keep the lung open. Intensive Care Med. 1992;18:319–21.

91. Lapinsky SE, Mehta S. Bench-to-bedside review: recruitment and recruiting maneuvers. Crit Care. 2005;9:60–5.

92. Tusman G, Böhm SH, Sipmann FS, Maisch S. Lung recruitment improves the efficiency of ventilation and gas exchange during one-lung ventilation anesthesia. Anesth Analg. 2004;98:1604–9.

93. Cinnella G, Grasso S, Natale C, et al. Physiological effects of a lung-recruiting strategy applied during one-lung ventilation. Acta Anaesthesiol Scand. 2008;52:766–75.

Anesthesia for Open Pulmonary Resection: A Systems Approach

23

E. Andrew Ochroch, Gavin Michael Wright,
and Bernhard J. C. J. Riedel

Key Points

- Perioperative morbidity and mortality are common following lung resection, with most deaths (>75%) attributed to major adverse pulmonary events (MAPE; including pneumonia, acute lung injury [ALI], and acute respiratory distress syndrome [ARDS]).

- Perioperative risk can be managed by dividing risk into two broad categories: iatrogenic risk and patient-attributed risk. Clinical care pathways manage iatrogenic risk, while perioperative strategies that allow identification and optimal management of high-risk patients manage patient-attributed risk. These factors will improve outcomes and reduce hospital costs.

- Patient safety and the delivery of quality care, with emphasis on systems improvement, have emerged as central tasks for healthcare providers. In fact, benchmarking of data will increasingly allow patients to identify institutions that deliver on the value proposition – providing medical care that measures up in safety and quality and yet is delivered at significantly lower costs.

E. A. Ochroch (✉)
Department of Anesthesiology and Critical Care,
University of Pennsylvania, Philadelphia, PA, USA
e-mail: ochrocha@uphs.upenn.edu

G. M. Wright
Department of Cardiothoracic Surgery, Royal Melbourne Hospital,
Parkville, VIC, Australia

Department of Surgery, University of Melbourne,
Melbourne, VIC, Australia

B. J. C. J. Riedel
Department of Anesthesiology, Perioperative and Pain Medicine,
Peter MacCallum Cancer Centre, Melbourne, VIC, Australia

University of Melbourne, Melbourne, VIC, Australia

General Concepts

Perioperative morbidity and mortality are common following lung resection (Table 23.1). Importantly, while the studies summarized in Table 23.1 highlight an increasing incidence of morbidity and mortality with increased volume of lung resected [1], these studies consistently report a need for improved predictors of adverse postoperative outcome. Further, major adverse pulmonary events (MAPE; including pneumonia, acute lung injury [ALI], and acute respiratory distress syndrome [ARDS]) have a high rate of mortality and contribute singularly to most (>75%) perioperative deaths. While a decline in adverse outcome has been witnessed over the last 50 years, it is important that we continue to seek strategies to improve perioperative outcome following open lung surgery. Recent strategies that have contributed to a reduction in the incidence and the mortality associated with ALI/ARDS include surgical attempts to limit the volume of lung resected (e.g., performing a sleeve resection rather than a pneumonectomy) and protective lung ventilation strategies (tidal volume reduction proportional to the number of segments resected) [2].

Strategies to further improve surgical outcome require a global approach, with implementation of (1) clinical care pathways that reduce iatrogenic risk and (2) perioperative strategies that focus on identifying and optimally managing the high-risk patient to reduce patient-attributed risk. Clinical care paths should embrace safety and quality initiatives, which when implemented within clinical practice should encompass improvements in reliability (reduced variability), processes, and performance and be combined with cost measures to assess the value of the care delivered. With society increasingly intent on actualizing the value proposition of healthcare, we are obligated to deliver optimized quality care within the constraints of cost [7]. Driven by the unsustainable growth in healthcare expenditure – accounting for 10–16% of the gross domestic product in developed nations – the need to improve quality and reduce costs has rapidly become the mantra of the healthcare industry.

© Springer Nature Switzerland AG 2019
P. Slinger (ed.), *Principles and Practice of Anesthesia for Thoracic Surgery*, https://doi.org/10.1007/978-3-030-00859-8_23

Table 23.1 Summary of key studies illustrating the incidence of perioperative morbidity and mortality associated with major lung resection

Author	Year	N	Morbidity	Mortality	Factors associated with mortality	Commentary
Kopec et al. [3]	1998		*All morbidities 40–60%*	*Right vs. left pneumonectomy 10–12% vs. 1–3.5%*		1. Review of literature on pneumonectomy. 2. Mortality has decreased significantly from 56.4% reported in www–1940.
Kutlu et al. [4]	1991–1997	1139		3.5%	*Cause of death* ALI/ARDS = 72.5%* Dysrhythmia = 12.5% Pneumonia = 5%* Pulmonary embolism = 5% Renal failure = 2.5% DIC = 2.5%	1. Review of all lung resections performed at an single institution. 2. While incidence of ALI/ARDS is low (3.9%), it is a leading cause of mortality. 3. >75%* of mortality is associated with major adverse pulmonary events.
Vaporciyan et al. [5]	2002	257	*MAPE only 12.8%*	*Overall mortality 6.2%*	*Mortality in patients without and with MAPE 2.1% vs. 39.3%*	1. Single institution review of pneumonectomy. 2. Smoking cessation within 1 month of surgery was only multivariate predictor of risk. 3. High mortality observed in patients that suffer a major adverse pulmonary event.
Dulu et al. [1]	2002–2004	2039	*Incidence of ALI/ ARDS 2.5%*	*Mortality associated with ALI/ARDS 40%*	*Incidence (and mortality) of ALI/ARDS by type of lung resection* Pneumonectomy: 7.9% (50%) Lobectomy: 2.96% (42%) Segmentectomy: 0.88% (22%)	1. Review of incidence of ALI/ARDS following lung resections performed at a single institution. 2. Increased incidence of ALI/ARDS with increasing lung volume resected. 3. High mortality in patients that suffer from ALI/ ARDS.
Tang et al. [2]	1991–1997 2000–2005	1376	*Incidence of ALI/ ARDS 3.2% 1.6%*	*Mortality associated with ALI/ARDS 72% 45%*	Pneumonectomy rate = 17.4% of resections Pneumonectomy rate = 6.4% of resections	1. Review of incidence of ALI/ARDS following lung resections performed at a single institution over two time periods. 2. High mortality in patients that suffering ALI/ ARDS. 3. Reduced incidence (and associated mortality) of ALI/ARDS after 2000 associated with two factors: (a) Aggressive strategies to avoid pneumonectomy. (b) Lung protective ventilation strategies (reduced tidal volume per number of resected segments).
Kozower et al. [6]	2002–2008	18,800		*Overall mortality 3.2%* *Composite major morbidity or mortality 8.6%*	68.3% thoracotomy 36.9% thoracoscopy Pneumonectomy rate 6%	1. STS database review. 2. 111 centers 3. Predictors of mortality include the following: Pneumonectomy ($p < 0.001$), bilobectomy ($p < 0.001$), American Society of Anesthesiology rating ($p < 0.018$), Zubrod performance status ($p < 0.001$), renal dysfunction ($p = 0.001$), induction chemoradiation therapy ($p = 0.01$), steroids ($p = 0.002$), age ($p < 0.001$), urgent procedures ($p = 0.015$), male gender ($p = 0.013$), forced expiratory volume in one second ($p < 0.001$), and body mass index ($p = 0.015$).

The Institute of Medicine's report on patient safety *To Err is Human: Building a Safer Health System* estimates that 100,000 people die each year from medical errors in US hospitals [8]. This report, a landmark study in modern medicine, is an important contributor to the current patient-safety movement, with patient safety and the delivery of quality care emerging as central issues in medicine and as central tasks for healthcare providers in the last decade. In fact, quality healthcare is now a worldwide goal. Consequently, an important paradigm shift occurred: with (1) emphasis shifting to systems improvement rather than exhortations to individual health professionals and (2) recognition that leadership in healthcare institutions is a key catalyst in improving patient safety and in the delivery of quality care. The Institute of Medicine defines "quality" as "the degree to which health services increase the likelihood of desired health outcomes, consistent with current professional knowledge" and as such recommends six standards of care (safe, effective, patient-centered, timely, efficient, and equitable) to achieve the delivery of quality healthcare [9].

Additionally, economic factors, such as reimbursement programs, market forces, and globalization of healthcare, will continue to drive the need to deliver quality care. Hospitals will increasingly compete for patients on the grounds of quality at local, regional, and global (medical tourism) levels. In this regard, reimbursement programs, such as pay for performance (P4P) or refusal of payment for preventable "never events," will increasingly be used to link patient outcomes with reimbursement. Benchmark data will increasingly allow patients to identify institutions that deliver on the value proposition – providing medical care that measures up in safety and quality at a lower cost.

A Systems Approach

Continued improvement in patient outcome is feasible when one understands and manages the risk types found within the complexity of a patient presenting for thoracic surgery. This complexity originates in the patient's disease process and associated comorbidities (patient-attributed risk; Fig. 23.1) and within the complexity of the healthcare system (iatrogenic risk). The majority of risk is derived from the burden of disease and the comorbidities that patients present with. However, iatrogenic risk, the risk of adverse outcome associated with therapy (medical, including anesthesia, or surgical therapy, or lack thereof, imposed by a third-party, the healthcare provider), remains sizeable, with an estimated 100,000

deaths occurring each year in the USA [8]. Importantly, this risk is largely preventable.

A strategy for understanding, examining, and improving care patterns, with the intended consequence of improved surgical outcome, and based on the two broad risk categories (iatrogenic and patient-attributed risk) is outlined in Fig. 23.2. This systems approach divides care into three broad areas based on decision points at Q1 and Q2.

Decision point Q1 delineates elective surgical care from emergent surgical care. While emergency procedures account for a small fraction of the thoracic surgical caseload, these patients nevertheless are often critically ill, have limited time for preoperative optimization, and are at significant risk for a protracted and costly length of hospital stay. Decision point Q2 delineates care into processes that (1) deliver the value proposition of the surgical procedure – delivering uncomplicated surgical outcome in a cost-effective manner through the implementation of clinical care pathways, thereby reducing iatrogenic risk – and (2) provide cost-effective perioperative risk stratification and optimization of high-risk patients, reducing patient-attributed risk and associated postoperative morbidity and mortality. The former processes are predominantly directed at the surgical disease and accompanying surgical procedure, while the latter are predominantly directed at the underlying disease burden and the medical comorbidities of the patient.

Patient Care Processes in Thoracic Anesthesia

The events involved between a patient presenting for thoracic surgery and having him/her discharged safely represent an extraordinarily complex system. This requires the collection, verification, and distribution of a large volume of information through multiple healthcare providers (including primary care physicians, pulmonologists, thoracic surgeons, oncologists, radiologists, cardiologists, nurse practitioners, and physiotherapists). Further complexity is added by the sophistication of the high acuity perioperative environment, with numerous perioperative physiological monitors and surgical instruments. A high volume of information must be processed in real time, communicated effectively throughout the operative team, and acted upon. Harm can originate at a multitude of levels [10]. The uncertainty and urgency inherent in the decision-making processes produce risk, which is compounded by external stressors, such as work load, fatigue, and a great degree of variability in organizational and/or environmental structures that support decision-making and physical tasks. After completion of the surgical procedure, patients then typically reside in the postanesthesia care unit where care decisions are divided between anesthesiologists, surgeons, and the acute pain

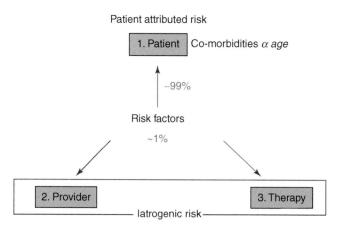

Fig. 23.1 Complexity and risk for adverse outcome originate in the patient's disease process and Associated comorbidities (patient-attributed risk) and within the complexity of the healthcare system (iatrogenic risk)

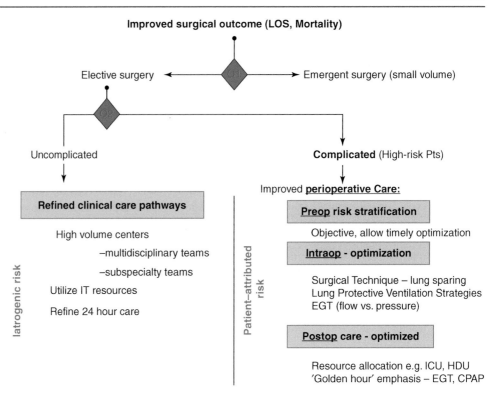

Fig. 23.2 A strategy for understanding, examining, and improving care patterns, with the intended consequence of improved surgical outcome. *CPAP* continuous positive airway pressure, *EGT* early goal-directed therapy, *HDU* high dependency unit, *ICU* intensive care unit, *IT* information technology, *LOS* length of stay, *postop* postoperative, *Q1 Q2* decision points

team, all of whom have ongoing responsibilities. Even when the patient is ensconced on the hospital ward, care for chest tubes, pulmonary toilet, X-ray follow-up, medication therapy, etc. requires a continuous flow of interactions and communication.

Recent progress in patient safety originates from the adoption of a systems analysis approach developed in other high-risk environments such as aviation. Vincent et al. [11] (among others) adopted these approaches for patient care (Table 23.2) and further modified these specifically to suite the perioperative care of the surgical patient (Table 23.3). Improved safety evolves from the study of this exhaustive list, which covers all aspects of the patient, the patient's interactions with the care team, the interaction among members of the care team, and the interactions of the patient and care team with the hospital environment. This has changed the focus of care from one of a surgeon's skill vs. the patient's disease to one of care that encompasses development of the care pathways that ensure consistent best practice regardless of the caregiver, individual performance within a team setting, optimal team coordination and communication, and the interaction of all of these aspects within the larger hospital organization/environment – all of which can help or hinder performance. Such approaches require a nonpunitive culture that promotes open dialog with a focus on improved patient outcomes.

Table 23.2 Framework of factors influencing clinical practice

Factor types	Influencing contributory factors
Institutional context	Economic and regulatory context
	National health service executive
	Clinical negligence scheme for trusts
Organizational and management factors	Financial resources and constraints
	Organizational structure
	Policy standards and goals
	Safety culture and priorities
Work environment factors	Staffing levels and skills mix
	Workload and shift patterns
	Design, availability, and maintenance of equipment
	Administrative and managerial support
Team factors	Verbal communication
	Written communication
	Supervision and seeking help
	Team structure (consistency, leadership, etc.)
Individual (staff) factors	Knowledge and skills
	Competence
	Physical and mental health
Task factors	Task design and clarity of structure
	Availability and use of protocols
	Availability and accuracy of test results
Patient factors	Condition (complexity and seriousness)
	Language and communication
	Personality and social factors

Reproduced from British Medical Journal. Vincent C, Taylor-Adams S, Stanhope N. 316; © 1998 with permission from BMJ Publishing Group LTD

Table 23.3 Principal features of the operation profile

Patient factors
   Principal complaint
   Comorbidities
   ASA, BMI, age, and other relevant clinical information
The surgical team
   Personnel
   Experience of previous work together
   Familiarity with procedure
   Fatigue, sleep loss, stress, etc.
Processes and procedures
   Adequacy of notes and management plan
   Consent and preparation
   Anesthetic procedures
Key operative events
   Blood loss
   Minor and major complications
   Error compensation and recovery
Flow of information regarding patient
   Adequacy of notes and consent
   Specific intraoperative communications
   Handover
Technical skills
   Ratings of good general surgical practice
   Ratings of operation-specific steps
   Identification of specific technical errors
Team performance and leadership
   Leadership
   Coordination between team members
   Willingness to seek advice and help
   Responsiveness and flexibility
Decision-making and situation awareness
   Patient limitations
   Operation limitations
   Surgeon's limitations
   Team limitations
The operative environment
   Availability and adequacy of equipment
   Availability of notes, records
   Noise and lighting
   Distractions
Interruptions
   Phone calls, messages, outside theater events, etc.

An important use of systems analysis to reduce medical errors focused on process improvement in transitions in care to decrease medical errors. In thoracic surgery the patient transitions from outpatient to preoperative holding, intraoperative care, PACU or ICU care, floor care, and then discharge/home care. Each instance of transition presents an opportunity for the failure to transfer critical information which may impact morbidity and mortality. While not yet studied in thoracic surgery, the I-PASS study focused on defining critical elements of transition of care and produced "bundles" of critical elements. The use of these bundles (a structured transition of care approach) at nine sites reduced

medical error from 24.5 to 18.8 per 100 admissions $p < 0.001$ and preventable adverse events from 4.7% to 3.3% per 100 admissions $p < 0.001$ [10]. The greater acuity of thoracic surgical patients should increase the impact of such improvements in care.

While there have been few specific studies of a systems approach in thoracic surgery, clear examples abound. Although controversial, increasing data support benefits through reduced morbidity and improved survival in patients having high-risk operations performed by subspecialty-trained surgeons [12, 13]. Such results are especially evident in esophageal cancer surgery, colorectal cancer surgery, and vascular surgery [12–16]. It is unclear if this is purely a volume effect, i.e., greater numbers of surgeries produce better results. A study of 40,460 thoracic surgeries captured by the 2007 Nationwide Inpatient Sample (NIS) indicated that volume only accounted for outcomes differences if analysis was done with center volume broken down into quartiles [17]. Similarly, no differences in outcome by center volume were found in an analysis of esophageal surgeries in the General Thoracic Surgery Database – a component of the Society of Thoracic Surgeons (STS) National (US) Database [18]. While the volume effect may speak for the technical proficiency of the surgeon, it is likely to also reflect on the wider care services provided by other team members, including anesthesiologists, intensive care physicians, nurses, physiotherapists, etc. The effect of wider care services has been demonstrated in patients requiring thoracotomy for lobectomy where defined clinical care pathways both improved outcomes and reduced hospital costs [19, 20]. These pathways have the further benefit of patient education, managing patient and family expectations, educating junior house staff and new care team members, and defining points of care and team interaction with the patient where data can be collected, analyzed, and benchmarked.

Care patterns and outcomes need to be assessed and examined both for benchmarks; to track changes from trends in technology, reimbursement, or patient issues; and to seek improvement in outcomes. These outcomes need to be examined locally and against national data such as the General Thoracic Surgery Database – a component of the Society of Thoracic Surgeons (STS) National (US) Database, which collected 9470 adult thoracic procedures between July 2012 and June 2016 from its 6000 participating surgeons and allied health professionals. Potential biases in these data include the voluntary reporting process and the fact that most of the participating centers are affiliated with surgical training and/or research institutions – with the potential for such institutions to have sicker or more complicated patients and thus worse outcomes if the data are not appropriately adjusted for risk. Mandatory reporting, such as the National Surgical

Quality Improvement Program (NSQIP) in the USA, may provide more reliable comparative data due to wider data capture, incorporating more diverse patients, and thereby facilitate risk adjustment.

Once the care pathway has been defined and the internally collected data have been reviewed and examined against external benchmark data, meaningful changes can then be implemented. For example, as a result of the NSQIP program, the changes implemented in the US Veterans Affairs hospital system decreased the 30-day morbidity from major surgery by 45% and decreased 30-day mortality by 27% [21, 22]. Such improvements promise expansion into other surgical avenues and potentially into outcomes other than morbidity and mortality that include patient and provider satisfaction with the care process.

Preoperative Care

In North America and Europe, the majority of patients present for open thoracic procedures with a confirmed diagnosis of cancer or an intrathoracic process suspicious for cancer. In contrast, patients in the developing world are likely to present with trauma or pulmonary infection. Patients also often present with comorbidities, especially smoking-related comorbidities that dramatically increase their risk for perioperative pulmonary and cardiac complications. Irrespective of the underlying disease mechanism, all patients require a thorough preoperative assessment to address and improve correctable physiological problems and to assure adequate physiological reserve following surgical intervention. The preoperative evaluation needs to be focused on preoperative risk stratification, identification of reversible pathologies, and decreasing the patient's risk through preoperative optimization (see Chap. 2 for a detailed review) [23]. Beyond reducing risk, preoperative interaction with the patient allows practitioners to mentally prepare patients for the rigors of recovery.

Preoperative smoking cessation and pulmonary rehabilitation have not been consistently noted to be effective in improving outcomes [24, 25]. A study of 7990 thoracic surgeries from 1999 to 2007 indicated a small mitigation of smoking risk with duration of cessation, although this could have been due to increased focus on outpatient pulmonary toilet [26]. Consequently, practitioners should ensure continuation of bronchodilator therapy throughout the perioperative period. Patients need to understand the importance of complying with their pulmonary toilet; moreover, it should be explained that even with aggressive postoperative epidural analgesia combined with multimodal therapy, visual analog pain scores with pulmonary toilet are typically 5 out of 10 for the first 5 postoperative days [27].

For patients with cardiovascular comorbidities, the acute introduction of beta-blocker therapy may increase the risk for cardiovascular harm [28, 29]. Similarly, randomized trials of coronary revascularization before major surgery have not shown any clear benefits [30–32]. As such, it is currently recommended that the preoperative evaluation of coronary artery disease should only be addressed in those patients with acute changes in symptoms while focusing on optimized medical therapy and exploring other cardioprotective strategies (e.g., statins) for the remaining patients with stable coronary disease.

If beta-blockers are indicated for intercurrent medical conditions, then these medications should be started well before rather than at the time of surgery. In cases where coronary heart disease is only recognized at the time of admission for elective surgery, results of the POISE trial suggest that while acute perioperative administration of beta-blocker therapy may confer cardioprotection, it increases the risk of stroke and all-cause mortality [28]. Further, beta-blocked patients seem to tolerate surgical anemia less than patients who are naïve to beta-blockers, resulting in increased adverse postoperative events [33].

Studies suggest that the pleiotropic effects (nonlipid-lowering effects, including anti-inflammatory effects and endothelial modulation) of statins improve outcomes in the perioperative period in patients undergoing major cardiac and noncardiac surgery [34, 35]. The best evidence comes from vascular surgery patients where preoperative fluvastatin, commenced at least 30 days before (and continued for at least 30 days after surgery), significantly reduced postoperative myocardial ischemia and death from cardiovascular causes, without adverse skeletal muscle or hepatic injury [35]. (This study was investigated due to a co-author's – Poldermans – nonconformity with consent procedures but was found to be valid.) [29] Specific to the thoracic surgery population, preoperative statin therapy is reported to result in a threefold reduction in the incidence of postoperative atrial fibrillation [36]. These pleiotropic effects of statin therapy may translate into perioperative protection of the heart, brain, and kidney for other major surgeries, but they cannot be currently recommended [29].

Antihypertensive medications (including beta-blockers), HMG Co-A reductase inhibitor (statin) therapy, and where possible antiplatelet therapy should be continued to avoid potential cardiovascular harm associated with drug withdrawal [37–39]. Controversy, however, surrounds the preoperative management of antiplatelet therapy, with increasing data supporting the continuation of clopidogrel and aspirin in the perioperative period to reduce both stroke and myocardial infarction [40]. Factors increasing the risk for such thrombotic adverse events include poor endothelialization of drug-eluting coronary stents, hypercoagulability induced by the surgical stress response, and a rebound response from the perioperative withdrawal of antiplatelet therapy. To prevent acute in-stent thrombosis, patients with bare metal and drug-eluting coronary stents should continue dual antiplatelet therapy for a minimum of 3 and 12 months, respectively, after stent placement, with consideration for lifelong anti-platelet monotherapy; thereafter patients at increased risk may require lifelong dual antiplatelet therapy. If possible, elective surgery should be performed beyond this 3- or 12-month window and strong consideration given to continue dual antiplatelet therapy, with a minimum of antiplatelet monotherapy with aspirin, throughout the perioperative period. This continuation protocol needs to be balanced against the risk of perioperative bleeding and the need for epidural analgesia.

Patient safety decisions need to be incorporated into the preoperative phase. There has been recent focus on a morning "huddle" in which the day's cases are discussed among surgeons, anesthesiologists, nurses, and technicians. This ensures proper equipment, identifies particular patient's risks (latex allergy), and helps to develop patient-specific multi-discipline plans. Although potentially impactful on safety, most of the data focuses on efficiency metrics. Intraoperative safety issues to be discussed include surgical site marking, surgical plan, allergies, patient-specific medical comorbidities, thromboembolic prophylaxis (sequential compression stockings or subcutaneous heparin), strategies to maintain normothermia, antibiotic administration within 1 h prior to incision, universal precautions (gown and gloves) as mandated for invasive procedures, and a type and screen for blood cross-matching sent to transfusion services.

Intraoperative Care

Operating room preparation needs to occur as with every case to ensure patient safety. In addition to a routine setup, typical airway management equipment includes methods of establishing (double lumen tubes [DLT], bronchial blockers, or Univent tubes) and verifying (pediatric fiber-optic bronchoscope) lung isolation. A circuit for delivering continuous positive airway pressure (CPAP) to the nondependent lung should be immediately available. Other devices that should be in the room include the following: a "bean bag" placed on the operating table prior to the patient's arrival; an arm holder for positioning the nondependent arm; warming devices such as intravenous fluid warmers and warm air blankets for maintaining normothermia in patients and thereby negating the adverse effect of hypothermia on hypoxic pulmonary vasoconstriction (HPV), coagulopathy, and wound healing; and mechanical compression devices to prevent thromboembolism.

Once consent is obtained and the patient has been properly identified and the surgical site marked, an intravenous catheter should ideally be placed in the hand/wrist/forearm of the operative (nondependent) side. The antecubital fossa is not ideal due to the position of the arms in the lateral decubitus position where the arms will be bent at 90° and the flow potentially inhibited. An 18-gauge intravenous catheter is sufficient for medication and fluid management since for a thoracotomy in a hemithorax that has not had previous surgery, chest tubes, trauma, or radiation therapy, the operative blood loss should be minimal. However, after induction of anesthesia, an additional intravenous cannula is typically placed in case of sudden unanticipated blood loss. This is especially mandatory in re-operative cases, cases where the patient received preoperative radiation therapy, or cases that require an extrapleural approach (e.g., extrapleural pneumonectomy for mesothelioma). If surgical dissection is required around the greater veins (vena cava or subclavian veins), contralateral access, central access, and/or lower extremity access should then be considered.

Paravertebral and epidural catheter placement is equally efficacious for postoperative analgesia [41]. Regional anesthesia is typically established in the preoperative area or in the operating room prior to induction, with the goal of establishing adequate analgesia prior to completion of the surgical procedure and emergence from anesthesia. Once the patient is positioned for regional anesthesia, noninvasive monitoring (pulse oximeter and blood pressure cuff) and nasal oxygen are applied, and sedation is then administered to facilitate regional anesthesia. Typical sedative regimens used to facilitate the induction of regional anesthesia include titrated doses of midazolam and/or fentanyl as dictated by patient anxiety and medical status. Dexmedetomidine is a viable alternative for sedation, especially if it is planned to be used as part of the general anesthetic technique or if awake fiber-optic bronchoscopy (usually for an anticipated difficult airway) is planned preceding the induction of general anesthesia.

After securing the regional anesthesia catheter, the patient is positioned in the supine position and the standard American Society of Anesthesiologists (ASA) monitors placed. The placement of the EKG leads requires an understanding of the surgical approach. For a thoracotomy, care should be taken to avoid trapping the electrodes and leads between the patient and the bed as this can lead to pressure necrosis. For a left-sided thoracotomy, the V_5 lead cannot be placed in its usual position over the fourth interspace in the anterior axillary line as this intrudes on the surgical field. It is typically placed in the V_1 position (second interspace, right of the sternum). These factors (modified lead placement and lateral decubitus positioning) are likely to reduce the sensitivity of such monitoring for ischemic events.

After all noninvasive monitors are secured, preoxygenation is commenced. Five minutes of tidal breathing preoxygenation compensates for delayed nitrogen washout in patients with chronic obstructive pulmonary disease (COPD) [42]. During this period, a preinduction arterial line can be placed if needed; however, in primary thoracotomy it is unclear if arterial line monitoring reduces risk. Placement of the arterial line is typically preferred in the dependent arm to avoid waveform damping by compression of the nondependent wrist by the overhead arm holder.

Induction agents are chosen in relation to the patient's medical status and are intended to blunt the sympathetic stimulation associated with laryngoscopy and intubation without producing deleterious hypotension. Propofol doses of 0.5–1 mg/kg can adequately ensure unconsciousness with minimal hemodynamic impact. Etomidate doses of 0.1–0.2 mg/kg are reasonable alternatives. A reduction in the dose of the induction agent, thereby avoiding hypotension, can be achieved by incorporating analgesic agents during induction and by ensuring that the peak effect of analgesia coincides with laryngoscopy. The onset of significant analgesia following intravenous fentanyl, sufentanyl, and remifentanil is noted to be 2–5 min [43]. Doses of fentanyl would typically be 2–4 µg/kg. Lidocaine 0.5–1 mg/kg can also be used for reducing this sympathetic response.

An understanding of the physiology of one-lung ventilation (OLV), the strategies for inducing OLV, and the means to address intraoperative challenges associated with OLV is required to improve operative efficiencies and patient outcomes. Patient safety can be advanced through the use of task trainers and simulations to improve skills in the use of double lumen tubes and bronchial blockers [44]. Bronchoscopic anatomy can be learned first on online simulations.

A plan to maintain a patent airway and adequate ventilation at all times will ensure maintenance of hyperoxia and normocarbia. To this effect, mask ventilation needs to be rapidly established after loss of consciousness and neuromuscular blockade rapidly induced – to accommodate the reduction in functional residual capacity (FRC) associated with smoking-related disease, which shortens the apneic oxygenation time in these patients. Sevoflurane is initially employed in patients with reactive airway disease until sufficient depth of anesthesia is obtained. No significant outcome differences have been established in terms of maintenance of anesthesia for currently used volatile agents, such as isoflurane, sevoflurane, and desflurane (see HPV).

If the patient is scheduled for a diagnostic bronchoscopy, a laryngeal mask airway (LMA) may be placed. This allows the upper airway to also be assessed for associated smoking-related laryngeal cancers. However, if the patient is scheduled for a mediastinoscopy, a standard single-lumen endotracheal tube (preferably 8.0 mm, internal diameter) may be preferred. Once bronchoscopy and mediastinoscopy are complete, lung isolation using a DLT or bronchial blocker needs to be implemented to facilitate the thoracotomy. The

endotracheal tube (DLT or single-lumen tube with bronchial blocker) should then be secured with tape to the nondependent side, allowing easy access to the tape if the tube needs to be repositioned while in the lateral decubitus position. The patient is then positioned in the lateral decubitus position, 100% FiO_2 maintained, and lung isolation then established. Proper positioning of the endotracheal tube should be reconfirmed after the patient's repositioning, because flexion or extension of the neck can potentially displace the endotracheal tube. The "tip of the tube follows the tip of the nose"; therefore, head extension causes the endotracheal tube to move proximally, and the endobronchial balloon can herniate across the main carina. Confirmation of tube position with fiber-optic bronchoscopy after placement and position change decreases the incidence of inadequate lung isolation.

The use of a left double lumen endotracheal tube for a left thoracotomy carries the increased risk of acute intraoperative hypoventilation if the endotracheal tube displaces proximally with the endobronchial balloon herniating across the carina, especially if lung retraction moves the left main stem bronchus caudad. This can also occur from overinflation of the endobronchial balloon. The astute anesthesiologist may notice decreased tidal volumes as the balloon partially obstructs the right main stem orifice. Minute ventilation alarms may be triggered if there is a partial occlusion, or the high-pressure alarms will be triggered if there is a total or near total occlusion. The anesthesiologist reacts based on the patient's oxygenation and the surgeon's flexibility. If the patient is appropriately oxygenated, then ventilation can be briefly suspended and the fiber-optic bronchoscope utilized to check tube position and the endobronchial cuff deflated prior to tube advancement. If the patient deoxygenates acutely to dangerously low levels, then quick communication should inform the surgeon of the urgent need to re-establish two-lung ventilation. This is achieved by re-establishing ventilation through both the tracheal and endobronchial lumens of the DLT and, importantly, by deflation of the endobronchial balloon. The endotracheal tube can then be repositioned and OLV re-established once oxygenation levels are satisfactory.

OLV strategies are covered in detail in Chap. 6. Briefly, the patient is maintained on 100% oxygen (or combined with nitrous oxide) during initial two-lung ventilation. This denitrogenation allows for faster deflation – through absorption atelectasis – of the nondependent (surgical) lung on the initiation of OLV. ALI increases with greater peak inspiratory pressures [45, 46]. Ventilation parameters during OLV therefore typically strive to reduce the risk of ALI associated with barotrauma or volutrauma through tidal volume reduction (<6 mL/kg), respiratory rate > 10 breaths per minute, I:E ratio of 1:2, and peak inspiratory pressure < 25 mmHg. Such a protective ventilatory strategy aims to maintain baseline

CO_2 levels or tolerate permissive hypercapnia (pH > 7.25) rather than mild hypocapnia. This protective ventilatory strategy is supported by evidence that reduced tidal volume (5 mL/kg) during OLV decreases the pro-inflammatory systemic response, improves lung function, and results in earlier extubation after esophagectomy [47]. Similarly, mechanical ventilation with lower tidal volumes (6 mL/kg and 10 cm H_2O positive end expiratory pressure; PEEP) after 5 h of two-lung mechanical ventilation is noted to induce lowered activation of bronchoalveolar coagulation, as reflected by reduced thrombin–antithrombin complexes, soluble tissue factor, and factor VIIa levels in lavage fluids when compared to higher tidal volumes (12 mL/kg ideal body weight) without PEEP [48, 49]. Inhalational agents tend to provide an inhibitory (protective) effect on inflammation during one-lung ventilation as compared to propofol [50].

In patients with significant COPD with a prolonged exhalation phase and CO_2 retention, the respiratory rate and I:E ratio need to be adjusted to avoid hyperexpansion from breath stacking. In patients with right ventricular dysfunction or pulmonary hypertension, ventilator parameters should aim to maintain hyperoxia and induce mild hypocarbia in an attempt to reduce pulmonary vasoconstriction and any further strain on the right heart.

Optimal ventilation can be achieved by maintaining an appropriate plane of anesthesia to decrease the risk of reactive airways, inducing neuromuscular blockade to prevent abdominal or chest wall contractions, suctioning the double lumen to prevent mucus plugs, and visual bronchoscopic checks of the tube placement to correct tube malposition, kinking, and misalignment.

Typically, for a patient on 100% oxygen, the initiation of OLV does not bring on any immediate changes except for changes in ventilatory pressures or parameters [51]. Oxygenation is initially maintained due to apneic oxygenation. The duration of apneic oxygenation is proportional to the FRC and dependent on oxygen utilization. This can last a few minutes in COPD patients with reduced FRC or longer (8–15 min) in healthy nonsmokers. Once the nondependent lung is bereft of oxygen, a shunt develops and hypoxemia can ensue. HPV (discussed below) is initiated by the mitochondria sensing decreased oxygen levels.

Should hypoxia develop during OLV, the first response should be to communicate this to the surgeon in case two-lung ventilation needs to be resumed. Delivery of 100% oxygen through a properly positioned endotracheal tube needs to be ensured. Assuming that the rate of descent of the saturation is not too rapid and the nadir is safe (moderate hypoxemia, 88–90% saturation), then the nadir can be tolerated for several minutes until HPV has a chance to decrease the shunt. If unsafe levels of hypoxemia are reached, then the shunt needs to be decreased. This can be achieved through the application of CPAP, with 100% O_2 delivery to the nondependent lung. PEEP to the dependent lung can eliminate atelectasis, but this typically has a lesser impact on saturation than does CPAP. Restoration of adequate cardiac output and blood pressure can also restore oxygenation by improving the blood flow (perfusion zones) and V/Q matching in the dependent lung. It is important to advise the surgeon to any changes in ventilation, particularly when they are dissecting around the hilum. Obviously, if the oxygen saturation falls to a dangerous level, then either two-lung ventilation needs to be resumed, or a temporary clamp on the pulmonary artery of the nondependent lung can be placed. While the temporary pulmonary artery clamp will significantly reduce the shunt, extreme care should be taken as it can incite right heart strain and right heart failure.

After positioning the patient, prior to surgery, the multidisciplinary (anesthesia, surgical, and nursing) team should "time out" and pause for open dialog to ensure that the correct patient, correct surgical side, sterility of instruments, and patient-safety procedures (including surgical site marking, thromboembolic prophylaxis, strategies to maintain normothermia, antibiotic administration within 1 h prior to incision, type and screen for blood cross-matching, correct surgical instruments, etc.) are verified and to provide an opportunity to address any potential concerns that need clarification or may harm the patient. In the future, computerized information technology (anesthesia information management systems, AIMS) will increasingly assist supportive decision-making, with smart alerts prompting for critical items such as timely antibiotic administration and risk prediction modeling, and allow benchmarking against national outcome databases.

At rest, the normal pulmonary vascular system is noted as a high-compliance, high-flow, low-pressure system. This contrasts the systemic circulation, which has much higher resting levels of arterial and venous tone. This difference stems partly from the anatomy because the pulmonary precapillary arterioles have a thinner media and less smooth muscle than their systemic counterparts. Furthermore, at rest, there are far more recruitable vessels in the pulmonary bed that allow dramatic increases in flow with minimal impact on pressure.

The difference between the systemic and arterial systems is also due to the way in which the pulmonary vascular endothelium responds to the challenges of hypoxia, i.e., hypoxic pulmonary vasoconstriction (HPV). This vasoconstriction is known as the Euler–Liljestrand reflex. While the basic mechanism of HPV is controversial [52], it appears that mitochondria play a key role as the primary sensors of hypoxia, with intracellular calcium levels increasing as a key response [53, 54]. Voltage-gated K^+ channels directly alter mitochondrial responses. L-type Ca^{2+} channels are facilitated by the depolarization of the K^+ channels, and they directly increase intracellular Ca^{2+}. Classical transient receptor potential channel 6 (TRPC6) also increases intracellular Ca^{2+} as do store-operated channels (SOC) and Na^+/Ca^{2+} exchangers (NCX) [53]. This rise in intracellular Ca^{2+} triggers further Ca^{2+} release from the sarcoplasmic reticulum via activation of the ryanodine receptors. The end result is constriction of the smooth muscle of the precapillary sphincters and pulmonary arterioles. This calcium-dependent vasoconstriction is the primary phase of HPV and lasts 15–30 min. The calcium-independent phase (the sustained phase) of pulmonary vascular constriction starts at 15 min and can last for several hours. It is highly dependent on RhoA/Rho kinase (ROCK)-mediated Ca^{2+} sensitization [55] and may play a key role in the development of pulmonary hypertension [56]. Interestingly, NO-induced relaxation and endothelin-1-induced vasoconstriction of pulmonary arteries has been demonstrated to be due to the regulation of ROCK-mediated Ca^{2+}-sensitization, rather than altered Ca^{2+} metabolism [57, 58].

End tidal CO_2 can influence HPV. Alveolar hypercapnia, but not arterial hypercapnia, can inhibit NO synthetase [59]. This inhibition augments the increase in pulmonary vascular tone following endothelin-induced vasoconstriction. Consequently, mild hypercapnia can reduce shunt. However, hypoventilation can worsen hypoxemia, as can right heart strain and decreasing cardiac output.

Anesthetics can influence pulmonary vascular function and inhibit HPV. Inhalational agents (halothane and enflurane and, to a lesser degree, isoflurane, desflurane, and sevoflurane) will inhibit HPV but at concentrations of greater than 1 MAC [60]. Propofol may have a less profound impact on HPV than the inhalational agents [61], but this effect is not significant when a BIS of 40–60 is targeted [62]. Opioids, benzodiazepines, and epidural and paravertebral analgesics/anesthetics have minimal impact. Normothermia, mild hypercapnia, and mild acidosis may enhance HPV. Direct vasodilators such as sodium nitroprusside and nitroglycerine should be avoided as they abolish HPV, thus increasing the shunt and causing hypoxemia [55, 60]. Antihypertensives such as beta-blockers, calcium channel blockers, and angiotensin-converting enzyme (ACE) inhibitors may theoretically reduce HPV but have minimal impact in clinical practice [35].

It is unlikely that the routine patient would tolerate the sole use of regional anesthesia, especially during an open thoracotomy. The techniques of general and epidural or paravertebral anesthesia often are combined to utilize the benefits of each. The relative contribution of each technique to combined anesthesia can vary. The regional block may either be used for postoperative analgesia or as the major anesthetic, with light general anesthesia used for amnesia and sedation. Regional block has the advantages of reduction in afterload, improved pulmonary function [63–67],

decreased incidence of venous thromboembolism [63, 68, 69], and suppression of the stress response [67, 70–73]. Potential disadvantages include the time required to establish the block, potential increased fluid requirements, relative decrease in blood pressure associated with sympathectomy, and the potential for adverse complications such as epidural hematoma.

A prospective, randomized, controlled clinical study has previously examined the effects of epidural anesthesia and postoperative analgesia on the postoperative morbidity rate in high-risk surgical patients [74]. Patients who received epidural anesthesia and analgesia had fewer overall complications and fewer cardiovascular or major infectious complications, lower urinary cortisol secretion (a marker of the stress response), and lower hospital costs [74]. Vital capacity and lung compliance are known to decrease after general anesthesia and neuromuscular blockade in patients undergoing thoracotomy. Epidural analgesia with light general anesthesia results in a comparatively lesser decrease in static compliance and fewer alterations in postoperative pulmonary function [75, 76]. The perioperative use of epidural anesthesia is also associated with fewer major postoperative infections. This may result from (1) the decreased duration of endotracheal intubation and mechanical ventilation, which diminishes many of the defense mechanisms against infection [77, 78]; (2) decreased duration of intensive care unit (ICU) stay postoperatively and reduced risks of nosocomial infection; (3) suppression of the endocrine stress response to the surgery, which has an inhibitory effect on the immune system; and (4) improved compliance with pulmonary toilet. Immune competence is better preserved postoperatively when epidural anesthesia is used compared with other anesthetic/analgesic techniques [70, 72, 73]. Epidural anesthesia is also reported to be associated with fewer cardiovascular complications, such as a lower incidence of congestive heart failure [75] and decreased size of myocardial infarctions, which are probably related to improved regional subendocardial perfusion [71, 79, 80]. Possible mechanisms for the improved function include afferent sensory blockade, decreased adrenergic tone, and coronary and systemic vasodilation with a reduction in cardiac preload and afterload [71, 79, 80].

The timing of initiation of regional anesthetic is a mildly contentious issue. There has been no consistent benefit from a preemptive analgesic approach when measuring long-term outcomes (chronic pain, survival, readmission, etc.) where the regional anesthetic is established well prior to surgical incision [27, 81]. Similarly, it remains unclear what the concentration of intraoperative local anesthetics should be, since concentrations of bupivacaine an order of magnitude apart (0.5–0.05%) have similar short- and long-term pain outcomes as well as similar morbidity and mortality [81–84]. It is considered that if an epidural is employed, a thoracic epidural and a combination of local anesthetics and opioids [85] are superior to local anesthetics or opioids alone. For paravertebral blockade there is no advantage of adding opioids to local anesthetics [86]. A real advantage of utilizing a combined regional and general anesthetic approach is the ability to limit the amount of inhaled anesthetics, thereby theoretically reducing the inhibition of HPV. The risk of hypotension is reduced with a paravertebral catheter as compared to an epidural catheter [87], but even with an epidural, it can be easily managed with alpha agonists and minimal fluid therapy.

Maintenance of anesthesia during thoracic surgery requires attention to the activities of the surgeon. Given the typically long time between induction and incision, epidural or paravertebral bupivacaine loaded after incision should blunt the majority of sympathetic stimulation from the incision and retractor insertion. Manipulation of visceral pleura and the bronchi, which have vagal and phrenic afferents, is not blocked by regional anesthesia; accordingly, these may require supplemental inhalational or intravenous agents.

Volatile, halogenated anesthetic drugs have several desirable properties for use during thoracic procedures. They decrease airway irritability and obtund airway reflexes in patients who usually have reactive airways, and they maintain adequate anesthesia while allowing increased inspired oxygen concentrations. They can be eliminated rapidly, allowing tracheal extubation in the operating room with less concern for postoperative respiratory depression. While it has not been definitively been shown to alter outcome, fluorinated inhalational agents inhibit pulmonary inflammation from lung surgery as compared to propofol [88]. Although volatile anesthetics allow high inspired O_2 concentrations, they may reduce PaO_2 by increasing the shunt caused by the partial inhibition of HPV. Because large intrapulmonary shunts are anticipated with the initiation of OLV, it is prudent to increase the inspired concentration of oxygen. Nitrous oxide should be avoided in patients who have marginal preoperative oxygenation or in those with large bullae and emphysematous lungs to avoid expansion of bullae by nitrous oxide.

The management of perioperative fluid therapy remains controversial without conclusive data to guide treatment [89]. The origins of the controversy stem from the significant risk of mortality in patients who develop ALI (previously also termed "post-pneumonectomy pulmonary edema") after thoracic surgery. Retrospective reviews have highlighted the possible role of fluid management in the development of ALI, with large volumes of crystalloid and blood component therapy predicting post-pneumonectomy pulmonary edema in regression analysis [90]. Obviously, these predictors can simply represent more complex surgery on sicker patients. However, typical guidelines that are pro-

mulgated suggest minimizing crystalloid therapy by not replacing the overnight losses, utilizing alpha agonists rather than fluid boluses to compensate for vasodilatation from regional anesthesia, and disregarding low urine output and consider utilizing appropriate blood transfusion to replace lost blood [45, 91]. These guidelines appear prudent, especially given that concomitant smoking-related cardiac disease can decrease systolic function and potentiate right heart strain from surgery and associated changes in pulmonary vascular resistance.

In brief, much data has been accumulated to suggest that perioperative ALI is an inflammatory response to perioperative stress [46, 92]. Regardless of the volume of fluid, 0.9% (normal) saline appears to induce a stress response in research settings [93]. However, since there are scant data to suggest that other balanced salt solutions would result in an improved outcome, the use of colloids to reduce overall extracellular fluid gain seems reasonable. The concern over the antiplatelet/antithrombotic effect of hydroxyethyl starch results from the effects of the early high-molecular-weight compounds, the so-called HES 200/0.5, when dosed greater than 15 mL/kg [94–96]. The newer formulation with small starch particles, the HES 130/0.42, has fewer risks and may be a better alternative to older HES formulations and large-volume crystalloid therapy for blood loss that needs replacement. Albumin therapy probably has an insignificant role in perioperative fluid management unless a large volume of pleural effusion or peritoneal effusion has been drained at the time of surgery [97, 98]. HES has not been shown to decrease mortality [99, 100].

Overall, perioperative fluid management goals for a lobectomy or pneumonectomy attempt to maintain a euvolemic state – favoring fluid restriction (~1.0–1.5 L total crystalloid) and the judicious use of vasoconstrictors such as phenylephrine to provide hemodynamic stability, in an attempt to preserve renal function. Although large volumes of blood loss are rare, any blood loss should be replaced with packed red blood cells. Fresh frozen plasma should only be considered when directed by perioperative testing indicating coagulopathy. Platelet therapy is rarely indicated except in the case of severe thrombocytopenia or perioperative platelet inhibitors associated with widespread oozing, where there are few other therapeutic choices available.

With restriction of fluid therapy comes a concern about renal damage [101]. A recent review indicates that patients who developed acute kidney injury (AKI) were significantly older and had a larger body mass index, higher ASA classification, lower preoperative hemoglobin concentration, higher serum creatinine, and lower glomerular filtration rate. Further AKI was seen in patients who received larger intraoperative volumes of crystalloid [101]. Consequently, AKI seems to be related to preoperative comorbidities and difficulty/duration of surgery.

Postoperative Care

On the basis of the evidence available showing improved postoperative outcomes with aggressive postoperative management in high-risk general surgical patients [102] and thoracic surgery patients [103], a decision-making algorithm may guide the need for elective admission into a high dependency unit (HDU) or ICU postoperatively [103]. Proposed criteria include the following: age > 70 years; those at increased risk of general anesthesia, as judged by ASA risk score, performance status scores, and cardiovascular risk assessment; and those patients with preexisting fibrotic lung disease. Patients undergoing OLV, especially with a predicted postoperative forced expiratory volume in one second (FEV_1) of less than 44%, and those undergoing extensive lymphatic dissection should be monitored closely for signs of ALI in the first 5 days postoperatively. These high-risk categories, together with any indication of postoperative complications such as bronchopleural fistula (BPF) or empyema, should mandate immediate transfer to the ICU.

Early identification of high-risk individuals will allow close monitoring and early institution of therapy during the "golden hours" immediately following surgery. Such therapy may include early goal-directed therapy with hemodynamic optimization, early institution of CPAP for hypoxemia, aggressive pain management, and early mobilization. Such strategies are expected to improve postoperative outcomes and shorten length of hospital stays.

Lung Cancer

Lung cancer is currently the most common cause of cancer mortality throughout the world, with 243,820 new cases diagnosed and 158,080 deaths reported in the USA in 2015 [104]. The World Health Organization (WHO) classification of lung tumors, revised most recently in 2015 [105], remains the foundation for lung carcinoma nomenclature. Lung cancer is divided into two broad categories: small cell lung carcinoma (SCLC, ~15–20%) and non-small cell lung carcinoma (NSCLC, ~80–85%). Less common are other types of cancers, e.g., bronchial carcinoid tumors. SCLC has been demonstrated to have a strong correlation with cigarette smoking [106]. NSCLC comprises several broad categories based on histology: adenocarcinoma (38–61%), squamous cell carcinoma (SCC, 21–38%), large cell carcinoma, pleomorphic carcinoma, and adenosquamous carcinoma [107, 108].

Intrathoracic Manifestations

The clinical manifestations of lung cancer are varied. Common symptoms include shortness of breath, hemoptysis, chest pain, and increasing dyspnea on exertion. Pleural effusions are a common but nonspecific finding observed on chest radiographs. Such effusions result from obstruction of lymphatic drainage or malignant extension of the tumor to the lung surface. Chest pain associated with lung cancer is generally a dull or mild nonspecific pain occurring ipsilateral to the tumor. Metastasis to the chest wall and ribs can result in local tenderness and pleuritic chest pain. Shoulder pain may result from tumor growth at the lung apex and invasion or encroachment of the brachial plexus (such as in superior sulcus or Pancoast tumors) or invasion of the phrenic nerve. Tumor extension into the pericardium can result in pericarditis, cardiac arrhythmias, and pericardial effusions that cause tamponade. In addition, superior vena cava obstruction by direct invasion or lymphatic metastases impedes venous return from the head and upper extremities. Other manifestations of lung cancer include neurologic symptoms caused by mechanical encroachment or invasion of the nerve plexus. Involvement of the brachial plexus may result in not only shoulder pain but also upper arm pain and weakness. Involvement of the phrenic nerve can lead to unilateral diaphragmatic dysfunction, and involvement of the recurrent laryngeal nerve is characterized by hoarseness of the voice.

Extrathoracic Metastatic Manifestations

Common extrathoracic sites of metastases include the lymph nodes, brain, bone, liver, skin, and adrenal glands [109]. The neurologic manifestations of metastatic brain tumors include hemiplegia, personality changes, cerebellar disturbances, seizures, headache, and confusion. Metastases to the bone occur primarily in the ribs, vertebra, humerus, and femur. Although metastases to the spinal cord and vertebral column are less common, they have implications for positioning and postoperative management of pain.

Extrathoracic Nonmetastatic Manifestations

The extrapulmonary manifestations of lung cancer affect the metabolic, neuromuscular, skeletal, dermatologic, vascular, and hematologic systems. Although uncommon, the systemic manifestations of such paraneoplastic syndromes, especially the metabolic and neuromuscular manifestations, and other nonspecific findings such as malaise, weight loss, and cachexia, may affect perioperative management and impact the patient's recovery and survival.

Metabolic manifestations result from endocrine secretions by the tumor as follows:

- Adrenal corticotrophic hormone (ACTH, Cushing's syndrome): most often associated with small cell carcinoma [110].

- Antidiuretic hormone (syndrome of excessive ADH): associated with small cell carcinoma; it may manifest as nausea, vomiting, anorexia, hyponatremia, seizures, or other neurologic disturbances [111].
- Serotonin (carcinoid syndrome): diagnosed by elevated 5-hydroxyindoleacetic acid (5-HIAA) [110].
- Parathyroid hormone-like polypeptide: associated with bronchogenic carcinoma; results in hypercalcemia and hypophosphatemia [112].
- Ectopic gonadotropin production and hypoglycemia are rare manifestations.

Neuromuscular manifestations are the most frequent extrathoracic nonmetastatic effects of lung cancer, most often associated with small cell carcinoma of the lung [109, 113]. The paraneoplastic myopathy, Eaton-Lambert syndrome, may appear as a myasthenic-like syndrome characterized by proximal muscle weakness, particularly of the pelvic and thigh muscles. The defect in neuromuscular transmission is a result of an antibody-mediated impairment in presynaptic neurocalcium channel activity, which reduces the release of acetylcholine [113]. Patients with this syndrome do not respond as well to anticholinesterase drugs as do patients with myasthenia gravis. In contrast, these patients exhibit an increased sensitivity to succinylcholine and non-depolarizing muscle relaxants.

Other neuromuscular manifestations include subacute cerebral degeneration, encephalomyelopathy, and polymyositis. The cause and the pathogenesis of these neuropathies are not completely understood. Immunologic factors are believed to be important in the pathogenic process, because antibody and T-cell responses are directed against shared antigens that are ectopically expressed by the tumor but otherwise exclusively expressed by the nervous system [114].

In general, these extrathoracic symptoms resolve, and laboratory studies return to normal after successful tumor resection.

Treatment Options

SCLC tumors often have distant metastases at the time of diagnosis and are therefore managed primarily by chemotherapy. Only ~50% of people with SCLC survive for 4 months without chemotherapy. With chemotherapy, their survival time is increased by four to five-fold. Chemotherapy may be given alone, as an adjuvant to surgical therapy, or in combination with radiotherapy. While a number of chemotherapeutic drugs have been developed, the platinum-based class of drugs has been the most effective in the treatment of lung cancers. Chemotherapy alone is not particularly effective in treating primary NSCLC, but prolongs survival when NSCLC has metastasized [115].

Radiation therapy may be employed as a treatment for both NSCLC and SCLC. Radiation therapy may be given as curative therapy, palliative therapy (using lower doses of radiation than with curative therapy), or adjuvant therapy in combination with surgery or chemotherapy. Radiation therapy can be administered if a person refuses surgery, if a tumor has spread to areas such as lymph nodes or the trachea – making surgical removal impossible, or if a person has other conditions that disallow major surgery. Radiation therapy generally only shrinks a tumor or limits its growth when given as a sole therapy; however, in 10–15% of patients, it leads to long-term remission and palliation of the cancer. Combining radiation therapy with chemotherapy can further prolong survival.

NSCLC tumors are more localized and thus better candidates than other types of tumors for curative resection. Surgical removal of the tumor is generally performed for limited-stage NSCLC (Stage I or some Stage II; see Chap. 2) [116]. About 10–35% of lung cancers can be removed surgically, but removal does not always result in a cure, since the tumors may already have spread microscopically and can recur. Lobectomy, the surgical removal of an anatomic lobe of a lung, is generally accepted as the optimal procedure for early-stage NSCLC because of its ability to preserve pulmonary function [116]. Limited (sub-lobar, segmentectomy) resection is increasingly used to treat patients who cannot tolerate a full lobectomy because of severely compromised pulmonary function, advanced age, or extensive medical comorbidities. Among people who have an isolated, node-negative lung cancer resected, the 5-year survival is now in the range of 47–92%, depending on size and degree of invasion [117]. In addition to surgery, adjuvant chemotherapy may be administered for selected patients with Stage IB, II, and IIIA disease for a 5-year absolute survival benefit of 5.4%. There are predictors of response to adjuvant chemotherapy. The morphology of the tumor, using the new WHO classification of lung adenocarcinoma, can predict response to adjuvant chemotherapy [118]. Gene expression profiles have also been developed from randomized trials of adjuvant chemotherapy to predict which early-stage lung cancers will have a poorer prognosis and a better response to adjuvant chemotherapy [119]. Many advances have been made on companion biomarkers and therapy in NSCLC. These are vital in a disease where even apparent curative surgery has a high relapse rate. The presence of specific genomic aberrations, specifically activating EGFR mutation and ALK or ROS1 gene rearrangements, predicts very high response rates with targeted therapies such as gefitinib and erlotinib (tyrosine kinase inhibitors of EGFR) and crizotinib (tyrosine kinase inhibitor of ALK) [120, 121]. Almost invariably, the tumors eventually become resistant to these therapies with time, due to the selection pressure of resistant clones within a notoriously heterogeneous tumor. Newer-generation tyrosine kinase inhibitors which target the common resistance mechanisms are currently in clinical trials.

The presence of PDL-1 expression and tumor-infiltrating lymphocytes (TILs) appears to predict response for the immune checkpoint inhibitors such as nivolumab and pembrolizumab, with an apparent durable remission in 15–20% of cases.

These advances and the improved surgical results over the last decade suggest that the nihilism associated with lung cancer [122] should be consigned to history and every endeavor should be made to resect lung cancers from patients with adequate physiologic reserves.

Anesthesia and Long-Term Cancer Outcomes

It is increasingly recognized that anesthetic factors (volatile agents, opioid analgesics, surgical neuroendocrine response, blood transfusion, etc.) may shift the balance toward the progression of residual disease after potentially curative cancer surgery [123, 124]. Anesthetics may inhibit both cellular and humoral immune functions through the impairment of neutrophil, macrophage, T-cell, and natural killer cell functions. Regional analgesia attenuates these adverse events by largely preventing the neuroendocrine surgical stress response and minimizing the amount of volatile anesthetic and opioids required. Preliminary animal and human data suggest that regional analgesia may reduce tumor recurrence after cancer surgery [124].

Other perioperative strategies that may impact long-term cancer outcomes seem to focus on anti-inflammatory pathways. Statins, via the inhibition of the rate-limiting step of the mevalonate pathway, have potential anticancer effects [125]. There is some evidence for the anticancer effects of statins in patients with esophageal [126] and lung cancer [127, 128]. Additionally, other agents with known anti-inflammatory effects also point to the potential for improved outcomes in cancer patients. In this regard, aspirin use is reported to be associated with prolonged survival in many types of cancer, but often only seen after many years of therapy [129], while the perioperative use of anti-inflammatory agents (Cox-II inhibitor use in lung cancer; aprotinin use in mesothelioma) [130, 131] is associated with improved postoperative survival. Moreover, the use of regional analgesia is commonly employed in the thoracic surgery population and has been associated with attenuation of metastasis and improvement in recurrence rates for some types of cancers [123, 124]. It is imperative that further research is conducted in this field as we strive to improve long-term outcomes.

Surgical Procedure

To allow anesthesiologists to function within the combined expertise of the multidisciplinary team and to ensure optimal patient safety and outcome, a thorough understanding of the salient features of procedure-specific issues is required.

Pulmonary Resection

In most thoracic surgery practices, approximately two-thirds of surgical interventions are related to the management of intrathoracic malignancy or clinical sequelae of cancer. Anatomic resections (segmentectomy, lobectomy, and pneumonectomy) are most commonly performed for lung cancer, while nonanatomic resections (wedge) are typically performed for pulmonary nodules with diagnostic or therapeutic intention. Lobectomy with mediastinal lymph node dissection remains the standard surgical recommendation for the technical management of lung cancer. Segmental resection is a sound oncological operation that is typically used in patients with smaller cancers and marginal pulmonary reserve, such as those patients with COPD [132]. Pneumonectomy offers some more unique possible challenges including a higher mortality rate. The mortality rate of pneumonectomy is 8–10% vs. 2% for lobectomy [133].

Pulmonary resections can be performed via an open, thoracoscopic, or robotic approach. The technical aspects of the resection are essentially identical regardless of the approach. Evolution of surgical technique and technical advances in electronics and instrumentation has renewed interest in thoracoscopy, especially video-assisted thoracic surgery (VATS) and robotic VATS. As such, thoracoscopy permits the visualization of the pulmonary cavity through several small portals. These portals provide access for the video camera and allow manipulation of thoracic structures and use of surgical instruments such as staplers, dissectors, coagulators, and lasers. Although initially used for only minor surgical procedures, the application of VATS and robotics has expanded considerably for both diagnostic and therapeutic procedures and increasingly utilized in anatomic (lobectomy, segmentectomy) and limited (wedge) resections in selected patients.

Data suggests that VATS procedures may offer advantages beyond open thoracotomy, including decreased postoperative pain, reduced pulmonary impairment, reduced postoperative morbidity, shortened hospital stay, and potentially improved 1-year survival [134, 135]. There is less evidence of benefit of robotic-assisted thoracic surgery, but it seems to be at least equivalent to VATS in outcomes as compared to open surgery [136]. If access is inadequate or if bleeding complications occur, a thoracoscopic approach is easily converted to a limited open thoracotomy. VATS procedures for larger resections such as lobectomy seem to derive benefit from more aggressive pain management strategies, and epidural techniques may be beneficial. As such, careful communication between surgeon, patient, anesthesiologist, and the acute pain service is warranted to determine the best pain management strategy for each patient.

A thorough physiological assessment with attention to physiological and cardiac reserve is required prior to proceeding with surgical therapy. Spirometry, quantitative ventilation-perfusion scanning, and exercise cardiopulmonary testing can be helpful to determine physiological reserve for resection considerations. When considering pulmonary resection, a postoperative predicted FEV_1 or D_LCO of greater that 40% is a general requirement for resection considerations. In this regard, for patients whose preoperative FEV_1 or D_LCO is less than 60% predicted, a quantitative lung scan is performed to determine the predicted postoperative lung function. If the predicted postoperative ppoFEV_1 or D_LCO is greater than 40%, then surgical resection is feasible. In patients with predicted postoperative FEV_1 or D_LCO less than 40%, additional workup with cardiopulmonary exercise testing is required to delineate patient risk. Adequate aerobic exercise capacity (preoperative VO_2 max > 15 mL/kg/min and predicted postoperative VO_2 max > 10 mL/kg/min or stair climb >3 flights of stairs – 54 steps) improves patients' safety of operation [137]. In those patients who fail to meet these criteria, alternatives to resection should be considered. Relative contraindications for pulmonary resection that point to inadequate pulmonary reserve include chronic oxygen use, severe hypercarbia ($PaCO_2$ > 55 mmHg), and moderate pulmonary hypertension (PA pressure greater than one-half systemic pressures).

Anesthetic management for pulmonary resection requires effective isolation of the operative lung, judicious fluid management, and an appropriate ventilation strategy of the dependent lung [138–140]. Intraoperative bleeding is not a common challenge; however, catastrophic hemorrhage can occur in association with pulmonary arterial injury. This necessitates that patients have preoperative typing and screening for potential transfusion, with good venous access and hemodynamic monitoring – typically an arterial line and two large peripheral cannulae. More central cancers generally increase the risk for an intraoperative event.

The primary cause of perioperative mortality of lung resection remains ALI which can be secondary to infection, transfusion-related, pulmonary embolism, but often there is no specific identifiable etiology. Two factors, intraoperative fluid administration and prolonged elevated airway pressures during OLV, have been consistently implicated with perioperative lung injury [138–140]. Optimal intraoperative management of these factors is thus required.

During the conduct of an anatomic pulmonary resection, three structures (the pulmonary artery, pulmonary vein, and bronchus) are identified and divided at the segmental level (segmentectomy), at the bronchial level (lobectomy), or at the main stem bronchus (pneumonectomy). Prior to division of any structure, there must be assurance that anesthetic "hardware" (endotracheal tubes, suction catheters, nasogastric tube, pulmonary arterial catheters) are absent from the site of resection. Additionally, during the conduct of a segmental resection or lobectomy, patency of the remaining airway must be confirmed prior to airway division. This requires temporary ventilation of the lung in the surgical field to ensure expansion of non-resected segments or lobes. Intraoperatively, chest drains are placed for perioperative management. During chest closure while the patient is still requiring positive-pressure ventilation, these drainage catheters should be placed to suction. Provided that postoperative air leak is minimal, most surgeons manage chest drainage tube without suction (i.e., "water seal") [141].

Regardless of the type of pulmonary resection performed, extubation should be planned following surgery. Adequate postoperative analgesia is required to optimize patient outcome by ensuring the patient can cough and has adequate tidal volumes with breathing. As a result, liberal use of thoracic epidural analgesia is encouraged. Resumption of spontaneous breathing will avoid possible lung barotrauma as well as the risk of bronchial stump disruption and resultant BPF formation. Attention to optimal analgesia, pulmonary toilet, and pleural space management is required to achieve optimal patient outcome. Regional analgesia with epidural catheter provides superior pain control and promotes effective pulmonary toilet. Early mobilization is required with ambulation initiated the first postoperative day. Most patients will have a component of underlying reactive airway disease, and regular administration of bronchodilator therapy is typically used. Awake, bedside bronchoscopy is used liberally for secretion management. Noninvasive ventilator support, such as CPAP or BiPAP, can be used, but more often, endotracheal intubation is optimal for postoperative respiratory failure so as to decrease risk of aspiration event and subsequent pneumonia.

Lobectomy

Lobectomy with mediastinal lymph node dissection remains the standard surgical recommendation for the technical management of lung cancer. Lobectomy, commonly performed via open thoracotomy or VATS, is associated with lower local tumor recurrence compared to lesser resections. An open thoracotomy is usually performed through a posterolateral thoracotomy incision, but anterolateral and muscle-sparing lateral incisions are used occasionally. In cases where the clinical staging of the lung cancer is advanced, an elective lobectomy may be converted to a bilobectomy or pneumonectomy during the operation. Potential intraoperative problems include damage to the airway while using lung isolation devices, potential for bleeding, and hypoxemia during OLV.

After the lobe and blood vessels have been dissected, a test maneuver is performed by the surgeon clamping the surgical bronchus and confirming that the correct lobe is extirpated. The anesthesiologist then unclamps the DLT on the respective side or, in the case of a bronchial blocker, deflates the blocker balloon and re-expands the lung with manual ventilation. During VATS lobectomy, reinflating the residual lobe may interfere with the surgical field, and so the anesthesiologist may be asked to fiber-optically inspect the bronchial tree to confirm patency of the bronchus of the noninvolved lobe. Once the lobectomy has been performed, the bronchial stump is usually tested with 30 cm H_2O positive pressure in the anesthetic circuit to detect the presence of air leaks. Following an uncomplicated lobectomy, the patient is usually extubated in the operating room, provided preoperative respiratory function is adequate. Emergence of the patient in a comfortable manner with good inspiratory effort and ability to cough requires aggressive postoperative analgesia, commonly achieved through the use of either a thoracic epidural or through a paravertebral analgesia technique.

Pancoast tumors are carcinomas of the superior sulcus of the lung and can invade/compress local structures including the lower brachial plexus, subclavian blood vessels, stellate ganglion (resulting in Horner's syndrome), and vertebrae. More complicated resection may entail a two-stage procedure with an initial operation for posterior instrumentation/stabilization of the spine. During lobectomy extensive chest wall resection may be required and massive transfusion is a possibility. Peripheral lines and monitoring should be placed in the contralateral arm due to frequent compression of the ipsilateral vessels during surgery.

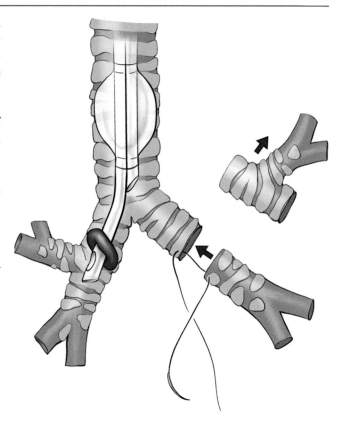

Fig. 23.3 Illustration of a sleeve resection for carcinoma of the left upper lobe, with reimplantation of the left lower lobe

Sleeve Lobectomy

Bronchogenic carcinoma is the most frequent indication for a sleeve lobectomy, followed by carcinoid tumors, endobronchial metastases, primary airway tumors, bronchial adenomas, and occasionally benign strictures. Sleeve lobectomy involving parenchyma-sparing techniques in patients with limited pulmonary reserve provides an alternative surgery for patients that cannot tolerate a pneumonectomy. The sleeve technique involves main stem bronchial resection without parenchymal involvement and possibly resection of pulmonary arteries to avoid pneumonectomy (Fig. 23.3). Sleeve resection, with reimplantation of the remaining lobe, associates with shorter periods of postoperative mechanical ventilation, shorter duration of ICU stay, fewer locoregional recurrences, and improved overall survival. Immediate and long-term survival is better after sleeve lobectomy compared with right pneumonectomy for comparable stages of right upper lobe cancer [142].

Ideally, patients undergoing sleeve lobectomy require lung isolation with a contralateral DLT or endobronchial tube, thereby improving surgical exposure for resection and reimplantation. High-frequency jet ventilation can be used for resections close to the tracheal carina. In rare cases a sleeve lobectomy may require transplant of vessels, thereby

necessitating temporary heparinization. In these cases, thoracic epidural catheters should not be manipulated for 24 h following heparin administration. During pulmonary arterioplasty uncontrollable bleeding may occur. For this reason, large bore intravenous catheters should be used. Patients undergoing sleeve lobectomy are usually extubated in the operating room before transfer to the postanesthesia recovery room.

Pneumonectomy

Complete removal of the lung is required when a lobectomy or its modifications (bilobectomy or sleeve lobectomy) are not adequate to remove the local disease and/or ipsilateral lymph node metastases. However, pneumonectomy offers more unique challenges, including a higher incidence of morbidity (cardiac complications, ALI, ARDS) and mortality (8–10% for pneumonectomy vs. 2% for lobectomy) [133]. The overall operative mortality correlates inversely with the surgical case volume [143].

The technical conduct of the resection is typical as with any pulmonary resection. The pneumonectomy is usually performed through a standard posterolateral incision. Following incision of the mediastinal pleura, the pulmonary artery, the superior and inferior pulmonary veins, and the main stem bronchus are evaluated for resectability. After all vessels are stapled, stapling of the bronchus occurs, and the entire lung is taken from the chest. A test for air leaks is generally performed at this point, and reconstruction of the bronchial stump is completed. The bronchial stump should be as short as possible to prevent a pocket for the collection of secretions.

Patients undergoing a pneumonectomy commonly receive a thoracic epidural catheter for postoperative analgesia, unless there is a contraindication. The placement of large bore intravenous lines is necessary in case blood products need to be administered. An invasive arterial line is placed for measurement of beat-to-beat blood pressure and to monitor arterial blood gases. A central venous pressure catheter is recommended to help guide intravascular fluid management, specifically in the postoperative period. Management of lung isolation in a pneumonectomy patient can be achieved with a DLT, bronchial blocker, or single-lumen endobronchial tube. When using a DLT for a pneumonectomy patient, it is preferable to use a device that does not interfere with the ipsilateral airway; however, the preference to use a left-sided DLT (or left-sided bronchial blocker) requires that during a left pneumonectomy, these devices are withdrawn prior to stapling the bronchus, in order to avoid accidental inclusion into the suture line.

Challenges can arise related to the empty hemithorax following pneumonectomy. There is no consensus among thoracic surgeons as to the best management of the post-pneumonectomy space. Some thoracic surgeons do not place a chest drain after a pneumonectomy, while others prefer a temporary drainage catheter to add or remove air. The removal of air, ranging from 0.75 to 1.5 L, is necessary to empty the chest and to keep the mediastinum and trachea "balanced" (in the midline). Some surgeons place a specifically designed post-pneumonectomy chest drainage system with both high- and low-pressure underwater relief valves to balance the mediastinum. A chest X-ray is mandatory after the patient arrives in the postanesthesia care unit or in the surgical ICU to assess for mediastinal shift. If suction is applied to an empty hemithorax or a chest drain is connected to a standard underwater seal system, it may cause mediastinal shift, impingement of venous return to the heart, and hemodynamic collapse. This requires correction with appropriate instillation or evacuation of air from the empty hemithorax. Although rare, cardiac herniation (more common following right pneumonectomy) can occur with catastrophic consequences and need for emergent correction.

The high morbidity and mortality associated with pneumonectomy are predominantly driven by ALI (also previously termed "post-pneumonectomy pulmonary edema"), culminating in respiratory failure. While the incidence of ALI after pneumonectomy is only 4%, the mortality rate associated with ALI is 30–50%.

The etiology for ALI seems multifactorial. In a retrospective report by Zeldin et al. [144], the risk factors that were identified for the development of ALI, previously termed "post-pneumonectomy pulmonary edema," were a right-sided pneumonectomy, increased perioperative intravenous fluid administration, and increased urine output in the postoperative period. However, close analysis of Zeldin's data reveals that only six out of ten cases had full intake and output data. A more recent study by Licker et al. has shown that the excessive administration of intravenous fluids in thoracic surgical patients (more than 3 L in the first 24 h) is an independent risk related to an ALI [139]. Further, the decrease in ventilatory function, increase in pulmonary artery pressure, and pulmonary vascular resistance (right ventricular afterload) may have a significant detrimental effect on right ventricular function [145].

Consequently, in an attempt to reduce high risk for perioperative morbidity and mortality following a pneumonectomy, perioperative management should focus on the judicious management of perioperative fluid therapy, tidal volumes during mechanical ventilation, and improved ICU strategies. In this regard, a retrospective review (Table 23.1) suggested that the incidence and mortality of ARDS after lung resection are declining and likely associated with more aggressive strategies to avoid pneumonectomy and greater attention to protective ventilation strategies during surgery and to improved ICU management of ARDS [2].

A retrospective report [146] involving 170 pneumonectomy patients showed that patients that received median tidal volumes greater than 8 mL/kg had a greater risk of respiratory failure in the postoperative period after pneumonectomy. In contrast, patients that received tidal volumes less than 6 mL/kg were at lower risk of respiratory failure. Schilling et al. [147] have shown that a tidal volume of 5 mL/kg during OLV significantly reduces the inflammatory response to alveolar cytokines. Considering these factors, it is prudent to use lower tidal volumes (i.e., 5–6 mL/kg, ideal body weight) in the pneumonectomy patient and limit peak and plateau inspiratory pressures (i.e., <30 and 25 cm H_2O) during OLV [138].

The presentation of ALI is biphasic, with intraoperative strategies (fluid restriction and lower tidal volumes) aimed at reducing the incidence of the primary form, which typically has a clinical onset during the first 72 h. The secondary, or late form, appears after 72 h and is usually related to other complications such as aspiration, BPF, or surgical complications. At the present time, only symptomatic management is appropriate for ALI, including fluid restrictions, diuretic administration, low ventilatory pressures and tidal volumes (if mechanical ventilation is used), and measures to decrease the pulmonary artery pressure.

Sleeve Pneumonectomy

Tumors involving the most proximal portions of the main stem bronchus and the carina may require a sleeve pneumonectomy. These are most commonly performed for right-sided tumors and can usually be performed without cardiopulmonary bypass via a right thoracotomy. A long single-lumen endobronchial tube can be advanced across into the left main stem bronchus during the period of tracheobronchial anastomosis. High-frequency positive-pressure ventilation has also been used for this procedure. Since the carina is surgically more accessible from the right side, left sleeve pneumonectomies are commonly performed as a two-stage operation, with a left thoracotomy to perform the pneumonectomy and a right thoracotomy to perform the carinal excision. The complication rate and mortality are higher, and the 5-year survival is significantly lower than for other pulmonary resections. Post-pneumonectomy pulmonary edema is particularly a problem following right sleeve pneumonectomy.

Limited Pulmonary Resections: Segmentectomy and Wedge Resection

Segmentectomy and wedge resection are limited pulmonary resections. Segmentectomy is a sound oncological operation that is typically used in patients with smaller cancers and marginal pulmonary reserve, such as those patients with COPD [132]. It entails an anatomic pulmonary resection of the pulmonary artery, vein, bronchus, and parenchyma of a particular segment of the lung. Lung cancers that are considered for limited resection are usually less than 3 cm in size, located in the periphery of the lung, and with regional lymph nodes free of metastatic cancer.

In contrast, a wedge resection is a nonanatomic removal of a portion of the lung parenchyma with a 1.5–2.0 cm margin and can be accomplished by open thoracotomy or VATS. Wedge resections are most commonly performed for diagnosis of lung lesions with unknown histology or as palliation in patients with metastatic lesions in the lungs from distant primary tumors.

A group of patients considered for limited pulmonary resection are those who develop a new primary lesion after a previous lobectomy or pneumonectomy. The patient with compromised lung function presents a greater risk in the intraoperative period (hypoxemia during OLV or prolonged intubation after surgery). Cerfolio [148] et al. reported that lung cancer patients with compromised pulmonary function can safely undergo limited pulmonary resection if selected appropriately. Segmentectomies and wedge resections can be performed with any of the standard thoracotomy or VATS incisions. Segments that are most commonly resected are the lingular and superior divisions of the left upper lobe and the superior segments of the lower lobes.

Anesthetic technique and monitoring are essentially the same as for larger pulmonary resections. In order to facilitate surgical exposure and achieve OLV, it is necessary to use either a DLT or a bronchial blocker. If the patient had a previous contralateral lobectomy or a pneumonectomy, selective lobar collapse with the use of a bronchial blocker will facilitate surgical exposure while maintaining oxygenation. In selected cases the combined use of a DLT and a bronchial blocker will allow selective lobar collapse/ventilation in the ipsilateral lung [149]. It is very important to use low tidal volumes (i.e., 3–5 mL/kg) during selective lobar ventilation, particularly in patients with previous pneumonectomy to prevent overinflation in the remaining lobes.

Segmentectomy plays a significant role in the management of patients with a second primary lung cancer. Many of these patients have previously undergone thoracic surgery; this includes previous lobectomy or pneumonectomy; therefore the potential for increased intraoperative bleeding is always a risk. In addition, because many of these patients have compromised lung function, early extubation may not be feasible. A common complication after surgery is an air leak. Chest tubes are placed to maximize postoperative expansion and minimize space complications. Suction and underwater seal chest drainage are used in the postoperative period.

Bronchopleural Fistula

BPF can result as a consequence of surgical therapy (Fig. 23.4) or from the complications of intrathoracic infection or malignancy (see also Chap. 43). The classic presentation is a patient who has undergone a resection 10–14 days previously, who feels unwell and who has developed a productive cough of "salmon-colored" sputum. Patients can succumb to the resultant soilage of the lung and pneumonitis. If surgical therapy is required for BPF, the surgeon and anesthesiologist must combine their efforts to prevent any further lung injury.

In order to achieve satisfactory and sustainable ventilation, the team must have a command of the airway options as well as knowledge of nonstandard ventilation strategies. Positive-pressure ventilation is achievable in patients with a small fistula. However, with larger fistula, the ability to ventilate without isolating the fistula may be limited, and maintaining spontaneous ventilation may be a requisite. The initial management of the fistula is indeed drainage of

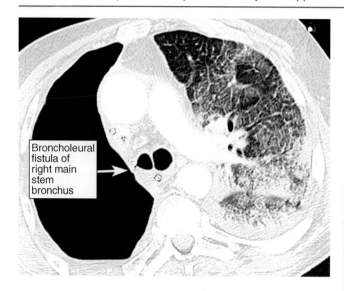

Fig. 23.4 CT image of a bronchopleural fistula in the right main stem bronchus, which developed after pneumonectomy, with accompanying pneumonitis in the contralateral lung

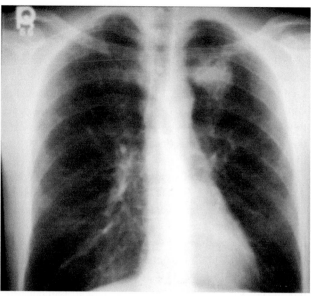

Fig. 23.5 Chest X-ray demonstrating a carcinoma of the left upper lobe

the infected pleural space. Patient positioning should be kept in mind, and the side of the fistula should be maintained in a dependent position. Surgical management of the fistula typically involves closure with vascularized flap coverage or window thoracostomy for drainage. Rarely, additional pulmonary parenchyma resection is required. As with tracheal surgical interventions, the use of jet ventilation and appropriate airway isolation strategies could potentially be necessary. Prompt discontinuation of positive-pressure ventilation is also required. In fact, if patients need positive-pressure ventilation in the presence of a BPF and this provides satisfactory ventilation and oxygenation, the surgical treatment of the BPF is relatively contraindicated.

Clinical Case Discussion

Case: A 68-year-old male presents for anesthesia. He has a 40-pack-year smoking history, hypertension controlled with diltiazem, and hypercholesterolemia controlled with simvastatin. He gives no history of exertional angina. The chest X-ray indicates a mass in the left upper lobe (Fig. 23.5), with absence of metastatic disease as assessed by computerized tomography and by a nuclear bone scan. Pulmonary function testing shows impaired function, characteristic of moderate COPD, with a negligible reversible component and a predicted postoperative FEV_1 of 48%.

Previous diagnostic bronchoscopy revealed encroachment of a non-small cell lung cancer onto the left main stem bronchus. Consequently, he is now scheduled for a

bronchoscopy, mediastinoscopy and left upper lobectomy with sleeve resection, and reattachment of the left lower lobe.

Questions

1. How does the mediastinoscopy alter perioperative management?
2. What airway management technique would be optimal?
3. What invasive monitoring is necessary?
4. Is there an optimal analgesic regimen?
5. Can perioperative fluid management affect outcome?
6. What ventilation strategy would promote optimal outcome?

Discussion

Given the rarity of blood loss requiring blood transfusion, an 18- or 16-gauge intravenous catheter, preferably placed in the nondependent hand, wrist, or forearm, would be appropriate. It is best to avoid the antecubital veins as the arms are bent at 90° when the patient is positioned in a lateral decubitus position, and this will hamper flow of the intravenous fluids. In anticipation of continuation to thoracotomy after mediastinoscopy, a thoracic epidural (alternatively, a paravertebral block) is placed in the T5–T8 region prior to induction. Standard noninvasive monitors will be used, with ECG leads placed as for any median sternotomy, thereby allowing the entire chest to be prepped in a sterile fashion in case an emergent sternotomy is required due to massive bleeding resulting from the mediastinoscopy.

After induction, tailored to the patient, the airway is secured using an 8.0-mm single-lumen endotracheal tube to facilitate bronchoscopy. A LMA can be used for bronchoscopy if mediastinoscopy is not required. The endotracheal tube is usually brought out to the side of the mouth closest to the anesthesia machine once the bed is turned 90° for mediastinoscopy.

Given the absence of significant cardiac disease, invasive monitoring, with placement of an arterial line, can be deferred until after the mediastinoscopy is completed, and the decision is made to proceed to a thoracotomy – based on the absence of mediastinal lymph node involvement by the cancer. Placement of the arterial line is preferred in the dependent radial artery. This allows vigilant hemodynamic monitoring since acute hemodynamic embarrassment often occurs during surgical manipulation and due to the risk of catastrophic pulmonary vasculature injury. Significant fluctuations in blood pressure are especially seen with left-sided procedures where compression of the heart may occur during surgical manipulation.

A right-sided DLT would be of greater advantage in this case. Since a thoracotomy with sleeve resection requires surgical reimplantation of the left lower lobe bronchus (Fig. 23.3), a left-sided DLT may hamper optimal surgical exposure. If intubation is profoundly difficult, to the point where even changing the endotracheal tube over a tube changer would place the patient at significant risk, then alternative strategies including placement of a left main stem bronchial blocker or advancement of the single-lumen endotracheal tube into the right main stem bronchus should be considered.

Clear communication between the surgical and anesthetic team is essential if the pulmonary artery requires resection and reconstruction. In this case blood products should be readily available in the operating room, and steps to reduce the pulmonary artery pressure should be implemented. Such steps may include increased oxygenation (FiO$_2$, 100%), moderate hypocarbia (P$_a$CO$_2$, 30–35 mmHg), an appropriately "deep" level of anesthesia, minimized use of phenylephrine (consider vasopressin if blood pressure is low), and inhaled epoprostenol therapy to the ventilated lung.

Timing of initiation of the epidural and the choice of neuraxial medications remains controversial. A common practice is to initiate the epidural prior to induction so that inhalational anesthetics can be reduced to levels where HPV is not hampered. The intraoperative use of the epidural also helps to minimize the use of systemic opioids to reduce the risk of postoperative respiratory depression. Typically, more concentrated local anesthetics (± opioids) are used intraoperatively and more dilute combinations of local anesthetics and opioids used postoperatively.

The management of perioperative fluid therapy remains a controversy without conclusive data to guide treatment. The origins of the controversy stem from the significant risk of mortality from patients who develop ALI after thoracic surgery, in particular, those that develop post-pneumonectomy pulmonary edema. Typical guidelines suggest minimizing crystalloid therapy to 1.0–1.5 L, as this may help to reduce post-lobectomy pulmonary edema and facilitate early postoperative extubation.

Ventilation parameters during OLV typically strive to reduce the risk of ALI associated with barotrauma or volutrauma through tidal volume reduction (<6 mL/kg), respiratory rate > 10 breaths per minute, I:E ratio of 1:2, and peak inspiratory pressure < 25 mmHg. Such a protective ventilatory strategy aims to maintain baseline CO$_2$ levels or tolerate permissive hypercapnia (pH >7.25) rather than mild hypocapnia. Importantly, prolonged positive-pressure ventilation may hamper the tenuous blood supply of the sleeve anastomosis and increase the risk for a BPF and its associated complications. As such, this necessitates that the overall anesthetic technique be tailored to afford prompt and comfortable extubation of the patient.

References

1. Dulu A, et al. Prevalence and mortality of acute lung injury and ARDS after lung resection. Chest J. 2006;130:73–8.
2. Tang SS, et al. The mortality from acute respiratory distress syndrome after pulmonary resection is reducing: a 10-year single institutional experience. Eur J Cardiothorac Surg. 2008;34:898–902.
3. Kopec SE, Irwin RS, Umali-Torres CB, Balikian JP, Conlan AA. The postpneumonectomy state. Chest J. 1998;114:1158–84.
4. Kutlu CA, Williams EA, Evans TW, Pastorino U, Goldstraw P. Acute lung injury and acute respiratory distress syndrome after pulmonary resection. Ann Thorac Surg. 2000;69:376–80.
5. Vaporciyan AA, et al. Incidence of major pulmonary morbidity after pneumonectomy: association with timing of smoking cessation. Ann Thorac Surg. 2002;73:420–6.
6. Kozower BD, et al. STS database risk models: predictors of mortality and major morbidity for lung cancer resection. Ann Thorac Surg. 2010;90:875–83.
7. Lighter DE. Advanced performance improvement in healthcare. Sudbury: Jones and Bartlett Publishers; 2010. p. 1–16.
8. Kohn LT, Corrigan JM, Donaldson MS. To err is human: building a safer health system. Washington, DC: National Academies Press; 2000.
9. Richardson WC, et al. Crossing the Quality Chasm: A New Health System for the 21st Century. Washington, DC: Institute of Medicine, National Academy Press; 2001.
10. Starmer AJ, et al. Changes in medical errors after implementation of a handoff program. N Engl J Med. 2014;371:1803–12.
11. Vincent C, Moorthy K, Sarker SK, Chang A, Darzi AW. Systems approaches to surgical quality and safety: from concept to measurement. Ann Surg. 2004;239:475–82. 00000658-200404000-00007 [pii].
12. Dimick JB, Pronovost PJ, Cowan JA, Lipsett PA. Surgical volume and quality of care for esophageal resection: do high-volume

hospitals have fewer complications? Ann Thorac Surg. 2003;75:337–41.

13. Chowdhury MM, Dagash H, Pierro A. A systematic review of the impact of volume of surgery and specialization on patient outcome. Br J Surg. 2007;94:145–61.

14. Dimick JB, Cowan JA Jr, Ailawadi G, Wainess RM, Upchurch GR Jr. National variation in operative mortality rates for esophageal resection and the need for quality improvement. Arch Surg. 2003;138:1305–9.

15. Dimick JB, Cowan JA Jr, Upchurch GR Jr, Colletti LM. Hospital volume and surgical outcomes for elderly patients with colorectal cancer in the United States. J Surg Res. 2003;114:50–6.

16. Verhoef C, van de Weyer R, Schaapveld M, Bastiaannet E, Plukker JTM. Better survival in patients with esophageal cancer after surgical treatment in university hospitals: a plea for performance by surgical oncologists. Ann Surg Oncol. 2007;14:1678–87.

17. Kozower BD, Stukenborg GJ. The relationship between hospital lung cancer resection volume and patient mortality risk. Ann Surg. 2011;254:1032–7.

18. Wright CD, Kucharczuk JC, O'brien SM, Grab JD, Allen MS. Predictors of major morbidity and mortality after esophagectomy for esophageal cancer: a Society of Thoracic Surgeons General Thoracic Surgery Database risk adjustment model. J Thorac Cardiovasc Surg. 2009;137:587–96.

19. Zehr KJ, Dawson PB, Yang SC, Heitmiller RF. Standardized clinical care pathways for major thoracic cases reduce hospital costs. Ann Thorac Surg. 1998;66:914–9.

20. Wright CD, et al. Pulmonary lobectomy patient care pathway: a model to control cost and maintain quality. Ann Thorac Surg. 1997;64:299–302.

21. Khuri SF. Quality, advocacy, healthcare policy, and the surgeon. Ann Thorac Surg. 2002;74:641–9.

22. Khuri SF, Daley J, Henderson WG. The comparative assessment and improvement of quality of surgical care in the Department of Veterans Affairs. Arch Surg. 2002;137:20–7.

23. Brunelli A, Kim AW, Berger KI, Addrizzo-Harris DJ. Physiologic evaluation of the patient with lung cancer being considered for resectional surgery: diagnosis and management of lung cancer: American College of Chest Physicians evidence-based clinical practice guidelines. Chest J. 2013;143:e166S–90S.

24. Ries AL, et al. The effects of pulmonary rehabilitation in the national emphysema treatment trial. Chest. 2005;128:3799–809.

25. Ries AL. Pulmonary rehabilitation and COPD. Respir Med. 2005;26:133–41.

26. Mason DP, et al. Impact of smoking cessation before resection of lung cancer: a Society of Thoracic Surgeons General Thoracic Surgery Database study. Ann Thorac Surg. 2009;88:362–71.

27. Ochroch EA, et al. Long-term pain and activity during recovery from major thoracotomy using thoracic epidural analgesia. Anesthesiology. 2002;97:1234–44.

28. Devereaux P, et al. POISE (PeriOperative ISchemic Evaluation) Investigators. Characteristics and short-term prognosis of perioperative myocardial infarction in patients undergoing noncardiac surgery: a cohort study. Ann Intern Med. 2011;154:523–8.

29. Nowbar AN, Cole GD, Shun-Shin MJ, Finegold JA, Francis DP. International RCT-based guidelines for use of preoperative stress testing and perioperative beta-blockers and statins in noncardiac surgery. Int J Cardiol. 2014;172:138–43.

30. Garcia S, et al. Usefulness of revascularization of patients with multivessel coronary artery disease before elective vascular surgery for abdominal aortic and peripheral occlusive disease. Am J Cardiol. 2008;102:809–13.

31. Garcia S, McFalls EO. CON: preoperative coronary revascularization in high-risk patients undergoing vascular surgery. Anesth Analg. 2008;106:764–6.

32. McFalls EO, et al. Predictors and outcomes of a perioperative myocardial infarction following elective vascular surgery in patients with documented coronary artery disease: results of the CARP trial. Eur Heart J. 2008;29:394–401.

33. Beattie WS, et al. Acute surgical anemia influences the cardioprotective effects of beta-blockade: a single-center, propensity-matched cohort study. Anesthesiology. 2010;112:25–33. https://doi.org/10.1097/ALN.0b013e3181c5dd81. 00000542-201001000-00013 [pii].

34. Hindler K, et al. Improved postoperative outcomes associated with preoperative statin therapy. Anesthesiology. 2006;105:1260–72; quiz 1289–90, 00000542-200612000-00027 [pii].

35. Schouten O, et al. Fluvastatin and perioperative events in patients undergoing vascular surgery. N Engl J Med. 2009;361:980–9.

36. Amar D, et al. Statin use is associated with a reduction in atrial fibrillation after noncardiac thoracic surgery independent of C-reactive protein. Chest. 2005;128:3421–7. 128/5/3421 [pii]. https://doi.org/10.1378/chest.128.5.3421.

37. Amar D. Beta-adrenergic blocker withdrawal confounds the benefits of epidural analgesia with sympathectomy on supraventricular arrhythmias after cardiac surgery. Anesth Analg. 2002;95:1119, author reply 1119.

38. Schouten O, et al. Effect of statin withdrawal on frequency of cardiac events after vascular surgery. Am J Cardiol. 2007;100:316–20. S0002-9149(07)00718-7 [pii]. https://doi.org/10.1016/j.amjcard.2007.02.093.

39. Rebound risk: aspirin and statin withdrawal. Consum Rep. 2005;70:48.

40. Collet JP, Montalescot G. Optimizing long-term dual aspirin/clopidogrel therapy in acute coronary syndromes: when does the risk outweigh the benefit? Int J Cardiol. 2009;133:8–17. S0167-5273(09)00013-8 [pii]. https://doi.org/10.1016/j.ijcard.2008.12.202.

41. Ding X, et al. A comparison of the analgesia efficacy and side effects of paravertebral compared with epidural blockade for thoracotomy: an updated meta-analysis. PLoS One. 2014;9:e96233.

42. Samain E, et al. [Monitoring expired oxygen fraction in preoxygenation of patients with chronic obstructive pulmonary disease]. Ann Fr Anesth Reanim. 2002;21:14–9.

43. Servin FS, Billard V. Remifentanil and other opioids. Handb Exp Pharmacol. 2008;(182):283–311.

44. Failor E, Bowdle A, Jelacic S, Togashi K. High-fidelity simulation of lung isolation with double-lumen endotracheal tubes and bronchial blockers in anesthesiology resident training. J Cardiothorac Vasc Anesth. 2014;28:865–9.

45. Slinger P. Update on anesthetic management for pneumonectomy. Curr Opin Anaesthesiol. 2009;22:31–7.

46. Bigatello LM, Allain R, Gaissert HA. Acute lung injury after pulmonary resection. Minerva Anestesiol. 2004;70:159–66.

47. Michelet P, et al. Protective ventilation influences systemic inflammation after esophagectomy: a randomized controlled study. Anesthesiology. 2006;105:911–9. 00000542-200611000-00011 [pii].

48. Choi G, et al. Mechanical ventilation with lower tidal volumes and positive end-expiratory pressure prevents alveolar coagulation in patients without lung injury. Anesthesiology. 2006;105:689–95. 00000542-200610000-00013 [pii].

49. Determann RM, et al. Ventilation with lower tidal volumes as compared with conventional tidal volumes for patients without acute lung injury: a preventive randomized controlled trial. Crit Care. 2010;14:R1. cc8230 [pii]. https://doi.org/10.1186/cc8230.

50. De Conno E, et al. Anesthetic-induced improvement of the inflammatory response to one-lung ventilation. Anesthesiology. 2009;110:1316–26.

51. Brassard C, Lohser J, Donati F, Bussieres J. Step-by-step clinical management of one-lung ventilation: continuing professional development. Can J Anesth. 2014;61:1003–21.

52. Swenson ER. Hypoxic pulmonary vasoconstriction. High Alt Med Biol. 2013;14:101–10.

53. Ward J, McMurtry I. Mechanisms of hypoxic pulmonary vasoconstriction and theirroles in pulmonary hypertension: new findings for an old problem. Curr Opin Pharmacol. 2009;9:1–10.

54. Dunham-Snary KJ, et al. Hypoxic pulmonary vasoconstriction: from molecular mechanisms to medicine. Chest. 2017;151:181–92.

55. Aaronson PI, et al. Hypoxic pulmonary vasoconstriction: mechanisms and controversies. J Physiol. 2006;570:53–8.

56. Rhodes CJ, Davidson A, Gibbs JSR, Wharton J, Wilkins MR. Therapeutic targets in pulmonary arterial hypertension. Pharmacol Ther. 2009;121:69–88.

57. Weigand L, Sylvester JT, Shimoda LA. Mechanisms of endothelin-1-induced contraction in pulmonary arteries from chronically hypoxic rats. Am J Physiol Lung Cell Mol Physiol. 2006;290:L284–90.

58. Jernigan NL, Walker BR, Resta TC. Chronic hypoxia augments protein kinase G-mediated Ca2+ desensitization in pulmonary vascular smooth muscle through inhibition of RhoA/Rho kinase signaling. Am J Physiol Lung Cell Mol Physiol. 2004;287:L1220–9.

59. Yamamoto Y, et al. Role of airway nitric oxide on the regulation of pulmonary circulation by carbon dioxide. J Appl Physiol. 2001;91:1121–30.

60. Nagendran J, Stewart K, Hoskinson M, Archer SL. An anesthesiologist's guide to hypoxic pulmonary vasoconstriction: implications for managing single-lung anesthesia and atelectasis. Curr Opin Anaesthesiol. 2006;19:34–43.

61. Abe K, Shimizu T, Takashina M, Shiozaki H, Yoshiya I. The effects of propofol, isoflurane, and sevoflurane on oxygenation and shunt fraction during one-lung ventilation. Anesth Analg. 1998;87:1164–9.

62. Pruszkowski O, et al. Effects of propofol vs sevoflurane on arterial oxygenation during one-lung ventilation. Br J Anaesth. 2007;98:539–44.

63. Popping DM, Elia N, Marret E, Remy C, Tramer MR. Protective effects of epidural analgesia on pulmonary complications after abdominal and thoracic surgery: a meta-analysis. Arch Surg. 2008;143:990–9; discussion 1000.

64. Groeben H. Epidural anesthesia and pulmonary function. J Anesth. 2006;20:290–9.

65. Moraca RJ, Sheldon DG, Thirlby RC. The role of epidural anesthesia and analgesia in surgical practice. Ann Surg. 2003;238:663–73.

66. Kehlet H, Wilmore DW. Multimodal strategies to improve surgical outcome. Am J Surg. 2002;183:630–41.

67. Grass JA. The role of epidural anesthesia and analgesia in postoperative outcome. Anesthesiol Clin North Am. 2000;18:407–28.

68. De Cosmo G, Aceto P, Gualtieri E, Congedo E. Analgesia in thoracic surgery: review. Minerva Anestesiol. 2009;75:393–400.

69. Guay J. The benefits of adding epidural analgesia to general anesthesia: a metaanalysis. J Anesth. 2006;20:335–40.

70. Holte K, Kehlet H. Effect of postoperative epidural analgesia on surgical outcome. Minerva Anestesiol. 2002;68:157–61.

71. Lewis KS, Whipple JK, Michael KA, Quebbeman EJ. Effect of analgesic treatment on the physiological consequences of acute pain. Am J Hosp Pharm. 1994;51:1539–54.

72. Kehlet H. The stress response to surgery: release mechanisms and the modifying effect of pain relief. Acta Chir Scand Suppl. 1989;550:22–8.

73. Hahnenkamp K, Herroeder S, Hollmann MW. Regional anaesthesia, local anaesthetics and the surgical stress response. Best Pract Res Clin Anaesthesiol. 2004;18:509–27.

74. Yeager MP, Glass DD, Neff RK, Brinck-Johnsen T. Epidural anesthesia and analgesia in high-risk surgical patients. Anesthesiology. 1987;66:729–36.

75. Clemente A, Carli F. The physiological effects of thoracic epidural anesthesia and analgesia on the cardiovascular, respiratory and gastrointestinal systems. Minerva Anestesiol. 2008;74:549–63.

76. Bromage P. Spirometery in assessment of analgesia after abdominal surgery. Br Med J. 1955;2:589–93.

77. Spray SB, Zuidema GD, Cameron JL. Aspiration pneumonia; incidence of aspiration with endotracheal tubes. Am J Surg. 1976;131:701–3.

78. Sackner MA, Hirsch J, Epstein S. Effect of cuffed endotracheal tubes on tracheal mucous velocity. Chest. 1975;68:774–7.

79. Chaney MA. Intrathecal and epidural anesthesia and analgesia for cardiac surgery. Anesth Analg. 2006;102:45–64.

80. Riedel BJ, Wright IG. Epidural anesthesia in coronary artery bypass grafting surgery. Curr Opin Cardiol. 1997;12:515–21.

81. Gottschalk A, Cohen SP, Yang S, Ochroch EA. Preventing and treating pain after thoracic surgery. Anesthesiology. 2006;104:594–600.

82. Grape S, Tramer MR. Do we need preemptive analgesia for the treatment of postoperative pain? Best Pract Res Clin Anaesthesiol. 2007;21:51–63.

83. Pogatzki-Zahn EM, Zahn PK. From preemptive to preventive analgesia. Curr Opin Anaesthesiol. 2006;19:551–5.

84. Ochroch EA, Gottschalk A. Impact of acute pain and its management for thoracic surgical patients. Thorac Surg Clin. 2005;15:105–21.

85. George MJ. The site of action of epidurally administered opioids and its relevance to postoperative pain management. Anaesthesia. 2006;61:659–64.

86. Davies RG, Myles PS, Graham JM. A comparison of the analgesic efficacy and side-effects of paravertebral vs epidural blockade for thoracotomy – a systematic review and meta-analysis of randomized trials. [erratum appears in Br J Anaesth. 2007;99(5):768]. British Journal of Anaesthesia. 2006;96:418–26.

87. Joshi GP, et al. A systematic review of randomized trials evaluating regional techniques for postthoracotomy analgesia. Anesth Analg. 2008;107:1026–40.

88. Sugasawa Y, et al. Effects of sevoflurane and propofol on pulmonary inflammatory responses during lung resection. J Anesth. 2012;26:62–9.

89. Chong PC, et al. Substantial variation of both opinions and practice regarding perioperative fluid resuscitation. Can J Surg. 2009;52:207–14.

90. Turnage WS, Lunn JJ. Postpneumonectomy pulmonary edema. A retrospective analysis of associated variables. Chest. 1993;103:1646–50.

91. Jackson TA, et al. Case 5-2007 postoperative complications after pneumonectomy: clinical conference. J Cardiothorac Vasc Anesth. 2007;21:743–51.

92. Jordan S, Mitchell JA, Quinlan GJ, Goldstraw P, Evans TW. The pathogenesis of lung injury following pulmonary resection. Eur Respir J. 2000;15:790–9.

93. Polubinska A, Breborowicz A, Staniszewski R, Oreopoulos DG. Normal saline induces oxidative stress in peritoneal mesothelial cells. J Pediatr Surg. 2008;43:1821–6.

94. Westphal M, et al. Hydroxyethyl starches: different products--different effects. Anesthesiology. 2009;111:187–202.

95. Boldt J. Modern rapidly degradable hydroxyethyl starches: current concepts. Anesth Analg. 2009;108:1574–82.

96. Boldt J. Saline versus balanced hydroxyethyl starch: does it matter? Curr Opin Anaesthesiol. 2008;21:679–83.

97. Ueda H, Iwasaki A, Kusano T, Shirakusa T. Thoracotomy in patients with liver cirrhosis. Scand J Thorac Cardiovasc Surg. 1994;28:37–41.

98. Ceyhan B, Celikel T. Serum-effusion albumin gradient in separation of transudative and exudative pleural effusions.[comment]. Chest. 1994;105:974–5.

99. Zarychanski R, et al. Association of hydroxyethyl starch administration with mortality and acute kidney injury in critically ill patients requiring volume resuscitation: a systematic review and meta-analysis. JAMA. 2013;309:678–88.

100. Taylor C, et al. Hydroxyethyl starch versus saline for resuscitation of patients in intensive care: long-term outcomes and cost-effectiveness analysis of a cohort from CHEST. Lancet Respir Med. 2016;4:818–25.

101. Ishikawa S, Griesdale DE, Lohser J. Acute kidney injury after lung resection surgery: incidence and perioperative risk factors. Anesth Analg. 2012;114:1256–62.

102. Older P, Hall A, Hader R. Cardiopulmonary exercise testing as a screening test for perioperative management of major surgery in the elderly. Chest. 1999;116:355–62.

103. Jordan S, Evans TW. Predicting the need for intensive care following lung resection. Thorac Surg Clin. 2008;18:61–9.

104. Siegel RL, Miller KD, Jemal A. Cancer statistics, 2016. CA Cancer J Clin. 2016;66:7–30.

105. Travis WD, et al. The 2015 World Health Organization classification of lung tumors: impact of genetic, clinical and radiologic advances since the 2004 classification. J Thorac Oncol. 2015;10:1243–60.

106. Maggiore C, et al. Histological classification of lung cancer. Rays. 2004;29:353–5.

107. Lortet-Tieulent J, et al. International trends in lung cancer incidence by histological subtype: adenocarcinoma stabilizing in men but still increasing in women. Lung Cancer. 2014;84:13–22.

108. Houston KA, Henley SJ, Li J, White MC, Richards TB. Patterns in lung cancer incidence rates and trends by histologic type in the United States, 2004–2009. Lung Cancer. 2014;86:22–8.

109. Beckles MA, Spiro SG, Colice GL, Rudd RM. Initial evaluation of the patient with lung cancer: symptoms, signs, laboratory tests, and paraneoplastic syndromes. Chest. 2003;123:97S–104S.

110. Amer KM, Ibrahim NB, Forrester-Wood CP, Saad RA, Scanlon M. Lung carcinoid related Cushing's syndrome: report of three cases and review of the literature. Postgrad Med J. 2001;77:464–7.

111. Radulescu D, Pripon S, Bunea D, Ciuleanu TE, Radulescu LI. Endocrine paraneoplastic syndromes in small cell lung carcinoma. Two case reports. J BUON. 2007;12:411–4.

112. Gerber RB, Mazzone P, Arroliga AC. Paraneoplastic syndromes associated with bronchogenic carcinoma. Clin Chest Med. 2002;23:257–64.

113. Pourmand R. Lambert-eaton myasthenic syndrome. Front Neurol Neurosci. 2009;26:120–5.

114. Darnell RB, Posner JB. Paraneoplastic syndromes affecting the nervous system. Semin Oncol. 2006;33:270–98.

115. D'addario G, et al. Platinum-based versus non-platinum-based chemotherapy in advanced non-small-cell lung cancer: a meta-analysis of the published literature. J Clin Oncol. 2005;23:2926–36.

116. Endo C, et al. Surgical treatment of stage I non-small cell lung carcinoma. Ann Thorac Cardiovasc Surg. 2003;9:283–9.

117. Goldstraw P, et al. The IASLC Lung Cancer Staging Project: proposals for the revision of the TNM stage groupings in the forthcoming (seventh) edition of the TNM Classification of malignant tumours. J Thorac Oncol. 2007;2:706–14.

118. Tsao M-S, et al. Subtype classification of lung adenocarcinoma predicts benefit from adjuvant chemotherapy in patients undergoing complete resection. J Clin Oncol. 2015;33:3439–46.

119. Der SD, et al. Validation of a histology-independent prognostic gene signature for early-stage, non–small-cell lung cancer including stage IA patients. J Thorac Oncol. 2014;9:59–64.

120. Fukuoka M, et al. Biomarker analyses and final overall survival results from a phase III, randomized, open-label, first-line study of gefitinib versus carboplatin/paclitaxel in clinically selected patients with advanced non–small-cell lung cancer in Asia (IPASS). J Clin Oncol. 2011;29:2866–74.

121. Solomon BJ, et al. First-line crizotinib versus chemotherapy in ALK-positive lung cancer. N Engl J Med. 2014;371:2167–77.

122. Chambers SK, et al. A systematic review of the impact of stigma and nihilism on lung cancer outcomes. BMC Cancer. 2012;12:184.

123. Gottschalk A, Sharma S, Ford J, Durieux ME, Tiouririne M. The role of the perioperative period in recurrence after cancer surgery. Anesth Analg. 2010;110:1636–43.

124. Myles PS, et al. Perioperative epidural analgesia for major abdominal surgery for cancer and recurrence-free survival: randomised trial. BMJ. 2011;342:d1491.

125. Nielsen SF, Nordestgaard BG, Bojesen SE. Statin use and reduced cancer-related mortality. N Engl J Med. 2012;367:1792–802.

126. Singh S, Singh AG, Singh PP, Murad MH, Iyer PG. Statins are associated with reduced risk of esophageal cancer, particularly in patients with Barrett's esophagus: a systematic review and meta-analysis. Clin Gastroenterol Hepatol. 2013;11:620–9.

127. Pelaia G, et al. Effects of statins and farnesyl transferase inhibitors on ERK phosphorylation, apoptosis and cell viability in non-small lung cancer cells. Cell Prolif. 2012;45:557–65.

128. Khurana V, Bejjanki HR, Caldito G, Owens MW. Statins reduce the risk of lung cancer in humans: a large case-control study of US veterans. Chest. 2007;131:1282–8. 131/5/1282 [pii]. https://doi.org/10.1378/chest.06-0931.

129. Rothwell PM, et al. Effect of daily aspirin on long-term risk of death due to cancer: analysis of individual patient data from randomised trials. Lancet. 2011;377:31–41.

130. Norman PH, et al. A possible association between aprotinin and improved survival after radical surgery for mesothelioma. Cancer. 2009;115:833–41. https://doi.org/10.1002/cncr.24108.

131. Norman P. Rofecoxib provides significant improvement in survival following lung resection for cancer. Anesthesiology. 2008;109:A1586.

132. Landreneau RJ, et al. Recurrence and survival outcomes after anatomic segmentectomy versus lobectomy for clinical stage I non–small-cell lung cancer: a propensity-matched analysis. J Clin Oncol. 2014;32:2449–55.

133. Allen MS, et al. Morbidity and mortality of major pulmonary resections in patients with early-stage lung cancer: initial results of the randomized, prospective ACOSOG Z0030 trial. Ann Thorac Surg. 2006;81:1013–9; discussion 1019–20, S0003-4975(05)01175-6 [pii]. https://doi.org/10.1016/j.athoracsur.2005.06.066.

134. Falcoz P-E, et al. Video-assisted thoracoscopic surgery versus open lobectomy for primary non-small-cell lung cancer: a propensity-matched analysis of outcome from the European Society of Thoracic Surgeon database. Eur J Cardiothorac Surg. 2016;49:602–9.

135. Bendixen M, Jørgensen OD, Kronborg C, Andersen C, Licht PB. Postoperative pain and quality of life after lobectomy via video-assisted thoracoscopic surgery or anterolateral thoracotomy for early stage lung cancer: a randomised controlled trial. Lancet Oncol. 2016;17:836–44.

136. Kent M, et al. Open, video-assisted thoracic surgery, and robotic lobectomy: review of a national database. Ann. Thorac. Surg. 2014;97:236–44.

137. O'doherty A, West M, Jack S, Grocott M. Preoperative aerobic exercise training in elective intra-cavity surgery: a systematic review. Br J Anaesth. 2013;110:679–89.

138. Kozian A, Schilling T. Protective ventilatory approaches to one-lung ventilation: more than reduction of tidal volume. Curr Anesthesiology Rep. 2014;4:150–9.

139. Licker M, Fauconnet P, Villiger Y, Tschopp JM. Acute lung injury and outcomes after thoracic surgery. Curr Opin Anaesthesiol.

2009;22:61–7. https://doi.org/10.1097/ACO.0b013e32831b466c. 00001503-200902000-00012 [pii].

140. Chau EHL, Slinger P. Seminars in cardiothoracic and vascular anesthesia. Los Angeles: SAGE Publications Sage CA. p. 36–44.

141. Madani A, et al. An enhanced recovery pathway reduces duration of stay and complications after open pulmonary lobectomy. Surgery. 2015;158:899–910.

142. Ludwig C, Stoelben E, Olschewski M, Hasse J. Comparison of morbidity, 30-day mortality, and long-term survival after pneumonectomy and sleeve lobectomy for non–small cell lung carcinoma. Ann Thorac Surg. 2005;79:968–73.

143. Finks JF, Osborne NH, Birkmeyer JD. Trends in hospital volume and operative mortality for high-risk surgery. N Engl J Med. 2011;364:2128–37.

144. Zeldin R, Normandin D, Landtwing D, Peters R. Postpneumonectomy pulmonary edema. J Thorac Cardiovasc Surg. 1984;87:359–65.

145. Foroulis CN, et al. Study on the late effect of pneumonectomy on right heart pressures using Doppler echocardiography. Eur J Cardiothorac Surg. 2004;26:508–14.

146. Fernández-Pérez ER, Keegan MT, Brown DR, Hubmayr RD, Gajic O. Intraoperative tidal volume as a risk factor for respiratory failure after pneumonectomy. Anesthesiology. 2006;105:14–8.

147. Schilling T, et al. The pulmonary immune effects of mechanical ventilation in patients undergoing thoracic surgery. Anesth Analg. 2005;101:957–65.

148. Cerfolio RJ, et al. Lung resection in patients with compromised pulmonary function. Ann Thorac Surg. 1996;62:348–51.

149. McGlade DP, Slinger PD. The elective combined use of a double lumen tube and endobronchial blocker to provide selective lobar isolation for lung resection following contralateral lobectomy. Anesthesiology. 2003;99:1021–2.

Anesthesia for Video-Assisted Thoracoscopic Surgery (VATS)

Edmond Cohen and Peter Slinger

Key Points

- VATS has been shown to decrease postoperative complications compared to open thoracotomy in high-risk patients.
- Limited options to treat hypoxemia during one-lung ventilation compared to open thoracotomy. CPAP interferes with surgical exposure during VATS.
- Priority on rapid and complete lung collapse.
- Decreased postoperative analgesic requirements compared to open thoracotomy.
- Small and/or deep parenchymal lesions can be located by CT-guided micro-coil placement preoperatively
- Uniportal VATS surgery may offer improved postoperative recovery.

Historical Considerations of Video-Assisted Thoracoscopy

Thoracoscopy involves intentionally creating a pneumothorax and then introducing an instrument through the chest wall to visualize the intrathoracic structures. Recent application of video cameras to thoracoscopes for high-definition magnified viewing coupled with the development of sophisticated surgical instruments and stapling devices has greatly expanded the endoscopist's ability to do increasingly more complex procedures by thoracos-

copy. It was widely believed that the first to perform a documented thoracoscopy using a Nitze cystoscope in a human patient was the Swedish internist Hans Christian Jacobaeus. Thoracoscopy, the introduction of an illuminated tube through a small incision made between the ribs, was first used in 1910 for the treatment of tuberculosis. In 1882 the tubercle bacillus was discovered by Koch, and Forlanini observed that tuberculous cavities collapsed and healed after patients developed a spontaneous pneumothorax. The technique of injecting approximately 200 cc of air under pressure to create an artificial pneumothorax became a widely used technique to treat tuberculosis [1].

Jacobaeus [2], however, was able to directly visualize pleural adhesions using thoracoscopy and described a method for cutting them to facilitate lung collapse. Closed intrapleural pneumolysis, also called the Jacobaeus operation, consisted in inserting a galvanocautery into the pleural cavity through another small opening in the chest wall and dividing the adhesions under thoracoscopic control. Thus the two-point entry technique of medical thoracoscopy was born.

After the introduction of tuberculostatic medications, this surgical approach was practically abandoned until the early 1990s when advancement in fiber-optic light transmission, image display, and instrumentation made video-assisted thoracoscopic surgery (VATS) possible. The improvements in video endoscopic surgical equipment and a growing enthusiasm for minimally invasive surgical approaches brought VATS to the practice of surgery for diagnostic and therapeutic procedures. Most of these procedures required general anesthesia and a well-collapsed lung and are an indication for one-lung ventilation (OLV).

A variety of medical and surgical procedures are performed by VATS [3] (see Table 24.1). The patient population tends to be either very healthy, undergoing diagnostic procedures, or high-risk patients who are undergoing VATS to avoid the risks of thoracotomy. Patients with advanced

E. Cohen
Department of Anesthesiology, Mount Sinai Hospital and School of Medicine, New York, NY, USA

P. Slinger (✉)
Department of Anesthesia, Toronto General Hospital, Toronto, ON, Canada
e-mail: peter.slinger@uhn.ca

© Springer Nature Switzerland AG 2019
P. Slinger (ed.), *Principles and Practice of Anesthesia for Thoracic Surgery*, https://doi.org/10.1007/978-3-030-00859-8_24

Table 24.1 Spectrum of minimally invasive thoracic surgical procedures

Diagnostic
  a. Pleural disease
     Biopsy, thoracentesis
  b. Staging
     Lung, pleural, esophageal cancer
  c. Parenchymal disease
     Fibrosis, solitary nodules, pneumonitis
  d. Mediastinal tumors
     Thymoma, lymphoma, sarcoma, germ cell
  e. Pericardial disease
     Pericarditis, tumors
Therapeutic
  a. Pleural disease
     Pleurodesis, decortication
  b. Parenchymal disease
     Wedge resection, segmentectomy, lobectomy, pneumonectomy, bleb/bullae resection, lung volume reduction
  c. Cardiovascular disease
     Pericardial window, valve repair, coronary artery bypass, arrhythmia ablation
  d. Mediastinal disease
     Tumor excision, thymectomy, chylothorax
  e. Esophageal surgery
     Vagotomy, myotomy, antireflux surgery, esophagectomy
  f. Sympathectomy
     Hyperhidrosis, reflex sympathetic dystrophy
  g. Spinal surgery

cardiopulmonary disease, malignancies, and heavy smoking history deserve an extensive preoperative evaluation and optimization since conversion to an open procedure is always a possibility. Intraoperative monitoring in these high-risk patients should be the same as for thoracotomy.

Medical Thoracoscopy This is mainly performed for diagnostic procedures. Initially it was limited to the use of a rigid thoracoscope; however with the introduction of optical fibers, it was expanded to include diagnostic procedures with flexible thoracoscopy. Unlike VATS, which consist of multiple access ports, medical thoracoscopy involves the insertion of an endoscope through a single entry port into the thoracic cavity and pleural space. Medical thoracoscopy is limited to diagnosis and biopsy of pleural disease, pleural effusions, infectious diseases, staging procedures, chemical pleurodesis, and occasionally for lung biopsy. It is often performed by the pulmonologist in the clinic rather than the operating room and is generally under local anesthesia. A small incision is made in thorough the lateral chest wall, and with the insertion of the instrument, fluid and biopsy specimens are easily obtained. Medical thoracoscopy has somewhat limited applications which are confined by the inability, in most cases, to perform more extensive therapeutic procedures such as wedge resection, lobectomy, or pneumonectomy.

Surgical Thoracoscopy VATS was introduced to thoracic surgical practice in the early 1990s and entails making multiple small incisions in the chest wall, which allow the introduction of a video camera and surgical instruments into the thoracic cavity through access ports. Most commonly, it is performed by a thoracic surgeon in the operating room under general anesthesia. In more recent years, surgical techniques, instruments, and video technology have improved to permit a wide variety of therapeutic procedures to be performed using VATS.

Indications

The proportion of thoracic procedures performed by VATS vs. thoracotomy has increased dramatically in the past decade. Currently, at one of the Author's (PS) institutions, approximately 70% of all lobectomies are performed by VATS. Previously, it was thought that survival after lung cancer surgery may be decreased with VATS due to incomplete resection. However, recently it has been shown that long-term survival is not decreased by VATS surgery vs. open thoracotomy [4].

Initially, when introduced to clinical practice, VATS was limited to diagnostics procedures of short duration and limited extension. Increased familiarity with thoracoscopic techniques, as with laparoscopic techniques, had enabled surgeons to perform almost any major thoracic surgical procedure in a minimally invasive manner. VATS operations can be used for all structures in the chest and are not limited to the lungs, pleura, and mediastinum.

Diagnostic Procedures

With VATS, diagnosis of pleural disease, thoracentesis, and pleural biopsy of a specific area under direct vision can be performed. In many cases this is indicated for an undiagnosed pleural effusion, in which the cytology is inconclusive. VATS for parenchymal lung pathology such as biopsy, wedge resection for solitary lung nodules or for diffuse interstitial lung disease is a common indication. In the past, such a diagnosis was possible only by subjecting the patient to an open thoracotomy, despite the associated morbidity, or the patient was treated empirically. VATS, which offers an extensive visualization of the entire chest cavity, essentially has replaced the traditional mini-thoracotomy particularly in cases where percutaneous needle aspiration biopsy is inconclusive. Other diagnostic procedures are performed on the mediastinum for biopsy of lymph nodes not accessible via traditional mediastinoscopy such as the subcarinal lymph nodes or for mediastinal masses, either primary or metastatic. This procedure is essential when staging of the disease needs to be established. It is also useful for assessing resectability, to exclude direct invasion of the mediastinal structures. Lymphomas or germ-cell tumors that require a tissue diagnosis may benefit from a VATS approach. Diagnostic procedures involving the pericardium, such as a pericardial biopsy and/or drainage of a pericardial effusion can be accomplished both for diagnosis and therapy with a VATS pericardial window.

Therapeutic Procedures

Pleural disease can be managed by VATS including pleurocentesis, pleural abrasion for recurrent pleural effusion from malignancy or pneumothorax, decortication, empyectomy, and lysis of adhesions. In the past, thoracotomy was performed for formal decortication to permit re-expansion of the lung. With VATS, thoracotomy can be avoided, particularly in the early stages of empyema. Malignant pleural effusions, particularly those with multiple loculated collections, are difficult to drain with tube thoracostomy and can be effectively treated with VATS.

Lung parenchymal disease such as wedge resection of a lesion, lobectomy or pneumonectomy can routinely be performed with VATS. These are better tolerated by the compromised patient with decreased pulmonary reserve [5]. VATS offers the opportunity to both diagnose and treat parenchymal lesions at the same time. Management of bullous disease, particularly giant bullae with significant compression of the adjacent lung, is frequently managed with VATS. Often these cases present with recurrent pneumothoraces or air leaks associated with apical blebs. Lung volume reduction (LVR) performed by VATS is better tolerated by the patient with severe emphysema (see also Chap. 46). Resection of mediastinal masses such as thymoma or mediastinal cyst or resection of posterior mediastinal neurogenic tumors, treatment of chylothorax by ligation of the thoracic duct, bilateral sympathectomy are all possible with VATS.

A variety of esophageal procedures can be performed minimally invasively. Vagotomy, Heller myotomy, antireflux procedures, or staging of esophageal cancer are common procedures done with VATS. Finally, the dissection of the thoracic esophagus in cases of esophagogastrectomy is increasingly performed with a combined VATS and laparotomy.

VATS sympathectomy is usually performed for hyperhidrosis or reflux sympathetic dystrophy. The sympathetic chain is visualized as it lies along the vertebral bodies. The magnification provided by VATS facilitates the procedure, which is usually done bilaterally during the same anesthetic.

Benefits

The incisions for VATS are usually 2–4 ports to allow for the passage of a video camera stapling device and forceps. Because the ribs are not spread, patients have lower narcotic requirements for postoperative pain, reduced shoulder dysfunction, and decreased time until return to preoperative activities. There is a reduced risk of respiratory depression, reduced risk of atelectasis due to splinting, or reduced ability to sustain deep breathing and reduction in retained secretions.

A propensity score matched study has shown that fewer patients had complications after VATS vs. open lobectomies [6] (see Table 24.2). Patients who are considered high risk for lobectomy via open thoracotomy, based on preoperative pulmonary function studies, were demonstrated not to have an increased risk compared to low-risk patients when the surgery was performed by VATS (see Fig. 24.1) [7]. COPD patients have been shown to have improved outcomes after lobectomy with VATS vs. open thoracotomy (see Table 24.3) [8]. A randomized study has shown that long-term postoperative pain after lobectomy is decreased in VATS

Table 24.2 Postlobectomy complications VATS vs. open thoracotomy

Outcome	VATS ($n = 122$)	Open ($n = 122$)	p value
Length of stay (days ± SD)	4.9 ± 2.4	7.2 ± 3.8	0.001
All complications	17%	28%	0.046
Atrial fibrillation	12%	16%	0.36
Prolonged air leaks	3.8%	5.7%	0.54
Pneumonitis	1.6%	4.1%	0.28

Based on data from Bendixen et al. [9]

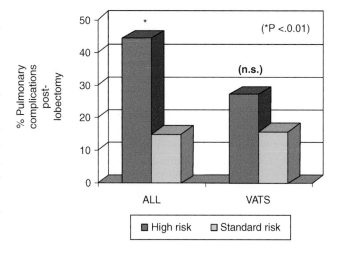

Fig. 24.1 The percentages of high-risk vs. standard-risk patients having postlobectomy pulmonary complications during the period 2002–2010. High risk was defined based on preoperative pulmonary function tests, cardiac function, and exercise performance. For VATS procedures, there was no statistically significant increase in complications for high-risk patients vs. standard-risk patients

Table 24.3 Postlobectomy complications in elderly patients

Outcome	VATS	Open	p value
Median length of stay (days)	5	6	0.001
No complications	72%	55%	0.04
Pulmonary	15%	33%	0.01
Cardiac	17%	23%	0.44

Based on data from Miyazaki et al. [10]

patient vs. thoracotomy patients [9]. VATS procedures seem to benefit elderly patients. A series of five nonagenarian patients has been published with successful lung cancer surgery by VATS [10]. Although decreased rates of complications are seen with lobectomies or wedge resections, this has not been evident for pneumonectomies [11].

Surgical Technique

VATS is performed usually in the lateral position through three to five entry ports created in the chest wall on the side of the pathology (see Fig. 24.2). A video camera is inserted to allow for direct visualization of the entrance of trocars into the thorax. The lung is collapsed on the ipsilateral side by passive elastic recoil equilibrium of intrapleural and atmospheric pressure occurs through the access port. If the lung is not adequately collapsed, the surgeon is not able to appreciate the surgical field and identify a lung lesion when it is not located on the surface of the lung. Additionally, placing a stapler suture on a lung that is only partially deflated may result in inadequate closure lines which may be the source of continuous air leak (see Fig. 24.3).

Although rarely used in thoracoscopic procedures, unlike laparoscopic procedures, some surgeons may elect to insufflate CO_2 gas into the ipsilateral hemithorax to assist in collapsing the lung and breaking adhesions and to maintain the pneumothorax. There is no good evidence that a CO_2 insufflation has any benefit. Insufflation of CO_2 into the ipsilateral hemithorax can be associated with hemodynamic compromise and significant hypotension since the chest is a closed cavity, and the increase in intra-thoracic pressure by insufflation of CO_2 will reduce venous return and cardiac output. The pressure inside the thorax must be measured and kept low. Keeping the intra-thoracic pressure below 10 cm of H_2O should minimize the negative hemodynamic effects. This is a period when communication between surgeon and anesthesiologist is crucial.

Anesthetic Management

After appropriate anesthesia and surgical evaluation, an anesthetic plan is devised to allow the patient to be safely anesthetized for the surgical procedure and to recover. Most patients find it reassuring to have a discussion with their anesthesiologist

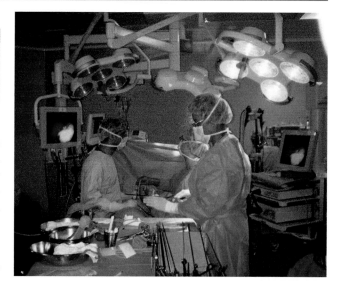

Fig. 24.2 Video-assisted thoracoscopic surgery as viewed from the foot of the operating table. A well-collapsed lung on the side of surgery is necessary for any major procedure

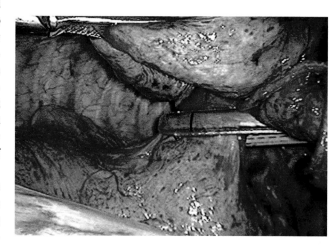

Fig. 24.3 A stapling devise is used to open the interlobar fissure as part of the initial surgical approach during a VATS lobectomy. If the lung is not well collapsed, there is an increased risk of air leaks from the staple lines

about the anesthetic and postoperative pain relief options. The choice of anesthetic technique is variable and dependent upon the wishes of the patient and the experience of the clinician. While simple diagnostic procedures can be performed under local anesthesia by infiltrating the chest wall accompanied by light sedation, more complex procedures that require sampling of tissue are best done under regional (epidural, intercostal blocks) or general anesthesia. The main disadvantage of local and regional anesthesia is that the patient is required to breathe spontaneously. While this is generally tolerated for brief periods of time, most VATS procedures today are performed under general anesthesia utilizing one-lung ventilation (OLV) techniques, which provides better exposure and guarantees a secure airway in the lateral decubitus position.

Each of the above techniques has its advantages and disadvantages. Decisions regarding postoperative pain relief should be made preoperatively. The management of an epidural vs. patient-controlled analgesia (PCA) vs. PRN medications given by the nurse with or without adjunctive agents is best evaluated on a daily basis by a specialist in the field of pain management. Additional considerations regarding postoperative pain management should be given to the likelihood of proceeding on to thoracotomy.

Local/Regional Anesthesia

The simplest technique is to use a local anesthetic to infiltrate the lateral thoracic wall and parietal pleura combined with appropriate sedation and supplemental oxygen. Preferably intercostal nerve blocks can be performed at the level of the incision(s) and at two interspaces above and below (see Chap. 59). Thoracic epidural anesthesia can also be used [12]. For VATS procedures under local or regional anesthesia, an ipsilateral stellate ganglion block is often performed to inhibit the cough reflex from manipulation of the hilum. To anesthetize the visceral pleura, topical local anesthetics can be applied. Intravenous sedation with propofol may be needed to supplement regional nerve blocks.

For VATS performed under local or regional anesthesia with the patient breathing without assistance, partial collapse of the lung on the operated side occurs when air is allowed to enter the pleural cavity. The resulting atelectasis may provide suboptimal surgical exposure. The major disadvantage to VATS under local or regional anesthesia is that the patient must breathe spontaneously. This is usually tolerated for short periods of time, but for major VATS procedures, a general anesthetic with OLV is a better choice.

The collapse of the lung provides the surgeon with a working space, and a chest tube is placed at the conclusion of the surgery. Changes in PaO2, PaCO2, and cardiac rhythm are usually minimal when the procedure is performed using local or regional anesthesia. With local anesthesia, the spontaneous pneumothorax is usually well tolerated because the skin and chest wall form a seal around the thoracoscope and limit the degree of lung collapse. Occasionally, however, the procedure is poorly tolerated, and general anesthesia must be induced. The insertion of a double-lumen tube (DLT) with the patient in the lateral position may be difficult, in which case the patient may be temporarily placed in the supine position for the intubation.

If general anesthesia is required, a DLT is preferable to a single-lumen tube because positive-pressure ventilation via a single-lumen tube would interfere with endoscopic visualization. In addition, if pleurodesis is being performed, general anesthesia through a DLT allows for re-controlled re-expansion of the lung. A regional approach is well suited to a patient who is motivated to maintain control of their environment, a surgeon who can work gently, and for a procedure that is short in duration. A benefit of regional anesthesia is that it wears off slowly over a few hours allowing for oral opioids and adjuvant analgesics to be added as needed with minimal discomfort to the patient. The risks of this approach include accidental intravenous, epidural or spinal injection with associated toxicity, or cardiopulmonary embarrassment. In experienced hands, complications are rare enough to allow for the routine use of regional anesthesia for minor VATS procedures. Because the patient is not under general anesthesia and local anesthetic has only been applied to the rib cage, the patients may complain of discomfort during manipulation of lung tissue with pain referred to the shoulder. Referred shoulder pain may be difficult to differentiate from the anginal discomfort of cardiac disease.

General Anesthesia

Indications for one-lung ventilation: "Lung isolation" includes the classical absolute indications for OLV, such as massive bleeding, pus, and alveolar proteinosis or bronchopleural fistula. The goal is to protect the non-diseased contralateral lung from contamination. "Lung separation," on the other hand, refers to cases with no risk of contamination to the dependent lung and is performed primarily to improve surgical exposure such as for VATS. The inability to completely deflate the non-dependent lung during VATS leads to poor surgical exposure, which in turn can jeopardize the success of the procedure, potentially requiring conversion to an open technique. Because of the increasing number of diagnostic and therapeutic procedures performed with VATS, the need to provide OLV has risen significantly.

Treatment of Hypoxemia During VATS The application of continuous positive airway pressure (CPAP) by oxygen insufflation to the non-ventilated lung has traditionally been accepted as the best maneuver to treat hypoxemia during OLV [13] (see also Chap. 6). This maneuver is well accepted during open thoracotomy. Unfortunately, the application of CPAP is poorly tolerated by the surgeon during VATS because of the obstruction of the surgical field by the partially inflated lung [14] (see Fig. 24.4). Since most patients will develop atelectasis in the ventilated dependent lung during general anesthesia in the lateral position (see Fig. 24.5), recruitment maneuvers [15] and the application of PEEP to the ventilated lung are useful in the majority of patients, except those with severe obstructive lung disease [16] (see Fig. 24.6). A useful method of improving oxygenation during

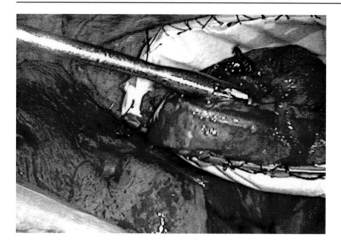

Fig. 24.4 During a VATS lobectomy, the excised lobe is placed in a retrieval bag before being removed through a small chest wall incision. Good collapse of the operative lung is required for the surgeon to perform this operation

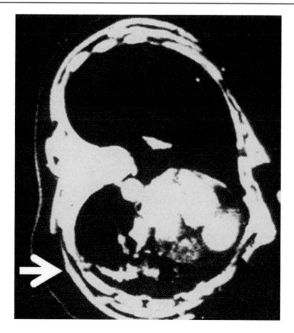

Fig. 24.5 Chest CT scan during general anesthesia in the lateral position. The white arrow points to a plaque of atelectasis in the dependent lung. Most patients develop atelectasis in the dependent lung during anesthesia

Fig. 24.6 A comparison of the effects of PEEP and CPAP on oxygenation during one-lung ventilation in patients with COPD (Capan) vs. normal pulmonary function (Fujiwara). PEEP improves PaO2 for most patients with normal pulmonary function during OLV (* significant improvement $p < 0.05$) but decreases PaO2 in patients with COPD. (Based on data from Refs. [13, 15])

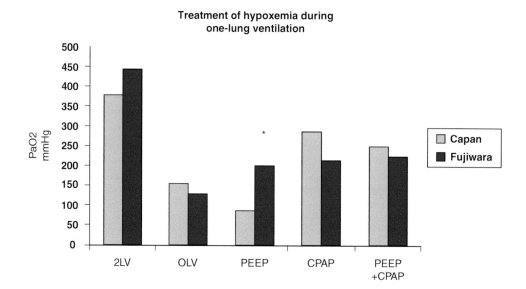

OLV for VATS is the bronchoscope-guided insufflation of oxygen into segments of the non-dependent lung remote to the site of surgery [17] (see Chap. 6, Fig. 6.10).

Improving Lung Collapse During VATS Since a collapsed immobile lung on the side of surgery is fundamental to VATS for major pulmonary resections, one of the anesthesiologists' responsibilities is to facilitate collapse of the non-ventilated lung. There are three basic maneuvers that will increase the rate of lung collapse:

1. Eliminate all nitrogen from the operative lung prior to the initiation of lung collapse. The poorly-soluble nitrogen in

air delays collapse in non-ventilated alveoli. Although the use of air-oxygen mixtures are desirable to prevent the development of atelectasis in the ventilated lung during one-lung anesthesia, if air is present in the non-ventilated lung at the start of OLV it will delay collapse [18] (see Chap. 6). It is best to ventilate with a FiO2 of 1.0 for a period of 3–5 min immediately prior to the start of OLV to denitrogenate the operative lung. After a recruitment maneuver of the ventilated dependent lung, air can then be reintroduced to the gas mixture after the start of OLV as tolerated, according to the arterial oxygen saturation.

2. Avoid entrainment of room air into the non-ventilated lung during closed-chest OLV. Many anesthesiologists

will begin OLV as soon as possible to encourage lung collapse prior to the start of surgery. However during closed-chest OLV, if the lumen of the DLT to the non-ventilated lung is open to atmosphere, passive paradoxical ventilation of the non-ventilated lung will occur (inspiration during the expiratory phase of the ventilated lung), and air will be drawn into the non-ventilated lung delaying collapse (see Fig. 24.7). It has been shown that these passive tidal volumes are approximately 130 ml/breath [19] which far exceeds the dead space of one side of a DLT (10–15 ml). These passive tidal volumes cease as soon as atmospheric pressure is allowed into the operative hemithorax.

3. Apply suction to the lumen of the DLT or bronchial blocker to the non-ventilated lung at the start of OLV. Low suction (−20 cmH2O) improves the rate of lung collapse for both open thoracotomy and VATS [20] (see Figs. 24.8). It is not clear whether the effect of suction is due to the negative pressure or simply due to a suction catheter preventing passive entrainment of air into the non-ventilated lung (see Fig. 24.9).

Verifying Patency of Other Bronchi During VATS Lobectomy During open thoracotomy for lobectomy, to ensure that the patency of a bronchus to a remaining lobe has not been compromised, the surgeon will often ask the anesthesiologist to temporarily re-inflate the non-ventilated lung

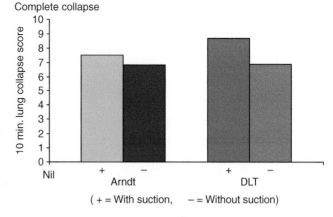

Effect of suction (-20 cmH20) on lung collapse

(+ = With suction,   − = Without suction)

Fig. 24.8 The application of low suction to the channel of a bronchial blocker (in this case the Arndt blocker) or to the lumen of the DLT to the non-ventilated lung significantly improves the speed of lung collapse measured both 10 min (shown here) and 20 min after the start of OLV. (Based on data from Ref. [20])

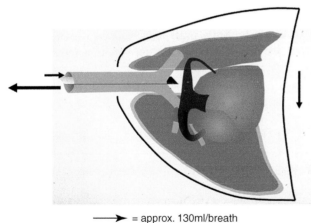

Passive paradoxical gas exchange in the non-ventilated lung during closed-chest one-lung ventilation

⟶ = approx. 130ml/breath

Fig. 24.7 Passive paradoxical gas exchange occurs in the non-ventilated lung during OLV if the chest is closed. As the mediastinum falls during exhalation of the ventilated lung, the resultant negative pressure in the non-ventilated hemithorax entrains room air into the non-ventilated lung if the lumen of the DLT is open to atmosphere. This air is then expired during the inspiration phase of the ventilated lung. The passive tidal volumes depend on the size of the patient and cease once the initial VATS port allows atmospheric pressure to equilibrate in the non-ventilated hemithorax. (Based on data from Ref. [19])

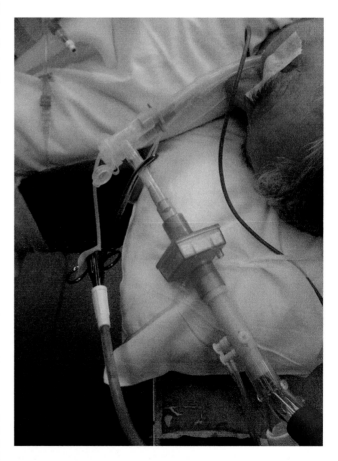

Fig. 24.9 Photograph of suction being applied via a catheter to the tracheal lumen of a left-sided DLT during a right-sided VATS procedure. Low suction (–20cmH2O) should be applied from the start of OLV until the non-ventilated lung is completely collapsed

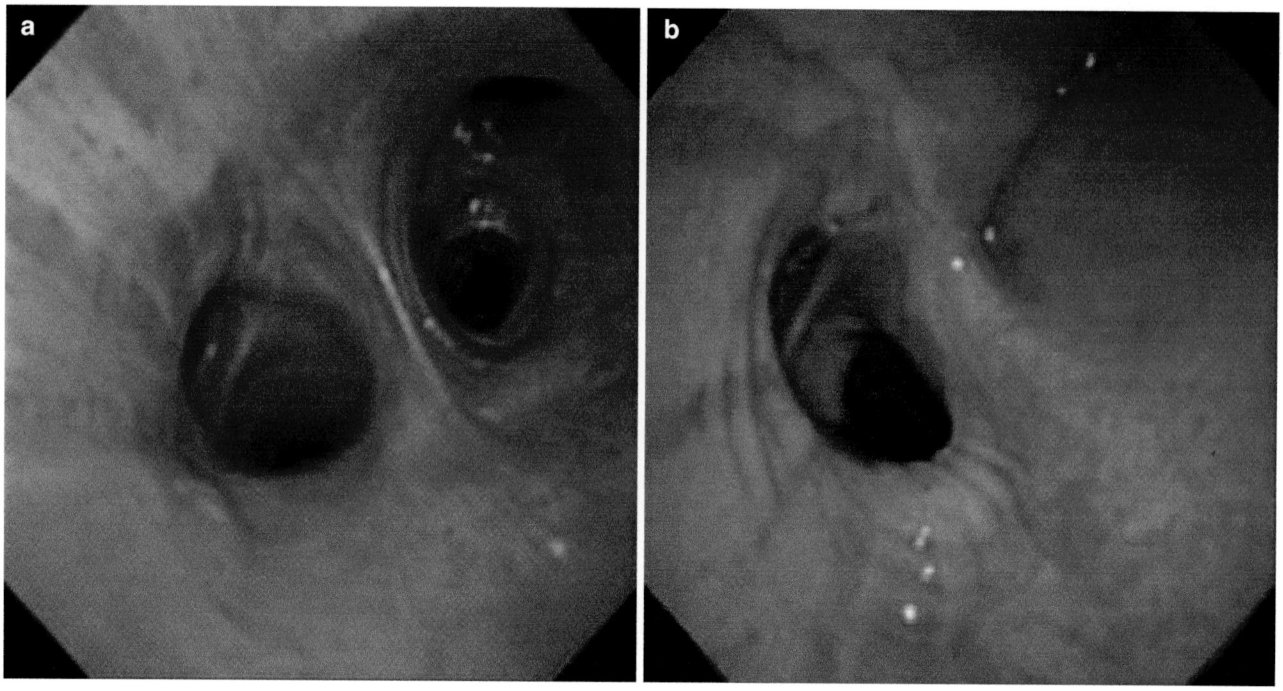

Fig. 24.10 (a) Normal anatomy of the secondary carina of the left lung as seen during fiber-optic bronchoscopy during VATS lobectomy. The left upper lobe orifice is at the upper right. The posterior wall of the mainstem bronchus is identified by the longitudinal elastic bundles, seen at 9 o'clock, which extend into the left lower lobe. (b) A surgical stapler has been applied to the left upper lobe bronchus. The anesthesiologist is asked to ensure that the bronchus to the left lower lobe remains patent, as seen in the photograph, prior to firing the stapler

after the stapling device has occluded the bronchus to the operative lobe or segment, just before the desired bronchus is cut and stapled. Re-inflation of the ipsilateral remaining lobe(s) ensures the patency of their bronchi. However, during a VATS resection, this maneuver impairs the surgeon's ability to visualize the surgical field and to proceed with the resection. To avoid this potential for compromise of non-involved bronchi during VATS, the anesthesiologist may be asked to perform fiber-optic bronchoscopy at this stage to ensure that the bronchi to the remaining ipsilateral lobe(s) are patent (see Fig. 24.10a, b). To perform this, the anesthesiologist needs a detailed knowledge endoscopic bronchial anatomy (see Chap. 17).

Lung Isolation The use of double-lumen tubes (DLT) has classically been considered the "gold standard" for achieving OLV. Proper position of the DLT or endobronchial blocker is often confirmed in the supine position, but it is when the patient has been placed in the lateral decubitus position that matters most since the surgery will take place in that position and dislocation during position changes are not uncommon. A study conducted by Narayanaswamy and colleagues [20] showed in 104 patients undergoing left-sided lung surgery that, in regards to quality of surgical exposure, there was no difference between the use of bronchial blockers (Arndt

wire-guided, Cohen Flexi-tip, Fuji Uniblocker) and a left-sided DLT. However, significant differences were found favoring the use of DLTs with regard to time to initial lung deflation and amount of repositioning required after initial placement of the lung isolation device. Since most VATS procedures require lung separation and not isolation, the insertion of a bronchial blocker to obtain OLV is an attractive alternative to a DLT, especially since multiple intubations of the trachea will not be necessary when using a bronchial blocker. Additionally, a difficult intubation is even more difficult much when using a DLT.

Management of OLV

Peak airway pressure, delivered tidal volume (spirometry), and the wave-form of the capnogram should be inspected to identify obstruction or reduced end-tidal carbon dioxide tension from inadequate gas exchange subsequent to DLT malposition. A peak airway pressure of up to 35 cmH_2O during OLV is acceptable. A sudden increase in the peak airway pressure (during volume-controlled ventilation) may be from DLT or endobronchial blocker dislocation. These tube or blocker movements are often a consequence of surgical manipulation. During pressure-controlled ventilation, this will present as a fall in tidal volume. When OLV is required, a FiO_2 of 1.0 provides the greatest margin of safety against hypoxemia. When using a FiO_2 of 1.0, assuming a typical HPV response, the expected PaO_2 during OLV should be between 150 and 210 mmHg. I typically ventilate OLV patients with a tidal volume of 6–7 ml/kg, PEEP 5 cm H_2O, and at a respiratory rate sufficient to maintain a $PaCO_2$ of 35 ± 3 mmHg. Following the initiation of OLV, PaO_2 can continue to decrease for up to 45 min; hence, a pulse oximeter is indispensable. Should hypoxia occur, proper positioning of the DLT should be reconfirmed using fiber-optic bronchoscopy.

Other Anesthetic Considerations for VATS In addition to the usual complications related to intrathoracic surgery and anesthesia, thoracoscopic procedures can be associated with massive hemorrhage and decreased inability to control large blood vessels. Maintaining stable hemodynamics can present a challenge until the surgeon gets control of the source of bleeding which may require conversion to an open thoracotomy. Therefore, large-bore intravenous catheters are even more critical for VATS procedures than open thoracotomy where the hilar blood vessels can be controlled easier. Bleeding can be from placement of trocars into the lung or great vessels

A false assumption that is made by patients coming for minimal invasive surgery is that the perioperative risk will also be "minimal." VATS is frequently described to the patient and their family as a simple entry into the chest. While VATS is associated with improved healing, lung function and shorter hospital length of stay, by no means should one be lured into thinking that the procedure is any less invasive than an open thoracotomy. Diagnostic VATS procedures are being increasingly performed on ASA III-IV patients, who historically would have been classified as inoperable using an open approach. An example would be a patient on the cardiac transplant list that needs a pre-transplant tissue diagnosis of a lung lesion seen on a preoperative chest X-ray. Consequently, very ill patients requiring flawless lung separation techniques, who expect an uneventful perioperative course, pose an increased stress for the anesthesia team.

Localization of Small Parenchymal Lesions

As imaging modalities improve, smaller lung lesions are detected at an early stage when surgical intervention may be optimal. Initially VATS procedures were considered unsuitable for small lesions deep in the parenchyma which needed to be localized by surgical palpation of the lung. A

number of techniques have been developed to identify these lesions before surgery so that they could be removed by VATS. These techniques include percutaneous CT-guided injection of the lesions with dye or placement of a hookwire. Preoperative CT-guided placement of micro-coils has proven to be the most useful of these techniques [21]. A micro-coil is placed adjacent to the lesion by radiology using CT guidance in the awake patient with local anesthesia and sedation. Anesthesia is then induced with one-lung ventilation. During VATS, intraoperative fluoroscopy is used to localize the lesion for resection. This technique has been shown to have a high success rate for removal of small lesions.

The specific anesthetic concern is that a significant number of these patients develop a small pneumothorax at the time of coil placement. All these patients should be assumed to have a potential bronchopleural fistula for purposes of anesthetic induction. Positive-pressure ventilation without lung isolation could lead to an ipsilateral tension pneumothorax. This Author's (PS) management is a modified rapid-sequence induction of anesthesia with a DLT. The position of the DLT is adjusted with fiber-optic bronchoscopy immediately after intubation. One-lung ventilation of the contralateral lung is then begun after confirmation of the DLT positon and inflation of the bronchial cuff.

Uniportal VATS

Initially, VATS procedures have been performed through 2–4 surgical ports. Over the past 7 years, the use of a single port for VATS procedures has become more widespread. The uniportal technique has now been extended to include lobectomies and even pneumonectomies [22]. The possible advantages include decreased postoperative pain and shorter length of stay. The uniportal procedure is performed with the patient in the standard lateral VATS positon with general anesthesia and one-lung ventilation (see Fig. 24.11). The single VATS port is placed through a 2–4 cm muscle-sparing incision in the 4th–6th intercostal space in the anterior axillary line. Like standard VATS, the uniportal technique can be used in non-intubated, spontaneously breathing patients (see also Chap. 25) [23].

Pain Management Techniques

Extensive discussion of the management of post-thoracotomy pain can be found in Chap. 59. A commonly cited advantage of VATS when compared to open thoracotomy is a reduction in postoperative pain. While this is true in a relative sense, VATS procedures are still associated with a significant amount of postoperative pain that is not only disturbing to

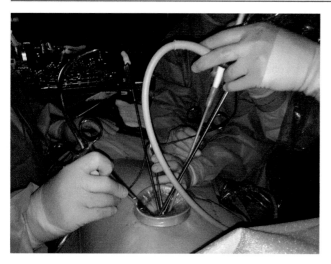

Fig. 24.11 Photograph of uniportal VATS surgery. The patient is in the right lateral position. Multiple surgical instruments can be passed through a single port. (Photograph courtesy of Dr. J Bussieres)

patients but may be associated with pain-related morbidities and prolonged hospital stays. The preponderance of literature suggests that VATS lung resection is associated with decreased postoperative pain compared with conventional thoracotomy. Sugiura and colleagues found a reduced duration of epidural catheter use, less narcotic use, decreased frequency of analgesic administration, and possibly a lower incidence of post-thoracotomy pain syndrome in patients undergoing VATS compared with those undergoing thoracotomy [20].

Thoracic epidural analgesia has a long track record of efficacy and safety and is considered by many anesthesiologists the gold standard in pain relief during the postoperative period for thoracotomy. However, the majority of VATS procedures are now performed with other types of regional block. While other forms of postoperative analgesia are possible, many are associated with unwanted side effects. Systemic opioids are respiratory depressive and inhibit the cough reflex. Nonsteroidal anti-inflammatory medication can inhibit coagulation and in isolation do not suffice to control the immediate postoperative pain experienced by this patient population. The utilization of paravertebral, serratus anterior plane, and erector spinae plane blocks has shown promise as an alternative to epidural analgesia.

The control of postoperative pain in patients after intrathoracic surgery is critical to the rehabilitation of their respiratory function. Postoperative pain in the chest wall can cause splinting which will impair couching, deep breathing leading to retention of secretions, and a decrease in FRC. These problems have been shown to be a source of great morbidity and should be managed aggressively. The options for postoperative pain management should begin preoperatively and not postoperatively. A frank discussion

with the patient will allow the patient to discuss their fears of anesthesia and postoperative pain. Pain control options include cognitive/behavioral (i.e., relaxation, distraction, and imagery techniques), intravenous administration of opioids and adjuvant agents (i.e., nonsteroidal anti-inflammatory drugs, tricyclic agents) on an "around the clock" and/or PRN basis, PCA intravenous pumps, neuraxial (epidural, intrathecal) agents (local anesthetics, opioids, ketamine, clonidine, alpha agonists), intermittent neural blockade (with local anesthetics, cryoprobe, neurolytic agents) or continuous neural blockade (with an intrapleural catheter), physical application of hot and cold compresses, or TENS (transcutaneous electrical nerve stimulation). The surgical technique plays a very important part in the level of pain the patient will have postoperatively. There should be less pain associated with a VATS vs. open thoracotomy since there is less chest wall muscle damage. Controversy exists whether thoracic epidural analgesia is necessary for procedures performed with VATS since the pain experience is less dominated by the incisional component, compared to a thoracotomy. Thoracoscopy pain reflects more the visceral, pleural, and diaphragmatic nociceptive components. Multimodal techniques involving a combination of intraoperative intercostal nerve blocks, pre- and postoperative oral anti-inflammatories, and postoperative intravenous patient-controlled opioid analgesia are common strategies for the majority of VATS patients in many centers. Thoracic epidural may be reserved for patients with severe pulmonary dysfunction who are at a high risk for postoperative respiratory complications.

Clinical Case Discussion

A 67-year-old male with a right upper lobe non-small cell lung tumor is scheduled for VATS right upper lobectomy (see Fig. 24.12). He has COPD, preoperative FEV_1 is 57% predicted, and DLCO is 60%. No other comorbidities. After intravenous induction of anesthesia, he is intubated with a left double-lumen tube. After turning the patient to the left lateral position and confirming the position of the double-lumen tube with fiber-optic bronchoscopy, one-lung anesthesia is begun with sevoflurane (1MAC) and a FiO_2 of 1.0, pressure-control ventilation, tidal volume 6 ml/kg, and resp. rate 12/min. When the surgeon places the VATS camera in the right chest, the lung is not completely collapsed. What can be done to improve lung collapse?

Answer: The position of the double-lumen tube should be reconfirmed with bronchoscopy. The adequacy of lung isolation should be confirmed by verifying that the inspired and expired tidal volumes of the left lung match using sidestream spirometry (the expired tidal volume is often a small percentage lower than the inspired volume due to the greater uptake of oxygen than the production of CO_2). The use of

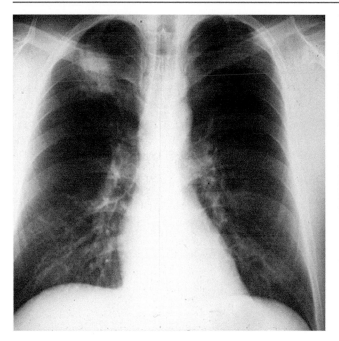

Fig. 24.12 Chest X-ray of a patient with a right upper lobe non-small cell lung cancer scheduled for VATS lobectomy. The patient has moderate COPD as evidenced by the hyperinflation of the lungs and the narrow cardiac silhouette

FiO2 1.0 to the operative lung prior to the initiation of one-lung ventilation will increase the rate of lung collapse, and a low suction (20 cmH20) applied to the non-ventilated lung will also speed collapse (see text).

With the onset of one-lung ventilation, the arterial oxygen saturation begins to slowly decrease. All other vital signs are stable: HR 78, BP 130/82, and PetCO2 32 mmHg. After 20 min of surgery, the SpO2 has fallen to 89% and continues to decline. What is the most appropriate next step?

Answer: After reconfirming the FiO2 and the correct position of the double-lumen tube with bronchoscopy, a recruitment maneuver of the left lung is performed, and PEEP 5cmH2O is added to the left lung. In spite of these therapies, the SpO2 continues to fall and is now 87%. The anesthesiologist suggests applying CPAP to the operative left lung. The surgeon is adamant that he/she will not be able to complete the operation as a VATS procedure if CPAP is necessary and will have to convert to an open thoracotomy.

Is there any other therapy that can improve oxygenation and will not interfere with surgical exposure?

Answer: Guided insufflation of oxygen at 5 L/min into the basilar segments of the right lower lobe is performed for 30 sec via the suction channel of the fiber-optic bronchoscope, while the surgeon monitors the insufflation using the VATS camera (see Chap. 6, Fig. 6.10). After partial re-inflation of the anterior and lateral basal segments of the right lower lobe, the SpO2 increases to 93% and surgery continues. The bronchoscopic segmental insufflation needed

Table 24.4 Management of hypoxemia during VATS

Severe or acute desaturation
Resume two-lung ventilation
Gradual desaturation
1. Assure FiO$_2$ = 1.0
2. Check double-lumen tube or bronchial blocker placement with fiber-optic bronchoscopy
3. Optimize cardiac output
4. Recruitment maneuver of the ventilated lung
5. Apply PEEP 5 cm H$_2$O to ventilated lung (except moderate–severe COPD patients)
6. Partial ventilation of the non-ventilated lung
(i) Segmental re-inflation (with fiber-optic bronchoscopy)
(ii) High-frequency jet ventilation

to be repeated once again 20 min later when the SpO2 fell to <90%. Surgery was completed without complication or conversion to open thoracotomy. Management of hypoxemia during VATS procedures is outlined in Table 24.4.

References

1. Sakula A. Carlo Forlanini, inventor of artificial pneumothorax for treatment of pulmonary tuberculosis. Thorax. 1983;38:326–32.
2. Jacobaeus HC. The cauterization of adhesions in artificial pneumothorax treatment of pulmonary tuberculosis under thoracoscopic control. Proc R Soc Med. 1923;16:45–62.
3. Fischer GW, Cohen E. An update on anesthesia for thoracoscopic surgery. Curr Opin Anaesthesiol. 2010;23:7–11.
4. Yang C, Kumar A, Klapper J, et al. A national analysis of long-term survival following thoracosopic versus open lobectomy for stage 1 non-small cell lung cancer. Ann Surg. 2017, Aug;9, epub ahead of print.
5. Demmy TL, Curtis JJ. Minimally invasive lobectomy directed toward frail and high-risk patients: a case-control study. Ann Thorac Surg. 1999;68:194–200.
6. Agostini P, Lugg S, Adams K, et al. Postoperative pulmonary complications and rehabilitation requirements following lobectomy. Interact Cardiovasc Thorac Surg. 2017;24:931–7.
7. Donahoe L, de Valence M, Atenafu E, et al. High risk for thoracotomy but not thoracoscopic lobectomy. Ann Thorac Surg. 2017;103:1730–5.
8. Jeon J, Kang C, Kim H-S, et al. Video-assisted thoracoscopic lobectomy in non-small cell lung cancer patients with chronic obstructive pulmonary disease. Eur J Cardiothorac Surg. 2014;45:640–5.
9. Bendixen M, Jorgensen O, Kronborg C, et al. Postoperative pain and quality of life after lobectomy. Lancet Oncol. 2016;17(6):836–44.
10. Miyazaki T, Yamasaki N, Tsuchiya A, et al. Pulmonary resection for lung cancer in nonagenerains. Ann Thorac Surg. 2014;20:s497–500.
11. Batoo A, Jahan A, Yang Z, et al. Thoracoscopic pneumonectomy: an 11-year experience. Chest. 2014;146:1300–9.
12. Williams A, Kay J. Thoracic epidural anesthesia for thoracoscopy, rib resection, and thoracotomy in a patient with a bronchopleural fistula postpneumonectomy. Anesthesiology. 2000;92:1482–4.
13. Capan LM, Turndorf H, Patel C, et al. Optimization of arterial oxygenation during one-lung anesthesia. Anesth Analg. 1980;59:847–51.

14. Thomsen RW. Mediastinoscopy and video-assisted thoracoscopic surgery: anesthetic pitfalls and complications. Semin Cardiothorac Vasc Anesth. 2008;12:128–32.

15. Tusman G, Bohm SH, Sipmann FS, Maisch S. Lung recruitment improves the efficiency of ventilation and gas exchange during one-lung ventilation anesthesia. Anesth Analg. 2004;98:1604–9.

16. Fujiwara M, Abe K, Mashimo T. The effect of positive end-expiratory pressure and continuous positive airway pressure on the oxygenation and shunt fraction during one-lung ventilation with propofol anesthesia. J Clin Anesth. 2001;13:473–7.

17. Ku CM, Slinger P, Waddell T. A novel method of treating hypoxemia during one-lung ventilation for thoracoscopic surgery. J Cardiothorac Vasc Anesth. 2009;23:850–2.

18. Ko R, McRae K, Darling G, et al. The use of air in the inspired gas mixture during two-lung ventilation delays lung collapse during one-lung ventilation. Anesth Analg. 2009;108:1092–6.

19. Pfitzner J, Peacock MJ, McAleer PT. Gas movement in the non-ventilated lung at the onset of single-lung ventilation for video-assisted thoracoscopy. Anaesthesia. 2000;54:437–43.

20. Narayanaswamy M, McRae K, Slinger P, et al. Choosing a lung isolation device for thoracic surgery: a randomized trial of three bronchial blockers versus double-lumen tubes. Anesth Analg. 2009;108:1097–101.

21. Donahoe L, Nguyen E, Chung T-B, et al. CT-guided microcoil VATS resection of lung nodules. J Thorac Dis. 2016;8:1986–94.

22. Ismail M, Swierzy M, Nachira D, et al. Uniportal video-assisted thoracic surgery for major lung resections. J Thorac Dis. 2017;9:885–97.

23. Irons J, Miles L, Klein A, et al. Intubated versus non-intubated general anesthesia for video-assisted thoracoscopic surgery. J Cardiothorac Vasc Anesth. 2017;31:411–7.

Anesthesia for Non-intubated Thoracic Surgery

25

Peter Slinger

Key Points

- The increasing use of VATS surgery has revived interest in non-intubated thoracic surgery.
- Recent advances in regional local anesthetic chest wall blocks have improved anesthesiologist's willingness to use non-intubated thoracic anesthesia.
- Improved methods of sedation have increased patients satisfaction with non-intubated thoracic anesthesia techniques.

Initial attempts at anesthesia for thoracic surgery in the late 1800s were all made with non-intubated patients breathing air-ether spontaneously through a mask. The lung collapse and pendelluft effect (see Chap. 1) when the surgeon opened the chest led to hypoxemia, hypercapnia, and hemodynamic instability [1]. The first major advance in thoracic anesthesia came in the first decade of 1900 when Sauerbruch developed the negative pressure chamber for thoracic anesthesia (see Fig. 25.1) [2]. Non-intubated patients continued to breathe air-ether spontaneously, but the negative pressure in the chamber (which excluded the patients head) prevented the lung in the open hemithorax from collapsing. However, this technique did not deal well with the problem of secretions. This was a major drawback since most of the chest surgery in the early part of the past century was for infectious causes.

As intubation, methods of lung isolation, and positive-pressure ventilation were developed, non-intubated thoracic anesthesia became very infrequent, although there were always case reports using spinal [3] or epidural [4] anesthesia. With the use of supplemental oxygen, the problem of hypoxemia is rarely an issue during non-intubated thoracic

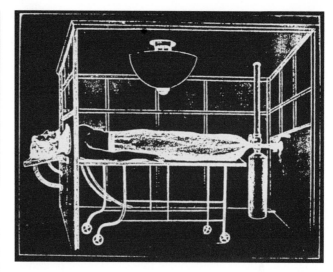

Fig. 25.1 The negative pressure chamber for thoracic anesthesia. Designed in 1900 by Sauerbruch. The patient's torso was placed in an airtight box along with the surgeon and nurse. Anesthesia was induced and maintained by breathing an air-ether mixture from a mask. The box was then evacuated to -10cmH2O pressure. When the surgeon opened the chest because of the pressure differential between the patient's lung and the box, the operative lung did not collapse. This apparatus was used in some centers until the 1930s but was replaced by endotracheal intubation and positive-pressure ventilation

anesthesia. During traditional one-lung ventilation, the positive pressure in the ventilated hemithorax tends to divert pulmonary blood flow to the non-ventilated lung and partially opposes the redistribution of blood flow by hypoxic pulmonary vasoconstriction in the non-ventilated lung (see Chap. 5). This effect is not seen when positive-pressure ventilation is avoided and arterial oxygenation is often equivalent or better with non-intubated techniques [5]. In 2010 Katlic and Facktor described 384 consecutive cases of VATS with local anesthesia and sedation. The patients ranged in age from 21 to 100 years (mean 67 years). Operations included pleural biopsy drainage with or without talc (244), drainage of empyema (74), lung biopsy (40), evacuation of hemothorax

P. Slinger (✉)
Department of Anesthesia, Toronto General Hospital, Toronto, ON, Canada
e-mail: peter.slinger@uhn.ca

© Springer Nature Switzerland AG 2019
P. Slinger (ed.), *Principles and Practice of Anesthesia for Thoracic Surgery*, https://doi.org/10.1007/978-3-030-00859-8_25

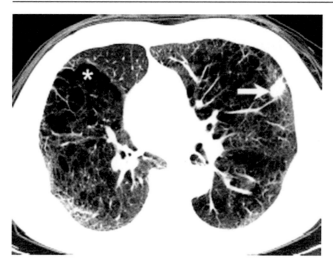

Fig. 25.2 Axial CT scan showing a solid 16 mm lung tumor in the left upper lobe (white arrow). The patient had previously undergone right upper lobectomy for lung cancer. Multiple emphysematous bullae can be seen in the left lower lobe (asterisk). Non-intubated thoracic anesthesia was used for a left segmentectomy. (Reproduced with permission from Ref. [8])

(13), pericardial window (7), drainage of lung abscess (2), treatment of chylothorax (2), treatment of pneumothorax (1), and biopsy of mediastinal mass (1). No patient required intubation or conversion to thoracotomy [6].

Since then the number of different types of thoracic procedures performed on non-intubated patients has expanded to include lobectomy, segmentectomy, and lung volume reduction. Almost any common thoracic surgical procedure has now been reported using non-intubated anesthesia. A meta-analysis comparing intubated to non-intubated VATS surgery has shown shorter surgical times, shorter hospital stays, and lower rates of postoperative complications with non-intubated anesthesia [7]. However, the majority of publications on non-intubated thoracic anesthesia come from a few centers, and there may be a degree of patient selection. Also, the learning curve of the anesthesiologist-surgeon team, prior to publication, is difficult to appreciate.

The potentially harmful effects of intubation, lung isolation, and positive-pressure ventilation can be avoided using non-intubated thoracic anesthesia. This may be applicable in patients who require lung surgery but have contralateral bullae or bronchial injuries (see Fig. 25.2) [8].

Techniques of Non-intubated Thoracic Anesthesia

Techniques of non-intubated thoracic anesthesia include a variety of methods of sedation or general anesthesia maintaining spontaneous ventilation [5]. Patients should receive supplemental oxygen to avoid hypoxemia. Patients may develop hypercapnia; however, mild hypercapnia is usually well tolerated. For patients who are hypercapnic at rest, the use of high-flow nasal oxygen (see Chap. 54) may be beneficial. Dexmedetomidine has been described to provide satisfactory sedation in combination with epidural anesthesia for VATS in patients with severe respiratory dysfunction [9]. If general anesthesia is selected, with either total intravenous or volatile anesthesia, a laryngeal mask airway is useful for non-intubated procedures. Regional anesthesia is commonly provided by either intercostal, paravertebral, or epidural blocks. Either of the two ultrasound-guided chest wall blocks (serratus anterior plane and erector spinae plane) (see Chap. 59) may be appropriate in some patients. A remifentanil infusion may be helpful in patients who are tachypneic without hypoxemia. Also, remifentanil may decrease the cough reflex. But the risk of apnea must be appreciated and ventilation closely monitored. For surgical procedures that involve manipulation near the hilum, coughing may be problematic. Chen et al. describe the use of an intrathoracic vagal block with 2–3 ml of 0.25% bupivacaine injected close to the vagus nerve at the level of the lower trachea in the right hemithorax or in the aortopulmonary window on the left [10]. This resulted in abolition of coughing for 3 h.

Conversion to General Anesthesia and Endotracheal Intubation

During non-intubated thoracic surgery, conversion to general anesthesia with endotracheal intubation may become necessary if there is persistent agitation, hypoxemia, tachypnea, hemodynamic instability, or hypercarbia [5]. Surgical problems which may lead to conversion include hemorrhage and adhesions. Since the patient is in the lateral position, airway access may be awkward. There are several options. Initial airway control may be achieved with a LMA. Then a fiberoptic bronchoscope can be passed through the LMA inside an Aintree tube exchange catheter (Cook Medical, Bloomington IN) which can be left in place to guide endotracheal intubation after the LMA is removed. After securing the airway with a single-lumen endotracheal tube (ETT), the options include proceeding with surgery using two-lung ventilation or, if one-lung ventilation is required, either to use a bronchial blocker via the ETT or to exchange the ETT for a double-lumen tube using a video laryngoscope and double-lumen tube exchange catheter (see Chaps. 16, 17, and 18).

Clinical Case Discussion

A 72-year-old male has developed a bronchopleural fistula 5 days postoperatively after an uncomplicated right pneumonectomy (see Fig. 25.3). The patient has been started on anti-

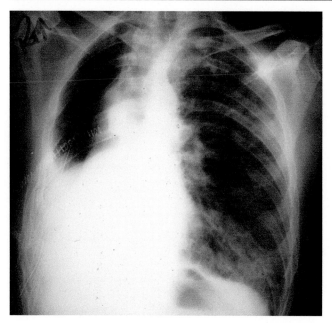

Fig. 25.3 Chest X-ray of a 72-year-old patient who developed a bronchopleural fistula after a right pneumonectomy

biotics and a chest drain inserted which drained 250 ml of fluid and showed a persistent air leak. The patient is not septic. The patient is scheduled to undergo thoracoscopy, rib resection, and insertion of a large-caliber drainage tube. The surgeon has requested that the airway not be instrumented due to the possibility of injury to the precarious bronchial stump.

How would you manage the anesthetic for this surgical procedure?

After placement of standard ASA monitors and an arterial line, a thoracic epidural catheter was placed by a paramedian technique at the T5-6 level. After a test dose of 3 ml lidocaine 2%, a mixture of bupivacaine 0.2% and fentanyl 10ug/ml was titrated in 2 ml aliquots (total dose 8 ml) until a sensory

block developed from T2-10. The patient was then started on an intravenous infusion of dexmedetomidine 0.7ug/kg/h and supplemental oxygen via a facemask and turned to the left lateral positon for surgery.

How would you manage this case if the patient was septic?

Because of the concern of the development of an epidural abscess in a septic patient, other types of nerve block may be optimal for this patient. Ultrasound-guided serratus anterior or erector spinae plane blocks may be considered in place of an epidural (see Chap. 59).

References

1. Mushin W, Rendell-baker L. The origins of Thoracic Anesthesia: Wood Library of Anesthesiology. Chicago, IL. 1953.
2. Sauerbruch F. Investigations concerning ventilation during lung surgery. Mitt Grenzgeb Med Chir. 1904;13:399.
3. Shields H. Spinal anesthesia for thoracic surgery. Anesth Analg. 1935;14:193.
4. Williams A, Kay J. Thoracic epidural anesthesia for thoracoscopy, rib resection and thoracotomy. Anesthesiology. 2000;92:1482–4.
5. Sunaga H, Blasberg J, Heerdt P. Anesthesia for non-intubated video-assisted thoracic surgery. Curr Opin Anaesthesiol. 2017;30:1–6.
6. Katlic M, Facktor M. Video-assisted thoracic surgery utilizing local anesthesia and sedation: 384 consecutive cases. Ann Thorac Surg. 2010;90:240–5.
7. Deng H-Y, Zhu Z-J, et al. Non-intubated video-assisted thoracoscopic surgery under loco-regional anesthesia for thoracic surgery: a meta-analysis. Interact Cardiovasc Thorac Surg. 2016;23:31–40.
8. Lu Y-F, Hung M-H, Hsu H-H, et al. Non-intubated thoracoscopic segmentectomy for second primary lung cancer in a patient with previous contra-lateral lobectomy and emphysematous bullae. J Cardiothorac Vasc Anesth. 2016;30:1639–40.
9. Iwata Y, Hamai Y, Koyama T. Anesthetic management of non-intubated video-assisted thoracoscopic surgery using epidural anesthesia and dexmedetomidine in three patients with severe respiratory dysfunction. J Anesth. 2016;30:324–7.
10. Chen K, Chen Y, Hung M, et al. Nonintubated thoracoscopic surgery for lung cancer using epidural anesthesia and intercostal blockade. J Thorac Dis. 2012;4:347–51.

Troubleshooting One-Lung Ventilation

26

Danielle Sophia Shafiepour

Key Points

- The perioperative hypoxemia that can accompany thoracic surgery is likely the principal contributor to cerebral desaturations that are observed during these cases and may be linked to adverse outcomes.
- There is no accepted "safe lower limit" for oxygen saturation during one-lung ventilation.
- During one-lung ventilation, a stepwise approach to hypoxia typically allows for the surgery to progress unhindered.
- Optimal V/Q matching during OLV requires that both perfusion to the ventilated lung and pulmonary vascular resistance (PVR) to the non-ventilated lung are maximized, while atelectasis in the ventilated lung is minimized.

Introduction

The introduction of reliable methods to isolate the operative lung and achieve one-lung ventilation has allowed for drastic advances in the field of thoracic surgery. Prior to this, attempts at thoracotomy were limited by the challenges of operating on a moving surgical field in a patient experiencing respiratory distress. These phenomena are the result of disrupting the pleural interface which exposes the pleural cavity to atmospheric pressure in a spontaneously breathing patient. The patient is prevented from generating negative pressure in the operative hemithorax despite diaphragmatic contraction, resulting in mediastinal shift downward with inspiration and

"Pendelluft" or paradoxical back and forth rebreathing of air from one lung to the other [1].

Prior to the use of routine fiberoscopy to confirm adequate lung isolation and the use of modern inhaled anesthetics that have less of an inhibitory action on hypoxic vasoconstriction, hypoxemia was a frequent complication of one-lung ventilation. Even with modern lung isolation and anesthetic techniques, however, significant desaturation may still occur in a proportion of patients and can prove to be quite a challenge for the anesthesia team. This chapter will discuss a stepwise approach to this problem, addressing the physiology that underlies hypoxia on one-lung ventilation. Troubleshooting the poorly deflated operative lung will also be covered.

Hypoxia

Permissive Hypoxia

Before tackling what to do about hypoxia during one-lung ventilation, it deserves to be noted that no safe lower limit of oxygen saturation (SpO_2) has been designated as an acceptable threshold during one-lung ventilation. The question is an important one, however, because unlike other clinical situations, the desaturation during one-lung ventilation is "iatrogenic" so to speak and typically entirely reversible by resuming two-lung ventilation. Naturally this is disruptive to the surgical procedure taking place, so in cases of hypoxia during one-lung ventilation, the burden remains with the anesthesiologist to decide how low is too low and at what point, when other manoeuvers fail, should one-lung ventilation be abandoned.

An evidence-based review of OLV management suggests titration of the inspired oxygen fraction (FiO_2) to target an SpO_2 of 92–96% to avoid both atelectasis and oxygen toxicity [2]. Saturations of 90% are often accepted in clinical

D. S. Shafiepour (✉)
Department of Anesthesiology, Montreal General Hospital, Montreal, QC, Canada
e-mail: Danielle.shafiepour@mcgill.ca

© Springer Nature Switzerland AG 2019
P. Slinger (ed.), *Principles and Practice of Anesthesia for Thoracic Surgery*, https://doi.org/10.1007/978-3-030-00859-8_26

429

practice, and even desaturations to the high 80s may be tolerated, ideally in the absence of significant comorbid disease.

Hyperoxia is increasingly recognized to contribute to pulmonary morbidity both through generation of absorption atelectasis and direct pulmonary toxicity, as well as systemic morbidity, with worse outcomes demonstrated in settings such as post-myocardial infarction or cardiac arrest [3, 4]. Interest has therefore emerged in the evaluation and adoption of a conservative or restrictive approach to oxygen therapy versus the more traditional liberal approach. Studies on outcomes in this area may allow for extrapolation to the thoracic surgery population and provide some further insight into the question of acceptable lower limits. A recent international multicenter randomized pilot study of mechanically ventilated ICU patients comparing liberal ($\geq 96\%$) and restrictive (88–92%) oxygen targets showed no difference in measures of organ dysfunction, ICU, or 90-day mortality between the groups despite a higher incidence of hypoxia (SpO_2 <88%) in the conservative group [5]. While these preliminary results are interesting, their extrapolation to the typical one-lung ventilation patient may be limited by the inclusion of patients with a wide variety of underlying critical illnesses including ARDS. Outcomes that are more relevant to the typical thoracic surgery population were not assessed, such as differences in postoperative neurocognitive testing scores. This approach also does not allow for an individualized management strategy, as likely the acceptable low SaO_2 differs between patients.

A small observational study exploring the cerebral oxygenation of patients undergoing thoracic procedures with one-lung ventilation demonstrated that patients spent a significant proportion of time with saturations considerably lower than their baseline on two lungs [6]. Important desaturations (>20% of baseline) occurred more frequently than those reported in non-thoracic surgery cohorts and were more common in patients who were elderly and heavier and had higher ASA scores. In other surgical populations, cerebral desaturations of this magnitude have been shown to correlate with adverse postoperative outcomes. The authors did not examine postoperative outcomes, however, and they used "baseline" values under anesthesia as opposed to preinduction which limits the validity of clinically significant desaturation cutoffs when comparing to other studies. Subsequent studies however have confirmed this observation and have found even higher rates of significantly decreased cerebral oxygenation during OLV [7–9]. In thoracic surgery patients, absolute cerebral oximetry levels of 65% have been correlated with increased postoperative organ dysfunction and complications, and the time spent at levels below 65% appears to correlate with worsened cognitive function at 24 h [8, 9]. Interestingly these cerebral desaturations are often not heralded by declines in SaO_2 or any other conventionally measured vital signs, but the authors point out that the lower

PaO_2 values without frank hypoxia during OLV may put these patients at risk for cerebral desaturation. Other mechanisms particular to the thoracic surgery setting have been proposed to possibly contribute to cerebral desaturation, such as changes in cardiac output with the lateral position and mediastinal shift and even a decrease in cerebral perfusion pressure due to elevated central venous pressure resulting from elevated pulmonary vascular resistance. A review on the subject of cerebral oximetry in thoracic anesthesia suggests that perioperative hypoxemia is most likely the principal contributor to cerebral desaturations during these cases [10]. Further work in this field may allow for a more individualized and targeted approach to oxygenation during OLV.

Management of Hypoxia

Ventilation of the Dependent Lung

Debates about optimal saturation during OLV aside, significant desaturation below 90% does still occur with enough frequency that the anesthesiologist taking care of thoracic surgical patients must have an approach when faced with this challenge. The typical pattern observed during OLV consists of a PaO_2 nadir 20–30 min after the initiation of OLV followed by a stabilization or increase thereafter. This is due to the biphasic nature of the hypoxic pulmonary vasoconstriction response that commences when moderate hypoxia is sustained [11]. In the event of an abrupt profound desaturation, restoring oxygenation is a priority, and two-lung ventilation should be resumed. This should be communicated to the surgeon who may have insight into the cause if the reason is a mechanical one, e.g., tube dislodgment or decreased cardiac output due to compression of the heart. The FiO_2 should be increased to 1.0, and the bronchial cuff of the double-lumen tube or the balloon on the blocker should be deflated. Frequently in this setting, failure of appropriate device placement may be to blame, and this can be verified and corrected bronchoscopically. For example, the cuff may have herniated over the carina to obstruct the trachea when ventilating through the tracheal lumen of a DLT or with a blocker, or a left DLT may have been positioned too far excluding part of the left lung when ventilating through the bronchial lumen. If these scenarios are eliminated as potential causes for desaturation, proceeding without lung isolation may be an option in some cases but is rarely a realistic choice particularly in video-assisted thoracoscopy which requires good lung isolation. A stepwise approach to improving oxygenation during OLV allows for continuation of surgery with OLV in the majority of cases.

During OLV, the primary mechanism responsible for hypoxia is the shunting of deoxygenated blood through the pulmonary circulation of the non-ventilated lung. This is worsened as atelectasis develops in the ventilated lung due to compression from the mediastinum and abdominal contents as well as absorption aggravated by the usually high inspired oxygen content. In order to optimize V/Q matching during OLV, both perfusion to the dependent lung and pulmonary vascular resistance (PVR) to the nondependent lung should be maximized. Lung volumes influence PVR in a hyperbolic manner with PVR at its highest at either extreme, total lung capacity (TLC) or residual volume (RV). Ideally the dependent lung should be kept as close to functional residual capacity (FRC) as possible. Any atelectasis that develops in this lung results in the end-expiratory volume trending toward RV in the absence of positive pressure to counteract this. Following lung isolation, a gentle manual recruitment maneuver is recommended, and the use of PEEP 3–10 cm H_2O has been recommended for ventilation of the dependent lung [2]. In the event of hypoxia, rerecruitment may be attempted; however there is no consensus on the optimal method to perform this maneuver. Brassard et al. recommend a gentle increase in pressure to 30 cm H_2O for at least 10 s [2]. Others have advocated cycling maneuvers with stepwise increases of PEEP and peak pressure. A rat model of acute lung injury demonstrated increased markers of injury after a continuous pressure of 30 cm H_2O maneuver vs a stepwise increase with the same time pressure product. Both methods yielded the same benefit with regard to oxygenation and pulmonary compliance [12]. During or immediately following a recruitment maneuver, it is common to see the saturation fall transiently as the perfusion is shifted momentarily to the non-ventilated lung.

The optimal level of PEEP depends on the individual patient, and it should be noted that both inadequate and excessive PEEP may worsen hypoxia. Inadequate PEEP will allow for development of atelectasis, and excessive PEEP may have adverse effects on the PVR, diverting blood to the non-ventilated lung and increasing shunt. Ideally PEEP should be titrated in order to optimize lung compliance. Ferrando et al. describe a more fine-tuned approach by performing a PEEP decrement trial at the initiation of OLV starting from 20 cm H_2O and decreasing by 2 cm H_2O each 2 min seeking the maximum dynamic compliance [13]. In their randomized comparison of this technique vs a control group with a fixed PEEP of 5 cm H2O, the study group showed improved oxygenation and compliance at the end of OLV. The average (optimal) PEEP in the decremental titration group was 10 cm H_2O.

The type of positive-pressure ventilation used appears to have little if any significant impact on hypoxia. A meta-analysis of six studies comparing VCV and PCV during OLV showed a statistically but not clinically significant difference in PaO_2/FiO_2 ratio in favor of PCV [14]. If hypoxia persists, an arterial gas should be sent to ensure ventilation is adequate as HPV in the non-ventilated lung may be impaired by

respiratory alkalosis, and significant respiratory acidosis may increase the PVR disproportionately in the ventilated lung as the non-ventilated lung is already vasoconstricted. Because of the high level of V/Q mismatch in the diseased lungs of many thoracic surgical patients, $EtCO_2$ may less reliably correlate with $PaCO_2$.

Management of the Non-ventilated Lung

If these measures do not adequately improve oxygenation, consideration should be given to applying continuous positive airway pressure (CPAP) with oxygen to the nondependent lung. The use of a PEEP valve with an oxygen source allows accurate measurement of the pressure applied. If not readily available, oxygen tubing with flows around 2 L/min may be attached to a double-lumen tube suction catheter advanced down the side of the nondependent lung, with a piece of tape partially occluding the thumb-control valve to control the amount of oxygen delivered (see Fig. 26.1). The lung should be observed in the field or on the VATS screen to assess for overinflation. To be most effective, CPAP should be preceded by a recruitment maneuver of the non-ventilated lung as atelectatic alveoli have a high opening pressure (>20 cm H_2O). This requires transient interruption of the surgical procedure, and for thoracoscopic procedures, even a small amount of CPAP may impair the surgical view. CPAP of only 2 cm H_2O has been demonstrated to improve oxygenation provided that it is applied after a recruitment maneuver [15].

Another method that has been described involves attaching a standard bacterial filter to the lumen of the DLT corresponding to the non-ventilated lung and attaching oxygen flowing at 2 L/min to the gas sampling port (see Fig. 26.2). When the open end of the filter is occluded manually for 2 s, approximately 66 mL of oxygen will enter the non-ventilated lung; in a series of 26 thoracotomy patients, only in 6 cases

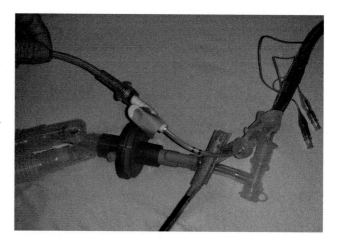

Fig. 26.1 This photograph illustrates the use of a double-lumen tube suction catheter to insufflate oxygen to the non-ventilated lung during OLV

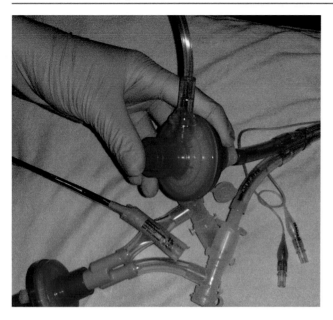

Fig. 26.2 This photograph illustrates the use of a breathing circuit filter to transiently insufflate small volumes of oxygen to the non-ventilated lung during OLV

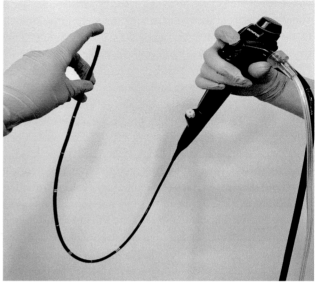

Fig. 26.3 This photograph illustrates the use of a bronchoscope with oxygen tubing attached to the suction port to selectively insufflate lobes or segments of the non-ventilated lung

did the surgeon notice the lung move, and in no cases did this negatively impact surgical exposure [16]. A case report describes successful treatment of hypoxia in a robotic VATS thymectomy using "high-frequency/small tidal volume" differential ventilation [17]. The procedure was performed in the semi-lateral position and was complicated by hypoxia that would not resolve with CPAP of 5 cm H_2O applied to the non-ventilated lung. Using a second circuit attached to the non-ventilated lung set to deliver tidal volumes of 60 mL at a rate of 35–40 breaths per minute, the authors describe successful oxygenation with no interference to the surgical procedure.

Other techniques allow for oxygen insufflation or ventilation to only part of the non-ventilated lung. Selective lobar collapse may be achieved by directing a bronchial blocker into a lobar bronchus which allows for ventilation to the remaining portions of that lung [18]. Naturally this comes at the expense of worsened surgical exposure. In some settings (patient with a previous contralateral pneumonectomy), this is the only alternative to intermittent apnea. Oxygen may also be intermittently insufflated selectively into segments or lobes of the operative lung that are remote from the surgical site [19]. This can be achieved by attaching oxygen tubing flowing at 5 L/min to the suction port of the bronchoscope and advancing the bronchoscope into, for example, the lower lobe during upper lobe surgery and pressing on the suction trigger for a couple of seconds (see Fig. 26.3). The surgeon should be warned before as the lung will move and visibility may still be impaired, but less so than with generalized CPAP. The surgeon can also direct the VATS cameras to the area being inflated and alert the anesthesiologist to any

overinflation observed as there is no pressure gauge and insufflation is being performed blindly. If hypoxia recurs after the oxygen is gradually absorbed, this maneuver may be repeated.

Regulation of Perfusion

In addition to ventilation strategies, the anesthesiologist should also be aware of the interaction between the circulatory system and hypoxia during OLV. The shunt fraction can be influenced by controlling the relative flow of blood to each lung. During a pulmonary resection, exclusion of the vessels to the soon-to-be resected lobe usually coincides with an improvement in saturation because of a decrease in the amount of shunt. If issues with hypoxia are communicated to the surgeons, they may be able to assist by accomplishing this more quickly. In the case of significant hypoxia, the surgeon may be able to partially or completely occlude the pulmonary artery on the operative side, bearing in mind that this will generate a significant increase in right ventricular afterload.

Acute changes in blood pressure and cardiac output are common in thoracic surgery, due, for example, to factors such as manipulation of the heart and great vessels by the surgeon or use of thoracic epidural boluses. Such changes should be sought when dealing with hypoxia during OLV as they may be contributory. Cardiac output influences saturation during OLV in two main ways. An increase can cause dilation of the pulmonary bed and increase perfusion to the non-ventilated lung, counteracting HPV and increasing the shunt fraction, thereby worsening oxygenation. This effect is counterbalanced however by the effect of increased cardiac output on mixed venous oxygen saturation (SvO_2). If oxygen consumption is relatively stable, an increase in CO will increase the SvO_2, and in the presence of significant shunting (as in OLV), this will have a positive effect on oxygenation. The overall effect is that both increasing and decreasing cardiac output can have detrimental effects and maintaining a normal cardiac output is optimal (see Chap. 5, Fig. 5.5).

Pharmacology

HPV is essential to minimize the degree of V/Q mismatch during OLV. Pharmacologic agents can either enhance or impair this response. Of particular relevance to the anesthetic setting, older volatile anesthetics (halothane, enflurane, and isoflurane) have been demonstrated to cause a dose-dependent reduction in the vasoconstrictive response to hypoxia with a 50% reduction at approximately 0.5 MAC units in in vitro animal studies [20]. A lesser magnitude of effect has been observed with in vivo animal studies suggesting a 21% reduction in response at 1 MAC for isoflurane [21]. Human studies of modern volatile agents do not support a large effect or a difference between agents with isoflurane, desflurane, or sevoflurane at doses up to 1 MAC [22, 23]. Previous comparisons of total intravenous anesthesia (TIVA) using propofol-narcotic combinations with sevoflurane and isoflurane have shown no significant difference in oxygenation with TIVA [24–26]. A recent RCT comparing desflurane-remifentanil and propofol-remifentanil calls this into question as the authors demonstrated a significant difference in PaO_2 values at all time points measured (15, 30, 45, and 60 min after initiation of OLV) [27]. An advantage of this study is its larger size compared to previous ones, as well as the duration of observation which suggests that a difference may have been missed before as one of the previously mentioned studies measured up to 10 min of OLV only. The study may be criticized however as the mean MAC in the desflurane group was 1.1 which seems high for a balanced anesthetic using remifentanil. The BIS target was lower in this study (30–50), and there was indeed more hypotension in the desflurane group which may have driven the difference in PaO_2 via the effect on SvO_2 as outlined above. It should be mentioned that volatiles, particularly sevoflurane, have been shown to have a protective effect during OLV, mitigating some of the alveolar and systemic inflammatory responses seen in this setting [28–30]. Taken together, the evidence to minimize volatile use to 1 MAC or less or abandon them in favor of a propofol anesthetic is not compelling. In the setting of refractory hypoxia, however, converting to a propofol-based anesthetic seems an acceptable move, but the benefit is unlikely to be large.

Conflicting results exist regarding an effect of thoracic epidural analgesia (TEA) on saturations during OLV. Two proposed mechanisms have been described to explain the potential influence of local anesthetics in the epidural space on hypoxia during OLV. First, if the cardiac output is allowed to fall with use of TEA, the SvO_2 may decrease and negatively impact oxygenation due to the presence of a large shunt as described earlier. Second, a decrease in sympathetic tone may decrease PVR in the nondependent lung therefore counteracting the HPV. In a small study where the mean blood pressure was comparable between the TEA group and the non-TEA group, there was no difference in PaO_2 [31]. Another study showed a nonsignificant trend to worsened PaO_2 with TEA, but there was also a nonsignificant trend to decreased blood pressure in the TEA group [32]. These studies would suggest that if cardiac output is maintained, TEA has little if any effect on PaO_2 during OLV. Others have found a decrease in PaO_2 and an increase in shunt fraction (Qs/Qt) with the use of TEA, which supports the second theory [33].

A recent interest has emerged in determining the effect of dexmedetomidine on oxygenation during OLV. Dexmedetomidine may potentially cause vasoconstriction through a direct peripheral alpha effect, but the central alpha-2 effect could result in vasodilation. Several groups have demonstrated a favorable effect of dexmedetomidine on oxygenation during OLV when combined with inhalational agents titrated to BIS values [34, 35]. A typical loading dose of 1 μg/kg was used followed by infusions that varied between 0.5 and 0.7 μg/kg/hr in different studies. The differences in PaO_2 were on the order of approximately 30 mm Hg at several time points in one study [34]. Interestingly another study specifically looking at patients with COPD demonstrated improved postoperative PaO_2/FiO_2 ratios and decreased ICU admission in the dexmedetomidine group [35]. Other proposed mechanisms include a reduction in inhalational agent requirement and a direct effect on pulmonary mechanics.

Another potential strategy to improve oxygenation during OLV is the selective delivery of vasodilators to the ventilated lung via the inhalational route, with or without concurrent administration of systemic vasoconstrictor drugs to enhance HPV in the non-ventilated lung. For example, the combination of 20 ppm inhaled nitric oxide (iNO), a selective pulmonary vasodilator, with almitrine, a systemic vasoconstrictor, has been demonstrated to improve oxygenation during OLV in humans [36]. The relative contribution of each drug is not certain, however, as iNO alone has not consistently been shown to improve oxygenation in this setting [37] and a small randomized study of almitrine alone did demonstrate improvement in PaO_2 during OLV [38]. Since almitrine, a respiratory stimulant, is no longer available in North America, these results are interesting more from a purely theoretical point of view; however interest in pharmacologically modulating the amount of shunt has led to research with other available medications.

In lung transplantation, use of inhaled prostaglandin E_1 (PGE_1) during implantation of the first lung (during OLV but after pulmonary artery clamping) has been demonstrated to lower pulmonary artery pressure (PAP) but also to improve the PaO_2/FiO_2 ratio by decreasing shunt wthin the ventilated lung. Presumably the drug preferentially vasodilated the better ventilated portions of the recipient's lung thereby optimizing V/Q matching [39]. Inhaled prostacyclin (PGI_2, commercially known as Flolan) is an appealing alternative to iNO for reducing PAP in heart and lung transplant patients as it can be easily delivered directly to a breathing circuit via nebulization and is much cheaper [40]. A case report describes a dramatic improvement in oxygenation observed with the combination of inhaled PGI_2 at a dose of 50 ng/kg/min and IV phenylephrine used in a hypoxic patient during OLV for a VATS procedure [41]. In my (albeit limited) experience, using this combination in hypoxic patients during OLV has led to a modest improvement in saturation shortly after initiation of the inhaled prostacyclin. Further research is needed in this area to confirm this effect and clarify the magnitude and time course.

Lung Collapse

Sometimes, despite adequate positioning of the lung isolation device, the deflation of the operative lung is suboptimal. Occasionally this may be worsened by adhesions in the chest cavity, but often it is due to the slow egress of air, particularly in patients with decreased lung elasticity as in the case of chronic obstructive pulmonary disease (COPD). This can be particularly problematic in VATS cases and may require conversion to an open technique if the surgical team is not able to fully visualize the relevant structures.

Certain strategies may be employed to avoid this issue. Prior to the initiation of OLV, the patient should be kept on an FiO_2 of 100% to ensure the elimination of nitrogen from the non-ventilated lung. After the pleural space equilibrates with atmospheric pressure on chest opening and the lung begins to collapse, the remaining gas will be absorbed much faster if the lung is filled with oxygen instead of air [42]. When using a bronchial blocker, the anesthesiologist should ensure that the blocker is inflated only after turning the ventilator to manual and allowing for a very long expiratory pause, ensuring that lung deflation is not commencing with the lung in a partially inflated state. Both of these maneuvers, the use of 100% FiO_2 and allowing for a prolonged expiration with no PEEP, will encourage atelectasis formation in the ventilated lung, so a recruitment maneuver may be performed after initiation of OLV and the FiO_2 titrated down as permitted.

In patients with significant obstructive pulmonary disease, it seems intuitive that the lung should be isolated immediately after positioning to allow time for deflation, particularly for VATS cases. An interesting consideration, however, is that prior to the chest being opened, this can lead to entrainment of nitrogen through the open end of the DLT due to cyclical changes in the pressure of the non-ventilated hemithorax that occur with ventilation of the dependent lung [43]. A proposed method to counteract this is connecting the non-ventilated lumen to an oxygen source, either via suction tubing passed down the lumen or an oxygen-filled reservoir bag.

A suction catheter on low suction (approximately -20 cm H_2O) may be applied to either a blocker or passed down the lumen of the DLT. This may serve to hasten lung collapse both by aspiration of gas from the lung and impeding the entrainment of nitrogen into the non-ventilated lung.

Case Discussion

Your next patient is a 65 year-old man awaiting a VATS right upper lobectomy for adenocarcinoma of the lung. He is 169 cm tall and weighs 74.0 kg. He has a preoperative FEV1 of 82% predicted with an obstructive FEV1/FVC ratio and a DLCO of 58%. He quit smoking 3 years ago and is on an ACE inhibitor for hypertension but has no other comorbidities. He climbs two flights of stairs without difficulty.

After a smooth induction and placement of your 39 Fr DLT, you turn the patient on his left side. Because of the obstructive lung disease, you isolate the lung early and pass a suction catheter down the tracheal lumen at 20 cm H_2O to encourage lung deflation. The ventilator is set at 15 × 380 with a PEEP of 5, and FiO_2 has been turned down to 80%. The surgery begins, and the surgeon is pleased with lung collapse. After 5 min, you notice that the saturation has fallen gradually and is now hovering at 87%.

1. Is this desaturation surprising in this case?
   - Early after lung isolation, desaturation may happen because of either tube malposition or because of the slow onset of HPV which has not kicked in fully yet. In this case risk factors include the fact that surgery is taking place on the right lung which implies a potentially larger shunt, and the poor preoperative DLCO which suggests that the PaO_2 prior to OLV may already be suboptimal. The patient is also taking a systemic vasodilator drug that can impair HPV.
2. Describe your management at this point.
   - The FiO_2 and flows should be turned up in order to deliver 100% oxygen. If it appears that the saturation is

falling precipitously, it would be prudent to notify the surgeon and resume TLV. Since the fall described here is gradual, bronchoscopy may be performed to confirm adequate tube positioning, and a stepwise approach to hypoxia on one lung can be performed.

3. The blue cuff is situated well beyond the carina but when scoping down the bronchial lumen, you note that you cannot see the left upper lobe bronchus suggesting that the tube is too far. A larger shunt is likely the cause of the hypoxia because of complete or partial exclusion of the left upper lobe which is not being ventilated due to mal-positioning of the tube. You reposition the tube under bronchoscopic guidance by entering the tracheal lumen, pulling the tube back and then confirming through the bronchial lumen that the tip is well situated in the left main bronchus. What do you do next?

   - Prior to resuming ventilation to the dependent lung, a manual recruitment maneuver may be performed with a gentle sustained pressure of 30 cm H_2O for 10 s, as the poorly ventilated left upper lobe has likely developed some atelectasis during this time. You may then proceed to titrate your FiO_2 down to aim for a saturation of 92–96%.

4. The saturation improves to 96% but 10 min later has drifted down again to 88%. Bronchoscopy confirms that the DLT is well positioned. How do you proceed?

   - Initial steps may include ruling out physiologic derangements that would impair saturation such as decreased perfusion or inadequate or over-ventilation. You may check for hypotension from surgical compression, hypovolemia, or excessive anesthesia and send an ABG to assess $PaCO_2$. An optimal ventilator strategy in the dependent lung is one that avoids the development of atelectasis but doesn't over distend alveoli to the point that PVR increases in that lung. Following another manual recruitment maneuver, a PEEP decrement trial may be employed, searching for the PEEP that provides optimal compliance. If more than one MAC of volatile is being used, a balanced technique should be employed, or TIVA may be considered if it is not possible to reduce the dose of volatile.
   - If the saturation has not improved, the surgeon should be made aware and a plan agreed upon. As this case is a VATS, the surgeon will likely be very reluctant to employ CPAP to the non-ventilated lung. They may in fact prefer intermittent gentle re-expansion with 100% oxygen, repeating as needed. An alternate approach would be using a bronchoscope with oxygen attached to the suction port to selectively insufflate the lower lobe segments. This needs to be done in collaboration

with the surgeons who can direct their cameras to observe the insufflated segment and avoid overdistension.

References

1. Maloney JV Jr, Schmutzer KJ, Raschke E. Paradoxical respiration and "pendelluft". J Thorac Cardiovasc Surg. 1961;41:291–8.
2. Brassard CL, Lohser J, Donati F, Bussieres JS. Step-by-step clinical management of one-lung ventilation: continuing professional development. Can J Anesth. 2014;61:1103–21.
3. Stub D, Smith K, Bernard S, et al. Air versus oxygen in ST-segment-elevation myocardial infarction. Circulation. 2015;131:2143–50.
4. Eastwood GM, Tanaka A, Espinoza ED, et al. Conservative oxygen therapy in mechanically ventilated patients following cardiac arrest: a retrospective nested cohort study. Resuscitation. 2016;101:108–14.
5. Panwar R, Hardie M, Bellomo R, et al. Conservative versus liberal oxygenation targets for mechanically ventilated patients. A pilot multicenter randomized controlled trial. Am J Respir Crit Care Med. 2016;193:43–51.
6. Tobias JD, Johnson GA, Rehman S, Fisher R, Caron N. Cerebral oxygenation monitoring using near infrared spectroscopy during one-lung ventilation in adults. J Minim Access Surg. 2008;4:104–7.
7. Hemmerling TM, Bluteau MC, Kazan R, Bracco D. Significant decrease of cerebral oxygen saturation during single-lung ventilation measured using absolute oximetry. Br J Anaesth. 2008;101:870–5.
8. Kazan R, Bracco D, Hemmerling TM. Reduced cerebral oxygen saturation measured by absolute cerebral oximetry during thoracic surgery correlates with postoperative complications. Br J Anaesth. 2009;103:811–6.
9. Tang L, Kazan R, Taddei R, Zaouter C, Cyr S, Hemmerling TM. Reduced cerebral oxygen saturation during thoracic surgery predicts early postoperative cognitive dysfunction. Br J Anaesth. 2012;108:623–9.
10. Mahal I, Davie SN, Grocott HP. Cerebral oximetry and thoracic surgery. Curr Opin Anaesthesiol. 2014;27:21–7.
11. Talbot NP, Balanos GM, Dorrington KL, Robbins PA. Two temporal components within the human pulmonary vascular response to ~2h of isocapnic hypoxia. J Appl Physiol. 2005;98:1125–39.
12. Silva PL, Moraes L, Santos RS, Samary C, Ramos MB, Santos CL, Morales MM, Capelozzi VL, Garcia CS, de Abreu MG, Pelosi P, Marini JJ, Rocco PR. Recruitment maneuvers modulate epithelial and endothelial cell response according to acute lung injury etiology. Crit Care Med. 2013;41:e256–65.
13. Ferrando C, Mugarra A, Gutierrez A, et al. Setting individualized positive end-expiratory pressure level with a positive end-expiratory pressure decrement trial after a recruitment maneuver improves oxygenation and lung mechanics during one-lung ventilation. Anesth Analg. 2014;118:657–65.
14. Kim KN, Kim DW, Jeong MA, Sin YH, Lee SK. Comparison of pressure-controlled ventilation with volume-controlled ventilation during one-lung ventilation: a systematic review and meta-analysis. BMC Anesthesiol. 2016;16(1):72.
15. Hogue CW Jr. Effectiveness of low levels of non-ventilated lung continuous positive airway pressure in improving oxygenation during one-lung ventilation. Anesth Analg. 1994;79:364.
16. Russell WJ. Intermittent positive airway pressure to manage hypoxia during one-lung anaesthesia. Anaesth Intensive Care. 2009;37(3):432–4.

17. Shoman BM, Ragab HO, Mustafa A, Mazhar R. High frequency/small tidal volume differential lung ventilation: a technique of ventilating the nondependent lung of one lung ventilation for robotically assisted thoracic surgery. Case Rep Anesthesiol. 2015;2015:631450., 3 p.

18. Campos JH. Effects on oxygenation during selective lobar versus total lung collapse with or without continuous positive airway pressure. Anesth Analg. 1997;85(3):583–6.

19. Ku CM, Slinger P, Waddell T. A novel method of treating hypoxemia during one-lung ventilation for thoracoscopic surgery. J Cardiothorac Vasc Anesth. 2009;37:432.

20. Marshall C, Lindgren L, Marshall BE. Effects of halothane, enflurane, and isoflurane on hypoxic pulmonary vasoconstriction in rat lungs in vitro. Anesthesiology. 1984;60:304.

21. Domino KB, Borowec L, Alexander CM, Williams JJ, Chen L, Marshall C, Marshall BE. Influence of isoflurane on hypoxic pulmonary vasoconstriction in dogs. Anesthesiology. 1986;64:423–9.

22. Wang JY, Russel GN, Page RD, et al. A comparison of the effects of sevoflurane and isoflurane on arterial oxygenation during one-lung anesthesia. Br J Anesth. 2000;81:850.

23. Wang JY, Russel GN, Page RD, et al. A comparison of the effects of desflurane and isoflurane on arterial oxygenation during one-lung ventilation. Anaesthesia. 2000;55:167.

24. Reid CW, Slinger PD, Lewis S. Comparison of the effects of propofol-alfentanil versus isoflurane anesthesia on arterial oxygenation during one-lung anesthesia. J Cardiothroac Vasc Anesth. 1996;10:860.

25. Pruszkowski O, Dalibon N, Moutafis M, Jugan E, Law-Koune JD, Laloë PA, Fischler M. Effects of propofol vs sevoflurane on arterial oxygenation during one-lung ventilation. Br J Anaesth. 2007;98(4):539–44.

26. Sharifian Attar A, Tabari M, Rahnamazadeh M, Salehi M. A comparison of effects of propofol and isoflurane on arterial oxygenation pressure, mean arterial pressure and heart rate variations following one-lung ventilation in thoracic surgeries. Iran Red Crescent Med J. 2014;16:e15809.

27. Cho YJ, Kim TK, Hong DM, Seo J-H, Bahk J-H, Jeon Y. Effect of desflurane-remifentanil vs. Propofol-remifentanil anesthesia on arterial oxygenation during one-lung ventilation for thoracoscopic surgery: a prospective randomized trial. BMC Anesthesiol. 2017;17(1):9.

28. Schilling T, Kozian A, Senturk M, et al. Effects of volatile and intravenous anesthesia on the alveolar and systemic inflammatory response in thoracic surgical patients. Anesthesiology. 2011;115:65–74.

29. De Conno E, Steurer M, Wittlinger M, et al. Anesthetic-induced improvement of the inflammatory response to one-lung ventilation. Anesthesiology. 2009;110:1316–26.

30. Potočnik I, Novak Janković V, Šostarič M, et al. Anti-inflammatory effect of sevoflurane in open lung surgery with one-lung ventilation. Croat Med J. 2014;55(6):628–37.

31. Casati A, Mascotto G, Iemi K, Nzepa-Batonga J, De Luca M. Epidural block does not worsen oxygenation during one-lung ventilation for lung resections under isoflurane/nitrous oxide anaesthesia. Eur J Anaesthesiol. 2005;22(5):363–8.

32. Ozcan PE, Senturk M, Sungur Ulke Z, et al. Effects of thoracic epidural anaesthesia on pulmonary venous admixture and oxygenation during one-lung ventilation. Acta Anaesthesiol Scand. 2007;51(8):1117–22.

33. Garutti I, Quintana B, Olmedilla L, Cruz A, Barranco M, Garcia de Lucas E. Arterial oxygenation during one-lung ventilation: combined versus general anesthesia. Anesth Analg. 1999;88:494–9.

34. Xia R, Yin H, Xia ZY, et al. Effect of intravenous infusion of dexmedetomidine combined with inhalation of isoflurane on arterial oxygenation and intrapulmonary shunt during single-lung ventilation. Cell Biochem Biophys. 2013;67:1547–50.

35. Lee SH, Kim N, Lee CY, Ban MG, Oh YJ. Effects of dexmedetomidine on oxygenation and lung mechanics in patients with moderate chronic obstructive pulmonary disease undergoing lung cancer surgery: a randomised double-blinded trial. Eur J Anaesthesiol. 2016;33:275–82.

36. Silva-Costa-Gomes T, Gallart L, Valle's J, et al. Low vs high-dose almitrine combined with nitric oxide to prevent hypoxia during open-chest one-lung ventilation. Br J Anaesth. 2005;95(3):410–6.

37. Schwarzkopf K, Klein U, Schreiber T, et al. Oxygenation during one-lung ventilation: the effects of inhaled nitric oxide and increasing levels of inspired fraction of oxygen. Anesth Analg. 2001;92(4):842–7.

38. Moutafis M, Liu N, Dalibon N, et al. The effects of inhaled nitric oxide and its combination with intravenous almitrine on Pao2 during one-lung ventilation in patients undergoing thoracoscopic procedures. Anesth Analg. 1997;85(5):1130–5.

39. Della Rocca G, Coccia C, Pompei L, et al. Inhaled aerosolized prostaglandin E1, pulmonary hemodynamics, and oxygenation during lung transplantation. Minerva Anestesiol. 2008;74(11):627–33.

40. Khan TA, Schnickel G, Ross D, et al. A prospective, randomized, crossover pilot study of inhaled nitric oxide versus inhaled prostacyclin in heart transplant and lung transplant recipients. J Thorac Cardiovasc Surg. 2009;138(6):1417–24.

41. Raghunathan K, Connelly NR, Robbins LD, Ganim R, Hochheiser G, DiCampli R. Inhaled epoprostenol during one-lung ventilation. Ann Thorac Surg. 2010;89(3):981–3.

42. Ko R, Mrae K, Darling G, et al. The use of air in the inspired gas mixture during two-lung ventilation delays lung collapse during one-lung ventilation. Anesth Analg. 2009;108:1092–6.

43. Pfitzner J, Peacock MJ, McAleer PT. Gas movement in the non-ventilated lung at the onset of single-lung ventilation for video-assisted thoracoscopy. Anaesthesia. 2000;54:437–43.

Intraoperative Extracorporeal Life Support for Thoracic and Airway Surgery

27

Daniel Sellers, Karen Lam, and Karen McRae

Abbreviations

ACT	Activated clotting time
APTT	Activated partial thromboplastin time
CPB	Cardiopulmonary bypass
ECLS	Extracorporeal life support
ECMO	Extracorporeal membrane oxygenation
FEV_1	Forced expiratory volume in 1 second
FVC	Forced vital capacity
HIT	Heparin-induced thrombocytopenia
ICU	Intensive care unit
INR	International normalised ratio
IVC	Inferior vena cava
OLV	One-lung ventilation
RA	Right atrium
SVC	Superior vena cava
SVR	Systemic vascular resistance
TEE	Transoesophageal echocardiography
TTE	Transthoracic echocardiography

D. Sellers
Department of Anesthesia and Pain Management,
Toronto General Hospital, University Health Network,
Toronto, ON, Canada
e-mail: daniel.sellers@uhn.ca

K. Lam
University of Toronto, Department of Anaesthesia,
Toronto, ON, Canada

K. McRae (✉)
Department of Anesthesia and Pain Management,
Toronto General Hospital, University Health Network,
Toronto, ON, Canada
e-mail: karen.mcrae@uhn.ca

Key Points
- Extracorporeal support is an established therapy in perioperative care of lung transplant recipients.
- New applications of intraoperative extracorporeal life support (ECLS) are increasingly being explored in thoracic surgery.
- In clinical scenarios which compromise oxygenation, VV-ECMO is most often used. These include procedures for patients with airway obstruction, require an open airway or have advanced lung disease.
- Surgery which will compromise cardiac function or great vessel flow is best supported by VA-ECMO. These include procedures for life-threatening mediastinal masses and locally advanced malignancies requiring resection of the atrium or great vessels.
- Unanticipated perioperative respiratory failure may require extracorporeal support.
- Meticulous and multidisciplinary preoperative assessment and planning are essential. The anaesthesiologist should understand the technical capability and limitations of the ECLS device.
- Critically ill patients may require cannulation of vessels under local anaesthesia, which may be technically challenging and uncomfortable but best done electively rather than emergently.
- ECLS applied to thoracic surgery is not as yet supported by strong medical evidence, but can be life-saving in individual cases.

Introduction

Extracorporeal life support (ECLS) encompasses a spectrum of temporary mechanical support for patients with heart or lung dysfunction that does not respond to traditional critical

© Springer Nature Switzerland AG 2019
P. Slinger (ed.), *Principles and Practice of Anesthesia for Thoracic Surgery*, https://doi.org/10.1007/978-3-030-00859-8_27

care therapy. The term ECMO (extracorporeal membrane oxygenation) is often used when the primary indication for support is failure of gas exchange. The physiologic goals vary with patient needs but may include oxygenation and CO_2 removal, increased oxygen delivery via improved perfusion and the provision of lung rest and cardiac unloading. ECLS is available in an increasing number of specialised centres and may be of short duration (hours) to facilitate a surgical procedure or provide support for prolonged periods (weeks to months).

The dramatic expansion of ECLS applications during the last decade is evidenced by an ever-increasing number of annual ECLS-related publications. It is a challenge for the interested clinician to keep up with the latest literature on the topic [1]. Use of ECLS for cardiac failure and cardiac procedures is beyond the scope of this chapter. The highest level of evidence for the clinical benefit of all the ECLS technologies in both respiratory and cardiac disease are randomised controlled trials of ECMO in acute respiratory distress syndrome (ARDS); all other applications are described in case series or cohort studies [2].

This chapter endeavours to provide the anaesthesiologist with a clear understanding of the nomenclature used to describe ECLS, the configurations of ECLS circuits and their physiological effects and the applications described for support of the thoracic surgical patient population both in the critical care unit and the operating room. Most applications in thoracic surgery require some degree of gas exchange support and therefore for the purposes of this chapter will be referred to as ECMO.

Brief History

ECMO first became an established practice in neonates with hyaline membrane disease and has been used in that context since the 1970s. In adults, although it had been occasionally reported as a rescue technique for the critically ill for decades, high mortality and significant neurological complication rate prevented its widespread use. However, interest was renewed in the intensive care population during the influenza outbreak of 2009 [3]. The CESAR trial demonstrated a 6-month survival benefit with ECMO use versus optimal conventional ventilator management of ARDS [4]. Additionally, streamlined ECLS technology has improved the feasibility of transporting critically ill patients from outside facilities to specialised ECLS-capable centres. In the last decade, ECMO has become a widely accepted supportive treatment for severe respiratory failure in the ICU. Improved survival has also been observed in end-stage lung disease patients supported with ECMO as a bridge to transplant and for severe primary graft dysfunction as a bridge to recovery. The growing experience of

thoracic surgical teams in operating on patients on ECMO, either from the ICU for diagnostic or therapeutic procedures or for lung transplantation, has meant that this form of support is increasingly for elective surgical situations where adequate gas exchange cannot be guaranteed. Historically, full cardiopulmonary bypass (CBP) has been the most typical form of extracorporeal mechanical and gas exchange support for complex thoracic surgery. Use of CPB has the known disadvantages of the need for full heparinisation, increased transfusion requirements, pump-related inflammatory response and the potential recirculation of tumour cells in oncology cases. Technological improvements offered by ECMO include the miniaturisation of circuits requiring lower priming volumes, limited air/blood contact by closed circuits without cardiotomy suction/reservoir and improved biocompatibility of material used in circuit components [5].

Components of the ECMO Circuit

The equipment used for mechanical cardiac or respiratory support have evolved from components of cardiopulmonary bypass for cardiac surgery. The original ECMO circuits used a CPB circuit stripped down to an oxygenator, pump, heating coil and minimal volume tubing, with no reservoir. There now exists a wide spectrum of different circuit configurations and cannulation options for mechanical support, but the basic components remain similar. It is important to understand the different components of the circuit being used, as they directly affect aspects of anaesthetic management such as oxygenation, anticoagulation, monitoring, transfusion, inotrope and volume status management (see Fig. 27.1).

Oxygenator

The oxygenator in an ECMO circuit channels blood down hollow fibres, with a counter current gas flow surrounding the fibres. Gases diffuse down concentration gradients, a similar mechanism to haemodialysis. The rate of gas exchange along the fibres can be controlled by altering the gas flow (sweep) and blood flow to change the partial pressure difference of oxygen and carbon dioxide across the membrane. Oxygenation is mainly a function of blood flow, while CO_2 removal can be modified by regulating the sweep. Modern membrane oxygenators are compact and have a very low resistance to flow. They are susceptible to fibrin clots making them first less efficient and then eventually fail; however, this usually occurs after weeks of support, and anticoagulation is used to delay this. In addition, their delicate structure makes them susceptible to trauma.

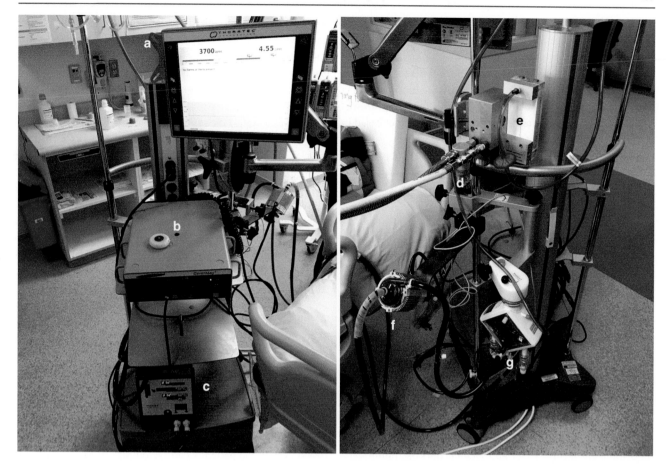

Fig. 27.1 Typical bedside ECLS circuit (back and front views shown). (**a**) Display with revolutions per minute, pump flow and resistance display (lower line). (**b**) Pump control terminal. (**c**) Oxygenator heater, (**d**) Air and oxygen wall gas inlet, (**e**) Sweep gas flowmeter, (**f**) Centrifugal pump, (**g**) Oxygenator (note oxygenated blood line marked with red tape)

Pump (When Applicable)

In CPB both roller pumps and centrifugal pumps are used. However, centrifugal pumps cause less haemolysis during long-term use, so in ECMO they are used almost exclusively. Centrifugal pumps are composed of a disposable cone which sits on top of a spinning magnet and rotate through magnetic coupling. The centrifugal force generated by this rotation causes a pressure difference across the cone which drives the blood flow. Pump flow is determined by this pressure difference, as well as preload and afterload, in a non-linear way. There is limited scope for the perfusionist to increase the cardiac output by turning up the revolutions per minute, as decoupling of the magnets can take place. Compared to CPB, the amount of flow is much more limited by technical design of the pump. Crucially, centrifugal pump flows are dependent on both preload and afterload conditions. If preload drops or the drainage line occludes, the centrifugal pump generates high negative pressures, and the cone slows down causing the flow to drop. This is seen clinically as "chugging" of the drainage line requiring restoration of patient volume to maintained desired flow. If afterload suddenly increases, the pressure difference across the pump drops and flow slows. Retrograde flow can happen, which would exsanguinate the patient or aspirate air from the reinfusion cannula site. If centrifugal pump flows drop too much, the perfusionist *must* clamp the arterial line and come off support altogether until the problem is rectified. This means that in a haemodynamic crisis, support may be suddenly terminated which can be difficult to manage.

Reservoir, Circuit and Connectors

A major step in the evolution of ECMO from CPB pumps was the removal of components such as the venous reservoir, three-way taps, stop cocks and shortening of lines. This has the effect of reducing the priming volume required for an ECMO circuit, minimising dilution. The use of heparin-bonded circuit components and removal of the large reservoir, filled with static blood often with an air/blood interface, means that the anticoagulation requirement is much lower (activated clotting times of 160–200 s compared to >400 s for CPB [6]). Since the ECMO circuit is completely closed, the risk of accidental air entrainment is much reduced (a requirement for long-term use). Unlike a CPB circuit, there are no infusion ports meaning that all drugs, blood products and replacement volume must be delivered by direct intravenous access into the patient. Shed blood must be processed in a cell saver prior to reinfusion.

ECMO Configurations

Configurations of ECMO

Several different ECMO configurations are possible, with varying levels of gas exchange capacity and haemodynamic support (summarised in Table 27.1).

Veno-venous ECMO

VV-ECMO is used in refractory respiratory failure and requires only peripherally placed venous catheters. Blood is drained from and reinfused into central veins. In the most common configuration with early use of VV-ECMO, deoxygenated blood drained via a femoral catheter was actively pumped though the membrane oxygenator and returned via a jugular catheter (Fig. 27.2). Oxygenated blood is reinfused into the right atrium (RA) and ejected into the pulmonary circulation by the patient's own cardiac output, mixing with the deoxygenated venous return. VV-ECMO has no direct effect on cardiac function; however, myocardial dysfunction

associated with hypoxia and respiratory acidosis will improve. Additionally, oxygenated blood entering the pulmonary circulation will reduce hypoxic pulmonary vasoconstriction, increasing the shunt fraction but decreasing right heart afterload. It is not unusual for depressed right ventricular function to improve after institution of VV-ECMO. In TEE assessment of the reinfusion cannula, the recommended position of the tip is in the RA just beyond the IVC/RA junction, a safe distance away from the intra-atrial septum and the tricuspid valve [9].

The development of bi-caval dual-lumen catheters allowed for inflow and outflow from a single percutaneous site, usually the right jugular vein (Fig. 27.4). Optimal cannula positioning is essential for good oxygenation; specifically, the infusion jet should be directed towards the tricuspid valve. TEE assessment of position and flow is very helpful, although fluoroscopy may also be used to guide venous catheter placement. By avoiding femoral cannulation, patient mobilisation is improved and participation in rehabilitation is possible, which is important in patients being bridged to transplant.

In VV-ECMO there is a functional dissociation of decarboxylation and oxygenation. Oxygenation varies primarily with blood flow through the membrane oxygenator, while CO_2 removal is dependent on the gas sweep past the membrane. Oxygenation also varies with the ratio of the circuit blood flow to the patient's cardiac output. Blood flow of 3–6 L/min is typically required to maintain acceptable oxygenation in patients with severe lung injury. The higher range of ECMO blood flow may be required to oxygenate an

Table 27.1 Extracorporeal life support configurations, indications and applications in thoracic surgery

Mode of ECLS	Hypercapnia	Hypoxia	RV failure	RV and LV failure	Applications in thoracic surgery
Low-flow VV-ECMO	Yes	No	No	No	Bridge to LTX
High-flow VV-ECMO	Yes	Yes	Rarely, only if ASD or PFO is present	No	Bridge to LTX LTX intraoperative Post-LTX – primary graft dysfunction Airway surgery Impossible one-lung ventilation Lung lavage
VA-ECMO	Yes	Yes	Yes	Yes	Bridge to LTX LTX intraoperative Myocardial dysfunction post-LTX or HLTX Airway surgery Mediastinal mass Lung resection involving the atrium or great vessels
AV-ECMO (pumpless)	Yes	No	No	No	Bridge to LTX Airway surgery Impossible one-lung ventilation
PA-LA Novalung (pumpless)	No	No	Yes	No	Bridge to LTX for PH

Adapted from Machuca et al. [7]

ASD indicates atrial septal defect, *AV* arteriovenous, *ECLS* extracorporeal life support, *ECMO* extracorporeal membrane oxygenation, *HLTX* heart-lung transplant, *LTX* lung transplant, *LV* left ventricular, *PA-LA* pulmonary artery to left atrium, *PFO* patent foramen ovale, *PH* pulmonary hypertension, *RV* right ventricle, *VA* veno-arterial, and *VV* veno-venous

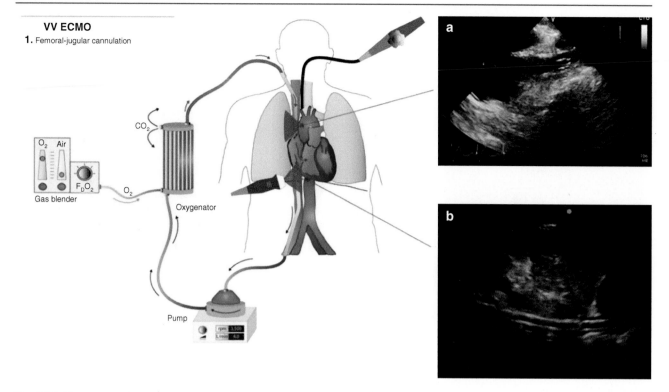

Fig. 27.2 Veno-venous (VV)-ECMO with drainage of deoxygenated blood from the inferior vena cava (IVC) via cannulation of a femoral vein and reinfusion of oxygenated blood into the superior vena cava (SVC) via cannulation of the jugular vein. Oxygenated blood is ejected into the pulmonary circulation by the patient's right heart function.

(**a**) Mid-oesophageal TEE view verifies the position of the outflow cannula in the SVC. (**b**) TTE subcostal view visualises the inflow cannula within the long axis of the IVC. (Adapted with permission from Doufle et al. [8])

unventilated surgical patient with a hyperdynamic circulation. If the lungs are not severely injured and can be partially ventilated with oxygen, oxygenation can be maintained with lower flows. Low-flow VV-ECMO via small-sized cannula can achieve blood flow of up to 1.0 L/min which is sufficient for CO2 removal but provides very little oxygenation [10].

Veno-arterial ECMO

VA-ECMO is used for cardiocirculatory support with or without respiratory failure. Blood is drained from the venous side and reinfused arterially; for peripheral VA-ECMO in adults, the femoral vessels are most often used for cannulation (Fig. 27.3). Blood drained from the RA is pumped through the membrane oxygenator and reinfused in the midaorta. Oxygenated blood mixes with the blood ejected from the heart with direct perfusion of the central organs. Physiological effects include unloading of the RV; when ECMO blood flows are high, much of the patient's venous return bypasses the pulmonary circulation. While organ perfusion pressure is improved, left ventricular afterload is increased as blood from the ECMO circuit is reinfused at arterial pressure. The cannula chosen should be large enough to allow VA-ECMO blood flow up to 2 L/min higher than the calculated cardiac output [11]. Because of the large size of

the femoral arterial cannula required, distal limb perfusion may be compromised, and a distal arterial perfusion catheter is routinely placed. Disadvantages of VA-ECMO include the risk of arterial cannulation: arterial injury, bleeding and embolism, distal limb ischemia and cardiac thrombus if low flows are maintained through the heart. TEE can be used to assessing the drainage cannula position, ideally in the lower part of the RA, and decompression of the right side of the heart, as well as overall heart function.

Central cannulation directly in the left atrium and ascending aorta enables placement of larger cannula and higher ECMO blood flows but requires an open chest and is generally reserved for operative cases that require haemodynamic support, including lung transplantation.

Patients on VV-ECMO for respiratory failure who subsequently develop haemodynamic instability can be supported by the addition of an arterial cannula for a hybrid configuration called veno-veno-arterial ECMO. Both venous catheters are used for drainage into a single ECMO circuit with reinfusion via a third (usually femoral) catheter.

AV-ECMO (Pumpless)

The Novalung interventional lung assist device (Novalung GmbH, Hechingen, Germany) is a low-resistance gas

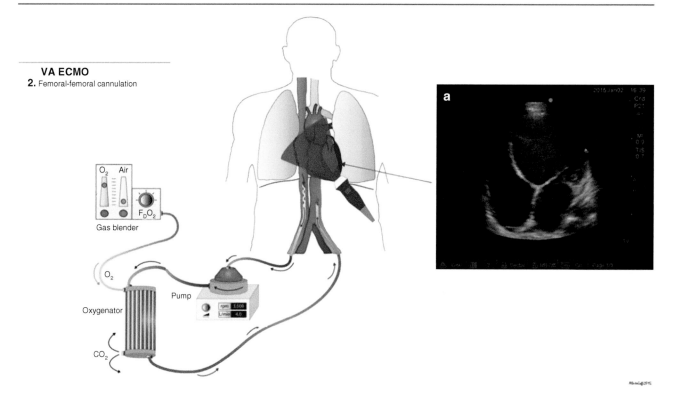

Fig. 27.3 Veno-arterial (VA)-ECMO with drainage of deoxygenated blood from the IVC via cannulation of a femoral vein and reinfusion of oxygenated blood into the ascending aorta via cannulation of a femoral artery. (**a**) Four-chamber view visualised by a TTE four-chamber view to assess cardiac function. (Adapted with permission from Doufle et al. [8])

exchanger designed for pulsatile blood flow driven by the patient's cardiac output. A drainage catheter is inserted into a femoral artery and reinfusion catheter into a femoral vein. The two are connected to the Novalung via a short, pumpless circuit. The blood flows generated are dependent on cardiac function and arterial blood pressure and are in the range of 1–2.5 L/min. This allows full decarboxylation, but only partial oxygenation, so this modality is particularly useful for treating hypercapnic respiratory failure [10].

Pumpless configurations have the advantage of greater portability and low priming volumes. They are practical for inter-hospital transport [12]. Once hypercarbia is controlled, many patients can be extubated, be mobilised and participate in rehabilitation [13].

PA-LA Novalung (Pumpless)

Another pumpless configuration is applicable only to patients with pulmonary hypertension and impending right heart failure. The Novalung is connected via a short tubing circuit between a drainage cannula placed directly into the main PA and reinfusion catheter inserted in the left atrium via the right upper pulmonary vein. High right-sided pressures drive the flow through the low-resistance Novalung. This oxygenated right to left shunt has the effect of unloading the RV, reduced septal shift, allowing better LV filling,

coronary perfusion and leading to improved RV function. This modality involves central cannulation via a sternotomy; patients who are awake but haemodynamically unstable may need femoral cannulation for peripheral VA-ECMO to safely tolerate the induction of general anaesthesia, with planned weaning when the right heart is decompressed. Intraoperative TEE does not direct the cannula positioning; however, it is vital for assessing adequate unloading of the RV and the status of LV function. It is crucial to verify that the LV is able to tolerate increased blood flow without failing. In the event of LV decompensation, longer-term VA-ECMO would be required. At the end of the procedure, the PA and LA cannulas are advanced through the skin of the upper abdomen and the chest closed. Used as a bridge to transplant, many patients can be extubated and subsequently mobilised [7, 14].

Applications in Thoracic Surgery

Lung Transplantation

ECMO is being used at an increasing number of specialised centres to bridge deteriorating patients with end-stage lung disease to lung transplant surgery. ECMO-bridged patients are at an increased risk of perioperative morbidity and mortality but do have an excellent 1-year survival (>90%) [2]. Given that without pre-transplant ECLS most of the ECMO-bridged patients would have died, this is increasingly an accepted practice. Many patients with hypercapnic respiratory failure can be bridged with pumpless AV-ECMO or preferably low-flow VV-ECMO. Those with significant hypoxia will require full-flow VV or if haemodynamically unstable peripheral VA-ECMO. In the subgroup with severe pulmonary hypertension, VA-ECMO or PA-LA Novalung is used [14].

Lung transplant surgery is characterised by dynamic haemodynamic and respiratory compromise, the most challenging being systemic hypotension, pulmonary hypertension and hypoxemia (see Chap. 47). ECMO is supplanting CBP as the favoured form of ECLS to stabilise patients. Typically, when ECMO is initiated intraoperatively, a VA-ECMO configuration via central cannulation sites is used. In a recent case-control cohort study of patients where cardiopulmonary support was used intraoperatively, those managed with ECMO had better early outcomes including duration of mechanical ventilation, ICU and hospital length of stay than patient who went on CBP. Blood product usage was significantly less in the ECMO patients [15].

VV-ECMO is the most common mode for preoperative bridging. When these patients undergo their transplant, some patients can be adequately supported with continued VV support. Many though require higher flows or increased haemodynamic support, often with a hybrid configuration. Patients who arrive in the operating room with a jugular dual-lumen catheter and with the addition of a central aortic catheter can receive veno-venous-arterial support with drainage via the bi-caval lumen and reinfusion of oxygenated blood into both the atrial lumen and into the aorta. Alternately, the VV-ECMO can be maintained unchanged via the jugular catheter, and additional central IVC and aortic cannulas can be placed as separate circuit for simultaneous VA-ECMO (personal communication Dr. Marcelo Cypel). The VV-ECMO is maintained during the surgery to avoid any thrombotic problem in the circuit and thus can be resumed postoperatively after weaning VA-ECMO if necessary.

Upon completion of the transplant, ECMO will be weaned for assessment of graft function. While desirable to decannulate the patient, the function of the allograft dictates the withdrawal of support. Some patients are decannulated of all extracorporeal support, patients with hypoxemia may be converted to VV, and those with pulmonary hypertension or severe myocardial dysfunction need continued VA-ECMO, requiring a later return to the operating room for decannulation. Any form of postoperative ECMO has the disadvantage of increased bleeding risk from continued anticoagulation after major surgery. Lung transplant recipients requiring ECMO for PGD have decreased survival as compared to those without PGD, but similar outcomes to patients with PGD managed without ECMO. Bridge to recovery support with VA-ECMO has a much higher 30-day mortality than VV-ECMO [2].

Airway Surgery

ECMO may be used to support patients with critical airway obstruction. Lesions above the larynx may be managed with awake fibre-optic intubation or tracheostomy under local anaesthesia. When severe obstruction is encountered below the larynx, while intubating the vocal cords may not be difficult, ventilation may be impossible. While some lesions may be managed by rigid bronchoscopy and debridement with intermittent ventilation (see Chaps. 11 and 13), extensive tracheal obstruction, need for prolonged debridement and significant bleeding into the airway present formidable problems. Historically, full CPB support was instituted via femoral venous and arterial catheters placed under local anaesthesia [16]. More recently, VV-ECMO support has been reported for endotracheal tumour resection [17, 18], dislodged stents [17, 19], foreign body removal [20], control of haemoptysis [21], debridement of papillomatosis [22] and relief of external compression [17, 23, 24] in adults. A variety of cannulation strategies have been reported: femoral and jugular single-lumen catheters [17, 20, 22] and bi-caval dual-lumen catheter in the right jugular vein [18, 24] have been described. Death as a result of post-resection haemoptysis has been reported likely exacerbated by anticoagulation for ECMO [17]. Relief of airway obstruction in small children has been performed with both VV- and VA-ECMO [25].

ECMO management has been reported after resuscitation from cardiopulmonary arrest due to airway obstruction; both VA [19] and VV [18] have been used. While VV support was successful in a hypoxic patient where haemodynamic stability had been restored, if there is postarrest myocardial dysfunction, VA-ECMO is a better choice. Both reports describe ECMO support during restoration of airway patency, conversion to conventional mechanical ventilation and a short period of observation for neurological sequelae, followed by successful extubation.

An additional challenge presented by tracheal resection and reconstruction is continued oxygenation and ventilation during the period with an open airway. Distal airway management often involves cross-field ventilation with an endotracheal tube or jet ventilation with a tracheal catheter, both of which may obstruct the surgical field (see Chap. 13). Complex reconstruction may be facilitated with ECMO support, as can open airway procedures in patients with limited respiratory reserve [26, 27]. Advanced tumours requiring extensive en bloc resection have been managed with VA-ECMO due to the need for vigorous retraction of the heart and great vessels. Both central and peripheral cannulation has been described [26]. VV-ECMO support is more often reported and is suitable for tracheal and carinal resection including carinal pneumonectomy [28–30]. An unusual case of repair of a complex tracheoesophageal fistula was reported using pumpless AV-ECMO, with a low-resistance circuit placed between femoral arterial and venous catheters for CO_2 removal. Apnoeic oxygenation was provided via a small endotracheal tube at the carina, allowing 12 h of surgery under without ventilation of the lungs [31]. Tracheal resection has also been described with AV-ECMO [32]. When VV-ECMO provides insufficient oxygenation during tracheal surgery, supplemental catheter oxygen insufflation had also been used [29].

Impossible One-Lung Ventilation

Patients under consideration for thoracic surgery may have limited pulmonary reserve, making oxygenation with one-lung ventilation impossible. Successful prior management of lung cancer may result in patients who have undergone pneumonectomy presenting with contralateral disease. Post-pneumonectomy patients have undergone contralateral wedge resection and segmentectomy for second malignancies [30, 33], VATS bullectomy [34] and esophagectomy [35] with VV-ECMO support. A low-flow VV-ECMO was noted to suffice in a subgroup of 3 of these patients undergoing segmentectomy. A dual-lumen catheter inserted in a femoral artery and an average of 1.6 L/min blood flow and sweep gas flow of 5 L/min through the oxygenator maintained stable blood gases for over 45 min. Pumpless AV-ECMO has also been used to facilitate wedge resection and decortication in post-pneumonectomy patients [32].

Patients who have advanced pulmonary parenchymal lung disease may present for vital thoracic surgery procedures; however, may not tolerate OLV. There are no guidelines to determine which patients will need extracorporeal support and who will tolerate the procedure without. Arterial P_aO_2 on two-lung ventilation, FEV_1/FVC ratio and side of operation are usually good predictors of hypoxia on OLV [36]; however, this information may be limited on critically ill patients and may not reflect new pulmonary co-morbidities such as empyema or an air leak. Patients for empyema surgery frequently have necrotising pneumonia or bronchiectasis, and VV-ECMO has been instituted intraoperatively to allow aggressive decortication of empyema [37]. The bilateral decortication of critically ill, VV-ECMO-dependent patients was proposed to be a crucial step in their weaning from ECMO, followed by successful extubation [38].

Patients with emphysema are prone to ruptured bullae and prolonged air leaks, and VATS resection of bullae has been

with both VV-ECMO support [30] and AV-ECMO [32]. In the late 1990s, elective intraoperative initiation of ECMO was used to support three COPD patients with severe hypercapnia undergoing LVRS, who therefore did not meet standard selection criteria for this procedure [39]. VA-ECMO was chosen due to the anticipated haemodynamic instability often seen with positive pressure of patients with pulmonary hyperinflation. This must be described as a controversial treatment plan as severe hypercapnia is a risk factor for perioperative mortality. This practice has not been reported by other groups. VV-ECMO has been used to facilitate LVRS/major bullectomy to liberate COPD patients from mechanical ventilation [40, 41].

Additionally, VV-ECMO has been used to enable patients with significant loss of lung parenchyma to tolerate resections: metastasectomy after prior extensive lung resection [30], bullectomy [42] and resection of aspergilloma [43] after scarring from tuberculosis have been reported.

Finally, patients with alveolar proteinosis with progressive hypoxia require whole lung lavage of both lungs with large volumes of saline to remove lipoprotein deposits. Classically, this has been done sequentially via a double-lumen tube, but severely affected patients may not tolerate this, and there are many case reports describing VV-ECMO support to enable lavage in this patient group [44–55].

Mediastinal Masses

Large masses occupying the anterior mediastinum have the potential to cause compression of great vessels and right atrium, causing reduction in preload and cardiac output. In the awake patient, the negative pressure generated by inspiration reduces this effect so that compression is minimal until surgical disease is advanced. However, this is abolished by muscle relaxants, and positive pressure ventilation can precipitate collapse of cardiac output and arrest. This is a particular risk for children with large anterior lymphomas. Historically, this has been treated with CPB support [56–59]. More recently, preinduction femoral VA-ECMO while maintaining spontaneous ventilation has been described in children [60] and adults [61]. The VA configuration is warranted by the potential for cardiovascular collapse. This is a well-known problem in thoracic anaesthesia, and the risk assessment for extracorporeal support is described in more detail in Chap. 14.

Advanced Surgical Resections

Late presentation of intrathoracic cancer with local invasion historically was deemed unresectable. However, tertiary referral centres are increasingly undertaking resection of advanced lung and oesophageal malignancies as part of multimodal therapy and reporting reasonable survival [62–72]. The most common extrapleural site of invasion for lung cancer is the left atrium. Resection requires clamping the affected area of the atrial wall, which causes haemodynamic instability which can be prolonged as a patch repair or primary closure of the atrium is required before the clamp can be released. This can be achieved in some cases without extracorporeal support [63, 73]. Resection of lung malignancies with reconstruction of the superior or inferior vena cava, left atrium, distal aorta and carina has been described with VA-ECMO support [71] as have oesophageal malignancies invading carina [5]. Cannulation sites are chosen according to the planned resection and may be central or peripheral [71]. Resection of complex thoracic malignancies with extension into the pulmonary trunk, the aortic arch or the heart requiring opening a cardiac chamber is only amenable to traditional CPB [71, 74–76].

Thoracic Emergencies

ECMO has been described as a life-saving emergency treatment of massive haemoptysis [21, 77, 78]. Intraoperative iatrogenic large vessel injury with massive bleeding is most often managed with CPB, which provides the advantages of rapid infusion, autotransfusion and delivery of cardioplegia for cardiac arrest or deep hypothermic circulatory arrest if needed [5]. In the event of pulmonary artery injury, the reduction of blood flow through the pulmonary trunk enables surgical repair [5, 79], whereas ECMO has been shown to be of benefit in a wide variety of tracheal injuries to facilitate tracheal repair and healing. These include iatrogenic injury, postoperative fistulae and trauma [27, 80].

ECMO for primary graft dysfunction is frequently required after lung transplantation, to support the lungs, while reperfusion injury abates but has also been instituted emergently for other perioperative aetiologies of lung failure. These include haemodynamic stabilisation in patients with acute severe pulmonary embolism [81] to allow pulmonary embolectomy [82, 83], reperfusion injury after pulmonary thromboendarterectomy [84–86] for chronic thromboembolic pulmonary hypertension and the indications and methodology of which have recently been reviewed [7]. Support for postoperative transfusion-associated lung injury (TRALI) is also well-described [87, 88]. The importance of advanced planning for emergencies and effective multidisciplinary team-working has recently been emphasised in maintaining good patient outcomes [5]. In addition, ECMO has been used outside the thoracic operating rooms

as part of resuscitation and surgical repair for thoracic trauma [37, 89–92].

The choice of VV- versus VA-ECMO in emergency circumstances is dependent on the need for primarily oxygenation versus the need for concomitant haemodynamic support. When urgent ECMO is instituted intraoperatively, available venous and arterial cannulation sites may be dictated by patient position and available vessels [5].

Preoperative Planning of ECMO

For any patient who requires extracorporeal support, the surgical checklist should include the planned ECMO configuration, cannulation sites, timing of cannulation (before or after induction of general anaesthesia) and anticipated timing of weaning and decannulation. Patient position and planned incision will influence cannulation sites [5]. If patients are transferred to the operating room already on ECMO, any required modification of support or additional cannulation should be discussed. This allows the anaesthesiologist to optimise intravenous and arterial access for monitoring and volume infusion.

Are the Proposed Vessels Big Enough?

The sizes of the cannulas currently available for ECMO are summarised in Table 27.2.

The size of the cannula required will depend on the patient's body surface area (aiming for 2.5 L/min/m^2), the achievable flow rate through the cannula without excessively high pressures (a technical property of the cannula available from the manufacturer). A large adult will need femoral vessels in the range of 8–10 mm in diameter, without atherosclerosis, stricture or tortuosity to be successful. This can be checked preoperatively with ultrasound or ultimately with angiography. Central cannulation typically allows placement of larger cannulas and consequently higher flows than peripheral ECMO.

Table 27.2 Sizes of currently available ECMO cannulas

Manufacturer	Central ECMO		Peripheral ECMO	
	Arterial Fr (mm)	Venous Fr (mm)	Arterial Fr (mm)	Venous Fr (mm)
Terumo	10–26 (3.3–8.7)	28–36 (9.3–12)	20–24 (6.7–8)	19–29 (6.3–9.7)
Medtronic	15–24 (5–8)	28–36 (9.3–12)	None	None
Maquet	20–24 (6.7–8)	32–36 (10.7–12)	15–29 (5–9.7)	19–29 (6.3–9.7)
Edwards	None	None	16–24 (5.3–8)	18–28 (6–9.3)

Note: dual-lumen cannulas are larger at 23–32 Fr (7.7–10.7 mm) [93]

Will the Patient Tolerate the Procedure?

An intrathoracic mass large enough to cause obstruction on induction may also cause positional symptoms, and such patients can often not lie flat for any length of time. Airway tumours also often cause positional dyspnoea. It is very difficult for the surgeon to insert these large cannulas into the groin with the patient in a semi-sitting position, and this must be done carefully to avoid iatrogenic vessel injury. In addition, even with meticulous local anaesthetic, the procedure can be painful for the patient as the cannulas are introduced and as the innervation of the vessels is visceral rather than somatic. Judicious sedation and analgesia may be helpful while maintaining respiratory drive and muscle strength. In the authors' experience, a vasovagal response to awake femoral cannulation can provoke cardiopulmonary arrest, so cannulation should only be done in a fully monitored setting with resuscitative drugs and equipment immediately available.

Are the Cannulas Correctly Positioned?

Malpositioned cannulas have the potential to become obstructed or create recirculation (see "Troubleshooting ECMO"), causing the patient to become hypoxic. The position can be checked with TEE or fluoroscopically. The chosen imaging modality should be in place prior to induction.

What Are the Risks of Anticoagulation, and How Should It Be Managed?

Once the cannulas are in place, the patient must be sufficiently anticoagulated to prevent thrombosis, either at the tips of the cannulas or in the circuit. This potentially has implications for neuraxial analgesia and surgical blood loss, which can be significant and rapid, so appropriate intravenous access should be gained prior to insertion.

Historically, the predominant causes of adverse outcome from ECMO on ICU patients with respiratory failure have been major bleeding requiring surgical intervention, and intracerebral haemorrhage, particularly in neonates. ICU patients on long-term ECMO have low platelet function and numbers, fibrinogen deficiency, loss of vitamin K-dependent clotting factors and acquired Von Willebrand's disease resulting in complex coagulopathy, which has been recently reviewed [94]. International guidelines from the Extracorporeal Life Support Organization (ELSO) [95] are summarised in Table 27.3. For CPB, anticoagulation practices are well-established [96], and a typical institutional protocol is given in Table 27.3 for comparison.

Table 27.3 Anticoagulation for ECMO and CPB

	ECMO (as per ELSO [95])	CPB
Unfractionated heparin bolus (units/kg)	50–100	300
Maintenance heparin	7.5–20 units/kg/hr	5000–10,000 unit boluses guided by ACT
ACT target (seconds)	180–220	480
Anti-Xa target (units/ml)	0.3–0.7	–
APTT range	1.5 x baseline	–
Fibrinogen target (mg/dl)	>150	>200
INR	<1.5	<1.5
Platelet target (1000 cells/mm^3)	>100	>75
Haematocrit (%)	35–40	24–28

It should be emphasised that the risk/benefit gained from anticoagulation in the intraoperative setting is potentially different, and these guidelines were not designed for short-term operative use. For example, the use of a heparin-bonded circuit can reduce the heparin requirement substantially for the first 6 h of its use [95]. This doesn't reduce the heparin requirement in the long term, but could substantially reduce the thrombosis risk in the intraoperative situation. Similarly, patients undergoing procedures with major blood loss will also be deficient in platelets, fibrinogen and other clotting factors, which will potentially prolong coagulation in the absence of heparin. There are multiple reports of surgical interventions with high bleeding risk using ECMO without heparin [21, 32, 33, 37, 38]. In our institution, we routinely target an ACT of 160–180 s for these reasons, checking at least every 30 min and giving small boluses of heparin as needed rather than running an infusion. We also routinely use ROTEM™ and platelet function assay, as an adjunct to ACT, to detect other potential causes of bleeding such as factor deficiency, platelet dysfunction or fibrinolysis.

Vascular Access

Two-cannula peripheral ECMO may use femoral vessels (often on both sides) or jugular and femoral vessels. A single-stage VV-ECMO cannula is usually placed in the right internal jugular, but axillary [97, 98] and supraclavicular cannulation sites have also been described [99, 100]. Placement of central lines should be planned in discussion with the surgeon, leaving the sites with the highest calibre for ECMO cannulas. If ECMO is already in place and central venous line placement is required, the potential for air entrainment is increased by the negative pressure generated by the drainage cannula. In VA-ECMO there is a risk of paradoxical arterial air embolism from venous bubbles, via the arterial return cannula (the ECMO circuit contains no bubble traps or filters).

Ventilation Strategies for ECMO

All configurations of ECMO are extremely efficient at clearing carbon dioxide, which means that in the ECMO patient the main determinant of p_aCO2 is sweep gas flow and carbon dioxide tension, not the patient's minute volume. Alveolar pO_2 is still important to preserve when possible, as it contributes to oxygenating the remaining pulmonary blood flow. Tidal volumes and respiratory rate can be reduced far beyond what is normally possible. Given the established link between mechanical ventilation and lung injury, particularly in thoracic surgery and one-lung ventilation [101, 102], it would seem prudent to adopt a lung-protective ventilation strategy even in patients without prior injury, with tidal volumes 6–8 ml/kg (ideal body weight) preventing volutrauma. Prevention of atelectasis with 5-10 mmHg of PEEP will reduce atelectotrauma. Reducing the ventilator rate to 6–10 breaths a minute will allow for reduction in ventilator mean pressures, and longer rise times, with consequent reduction in strain forces which may be associated with acute lung injury. High alveolar oxygen tensions can exacerbate perioperative lung injury, so titrating FiO2 as low as saturations allow is advisable [103].

The efficacy of ECMO means that the patient can receive little to no ventilation and remain stable – so "ultraprotective" lung ventilation has been advocated for the ARDS patient group [104]. This comprises tidal volumes of less than 4 ml/kg, with PEEP >10 mmHg and a respiratory rate of 6 breaths/minute. The degree of protection is not mandatory for the perioperative patient, but is easy to achieve with ECMO support.

Monitoring Patients on ECMO

Monitoring considerations for patients on ECMO in the ICU has recently been authoritatively reviewed, with particular emphasis on the importance of TEE for cannula positioning [9]. Arterial lines are best placed in the right arm to measure pressure and P_aO_2 downstream from the brachiocephalic artery, which correlates most closely with conditions in the right carotid artery and coronary arteries. Central venous line location most likely will be dictated by the surgical incision, but care should be taken not to advance the tip of the catheter too far into the central circulation, so that it is not aspirated into the lumen of the ECMO cannula. Once the ECMO is started, central venous pressure monitoring may not be reliable. Pulmonary artery (PA) catheters may be very difficult to insert if upper body ECMO cannulas are already in place, both in terms of passing the catheter through the occupied SVC and in floating into the right heart with ongoing drainage into the ECMO circuit. It is possible for the PA catheter balloon to be aspirated into a drainage cannula and occlude it

completely. Seeing a pulsatile PA tracing is a reassuring sign that volume replacement is adequate.

Peripheral saturation probes should be placed on the right hand, to guard against diffusion hypoxia. Consideration should be given to cerebral saturation monitoring with near-infrared spectroscopy, as an indicator of cerebral hypoxia. In a short retrospective case series using this monitor, Wong et al. found a 100% rate of cerebral desaturation on initiation of ECMO, 80% of which were reversible with changes in haemodynamic management [105].

Troubleshooting ECMO

Hypoxia

Flows Are Insufficient

VV-ECMO is dependent on sufficient venous blood flow through the oxygenator before returning it to the right atrium. If flow through the oxygenator is much less than the total cardiac output, the difference will pass through the unventilated pulmonary circulation, and the arterial saturation will be reduced by this mixing. In severe respiratory failure, VV-ECMO flows of 60% of cardiac output are required to maintain an SpO_2 over 90% [106]. The solution is to oxygenate via the lungs if possible, optimise venous drainage, increase the ECMO flows if possible, increase the sweep gas to ensure full oxygenation of the return blood and if necessary reduce the cardiac output. When this problem occurs on the ICU, beta-blockers are occasionally used, but their use should only be considered carefully in the unstable patient in the operating room.

Recirculation

In VV-ECMO, recirculation of blood between the reinfusion and drainage catheters can occur. The intent is for the oxygenated return blood to pass through the tricuspid valve; therefore, the reinfusion ports should be in the right atrium. Oxygenated reinfused blood may flow into a single-lumen drainage catheter if the catheters are too close together. Recirculation can also occur with bi-caval dual-lumen catheters particularly if malpositioned and when higher flow rates are used but is less common than with two cannula configurations [107]. Echocardiography using colour Doppler can be useful for assessing ECMO cannula positions and direction of flows. The IVC cannula should be below the hepatic vein, SVC cannula should be at the SVC-RA border, and double-lumen cannulas should have the return port pointed at the tricuspid valve.

Differential Hypoxia/Watershed Phenomenon

In peripheral VA-ECMO, oxygenated arterial flow is retrograde from the femoral arterial reinfusion catheter back to

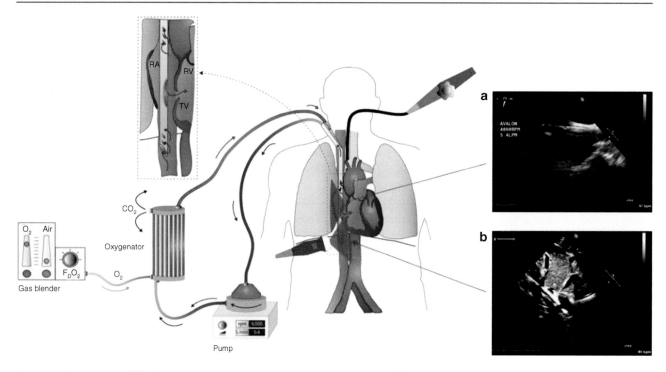

Fig. 27.4 Veno-venous (VV)-ECMO via a bi-caval dual-lumen cathe-ter inserted via the jugular vein. Deoxygenated blood is aspirated via holes located in the drainage lumen of the catheter: proximally in the SVC and distally in the IVC. Oxygenated blood is reinfused via the atrial lumen with infusion port oriented towards the tricuspid valve (inset). (**a**) TEE mid-oesophageal bi-caval view of the cannula within the right atrium. (**b**) TTE subcostal view of the injection port facing the tricuspid valve and the tip of the cannula within the IVC. (Adapted with permission from Doufle et al. [8])

the aortic arch. Reinfused blood competes with anterograde (deoxygenated) cardiac output ejected from the left ventri-cle. This means that while the lower body is perfused with highly oxygenated blood, there may be ongoing upper body hypoxia (see Fig. 27.4). Importantly, this may result in deox-ygenated blood flow to the brain and coronary arteries [11]. This is a particular risk in the patient with poor lung function in the presence of preserved myocardial function. The solu-tion is to increase ECMO blood flow: the effect of this is twofold, and it will reduce pulmonary blood flow while increasing the ECMO flow itself. The replacement of inotro-pes by purely vasopressor medications may also be helpful (Fig. 27.5).

Hypotension

VA-ECMO Flows Are Insufficient
Check the drainage cannula: if it is chugging, flow may be obstructed (ask surgeon to check), the line may be kinked (perfusionist can check), the patient's great veins are com-pressed (e.g. by extrinsic pressure or retraction), or the patient may be hypovolemic. Intravascular volume status is the responsibility of the anaesthesiologist, and volume must

be delivered intravenously as the perfusionist has no reservoir. Check the reinfusion cannula; low flows can occur if the line is kinked or cannula is misplaced.

The Patient's Afterload Is Too Low
Support of the patient's SVR on ECMO is the responsibility of the anaesthesiologist, requiring infusion of vasopressors via a central venous line separate from the ECLS device. In addition, the ECMO flows vary with the level of support required and surgical manipulation. Inotropy is frequently required.

Weaning ECMO

VA-ECMO

At the end of the surgical procedure, if ECMO support is not planned into the postoperative period, VA-ECMO can be weaned by sequentially dropping the flows on the pump over a period of 10–20 min, with the lungs well recruited, suctioned and ventilated at protective tidal volumes. In preparation for this, the anaesthesiologist must ensure ade-quate filling, afterload and inotropy and be prepared to react

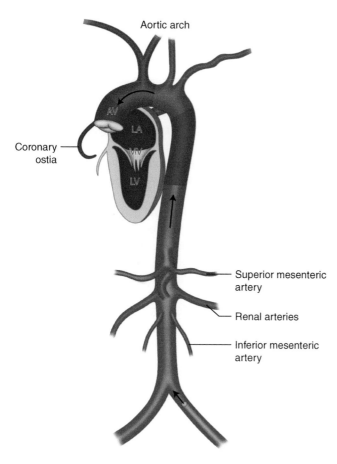

Fig. 27.5 Differential hypoxia or the watershed phenomenon. In peripheral VA-ECMO, oxygenated blood reinfused into the descending aorta mixes with blood ejected from the left ventricle. The mixing point (or watershed) is typically located at the base of the aortic root but will vary depending on the ECMO flows and the patient's cardiac output. In situations of severe lung injury with preserved myocardial function, deoxygenated blood ejected from the heart can force the watershed distally, resulting in hypoxemia of the heart and brain. The SaO2 in the right arm will be lower than the other limbs. This phenomenon is alternately called the "harlequin syndrome"

quickly to deterioration. The right heart in particular is at risk of failure, as no cardioprotection is used during ECMO, and coronary perfusion may be threatened by the watershed phenomenon as described above. Pulmonary vascular resistance may be altered by the surgical procedure, and clots can form in the relatively empty heart on ECMO. A thorough TEE evaluation prior to and during weaning ECMO, monitoring right ventricular size and function in real time as flows are reduced, should be considered. Once flows are down to around 1 L/min, the ECMO pump is stopped altogether and the arterial line clamped. This process often reveals hypovolemia, which the anaesthesiologist should be prepared to treat. If the patient remains stable and the arterial blood gas is adequate after 5 min, the patient can be decannulated.

VV-ECMO

Weaning VV-ECMO takes place with full flows running and the sweep gas speed and FiO_2 slowly being reduced. This gradually reduces the diffusion gradient of oxygen and carbon dioxide across the oxygenator membrane to zero, allowing the lungs to take over the process of gas exchange. Since flows are maintained, this process can be done slowly if necessary, with time for serial arterial blood gases, suctioning, bronchoscopy, recruitment manoeuvres and trials of high PEEP to optimise gas exchange. If blood gases remain good on low sweep flows, the pump can be stopped, and decannulation can take place.

Complications of ECLS

Most of the studies describing ECMO complications (see Table 27.4) have been in ICU populations, where ECMO use lasts for weeks rather than hours. The extent to which these risks can be extrapolated to short-term intraoperative use is unknown. Acute kidney injury, haemolysis and HIT are all

Table 27.4 Complications of long-term ECMO in adult ICU patients [98, 108–115]

Complication	Incidence	Notes
Acute kidney injury	70–85%	Very high rate due to pre-existing critical illness
Arrhythmia	15%	
Haemorrhage	Overall: 10–30% GI:4–6% Cannulation site: 15–20% Surgical site: 14–20% Intracerebral: 2–4% Pulmonary: 3–7%	
Seizure	1–2%	
Cerebral infarct	2–4%	
Systemic embolism	8%	Rate of cannula-tip thrombosis is as high as 85% but occurs after weeks of treatment
Haemolysis	6–7%	
Heparin-induced thrombocytopenia (HIT)	1–5%	Occurs 5–14 days post exposure to unfractionated heparin
Circuit clotting	2–19%	Varies according to component; may be less with heparin-bonded circuits
Air embolism	2%	
Oxygenator failure	16%	Usually chronic due to subclinical thrombosis
Vascular complications	<5%	For example, distal ischemia, dissection, pseudoaneurysm

complications of long-term ECMO use and are unlikely relevant intraoperative considerations. Incidence of infection is also correlated to the duration of ECMO [116]. In intraoperative ECMO, cannulation and surgical site haemorrhage, thrombotic events and vascular complications are probably the most relevant issues.

Neurological complications in ECMO are insidious and therefore potentially more common than Table 27.4 would suggest. For example, in a retrospective case series of adults who received ECMO for an average of 91 h, 50% suffered a variety of complications including subarachnoid haemorrhage, watershed ischemia and hypoxic-ischemic encephalopathy [117]. Overt stroke was rarely clinically diagnosed, in keeping with a rate of 2–4% as above, but nine out of ten patients who died had cerebral infarcts on autopsy. Similarly, in an autopsy study of patients who received emergency ECMO post cardiotomy, Rastan et al. [118] found an unrecognised cerebral infarct rate of 9%, unrecognised venous thromboembolism in 32% and unrecognised systemic embolism in 31%. In total 69–75% of long-term ECMO recipients were having subclinical thrombosis on autopsy [118, 119]. In addition, the rate of gaseous microembolism during ECMO support rivals that of CPB, with intravenous injections being the most common culprit, with potential for postoperative neurological morbidity [120]. For the perioperative context, simple maintenance of peripheral saturation and blood pressure are not necessarily sufficient to ensure adequate oxygen delivery to the brain – some form of active cerebral monitoring, such as near-infrared spectroscopy, should be considered [9, 105].

Fatal air embolism has been reported associated with performance of tracheostomy while on high-flow VV-ECMO with drainage via a bi-caval dual-lumen jugular catheter [121]. Inadvertent breach of the neck veins enabled the negative pressure in the SVC to aspirate air into the ECMO circuit. Suggested measures for avoiding this complication include temporary reduction of ECMO flows, performance of tracheotomy with the patient in a head down position and coverage of the puncture sites with wet compresses. The risk of air embolism by a similar mechanism could occur during placement of upper body central venous lines.

Clinical Case Discussion

A 54-year-old man with relapsing polychondritis presented for elective rigid bronchoscopy and tracheal stent repositioning. His original silicone stent was placed 3 years ago for tracheomalacia. He had stridor on forceful inhalation from suspected granulation tissue distal to the stent, but no stridor at rest. He is able to lie supine with no dyspnoea. He had a history of well-controlled hypertension and stable ankylos-

ing spondylitis treated with prednisone and adalimumab. He had normal cardiac function and no valvular lesions. His airway examination revealed Mallampati I view with unrestricted cervical spine motion. He underwent a titrated intravenous induction and was maintained on a propofol and remifentanil infusion with muscle relaxation and intermittent jet ventilation. Rigid bronchoscopy and debridement of granulation tissue were performed. The stent was unable to be removed after multiple attempts and was ultimately pushed further distally over the area of granulation. At the end of the case, a mucosal tear of the posterior mid-trachea was noted.

On emergence, the patient had acute stridor and hypoxemia, requiring urgent reinduction and positive pressure ventilation. Repeat rigid bronchoscopy was performed and a Y-stent was inserted at the carina. The patient developed subcutaneous emphysema of the upper chest and neck. There was suspected perforation of one arm of the Y-stent through the trachea into the mediastinum. The stent was removed, and a tear could be seen from the mid-trachea extending into the left mainstem bronchus just distal to the carina.

The thoracic surgeons proposed to repair the tracheal tear via right thoracotomy.

What is your anesthetic plan for converting to thoracotomy?

During positioning and exposure of the left thorax, the goals are to provide gas exchange while avoiding high airway pressures and expansion of the mediastinal emphysema. Our patient was intubated orotracheally with an endobronchial tube with a narrow cuff placed just below the vocal cords and above the area of airway disruption to avoid pressure on the area. We maintained the patient asleep on total intravenous anaesthesia as volatile agents could not be reliably delivered during the complex lung isolation. A radial arterial line and right internal jugular central venous catheter were placed.

What are the options for oxygenating and ventilating this patient during repair of the trachea and left mainstem bronchus?

Due to the location of the tear, oxygenation via a right- or left-sided double-lumen tube or endobronchial tube would be impossible. Likewise, cross-field ventilation from an endobronchial tube placed directly into the right mainstem bronchus would be interrupted almost continuously to allow for repair of the tear. Therefore, veno-arterial extracorporeal membrane oxygenation (ECMO) was initiated via femoral cannulation to provide continuous gas exchange, allowing the surgeons full access to open and repair the trachea and bronchus. After cannulation and heparinisation, the patient's oxygenation improved on flows of 2–4 L/min. He was placed in the left lateral decubitus position, the right chest was opened and the trachea, and bronchi were repaired with both lungs collapsed. A Y-stent is inserted at the carina. The lungs were re-expanded with positive pressure through the endotracheal tube and new stent, and water sealing test with Valsalva did not reveal any leaks. Chest tubes were placed in the right hemithorax and the chest was closed.

How will you wean ECMO support, and what are the postoperative considerations?

The ECMO flows were weaned to 1.5 L/min and the patient was decannulated after good oxygenation and blood chemistry were confirmed. The patient was transferred to the ICU intubated. He was neurologically intact, but failed extubation twice due to hospital-acquired pneumonia and difficulty clearing secretions. He eventually required tracheostomy. He left the ICU on postoperative day 18 and was discharged home on day 45 with a speaking tracheostomy.

Summary

As the technical frontiers of thoracic procedures are pushed ever forwards by our surgical colleagues, demand for intraoperative ECLS may be predicted to increase. It is unlikely that preinduction provision of mechanical support will ever become routine, and any procedure major enough to require it should not be taken lightly; however, with the help of the principles outlined in this chapter, they can at least feel within our envelope of comfort and experience.

References

1. Squiers JJ, Lima B, DiMaio JM. A call for standardized end point definitions regarding outcomes of extracorporeal membrane oxygenation. J Thorac Cardiovasc Surg. 2017;153(1):147–8.
2. Squiers JJ, Lima B, DiMaio JM. Contemporary extracorporeal membrane oxygenation therapy in adults: fundamental principles and systematic review of the evidence. J Thorac Cardiovasc Surg. 2016;152(1):20–32.
3. Dalton HJ. Extracorporeal life support: moving at the speed of light. Respir Care. 2011;56(9):1445–53.
4. Peek GJ, Mugford M, Tiruvoipati R, Wilson A, Allen E, Thalanany MM, et al. Efficacy and economic assessment of conventional ventilatory support versus extracorporeal membrane oxygenation for severe adult respiratory failure (CESAR): a multicentre randomised controlled trial. Lancet (London, England). 2009;374(9698):1351–63.
5. Machuca TN, Cypel M, Keshavjee S. Cardiopulmonary bypass and extracorporeal life support for emergent intraoperative thoracic situations. Thorac Surg Clin. 2015;25(3):325–34.
6. Esper SA, Levy JH, Waters JH, Welsby IJ. Extracorporeal membrane oxygenation in the adult: a review of anticoagulation monitoring and transfusion. Anesth Analg. 2014;118(4):731–43.
7. Machuca TN, de Perrot M. Mechanical support for the failing right ventricle in patients with precapillary pulmonary hypertension. Circulation. 2015;132(6):526–36.
8. Doufle G, Roscoe A, Billia F, Fan E. Echocardiography for adult patients supported with extracorporeal membrane oxygenation. Crit Care. 2015;19:326.
9. Doufle G, Ferguson ND. Monitoring during extracorporeal membrane oxygenation. Curr Opin Crit Care. 2016;22(3):230–8.
10. Gattinoni L, Carlesso E, Langer T. Clinical review: extracorporeal membrane oxygenation. Crit Care. 2011;15(6):243.
11. Reeb J, Olland A, Renaud S, Lejay A, Santelmo N, Massard G, et al. Vascular access for extracorporeal life support: tips and tricks. J Thorac Dis. 2016;8(Suppl 4):S353–63.
12. Zimmermann M, Bein T, Philipp A, Ittner K, Foltan M, Drescher J, et al. Interhospital transportation of patients with severe lung failure on pumpless extracorporeal lung assist. Br J Anaesth. 2006;96(1):63–6.
13. Schellongowski P, Riss K, Staudinger T, Ullrich R, Krenn CG, Sitzwohl C, et al. Extracorporeal CO2 removal as bridge to lung transplantation in life-threatening hypercapnia. Transpl Int. 2015;28(3):297–304.
14. de Perrot M, Granton JT, McRae K, Cypel M, Pierre A, Waddell TK, et al. Impact of extracorporeal life support on outcome in patients with idiopathic pulmonary arterial hypertension awaiting lung transplantation. J Heart Lung Transplant. 2011;30(9):997–1002.
15. Machuca TN, Collaud S, Mercier O, Cheung M, Cunningham V, Kim SJ, et al. Outcomes of intraoperative extracorporeal membrane oxygenation versus cardiopulmonary bypass for lung transplantation. J Thorac Cardiovasc Surg. 2015;149(4):1152–7.
16. Jensen V, Milne B, Salerno T. Femoral-femoral cardiopulmonary bypass prior to induction of anaesthesia in the management of upper airway obstruction. Can Anaesth Soc J. 1983;30(3 Pt 1):270–2.
17. Hong Y, Jo KW, Lyu J, Huh JW, Hong SB, Jung SH, et al. Use of venovenous extracorporeal membrane oxygenation in central airway obstruction to facilitate interventions leading to definitive airway security. J Crit Care. 2013;28(5):669–74.
18. Ko M, dos Santos PR, Machuca TN, Marseu K, Waddell TK, Keshavjee S, et al. Use of single-cannula venous-venous extracorporeal life support in the management of life-threatening airway obstruction. Ann Thorac Surg. 2015;99(3):e63–5.
19. Willms DC, Mendez R, Norman V, Chammas JH. Emergency bedside extracorporeal membrane oxygenation for rescue of acute tracheal obstruction. Respir Care. 2012;57(4):646–9.
20. Higashi K, Takeshita J, Terasaki H, Tanoue T, Esaki K, Sakamoto M, et al. A case of acute airway obstruction with sharp sawdust particles, successfully treated by extracorporeal lung assist. Kokyu To Junkan. 1989;37(3):329–33.
21. Park JM, Kim CW, Cho HM, Son BS, Kim DH. Induced airway obstruction under extracorporeal membrane oxygenation during treatment of life-threatening massive hemoptysis due to severe blunt chest trauma. J Thorac Dis. 2014;6(12):E255–8.
22. Smith IJ, Sidebotham DA, McGeorge AD, Dorman EB, Wilsher ML, Kolbe J. Use of extracorporeal membrane oxygenation during resection of tracheal papillomatosis. Anesthesiology. 2009;110(2):427–9.
23. Fung R, Stellios J, Bannon PG, Ananda A, Forrest P. Elective use of veno-venous extracorporeal membrane oxygenation and high-flow nasal oxygen for resection of subtotal malignant distal airway obstruction. Anaesth Intensive Care. 2017;45(1):88–91.
24. Natt B, Knepler J Jr, Kazui T, Mosier JM. The use of extracorporeal membrane oxygenation in the bronchoscopic management of critical upper airway obstruction. J Bronchology Interv Pulmonol. 2017;24(1):e12–e4.
25. Park AH, Tunkel DE, Park E, Barnhart D, Liu E, Lee J, et al. Management of complicated airway foreign body aspiration using extracorporeal membrane oxygenation (ECMO). Int J Pediatr Otorhinolaryngol. 2014;78(12):2319–21.
26. Lang G, Ghanim B, Hotzenecker K, Klikovits T, Matilla JR, Aigner C, et al. Extracorporeal membrane oxygenation support for complex tracheo-bronchial procedures. Eur J Cardiothorac Surg. 2015;47(2):250–5. discussion 6

27. Johnson AP, Cavarocchi NC, Hirose H. Ventilator strategies for VV ECMO management with concomitant tracheal injury and H1N1 influenza. Heart Lung Vessel. 2015;7(1):74–80.

28. Kim CW, Kim DH, Son BS, Cho JS, Kim YD, I H, et al. The feasibility of extracorporeal membrane oxygenation in the variant airway problems. Ann Thorac Cardiovasc Surg. 2015;21(6):517–22.

29. Keeyapaj W, Alfirevic A. Carinal resection using an airway exchange catheter-assisted venovenous ECMO technique. Can J Anaesth. 2012;59(11):1075–6.

30. Redwan B, Ziegeler S, Freermann S, Nique L, Semik M, Lavae-Mokhtari M, et al. Intraoperative veno-venous extracorporeal lung support in thoracic surgery: a single-centre experience. Interact Cardiovasc Thorac Surg. 2015;21(6):766–72.

31. Walles T, Steger V, Wurst H, Schmidt KD, Friedel G. Pumpless extracorporeal gas exchange aiding central airway surgery. J Thorac Cardiovasc Surg. 2008;136(5):1372–4.

32. Wiebe K, Poeling J, Arlt M, Philipp A, Camboni D, Hofmann S, et al. Thoracic surgical procedures supported by a pumpless interventional lung assist. Ann Thorac Surg. 2010;89(6):1782–7. discussion 8

33. Gillon SA, Toufektzian L, Harrison-Phipps K, Puchakayala M, Daly K, Ioannou N, et al. Perioperative extracorporeal membrane oxygenation to facilitate lung resection after contralateral pneumonectomy. Ann Thorac Surg. 2016;101(3):e71–3.

34. Oey IF, Peek GJ, Firmin RK, Waller DA. Post-pneumonectomy video-assisted thoracoscopic bullectomy using extracorporeal membrane oxygenation. Eur J Cardiothorac Surg. 2001;20(4):874–6.

35. Schiff JH, Koninger J, Teschner J, Henn-Beilharz A, Rost M, Dubb R, et al. Veno-venous extracorporeal membrane oxygenation (ECMO) support during anaesthesia for oesophagectomy. Anaesthesia. 2013;68(5):527–30.

36. Slinger P, Suissa S, Adam J, Triolet W. Predicting arterial oxygenation during one-lung ventilation with continuous positive airway pressure to the nonventilated lung. J Cardiothorac Anesth. 1990;4(4):436–40.

37. Brenner M, O'Connor JV, Scalea TM. Use of ECMO for resection of post-traumatic ruptured lung abscess with empyema. Ann Thorac Surg. 2010;90(6):2039–41.

38. Bressman M, Raad W, Levsky JM, Weinstein S. Surgical therapy for complications of pneumonia on extracorporeal membrane oxygenation can improve the ability to wean patients from support. Heart Lung Vessel. 2015;7(4):330–1.

39. Tsunezuka Y, Sato H, Tsubota M, Seki M. Significance of percutaneous cardiopulmonary bypass support for volume reduction surgery with severe hypercapnia. Artif Organs. 2000;24(1):70–3.

40. Li X, He H, Sun B. Veno-venous extracorporeal membrane oxygenation support during lung volume reduction surgery for a severe respiratory failure patient with emphysema. J Thorac Dis. 2016;8(3):E240–3.

41. Redwan B, Ziegeler S, Semik M, Fichter J, Dickgreber N, Vieth V, et al. Single-site cannulation venovenous extracorporeal CO2 removal as bridge to lung volume reduction surgery in end-stage lung emphysema. ASAIO J. 2016;62(6):743–6.

42. Kim JD, Ko ES, Kim JY, Kim SH. Anesthesia under cardiopulmonary bypass for video assisted thoracoscopic wedge resection in patient with spontaneous pneumothorax and contralateral post-tuberculosis destroyed lung. Korean J Anesthesiol. 2013;65(2):174–6.

43. Julien F, Mosolo A, Hubsch JP, Souilhamas R, Safran D, Cholley B. Respiratory support using veno-venous ECMO during lung resection for aspergilloma. Ann Fr Anesth Reanim. 2010;29(9):645–7.

44. Sivitanidis E, Tosson R, Wiebalck A, Laczkovics A. Combination of extracorporeal membrane oxygenation (ECMO) and pulmo-

nary lavage in a patient with pulmonary alveolar proteinosis. Eur J Cardiothorac Surg. 1999;15(3):370–2.

45. Sihoe AD, Ng VM, Liu RW, Cheng LC. Pulmonary alveolar proteinosis in extremis: the case for aggressive whole lung lavage with extracorporeal membrane oxygenation support. Heart Lung Circ. 2008;17(1):69–72.

46. Krecmerova M, Mosna F, Bicek V, Petrik F, Grandcourtova A, Lekes M, et al. Extracorporeal membrane oxygenation to support repeated whole-lung lavage in a patient with pulmonary alveolar proteinosis in life threatening dyspnoe – a case report. BMC Anesthesiol. 2015;15:173.

47. Kim KH, Kim JH, Kim YW. Use of extracorporeal membrane oxygenation (ECMO) during whole lung lavage in pulmonary alveolar proteinosis associated with lung cancer. Eur J Cardiothorac Surg. 2004;26(5):1050–1.

48. Kaya FN, Bayram AS, Kirac F, Basagan-Mogol E, Goren S. Abstract OR001: extracorporeal membrane oxygenation to support whole lung lavage in a patient with pulmonary alveolar proteinosis. Anesth Analg. 2016;123(3 Suppl 2):1.

49. Hurrion EM, Pearson GA, Firmin RK. Childhood pulmonary alveolar proteinosis. Extracorporeal membrane oxygenation with total cardiopulmonary support during bronchopulmonary lavage. Chest. 1994;106(2):638–40.

50. Hasan N, Bagga S, Monteagudo J, Hirose H, Cavarocchi NC, Hehn BT, et al. Extracorporeal membrane oxygenation to support whole-lung lavage in pulmonary alveolar proteinosis: salvage of the drowned lungs. J Bronchology Interv Pulmonol. 2013;20(1):41–4.

51. Guo WL, Chen Y, Zhong NS, Su ZQ, Zhong CH, Li SY. Alveolar proteinosis in extremis: a critical case treated with whole lung lavage without extracorporeal membrane oxygenation. Int J Clin Exp Med. 2015;8(10):19556–60.

52. Cohen ES, Elpern E, Silver MR. Pulmonary alveolar proteinosis causing severe hypoxemic respiratory failure treated with sequential whole-lung lavage utilizing venovenous extracorporeal membrane oxygenation: a case report and review. Chest. 2001;120(3):1024–6.

53. Chauhan S, Sharma KP, Bisoi AK, Pangeni R, Madan K, Chauhan YS. Management of pulmonary alveolar proteinosis with whole lung lavage using extracorporeal membrane oxygenation support in a postrenal transplant patient with graft failure. Ann Card Anaesth. 2016;19(2):379–82.

54. Cai HR, Cui SY, Jin L, Huang YZ, Wang ZY, Cao B, et al. Pulmonary alveolar proteinosis treated with whole-lung lavage utilizing extracorporeal membrane oxygenation: a case report and review of literatures. Chin Med J (Engl). 2004;117(11):1746–9.

55. Cai HR, Cui SY, Jin L, Huang YZ, Cao B, Wang ZY, et al. Pulmonary alveolar proteinosis treated with whole-lung lavage utilizing extracorporeal membrane oxygenation: a case report and review. Zhonghua Jie He He Hu Xi Za Zhi. 2005;28(4):242–4.

56. Asai T. Emergency cardiopulmonary bypass in a patient with a mediastinal mass. Anaesthesia. 2007;62(8):859–60.

57. Said SM, Telesz BJ, Makdisi G, Quevedo FJ, Suri RM, Allen MS, et al. Awake cardiopulmonary bypass to prevent hemodynamic collapse and loss of airway in a severely symptomatic patient with a mediastinal mass. Ann Thorac Surg. 2014;98(4):e87–90.

58. Sendasgupta C, Sengupta G, Ghosh K, Munshi A, Goswami A. Femoro-femoral cardiopulmonary bypass for the resection of an anterior mediastinal mass. Indian J Anaesth. 2010;54(6):565–8.

59. Tempe DK, Arya R, Dubey S, Khanna S, Tomar AS, Grover V, et al. Mediastinal mass resection: Femorofemoral cardiopulmonary bypass before induction of anesthesia in the management of airway obstruction. J Cardiothorac Vasc Anesth. 2001;15(2):233–6.

60. Wickiser JE, Thompson M, Leavey PJ, Quinn CT, Garcia NM, Aquino VM. Extracorporeal membrane oxygenation (ECMO) ini-

tiation without intubation in two children with mediastinal malignancy. Pediatr Blood Cancer. 2007;49(5):751–4.

61. Felten ML, Michel-Cherqui M, Puyo P, Fischler M. Extracorporeal membrane oxygenation use for mediastinal tumor resection. Ann Thorac Surg. 2010;89(3):1012.

62. de Perrot M, Fadel E, Mussot S, de Palma A, Chapelier A, Dartevelle P. Resection of locally advanced (T4) non-small cell lung cancer with cardiopulmonary bypass. Ann Thorac Surg. 2005;79(5):1691–6. discussion 7

63. Galvaing G, Tardy MM, Cassagnes L, Da Costa V, Chadeyras JB, Naamee A, et al. Left atrial resection for T4 lung cancer without cardiopulmonary bypass: technical aspects and outcomes. Ann Thorac Surg. 2014;97(5):1708–13.

64. Langer NB, Mercier O, Fabre D, Lawton J, Mussot S, Dartevelle P, et al. Outcomes after resection of T4 non-small cell lung cancer using cardiopulmonary bypass. Ann Thorac Surg. 2016;102(3):902–10.

65. Belov YV, Komarov RN, Parshin VD, Yavorovsky AG, Chernyavsky SV, Mnatsakanyan GV. Right-sided pneumonectomy with left atrium resection under cardiopulmonary bypass in the patient with lung cancer (the first case in Russia). Khirurgiia (Mosk). 2017;(1):78–81.

66. Ferguson ER Jr, Reardon MJ. Atrial resection in advanced lung carcinoma under total cardiopulmonary bypass. Tex Heart Inst J. 2000;27(2):110–2.

67. Hasegawa S, Bando T, Isowa N, Otake Y, Yanagihara K, Tanaka F, et al. The use of cardiopulmonary bypass during extended resection of non-small cell lung cancer. Interact Cardiovasc Thorac Surg. 2003;2(4):676–9.

68. Kugai T, Kinjyo M, Hosokawa Y. The combined resection of left atrium for advanced lung cancer on cardiopulmonary bypass: a case report. Kyobu Geka. 1996;49(9):738–41.

69. Marseu K, Minkovich L, Zubrinic M, Keshavjee S. Anesthetic considerations for pneumonectomy with left atrial resection on cardiopulmonary bypass in a patient with lung cancer: a case report. A A Case Rep. 2017;8(3):61–3.

70. Shimizu J, Ikeda C, Arano Y, Adachi I, Morishita M, Yamaguchi S, et al. Advanced lung cancer invading the left atrium, treated with pneumonectomy combined with left atrium resection under cardiopulmonary bypass. Ann Thorac Cardiovasc Surg. 2010;16(4):286–90.

71. Lang G, Taghavi S, Aigner C, Charchian R, Matilla JR, Sano A, et al. Extracorporeal membrane oxygenation support for resection of locally advanced thoracic tumors. Ann Thorac Surg. 2011;92(1):264–70.

72. Byrnes J, Leacche M, Adnithotri A, Paul S, Bueno R, Mathisen D, et al. The use of cardiopulmonary bypass during resection of locally advanced thoracic malignancies. Chest. 2004;125(4):1581–6.

73. Shirakusa T, Kimura M. Partial atrial resection in advanced lung carcinoma with and without cardiopulmonary bypass. Thorax. 1991;46(7):484–7.

74. Kobayashi S, Sawabata N, Araki O, Karube Y, Seki N, Tamura M, et al. Dissection of a mediastinal mature teratoma requires replacement of the ascending aorta during cardiopulmonary bypass. J Thorac Cardiovasc Surg. 2007;134(5):1371–2.

75. Agathos EA, Lachanas E, Karagkiouzis G, Spartalis E, Tomos P. Cardiopulmonary bypass assisted resection of mediastinal masses. J Card Surg. 2012;27(3):338–41.

76. Mei J, Pu Q, Zhu Y, Ma L, Ren F, Che G, et al. Reconstruction of the pulmonary trunk via cardiopulmonary bypass in extended resection of locally advanced lung malignancies. J Surg Oncol. 2012;106(3):311–5.

77. Abrams D, Agerstrand CL, Biscotti M, Burkart KM, Bacchetta M, Brodie D. Extracorporeal membrane oxygenation in the management of diffuse alveolar hemorrhage. ASAIO J. 2015;61(2):216–8.

78. Patel JJ, Lipchik RJ. Systemic lupus-induced diffuse alveolar hemorrhage treated with extracorporeal membrane oxygenation: a case report and review of the literature. J Intensive Care Med. 2014;29(2):104–9.

79. Abbas AE. Traumatic injury of the pulmonary artery: transection, rupture, pseudoaneurysm, or dissection? Sometimes semantics do matter. J Thorac Cardiovasc Surg. 2016;152(5):1437–8.

80. Jeng EI, Piovesana G, Taylor J, Machuca TN. Extracorporeal membrane oxygenation to facilitate tracheal healing after oesophagogastric catastrophe. Eur J Cardiothorac Surg. 2018;53(1):288–9.

81. Weinberg A, Tapson VF, Ramzy D. Massive pulmonary embolism: extracorporeal membrane oxygenation and surgical pulmonary embolectomy. Semin Respir Crit Care Med. 2017;38(1):66–72.

82. Lebreton G, Bouabdallaoui N, Gauduchon L, Mnif MA, Roques F. Successful use of ECMO as a bridge to surgical embolectomy in life-threatening pulmonary embolism. Am J Emerg Med. 2015;33(9):1332 e3–4.

83. Kawahito K, Murata S, Ino T, Fuse K. Angioscopic pulmonary embolectomy and ECMO. Ann Thorac Surg. 1998;66(3):982–3.

84. Berman M, Tsui S, Vuylsteke A, Snell A, Colah S, Latimer R, et al. Successful extracorporeal membrane oxygenation support after pulmonary thromboendarterectomy. Ann Thorac Surg. 2008;86:1261–7.

85. Caridi-Scheible ME, Blum JM. Use of Perfluorodecalin for Bronchoalveolar lavage in case of severe pulmonary hemorrhage and extracorporeal membrane oxygenation: a case report and review of the literature. A A Case Rep. 2016;7(10):215–8.

86. Chacon-Alves S, Perez-Vela JL, Grau-Carmona T, Dominguez-Aguado H, Marin-Mateos H, Renes-Carreno E. Veno-arterial ECMO for rescue of severe airway hemorrhage with rigid bronchoscopy after pulmonary artery thromboendarterectomy. Int J Artif Organs. 2016;39(5):242–4.

87. Kuroda H, Masuda Y, Imaizumi H, Kozuka Y, Asai Y, Namiki A. Successful extracorporeal membranous oxygenation for a patient with life-threatening transfusion-related acute lung injury. J Anesth. 2009;23(3):424–6.

88. Lee AJ, Koyyalamudi PL, Martinez-Ruiz R. Severe transfusion-related acute lung injury managed with extracorporeal membrane oxygenation (ECMO) in an obstetric patient. J Clin Anesth. 2008;20(7):549–52.

89. Incagnoli P, Blaise H, Mathey C, Vinclair M, Albaladejo P. Pulmonary resection and ECMO: a salvage therapy for penetrating lung trauma. Ann Fr Anesth Reanim. 2012;31(7–8):641–3.

90. Swol J, Cannon JW, Napolitano LM. ECMO in trauma: what are the outcomes? J Trauma Acute Care Surg. 2017;82(4):819–20.

91. Zhou R, Liu B, Lin K, Wang R, Qin Z, Liao R, et al. ECMO support for right main bronchial disruption in multiple trauma patient with brain injury – a case report and literature review. Perfusion. 2015;30(5):403–6.

92. Jacobs JV, Hooft NM, Robinson BR, Todd E, Bremner RM, Petersen SR, et al. The use of extracorporeal membrane oxygenation in blunt thoracic trauma: a study of the extracorporeal life support organization database. J Trauma Acute Care Surg. 2015;79(6):1049–53. discussion 53-4

93. Pavlushkov E, Berman M, Valchanov K. Cannulation techniques for extracorporeal life support. Ann Transl Med. 2017;5(4):70.

94. Raiten JM, Wong ZZ, Spelde A, Littlejohn JE, Augoustides JGT, Gutsche JT. Anticoagulation and transfusion therapy in patients requiring extracorporeal membrane oxygenation. J Cardiothorac Vasc Anesth. 2017;31(3):1051–9.

95. Organization ELS. ELSO anticoagulation guidelines. Ann Arbor, Michigan: Extracorporeal Life Support Organization; 2014.

96. O'Carroll-Kuehn BU, Meeran H. Management of coagulation during cardiopulmonary bypass. Contin Educ Anaesth Crit Care Pain. 2007;7(6):195–8.

97. Joffre J, Preda G, Arrive L, Maury E. Fatal aortic dissection during ECMO axillary cannulation confirmed by postmortem CT angiography. Am J Respir Crit Care Med. 2017;195:953.

98. Roussel A, Al-Attar N, Khaliel F, Alkhoder S, Raffoul R, Alfayyadh F, et al. Arterial vascular complications in peripheral extracorporeal membrane oxygenation support: a review of techniques and outcomes. Future Cardiol. 2013;9(4):489–95.

99. Bojic A, Steiner I, Gamper J, Schellongowski P, Lamm W, Hermann A, et al. The supraclavicular approach to the subclavian vein as an alternative venous access site for ECMO cannulae? A retrospective comparison. ASAIO J. 2017;63:679.

100. Banfi C, Pozzi M, Brunner ME, Rigamonti F, Murith N, Mugnai D, et al. Veno-arterial extracorporeal membrane oxygenation: an overview of different cannulation techniques. J Thorac Dis. 2016;8(9):E875–e85.

101. Slinger P, Kilpatrick B. Perioperative lung protection strategies in cardiothoracic anesthesia: are they useful? Anesthesiol Clin. 2012;30(4):607–28.

102. Adeniji K, Steel AC. The pathophysiology of perioperative lung injury. Anesthesiol Clin. 2012;30(4):573–90.

103. Kilpatrick B, Slinger P. Lung protective strategies in anaesthesia. Br J Anaesth. 2010;105(Suppl 1):i108–16.

104. Schmidt M, Pellegrino V, Combes A, Scheinkestel C, Cooper DJ, Hodgson C. Mechanical ventilation during extracorporeal membrane oxygenation. Crit Care. 2014;18(1):203.

105. Wong JK, Smith TN, Pitcher HT, Hirose H, Cavarocchi NC. Cerebral and lower limb near-infrared spectroscopy in adults on extracorporeal membrane oxygenation. Artif Organs. 2012;36(8):659–67.

106. Formica F, Avalli L, Colagrande L, Ferro O, Greco G, Maggioni E, et al. Extracorporeal membrane oxygenation to support adult patients with cardiac failure: predictive factors of 30-day mortality. Interact Cardiovasc Thorac Surg. 2010;10(5):721–6.

107. Xie A, Yan TD, Forrest P. Recirculation in venovenous extracorporeal membrane oxygenation. J Crit Care. 2016;36:107–10.

108. Kilburn DJ, Shekar K, Fraser JF. The complex relationship of extracorporeal membrane oxygenation and acute kidney injury: causation or association? Biomed Res Int. 2016;2016:1094296.

109. Makdisi G, Wang IW. Extra corporeal membrane oxygenation (ECMO) review of a lifesaving technology. J Thorac Dis. 2015;7(7):E166–76.

110. Ventetuolo CE, Muratore CS. Extracorporeal life support in critically ill adults. Am J Respir Crit Care Med. 2014;190(5):497–508.

111. Turner DA, Cheifetz IM. Extracorporeal membrane oxygenation for adult respiratory failure. Respir Care. 2013;58(6):1038–52.

112. Pollak U, Yacobobich J, Tamary H, Dagan O, Manor-Shulman O. Heparin-induced thrombocytopenia and extracorporeal membrane oxygenation: a case report and review of the literature. J Extra Corpor Technol. 2011;43(1):5–12.

113. Sy E, Sklar MC, Lequier L, Fan E, Kanji HD. Anticoagulation practices and the prevalence of major bleeding, thromboembolic events, and mortality in venoarterial extracorporeal membrane oxygenation (VA-ECMO): a systematic review and meta-analysis. J Crit Care. 2017;39:87–96.

114. Menaker J, Tabatabai A, Rector R, Dolly K, Kufera J, Lee E, et al. Incidence of cannula associated deep vein thrombosis after venovenous ECMO. ASAIO J. 2017;63:588.

115. Petricevic M, Milicic D, Boban M, Mihaljevic MZ, Baricevic Z, Kolic K, et al. Bleeding and thrombotic events in patients undergoing mechanical circulatory support: a review of literature. Thorac Cardiovasc Surg. 2015;63(8):636–46.

116. Biffi S, Di Bella S, Scaravilli V, Peri AM, Grasselli G, Alagna L, et al. Infections during extracorporeal membrane oxygenation: epidemiology, risk factors, pathogenesis and prevention. Int J Antimicrob Agents. 2017;50(1):9–16.

117. Mateen FJ, Muralidharan R, Shinohara RT, Parisi JE, Schears GJ, Wijdicks EF. Neurological injury in adults treated with extracorporeal membrane oxygenation. Arch Neurol. 2011;68(12):1543–9.

118. Rastan AJ, Lachmann N, Walther T, Doll N, Gradistanac T, Gommert JF, et al. Autopsy findings in patients on postcardiotomy extracorporeal membrane oxygenation (ECMO). Int J Artif Organs. 2006;29(12):1121–31.

119. Reed RC, Rutledge JC. Laboratory and clinical predictors of thrombosis and hemorrhage in 29 pediatric extracorporeal membrane oxygenation nonsurvivors. Pediatr Dev Pathol. 2010;13(5):385–92.

120. Jiao Y, Gipson KE, Bonde P, Mangi A, Hagberg R, Rosinski DJ, et al. Quantification of postmembrane gaseous microembolization during venoarterial extracorporeal membrane oxygenation. ASAIO J. 2018;64(1):31–7.

121. Lother A, Wengenmayer T, Benk C, Bode C, Staudacher DL. Fatal air embolism as complication of percutaneous dilatational tracheostomy on venovenous extracorporeal membrane oxygenation, two case reports. J Cardiothorac Surg. 2016;11(1):102.

Part VII

Applications of Ultrasound in Thoracic Anesthesia

Pulmonary Ultrasound

28

Nathan Ludwig and Ahmed F. Hegazy

Key Points
- Pulmonary ultrasound is a powerful bedside tool that anesthesiologists can use to expeditiously guide patient management decisions in the perioperative period.
- Ultrasonographic lung and pleural patterns such as A-lines, B-lines, lung sliding, and consolidation can be easily recognized by the anesthesiologist with basic ultrasound training. In the appropriate clinical setting, these can provide diagnostic evidence of pulmonary edema, atelectasis, pneumothorax, pneumonia, or normal lung aeration.
- Pulmonary ultrasound can help narrow the differential diagnosis in patients with undifferentiated respiratory failure, help assess the size and significance of pleural effusions, and aid in lung recruitment and ventilator management in the perioperative setting.
- Pulmonary ultrasound can be incorporated into a more general ultrasound assessment of the trauma or shock patient.

Introduction

The advancement of clinical ultrasound technology and reduction in costs have led to its widespread adoption in the clinical practice of anesthesiology. Most anesthesiologists have become comfortable with the use of ultrasound in vascular access. Ultrasound-based regional anesthesia has become commonplace, replacing and/or complementing landmark and nerve stimulator-based techniques. In addition, point-of-care echocardiography is becoming more commonly used by both cardiac- and noncardiac-trained anesthesiologists as a monitor of heart function, valvular performance, and fluid status. Using this experience and knowledge as a starting point, anesthesiologists can easily incorporate pulmonary ultrasound into their practice. When used in conjunction with physical examination and other imaging modalities, pulmonary ultrasound is a powerful technique that can aid in the diagnosis and management of patients in respiratory failure.

Ultrasound Physics

It can be argued that an advanced knowledge of ultrasound physics is unnecessary for the average clinician to incorporate ultrasound into their practice. A basic understanding of ultrasound physics, however, is useful in understanding how to optimize your image, interpret artifacts, as well as recognize the limitations of different ultrasound transducers. This chapter will review what the authors feel is essential knowledge for frontline clinicians to preform and interpret pulmonary ultrasound [1, 2].

Put simply, ultrasound transducers convert electrical energy into mechanical energy with the use of vibrating piezoelectric crystals. This leads to the creation of ultrasonic waves that penetrate body tissues and are reflected back to the transducer. The reflected waves are then reconverted into an electric signal that is processed and displayed as an image.

Electronic Supplementary Material The online version of this chapter (https://doi.org/10.1007/978-3-030-00859-8_28) contains supplementary material, which is available to authorized users.

N. Ludwig (✉)
Department of Anesthesiology, Western University, London Health Sciences, London, ON, Canada
e-mail: nludwig2@uwo.ca

A. F. Hegazy
Departments of Anesthesiology and Critical Care Medicine, Western University, London Health Sciences, London, ON, Canada

Body tissues vary in the resistance they offer to ultrasound waves, described mathematically as their acoustic impedance. Bone offers very high resistance to ultrasound waves, and most of the ultrasound wave is reflected off the bone surface. It is therefore very common to see complete darkness below ribs in a phenomenon called acoustic shadowing or attenuation artifact (Video 28.1). In contrast, adipose tissue and muscle have a low impedance, and therefore ultrasound waves can easily be transmitted through these tissues, and visualization of deeper structures is often possible. Knowledge of how ultrasound waves interact with various body tissues is useful to the sonographer as it allows for an understanding of why it is critically important to position the transducer correctly in the intercostal spaces during pulmonary ultrasound.

When ultrasound waves encounter an interface between two tissue planes that vary in their acoustic impedance, reflection of waves back to the transducer occurs. It is possible for a wave to reflect back and forth between two surfaces in the body or between one surface and the transducer. Sound waves bouncing back and forth between a tissue surface and the transducer produce what is called reverberation artifact (Fig. 28.1). Reverberations can be of significant diagnostic value and produce a sonographic pattern known as A-lines (described later in this chapter). An ultrasound beam trapped in a pocket of fluid will vibrate within that pocket, causing a constant energy return to the transducer (Fig. 28.2). This constant energy return will produce what is known as a ring down or comet-tail artifact. Comet tails are

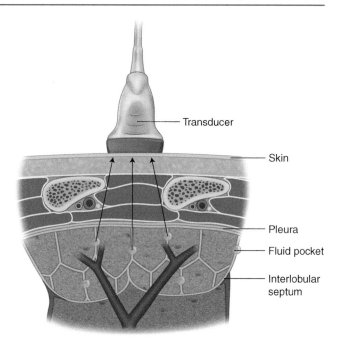

Fig. 28.2 Comet-tail artifact. An ultrasound beam trapped in a fluid pocket in the interlobular septum leads to a constant energy return to the transducer. The resultant comet-tail artifact in pulmonary ultrasound is referred to as B-lines

also of diagnostic significance and produce a sonographic pattern called B-lines (also described later in this chapter).

Transducers

In order to save costs, many clinical departments will purchase ultrasound machines with multiple transducers, commonly known as probes. This allows for the same machine to be used in a wide range of clinical uses. It is essential that the clinician understands the utility and limitations of the various transducers. Portable bedside ultrasound machines typically come with some combination of linear, curvilinear, and phased array transducers. All three of these transducer types can be used in pulmonary ultrasound.

Linear transducers are probably most familiar to anesthesiologists as they are used frequently for regional anesthesia and vascular access. These are high-frequency probes that provide excellent resolution for superficial structures like the pleural line. High-frequency ultrasound waves, however, undergo very rapid attenuation making linear probes a very poor choice when trying to visualize deeper structures. By contrast, curvilinear probes are low frequency, with less ultrasound attenuation and greater capability of visualizing deeper lung structures. They have a much larger footprint, however, and, when used for pulmonary ultrasound, will always show rib shadows within the scanning sector. Phased array probes are also low-frequency probes but with a flat and much

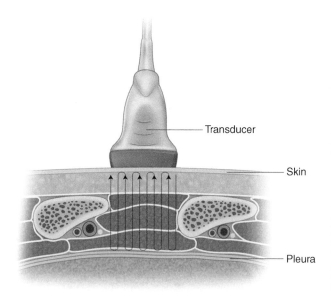

Fig. 28.1 Reverberation artifact. Reflection of ultrasound waves between the transducer and the pleural line leads to the generation of multiple horizontal lines on the screen, equidistant between the transducer and the pleura. In pulmonary ultrasound, this artifact is called A-lines

smaller footprint. This small footprint fits nicely between the ribs, making these probes ideal for thoracic scanning. In addition, phased array probes are capable of producing high frame rates providing good visualization of rapidly moving structures like the heart. They have therefore been the probe of choice for echocardiography applications since their inception. This fast frame rate, however, comes at a cost of a lower spatial resolution than its curvilinear counterpart. The curvilinear probe is therefore superior to the phased array probe at visualizing needles in deeper tissue planes (e.g., real-time ultrasound-guided pleural drainage). An understanding of the advantages and limitations of each transducer is essential when attempting to examine the lungs and pleura. Table 28.1 demonstrates the various transducer characteristics and their appropriate uses in pulmonary ultrasound.

Ultrasound Nomenclature

Some basic knowledge of ultrasound terminology is necessary to communicate findings effectively. The near field describes superficial structures displayed at the top of the screen. The far field describes deeper structures that are displayed at the bottom of the screen. Structures can be described based on how well they reflect or transmit ultrasound waves. Hyperechoic structures are very strong reflectors of ultrasound waves and therefore appear white on the screen (e.g., bone surface). Anechoic structures do not reflect ultrasound waves and thus appear black on the screen (e.g., fluid). Hypoechoic structures are partial reflectors of ultrasound waves and therefore appear gray on the screen (e.g., adipose tissue or muscle) [3].

Table 28.1 Transducers used in pulmonary ultrasound

Transducer	Linear transducer	Curvilinear transducer	Phased array transducer
Photo			
Image produced			
Frequency	High frequency (5–15 MHz)	Low frequency (2–5 MHz)	Low frequency (2–5 MHz)
Resolution and depth of penetration	Excellent axial resolution but limited depth of penetration (up to 6 cm)	Lower axial resolution but greater depth of penetration (up to 35 cm)	Lower axial resolution but greater depth of penetration(up to 35 cm)
Scanning beam	Straight scanning beam (produces rectangular image)	Divergent scanning beam (produces a sector shaped image)	Divergent scanning beam(produces a sector shaped image)
Footprint	Small linear footprint	Large curved footprint	Small flat footprint
Frame rate	Fast frame rate	Slow frame rate but better spatial resolution	Fast frame rate at the cost of lower spatial resolution
Uses (diagnostic)	Used for imaging the pleural line	Used for pleural and lung parenchymal assessments	Used for pleural and lung parenchymal assessments
Uses (procedural)	Adequate needle visualization only in superficial tissue planes	Adequate needle visualization in deeper tissue planes (e.g., real-time ultrasound-guided pleural drainage)	Inadequate needle visualization in tissue planes

Clinical Environment

The clinician using pulmonary sonography must be self-sufficient in setting up a suitable clinical environment for examination. Typically, the clinician stands or sits on one side of the patient. It is easiest to have the machine on the same side of the bed as the sonographer as to allow for independent control of the machine settings. To the maximum extent possible, maintain privacy by exposing the patient only as necessary. It is useful to have a supply of clean towels to clean up ultrasound gel after the imaging is done. Gel is necessary to maintain good contact and to avoid air in the probe/patient interface. Donning the appropriate personal protective equipment may be necessary for patients with contact, droplet, or airborne precautions. The machine and transducers require cleaning after each patient use as per the hospital and manufacturer recommendations.

Pulmonary ultrasound is often done with the patient in the supine position, though limited scans are often done in the sitting position as well. It is often necessary to move the patient to lateral position for imaging of posterior structures. Abduction of the arm can be useful to expose the entire hemithorax for examination. Space limitations, in many clinical environments, often require the clinician to become comfortable with imaging using either hand.

Image Acquisition

For any pulmonary ultrasound, the probe index mark should always be oriented in a cephalad direction. At a minimum, a three-zone examination of each hemithorax should be performed as outlined in the seminal works of Lichtenstein [4, 5]. The authors of this chapter however recommend obtaining a four-zone examination of each hemithorax whenever possible. These images are digitally stored and labeled as shown in Table 28.2. We choose to label the images with acronyms that describe the physical location. The left ante-

Table 28.2 Scanning points in the left hemithorax. The exam is then repeated in the contralateral hemithorax with appropriate labeling. Throughout the exam, the transducer index mark is maintained in a cephalad direction

Left anterior chest wall (LACW) Transducer is placed in the midclavicular line at approximately the second or third intercostal space. This corresponds to the left (or right) upper lobe of the lung	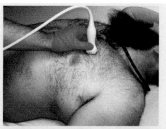
Left anterior axillary line (LAAXL) Transducer is moved to the fourth or fifth intercostal space in the anterior axillary line. This corresponds to the lingula on the left or the right middle lobe on the right	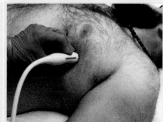
Left costophrenic angle (LCOSTO) Transducer is placed in the midaxillary line along the diaphragm-lung interface. This corresponds to the left (or right) lower lobe of the lung	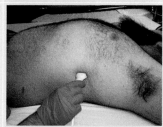
Left posterolateral alveolar pleural syndrome (LPLAPS) The transducer is moved posteriorly, along the diaphragm, to the posterior axillary line. It is often necessary to rotate the patient to the opposite side for adequate examination. This point corresponds to the left (or right) posterior basal segments. In the supine patient, this is the most dependent portion of the lung	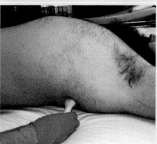

rior chest wall is labeled LACW, which corresponds anatomically to the left upper lobe. The left anterior axillary line is labeled LAAXL, which corresponds to the lingula (left) or right middle lobe on the right. The left costophrenic angle is labeled LCOSTO, which corresponds with the left lower lobe. PLAPS (posterolateral alveolar pleural syndrome), as described by Lichtenstein et al., is the label we use for the last point [4]. The PLAPS point corresponds to the posterior basal segments and, in the supine patient, is the most dependent point in the lung. Slight tilting of the patient into the lateral position is sometimes required to image the PLAPS point.

The examination is then repeated on the contralateral side, using a similar labeling scheme for the right side. Analogous to a stethoscope examination of the chest, additional points can be examined on either side if the clinician feels there is additional information to be gained.

There is a learning curve associated with image optimization. This involves slight adjustments of the imaging hand by the sonographer as well as interaction with the machine settings. Adjusting your probe position until a certain lung aeration pattern (A-lines or B-lines) is obtained is sometimes necessary. A common language is useful in describing movements of the probe on the patient's body, especially when giving suggestions to a medical trainee new to sonography. We commonly describe three hand motions of the transducer: sliding, rotating, and tilting. Sliding describes moving the transducer in a particular direction "slide superiorly" while keeping the angle of the interaction between traducer and the patient fixed. Rotating the probe describes keeping the transducer position fixed while turning its central axis, like turning a screw "rotate clockwise." Tilting the probe describes adjustments to the angle of the interaction between the transducer and the patient both in the long and short axis of the transducer "tilt superiorly or inferiorly or tilt right or left."

Machine Settings

Adjusting the imaging settings is useful to optimize the images obtained. The first setting to consider is the exam type preset also called the machine mode. Many modern ultrasound machines have a specific lung mode. If this is unavailable, an abdominal mode is sufficient. The cardiac preset is not ideal as it sacrifices resolution, to detect fast tissue movements (as is appropriate for echocardiography).

Both lung and abdominal modes display ultrasound images using the "radiology convention." The orientation mark in the radiology convention displays on the left side of the screen. While acquiring lung and pleural images, the transducer index mark should always be directed cephalad. The orientation mark on the screen would, therefore, always represent the superior (cranial) aspect of the body. This contrasts with the cardiology convention, which displays the orientation mark on the right side of the screen. This can be quite confusing to novices as it is fairly routine to use the phased array transducer for both echocardiography (using the cardiology convention) and pulmonary ultrasound (using the radiology convention). Changing the machine preset to "lung" or "abdominal" mode is therefore necessary prior to starting a pulmonary ultrasound examination, both to optimize image quality and change the display to the standard radiology convention.

Adjustment of depth and gain is often necessary to optimize the images obtained. When examining the anterior pleural line, the required depth is usually very superficial. Setting the exam depth to 4–6 cm will optimize image resolution and make pleural sliding very apparent. When examining lung parenchyma using a low-frequency probe, however, a depth of at least 15 cm is recommended. Most images in pulmonary ultrasound are taken in 2D mode though M-mode has significant utility as well. Doppler modes are rarely needed in pulmonary ultrasound.

Lung Sliding, Lung Pulse, and Lung Point

A pulmonary ultrasound finding that is the result of the interaction between the visceral and parietal pleura during respiration is termed lung sliding. This is often visualized as a subtle to-and-fro movement (or shimmering) of the pleural line with each inspiration and expiration (Video 28.1). A positive finding of lung sliding indicates contact between the two pleural linings and rules out the presence of air or fluid between them. By examining the nondependent areas of each hemithorax and confirming the presence of lung sliding throughout, pneumothorax is ruled out with 100% sensitivity [6].

Pleural movement that is the result of a transmitted cardiac activity results in a similar interaction between the layers of the pleura. This is referred to as the lung pulse and is usually observed as a pleural shimmering of a faster rate (coinciding with the heart rate) more in the left hemithorax (Video 28.2). A pneumothorax will typically act as an air cushion, preventing transmission of these cardiac oscillations to the parietal pleura. Demonstration of a lung pulse at the pleural line therefore rules out a pneumothorax, at the site of probe application.

2D images of lung sliding can be created using either a high-frequency linear transducer or a low-frequency (phased array or curvilinear) transducer. As a matter of efficiency, a low-frequency transducer is commonly used for the entire examination – visualizing lung sliding before moving on to the deeper structures. However, more detailed images of the presence or absence of lung sliding can be created using the high-frequency linear probe.

Lung sliding can be further confirmed using M-mode (motion mode). The presence of movement below the pleural line during normal respiration gives a characteristic sand-like appearance, while the tissues above the pleural line remain relatively static and appear as straight lines. This characteristic pattern is known as the "seashore sign" (Fig. 28.3). Conversely, the absence of lung sliding or lung pulse at the pleural line results in an M-mode image of multiple static horizontal lines both above and below the pleural line. This is sometimes referred to as the "bar code" or "stratosphere sign" (Fig. 28.4).

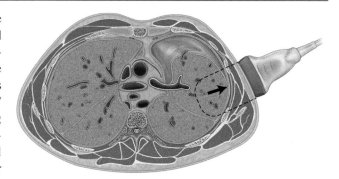

Fig. 28.5 Lung point. The point of separation between the visceral and the parietal pleura is demonstrated. Despite this finding being very specific to pneumothorax, locating this point of separation may be challenging

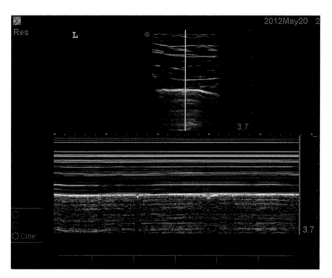

Fig. 28.3 M-mode of the pleura showing the seashore sign. The "sandy" appearance underneath the pleural line indicates the presence of lung sliding (seashore sign). Image captured using a linear transducer

As mentioned, the presence of lung sliding is a very powerful finding, ruling out a pneumothorax with 100% sensitivity. The absence of lung sliding however (Video 28.3) is not specific to pneumothorax. In essence, any condition preventing movement of the visceral against the parietal pleura (as occurs with normal respiration) will cause absent lung sliding. Apnea, non-ventilated lungs with massive atelectasis, mainstem intubation, and lobar pneumonia are among the possible culprits. In addition, sliding is absent post-pleurodesis. In the right clinical context, absent lung sliding is very suggestive of a pneumothorax, but the differential diagnosis of this ultrasound finding is quite broad [7].

In the absence of lung sliding, the detection of a lung point can help diagnose a pneumothorax. A lung point is an image that captures the transition point between normal lung sliding and the absence of lung sliding (Video 28.4). Anatomically, this represents the point where the visceral and parietal pleura start separating in a pneumothorax (Fig. 28.5). As an ultrasound finding, it is 100% specific for a pneumothorax. In the setting of a significant pneumothorax, however, the lung point may be very posteriorly located or, in cases of large circumferential pneumothorax, nonexistent. In these circumstances, it may be very difficult, time-consuming, and sometimes impossible to find. The authors of this chapter, therefore, do not advocate searching for a lung point on a routine basis. In an unstable patient with clinical findings suggestive of a pneumothorax, absent lung sliding should trigger immediate decompression. Searching for a lung point in such a critical situation is not appropriate and may delay time-sensitive management.

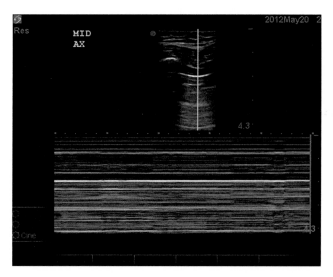

Fig. 28.4 M-mode of the pleura showing the stratosphere or bar code sign. The static appearance of straight lines underneath the pleura indicates the absence of lung sliding (stratosphere or bar code sign). Image captured using a linear transducer

A-Lines, B-Lines, and Consolidation Patterns

A central concept in the assessment of lung parenchyma by ultrasound is the assessment of the presence of A-lines and B-lines [8]. A-lines are the result of reverberation artifacts

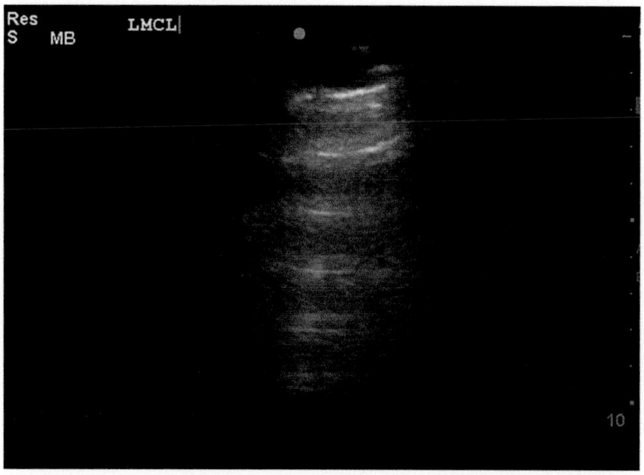

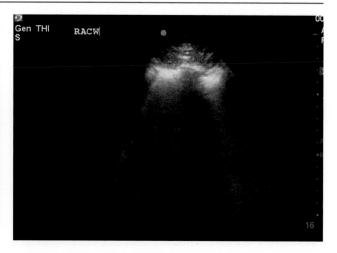

Fig. 28.6 A-line artifact. A-lines appear as horizontal, equidistant, repetitious lines parallel to the pleural surface. In the presence of lung sliding, they indicate normal lung aeration at the point of probe placement

Fig. 28.7 B-line artifact. B-lines appear as vertical, hyperechoic lines emanating from the pleural surface and extending to the end of the screen. B-line patterns indicate abnormal lung aeration at the point of probe placement

resulting from the reflection of ultrasound waves between the pleura and the ultrasound transducer (Fig. 28.1). They are therefore seen as equidistant horizontal hyperechoic lines below the pleural line (Fig. 28.6). The presence of A-lines suggests an absence of significant alveolar/interstitial edema and the absence of lung consolidation. Visualization of one or more A-lines therefore indicates normal lung aeration at the point of probe placement. Furthermore, sonographically normal lungs are defined as having lung sliding throughout with bilateral A-line predominance. Depending on the depth visualized on the screen, it is often possible to view multiple A-lines that are equidistant below the pleural line. However, the number of A-lines does not provide any additional diagnostic information.

In contrast B-lines are the results of a ring down or comet-tail artifact originating from the subpleural lung parenchyma (Fig. 28.2). B-lines are described as hyperechoic, vertical, laser-like lines that travel down to the bottom of the screen (Fig. 28.7). These commonly reflect the presence of pockets of fluid in the interlobular septa and indicate pulmonary edema. Other pathological processes that may cause the accumulation of protein, connective tissue, cells, or blood in the interlobular septa will also produce a sonographic B-line pattern. These include pneumonia, pulmonary fibrosis, pulmonary contusions, and lung neoplasms. Lastly, subsegmental atelectasis may produce localized B-lines, especially in the dependent portions of the lungs [9, 10].

B-lines have several defining features that are important to note. B-lines originate from the pleural line, extend to the

periphery of the far field without fading, and move synchronously with lung sliding (Video 28.5). B-lines also dominate over A-lines, and when both are visible, B-lines will obliterate A-lines to reach the end of the screen. It is not uncommon to see a few scattered B-lines even in healthy aerated lungs. As a clinical threshold, however, three or more B-lines present in one field of view or a large coalescence of B-lines is considered pathological [4].

It is important to distinguish B-lines from Z-lines. Z-lines are short faint vertical lines that attenuate before reaching the end of the screen, do not obliterate A-lines, and are independent of lung sliding. Z-lines are a common artifact that is devoid of any pathological significance and should be disregarded [11].

If it is not possible to see either an A-line pattern or B-line pattern, it is likely that the transducer is not perpendicular to the pleura. In order to generate a reverberation A-line artifact, it is important to acknowledge that the ultrasound beam needs to fall perpendicular on the pleural surface. It may be necessary to adjust the angle of the probe by means of sliding and tilting as described above, until either an A- or B-line artifact pattern is generated.

A third pattern that can be identified is that of pulmonary consolidation. It is common to identify consolidated lung in the dependent regions in patients that have been ventilated for long periods of time. By ultrasound, a consolidated lung has a tissue density that appears similar to the liver. Some have called this appearance "hepatized lung" (Fig. 28.8). The differential diagnosis of lung consolidation includes lobar atelectasis and pneumonia [12].

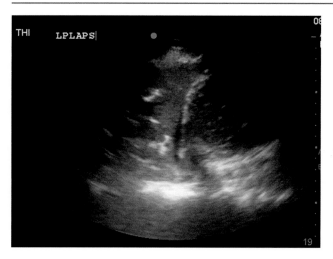

Fig. 28.8 Hepatized lung. Consolidated lung takes the appearance of a solid organ or a liver-like appearance, hence the name "hepatized lung." Note the small rim of pleural effusion inferior the lung

Table 28.3 Differential diagnosis of lung ultrasound findings in patients with respiratory failure

A-lines with lung sliding	Bilateral diffuse B-lines	Consolidation
COPD Asthma exacerbation Pulmonary embolism Extrathoracic process (e.g., acidosis)	Pulmonary edema (homogeneous B-lines) ARDS (heterogeneous B-line pattern)	Pneumonia (late/severe) Lobar atelectasis ormucus plug (late) Compressive atelectasis (due to large pleural effusion)
A-lines with absent lung sliding	**Unilateral or localized B-lines**	
Pneumothorax Mainstem intubation Post-pleurodesis Post pneumonectomy Lobar atelectasis or mucus plug (early)	Pneumonia (early/mild) Pulmonary contusions Lung neoplasm Subsegmental atelectasis	

Clinical Applications

Assessment of the Patient in Undifferentiated Respiratory Failure

Frontline clinicians know that there can be at times diagnostic uncertainty to the cause of respiratory failure despite a properly conducted history, physical examination, and chest radiograph. Pulmonary ultrasound is a modality that can provide additional and often diagnostic information. It can be conducted rapidly, and once it becomes part of routine practice, it can even be done while conducting the patient history and physical examination.

As a bedside diagnostic tool, we find it often provides an opportunity to develop positive physician-patient interactions. This is perhaps the most underappreciated aspect of point-of-care ultrasound in general. Patients seem to appreciate their physician spending time at the bedside, as opposed to spending time reviewing test results or radiographs. If it is appropriate, the patient can even be shown in real time their pathology. Table 28.3 lists the differential diagnosis of respiratory failure in patients with a predominantly A-line, B-line, and consolidation pattern.

It is important to conduct a thorough examination bilaterally. The presence of unilateral findings, such as unilateral B-lines, or unilateral absence of lung sliding can help localize pathology such as pneumonia or pneumothorax, respectively [7].

Respiratory failure with an ultrasound pattern of bilateral A-line predominance is analogous to respiratory failure with a normal chest X-ray. This is usually secondary to nonparenchymal lung disease, e.g., chronic obstructive pulmonary disease (COPD) exacerbations, acute asthma exacerbations, and pulmonary embolism. In these clinical scenarios, the utility of pulmonary ultrasound is in ruling out other causes of dyspnea. The additional ultrasound skill of detecting deep vein thrombosis by ultrasound is also a useful skill in the workup of dyspnea [4].

Assessment of Pneumothorax

As described above the presence of a pneumothorax can be assessed by the presence or absence of lung sliding. In the unstable patient with cardiovascular or respiratory compromise, there is often a clinical need to rule out a large pneumothorax. This can be accomplished with pulmonary ultrasound in a more time-efficient manner than a chest X-ray and with greater confidence than clinical exam alone.

If present in the supine patient, a physiologically significant pneumothorax is unlikely to be present only in the anterior chest. A positive finding of lung sliding rules out a pneumothorax within the field of view of the transducer [6]. In a time-efficient manner, the clinician can examine significant portions of the anterior chest wall bilaterally and rule out a large pneumothorax as a cause of cardiac or respiratory compromise.

Additional diagnostic certainty can be gained by the presence of B-lines. B-lines are not present when there is a pneumothorax within the field of view. Using CT imaging as a control in 73 ICU patients, Lichtenstein et al. showed that the presence of B-lines ruled out a pneumothorax with a 100% negative predictive value [13]. Lastly, another finding used to rule out a pneumothorax at the site of probe application is a lung pulse [14].

As described above, the presence of a lung point may be used to rule in/diagnose a pneumothorax. In an ICU study of 66 cases of pneumothorax and 233 controls, the presence of a lung point had a sensitivity of 66% and 100% specificity [15]. Although a very specific finding, being unable to elicit a lung point does not rule out a pneumothorax.

The ultrasound assessment of pneumothorax is helpful tool in trauma patients [16]. It can be completed in the trauma bay, while resuscitation is ongoing and while other diagnostic modalities are also being employed. This may allow for faster diagnosis without patient transfer to the CT scanner for the diagnosis of occult pneumothorax missed by chest radiographs. In a recent review of the trauma literature, the sensitivity of ultrasound to detect pneumothorax ranged from 86 to 98%, while the specificity ranged from 97 to 100%. For comparison, this review found the sensitivity of chest radiographs in the diagnosis of pneumothorax to be only 28–75% [17].

Assessment of Pulmonary Edema and Fluid Tolerance

Patients in shock states are often given large volumes of fluid resuscitation as a matter of course. Pulmonary ultrasound presents a means of interval scanning of the lungs to determine if the presence of pulmonary edema is developing. After a baseline scan is taken and further fluid resuscitation is given, the lungs can be reexamined to look for the interval development of B-lines. If an A-line pattern is dominant and the patient is still in a shock state, this would indicate fluid tolerance and serve as an invitation for further fluid administration. If, however, there has been an interval development of B-lines, this finding may give the clinician a signal to stop giving additional fluid and instead utilize other means of hemodynamic support. The concept of fluid tolerance should not be confused with fluid responsiveness. Whereas fluid tolerance is a marker of pulmonary edema, fluid responsiveness indicates an increase in cardiac output as the result of fluid resuscitation.

The presence of A-lines has been correlated with a low pulmonary artery occlusion pressure (PAOP) in certain conditions. In a study of ICU patients with septic shock, Lichtenstein et al. found that the presence of an A-line dominant pattern was associated with a PAOP <18 mmHg, while a B-line dominance, however, was observed in a wide range of PAOP patterns [8]. In a more recent study of mixed ICU patients, the presence of B-lines was shown to correlate with extravascular lung water as measured by the transpulmonary thermodilution method (PiCCO system). In this study, however, A-lines were found to be predictive of a low PAOP (<18 mmHg) only in patients with a normal ejection fraction [18].

Previous attempts have been made to incorporate findings from pulmonary ultrasound with point-of-care echocardiography to develop protocols for the management of shock patients [5, 19]. In the critically ill patient with cardiorespiratory failure, it is unlikely that pulmonary ultrasound alone will provide a complete clinical picture. Incorporating pulmonary ultrasound with assessments of LV size and function, RV size and function, and IVC dynamics allows for a more thorough assessment of patient status. For this reason, we incorporate pulmonary ultrasound findings with bedside echocardiography findings, and we encourage our trainees to do the same.

When a patient is being diuresed during the de-resuscitation phase of shock, the presence or absence of B-lines can also be useful. In a patient that cannot be weaned from ventilatory support, the presence of B-lines may indicate the need for continued/additional diuresis. The absence of B-lines may lead the clinician to look for additional causes of respiratory failure such as those listed in Table 2.3. At a minimum, the use of pulmonary ultrasound in the ICU setting has been shown to minimize the need for radiographs and CTs [20].

Assessment for the Presence of Pneumonia and Atelectasis

The presence of pneumonia can create a wide range of pulmonary ultrasound findings. It can present as B-lines (unilateral or bilateral) or consolidated "hepatized" lung tissue, with or without lung sliding [4]. The presence of dynamic air bronchograms can often be seen, but they are not specific to pneumonia (Video 28.6). In a recent systematic review, the sensitivity and specificity of pulmonary ultrasound for the diagnosis of pneumonia were 85% and 93%, respectively [21].

Consolidation patterns secondary to atelectasis are extremely common in patients undergoing long-term ventilation, especially those with dependent pleural effusions. Even patients undergoing short-term ventilation for surgical procedures have atelectasis that can be detected by ultrasound [22]. Tusman et al. published a suggested protocol for using lung ultrasound to titrate recruitment maneuvers and PEEP to minimize atelectasis and ventilator-associated lung injury [23, 24]. Once atelectasis is confirmed by ultrasound, recruitment maneuvers are done with a stepwise increase in pressure in order to determine the opening pressure of the lungs. Following this, PEEP is decreased incrementally to until the reappearance of atelectatic lung by ultrasound. The level of PEEP is then chosen to be 2 cm H20 above this closing pressure.

Assessment of Acute Respiratory Distress Syndrome

The B-line appearance pattern created by cardiogenic edema differs from that of acute respiratory distress syndrome

(ARDS). While the B-line pattern associated with cardiogenic pulmonary edema is fairly uniform throughout the chest, ARDS sonography findings are less homogeneous with spared areas of A-line dominance, other areas with significant B-lines, areas with consolidation (usually dependent), and pleural line abnormalities [25]. In patients presenting with undifferentiated respiratory failure, pulmonary ultrasound has been validated as a diagnostic tool, differentiating both clinical entities (ARDS vs. cardiogenic pulmonary edema) with good discriminatory power [26]. Furthermore, pulmonary ultrasound may be of potential value in assessing the effectiveness of positive end expiratory pressure (PEEP) titrations and lung recruitment maneuvers in hypoxemic mechanically ventilated patients [27].

Assessment of Pleural Effusions

Point-of-care ultrasound very accurately distinguishes pleural from parenchymal pathology and is therefore of great value in patients with undifferentiated lung field opacification on chest X-ray. In addition, patients presenting with acute respiratory failure may benefit from an expedited ultrasound diagnosis and quantification of a pleural effusion, knowledge of which has immediate clinical applications. Lastly, ultrasound allows for safe pleural drainage at the bedside and can be used to demarcate the pleural space boundaries and guide needle placement. Assessment of pleural effusions is therefore an important skill to master and is relatively easy to learn for the novice sonographer [28].

Unlike assessment of lung aeration, where generation of artifact is the goal, pleural effusions are directly and very easily visualized with ultrasound. Fluid is generally a very good transmitter of ultrasound with very little of the incident ultrasound beam being reflected back to the probe. Pleural effusions therefore appear anechoic (black) on ultrasound, in contrast with their surrounding anatomical structures.

On ultrasound, three criteria must be fulfilled to make the diagnosis of a pleural effusion [29]. First, it must be identified as an anechoic space. Second, this anechoic space must be within the typical anatomical boundaries. The surrounding chest wall, lungs, and diaphragm must be clearly identified, and the fluid collection must be clearly visible above, and not below, the diaphragm (Fig. 28.9). Third, a dynamic component for the fluid boundaries must be demonstrated. This includes the lungs flapping in this space or diaphragmatic descent underneath the fluid with every respiration (Video 28.7).

It is possible to estimate the volume of pleural fluid in mechanically ventilated patients, using ultrasound [30]. In supine position, with a mild trunk elevation at 15°, an ultrasound view of the pleural fluid between the base of the lung and the diaphragm is obtained. Then the maximal distance

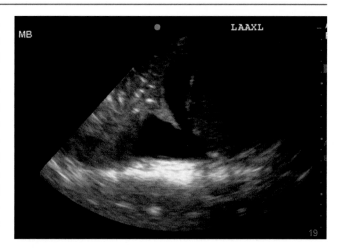

Fig. 28.9 Pleural effusion. Pleural fluid appears anechoic (black), within typical anatomical boundaries (lungs superior and diaphragm inferior), and has dynamic features

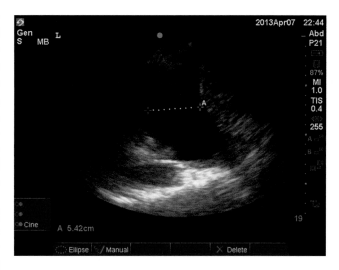

Fig. 28.10 Pleural effusion quantification. Measurement of the maximal subpulmonic distance between the visceral pleura (at the base of the lung) and parietal pleura (above the diaphragm). Distance measured = 54 mm. In this patient, pleural effusion volume estimation = 54 * 20 = 1080 ml

between the diaphragm surface (parietal pleura) and the base of the lung (visceral pleura) is measured (Fig. 28.10). Pleural fluid volume is then calculated using the equation:

Pleural Fluid Volume (Ml) = Maximal Subpulmonic Distance (Mm) * 20

A 2D examination of the pleural fluid can provide important insight into the character of the effusion. Transudative effusions usually appear completely anechoic, with no evidence of cellular material or debris in the pleural fluid. Conversely, presence of echogenic components in an effusion is strongly suggestive of an exudative process. Observing swirling

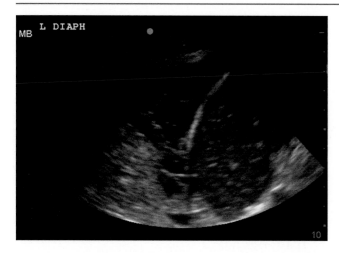

Fig. 28.11 Complex pleural effusion with septations. Septations within a pleural effusion indicate complexity and are better detected by ultrasound than CT scan. Septations and fibrin strands predict longer chest drainage times, potential need for intrapleural fibrinolytics, longer hospitalization, and greater potential for surgical intervention for adequate drainage. Early thoracic surgery consultation is warranted

debris in the pleural fluid with heart contractions or respiratory movements has been named the "plankton sign" and is evidence of an exudative effusion (Video 28.8). Other findings suggestive of a complex exudative effusion include the presence of septations (Fig. 28.11), fibrin strands, loculations, and layering of the effusion fluid into two layers of different densities. This layering is sometimes observed with empyema and hemothorax (hematocrit sign). Septations and fibrin strands are detected more readily with ultrasound than CT scan, and their presence is predictive of the need for longer periods of chest drainage, longer hospital stays, higher incidence of requiring intrapleural fibrinolytics, and higher chance of needing surgery for adequate drainage [31, 32]. We therefore recommend involving thoracic surgery early in the management of all sonographically complex pleural effusions.

Assessment of Respiratory Complications Post-brachial Plexus Blockade

Brachial plexus blockade is associated with the pulmonary complications of phrenic nerve blockade and pneumothorax, with the interscalene approach particularly associated with phrenic nerve blockade and the supraclavicular approach with pneumothorax [33]. Immediate onset of respiratory distress in a patient undergoing these blocks should lead the clinician to consider these two diagnoses. Pneumothorax can be ruled out by the methods mentioned in this chapter. Diaphragmatic weakness associated with phrenic nerve blockade is more complicated to assess. Simple assessments of lung sliding are not sufficient to assess for phrenic nerve

blockade as pleural movement is the result of all total function of all the respiratory muscles. Assessments of diaphragmatic excursion and diaphragm thickening with respiration are therefore required [34, 35].

Case Presentation

The postanesthesia care unit (PACU) nurse asks for your help. A 55-year-old lady underwent a left video-assisted thoracoscopic surgery (VATS) talc pleurodesis for a chronic left pleural effusion, 2 h earlier, and has since been in the PACU with high oxygen requirements. The nurse mentions that all attempts at weaning her oxygen requirements to get her ready for ward transfer have been unsuccessful and she currently remains on an FiO2 of 0.6 by face mask. Her past medical history is significant for an ischemic cardiomyopathy with an estimated left ventricular ejection fraction of 35%. The anesthesiologists' records document stable hemodynamics throughout the procedure, minimal blood loss, and a slight positive fluid balance of only 500 ml.

The patient appears to be fully awake and has good motor strength. Her BP is 105/60 mmHg, HR 82 beats/min, and her SpO2 92%. A portable chest X-ray, performed in PACU, was inconclusive (Fig. 28.12). A lung and pleural ultrasound is performed to further delineate the cause of her hypoxemia.

Case Resolution

Using a phased array transducer, her nonoperative right lung was scanned at two points: the anterior chest wall (Video

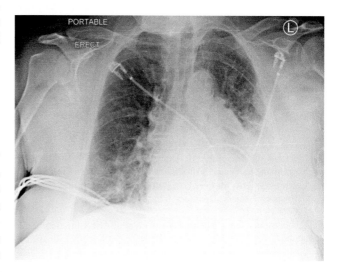

Fig. 28.12 Plain portable chest X-ray of patient with undifferentiated hypoxia. Plain chest radiograph suggestive, but not conclusive, of pulmonary edema. As a modality, the sensitivity of plain chest X-rays in pulmonary edema detection is 50–68%

28.9) and the anterior axillary line (Video 28.10). Due to the surgical dressing covering large portions of her operative side, only her nonoperative side was scanned. Acquired images demonstrated a diffuse B-line pattern, consistent with an interstitial alveolar syndrome. With a working diagnosis of pulmonary edema, furosemide 40 mg was administered intravenously. Over the next 90 min, the patient diuresed 800 ml of urine, and her oxygen requirements were weaned to 3 L/min oxygen by nasal prongs. After meeting PACU discharge criteria, the patient was transferred safely to the ward.

The sensitivity of ultrasound in detecting pulmonary edema far surpasses that of plain chest X-rays (100% vs. 65%) [36, 37]. As a modality, ultrasound is quick and easy to use at the bedside and can be used either to make a diagnosis or, in this case, confirm a clinical suspicion. B-lines are defined as vertical hyperechoic comet tails that (a) emanate from the pleural line, (b) extend all the way to the end of the screen, (c) move with lung sliding, and (d) dominate over any other aeration patterns (i.e., dominate over A-lines). A clinically significant B-line pattern indicative of an interstitial syndrome is present when three or more B-lines or a coalescence of B-lines is visible on the same screen. The differential diagnosis for B-line predominance includes pulmonary edema, ARDS, early pneumonia, and subsegmental atelectasis. In this case, the relatively uniform B-line presence throughout the anterior and lateral chest was diagnostic of pulmonary edema.

This case highlights the value of ultrasound in dismissing diagnostic uncertainties. In general, the indications of perioperative ultrasound include assessing undifferentiated hypoxia, evaluating undifferentiated opacities on chest X-rays, and determining the safety of further fluid resuscitation. Point-of-care ultrasound empowers clinicians to make diagnoses at the bedside and may therefore expedite appropriate management and improve timely patient care.

References

1. Shriki J. Ultrasound physics. Crit Care Clin. 2014;30(1):1–24. v
2. Enriquez JL, Wu TS. An introduction to ultrasound equipment and knobology. Crit Care Clin. 2014;30(1):25–45. v
3. Ihnatsenka B, Boezaart AP. Ultrasound: basic understanding and learning the language. Int J Shoulder Surg. 2010;4(3):55–62.
4. Lichtenstein DA, Mezière GA. Relevance of lung ultrasound in the diagnosis of acute respiratory failure: the BLUE protocol. Chest. 2008;134(1):117–25.
5. Lichtenstein DA. BLUE-protocol and FALLS-protocol: two applications of lung ultrasound in the critically ill. Chest. 2015;147(6):1659–70.
6. Lichtenstein DA, Menu Y. A bedside ultrasound sign ruling out pneumothorax in the critically ill. Lung sliding. Chest. 1995;108(5):1345–8.
7. Lichtenstein DA. Lung ultrasound in the critically ill. Ann Intensive Care. 2014;4(1):1.
8. Lichtenstein DA, Mezière GA, Lagoueyte J-F, Biderman P, Goldstein I, Gepner A. A-Lines and B-Lines. Chest. 2009;136(4):1014–20.
9. Volpicelli G, Elbarbary M, Blaivas M, Lichtenstein DA, Mathis G, Kirkpatrick AW, et al. International evidence-based recommendations for point-of-care lung ultrasound. Intensive Care Med. 2012;38(4):577–91.
10. Soldati G, Inchingolo R, Smargiassi A, Sher S, Nenna R, Inchingolo CD, et al. Ex vivo lung sonography: morphologic-ultrasound relationship. Ultrasound Med Biol. 2012;38(7):1169–79.
11. Lichtenstein DA, Mezière G, Lascols N, Biderman P, Courret J-P, Gepner A, et al. Ultrasound diagnosis of occult pneumothorax. Crit Care Med. 2005;33(6):1231–8.
12. Mayo PH, Doelken P. Pleural ultrasonography. Clin Chest Med. 2006;27(2):215–27.
13. Lichtenstein D, Meziere G, Biderman P, Gepner A. The comet-tail artifact: an ultrasound sign ruling out pneumothorax. Intensive Care Med. 1999;25(4):383–8.
14. Volpicelli G. Sonographic diagnosis of pneumothorax. Intensive Care Med. 2011;37(2):224–32.
15. Lichtenstein D, Meziere G, Biderman P, Gepner A. The "lung point": an ultrasound sign specific to pneumothorax. Intensive Care Med. 2000;26(10):1434–40.
16. Nandipati KC, Allamaneni S, Kakarla R, Wong A, Richards N, Satterfield J, et al. Extended focused assessment with sonography for trauma (EFAST) in the diagnosis of pneumothorax: experience at a community based level I trauma center. Injury. Elsevier Ltd. 2011;42(5):511–4.
17. Gentry Wilkerson R, Stone MB. Sensitivity of bedside ultrasound and supine anteroposterior chest radiographs for the identification of pneumothorax after blunt trauma. Acad Emerg Med. 2010;17(1):11–7.
18. Volpicelli G, Skurzak S, Boero E, Carpinteri G, Tengattini M, Stefanone V, et al. Lung ultrasound predicts well extravascular lung water but is of limited usefulness in the prediction of wedge pressure. Anesthesiology. 2014;121(2):320–7.
19. Lee CWC, Kory PD, Arntfield RT. Development of a fluid resuscitation protocol using inferior vena cava and lung ultrasound. J Crit Care. 2016;31(1):96–100.
20. Peris A, Tutino L, Zagli G, Batacchi S, Cianchi G, Spina R, et al. The use of point-of-care bedside lung ultrasound significantly reduces the number of radiographs and computed tomography scans in critically ill patients. Anesth Analg. 2010;111(3):687–92.
21. Alzahrani SA, Al-Salamah MA, Al-Madani WH, Elbarbary MA. Systematic review and meta-analysis for the use of ultrasound versus radiology in diagnosing of pneumonia. Crit Ultrasound J. 2017;9(1):6.
22. Monastesse A, Girard F, Massicotte N, Chartrand-Lefebvre C, Girard M. Lung ultrasonography for the assessment of perioperative atelectasis: a pilot feasibility study. Anesth Analg. 2017;124(2):494–504.
23. Tusman G, Acosta CM, Nicola M, Esperatti M, Bohm SH, Suarez-Sipmann F. Real-time images of tidal recruitment using lung ultrasound. Crit Ultrasound J. 2015;7(1):19.
24. Tusman G, Acosta CM, Costantini M. Ultrasonography for the assessment of lung recruitment maneuvers. Crit Ultrasound J. 2016;8(1):8.
25. Copetti R, Soldati G, Copetti P. Chest sonography: a useful tool to differentiate acute cardiogenic pulmonary edema from acute respiratory distress syndrome. Cardiovasc Ultrasound. 2008;6:16.
26. Schmickl CN, Pannu S, MO A-Q, Alsara A, Kashyap R, Dhokarh R, et al. Decision support tool for differential diagnosis of acute respiratory distress syndrome (ARDS) vs cardiogenic pulmonary edema (CPE): a prospective validation and meta-analysis. Crit Care. 2014;18(6):659.

27. Bouhemad B, Mongodi S, Via G, Rouquette I. Ultrasound for "lung monitoring" of ventilated patients. Anesthesiology. 2015;122(2):437–47.

28. Soni NJ, Franco R, Velez MI, Schnobrich D, Dancel R, Restrepo MI, et al. Ultrasound in the diagnosis and management of pleural effusions. J Hosp Med. 2015;10(12):811–6.

29. Mayo PH, Beaulieu Y, Doelken P, Feller-Kopman D, Harrod C, Kaplan A, et al. American College of Chest Physicians/La Societe de Reanimation de Langue Francaise statement on competence in critical care ultrasonography. Chest. 2009;135(4):1050–60.

30. Balik M, Plasil P, Waldauf P, Pazout J, Fric M, Otahal M, et al. Ultrasound estimation of volume of pleural fluid in mechanically ventilated patients. Intensive Care Med. 2006;32(2):318–21.

31. McLoud TC, Flower CD. Imaging the pleura: sonography, CT, and MR imaging. AJR Am J Roentgenol. 1991;156(6):1145–53.

32. Chen KY, Liaw YS, Wang HC, Luh KT, Yang PC. Sonographic septation: a useful prognostic indicator of acute thoracic empyema. J Ultrasound Med. 2000;19(12):837–43.

33. Mian A, Chaudhry I, Huang R, Rizk E, Tubbs RS, Loukas M. Brachial plexus anesthesia: a review of the relevant anatomy, complications, and anatomical variations. Clin Anat. 2014;27(2):210–21.

34. Umbrello M, Formenti P. Ultrasonographic assessment of diaphragm function in critically ill subjects. Respir Care. 2016;61(4): 542–55.

35. Haskins SC, Tsui BC, Nejim JA, Wu CL, Boublik J. Lung ultrasound for the regional anesthesiologist and acute pain specialist. Reg Anesth Pain Med. 2017;42(3):289–98.

36. Lichtenstein D, Meziere G. A lung ultrasound sign allowing bedside distinction between pulmonary edema and COPD: the comet-tail artifact. Intensive Care Med. 1998;24(12): 1331–4.

37. Cardinale L, Priola AM, Moretti F, Volpicelli G. Effectiveness of chest radiography, lung ultrasound and thoracic computed tomography in the diagnosis of congestive heart failure. World J Radiol. 2014;6(6):230–7.

Ultrasound for Vascular Access

29

James P. Lee, Joshua M. Zimmerman,
and Natalie A. Silverton

Key Points
- The use of ultrasound for vascular access has been shown to decrease complications and improve success rates.
- Current guidelines recommend the use of ultrasound for central venous cannulation of the internal jugular vein, but ultrasound can be used to facilitate subclavian vein and femoral vein cannulation as well.
- Anatomic relationships are important to learn with ultrasound, but anatomic variability exists; therefore care must be taken to distinguish arterial from venous structure with ultrasound prior to cannulation. Venous structures are often thin walled and easily collapsible with flow in both systole and diastole. Arterial structures have thicker walls and visually pulsatile due to systolic flow.
- The internal jugular vein (IJV) runs vertically in the neck from the jugular foramen at the base of the skull until it joins the subclavian vein (SCV) within the chest to form the innominate or brachiocephalic vein. The right and left brachiocephalic veins then join to form the superior vena cava (SVC) which drains into the right atrium of the heart.

- The IJV can be visualized in short axis or long axis. The advantage of short axis imaging is that the image allows for visualization of surrounding anatomic structures such as the carotid artery. The advantage of long axis imaging is that the needle can be introduced "in plane" allowing for visualization of the entire needle tip.
- The SCV is a continuation of the axillary vein from the deltopectoral groove to where it joins the IVJ to form the innominate vein. The SCV can be accessed on either side of the clavicle, and both infraclavicular and supraclavicular techniques can be visualized with ultrasound.
- Femoral vein (FV) cannulation is often used in emergencies when rapid access is needed or if IJV/SCV cannulation is impossible or contraindicated. Ultrasound can be used to facilitate FV cannulation with either a short axis or long axis technique.
- Although the landmark and palpation technique for radial artery catheterization is the mostly widely used technique, ultrasound may be used for difficult access or in cases where first-pass success is desired.

Electronic Supplementary Material The online version of this chapter (https://doi.org/10.1007/978-3-030-00859-8_29) contains supplementary material, which is available to authorized users.

J. P. Lee
Department of Anesthesiology, University of Utah School of Medicine, Salt Lake City, UT, USA

J. M. Zimmerman
University of Utah School of Medicine, Salt Lake City, UT, USA

N. A. Silverton (✉)
Department of Anesthesiology, University of Utah, Salt Lake City, UT, USA
e-mail: natalie.silverton@hsc.utah.edu

Introduction

Since its introduction into clinical practice in the 1970s, the use of ultrasound has grown substantially. Ultrasound today has better resolution and is more compact, user friendly, and affordable than it was in the past. One of the more widely accepted applications of ultrasound in medical practice is its use for vascular access. Central venous catheters (CVC) are placed for hemodynamic monitoring, fluid management, renal replacement therapy, drug therapy, cardiac pacemaker placement, and total parenteral nutrition. In this chapter we will discuss the use of ultrasound for the placement of CVCs

P. Slinger (ed.), *Principles and Practice of Anesthesia for Thoracic Surgery*, https://doi.org/10.1007/978-3-030-00859-8_29

and radial artery catheters. Ultrasound for vascular access is most commonly used for internal jugular vein (IJV) cannulation. Increasingly, however, this technique is being applied to femoral vein (FV) and, more recently, subclavian vein (SCV) cannulation. We will describe ultrasound techniques for each of these access sites as well as the use of ultrasound for radial artery cannulation as the latter is also a common practice.

Why Use Ultrasound?

The Seldinger technique for vascular access was first described in 1953 [1]. What we now consider the traditional "landmark" techniques for SCV and IJV cannulations were developed shortly thereafter [2, 3]. As these techniques preceded the routine use of ultrasound, they relied solely on the anatomic relationships of vascular structures to fixed landmarks on the surface anatomy such as the clavicle and the sternocleidomastoid muscle. These techniques assumed a minimal variation in anatomy between patients. Today, from ultrasound-based studies of anatomy, we know that this assumption is not valid and can lead to an increased incidence of complications such as nerve injury, pneumothorax, hemothorax, or accidental arterial puncture [4–6]. Overall, the risk of mechanical complication with central venous cannulation (internal jugular, subclavian, and femoral) is 5–19% [7]. A recent Cochrane review of 35 randomized controlled trials and over 5000 patients concluded that the use of ultrasound for IJV cannulation was associated with a significant reduction in the incidence of accidental carotid puncture (relative risk reduction 72%) and in overall complications (relative risk reduction 71%) [8]. Ultrasound has also been associated with a decreased incidence of inadvertent subclavian artery and femoral artery puncture [9, 10]. Faster access times as well as higher first-pass and overall success rates have been reported with ultrasound-guided cannulation of all three vessels, even in emergent situations such as ongoing CPR [9–12].

Because of the strength of the evidence for the use of ultrasound in vascular access, the most recent practice guidelines from the American Society of Anesthesiologists recommend that when available, real-time ultrasound should be used for IJV cannulation (*category A1/A2 evidence*) and FV cannulation (*category A3 evidence*) [13]. Although their recommendations were "equivocal" for the use of ultrasound for SCV cannulation, they did present evidence that this technique reduces inadvertent arterial puncture, the incidence of hematomas, as well as shorter access times and higher success rates (*category A2 evidence*) [13]. The use of real-time ultrasound for central venous catheter placement has also been advocated by the

American College of Surgeons [14] and Society of Critical Care Medicine [15].

Despite these guidelines and the evidence that supports them, a 2006 survey of anesthesia providers suggested that 67% have never or almost never use ultrasound for IJV cannulation. The most common reason listed as to why ultrasound was not used is it is not "necessary" [16]. More recently, a 2014 survey of emergency physicians reported that 44% "never use ultrasound when placing CVCs." The most common reason cited was lack of training, followed by the perception that ultrasound was too time consuming and the lack of equipment [17].

Which Ultrasound Probe Should I Use?

Ultrasound probes used today come in a variety of sizes, shapes, and frequencies.

The three major types of ultrasound probes, phased array, curvilinear, and the linear probe, are all used for different purposes and cannot easily be interchanged. The phased array and curvilinear probes are lower-frequency probes designed to image structures deep within the body such as the heart, gallbladder, intra-abdominal aorta, or bladder. The standard linear array probe uses high-frequency ultrasound crystals (5–13 MHz) linearly arranged on a flat footprint, thus producing sound waves in a straight line. The result is high-resolution imaging of superficial structures displayed in a rectangular image. The higher frequencies of the linear probe allow for improved image resolution but at the cost of decreased tissue penetration. Thus it is recommended to use a higher-frequency probe during vascular access as the vascular targets are usually less than 5 cm from the skin surface and image quality will be improved.

Before Placing the Probe: A Word About Aseptic Technique

Care should be taken to place a central venous catheter in an aseptic manner. The 2011 CDC recommendations for the prevention of intravascular catheter-related infections can be summarized as follows [18]. The patient's skin should first be cleaned with an antiseptic agent, as described by the CDC guidelines. The patient should then be draped in a standard sterile fashion. The provider should perform proper hand hygiene and use barrier precautions such as a cap, mask, a sterile gown, and sterile gloves. The ultrasound probe should be placed into a sterile sheath, and sterile gel should be used in the field. Care should be taken to not contaminate the field or the operator during the placement of sterile sheath onto the ultrasound probe.

Image Optimization

When performing ultrasound-guided vascular access, the probe and screen display are best oriented anatomically, that is, similar to that which is seen from the vantage point of the operator. Accordingly the left side of the probe and the image on the screen should correspond to the left side of the operator. Each probe has an indicator (usually a dot, a line, or a small LED) to identify probe laterality. A corresponding indicator dot is often displayed on the screen. Laterality can also be determined by applying external pressure to one side of the probe while simultaneously visualizing the display screen.

Once the laterality of the probe and image has been determined, the operator should adjust the depth appropriately so that the entire vein and surrounding vascular structures are visualized. The gain on the ultrasound machine should be adjusted in order to make the center of the vascular structures dark (echo lucent) and the surrounding structures appropriately bright. If the gain is increased too much (over-gained), the surrounding structures will be displayed overly bright and may make visualization of the vascular structures difficult.

Distinguishing the Vein from the Artery

With ultrasound, both veins and arteries will appear as dark (echo lucent) round structures with brighter (echo dense) borders. Veins are usually fully collapsible when pressure is applied to it by the ultrasound probe, while the arteries are often rounder in shape, more pulsatile, and not fully collapsible. Valves may also be visualized in the vein but not in the artery. Color flow Doppler may be used to determine pulsatility and the direction of flow, but the latter must be used with caution as the color displayed on the monitor (red versus blue) depends on probe orientation and may fool the beginning practitioner. Venous flow occurs in systole and diastole, whereas arterial flow is predominately in systole.

Limitations of Ultrasound Technique

Static imaging is a type of "X marks the spot" technique where ultrasound is used to mark the location of the vein prior to sterile prepping and draping. While this technique is still advocated by the American Society of Anesthesiologists [13], the use of real-time ultrasound has been shown to improve first-pass success and overall success [12]. Real-time ultrasound, however, requires some degree of practice and technical skill as simultaneous manipulation of the probe with one hand and the needle with the other hand is required.

It is also important to remember that the image displayed is in two dimensions, while the needle tip trajectory toward the vessel is a three-dimensional path. When the image is displayed in short axis (Fig. 29.1a), the shaft of the needle cannot be easily distinguished from the needle tip. Past pointing occurs when the needle tip crosses through and past the ultrasound beam because the needle shaft seen on the ultrasound screen is mistaken for the needle tip. Figure 29.1a

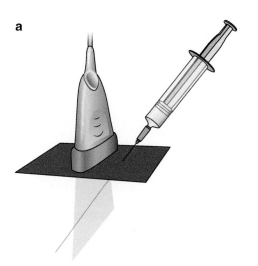
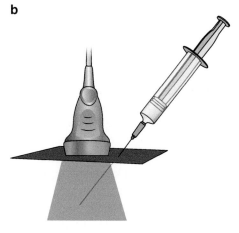

Fig. 29.1 Illustrates the technique of ultrasound imaging in short axis (**a**) and long axis (**b**). Note how in the short axis imaging (**a**) the needle tip is well beyond the ultrasound beam and out of the plane of the image. In the long axis imaging (**b**), the entire needle trajectory and needle tip are visualized

illustrates how the needle tip is no longer visualized and is actually deeper than seen on the display screen. In order to prevent past pointing, the operator can move the probe along the skin surface to ensure that the needle tip is always visualized as the needle is driven toward the target of interest. Alternatively, a long axis technique can be used to visualize the needle tip through its entire trajectory (Fig. 29.1b). Complications of unrecognized past pointing include inadvertent arterial puncture, pneumothorax, and damage to surrounding structures.

Summary

Ultrasound guidance has become the standard of care for IJ vein cannulation, and its use in vascular access in general is increasing. The advantage to using ultrasound is the ability to visualize the vessel of interest and surrounding structures. Ultrasound has been shown to decrease complications and improve success rates for central line placement, but the technique requires some acquired skill and practice in order to accurately visualize needle tip placement in real time. In this chapter, we will discuss the use of ultrasound for IJV, SCV, FV, and radial artery cannulation as these are the most common uses of this technology in daily practice.

Ultrasound for Internal Jugular Vein Cannulation

Anatomy

The internal jugular vein (IJV) runs vertically in the neck from the jugular foramen at the base of the skull until it joins the subclavian vein (SCV) within the chest to form the innominate or brachiocephalic vein. The right and left brachiocephalic veins then join to form the superior vena cava (SVC) which drains into the right atrium of the heart (Fig. 29.2a). The IJV lies within the carotid sheath along with the carotid artery (CA) and vagus nerve. Normally, the IJV is found anterior and lateral to the CA, but the anatomic variation among patients can be considerable, and frequently the IJV lies outside the path predicted by a landmark technique [4–6].

Sedillot's triangle is the anatomical landmark for IJV cannulation and is bounded by the sternal and clavicular heads of the sternocleidomastoid muscle medially and laterally, respectively, and the clavicle inferiorly. The IJV is found at the apex of this triangle, and this is a good starting point for initial ultrasound probe placement. Initial ultrasound images of the neck should show two dominant echo-lucent vessels in short axis representing the CA and IJV (Fig. 29.2b). The CA and IJV should be clearly distinguished with the CA having

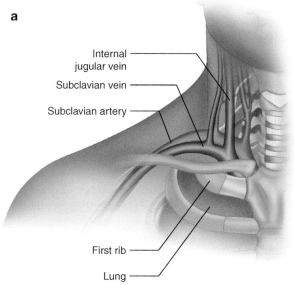

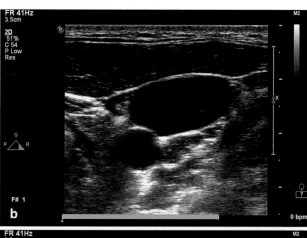

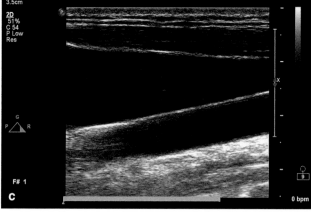

Fig. 29.2 Illustrates the anatomy of the internal jugular vein and its relationship to the carotid artery and subclavian vein (**a**). Ultrasound imaging of the internal jugular vein (IJV) and carotid artery (CA) is demonstrated in short axis (**b**) and in long axis (**c**)

a more circular shape, being less compressible, and having more pulsatile flow. The IJV is often larger and more lateral, but this is not always the case.

After adjustment for the appropriate depth and gain, and once the identity of the two major vessels is determined, the ultrasound probe should be moved up and down the neck to identify the ideal cannulation site. Because the relative anatomic relationship between the CA and the IJV changes throughout the neck from superior to inferior (Video 29.1), there may be some locations on the neck where the relationship is more favorable (i.e., the CA and the IVJ are separated anatomically with little overlap). Other considerations for cannulation site placement are the location of the external jugular vein (often found anterior and in the path of cannulation if the puncture site is too superior) and the increased likelihood of pneumothorax or inadvertent brachiocephalic, subclavian, or even aortic injury if the puncture site is too inferior [19].

Short Axis Technique

In this section we will describe the standard short axis approach to ultrasound-guided IJV cannulation. After the appropriate anatomy is identified and the cannulation site is determined (see above), lidocaine can be used to anesthetize the skin in awake patients. While the lidocaine needle can be visualized with ultrasound and this may help prevent inadvertent intravascular injection of lidocaine, finder needles in the traditional sense are not necessary with ultrasound.

The ideal needle puncture site is approximately the same distance back from the probe as the depth of the IJV when the needle is advanced at a 45-degree angle (Video 29.1). Using this triangulation technique will help facilitate finding the needle tip within the ultrasound beam. The depth of the IJV is usually 1–1.5 cm below the surface of the skin, but in larger patients with deeper vessels, the entrance point of the needle should either be farther from the transducer or the needle trajectory will need to be steeper in order to avoid past pointing the needle beyond the beam of the ultrasound (Fig. 29.1a). With traditional landmark technique, the needle direction after entering the skin was to point laterally toward the ipsilateral nipple. In a similar manner, with ultrasound technique, the needle should enter the skin on the medial side of the IJV and then advanced laterally toward the center of the vessel. This medial to lateral trajectory is meant to reduce the risk of inadvertent puncture of the more medial CA.

As mentioned above, the major limitation of the short axis technique is the difficulty of needle tip identification and the potential past pointing (Fig. 29.1a). One method to improve needle tip visualization is to move the transducer up and down the neck slightly to identify the most distal end of the needle and then to progressively move the ultrasound

transducer toward the patient's feet as the needle is advanced. Ultimately as the needle is advanced, tenting of the anterior wall of the IJV is seen. This confirms placement of the needle tip and can be used to modify placement such that the needle is in the center of the vessel. Subsequently, the vessel can be either punctured in short axis or the transducer can be turned 90° to confirm needle tip placement in long axis as the needle punctures the vessel (Video 29.1).

Long Axis Technique

Although multiple studies have shown that ultrasound guidance increases first-pass success rate and decreases complications [5, 6, 12, 20], the incidence of inadvertent CA puncture is still as high as 4% [21–23]. Part of the reason for the continued risk of CA puncture even with ultrasound guidance is the inability to accurately visualize the needle tip while using the short axis technique above. One alternative is to rotate the ultrasound transducer 90°, thereby using a long axis or in-plane technique (Fig. 29.1b). The advantage to the long axis technique is that not only can the needle tip can be visualized as it punctures the vessel but also the tip of the needle can then be precisely placed in the center of the lumen avoiding "back walling" of the needle or injury to the posterior surface of the IJV.

Studies suggest that "back walling" or puncture of the posterior surface of the IJV occurs in 34–64% of procedures [24, 25]. Injury to the posterior wall of the IJV may cause neck hematoma or thrombus. In theory direct visualization of the needle tip will reduce this complication, and there is some limited evidence to support this, although large randomized studies have not been performed [26].

With the long axis technique, it is helpful to identify the CA and IJV in short axis initially as above and then centering the probe over the IJV, rotating the probe 90° to view the vessel in long axis (Fig. 29.2c and Video 29.2). The needle is then introduced in the plane of the ultrasound (Fig. 29.1b) and can be visualized in its entirety as it is advanced. Once the needle punctures the vessel, the needle tip can be precisely placed in the middle of the vessel which facilitates smooth wire placement.

The major disadvantage of the long axis technique is that while the IJV and needle are well visualized, the CA is often no longer visible. This should not matter as long as the IJV was clearly identified in the short axis view initially. A second disadvantage is that the relative medial vs lateral location of IJV puncture is difficult to determine because the probe is now oriented vertically. One way to circumvent this problem is to start in short axis and to continue advancing the needle until there is tenting of the IJV in a central location. At this point the transducer can be rotated 90°, and the needle tip can be visualized and advanced into the vessel in long axis (Video 29.1). A second alternative is to use a "medial-oblique" approach as described by Dilisio et al. [27]. Here the ultrasound transducer is rotated only 30° to create a hybrid short/long axis view.

Wire Confirmation, Trouble Shooting, and Complications

Once the IJV is punctured, the next step in the Seldinger technique is to advance a guidewire through the needle. The needle is then removed, and after confirmation of the guidewire in the vein, the central venous cannula is introduced over the guidewire. The most reliable means of guidewire confirmation is with the use of concomitant transesophageal echocardiography (TEE) demonstrating the "J" of the wire in the right atrium. This is particularly convenient in line placement for cardiac surgery as TEE is used in many of these procedures. Transthoracic echocardiography (TTE) can also be used for this purpose with the guidewire visualized in the right atrium or inferior vena cava using a subcostal view [28]. If TEE or TTE is not part of the procedure or treatment plan, however, it is possible to visualize the guidewire in the IJV distal to the insertion point either in short or long axis. The guidewire can then be followed inferiorly and sometimes can be seen beneath the clavicle entering the brachiocephalic vein. Because of the close proximity of the proximal IJV and brachiocephalic vein to the innominate and subclavian arteries, however, confirmation using this technique does not exclude inadvertent arterial puncture within the chest. The best means of venous confirmation without the use of TEE or TTE is therefore not ultrasound but pressure monitoring either directly or through column manometry [19].

One of the more common frustrating experiences of trainees is difficult guidewire placement after a seemingly uneventful IJV puncture under ultrasound. Sometimes patients have vascular anomalies, strictures, or obstructions that prevent direct access to the right atrium from the IJV. Most times, however, the patient has no such history and still guidewire placement is difficult. Often in these cases, if the ultrasound probe is placed back on the neck and the needle is visualized again in long axis, it may be determined that the needle is up against the posterior wall of the IJV. When this occurs, blood will still draw easily from the needle, but the guidewire will not advance. If this problem is identified with a long axis view, the needle can simply be withdrawn slightly until it is again visualized in the center of the vessel and the guidewire will often go more smoothly.

Finally, ultrasound can be used to diagnose complications associated with central line placement. In some patients who have had multiple catheter placements or prior dialysis, IJV thrombus, strictures, or anomalies can be identified and avoided prior to cannulation. Neck hematomas from posterior wall or CA puncture can be easily visualized. After central line placement, the high-frequency linear probe can also then be placed on the chest, and pneumothorax can be excluded by visualization of lung sliding, lung pulse, or B lines, the description of which is beyond the scope of this chapter but is further described in Chap. 28.

Summary

Real-time ultrasound guidance for IJV central venous catheter placement has become the standard of care because it is easy to use and has been shown to improve first-pass success and reduce complications. Visualization of the IJV and CA can be accomplished with a short axis, a long axis, or a combination of both techniques. Although the long axis technique for IJV cannulation offers the advantage of needle tip visualization, the technique is more difficult to master technically, and this may limit first-pass success and lengthen procedural time compared to the short axis technique [29].

Regardless of the technique, however, the important steps to safe cannulation include confirming the anatomy, visualizing the needle tip, confirming guidewire placement, and confirming venous puncture. Ultrasound can also be used for troubleshooting difficult guidewire placement and complications such as hematoma or pneumothorax.

Ultrasound for Subclavian Vein Cannulation

Anatomy

The subclavian vein (SCV) is a continuation of the axillary vein, running from the lateral border of the first rib until it joins the IJV to form the brachiocephalic vein (Fig. 29.3a). In a recent multicenter randomized controlled trial, SCV cannulation was associated with a lower risk of infection and symptomatic thrombosis than IJV or femoral catheterization [30]. Anatomic landmarks for SCV include the deltopectoral groove and the junction of the middle to inner 1/3 of the clavicle where it enters the thorax. The SCV lies anterior and inferior to the subclavian artery (SCA) with the insertion of the anterior scalene muscle in between them. Other important surrounding structures include the brachial plexus, the pleura, and the thoracic duct (for left SCV).

Figure 29.3b shows an ultrasound image of the SCV and SCA in short axis. To generate this image, the ultrasound probe is placed on the chest approximately 1–2 cm lateral to the junction between the medial and middle 1/3 of the clavicle as would be recommended for needle placement using the landmark technique. The probe is oriented perpendicular to the clavicle with the marker pointed toward the patient's head. The right side of the screen is superior and the left side is inferior. Here the SCV can be identified as the round echo-lucent vessel inferior to the SCA and superior and anterior to the white pleural line. The SCV should be differentiated from the SCA with the SCV as more inferior compared to the SCA, less pulsatile, and more compressible.

Infraclavicular Approach

Although the current standard of care for SCV cannulation is a landmark approach, interest in ultrasound for SCV access is increasing because of the added margin of safety it provides. In a landmark approach, the junction of the medial and middle 1/3 of the clavicle is identified, and the needle enters the skin 1–2 cm inferior and lateral to that point. The needle is then directed superficially toward the suprasternal notch until it butts against the clavicle. The needle is then redirected posteriorly to dive just under the clavicle to access the SVC. While this technique is often successful, the incidence of pneumothorax is higher than IJV cannulation [30] because the technique is blind and the pleura is often adjacent to the SCV. To avoid pneumothorax, the needle is placed just underneath the clavicle, a practice which often makes subsequent wire placement, dilation, and catheter placement difficult.

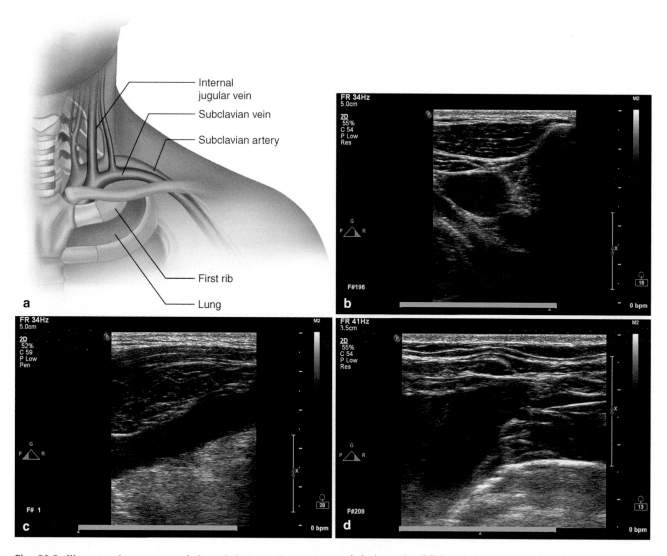

Fig. 29.3 Illustrates the anatomy of the subclavian vein and its relationship to the subclavian artery, clavicle, and lung (**a**). Ultrasound imaging of the subclavian vein is demonstrated in short axis (**b**) and long axis (**c**). It is important to note the close relationship between the subclavian vein (SCV), subclavian artery (SCA), and pleural line. Ultrasound imaging of the subclavian vein (SCV) from a supraclavicular approach (**d**) also illustrates the proximity of the subclavian vein (SCV) and the innominate vein (InV) to the pleura

When using ultrasound, the probe is placed on the chest just inferior to the clavicle approximately over the site of needle puncture for the landmark technique. As described above, the SCV and SCA can be identified in short axis, and the ultrasound probe can then be centered over the SCV (Fig. 29.3b). Turning the probe 90° counterclockwise will then create a long axis view of the SCV (Fig. 29.3c). The identity of the SCV should then be confirmed by angling the probe toward the head of the patient and visualizing the pulsating SCA in long axis and then angling the probe back toward the feet and visualizing the compressible SCV. At this point the probe will be at an oblique angle to the clavicle, parallel with the deltopectoral groove (Video 29.3). The needle can then be introduced from the distal end of the ultrasound probe and the entire shaft, and needle tip can be visualized in plane of the ultrasound as it is advanced into the SCV. Depending on the size of the patient and footprint of the ultrasound probe, the actual puncture site of the vessel may technically be in the axillary vein rather than the SCV. This should be kept in mind when determining the depth of the catheter with final placement as the entrance point of the catheter may be several centimeters more distal than standard SCV placement.

Compared to a landmark technique, ultrasound-guided SCV cannulation has been associated with reduced complications and decreased numbers of attempts [11]. A short axis technique for SCV cannulation has been described as well. As in IJV cannulation, the long axis technique has the advantage of needle tip visualization, which is particularly important with SCV cannulation because of the close proximity of the SCV to the pleura. The short axis technique has been associated with a significantly higher rate of posterior wall puncture than the long axis technique [26]. The long axis technique, however, maybe technically more difficult than the short axis technique and is associated with longer procedure time and lower first-pass success rates [31].

Supraclavicular Approach

An alternative to the traditional infraclavicular technique is the supraclavicular approach. First described in 1965 [2], the supraclavicular approach to the SCV has a number of advantages such as a straighter path to the superior vena cava, less proximity to the pleura, and the ability to keep the catheter out of the surgical field during cardiac or thoracic surgery [32, 33].

With the landmark approach for supraclavicular SCV cannulation, the needle is inserted above the clavicle, just lateral to the sternocleidomastoid muscle, and advanced superficially toward the suprasternal notch. The goal is to puncture the SCV just before it joins the IJV to form the brachiocephalic vein [34]. Figure 29.3 illustrates the close

relationship between the SCV, SCA, brachial plexus, and the upper dome of the pleura highlighting the potential for complications with a blind technique. An ultrasound-guided approach has been described for supraclavicular SCV cannulation that may reduce the risk of inadvertent arterial puncture, brachial plexus injury, or pneumothorax [35–38].

Similar to the IJV and infraclavicular ultrasound techniques, the probe is placed just proximal to the needle insertion site used for the landmark approach. For supraclavicular SCV cannulation, the probe is placed just above the clavicle and directly over the sternocleidomastoid muscle. Alternatively, the ultrasound probe can be placed on the neck as one would do with IJV cannulation and then the IJV can be followed down the neck until it joins the SCV. With this technique, the IJV will be seen in short axis, and the SCV and brachiocephalic vein will be seen in long axis (Fig. 29.3d).

Some authors recommend using a special probe for the supraclavicular SCV technique, either an endocavitary probe [35] or a "hockey stick" probe [38]. While these small probes may be convenient in the small space of the supraclavicular fossa, a standard high-frequency linear probe can be used as well. Once the SCV is visualized in long axis just below the clavicle, an in-plane technique can be used for needle guidance. Head-to-head comparisons of the supraclavicular and infraclavicular techniques have suggested that the supraclavicular approach may result in better imaging of the SCV, shorter mean puncture times, fewer attempts, and less guidewire misplacement [37, 39].

Wire Confirmation, Trouble Shooting, and Complications

As with IJV cannulation, the Seldinger technique is the most widely used technique for SCV central line placement. Accordingly, after accessing the vein with the needle, the next step is wire placement. The advantage of using real-time ultrasound for SCV cannulation is that the ultrasound can also be used to confirm the path of the wire into the brachiocephalic vein than retrograde up into the IJV. Other complications such as inadvertent arterial placement, hematoma, and even pneumothorax can also be evaluated using real-time ultrasound.

Summary

While the traditional landmark approach is still widely used, there is increasing interest in the use of real-time ultrasound for SCV cannulation. The ultrasound technique for the SCV is easy to learn and allows direct visualization of surrounding structures such as the SCA, the brachial plexus, and the pleura so that they can be avoided, and this technique may be associated with a reduced risk of arterial puncture and/or hematoma [9]. The SCV can be accessed either from a supraclavicular or an infraclavicular approach, both of which can be performed with real-time ultrasound guidance. Perhaps the biggest advantage of ultrasound guidance for SCV cannulation is the ability to immediately identify complications such as inadvertent arterial placement, hematoma, wire misdirection, or pneumothorax. Based on these advantages, it is likely that the use of ultrasound for SCV cannulation will continue to increase.

Ultrasound for Femoral Vein Cannulation

Anatomy

Although associated with increased risk of infection and thrombosis in some studies [30], femoral vein (FV) cannulation is often used in emergencies when rapid access is needed or if IJV/SCV cannulation is impossible or contraindicated. The FV is part of the neurovascular bundle that lies within the femoral triangle. The borders of the femoral triangle are the inguinal ligament superiorly, the adductor longus muscle medially, and the sartorius muscle laterally. Inside the triangle, the FV and femoral artery (FA) run within the femoral sheath with the femoral nerve just outside and lateral to the sheath (Fig. 29.4a).

With a landmark technique for FV access, the FA is palpated immediately below the inguinal ligament. The FV is then found approximately 0.5 cm medial to this point. Care must be taken to access the FV distal to the inguinal ligament in order to compress the vessel adequately to prevent hematoma formation either with posterior wall puncture and hematoma or with catheter removal. Placement too far below the inguinal ligament, however, increases the risk of inadvertent arterial puncture, as in the more distal portion of the thigh; the FV becomes posterior to the FA rather than medial to it.

Ultrasound Technique

Real-time ultrasound-guided FV cannulation has been associated with improved first time and overall success rate compared with traditional landmark technique [9], particularly when placed during CPR [10]. As with IJV cannulation, the ultrasound probe is placed on the skin in the same location as described by the landmark technique. For the FV, ideal probe placement is over the femoral triangle just inferior to the inguinal ligament. With a short axis technique, the FA can easily be identified as a round echo-lucent pulsating structure

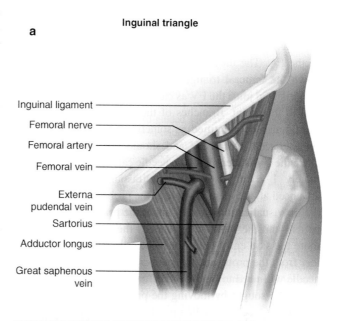

Inguinal triangle

Inguinal ligament —
Femoral nerve —
Femoral artery —
Femoral vein —
Externa pudendal vein —
Sartorius —
Adductor longus —
Great saphenous vein —

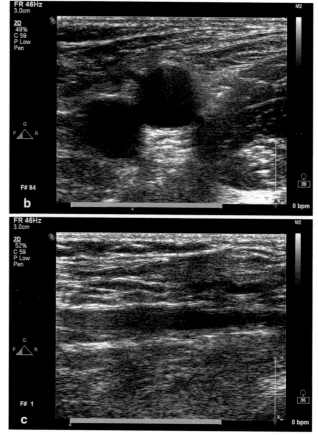

Fig. 29.4 Illustrates the anatomy of the femoral vein (**a**). Ultrasound imaging of the femoral vein in short axis (**b**) and long axis (**c**). It is important to note the close relationship between the femoral vein (FV), femoral artery (FA), and femoral nerve (FN)

jugular vein central catheters using ultrasound guidance. Crit Care Med. 2009;37(8):2345–9. quiz 2359.

26. Vogel JA, Haukoos JS, Erickson CL, Liao MM, Theoret J, Sanz GE, Kendall J. Is long-axis view superior to short-axis view in ultrasound-guided central venous catheterization? Crit Care Med. 2015;43(4):832–9.

27. Dilisio R, Mittnacht AJ. The "medial-oblique" approach to ultrasound-guided central venous cannulation--maximize the view, minimize the risk. J Cardiothorac Vasc Anesth. 2012;26(6):982–4.

28. Arellano R, Nurmohamed A, Rumman A, Day AG, Milne B, Phelan R, Tanzola R. The utility of transthoracic echocardiography to confirm central line placement: an observational study. Can J Anaesth. 2014;61(4):340–6.

29. Chittoodan S, Breen D, O'Donnell BD, Iohom G. Long versus short axis ultrasound guided approach for internal jugular vein cannulation: a prospective randomised controlled trial. Med Ultrason. 2011;13(1):21–5.

30. Parienti JJ, Mongardon N, Megarbane B, Mira JP, Kalfon P, Gros A, Marque S, Thuong M, Pottier V, Ramakers M, et al. Intravascular complications of central venous catheterization by insertion site. N Engl J Med. 2015;373(13):1220–9.

31. Vezzani A, Manca T, Brusasco C, Santori G, Cantadori L, Ramelli A, Gonzi G, Nicolini F, Gherli T, Corradi F. A randomized clinical trial of ultrasound-guided infra-clavicular cannulation of the subclavian vein in cardiac surgical patients: short-axis versus long-axis approach. Intensive Care Med. 2017;43:1594.

32. Patrick SP, Tijunelis MA, Johnson S, Herbert ME. Supraclavicular subclavian vein catheterization: the forgotten central line. West J Emerg Med. 2009;10(2):110–4.

33. Kocum A, Sener M, Caliskan E, Bozdogan N, Atalay H, Aribogan A. An alternative central venous route for cardiac surgery: supraclavicular subclavian vein catheterization. J Cardiothorac Vasc Anesth. 2011;25(6):1018–23.

34. Brahos GJ. Central venous catheterization via the supraclavicular approach. J Trauma. 1977;17(11):872–7.

35. Mallin M, Louis H, Madsen T. A novel technique for ultrasound-guided supraclavicular subclavian cannulation. Am J Emerg Med. 2010;28(8):966–9.

36. Takechi K, Tubota S, Nagaro T. Ultrasound-guided in-plane supraclavicular approach for central venous catheterisation in patients with underlying bleeding disorders. Anaesth Intensive Care. 2011;39(6):1156–8.

37. Byon HJ, Lee GW, Lee JH, Park YH, Kim HS, Kim CS, Kim JT. Comparison between ultrasound-guided supraclavicular and infraclavicular approaches for subclavian venous catheterization in children--a randomized trial. Br J Anaesth. 2013;111(5):788–92.

38. Saini V, Samra T. Ultrasound guided supraclavicular subclavian cannulation: a novel technique using "hockey stick" probe. J Emerg Trauma Shock. 2015;8(1):72–3.

39. Thakur A, Kaur K, Lamba A, Taxak S, Dureja J, Singhal S, Bhardwaj M. Comparative evaluation of subclavian vein catheterisation using supraclavicular versus infraclavicular approach. Indian J Anaesth. 2014;58(2):160–4.

40. Shiloh AL, Savel RH, Paulin LM, Eisen LA. Ultrasound-guided catheterization of the radial artery: a systematic review and meta-analysis of randomized controlled trials. Chest. 2011;139(3):524–9.

41. Tada T, Amagasa S, Horikawa H. Usefulness of ultrasonic two-way Doppler flow detector in percutaneous arterial puncture in patients with hemorrhagic shock. J Anesth. 2003;17(1):70–1.

42. Shiver S, Blaivas M, Lyon M. A prospective comparison of ultrasound-guided and blindly placed radial arterial catheters. Acad Emerg Med. 2006;13(12):1275–9.

43. Sandhu NS, Patel B. Use of ultrasonography as a rescue technique for failed radial artery cannulation. J Clin Anesth. 2006;18(2):138–41.

Intraoperative Transesophageal Echocardiography for Thoracic Surgery

30

Massimiliano Meineri

Abbreviations

TEE	Transesophageal echocardiography		
3D TEE	Three-dimensional transesophageal echocardiography		
TTE	Transthoracic echocardiography		
Anatomy		*TEE views*	
LV	Left ventricle	TG SAX	Transgastric short axis view
RV	Right ventricle	ME 4C	Mid-esophageal four chamber view
LA	Left atrium	ME 2C	Mid-esophageal two chamber view
RA	Right atrium	ME RV In-Out	Mid-esophageal right ventricle inflow-outflow view
LVOT	Left ventricular outflow tract	ME BiC	Mid-esophageal bicaval view
RVOT	Right ventricular outflow tract	ME Asc Ao SAX	Mid-esophageal ascending aorta short axis view
PFO	Patent foramen ovale	UE Ao Arch SAX	Upper esophageal aortic arch short axis view
TV	Tricuspid valve	*Measures*	
PV	Pulmonic valve	LVEDD	Left ventricular end-diastolic diameter
IAS	Interatrial septum	LVESD	Left ventricular end-systolic diameter
IVS	Interventricular septum	LVEDA	Left ventricular end-diastolic diameter
IVC	Inferior vena cava	LVESA	Left ventricular end-systolic area
SVC	Superior vena cava	LVEDV	Left ventricular end-diastolic volume
PA	Pulmonary artery	LVESV	Left ventricular end-systolic volume

RPA	Right pulmonary artery	RVEDA	Right ventricular end-diastolic area
LPA	Left pulmonary artery	FS	Fractional shortening
PV	Pulmonary veins	FAC	Fractional area change
LUPV	Left upper pulmonary vein	LVEF	Left ventricular ejection fraction
LLPV	Left lower pulmonary vein	SV	Stroke volume
RUPV	Right upper pulmonary vein	TAPSE	Tricuspid valve annular plane systolic excursion
RLPV	Right lower pulmonary vein	TR	Tricuspid regurgitation
		RVSP	Right ventricular systolic pressure

Key Points

- Despite its intuitive advantages, the use of TEE in non-cardiac surgery is still limited by the availability of trained anesthesiologists. In fact, very few studies have looked at the impact of intraoperative TEE in non-cardiac surgery on patients' outcomes.
- TEE is a considered a safe technique. However, despite its relative noninvasiveness, it carries potentially severe complications and needs to be supported by congruent indications.
- Basic hemodynamic monitoring can be easily achieved with TEE. Qualitative and quantitative assessments of right and left ventricular function are feasible and can be integrated as a complete standard in intraoperative hemodynamic monitoring.
- TEE for lung transplant, while standard of care in many centers, is not specifically recommended by current guidelines. TEE provides ideal intraoperative hemodynamic monitoring, and it allows the assessment of all vascular anastomoses immediately after the reperfusion of the graft.

Electronic Supplementary Material The online version of this chapter (https://doi.org/10.1007/978-3-030-00859-8_30) contains supplementary material, which is available to authorized users.

M. Meineri (✉)
Department of Anesthesia, Toronto General Hospital, University of Toronto, Toronto, ON, Canada
e-mail: Massimiliano.meineri@uhn.ca

- TEE has a promising role in the diagnosis and follow-up of both acute and chronic pulmonary embolisms. TEE can easily detect and monitor the effects of acute and chronic pressure overload on the right ventricle and can rule out dangerous intracardiac shunts. These characteristics make it a powerful tool for intraoperative monitoring during pulmonary embolectomy and endarterectomy surgeries.
- The ability to image cardiac structures with a high spatial resolution makes TEE suitable for assessing the effect of mediastinal masses on cardiac chambers. TEE may also provide useful information to guide surgical resection.

Introduction

The use of TEE outside of the cardiac operating room has significantly increased over the last few years. Thoracic surgery is naturally becoming an exciting field for the application of this powerful technology for more than one reason. In fact, in many institutions cardiac anesthetists, most of whom are TEE trained, provide their services to thoracic surgery. Moreover, the physiology of cardiopulmonary interaction, the growing number of combined cardiothoracic operations, and the increasing complexity of patients' pathologies create the need for the complete intraoperative monitoring of cardiac function.

Guidelines for the use of TEE for intraoperative hemodynamic monitoring of non-cardiac surgery are very vague and make its practice around the world very variable. As the use of the pulmonary artery catheter is falling out of fashion, intraoperative TEE is becoming a reliable and even more powerful alternative [1].

Indications for TEE in Thoracic Surgery

Indications for TEE during thoracic surgery do not differ from other non-cardiac indications, and it is limited to "when the surgery or the patient's cardiovascular morbidities may result in severe hemodynamic pulmonary or neurological compromise" [2]. Currently, there are no scoring systems suggesting how to identify, at baseline, patients who may fit into this category. Thus, the use of TEE outside of cardiac anesthesia remains heavily based on single center resources and practice. Based on current evidence, the aim of a TEE exam during major thoracic surgery should be directed toward identification of atrial septal defect, myocardial ischemia, hypovolemia, pericardial tamponade, thromboembolic events (Category B2 evidence: high agreement members

opinion), pericardial effusion, tamponade, and intrapulmonary emboli in other major surgery (i.e., lung, renal, abdominal, and head/neck/chest wall surgeries) (Category B3 evidence: intermediate agreement members opinion).

However, current guidelines suggest TEE should be performed in all open-heart surgery. Pulmonary embolectomy and lung transplant may be considered an intracardiac procedure as they involve great vessels and often the use of mechanical circulatory support.

None of the studies used to gage recommendations was specifically conducted in thoracic surgery, and some included cardiac surgical patients [3, 4]; however the care of thoracic surgery patients may share common scenarios with other surgical settings. The lack of outcome trials looking at the impact of the use of intraoperative TEE in non-cardiac surgery makes it still an interesting field for future research.

The impact of emergent TEE in the course of cardiac arrest in non-cardiac patients has been specifically assessed in the operating room [5], as well as during in-hospital resuscitation [6]. In both settings, TEE has been reported to provide prompt diagnosis of the cause of circulatory arrest in 64–86% of the cases and to guide new surgical intervention in 54% of the patients. The ability of TEE to identify the etiology of cardiac arrest has been quantified with a sensitivity and specificity of 90 and 50%, respectively [6] (Table 30.1). The release of new portable TEE equipment and the fact that TEE does not interfere with cardiopulmonary resuscitation (CPR) make TEE suitable to be integrated into advanced cardiac life support algorithms.

In North America, the need for TEE-certified anesthesiologists [7] and the availability of TEE equipment are the main limitations to the routine use of TEE outside of the cardiac operating room. Some authors have suggested that the use of a simplified focused TEE examination for transplant surgery may be adequate [8]. The American National Board of Echocardiography has introduced a new certification process in basic perioperative TEE [9] that will potentially expand the use of TEE as an intraoperative monitoring tool.

Safety and Complications of TEE Probe Insertion

Although none of the studies mentioned above reported any complication related to the use of TEE, the insertion and manipulation of the TEE probe is not free of risks [10]. Major complications in the use of TEE have been described and include esophageal dissection [11] and perforation [12].

Two large retrospective reviews on cardiac surgical patients undergoing intraoperative TEE reported incidences of major complications, respectively, of 0.2% of

Table 30.1 Use of TEE in non-cardiac surgery

Author/year	Number of patients	Indication	Type of surgery	Type of study	Change hemodynamic management	Change surgical management
Canthy/2009	13	I 4 (30%) II 9 (70%)	Gynecology, neurosurgery	Retrospective	9/13 (69%)	2/13 (14%)
Schulmeyer/2006	98	II 98 (100%)	Abdominal, gynecology, urology	Prospective	47/98 (48%)	3/98 (3%)
Hofer/2004	99	II 99 (100%)	Vascular, lung transplant, liver transplant, thoracic, orthopedic, reconstructive	Prospective cohort	54/99 (55%)	3/99 (3%)
Denault/2002	155	I 44 (28%) II 57 (37%) III 54 (35%)	Vascular, neurosurgery, lung transplant	Retrospective	43/155 (27%)	10/155 (6%)
Suriani/1998	123	II 123 (100%)	Vascular, abdominal, hepatic, thoracic, head and neck, urology	Retrospective	78/123 (63%)	2/123 (1%)
Kolev/1998	224	I 48 (26%), II 151 (67%) III 15 (7%)	Cardiac 155 (69%), non-cardiac 69 (31%)	Prospective multicenter cohort	25% of all interventions were uniquely based on TEE	9/224 (4%)
Brandt/1998	66	I 66 (100%)	Cardiac and non-cardiac	Retrospective	53 (80%)	15 (23%)

patients with no associated deaths [13] and of 0.1% with a mortality of 0.02% [14].

A careful assessment of the potential benefit of an intra-operative TEE exam against its potential complications must be performed in each patient.

Preoperative assessment is very important, and patient consent should be obtained whenever possible. A patient's history should be reviewed in order to rule out gastroesophageal pathology. Esophageal narrowing should always be suspected with the presence of dysphagia. A radiological barium swallowing study remains the gold standard to rule out esophageal strictures [10] and should be performed whenever there is clinical suspicion.

The TEE probe should always be gently manipulated, and any force should be avoided in case of resistance to advancement into the esophagus. Esophageal perforation or tear may present soon after the removal of the probe with profuse bleeding from the pharynx or from a nasogastric tube and can present over 48 h after probe insertion [14].

Intubation of the esophagus, in the anesthetized patient, can be performed under direct vision or blindly with the help of jaw thrust maneuver. Esophageal intubation is a strong stimulus, and adequate depths of anesthesia and muscle paralysis are necessary to minimize the hemodynamic impact. It is a standard practice in many centers to insert the TEE probe right after the placement of the endotracheal tube.

To minimize the risk of esophageal injury, the use of a pediatric TEE probe (Fig. 30.1) should be considered in very small-sized adults.

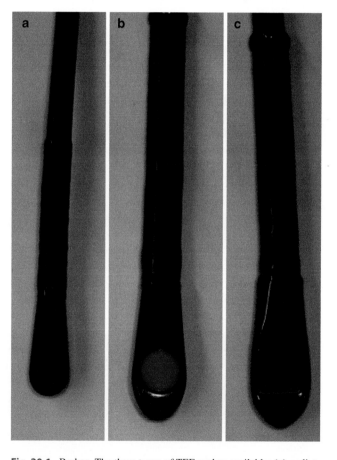

Fig. 30.1 Probes. The three types of TEE probes available: (**a**) pediatric, (**b**) adult Omniprobe, (**c**) adult 3D

Basic Hemodynamic Assessment

A complete intraoperative TEE assessment comprises the use of an omniplane TEE probe and the analysis of 28 standard TEE views [15]. It should be performed at baseline and requires an expertise in TEE. Current guidelines do not specify how often a complete exam should be repeated during the course of surgery and what views should be used for intraoperative hemodynamic monitoring.

After a complete baseline exam, many authors [3, 16–18] chose to leave the TEE probe in the stomach and use the transgastric short axis view (TG SAX) for the continuous assessment of LV function.

Visual analysis of the short axis of the LV in the TG SAX view provided adequate qualitative, online assessment of LV and RV function as well as an estimated volume status in many studies [3, 16–18].

TEE has been reported to predict postoperative myocardial infarction in patients following surgical myocardial revascularization [19], but its role in the detection of intraoperative myocardial ischemia in non-cardiac surgery has been heavily questioned by negative studies [20].

A simplified approach to intraoperative TEE hemodynamic monitoring identifies five possible hemodynamic states [21] (Table 30.2): normal, hypovolemia, LV systolic failure, LV diastolic failure, and right ventricular (RV) failure.

The differential diagnosis of hemodynamic status can be easily accomplished by combining the assessment of LV and RV function with the estimation of left atrial (LA) pressure.

An easy way of visually assessing LA pressure in mechanically ventilated patients is to determine the movement of the interatrial septum during the respiratory cycle [22] (Fig. 30.2). A fixed septum that never shifts left and right is a sign of increased LA pressure; this technique has been successfully validated against invasive monitoring [23]. We will discuss the assessment of LV and RV function in detail in the next paragraphs.

It has been reported that novices can achieve adequate confidence in assessing basic hemodynamics after a minimum number of supervised studies [24].

Assessment of Left Ventricular (LV) Function

Assessment of LV function includes assessments of the LV preload, global, and regional systolic function and diastolic function.

For the basic assessment of LV function [25], three standard views must be obtained: TG SAX, mid-esophageal four-chamber view (ME 4C), and mid-esophageal two-chamber view (ME 2C) (Fig. 30.3).

The LV end-diastolic volume (LVEDV) is the best estimate of LV preload [21, 26]. LVEDV can be easily estimated by the linear measurement of the LV infero-anterior end-diastolic diameter (LVEDD) or, more precisely, the LV end-diastolic area (LVEDA) in the TG SAX view [27] (Fig. 30.4). Complete emptying of the LV with virtualization of the LV cavity at end-systole is also a sign of decreased preload.

Table 30.2 Hemodynamic status

Status	LV EDV	LV systolic function	LV diastolic function	RV systolic function	IAS in Systole
Normal	Normal	Normal	Normal	Normal	Swing
Hypovolemia	Decreased	Normal or increased	Normal	Normal	Swing
LV failure	Increased	Decreased	Normal or abnormal	Normal	Fixed
LV diastolic failure	Decreased	Normal	Abnormal	Normal	Fixed
RV failure	Decreased	Normal	Normal or abnormal	Decreased	Fixed

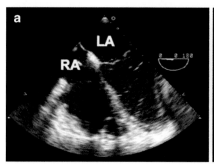 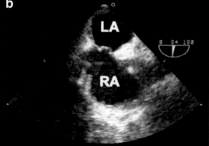 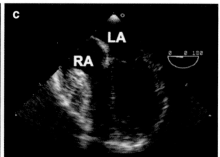

Fig. 30.2 Interatrial septum shift. In mechanically ventilated patients, the movement of the interatrial septum (IAS) during the respiratory cycle reflects the pressure in the atrial chambers. High LA pressure results in a right bulge of the IAS that remains immobile during the respiratory cycle (**a**). Low LA pressure allows left and right IAS shifting that often presents as a "wrinkled" IAS (**b**). A fixed left bulge is characteristic of high RA pressure(**c**)

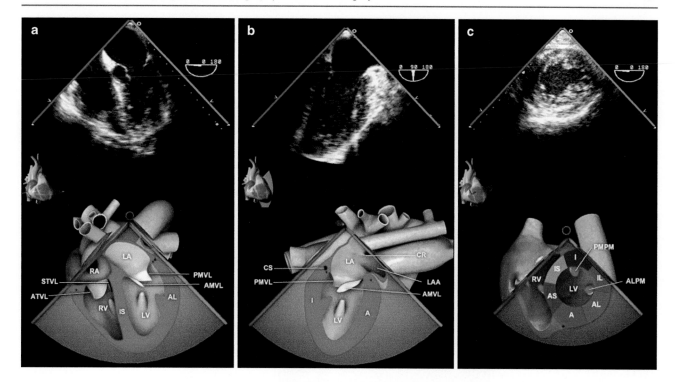

Fig. 30.3 LV views. Assessment of the left ventricular function requires obtaining the following three standard views: mid-esophageal four-chamber view (**a**), mid-esophageal two-chamber view (**b**), trans-gastric left ventricular mid short axis view (**c**). (Courtesy of Michael Corrin (http://pie.med.utoronto.ca/TEE))

The LV ejection fraction (LVEF) is the percentage change in LV volume during the cardiac cycle and reflects the global LV systolic function. It is defined by the equation,

LVEF = [(LVEDV-LVESV)/LVEDV] × 100, where LVESV is the LV end-systolic volume.

TG SAX allows the visual assessment of global LV systolic function and was shown to correlate well with measured LVEF even when assessed by novices [28].

The quantification of LV function can be done in one (measuring diameters), two (measuring areas), or three dimensions (measuring volumes) (Fig. 30.4).

Linear measurement of LV function consists of the measurement of fractional shortening or the percentage of change in the LV diameter during the cardiac cycle. It can be achieved by tracing a line across the maximum LV diameter in the TG SAX view, and, although based on the movement of two points in the entire LV, it correlates with LV EF.

In the same view, the fractional area change (FAC), or the percentage change in the LV cross-sectional area during the cardiac cycle, can be measured. It is easily obtained by tracing the endocardial border of the LV in the end-systolic and the end-diastolic frames. FAC is easy to calculate and correlates well with the ejection fraction. Automatic endocardial border detection and automatic continuous FAC calculation software has been developed for continuous intraoperative monitoring but, after successful testing [29], never became widely used.

Global LV function can also be assessed by deriving the LV stroke volume (SV) from the Doppler measurement of the blood flow at the level of the LV outflow tract (LVOT) [30]. This technique is complex and may underestimate LV SV by underestimating the flow across the LVOT due to the malalignment of the Doppler beam and the LVOT flow.

LV volumes can be measured using the biplane method of the disks (modified Simpson's rule). It is based on the concept of dividing the LV cavity into a stack of 20 ellipsoids whose height is directly related to the length on the LV. After manually tracing the endocardial border in the end-diastolic and the end-systolic frames of a ME 2C and a ME4C view, the modern echocardiographic machine automatically calculates LVEDV, LVESV, SV, and EF. This method is considered the gold standard [25], but it is time-consuming, requires good quality images, and necessitates experience with the technology.

To standardize the assessment of LV regional wall motion, the American Society of Echocardiography (ASE) classification divided the LV into 17 segments (Fig. 30.5) [31]. The segments are grouped into three levels, namely, the basal (six), mid-ventricular (six), and apical (four), plus an apical cap. For a complete assessment of LV regional wall motion, all segments should be displayed and individually assessed according to a rating scale (Table 30.3).

Fig. 30.4 Common methods and normals for quantification of LV function

Measure	Formula	Normal values
Fractional shortening (FS) 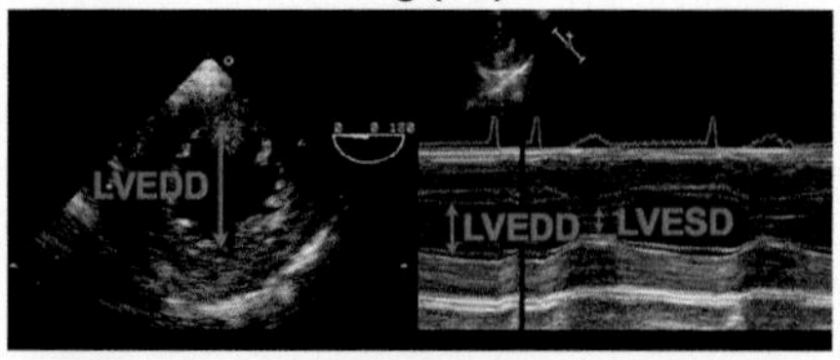 	[(LVEDD-LVESD)/ LVEDD]×100	FS: 25–45 % LVEDD: 4–5 cm
Fractional area change (FAC) 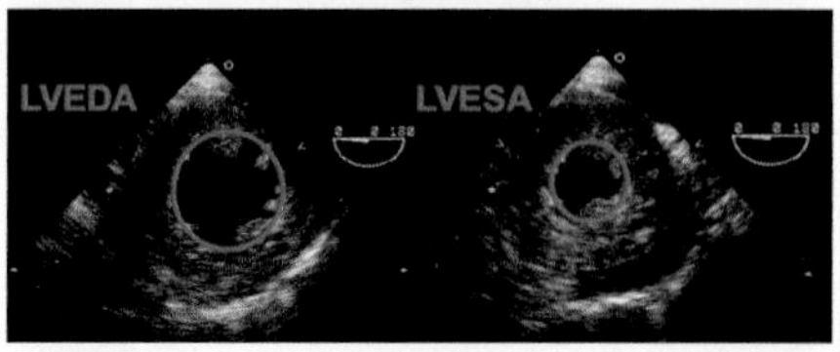 	[(LVEDA-LVESA)/ LVEDA]×100	FAC: >55% LVEDA: 8–12 cm^2
Ejection fraction (EF) 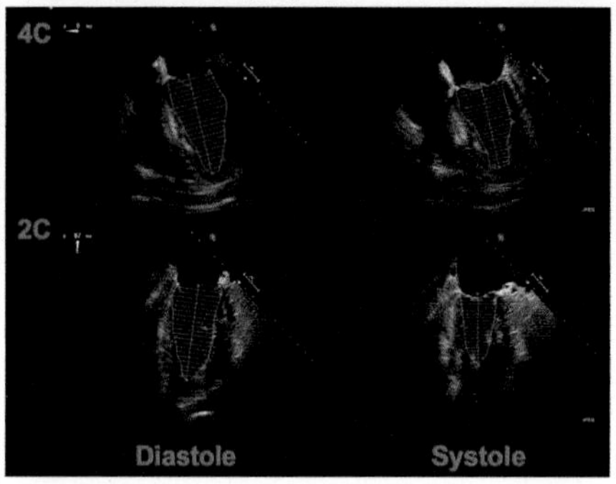 	Automatically calculated based on Simpson's rule	EF: >55%
Stroke volume (SV) 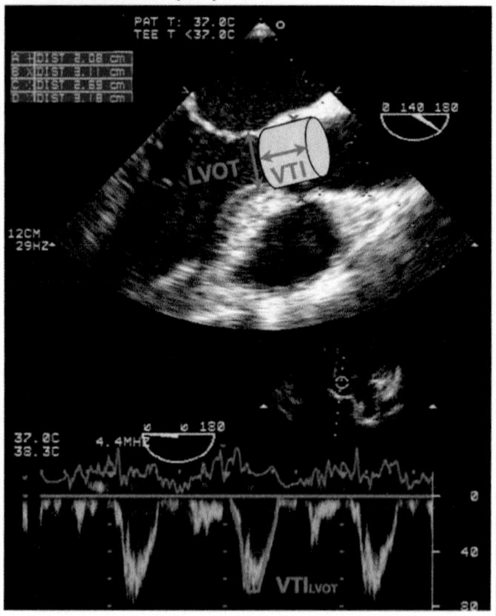 	TT(d_{LVOT}) × VTI_{LVOT}	SV: 50–70 ml

All of the segments are attributed to the main coronary arteries (Fig. 30.5); thus, the analysis of segmental wall motion may allow the localization of individual coronary stenosis [25].

The TG SAX view allows the simultaneous visualization of the territories of the three main coronary arteries.

The quantitative assessment of diastolic dysfunction is complex and requires the assessment of multiple measures [32].

The advent of 3D TEE technology [33] offered the ability of directly and accurately measuring LV volumes [34, 35].

High-quality images of the LV are necessary and currently require the acquisition of a 3D dataset over four or eight heartbeats [36]. The acquired 3D volume "block" will subsequently be analyzed using an off-line quantification software (Philips QLab™, Tomtec™).

Fig. 30.5 17 Segment model and coronary distribution. The diagram explains which left ventricular segments are seen in the most common TEE views of the LV (**a**). The relative coronary distribution is displayed in panel **b**. (Photo is courtesy of GM Busato)

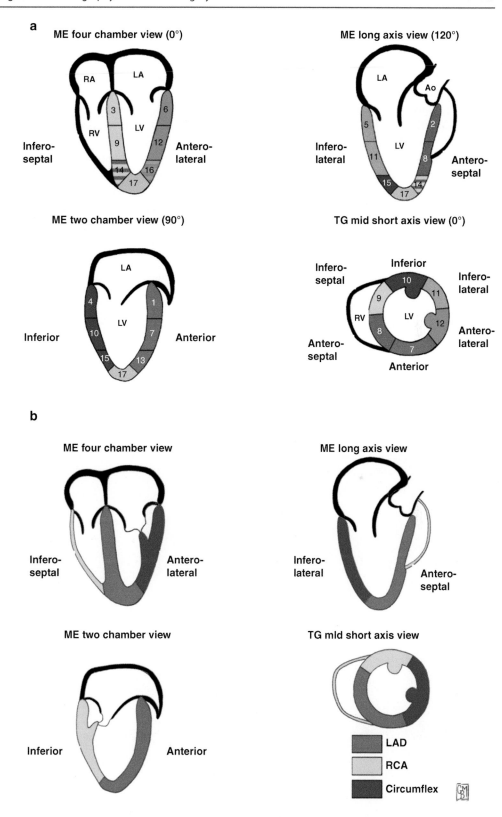

The current software offers a semiautomatic method for the 3D reconstruction of the LV: given six anatomical landmarks on three orthogonal cuts of the full-volume scan of the LV on the systolic and the diastolic frames, the software elaborates a moving 3D cast of the LV cavity. The change in global LV volume is immediately displayed on a graphic plot of the LV volume/time, together with measured LVEDV, LVESV, LVSV, and LVEF.

To allow the assessment of regional LV wall motion, the 3D cast of the LV cavity is divided into 17 pyramids according to the ASE 17 segment model [25], and the change in volume of each pyramid is plotted over time.

The volume/time plots of all segments are superimposed, allowing the assessment of dyssynchrony.

The validity of 3D TEE in assessing LV dyssynchrony has been extensively tested [37, 38] (Fig. 30.6).

The limitation of current 3D technology is the fact that it is not real time and requires an expertise in acquiring and manipulating the datasets. Until newer, more powerful machines will allow automatic LV reconstruction, the role of 3D TEE for the intraoperative monitoring of LV function seems to be limited.

Intraoperative diastolic dysfunction [39] seems to correlate with poor postoperative outcome in non-cardiac surgery [40]. It is unclear how to manage low grades of intraoperative diastolic dysfunction.

However, for a basic hemodynamic assessment, it is important to recognize an increased atrioventricular gradient that corresponds to a severe degree of diastolic dysfunction.

As simplified approach to the assessment of diastolic function allowed grading of dysfunction in patients undergoing coronary revascularization and correlated with short- and long-term outcome [41]. It is based on mitral inflow early wave (E) peak and lateral MV annulus tissue Doppler early wave (E') velocities. $E' < 10$ cm/s defines DD. E/E' is used to grade DD severity: $E/E' < 8$, mild; E/E' 9–12, moderate; and $E/E' > 13$, severe.

Assessment of Right Ventricular (RV) Function

RV dysfunction is very common in patients with severe pulmonary disease [42]. TEE allows prompt diagnosis of

Table 30.3 LV wall motion

Definition	Standard terminology	Sign
Normal movement	Normal	++
Decreased movement	Hypokinetic	+
No movement	Akinetic	0
Outward bulging in systole	Dyskinetic	–
Fixed outward bulging	Aneurysmal	– –

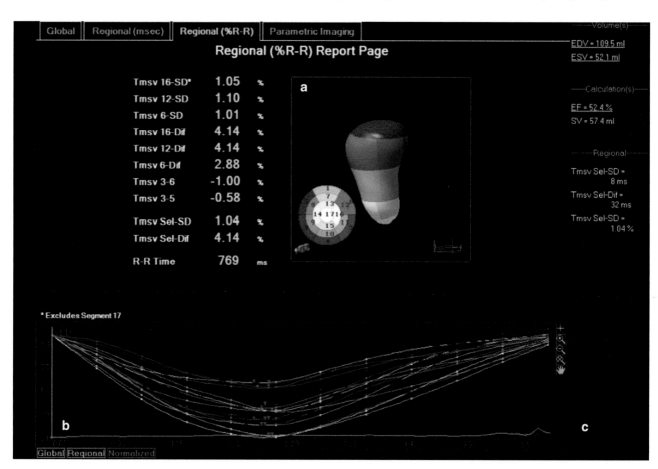

Fig. 30.6 3D TEE LV assessment. Panel **a** displays the left ventricular (LV) cast. The LV cavity is divided into 17 wedges each corresponding to one of the 17 segments. The change in shape of each on the 17 segments is plotted over time (**b**). The LV end-diastolic volume, end-systolic volume, and ejection fraction are automatically measured (**c**)

RV dysfunction but requires an understanding of the pathophysiology of RV dysfunction and the complex 3D RV anatomy [43].

RV dysfunction is characterized by increased RA pressure, venous stasis, low cardiac output, LV diastolic dysfunction, and decreased LV preload [44]. It can be the result of RV pressure or volume overload and RV ischemia. The assessment of RV function includes assessments of the RV morphology and RV systolic function [45].

The right ventricle has a complex 3D architecture as it wraps around a conical LV. The RV can anatomically be divided into three parts: the inlet, composed by the tricuspid valve (TV), the chordae, and the papillary muscles; the trabeculated muscular apex; and the outlet, composed by the smooth muscle outflow tract (RVOT).

The distinctive anatomical features of the RV are a prominent muscular band from the free wall to the IVS, the proximity of the RV apex (moderator band), the more apical attachment of the septal leaflet of the tricuspid valve (TV) in comparison to the anterior leaflet of the mitral valve (MV), and the presence of more than two papillary muscles [46, 47].

The RV is a thin-walled structure, usually exposed to low pressures. The RV is very compliant and sensitive to changes in afterload; an acute increase in afterload results in RV dilatation. Chronic RV pressure overload causes concentric hypertrophy.

The basic TEE assessment of RV function requires the collection of the following three standard views: ME 4C, TG SAX, and mid-esophageal RV inflow-outflow (ME RV in-out) (Fig. 30.7).

The ME 4C view displays the triangular-shaped RV long axis. In this view the RV end-diastolic area (RVEDA) can be measured and compared to the LV EDA (Fig. 30.8a). A nor-

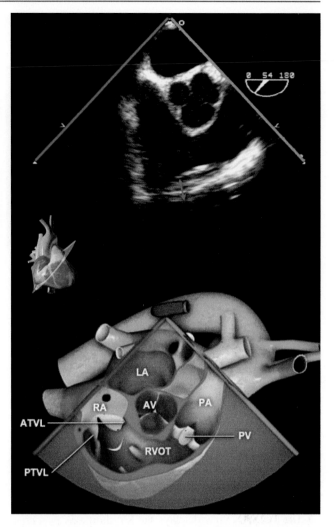

Fig. 30.7 RV inflow-outflow view. In this view the ultrasound beam cuts the RV through its entire length. The arrow indicates RV wall thickness. (Photo is courtesy of Michael Corrin (http://pie.med.utoronto.ca/TEE))

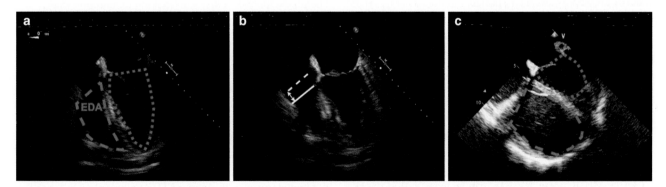

Fig. 30.8 Assessment of RV function. In the mid-esophageal four-chamber view, the right ventricle (RV) end-diastolic area can be measured and compared to LV EDA (**a**). The systolic displacement of the tricuspid valve annulus (TAPSE) (arrow) reflects RV function (**b**). With dilatation, the RV cavity loses its triangular shape and takes over the apex of the heart (**c**)

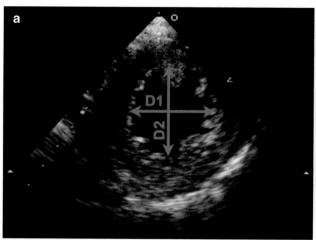

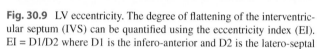

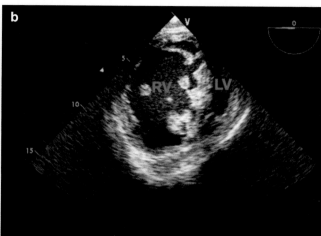

Fig. 30.9 LV eccentricity. The degree of flattening of the interventricular septum (IVS) can be quantified using the eccentricity index (EI). EI = D1/D2 where D1 is the infero-anterior and D2 is the latero-septal LV diameters (**a**). With RV dilatation flattening of the IVS results in a "D"-shaped LV gross section (**b**)

mal RVEDA/LVEDA is <0.6, and a RVEDA/ LVEDA >1 indicates severe RV dilatation [46]. In the same view, we can observe that, as the RV dilates, it loses its triangular shape, and when it is as big as the LV, it starts to share the apex of the heart, to finally take over with severe dilatation [48] (Fig. 30.8c).

The ME RV in-out view displays the RV crescent shape. In this view, the RV inlet, free wall, and outflow tract can be seen; linear measures include the RVOT diameter and the thickness of the RV free wall. A free wall thickness >5 mm at end diastole indicates RV hypertrophy [31].

The TG SAX view displays the RV short axis as a crescent shape attached to a circular LV. With RV pressure overload, RV dilatation displaces the interventricular septum (IVS) toward the left. Distortion of the IVS is measured by the LV eccentricity index, which is the ratio of the LV inferoanterior and septo-lateral LV short axis diameters (Fig. 30.9a). With severe RV dilatation, the LV loses its circular shape and instead becomes D-shaped (eccentricity index >1) (Fig. 30.9b).

RV ejection is generated by three separate mechanisms: inward movement of the RV free wall, apical displacement of the TV annulus, and traction of the free wall by contraction of the LV [49].

Qualitative assessment of RV function consists of visual determination of inward movement of the RV free wall in the ME 4C and the ME RV in-out views (Fig. 30.8).

In the ME 4C view, RV FAC can be measured as the percentage of change of the RV area during the cardiac cycle. RV FAC well correlates with the RV EF measured by cardiac MRI [50]. The predominant motion of RV free wall movement is a sequential longitudinal shortening from the inflow portion of the RV to the infundibulum which can be measured with modern technology by tracking the displacement of RV free wall muscle speckles (speckle tracking). In the ME 4C view, speckle tracking of the RV free wall allows measurement of the percentage of muscle shortening known as strain [51]. This is becoming an accurate quantification of RV function with a normal value >20% that has shown promising prognostic value in the cardiac surgical population [52] (Fig. 30.10).

In the same view, the TV annular plane systolic excursion (TAPSE) can be determined (Fig. 30.8b). In a normal heart, TAPSE is 1.5–2.0 cm, and a TAPSE <1.5 is associated with a poor outcome in patients with heart failure [53]. However, the TV annulus moves in a plane that is almost perpendicular to the TEE ultrasound beam, and this makes the accurate measurement of TAPSE with TEE very difficult.

A recent work further highlighted these limitations in a direct comparison with transthoracic echocardiography and suggested the use of speckle tracking technology [54].

The dilatation of the RV results in TV annular dilatation and regurgitation (TR) [55]. The severity of TR is not directly related to the severity of RV dysfunction. As the RV function deteriorates, the ability of RV to generate pressure is impaired; thus, a large, turbulent TR jet may turn into a low-velocity, laminar flow. In contrast, with RV remodeling following the treatment of RV pressure overload using, for example, pulmonary endarterectomy (PEA), an improvement in TR is observed [56].

Due to the complex shape of the RV, the RV volumes cannot be measured with standard TEE using polygonal models, as are commonly used for the LV.

Real-time 3D TEE overcomes some of the limitations of 2D TEE. A full-volume 3D dataset of the RV is obtained over multiple subsequent heartbeats. The 3D block obtained can then be used for the off-line measurement of right ventricular volume and function using special analytical soft-

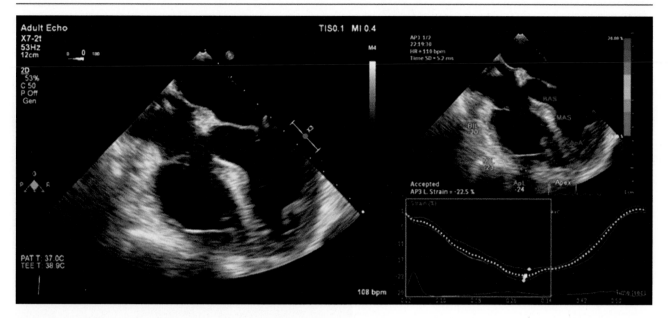

Fig. 30.10 TEE RV strain. Measurement of RV free wall strain. A ME 4C view was analyzed using the LV strain software, and the ME LAX model was applied to the RV to maintain the lateral and septal wall nomenclature. The septum was excluded from the analysis, and a global longitudinal strain was measured at 22.5%, which is considered within normal range

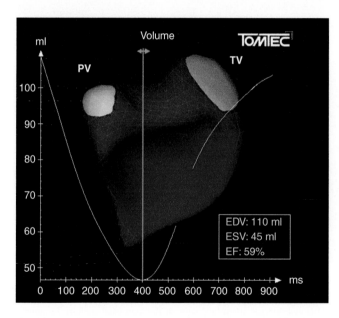

Fig. 30.11 3D TEE RV assessment. 4D RV-Function© application (TomTec Imaging Systems GmbH, Munich, Germany) allows off-line processing of 3D TEE datasets and semiautomatic reconstruction of the RV cavity. In the RV cast tricuspid annulus (TV) and pulmonary valve annulus (PV) can be recognized

ware (4D RV-Function© application; TomTec Imaging Systems GmbH, Munich, Germany). 4D RV-Function© software allows the creation of a cast of the RV cavity and provides automatic measurement of RV volumes and EF (Fig. 30.11).

The feasibility of intraoperative RT 3D TEE has been reported [57]; however, all the literature assessing the accuracy of this technique is based on transthoracic echocardiography (TTE) [58–60] with good correlation with cardiac MRI [58, 59] with better reproducibility than 2D TTE [59] for the assessment of right ventricular volume and function in adults and children [61].

TEE Assessment of PFO

Patent foramen ovale (PFO) is the result of the lack of fusion of the two interatrial septal flaps, the septum primum (left side) and the septum secundum (right side) (Fig. 30.12a). Until birth, an orifice in the septum secundum, covered by a mobile septum primum, allows maternal circulation through the heart.

At birth, as the left atrial pressure overcomes the right atrial pressure, the functional closure of the foramen ovale occurs. Through the years, a permanent fusion of the two flaps will seal the defect.

PFO is relatively common in the general population and is found in about 25% of autopsies [62].

TEE is the gold standard for the detection of PFO, with sensitivity between 80% and 100% and specificity of 100% [63–65].

To rule out the presence of a PFO, the TEE exam should focus on the careful inspection of the interatrial septum (IAS) in the ME 4C view. Once the IAS is visualized, the probe is rotated toward the right to bring the IAS into the middle of the screen. Given the normally small size, a PFO is unlikely noticed as a gap upon 2D examination. The color Doppler volume is then positioned to cover the IAS, and the

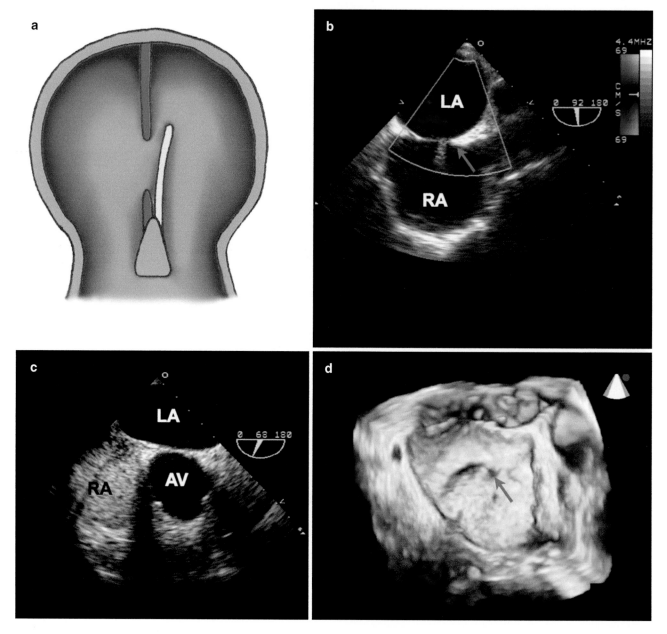

Fig. 30.12 Patent foramen ovale. Patent foramen ovale (PFO) is the result of lack of fusion of the septum primum (left side) and septum secundum (right side) (**a**) (Photo is courtesy of GM Busato). Color Doppler allows identification of flow across a PFO that commonly cre-ates a small left-to-right shunt (**b**). Agitated saline is the contrast medium of choice to confirm and detect the presence of PFO(**c**). 3D TEE can provide an en face view of the interatrial septum. In panel **d** the PFO is seen from the left atrial side

Nyquist limit is adjusted to 45–55 cm/s (Fig. 30.12b). While maintaining the IAS in the middle of the screen, the omnip-lane angle is rotated to slowly scan through the IAS from 0 to 120–130°.

To increase the sensitivity of the exam, a contrast study should be done. This consists of injecting an agitated saline solution through a central or a peripheral line and visualizing the shunt of air bubbles across the IAS.

Normally, the left atrial pressure is higher than that of the right atrial pressure, and even with the injection of agitated saline, a shunt across the IAS cannot be seen. Provocative

maneuvers such as a Valsalva or cough are used at the time of injection in order to increase the right atrial pressure [66] (Fig. 30.12c).

In the operating room on a ventilated patient, the sudden termination of a lung recruitment maneuver can cause an increase in the venous return and a subsequent increase in RA pressure. Thus, it is important to assess the transit of the contract in the atria right at the end of a breath-hold.

A PFO is normally a benign cardiac abnormality, and in many patients, it may remain undiagnosed for their entire life. Factors that determine the clinical significance of a PFO are size, cryptogenic strokes, RA to LA pressure gradient, and flow from the inferior vena cava (IVC).

Smaller PFOs are less likely to be the cause of any symptoms, but they potentially allow paradoxical embolism, which may result in stroke [67]. The closure of the PFO in these circumstances has to be considered as part of the prevention strategy.

With normal RA and LA pressures, a PFO results in a left-to-right shunt. All causes of increased RA pressure can revert the left-to-right shunt and result in hypoxia. An increase in RA pressure is very common in the thoracic surgical population with pulmonary disease and increased RV pressure overload. During major thoracic procedures such as lung transplant surgery, the clamping of the pulmonary artery results in a sudden increase in RV pressure that is reflected in the RA and can cause a hypoxic right-to-left shunt.

A diversion of the IVC flow toward the PFO due to altered anatomy has been described [68] after right pneumonectomy and can be the cause of otherwise unexpected severe hypoxia.

Percutaneous closure of the PFO has become the procedure of choice given its safety and minimal invasiveness [69]. On the other hand, the surgical closure of PFO, although a simple procedure, requires opening the heart chambers under cardiopulmonary bypass.

During thoracic surgery, each patient with an intraoperative TEE diagnosis of PFO should be individually assessed. The detection of a continuous or intermittent right-to-left shunt may direct PFO closure, especially if the procedure involves the use of cardiopulmonary bypass (CPB) anyway.

The best surgical management in the case of incidental intraoperative PFO finding in asymptomatic patients is not clear. In fact, a recent study [70] showed a cardiac surgical population with worse neurological outcomes after surgical PFO closure.

Specific Applications

Lung Transplant

The number of lung transplants has been increasing due to the increased demand for lung transplantation and the use of new techniques to expand the pool of donors [71, 72].

The increase in recipient ages and comorbidities makes optimal intraoperative anesthetic management more challenging. Cardiac abnormalities are commonly associated with severe pulmonary hypertension [73]. Coronary artery disease is present in up to 30% of patients with end-stage lung disease [74], and it is not uncommon for surgical coronary revascularization to be performed at the time of lung transplant.

Extracorporeal membrane oxygenators (ECMO) [75] and pumpless extracorporeal lung support (Novalung™) [76] have been increasingly used as bridges to transplantation (see Chap. 47).

Although its impact on patient outcome is not clear, TEE provides ideal intraoperative monitoring in the course of lung transplant [8]. Current guidelines do not specifically mention this procedure as an indication for TEE; however, it may fall under the category of open-heart surgery [77]. Older ASE guidelines considered the use of TEE for lung transplant surgery as a Category II indication, as lung transplant recipients are at high risk for intraoperative hemodynamic compromise and for problems with surgical anastomoses [78].

Table 30.4 summarizes the focus of the intraoperative TEE examination at different stages of the lung transplant.

The only direct contraindication to the insertion of the TEE probe in end-stage lung disease may be scleroderma, as it is associated in up to 30% of cases with esophageal strictures [79].

Some authors [8] have suggested inserting the TEE probe at the time of endotracheal intubation, as TEE may provide prompt diagnosis of the hemodynamic instability not uncommon immediately after the induction of anesthesia for lung transplant surgery [80]. The TEE examination should be started as soon as possible after induction, as the prolonged use of electrocautery after skin incision causes artifacts, making the interpretation of TEE images very difficult.

The TEE exam should first confirm the preoperative findings, as a significant amount of time may have passed from the preoperative assessment to the day of surgery.

The baseline TEE assessment should include a complete examination with special attention to RV function and the presence of intracardiac shunts. As previously discussed, a benign left-to-right shunt, such as a small PFO, may revert and cause hypoxia during the course of surgery as the right-

Table 30.4 TEE for lung transplant

Induction	Dissection	PA clamping	Graft reperfusion	Post-implant
TR and RVSP	LV, RV filling, and function	RV function	Intracardiac air and LV function	TR and RVSP
Pulmonary veins				RV, LV function
LV, RV function				Pulmonary veins (all four) and pulmonary artery:
IAS: R/O PFO and intracardiac shunts				R/O stenosis/thrombosis

sided pressure increases after the clamping of the pulmonary artery (PA) or during the manipulation of the heart. The surgeon may decide for the elective use of CPB in these circumstances to repair the PFO.

TEE assessment of extracorporeal devices requires an understanding of the basic circuits and surgical cannulation techniques. The use of TEE for this specific indication is not considered by current ASE guidelines.

Novalung™ is in interventional lung assist device, a pumpless membrane oxygenator, used in severe respiratory failure to provide CO_2 removal and oxygenation. The inflow cannula is placed percutaneously into the femoral artery and provides arterial blood flow to an oxygenator as the outflow cannula returns the oxygenated blood to the femoral vein. Normally the short Novalung™ cannulas are not seen with TEE. In the presence of severe RV pressure overload and hypoxia, Novalung™ has successfully been implanted between the main PA and the left upper pulmonary vein, creating a septostomy-like shunt [76]. In these circumstances, TEE can easily visualize the cannulas and assess the flow (Fig. 30.13).

Whenever respiratory insufficiency is associated with heart failure, the use of ECMO becomes mandatory. An inflow cannula provides venous blood to an oxygenator that is pumped back to the patient's artery or vein by a centrifugal pump. Femoral or jugular vessels are commonly used for cannulation, which can be performed percutaneously [81]. While the short arterial cannula cannot usually be seen by TEE when inserted peripherally, TEE becomes crucial for guiding the positioning of the long venous cannulas, specifically when using the jugular Avalon™ cannula [82].

Malpositioning of the venous cannula would result in impaired venous return and an inability to provide adequate arterial blood. In lung transplant recipients, TEE should assess the position and patency of the venous cannula at baseline and, when still necessary, after CPB.

During dissection of the native lungs, significant mechanical compression of the heart and distortion of great vessels can cause hemodynamic instability. TEE can promptly exclude other causes of hypotension, and manual compression of the heart chambers can easily be detected.

The use of CPB for lung transplantation, although not associated with increased mortality [83], certainly carries significant adverse effects such as systemic inflammatory syndrome and coagulopathy [84].

One indication for the elective use of CPB during lung transplantation is the need for simultaneous open-heart procedures. Given the lack of guidelines, the threshold for the use of CPB for lung transplant varies among different institutions. CPB is used in the presence of an occurrence of acute circulatory failure that usually presents as severe right ventricular failure at clamping of the PA. In these circumstances, TEE is a very sensitive tool for assessing RV function in real time [48, 85], can detect early signs of RV failure after manual clamping of the PA, and can prompt the use of CPB, thereby avoiding dangerous circulatory collapse [86].

After the completion of graft anastomoses, it is not uncommon to observe hypotension and ventricular failure at the unclamping of arterial and venous anastomoses. TEE commonly reveals a flush of air bubbles from the transplanted lung into the LV at this phase of the operation. Coronary air embolism, hypothermia, and metabolites from the preservative solution may cause severe LV failure at this stage.

TEE will assist weaning from CPB, as for all cardiac procedures, by monitoring the proper de-airing of the heart chambers and guiding the hemodynamic management. TEE allows the prompt diagnosis of post-CPB dynamic LV outflow tract obstruction and is very useful in guiding hemodynamic management in this condition [87].

Severe pulmonary hypertension and RV failure have been observed after the administration of protamine; TEE is thus critical in monitoring RV function should, at this time and whenever during the course of the surgery, treatment with pulmonary vasodilators became necessary [88].

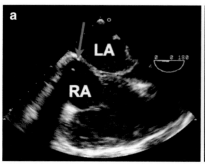 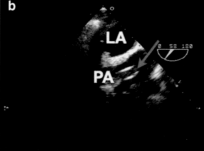 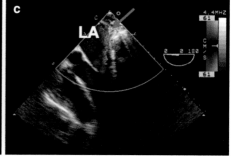

Fig. 30.13 Cannulas. TEE allows assessment of atrial cannulas for ECMO or Novalung. (**a**) the arrow indicates the ECMO venous cannula in the right atrium. When the Novalung™ is used for central bypass and decompression of the right heart chambers, the inflow cannula (flow to the Novalung) is placed in the pulmonary artery (PA) (**b**), and the outflow cannula (return to the patient) is positioned in a pulmonary vein (here the left upper pulmonary vein) and drains into the left atrium (LA) (**c**)

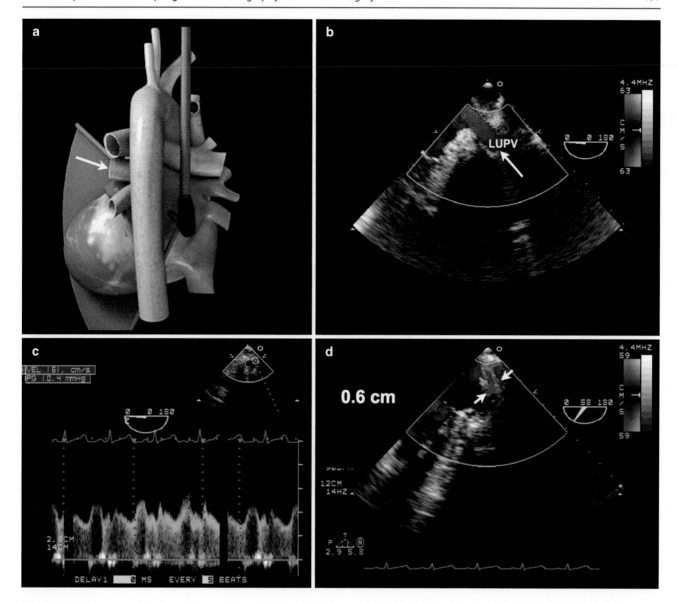

Fig. 30.14 TEE view of the pulmonary veins. After double-lung transplant the four pulmonary veins should be examined (**a**). The left upper pulmonary vein (arrow) is the easiest to image (**b**). Turbulent flow may correlate with narrowing (**d**) and normally leads to flow acceleration (**c**). (Modified from http://pie.med.utoronto.ca/TEE)

Following reperfusion of the grafts, a complete exam should be repeated. A lack of improvement of RV function following lung transplant has been associated with a poor outcome [89].

The visualization and measurement of flow in all of the pulmonary veins and pulmonary arteries is mandatory at this stage of surgery [90] and requires advanced TEE skills.

The proximal portion of the main pulmonary artery is seen with the PV and RVOT in the ME RV in-out view; in this view, its proximal diameter can be measured. Two other views should be used to assess the pulmonary artery: the mid-esophageal ascending aorta short axis (ME Asc Ao SAX) and the upper esophageal aortic arch short axis (UE Ao Arch Sax) (Fig. 30.14).

The ME Asc Ao SAX displays the PA long axis at its bifurcation and the right PA (RPA). The left PA (LPA) is rarely seen as it is shadowed by the left main stem bronchus. In this view, the diameter of the PA anastomosis and the type of flow (laminar vs. turbulent) can be assessed. The UE Ao Arch Sax view shows the long axis of the PA, the bifurcation, and the RPA, and it allows optimal alignment of the Doppler beam to the PA flow and the measurement of the flow velocity. Whenever the quality of TEE images is suboptimal or LPA could not be displayed, pericardial echocardiography should be considered [91].

Pulmonary veins can be seen starting from two standard views: ME 2C and the mid-esophageal bicaval view (ME

BiC). From the ME 2C view while slightly pulling the TEE probe, we can visualize the left upper pulmonary vein (LUPV) that lies right above the LA appendage. By advancing the probe 1–2 cm, the left lower pulmonary vein (LLPV) can be visualized. LLPV is more difficult to see and often merges with the LUPV to form a common vessel. By rotating the probe toward the right, the right upper pulmonary vein (RUPV) is visualized as it enters the LA just above the SVC. By advancing the probe and slightly rotating it to the right, the right lower pulmonary vein (RLPV) can be seen. In all of the mentioned views, the diameter as well as the flow of all PV can be measured. The stenosis and thrombo-

sis of pulmonary venous (PV) anastomoses have been reported by several authors [92], with incidences of PA stenosis around 7% [93] and PV stenosis around 10% [94]. A diameter <5 mm and a peak systolic velocity >1 m/s are considered a cutoff for the definition of PV stenosis [92] (Fig. 30.15).

The gold standard for the diagnosis of PV stenosis and thrombosis remains angiography.

Epicardial echocardiography has also been suggested as an effective alternative to TEE in the assessment of pulmonary venous anastomoses specially when the TEE images are suboptimal [95].

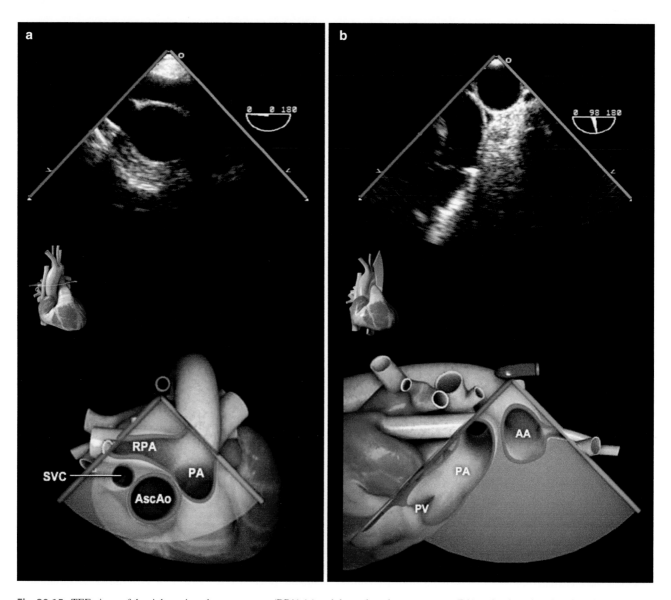

Fig. 30.15 TEE views of the right main pulmonary artery (RPA) (**a**) and the main pulmonary artery (PA) and pulmonic valve (PV) (**b**). (Modified from http://pie.med.utoronto.ca/TEE)

Heart-Lung Transplant

Heart-lung transplant is offered to some patients with congenital heart disease and/or pulmonary hypertension [96]. These patients may present to the operating room with ECMO or Novalung™. The aim of the TEE examination is to guarantee the safe transition to full CPB.

The baseline assessment includes assessments of the cannulas' positioning and flows. The surgery consists of the en bloc transplant of heart and lungs requiring four anastomoses: the trachea, ascending aorta, and inferior and superior vena cava. After weaning from CPB, flow in the IVC and SVC rules out stenoses [97]. In these cases, there is no risk of the stenosis of the pulmonary vein and PA anastomoses as they are not affected by the surgery.

Prolonged CPB may lead to significant edema of the heart and mediastinal structures; RV compression and hypotension may prevent chest closure after heart-lung transplant.

Pulmonary Embolism

The use of TEE for pulmonary embolectomy is not specifically mentioned by current SCA/ASA guidelines [2]. Although there are no outcome studies available assessing this specific application of TEE, it has been successfully used in the diagnosis of acute pulmonary embolism (PE) both in the operating room [98] and in the course of cardiopulmonary resuscitation [99].

Surgical pulmonary embolectomy is more often performed in tertiary care centers and consists of suctioning the fresh thrombi from the main PA on CPB and often positioning of an IVC filter [100].

Chronic PE leads to pulmonary hypertension and ultimately RV failure. Pulmonary thromboendarterectomy (PTE) is considered the definite treatment of pulmonary hypertension in these circumstances. It is commonly per-

formed on CPB with deep hypothermic circulatory arrest and consists of the removal of thrombi and a thorough endarterectomy of the pulmonary circulation [101]. TEE is commonly a part of the intraoperative monitoring for both procedures [102]. Table 30.5 summarizes the focus of intraoperative TEE for PTE.

A complete TEE examination is performed at baseline, and it is focused on the detection of thrombi, the assessment of RV function, and the exclusion of other causes of pulmonary hypertension.

TEE can easily see fresh thrombi in the inferior vena cava, RA, RV, and proximal PA (Fig. 30.16). The presence of free-floating thrombi in the RA is associated with PE in the great majority of patients [103].

However, the ability of TEE in localizing thrombi in the pulmonary circulation is limited by the fact that TEE can only image the proximal pulmonary circulation and that the LPA is often completely shadowed by the left main stem bronchus. PE causes RV pressure overload that manifests with PA, RV dilatation, and TR [45] (Figs. 30.17 and 30.18). RV dysfunction in the course of PE has found to be associated with poor in-hospital outcomes [104]. The assessment of PFO is crucial due to the high risk of paradoxical emboli and, when present, predisposes to poor outcomes [105].

Basic grading of TR at baseline is very important, and it can be performed in the ME 4C and the RV in-out views. It consists of tracing the area of the TR jet and measuring the

Table 30.5 TEE for pulmonary embolectomy

Induction	Weaning from CPB	PA clamping
TR and RVSP	De-airing of RV and LV	TR and RVSP
Pulmonary artery Doppler profile		RV function
	RV, LV function	R/O PA clots
LV, RV function		
IAS: R/O PFO and intracardiac shunts		
R/O clots in RA, RV, and PA		

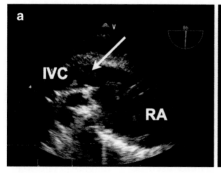
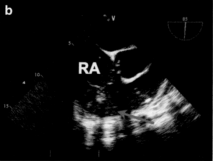
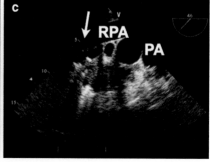

Fig. 30.16 Pulmonary embolism. Presence of thrombi (arrow) in the inferior vena cava (**a**) and right ventricle (arrow) (**b**) very often correlates with pulmonary embolism (**c**)

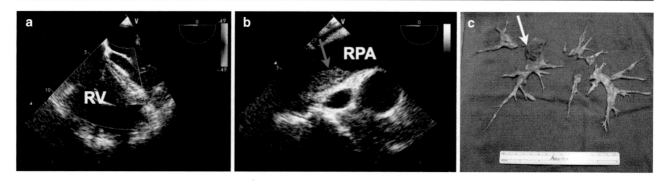

Fig. 30.17 Chronic pulmonary embolism. Chronic pulmonary embolism results in pulmonary hypertension and right ventricular overload and dilatation (**a**). TEE can detect thrombi in the right PA (**b**, arrow). Pulmonary endarterectomy consists in removal of thrombi (arrow) and thorough endarterectomy of the pulmonary circulation (**c**). (Photo is courtesy of Dr. M. De Perrot)

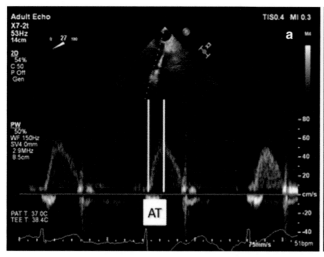
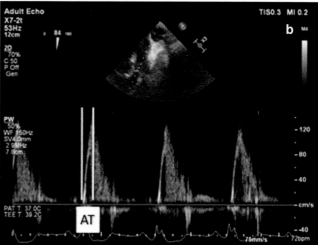

Fig. 30.18 Pulmonary hypertension. Pulsed wave Doppler interrogation of the main pulmonary artery in the UE aortic arch SAX view. Normal pulmonary artery pressure presents with an acceleration time (AT) (time from zero to peak velocity) > 100 ms (**a**). Pulmonary hypertension presents with an AT <100 ms (**b**)

TR jet width at the level of the TV leaflets (vena contracta) [106]. In the ME RV in-out view, Doppler measurement of the TV regurgitant jet peak velocity allows the calculation of the RV end-systolic pressure (RVSP). Due to the malalignment of the Doppler beam and the TR jet, the RVSP is often underestimated with TEE.

Assessment of pulmonary artery flow Doppler trace allows quantification of main pulmonary artery pressures. An increase in the upstroke slope with shortening of time to reach the peak velocity is consistent with increase in pulmonary artery pressures [107] (Fig. 30.19). Pointy traces with high peak velocity are typical in this patients' population where it is also not uncommon to identify a systolic notch. The presence of a notch seems to correlate with severely increased pulmonary vascular resistances.

At separation from cardiopulmonary bypass, TEE is used to guide the careful de-airing of the heart chambers and for hemodynamic management [107]. Preoperative late notching (later than mid ejection), calculated as a notch ratio

(NR) < 1, has been associated with worse postoperative outcome, likely related to more advanced disease [108] (Fig. 30.19).

A complete exam is then repeated at the end of the surgery and is needed to grade RV function, TR, and RVSP.

Improvements in RV function and TR are signs of a successful surgery; in contrast, the persistence of RV dysfunction and the lack of improvement in TR do not constitute a reason for further surgery, as remodeling of the RV and improvement in TR often take weeks after PTE [109, 110].

Lung and Mediastinal Masses

TEE has been successfully used in the diagnosis and management of mediastinal masses:

TEE allowed the incidental diagnosis of mediastinal tumors in patients referred for drainage of pericardial effusion [110, 111]; TEE identified the presence of surgical

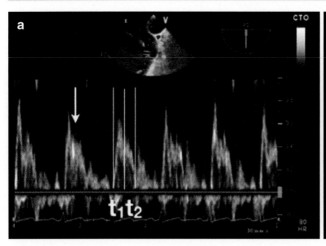
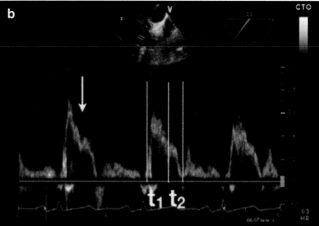
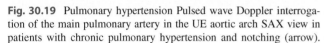

Fig. 30.19 Pulmonary hypertension Pulsed wave Doppler interrogation of the main pulmonary artery in the UE aortic arch SAX view in patients with chronic pulmonary hypertension and notching (arrow). Notching ratio (NR) is calculated as t_1/t_2. Early notching (NR < 1) (**a**) correlates with less advanced disease and better post endarterectomy outcome compared to late (NR > 1) (**b**) notching

sponges [112] and led to the diagnosis of esophageal cancer [113]; and finally, the resection of large anterior [114] and middle [115] mediastinal tumors greatly benefited from intraoperative TEE.

TEE can assess all cardiac chambers and may define extrinsic compression and tumor invasion. As previously reported [111], the presence of mediastinal masses predisposes to circulatory collapse at the induction of anesthesia, which is a Category I indication for the use of TEE.

In patients with cancer of the left lung, TEE has been used in the preoperative assessment of the invasion of the thoracic aortic wall and showed very high sensitivity when compared to CT scan [116].

Clinical Case Discussion

Case: A 54-year-old female presents for double lung transplantation. The patient has a history of end-stage lung disease secondary to bronchiolitis obliterans. Preoperative echocardiogram showed normal RV and LV function, normal valves, and RVSP of 34 mmHg. MUGA confirmed good LV function and excluded myocardial ischemia. After a smooth induction of anesthesia, a TEE probe is inserted. The ME 4C view is displayed. Color Doppler analysis is performed on the MV (Video. 30.1).

- Is there anything abnormal with the MV?
  - The base of the posterior mitral valve leaflet is calcified, a mass attached to its atrial aspect (arrow).
- What could be the differential diagnosis of this pathology?
  - Thrombus, infective vegetation, or tumor.
- What should be done to better assess the MV?

- Obtain multiple views of the mitral valve with and without color Doppler.
- What may be the surgical implications of this finding?
  - Use cardiopulmonary bypass to surgically explore the mitral valve and eventually perform valve surgery. Gentle manipulation of the heart should prevent dislodging of the mass attached to the mitral valve. A double lung transplant is performed without CPB. No surgery is performed on the MV nor is it surgically inspected.
- What should be the focus of immediate post-CPB TEE exam?
  - Assess mitral valve for regurgitation and mass on the posterior leaflet.

After weaning from CPB, the patient is hypotensive regardless of high doses of inotropes.

TEE shows the abnormal flow in the LVOT and severe MR (Video 30.2).

- What is happening?
  - This is a case of dynamic LVOT obstruction and systolic motion of the anterior mitral valve leaflet with severe mitral regurgitation. The hyperdynamic, hypertrophic left ventricle generates a high pressure gradient across the LVOT and for a Bernoulli effect sucks in the anterior leaflet of the mitral valve.
- What is the treatment?
  - Volume load, avoid inotropes, and administer short-acting beta-blockers and vasopressor.
  - The postoperative course is complicated by decreased level of consciousness. Seven days postoperatively a CT scan of the brain showed multiple strokes. We cannot exclude that embolization of material from the MV mass may have contributed to the clinical picture.

References

1. Mahmood F, Christie A, Matyal R. Transesophageal echocardiography and noncardiac surgery. Semin Cardiothorac Vasc Anesth. 2008;12:265–89.

2. American Society of A, Society of Cardiovascular Anesthesiologists Task Force on Transesophageal E. Practice guidelines for perioperative transesophageal echocardiography. An updated report by the American Society of Anesthesiologists and the Society of Cardiovascular Anesthesiologists Task Force on Transesophageal Echocardiography. Anesthesiology. 2010;112:1084–96.

3. Kolev N, Brase R, Swanevelder J, et al. The influence of transoesophageal echocardiography on intra-operative decision making. A European multicentre study. European Perioperative TOE Research Group. Anaesthesia. 1998;53:767–73.

4. Brandt RR, Oh JK, Abel MD, Click RL, Orszulak TA, Seward JB. Role of emergency intraoperative transesophageal echocardiography. J Am Soc Echocardiogr. 1998;11:972–7.

5. Memtsoudis SG, Rosenberger P, Loffler M, et al. The usefulness of transesophageal echocardiography during intraoperative cardiac arrest in noncardiac surgery. Anesth Analg. 2006;102:1653–7.

6. van der Wouw PA, Koster RW, Delemarre BJ, de Vos R, Lampe-Schoenmaeckers AJ, Lie KI. Diagnostic accuracy of transesophageal echocardiography during cardiopulmonary resuscitation. J Am Coll Cardiol. 1997;30:780–3.

7. Cahalan MK, Abel M, Goldman M, et al. American Society of Echocardiography and Society of Cardiovascular Anesthesiologists task force guidelines for training in perioperative echocardiography. Anesth Analg. 2002;94:1384–8.

8. Serra E, Feltracco P, Barbieri S, Forti A, Ori C. Transesophageal echocardiography during lung transplantation. Transplant Proc. 2007;39:1981–2.

9. Muller-Redetzky HC, Felten M, Hellwig K, et al. Increasing the inspiratory time and I:E ratio during mechanical ventilation aggravates ventilator-induced lung injury in mice. Crit Care. 2015; 19:23.

10. Côté G, Denault A. Transesophageal echocardiography-related complications. Can J Anaesth. 2008;55:622–47.

11. El-Chami MF, Martin RP, Lerakis S. Esophageal dissection complicating transesophageal echocardiogram--the lesson to be learned: do not force the issue. J Am Soc Echocardiogr. 2006;19:579. e575–577.

12. Augoustides JG, Hosalkar HH, Milas BL, Acker M, Savino JS. Upper gastrointestinal injuries related to perioperative transesophageal echocardiography: index case, literature review, classification proposal, and call for a registry. J Cardiothorac Vasc Anesth. 2006;20:379–84.

13. Kallmeyer IJ, Collard CD, Fox JA, Body SC, Shernan SK. The safety of intraoperative transesophageal echocardiography: a case series of 7200 cardiac surgical patients. Anesth Analg. 2001;92:1126–30.

14. Piercy M, McNicol L, Dinh DT, Story DA, Smith JA. Major complications related to the use of transesophageal echocardiography in cardiac surgery. J Cardiothorac Vasc Anesth. 2009;23:62–5.

15. Hahn RT, Abraham T, Adams MS, et al. Guidelines for performing a comprehensive transesophageal echocardiographic examination: recommendations from the American Society of Echocardiography and the Society of Cardiovascular Anesthesiologists. J Am Soc Echocardiogr. 2013;26:921–64.

16. Denault AY, Couture P, McKenty S, et al. Perioperative use of transesophageal echocardiography by anesthesiologists: impact in noncardiac surgery and in the intensive care unit. Can J Anaesth. 2002;49:287–93.

17. Schulmeyer MC, Santelices E, Vega R, Schmied S. Impact of intraoperative transesophageal echocardiography during noncardiac surgery. J Cardiothorac Vasc Anesth. 2006;20:768–71.

18. Hofer CK, Zollinger A, Rak M, et al. Therapeutic impact of intraoperative transoesophageal echocardiography during noncardiac surgery. Anaesthesia. 2004;59:3–9.

19. Comunale ME, Body SC, Ley C, et al. The concordance of intraoperative left ventricular wall-motion abnormalities and electrocardiographic S-T segment changes: association with outcome after coronary revascularization. Multicenter Study of Perioperative Ischemia (McSPI) Research Group. Anesthesiology. 1998;88:945–54.

20. Eisenberg MJ, London MJ, Leung JM, et al. Monitoring for myocardial ischemia during noncardiac surgery. A technology assessment of transesophageal echocardiography and 12-lead electrocardiography. The Study of Perioperative Ischemia Research Group. JAMA. 1992;268:210–6.

21. Royse CF. Ultrasound-guided haemodynamic state assessment. Best Pract Res Clin Anaesthesiol. 2009;23:273–83.

22. Kusumoto FM, Muhiudeen IA, Kuecherer HF, Cahalan MK, Schiller NB. Response of the interatrial septum to transatrial pressure gradients and its potential for predicting pulmonary capillary wedge pressure: an intraoperative study using transesophageal echocardiography in patients during mechanical ventilation. J Am Coll Cardiol. 1993;21:721–8.

23. Royse CF, Royse AG, Soeding PF, Blake DW. Shape and movement of the interatrial septum predicts change in pulmonary capillary wedge pressure. Ann Thorac Cardiovasc Surg. 2001;7: 79–83.

24. Royse CF, Seah JL, Donelan L, Royse AG. Point of care ultrasound for basic haemodynamic assessment: novice compared with an expert operator. Anaesthesia. 2006;61:849–55.

25. Lang RM, Badano LP, Mor-Avi V, et al. Recommendations for cardiac chamber quantification by echocardiography in adults: an update from the American Society of Echocardiography and the European Association of Cardiovascular Imaging. Eur Heart J Cardiovasc Imaging. 2015;16:233–70.

26. Della Rocca G, Costa MG, Coccia C, et al. Continuous right ventricular end-diastolic volume in comparison with left ventricular end-diastolic area. Eur J Anaesthesiol. 2009;26:272–8.

27. Scheuren K, Wente MN, Hainer C, et al. Left ventricular end-diastolic area is a measure of cardiac preload in patients with early septic shock. Eur J Anaesthesiol. 2009;26:759–65.

28. Hope MD, de la Pena E, Yang PC, Liang DH, McConnell MV, Rosenthal DN. A visual approach for the accurate determination of echocardiographic left ventricular ejection fraction by medical students. J Am Soc Echocardiogr. 2003;16:824–31.

29. Spencer KT, Lang RM, Kirkpatrick JN, Mor-Avi V. Assessment of global and regional left ventricular diastolic function in hypertensive heart disease using automated border detection techniques. Echocardiography. 2003;20:673–81.

30. London MJ. Assessment of left ventricular global systolic function by transoesophageal echocardiography. Ann Card Anaesth. 2006;9:157–63.

31. Lang RM, Bierig M, Devereux RB, et al. Recommendations for chamber quantification: a report from the American Society of Echocardiography's Guidelines and Standards Committee and the Chamber Quantification Writing Group, developed in conjunction with the European Association of Echocardiography, a branch of the European Society of Cardiology. J Am Soc Echocardiogr. 2005;18:1440–63.

32. Nagueh SF, Appleton CP, Gillebert TC, et al. Recommendations for the evaluation of left ventricular diastolic function by echocardiography. J Am Soc Echocardiogr. 2009;22:107–33.

33. Fischer GW, Salgo IS, Adams DH. Real-time three-dimensional transesophageal echocardiography: the matrix revolution. J Cardiothorac Vasc Anesth. 2008;22:904–12.

34. Mor-Avi V, Jenkins B, Kuhl H, et al. Real-time 3D echocardiographic quantification of left ventricular volumes: multicenter study

for validation with magnetic resonance imaging and investigation of surces of error. JACC Cardiovasc Imaging. 2008;1:413–23.

35. Pouleur AC, le Polain de Waroux JB, Pasquet A, et al. Assessment of left ventricular mass and volumes by three-dimensional echocardiography in patients with or without wall motion abnormalities: comparison against cine magnetic resonance imaging. Heart. 2008;94:1050–7.

36. Salgo IS. Three-dimensional echocardiographic technology. Cardiol Clin. 2007;25:231–9.

37. Vieira ML, Cury AF, Naccarato G, et al. Analysis of left ventricular regional dyssynchrony: comparison between real time 3D echocardiography and tissue Doppler imaging. Echocardiography. 2009;26:675–83.

38. Liodakis E, Al Sharef O, Dawson D, Nihoyannopoulos P. The use of real time three dimensional echocardiography for assessing mechanical synchronicity. Heart. 2009;95(22):1865–71.

39. Nagueh SF, Smiseth OA, Appleton CP, et al. Recommendations for the evaluation of left ventricular diastolic function by echocardiography: an update from the American Society of Echocardiography and the European Association of Cardiovascular Imaging. J Am Soc Echocardiogr. 2016;29:277–314.

40. Matyal R, Hess PE, Subramaniam B, et al. Perioperative diastolic dysfunction during vascular surgery and its association with postoperative outcome. J Vasc Surg. 2009;50:70–6.

41. Swaminathan M, Nicoara A, Phillips-Bute BG, et al. Utility of a simple algorithm to grade diastolic dysfunction and predict outcome after coronary artery bypass graft surgery. Ann Thorac Surg. 2011;91:1844–50.

42. Vizza CD, Lynch JP, Ochoa LL, Richardson G, Trulock EP. Right and left ventricular dysfunction in patients with severe pulmonary disease. Chest. 1998;113:576–83.

43. Rudski LG, Lai WW, Afilalo J, et al. Guidelines for the echocardiographic assessment of the right heart in adults: a report from the American Society of Echocardiography endorsed by the European Association of Echocardiography, a registered branch of the European Society of Cardiology, and the Canadian Society of Echocardiography. J Am Soc Echocardiogr. 2010;23:685–713; quiz 786-688.

44. Pedoto A, Amar D. Right heart function in thoracic surgery: role of echocardiography. Curr Opin Anaesthesiol. 2009;22: 44–9.

45. Haddad F, Doyle R, Murphy DJ, Hunt SA. Right ventricular function in cardiovascular disease, part II: pathophysiology, clinical importance, and management of right ventricular failure. Circulation. 2008;117:1717–31.

46. Vieillard-Baron A. Assessment of right ventricular function. Curr Opin Crit Care. 2009;15:254–60.

47. Davlouros PA, Niwa K, Webb G, Gatzoulis MA. The right ventricle in congenital heart disease. Heart. 2006;92(Suppl 1):i27–38.

48. Haddad F, Couture P, Tousignant C, Denault AY. The right ventricle in cardiac surgery, a perioperative perspective: I. anatomy, physiology, and assessment. Anesth Analg. 2009;108:407–21.

49. Haddad F, Hunt SA, Rosenthal DN, Murphy DJ. Right ventricular function in cardiovascular disease, part I: anatomy, physiology, aging, and functional assessment of the right ventricle. Circulation. 2008;117:1436–48.

50. Anavekar NS, Gerson D, Skali H, Kwong RY, Yucel EK, Solomon SD. Two-dimensional assessment of right ventricular function: an echocardiographic-MRI correlative study. Echocardiography. 2007;24:452–6.

51. Silverton N, Meineri M. Speckle tracking strain of the right ventricle: an emerging tool for intraoperative echocardiography. Anesth Analg. 2017;125:1475.

52. Duncan AE, Sarwar S, Kateby Kashy B, et al. Early left and right ventricular response to aortic valve replacement. Anesth Analg. 2015;

53. Meluzin J, Spinarova L, Hude P, et al. Prognostic importance of various echocardiographic right ventricular functional parameters in patients with symptomatic heart failure. J Am Soc Echocardiogr. 2005;18:435–44.

54. Markin NW, Chamsi-Pasha M, Luo J, et al. Transesophageal speckle-tracking echocardiography improves right ventricular systolic function assessment in the perioperative setting. J Am Soc Echocardiogr. 2017;30:180–8.

55. Fukuda S, Gillinov AM, McCarthy PM, et al. Determinants of recurrent or residual functional tricuspid regurgitation after tricuspid annuloplasty. Circulation. 2006;114:I582–7.

56. Rogers JH, Bolling SF. The tricuspid valve: current perspective and evolving management of tricuspid regurgitation. Circulation. 2009;119:2718–25.

57. Fusini L, Tamborini G, Gripari P, et al. Feasibility of intraoperative three-dimensional transesophageal echocardiography in the evaluation of right ventricular volumes and function in patients undergoing cardiac surgery. J Am Soc Echocardiogr. 2011;24: 868–77.

58. Niemann PS, Pinho L, Balbach T, et al. Anatomically oriented right ventricular volume measurements with dynamic three-dimensional echocardiography validated by 3-Tesla magnetic resonance imaging. J Am Coll Cardiol. 2007;50:1668–76.

59. Gopal AS, Chukwu EO, Iwuchukwu CJ, et al. Normal values of right ventricular size and function by real-time 3-dimensional echocardiography: comparison with cardiac magnetic resonance imaging. J Am Soc Echocardiogr. 2007;20:445–55.

60. Kjaergaard J, Petersen CL, Kjaer A, Schaadt BK, Oh JK, Hassager C. Evaluation of right ventricular volume and function by 2D and 3D echocardiography compared to MRI. Eur J Echocardiogr. 2006;7:430–8.

61. Lu X, Nadvoretskiy V, Bu L, et al. Accuracy and reproducibility of real-time three-dimensional echocardiography for assessment of right ventricular volumes and ejection fraction in children. J Am Soc Echocardiogr. 2008;21:84–9.

62. Hagen PT, Scholz DG, Edwards WD. Incidence and size of patent foramen ovale during the first 10 decades of life: an autopsy study of 965 normal hearts. Mayo Clin Proc. 1984;59:17–20.

63. Schneider B, Zienkiewicz T, Jansen V, Hofmann T, Noltenius H, Meinertz T. Diagnosis of patent foramen ovale by transesophageal echocardiography and correlation with autopsy findings. Am J Cardiol. 1996;77:1202–9.

64. Konstadt SN, Louie EK, Black S, Rao TL, Scanlon P. Intraoperative detection of patent foramen ovale by transesophageal echocardiography. Anesthesiology. 1991;74:212–6.

65. Di Tullio M, Sacco RL, Venketasubramanian N, Sherman D, Mohr JP, Homma S. Comparison of diagnostic techniques for the detection of a patent foramen ovale in stroke patients. Stroke. 1993;24:1020–4.

66. Woods TD, Patel A. A critical review of patent foramen ovale detection using saline contrast echocardiography: when bubbles lie. J Am Soc Echocardiogr. 2006;19:215–22.

67. Thaler DE, Saver JL. Cryptogenic stroke and patent foramen ovale. Curr Opin Cardiol. 2008;23:537–44.

68. Smeenk FW, Postmus PE. Interatrial right-to-left shunting developing after pulmonary resection in the absence of elevated right-sided heart pressures. Review of the literature. Chest. 1993;103:528–31.

69. Carroll JD, Dodge S, Groves BM. Percutaneous patent foramen ovale closure. Cardiol Clin. 2005;23:13–33.

70. Krasuski RA, Hart SA, Allen D, et al. Prevalence and repair of intraoperatively diagnosed patent foramen ovale and association with perioperative outcomes and long-term survival. JAMA. 2009;302:290–7.

71. Cypel M, Yeung JC, Hirayama S, et al. Technique for prolonged normothermic ex vivo lung perfusion. J Heart Lung Transplant. 2008;27:1319–25.

72. Cypel M, Sato M, Yildirim E, et al. Initial experience with lung donation after cardiocirculatory death in Canada. J Heart Lung Transplant. 2009;28:753–8.

73. Gorcsan J 3rd, Edwards TD, Ziady GM, Katz WE, Griffith BP. Transesophageal echocardiography to evaluate patients with severe pulmonary hypertension for lung transplantation. Ann Thorac Surg. 1995;59:717–22.

74. Izbicki G, Ben-Dor I, Shitrit D, et al. The prevalence of coronary artery disease in end-stage pulmonary disease: is pulmonary fibrosis a risk factor? Respir Med. 2009;103:1346–9.

75. Jackson A, Cropper J, Pye R, Junius F, Malouf M, Glanville A. Use of extracorporeal membrane oxygenation as a bridge to primary lung transplant: 3 consecutive, successful cases and a review of the literature. J Heart Lung Transplant. 2008;27:348–52.

76. Strueber M. Extracorporeal support as a bridge to lung transplantation. Curr Opin Crit Care. 2010;16(1):69–73.

77. Cahalan MK, Stewart W, Pearlman A, et al. American Society of Echocardiography and Society of Cardiovascular Anesthesiologists task force guidelines for training in perioperative echocardiography. J Am Soc Echocardiogr. 2002;15:647–52.

78. Practice guidelines for perioperative transesophageal echocardiography. A report by the American Society of Anesthesiologists and the Society of Cardiovascular Anesthesiologists Task Force on Transesophageal Echocardiography. Anesthesiology. 1996;84:986–1006.

79. Ebert EC. Esophageal disease in scleroderma. J Clin Gastroenterol. 2006;40:769–75.

80. Della Rocca G, Brondani A, Costa MG. Intraoperative hemodynamic monitoring during organ transplantation: what is new? Curr Opin Organ Transplant. 2009;14:291–6.

81. Marasco SF, Lukas G, McDonald M, McMillan J, Ihle B. Review of ECMO (extra corporeal membrane oxygenation) support in critically ill adult patients. Heart Lung Circ. 2008;17(Suppl 4):S41–7.

82. Doufle G, Roscoe A, Billia F, Fan E. Echocardiography for adult patients supported with extracorporeal membrane oxygenation. Crit Care. 2015;19:326.

83. Gammie JS, Cheul Lee J, Pham SM, et al. Cardiopulmonary bypass is associated with early allograft dysfunction but not death after double-lung transplantation. J Thorac Cardiovasc Surg. 1998;115:990–7.

84. Paradela M, Gonzalez D, Parente I, et al. Surgical risk factors associated with lung transplantation. Transplant Proc. 2009;41:2218–20.

85. Haddad F, Couture P, Tousignant C, Denault AY. The right ventricle in cardiac surgery, a perioperative perspective: II. Pathophysiology, clinical importance, and management. Anesth Analg. 2009;108:422–33.

86. Subramaniam K, Yared JP. Management of pulmonary hypertension in the operating room. Semin Cardiothorac Vasc Anesth. 2007;11:119–36.

87. Murtha W, Guenther C. Dynamic left ventricular outflow tract obstruction complicating bilateral lung transplantation. Anesth Analg. 2002;94:558–9; table of contents.

88. Granton J, Moric J. Pulmonary vasodilators--treating the right ventricle. Anesthesiol Clin. 2008;26:337–53. vii.

89. Katz WE, Gasior TA, Quinlan JJ, et al. Immediate effects of lung transplantation on right ventricular morphology and function in patients with variable degrees of pulmonary hypertension. J Am Coll Cardiol. 1996;27:384–91.

90. Hausmann D, Daniel WG, Mugge A, et al. Imaging of pulmonary artery and vein anastomoses by transesophageal echocardiography after lung transplantation. Circulation. 1992;86:II251–8.

91. Reeves ST, Glas KE, Eltzschig H, et al. Guidelines for performing a comprehensive epicardial echocardiography examination: recommendations of the American Society of Echocardiography and the Society of Cardiovascular Anesthesiologists. J Am Soc Echocardiogr. 2007;20:427–37.

92. Gonzalez-Fernandez C, Gonzalez-Castro A, Rodriguez-Borregan JC, et al. Pulmonary venous obstruction after lung transplantation. Diagnostic advantages of transesophageal echocardiography. Clin Transplant. 2009;23(6):975–80.

93. Michel-Cherqui M, Brusset A, Liu N, et al. Intraoperative transesophageal echocardiographic assessment of vascular anastomoses in lung transplantation. A report on 18 cases. Chest. 1997;111:1229–35.

94. Schulman LL, Anandarangam T, Leibowitz DW, et al. Four-year prospective study of pulmonary venous thrombosis after lung transplantation. J Am Soc Echocardiogr. 2001;14:806–12.

95. Felten ML, Michel-Cherqui M, Sage E, Fischler M. Transesophageal and contact ultrasound echographic assessments of pulmonary vessels in bilateral lung transplantation. Ann Thorac Surg. 2012;93:1094–100.

96. Hunt SA, Abraham WT, Chin MH, et al. 2009 focused update incorporated into the ACC/AHA 2005 Guidelines for the Diagnosis and Management of Heart Failure in adults: a report of the American College of Cardiology Foundation/American Heart Association Task Force on Practice Guidelines: developed in collaboration with the International Society for Heart and Lung Transplantation. Circulation. 2009;119:e391–479.

97. Jacobsohn E, Avidan MS, Hantler CB, Rosemeier F, De Wet CJ. Case report: inferior vena-cava right atrial anastomotic stenosis after bicaval orthotopic heart transplantation. Can J Anaesth. 2006;53:1039–43.

98. Rosenberger P, Shernan SK, Mihaljevic T, Eltzschig HK. Transesophageal echocardiography for detecting extrapulmonary thrombi during pulmonary embolectomy. Ann Thorac Surg. 2004;78:862–6; discussion 866.

99. Comess KA, DeRook FA, Russell ML, Tognazzi-Evans TA, Beach KW. The incidence of pulmonary embolism in unexplained sudden cardiac arrest with pulseless electrical activity. Am J Med. 2000;109:351–6.

100. Aklog L, Williams CS, Byrne JG, Goldhaber SZ. Acute pulmonary embolectomy: a contemporary approach. Circulation. 2002;105:1416–9.

101. Thistlethwaite PA, Kaneko K, Madani MM, Jamieson SW. Technique and outcomes of pulmonary endarterectomy surgery. Ann Thorac Cardiovasc Surg. 2008;14:274–82.

102. Lengyel M. The role of transesophageal echocardiography in the management of patients with acute and chronic pulmonary thromboembolism. Echocardiography. 1995;12:359–66.

103. Chartier L, Bera J, Delomez M, et al. Free-floating thrombi in the right heart: diagnosis, management, and prognostic indexes in 38 consecutive patients. Circulation. 1999;99:2779–83.

104. Ribeiro A, Lindmarker P, Juhlin-Dannfelt A, Johnsson H, Jorfeldt L. Echocardiography Doppler in pulmonary embolism: right ventricular dysfunction as a predictor of mortality rate. Am Heart J. 1997;134:479–87.

105. Konstantinides S, Geibel A, Kasper W, Olschewski M, Blumel L, Just H. Patent foramen ovale is an important predictor of adverse outcome in patients with major pulmonary embolism. Circulation. 1998;97:1946–51.

106. Zoghbi WA, Enriquez-Sarano M, Foster E, et al. Recommendations for evaluation of the severity of native valvular regurgitation with two-dimensional and Doppler echocardiography. J Am Soc Echocardiogr. 2003;16:777–802.

107. Tousignant C, Van Orman JR. Pulmonary artery acceleration time in cardiac surgical patients. J Cardiothorac Vasc Anesth. 2015;29:1517–23.

108. Hardziyenka M, Reesink HJ, Bouma BJ, et al. A novel echocardiographic predictor of in-hospital mortality and mid-term hae-

modynamic improvement after pulmonary endarterectomy for chronic thrombo-embolic pulmonary hypertension. Eur Heart J. 2007;28:842–9.

109. D'Armini AM, Zanotti G, Ghio S, et al. Reverse right ventricular remodeling after pulmonary endarterectomy. J Thorac Cardiovasc Surg. 2007;133:162–8.

110. Brooker RF, Zvara DA, Roitstein A. Mediastinal mass diagnosed with intraoperative transesophageal echocardiography. J Cardiothorac Vasc Anesth. 2007;21:257–8.

111. Lin CM, Hsu JC. Anterior mediastinal tumour identified by intraoperative transesophageal echocardiography. Can J Anaesth. 2001;48:78–80.

112. Tsutsui JM, Hueb WA, Nascimento SA, Borges Leal SM, de Andrade JL, Mathias W Jr. Detection of retained surgical sponge

by transthoracic and transesophageal echocardiography. J Am Soc Echocardiogr. 2003;16:1191–3.

113. Shah A, Tunick PA, Greaney E, Pfeffer RD, Kronzon I. Diagnosis of esophageal carcinoma because of findings on transesophageal echocardiography. J Am Soc Echocardiogr. 2001;14:1134–6.

114. Redford DT, Kim AS, Barber BJ, Copeland JG. Transesophageal echocardiography for the intraoperative evaluation of a large anterior mediastinal mass. Anesth Analg. 2006;103:578–9.

115. DeBoer DA, Margolis ML, Livornese D, Bell KA, Livolsi VA, Bavaria JE. Pulmonary venous aneurysm presenting as a middle mediastinal mass. Ann Thorac Surg. 1996;61:1261–2.

116. Schroder C, Schonhofer B, Vogel B. Transesophageal echographic determination of aortic invasion by lung cancer. Chest. 2005;127:438–42.

Anesthesia for Patients with End-Stage Lung Disease

31

Florin Costescu and Martin Ma

Key Points

- Preoperative optimization with pulmonary rehabilitation, smoking cessation, and education can improve surgical outcomes in patients with end-stage lung disease (ESLD).
- ESLD is associated with a high incidence of pulmonary hypertension and right ventricular dysfunction. The anesthetic goals for these patients include optimizing preload, maintaining a low normal heart rate, maintaining contractility, decreasing pulmonary vascular resistance, and ensuring systemic pressures that are greater than pulmonary pressures.
- Compared with general anesthesia, regional anesthesia and analgesia may reduce the risk of pulmonary complications and perioperative morbidity.
- Even mild pulmonary insults will be poorly tolerated by patients with ESLD. Ventilation strategies that utilize low tidal volumes and low airway pressures may reduce the risk of volutrauma, barotrauma, and acute lung injury.
- Intraoperative management can facilitate early recovery and early tracheal extubation after general anesthesia. Short-acting anesthetic agents are recommended. As elimination of inhalational agents is impaired by ESLD, total intravenous anesthesia (TIVA) may be preferred. Maintenance of normothermia will avoid increases in ventilatory demand associated with postoperative shivering.

- Effective postoperative analgesia is essential in patients with ESLD. Regional analgesia is preferred over parenteral opioid analgesics. Adjuvant pain medications which have an opioid-sparing effect should be used.
- Chronic obstructive pulmonary disease is a common cause of ESLD. Severe airflow obstruction results in a high risk of air trapping, pneumothorax, and dynamic hyperinflation. In addition to aggressive bronchodilation, ventilation with low inspiratory/expiratory ratios (1:3 to 1:4.5) and low respiratory rates (6–10/min) will optimize expiratory airflow.
- Cystic fibrosis is a multisystemic disease that results in abnormally viscous secretions. Inability to clear pulmonary secretions results in airflow obstruction and chronic infection. Management focuses on improving sputum clearance and minimizing airway obstruction.
- The interstitial lung diseases cause lung restriction and are characterized by chronic inflammation and fibrosis. Ventilation strategies that minimize tidal volume and airway pressures should be used.

F. Costescu
Department of Anesthesia, McGill University Health Centre – Montreal General Hospital, Montreal, QC, Canada

M. Ma (✉)
Department of Anesthesia and Pain Management, University Health Network, Toronto General Hospital, Toronto, ON, Canada
e-mail: martin.ma@uhn.ca

Introduction

Providing a safe anesthetic for patients with end-stage lung disease (ESLD) is a challenge. Postoperative pulmonary complications (PPCs) are poorly tolerated in this group of patients and can result in significant morbidity and mortality. Ideally, efforts to minimize this risk begin in the preoperative period with patient education, smoking cessation counseling, and pulmonary rehabilitation programs. Although this is not always possible, participation in these programs can reduce perioperative complications. Intraoperatively, problems may include inadequate oxygenation and ventilation, as well as barotrauma, volutrauma, and acute lung injury (ALI). In this high-risk patient population, an anesthetic technique that facilitates early recovery and tracheal extubation is also of key importance. Optimal perioperative management of patients with ESLD requires a multidisciplinary approach that includes respirologists, surgeons, nurses, physiotherapists, respiratory therapists, and of course anesthesiologists. This chapter begins with an overview of the management considerations that are applicable to all patients with ESLD. This discussion is summarized in Table 31.1. Specific considerations for the most common causes of ESLD including chronic obstructive lung disease (COPD), cystic fibrosis (CF), and interstitial lung diseases (ILDs) are then outlined.

Preoperative Optimization

Smoking Cessation

The link between smoking and increased perioperative morbidity is well established in the literature. Smoking increases the relative risk of postoperative pulmonary complications by up to six times [1]. A common concern is the increased risk of laryngospasm and bronchospasm. High levels of carbon monoxide limit the ability of hemoglobin to bind and transport oxygen, predisposing surgical patients to an increased risk of tissue hypoxia. Smoking increases airway mucous production and impairs ciliary function resulting in poor sputum clearance. This, in combination with smoke-induced impairment of immune function, increases the likelihood of developing postoperative pneumonia. The long-term pulmonary consequence of smoking is worsening airway obstruction as measured by the forced expired volume in 1 s (FEV_1) [2]. Although cessation will not reverse

the degree of airway obstruction caused by smoking, it does reduce the rate at which FEV_1 subsequently declines (Fig. 31.1). Nicotine causes direct coronary vasoconstriction as well as an increase in the rate-pressure product. This contributes to the observation that smokers with no history of coronary artery disease have significantly more episodes of ST segment depression during surgery than nonsmokers [3]. Other concerns include impaired wound healing, surgical

Table 31.1 Summary of anesthetic management for patients with end-stage lung disease (ESLD)

Optimization	Encourage smoking cessation
	Enroll patients in pulmonary rehabilitation
	Educate patients on postoperative chest physiotherapy
	Ensure preoperative use of routine bronchodilators
Anesthesia	Patients may have pulmonary hypertension (see Table 31.4)
	Regional anesthesia and analgesia will minimize the risk of postoperative pulmonary complications
	Judiciously titrate short- or intermediate-acting neuromuscular blockers and ensure complete reversal before extubation
	Minimize fluid administration as clinically appropriate
	Emergence is more predictable with short-acting agents and total intravenous anesthesia (TIVA)
	Maintain normothermia
	Avoid prophylactic insertion of nasogastric tubes
Ventilation	Use lung protective ventilation with low tidal volume (6–8 mL/kg of predicted body weight)
	Maintain airway pressures as low as possible
Postoperative care	Patients will require care in a monitored setting postoperatively (e.g., step-down unit, intensive care unit)
	Encourage early mobilization, incentive spirometry, and chest physiotherapy
	Minimize opioid use while maximizing nonopioid pain medications

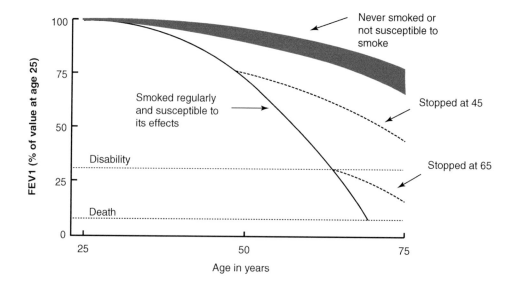

Fig. 31.1 Decline in FEV_1 with age and smoking. (Reprinted from Kemp et al. [2]. © 2009 with permission from Elsevier)

Table 31.2 Reversible effects of smoking

Respiratory	
↑ Carbon monoxide	
↑ Mucous production	↑ Risk of hypoxia
↓ Ciliary function	↑ Risk of pulmonary infections
↓ Immune function	
↑ Airway reactivity	↑ Risk of bronchospasm
Cardiac	
↑ Rate-pressure product	↑ Risk of myocardial ischemia
↑ Myocardial O_2 consumption	
Coronary vasoconstriction	
Hematologic	
↓ Macrophage function	↓ Immune function
↑ Platelet aggregation	↑ Risk of thrombosis
↑ Coagulation	
Impaired wound healing	

site infections, and perioperative venous thrombosis secondary to a procoagulant state caused by nicotine. The reversible effects of smoking are summarized in Table 31.2. Given the potential perioperative cardiorespiratory complications of smoking, preoperative cessation is important for patients with ESLD.

The long-term benefits of smoking cessation are undisputed, but the minimum duration of preoperative abstinence necessary to decrease the risk of postoperative complications is unclear. Despite earlier concerns about increased risk of postoperative pulmonary complications after short-term (< 4–8 weeks) preoperative smoking cessation [4, 5], more recent studies have not demonstrated this paradoxical response [6]. Data from randomized trials show a clear reduction in postoperative pulmonary complications and wound healing complications with preoperative smoking cessation interventions [7–9]. Moreover, multiple studies have shown that preoperative interventions may provide long-term benefits with increased smoking abstinence rates at 1 year follow-up [8, 10]. There is now wide consensus that the preoperative period is an excellent opportunity to promote smoking cessation, especially since the reduction in perioperative complications may provide additional motivation for patients to quit [11]. Interventions aimed at reducing or stopping cigarette use should be implemented as early as possible to have an impact on perioperative outcomes.

Effective interventions to assist patients who wish to quit smoking include medical counseling and pharmacotherapy such as nicotine replacement therapy, bupropion, and varenicline [8]. In one study, 120 smokers scheduled for elective orthopedic surgery were randomized to an intervention group including counseling and nicotine replacement therapy for 6–8 weeks or a control group [7]. In the intervention group, 89% of the analyzed patients either quit or reduced smoking by more than 50%, in contrast to only 8% in the control group. The intervention group had significantly less overall postoperative complications (18% vs. 52%, $p = 0.0003$) and less wound-related complications (5% vs. 31%, $p = 0.001$). A multicenter trial randomized 286 smokers scheduled for elective surgery to a 12-week course of varenicline starting 1 week before surgery or placebo [12]. All patients received smoking cessation counseling. At 12 months, 36.4% of patients in the varenicline group were abstinent vs. 25.2% in the placebo group ($p = 0.04$). There were no statistically significant differences in postoperative complications between the groups, but more patients receiving varenicline reported nausea.

Pulmonary Rehabilitation

Many patients with ESLD are at risk of progressive deconditioning related to dyspnea, decreased physical activity, and decreased cardiopulmonary capacity, all of which contribute to a downward cycle of worsening in dyspnea and quality of life. Pulmonary rehabilitation is a comprehensive multidisciplinary therapeutic intervention which includes exercise training, nutritional support, education, and psychological support aimed at breaking this cycle [13]. One of the key elements of pulmonary rehabilitation is improvement in muscle function and exercise capacity through both aerobic and strength training. For any given activity, this translates into decreased lactic acid production, decreased carbon dioxide (CO_2) production, and thus, decreased ventilatory demand [14, 15]. Although this benefits all patients with ESLD, it is particularly relevant to those with COPD in whom hyperventilation causes inadequate expiratory time, dynamic hyperinflation, and worsened dyspnea. The educational component of pulmonary rehabilitation aims to improve the patient's understanding of the disease and its management. Common themes include smoking cessation, the early detection and treatment of pulmonary exacerbations, the role of exercise in improving function, and promoting compliance with therapy. ESLD is often associated with poor nutritional status which results in muscle catabolism. In and of itself, aggressive nutritional support in patients with advanced lung disease has not led to clinically relevant improvements in functional outcome [16–18]. When used in conjunction with exercise, nutritional support may improve lean muscle mass function and improve exercise performance [19].

Pulmonary rehabilitation programs have been studied most extensively in COPD patients and have been shown to significantly improve exercise capacity and health-related quality of life while reducing the severity of dyspnea [18, 19]. In a recent meta-analysis of 65 randomized controlled trials involving 3822 COPD patients, pulmonary rehabilitation programs significantly improved exercise capacity and increased the 6-min walk distance by 44 m. Dyspnea, fatigue, and emotional function were also significantly improved [20].

Although the impact of pulmonary rehabilitation is less well studied for other forms of ESLD, current evidence suggests that it is beneficial. A meta-analysis of five randomized trials including 162 patients with interstitial lung disease showed a significant and clinically important short-term improvement in 6-minute walk test by 44 m and peak oxygen consumption (VO_2 max) by 1.24 mL/kg/min. There were also significant improvements in dyspnea and quality of life. Long-term outcome data is still limited [21]. In patients with cystic fibrosis, some randomized trials have shown improved exercise capacity and quality of life after training programs [22], but these results are not consistent across studies [23]. A meta-analysis of 21 randomized trials including 772 patients with asthma concluded that physical training significantly improved maximal heart rate and VO_2 max, but had no effect on pulmonary function tests [24]. Some trials found a significant improvement in quality of life and reduced psychosocial distress in this patient population [25, 26]. In a small study of 25 patients with pulmonary hypertension, an exercise program reduced New York Heart Association dyspnea scores and improved 6-min walk test results [27]. Current evidence-based guidelines strongly recommend pulmonary rehabilitation programs for patients with COPD and other causes of ESLD [19].

In the preoperative setting, pulmonary rehabilitation is mandatory for patients undergoing lung volume reduction surgery (LVRS) and lung transplantation. For these high-risk procedures, successful completion of pulmonary rehabilitation is used not only as a marker for patient motivation and therapy compliance but also as a risk assessment tool. For example, the National Emphysema Treatment Trial (NETT) found that patients with primarily upper lobe emphysema and low maximal workload after rehabilitation benefited from LVRS. In comparison, patients with non-upper lobe emphysema and high maximal workload following rehabilitation have higher mortality rates with LVRS than conservative management with medical therapy only [28].

There is a growing interest in establishing whether preoperative pulmonary rehabilitation may play a role in either (1) improving exercise reserve sufficiently to enable borderline operative candidates to undergo surgery or (2) improving perioperative outcome. Patient suitability for lung resection is commonly based upon three factors: respiratory mechanics, lung parenchymal function, and cardiopulmonary reserve. While lung function is relatively fixed, cardiopulmonary reserve can be improved. In a small pilot study, eight COPD patients with resectable lung cancers were denied surgery as a result of poor pulmonary function (mean preoperative $FEV_1\%$ predicted = 40%). Following 4 weeks of pulmonary rehabilitation, all eight patients successfully had a lobectomy [29]. In another study, 12 patients scheduled for lung resection with a VO_2 max ≤15 mL/kg/min underwent a 4-week pulmonary rehabilitation program. Preoperative VO_2 max improved by a mean of 2.8 mL/kg/min, and 11 patient underwent lung resection without perioperative mortality [30]. A randomized trial of 40 patients undergoing lobectomy showed improved postoperative VO_2 max in patients who had preoperative high-intensity training compared to controls [31]. With respect to improving patient outcome, the role of preoperative pulmonary rehabilitation has been examined in one small study of 45 patients with COPD undergoing coronary artery bypass grafting. Pulmonary rehabilitation led to significantly lower postoperative ventilation times, postoperative complications, and hospital length of stay [32]. Although the preoperative role of pulmonary rehabilitation appears promising, there is currently very little clinical evidence to support or refute its use for improving postoperative clinical outcomes.

Medical Optimization

To minimize the risk of perioperative pulmonary complications, care must be taken to ensure that patients with ESLD are medically optimized prior to elective surgery. Bronchospasm and difficulty in clearing sputum are common problems in patients with COPD, bronchiectasis, and CF and may contribute to the development of hypoxia, atelectasis, and pneumonia. This risk may be decreased with the use of maximal bronchodilator and inhaled glucocorticoid therapy in the immediate preoperative period. During an acute exacerbation, patients may benefit from aggressive antibiotics or antivirals targeting likely infectious pathogens, and strong consideration should be made to postponing elective surgery (typically for 6 weeks). The development of pulmonary hypertension is a concern for all patients with ESLD. Appropriate medical therapy to minimize pulmonary artery pressure (PAP) and improve right ventricular function such as long-term supplemental oxygen, careful diuretic therapy, and advanced therapy agents should be instituted as indicated prior to surgery. In general, advanced therapeutic agents such as calcium channel blockers, prostacyclin agonists, endothelin receptor antagonists, and NO-cGMP enhancers are used in patients with Group 1 pulmonary arterial hypertension (see Table 31.3) but may be harmful for other groups (see Chap. 34). Riociguat, a guanylate cyclase stimulant, can also be considered in the management of patients with chronic thromboembolic pulmonary hypertension (Group 4) (see Chap. 49).

Table 31.3 Classification of pulmonary hypertension – 5th World Symposium on Pulmonary Hypertension [33]

1. Pulmonary arterial hypertension (PAH)
  1.1. Idiopathic PAH
  1.2. Heritable
     1.2.1. Bone morphogenetic protein receptor type II gene abnormality
     1.2.2. Other genetic mutations: ALK-1, ENG, SMAD9, CAV1, KCNK3
     1.2.3. Unknown
  1.3. Drug- and toxin-induced
  1.4. Associated with
     1.4.1. Connective tissue diseases
     1.4.2. HIV infection
     1.4.3. Portal hypertension
     1.4.4. Congenital heart diseases
     1.4.5. Schistosomiasis
1' Pulmonary veno-occlusive disease and/or pulmonary capillary hemangiomatosis
1"Persistent pulmonary hypertension of the newborn
2. Pulmonary hypertension due to left heart disease
  2.1 Left ventricular systolic dysfunction
  2.2 Left ventricular diastolic dysfunction
  2.3 Valvular disease
  2.4 Congenital/acquired left heart inflow/outflow tract obstruction and congenital cardiomyopathies
3. Pulmonary hypertension due to lung diseases and/or hypoxia
  3.1. Chronic obstructive pulmonary disease
  3.2. Interstitial lung disease
  3.3. Other pulmonary diseases with mixed restrictive and obstructive pattern
  3.4 Sleep-disordered breathing
  3.5 Alveolar hypoventilation disorders
  3.6 Chronic exposure to high altitude
  3.7 Developmental lung diseases
4. Chronic thromboembolic pulmonary hypertension
5. Pulmonary hypertension with unclear multifactorial mechanisms
  5.1 Hematologic disorders: chronic hemolytic anemia, myeloproliferative disorders, splenectomy
  5.2 Systemic disorders: sarcoidosis, pulmonary histiocytosis, lymphangioleiomyomatosis
  5.3 Metabolic disorders: glycogen storage disease, Gaucher disease, thyroid disorders
  5.4 Others: tumoral obstruction, fibrosing mediastinitis, chronic renal failure, segmental pulmonary hypertension

Adapted from Simonneau et al. [33] with the permission from Elsevier

Chest Physiotherapy

Impaired mucociliary clearance, decreased lung volumes, atelectasis, bed rest, diaphragmatic dysfunction, shallow breathing, and pain all contribute to the development of postoperative pulmonary complications. Various forms of chest physiotherapy including incentive spirometry, cough/deep breathing exercises, intermittent positive pressure breathing, and continuous positive airway pressure have been used with equal efficacy to minimize this risk [34]. In one study, 174 patients undergoing major abdominal surgery were random-

ized to either intervention with postoperative chest physiotherapy or control. Chest physiotherapy significantly reduced the incidence of both pneumonia and all pulmonary complications (6% vs. 27%; $p < 0.001$) [35].

The benefit of chest physiotherapy is even greater when patients participate in an intensive chest physiotherapy education session preoperatively. In a randomized controlled trial, 279 patients undergoing coronary artery bypass grafting were randomized to either "intensive muscle training" (IMT) or the control group. IMT program trained patients daily for a minimum of 2 weeks preoperatively in breathing exercises, forced exhalation techniques, and the use of inspiratory spirometry. The control group received instruction on deep breathing maneuvers, coughing, and early ambulation on the day prior to surgery. Postoperative management of both groups was similar and consisted of incentive spirometry, chest physiotherapy, and mobilization. Compared with postoperative physiotherapy only, IMT further reduced the incidence of postoperative pulmonary complications (18% vs. 48%, $p = 0.02$) and pneumonia (6.5% vs. 16.1%; $p = 0.01$) by approximately 60% [36]. These findings have been confirmed in a recent review of randomized trials [37]. The reduction in pulmonary complications with preoperative physiotherapy education and training may relate to improved compliance and performance in the postoperative period [38].

General Considerations

Preoperative Assessment

The primary focus of the preoperative evaluation in patients with ESLD is the respiratory and cardiac systems. A history of patient symptoms, functional status, and activities of daily living, not to mention the physical examination, can be a valuable source of information. As discussed in Chap. 2, the patient's respiratory function needs to be assessed in terms of (1) respiratory mechanics, (2) lung parenchymal function, and (3) cardiopulmonary reserve. In this regard, pulmonary function testing is essential in determining the intraoperative management and postoperative disposition of patients with advanced lung disease. While a detailed history is often sufficient for estimating cardiopulmonary reserve, formal exercise testing or a 6-min walk test can be used to provide a quantitative assessment. In patients with ESLD, a preinduction arterial blood gas should be drawn to establish the patient's baseline P_aO_2 and P_aCO_2. This will help guide the intraoperative management, including mechanical ventilation and monitoring, as well as postoperative care.

The preoperative workup of patients with ESLD routinely includes a recent echocardiogram to assess right ventricular size, thickness, and function. Echocardiography can also identify signs of right ventricular pressure or volume over-load, as well as the presence of intracardiac lesions which may cause right to left shunting in the face of elevated right-sided pressures. It can also rule out other pathologies that may contribute to pulmonary hypertension such as valvu-lopathies or left ventricular dysfunction. Multiple echocar-diographic parameters have demonstrated the prognostic value of echocardiography in patients with pulmonary hypertension and right ventricular dysfunction [39]. However, while echocardiography is a common first-line tool in the assessment of pulmonary hypertension, it can be limited by uninterpretable tracings in a significant proportion of patients and a relatively low sensitivity (60–87%) and specificity (74–79%) [39]. In patients with parenchymal lung disease, the echocardiography images may also be suboptimal.

Nocturnal Hypoxemia

Sleep, even in normal individuals, is associated with physi-ologic changes in respiratory function. During all stages of sleep, the effectiveness of chemoreceptors and mechanore-ceptors is reduced which leads to lower minute ventilation. This is particularly pronounced during rapid eye movement sleep. Decreased muscle contractility of the diaphragm as well as the accessory muscles further reduces the ventilatory response and contributes to the rapid shallow breathing observed during sleep.

Normal fluctuations in the circadian rhythm also cause nocturnal bronchoconstriction. These changes, which are summarized in Fig. 31.2, result in a hypoventilation, decreased functional residual capacity (FRC), and increased ventilation–perfusion (V/Q) mismatch [40, 41]. In normal

individuals, this translates into an 8–10 mmHg drop in over-night P_aO_2 (arterial partial pressure of oxygen) levels [41].

The potential adverse cardiac (e.g., worsened pulmonary hypertension, RV failure, arrhythmia), neurologic, and hematologic (e.g., polycythemia) effects of nocturnal hypox-emia are particularly worrisome in patients with low daytime oxygen saturation. Though best studied in COPD and CF populations, other causes of ESLD including ILDs and pri-mary pulmonary hypertension have also been associated with higher rates of nocturnal hypoxemia [41–44]. These pathophysiologic processes are of particular concern in the perioperative period, as further fall in FRC and the use of opioid analgesia places these patients at high risk of severe hypoxemia during sleep. Although oxygen therapy is used successfully to minimize the incidence of desaturation over-night, there is no clear evidence that treatment of isolated nocturnal hypoxemia improves mortality [40, 45]. In some patients oxygen therapy may exacerbate the degree of hypercapnia.

Pulmonary Hypertension and Right Ventricular Function

Although primary pulmonary hypertension may in and of itself be a cause of ESLD, this is a rare condition that has an incidence of only 1–2 per million [46, 47]. Much more com-monly, pulmonary hypertension is the result of ESLD and chronic hypoxemia. The most recent classification of pulmo-nary hypertension is detailed in Table 31.3. While estimates vary widely depending on disease severity and the method of measurement, the prevalence of pulmonary hypertension (mean PAP >25 mmHg) in advanced COPD, IPF, and CF ranges from 35% to 50% [48–50]. As PAPs rise, evidence of cor pulmonale develops as increased strain causes the right ventricle to hypertrophy. As the disease process worsens, the limited ability of the right ventricle to compensate is over-whelmed, which leads to right ventricular dilation and dys-function. In the United States, cor pulmonale accounts for 10–30% of all heart failure admissions, of which 84% are secondary to COPD [48]. The risk of right ventricular isch-emia is also increased. The right ventricle is normally per-fused throughout the cardiac cycle. However, the increased right ventricular transmural and intracavitary pressures asso-ciated with pulmonary hypertension may restrict perfusion of the right coronary artery during systole, especially if PAPs approach systemic levels.

The impact of pulmonary hypertension on right ventricu-lar dysfunction has several anesthetic implications. The car-diac goals are similar to other conditions in which cardiac output is relatively fixed. These are summarized in Table 31.4. Care should be taken to avoid physiologic states which will worsen pulmonary hypertension such as hypoxemia, hyper-

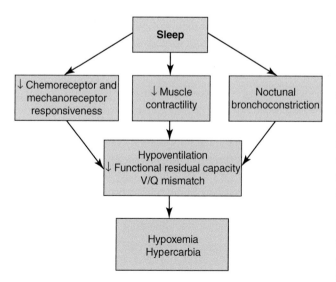

Fig. 31.2 The effects of sleep on breathing

Table 31.4 Anesthetic goals in pulmonary hypertension

Optimize preload	Hypovolemia will further impair cardiac output
	Hypervolemia will precipitate right ventricular failure and impair LV filling
Maintain a low normal HR	Tachycardia will impair ventricular filling and cardiac output
Maintain RV contractility	Consider inotropes including epinephrine, norepinephrine, dobutamine, and phosphodiesterase inhibitors
Maintain or ↓ PVR	Avoid physiologic states that ↑ PVR (hypoxia, hypercarbia, acidosis, hypothermia, high airway pressures, atelectasis)
	Avoid nitrous oxide
	Consider using intravenous dobutamine, phosphodiesterase inhibitors, or prostaglandins
	Consider using inhaled prostaglandins, nitric oxide, or phosphodiesterase inhibitors
Maintain or ↑ SVR	To maintain RV perfusion, SBP > PAP must be maintained
	Consider using vasopressors including norepinephrine, phenylephrine, and vasopressin

carbia, acidosis, and hypothermia. Conditions which impair right ventricular filling such as tachycardia and arrhythmias may not be well tolerated. Ideally, under anesthesia, right ventricular contractility and systemic vascular resistance (SVR) are maintained or increased, while pulmonary vascular resistance (PVR) decreases. This would ensure forward flow and minimize the risk of right ventricular ischemia. In practice, these goals can be a challenge to achieve because anesthetics are commonly associated with a decrease in SVR and a variable effect on PVR (e.g., propofol, thiopental, inhalational agents) [51]. Ketamine may be an interesting exception. Known for its sympathomimetic effects, ketamine increases cardiac contractility and SVR. However, its effect on PVR is controversial. Though concern is often raised over ketamine's potential to worsen pulmonary hypertension [52, 53], some animal in vitro and human clinical studies have suggested that it may decrease PVR or at least maintain pulmonary to systemic vascular resistance ratio [46, 51, 54, 55]. Anecdotally, at the authors' institution, ketamine is commonly and safely used to induce patients with severe pulmonary hypertension. Inotropes such as dobutamine and phosphodiesterase inhibitors (e.g., milrinone) will improve right ventricular function while reducing PVR. However, they also cause a significant decrease in systemic vascular tone, which may reduce right ventricular coronary perfusion pressure.

To maintain a systemic blood pressure (SBP) that is greater than the pulmonary, vasopressors such as phenylephrine or norepinephrine are commonly used. Of the two, norepinephrine is better suited in pulmonary hypertension because it maintains cardiac index and decreases the ratio of PAP to SBP [46, 51]. In contrast, phenylephrine causes the cardiac index to drop, while the PAP/SBP ratio remains the

same. Increasingly, vasopressin is also being used to maintain systemic pressures. Vasopressin appears to significantly increase SBP without affecting PAPs in patients with pulmonary hypertension (Fig. 31.3) [56–58]. In a study of isolated human radial and pulmonary arteries, norepinephrine and phenylephrine had concentration-dependent vasoconstricting effects on both radial and pulmonary arteries, whereas vasopressin had similar effect and potency on radial arteries but no effect on pulmonary arteries [59]. Vasopressin has also been associated with less arrhythmias when compared to norepinephrine [60]. In patients with severe pulmonary hypertension, selective pulmonary vasodilators including inhaled nitric oxide and inhaled prostaglandins should be considered. The effects of medications on PVR are discussed in greater detail in Chap. 9.

The extreme ends of patient lung volumes can cause compression of the extraalveolar and alveolar vessels, both of which contribute to an increased PVR (see Fig. 4.5). As a result, a ventilation strategy that avoids atelectasis as well as lung hyperinflation should be employed.

Intraoperative Monitoring

ESLD is frequently associated with a large arterial–end tidal CO_2 gradient. Placement of an arterial line facilitates intraoperative blood gas sampling to ensure adequate oxygenation and ventilation. In patients with pulmonary hypertension, continuous blood pressure monitoring is also reassuring. A central line is useful in monitoring and managing patients with moderate-to-severe pulmonary hypertension. Pulmonary artery catheters (PAC) may be of use in patients with PAPs which approach system pressures. However, the utility of PACs is controversial. From a large randomized trial, the use of PAC in ASA III and IV patients undergoing urgent or elective non-cardiac surgery showed no effect on mortality or the incidence of postoperative pneumonia [61]. However, no studies have specifically looked at the perioperative use of PACs in patients with pulmonary hypertension. We routinely place PACs in patients with severe pulmonary hypertension undergoing major surgery as it provides valuable information on the pulmonary to systemic pressure ratio, the cardiac output, and can help guide hemodynamic management. It is important to note that PAC use in patients with pulmonary hypertension is associated with a higher risk of pulmonary artery rupture.

General Versus Regional Anesthesia

Whether surgical outcomes are altered by the use of general or regional anesthesia has been a topic of debate for decades. Although the role regional anesthesia plays in

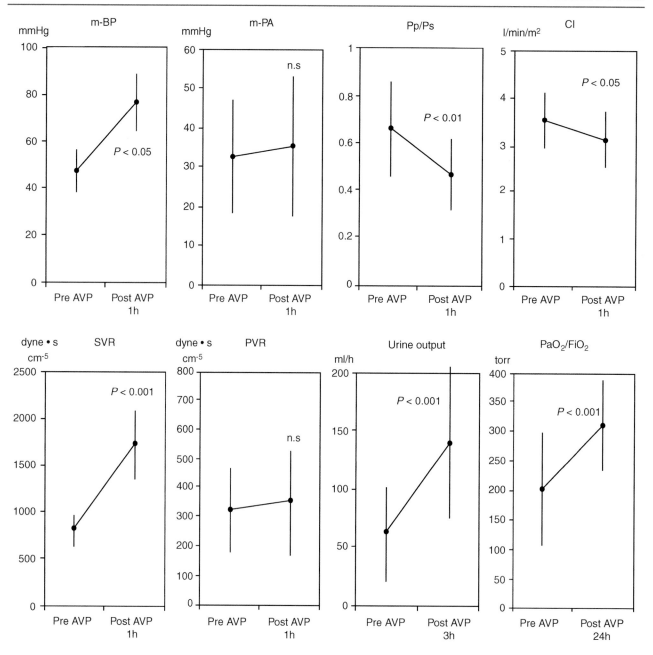

Fig. 31.3 Effect of arginine vasopressin (AVP) on mean systemic blood pressure (mSBP), mean pulmonary artery pressure (mPAP), pulmonary artery pressure/systemic blood pressure (Pp/Ps), cardiac index (CI), SVR, PVR, urine output, and P_aO_2/FiO_2 (Reprinted from Tayama et al. [56]. © 2007 with permission)

reducing mortality, deep vein thrombosis, pulmonary embolism, cardiac ischemia, and blood loss remains controversial, current evidence suggests intraoperative neuraxial anesthesia followed by postoperative neuraxial analgesia reduces the incidence of postoperative pulmonary complications [62–69]. In a meta-analysis of randomized trials, neuraxial anesthesia significantly reduced the risk of pneumonia by 39% and postoperative respiratory depression by 59% [62]. This may occur because general anesthesia decreases the number and activity of alveolar macrophages and inhibits mucociliary clearance, thereby increasing the risk of pulmonary infection [70]. General anesthesia also causes atelectasis in dependent areas of lung, decreased FRC, and an increase in V/Q mismatching, all of which contribute to the development of hypoxia. Following thoracic or upper abdominal surgery, atelectasis and the reduction in FRC may persist for up to 2 weeks as a result of postoperative diaphragmatic dysfunction. Though the precise mechanism is unclear, this dysfunction appears to result from reflex inhibition of the phrenic nerve secondary to irritation of splanchnic afferents or visceral pain. There is evidence that postoperative epidural analgesia blocks the stimulus for the reflex inhibition and restores normal diaphragm function [70–72].

Park et al. randomized 1021 ASA III or IV patients undergoing intraabdominal aortic, gastric, biliary, or colon operations to receive either (1) general anesthesia and systemic morphine for postoperative pain control or (2) epidural anesthesia combined with a light general anesthesia and epidural morphine for postoperative pain. Overall, no difference in death or major complications were noted, although the epidural group did have a lower incidence of respiratory failure that approached significance ($P=0.06$). In a subgroup analysis of the 374 patients who underwent aortic surgery, epidural anesthesia did significantly reduce the incidence of myocardial infarction, stroke, and respiratory failure (14% vs. 28%; $P<0.01$) [63]. The subgroup analysis also showed a trend toward lower rates of pneumonia (51% vs. 71%; $P=0.06$). In another large trial by Rigg et al., 915 patients with one of nine high-risk comorbid states were randomized to receive either (1) general anesthesia and postoperative pain control with parenteral opioids or (2) combined epidural/general anesthesia and postoperative epidural analgesia. All patients had major abdominal surgery. Of the measured endpoints, the only difference was a reduction in respiratory failure in the epidural group (23.3% vs. 30.2%; $P=0.02$) [64].

The improved respiratory outcomes associated with regional anesthesia and analgesia are particularly important in patients with preexisting lung disease for whom the risk of developing a postoperative pulmonary complication is increased tenfold [73]. Moreover, patients with ESLD may be inherently more challenging to extubate following surgery and may require a prolonged ventilator wean. In recent years, the desire to avoid general anesthesia in severely compromised respiratory patients has led to several reports of neuraxial blockade being used as the sole anesthetic for intraabdominal procedures. Van Zundert et al. [74] have successfully used a combined spinal–epidural placed at the T10 interspace to anesthetize a 47-year-old man with α-1-antitrypsin deficiency ($FEV_1/FVC=19\%$) for a laparoscopic cholecystectomy. Savas et al. [73] have reported using epidural anesthesia to facilitate awake surgery for sigmoidectomy, open cholecystectomy, incisional hernia repair, and laparoscopic inguinal hernia repair in patients with severe COPD.

To date, only a few studies have specifically compared regional anesthesia vs. general anesthesia outcomes in patients with advanced lung disease [68, 75–77]. In a retrospective cohort study examining data from the American College of Surgeons National Surgical Quality Improvement Program (ACS-NSQIP), 2644 COPD patients were propensity-matched for comorbidities, level of dyspnea, history of bleeding disorder, and primary surgical procedure [68]. Patients who had general anesthesia as their primary anesthetic technique compared to those having regional anesthesia had higher incidence of postoperative pneumonia (3.3% vs. 2.3%, $P = 0.0384$), prolonged ventilator dependence (2.1% vs. 0.9%, $P = 0.0008$), and unplanned postoperative intubation (2.6% vs. 1.8%, $P = 0.0487$). Thirty-day mortality was similar (2.7% vs. 3.0%, $P = 0.6788$).

Ventilation and ESLD

In the last two decades, the influence of ventilation strategy on acute respiratory distress syndrome (ARDS) has become clearer. The transition from high tidal volume (V_T) ventilation [$V_T = 10$–12 mL/kg predicted body weight (PBW)] and zero end-expiratory pressure (ZEEP) to low V_T lung ventilation ($V_T = 6$ mL/kg PBW) with positive end-expiratory pressure (PEEP) has improved survival and become a standard therapy in the management of patients with ARDS in the intensive care setting [78]. Whether patients without ARDS may also benefit from a low V_T ventilation strategy intraoperatively has been a subject of increasing interest and debate. The largest trial to date randomized 400 patients at intermediate to high risk of PPCs undergoing major elective abdominal surgery to either intraoperative protective lung ventilation (V_T of 6–8 mL/kg of PBW, PEEP of 6–8 cmH$_2$O, and recruitment maneuvers (RM) every 30 min) or non-protective lung ventilation (V_T of 10–12 mL/kg of PBW, no PEEP, and no RM) [79]. The primary outcome, which was a composite of major pulmonary (pneumonia or need for mechanical ventilation) and extrapulmonary complications (sepsis or death) occurring within seven postoperative days, was lower in the protective ventilation group (10.5% vs. 27.5% $p = 0.001$). The patients in the protective ventilation group had significantly lower rates of pneumonia, atelectasis, need for noninvasive mechanical ventilation, and sepsis. There was no difference in mortality between the groups.

More recent evidence suggests that the most important parameter associated with improved outcomes may be the use of low driving pressure [80]. Driving pressure is the difference between the PEEP and the plateau pressure. Neto et al. performed a meta-analysis of 2250 patients from 17 randomized controlled trials comparing intraoperative protective ventilation vs. conventional ventilation [81]. A multivariate analysis found that the only parameters associated with PPCs were static compliance and driving pressure. Surprisingly, V_T and PEEP were not independently associated with a reduced PPC rate. Moreover, in some patients, they found that increasing levels of PEEP actually lead to an increase in driving pressure, which in turn was associated with a greater risk of PPCs ($OR = 3.11$, $p = 0.006$). Presumably, in patients with minimal atelectasis, recruitment with PEEP resulted in overdistension of alveoli and a shift to a steeper portion of the respiratory compliance curve. In patients where increasing the PEEP either decreased or did not affect the driving pressure, the risk of PPCs was unchanged.

No study has specifically addressed how patients with end-stage lung disease should be ventilated intraoperatively. In spite of this paucity of evidence, we believe it is prudent to apply principles of lung protective ventilation to this population while keeping in mind the specific pathophysiologic processes at play for each disease (see sections on specific diseases in this Chapter). However, the recent literature gives us clues that a "magical recipe" of blindly applying a predetermined V_T, PEEP, F_iO_2, and RM may not achieve the best possible outcomes. An individualized approach that accounts for the patient's pathophysiology, lung and respiratory system compliance, amount of recruitable atelectatic alveoli, surgical requirements, and the interplay of other organ systems may improve outcomes.

Minimally Invasive Surgery

Key advantages of minimally invasive surgical procedures include reduced postoperative pain and an earlier return to baseline activities. For cholecystectomy and colorectal bowel resection, laparoscopic surgery results in less compromise of FEV_1 and forced vital capacity (FVC), as well as a lower incidence of atelectasis on postoperative chest X-rays. In spite of these improved clinical measures, a significant difference in postoperative pulmonary complications has not been demonstrated [82, 83]. However, the anesthetic management of patients with ESLD undergoing laparoscopic surgery can be challenging. Laparoscopy causes a decrease in FRC, which results in atelectasis and hypoxemia. Insufflation of CO_2 contributes to hypercarbia and respiratory acidosis. Although this is commonly controlled with increases in minute ventilation, this intervention may be of limited value in patients with abnormal lung mechanics and impaired gas exchange. In the rare circumstance where patients with ESLD require awake laparoscopy under regional anesthesia, the additional CO_2 load may precipitate respiratory failure. The development of hypoxia, hypercarbia, and acidosis (all of which contribute to pulmonary vasoconstriction) can also significantly worsen the degree of pulmonary hypertension and right heart failure. As a result, ventilatory parameters and cardiac function must be carefully monitored, especially during abdominal CO_2 insufflation. If respiratory or cardiac decompensation occurs, abortion of the procedure or conversion to an open surgery should be considered.

Optimizing Emergence

Temperature monitoring should be used in patients with ESLD. Postoperative hypothermia and shivering significantly increase oxygen consumption and carbon dioxide production. Such an increase in ventilatory demand is poorly tolerated in ESLD and may lead to respiratory failure. Intraoperative maintenance of normothermia with warming blankets and fluid warmers is extremely important.

While a variety of techniques and drugs may be used to safely induce and maintain anesthesia in patients with ESLD, agents with a short duration of action are preferred to minimize the risk of respiratory compromise at emergence. These patients are particularly sensitive to respiratory depressants such as benzodiazepines and opioids, and thus, these drugs should be used sparingly. Drugs which bronchodilate and do not inhibit hypoxic pulmonary vasoconstriction (HPV) are also favored. In this respect, the newer inhalational agents, such as sevoflurane or desflurane, are well suited for most patients. However, as a result of diffusion abnormalities and ventilation–perfusion mismatch, the elimination of inhalational agents may be unpredictable in patients with ESLD and result in delayed awakening. In patients with baseline hypoxia and/or bullous disease, nitrous oxide should be avoided. Total intravenous anesthesia (TIVA) is an excellent alternative to inhalational anesthesia for maintenance. Intravenous anesthetics do not affect HPV and lead to a timely awakening once turned off, especially when short-acting drugs such as propofol or remifentanil are used. While ketamine offers several distinct advantages including bronchodilation, preserved respiratory effort, and analgesic properties, it is associated with a 20–30% risk of postoperative hallucinations and nightmares and should be used cautiously [52, 84].

Postoperative Management

In patients with limited pulmonary reserve, effective postoperative pain management is essential. Splinting as a result of poorly controlled pain, especially from thoracic and abdominal surgery, can contribute to increased pulmonary complications including respiratory failure. In patients without contraindications, multimodal analgesic adjuvants including acetaminophen and nonsteroidal antiinflammatory drugs should be used. Although parenteral opioid use is effective in blunting pain, the amount needed following a thoracotomy or laparotomy may cause significant sedation and hypoventilation. Clearly, this is undesirable in patients with ESLD, especially those at risk of nocturnal hypoxemia. In comparison, a well-functioning regional block (e.g., thoracic epidural, paravertebral block) consistently provides superior analgesia and improves postoperative outcomes [64, 68, 69, 85, 86]. In patients with severely compromised respiratory function, the use of regional analgesia in minimally invasive surgeries such as video-assisted thoracoscopic surgery or laparoscopy should be considered. For instance, epidural analgesia is standard for our patients with COPD undergoing video-assisted thoracoscopic lung volume reduction surgery. A complete discussion regarding postoperative analgesia is found in Chap. 59.

Although nasogastric tubes are often routinely placed intraoperatively to facilitate gastric decompression after surgery, this practice is associated with an increased risk of atelectasis and pneumonia. In a meta-analysis of 24 studies, routine nasogastric tube use was associated with a statistically significant increased risk of pulmonary complications (OR = 1.4; 95% CI = 1.08–1.93) [87]. Accordingly, the use of postoperative nasogastric tubes should be avoided when possible.

Chronic Obstructive Pulmonary Disease

Chronic obstructive pulmonary disease (COPD) is defined by the Global Initiative for Chronic Obstructive Lung Disease (GOLD) as *a common preventable and treatable disease, characterized by persistent respiratory symptoms and airflow limitation that is due to airway and/or alveolar abnormalities usually caused by significant exposure to noxious particle or gases* [88]. It is associated with chronic inflammation, parenchymal destruction, and enhanced airway reactivity that are not fully reversible. Though most commonly associated with chronic bronchitis and emphysema, the COPD spectrum also includes asthma, between which there can be considerable clinical overlap. COPD is a major cause of morbidity and mortality worldwide, affecting 5–12% of the population, and is responsible for around three million deaths each year globally. It is expected to become the third leading cause of death by 2020.

Diagnosis and Staging of COPD

COPD should be considered in any patient who has dyspnea, chronic cough or sputum production, and/or a history of exposure to relevant risk factors. The diagnosis is confirmed with spirometry if the post-bronchodilator FEV_1 to FVC ratio is less than 0.7. The $FEV_1\%$ predicted is then used to stratify patients into one of four disease stages, as outlined in Table 31.5. Although $FEV_1\%$ predicted can also be used to predict survival rates, the BODE index – a composite score that includes measures of body mass index (B), airflow obstruction (O), dyspnea (D), and exercise capacity (E) – has been shown to be a better

Table 31.5 The GOLD classification of COPD based on post-bronchodilator spirometry

GOLD I	Mild	FEV_1/FVC <70%
		FEV_1 ≥80% predicted
GOLD II	Moderate	FEV_1/FVC <70%
		50% ≤ FEV_1 <80% predicted
GOLD III	Severe	FEV_1/FVC <70%
		30% ≤ FEV_1 <50% predicted
GOLD IV	Very severe	FEV_1/FVC <70%
		FEV_1 <30% predicted

Table 31.6 Variables and point values used for the computation of the BODE index

| Variable | Points on BODE index | | | |
	0	1	2	3
Body mass index	>21	≤21		
Airflow obstruction – $FEV_1\%$ predicted	≥65	50–64	36–49	≤35
Modified medical research council dyspnea scale	0–1	2	3	4
Exercise – Distance walked in 6 min (m)	≥350	250–349	150–249	≤149

predictor of patient survival [89]. On the basis of patient investigations and clinical status, each variable is assigned a point value according to Table 31.6. Adding these points together gives the BODE index, which can range from 0 to 10. The Kaplan–Meier survival curves based on BODE index and FEV_1 are illustrated in Fig. 31.4. The improved accuracy of the BODE index over FEV_1 alone in predicting patient survival reflects the reality that COPD is more than a pulmonary disease and that its outcome is closely related to systemic factors, including cardiopulmonary reserve.

Etiology of COPD

The development of COPD is strongly associated with exposure to noxious gases and particles. By far the most important risk factor for developing COPD is the amount and duration of cigarette smoking, which accounts for 75–90% of all cases in western nations [2, 90]. Worldwide, however, the use of biomass fuel (wood, charcoal, vegetable matter, animal dung) for heating and cooking is a significant risk factor for COPD. In fact, compared to the number of cigarette smokers, nearly three times as many people are exposed to biomass smoke [90]. The WHO estimates that 22% of COPD is attributable to biomass smoke [2]. Other significant contributors include air pollution, occupational exposure, and a history of pulmonary tuberculosis [90]. The inhalation of noxious fumes triggers macrophages and neutrophils to release inflammatory mediators, cytokines, as well as proteases. Although proteases play an important role in preventing infection, they can also cause damage to lung tissue. The latter is normally prevented by the presence of antiproteases enzymes such as α-1 antitrypsin. However, chronic inflammation and inactivation of antiproteases by oxidants lead to an imbalance resulting in unopposed protease activity. Long-term exposure to this process leads to fibrosis of the airway as well as destruction of alveoli [91]. The pathogenesis of COPD is summarized in Fig. 31.5.

COPD may also result from a number of genetic abnormalities, of which α-1 antitrypsin deficiency is the most well-known. Over 100 alleles have been identified for α-1

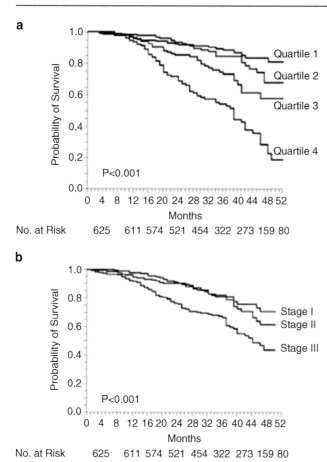

Serpine2, etc.) have been linked to increased risk of COPD in smokers.

COPD has also been associated with childhood pulmonary illnesses such as neonatal bronchopulmonary dysplasia and persistent asthma [93].

Causes of Expiratory Flow Obstruction

Expiratory flow limitation results from compression of the airways by intrathoracic pressure. In normal individuals, this only occurs during forced expiration. The mechanism for this is shown in Fig. 31.6. Prior to inspiration and the initiation of flow, the airway pressure is zero throughout. With a resting intrapleural pressure of −5 cm water, a transmural pressure of 5 cm water maintains airway patency (Fig. 31.6a). With normal inspiration, both intrapleural and alveolar pressures decrease by 3 cm water, and flow begins (Fig. 31.6b). Although this pressure is transmitted into the airway, its magnitude progressively declines because of airway resistance. Assuming an airway pressure of −1 cm water during inspiration, then the airway is kept open by 7 cm water. At end-inspiration, the airway pressures return to zero as flow ceases (Fig. 31.6c). During exhalation an increase in both intrapleural and alveolar pressures occurs. As with inhalation, the transmitted pressure from the alveoli drops within the airway as a result of resistance. With quiet exhalation, the passive return of the lung and chest wall to their equilibrium positions generates a pressure of 3 cm water within the intrapleural space and alveoli (Fig. 31.6d). As a result, the pressure within the airway always exceeds the intrapleural pressure. In this example, pressures may increase up to 8 cm water without causing airway collapse. However, higher pressures associated with forced expiration will lead to airway compression when the intraluminal pressure drops below the intrapleural pressure. This is called the equal pressure point (EPP). Beyond this, further increases in expiratory effort (which will also increase intrapleural pressure) will only contribute to flow limitation and airway collapse. For example, if both intrapleural and alveolar pressures increase by 24 cm water during forced expiration, then the EPP occurs at 16 cm water, below which airway collapse will occur (Fig. 31.6e). The effective driving pressure is therefore alveolar minus intrapleural pressure.

Factors that contribute to worsening flow limitation in patients with COPD are summarized in Table 31.7. Causes that may respond to intervention include active bronchospasm and airway obstruction by secretions. The loss of elastic recoil observed in emphysema results in less negative intrapleural pressures and reduces the outward traction normally exerted by lung parenchyma on the airway. This lowers the transmural pressure which keeps the airway open as well as the effective driving pressure. In our COPD example shown in Fig. 31.7a, the intrapleural and the transmural pres-

Fig. 31.4 Kaplan–Meier survival curves for the four quartiles of the BODE index (**a**) and the three stages of severity of chronic obstructive pulmonary disease as defined by the American Thoracic Society (**b**). In (**a**), quartile 1 is a score of 0–2, quartile 2 is a score of 3–4, quartile 3 is a score of 5–6, and quartile 4 is a score of 7–10. Survival differed significantly among the four groups ($P < 0.001$ by the log-rank test). In (**b**), stage I is defined by a forced expiratory volume in 1 s (FEV_1) that is more than 50% of the predicted value, stage II by an FEV_1 that is 36–50% of the predicted value, and stage III by an FEV_1 that is no more than 35% of the predicted value. Survival differed significantly among the three groups ($P < 0.001$ by the log-rank test). (Reproduced with permission from Celli et al. [89]. © 2004 Massachusetts Medical Society. All rights reserved)

antitrypsin, the most common of which are the normal allele "M" and the abnormal alleles "S" and "Z." Although, only one normal allele ("M") is needed to produce the normal phenotype, heterozygote individuals ("MZ" or "MS") tend to produce 65% less α-1 antitrypsin than normal individuals ("MM") [2, 92]. The abnormal homozygote ("ZZ") which results in no α-1 antitrypsin production occurs with a prevalence between 1/1575 and 1/5097 and accounts for 2–3% of COPD [92]. While the disease onset varies, it is usually evident by the fourth or fifth decade and even earlier in those who smoke [2]. In contrast to normal "MM" individuals who preferentially develop emphysematous changes in the apices, the distribution of emphysema in α-1 antitrypsin tends to be relatively homogeneous. Other genetic abnormalities (e.g., polymorphisms of TGF β1,

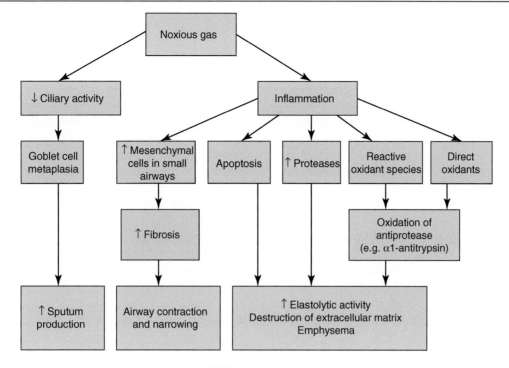

Fig. 31.5 Pathogenesis of chronic obstructive lung disease (COPD)

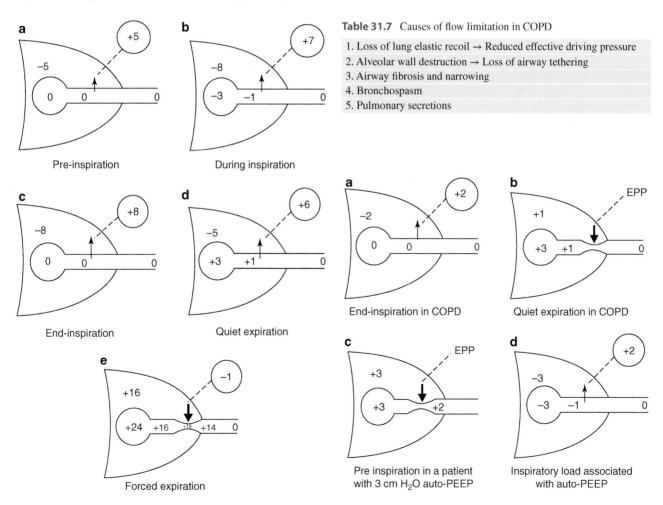

Table 31.7 Causes of flow limitation in COPD

1. Loss of lung elastic recoil → Reduced effective driving pressure
2. Alveolar wall destruction → Loss of airway tethering
3. Airway fibrosis and narrowing
4. Bronchospasm
5. Pulmonary secretions

Fig. 31.6 The effect of intrapleural and alveolar pressures on airway patency. (Adapted from West [94])

Fig. 31.7 The effect of intrapleural and alveolar pressures on airway patency in patients with COPD. *EPP* equal pressure point

sure at end-inspiration is −2 cm water, 6 cm water less negative than in a normal individual (see Fig. 31.6c). The propensity for airway collapse is accentuated by inflammatory and fibrotic changes which lead to contraction and narrowing of the small airways. As a result, even normal pressure increases of 3 cm water associated with quiet expiration may result in flow limitation in patients with severe COPD (Fig. 31.7b).

Dynamic Hyperinflation

In COPD individuals, acute worsening of flow limitation may be precipitated by increased respiratory rates, physical activity, or COPD exacerbations. When flow limitation occurs, individuals with COPD are unable to exhale fully to FRC before their next inspiration. The positive pressure within the lung segments with air trapping is referred to interchangeably as auto-PEEP or intrinsic PEEP ($PEEP_i$). With each subsequent inspiration, "breath stacking" occurs, and the alveoli become progressively more hyperinflated as auto-PEEP accumulates. Initially, auto-PEEP may improve respiratory mechanics and minimize the effect of flow limitation. Since patients with COPD generally expire along the maximum flow–volume loop envelop at rest, they have very limited ability to further increase expiratory flow (see Fig. 31.8) [95]. In this setting, low levels of auto-PEEP help to temporarily improve ventilation by increasing the effective driving pressure and thus expiratory flows.

However, as dynamic hyperinflation worsens, the work of breathing increases dramatically. There are two reasons for this. First, for inspiratory flow to occur, the alveolar pressure must be less than the atmospheric pressure. In normal individuals, this involves minimal effort. When auto-PEEP is present, an equivalent (and potentially large) amount of inspiratory pressure must be generated before airflow even begins. In essence, auto-PEEP is an additional inspiratory load [2, 96]. For example, if 3 cm water of auto-PEEP is present (Fig. 31.7c), then a typical inhalational effort of −3 cm water (see Fig. 31.6a, b) would only drop the alveolar pressure to atmospheric pressure. As a result, despite the pressure change, no inspiratory airflow would occur. In this example, to produce the −3 cm water pressure change required for a normal tidal volume breath (Fig. 31.6a, b), the COPD patient needs to generate an inspiratory pressure of −6 cm water (Fig. 31.7d). Second, dynamic increases in the end-expiratory lung volume results in each tidal volume breath shifting rightward of the flat portion of the volume–pressure compliance curve (see Fig. 31.9) [2, 95, 96]. This increases the work of breathing since a greater pressure must be generated in order to maintain a given tidal volume. Hyperinflation also leads to shortening of the inspiratory muscles, including the diaphragm. This mechanical disadvantage results in functional muscle weakness. Consequently, patients who develop dynamic hyperinflation experience significant dyspnea, respiratory distress, and muscle fatigue.

Hemodynamic instability is also common with high levels of dynamic hyperinflation. Increased intrathoracic pressure associated with auto-PEEP reduces the pressure gradient for venous return into the thorax and also causes direct compression of the ventricles, both of which decrease preload and impair diastolic filling. High auto-PEEP will also

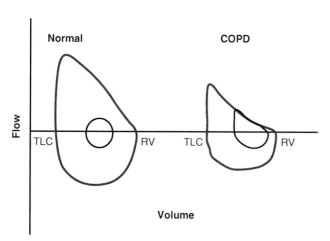

Fig. 31.8 Examples of flow–volume loops obtained in a healthy subject and a patient with COPD. The *black lines* represent the flow–volume loops at rest. The *gray lines* represent the maximal inspiratory and expiratory flow–volume loops. (Adapted from Pepin et al. [95])

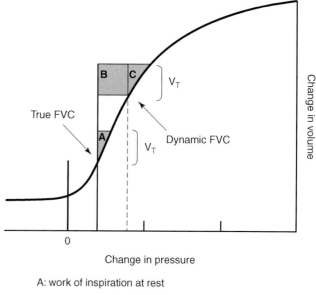

A: work of inspiration at rest

B: work of overcoming PEEPi

C: work of inspiration at dynamic FRC

Fig. 31.9 Compliance curve of the lung. (Reprinted from Kemp et al. [2]. © 2009 with permission from Elsevier)

increase PVR which may precipitate right ventricular dysfunction. In extreme cases, dynamic hyperinflation can cause cardiac arrest and subsequently impair resuscitation. The "Lazarus syndrome," in which patients recover from a cardiac arrest only after resuscitative efforts and positive pressure ventilation are stopped, has been attributed to resolving dynamic hyperinflation [97].

During anesthesia, dynamic hyperinflation commonly presents with increasing airway pressures and severe hypotension shortly after induction when manual or mechanical ventilation is initiated. Other complications that may produce similar clinical findings include tension pneumothorax, anaphylaxis, and cardiac ischemia. When dynamic hyperinflation is suspected, the anesthetic circuit should be disconnected from the patient to permit full exhalation.

Intraoperatively, the buildup of intrinsic PEEP can be difficult to assess. Ideally, the magnitude of auto-PEEP is measured directly at end-expiration, with an end-expiratory gas flow pause. While this function is commonly found on intensive care ventilators, it is rarely available on anesthesia gas machines. However, the presence of intraoperative breath stacking can be indirectly assessed by capnography and spirometry loops. The capnograph tracing normally plateaus at the end of a fully exhaled breath, reflecting a constant alveolar concentration of CO_2. In obstructive diseases, although the capnograph commonly upslopes as a result of air from dead space diluting the exhaled CO_2 concentration, the capnograph will still plateau when exhalation is complete. If the next breath is initiated before the CO_2 plateaus, the presence of auto-PEEP should be suspected [98]. Similarly, the presence of air trapping may be inferred from flow–volume loops when the expiratory flow does not drop to zero before the next breath (see Fig. 6.6).

Respiratory Drive in COPD

The control of ventilation is primarily regulated by the arterial partial pressure of carbon dioxide ($PaCO_2$), with each 1 mmHg rise increasing minute ventilation by 2–3 L/min [99, 100]. However, this relationship is self-limiting. Within the central nervous system (CNS), severe hypercapnia and acidosis are associated with increased glutamine and gamma-aminobutyric acid (GABA) and decreased glutamate and aspartate levels. These changes result in a decreased level of consciousness, as well as reduced minute ventilation and inspiratory drive [101]. Typically, these CNS effects manifest when the $PaCO_2$ is greater than 60–70 mmHg. In patients with chronic hypercapnia that is compensated by an increase in bicarbonate, even higher $PaCO_2$ levels may be tolerated before respiratory depression occurs. In comparison with the linear minute ventilation response to $PaCO_2$, decreases in the P_aO_2 lead to an exponential increase in minute ventilation only when levels fall below 60 mmHg.

Patients with severe COPD often have an elevated $PaCO_2$ at rest. Retention of carbon dioxide occurs because these patients are unable to maintain sufficient respiratory work to keep their $PaCO_2$ at normal levels. In these patients, clinicians have observed that oxygen administration can worsen the degree of hypercapnia. Traditionally, clinicians believed that patients with chronic hypercapnia had a blunted ventilatory response to increased $PaCO_2$ and were dependent on hypoxic drive to breath. Supplemental oxygen would therefore inhibit hypoxic drive and decrease minute ventilation. While this explanation is valid, its contributing role to the overall increase in $PaCO_2$ is overstated. In one study of patients with COPD in acute respiratory failure, oxygen administration at 5 L/min only reduced the respiratory rate and the minute ventilation by 14% – an insufficient drop to account for the entire rise in $PaCO_2$. Moreover, while ventilatory drive was reduced following oxygen supplementation, it remained three times greater than in normal individuals [102]. In another study, the rise in $PaCO_2$ that could be attributable to decreased minute ventilation was only 22%. In comparison, 48% of the $PaCO_2$ increase was attributed to an increase in dead-space ventilation, and 30% resulted from reduced Haldane effect [103]. In patients with COPD, the degree of V/Q mismatching and dead-space ventilation is minimized by HPV which redirects blood away from poorly ventilated to well-ventilated areas. The use of supplemental oxygen hinders this effect, resulting in increased dead-space ventilation and reduced CO_2 elimination. The Haldane effect describes the enhanced dissociation of CO_2 from red blood cells caused by the oxygenation of hemoglobin. Oxygenated hemoglobin has a much lower affinity for CO_2 than deoxygenated hemoglobin. As a result, deoxygenated hemoglobin facilitates the loading of CO_2 from peripheral tissue, while the oxygenation of hemoglobin in the lungs leads to offloading. The magnitude of the Haldane effect is proportional to the difference between the mixed venous oxygen saturation and the arterial oxygen saturation. In other words, more CO_2 is released in the lungs when the mixed venous–arterial gradient is large. In COPD patients, the use of high-inspired fractions of oxygen (FiO_2) leads to a significant increase in the mixed venous oxygen saturation, which limits the ability of hemoglobin to bind and eliminate CO_2 from the periphery.

In spite of the potential increase in $PaCO_2$ associated with the administration of oxygen to patients with COPD, titrated oxygen therapy must be used to avoid hypoxia. In patients with acute respiratory failure, the reduction in ventilatory drive associated with oxygen administration may actually be of benefit. A lower respiratory rate minimizes the risk of dynamic hyperinflation, the work of breathing, and the potential for respiratory muscle fatigue. Patients requiring supplemental oxygen need to be closely monitored for signs of CNS depression and CO_2 narcosis. The P_aO_2 and the $PaCO_2$ should be frequently checked. For most patients, titrating the FiO2 to maintain an O_2 saturation of 88–92% is usually sufficient [88].

Bullae

Bullae are cystic air spaces in the lung parenchyma with a diameter greater than 1 cm. Most commonly, bullae develop as a result of worsening emphysematous disease. Bullae form when there is a loss of structural support tissue within a localized area. Preserved elastic recoil of the surrounding lung tissue places outward traction on bulla, causing it to enlarge. This results in the characteristic "inflated" look of bullae on chest X-rays and computed tomography scans. Although bullae appear to compress adjacent lung segments, direct measurements have conclusively shown that they are not under positive pressure [104]. Perhaps surprisingly, bullae do not contribute significantly to increased dead-space ventilation. In spite of unimpeded communication between the airways and bullae, very little airflow occurs. The lack of elastic recoil essentially prevents fully expanded bullae from emptying during exhalation or from filling any further during inhalation. In addition, because bullae are relatively avascular, they do not participate in gas exchange. In patients with large bullae occupying more than a third of the hemithorax (i.e., "giant bullae"), a mixed restrictive–obstructive disease pattern may emerge as the volume available to the nonbullous lung segments is reduced. The loss of structural integrity within bullae predisposes patients to serious complications including rupture, tension pneumothorax, and bronchopleural fistula. Although the risk of these adverse events is increased with positive pressure ventilation, it may be safely used so long as the airway pressures are kept low. Chest tube insertion and lung isolation may be required should these complications arise.

Ventilation Strategies in Patients with Obstructive Disease

Providing effective mechanical ventilation for patients with severe COPD can be challenging. Key goals, which at times conflict, include (1) avoiding dynamic hyperinflation, (2) avoiding barotrauma and volutrauma, and (3) maintaining adequate oxygenation and ventilation. As previously discussed, dynamic hyperinflation occurs when inadequate expiratory time leads to breath stacking. This risk can be minimized by using low I/E ratios in the range of 1:3 to 1:5, as well as low respiratory rates. This may result in lower minute ventilation and cause hypercarbia and hypoxia, both of which worsen pulmonary hypertension and right ventricular strain. Higher tidal volumes may improve these gas exchange abnormalities, but this may significantly increase airway pressures and expose patients to a higher risk of volutrauma or barotrauma.

In spontaneously breathing patients with obstructive lung disease, applying extrinsic PEEP that is equal to or less than the patient's auto-PEEP has been shown to reduce the work of breathing associated with air trapping. In contrast, for mechanically ventilated patients, the use of extrinsic PEEP in patients with obstructive disease is controversial. Theoretical advantages of applying extrinsic PEEP include maintaining alveoli open in areas of more normal lung mechanics and keeping small and easily collapsible airways patent, thereby reducing expiratory flow limitation. While extrinsic PEEP improves gas exchange and hemodynamics in some studies, others have demonstrated a worsening of expiratory airflow [98]. In one study of eight patients, Caramez et al. [105] examined the effect of increasing extrinsic PEEP from 0% to 150% of intrinsic PEEP using four different ventilatory settings. Using total PEEP, FRC, and plateau pressure as markers of expiratory flow limitation, the pooled data reliably showed a biphasic response with either no change or a slight increase in flow limitation when extrinsic PEEP was less than intrinsic PEEP, followed by a sharp rise once intrinsic PEEP was exceeded. However, when individual patient data were examined, three different responses to external PEEP were noted (see Fig. 31.10). In five patients, the use of external PEEP reduced air trapping and hyperinflation during at least one of the four ventilatory settings. Unfortunately, patient response to extrinsic PEEP was unpredictable and appeared to be independent of the disease, mechanics, or ventilation parameters. In another study by Jolliet et al. [106], the use of extrinsic PEEP at 80% of intrinsic PEEP significantly reduced the degree of intrinsic PEEP (7.8–4.4 cm H_2O; $P < 0.001$) as well as the volume of air trapping (216–120 mL; $P < 0.001$). In spite of these improvements, no change in hemodynamic parameters (mean arterial pressure and cardiac output) or gas exchange (P_aO_2 and $PaCO_2$) was noted. Clinical relevance aside, it is dif-

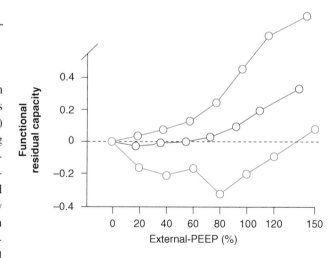

Fig. 31.10 The three potential responses in FRC when external PEEP (represented as a percentage of PEEPi measured at zero external PEEP) is applied. *Blue* is biphasic response; *green* is classic overinflation response; and *red* is paradoxic response

ficult to accurately measure the degree of intrinsic PEEP intra-operatively, and thus, select a level of extrinsic PEEP that does not exceed it. Extrinsic PEEP that is greater than intrinsic PEEP will worsen expiratory flow and increase hyperinflation. Given the limited evidence of benefit, the inability to define a clear expiratory PEEP target, and the risk of exacerbating air trapping, extrinsic PEEP in mechanically ventilated patients with obstructive lung disease should be minimized.

Cystic Fibrosis

Cystic fibrosis (CF) is an autosomal recessive disorder that results in impaired transport of sodium, chloride, and water across epithelial tissue. This leads to abnormally viscous secretions which can cause obstruction of the respiratory tracts, pancreas, biliary system, intestines, and sweat glands. The organ systems that are affected are summarized in Table 31.8. Though most commonly associated with Caucasians (1:3000), the disease also affects Hispanics (1:9500), African Americans (1:15,300), and Asian Americans (1:32,100) [107]. With improved medical care over the last half century, the prognosis for patients with CF has improved dramatically, and the median predicted sur-

Table 31.8 Clinical manifestations of cystic fibrosis

Organ system	Clinical features
Pulmonary	Impaired clearance of viscous secretions, mucous plugging
	Obstructive lung disease
	Bronchiectasis
	Reactive airways
	Hemoptysis
	Recurrent infections and chronic colonization (*S. aureus, H. influenzae, Aspergillus, B. cepacia*)
Cardiac	Pulmonary hypertension and right ventricular failure
Hepato-biliary	Impaired biliary drainage, cholelithiasis, cholecystitis
	Fatty liver, cirrhosis → portal hypertension, esophageal varices, coagulopathy
	Hepatosplenomegaly → sequestration of platelets → thrombocytopenia
Pancreas	Obstruction of pancreatic duct → pancreatitis
	Exocrine dysfunction → ↓ pancreatic enzymes → malabsorption of vitamins A, D, E, K → impaired synthesis of coagulation factors
	Endocrine dysfunction → glucose intolerance, CF-related diabetes
Gastrointestinal tract	Distal intestinal obstructive syndrome
	Gastroesophageal reflux disease → micro-aspirations
Ears, nose, throat	Large nasal polyps
	Sinusitis
Musculoskeletal	Decreased bone mineral density → fractures, kyphoscoliosis
	Hypertrophic osteoarthropathy

vival age was 41.6 years in 2015 (Fig. 31.11). The early mortality of CF is primarily the result of pulmonary complications, which include pneumothorax, massive hemoptysis, severe respiratory infections, and respiratory failure [108–110].

Pulmonary Manifestations of CF

As with COPD, CF is characterized primarily by airflow obstruction, although varying degrees of restriction can also occur. Early in the disease, expiratory flow limitation is caused by the accumulation of thick dehydrated mucous in the respiratory tract that is difficult to expectorate. Inability to clear the thick purulent secretions enhances bacterial growth, and as the disease advances, colonization of the airways with *Pseudomonas aeruginosa* and *Staphylococcus aureus* is considered normal. Infection with other bacteria, though less common, is often much more serious. For instance, *Burkholderia cepacia* is associated with rapid deterioration of pulmonary function, uncontrolled bronchopneumonia, and death. Although infection results in a massive influx of inflammatory cells into the airways, this immune response is ineffective once bacterial infection is established and actually contributes to disease progression. Elastase released by neutrophils overwhelms the antiprotease mechanisms of the lung resulting in inflammatory destruction of airway supportive tissue, increased airway collapsibility during expiration, the development of bronchiectasis, and worsened airway obstruction. As a consequence of these airway changes, ciliary function is impaired, further limiting the patient's ability to clear secretions. In some, reactive airway disease may also contribute to the airflow obstruction. As with other causes of obstructive lung disease, patients with CF are at increased risk of dynamic hyperinflation and pneumothorax. Strategies that maintain low airway pressures and long expiratory times should be considered during mechanical ventilation. Chronic infection and inflammation also leads to increased airway vascularity through both bronchial artery hypertrophy and angiogenesis. The system of enlarged, dilated, and tortuous vessels that develops is highly susceptible to trauma, and as a result, hemoptysis is common in patients with CF. Although most episodes of hemoptysis are self-resolving, some patients may require bronchial artery embolization or even surgical intervention [111]. In patients with hemoptysis requiring a general anesthetic, positive pressure ventilation may increase airway wall tension and precipitate massive hemoptysis. In one case report of 12 patients undergoing bronchial artery embolization who were managed with general anesthesia and intubation, three developed massive hemoptysis and died. In contrast, none of the eight patients managed with sedation developed massive hemoptysis [112].

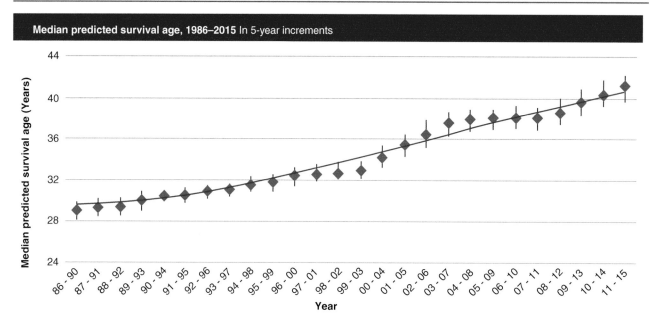

Fig. 31.11 Median predicted survival age from 1986 to 2015 by 5-year increments. (Adapted from Cystic Fibrosis Foundation Patient Registry Annual Data Report 2015)

Management of CF

Effective sputum elimination is a key goal in the long-term management of CF. A long-standing practice used to facilitate this is chest physiotherapy. Traditionally, this consisted of chest percussion with postural drainage. However, as more patients with CF survive into adulthood, there has been a shift toward forms of physiotherapy that can be performed independently. These alternatives range from simple breathing and coughing techniques to the use of medical devices of varying complexity [113]. Although chest physiotherapy is considered standard care, the number of quality trials examining its efficacy is limited. Inhaled DNase I, a human recombinant enzyme that can decrease sputum viscosity by hydrolyzing extracellular DNA, has been shown to improve pulmonary function and reduce the incidence of pulmonary exacerbations. In a randomized controlled trial of 968 patients with CF, twice daily use of DNase I improved FEV_1 by approximately 6% ($p<0.01$) and reduced the risk of pulmonary exacerbations by 37% ($p<0.01$) [114]. Sputum viscosity can also be reduced by using inhaled hypertonic saline which osmotically draws water from the airway mucosa into the lumen. In a study of 164 patients, this therapy reduced the risk of pulmonary exacerbations by 56% ($p = 0.02$) [115].

CFTR modulators are a new class of medication developed to directly improve the function of the defective cystic fibrosis transmembrane regulator protein. They have been shown in randomized trials to improve PFTs and reduce pulmonary exacerbations [116, 117]. Unfortunately, these medications are only approved for specific genetic mutations, and not all CF patients benefit from it.

To optimize patients with CF for anesthesia, chest physiotherapy should be performed immediately prior to surgery. In patients who were prescribed inhaled DNase I and hypertonic saline, these should also be administered. Both during anesthesia and in the postoperative period, the viscosity of pulmonary secretions can be minimized by humidifying the inspired gases. Patient volume status needs to be carefully monitored to avoid both hypovolemia which may worsen secretion tenacity and hypervolemia which may trigger heart failure. Drugs which may either increase pulmonary secretions (e.g., ketamine) or contribute to increased sputum viscosity (e.g., anticholinergics) are relatively contraindicated. Although supraglottic airways have been successfully used in patients with CF requiring general anesthesia, intubation with a large-sized endotracheal tube is usually preferred because it permits better control of ventilation and it facilitates endobronchial toileting with a suction catheter and/or fiber-optic bronchoscopy. When appropriate, the use of regional anesthesia and opioid-sparing adjuvant medications for management of postoperative pain is preferred. In addition to generalized respiratory depression, opioids may diminish the cough reflex and thus sputum clearance.

Extrapulmonary Manifestations of CF

Of the organ systems that are affected by CF, gastrointestinal dysfunction is particularly relevant to the anesthesiologist. Compared to normal individuals, gastroesophageal reflux is six to eight times more common in patients with CF and may contribute to worsening respiratory symptoms [118]. Reflux symptoms should be treated aggressively, and precautions that minimize gastric acidity as well as the risk of aspiration should be considered during anesthesia (e.g., antacids, rapid sequence intubation). The buildup of thick secretions within the intestinal tract of patients with CF results in an increased risk of constipation and bowel obstruction. The use of narcotics may further exacerbate the potential for this complication. Though uncommon, patients with CF may develop a coagulopathy and have an increased risk of bleeding as a result of biliary duct obstruction. Generally, this only causes asymptomatic liver dysfunction. However, as the life expectancy of CF increases, the development of advanced liver disease and cirrhosis may produce complications such as bleeding from esophageal varices, impaired synthesis of coagulation factors, and thrombocytopenia secondary to hepatosplenomegaly. In addition, pancreatic exocrine insufficiency which results in malabsorption of protein, fat, as well as the fat-soluble vitamins is present in 85% of patients with CF [109]. Without supplementation, this causes a deficiency in vitamin K, an important precursor for the synthesis of coagulation factors X, IX, VII, and II. Pancreatic endocrine function may also be affected by CF. Approximately 75% of patients show evidence of glucose intolerance, while 10% develop CF-related diabetes mellitus.

Pregnancy and CF

The improved life expectancy associated with CF over the past few decades has led to a rise in the number of patients presenting for medical care while pregnant. In contrast to males with CF, of whom 95% are infertile, the fertility of young women with CF is almost unaffected [107, 119]. However, pregnancy is associated with a several physiologic changes that may stress the respiratory status of patients with CF. These include an increased oxygen consumption of 30–60%, an increased respiratory rate, decreased chest wall compliance, and decreased FRC. Patients with CF are also exposed to an increased risk of respiratory infection because pregnancy results in a state of relative immunosuppression, and maintenance chest physiotherapy becomes more difficult to perform. A recent observational study that included over 1100 CF parturients demonstrated an increased risk of peripartum mortality, need for mechanical ventilation, pneumonia, acute renal failure, and preterm labor when compared to parturients without CF [120].

The anesthetic management for this patient group follows the same principles already discussed for ESLD. In patients who require a cesarean section, the high risk of desaturation and difficult intubation associated with pregnancy combined with the respiratory impairment of CF strongly favors the use of regional anesthesia over general anesthesia. However, an inadvertent high block will also interfere with ventilation. Although spinal anesthesia is commonly used, the downside

to a rapid onset dense block is that it can also cause significant vasodilation. In patients with pulmonary hypertension, large decreases in systemic pressure may precipitate right ventricular ischemia. A titrated epidural results in less hemodynamic instability and greater control over block level and provides superior postoperative pain management. Following delivery, uterotonic agents such as oxytocin and methylergonovine should be administered cautiously because they may cause significant hemodynamic derangements including tachycardia, hypotension, or vasoconstriction. 15-Methyl prostaglandin F2-α (Hemabate) not only increases PVR but can also result in significant bronchospasm and should be avoided in patients with CF. Misoprostol, a prostaglandin E1 analog, may have a more favorable side effect profile in patients with cardiorespiratory disease.

Interstitial Lung Diseases

Interstitial lung diseases (ILDs) are a heterogeneous group of disorders associated with inflammation and fibrosis of the lung parenchyma. ILDs are characterized by restrictive physiology on PFTs and are usually differentiated from extrapulmonary restrictive respiratory diseases by an impaired diffusing capacity for carbon monoxide (DLCO). As with COPD and CF, inflammation plays an integral role in ILDs. However, the inflammation associated with ILDs results predominately in diffuse scarring and fibrosis of the alveolar walls and small airways, as opposed to tissue destruction. The factors which influence whether inflammation will precipitate one outcome vs. the other are unclear. About 35% of ILDs are attributable to an identifiable cause such as exposure to inorganic dust, organic antigen, drugs, or radiation. In the remaining 65% of patients, even though the disease pattern may be given a specific name, the inciting agent resulting in ILDs is unknown (Table 31.9).

Confirming the diagnosis can be challenging and may require a multidisciplinary approach involving experienced respirologists, radiologists, and pathologists, taking into account clinical, radiologic (reticular pattern on chest radiography, disease-specific interstitial opacities on computed tomography), physiologic (restrictive lung function, impaired DLCO), and pathologic (lung biopsy, bronchoalveolar lavage) evidence.

Pulmonary Manifestations of ILDs

As a consequence of inflammation and fibrosis of the alveolar walls, the elastic recoil of the lungs increases, they become less distensible, and lung volumes contract. Early in the disease, despite decreased maximal voluntary ventilation, patients adapt to lower tidal volumes by increasing their

References

1. Bluman LG, Mosca L, Newman N, et al. Preoperative smoking habits and postoperative pulmonary complications. Chest. 1998;113:883–9.
2. Kemp SV, Polkey MI, Shah PL. The epidemiology, etiology, clinical features, and natural history of emphysema. Thorac Surg Clin. 2009;19(2):149–58.
3. Fischer SP, Bader AM, Sweitzer BJ. Preoperative evaluation. In: Miller RD, Eriksson LI, Fleisher LA, Wiener-Kronish JP, Young WL, editors. Miller's anesthesia. 7th ed. Philadelphia: Churchill Livingstone; 2009. p. 1022.
4. Warner MA, Offord KP, Warner ME, et al. Role of preoperative cessation of smoking and other factors in postoperative pulmonary complications: a blinded prospective study of coronary artery bypass patients. Mayo Clin Proc. 1989;64(6):609–16.
5. Nakagawa M, Tanaka H, Tsukuma H. Relationship between the duration of the preoperative smoke-free period and the incidence of postoperative pulmonary complications after pulmonary surgery. Chest. 2001;120:705–10.
6. Wong J, Lam DP, Abrishami A, Chan MTV, Chung F. Short-term preoperative smoking cessation and postoperative complications: a systematic review and meta-analysis. Can J Anesth. 2012;59:268–79.
7. Møller AM, Villebro N, Tom Pedersen T, Tønnesen H. Effect of preoperative smoking intervention on postoperative complications: a randomised clinical trial. Lancet. 2002;359:114–7.
8. Thomsen T, Villebro N, Møller AM. Interventions for preoperative smoking cessation. Cochrane Database Syst Rev. 2014;3:CD002294.
9. Thomsen T, Tønnesen H, Møller AM. Effect of preoperative smoking cessation interventions on postoperative complications and smoking cessation. Brit J Surg. 2009;96:451–61.
10. Lee SM, Landry J, Jones PM, Buhrmann O, Morley-Forster P. Long-term quit rates after a perioperative smoking cessation randomized controlled trial. Anesth Analg. 2015;120:582–7.
11. ASA task force on smoking cessation. Statement on smoking cessation. 2008.
12. Wong J, Abrishami A, Yang Y, Zaki A, Friedman Z, Selby P, et al. A perioperative smoking cessation intervention with varenicline - a double-blind, randomized, placebo-controlled trial. Anesthesiology. 2012;117:755–64.
13. Spruit MA, Singh SJ, Garvey C, ZuWallack R, Nici L, Rochester C, et al. ATS/ERS Task Force on Pulmonary Rehabilitation. An Official American Thoracic Society/European Respiratory Society Statement: key concepts and advances in pulmonary rehabilitation. Am J Respir Crit Care Med 2013;188(8):e13–64.
14. Casaburi R, Patessio A, Ioli F, et al. Reductions in exercise lactic acidosis and ventilation as a result of exercise training in patients with obstructive lung disease. Am Rev Respir Dis. 1991;143(1):9–18.
15. Meyer T, Faude O, Scharhag J, et al. Is lactic acidosis a cause of exercise induced hyperventilation at the respiratory compensation point? Br J Sports Med. 2004;38(5):622–5.
16. Kesten S. Pulmonary rehabilitation and surgery for end-stage lung disease. Clin Chest Med. 1997;18(2):173–81.
17. Donahoe M. Nutritional support in advanced lung disease. The pulmonary cachexia syndrome. Clin Chest Med. 1997;18(3):547–61.
18. Casaburi R, ZuWallack R. Pulmonary rehabilitation for management of chronic obstructive pulmonary disease. N Engl J Med. 2009;360(13):1329–35.
19. Ries AL, Bauldoff GS, Carlin BW, et al. Pulmonary rehabilitation: joint ACCP/AACVPR evidence-based clinical practice guidelines. Chest. 2007;131(5 Suppl):4S–2.
20. McCarthy B, Casey D, Devane D, Murphy K, Murphy E, Lacasse Y. Pulmonary rehabilitation for chronic obstructive pulmonary disease. Cochrane Database Syst Rev. 2015;2:CD003793.
21. Dowman L, Hill CJ, Holland AE. Pulmonary rehabilitation for interstitial lung disease. Cochrane Database Syst Rev. 2014;10:CD006322.
22. Klijn PHC, Oudshoorn A, van der Ent CK, van der NET J, Kimpen JL, Helders PJM. Effects of anaerobic training in children with cystic fibrosis – a randomized controlled study. Chest. 2004;125:1299–305.
23. Radtke T, Nolan SJ, Hebestreit H, Kriemler S. Physical exercise training for cystic fibrosis. Cochrane Database Syst Rev. 2015;6:CD002768.
24. Carson KV, Chandratilleke MG, Picot J, Brinn MP, Esterman AJ, Smith BJ. Physical training for asthma. Cochrane Database Syst Rev. 2013;9:CD001116.
25. Mendes FAR, Goncalves RC, Nunes MPT, Saraiva-Romanholo BM, Cukier A, Stelmach R, et al. Effects of aerobic training on psychosocial morbidity and symptoms in patients with asthma - a randomized clinical trial. Chest. 2010;138(2):331–3.
26. Turner A, Eastwood P, Cook A, Jenkins S. Improvements in symptoms and quality of life following exercise training in older adults with moderate/severe persistent asthma. Respiration. 2011;81:302–10.
27. Uchi M, Saji T, Harada T. Feasibility of cardiopulmonary rehabilitation in patients with idiopathic pulmonary arterial hypertension treated with intravenous prostacyclin infusion therapy. J Cardiol. 2005;46(5):183–93.
28. National Emphysema Treatment Trial Research Group. A randomized trial comparing lung-volume–reduction surgery with medical therapy for severe emphysema. N Engl J Med. 2003;348:2059–73.
29. Cesario A, Ferri L, Galetta D, et al. Pre-operative pulmonary rehabilitation and surgery for lung cancer. Lung Cancer. 2007;57(1):118–9.
30. Bobbio A, Chetta A, Ampollini L, Primomo GL, Internullo E, Carbognani P, et al. Preoperative pulmonary rehabilitation in patients undergoing lung resection for non-small cell lung cancer. Eur J Cardiothorac Surg. 2008;33:95–8.
31. Stefanelli F, Meoli I, Cobuccio R, Curcio C, Amore D, Casazza D, et al. High-intensity training and cardiopulmonary exercise testing in patients with chronic obstructive pulmonary disease and non-small-cell lung cancer undergoing lobectomy. Eur J Cardiothorac Surg. 2013;44:e260–5.
32. Rajendran AJ, Pandurangi UM, Murali R, et al. Pre-operative short term pulmonary rehabilitation for patients of chronic obstructive pulmonary disease undergoing coronary artery bypass graft surgery. Indian Heart J. 1998;50(5):531–4.
33. Simonneau G, Gatzoulis MA, Adatia I, Celermajer D, Denton C, Ghofrani A, et al. Updated clinical classification of pulmonary hypertension. J Am Coll Cardiol. 2013;62:D34–41.
34. Lawrence VA, Cornell JE, Smetana GW. Strategies to reduce postoperative pulmonary complication after noncardiothoracic surgery: systemic review for the American College of Physicians. Ann Intern Med. 2006;144:596–608.
35. Olsen MF, Hahn I, Nordgren S, et al. Randomized controlled trial of prophylactic chest physiotherapy in major abdominal surgery. Br J Surg. 1997;84:1535–8.
36. Hulzebos EH, Helders PJ, Favié NJ, et al. Preoperative intensive inspiratory muscle training to prevent postoperative pulmonary complications in high-risk patients undergoing CABG surgery: a randomized clinical trial. JAMA. 2006;296(15):1851–7.
37. Katsura M, Kuriyama A, Takeshima T, Fukuhara S, Furukawa TA. Preoperative inspiratory muscle training for postoperative pulmonary complications in adults undergoing cardiac and major abdominal surgery. Cochrane Database Syst Rev. 2015;10:CD010356.
38. Warner DO. Preventing postoperative pulmonary complications. Anesthesiology. 2000;92:1467–72.
39. Bossone E, Ferrara F, Grunig E. Echocardiography in pulmonary hypertension. Curr Opin Cardiol. 2015;30:574–86.

40. Gay PC. Chronic obstructive pulmonary disease and sleep. Respir Care. 2004;49:39–51.

41. Bhullar S, Phillips B. Sleep in COPD patients. COPD. 2005;2:355–61.

42. Rafanan AL, Golish JA, Dinner DS, et al. Nocturnal hypoxemia is common in primary pulmonary hypertension. Chest. 2001;120:894–9.

43. Agarwal S, Richardson B, Krishnan V, et al. Interstitial lung disease and sleep: what is known? Sleep Med. 2009;10:947–51.

44. Milross MA, Piper AJ, Dobbin CJ, et al. Sleep disordered breathing in cystic fibrosis. Sleep Med Rev. 2004;8:295–308.

45. Schneider H. Sleep-related breathing disorders in COPD. In: Stoller JK, Badr MS, Hollingsworth H, Eichler AF, editors. UpToDate. Waltham: UpToDate; 2017.

46. Fischer LG, Van Aken H, Bürkle H. Management of pulmonary hypertension: physiological and pharmacological considerations for anesthesiologists. Anesth Analg. 2003;96(6): 1603–16.

47. Blaise G, Langleben D, Hubert B. Pulmonary arterial hypertension: pathophysiology and anesthetic approach. Anesthesiology. 2003;99(6):1415–32.

48. Rovedder PM, Ziegler B, Pinotti AF, et al. Prevalence of pulmonary hypertension evaluated by Doppler echocardiography in a population of adolescent and adult patients with cystic fibrosis. J Bras Pneumol. 2008;34(2):83–90.

49. Han MK, McLaughlin VV, Criner GJ, et al. Pulmonary diseases and the heart. Circulation. 2007;116(25):2992–3005.

50. Andersen KH, Iversen M, Kjaergaard J, Mortensen J, Nielsen-Kudsk JE, Bendstrup E, et al. Prevalence, predictors, and survival in pulmonary hypertension related to end-stage chronic obstructive pulmonary disease. J Heart Lung Transplant. 2012;31: 373–80.

51. Subramaniam K, Yared JP. Management of pulmonary hypertension in the operating room. Semin Cardiothorac Vasc Anesth. 2007;11:119–36.

52. Stoelting RK, Hillier SC. Nonbarbituate intravenous anesthetic drugs. In: Stoelting RK, Hillier SC, editors. Pharmacology and physiology in anesthesia practice. 4th ed. Philadelphia: Lippincott Williams & Wilkins; 2006. p. 155–79.

53. Fox C, Kalarickal PL, Yarborough MJ, et al. Perioperative management including new pharmacological vistas for patients with pulmonary hypertension for noncardiac surgery. Curr Opin Anaesthesiol. 2008;21:467–72.

54. Friesen RH, Williams GD. Anesthetic management of children with pulmonary arterial hypertension. Paediatr Anaesth. 2008;18:208–16.

55. Friesen RH, Twite MD, Nichols CS, Cardwell KA, Pan Z, Darst JR, et al. Hemodynamic response to ketamine in children with pulmonary hypertension. Paediatr Anaesth. 2016;26:102–8.

56. Tayama E, Ueda T, Shojima T, et al. Arginine vasopressin is an ideal drug after cardiac surgery for the management of low systemic vascular resistant hypotension concomitant with pulmonary hypertension. Interact Cardiovasc Thorac Surg. 2007;6:715–9.

57. Price LC, Forrest P, Sodhi V, et al. Use of vasopressin after Caesarean section in idiopathic pulmonary arterial hypertension. Br J Anaesth. 2007;99:552–5.

58. Smith AM, Elliot CM, Kiely DG, et al. The role of vasopressin in cardiorespiratory arrest and pulmonary hypertension. QJM. 2006;99:127–33.

59. Currigan DA, Hughes RJA, Wright CE, Angus JA, Soeding PF. Vasoconstrictor responses to vasopressor agents in human pulmonary and radial arteries an in vitro study. Anesthesiology. 2014;121:930–6.

60. Hajjar LA, Vincent JL, Galas FRBG, Rhodes A, Landoni G, Osawa EA, et al. Vasopressin versus norepinephrine in patients with vasoplegic shock after cardiac surgery the VANCS randomized controlled trial. Anesthesiology. 2017;126:85–93.

61. Sandham JD, Hull RD, Brant RF, et al. A randomized, controlled trial of the use of pulmonary-artery catheters in high-risk surgical patients. N Engl J Med. 2003;348:5–14.

62. Rodgers A, Walker N, Schug S, et al. Reduction of postoperative mortality and morbidity with epidural or spinal anaesthesia: results from overview of randomised trials. BMJ. 2000;321:1493.

63. Park WY, Thompson JS, Lee KK. Effect of epidural anesthesia and analgesia on perioperative outcome: a randomized, controlled Veterans Affairs cooperative study. Ann Surg. 2001;234:560–9.

64. Rigg JR, Jamrozik K, Myles PS, et al. Epidural anaesthesia and analgesia and outcome of major surgery: a randomised trial. Lancet. 2002;359:1276–82.

65. Tziavrangos E, Schug SA. Regional anaesthesia and perioperative outcome. Curr Opin Anaesthesiol. 2006;19:521–5.

66. Gulur P, Nishimori M, Ballantyne JC. Regional anaesthesia versus general anaesthesia, morbidity and mortality. Best Pract Res Clin Anaesthesiol. 2006;20:249–63.

67. Breen P, Park KW. General anesthesia versus regional anesthesia. Int Anesthesiol Clin. 2002;40:61–71.

68. Hausman MS Jr, Jewell ES, Engoren M. Regional versus general anesthesia in surgical patients with chronic obstructive pulmonary disease: does avoiding general anesthesia reduce the risk of postoperative complications? Anesth Analg. 2015;120:1405–12.

69. Popping DM, Elia N, Van Aken HK, Marret E, Schug SA, Kranke P, et al. Impact of epidural analgesia on mortality and morbidity after surgery - systematic review and meta-analysis of randomized controlled trials. Ann Surg. 2014;259:1056–67.

70. Rock P, Rich PB. Postoperative pulmonary complications. Curr Opin Anaesthesiol. 2003;16:123–31.

71. Kozian A, Schilling T, Hachenberg T. Non-analgetic effects of thoracic epidural anaesthesia. Curr Opin Anaesthesiol. 2005; 18:29–34.

72. Drummond GB. Diaphragmatic dysfunction: an outmoded concept. Br J Anaesth. 1998;80:277–80.

73. Savas JF, Litwack R, Davis K, et al. Regional anesthesia as an alternative to general anesthesia for abdominal surgery in patients with severe pulmonary impairment. Am J Surg. 2004;188(5):603–5.

74. van Zundert AA, Stultiens G, Jakimowicz JJ, et al. Segmental spinal anaesthesia for cholecystectomy in a patient with severe lung disease. Br J Anaesth. 2006;96:464–6.

75. Kalko Y, Ugurlucan M, Basaran M, et al. Epidural anaesthesia and mini-laparotomy for the treatment of abdominal aortic aneurysms in patients with severe chronic obstructive pulmonary disease. Acta Chir Belg. 2007;107(3):307–12.

76. Tarhan S, Moffitt EA, Sessler AD, Douglas WW, Taylor WF. Risk of anesthesia and surgery in patients with chronic bronchitis and chronic obstructive pulmonary disease. Surgery. 1973;74:720–6.

77. van Lier F, van der Geest PJ, Hoeks SE, van Gestel YRBM, Hol JW, Sin DD, et al. Epidural analgesia is associated with improved health outcomes of surgical patients with chronic obstructive pulmonary disease. Anesthesiology. 2011;115:315–21.

78. Amato MB, Barbas CS, Medeiros DM, et al. Effect of a protective-ventilation strategy on mortality in the acute respiratory distress syndrome. N Engl J Med. 1998;338:347.

79. Futier E, Constantin JM, Paugam-Burtz C, Pascal J, Eurin M, Neuschwander A, IMPROVE Study Group. A trial of intraoperative low-tidal-volume ventilation in abdominal surgery. N Engl J Med. 2013;369:428–37.

80. Amato MBP, Meade MO, Slutsky AS, Brochard L, Costa ELV, Schoenfeld DA, et al. Driving pressure and survival in the acute respiratory distress syndrome. N Engl J Med. 2015;372:747–55.

81. Neto AS, Hemmes SNT, Barbas CSV, Beiderlinden M, Fernandez-Bustamante A, Futier E, et al. Association between driving pressure and development of postoperative pulmonary complications in patients undergoing mechanical ventilation for general anaesthesia: a meta-analysis of individual patient data. Lancet Respir Med. 2016;4:272–8034.

82. Lawrence VA, Cornell JE, Smetana GW, et al. Strategies to reduce postoperative pulmonary complications after noncardiothoracic surgery: systematic review for the American College of Physicians. Ann Intern Med. 2006;144:596–608.

83. Abraham NS, Young JM, Solomon MJ. Meta-analysis of short-term outcomes after laparoscopic resection for colorectal cancer. Br J Surg. 2004;91:1111–24.

84. Avidan MS, Maybrier HR, Abdallah AB, Jacobsohn E, Vlisides PE, Pryor KO, et al. PODCAST Research Group. Intraoperative ketamine for prevention of postoperative delirium or pain after major surgery in older adults: an international, multicentre, double-blind, randomised clinical trial. Lancet 2017;390: 267–75.

85. Conacher ID, Slinger PD. Pain management. In: Kaplan JA, Slinger PD, editors. Thoracic anesthesia. 3rd ed. Philadelphia: Churchill Livingstone; 2003. p. 436–62.

86. Groeben H. Epidural anesthesia and pulmonary function. J Anesth. 2006;20:290–9.

87. Nelson R, Edwards S, Tse B. Prophylactic nasogastric decompression after abdominal surgery. Cochrane Database Syst Rev 2007;3:CD004929.

88. Global initiative for chronic obstructive lung disease – global strategy for the diagnosis, management and prevention of chronic obstructive pulmonary disease – 2017 Report. www.goldcopd.org. Accessed on 26 March 2017.

89. Celli BR, Cote CG, Marin JM, et al. The body-mass index, airflow obstruction, dyspnea, and exercise capacity index in chronic obstructive pulmonary disease. N Engl J Med. 2004;350:1005–12.

90. Salvi SS, Barnes PJ. Chronic obstructive pulmonary disease in non-smokers. Lancet. 2009;374:733–43.

91. Spurzem JR, Rennard SI. Pathogenesis of COPD. Semin Respir Crit Care Med. 2005;26:142–53.

92. Stroller J. Clinical manifestations, diagnosis, and natural history of alpha-1 antitrypsin deficiency. In: Barnes PJ, Hollingsworth H, editors. UpToDate. Waltham: UpToDate; 2017.

93. McGeachie MJ, Yates KP, Zhou X, Guo F, Sternberg AL, Van Natta ML, et al. CAMP Research Group. Patterns of growth and decline in lung function in persistent childhood asthma. N Engl J Med. 2016;374:1842–52.

94. West JB. Mechanics of breathing. In: West JB, editor. Respiratory physiology. 5th ed. Baltimore: Williams & Wilkins; 1990. p. 117–32.

95. Pepin V, Saey D, Laviolette L, Maltais F. Exercise capacity in chronic obstructive pulmonary disease: mechanisms of limitation. COPD. 2007;4:195–204.

96. O'Donnell DE, Parker CM. COPD exacerbations-3: pathophysiology. Thorax. 2006;61:354–61.

97. Ben-David B, Stonebreaker VC, Hershman R. Survival after failed intraoperative resuscitation: a case of "Lazarus syndrome". Anesth Analg. 2001;92:690–2.

98. Edrich T, Sadovnikoff N. Anesthesia for patients with severe chronic obstructive pulmonary disease. Curr Opin Anaesthesiol. 2010;23:18–24.

99. West JB. Control of ventilation. In: West JB, editor. Respiratory physiology. 5th ed. Baltimore: Williams & Wilkins; 1990. p. 117–32.

100. Hirshman CA, McCullough RE, Weil JV. Normal values for hypoxic and hypercapnic ventilatory drives in man. J Appl Physiol. 1975;38:1095–8.

101. Feller-Kopman DJ, Schwartzstein RM. In: Stoller JK, editor. Mechanisms, causes and effects of hypercapnia. Waltham: UpToDate; 2017.

102. Aubier M, Murciano D, Fournier M, et al. Central respiratory drive in acute respiratory failure of patients with chronic obstructive pulmonary disease. Am Rev Respir Dis. 1980;122:191–9.

103. Aubier M, Murciano D, Milic-Emili J, et al. Effects of the administration of O_2 on ventilation and blood gases in patients with chronic obstructive pulmonary disease during acute respiratory failure. Am Rev Respir Dis. 1980;122: 747–54.

104. Morgan MD, Edwards CW, Morris J, et al. Origin and behaviour of emphysematous bullae. Thorax. 1989;44:533–8.

105. Caramez MP, Borges JB, Tucci MR, et al. Paradoxical responses to positive end-expiratory pressure in patients with airway obstruction during controlled ventilation. Crit Care Med. 2005;33:1519–28.

106. Jolliet P, Watremez C, Roeseler J, et al. Comparative effects of helium-oxygen and external positive end-expiratory pressure on respiratory mechanics, gas exchange, and ventilation-perfusion relationships in mechanically ventilated patients with chronic obstructive pulmonary disease. Intensive Care Med. 2003;29:1442–50.

107. Karlet MC. An update on cystic fibrosis and implications for anesthesia. AANA J. 2000;68:141–8.

108. Howell PR, Kent N, Douglas MJ. Anaesthesia for the parturient with cystic fibrosis. Int J Obstet Anesth. 1993;2: 152–8.

109. Walsh TS, Young CH. Anaesthesia and cystic fibrosis. Anaesthesia. 1995;50:614–22.

110. Cystic Fibrosis Foundation Patient Registry Annual Data Report 2015.

111. Stenbit A, Flume PA. Pulmonary complications in adult patients with cystic fibrosis. Am J Med Sci. 2008;335:55–9.

112. McDougall RJ, Sherrington CA. Fatal pulmonary haemorrhage during anaesthesia for bronchial artery embolization in cystic fibrosis. Paediatr Anaesth. 1999;9:345–8.

113. Simon RH. Cystic fibrosis: overview of the treatment of lung disease. In: Mallory GB, Hopin AG, editors. UpToDate. Waltham, MA: UpToDate; 2017.

114. Fuchs HJ, Borowitz DS, Christiansen DH, et al. Effect of aerosolized recombinant human DNase on exacerbations of respiratory symptoms and on pulmonary function in patients with cystic fibrosis. The Pulmozyme Study Group. N Engl J Med. 1994;331:637–42.

115. Elkins MR, Robinson M, Rose BR, et al. A controlled trial of long-term inhaled hypertonic saline in patients with cystic fibrosis. N Engl J Med. 2006;354:229–40.

116. Ramsey BW, Davies J, McElvaney NG, Tullis E, Bell SC, Drevinek P, et al. A CFTR potentiator in patients with cystic fibrosis and the G551D mutation. N Engl J Med. 2011;365: 1663–72.

117. Wainwright CE, Elborn JS, Ramsey BW, Marigowda G, Huang X, Cipolli M, et al. Lumacaftor–Ivacaftor in patients with cystic fibrosis homozygous for Phe508del CFTR. N Engl J Med. 2015;373:220–31.

118. Sabharwal S, Borowitz D. Cystic fibrosis: overview of gastrointestinal disease. In: Mallory GB, Heyman MB, Hoppin AG, editors. UpToDate. Waltham: UpToDate; 2017.

119. Tonelli MR, Aitken ML. Pregnancy in cystic fibrosis. Curr Opin Pulm Med. 2007;13:537–40.

120. Patel EM, Swamy GK, Heine RP, Kuller JA, James AH, Grotegut CA. Medical and obstetric complications among pregnant women with cystic fibrosis. Am J Obstet Gynecol. 2015;212: 98.e1–9.

121. King Jr TE, Bradford WZ, Castro-Bernardini S, Fagan EA, Glaspole I, Glassberg MK, et al. ASCEND Study Group. A phase 3 trial of pirfenidone in patients with idiopathic pulmonary fibrosis. N Engl J Med. 2014;370:2083–92.

122. Richeldi L, du Bois RM, Raghu G, Azuma A, Brown KK, Costabel U, et al. INPULSIS trial investigators. Efficacy and

safety of nintedanib in idiopathic pulmonary fibrosis. N Engl J Med. 2014;370:2071–82.

123. Carron M, Marchet A, Ori C. Supreme laryngeal mask airway for laparoscopic cholecystectomy in patient with severe pulmonary fibrosis. Br J Anaesth. 2009;103:778–9.

124. Schure AY, Holzman RS. Anesthesia in a child with severe restrictive pulmonary dysfunction caused by chronic graft-versus-host disease. J Clin Anesth. 2000;12:482–6.

125. Kayatta MO, Ahmed S, Hammel JA, Fernandez F, Pickens A, Miller D, et al. Surgical biopsy of suspected interstitial lung disease is superior to radiographic diagnosis. Ann Thorac Surg. 2013;96:399–401.

126. Hutchinson JP, Fogarty AW, McKeever TM, Hubbard RB. In-hospital mortality after surgical lung biopsy for interstitial lung disease in the United States - 2000 to 2011. Am J Respir Crit Care Med. 2016;193:1161–7.

127. Kumar P, Goldstraw P, Yamada K, Nicholson AG, Wells AU, Hansell DM, et al. Pulmonary fibrosis and lung cancer: risk and benefit analysis of pulmonary resection. J Thorac Cardiovasc Surg. 2003;125:1321–7.

128. Sato T, Teramukai S, Kondo H, Watanabe A, Ebina M, Kishi K, et al. Japanese Association for Chest Surgery. Impact and predictors of acute exacerbation of interstitial lung diseases after pulmonary resection for lung cancer. J Thorac Cardiovasc Surg. 2014;147:1604–11.

Thoracic Surgery in the Elderly

32

Maria D. Castillo, Jeffrey Port, and Paul M. Heerdt

Key Points

- As the population ages, increasing numbers of elderly patients will present for thoracic surgery.
- Physiologic changes that occur with advanced age result in a decline of maximal reserves, affecting the patient's ability to cope with the stress of surgery. Increased age is also associated with an increase in the number of comorbidities.
- Elderly patients with cancer may still stand to benefit from surgery, since survival rates for lung and esophageal cancer are very low without surgical resection.
- Perioperative morbidity and mortality is more closely associated with preoperative health status and tumor stage than chronological age.
- Minimally invasive surgical techniques such as video-assisted thoracoscopic surgery (VATS) have been shown to be an effective approach for surgical resection of cancer.
- Because better postoperative pulmonary function, less postoperative pain, and fewer complications were shown for patients who underwent VATS compared to those who underwent thoracotomy for lobectomy, VATS may be a good choice for patients of advanced age due to their decreased physiologic reserves.
- Careful preoperative assessment and postoperative care are essential in this surgical population due to their diminished ability to handle the stress of surgery.

M. D. Castillo
Department of Anesthesiology, Mt. Sinai College of Medicine, New York, NY, USA

J. Port
Department of Cardiothoracic Surgery, Weill Medical College of Cornell University, New York, NY, USA

P. M. Heerdt (✉)
Department of Anesthesiology, Yale University School of Medicine, New Haven, CT, USA
e-mail: paul.heerdt@yale.edu

Introduction

Demographic projections indicate that by the year 2030, the number of US citizens over the age of 65 will exceed 70 million, with those over 80 years of age comprising about 5% of the total population [1]. Currently, centenarians are the fastest growing segment of the population, a phenomenon that underscores the public health issues presented by an aging citizenry [1–3].

Lung cancer, the major reason for most thoracic surgery and the primary focus of this chapter, is particularly prominent in the elderly. As such, anesthesiologists are increasingly presented with the task of caring for patients exhibiting not only the normal physiological changes associated with aging but also a wide range of age-related comorbidities. In that fundamental aspects of preoperative evaluation, anesthetic pharmacology, and postoperative management are reviewed in other sections, this chapter shall primarily focus on the cardiopulmonary and hepatorenal ramifications of aging, the impact of aging on the thoracic surgical population, the risk–benefit relationship of thoracic surgery for the treatment of cancer in the elderly, and the emerging role of minimally invasive surgical techniques.

Physiology of Aging

Appreciation of the fact that the elderly population is expanding in both size and range underscores the importance of understanding the physiology of senescence. Ultimately, perioperative management of the elderly thoracic surgical candidate is often more complex than that of younger patients due to both the physiologic changes associated with advanced age and the increased incidence of comorbidities, particularly cardiovascular pathology and chronic obstructive pulmonary disease (COPD). In general, as people age, their maximal physiologic reserves decline, potentially limiting their ability to respond adequately to the stress presented by a major operation or acute illness. Functionally, elderly patients may experience symptoms indicative of pathology that are blunted or diminished in intensity, are atypical, or may be misdiagnosed as simply due to "old age" [4].

Cardiovascular

A variety of molecular and structural changes occur within the aorta, myocardium, and cardiac conduction system that are, at least in part, interrelated and adaptive within certain limits [5–7] (Table 32.1). For example, aging is associated with an increase in left ventricular (LV) afterload due to an increase in the stiffness of large elastic arteries and the resultant increased pulse wave velocity. Advanced age is also associated with increased LV mass secondary to myocyte hypertrophy, myocardial fibrosis, and valvular sclerosis and calcification. Vascular stiffness occurs secondary to the breakdown of elastin and collagen. Accompanying these structural changes are subcellular alterations in myocyte calcium cycling that allow the ventricle to maintain tension against the increased afterload for a longer period of time [6]. However, while this adaptation can be beneficial under

some conditions, it can be maladaptive in others, such as tachycardia, when delayed relaxation can impede chamber filling. Superimposed on the direct changes that occur in the heart and circulation is a dampening of homeostatic reflexes that can serve to amplify the functional impact of an age-related decline in cardiovascular reserve [6].

Pulmonary

In general, the aging process is associated with alterations in the lung parenchyma, the chest wall "bellows" function, and central regulation of respiration (Table 32.2). Not surprisingly, respiratory complications are a major cause of morbidity and mortality after thoracic surgery. However, risk generalizations regarding the elderly population are difficult due to wide differences in functional status, largely reflecting the overlay of pathologic changes (i.e., COPD)

Table 32.1 Cardiovascular changes with aging

Cardiac	Left ventricular hypertrophy – increased mass and decreased compliance
	Increased fatty infiltration, fibrosis, amyloid, and altered collagen cross-linking
	Increased risk of conduction defects
	Increased stroke work
	Slower myocardial relaxation (decreased lusitropy)
Vascular	Increased characteristic impedance and peripheral vascular resistance
	Increased incidence of coronary artery disease, plaques, calcified lesions, and fixed stenoses
	Decreased arterial elasticity with increased pulse pressure
	Aortic dilation with decreased compliance and higher wall tension
Reflex regulation	Decreased baroreceptor sensitivity
	Diminished myocardial chronotropic and inotropic response to catecholamines
	Decreased maximal cardiac output and heart rate
	Decreased autonomic control of peripheral vascular resistance

Adapted from Castillo and Heerdt [7]

Table 32.2 Respiratory changes with aging

Structural	Decreased number of alveoli
	Decreased number of lung capillaries
	Decreased elastic recoil, causing easier collapse of peripheral airways
	Decreased airway size
	Decreased alveolar–capillary surface area
	Decreased negative intrapleural pressure
	Weakening of respiratory muscles
	Stiffer chest wall due to fibrosis and calcification
Secretory and immune	Less efficient mucociliary transport
	Less sensitive protective airway reflexes
	Diminished delayed-type hypersensitivity response to foreign antigens
	Increased response to autologous antigens
	Decreased polymorphonuclear leukocyte function
Central regulation	Blunted ventilatory response to hypoxia
	Blunted ventilatory response to hypercarbia
	Increased periodic breathing during sleep
Functional manifestations	Increased functional residual capacity (FRC)
	Increased air trapping
	Decreased forced expiratory volume exhaled in 1 s (FEV1)
	Decreased forced vital capacity (FVC)
	Decreased diffusing capacity
	Decreased venous blood oxygenation
	Increased closing capacity
	Decreased maximal voluntary ventilation (MVV)
	Increased work of breathing
	Widened alveolar–arterial gradient for oxygen
	Increased dead space fraction
	Increased ventilation–perfusion mismatch
	Increased propensity for infection
	Decreased resting PaO_2

Adapted from Castillo and Heerdt [7]

on basic age-related changes. Thus, functional status clearly determines perioperative risk more than age alone [4]. Nonetheless, all elderly patients – regardless of functional status – will exhibit structural, secretory, and regulatory changes that can affect both ventilation and respiration [7, 8]. The integration of these changes with perioperative events can impact even short-term outcomes. For example, if an 80-year-old begins to shiver in response to hypothermia following a thoracotomy, the ability to compensate for increased carbon dioxide production is dampened intrinsically by reduced responsiveness of the central nervous system to drive ventilation coupled with impaired chest wall mechanics and alveolar gas exchange. Superimposed on these effects are the extrinsic effects of opiates to further depress central responsiveness and the added mechanical deficit imposed by thoracotomy. Ultimately, the patient is placed at increased risk of developing significant hypercarbia.

Hepatorenal

Aging produces progressive changes in the liver and kidneys (Table 32.3) that can have a profound effect on drug metabolism and clearance [5]. By the age of 80 years, liver size decreases by as much as 40%, and renal tissue mass has decreased by 30% [9]. At the same time, age-related changes in the perfusion patterns of organs in the body result in decreased blood flow to the liver and kidneys [9]. Ultimately, the decrease in size and perfusion of the liver can affect the plasma clearance of opiates, barbiturates, benzodiazepines, propofol, etomidate, most nondepolarizing relaxants, and other drugs metabolized by the liver [5]. Tissue atrophy and reduced renal blood flow result in decreased glomerular filtration rate, creatinine clearance, renal functional reserve, responsiveness to antidiuretic hormone, and increased susceptibility to renal ischemia and acute renal failure. These age-related changes result in the prolongation of the elimination half-time of drugs and metabolites requiring renal clearance. As people age, there is also increasing variability in

Table 32.3 Hepatorenal changes with aging

Hepatic	Decreased liver size
	Decreased perfusion
	Decreased synthetic and metabolic capacity
Renal	Decreased renal tissue mass
	Decreased perfusion
	Decreased glomerular filtration rate and functional reserve
	Decreased creatinine clearance
	Decreased response to antidiuretic hormone
	Decreased ability to conserve sodium or concentrate urine
	Increased number of nonfunctional glomeruli
	Increased susceptibility to renal ischemia and renal failure

individually calculated pharmacokinetic parameters, such that the clearance of drugs may vary greatly among elderly patients [10].

Nervous System

As with other aspects of senescence, cognitive function shows a great deal of variation in terms of baseline deficit and reserve. Recent data have highlighted the association between postoperative delirium and long-term outcome, underscoring the concept that even short-term cognitive impairment may reflect more systemic deficits. While there are considerable data regarding postoperative delirium in cardiac surgical patients subject to microembolic insults to the brain as the result of manipulation of the heart and aorta [11], other reports have focused on implications in noncardiac surgical patients. Robinson et al. [12] published a study of 144 patients over the age of 50 – of which over half underwent noncardiac thoracic surgery – that found a 44% incidence of delirium when a series of functional and cognitive assessments were carefully applied. The average time to onset was 2.1 ± 0.9 days with a duration of 4.0 ± 5.1 days. Risk factors included increasing age, hypoalbuminemia, anemia, intraoperative hypotension, history of alcohol abuse, and comorbid conditions, along with pre-existing dementia and impaired functional status. Importantly, the presence of delirium was associated with an increased length of hospital stay, a higher incidence of post-discharge institutionalization, and a higher 6-month mortality.

Aging and the Thoracic Surgical Population

Although cancer can occur at any age, it disproportionately strikes the elderly. Cancer is the leading cause of death among people aged 60–79 and the second leading cause of death in those aged 80 and older [2]. Data indicate that persons older than 65 have a 9.8-fold increased incidence of cancer compared with those younger than 65 [3], and the National Cancer Institute Surveillance, Epidemiology, and End Results (SEER) Program revealed that 56% of all newly diagnosed cancer patients were over 65 years of age [1]. Consistent with the overall aging of the population and the trend toward increasing age at the time of cancer diagnosis is an increase in the absolute number of elderly patients presenting with potentially resectable malignancy. For lung cancer in particular, the median age of patients presenting for surgical resection is now in excess of 70 years [2].

Other factors are also increasing the number of aged patients undergoing surgical treatment. For example, projections suggest that the incidence of lung cancer in women will soon equal that of men with a presumptive increase in the number of elderly women presenting for lung resection [13]. Similarly, neoadjuvant chemotherapy and radiation in patients with locally advanced stage III non-small cell lung cancer (NSCLC) are expanding the range of patients who are candidates for surgical resection. Support for this trend can be found in studies that demonstrated a significant survival advantage in patients undergoing preoperative chemotherapy followed by surgery compared to those undergoing surgery alone [14–18]. Emerging data suggests that even elderly patients who receive neoadjuvant therapy for esophageal cancer do not have significantly increased mortality or major complications after esophagectomy despite the insult of both laparotomy and thoracotomy [19].

The Risk-Benefit Relationship of Surgical Intervention in the Elderly

Surgical resection remains the treatment of choice for early-stage lung cancer, yet several reports have presented variable results for resection in the elderly. Based on these data and the fact that the elderly will present with significant comorbidities, clinicians have traditionally offered less aggressive treatment to this group, with some even recommending a nonoperative approach or less than an anatomic resection. However, advances in perioperative care and in surgical technique have now encouraged many to offer surgical resection to the aged population. Ultimately, the fundamental question for many patients is how the risk of surgery compares to that of other interventions or no intervention at all. Current data indicate that at initial diagnosis elderly patients tend to have earlier stage lung cancer than younger patients [20]. In addition, they tend to have a higher incidence of squamous cell lung cancers with a clinically reduced growth rate and metastatic potential. Nonetheless, these data need to be interpreted in the context of operative risk and what "long term" may mean to an 85-year-old.

Age-Related Perioperative Morbidity and Mortality

For patients aged ≥70, Birim et al. [21] concluded from a retrospective study that operative morbidity and mortality are low enough to justify pulmonary resection for cancer. In this population, surgery was associated with a hospital mortality rate of 3.2% (relative to the common rate of ~1.5% reported for patients less than 65) along with minor and major complication rates of 51 and 13%, respectively, the most frequent events being arrhythmia (31%) and air leak lasting >5 days (21%). Five- and 10-year survival rates were 37 and 15%, respectively, with smoking, COPD, and pathologic stage significant risk factors in overall survival. In

patients aged 80 and older, data from The Lung Cancer Study published in 1983 indicate that rates of complication and mortality for octogenarians are substantially higher than for the under 65 group (mortality rate of 8.1 vs. 1.6%) [22]. However, more recent studies suggest improvement in the results of lung resection in octogenarians [23–36]. In 1998, the Japanese Association of Chest Surgery reported a mortality rate of only 2.2% in a sample of 225 octogenarians undergoing lung cancer resection [37], while other series [27–36, 38–43] found a mortality of less than 5% (Tables 32.4 and 32.5). Results of a retrospective cohort study of 68 octogenarians with NSCLC who underwent lung resection reinforced that health status and tumor stage are more important than chronologic age with regard to outcome and survival rate [41]. In this study, ASA classification, forced expiratory volume in 1 s (FEV1) of less than 1.5 L, and stage of disease were strong, independent predictors of long-term survival. Similarly, in a study of octogenarians who were offered surgical resection, the mortality was 1.6% and overall 5-year survival for stage 1a patients was 82% [42]. Miyazaki and colleagues reported a series of five cases of pulmonary resection for lung cancer in carefully selected nonagenarians. Each patient survived the perioperative period, with two of the five experiencing minor complications. One patient died of a fatal arrhythmia, one patient had a local recurrence of tumor, and the remaining patients survived throughout the follow-up period [43]. Somewhat surprisingly, several recent studies of patients undergoing esophagectomy for esophageal cancer report that outcomes for elderly patients, including mortality, postoperative complications, and long-term results, are also similar to those for younger patients [45–50].

Risk and Oncological Outcome

Compared to a younger patient, an elderly person may value different goals of therapy. As the risks of surgical intervention increase along with severity of comorbid conditions, the patient's priorities may shift. Long-term survival may become less important than relief of symptoms, quality of life, and maintaining level of functioning. Accordingly, elderly patients may be less inclined to accept the risks of a major surgery, even if it might be curative, in favor of less invasive alternatives [4]. However, there being such variation in functional status among elderly patients, major surgical procedures that are potentially curative may be perfectly reasonable for many patients particularly when considered in light of data suggesting that average life expectancies for 70-year-old men and women are currently an additional 14.4 and 16.6 years, respectively. For 85-year-old men and women, they may expect an additional 5.9 and 7.0 years, respectively, and even the 100-year-old person may expect an additional

Table 32.4 Reported morbidity and mortality with surgical resection in the elderly

Source	Number of patients	Procedures	Morbidity (minor and major) (%)	Mortality (%)	Mean age
Onaitis et al. [38]	500	VATS lobectomy	20	1.2	65
McKenna et al. [39]	1100	VATS lobectomy	15.3	0.8	71
McVay et al. [40]	159	VATS153 Lobectomy 3 Bilobectomy 3 Pneumonectomy 3	18	1.8	83
Matsuoka et al. [41]	40	16 lobectomy 12 segmentectomy 12 wedge resections	20	0	82
Port et al. [42]	61	46 lobectomy 6 segmentectomy 5 wedge resections 4 pneumonectomy	38	1.6	82
Brock et al. [44]	68	47 lobectomy 11 wedge resections 5 segmentectomy 4 bilobectomy 1 pneumonectomy	44	8.8	82
Koizumi et al. [70]	32	17 VATS lobectomy 15 thoracotomy lobectomy	56	12.5	82
Aoki et al. [78]	35	25 standard or extended lobectomy 10 wedge resections	60	0	80
Pagni et al. [51]	54	43 lobectomy 2 extended lobectomy 2 bilobectomy 3 segmentectomy 3 wedge resections 1 pneumonectomy	42	3.7	82

Table 32.5 Reported morbidity and mortality with surgical resection in the octogenarians

Source	Number of patients	Mean age	Morbidity (minor and major) (%)	Mortality (%)	5-year survival (%)
Feczko et al. [27]	45	82.2	62	2	52
Tutic-Horn et al. [28]	88	82	58	1.1	45
Port et al. [29]	121	82	53.7	1.7	56.6
Okada et al. [30]	44	81.8	20	0	44.9
Dell'Amore et al. [31]	73	81.8	41	2.7	78
Matsuoka et al. [32]	174	82.6	24.3	1.15	48.3
Fanucchi et al. [33]	82	81	30	2.4	36
Zhang et al. [34]	52	83.6	44.2	3.8	19.1
Srisomboon et al. [35]	24	(>80)	29	4	74
Miura et al. [36]	49	83	40.8	4.1	53.1

2 years of life, on average [51, 52]. Nonetheless, with increasing age, the absolute gain in life expectancy from surgical treatment clearly diminishes. However, the life expectancy among patients with lung cancer that is not surgically managed is so low that resection for an 85-year-old patient may still result in an appreciable prolongation of life. For example,

impression that the life expectancy of an octogenarian with lung cancer is limited by death from natural causes is not supported by the US census data. In fact, the average life expectancy for an 80-year-old living in the United States is now an impressive 8.6 years. This translates into an overall 5-year survival for an age-matched population of 80%, as calculated from life tables. Furthermore, the majority of this time is anticipated to be years of active and independent life. Given these facts, it seems likely that the greatest impact on an elderly patient's survival and quality of life would be their cancer-related mortality rather than their age. This prospect is highlighted by the results of a retrospective review of 49 patients with early stage disease who either refused surgery or whose comorbid conditions rendered surgery unreasonable and experienced a survival time of only 14 months [53]. A meta-analysis of patients enrolled in trials for computed tomography screening that did not receive surgical therapy for their stage I disease produced similar findings [54], and a study of elderly subjects with stage I and II NSCLC receiving radiation alone revealed 2- and 5-year survival rates of only 40% and 16%, respectively [55]. On the whole, these data indicate that early stage lung cancer is a fatal disease and suggest that for patients with lung cancer who are over 80 years old, the majority of deaths will be related to the progression of lung cancer rather than other causes.

The Emerging Role of Minimally Invasive Surgical (MIS) Techniques

In that there is an association between the magnitude of pulmonary resection and postoperative complications in elderly subjects, some surgeons advocate "less invasive" lung-sparing techniques such as wedge resection and segmentectomy for the treatment of pulmonary malignancy whenever possible [56]. While controversy exists as to whether these procedures, which still involve at least a limited thoracotomy, carry a higher risk of local recurrence, Mery et al., using data from the SEER database, found that, among patients age 75 or older, there was no difference in overall survival time between patients undergoing lobectomy and those undergoing limited resection [20].

Both the scientific literature and lay press contain a wide variety of publications relating to VATS as a truly "minimally invasive" approach to the treatment of lung cancer and as an adjunct in the treatment of esophageal cancer. Published data suggest that relative to thoracotomy, VATS patients experience shorter chest tube duration, shorter postoperative hospital stays, lower narcotic requirements for postoperative pain, and reduced shoulder dysfunction [57]. Similarly, patients who had VATS lobectomy reported less postoperative pain, decreased time until return to preoperative activities, and higher satisfaction with the results of surgery than those patients undergoing conventional thoracotomy [58]. In addition, there was a lower observed incidence of postoperative confusion [59], which has been associated with increased postoperative morbidity and mortality. VATS lobectomy patients also appear to return to their oncologists for adjuvant chemotherapy more readily. A recent review of 1100 VATS lobectomies with either lymph node sampling or dissection for patients with a mean age of 71.2 years demonstrated low rates of mortality (<1%) and morbidity, with 84.7% of patients exhibiting no significant complications [39]. For esophagectomy, several minimally invasive approaches have been developed, including those incorporating thoracoscopy and/or laparoscopy into a typical three-stage Ivor Lewis operation, approaches incorporating laparoscopy for a transhiatal approach, and those incorporating robotics. Emerging data support the oncological efficacy of these approaches [60, 61]. Galvani et al. reported experiences with robotically assisted laparoscopic transhiatal esophagectomy, suggesting that this approach is safe and effective [62].

Despite favorable perioperative outcome data, questions remain as to whether lobectomy via thoracotomy and VATS are equivalent therapeutic interventions for cancer. However, a series of 159 VATS lobectomies for stage I and II NSCLC revealed long-term outcomes and local recurrence rates that were at least equivalent to those of open thoracotomy [63], and a prospective, randomized trial of 100 patients with stage IA NSCLC concluded that long-term survival and local recurrence rates after VATS lobectomy were comparable to those for open thoracotomy [64]. Another study actually reported better 5-year survival rate of stage I lung cancer after VATS vs. thoracotomy perhaps due in part to superior postoperative pulmonary function [65]. Several other studies reported similar outcomes [66–69]. For the geriatric population, a retrospective study of 32 lobectomy patients aged 80 years or older (17 VATS, 15 thoracotomies) also demonstrated better 5-year survival following VATS [70]. A recent review of our own data related to VATS lobectomy in octogenarians revealed patients had a significantly decreased length of ICU and hospital stay as well as a decreased complication rate when compared to those who underwent open thoracotomy [29]. Interestingly, significantly fewer patients required discharge to a formal rehabilitation center and were discharged to home.

To date, most large reports show that across all age groups, VATS for lobectomy is safe, with morbidity rates in some reports lower than seen historically with thoracotomy. Other data suggest that pulmonary function as measured by vital capacity and FEV1 may be better preserved in patients undergoing VATS rather than thoracotomy [65]. Kirby et al. [71] reported that, while they found no difference in intraoperative time, blood loss, or length of hospital stay between patients who underwent VATS vs. thoracotomy, the thoracotomy group did experience significantly more postoperative complications, most notably prolonged air leaks.

The prospect of superior pulmonary function following VATS relative to thoracotomy has particular significance in the elderly population. To determine if the VATS approach for lobectomy offers specific advantages over thoracotomy in the elderly, retrospective studies have compared the two in aged patient populations. Jaklitsch reported that VATS procedures for patients ≥65 years of age resulted in superior 30-day operative mortality, which was essentially unrelated to age, and a decreased length of hospital stay compared to previous reports for standard thoracotomy [59]. More recently, Cattaneo et al. analyzed the incidence and grade of postoperative complications in patients ≥70 years of age undergoing a VATS approach vs. a thoracotomy for lobectomy [72]. The two groups were identically matched for age, gender, comorbidities, and clinical stage. This study found that VATS resulted in a lower overall complication rate, less pulmonary morbidity, and a decreased median length of stay. In addition, the severity of complications were less in the VATS group, suggesting that the minimally invasive approach can lead to better tolerance in a high-risk, elderly population.

Whether there are cardiovascular benefits to VATS lobectomy remains unclear. Multiple studies have established the relationship between age and the occurrence of atrial fibrillation following lobectomy, with recent data indicating an incidence of 27% in patients over the age of 60 when continuous telemetry is used for diagnosis [73]. Two large series have reported lower than expected rates of postoperative atrial fibrillation following VATS lobectomy relative to thoracotomy, ranging from 2.9% to 10% [38, 39]. However, neither study used routine postoperative telemetry in the highest risk patients, i.e., elderly patients, and likely underreported asymptomatic episodes of atrial fibrillation. In contrast, a matched, case-control study by Park et al. comparing 244 patients undergoing lobectomy by either VATS or thoracotomy [74] showed no difference in the rate of postoperative atrial fibrillation with VATS patients exhibiting a 12% rate of postoperative atrial fibrillation compared to 16% for thoracotomy patients ($p = 0.36$). Predictably, in both groups patients experiencing atrial fibrillation were significantly older (median 72 years) than those who did not develop the arrhythmia (median 66 years).

Preoperative Evaluation and Postoperative Care

Although the fundamentals of preoperative evaluation outlined elsewhere in the text remain appropriate, aspects of perioperative assessment and planning take on increased importance and/or require different interpretation in the elderly.

Preoperative Assessment

Current guidelines developed by the American College of Chest Physicians for preoperative assessment of patients considered for thoracic surgery begins with a physical exam combined with cardiovascular evaluation and spirometry [75]. Given the lung parenchymal changes associated with aging and propensity for obstructive physiology, measurement of diffusion capacity (DLCO) is important, particularly for patients with clinical signs of dyspnea out of proportion to the spirometry results. In patients with an FEV1 or DLCO <80% of predicted – a relatively common finding in the elderly – estimated postoperative FEV1 and DLCO values should be calculated as described in Chap. 2. Estimated postoperative values for either variable of <40% is a significant negative predictor of outcome in all patients and may be even more relevant in the aged due to the expected changes in intrinsic pulmonary reserve associated with senescence. Importantly, results need to be interpreted in the context of a patient's clinical presentation; a low FEV1 in a patient with a large left main stem bronchus tumor should be regarded differently than a patient who has a similarly low value and a small peripheral lesion.

Guidelines suggest that further definition of a patient's risk with cardiopulmonary exercise testing and estimation of maximal oxygen consumption (VO_2 max) is often valuable. A VO_2 max <15 mL/kg/min is a negative predictor for outcome. If cardiopulmonary exercise testing is not available, other surrogates can be performed and include stair climbing, shuttle walk, and the 6-min walk. If a patient cannot climb one flight of stairs or perform 25 shuttles, usually their VO_2 max will be <10 mL/kg/min. However, while exercise testing is a potentially powerful tool, it is not always applicable in the geriatric population due to the presence of comorbidities such as arthritis or peripheral vascular disease that limit mobility independent of VO_2 max.

In the elderly population, it is also important to identify factors such as dementia, undernutrition, thromboembolic disorders, subclinical diabetes, thyroid disorders, and renal insufficiency. For many patients, perioperative risk can be reduced by modest exercise along with nutritional and hormonal optimization. However, unlike recommendations published nearly 20 years ago suggesting 8 weeks of optimization prior to surgery [76], in the current environment, and in the setting of progressive malignancy, the time available for meaningful preoperative optimization is often quite short.

Postoperative Planning

In the absence of severe pre-existing critical illness or profound intraoperative complications, diagnostic and staging procedures such as bronchoscopy, cervical mediastinoscopy, and potentially even minimally invasive wedge biopsies may be performed as outpatients, even in elderly patients. Following VATS or open lobectomy and even pneumonectomy, elderly patients generally are candidates for standard admission to postoperative acute care units [77]. Alternatively, after more extensive procedures such as bilobectomy, esophagectomy, or resection of a large or adherent mediastinal mass, ICU admission is often desirable due to the increased potential for major respiratory and cardiovascular postoperative complications.

It is also important to consider discharge planning even during the initial preoperative visit in the elderly population. For example, it is necessary to consider who will be providing support for the patient following discharge and where this care will take place. Many patients who are entirely self-sufficient preoperatively may not be able to care for themselves for a period of time postoperatively, and as such, early discharge planning becomes critical.

Conclusion

As the population ages, increasing numbers of elderly people will present with lung cancer. Due to recent advances in neoadjuvant therapies and accumulating data demonstrating a

39. McKenna RJ Jr, Houck W, Fuller CB. Video-assisted thoracic surgery lobectomy: experience with 1, 100 cases. Ann Thorac Surg. 2006;81(2):421–5.

40. McVay CL, Pickens A, Fuller C, et al. VATS anatomic pulmonary resection in octogenarians. Am Surg. 2005;71(9):791–3.

41. Matsuoka H, Okada M, Sakamoto T, Tsubota N. Complications and outcomes after pulmonary resection for cancer in patients 80 to 89 years of age. Eur J Cardiothorac Surg. 2005;28(3):380–3.

42. Port JL, Kent M, Korst RJ, et al. Surgical resection for lung cancer in the octogenarian. Chest. 2004;126(3):733–8.

43. Miyazaki T, Yamasaki N, Tsuchiya T, et al. Pulmonary resection for lung cancer in nonagenarians: a report of five cases. Ann Thorac Cardiovasc Surg. 2014;20(Suppl):497–500.

44. Brock MV, Kim MP, Hooker CM, et al. Pulmonary resection in octogenarians with stage I nonsmall cell lung cancer: a 22-year experience. Ann Thorac Surg. 2004;77(1):271–7.

45. Internullo E, Moons J, Nafteux P, et al. Outcome after esophagectomy for cancer of the esophagus and GEJ in patients aged over 75 years. Eur J Cardiothorac Surg. 2008;33(6):1096–104.

46. Perry Y, Fernando HC, Buenaventura PO, et al. Minimally invasive esophagectomy in the elderly. JSLS. 2002;6(4):299–304.

47. Nguyen NT, Hinojosa MW, Smith BR, et al. Minimally invasive esophagectomy: lessons learned from 104 operations. Ann Surg. 2008;248(6):1081–91.

48. Ruol A, Portale G, Zaninotto G, et al. Results of esophagectomy for esophageal cancer in elderly patients: age has little influence on outcome and survival. J Thorac Cardiovasc Surg. 2007;133(5):1186–92.

49. Morita M, Egashira A, Yoshida R, et al. Esophagectomy in patients 80 years of age and older with carcinoma of the thoracic esophagus. J Gastroenterol. 2008;43(5):345–51.

50. Alibakhshi A, Aminian A, Misharifi R, et al. The effect of age on the outcome of esophageal cancer surgery. Ann Thorac Med. 2009;4(2):71–4.

51. Pagni S, McKelvey A, Riordan C, et al. Pulmonary resection for malignancy in the elderly: is age still a risk factor? Eur J Cardiothorac Surg. 1998;14(1):40–4.

52. Arias E, Heron M, Xu J. United States life tables, 2013. Natl Vital Stat Rep. 2017;66(3):1–64.

53. McGarry RC, Song G, des Rosiers P, et al. Observation-only management of early stage, medically inoperable lung cancer: poor outcome. Chest. 2002;121:1155–8.

54. Flehinger BJ, Kimmel M, Melamed MR. The effect of surgical treatment on survival from early lung cancer: implications for screening. Chest. 1992;101:1013–8.

55. Furuta M, Hayakawa K, Katano S, et al. Radiation therapy for stage I-II non-small cell lung cancer in patients aged 75 years and older. Jpn J Clin Oncol. 1996;26:95–8.

56. Wiener DC, Argote-Greene LM, Ramesh H, et al. Choices in the management of asymptomatic lung nodules in the elderly. Surg Oncol. 2004;13(4):239–48. Review

57. Landreneau RJ, Hazelrigg SR, Mack MJ, et al. Postoperative pain-related morbidity: video-assisted thoracic surgery versus thoracotomy. Ann Thorac Surg. 1993;56(6):1285–9.

58. Sugiura H, Morikawa T, Kaji M, et al. Long-term benefits for the quality of life after video-assisted thorascopic lobectomy in patients with lung cancer. Surg Laparosc Endosc Percutan Tech. 1999;9(6):403–8.

59. Jaklitsch MT, DeCamp MM, Liptay MJ, et al. Video-assisted thoracic surgery in the elderly. A review of 307 cases. Chest. 1996;110:751–8.

60. Schoppmann SF, Prager G, Langer F, et al. Fifty-five minimally invasive esophagectomies: a single centre experience. Anticancer Res. 2009;29(7):2719–25.

61. Braghetto I, Csendes A, Cardemil G, et al. Open transthoracic or transhiatal esophagectomy versus minimally invasive esophagectomy in terms of morbidity, mortality and survival. Surg Endosc. 2006;20(11):1681–6.

62. Galvani CA, Goodner MV, Moser F, et al. Robotically assisted laparoscopic transhiatal esophagectomy. Surg Endosc. 2008;22(1):188–95.

63. Walker WS, Codispoti M, Soon SY, et al. Long-term outcomes following VATS lobectomy for non-small cell bronchogenic carcinoma. Eur J Cardiothorac Surg. 2003;23(3):397–402.

64. Sugi K, Kaneda Y, Esato K. Video-assisted thoracoscopic lobectomy achieves a satisfactory long-term prognosis in patients with clinical stage IA lung cancer. World J Surg. 2000;24(1):27–30.

65. Kaseda S, Aoki T, Hangai N, Shimizu K. Better pulmonary function and prognosis with video-assisted thoracic surgery than with thoracotomy. Ann Thorac Surg. 2000;70(5):1644–6.

66. Daniels LJ, Balderson SS, Onaitis MW, D'Amico TA. Thoracoscopic lobectomy: a safe and effective strategy for patients with stage I lung cancer. Ann Thorac Surg. 2002;74(3):860–4.

67. Thomas P, Doddoli C, Yena S, et al. VATS is an adequate oncological operation for stage I non-small cell lung cancer. Eur J Cardiothorac Surg. 2002;21(6):1094–9.

68. Ohtsuka T, Nomori H, Horio H, et al. Is major pulmonary resection by video-assisted thoracic surgery an adequate procedure in clinical stage I lung cancer? Chest. 2004;125(5):1742–6.

69. Gharagozloo F, Tempesta B, Margolis M, Alexander EP. Video-assisted thoracic surgery lobectomy for stage I lung cancer. Ann Thorac Surg. 2003;76:10009–15.

70. Koizumi K, Haraguchi S, Hirata T, et al. Lobectomy by video-assisted thoracic surgery for lung cancer patients aged 80 years or more. Ann Thorac Cardiovasc Surg. 2003;9(1):14–21.

71. Kirby TJ, Mack MJ, Landreneau RJ, Rice TW. Lobectomy-video-assisted thoracic surgery versus muscle-sparing thoracotomy: a randomized trial. J Thorac Cardiovasc Surg. 1995;109:997–1002.

72. Cattaneo SM, Park BJ, Wilton AS, et al. Use of video-assisted thoracic surgery for lobectomy in the elderly results in fewer complications. Ann Thorac Surg. 2008;85(1):231–5.

73. Amar D, Zhang H, Heerdt PM, et al. Statin use is associated with a reduction in atrial fibrillation after noncardiac thoracic surgery independent of C-reactive protein. Chest. 2005;128(5):3421–7.

74. Park BJ, Zhang H, Rusch VW, Amar D. Video-assisted thoracic surgery does not reduce the incidence of postoperative atrial fibrillation after pulmonary lobectomy. J Thorac Cardiovasc Surg. 2007;133:775–9.

75. American College of Chest Physicians, Colice GL, Shafazand S, Griffin JP, et al. Physiologic evaluation of the patient with lung cancer being considered for resectional surgery: ACCP evidence-based clinical practice guidelines (2nd edition). Chest. 2007;132(3 Suppl):161S–77.

76. King MS. Preoperative evaluation of the elderly. J Am Board Fam Pract. 1991;4(4):251–8.

77. Pedoto A, Heerdt PM. Postoperative care after pulmonary resection: postanesthesia care unit versus intensive care unit. Curr Opin Anaesthesiol. 2009;22(1):50–5.

78. Aoki T, Yamato Y, Tsuchida M, et al. Pulmonary complications after surgical treatment of lung cancer in octogenarians. Eur J Cardiothorac Surg. 2000;18(6):662–5.

Thoracic Anesthesia for Morbidly Obese Patients and Obese Patients with Obstructive Sleep Apnea

33

George W. Kanellakos and Jay B. Brodsky

Key Points

- A patient with a BMI >30 kg/m^2 is considered obese. A patient with a BMI >40 kg/m^2 is morbidly obese (also known as Obesity Class III). Super-obesity refers to a patient with a BMI >50 kg/m^2.
- Morbid obesity (MO) is associated with medical conditions, including hypertension, type II diabetes mellitus, cardiovascular disease, obstructive sleep apnea (OSA), and obesity hypoventilation syndrome (OHS).
- Moderate to severe OSA is present in more than 50% of MO patients and is often unrecognized. The best screening tool for identifying patients with OSA is the STOP-Bang questionnaire. In the absence of a definitive diagnosis by polysomnography (PSG), all MO patients should be managed as if they have OSA.
- Anesthesiologists should have a high index of suspicion for the presence of OHS. Patients with OHS have a greater risk of cardiovascular problems and pulmonary hypertension.
- Preoperatively, treatment with continuous positive airway pressure (CPAP) can significantly improve OSA symptoms. The patient should bring their CPAP equipment to the hospital for use during their postoperative recovery.
- Many MO patients are difficult to ventilate by mask, but tracheal intubation by direct laryngoscopy is usually successful.

- The best preoperative predictors of potential problems with tracheal intubation in MO patients are high Mallampati (III or IV) score and increased neck circumference (>48 cm men, >40 cm women).
- A supine obese patient should not be allowed to breathe without assistance. All MO patients should be positioned in the "head-elevated laryngoscopy position" (HELP) prior to induction of anesthesia.
- Depressant medications should be avoided preoperatively as they can decrease ventilatory responsiveness to hypoxemia and hypercarbia and can cause airway collapse in the presence of OSA.
- Regional anesthesia techniques should be used when possible, including epidural or paravertebral analgesia for thoracic procedures.
- Obese patients are not at increased risk for gastric aspiration, and therefore rapid sequence induction is usually unnecessary.
- MO patients tolerate one-lung ventilation (OLV) in the lateral position but are unlikely to tolerate it in the supine position.
- For MO patients lean body weight (LBW) should be calculated for dosing of induction and opioid agents, IBW for non-depolarizing neuromuscular agents, and TBW for succinylcholine.
- MO patients can develop rhabdomyolysis (RML) after long-duration procedures. Any associated myoglobinuria can lead to acute renal failure. RML is treated by aggressive IV fluid administration.

G. W. Kanellakos
Department of Anesthesia, Pain Management & Perioperative Medicine, Dalhousie University, Halifax, NS, Canada
e-mail: george.kanellakos@dal.ca

J. B. Brodsky (✉)
Department of Anesthesia, Perioperative and Pain Medicine, Stanford University Medical Center, Stanford, CA, USA
e-mail: Jbrodsky@stanford.edu

Introduction

Advances in airway techniques, new drugs, and equipment have enabled anesthesiologists to manage even the most complex thoracic surgical patient. One group of patients,

© Springer Nature Switzerland AG 2019
P. Slinger (ed.), *Principles and Practice of Anesthesia for Thoracic Surgery*, https://doi.org/10.1007/978-3-030-00859-8_33

Table 33.1 Modified World Health Organization body mass index (BMI) classification

BMI (kg/m^2)	Classification
Below 18.5	Underweight
18.5–24.9	Normal weight (Ideal body weight)
25.0–29.9	Pre-obesity (overweight)
30.0–34.9	Obesity Class I (obese)
35.0–39.9	Obesity Class II (obese)
Above 40	Obesity Class III (morbid obesity)

those with morbid obesity (MO), can be especially challenging. Throughout the world, obesity levels over the past two decades have reached epidemic levels [1]. Extremely obese patients now routinely present to the operating for surgery [2]. MO patients differ from their normal-weight counterparts due to alterations in their anatomy and physiology [3]. They often have significant comorbid medical conditions that can complicate their operative course and increase the risks of postoperative problems. Obstructive sleep apnea (OSA), which is very common in obesity, further contributes to the complexity of managing these patients.

Obesity is usually described by body mass index (BMI). BMI is calculated by dividing patient weight in kilograms (kg) by the square of their height in meters (m), expressed as BMI = kg/m^2. BMI is an indirect estimation of obesity since it considers any increase in weight, not just increases in adipose tissue. Obesity definitions have changed over the years. The current BMI categories are listed in Table 33.1 [4]. Based on these definitions, more than one third of American adults are obese (BMI >30 kg/m^2), and almost 5% are MO (BMI >40 kg/m^2) [5]. The population with extreme weight has been increasing fastest [6, 7], and a new BMI category termed super-obesity is now used to describe larger patients (BMI >50 kg/m^2).

This chapter will describe the perioperative anesthetic considerations for the obese thoracic surgical patient. To date a limited number of reviews on this topic have been published [2, 8]. Most recommendations for obese patients undergoing thoracic surgery are derived from studies of patients undergoing other types of surgery, particularly weight loss operations.

Preoperative Considerations

A thorough preoperative assessment is indicated for every surgical patient. For the MO patient, the anesthesiologist must consider the associated comorbid conditions associated with extreme obesity (including hypertension and cardiovascular disease, type II diabetes, OSA and OHS, osteoarthritis), in addition to the medical indication for surgery. The specific preoperative management of each of these medical comorbidities is beyond the scope of this chapter, and the reader is referred to reviews on the subject [3, 9, 10].

Weight

Preoperative documentation of the MO patient's height and weight is extremely important for optimal pharmacologic management. Anesthetic drugs are usually administered by patient weight, either total body weight (TBW), ideal body weight (IBW), or lean body weight (LBW). Clinical trials during drug development usually have not included obese and MO subjects, so drug dosing in these patients based solely on actual or TBW can lead to overdosing, complicating perioperative management.

IBW is a measure initially derived by life insurance companies in the 1940s to describe the weight for a man or woman of a specific height that was statistically associated with maximum life expectancy. Accepted values for IBW have increased over the past seven decades since patients are now living longer despite significant increases in their average weight. In normal-weight patients TBW approximates IBW, that is, "normal" weight ranges between ± 10% of IBW. For drug dosing IBW can be estimated for both men and women using the formula, IBW = 22 × (height in meters)^2 [11].

LBW includes the weight of muscles, bones, tendons, ligaments, and body water. It is equal to actual weight (TBW) minus the weight of fat. LBW in nonobese patients should be about 80% TBW for males and 75% TBW for females. LBW and TBW both increase as a patient gets heavier since there are increases in the muscle and body water in addition to the much larger increases in adipose tissue. LBW can account for as much as 20–40% of the excess TBW [12, 13]. LBW is difficult to measure clinically, but it can be calculated by several formulas. Most formulas for LBW fail when applied to the extremely obese population. Equations 33.1 and 33.2 [14] are used to accurately estimate LBW (Fat Free Mass) in obesity:

$$T_o = \frac{Q_o}{D} = \frac{6000}{400,000} = 0.015 \, \text{years} = 5.475 \, \text{days} \tag{33.1}$$

$$T_o = \frac{Q_o}{D} = \frac{6000}{400,000} = 0.015 \, \text{years} = 5.475 \, \text{days} \tag{33.2}$$

For clinical anesthetic drug dosing, LBW can be roughly estimated in a MO patient simply by their IBW + 20–30%.

Pulmonary Function

Excess body fat significantly reduces chest wall and total pulmonary compliance. Airway resistance and work of breathing are increased in the spontaneously breathing MO patient. Preoperatively, spirometry usually reveals a restrictive defect with decreases in functional residual capacity (FRC), mainly expiratory reserve volume (ERV), associated with small airway collapse during tidal breathing. These changes result in ventilation/perfusion (V/Q) mismatch, an elevated shunt fraction, and relative hypoxemia [15].

Preoperative pulmonary function testing has been used to predict which patients can safely tolerate lung resection [16, 17]. The minimum values of at least 40% FEV_1 and 40% diffusion capacity may not be useful in the MO patient since these measurements are not indexed to weight. No predictive baseline spirometry studies for MO patients undergoing lung resection are available. However, as BMI increases, postoperative FEV_1 and FVC values decrease proportionally [18]. For example, following abdominal surgery MO patients experience significantly more atelectasis, greater decreases in FRC, and lower P_aO_2 values than matched normal-weight patients. Therefore, it is very likely, but still unproven, that MO patients also experience greater reductions in pulmonary function following thoracic operations than nonobese patients.

Obstructive Sleep Apnea

OSA is characterized by repetitive collapse of the upper airway during sleep, which results in complete cessation (apnea) or near complete cessation (hypopnea) of airflow. Apnea is defined as a total lack of airflow lasting at least 10 s. Hypopnea is a decrease of $\geq 50\%$ in airflow or $\leq 50\%$ decrease for at least 10 s. These events are associated with either arousal from sleep or oxygen desaturation of $\geq 3\%$ [19]. If there is increasing respiratory effort, the apnea is described as "obstructive," whereas in central sleep apnea, there is no breathing effort. Besides snoring, frequent awakenings, and apnea periods during sleep, OSA patients often have a history of daytime drowsiness, morning headaches, irritability, personality changes, depression, cognitive impairment, and visual incoordination. Severe OSA is associated with sleep fragmentation, transient hypoxemia and hypercapnia, large negative intrathoracic pressure swings, and marked elevations in blood pressure [20].

OSA is formally diagnosed by a "sleep study" (polysomnography, PSG). The apnea index (AI) is the number of apneas/hour of total sleep time. The hypopnea index (HI) is the number of hypopneas/hour of total sleep time. The sum of the AI and HI is the apnea-hypopnea index (AHI) [19]. The arousal index (ARI) is the number arousals/hour of total sleep that do not meet the definitions of apneas or hypopneas. The combination of ARI and AHI is the respiratory disturbance index (RDI), a measure that significantly correlates with excessive daytime sleepiness. An AHI >5 in combination with clinical symptoms is diagnostic of OSA.

The prevalence of moderate to severe OSA (apnea-hypopnea index (AHI) ≥ 15 events/hour) in the general population is 10–20% [21] and as high as 70% in MO

Table 33.2 STOP and STOP-Bang questionnaires sensitivity and specificity in surgical patients

	STOP questionnaire		STOP-Bang questionnaire	
	Sensitivity (%)	Specificity (%)	Sensitivity (%)	Specificity (%)
OSA (AHI >5)	65.6	60	84	56.4
OSA (AHI >15)	74	53	93	43
OSA (AHI >30)	80	49	100	37

Adapted from Chung et al. [24]

patients undergoing bariatric surgery [22]. Another study quotes the rate of OSA in MO patients to be 84% (AHI >5), 47% (AHI >15), and 27% (AHI >30) [23]. There have been many screening tools proposed for identifying OSA. The STOP and STOP-Bang questionnaires [24] are currently used in anesthetic practice. The STOP questionnaire includes four questions related to snoring, tiredness, observed apnea, and high blood pressure. The STOP-Bang questionnaire has four additional demographic questions: BMI, age, neck circumference, and male gender. The published sensitivity and specificity of the STOP and STOP-Bang questionnaires are given in Table 33.2. The probability of OSA being present increases as the STOP-Bang score increases. The ease of use and high level of sensitivity have resulted in the questionnaire being widely used as screening tool in preoperative clinics and is especially useful if a PSG is not obtained.

Patients with OSA also have metabolic changes. Intermittent hypercapnia secondary to nocturnal and even daytime obstructive apnea or hypoventilation may lead to elevation in serum bicarbonate levels as a compensatory mechanism for acute respiratory acidosis. Bicarbonate elevation correlates with AHI, and when used in conjunction with the STOP-Bang score, the specificity of the presence of moderate to severe OSA significantly increases [25].

Identifying patients who have OSA has important perioperative implications. Intermittent nocturnal sympathetic activation from hypoxemia and hypercarbia causes systemic hypertension. Recurrent hypoxic pulmonary vasoconstriction eventually results in pulmonary hypertension and right and left ventricular hypertrophy. OSA patients may have a higher rate of complications, including difficult intubation, difficult bag-mask ventilation, cardiopulmonary complications, unexpected reintubation, and ICU admission [26–28].

Continuous positive airway pressure (CPAP) is used to treat moderate to severe OSA. CPAP provides a pneumatic stent that opens the upper airway and maintains its patency. For patients requiring high levels of CPAP or those with chronic obstructive pulmonary disease as occurs in many thoracic surgical patients, bi-level positive airway pressure (BIPAP) is used since it allows for independent adjustment

pharyngeal space secondary to fat deposition in the pharyngeal wall, which can make airway access and bag-mask ventilation difficult. The patient's airway and anatomy should be closely examined. Airway management of MO patient has been reviewed elsewhere [43, 44].

The American Society of Anesthesiologists Task Force defines a difficult airway as the "clinical situation in which a conventionally trained anesthesiologist experiences problems with (a) face mask ventilation of the upper airway or (b) tracheal intubation or both" [45].

The criteria used to define difficult mask ventilation usually include failure to maintain oxygen saturation (SpO_2) >92%, the need for two providers, and/or complete inability to mask ventilate. Increased BMI and a history of OSA are each independent predictors for difficult mask ventilation [46], and there is general acceptance that MO patients, especially when supine, are more difficult to ventilate by mask than normal-weight patients. Age 49 years, short neck, and neck circumference are additional factors that have been identified as independent predictive factors for difficult bag-mask ventilation [47].

Numerous studies have considered tracheal intubation in the MO population. The view obtained during direct laryngoscopy is usually used as a measure for difficult or failed intubation; however, an ETT may be easy to place despite a poor laryngoscopic view, and even with a reasonable view there can be difficulty passing a tube. In MO patients video-laryngoscopy improves intubation conditions [48] and reduces hypoxic events during induction [49]. The best preoperative predictors of potential problems with tracheal intubation are Mallampati score (III/IV) and increased neck circumference [50].

The standard sniffing position for tracheal intubation is achieved in nonobese patients by raising their occiput 8–10 cm with a pillow or headrest. Obese patients require much greater elevation of their head, neck, and shoulders (HELP) to produce the same alignment of axes for intubation [38]. In studies of MO patients where the head position is suboptimal, which is not in the HELP, there are higher incidences of grade 3 and 4 Cormack-Lehane views potentially increasing difficulty with direct laryngoscopy [51]. Video-laryngoscopy for routine tracheal intubation has presumably led to better visualization of the glottis in MO patients [52]. In patients who are anesthetized and in whom a difficult laryngoscopy is encountered, an alternative method to securing the airway could involve passing a single-lumen endotracheal tube (ETT) through a laryngeal mask with the aid of a flexible fiberoptic bronchoscope [53, 54].

Certain clinical features are more likely to be present in obese or MO patients in whom direct laryngoscopy is difficult. As mentioned, high Mallampati score, large neck circumference, and excessive pretracheal adipose tissue may make laryngoscopy more difficult in some MO patients [50,

55]. However, increasing weight alone has never been correlated with increasing difficulty with tracheal intubation. BMI has no direct influence on difficult laryngoscopy, and rates of successful tracheal intubation in these MO patients are similar to those in nonobese patients [50, 56, 57]. In a small subset of male, MO patients with short wide necks, OSA, and high Mallampati scores direct laryngoscopy may be more difficult, and video-laryngoscopy should be considered for these patients. Anesthesiologists should always proceed with caution in any MO patient since difficulty with bag-mask ventilation is very common and all obese patients have a short SAT following muscle paralysis for laryngoscopy.

For most MO patients, an IV anesthetic induction with propofol and succinylcholine is the best means for securing the airway. Rocuronium can be used, but only if sugammadex is immediately available. Formally, a rapid sequence induction (RSI) was believed to be necessary for all MO patients because of the misperception that obesity increased risk for aspiration and pulmonary injury during anesthetic induction. It is now felt that most MO patients are at no greater risk than normal-weight patients. Obese patients that are at higher risk for gastric acid aspiration are those with a history of severe GERD and diabetic gastroparesis and patients who have previously undergone gastric banding procedures [58]. For these patients a RSI is still recommended. RSI is not without risks (awareness, under- and overdosing of drugs, impaired visualization during laryngoscopy, SpO_2 desaturation), and these risks are potentially greater than the low risk of aspiration.

In summary, for MO obese patients, induction of anesthesia and tracheal intubation should include placing the patient in a head-up position, adequate preoxygenation until end-tidal oxygen concentration is >80%, administration of fast-acting opioids to supplement the anesthetic induction agent, titration of the induction agent until loss of consciousness is achieved, avoidance of cricoid pressure (if possible), and continued bag-mask positive pressure ventilation following the administration of a neuromuscular blocking agent until the patient is fully paralyzed and ready for tracheal intubation. Bag-mask ventilation can be difficult and gastric insufflation from ineffective mask ventilation can increase the risk of regurgitation and acid aspiration. A second person experienced with airway management, preferably another anesthesiologist, should always be readily available to assist when difficulty is encountered.

Lung Separation

Safe and dependable isolation and selective ventilation of the lungs are essential for the practice of modern thoracic anesthesia. Lung separation is accomplished with either a DLT or with a balloon-tipped BB. There is no "best" method for lung separation, and choice of technique depends on the specific surgical requirements, the patient's airway, and the individual anesthesiologist's preferences and experience [59]. Despite the technical aspects of placing any airway device, it has also been shown that one of the most significant barriers to successful lung separation is the operator's knowledge of bronchial anatomy [60, 61]. Bronchoscopic tracheobronchial anatomy can be reviewed using an online simulator at www.thoracicanesthesia.com or www.pie.med.utoronto.ca/VB or in published illustrations [61].

Direct laryngoscopy and successful placement of a DLT or ETT should be no different in obese and normal-weight patients, provided the obese patient is appropriately positioned for laryngoscopy. In both normal-weight patients [62] and obese patients [63], tracheal intubation is usually more difficult using a DLT than with a single-lumen tube.

When problematic laryngoscopy is anticipated, or if difficulty is experienced when attempting to place a DLT, an ETT can be inserted using either a gum elastic bougie as a guide, through any of several laryngeal mask airways (LMAs) using fiberoptic bronchoscopy, or with any other intubation adjunct such as a Trachlight® [53, 54]. Once the ETT is in place, a BB can be used through the ETT, or alternatively a 100-cm long airway exchange catheter can be employed to change from the ETT to a DLT. A DLT can even be placed directly by fiberoptic bronchoscopy [64].

When tube exchange is not practical, lung isolation can always be achieved with a BB through the ETT. BB may be a better choice for those MO patients with high Mallampati score and thick necks with a potential "difficult" airway. The quality of lung collapse is unaffected whether a BB or DLT is used [59]. If postoperative ventilation is planned, it may be safer to avoid a DLT entirely and use a BB through an ETT since changing tubes at the completion of surgery can be potentially dangerous in MO patients.

Prior to intubation the patient's chest radiograph or CT scan should be examined to determine the tracheobronchial anatomy and airway diameters [65]. Unlike chronic obstructive lung disease, which results in a dilation of trachea and bronchi, a similar effect does not occur for the restrictive lung disease associated with obesity. Relatively, small tracheas are often found in very large patients. Even if a smaller DLT needs to be used, airway resistance is not a concern. Contrary to popular belief, most sizes of DLTs have reduced airflow resistance compared to ETTs [66].

One-Lung Ventilation

Hypoxemia during OLV is significantly affected by patient positioning. Normal-weight patients undergoing OLV in the supine position have significantly lower arterial oxygen ten-

sions than when the same patient is in lateral position [67]. For patients undergoing thoracotomy in the supine, the semi-lateral decubitus, and the lateral decubitus positions, oxygenation progressively decreases with time after the start of OLV. OLV in the supine position is associated with the highest incidence of hypoxemia, usually occurring approximately 10 min after initiating OLV with 100% oxygen [68]. Although MO patients maintain adequate oxygenation during OLV in the lateral position, they are much less likely to tolerate OLV in the supine position. Basilar atelectasis is present in supine MO patients preoperatively and worsens following induction of general anesthesia. MO patients benefit from lung recruitment maneuvers following induction of anesthesia, particularly prior to the institution of OLV [69]. Due to the presence of more atelectasis in dependent lung areas than normal-weight patients, recruitment maneuvers and PEEP are required for maintaining adequate oxygenation [70, 71]. Despite this, arterial oxygen tension in MO patients remains significantly lower during OLV than normal-weight patients [72]. Successful OLV in MO patients is technically possible in the lateral position if the panniculus can fall away from the body, therefore unloading the dependent diaphragm (Fig. 33.3).

For all patients, including the MO patients, lung protective ventilation strategies are practiced during OLV [73, 74]. Traditional ventilation parameters (large tidal volume with no recruitment or PEEP) may contribute to the development of ARDS and other postoperative pulmonary complications [75–77], even in patients without preexisting lung disease [78, 79]. Ventilation with tidal volumes as high as 13 mL/kg (IBW) during OLV do not improve oxygenation and can

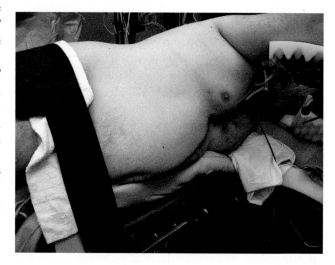

Fig. 33.3 Successful one-lung ventilation (OLV) in MO patients is technically possible in the lateral position if the panniculus can fall away from the body unloading the dependent diaphragm. MO patients are much less likely to tolerate OLV in the supine position since many patients already have reduced FRC and are relatively hypoxemic even during two-lung ventilation when they lie flat

result in excessively high peak pressures [80]. In the MO population, estimating tidal volumes based on actual weight (TBW) or height is a risk factor for delivering excessively high tidal volumes during mechanical ventilation [81, 82]. As with normal-weight patients, tidal volumes during OLV should be based on IBW (4–6 mL/kg IBW).

High peak inspiratory pressures secondary to restriction of chest wall and diaphragmatic excursion and the narrow single lumen of a DLT can further limit volume-controlled mechanical ventilation during OLV. Pressure-controlled ventilation during OLV can improve oxygenation and decrease peak pressures in normal-weight patients [83]. Pressure-limited OLV may have an application in the MO population, but if too low tidal volume is delivered to a patient with an already low FRC, hypoxemia will worsen. PEEP is beneficial during two-lung ventilation in MO patients. During OLV, a mild to moderate level of PEEP to the single ventilated dependent lung has been shown to improve oxygenation if it does not exceed the lower inflection point of the alveolar pressure-volume loop. High PEEP results in increased pulmonary vascular resistance thereby increasing shunt fraction and worsening hypoxemia [84].

Anesthetic Drugs/Maintenance of Anesthesia

MO patients should be managed as if they have OSA. When practical, opioid-sparing anesthetic techniques, including regional anesthesia, should be used. Short-acting anesthetic and analgesic agents are appropriate choices for the MO patient. All opioids have respiratory depressant properties, and IV administration should be carefully titrated according to individual patient needs. Remifentanil is administered based on LBW in MO patients.

Some anesthesiologists prefer a total intravenous anesthesia (TIVA) technique with propofol and remifentanil, while most find an inhalational technique combined with epidural analgesia best for thoracotomy. In a study of 120 MO patients [85], neither technique was associated with intraoperative awareness.

In current anesthetic practice, propofol is the induction agent of choice for surgical patients, including MO patients. In theory, a lipid-soluble agent like propofol should be dosed according to TBW, but if this was followed in MO patients, such large doses could result in cardiovascular collapse, particularly in the fluid restricted thoracotomy patient. For MO patients, the induction dose of propofol is based on LBW [36].

Succinylcholine should be used for tracheal intubation in the MO patient. The concentration of pseudocholinesterase, the enzyme that metabolizes succinylcholine, increases with increasing weight. A 1 mg/kg TBW dose of succinylcholine provides a rapid and profound neuromuscular block and better intubating conditions than non-depolarizing muscle blockers. Rocuronium can be used, but only if sugammadex

is available. Non-depolarizing muscle relaxants are initially dosed based on LBW, and a neuromuscular monitor is used to guide additional dosing.

When considering volatile anesthetics, isoflurane is more lipophilic than desflurane or sevoflurane, making it more soluble in adipose tissue. Desflurane and sevoflurane have each been marketed as anesthetics for MO patients. However, in obese patients, fat is poorly perfused and comparable recovery times with both agents have been reported in obese and nonobese subjects after anesthetic procedures lasting 2–4 h. There are no clinical differences in emergence and recovery profiles in MO patients receiving either desflurane or sevoflurane when anesthetic concentration is carefully titrated [86]. However, a meta-analysis review on the topic found that patients given desflurane took less time to emerge from anesthesia; that is, they took less time to respond to commands to open their eyes, to squeeze the investigator's hand, to be prepared for tracheal extubation, and to state their name. There were no differences in hemodynamics and respiratory function perioperatively using either agent [87]. There were no significant differences in postanesthesia care unit discharge times, nausea, or analgesic requirement [88]. Despite claims to the contrary, there is no clear advantage between any of the inhalational anesthetics in MO patients [89].

Intravenous Fluid Management

Routine clinical practice is to restrict IV fluid to reduce the incidence of postoperative pulmonary edema after lung resection [90]. Therefore, perioperative assessment of blood volume (BV) is particularly critical for patients undergoing thoracotomy. The mean value for BV in normal-weight adults is usually given as 70 mL/kg, but this value cannot be used for obese and MO patients. With progressive increase in BMI, total circulating BV also increases, but BV measured as mL/kg TBW decreases in a nonlinear manner [91]. Using 70 mL/kg will overestimate BV in MO patients and can lead to underadministration of crystalloids, colloids, and red blood cells in the event of massive fluid translocation and/or hemorrhage.

Emergence and Extubation

Early extubation of the trachea at the completion of pulmonary resection lowers the risk of bronchial stump disruption and pulmonary air leaks secondary to positive pressure ventilation and airway tube trauma. In normal patients, a DLT can be removed while the patient is still in the lateral position, followed by assisted mask ventilation until the patient is fully awake. In the MO patient, especially one with OSA, mask ventilation in the lateral position can be difficult. Tracheal extubation in a MO patient should be performed with the patient in HELP and the operating room table in the RTP to optimize ventilation and to allow access to the airway if reintubation becomes necessary.

A MO patient must be sufficiently awake and have a regular respiratory pattern before the trachea is extubated. Although it is rarely necessary, a DLT can be replaced with an ETT via an airway exchange catheter, and the patient can then be allowed to emerge from anesthesia. Alternatively, after deflating both the tracheal and bronchial cuffs and withdrawing the tube until the endobronchial segment is in the trachea, the tracheal cuff can be reinflated and the DLT used as a single-lumen tube. A DLT completely in the trachea is less stimulating than one still in the bronchus. Even when a DLT remains in the bronchus, it is tolerated by patients, and most anesthesiologists elect to keep the DLT in place. The tube is removed after routine criteria for extubation have been met.

It has been suggested that noninvasive positive pressure ventilation (NIPPV) be employed to reduce post-extubation complications. A Cochrane Database review demonstrated that there was no additional benefit of using NIPPV in postoperative pulmonary resection [92]. Outcomes such as pulmonary complications, rate of reintubation, mortality, rate of non-pulmonary complications, postoperative consumption of antibiotics, length of intensive care unit stay, length of hospital stay, and adverse effects related to NIPPV were analyzed. Based on low to moderate quality evidence, the authors concluded that more studies were needed to establish this conclusion with greater certainty.

Despite these findings, for the MO patient who has been using CPAP or BIPAP preoperatively, these devices should be available and used immediately after tracheal extubation to stent the upper airway, to reduce the work of breathing, and to improve tidal volume and gas exchange [22]. The noninvasive Boussignac mask-CPAP (BCPAP) system does not require a mechanical ventilator and is very helpful in maintaining satisfactory oxygenation in spontaneously breathing MO surgical patients [93, 94]. Supplemental oxygen should always be administered, but used with caution as oxygen therapy can increase the AHI, hypoventilation, and P_aCO_2 levels in a patient with OHS. Continuous, noninvasive, transcutaneous carbon dioxide ($P_{tc}CO_2$) monitoring is accurate and has been applied to MO patients, especially those with OSA and OHS to evaluate abnormalities in their alveolar ventilation [95].

Postoperative Pain Control

Satisfactory post-thoracotomy analgesia is extremely important to maximize lung function, particularly in the MO patient who has restricted lung function prior to surgery.

Epidural opioid analgesia, with or without local anesthetic, when compared to IV opioids reduces pain, improves pulmonary function and oxygenation and reduces post-thoracotomy complications [96]. Local anesthetics given epidurally also supplement general anesthesia and reduce opioid requirements during surgery. Postoperative pain control for thoracotomy is covered in detail elsewhere in this book.

In the postoperative period, it is known that lung volumes are significantly reduced. Lung volumes in obese patients are probably reduced even further. Although the effects of thoracic epidural analgesia (TEA) compared to conventional opioid-based analgesia in postoperative spirometry has not been studied in obese patients undergoing thoracotomy, it has in laparotomy patients [18]. Perioperative spirometry values decreased significantly with increasing BMI, with the greatest reduction in vital capacity immediately after tracheal extubation. The effects were less in all patients receiving TEA, but in obese patients (BMI >30 kg/m2), the difference in vital capacity was significantly more pronounced than in normal patients. Recovery of spirometry values was significantly quicker in patients receiving TEA, particularly in the obese patients.

With epidural analgesia, any postoperative hypotension and/or motor blockade from the local anesthetic will limit the MO patient's ability to ambulate increasing their already greater risk for pulmonary embolism. A Cochrane review revealed that continuous thoracic paravertebral (PVB) analgesia is as effective as epidural analgesia in managing post-thoracotomy incisional pain [97] and is associated with a lower incidence of complications, including fewer pulmonary complications, less nausea and vomiting, less hypotension, and fewer failed blocks than epidural analgesia [98]. Unlike epidural analgesia, paravertebral analgesia only blocks the operative side and ipsilateral parasympathetic chain. In some studies, the stress response to surgery with PVB is reduced more than what is achieved by epidural analgesia [99]. As evidence for the effectiveness of PVB grows, some predict that it will likely replace epidural analgesia as the preferred method of post-thoracotomy pain control [100, 101].

Early institution of postoperative multimodal analgesic regimens that can include local anesthetics, interpleural local anesthetic infusions, nonsteroidal anti-inflammatory agents, and other synergistic drugs to reduce the respiratory depressant effects of centrally acting agents is indicated for MO patients with OSA. Alpha-2 agonists (clonidine, dexmedetomidine) do not depress respiration and have analgesic properties and have been used as adjuncts to epidural local anesthetics for post-thoracotomy analgesia [102].

Complications

Studies have reported that extremely obese patients undergoing cardiac surgical procedures have longer recovery times and a greater incidence of postoperative complications and mortality than normal-weight patients [103]. Although the same may be true for MO patients undergoing thoracotomy, there have been few outcome studies to corroborate this. Most published post-thoracotomy outcome studies have considered obese (BMI >30 kg/m²) and not MO or super-obese patients [104]. One recent study did find a weak correlation between obesity (BMI >30 kg/m²) and increased length of hospital stay after thoracic surgery [105]. It is interesting to note that there was a much higher association of complications in low BMI (<18.5 kg/m²) patients following thoracotomy. Many other large series of patients undergoing non-thoracic operations have reported similar results, that is, obesity (BMI >30 kg/m²) is not a major risk factor but low BMI (<18.5 kg/m²) is highly associated with surgical complications and death [70]. This association has been referred to as the "obesity paradox" [106].

The risk of postoperative thromboembolism, atelectasis, and pneumonia is believed to be greater in MO surgical patients undergoing non-thoracic operations [107]. Presumably, the same is true for similar size patients undergoing thoracic surgery, but once again, no studies are available that can document this concern.

There is one postoperative complication that is now recognized as relatively common in MO surgical patients but rare in normal-weight patients. Rhabdomyolysis (RML) results from pressure injury to skeletal muscle due to prolonged stasis in a non-physiologic position, such as the lateral decubitus position [108]. Long-duration surgery is the major risk factor, but other factors include super-obesity, male patients, and a history of hypertension, diabetes and/or peripheral vascular disease. Intraoperative padding of all pressure points and close attention to patient positioning are essential to prevent RML, pressure ulcers, and neurologic damage in MO patients. Injured muscle releases myoglobin, electrolytes, and protein into the systemic circulation. Myoglobinuria can lead to acute renal failure (ARF), and electrolyte disturbances can cause dysrhythmias and even cardiac arrest. Local signs and symptoms of RML are nonspecific and include pain, tenderness, swelling, bruising, and weakness. Complaints of numbness and muscular pain are almost always present, but epidural analgesia can mask symptoms and delay diagnosis.

Myoglobinuria usually presents as "tea" or brown-colored urine. The primary diagnostic indicator of RML is elevated serum creatine phosphokinase (CPK) levels. A MO patient who complains of buttock, hip, or shoulder pain in the postoperative period and who has a serum CPK level >1,000 IU/L is considered to have RML. Treatment should be instituted once CPK levels increase beyond 5,000 IU/L. Although intraoperative fluid replacement can reduce the risk of postoperative RML, fluid replacement is usually restricted during pulmonary resections. However, once a diagnosis of RML is made, aggressive hydration with large volumes of intravenous fluids and administration of diuretics are required to flush myoglobin from the kidneys.

Surgical Issues

Operative exposure in a MO patient may be less than optimal as the usual lateral decubitus position with extreme table flexion may not result in an adequate opening of the chest wall. Exposure is further compromised by increased chest wall thickness. Soft-tissue thickness also becomes important during video-assisted thoracoscopy (VATS) procedures since longer instruments are needed and range of motion may be limited. Unsatisfactory conditions for VATS can lead to more frequent conversion to thoracotomy, but once again, it is unclear as to whether this complication occurs more often in MO patients. The possibility of changing from VATS to open thoracotomy has important implications since it raises issues as to whether an epidural catheter should be placed preoperatively in a "technically difficult" VATS patient when there is a high likelihood of proceeding to thoracotomy. If the surgeon can place paravertebral catheters for postoperative pain control, the concern for unnecessary epidural placement is alleviated.

Conclusion

MO patients comprise an ever-increasing percentage of the thoracic surgical population. Obesity is not a contraindication to thoracic surgery; however, given the potential problems of extreme obesity, thorough perioperative planning is critical to prevent problems. There is a paucity of published studies involving MO thoracic surgical patients, so current anesthetic management is based on experience from obese patients undergoing non-thoracic surgical procedures. Research to further refine specific anesthetic management strategies for MO thoracic surgery patients is needed.

Clinical Case Discussion

Case A 56-year-old, 180 cm, 148 kg (BMI 46 kg/m²) man with lung cancer is scheduled for a right-upper lobectomy. He is active and reports no limitations to his ability to work in the construction industry. His medical problems include mild hypertension and type-2 diabetes mellitus. He has never been hospitalized and has no history of previous surgery. During his preoperative examination, his wife says that he snores loudly at night. He has never had a formal sleep study (polysomnography, PSG). On examination, he has a grade III Mallampati airway with a neck circumference of 50 cm. The patient and his surgeon want to proceed with his surgery as soon as possible.

Preoperative Management

What further studies are needed?

- Although spirometry may be useful, it is doubtful that it would demonstrate an inability for this patient to tolerate the surgery since he is active and has no respiratory impairment. Pulmonary function studies in MO patients demonstrate a reduction in lung volume (mainly FRC) and a restrictive breathing pattern.

Should the patient undergo a preoperative PSG study?

- Given the patient's BMI (46 kg/m^2) and history of snoring, it is more likely than not that he has obstructive sleep apnea (OSA). The patient is positive for 6/8 questions on his STOP-Bang assessment (snoring, hypertension, BMI, age, neck circumference, and male). Although a PSG test would confirm the diagnosis, even without testing this patient (and most MO patients) should be treated as if they have OSA.

Should the surgery be postponed while the patient is placed on CPAP?

- This patient is anxious to proceed with the surgery immediately. Several weeks of preoperative CPAP therapy might be helpful, but surgery will be delayed. Many patients do not tolerate CPAP, and he may refuse to wear the device.

In addition to a routine ECG, does his cardiac status require further evaluation?

- A stress echocardiogram would be informative given his age and comorbidities, but it is not essential since he has a high exercise tolerance and is active. The majority of MO surgical patients do not need an extensive preoperative cardiac workup.

What needs to be done prior to induction of anesthesia?

- In the preoperative area, unless the patient is extremely anxious, sedation should be avoided. Midazolam, 1-2 mg IV, can be given, but no opioid premedication.
- Since a thoracotomy is planned, a thoracic epidural (TEA) should be placed for intra- and postoperative analgesia. A continuous paravertebral block (PVB) is alternative with the advantage being it would have a better postoperative profile (less hypotension and absence of motor blockade) than a TEA. It is important that all perioperative opioids, including postoperative PCA opioids, be kept to a minimum in this MO patient with OSA.

- An arterial line should be placed to obtain a baseline blood gas and for intra- and postoperative monitoring.
- On arrival in the operating room, he should not be allowed to lie flat since this will lead to further reductions in his FRC and decrease in safe apnea time (SAT). He should be positioned on the operating table with his upper body elevated by pillows and blankets in the "head-elevated laryngoscopy position" (HELP).

Intraoperative Management

How should the patient's airway be intubated?

- A potentially difficult intubation is always possible, especially since his preoperative assessment demonstrated a high Mallampati score and large neck circumference. The choice of proceeding with a conventional IV anesthetic induction and direct laryngoscopy, video-laryngoscopy, or even an "awake" fiberoptic intubation is up to the confidence and experience of the anesthesiologist. With the availability of video-laryngoscopes, fiberoptic bronchoscopy for intubation (which often requires sedation) is seldom required. Video-laryngoscopes can be used to intubate the trachea with a double-lumen tube (DLT) or with an endotracheal tube (ETT). However, a second trained physician or nurse should always be immediately available to assist with bag-mask ventilation (which is frequently difficult in MO patients) and/or with airway intubation.
- The patient should be preoxygenated with 100% oxygen until his end-tidal oxygen is >80%. A true "rapid sequence induction" is not needed since this patient has no risk factors for aspiration. The patient should be ventilated by mask once rendered apneic to increase his SAT until laryngoscopy is initiated.
- If an IV induction is chosen, we prefer propofol and succinylcholine. Rocuronium can be used, but only if sugammadex is available. Succinylcholine provides better relaxation for tracheal intubation.
- If with direct laryngoscopy the patient has a favorable Cormack-Lehane grade view, a left DLT could be placed and checked with flexible bronchoscopy.
- For more difficult views, a gum elastic bougie could be inserted through the glottis, followed by an ETT over the bougie. If intubation by direct or video-laryngoscopy and a bougie is not possible, an LMA could be placed, and a fiberoptic bronchoscope could then be used to intubate the trachea. Once the airway is secured, lung separation can then be accomplished with either a bronchial blocker through the ETT, or the ETT can be replaced with a DLT using a long airway exchange catheter (AEC).

Is there a better technique for one-lung ventilation – total IV anesthesia (TIVA) or inhalation technique?

- Although TIVA has theoretic advantages (less depression of hypoxic vasoconstrictive reflex), clinically there is no difference in oxygenation during one-lung ventilation using either technique.
- Long acting opioids should be avoided during surgery with either technique.
- Lung size does not increase with obesity. Tidal volume during volume-controlled OLV should be based on ideal body weight (4–6 mL/kg IBW) and not actual weight. Plateau pressure during pressure-controlled ventilation should not exceed 30 cm H_2O.
- CPAP to the non-ventilated lung is useful to maintain oxygenation. PEEP to the ventilated lung should also be used.

Postoperative Management

What if the patient complains of pain, even with a functioning TEA or PVB?

- Supplemental IV opioid analgesia should be kept to a minimum; multimodal analgesic techniques should be used both intra- and postoperatively.

How do you manage postoperative oliguria?

- The differential diagnosis includes hypovolemia from the routine practice of fluid restriction during thoracotomy and/or rhabdomyolysis, which is relatively frequent in MO patients. In either case, additional IV fluid administration is indicated.
- A serum CPK level should be obtained to rule out renal failure secondary to rhabdomyolysis. Clinically significant rhabdomyolysis results in myoglobinuria. This usually doesn't occur unless the CPK level is >5,000 IU/L, but aggressive fluid therapy should be instituted if the CPK level is >1,000 IU/L, a level diagnostic of RML.

References

1. Finucane MM, Stevens GA, Cowan MJ, Danaei G, Lin JK, Paciorek CJ, et al. National, regional, and global trends in body-mass index since 1980: systematic analysis of health examination surveys and epidemiological studies with 960 country-years and 9·1 million participants. Lancet. 2011;377(9765):557–67.
2. Lohser J, Kulkarni V, Brodsky JB. Anesthesia for thoracic surgery in morbidly obese patients. Curr Opin Anaesthesiol. 2007;20(1):10–4.
3. Bray GA, Kim KK, Wilding JPH. Obesity: a chronic relapsing progressive disease process. A position statement of the World Obesity Federation. Obes Rev. 2017;18(7):715–23.
4. Flegal KM, Kit BK, Orpana H, Graubard BI. Association of all-cause mortality with overweight and obesity using standard body mass index categories: a systematic review and meta-analysis. JAMA. 2013;309(1):71–82.
5. Yang L, Colditz GA. Prevalence of Overweight and Obesity in the United States, 2007–2012. JAMA Intern Med. 2015;175(8):1412–3.
6. Sturm R. Increases in morbid obesity in the USA: 2000-2005. Public Health. 2007;121(7):492–6.
7. Sturm R, Hattori A. Morbid obesity rates continue to rise rapidly in the United States. Int J Obes. 2013;37(6):889–91.
8. Campos JH, Ueda K. Lung separation in the morbidly obese patient. Anesthesiol Res Pract. 2012;2012:207598.
9. Schumann R, Jones SB, Cooper B, Kelley SD, Bosch MV, Ortiz VE, et al. Update on best practice recommendations for anesthetic perioperative care and pain management in weight loss surgery, 2004-2007. Obesity (Silver Spring). 2009;17(5):889–94.
10. Ortiz VE, Kwo J. Obesity: physiologic changes and implications for preoperative management. BMC Anesthesiol. 2015;15:97.
11. Lemmens HJ, Brodsky JB, Bernstein DP. Estimating ideal body weight--a new formula. Obes Surg. 2005;15(7):1082–3.
12. Hanley MJ, Abernethy DR, Greenblatt DJ. Effect of obesity on the pharmacokinetics of drugs in humans. Clin Pharmacokinet. 2010;49(2):71–87.
13. Cheymol G. Effects of obesity on pharmacokinetics implications for drug therapy. Clin Pharmacokinet. 2000;39(3):215–31.
14. Janmahasatian S, Duffull SB, Ash S, Ward LC, Byrne NM, Green B. Quantification of lean bodyweight. Clin Pharmacokinet. 2005;44(10):1051–65.
15. Pelosi P, Croci M, Ravagnan I, Tredici S, Pedoto A, Lissoni A, et al. The effects of body mass on lung volumes, respiratory mechanics, and gas exchange during general anesthesia. Anesth Analg. 1998;87(3):654–60.
16. Licker MJ, Widikker I, Robert J, Frey JG, Spiliopoulos A, Ellenberger C, et al. Operative mortality and respiratory complications after lung resection for cancer: impact of chronic obstructive pulmonary disease and time trends. Ann Thorac Surg. 2006;81(5):1830–7.
17. Slinger PD, Johnston MR. Preoperative assessment: an anesthesiologist's perspective. Thorac Surg Clin. 2005;15(1):11–25.
18. von Ungern-Sternberg BS, Regli A, Reber A, Schneider MC. Effect of obesity and thoracic epidural analgesia on perioperative spirometry. Br J Anaesth. 2005;94(1):121–7.
19. Stierer T, Punjabi NM. Demographics and diagnosis of obstructive sleep apnea. Anesthesiol Clin North Am. 2005;23(3):405–20. v.
20. Crummy F, Piper AJ, Naughton MT. Obesity and the lung: 2. Obesity and sleep-disordered breathing. Thorax. 2008;63(8):738–46.
21. Peppard PE, Young T, Barnet JH, Palta M, Hagen EW, Hla KM. Increased prevalence of sleep-disordered breathing in adults. Am J Epidemiol. 2013;177(9):1006–14.
22. Frey WC, Pilcher J. Obstructive sleep-related breathing disorders in patients evaluated for bariatric surgery. Obes Surg. 2003;13(5):676–83.
23. Chung F, Yang Y, Liao P. Predictive performance of the STOP-Bang score for identifying obstructive sleep apnea in obese patients. Obes Surg. 2013;23(12):2050–7.
24. Chung F, Abdullah HR, Liao P. STOP-Bang Questionnaire: A Practical Approach to Screen for Obstructive Sleep Apnea. Chest. 2016;149(3):631–8.
25. Chung F, Chau E, Yang Y, Liao P, Hall R, Mokhlesi B. Serum bicarbonate level improves specificity of STOP-Bang screening for obstructive sleep apnea. Chest. 2013;143(5):1284–93.
26. Corso RM, Petrini F, Buccioli M, Nanni O, Carretta E, Trolio A, et al. Clinical utility of preoperative screening with STOP-Bang questionnaire in elective surgery. Minerva Anestesiol. 2014;80(8):877–84.
27. Vasu TS, Doghramji K, Cavallazzi R, Grewal R, Hirani A, Leiby B, et al. Obstructive sleep apnea syndrome and postoperative com-

plications: clinical use of the STOP-BANG questionnaire. Arch Otolaryngol Head Neck Surg. 2010;136(10):1020–4.

28. Chia P, Seet E, Macachor JD, Iyer US, Wu D. The association of pre-operative STOP-BANG scores with postoperative critical care admission. Anaesthesia. 2013;68(9):950–2.

29. Couch ME, Senior B. Nonsurgical and surgical treatments for sleep apnea. Anesthesiol Clin North Am. 2005;23(3):525–34. vii.

30. Practice guidelines for the perioperative management of patients with obstructive sleep apnea: an updated report by the American Society of Anesthesiologists Task Force on Perioperative Management of patients with obstructive sleep apnea. Anesthesiology. 2014;120(2):268–86.

31. Corso R, Russotto V, Gregoretti C, Cattano D. Perioperative management of obstructive sleep apnea: a systematic review. Minerva Anestesiol. 2018;84(1):81–93.

32. Mokhlesi B. Obesity hypoventilation syndrome: a state-of-the-art review. Respir Care. 2010;55(10):1347–62. discussion 63-5.

33. Alpert MA, Lavie CJ, Agrawal H, Aggarwal KB, Kumar SA. Obesity and heart failure: epidemiology, pathophysiology, clinical manifestations, and management. Transl Res. 2014;164(4): 345–56.

34. Sidana J, Aronow WS, Ravipati G, Di Stante B, McClung JA, Belkin RN, et al. Prevalence of moderate or severe left ventricular diastolic dysfunction in obese persons with obstructive sleep apnea. Cardiology. 2005;104(2):107–9.

35. Ingrande J, Lemmens HJ. Dose adjustment of anaesthetics in the morbidly obese. Br J Anaesth. 2010;105(Suppl 1):i16–23.

36. Ingrande J, Brodsky JB, Lemmens HJ. Lean body weight scalar for the anesthetic induction dose of propofol in morbidly obese subjects. Anesth Analg. 2011;113(1):57–62.

37. Altermatt FR, Muñoz HR, Delfino AE, Cortínez LI. Preoxygenation in the obese patient: effects of position on tolerance to apnoea. Br J Anaesth. 2005;95(5):706–9.

38. Collins JS, Lemmens HJ, Brodsky JB, Brock-Utne JG, Levitan RM. Laryngoscopy and morbid obesity: a comparison of the "sniff" and "ramped" positions. Obes Surg. 2004;14(9):1171–5.

39. Perilli V, Sollazzi L, Modesti C, Sacco T, Bocci MG, Ciocchetti PP, et al. Determinants of improvement in oxygenation consequent to reverse Trendelenburg position in anesthetized morbidly obese patients. Obes Surg. 2004;14(6):866–7.

40. Dixon BJ, Dixon JB, Carden JR, Burn AJ, Schachter LM, Playfair JM, et al. Preoxygenation is more effective in the 25 degrees head-up position than in the supine position in severely obese patients: a randomized controlled study. Anesthesiology. 2005;102(6):1110–5. discussion 5A

41. Boyce JR, Ness T, Castroman P, Gleysteen JJ. A preliminary study of the optimal anesthesia positioning for the morbidly obese patient. Obes Surg. 2003;13(1):4–9.

42. Brunette KE, Hutchinson DO, Ismail H. Bilateral brachial plexopathy following laparoscopic bariatric surgery. Anaesth Intensive Care. 2005;33(6):812–5.

43. Langeron O, Birenbaum A, Le Saché F, Raux M. Airway management in obese patient. Minerva Anestesiol. 2014;80(3):382–92.

44. Kristensen MS. Airway management and morbid obesity. Eur J Anaesthesiol. 2010;27(11):923–7.

45. Apfelbaum JL, Hagberg CA, Caplan RA, Blitt CD, Connis RT, Nickinovich DG, et al. Practice guidelines for management of the difficult airway: an updated report by the American Society of Anesthesiologists Task Force on Management of the Difficult Airway. Anesthesiology. 2013;118(2):251–70.

46. Kheterpal S, Han R, Tremper KK, Shanks A, Tait AR, O'Reilly M, et al. Incidence and predictors of difficult and impossible mask ventilation. Anesthesiology. 2006;105(5):885–91.

47. Cattano D, Katsiampoura A, Corso RM, Killoran PV, Cai C, Hagberg CA. Predictive factors for difficult mask ventilation in the obese surgical population. F1000Res. 2014;3:239.

48. Marrel J, Blanc C, Frascarolo P, Magnusson L. Videolaryngoscopy improves intubation condition in morbidly obese patients. Eur J Anaesthesiol. 2007;24(12):1045–9.

49. Ndoko SK, Amathieu R, Tual L, Polliand C, Kamoun W, El Housseini L, et al. Tracheal intubation of morbidly obese patients: a randomized trial comparing performance of Macintosh and Airtraq laryngoscopes. Br J Anaesth. 2008;100(2):263–8.

50. Brodsky JB, Lemmens HJ, Brock-Utne JG, Vierra M, Saidman LJ. Morbid obesity and tracheal intubation. Anesth Analg. 2002;94(3):732–6. table of contents.

51. Keller C, Brimacombe J, Kleinsasser A, Brimacombe L. The Laryngeal Mask Airway ProSeal(TM) as a temporary ventilatory device in grossly and morbidly obese patients before laryngoscope-guided tracheal intubation. Anesth Analg. 2002;94(3):737–40. table of contents.

52. Lewis SR, Butler AR, Parker J, Cook TM, Smith AF. Videolaryngoscopy versus direct laryngoscopy for adult patients requiring tracheal intubation. Cochrane Database Syst Rev. 2016;11:CD011136.

53. Dhonneur G, Ndoko SK, Yavchitz A, Foucrier A, Fessenmeyer C, Pollian C, et al. Tracheal intubation of morbidly obese patients: LMA CTrach vs direct laryngoscopy. Br J Anaesth. 2006;97(5): 742–5.

54. Combes X, Sauvat S, Leroux B, Dumerat M, Sherrer E, Motamed C, et al. Intubating laryngeal mask airway in morbidly obese and lean patients: a comparative study. Anesthesiology. 2005;102(6):1106–9. discussion 5A.

55. Gonzalez H, Minville V, Delanoue K, Mazerolles M, Concina D, Fourcade O. The importance of increased neck circumference to intubation difficulties in obese patients. Anesth Analg. 2008;106(4):1132–6. table of contents.

56. Ezri T, Medalion B, Weisenberg M, Szmuk P, Warters RD, Charuzi I. Increased body mass index per se is not a predictor of difficult laryngoscopy. Can J Anaesth. 2003;50(2):179–83.

57. Meyer RJ. Obesity and difficult intubation. Anaesth Intensive Care. 1994;22(3):314–5. author reply 6.

58. Jean J, Compère V, Fourdrinier V, Marguerite C, Auquit-Auckbur I, Milliez PY, et al. The risk of pulmonary aspiration in patients after weight loss due to bariatric surgery. Anesth Analg. 2008;107(4):1257–9.

59. Narayanaswamy M, McRae K, Slinger P, Dugas G, Kanellakos GW, Roscoe A, et al. Choosing a lung isolation device for thoracic surgery: a randomized trial of three bronchial blockers versus double-lumen tubes. Anesth Analg. 2009;108(4): 1097–101.

60. Campos JH, Hallam EA, Van Natta T, Kernstine KH. Devices for lung isolation used by anesthesiologists with limited thoracic experience: comparison of double-lumen endotracheal tube, Univent torque control blocker, and Arndt wire-guided endobronchial blocker. Anesthesiology. 2006;104(2):261–6. discussion 5A.

61. Campos JH. Update on tracheobronchial anatomy and flexible fiberoptic bronchoscopy in thoracic anesthesia. Curr Opin Anaesthesiol. 2009;22(1):4–10.

62. Campos JH. Which device should be considered the best for lung isolation: double-lumen endotracheal tube versus bronchial blockers. Curr Opin Anaesthesiol. 2007;20(1):27–31.

63. Campos JH, Hallam EA, Ueda K. Lung isolation in the morbidly obese patient: a comparison of a left-sided double-lumen tracheal tube with the Arndt® wire-guided blocker. Br J Anaesth. 2012;109(4):630–5.

64. Shulman MS, Brodsky JB, Levesque PR. Fibreoptic bronchoscopy for tracheal and endobronchial intubation with a double-lumen tube. Can J Anaesth. 1987;34(2):172–3.

65. Brodsky JB, Lemmens HJ. Tracheal width and left double-lumen tube size: a formula to estimate left-bronchial width. J Clin Anesth. 2005;17(4):267–70.

66. Slinger PD, Lesiuk L. Flow resistances of disposable double-lumen, single-lumen, and Univent tubes. J Cardiothorac Vasc Anesth. 1998;12(2):142–4.

67. Bardoczky GI, Szegedi LL, d'Hollander AA, Moures JM, de Francquen P, Yernault JC. Two-lung and one-lung ventilation in patients with chronic obstructive pulmonary disease: the effects of position and F(IO)2. Anesth Analg. 2000;90(1):35–41.

68. Watanabe S, Noguchi E, Yamada S, Hamada N, Kano T. Sequential changes of arterial oxygen tension in the supine position during one-lung ventilation. Anesth Analg. 2000;90(1):28–34.

69. Henzler D, Rossaint R, Kuhlen R. Is there a need for a recruiting strategy in morbidly obese patients undergoing laparoscopic surgery? Anesth Analg. 2004;98(1):268. author reply -9.

70. Aldenkortt M, Lysakowski C, Elia N, Brochard L, Tramèr MR. Ventilation strategies in obese patients undergoing surgery: a quantitative systematic review and meta-analysis. Br J Anaesth. 2012;109(4):493–502.

71. Pelosi P, Ravagnan I, Giurati G, Panigada M, Bottino N, Tredici S, et al. Positive end-expiratory pressure improves respiratory function in obese but not in normal subjects during anesthesia and paralysis. Anesthesiology. 1999;91(5):1221–31.

72. Brodsky JB, Wyner J, Ehrenwerth J, Merrell RC, Cohn RB. One-lung anesthesia in morbidly obese patients. Anesthesiology. 1982;57(2):132–4.

73. Fernandez-Bustamante A, Hashimoto S, Serpa Neto A, Moine P, Vidal Melo MF, Repine JE. Perioperative lung protective ventilation in obese patients. BMC Anesthesiol. 2015;15:56.

74. Lohser J. Evidence-based management of one-lung ventilation. Anesthesiol Clin. 2008;26(2):241–72.

75. Brower RG, Matthay MA, Morris A, Schoenfeld D, Thompson BT, Wheeler A, et al. Ventilation with lower tidal volumes as compared with traditional tidal volumes for acute lung injury and the acute respiratory distress syndrome. N Engl J Med. 2000;342(18):1301–8.

76. Hemmes SN, Gama de Abreu M, Pelosi P, Schultz MJ, Anaesthesiology PNIftCTNotESo. High versus low positive end-expiratory pressure during general anaesthesia for open abdominal surgery (PROVHILO trial): a multicentre randomised controlled trial. Lancet. 2014;384(9942):495–503.

77. Petrucci N, De Feo C. Lung protective ventilation strategy for the acute respiratory distress syndrome. Cochrane Database Syst Rev. 2013;2:CD003844.

78. Serpa Neto A, Cardoso SO, Manetta JA, Pereira VG, Espósito DC, Pasqualucci MO, et al. Association between use of lung-protective ventilation with lower tidal volumes and clinical outcomes among patients without acute respiratory distress syndrome: a meta-analysis. JAMA. 2012;308(16):1651–9.

79. Futier E, Constantin JM, Paugam-Burtz C, Pascal J, Eurin M, Neuschwander A, et al. A trial of intraoperative low-tidal-volume ventilation in abdominal surgery. N Engl J Med. 2013;369(5):428–37.

80. Bardoczky GI, Yernault JC, Houben JJ, d'Hollander AA. Large tidal volume ventilation does not improve oxygenation in morbidly obese patients during anesthesia. Anesth Analg. 1995;81(2):385–8.

81. Jaber S, Coisel Y, Chanques G, Futier E, Constantin JM, Michelet P, et al. A multicentre observational study of intra-operative ventilatory management during general anaesthesia: tidal volumes and relation to body weight. Anaesthesia. 2012;67(9):999–1008.

82. Fernandez-Bustamante A, Wood CL, Tran ZV, Moine P. Intraoperative ventilation: incidence and risk factors for receiving large tidal volumes during general anesthesia. BMC Anesthesiol. 2011;11:22.

83. Sentürk NM, Dilek A, Camci E, Sentürk E, Orhan M, Tuğrul M, et al. Effects of positive end-expiratory pressure on ventilatory and

oxygenation parameters during pressure-controlled one-lung ventilation. J Cardiothorac Vasc Anesth. 2005;19(1):71–5.

84. Michelet P, Roch A, Brousse D, D'Journo XB, Bregeon F, Lambert D, et al. Effects of PEEP on oxygenation and respiratory mechanics during one-lung ventilation. Br J Anaesth. 2005;95(2):267–73.

85. Gaszyński T, Wieczorek A. A comparison of BIS recordings during propofol-based total intravenous anaesthesia and sevoflurane-based inhalational anaesthesia in obese patients. Anaesthesiol Intensive Ther. 2016;48(4):239–47.

86. Arain SR, Barth CD, Shankar H, Ebert TJ. Choice of volatile anesthetic for the morbidly obese patient: sevoflurane or desflurane. J Clin Anesth. 2005;17(6):413–9.

87. Ozdogan HK, Cetinkunar S, Karateke F, Cetinalp S, Celik M, Ozyazici S. The effects of sevoflurane and desflurane on the hemodynamics and respiratory functions in laparoscopic sleeve gastrectomy. J Clin Anesth. 2016;35:441–5.

88. Liu FL, Cherng YG, Chen SY, Su YH, Huang SY, Lo PH, et al. Postoperative recovery after anesthesia in morbidly obese patients: a systematic review and meta-analysis of randomized controlled trials. Can J Anaesth. 2015;62(8):907–17.

89. Brodsky JB, Lemmens HJ, Saidman LJ. Obesity, surgery, and inhalation anesthetics -- is there a "drug of choice"? Obes Surg. 2006;16(6):734.

90. Slinger PD. Perioperative fluid management for thoracic surgery: the puzzle of postpneumonectomy pulmonary edema. J Cardiothorac Vasc Anesth. 1995;9(4):442–51.

91. Lemmens HJ, Bernstein DP, Brodsky JB. Estimating blood volume in obese and morbidly obese patients. Obes Surg. 2006;16(6):773–6.

92. Torres MF, Porfirio GJ, Carvalho AP, Riera R. Non-invasive positive pressure ventilation for prevention of complications after pulmonary resection in lung cancer patients. Cochrane Database Syst Rev. 2015;9:CD010355.

93. Gaszynski T, Tokarz A, Piotrowski D, Machala W. Boussignac CPAP in the postoperative period in morbidly obese patients. Obes Surg. 2007;17(4):452–6.

94. Neligan PJ, Malhotra G, Fraser M, Williams N, Greenblatt EP, Cereda M, et al. Continuous positive airway pressure via the Boussignac system immediately after extubation improves lung function in morbidly obese patients with obstructive sleep apnea undergoing laparoscopic bariatric surgery. Anesthesiology. 2009;110(4):878–84.

95. Dion JM, McKee C, Tobias JD, Herz D, Sohner P, Teich S, et al. Carbon dioxide monitoring during laparoscopic-assisted bariatric surgery in severely obese patients: transcutaneous versus end-tidal techniques. J Clin Monit Comput. 2015;29(1):183–6.

96. Wu CL, Cohen SR, Richman JM, Rowlingson AJ, Courpas GE, Cheung K, et al. Efficacy of postoperative patient-controlled and continuous infusion epidural analgesia versus intravenous patient-controlled analgesia with opioids: a meta-analysis. Anesthesiology. 2005;103(5):1079–88. quiz 109-10.

97. Yeung JH, Gates S, Naidu BV, Wilson MJ, Gao SF. Paravertebral block versus thoracic epidural for patients undergoing thoracotomy. Cochrane Database Syst Rev. 2016;2:CD009121.

98. Davies RG, Myles PS, Graham JM. A comparison of the analgesic efficacy and side-effects of paravertebral vs epidural blockade for thoracotomy--a systematic review and meta-analysis of randomized trials. Br J Anaesth. 2006;96(4):418–26.

99. Richardson J, Sabanathan S, Jones J, Shah RD, Cheema S, Mearns AJ. A prospective, randomized comparison of preoperative and continuous balanced epidural or paravertebral bupivacaine on postthoracotomy pain, pulmonary function and stress responses. Br J Anaesth. 1999;83(3):387–92.

100. Chelly JE. Paravertebral Blocks. Anesthesiol Clin. 2012;30(1):75–90.

101. Conlon NP, Shaw AD, Grichnik KP. Postthoracotomy Paravertebral Analgesia: Will It Replace Epidural Analgesia? Anesthesiol Clin. 2008;26(2):369–80.

102. Hofer RE, Sprung J, Sarr MG, Wedel DJ. Anesthesia for a patient with morbid obesity using dexmedetomidine without narcotics. Can J Anaesth. 2005;52(2):176–80.

103. Tyson GH, Rodriguez E, Elci OC, Koutlas TC, Chitwood WR, Ferguson TB, et al. Cardiac procedures in patients with a body mass index exceeding 45: outcomes and long-term results. Ann Thorac Surg. 2007;84(1):3–9. discussion.

104. Smith PW, Wang H, Gazoni LM, Shen KR, Daniel TM, Jones DR. Obesity does not increase complications after anatomic resection for non-small cell lung cancer. Ann Thorac Surg. 2007;84(4):1098–105. discussion 105-6.

105. Suemitsu R, Sakoguchi T, Morikawa K, Yamaguchi M, Tanaka H, Takeo S. Effect of body mass index on perioperative complications in thoracic surgery. Asian Cardiovasc Thorac Ann. 2008;16(6):463–7.

106. Mariscalco G, Wozniak MJ, Dawson AG, Serraino GF, Porter R, Nath M, et al. Body Mass Index and Mortality Among Adults Undergoing Cardiac Surgery: A Nationwide Study With a Systematic Review and Meta-Analysis. Circulation. 2017;135(9):850–63.

107. Davenport DL, Xenos ES, Hosokawa P, Radford J, Henderson WG, Endean ED. The influence of body mass index obesity status on vascular surgery 30-day morbidity and mortality. J Vasc Surg. 2009;49(1):140–7. 7.e1; discussion 7.

108. Kong SS, Ho ST, Huang GS, Cherng CH, Wong CS. Rhabdomyolysis after a long-term thoracic surgery in right decubitus position. Acta Anaesthesiol Sin. 2000;38(4):223–8.

Pulmonary Resection in the Patient with Pulmonary Hypertension

34

Alexander Huang and Katherine Marseu

Key Points

- Pulmonary resection in the presence of pulmonary hypertension has been associated with increased risk for perioperative morbidity and mortality; however, advances in assessment, treatment, and intraoperative management have made surgery in these patients feasible.
- Preoperative assessment of these patients requires a multidisciplinary approach and various diagnostic tests to assess severity and determine appropriate treatment. This should be optimized preoperatively.
- The anesthetic goals for these patients include optimizing preload, maintaining a low-normal heart rate, maintaining contractility, decreasing pulmonary vascular resistance, and ensuring systemic pressures are greater than pulmonary pressures.
- Intraoperative monitoring should include invasive blood pressure monitoring and potentially the use of a pulmonary artery catheter and/or transesophageal echocardiography. The use of advanced monitors such as pulmonary artery catheters or transesophageal echocardiography should be decided on a case-by-case basis.
- Understanding of the interaction between anesthetic agents and pulmonary vascular physiology is of key importance. Volatile agents may impair right ventricular function and should be used with care. Ketamine has been shown to be safe for use in pulmonary hypertension.
- Inhaled nitric oxide and prostanoids are potentially useful adjuncts in the management of pulmonary pressures intraoperatively.
- Effective pain management is of utmost importance in patients with pulmonary hypertension presenting for pulmonary resection. Epidurals are effective and may reduce pulmonary complications as well as overall mortality but require close monitoring due to their potentially significant hemodynamic effects. Paravertebral catheters are also an alternative.
- Postoperative arrhythmias, acute pulmonary hypertension, and right heart failure are potential complications post-pulmonary resection and necessitate postoperative monitoring in a step-down or critical care unit for these patients.

Abbreviations

ARDS	Acute respiratory distress syndrome
ECG	Electrocardiogram
ECMO	Extracorporeal membrane oxygenation
ERA	Endothelin receptor antagonist
iNO	Inhaled nitric oxide
NYHA	New York Heart Association
OLV	One-lung ventilation
PAC	Pulmonary artery catheter
PAP or PA pressure	Pulmonary artery pressure
PCA	Patient-controlled analgesia
PDE-5	Phosphodiesterase-5
PGI_2	Prostacyclin
RHC	Right heart catheterization
RVSP	Right ventricular systolic pressure
SPAP	Systolic pulmonary artery pressure
TEE	Transesophageal echocardiography

A. Huang (✉) · K. Marseu
Department of Anesthesia and Pain Management, Toronto General Hospital, University Health Network and University of Toronto, Toronto, ON, Canada
e-mail: Alexander.Huang@uhn.ca

© Springer Nature Switzerland AG 2019
P. Slinger (ed.), *Principles and Practice of Anesthesia for Thoracic Surgery*, https://doi.org/10.1007/978-3-030-00859-8_34

TTE   Transthoracic echocardiography
VATS   Video-assisted thoracoscopic surgery
WHO   World Health Organization

Introduction

Pulmonary hypertension is defined as a resting mean pulmonary artery pressure of $\geq$25 mmHg [1] and carries with it significant implications for the patient presenting for thoracic surgery. Pulmonary hypertension is often associated with significant end-stage lung disease and can also be associated with numerous extrapulmonary diseases. The classification of pulmonary hypertension was most recently updated in 2013 to reflect five groups of disorders that cause it [2] (Table 34.1). Presently, pulmonary hypertension is thought to have a global prevalence of 1%; however, this may increase to as high as 10% in those greater than 65 years of age [3]. Typically, for the anesthetist, there are two main types of pulmonary hypertension: pulmonary hypertension related to left-heart disease and pulmonary hypertension related to lung disease (Table 34.2). Currently, with improved diagnostic testing and therapies, it is no longer uncommon for patients with pulmonary hypertension to present to the operating room for surgery. This chapter will consider the perioperative risk profile of patients with pulmonary hypertension presenting for lung resection surgery. It will then discuss the preoperative assessment, intraoperative, and postoperative management of this population.

Perioperative Risk

The increased risk in perioperative morbidity and mortality associated with pulmonary hypertension has been well-documented in the literature. Studies in the non-cardiac surgical population have demonstrated that these patients are at increased risk for perioperative heart failure, hemodynamic instability, sepsis, and respiratory failure. Furthermore, pulmonary hypertension patients require longer durations of mechanical ventilation and longer intensive care and hospital admissions [4, 5]. Higher pulmonary-to-systemic systolic pressure ratios are also associated with higher perioperative mortality [6]. In the literature, the morbidity and mortality in pulmonary hypertension patients presenting for non-cardiac surgery have been reported to be 14–42% and 1–18%, respectively [7]. Overall, patients with pulmonary hypertension present a significant challenge in the perioperative period.

Table 34.1 World Health Organization classification of pulmonary hypertension

1 Pulmonary arterial hypertension (PAH)
1.1 Idiopathic PAH
1.2 Heritable
1.2.1 Bone morphogenetic protein receptor type II gene abnormality
1.2.2 Other genetic mutations: ALK-1, ENG, SMAD9, CAV1, KCNK3
1.2.3 Unknown
1.3 Drug- and toxin-induced
1.4 Associated with
1.4.1 Connective tissue diseases
1.4.2 HIV infection
1.4.3 Portal hypertension
1.4.4 Congenital heart diseases
1.4.5 Schistosomiasis
1' Pulmonary veno-occlusive disease and/or pulmonary capillary hemangiomatosis
1" Persistent pulmonary hypertension of the newborn
2 Pulmonary hypertension due to left heart disease
2.1 Left ventricular systolic dysfunction
2.2 Left ventricular diastolic dysfunction
2.3 Valvular disease
2.4 Congenital/acquired left heart inflow/outflow tract obstruction and congenital cardiomyopathies
3 Pulmonary hypertension due to lung diseases and/or hypoxia
3.1 Chronic obstructive pulmonary disease
3.2 Interstitial lung disease
3.3 Other pulmonary diseases with mixed restrictive and obstructive pattern
3.4 Sleep-disordered breathing
3.5 Alveolar hypoventilation disorders
3.6 Chronic exposure to high altitude
3.7 Developmental lung diseases
4 Chronic thromboembolic pulmonary hypertension
5 Pulmonary hypertension with unclear multifactorial mechanisms
5.1 Hematologic disorders: chronic hemolytic anemia, myeloproliferative disorders, splenectomy
5.2 Systemic disorders: sarcoidosis, pulmonary histiocytosis, lymphangioleiomyomatosis
5.3 Metabolic disorders: glycogen storage disease, Gaucher disease, thyroid disorders
5.4 Others: tumoral obstruction, fibrosing mediastinitis, chronic renal failure, segmental pulmonary hypertension

Reproduced from Simonneau et al. [2] with permission from Elsevier

Table 34.2 Modified classification of pulmonary hypertension for anesthesia

Left heart disease	Lung disease
Systolic dysfunction	Pulmonary vascular disease
Diastolic dysfunction	Chronic lung disease, hypoxemia, sleep apnea
Mitral valvular disease: stenosis, regurgitation	Thromboembolic pulmonary hypertension
Congenital cardiac disease	Miscellaneous: autoimmune, metabolic

General indications for pulmonary resection include procedures for diagnosis (e.g., open lung biopsies for tumors and pulmonary fibrosis) or treatment of malignancy, congenital abnormalities, infection, and trauma. As mentioned previously, it is not unusual for elevated pulmonary arterial pressures to coexist with lung disease. Historically, lung resection surgery has been cautioned and discouraged in patients with pulmonary hypertension [8]. In small studies and case reports examining patients undergoing pulmonary resection, the presence of pulmonary hypertension was associated with increased morbidity and mortality (by 50% and 25%, respectively, in one small study) [9]. Significant bleeding [10, 11], increases in pulmonary artery pressures postoperatively [12], and right ventricular failure [13] have all been reported. However, more recently, Wei and colleagues retrospectively examined 298 patients (19 with pulmonary hypertension) undergoing pulmonary resection for lung cancer. In this study, the presence of pulmonary hypertension was not associated with increased morbidity or mortality as compared to non-pulmonary hypertension patients [14]. Though small, this study suggests the feasibility of safely conducting lung resections in this population.

The implications of lung resection surgery on the pathophysiology of underlying pulmonary hypertension must also be considered. The loss of lung parenchyma carries with it a loss of pulmonary vasculature, which can result in increased pulmonary vascular resistance. Pneumonectomy has been shown to produce significant right ventricular dysfunction in the immediate postoperative period [15, 16], as well as up to 4 years after surgery [17]. The etiology of this dysfunction is presumed to be due to increased right ventricular afterload. Pulmonary artery systolic pressures measured by Doppler echocardiography have also been shown to be elevated after pneumonectomy [17]. The literature remains inconsistent and unclear regarding the effects of subtotal pulmonary resections (lobectomies, segmentectomies, and wedge resections) on pulmonary arterial pressures [18]. However, the majority of published studies on the subject have involved patient populations without pulmonary hypertension. Presumably, the effect of pulmonary resection on existing pulmonary hypertension (as well as existing right heart dysfunction) is likely to be more significant and warrants additional concern by the anesthesiologist.

Preoperative Assessment

The preoperative assessment of patients presenting for thoracic surgery is discussed in great detail in Chap. 2 and can be applied to the patient with known or suspected pulmonary hypertension.

History, Physical Exam, and Investigations

Patients with known or suspected pulmonary hypertension commonly present with dyspnea and fatigue. Patients may also report additional symptoms, including presyncope, syncope, angina, and symptoms of right heart failure (peripheral edema, abdominal distension, and anorexia), which may reflect disease progression and severity. Unfortunately, these symptoms are vague and nonspecific and are often attributable to more common cardiopulmonary diagnoses. Furthermore, such symptoms are common in patients presenting for thoracic surgery, in general, and make identification of undiagnosed pulmonary hypertension challenging. Additional features on history such as orthopnea or paroxysmal nocturnal dyspnea (left-sided heart disease), arthralgias or skin changes (rheumatologic or connective tissue disorder), or snoring or observed apnea (obstructive sleep apnea) may also aid in evaluation or provide a unifying diagnosis.

In patients with known pulmonary hypertension, the development of symptoms of right heart failure is a means of gauging a patient's clinical status over time. The World Health Organization (WHO) has also developed a classification of functional status of patients with pulmonary hypertension [19] based on the New York Heart Association (NYHA) system (Table 34.3), which is also useful for assessing disease severity, progression, and response to treatment. The WHO/NYHA functional status has been shown to strongly correlate with long-term survival in patients with idiopathic pulmonary hypertension [20].

Beyond history and physical examination, the assessment of the patient with suspected or confirmed pulmonary hypertension presenting for thoracic surgery should also include a

Table 34.3 World Health Organization classification of functional status of patients with pulmonary hypertension

Class	Description
I	Patients with pulmonary hypertension in whom there is no limitation of usual physical activity; ordinary physical activity does not cause increased dyspnea, fatigue, chest pain, or presyncope
II	Patients with pulmonary hypertension who have mild limitation of physical activity. There is no discomfort at rest, but normal physical activity causes increased dyspnea, fatigue, chest pain, or presyncope
III	Patients with pulmonary hypertension who have a marked limitation of physical activity. There is no discomfort at rest, but less than ordinary activity causes increased dyspnea, fatigue, chest pain, or presyncope
IV	Patients with pulmonary hypertension who are unable to perform any physical activity at rest and who may have signs of right ventricular failure. Dyspnea and/or fatigue may be present at rest, and symptoms are increased by almost any physical activity

Reproduced from Barst et al. [19] with permission from Elsevier

chest X-ray and electrocardiogram (ECG). A chest X-ray not only allows for assessment of lung parenchyma and the specific lesion being operated on (e.g., tumor) but may also demonstrate features consistent with elevated pulmonary artery pressures such as prominent pulmonary arteries or right ventricular enlargement. The ECG may provide features suggestive or supportive of pulmonary hypertension including right ventricular hypertrophy or a right axis-deviation. Neither a chest X-ray nor ECG possess sufficient specificity or sensitivity to rule in or rule out pulmonary hypertension.

Transthoracic echocardiography (TTE) has rapidly become the investigation of choice for both screening and follow-up of patients with pulmonary hypertension, given its availability and noninvasiveness. TTE allows for the estimation of the right ventricular systolic pressure (RVSP), which closely approximates the systolic pulmonary artery pressure (SPAP) in the absence of pulmonary outflow obstruction. The RVSP measured by echocardiography has been shown to have moderate to strong correlation to the SPAP measured through right heart catheterization (correlation coefficient $R = 0.57$–0.93) [19]. However, in some cases, RVSP measurements done using TTE may deviate from SPAP values derived by right heart catheterization by as much as 10 mmHg in many patients, with a tendency to underestimate the true SPAP [21]. Furthermore, there is large variation in the sensitivity and specificity of TTE in the diagnosis of pulmonary hypertension, which has been shown to be 79–100% and 60–98%, respectively [22]. Additional echocardiography features include right ventricular dilatation or hypertrophy, right ventricular dysfunction, right atrial enlargement, the presence of significant tricuspid regurgitation, interventricular septal flattening, as well as the presence of pericardial effusions. The presence of these features has been associated with worse prognosis in pulmonary hypertension patients [22].

Right heart catheterization (RHC) remains the gold standard in terms of assessment and diagnosis of pulmonary hypertension. RHC allows for the measurement of pulmonary artery pressures (required for the formal diagnosis of pulmonary hypertension) as well as pulmonary vascular resistance. Additional useful information can be derived from RHC, including estimation of right heart pressures (right ventricular and right atrial pressures), pulmonary capillary wedge pressures, cardiac output, and pulmonary vasoreactivity.

In addition to the testing described above, other investigations may be necessary depending on the specific indication for pulmonary resection. Detailed discussion of these additional tests can be reviewed in Chap. 2.

Treatment and Consultations

The management and treatment of pulmonary hypertension requires a multidisciplinary approach and is a topic well beyond the scope of this chapter. However, the thoracic anesthetist should have a basic understanding of the management of pulmonary hypertension patients and the relevant perioperative implications of pulmonary hypertension treatment. All patients with significant pulmonary hypertension should ideally have consultation and ongoing follow-up with a pulmonary hypertension specialist and, if applicable, a specialist for the management of the underlying cause of their pulmonary hypertension (e.g., a cardiologist for left-sided heart disease, a rheumatologist for connective tissue disorders). Perioperative management should include consultation with these specialists to ensure proper optimization prior to presenting to the operating room.

Specific management of pulmonary hypertension is dependent on the underlying cause; however, pharmacologic management may involve the use of vasodilators, diuretics, steroids, and immune suppressants, as well as anticoagulants. Perioperative management of these pharmacologic regimens may be complex.

Pulmonary vasodilating agents, such as endothelin receptor antagonists, prostanoids, and phosphodiesterase-5 inhibitors, can be used alone or in combination in the management of pulmonary arterial hypertension (Group 1).

Endothelin receptor antagonists (ERAs) target the endothelin-1 receptor, which mediates vasoconstriction and plays a significant role in the pathogenesis of pulmonary arterial hypertension [23]. Commonly used preparations include bosentan, ambrisentan, and macitentan, all of which are administered orally. While generally well-tolerated, hepatotoxicity and the development of transaminitis are well-known adverse effects of ERAs and should be screened shortly after initiation [24]. Other less common but significant adverse effects include anemia and hypotension.

Prostanoids are prostacyclin analogues and exhibit potent vasodilating effects mediated through increasing intracellular cyclic adenosine monophosphate [25]. Presently, three prostacyclin analogues are available: epoprostenol (continuous intravenous infusion), treprostinil (continuous subcutaneous infusion), and iloprost (inhalational administration). The relatively short half-lives of these agents necessitate continuous or frequent administration. Epoprostenol's half-life is less than 5 min, and thus therapy requires continuous intravenous infusion via a portable infusion pump. The half-lives of treprostinil and iloprost are approximately 45–60 min [26]. Abrupt discontinuation of prostanoid therapy can result in life-threatening rebound of pulmonary hypertension. Additional concerns regarding prostanoids include the potential for systemic hypotension, as well as increased bleeding risk due to prostanoid-mediated inhibition of platelet aggregation [27].

Phosphodiesterase-5 (PDE-5) inhibitors were initially introduced for the management of erectile dysfunction but have found a significant role in the management of pulmonary arterial hypertension. PDE-5 is predominantly found in the lungs, and its inhibition prevents the breakdown of cyclic guanosine monophosphate (cGMP) [28]. cGMP potentiates the vasodilatory effects of nitric oxide, producing pulmonary vasodilation. Oral preparations of PDE-5 inhibitors include sildenafil and tadalafil. These agents are generally well-tolerated and produce minor adverse effects such as headaches, flushing, and dyspepsia [24].

In general, these agents (especially prostanoids) are continued in the perioperative period; however, adjustment of doses and dosing may need to occur and should be managed by an experienced prescriber.

Intraoperative Management

An understanding of the pathophysiology of pulmonary hypertension and its implications for general anesthesia is of utmost importance when managing the patient with pulmonary hypertension presenting for pulmonary resection. Right ventricular failure and resulting cardiovascular collapse secondary to pulmonary hypertension present the greatest risk in the perioperative period. The right ventricle

normally receives perfusing blood flow during both systole and diastole. However, elevated pulmonary arterial pressures produce increased right ventricular transmural and intracavitary pressures, which can limit ventricular perfusion during systole and result in RV ischemia [29]. Hypotension is poorly tolerated in significant pulmonary hypertension, as well as conditions impairing right ventricular filling, such as tachycardia and arrhythmias. Low systemic to pulmonary pressure ratios are associated with poorer outcomes and should be avoided intraoperatively. The pathophysiologic processes involved in right ventricular failure in the setting of increased right ventricular afterload (pulmonary hypertension) are shown in Fig. 34.1. In addition, care needs to be taken to prevent conditions which would worsen pulmonary arterial pressures, including hypoxemia, hypercarbia, hypothermia, acidosis, and elevated alveolar pressures.

The ideal anesthetic would maintain or enhance right ventricular function and systemic vascular resistance while decreasing pulmonary vascular resistance. However, in practice, this is challenging to achieve in the operating room. A summary of hemodynamic and ventilation goals is shown in Table 34.4.

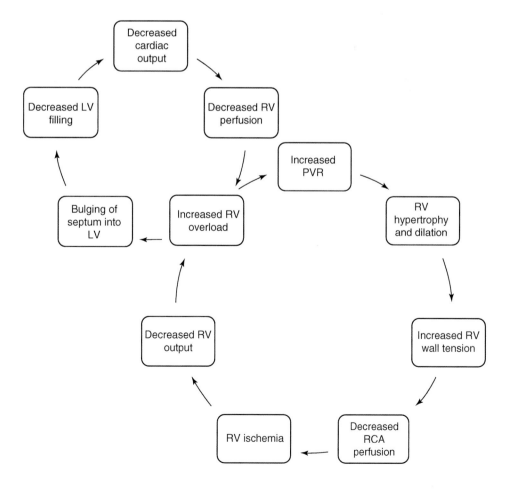

Fig. 34.1 Pathophysiologic mechanisms in right-sided heart failure. PVR pulmonary vascular resistance, RCA right coronary artery. (Reprinted from Wilcox et al. [29] with permission from Elsevier)

Table 34.4 Hemodynamic and ventilatory goals during anesthesia for pulmonary hypertension

Parameter	Goals
Hemodynamic conditions	
Preload	Avoidance of hypervolemia – precipitates RV failure
	Avoidance of hypovolemia – impairs stroke volume and cardiac output
	Hypovolemia is better tolerated
Afterload	Maintain a systemic systolic blood pressure greater than the pulmonary systolic pressure to maintain right ventricular perfusion
	Vasopressors may be used to achieve this
Right ventricular contractility	Avoid excessive myocardial depression (choice of anesthetic agent)
	Consider use of inotropes when needed
Heart rate	Normal heart rate – avoid tachycardia, which impairs right ventricular filling and cardiac output
Pulmonary vascular resistance	Avoid precipitants of increased pulmonary vascular resistance (hypoxia, hypercarbia, acidosis, hypothermia, increased sympathetic tone)
Ventilatory conditions	
Optimize oxygenation	Maintain higher FiO_2 as needed to avoid hypoxia
	Careful PEEP titration
CO_2	Target normocapnia to mild hypocapnia (pCO_2 30–35)
pH	Normal pH
	Mild alkalosis promotes pulmonary vasodilation
Airway pressure	Minimize peak inspiratory pressure as much as possible
	Peak inspiratory pressure <30 mmHg
	Avoid excessive PEEP

Premedication

The perioperative period is a stressful time for all patients, and many centers routinely provide patients with the option of an anxiolytic administered in a preoperative area. Care and attentiveness should be taken when administering sedating agents (such as benzodiazepines) to patients with pulmonary hypertension preoperatively, which is a period where continuous monitoring is not always available. Preoperative anxiolytics often have a sedating effect which can result in hypoventilation leading to hypercarbia and, in some cases, hypoxia. These two conditions can precipitate significant increases in pulmonary vascular resistance, which can be life-threatening. Sedative premedication should be used cautiously, or avoided completely, in the patient with significant pulmonary hypertension. If required, continuous hemodynamic monitoring, as well as supplemental oxygen, should be considered and readily available.

Intraoperative Monitoring

Intrathoracic surgery, including surgery for pulmonary resection, requires an increased level of intraoperative monitoring.

Routine noninvasive monitors, including 5-lead ECG, pulse oximetry, capnography, temperature, and noninvasive blood pressure monitoring, are complemented by invasive blood pressure monitoring. In patients presenting for thoracic surgery, invasive blood pressure monitoring via an intra-arterial catheter is routinely done prior to induction of anesthesia at the authors' institution. This allows for continuous monitoring of systemic blood pressure during induction and maintenance of anesthesia. Of equal importance, invasive blood pressure monitoring allows regular sampling of arterial blood gases to assess oxygenation and ventilation.

Central venous access should be considered in patients with significant pulmonary hypertension, evidence of right ventricular dysfunction, or for major pulmonary resections, as it allows for infusions of vasopressors and inotropes (discussed further below). Central venous access also allows for the insertion of a pulmonary artery catheter (PAC), which in turn allows for continuous measurement of pulmonary arterial pressures and determination of cardiac output. The use of PACs for intraoperative and perioperative monitoring has been subject to significant controversy in the literature. One large observational study determined that the perioperative use of PACs in patients presenting for non-cardiac surgery was associated with an increased risk of postoperative cardiac (myocardial infarction, angina, cardiogenic shock, ventricular fibrillation/tachycardia, cardiac arrest, or complete heart block) and non-cardiac (pulmonary embolism, non-cardiogenic pulmonary edema, prolonged mechanical ventilation, pneumonia, renal failure, stroke, or GI bleeding) morbidity [30]. A subsequent prospective randomized controlled study involving high-risk non-cardiac surgery patients found that the use of a PAC conferred no benefit in terms of overall mortality or cardiac and non-cardiac morbidity [31]. However, thoracic surgery patients made up only a small minority of the studied population in both studies and neither specifically assessed for pulmonary hypertension and its implications. Unfortunately, there is no large study investigating the use of PACs in thoracic (pulmonary resection or otherwise) surgery.

Given the lack of alternative means to continuously monitor pulmonary artery pressures intraoperatively, the use of PACs in patients presenting for pulmonary resection should strongly be considered in the setting of significant pulmonary hypertension and especially in patients where pulmonary artery pressures approach or exceed systemic pressures. The interpretation of PAC data can be challenging and misleading in patients with pulmonary hypertension, even for experienced clinicians [32]. Elevated and increasing pulmonary artery pressures are universally an indicator of worsening clinical status. However, decreasing pressure can indicate a desirable reduction in pulmonary artery pressures or impending right ventricular failure and subsequent cardiovascular collapse. As such, PAC data must be interpreted in the context of other hemodynamic indices such as arterial blood pressure, cardiac output, and central venous pressures. It should also be noted that the use of a PAC is not without risk, as pulmonary hypertension is a known risk factor for PAC-associated pulmonary artery rupture, which is an exceedingly rare (incidence 0.03–0.2%) but highly fatal (mortality ~ 70%) complication [33].

Intraoperative transesophageal echocardiography (TEE) is a monitoring tool that is growing in terms of availability and utility, particularly in the setting of assessment of dynamic ventricular function (see also Chap. 30). Intraoperative TEE has been recurrently shown to enhance and influence therapeutic decision-making in the OR during surgery [34, 35]. The American Society of Anesthesiologists recommends the use of intraoperative TEE during non-cardiac surgery "when the nature of the planned surgery or the patient's known or suspected cardiovascular pathology might result in severe hemodynamic, pulmonary, or neuro-logic compromise" [36]. As right ventricular failure in the context of worsening pulmonary hypertension is a major concern in the intraoperative period, the utility of TEE in assessment of right ventricular function is of growing inter-est. The use of TEE as a monitor intraoperatively in the patient with pulmonary hypertension allows for assessment of baseline right ventricular function and the presence of sig-nificant right ventricular dysfunction, which has been shown to be an important prognostic indicator in cardiac surgery [37]. However, unlike the left ventricle, where continuous TEE monitoring of function can be reasonably performed through a single view, the complex and irregular structure of the right ventricle requires multiple views to assess changes in regional function. As such, continuous monitoring with concurrent management of the potentially failing right ven-tricle in the setting of worsening pulmonary hypertension may be impractical for the lone care provider. The advent of new three-dimensional TEE technology has allowed for rapid and accurate assessment of right ventricular function in a matter of minutes [38] and may eventually evolve to allow for simple, reliable, and continuous monitoring of right ven-tricular function in the OR.

Anesthetic Management

The pharmacology and physiologic effects of commonly used anesthetic agents make induction and maintenance of anesthesia in the patient with pulmonary hypertension chal-lenging. The ideal anesthetic agent(s) would provide deep anesthesia while maintaining cardiac performance (specifi-cally that of the right ventricle) and systemic vascular resis-tance while reducing pulmonary vascular resistance. In practice, commonly used agents generally produce impair-ment in cardiac contractility and reduced systemic vascular

resistance while having variable or unclear effects on pulmo-nary vascular resistance.

Intravenous Agents

The use of intravenous agents in the anesthetic management of patients presenting to the OR is near ubiquitous. The growing number of pharmacologic agents available, as well as their varying pharmacodynamic effects, warrants closer examination, especially in the context of the deranged car-diorespiratory physiology involved in pulmonary hyperten-sion patients.

Propofol is among the most commonly used intravenous agents for both the induction and maintenance of anesthesia. The effect of propofol on pulmonary vascular tone is unclear; however, animal studies have shown that in the setting of increased adrenergic activity, administration of propofol has a vasoconstricting effect on pulmonary vasculature [39, 40]. However, in a human model, administration of propofol in normoxic conditions had a vasodilatory effect in the pulmo-nary vasculature [41], raising questions regarding propofol's true effect. What is clear, however, is that propofol exhibits depressant effects on both myocardial function and systemic vascular resistance. Both effects can impair right ventricular function, either directly or by reducing coronary perfusion to the right ventricle through reduced systemic pressures. As such, caution should be exercised when using propofol in the patient with pulmonary hypertension, especially if right ven-tricular dysfunction is present.

Etomidate is a less commonly used intravenous induction agent with a neutral hemodynamic profile, allowing for pre-served right ventricular function and perfusion. Furthermore, in vitro human pulmonary artery models have suggested some vasodilatory effects on the pulmonary vasculature [41]. While these properties would make etomidate the ideal induction agent in the patient with pulmonary hypertension, a recently published retrospective analysis looking at over 31,000 patients (ASA III–IV patients) found that the use of etomidate was associated with increased 30-day mortality and cardiovascular morbidity as compared to patients receiv-ing propofol [42]. While the study did not specifically include patients with pulmonary hypertension or those undergoing thoracic surgery, the results do raise concerns regarding the safety of etomidate in higher-risk patients.

Ketamine is an NMDA-receptor antagonist with activity at other sites, including opioid, acetylcholine, norepineph-rine, dopamine, and serotonin receptors. As such, ketamine possesses many attractive features for an intravenous agent, including its sympathomimetic effects producing increased myocardial contractility and systemic vascular resistance, as well as bronchodilator, analgesic, and antidepressant effects [43, 44]. There is much controversy surrounding the effects of ketamine on pulmonary pressures, as early studies investi-gating the drug's cardiovascular effects demonstrated significant increases in both pulmonary artery pressures and pulmonary vascular resistance [45, 46]. As such, the prevailing opinion was that ketamine should be avoided in patients with pulmonary hypertension. However, these early studies did not control for hypercarbia or hypoxia, two key triggers for pulmonary vasoconstriction [47]. More recently, human and animal studies have demonstrated that the use of ketamine, when controlling for ventilation, oxygenation, and acid-base status, does not increase pulmonary vascular resistance [48], is safe when used in patients with pulmonary hypertension [49], and may produce pulmonary vasodilation [50]. Of note, at the authors' institution, ketamine is routinely used in patients with significant pulmonary hypertension and right ventricular dysfunction presenting for cardiac, thoracic, and lung transplantation procedures.

Benzodiazepines and opioids are often used in conjunction with intravenous induction agents and produce minimal hemodynamic effects beyond their attenuation of sympathetic tone [7].

Volatile Anesthetics

Modern volatile anesthetics are commonly used to maintain general anesthesia intraoperatively. While much of the literature surrounding the cardiovascular effects of volatile anesthetics (specifically desflurane, isoflurane, and sevoflurane) has focused on their impact on left ventricular function, there is some suggestion that volatile agents produce significant effects on right ventricular performance as well. Animal studies have shown that sevoflurane, isoflurane, and desflurane all produce depression of right ventricular contractility, with sevoflurane effects being quite significant [51–53]. Furthermore, sevoflurane appears to produce greater reductions in systemic vascular resistance, without altering pulmonary vascular resistance [53]. This creates an unfavorable pulmonary-to-systemic pressure ratio relative to desflurane, in which systemic vascular resistance tends to be maintained with only a small increase in pulmonary pressures [51].

Vasopressor Agents

Due to the importance of preserved systemic pressures in maintaining right ventricular perfusion, vasopressor agents are useful in the intraoperative management of patients with pulmonary hypertension. As previously mentioned, the maintenance of a high ratio of systemic pressures to pulmonary pressures is important in avoiding deterioration in hemodynamics. Commonly used vasopressor agents, including phenylephrine, norepinephrine, and vasopressin have all been shown to exert different effects on hemodynamic parameters, including systemic and pulmonary pressures.

An early animal model demonstrated that commonly used agents, including phenylephrine, norepinephrine, and epinephrine, all increased systemic and pulmonary pressures to varying degrees while largely preserving pulmonary vascular

resistance [54]. Norepinephrine, in addition to its vasoconstricting effects, has β-1 receptor-mediated inotropic effects, which appear to improve right ventricular-pulmonary arterial coupling while maintaining cardiac output and right ventricular performance [55]. Animal models have also demonstrated that in doses less than 0.5 ug/kg/min, norepinephrine has minimal effects on pulmonary vascular resistance [56]. In contrast, phenylephrine has been shown to exert negative effects on right ventricular function in pulmonary hypertension patients by increasing pulmonary vascular resistance [57].

Perioperatively, in patients with pulmonary hypertension presenting for cardiac surgery, both norepinephrine and phenylephrine were shown to increase systemic and pulmonary pressures, however with distinct differences in hemodynamic parameters. Norepinephrine use resulted in a reduction of pulmonary arterial pressure to systemic blood pressure ratio without reducing cardiac index. Conversely, use of phenylephrine resulted in preservation of the pulmonary arterial pressure to systemic blood pressure ratio while reducing cardiac index [139]. These results suggest that norepinephrine is preferable to phenylephrine in the treatment of hypotension in pulmonary hypertension patients.

The effect of vasopressin on pulmonary arterial pressure has been subject to significant debate. In experimental animal models, vasopressin has been demonstrated to result in both pulmonary vasoconstriction [58] and pulmonary vasodilation [59, 60], leading to significant confusion. The absence of vasopressin receptors in human pulmonary vasculature has been widely posited, and recently, an experimental model using human radial and pulmonary arteries has demonstrated that while vasopressin exhibits a potent vasoconstricting effect in radial vessels, it had no effect on pulmonary vascular tone [61]. Subsequent to this finding, numerous publications have demonstrated consistent improvement in systemic blood pressures with minimal effect on pulmonary arterial pressures in hypotensive patients with pulmonary hypertension that are treated with vasopressin [62, 63]. These properties make vasopressin another valuable agent in the management of hypotension in pulmonary hypertension patients.

Vasodilator Agents

In addition to the use of agents to maintain systemic blood pressure intraoperatively, the use of vasodilating agents in order to decrease pulmonary vascular resistance has also garnered significant interest, particularly agents such as inhaled nitric oxide (iNO), milrinone, and prostaglandins.

iNO had garnered significant interest in the areas of acute respiratory distress syndrome (ARDS), heart and lung transplantation, and right ventricular failure, with mixed success [64–66]. Mechanistically, iNO is delivered noninvasively, or through a ventilator circuit, and is directed toward preferentially ventilated alveoli. Through its vasodilatory effects, iNO theoretically improves alveolar gas exchange and reduces pulmonary vascular resistance without resulting in systemic hypotension – all desirable in pulmonary hypertension. Clinically, dose ranges of 10–40 ppm are typically administered [67]. In the setting of right heart failure due to pulmonary hypertension, the use of iNO has been mixed and varies from patient to patient, as well as clinical scenario [68, 69]. One study [70] has examined the use of iNO (40 ppm) in thoracic surgery patients during one-lung ventilation and demonstrated that improvements in pulmonary vascular resistance and hypoxia during one-lung ventilation were only seen in patients with preexisting pulmonary hypertension. Unfortunately, due to the significant cost, as well as the advent of other alternative pulmonary vasodilators, intraoperative use of iNO has limited usage. However, given its mechanism of action, as well as the potential benefits during one-lung ventilation, iNO should be given consideration during the management of the patient with pulmonary hypertension presenting to the operating room.

Milrinone is a phosphodiesterase-3 inhibitor with both inotropic and vasodilatory effects when administered intravenously. Due to its effect of reducing both pulmonary and systemic vascular resistances, intravenous milrinone has limited effectiveness in right heart dysfunction related solely to pulmonary hypertension and often requires the concomitant administration of a vasopressor to counter the resulting hypotension. However, milrinone has demonstrated usefulness in patients with biventricular failure in the setting of pulmonary hypertension [71]. Administration of milrinone for pulmonary vasodilation in an inhaled form has gained significant interest recently, particularly in cardiac surgery. In patients with pulmonary hypertension presenting for cardiac surgery involving cardiopulmonary bypass, administration of inhaled milrinone (5 mg) prior to bypass was associated with reductions in pulmonary arterial pressures, enhancement of cardiac output, and minimal effect on mean arterial pressures [72, 73]. Unfortunately, there were no significant improvements in terms of intraoperative or postoperative complications (including right ventricular failure) in patients receiving inhaled milrinone. In addition, the combination of inhaled milrinone and inhaled prostacyclin appears to have an additive effect on pulmonary vasodilation [74]. Presently, there are no studies investigating the use of inhaled milrinone in the thoracic surgery population; however, given the favorable hemodynamics observed in the cardiac surgery population, it presents a potentially attractive option for pulmonary resection surgeries.

As previously discussed, prostanoids have an important role in the management of pulmonary arterial hypertension and are available in intravenous and inhaled formulations that can be used intraoperatively. Animal models for one-lung ventilation have demonstrated that both aerosolized and intravenous administration of prostacyclin (PGI_2)

reduce pulmonary arterial pressures [75]. While intravenous infusion of PGI_2 resulted in notable reduction in systemic vascular resistance, aerosolized PGI_2 produced selective pulmonary vasodilation. Similarly, intravenous prostaglandin E_1, a short-acting prostaglandin with pulmonary metabolism, administration during one-lung ventilation of pigs produced reductions in pulmonary vascular resistance and pulmonary arterial pressures but failed to demonstrate selective pulmonary vasodilation [76]. In the intraoperative setting, inhaled prostacyclin has been used in cardiac surgery patients with pulmonary hypertension with significant effect in terms of reducing pulmonary arterial pressures with minimal alterations in systemic blood pressure [77, 78]. Inhaled prostacyclin has also been used in the management of pulmonary hypertension during lung transplantation [79], as well as hypoxemia during one-lung ventilation for video-assisted thoracoscopic surgery in a patient without pulmonary hypertension [80]. As previously mentioned, while the use of prostanoids has been shown to significantly reduce pulmonary pressures in pulmonary hypertension patients, there is considerable uncertainty with respect to their effect on platelet function and bleeding risk, which needs to be considered in the intraoperative setting.

Analgesia

Analgesic strategies for pulmonary resection surgeries are typically determined based on the type of incision (thoracotomy vs video-assisted thoracoscopic surgery (VATS)) as well as patient-specific considerations, including decreased pulmonary reserve or a history of chronic pain or opioid use. At the authors' institution, analgesia for surgeries done using VATS are managed postoperatively with a combination of intercostal nerve blocks administered by the surgeon prior to chest closure and intravenous patient-controlled analgesia (PCA). In patients undergoing a thoracotomy without any contraindications, our practice is to provide patient-controlled epidural analgesia using a thoracic epidural placed prior to the induction of anesthesia.

Epidural analgesia carries a number of benefits, including enhanced analgesia compared to intravenous PCA [81–83]. Furthermore, it has been established that the use of epidural analgesia for major surgery, including thoracic surgery, is associated with reduced cardiovascular and pulmonary complications [84], as well as overall mortality [85]. Also of importance, the use of a thoracic epidural does not impact oxygenation during one-lung ventilation [86]. The beneficial effects on cardiorespiratory morbidity may be particularly important for high-risk patients such as those with pulmonary hypertension presenting for thoracic surgery. However, the relationship between the

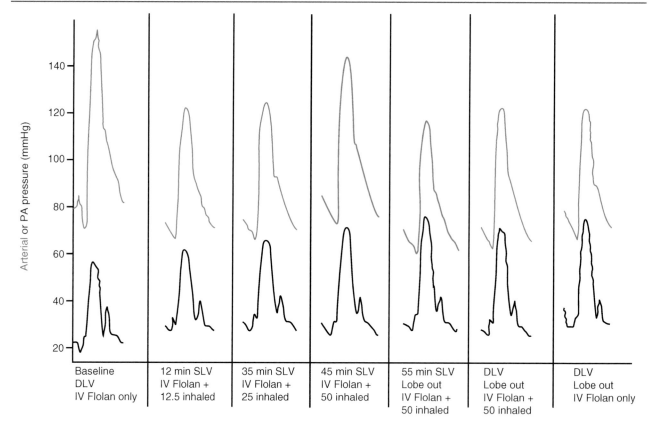

Fig. 34.3 Representative tracings of systemic and pulmonary arterial pressures during lung lobectomy in a patient with preexisting PAH. Representative simultaneous tracings of systemic arterial and pulmonary arterial (PA) pressures during lung lobectomy in a patient with preexisting PAH who was receiving intravenous (IV) Flolan (epoprostenol) preoperatively. With the transition from double-lung ventilation (DLV) to single-lung ventilation (SLV), the IV Flolan dose was decreased and inhaled Flolan initiated in order to maximize vascular dilation of the ventilated lung and potentially lessen the deleterious effects of systemic Flolan on hypoxic pulmonary vasoconstriction. Following lung resection and resumption of the preoperative Flolan dose, PA pressure remained elevated relative to baseline. (Reprinted from McGlothlin et al. [97] with permission from Elsevier)

Use of Extracorporeal Support for Pulmonary Resection (See Also Chap. 27)

There is growing use of extracorporeal life support, specifically extracorporeal membrane oxygenation (ECMO) in a variety of settings, including ARDS, cardiac failure, and transplantation. The use of extracorporeal support, such as ECMO or full cardiopulmonary bypass, during pulmonary resection surgery has been described in the literature, predominantly in cases involving large masses with significant cardiorespiratory compromise or procedures requiring tracheal or carina resection [120–123]. In patients with pulmonary hypertension, use of venoarterial ECMO allows for optimal gas exchange, as well as maintenance of cardiac output and coronary perfusion without increasing pulmonary pressures. Extracorporeal life support is presently limited to specialized centers and requires anticoagulation during its use which increases the risk for bleeding. Its use in pulmonary resection in the patient with pulmonary hypertension is presently not well-described in the literature and, however, presents an option requiring further investigation.

Postoperative Management

Postoperatively, patients presenting for pulmonary resection with significant pulmonary hypertension warrant admission to a unit with a higher-than-usual level of monitoring and care. Because of the significant cardiorespiratory compromise and the increased risk of postoperative complications, pulmonary hypertension patients require a postoperative setting capable of frequent, if not continuous, monitoring by skilled and experienced nursing care. Typically, this is an intensive care unit or a step-down unit with the ability to manage patients with invasive cardiovascular monitoring (such as invasive blood pressure monitoring, central venous pressure monitoring, or pulmonary artery catheters), patients who may require postoperative mechanical ventilation, and patients who require pharmacologic support with vasopressors, inotropes, or pulmonary vasodilators [7, 97]. It has been advocated that this should be a standard of care, irrespective of the intraoperative course [124].

In non-cardiac surgery, respiratory failure and right ventricular failure have been identified as the most common contributors to early (less than 30 days) postoperative mortality among patients with pulmonary hypertension [6]. With respect to reducing the risk of pulmonary complications that may contribute to respiratory failure, a number of strategies have been shown to be of benefit, including chest physiotherapy, continuous positive airway pressure, and incentive spirometry. In upper abdominal and thoracic surgery, use of these techniques may reduce pulmonary complications by half [125–127]. Chest physiotherapy and continuous positive airway pressure may not be widely available and may pose some safety concerns in the frail or borderline patient with pulmonary hypertension. Incentive spirometry is an easy and inexpensive way of encouraging deep breathing and lung expansion [128]. As previously mentioned, excessive fluid administration can increase the risk of postoperative pulmonary and cardiac complications, and the rational fluid management strategy used intraoperatively should be continued in the postoperative period as well.

Right ventricular failure is a major cause of postoperative mortality in pulmonary hypertension patients, with one study citing it as a contributor to mortality in 50% of cases [6]. The potential causes of right ventricular failure are numerous and, in the immediate postoperative period, include pulmonary embolism, infection, bleeding/anemia, arrhythmias, and acute worsening of pulmonary hypertension. Among these causes, pulmonary embolism and infection should be protected against with appropriate intra- and postoperative prophylaxis. Ongoing bleeding and resulting anemia should be identified and addressed immediately, as hypovolemia and anemia both increase myocardial (specifically right ventricular) work and may be poorly tolerated.

Postoperative arrhythmias, specifically atrial tachyarrhythmias, are common after thoracic surgery and occur most frequently on postoperative days 2 and 3 [129]. Atrial fibrillation and flutter are both associated with right ventricular failure, clinical deterioration, and death and require immediate management [130]. In unstable patients, electrical cardioversion is the treatment of choice and should not be delayed [129, 130]. In terms of pharmacologic management of the stable patient with an atrial tachyarrhythmia, beta-blockers and calcium channel blockers should be used with caution, as their potential for reducing myocardial contractility and vasodilating effects may be poorly tolerated in pulmonary hypertension patients [97, 131]. Instead, amiodarone and/or digoxin may be considered for rhythm and/or rate control in these cases. Intravenous magnesium is another option commonly recommended in the literature for both treatment and prophylaxis of atrial arrhythmias post-thoracic surgery [129, 132], and at the authors' institution, lung resection patients are typically given 2.5–5 g of intravenous magnesium sulfate by slow infusion intraoperatively for arrhythmia prophylaxis. Care should be exercised, however, as rapid administration of magnesium can produce significant hypotension.

Worsening pulmonary hypertension is another potential cause of right ventricular failure post-lung resection and should be closely monitored for postoperatively. There are multiple mechanisms for worsening pulmonary pressures including increased right ventricular afterload following resection of a significant amount of lung parenchyma. This has been observed post-pneumonectomy [15, 16] but less so after subtotal lung resections [18]. Precipitants of pulmonary vasoconstriction, including acidosis, hypercarbia, hypoxia, hypothermia, and pain, should also be avoided in the postoperative period [133]. Patients who were previously managed on pulmonary vasodilators preoperatively should resume their pulmonary hypertension treatment as early as possible postoperatively to prevent rebound pulmonary hypertension. In patients who required pulmonary vasodilators intraoperatively, this may need to be continued postoperatively for a period of time and carefully weaned. Oral PDE-5 inhibitors have been shown to be very useful in weaning patients from iNO and preventing rebound pulmonary hypertension [134–137].

Finally, optimal pain management is important postoperatively. Inadequate pain control can exacerbate pulmonary hypertension [124, 138]. As previously discussed, thoracic epidurals, paravertebral blocks, and systemic opioids are all commonly used strategies, with thoracic epidurals demonstrating potential reduction in pulmonary complications and mortality [84, 85]. Admission to a postoperative area with higher monitoring capabilities is also important for initial pain management, as all analgesic strategies carry significant potential risk in pulmonary hypertension patients. Specifically, thoracic epidurals and paravertebral blocks may produce significant hypotension requiring vasopressors to manage, and systemic opioids can produce hypoventilation leading to hypercarbia and hypoxia that should be identified and addressed quickly. Furthermore, analgesia post-pulmonary resection should be done under the guidance of an acute pain service.

Conclusion

The patient with pulmonary hypertension has historically presented a significant challenge perioperatively, with a high risk for morbidity and mortality often precluding surgery. Improvements in diagnosis and management of pulmonary hypertension, in general as well as within the operating room, have allowed for safe management of these patients during the pulmonary resection surgery. However, significant risk remains, and the thoracic anesthetist must be knowledgeable and vigilant with respect to the assessment and management of these patients. This includes an understanding of the various etiologies of pulmonary hypertension and their pharmacologic management, as well as the intraoperative strategies (monitoring, pharmacology, ventilation, etc.) that are available to assist with preservation of right heart function and minimization of increases in pulmonary pressures during one-lung ventilation. Furthermore, effective postoperative analgesia is highly important in these patients. While pulmonary resection in patients with pulmonary hypertension is feasible, it should be done in a center with experienced care providers and with appropriate postoperative monitoring facilities.

Clinical Case Discussion

A 68-year-old woman is scheduled to undergo pulmonary resection for a recently diagnosed lung cancer. She initially presented with a worsening cough and shortness of breath, prompting a chest X-ray by her primary care physician. A right-sided lung lesion was seen, leading to additional investigations. A CT scan and CT-guided biopsy revealed a 3 cm × 5 cm × 3 cm right lower lobe mass, with pathology-confirmed squamous cell carcinoma.

Her past medical history includes 40 pack-year smoking history – she has quit smoking since her diagnosis, a few weeks ago. Her other past medical history includes hypertension, hypercholesterolemia, mild gastroesophageal reflux disease, and osteoarthritis of the hips and knees. She has a long-standing history of NYHA 2–3 dyspnea, preceding her recent cancer diagnosis.

She has been referred to a thoracic surgeon for management and has been offered a right lower lobectomy by video-assisted thoracoscopic surgery, possibly open.

What preoperative investigations should be arranged for this patient?

1. Pulmonary function testing:
   (a) FEV$_1$ 70% predicted [ppoFEV$_1$ 50%]
   (b) FEV$_1$/FVC < 70%
   (c) DLCO 65% predicted [ppoDLCO 46%]
2. Six-minute walk test: 400 m walked, 80% predicted distance. Noted dyspnea during the testing, with desaturation events to as low as 88% on room air.
3. Arterial blood gas (on room air): pH 7.35, pCO$_2$ 48, pO$_2$ 70.
4. CT thorax: no significant bullous disease but evident diffuse centrilobular emphysema. The right lower lobe lesion in question is also seen.
5. Metastatic workup: no evidence of metastases.
6. ECG: sinus rhythm.
7. TTE: normal left ventricular size and function, with evidence of diastolic dysfunction. Mild right ventricular enlargement with low-normal function. There is mild tricuspid regurgitation with a right ventricular systolic pressure calculated at 55 mmHg. There are no other significant

valvulopathy. Her blood pressure during the TTE was 140/92.
8. V/Q study: demonstrates preferential perfusion to the left lung (60%) relative to the right lung (40%).
9. Right heart catheterization: see below.

The investigations above reveal several key pieces of information. Pulmonary function testing shows abnormal spirometry consistent with moderate COPD. The DLCO is also abnormal, consistent with a diagnosis of COPD. The predicted postoperative values for the proposed procedure remain acceptable to proceed, however. Her 6-min walk test is suggestive of reduced cardiopulmonary reserve and may warrant further investigations to assess this. Her room air arterial blood gas is consistent with her underlying diagnosis of COPD. Her imaging and ECG are within expected parameters.

The decision to request further cardiac testing (an echocardiogram) is reasonable, given her cardiac risk factors (smoking history, hypertension, hyperlipidemia) and limited exercise ability due to dyspnea (with a limited 6-min walk test performance). Noninvasive stress testing is likely appropriate/indicated as well. Her TTE result shows clear evidence of pulmonary hypertension (elevated RVSP) with secondary signs of pulmonary hypertension (RV enlargement and impaired systolic function). Given the absence of any history or testing results suggestive of an alternative diagnosis, the underlying cause of her elevated pulmonary pressures is likely to be COPD.

The decision of whether to pursue further invasive cardiac testing, specifically a right heart catheterization, is debatable. The TTE findings are highly suggestive of pulmonary hypertension, and right heart catheterization may not provide additional information that would influence decision-making. While not as accurate as with right heart catheterization, her pulmonary-to-systemic systolic pressure ratios based on TTE remain less than 0.5, which is also reassuring. Noninvasive stress testing may be a more appropriate direction for further testing at this point, with any abnormalities observed prompting left- and right heart catheterization.

A ventilation-perfusion study was done to assess differential lung perfusion and is useful to determine tolerance of one-lung ventilation intraoperatively. The preferential perfusion of the left lung in this case is reassuring, as the risk for hypoxia and rising pulmonary pressures intraoperatively is likely lower despite the expected need to perform one-lung ventilation of the left lung. This is not an absolute predictor, however.

How do you rationalize the information provided by the investigations above? Do you proceed with the case?

This patient presents with a lung malignancy for resection. Her preoperative testing is suggestive of moderate COPD and reduced exertional tolerance and cardiopulmonary reserve. Additionally, her echocardiogram shows clear evidence of pulmonary hypertension, likely related to her long-standing COPD. All of these findings are suggestive of an above-average risk for morbidity and mortality, based on the evidence in the literature concerning perioperative management of pulmonary hypertension patients [4–7].

However, recent evidence has shown that pulmonary resection in the setting of pulmonary hypertension (by TTE-based diagnosis) is not an absolute contraindication to surgery [14]. Given the presence of a single-lung lesion with no metastases, surgery presents a curative option for this patient. Additionally, the remainder of her workup would be considered acceptable for proceeding with surgery in the absence of pulmonary hypertension.

As such, proceeding with the proposed resection with caution is acceptable. A clear plan and discussion involving the patient and surgeon should be had prior to presenting to the operating room to discuss the elevated risk and the need for specialized intraoperative and postoperative monitoring. There should be a low threshold to abort the procedure should issues with pulmonary hypertension arise intraoperatively despite the adequate precautions and management.

What intraoperative monitoring should be available for this procedure?

Routine noninvasive monitors, including 5-lead ECG, pulse oximetry, capnography, temperature, and invasive and noninvasive blood pressure monitoring, are required for any pulmonary resection procedure. Invasive blood pressure monitoring is of critical importance in the patient with pulmonary hypertension, as it allows for accurate beat-to-beat blood pressure monitoring and facilitates arterial blood gas sampling for assessment of oxygenation and ventilation. Central venous access is recommended for this procedure, as management of hemodynamics with vasoactive substances will likely be required.

Pulmonary artery pressures should be monitored during this procedure, given the need to promptly address any acute rises in pulmonary pressures. The most common options for assessment of pulmonary pressures (and right heart function) are a pulmonary artery catheter or TEE. The decision of which option to employ, if not both, should be based on availability as well as potential risks and benefits as they pertain to this patient.

Typically, PACs are readily available and allow for continuous measurement of pulmonary pressures. In conjunction with invasive blood pressure monitoring, the pulmonary-to-systemic pressure ratio can be easily determined and optimally maintained. This patient has no contraindications to a PAC. However, interpretation of PAC data can be challenging. Furthermore, PACs do not provide direct monitoring of right ventricular functioning. Increases in PA pressures are undesirable but may be tolerated by a well-compensated right ventricle. Conversely, reductions in PA

pressures may represent improvement in pulmonary vascular resistance or impending right ventricular failure and need to be interepreted in conjunction with other available parameters such as CVP and systemic blood pressure.

The availability of intraoperative TEE is increasing, but remains a significant barrier to its usage in non-cardiac surgery. TEE allows for monitoring of right ventricular function intraoperatively, which would be beneficial in this scenario, as preexisting right ventricular enlargement and impairment are present. Furthermore, TEE allows for assessment of global cardiac function. Potential limitations of TEE in this scenario, in addition to availability, include limited ability to assess pulmonary pressures directly, as RVSPs can be calculated, but not on a continuous basis. Furthermore, assessment of right ventricular function requires multiple TEE views, again making timely continuous monitoring difficult. Additionally, assessment of TEE views in the lateral position (as required for a thoracotomy or VATS) may be technically challenging.

Should an epidural be placed in this patient?

Given that the proposed pulmonary resection is planned as a VATS procedure, an epidural would typically not be offered to this patient. However, consideration may be given to an epidural (or paravertebral catheter) given the above-average risk for complications postoperatively associated with this patient. Epidurals provide superior analgesia compared to intravenous PCA and have been associated with reduced pulmonary complications and mortality [84, 85]. While this patient has acceptable predicted postoperative FEV_1 and DLCO, optimization of her pulmonary mechanics remains necessary given her pulmonary hypertension. The potential benefits related to an epidural need to be weighed against the potential for complications related to an epidural, as well as the potential for hypotension and possible cardiac dysfunction secondary to neuraxial blockade.

The decision to offer an epidural should also take into consideration the risks and benefits discussed above, as well as the risk for conversion to a thoracotomy (requiring a discussion with the surgeon), and patient preferences.

What strategies should be employed to prevent or manage rises in pulmonary artery pressures intraoperatively?

Rises in pulmonary artery pressures should be identified and dealt with immediately. Optimization of ventilation parameters, hemodynamics, and pharmacologic interventions should all be considered for this patient.

Transition from ventilation with two lungs to one-lung ventilation is a period associated with many potential triggers for worsening pulmonary artery pressures, specifically hypoxia and hypercarbia. For this patient, a lung-protective strategy employing higher F_iO_2 should be used to optimize ventilation of the left lung. To minimize the risk of hypoxia and avoid significant hypercarbia, the F_iO_2 should be maintained at 1.0 when initiating OLV. A tidal volume of 4–6 mL/kg should be maintained, with the respiratory rate adjusted to target a $P_aCO_2 < 30$–40 mmHg. Normocapnia (or slight hypocapnia) is ideal; however, aggressive ventilation (higher tidal volumes or higher respiratory rates) can produce higher peak airway pressures leading to worsening pulmonary vascular resistance. The P_aCO_2 can be set to maintain a pH of greater than 7.2, provided there is no significant coexisting metabolic acidosis. The use of PEEP should be titrated carefully (0–10 cmH$_2$O), to maintain peak airway pressures below 30–35 cmH$_2$O, and may not be necessary in this patient, as obstructive lung disease tends to create intrinsic PEEP.

Maintenance of the pulmonary-to-systemic systolic pressure ratio at its baseline is also important intraoperatively, and higher ratios are associated with worse outcomes [6]. This can be achieved through augmentation of the systemic systolic pressure or by reducing pulmonary vascular resistance. Norepinephrine and vasopressin are the ideal vasopressors of choice to increase systemic vascular resistance and maintain right ventricular perfusion and cardiac output. Either agent should be started early should systemic pressure begin to drop with initiation of OLV. The use of pulmonary vasodilators should also be considered if pulmonary pressures increase significantly during the case. Consideration should be given to initiating iNO or epoprostenol IV to address this. iNO may be preferred, as its pulmonary selectivity means it can be initiated before OLV has started, and is unlikely to produce systemic vasodilation. iNO should be titrated to a maximum dose of 40 ppm before a second agent (such as epoprostenol IV) is added.

The threshold of concern for the absolute PA pressure, or pulmonary-to-systemic pressure ratio, is not well-defined in the literature but should take into account the patient's baseline ratio, in this case less than 0.5, and the right ventricular response to increased PA pressures. Continuous PA pressure monitoring using a PAC allows for the former, while TEE is more advantageous to assess the latter. For this patient, two scenarios should prompt discussion regarding aborting the case. First, a continually rising pulmonary-to-systemic ratio beyond 0.5 despite the use of systemic vasopressors and pulmonary vasodilators is highly concerning, given her preoperative baseline. Second, any PA pressure producing signs of RV dysfunction (based on TEE imaging or reduced PA pressures, rising CVP, and hypotension) that does not respond to vasopressors or pulmonary vasodilation is also a cause for alarm. At this point, two-lung ventilation should be restored (if possible), and a discussion about whether to proceed should occur.

The impact of surgical approach for the proposed pulmonary resection should also be considered. There is no evidence in the literature examining outcomes of VATS vs thoracotomy in pulmonary hypertension patients; however, both have been done successfully. A VATS approach is advantageous, since it produces less postoperative pain and, however, is more dependent on effective OLV and may be associated with longer operative time. A thoracotomy for this patient would necessitate a well-functioning epidural for postoperative pain but may allow for better surgical exposure and shorter periods of OLV. Improved surgical exposure through a thoracotomy also allows for advanced ventilation techniques (selective lobar ventilation, application of CPAP) that may be helpful for ventilation. For this patient, a discussion with the surgeon regarding surgical approach should occur preoperatively. It may be reasonable to attempt the procedure with VATS initially while having a low threshold to convert to an open thoracotomy should the surgeon believe this would expedite the surgery.

Where should this patient be admitted to postoperatively?

This patient requires admission to a unit with increased monitoring postoperatively, irrespective of intraoperative course. This should be a step-down unit at the very least; however, the need for intraoperative vasopressor or pulmonary vasodilator use should prompt admission to an intensive care unit.

References

1. Hoeper MM, Bogaard HJ, Condliffe R, Frantz R, Khanna D, Kurzyna M, et al. Definitions and diagnosis of pulmonary hypertension. J Am Coll Cardiol Elsevier Inc. 2013;62(S):D42–50.
2. Simonneau G, Gatzoulis MA, Adatia I, Celermajer D, Denton C, Ghofrani A, et al. Updated clinical classification of pulmonary hypertension. J Am Coll Cardiol. Elsevier Inc. 2013;62(S):D34–41.
3. Hoeper MM, Humbert M, Souza R, Idrees M, Kawut SM, Sliwa-Hahnle K, et al. A global view of pulmonary hypertension. Lancet Respir Med Elsevier Ltd. 2016;4(4):306–22.
4. Kaw R, Pasupuleti V, Deshpande A, Hamieh T, Walker E, Minai OA. Pulmonary hypertension: an important predictor of outcomes in patients undergoing non-cardiac surgery. Respir Med Elsevier Ltd. 2011;105(4):619–24.
5. Lai HC, Lai HC, Wang KY, Lee WL, Ting CT, Liu TJ. Severe pulmonary hypertension complicates postoperative outcome of non-cardiac surgery. Br J Anaesth. 2007;99(2):184–90.
6. Ramakrishna G, Sprung J, Ravi BS, Chandrasekaran K, MD MG. Impact of pulmonary hypertension on the outcomes of noncardiac surgery. J Am Coll Cardiol. Elsevier Masson SAS. 2005;45(10):1691–9.
7. Pilkington SA, Taboada D, Martinez G. Pulmonary hypertension and its management in patients undergoing non-cardiac surgery. Anaesthesia. 2014;70(1):56–70.
8. Nicod P, Moser KM. Primary pulmonary hypertension. The risk and benefit of lung biopsy. Circulation. 1989;80(5):1486–8.
9. Kreider ME, Hansen-Flaschen J, Ahmad NN, Rossman MD, Kaiser LR, Kucharczuk JC, et al. Complications of video-assisted thoracoscopic lung biopsy in patients with interstitial lung disease. Ann Thorac Surg. 2007;83(3):1140–4.
10. Hasegawa S, Isowa N, Bando T, Wada H. The inadvisability of thoracoscopic lung biopsy on patients with pulmonary hypertension. CHEST The American College of Chest Physicians. 2016;122(3):1067–8.
11. Heller AR. A fine balance--one-lung ventilation in a patient with Eisenmenger syndrome. Br J Anaesth. 2004;92(4):587–90.

12. Cheng DC, Edelist G. Isoflurane and primary pulmonary hypertension. Anaesthesia. 1988;43(1):22–4.
13. Ichinokawa M, Hida Y, Kaga K, Kawada M, Niizeki H, Kondo S. A case of primary pulmonary hypertension with pulmonary tumor. Ann Thorac Cardiovasc Surg. 2010;16(4):270–2.
14. Wei B, D'Amico T, Samad Z, Hasan R, Berry MF. The impact of pulmonary hypertension on morbidity and mortality following major lung resection. Eur J Cardiothorac Surg. 2014;45(6):1028–33.
15. Ota T, Okada M, Matsuda H, Okada K, Ishii N. Right ventricular dysfunction after major pulmonary resection. J Thorac Cardiovasc Surg. 1994;108(3):503–11.
16. Kowalewski J, Brocki M, Dryjański T, Kaproń K, Barcikowski S. Right ventricular morphology and function after pulmonary resection. Eur J Cardiothorac Surg. 1999;15(4):444–8.
17. Venuta F, Sciomer S, Andreetti C, Anile M, De Giacomo T, Rolla M, et al. Long-term Doppler echocardiographic evaluation of the right heart after major lung resections. Eur J Cardiothorac Surg. 2007;32(5):787–90.
18. Pedoto A, Amar D. Right heart function in thoracic surgery: role of echocardiography. Curr Opin Anaesthesiol. 2009;22(1):44–9.
19. Barst RJ, McGoon M, Torbicki A, Sitbon O, Krowka MJ, Olschewski H, et al. Diagnosis and differential assessment of pulmonary arterial hypertension. J Am Coll Cardiol. Elsevier Masson SAS. 2004;43(12):S40–7.
20. McLaughlin VV. Survival in primary pulmonary hypertension: the impact of epoprostenol therapy. Circulation. 2002;106(12):1477–82.
21. Fisher MR, Forfia PR, Chamera E, Housten-Harris T, Champion HC, Girgis RE, et al. Accuracy of Doppler echocardiography in the hemodynamic assessment of pulmonary hypertension. Am J Respir Crit Care Med. 2009;179(7):615–21.
22. Bossone E, D'Andrea A, D'Alto M, Citro R, Argiento P, Ferrara F, et al. Echocardiography in pulmonary arterial hypertension: from diagnosis to prognosis. J Am Soc Echocardiogr. Elsevier Inc. 2013;26(1):1–14.
23. Luscher TF, Barton M. Endothelins and endothelin receptor antagonists : therapeutic considerations for a novel class of cardiovascular drugs. Circulation. 2000;102(19):2434–40.
24. Frumkin LR. The pharmacological treatment of pulmonary arterial hypertension. Pharmacol Rev. 2012;64(3):583–620.
25. Montani D, Gunther S, Dorfmüller P, FDR P, Girerd B, Garcia G, et al. Pulmonary arterial hypertension. Orphanet J Rare Dis. 2013;8(1):1–1.
26. Badesch DB, McLaughlin VV, Delcroix M, Vizza C, Olschewski H, Sitbon O, et al. Prostanoid therapy for pulmonary arterial hypertension. J Am Coll Cardiol Elsevier Masson SAS. 2004;43(12):S56–61.
27. LeVarge B. Prostanoid therapies in the management of pulmonary arterial hypertension. TCRM. 2015;11:535–13.
28. Wilkins MR, Wharton J, Grimminger F, Ghofrani HA. Phosphodiesterase inhibitors for the treatment of pulmonary hypertension. Eur Respir J. 2008;32(1):198–209.
29. Wilcox SR, Kabrhel C, Channick RN. Pulmonary hypertension and right ventricular failure in emergency medicine. Ann Emerg Med. 2015;66(6):619–28.
30. Polanczyk CA, Rohde LE, Goldman L, Cook EF, Thomas EJ, Marcantonio ER, et al. Right heart catheterization and cardiac complications in patients undergoing noncardiac surgery: an observational study. JAMA. 2001;286(3):309–14.
31. Sandham JD, Hull RD, Brant RF, Knox L, Pineo GF, Doig CJ, et al. A randomized, controlled trial of the use of pulmonary-artery catheters in high-risk surgical patients. N Engl J Med. 2003;348(1):5–14.
32. Marik PE. Obituary: pulmonary artery catheter 1970 to 2013. Ann Intensive Care. 2013;3(1):38.
33. Kalra A, Heitner S, Topalian S. Iatrogenic pulmonary artery rupture during swan-Ganz catheter placement--a novel therapeutic approach. Catheter Cardiovasc Interv. 2013;81(1):57–9.
34. Kolev N, Brase R, Swanevelder J, Oppizzi M, Riesgo MJ, van der Maaten JM, et al. The influence of transoesophageal echocardiography on intra-operative decision making. A European multicentre study. European perioperative TOE research group. Anaesthesia. 1998;53(8):767–73.
35. Hofer CK, Zollinger A, Rak M, Matter-Ensner S, Klaghofer R, Pasch T, et al. Therapeutic impact of intra-operative transoesophageal echocardiography during noncardiac surgery. Anaesthesia. 2004;59(1):3–9.
36. American Society of Anesthesiologists and Society of Cardiovascular Anesthesiologists Task Force on Transesophageal Echocardiography. Practice guidelines for perioperative transesophageal echocardiography. An updated report by the American Society of Anesthesiologists and the Society of Cardiovascular Anesthesiologists Task Force on transesophageal echocardiography. Anesthesiology. 2010;112:1084–96.
37. Ternacle J, Berry M, Cognet T, Kloeckner M, Damy T, Monin JL, et al. Prognostic value of right ventricular two-dimensional global strain in patients referred for cardiac surgery. J Am Soc Echocardiogr Elsevier Inc. 2013;26(7):721–6.
38. Ostenfeld E, Flachskampf FA. Assessment of right ventricular volumes and ejection fraction by echocardiography: from geometric approximations to realistic shapes. Echo Res Pract. 2015;2(1):R1–R11.
39. Edanaga M, Nakayama M, Kanaya N, Tohse N, Namiki A. Propofol increases pulmonary vascular resistance during alpha-adrenoreceptor activation in normal and monocrotaline-induced pulmonary hypertensive rats. Anesth Analg. 2007;104(1):112–8.
40. Kondo U, Kim SO, Nakayama M, Murray PA. Pulmonary vascular effects of propofol at baseline, during elevated vasomotor tone, and in response to sympathetic alpha- and beta-adrenoreceptor activation. Anesthesiology. 2001;94(5):815–23.
41. Ouédraogo N, Mounkaïla B, Crevel H, Marthan R, Roux E. Effect of propofol and etomidate on normoxic and chronically hypoxic pulmonary artery. BMC Anesthesiol. 2006 Mar;6(1):715–0.
42. Komatsu R, You J, Mascha EJ, Sessler DI, Kasuya Y, Turan A. Anesthetic induction with etomidate, rather than propofol, is associated with increased 30-day mortality and cardiovascular morbidity after noncardiac surgery. Anesth Analg. 2013;117(6):1329–37.
43. Kohrs R, Durieux ME. Ketamine: teaching an old drug new tricks. Anesth Analg. 1998;87(5):1186–93.
44. Iadarola ND, Niciu MJ, Richards EM, Vande Voort JL, Ballard ED, Lundin NB, et al. Ketamine and other N-methyl-D-aspartate receptor antagonists in the treatment of depression: a perspective review. Ther Adv Chronic Dis. 2015;6(3):97–114.
45. Gooding JM, Dimick AR, Tavakoli M, Corssen G. A physiologic analysis of cardiopulmonary responses to ketamine anesthesia in noncardiac patients. Anesth Analg. 1977;56(6):813–6.
46. Tweed WA, Minuck M, Mymin D. Circulatory responses to ketamine anesthesia. Anesthesiology. 1972;37(6):613–9.
47. Maxwell BG, Jackson E. Role of ketamine in the management of pulmonary hypertension and right ventricular failure. J Cardiothorac Vasc Anesth Elsevier Inc. 2012;26(3):e24–5.
48. Williams GD, Philip BM, Chu LF, Boltz MG, Kamra K, Terwey H, et al. Ketamine does not increase pulmonary vascular resistance in children with pulmonary hypertension undergoing sevoflurane anesthesia and spontaneous ventilation. Anesth Analg. 2007;105(6):1578–84.
49. Williams GD, MAAN H, Ramamoorthy C, Kamra K, BRATTON SL, BAIR E, et al. Perioperative complications in children with pulmonary hypertension undergoing general anesthesia with ketamine. Pediatr Anesth. 2010;20(1):28–37.
50. Kaye AD, Banister RE, Fox CJ, Ibrahim IN, Nossaman BD. Analysis of ketamine responses in the pulmonary vascular bed of the cat. Crit Care Med. 2000;28(4):1077–82.

51. Kerbaul F, Rondelet B, Motte S, Fesler P, Hubloue I, Ewalenko P, et al. Isoflurane and desflurane impair right ventricular-pulmonary arterial coupling in dogs. Anesthesiology. 2004;101(6):1357–62.

52. Kerbaul F, Bellezza M, Mekkaoui C, Feier H, Guidon C, Gouvernet J, et al. Sevoflurane alters right ventricular performance but not pulmonary vascular resistance in acutely instrumented anesthetized pigs. J Cardiothorac Vasc Anesth. 2006;20(2):209–16.

53. Blaudszun G, Morel DR. Superiority of desflurane over sevoflurane and isoflurane in the presence of pressure-overload right ventricle hypertrophy in rats. Anesthesiology. 2012;117(5):1051–61.

54. Pearl RG, Maze M, Rosenthal MH. Pulmonary and systemic hemodynamic effects of central venous and left atrial sympathomimetic drug administration in the dog. J Cardiothorac Anesth. 1987;1(1):29–35.

55. Price LC, Wort SJ, Finney SJ, Marino PS, Brett SJ. Pulmonary vascular and right ventricular dysfunction in adult critical care: current and emerging options for management: a systematic literature review. Crit Care BioMed Central. 2010;14(5):R169.

56. Kerbaul F, Rondelet B, Motte S, Fesler P, Hubloue I, Ewalenko P, et al. Effects of norepinephrine and dobutamine on pressure load-induced right ventricular failure. Crit Care Med. 2004;32(4):1035–40.

57. Rich S, Gubin S, Hart K. The effects of phenylephrine on right ventricular performance in patients with pulmonary hypertension. Chest J. 1990;98(5):1102–6.

58. Leather HA, Segers P, Berends N, Vandermeersch E, Wouters PF. Effects of vasopressin on right ventricular function in an experimental model of acute pulmonary hypertension. Crit Care Med. 2002;30(11):2548–52.

59. Eichinger MR, Walker BR. Enhanced pulmonary arterial dilation to arginine vasopressin in chronically hypoxic rats. Am J Phys. 1994;267(6 Pt 2):H2413–9.

60. Walker BR, Haynes J, Wang HL, Voelkel NF. Vasopressin-induced pulmonary vasodilation in rats. Am J Phys. 1989;257(2 Pt 2):H415–22.

61. Currigan DA, Hughes RJA, Wright CE, Angus JA, Soeding PF. Vasoconstrictor responses to vasopressor agents in human pulmonary and radial arteries: an in vitro study. Anesthesiology. 2014;121(5):930–6.

62. Mizota T, Fujiwara K, Hamada M, Matsukawa S, Segawa H. Effect of arginine vasopressin on systemic and pulmonary arterial pressure in a patient with pulmonary hypertension secondary to pulmonary emphysema: a case report. JA Clinical Reports. 2017;3(1):1–4.

63. Tayama E, Ueda T, Shojima T, Akasu K, Oda T, Fukunaga S, et al. Arginine vasopressin is an ideal drug after cardiac surgery for the management of low systemic vascular resistant hypotension concomitant with pulmonary hypertension. Interact Cardiovasc Thorac Surg. 2007;6(6):715–9.

64. Creagh-Brown BC, Griffiths MJD, Evans TW. Bench-to-bedside review: inhaled nitric oxide therapy in adults. Crit Care. 2009;13(3):221.

65. Adhikari NKJ, Dellinger RP, Lundin S, Payen D, Vallet B, Gerlach H, et al. Inhaled nitric oxide does not reduce mortality in patients with acute respiratory distress syndrome regardless of severity: systematic review and meta-analysis. Crit Care Med. 2014;42(2):404–12.

66. Meade MO, Granton JT, Matte-Martyn A, McRae K, Weaver B, Cripps P, et al. A randomized trial of inhaled nitric oxide to prevent ischemia–reperfusion injury after lung transplantation. Am J Respir Crit Care Med. 2003;167(11):1483–9.

67. Sim J-Y. Nitric oxide and pulmonary hypertension. Korean J Anesthesiol. 2010;58(1):4–11.

68. Skhiri M, Hunt SA, Denault AY, Haddad F. Evidence-based management of right heart failure: a systematic review of an empiric field. Rev Esp Cardiol. 2010;63(4):451–71.

69. King R, Esmail M, Mahon S, Dingley J, Dwyer S. Use of nitric oxide for decompensated right ventricular failure and circulatory shock after cardiac arrest. Br J Anaesth. 2000;85(4):628–31.

70. Rocca GD, Passariello M, Coccia C, Costa MG, Di Marco P, Venuta F, et al. Inhaled nitric oxide administration during one-lung ventilation in patients undergoing thoracic surgery. J Cardiothorac Vasc Anesth. 2001;15(2):218–23.

71. Eichhorn EJ, Konstam MA, Weiland DS, Roberts DJ, Martin TT, Stransky NB, et al. Differential effects of milrinone and dobutamine on right ventricular preload, afterload and systolic performance in congestive heart failure secondary to ischemic or idiopathic dilated cardiomyopathy. Am J Cardiol. 1987;60(16):1329–33.

72. Laflamme M, Perrault LP, Carrier M, Elmi-Sarabi M, Fortier A, Denault AY. Preliminary experience with combined inhaled milrinone and prostacyclin in cardiac surgical patients with pulmonary hypertension. J Cardiothorac Vasc Anesth. 2015;29(1):38–45.

73. Denault AY, Bussières JS, Arellano R, Finegan B, Gavra P, Haddad F, et al. A multicentre randomized-controlled trial of inhaled milrinone in high-risk cardiac surgical patients. Can J Anaesth. 2016;63(10):1140–53.

74. Haraldsson Å, Kieler-Jensen N, Ricksten SE. The additive pulmonary vasodilatory effects of inhaled prostacyclin and inhaled milrinone in postcardiac surgical patients with pulmonary hypertension. Anesth Analg. 2001;93(6):1439–45. –tableofcontents.

75. Bund M, Henzler D, Walz R, Rossaint R, Piepenbrock S, Kuhlen R. Aerosolized and intravenous prostacyclin during one-lung ventilation. Hemodynamic and pulmonary effects. Anaesthesist Springer-Verlag. 2004;53(7):612–20.

76. Bund M, Henzler D, Walz R, Rossaint R, Piepenbrock S. Cardiopulmonary effects of intravenous prostaglandin E 1 during experimental one-lung ventilation. Thorac Cardiovasc Surg. 2006;54(5):341–7.

77. Haché M, Denault A, Bélisle S, Robitaille D, Couture P, Sheridan P, et al. Inhaled epoprostenol (prostacyclin) and pulmonary hypertension before cardiac surgery. J Thorac Cardiovasc Surg. 2003;125(3):642–9.

78. Jerath A, Srinivas C, Vegas A, Brister S. The successful management of severe protamine-induced pulmonary hypertension using inhaled prostacyclin. Anesth Analg. 2010;110(2):365–9.

79. Rocca Della G, Coccia C, Costa MG, Pompei L, Pietropaoli P. Inhaled prostacyclin during anaesthesia for lung transplantation. Eur J Anaesthesiol. 2000;17(Supplement 19):130.

80. Raghunathan K, Connelly NR, Robbins LD, Ganim R, Hochheiser G, DiCampli R. Inhaled epoprostenol during one-lung ventilation. ATS Elsevier Inc. 2010;89(3):981–3.

81. Wu CL, Cohen SR, Richman JM, Rowlingson AJ, Courpas GE, Cheung K, et al. Efficacy of postoperative patient-controlled and continuous infusion epidural analgesia versus intravenous patient-controlled analgesia with opioids: a meta-analysis. Anesthesiology. 2005;103(5):1079–88. –quiz1109–10.

82. Block BM, Liu SS, Rowlingson AJ, Cowan AR, Cowan JA, Wu CL. Efficacy of postoperative epidural analgesia: a meta-analysis. JAMA. 2003;290(18):2455–63.

83. Dolin SJ, Cashman JN, Bland JM. Effectiveness of acute postoperative pain management: I. evidence from published data. Br J Anaesth. 2002;89(3):409–23.

84. Pöpping DM, Elia N, Marret E, Remy C, Tramèr MR. Protective effects of epidural analgesia on pulmonary complications after abdominal and thoracic surgery: a meta-analysis. Arch Surg. 2008;143(10):990–9. –discussion1000.

85. Pöpping DM, Elia N, Van Aken HK, Marret E, Schug SA, Kranke P, et al. Impact of epidural analgesia on mortality and morbidity after surgery. Ann Surg. 2014;259(6):1056–67.

86. Ozcan PE, Sentürk M, Sungur Ulke Z, Toker A, Dilege S, Ozden E, et al. Effects of thoracic epidural anaesthesia on pulmonary venous

admixture and oxygenation during one-lung ventilation. Acta Anaesthesiol Scand. 2007;51(8):1117–22.

87. Miró M, Sanfilippo F, Pérez F, García Del Valle S, Gómez-Arnau JI. Influence of the thoracic epidural anesthesia on the left ventricular function: an echocardiographic study. Minerva Anestesiol. 2017;83(7):695–704.

88. Schmidt C, Hinder F, Van Aken H, Theilmeier G, Bruch C, Wirtz SP, et al. The effect of high thoracic epidural anesthesia on systolic and diastolic left ventricular function in patients with coronary artery disease. Anesth Analg. 2005;100(6):1561–9.

89. Clemente A, Carli F. The physiological effects of thoracic epidural anesthesia and analgesia on the cardiovascular, respiratory and gastrointestinal systems. Minerva Anestesiol. 2008;74(10):549–63.

90. Rex S, Missant C, Segers P, Wouters PF. Thoracic epidural anesthesia impairs the hemodynamic response to acute pulmonary hypertension by deteriorating right ventricular–pulmonary arterial coupling. Crit Care Med. 2007;35(1):222–9.

91. Missant C, Rex S, Claus P, Derde S, Wouters PF. Thoracic epidural anaesthesia disrupts the protective mechanism of homeometric autoregulation during right ventricular pressure overload by cardiac sympathetic blockade: a randomised controlled animal study. Eur J Anaesthesiol. 2011;28(7):535–43.

92. Wink J, de Wilde RBP, Wouters PF, van Dorp ELA, Veering BT, Versteegh MIM, et al. Thoracic epidural anesthesia reduces right ventricular systolic function with maintained ventricular-pulmonary coupling. Clinical perspective. Circulation. 2016;134(16):1163–75.

93. Yeung JH, Gates S, Naidu BV, Wilson MJA, Gao Smith F. Paravertebral block versus thoracic epidural for patients undergoing thoracotomy. Gao Smith F, editor. Cochrane Database Syst Rev. Chichester, UK: John Wiley & Sons, Ltd. 2016;2(4):CD009121.

94. Daly DJ, Myles PS. Update on the role of paravertebral blocks for thoracic surgery: are they worth it? Curr Opin Anaesthesiol. 2009;22(1):38–43.

95. Grider JS, Mullet TW, Saha SP, Harned ME, Sloan PA. A randomized, double-blind trial comparing continuous thoracic epidural bupivacaine with and without opioid in contrast to a continuous paravertebral infusion of bupivacaine for post-thoracotomy pain. J Cardiothorac Vasc Anesth. 2012;26(1):83–9.

96. Pintaric TS, Potocnik I, Hadzic A, Stupnik T, Pintaric M, Novak JV. Comparison of continuous thoracic epidural with paravertebral block on perioperative analgesia and hemodynamic stability in patients having open lung surgery. Reg Anesth Pain Med. 2011;36(3):256–60.

97. McGlothlin D, Ivascu N, Heerdt PM. Anesthesia and pulmonary hypertension. Prog Cardiovasc Dis. 2012;55(2):199–217.

98. Strumpher J, Jacobsohn E. Pulmonary hypertension and right ventricular dysfunction: physiology and perioperative management. YJCAN Elsevier Inc. 2011;25(4):687–704.

99. Şentürk M, Slinger P, Cohen E. Intraoperative mechanical ventilation strategies for one-lung ventilation. Best Pract Res Clin Anaesthesiol Elsevier Ltd. 2015;29(3):357–69.

100. Brassard CL, Lohser J, Donati F, Bussières JS. Step-by-step clinical management of one-lung ventilation: continuing professional development. Can J Anaesth. 2014;61(12):1103–21.

101. Magnusson L, Spahn DR. New concepts of atelectasis during general anaesthesia. Br J Anaesth. 2003;91(1):61–72.

102. Roberts DH, Lepore JJ, Maroo A, Semigran MJ, Ginns LC. Oxygen therapy improves cardiac index and pulmonary vascular resistance in patients with pulmonary hypertension. Chest. 2001;120(5):1547–55.

103. Gordon JB, Rehorst-Paea LA, Hoffman GM, Nelin LD. Pulmonary vascular responses during acute and sustained respiratory alkalosis or acidosis in intact newborn piglets. Pediatr Res. 1999;46(6):735–41.

104. Moreira GA, O'Donnell DC, Tod ML, Madden JA, Gordon JB. Discordant effects of alkalosis on elevated pulmonary vascular resistance and vascular reactivity in lamb lungs. Crit Care Med. 1999;27(9):1838–42.

105. Doras C, Le Guen M, Peták F, Habre W. Cardiorespiratory effects of recruitment maneuvers and positive end expiratory pressure in an experimental context of acute lung injury and pulmonary hypertension. BMC Pulm Med BioMed Central. 2015;15(1):82.

106. Takeuchi M, Imanaka H, Tachibana K, Ogino H, Ando M, Nishimura M. Recruitment maneuver and high positive end-expiratory pressure improve hypoxemia in patients after pulmonary thromboendarterectomy for chronic pulmonary thromboembolism. Crit Care Med. 2005;33(9):2010–4.

107. Hwang W, Jeon J. The effect of iloprost on arterial oxygenation during one-lung ventilation. Eur Respir J. 2016;48(suppl 60):OA1987.

108. Hill LL, Pearl RG. Combined inhaled nitric oxide and inhaled prostacyclin during experimental chronic pulmonary hypertension. J Appl Physiol. 1999;86(4):1160–4.

109. Flondor M, Merkel M, Hofstetter C, Irlbeck M, Frey L, Zwissler B. The effect of inhaled nitric oxide and inhaled iloprost on hypoxaemia in a patient with pulmonary hypertension after pulmonary thrombarterectomy. Anaesthesia. 2006;61(12):1200–3.

110. Hughes CG, Weavind L, Banerjee A, Mercaldo ND, Schildcrout JS, Pandharipande PP. Intraoperative risk factors for acute respiratory distress syndrome in critically ill patients. Anesth Analg. 2010;111(2):464–7.

111. Chau EHL, Slinger P. Perioperative fluid management for pulmonary resection surgery and esophagectomy. Semin Cardiothorac Vasc Anesth. 2014;18(1):36–44.

112. Licker M, de Perrot M, Spiliopoulos A, Robert J, Diaper J, Chevalley C, et al. Risk factors for acute lung injury after thoracic surgery for lung cancer. Anesth Analg. 2003;97(6):1558–65.

113. Vaporciyan AA, Rice D, Correa AM, Walsh G, Putnam JB, Swisher S, et al. Resection of advanced thoracic malignancies requiring cardiopulmonary bypass. Eur J Cardiothorac Surg. 2002;22(1):47–52.

114. Slinger P, Kilpatrick B. Perioperative lung protection strategies in cardiothoracic anesthesia. Anesthesiol Clin. 2012;30(4):607–28.

115. Assaad S, Popescu W, Perrino A. Fluid management in thoracic surgery. Curr Opin Anaesthesiol. 2013;26(1):31–9.

116. Kozian A, Schilling T, Röcken C, Breitling C, Hachenberg T, Hedenstierna G. Increased alveolar damage after mechanical ventilation in a porcine model of thoracic surgery. J Cardiothorac Vasc Anesth. 2010;24(4):617–23.

117. Arslantas MK, Kara HV, Tuncer BB, Yildizeli B, Yuksel M, Bostanci K, et al. Effect of the amount of intraoperative fluid administration on postoperative pulmonary complications following anatomic lung resections. J Thorac Cardiovasc Surg Elsevier Inc. 2015;149(1):314–20. 321.e1.

118. Rocca GD, Vetrugno L. Fluid therapy today: where are we? Turk J Anaesth Reanim. 2016;44(5):233–5.

119. Licker M, Triponez F, Ellenberger C, Karenovics W. Fluid therapy in thoracic surgery: a zero-balance target is always best! Turk J Anaesth Reanim. 2016;44(5):227–9.

120. Rinieri P, Peillon C, Bessou JP, Veber B, Falcoz PE, Melki J, et al. National review of use of extracorporeal membrane oxygenation as respiratory support in thoracic surgery excluding lung transplantation. Eur J Cardiothorac Surg. 2014;47(1):87–94.

121. Rosskopfova P, Perentes JY, Ris H-B, Gronchi F, Krueger T, Gonzalez M. Extracorporeal support for pulmonary resection: current indications and results. World J Surg Oncol. 2016; 14:1–10.

122. Lei J, Su K, Li XF, Zhou YA, Han Y, Huang LJ, et al. ECMO-assisted carinal resection and reconstruction after left pneumonectomy. J Cardiothorac Surg 5th ed. 2010;5(1):89.

123. Lang G, Ghanim B, Hotzenecker K, Klikovits T, Matilla JR, Aigner C, et al. Extracorporeal membrane oxygenation support for complex tracheo-bronchial procedures. Eur J Cardiothorac Surg. 2015;47(2):250–6.

124. Ross AF, Ueda K. Pulmonary hypertension in thoracic surgical patients. Curr Opin Anaesthesiol. 2010;23(1):25–33.

125. Warner DO. Preventing postoperative pulmonary complications. Anesthesiology. 2000;92(5):1467–72.

126. Lawrence VA. Strategies to reduce postoperative pulmonary complications after noncardiothoracic surgery: systematic review for the American College of Physicians. Ann Intern Med. 2006;144(8):596.

127. Smetana GW. Postoperative pulmonary complications: an update on risk assessment and reduction. Cleve Clin J Med. 2009;76(Suppl_4):S60–5.

128. Marseu K, Slinger P. Peri-operative pulmonary dysfunction and protection. Anaesthesia 1st ed. 2016;Suppl 1(S1):46–50.

129. Fernando HC, Jaklitsch MT, Walsh GL, Tisdale JE, Bridges CD, Mitchell JD, et al. The Society of Thoracic Surgeons practice guideline on the prophylaxis and management of atrial fibrillation associated with general thoracic surgery: executive summary. Ann Thorac Surg. 2011;92(3):1144–52.

130. Olsson KM, Nickel NP, Tongers J, Hoeper MM. Atrial flutter and fibrillation in patients with pulmonary hypertension. Int J Cardiol. 2013;167(5):2300–5.

131. Peacock A, Ross K. Pulmonary hypertension: a contraindication to the use of -adrenoceptor blocking agents. Thorax BMJ Publishing Group Ltd. 2010;65(5):454–5.

132. Frendl G, Sodickson AC, Chung MK, Waldo AL, Gersh BJ, Tisdale JE, et al. 2014 AATS guidelines for the prevention and management of perioperative atrial fibrillation and flutter for thoracic surgical procedures. J Thorac Cardiovasc Surg. 2014;148(3):e153–93.

133. Fischer LG, Aken HV, Bürkle H. Management of pulmonary hypertension: physiological and pharmacological considerations for anesthesiologists. Anesth Analg. 2003;96(6):1603–16.

134. Trachte AL, Lobato EB, Urdaneta F, Hess PJ, Klodell CT, Martin TD, et al. Oral sildenafil reduces pulmonary hypertension after cardiac surgery. Ann Thorac Surg. 2005;79(1):194–7.

135. Elias S, Sviri S, Orenbuch-Harroch E, Fellig Y, Ben-Yehuda A, Fridlender ZG, et al. The use of sildenafil to facilitate weaning from inhaled nitric oxide (iNO) and mechanical ventilation in a patient with severe secondary pulmonary hypertension and a patent foramen Ovale. Respir Care. 2011;56(10):1611–3.

136. Lee JE, Hillier SC, Knoderer CA. Use of sildenafil to facilitate weaning from inhaled nitric oxide in children with pulmonary hypertension following surgery for congenital heart disease. J Intensive Care Med. 2008;23(5):329–34.

137. Namachivayam P, Theilen U, Butt WW, Cooper SM, Penny DJ, Shekerdemian LS. Sildenafil prevents rebound pulmonary hypertension after withdrawal of nitric oxide in children. Am J Respir Crit Care Med. 2006;174(9):1042–7.

138. Fischer GW, Cohen E. An update on anesthesia for thoracoscopic surgery. Curr Opin Anaesthesiol. 2010;23(1):7–11.

139. Y. L. Kwak, C. S. Lee, Y. H. Park, Y. W. Hong, (2002) The effect of phenylephrine and norepinephrine in patients with chronic pulmonary hypertension*. Anaesthesia 57(1):9–14.

140. Xibing Ding, Shuqing Jin, Xiaoyin Niu, Hao Ren, Shukun Fu, Quan Li, Giovanni Landoni, (2014) A Comparison of the Analgesia Efficacy and Side Effects of Paravertebral Compared with Epidural Blockade for Thoracotomy: An Updated Meta-Analysis. PLoS ONE 9(5):e96233.

Part IX

Complex Thoracic Surgical Procedures

Surgery of the Chest Wall and Diaphragm

35

Peter Slinger

Key Points
- Surgery for benign chest wall deformities is most commonly performed for cosmetic reasons but in some cases for restrictive respiratory or cardiac symptoms.
- Postexcision, chest wall defects larger than 5 cm will require reconstruction to diminish paradoxical motion and impaired gas exchange.
- All full-thickness diaphragm defects should be repaired when diagnosed to prevent late onset of perforation or strangulation of abdominal contents in the chest.
- Diaphragm eventration requires repair only for symptoms of impaired gas exchange.

Chest Wall Surgery

Tumors

Benign tumors of the chest wall include chondromas, osteochondromas, fibrous dysplasia, and desmoid tumors. Because it is often not possible at the time of surgery to be certain of the pathology, benign tumors are treated the same as malignant tumors with wide excisions. Malignant tumors of the chest wall include soft tissue sarcomas, chondrosarcomas, and other varieties of sarcoma. They are excised with wide margins of at least 4 cm including several partial ribs above and below for rib lesions. For sternal lesions, a sternotomy with corresponding resection of bilateral adjacent costal arches is performed.

P. Slinger (✉)
Department of Anesthesia, Toronto General Hospital, Toronto, ON, Canada
e-mail: peter.slinger@uhn.ca

Defects of the chest wall less than 5 cm are usually closed primarily and not reconstructed. Defects larger than 5 cm in any diameter are reconstructed with a synthetic mesh. Soft tissue reconstruction of larger defects may include a flap of the latissimus dorsi, pectoralis major, rectus abdominis, or other muscles and/or omentum [1].

Anesthetic considerations for excision of chest wall tumors include possible invasive or compressive effects of the tumor on intrathoracic cardiovascular or respiratory structures (see Fig. 35.1). Postoperative pain and respiratory limitation is a major problem following excision of large chest wall tumors. Thoracic epidural analgesia may be indicated for patients with borderline preoperative respiratory function.

Congenital Deformities

The commonest congenital deformity of the chest wall presenting for surgery is pectus excavatum (see Fig. 35.2). This is a posterior angulation of the lower sternum and adjacent ribs. The severity can be assessed on chest imaging by the "pectus index" which is the distance ratio of the transverse chest diameter to the shortest distance between the posterior sternum and the anterior border of the spine. In normal individuals this ratio is approximately 2.5, and in patients with pectus excavatum, it typically exceeds 3.5. It may be associated with scoliosis or Marfan's syndrome. Pulmonary function tests generally show a mild restrictive pattern; however this does not improve significantly after repair [2]. However, repair of the deformity does improve exercise capacity secondary to improved cardiac output and stroke volume.

There are several different surgical procedures used to correct pectus excavatum. Most open procedures involve resection of the costal cartilages at the site of the deformity, an osteotomy of the sternum, and internal fixation or stabilization (see Fig. 35.3). In children and younger adolescents,

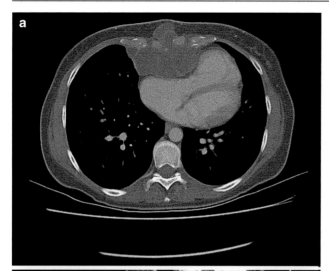

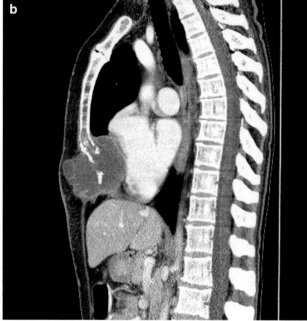

Fig. 35.1 Transverse (**a**) and sagittal (**b**) CT scan views of a patient with a chondrosarcoma of the lower sternum. The tumor is compressing the right ventricle

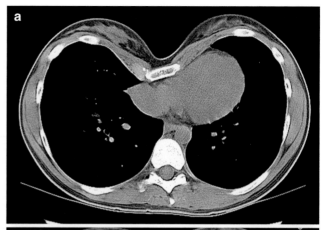

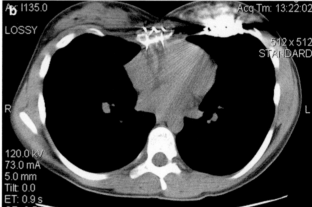

Fig. 35.2 Transverse CT scans of a patient with pectus excavatum. (**a**) Preoperative. The sternum is compressing the right ventricle. (**b**) Postoperative. Internal fixation of the sternum and a portion of the pectus bar attached to the ribs of the left chest can be seen

there is the option of a minimally invasive procedure with the insertion of a Nuss bar to elevate the sternum [3].

A variety of other less common congenital chest deformities such as pectus carinatum and Poland syndrome also can present for surgery. Anesthetic considerations for pectus excavatum and these other deformities are essentially identical to those for excision of chest wall tumors.

Thoracic Outlet Syndrome

Thoracic outlet syndrome refers to compression of the subclavian vessels and/or brachial plexus at the superior aperture of the chest. It may or may not be associated with the presence of a cervical rib. The compression is mainly

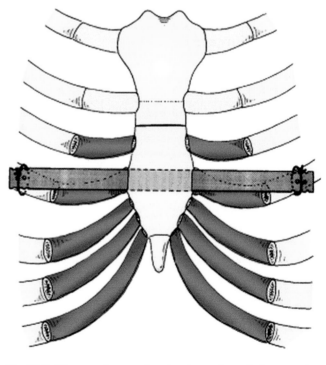

Fig. 35.3 Diagram of a pectus bar placed posterior to the lower portion of the sternum during open surgery for repair of pectus excavatum. (Reprinted from [5]. © Elsevier 2008, with permission)

caused by the first rib. Patients present with a variety of peripheral neurological or vascular symptoms which may include positional pain and paresthesia, commonly in the C8-T1 distributions of the medial hand and arm. Confirmation of the diagnosis may require nerve conduction studies or angiography. Treatment is initially conservative with physiotherapy. In refractory cases excision of the first rib and/or a cervical rib may be indicated. Surgery is via an extra-thoracic approach, and anesthetic concerns are similar to those for other types of head and neck procedures.

Diaphragm Surgery

Hernia

Repair of congenital diaphragmatic hernia in infants is discussed in Chap. 50. Adults may also present for repair of congenital or acquired defects of the diaphragm. Congenital malformations of the diaphragm in adults may be diagnosed incidentally on chest imaging or may cause a variety of compressive symptoms due to the intrathoracic mass of gastrointestinal contents. The commonest site for herniation of abdominal contents into the chest is through the esophageal hiatus (see Fig. 35.4). Other sites include the Bochdalek foramen (usually on the left side) and Morgagni foramen (usually on the right; see Fig. 35.5). An acquired hernia may be due to sudden severe blunt abdominal trauma. Occasionally these may present late, long after the initial trauma. All dia-

phragmatic hernias should be repaired when diagnosed due to the possibility of strangulation or perforation of bowel in the chest. Repairs are most commonly performed by laparotomy or laparoscopy. Anesthetic concerns for hiatal hernias are similar to those for other types of benign esophageal disease (see Chap. 38) specifically, an increased risk of aspiration on induction.

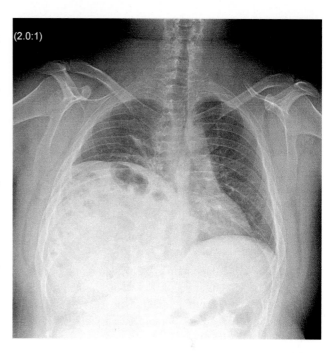

Fig. 35.5 Chest X-ray of an adult presenting for repair of a hernia of bowel into the right chest via the foramen of Morgagni

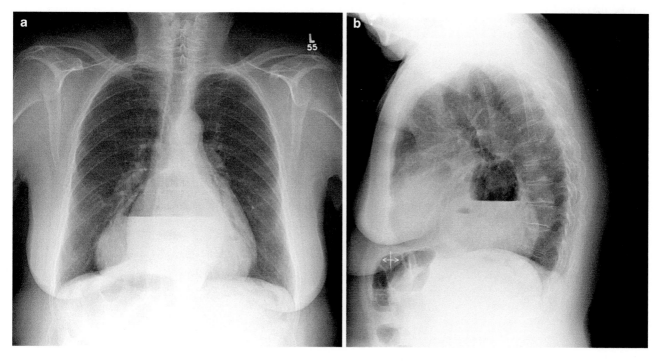

Fig. 35.4 (**a**) PA and (**b**) lateral chest X-rays of a patient with an intrathoracic stomach which has herniated through the esophageal hiatus of the diaphragm. The risk of aspiration of gastric contents during induction of anesthesia can be appreciated

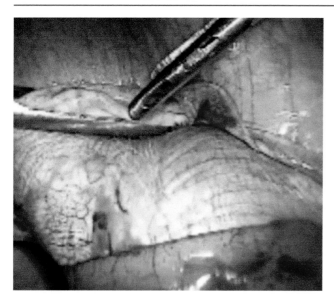

Fig. 35.6 Thoracoscopic plication of the diaphragm during one-lung ventilation

Eventration

Eventration of the diaphragm is an elevation of a portion of the diaphragm due to an incomplete development of part of the musculature. The differential diagnosis is a paralysis of the diaphragm. Causes of phrenic nerve paralysis such as lung cancer must be ruled out. Most cases of eventration in adult life are treated conservatively. Severe dyspnea or orthopnea may be an indication for surgery. Surgical repair is by plication of the involved portion of the diaphragm; this can be performed with a minimally invasive approach [4] (see Fig. 35.6).

References

1. Pairolero PC, Arnold PG. Chest wall tumors: experience with 100 consecutive patients. J Thorac Cardiovasc Surg. 1985;90:367–73.
2. Morshuis W, Folgering H, Barentsz J, et al. Pulmonary function before surgery for pectus excavatum and at long-term follow-up. Chest. 1994;105:1646–52.
3. Park HJ, Lee SY, Lee CS, et al. The Nuss procedure for pectus excavatum. Ann Thorac Surg. 2004;77:289–95.
4. Huttl TP, Wichmann MW, Reichart B, et al. Laparoscopic diaphragmatic plication. Surg Endosc. 2004;18:547–51.
5. Kucharczuk J. Surgery of pectus deformities. In: Patterson GA, editor. Pearson's thoracic and esophageal surgery. 3rd ed. Amsterdam: Elsevier. 2008; p. 1333.

Extrapleural Pneumonectomy

Ju-Mei Ng

Key Points
- Extrapleural pneumonectomy is a formidable surgical procedure performed on patients with limited life expectancy. Anesthetic management may contribute to containment of perioperative morbidity and mortality through the control of intraoperative physiologic disruptions and postoperative pain and an appreciation of the associated postoperative complications to affect early intervention.
- Beyond standard anesthetic management issues for pneumonectomy, there exist a number of important "EPP-specific" anesthetic concerns. These include significantly greater blood loss, more delicate management of intravascular fluid and blood components, greater operative impairment of venous return, high probability of dysrhythmias, and greater potential for hemodynamic instability related to pericardial window and its patch.
- Common causes of hypotension during EPP include compression of the heart or great vessels by tumor or surgical pressure/retraction, blood loss and/or inadequate fluid resuscitation, and thoracic epidural sympathetic blockade.
- No single anesthetic recipe is of proven superiority for either EPP or lung resection surgery in general. The priority for early extubation favors the use of short-acting modern inhalational and intravenous agents, with limited use of traditional parenteral narcotics. Thoracic epidural analgesia is widely employed intraoperatively to facilitate extubation at the conclusion of surgery by providing dense analgesia without depression of sensorium or respiratory drive.
- Fluid management remains a challenge due to the increased blood loss in EPP, hemodynamic instability, renal toxicity of chemotherapy agents, and the potential for exacerbation of acute lung injury.

Introduction

Extrapleural pneumonectomy (EPP), the en bloc resection of the lung, parietal and visceral pleurae, pericardium, and diaphragm, is a formidable surgical procedure. First described for the treatment of tuberculous empyema, it is currently typically performed for local control of malignant pleural mesothelioma (MPM). It may also be applied to other malignancies or infections involving or obliterating the pleural space, including thymoma and non-small cell lung cancer (NSCLC) [1]. Although there has been a dramatic reduction in perioperative mortality from 31% reported in the 1970s [2] to a recent systematic review demonstrating mortality ranging from 0% to 11.8% [3], postoperative major morbidity remains high (12.5–48%). Higher center volume may be associated with decreased mortality and morbidity after surgery for MPM [4]. Currently, EPP and the lung-sparing alternative, pleurectomy/decortication (P/D), are considered by many to have a critical role in the multimodality treatment of MPM [4–9]. This chapter will discuss the important "EPP-specific" anesthesia concerns [10, 11], including intraoperative intracavitary hyperthermic chemotherapy (IOHC), which is being applied in a few centers for better control of local disease in MPM.

J.-M. Ng (✉)
Department of Anesthesiology, Perioperative and Pain Medicine, Brigham and Women's Hospital, Boston, MA, USA
e-mail: jng1@bwh.harvard.edu

P. Slinger (ed.), *Principles and Practice of Anesthesia for Thoracic Surgery*, https://doi.org/10.1007/978-3-030-00859-8_36

Malignant Pleural Mesothelioma and Pleural Dissemination of Malignancy

MPM arises on the pleural surface of the chest wall, lung, pericardium, or diaphragm, tends to spread or recur locoregionally, and is generally fatal within a year of diagnosis [12]. Its etiologic link to asbestos exposure has been established [13], but not all patients with mesothelioma have a history of asbestos exposure, and other etiologies have been postulated [14]. The annual incidence of mesothelioma in the United States is estimated to be approximately 3300 cases per year [15]; this incidence of mesothelioma peaked around the year 2000 and is now declining, secondary to control of exposure to asbestos. No single modality of treatment significantly improves median survival beyond 12 months. EPP offers the most complete cytoreduction, but recurrence occurs locoregionally. Multimodality approaches, combining cytoreduction by P/D or EPP, with chemotherapy, radiotherapy, or photodynamic therapy have been evaluated in various combinations recently, with reported improved survival statistics [3–8]. The control of locally advanced disease in thymoma, sarcoma, and NSCLC has been reported with variable success. EPP in Stage IVa thymoma or Stage IV NSCLC (often combining induction chemotherapy and/or adjuvant radiation) has a 5-year survival of 53–78% and 24–55%, respectively [1]. But reports are sparse with mainly small cohorts of patients. With the exception of IOHC, these multimodality treatment therapies generally do not greatly impact anesthetic management of EPP.

Intraoperative Intracavitary Heated Chemotherapy

The intraoperative application of chemotherapy (usually cisplatin) to address microscopic disease remaining in the empty hemithorax prior to closure has important implications on anesthetic management. Intracavitary application targets the chemotherapy directly at the sites of recurrence (including the abdomen), with higher doses than would be tolerated systemically. Heating the chemotherapy agent increases tumoricidal activity by increasing the permeability and metabolic activity of the cells [16].

Surgical Considerations

The *technique* of *EPP* [17] consists of several basic steps:

1. *Incision and exposure of the parietal pleura*
   An extended posterolateral thoracotomy with resection of the 6th rib is the most common approach.

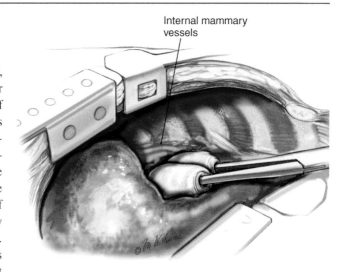

Internal mammary vessels

Fig. 36.1 Blunt anterior parietal dissection with identification of the internal mammary vessels. (Reprinted with permission from Marcia Williams Medical and Scientific Illustration [17])

2. *Extrapleural dissection to separate the tumor from the chest wall*
3. *En bloc resection of the lung, pleura, pericardium, and diaphragm with division of the hilar structures*
   A combination of blunt and sharp extrapleural dissection is initiated anterolaterly and advanced to and over the apex, to bring the tumor down from the posterior and superior mediastinum (Fig. 36.1).
   - Beware of injury to the internal mammary vessels/grafts and subclavian vessels during dissection anteriorly and at the apex, respectively, as well as traction injury to the azygous vein and superior vena cava in the superior mediastinum.
   - In addition, during left EPP, injury may occur to the intercostal arteries, thoracic duct, and recurrent laryngeal nerve.

   Posterior dissection is then performed and the esophagus dissected away from the tumor. The diaphragm is avulsed circumferentially (Fig. 36.2) and dissected bluntly from the underlying peritoneum (Fig. 36.3), and the pericardium is opened.
   - During division of the medial aspect of the diaphragm, the inferior vena cava may be injured or torsed.

   The main pulmonary artery (PA) and pulmonary veins are then dissected, isolated, and stapled extra- or intrapericardially. After the main bronchus is dissected as far as the carina, the bronchial stapler is fired under direct visualization with the fiber-optic video bronchoscope to assure a short bronchial stump. Bleeding from numerous exposed vessels on the inner thoracic cavity is temporized by packing, but definitive hemostasis is not sought until the specimen is removed.

4. *Radical lymph node dissection*
   Radical mediastinal lymph node dissection is performed, followed by reinforcement of the bronchial stump. The

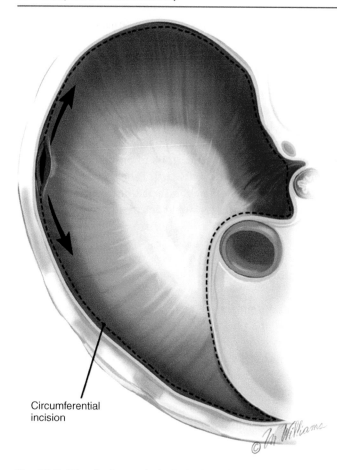

Circumferential
incision

Fig. 36.2 The diaphragm is incised circumferentially. (Reprinted with permission from Marcia Williams Medical and Scientific Illustration [17])

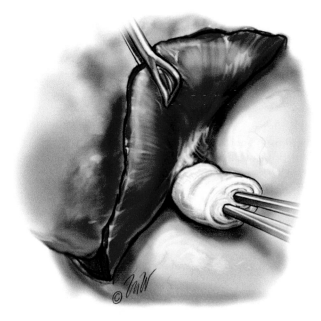

Fig. 36.3 The diaphragm is dissected bluntly from the underlying peritoneum. (Reprinted with permission from Marcia Williams Medical and Scientific Illustration [17])

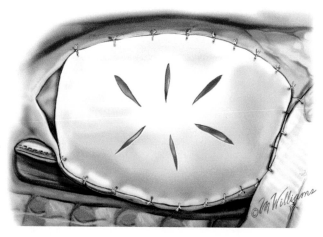

Fig. 36.4 Reconstruction with diaphragmatic and fenestrated pericardial patches which prevent herniation. (Reprinted with permission from Marcia Williams Medical and Scientific Illustration [17])

hemithorax is then irrigated with warm saline and water (wash phase) to remove and osmotically lyse residual microscopic tumor.

4. *Optional administration of IOHC*
5. *Reconstruction of the diaphragm and pericardium* (Fig. 36.4)

The last step is reconstruction of the diaphragm and pericardium using a prosthetic such as Gore-Tex DualMesh (W.L. Gore and Associates, Inc., Flagstaff, Arizona). These patches prevent subsequent herniation of abdominal contents and cardiac herniation into the empty hemithorax.

Technique of IOHC

Two perfusion cannulae (inflow and outflow) are placed within the open hemithorax after tumor resection and hemostasis. Chemotherapy in dialysate maintained at 42 °C is circulated via a pump for 60 min. The volume of perfusate is adjusted to keep the hemithorax full, which maximizes surface area contact between residual microscopic tumor cells and a high local concentration of cisplatin. Systemic administration of cytoprotectants is performed either before or after the chemotherapy administration depending on the agent used (Table 36.1); the timing is important to maximize tumorigenicity while sparing renal function [7]. Sodium thiosulfate covalently binds and inactivates cisplatin in the blood. Amifostine (Ethyol, Alza Pharmaceuticals – USA), which exhibits 100-fold preferential uptake by normal cells and salvages intracellular free radicals, has also been used. Amifostine may cause hypotension with rapid administration.

Table 36.1 Renal protective strategies for EPP with intraoperative intracavitary hyperthermic chemotherapy (IOHC) with cisplatin (Brigham and Women's Hospital Protocol)

Admission day before surgery for intravenous hydration
7-day hold of nonsteroidal anti-inflammatory drugs
Pretreatment with intravenous amifostine (30 mins prior to IOHC) and 2nd dose 2 h later (910 mg/m² and 500 mg/m²)
Intravenous sodium thiosulfate following IOHC (4 g/m² bolus, 12 g/m² over 6 h)
Liberalized IV hydration and assiduous avoidance of systemic hypotension during and after IOHC
Urine alkalinization (NaHCO₃ 45 mEq/h × 2 h, 22.5 mEq/h)

Table 36.2 Suggested exclusion criteria for EPP

Karnofsky performance status <70%
Abnormal creatinine
Abnormal liver function tests
Evidence of unresectability by CT, MRI, echocardiogram
Room air $PaCO_2$ > 45 mmHg
Room air PaO_2 < 65 mmHg
Left ventricular ejection fraction <45%
Predicted postoperative FEV_1 < 1 L[a]

Karnofsky score 70 – Care for self: unable to carry on normal activity or do active work

CT computed tomography, *MRI* magnetic resonance imaging, *FEV₁* forced expiratory volume in 1 s

[a]Patients with predicted postoperative FEV_1 < 2 L are recommended to undergo quantitative radionuclide ventilation-perfusion scanning

Patient Selection

Critical to risk reduction, general exclusion criteria utilized by the surgical group with the most favorable published survival statistics [5] are listed in Table 36.2. Patients with a predicted postoperative forced expiratory volume in 1 s (ppoFEV₁) or less than 0.8 L are considered for P/D, rather than EPP.

Preoperative Patient Preparation

An awareness of the perceived cardiopulmonary reserve, the anatomical extent and impact of the tumor, and coexisting disease states allows the anesthesiologist to tailor invasive monitors, lines, and anesthetic plan to preempt or efficiently respond to problems. If IOHC is planned, renal protection strategies begin preoperatively with hydration and the withholding of nonsteroidal anti-inflammatory medications (Table 36.1).

Cardiopulmonary Risk Assessment

The assessment of cardiopulmonary reserve is especially difficult. Measurements traditionally employed to predict post-

thoracotomy pulmonary complications include ppoFEV₁, maximal oxygen consumption (VO₂max), and diffusing capacity for carbon monoxide (DL_CO) [18]. Preoperative transthoracic echocardiograms are routine, and cardiac stress and right heart catheterization are utilized if there is evidence of ventricular dysfunction or pulmonary hypertension, respectively. History, physical examination, and echocardiography will reflect cardiac functional status but may not predict the response to the stress of pneumonectomy in the setting of major fluid shifts [19]. Patients with a history of recent myocardial infarction in the last 3 months or life-threatening arrhythmias would be considered for P/D rather than EPP.

Radiologic Studies

Computed tomography and magnetic resonance imaging (MRI) of the chest play an important role in assessing tumor invasion of the chest wall, vertebrae, diaphragm, and mediastinal structures. They are used for staging and/or to assess tumor resectability [20]. The anesthetic implications include safe placement of epidural catheters at the thoracic region, level and site of intravenous access, quantity of blood and blood products available, and the potential necessity for cardiopulmonary bypass during resection.

Anesthetic Considerations

Specific Anesthetic Issues for EPP

Beyond the standard management issues for pneumonectomy [21], important "EPP-specific" anesthesia concerns are shown in Table 36.3.

Table 36.3 Anesthetic issues for extrapleural pneumonectomy

Significantly greater blood loss compared to pneumonectomy
More delicate management of intravascular fluid and blood components
Greater operative impairment of venous return
Greater danger of surgical disruption of major vascular structures
More complex and variable physiology of the nonoperative lung (restrictive and obstructive)
High probability for disruption of internal mammary artery coronary grafts (if present)
High probability of dysrhythmias
Frequent "pseudo-ischemic" ST changes on EKG during wash phase
Greater potential for hemodynamic instability related to pericardial window and its patch
Greater postoperative pain and pulmonary dysfunction related to the larger incision

Lines and Monitors

Generous intravenous access is paramount, and blood should be available in the operating room. If the superior vena cava is in jeopardy, lower extremity intravenous access is mandatory. A nasogastric tube aids posterior esophageal dissection intraoperatively and gastric decompression (and the prevention of gastric acid aspiration) postoperatively. Invasive monitors (arterial and central venous lines) are routine. The site of central venous access is important, as the potential for causing a pneumothorax in the nonoperative lung has to be weighed against injury to the subclavian vein during surgical dissection on the operative side.

Although pulmonary artery (PA) catheters have potential interpretation pitfalls during pneumonectomy [22, 23], they may be useful for postoperative fluid and right heart management issues. Transesophageal echocardiography (TEE) is a more powerful and reliable monitor of right and left ventricular filling and function and is a more sensitive monitor of myocardial ischemia, particularly during left EPP when the surgical incision precludes appropriate EKG lead placement. However, there is no direct evidence of improved outcome, and the cost and need of technical expertise make this tool worthwhile only in selected cases.

Choice of Anesthesia

No single anesthetic recipe is of proven superiority for either EPP or lung resection surgery in general. The priority for early extubation favors the use of short-acting modern inhalational and intravenous agents, with limited use of traditional parenteral narcotics.

Thoracic Epidural Analgesia

Despite emerging promising regional techniques for post-thoracotomy analgesia, thoracic epidural analgesia (TEA) remains the technique of choice for EPP. TEA reduces perioperative pulmonary [24] and cardiac complications [25, 26], including pulmonary infections, atelectasis, myocardial infarction, and the incidence of supraventricular tachyarrhythmias post-thoracotomy. TEA is widely employed intra- and postoperatively for EPP. It also facilitates extubation at the conclusion of surgery by providing dense analgesia without depression of sensorium or respiratory drive.

The sympatholytic effects of TEA may complicate hemodynamic management if dense blockade is imposed during or prior to the dissection phase of EPP. It is therefore common to initiate bolus dosing of the epidural catheter later in the surgery. Ultimately, solutions and infusion rates are individualized to address catheter insertion site, hypotension, pruritus, nausea, opioid tolerance, sedation, or other side effects.

One-Lung Anesthesia

Lung Isolation Techniques

Lung isolation to facilitate surgical exposure may be achieved using either a double-lumen endotracheal tube (DLT) or a bronchial blocker. For EPP, DLTs allow rapid ventilation or collapse of either lung, effective suctioning, and uninterrupted lung isolation at the time of surgical cross clamp. We favor a left-sided DLT is for a right EPP (and vice versa). There is no hardware present in the operative bronchus, and compared to a bronchial blocker, a left-sided DLT is less likely to be dislodged with surgical manipulation. Although right-sided DLTs have a smaller margin of safety (due to short right upper lobe anatomy), this is rarely an impediment to their effective use. When an anomalously high right upper lobe precludes an effective air seal at the bronchial cuff, this is easily remedied by passing a blocker down the tracheal lumen [27]. Blockers are principally used for left-sided EPP in patients with difficult airway anatomy and withdrawn prior to stapling the bronchus in order to avoid accidental inclusion into the suture line.

Optimizing Oxygenation During One-Lung Ventilation (OLV)

"Lung-protective" (low tidal volume 5–6 ml/kg, limiting peak airway pressure <35 cmH$_2$O, and dependent lung positive end-expiratory pressure (PEEP)) ventilation with the intention of limiting dependent lung volutrauma and atelectasis is important [28]. Recruitment maneuvers (RM) and reducing FiO$_2$ < 1.0 when tolerated may be employed.

EPP patients, during OLV in the lateral decubitus position, often exhibit an element of restrictive physiology in the dependent lung imposed by the weight of the tumor and surgical pressure during dissection. Frequent large changes in compliance require vigilance to prevent high airway pressures or volumes (depending on the mode of ventilation). During intracavitary lavage, where a perfusate of cisplatin exerts weight on the mediastinum, both RM and PEEP are important to prevent atelectasis. In addition, dependent lung pneumothorax may easily occur during dissection of large tumors and will require surgical decompression. The IOHC fluid may accumulate in the dependent thorax if the pleural defect is not adequately repaired.

Despite a greater propensity for dependent lung atelectasis and possibly increased nondependent lung shunt (inhibition of hypoxic pulmonary vasoconstriction due to more vigorous surgical manipulation), hypoxemia during OLV for EPP is unusual. This is because the best predictor of oxygen desaturation during OLV is increased (>55% of cardiac output) blood flow to the operative lung, which is seldom the case in MPM [29].

Hemodynamic Management

Hypertension

Hypertension should be avoided during the dissection phase, as it will greatly exacerbate bleeding from the innumerable avulsed chest wall veins. It may also be an issue when the specimen is removed and venous return to the heart is suddenly unimpeded.

Hypotension

This is more frequent, and its treatment should reflect its etiology whenever possible (Table 36.4). Reduced venous return is the most common mechanism, caused by mechanical pressure on the mediastinum during dissection or torsion of great vessels. Critical phases of surgery when venous return is most threatened include the induction, dissection, and terminal repositioning phases. Vasodilation from hyperthermia during IOHC may occur as core temperatures not uncommonly exceed 38 °C.

Induction

Preemptive vasoconstricting agents and judicious selection of induction agents/doses are particularly indicated for patients with large tumor burdens, large effusions, or radiographic evidence of cardiac or major vessel impingement. Often, the thoracic epidural test-dose effect is still peaking at the time of induction, potentially further increasing compensatory vasoconstrictor requirements.

Dissection Phase

Venous return is impeded by blood loss, insensible losses, and variable degrees of compression from the tumor, retractors, and blunt dissection pressure. The temptation to correct venous return by enthusiastic crystalloid volume expansion is to be resisted. Judicious use of vasopressors, together with blood products when appropriate, will temporize until the specimen is removed. Communication with the surgeon during this phase is paramount, and a coordinated effort is necessary to maintain forward progress with acceptable hemodynamics. A low threshold for administration of blood during this phase often proves strategic. When the specimen is removed, venous return, hemodynamics, and respiratory compliance should normalize. Persistent hypotension at this stage suggests hypovolemia.

Repositioning and Emergence

Herniation of the heart (particularly with right EPP), with torsion of great vessels and circulatory arrest, may abruptly occur upon resumption of the supine position at the end of surgery. Immediate return to the lateral position is the appropriate reflex response. This usually improves hemodynamic parameters, while preparation for reoperation is made if necessary.

The diagnosis is less obvious when only moderate hypotension occurs at this juncture. Culprits include partial cardiac herniation (loose or partially ruptured pericardial patch), tamponade (tight pericardial patch or retained pericardial effusion), inferior vena cava impingement (tight right diaphragmatic patch), hypovolemia, and deviated mediastinum, among others.

Reduced venous return is the common mechanistic denominator. A sluggish response to fluid boluses and vasopressors suggests that mechanical impediments to venous return should be ruled out before leaving the operating room. Aggressive bolus dosing of the epidural in anticipation of emergence may contribute to diagnostic confusion. A portable chest radiograph is usually helpful in ruling out partial cardiac herniation or guiding medialization of the mediastinum by withdrawal of air from the chest drain. TEE may assist in the diagnosis.

Fluid Management

Average estimated intraoperative blood loss during EPP in the best of surgical hands is approximately 0.5–1.5 L. Most of this occurs in a gradual, continuous fashion during the processes of blunt separation of the parietal pleura from the chest wall, although catastrophic bleeding can occur from major vessels during dissection of the hilum or at the apex. Monitoring of the extent of blood loss requires vigilance and communication with the surgeons.

Antifibrinolytics have not been shown to reduce packed red blood cell requirements in EPP surgery [30]. As with any pneumonectomy, excessive crystalloid is to be avoided as it may exacerbate the pulmonary edema of post-lung resection acute lung injury. Fluid management thus becomes a balancing act in the setting of significant hemodynamic swings

Table 36.4 Causes of hypotension during EPP

Common	Compression of the heart or great vessels by tumor or surgical pressure/retraction
	Blood loss/inadequate fluid resuscitation
	Thoracic epidural sympathetic blockade
Uncommon	Air-trapping ("auto-PEEP")
	Tension pneumothorax
	Drugs (vasodilators/negative inotropes)
	Right heart dysfunction/failure
	Cardiac herniation
	Tight pericardial patch
	Shifted mediastinum following closure
	Myocardial ischemia
	Dysrhythmias
	Embolic events
	Transfusion reactions
	Drug reactions
	Sepsis

with intermittently moderate-to-major episodes of blood loss. This balance shifts in favor of more liberal fluid administration in patients receiving IOHC, out of concern for nephrotoxicity.

Central venous pressure measurements, PA occlusion pressures, or observance of respiratory variation on arterial line tracings may be unreliable indicators of intravascular volume during manipulation of weighty tumors, with the chest open to atmosphere. Attention to the surgical field (including the fullness of the heart), urine output, blood gas and hematocrit results, and occasionally TEE are helpful guides.

Postpneumonectomy Pulmonary Edema (PPE)

An emphasis is made on discriminating between hypovolemia and impairments of venous return out of concerns that unnecessary volume resuscitation may contribute to PPE. Pulmonary edema of the remaining lung following pneumonectomy occurs in 2–4% of patients and carries mortality in excess of 50% [31]. The incidence in EPP may be as high as 5–8% [32, 33], which may be in part due to the greater fluid shifts associated with EPP. It is apparent that in the presence of the increased pulmonary capillary permeability in acute lung injury, unnecessary crystalloid or colloid administration will exacerbate the degree of edema and hypoxemia. This is the basis for the widely adhered to practice of conservative (restrictive) fluid management for pneumonectomy patients [21] and highlights the importance of close attention to the matching of fluid administration to blood loss in EPP patients.

Cardiovascular Considerations

Dysrhythmias
The incidence of supraventricular dysrhythmias (SVD) after EPP is higher (21–44%) [4, 5, 7, 32, 34, 35] than for standard

pneumonectomy (13–20%) [35, 36]. Thoracic epidural blockade with bupivacaine has been shown to reduce the incidence of perioperative SVD compared to equianalgesic epidural narcotics [26], and there is increasing evidence that medical prophylaxis (amiodarone, beta-blockers, magnesium and calcium channel blockers) is effective in preventing postoperative atrial fibrillation after general thoracic surgery [37]. Although there may be currently inadequate evidence to recommend routine prophylaxis against AF for all patients undergoing lung surgery, it is reasonable to administer diltiazem to those patients with preserved cardiac function not taking beta-blockers preoperatively in intermediate to high-risk patients [37].

It is uncommon for routine prophylaxis against SVD for EPP but important to avoid withdrawal of beta-adrenergic blocking drugs, if they are in use. Intraoperative dysrhythmias are generally triggered by mechanical irritation and do not appear to predict postoperative SVD. EKG leads should be attached to a ready defibrillator to provide the capability of synchronized electrical cardioversion intraoperatively.

Myocardial Ischemia
Myocardial ischemia may be difficult to detect during EPP as alterations in the position of the heart relative to the surface EKG lead positions would be expected to alter their sensitivity. During left-sided thoracotomies, it is not practical to monitor lead V-5. When myocardial ischemia is suspected, TEE should be employed.

Dramatic ST segment elevations may occur during the wash phase. These tend to occur with irrigation, correct promptly with cessation, and are not associated with other hemodynamic alterations suggestive of myocardial ischemia (Fig. 36.5), most likely representing nonischemic electrophysiologic changes related to focal myocardial warming or surface electrolyte changes [38]. No treatment is necessary unless they persist, produce hemodynamic instability, or are confirmed to be associated with wall motion abnormalities by TEE.

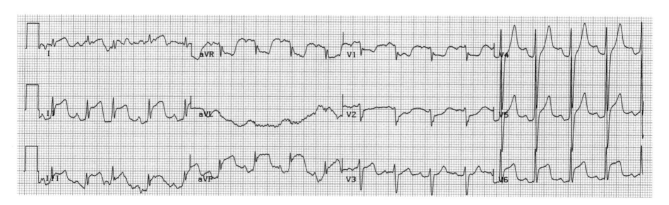

Fig. 36.5 The EKG obtained during wash phase with warm water, following removal of the specimen (including pericardium). Concurrent TEE revealed no global or regional wall motion abnormalities. The EKG rapidly normalized following termination of irrigation

Perioperative Pain Management

There is increasing evidence that TEA with local anesthetics and opioids is superior in the control of dynamic pain, plays a key role in early extubation and mobilization, reduces postoperative pulmonary complications, and has the potential to decrease the incidence of post-thoracotomy pain syndrome. For EPP, although a bolus dose of local anesthetic may be administered prior to surgical incision, the risk of hemodynamic instability usually precludes continuous intraoperative dense neuraxial blockade. Nonetheless, it is vital to aggressively control acute postoperative pain [39, 40].

Preexisting pain related to mesothelioma is not uncommon and frequently treated with opioids. Tolerance may occur after 1–2 weeks of treatment, and such patients present a challenge in terms of postoperative pain control and physiologic withdrawal. Patients on chronic opioids presenting for EPP would generally receive an opioid-free epidural infusion, with additional patient-controlled systemic opioids prescribed to minimize the occurrence of withdrawal. Ketamine may be a useful adjunct [41].

Early Postoperative Considerations

Depending on center experience, majority of patients may be weaned and extubated in the operating room. This minimizes duration of positive pressure on the bronchial stump and avoids the potential problems of ventilator-associated alveolar barotrauma and infection. Prudence is advised in difficult or complicated EPP with increased transfusion requirement or excessive fluid administration in the IOHC cases.

Management of the Ipsilateral Thoracic Space

In addition to the potential for cardiac herniation and its hemodynamic consequences (described earlier), rapid filling of the empty hemithorax with fluid, blood, or abdominal contents from a ruptured diaphragmatic patch can also compromise cardiorespiratory function. Air/fluid is removed from the chest drain at the end of surgery in an attempt to medialize the mediastinum. This is an imprecise process, and a chest radiograph is obtained on arrival in the ICU to assess mediastinal position. Intrathoracic pressure monitoring may guide intermittent fluid evacuation of the pneumonectomy space [42]. This prevents rapid accumulation resulting in respiratory compromise while avoiding contralateral lung hyperexpansion, compromised venous return, and hypotension with excessive and/or rapid removal.

Other Issues Specific to EPP

- Patients who have undergone IOHC receive liberal fluids for the initial 24 h as part of the renal protection strategy (Table 36.1).

- Standard chest compression is ineffective in EPP patients because the mediastinum is dynamic and shifts to the empty hemithorax.

Conclusion

EPP is a radical and aggressive surgery, which presents a great challenge to the thoracic anesthesiologist. Besides standard anesthesia concepts for pneumonectomy, management involves an understanding of the technique of EPP, common intraoperative physiologic disruptions, and anticipated complications. Emerging multimodality treatments for MPM have additional anesthetic implications. One of those, IOHC, is discussed in the context of general EPP-specific anesthetic issues.

Clinical Case Discussion

Case
A 50 year-old male is scheduled for right extrapleural pneumonectomy. The diagnosis of mesothelioma was made on pleural biopsy, and he has completed six cycles of chemotherapy. He is a nonsmoker, and apart from well-controlled hypertension, he has no other significant comorbidities.

Questions

1. *Apart from routine preoperative assessment for pulmonary resection:*
   (a) Are any specialized cardiac and pulmonary function tests indicated?
      - Echocardiography commonly used to assess cardiac function.
      - Stress test only when history, examination, and echocardiography suggest significant cardiac disease.
      - FEV_1, DL_{CO}, and exercise capacity routinely assessed.
      - Ventilation/perfusion scans recommended if $FEV_1 < 2$ L.
      - Predicted postoperative $FEV_1 < 1$ L may preclude EPP.
   (b) What is the importance of radiologic investigations?
      - Surgical staging and tumor resectability.
      - Anesthetic implications include safe placement of epidural catheters at the thoracic region, level of intravenous access, quantity of blood and blood products available, and the potential necessity for cardiopulmonary bypass during resection.

Table 36.5 Hypotension during critical phases of surgery

Phase	Mechanism(s)	Management strategy

Induction	Reduced venous return
	  Vasodilation (induction agents, epidural)
	  Exacerbation of tumor compressive effects by the decrease in FRC
	  Loss of "thoracic pump" of spontaneous ventilation
	  Positive pressure ventilation
		Preemptive vasoconstricting agents and judicious selection of induction agents/doses are particularly indicated for patients with large tumor burdens, large effusions, or radiographic evidence of cardiac or major vessel impingement

Dissection	Blood loss
	Insensible losses
	Variable degrees of compression from the tumor, retractors, and blunt dissection pressure
		Communication with the surgeon is paramount
		  Judicious use of vasopressors
		  A low threshold for administration of blood and products when appropriate

Repositioning and emergence	Circulatory arrest
	  Herniation of the heart (particularly with right EPP), with torsion of the SVC and IVC
	Moderate hypotension
	  Partial cardiac herniation (loose or partially ruptured pericardial patch)
	  Tamponade (tight pericardial patch)
	  Hypovolemia
	  Deviated mediastinum
	  Aggressive bolus dosing of the epidural in anticipation of emergence
		Immediate return to the lateral position
		A sluggish response to fluid boluses and vasopressors suggests that mechanical impediments to venous return should be ruled out
		A portable chest radiograph is usually helpful in ruling out partial cardiac herniation or guiding medialization of the mediastinum

2. *How is an extrapleural pneumonectomy different from pneumonectomy?*
   - See Table 36.3.
3. *What are the common causes of hypotension and the management strategies?* (Table 36.5)
4. *How would the application of intraoperative intracavitary heated chemotherapy affect the anesthetic management?*
   - Renal protective strategies should be employed (Table 36.1).
   - Restrictive physiology exhibited by EPP patients during one-lung ventilation is exacerbated by the weight of the perfusate, and positive end-expiratory pressure is especially important to prevent atelectasis.
   - Fluid management is delicate balance between renal protection and the potential for exacerbation of acute lung injury in fluid overload.

References

1. Wolf AS, Flores RM. Extrapleural pneumonectomy for pleural malignancies. Thorac Surg Clin. 2014;24:471–5.
2. Butchart EG, Ashcroft T, Barnsley WC, Holden MP. Pleuropneumonectomy in the management of diffuse malignant mesothelioma of the pleura. Experience with 29 patients. Thorax. 1976;31(1):15–24.
3. Cao CQ, Yan TD, Bannon PG, McCaughan BC. A systematic review of extrapleural pneumonectomy for malignant pleural mesothelioma. J Thorac Oncol. 2010;5:1692–703.
4. Burt BM, Cameron RB, Mollberg NM, Kosinski AS, Schipper PH, Shrager JB, et al. Malignant pleural mesothelioma and the Society of Thoracic Surgeons database: an analysis of surgical morbidity and mortality. J Thorac Cardiovasc Surg. 2014;148:30–5.
5. Sugarbaker DJ, Jaklitsch MT, Bueno R, Richards W, Lukanich J, Mentzer SJ, et al. Prevention, early detection, and management of complications after 328 consecutive extrapleural pneumonectomies. J Thorac Cardiovasc Surg. 2004;128(1):138–46.
6. Sugarbaker DJ, Flores RM, Jaklitsch MT, Richards WG, Strauss GM, Corson JM, et al. Resection margins, extrapleural nodal status, and cell type determine postoperative long-term survival in trimodality therapy of malignant pleural mesothelioma: results in 183 patients. J Thorac Cardiovasc Surg. 1999;117(1):54–63. discussion 63-5.
7. Tilleman TR, Richards WG, Zellos L, Johnson BE, Jaklitsch MT, Mueller J, et al. Extrapleural pneumonectomy followed by intracavitary intraoperative hyperthermic cisplatin with pharmacologic cytoprotection for treatment of malignant pleural mesothelioma: a phase II prospective study. J Thorac Cardiovasc Surg. 2009;138(2):405–11.
8. Rusch V, Baldini EH, Bueno R, De Perrot M, Flores R, Hasegawa S, et al. The role of surgical cytoreduction in the treatment of malignant pleural mesothelioma: meeting summary of the international mesothelioma interest group congress, September 11-14, 2012, Boston, Mass. J Thorac Cardiovasc Surg. 2013;145(4):909–10.
9. Cao C, Tian D, Manganas C, Matthews P, Yan TD. Systematic review of trimodality therapy for patients with malignant pleural mesothelioma. Ann Cardiothorac Surg. 2012;1(4):428–37.
10. Hartigan PM, Ng JM. Anesthetic strategies for patients undergoing extrapleural pneumonectomy. Thorac Surg Clin. 2004;14(4):575–83, xi.
11. Ng JM, Hartigan PM. Anesthetic management of patients undergoing extrapleural pneumonectomy for mesothelioma. Curr Opin Anaesthesiol. 2008;21(1):21–7.
12. Zellos L, Christiani DC. Epidemiology, biologic behavior, and natural history of mesothelioma. Thorac Surg Clin. 2004;14(4):469–77, viii.
13. Wagner JC, Sleggs CA, Marchand P. Diffuse pleural mesothelioma and asbestos exposure in the North Western Cape Province. Br J Ind Med. 1960;17:260–71.
14. Carbone M, Kratzke RA, Testa JR. The pathogenesis of mesothelioma. Semin Oncol. 2002;29(1):2–17.
15. Teta MJ, Mink PJ, Lau E, Sceurman BK, Foster ED. US mesothelioma patterns 1973-2002: indicators of change and insights into background rates. Eur J Cancer Prev. 2008;17(6):525–34.

16. Carroll N, Mohamed F, Sugarbaker P. Hyperthermic chemoper-fusion, and postoperative chemotherapy: The National Cancer Institute and Washington hospital center experience. In: Pass H, Vogelzang N, Carbone M, editors. Malignant mesothelioma: advances in pathogenesis, diagnosis and translational therapies. New York: Springer; 2005. p. 732–54.

17. Lee JM, Sugarbaker DJ. Extrapleural pneumonectomy for pleural malignancies. In: Sugarbaker DJ, Bueno R, Colson YL, Jaktlisch MT, Krasna MJ, Mentzer SJ, editors. Adult chest surgery. 2nd ed. New York: McGraw-Hill Professional; 2015. p. 998–1009.

18. Reilly JJ Jr. Evidence-based preoperative evaluation of candidates for thoracotomy. Chest. 1999;116(6 Suppl):S474–6.

19. Amar D, Burt ME, Roistacher N, Reinsel RA, Ginsberg RJ, Wilson RS. Value of perioperative Doppler echocardiography in patients undergoing major lung resection. Ann Thorac Surg. 1996;61(2):516–20.

20. Gill RR, Gerbaudo VH, Sugarbaker DJ, Hatabu H. Current trends in radiologic management of malignant pleural mesothelioma. Semin Thorac Cardiovasc Surg. 2009;21(2):111–20.

21. Slinger P. Update on anesthetic management for pneumonectomy. Curr Opin Anaesthesiol. 2009;22(1):31–7.

22. Wittnich C, Trudel J, Zidulka A, Chiu RC. Misleading "pulmonary wedge pressure" after pneumonectomy: its importance in postoperative fluid therapy. Ann Thorac Surg. 1986;42(2):192–6.

23. Brister NW, Barnette RE, Kim V, Keresztury M. Anesthetic considerations in candidates for lung volume reduction surgery. Proc Am Thorac Soc. 2008;5(4):432–7.

24. Ballantyne JC, Carr DB, deFerranti S, Suarez T, Lau J, Chalmers TC, et al. The comparative effects of postoperative analgesic therapies on pulmonary outcome: cumulative meta-analyses of randomized, controlled trials. Anesth Analg. 1998;86(3):598–612.

25. Beattie WS, Badner NH, Choi P. Epidural analgesia reduces postoperative myocardial infarction: a meta-analysis. Anesth Analg. 2001;93(4):853–8.

26. Oka T, Ozawa Y, Ohkubo Y. Thoracic epidural bupivacaine attenuates supraventricular tachyarrhythmias after pulmonary resection. Anesth Analg. 2001;93(2):253–9. 1st contents page.

27. Nino M, Body SC, Hartigan PM. The use of a bronchial blocker to rescue an ill-fitting double-lumen endotracheal tube. Anesth Analg. 2000;91(6):1370–1, TOC.

28. Senturk M, Slinger P, Cohen E. Intraoperative mechanical ventilation strategies for one-lung ventilation. Best Prac Res Clin Anaesthesiol. 2015;29(3):357–69.

29. Hurford WE, Kolker AC, Strauss HW. The use of ventilation/perfusion lung scans to predict oxygenation during one-lung anesthesia. Anesthesiology. 1987;67(5):841–4.

30. Bakaeen F, Rice D, Correa AM, Walsh GL, Vaporciyan AA, Putnam JB, et al. Use of aprotinin in extrapleural pneumonectomy: effect on hemostasis and incidence of complications. Ann Thorac Surg. 2007;84(3):982–6.

31. Slinger PD. Perioperative fluid management for thoracic surgery: the puzzle of postpneumonectomy pulmonary edema. J Cardiothorac Vasc Anesth. 1995;9(4):442–51.

32. Schipper PH, Nichols FC, Thomse KM, Deschamps C, Cassivi SD, Allen MS, et al. Malignant pleural mesothelioma: surgical management in 285 patients. Ann Thorac Surg. 2008;85(1):257–64.

33. Stewart DJ, Martin-Ucar AE, Edwards JG, West K, Waller DA. Extra-pleural pneumonectomy for malignant pleural mesothelioma: the risks of induction chemotherapy, right-sided procedures and prolonged operations. Eur J Cardiothorac Surg. 2005;27(3):373–8.

34. de Perrot M, McRae K, Anraku M, Karkouti K, Waddell TK, Pierre AF, et al. Risk factors for major complications after extrapleural pneumonectomy for malignant pleural mesothelioma. Ann Thorac Surg. 2008;85(4):1206–10.

35. Passman RS, Gingold DS, Amar D, Lloyd-Jones D, Bennett CL, Zhang H, et al. Prediction rule for atrial fibrillation after major noncardiac thoracic surgery. Ann Thorac Surg. 2005;79(5):1698–703.

36. Roselli EE, Murthy SC, Rice TW, Houghtaling PL, Pierce CD, Karchmer DP, et al. Atrial fibrillation complicating lung cancer resection. J Thorac Cardiovasc Surg. 2005;130(2):438–44.

37. Frendl G, Sodickson AC, Chung MK, Waldo AL, Gersh BJ, Tisdale JE, et al. 2014 AATS guidelines for the prevention and management of perioperative atrial fibrillation and flutter for thoracic surgical procedures. Executive summary. J Thorac Cardiovasc Surg. 2014;148(3):772–91.

38. Brown MJ, Brown DR. Thoracic cavity irrigation: an unusual cause of acute ST segment increase. Anesth Analg. 2002;95(3):552–4, table of contents.

39. Obata H, Saito S, Fujita N, Fuse Y, Ishizaki K, Goto F. Epidural block with mepivacaine before surgery reduces long-term postthoracotomy pain. Can J Anaesth. 1999;46(12):1127–32.

40. Senturk M, Ozcan PE, Talu GK, Kiyan E, Camci E, Ozyalcin S, et al. The effects of three different analgesia techniques on long-term postthoracotomy pain. Anesth Analg. 2002;94(1):11–5, table of contents.

41. Suzuki M, Haraguti S, Sugimoto K, Kikutani T, Shimada Y. Sakamoto A. Low-dose intravenous ketamine potentiates epidural analgesia after thoracotomy. Anesthesiology. 2006;105(1):111–9.

42. Wolf AS, Daniel J, Sugarbaker DJ. Surgical techniques for multimodality treatment of malignant pleural mesothelioma: extrapleural pneumonectomy and pleurectomy/decortication. Semin Thorac Cardiovasc Surg. 2009;21(2):132–48.

Pancoast Tumors and Combined Spinal Resections

37

Valerie W. Rusch, Ilya Laufer, Mark Bilsky, Alexandra Lewis, and David Amar

Key Points

- Pancoast tumors are very challenging lung cancers to treat because they involve vital structures including the brachial plexus, subclavian vessels, and spine.
- Multimodality management with induction chemoradiotherapy is now the standard of care.
- Preoperative planning between thoracic surgery, anesthesiology, and neurosurgery, including lung isolation technique, invasive hemodynamic monitoring, need for neurophysiologic monitoring, and a pain management plan, is essential.
- Surgical approach is determined by the anatomic location of the tumor and is performed from either a posterior or anterior approach or both.
- Because subclavian artery and vein involvement may require resection of these vessels, adequate intravascular monitoring and access must be planned.
- Pain control, pulmonary toilet, and physical therapy are key to achieving satisfactory postoperative recovery.

Introduction

Pancoast tumors, properly known as superior sulcus carcinomas, are a particularly challenging form of non-small cell lung cancer (NSCLC) to treat surgically because they commonly invade vital structures within and near the thoracic inlet. Invasion of the brachial plexus, subclavian vessels, and spine by direct tumor extension necessitates careful preoperative planning by surgeons and anesthesiologists. Originally described in 1924 [1] and again in 1932 [2], by Henry K. Pancoast, a radiologist at the University of Pennsylvania, this subset of NSCLC was considered inoperable, and thus fatal, for nearly two decades until the late 1950s when the combination of radiotherapy and surgery offered some curative hope. Pancoast's description of an apical chest tumor associated with shoulder and arm pain, a Horner's syndrome, and atrophy of the hand muscles describes the constellation of signs and symptoms of the syndrome that has come to bear his name.

Anatomy of Pancoast Tumors

An understanding of the anatomy of the superior sulcus is essential for the diagnosis and treatment of Pancoast tumors. The pulmonary sulcus is anatomically synonymous with the costovertebral gutter (the junction of the ribs to the vertebral column) in the posterior aspect of the chest and spans the thorax from the first rib down to the diaphragm. The superior pulmonary sulcus encompasses the most apical aspect of the gutter. Thus, a Pancoast tumor is a NSCLC arising in the apex of the lung located within the costovertebral gutter that causes constant pain due to local invasion into any of the following structures: the chest wall, spine, intercostal nerves, brachial plexus, subclavian vessels, sympathetic trunk, and stellate ganglion. The classic symptoms associated with Pancoast tumors are directly related to the structures compromised by this apicocostovertbral tumor. For instance,

V. W. Rusch (✉)
Thoracic Service, Department of Surgery, Memorial Sloan Kettering Cancer Center, New York, NY, USA
e-mail: ruschv@mskcc.org

I. Laufer · M. Bilsky
Department of Neurosurgery, Memorial Sloan Kettering Cancer Center, New York, NY, USA

A. Lewis
Department of Anesthesiology, Memorial Sloan Kettering Cancer Center, New York, NY, USA

D. Amar
Department of Anesthesiology and Critical Care Medicine, Memorial Sloan Kettering Cancer Center, New York, NY, USA

© Springer Nature Switzerland AG 2019
P. Slinger (ed.), *Principles and Practice of Anesthesia for Thoracic Surgery*, https://doi.org/10.1007/978-3-030-00859-8_37

shoulder pain is due to a combination of local invasion into the chest wall and intercostal nerves. Unrelenting pain radiating down the ulnar surface of the arm and 4th and 5th fingers results from T1 nerve root involvement, and motor weakness in the hand indicates C8 involvement. A Horner's syndrome is produced by tumor impingement on the sympathetic chain and stellate ganglion, structures located in the posterior aspect of the superior sulcus. Because some superior sulcus NSCLCs involve the subclavian vessels rather than the paravertebral area, the classification of a NSCLC as a Pancoast tumor has expanded to include all tumors of the superior sulcus whether or not there is involvement of the brachial plexus or stellate ganglion. NSCLCs located in the apex of the chest that involve the second rib or lower are not considered Pancoast tumors and are generally termed apical lung cancers.

The thoracic inlet is perhaps the most important anatomic area to understand when treating Pancoast tumors because this anatomic region encompasses crucial neurovascular structures and musculoskeletal elements and symptoms are directly related to the location of these tumors and their involvement of these structures. The surgical resection of superior sulcus tumors requires an intricate knowledge of these anatomic relationships and the consequences of resection, need for reconstruction, and risks of injury to the patient. The thoracic inlet is the superior aperture of the thoracic cavity bounded by the first thoracic vertebra (T1) posteriorly, the first ribs laterally, and the superior border of the manubrium anteriorly (Fig. 37.1) [3]. The root of the neck lies just superior to the thoracic inlet with the brachial plexus located in a superolateral position between the anterior and middle scalene muscles, superior to the first rib.

The thoracic inlet can be separated into three distinct compartments based on the insertion of the anterior and middle scalene muscles on the first rib and the posterior scalene muscle on the second rib. The anterior compartment is located in front of the anterior scalene muscle and contains the sternocleidomastoid and omohyoid muscles, the subclavian and internal jugular veins, and their branches. Tumors in this location tend to invade the first intercostal nerve and first rib resulting in pain in the upper and anterior chest wall (Fig. 37.2a, b). The middle compartment, located between the anterior and middle scalene muscles, includes the subclavian artery, the trunks of the brachial plexus, and the phrenic nerve that lies on the anterior surface of the anterior scalene muscle (Fig. 37.3). Tumors found in the middle compartment may invade the anterior scalene muscle, the phrenic nerve, the subclavian artery, and the trunks of the brachial plexus and middle scalene muscle. These tumors tend to present with signs and symptoms related to direct compression or infiltration of the brachial plexus such as pain and paresthesias in the ulnar distribution. The posterior compartment contains the nerve roots of the bra-

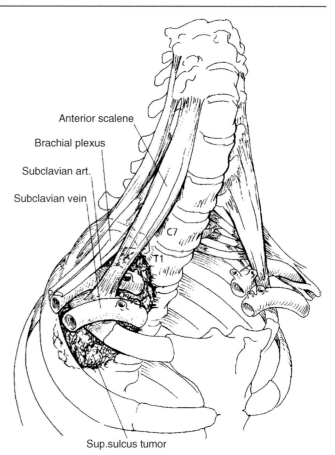

Fig. 37.1 The structure of the thoracic inlet. (From Nesbitt et al. Ref. [3], used with permission)

chial plexus, the stellate ganglion and the vertebral column, the posterior aspect of the subclavian artery, the paravertebral sympathetic chain, and the paravertebral musculature. Tumors in the posterior inlet can invade the transverse processes and vertebral bodies, as well as the spinal foramina (Fig. 37.4a, b), and be associated with neuromuscular pathology such as a Horner's syndrome (ptosis, miosis, and anhydrosis) and brachial plexopathy (weakness of the intrinsic muscles of the hand), paralysis of the flexors of the digits resembling a "claw hand," and diminished sensation over the medial side of the arm, forearm, and hand (related to C8 and T1 destruction).

Initial Assessment

Superior sulcus tumors or masses associated with chest and arm pain may be due to other pathologic processes including infectious conditions like tuberculosis or other malignant disorders including lymphoma, primary chest wall tumors, or metastatic disease from other neoplasms (Table 37.1) [4]. Therefore a diagnosis of NSCLC must be confirmed before instituting definitive therapy. This is best accomplished by

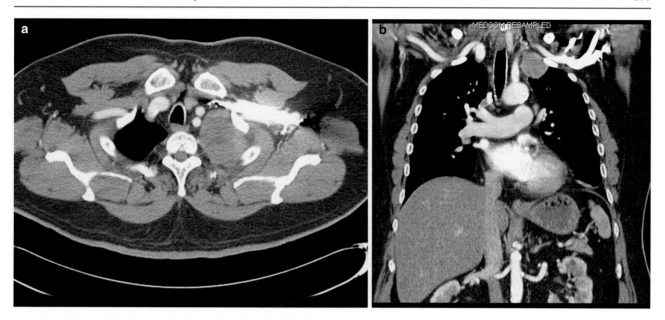

Fig. 37.2 (**a**, **b**) Left Pancoast tumor, clinical stage T3 filling superior sulcus but not invading spine or involving subclavian vessels (**a**). The extent of the tumor is also well defined on the coronal view of the CT scan

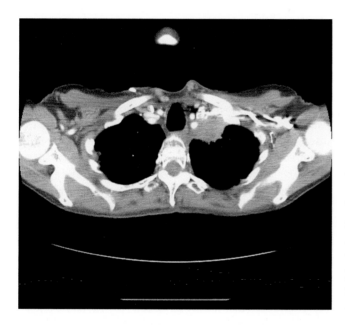

Fig. 37.3 Anteriorly located left Pancoast tumor involving subclavian vessels requiring anterior "Dartevelle" approach to resection

transthoracic fine needle aspiration (FNA) or core needle biopsy.

Once a diagnosis of NSCLC has been made, the extent of disease should be evaluated before surgical resection is considered. Patients are evaluated with a computed tomography (CT) of the chest and upper abdomen with intravenous contrast, including the adrenals, whole-body positron-emission tomography (FDG-PET), and a brain magnetic resonance imaging (MRI) to exclude metastatic disease in extrathoracic sites as well as in the mediastinum. Pancoast tumors are, by

definition, at least stage IIB lung cancers, with a significant risk of mediastinal nodal involvement approaching 10 to 20% of patients [5]. Because Pancoast tumors with mediastinal nodal involvement (N2 or N3 disease) have markedly worse survival than those that are N0 or N1, further staging by endobronchial ultrasound (EBUS) and/or mediastinoscopy should be considered if CT and PET suggest mediastinal nodal disease [6].

Due to the unique anatomic position of these tumors, diagnostic imaging with contrast MRI plays an essential role in defining the extent of local invasion and thus, resectability. The brachial plexus, subclavian vessels, vertebrae, and neural foramina are best visualized well with this modality. T1 involvement and resection are well tolerated; however, resection of the C8 nerve root and lower trunk of the brachial plexus generally leads to permanent loss of intrinsic hand function and lower arm function. Radiographic evidence of spine involvement, or neurologic symptoms and signs suggestive of nerve root or brachial plexus pathology, necessitates joint evaluation of these patients by a thoracic surgeon and a spine surgeon. At Memorial Sloan Kettering, the treatment of all Pancoast tumors is planned jointly by the thoracic surgeon and spine neurosurgeon.

Multimodality Treatment

From the late 1950s to the present day, the therapeutic approach to Pancoast tumors has evolved into a multidisciplinary and multimodality treatment regimen that includes induction chemoradiotherapy and resection. In 1956, Chardack and MacCallum described successful treatment of

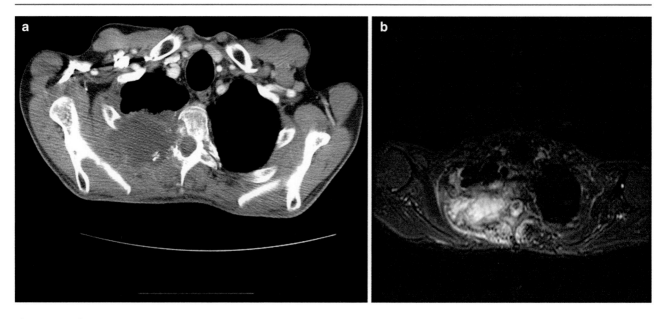

Fig. 37.4 (**a**, **b**) Right Pancoast tumor invading chest wall and destroying adjacent vertebral body as shown on CT (**a**) and MR (**b**) scans

Table 37.1 Causes of Pancoast's syndrome

Neoplastic	
Lung neoplasms	Primary bronchogenic
	Adenoid cystic carcinomas
	Hemangiopericytoma
	Mesothelioma
Metastatic neoplasms	Laryngeal cancer
	Cervical cancer
	Uroepithelial cancer
	Thyroid cancer
Hematologic neoplasms	Lymphoma
	Plasmacytoma
Infectious	
Bacterial	Staphylococcal pneumonia
	Pseudomonal pneumonia
	Actinomycosis
Fungal	Aspergillosis
	Cryptococcosis
	Tuberculosis
Parasitic	Hydatid cyst

a Pancoast tumor by en bloc resection of the right upper lobe, chest wall, and nerve roots followed by adjuvant radiotherapy leading to a 5-year survival in that patient [7]. In 1961, Shaw and colleagues reported their experience with a patient who presented with Pancoast's syndrome but became symptom-free after 30 Gy of radiotherapy and then went on to a successful resection. This treatment strategy was then applied to 18 more patients with good local control and better than expected long-term survival [8]. The Shaw and Paulson approach, based on induction radiotherapy and en bloc resection, then became the standard of care for Pancoast tumors. During the next 30 years, the basic approach to treat-

ment remained unchanged. The largest retrospective study published to date, from Memorial Sloan Kettering Cancer Center, defined negative prognostic factors including mediastinal lymph node metastases, N2 disease, vertebral and subclavian vessel involvement, and incomplete resection [6]. Complete (R0) resection was achieved in only 64% of patients with T3N0 disease and 39% of patients with T4N0 disease, and locoregional relapse was the most common site of tumor recurrence. Anatomic lobectomy was associated with a better outcome than sublobar resection, and intraoperative brachytherapy did not enhance overall survival [9]. This retrospective study documented the results of "standard" treatment for resectable Pancoast tumors during a nearly 40-year period and emphasized the need for novel approaches that would improve both local control and survival.

Because combined modality therapy was increasingly being used for other locally advanced NSCLC subsets (e.g., stage IIIA (N2) disease) [10], induction chemoradiotherapy followed by surgical resection was studied in a large North American prospective multi-institutional phase II trial for Pancoast tumors (T3–4 N0-1M0 tumors) [11]. A total of 110 eligible patients were enrolled on this study and received induction therapy using 2 cycles of cisplatin and etoposide chemotherapy along with 45 Gy of concurrent radiotherapy. Patients with stable or responding disease then underwent thoracotomy and resection followed by two more cycles of chemotherapy. Induction therapy was well tolerated allowing 75% of enrolled patients to go on to thoracotomy. R0 resection was achieved in 91% of T3 and 87% of T4 tumors. Approximately 1/3 of patient had no residual viable tumors, 1/3 had minimal residual microscopic disease, and 1/3 had gross residual tumor on final pathology. Patients who had a R0 resection experienced a 53 percent survival at 5 years, and the most common sites of relapse were distant rather than locoregional. Several more recent studies, including a multicenter prospective clinical trial from Japan, confirm these results [12–16] and establish induction chemoradiotherapy and surgery as standard care for resectable Pancoast tumors.

Surgical Approaches to Resection

The goal of any cancer operation is the complete resection of the tumor with negative margins. In the case of Pancoast tumors, due to their unique location at the apex of the chest and at times their involvement of the thoracic inlet, complete resection is challenging and usually includes the upper lobe, involved chest wall with or without the subclavian vessels, portions of the vertebral column and T1 nerve root, and dorsal sympathetic chain. Pancoast tumors may be approached through an extended high posterolateral thoracotomy incision (Paulson's approach) or through an anterior approach popularized by Dartevelle.

Posterior Approach

The patient is positioned in the lateral decubitus position but rotated slightly anteriorly to provide exposure to the paravertebral region (Fig. 37.5) [17]. A standard posterolateral thoracotomy is performed in the 5th intercostal and the chest explored to make sure that there is no evidence of metastatic disease. If the tumor appears resectable, the incision is extended superiorly to the base of the neck following a line midway between the spinous process and the edge of the scapula (Fig. 37.5). Extension of the incision anteriorly around the anterior border of the scapula up toward the axilla can also be used to enhance exposure. The scapula is elevated away from the chest wall with either a rib-spreading retractor or internal mammary retractor with good visualization of the apex of the chest. The scalene muscles are detached from the first and second ribs and the first rib exposed. Involved ribs are divided anteriorly to allow for a 4 cm margin away from the tumor. Dissection is carried along the superior border of the first rib subperiosteal plane in anterior to posterior direction. To facilitate the posterior dissection, the erector spinae muscles are retracted off the thoracic spine allowing for visualization of the costovertebral gutter. To provide an adequate posterior margin, the transverse processes and rib heads are usually resected en bloc. Anterior division of the ribs facilitates the disarticulation of the chest wall from vertebral column and when possible should be performed prior to sectioning of the transverse

processes. Palpation of the interarticularis (i.e., lateral border of the facet joint) defines the medial border of transverse process osteotomy. The osteotomy is generally performed using a curved osteotome, which is used to transect the transverse processes and costovertebral joint. The chest wall can then be retracted laterally and anteriorly, allowing visualization of the intercostal nerves, which are meticulously ligated before division to prevent leak of cerebrospinal fluid. Bleeding near the neural foramina is carefully controlled with bipolar electrocautery. Thoracic nerve roots below T1 are generally transected without neurologic sequelae. Since the T1 nerve root provides motor innervation to the hand, it is examined for tumor involvement and only ligated in cases of tumor invasion. Division of the T1 nerve root may cause mild weakness of the intrinsic muscles of the hand, but division of the C8 nerve root will result in permanent paralysis. Frozen sections are used liberally during the operation to determine the necessary extent of resection. Dissection and ligation of the nerve roots usually represent the final step of disarticulation of the chest wall from the spine. After the chest wall resection is completed, the detached chest wall is allowed to fall into the chest cavity and an upper lobectomy and mediastinal lymph node dissection is completed in the standard fashion. Reconstruction of the chest wall is not necessary unless the defect created is larger than the first three ribs in which case the angle of the scapula can herniate into the chest cavity causing pain and impaired movement. If a chest wall reconstruction is needed, a 2-mm-thick Gore-Tex patch (WL Gore, Flagstaff, AZ, USA) is sutured to the margins of resection under tension and secured in place.

Tumors Involving the Vertebral Bodies and Epidural Region

Vertebral body invasion by Pancoast tumors is not necessarily a contraindication to surgical resection. The development of better instrumentation for spine stabilization now permits a more aggressive approach to these tumors [17, 18]. Currently, with multimodality therapy, T4 lesions with vertebral body or epidural extension can be considered for resection with curative intent. At Memorial Sloan Kettering Cancer Center, spine MRI images are used to divide tumors into four classes, A–D, based on the degree of spinal column and neural tube involvement [17]. Class A and B tumors are T3 lesions that are amenable to complete R0 resection. Class A tumors involve only the periosteum of the vertebral bodies, and class B tumors are limited to the rib heads and distal neural foramina (Fig. 37.6). Class C and D tumors are T4 lesions that are not amenable to en bloc resection but can still be completely resected. Class C tumors extended into the neural foramina, limited or no vertebral body involvement but do have unilateral epidural compression. Class D tumors

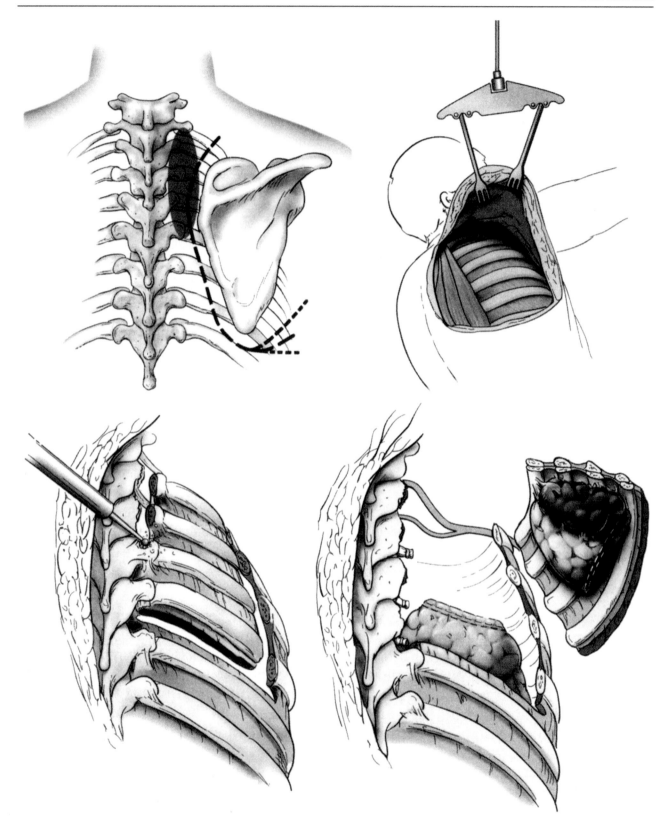

Fig. 37.5 Artist's illustration of a posterolateral thoracotomy. Upper left: incision is made midway between the spinous processes and medial border of the scapula and extending over the inferior border. Upper right: The rhomboid and levator scapulae muscles are sectioned to elevate the scapula from the chest wall by using a mammary self-retaining retractor. Lower left: The paraspinal muscles are dissected to expose the junction of the laminae and transverse processes. The drill is used to resect the transverse processes distal to the pedicle to expose the neural foramen. For a Type C resection, the laminae, facet joints, and pedicles are resected to expose the lateral dura. Lower right: the chest wall is then pushed forward, and the nerve roots are ligated at the distal neural foramen. En bloc chest wall and tumor resection are accomplished. (From Bilsky et al. Ref. [17], used with permission)

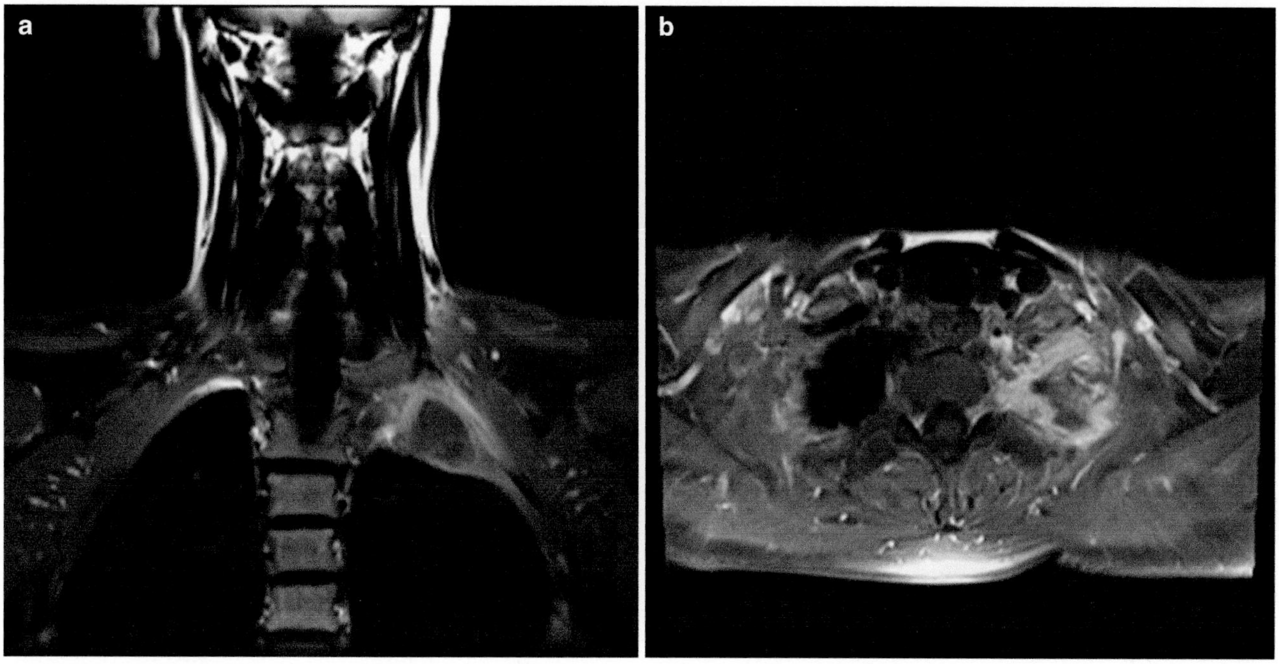

Fig. 37.6 Class B tumor (Figure 6A) with invasion of the rib head and neural foramen (Figure 6B). Patient underwent R0 excision using the posterior thoracotomy

involve the vertebral column, either the vertebral body and/or lamina with or without epidural compression. Class A and B and some class C tumors can be approached through posterolateral thoracotomy. A high-speed drill is used to remove involved vertebral bodies. The junction between the vertebral body and the pedicle provides an important landmark for vertebral body removal, signaling proximity to the spinal cord. The posterior longitudinal ligament is removed and provides a margin on the anterior dura. The disc spaces adjacent to the tumor are exenterated in order to aid in spinal fixation. Anterior reconstruction alone is sufficient for resections of one to two vertebral bodies. Autologous bone from the iliac crest or non-diseased rib, allograft fibula, methymethacrylate with Steinman pins, or corpectomy cages can all be used for reconstruction. Anterior approach provides very limited access to the T1 and T2 vertebrae and epidural space. Therefore patients requiring any degree of epidural decompression in the upper thoracic spine generally undergo posterior approach surgery along with the anterior approach. Furthermore, tumors with significant extension into the vertebral body place patients at high risk of postoperative mechanical instability, especially since the supporting chest wall is removed. Such patients may benefit from long-segment posterolateral spinal instrumentation and fusion in order to avoid development of debilitating deformity.

Class D tumors that involve the posterior elements (spinous process, laminae, and pedicles) are resected through a combined anterior/posterior approach. During the first stage of the operation, patients are positioned prone and a poste-rior midline incision made. Subperiosteal dissection is used to expose the level of the tumor along with several levels above and below the tumor in order to permit placement of posterior spinal instrumentation. The involved areas of the spinous process, laminae, and pedicles are resected. Epidural tumor is dissected off the dura and a multilevel resection of affected nerve roots done. Posterior fixation is accomplished in order to maintain coronal and sagittal stability (Fig. 37.7). If soft tissue over the reconstruction is inadequate, muscle flap rotation by a plastic surgeon can be done to reduce the risk of skin breakdown and infection of the spine hardware [18, 19]. Once the posterior resection and reconstruction are complete, the incision is closed, the patient turned to the lateral decubitus position, a posterolateral thoracotomy performed, and the lung and chest wall resection completed. The proximity and the parallel orientation of the thoracotomy and midline incisions result in a challenging environment for wound healing, and low threshold for plastic surgery consultation is recommended.

Anterior Approaches

Pancoast tumors that involve the subclavian vessels are best approached anteriorly. Although several different approaches have been described [20–25], the anterior transcervical approach, originally described by Dartevelle and modified by others [26], is considered the standard approach for this subset of Pancoast tumors.

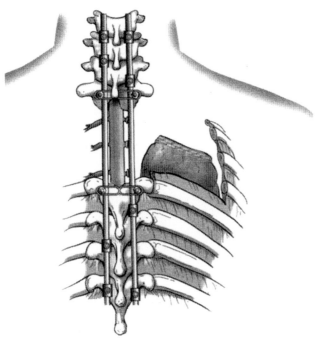

Fig. 37.7 Artist's illustration depicting a posterolateral transpedicular approach for class D tumor with bilateral posterior segmental fixation. (From Bilsky et al. Ref. [17], used with permission)

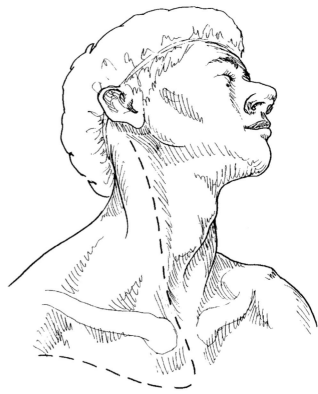

Fig. 37.8 An anterior transcervical incision is made and curved under the head of the clavicle in an L-fashion. (From Nesbitt et al. Ref. [3], used with permission)

The patient is positioned supine with the neck hyperextended and the head turned to the opposite side of the lesion [27, 28]. An inverted L-shaped incision is carried down the anterior border of the sternocleidomastoid muscle and extended below the clavicle to the level of the second intercostal space and then turned horizontally following a parallel line below the clavicle to the deltopectoral groove (Fig. 37.8). The sternal attachment of the sternocleidomastoid is divided along with the insertion of the pectoralis major. A myocutaneous flap is then folded laterally exposing the thoracic inlet. The scalene fat pad is excised and sent for frozen section to determine lymph node involvement. If the tumor is deemed resectable, the upper part of the manubrium is divided and the incision carried into the second intercostal space via an L-shaped incision. The involved section of the subclavian vein is resected but not reconstructed (collateral venous flow around this area being sufficient).

Next, the anterior scalene muscle is divided either at its insertion onto the first rib. The phrenic nerve is identified and preserved. The subclavian artery is resected and reconstructed with a 8 or 10 mm polytetrafluoroethylene (PTFE) graft (Fig. 37.9). The middle scalene muscle is detached above its insertion on the first rib to expose the C8 and T1 nerve roots. These are dissected in a lateral to medial direction up to the confluence of the lower trunk and brachial plexus. The ipsilateral prevertebral muscles and paravertebral sympathetic chain and stellate ganglion are then resected off the anterior aspect of the vertebral bodies of C7 and T1.

The T1 nerve root is commonly divided just lateral to the T1 intervertebral foramen.

Attention can now be placed on the chest wall resection. The anterolateral arch of the first rib is divided at the costochondral junction, and the second rib is divided at its midpoint. The third rib is dissected on its superior border in a posterior direction toward the costovertebral angle, and the first two through three ribs are disarticulated from the transverse processes. From this cavity, an upper lobectomy is completed. If exposure for the lobectomy and chest wall resection is inadequate, the anterior incision is closed and the patient turned into the lateral decubitus position. The remainder of the resection can then be performed via a posterolateral thoracotomy incision.

Anesthetic Considerations

Lung isolation with a left-sided double-lumen tube or right-sided bronchial blocker can be used depending on surgeon and anesthesiologist experience and preference. Intra-arterial blood pressure monitoring and large bore IV access should be placed on the opposite side of the tumor. If there is potential for SVC or innominate vein resection, venous access via the femoral region or lower extremity is advisable. Central

Fig. 37.9 The phrenic nerve and subclavian vein are retracted. The anterior scalene muscle is divided to expose the subclavian artery. (From Nesbitt et al. Ref. [3], used with permission)

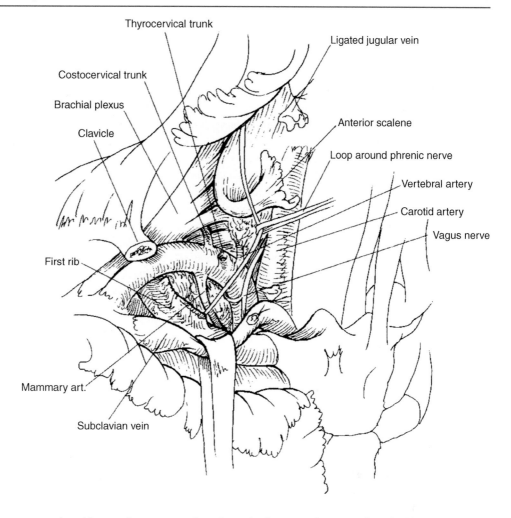

venous catheterization on the nonoperative side may be considered if adequate IV access is unavailable or if the patient's cardiovascular reserve is limited and perioperative use of vasoactive agents is anticipated. There are sparse data on whether to employ neurophysiologic monitoring during resection of Pancoast tumors. In the case of thoracic and thoracoabdominal aortic aneurysm repair where spinal cords ischemia is a devastating complication, a recent prospective series of 233 patients demonstrated that normal somatosensory and motor evoked potential monitoring intraoperatively had a strong negative predictive value indicating that patients without signal loss are unlikely to awake with a neurologic deficit, whereas irreversible changes on monitoring were significantly associated with immediate postoperative neurologic deficit [29]. If spine stabilization is required, it is our practice to employ somatosensory and motor evoked potential monitoring intraoperatively. The cause of reversible changes during surgery is often due to compression of segmental spinal arteries or spinal cord hypoperfusion. Both of these situations can lead to spinal cord infarction unless corrected usually by pharmacologically elevating the patient's blood pressure. During neurophysiologic monitoring, the use of inhalation agents can depress the amplitude

and prolong the latency of measured evoked potentials. It is generally accepted that a decrease in amplitude by >50% and an increase in latency are defined as clinically significant [30]. Therefore, it is customary to employ minimal inhalation anesthesia balanced by total intravenous anesthetic regimens with Bispectral brain monitoring when feasible.

Since lobectomy or pneumonectomy is needed in some cases, protective one-lung ventilation and judicious fluid administration are recommended due to the risk of postoperative pulmonary edema and respiratory distress in these patients. Trends in pulse pressure variation (PPV) can be used noninvasively to assess fluid status during anesthesia and one-lung ventilation during thoracic surgery. A very small study suggested that PPV can predict fluid responsiveness under protective lung ventilation (FiO2 1.0, tidal volume 6 mL/kg, PEEP 5 mmHg) compared to conventional one-lung ventilation (FiO2 1.0, tidal volume 10 mL/kg, no PEEP), and its use may improve hemodynamic conditions in individual patients [31]. Other traditional methods of assessing fluid status include traditional hemodynamic parameters and urine output. Despite knowing that a patient may be relatively dry, this is often our choice in the management of lung resection patients.

While fluid management is complex, pain management poses a significant challenge for the anesthesiologist. Pain control must be accomplished, usually with an epidural catheter, in order to aid in early mobilization, pulmonary toilet, and chest physiotherapy. It is strongly advised to consider a multimodal pain regimen along with epidural analgesia. Preoperative medications with gabapentin or pregabalin are reasonable to manage neuropathic pain. The use of non-opioid adjuvants, like intravenous dexmedetomidine and ketamine, may reduce intraoperative opioid requirements. While there are limited and conflicting studies on the use of dexmedetomidine for neuromonitoring, a low-dose infusion without a loading dose may prevent intraoperative hypotension and minimize changes in evoked potentials. Dexmedetomidine as an adjuvant to desflurane and remifentanil anesthesia, at target plasma concentration of up to 0.6 ng/ml, has not been shown to change SSEPs or MEPs response during complex spinal surgery by any clinical significant amount [32]. Unlike dexmedetomidine, ketamine achieves greater hemodynamic stability with minimal effect on mean arterial pressure and heart rate. The advantage of ketamine is its dual property as a potent analgesic and an anesthetic agent, which can cause increases in the amplitude of somatosensory and motor evoked potentials. While the use of ketamine and dexmedetomidine is gaining wide acceptance as adjuvants during neuromonitoring, the use of intravenous lidocaine during surgery is emerging as a reasonable option for patients ineligible for an epidural catheter. Lidocaine has been shown to depress the amplitude and prolong the latency of SSEPs, but the SSEP waveforms remain preserved and interpretable when used as a part of a narcotic-based anesthetic [33]. Acetaminophen and non-steroidal anti-inflammatory agents are routinely administered, and their use is strongly advised in the absence of renal or hepatic dysfunction.

In complex chronic pain patients, it is strongly recommended to involve a pain specialist to assist with intraoperative and postoperative pain control. Patients with chronic pain will likely have opioid tolerance, thus requiring a careful multimodal approach that might include epidural analgesia, intravenous ketamine infusion, and the addition of methadone in extreme cases.

Postoperative Considerations

The most common postoperative complications are respiratory (atelectasis, pneumonia) and are related to the extent of the incision and associated pain. Adequate pain control and intensive respiratory care are pivotal to preventing these problems. The patient should be mobilized the first postoperative day with attention to chest physiotherapy. Awake bronchoscopic suctioning may be required to clear retained secretions in those patients who have an ineffective cough. Other postoperative complications are those usually seen after pulmonary resection, including supraventricular cardiac dysrhythmias, bleeding, wound infection, or empyema. Chylothoraces can occur in patients who had had extensive resections in the paravertebral region (either right- or left-sided). Infection of the hardware used for spine stabilization is an uncommon but very serious adverse event that may require reoperation and drainage.

Clinical Case Discussion

Case: A 50-year-old man with a recent history of dyspnea on exertion and recurrent pneumonias for the past year is scheduled for surgical resection of a large apical right lung mass (Fig. 37.4a). He is a former 40 pack-year smoker. He has moderately severe but clinically stable multiple sclerosis. He reports pain in his shoulder radiating down his arm but has normal strength and function in his right hand. CT scan, PET scan, and MRI have been done and suggest no evidence of metastatic disease but extension into the paravertebral area and spine.

Questions

1. What position(s) will the patient be in for resection?
2. What is your plan for intravascular monitoring and access?
3. Do you think a chest wall reconstruction will be necessary?
4. If the vertebral bodies are involved, what other exposure is necessary?
5. What strategy do you have for fluid management and postoperative pain control?

Discussion

Based on the history and preoperative imaging, this patient has a superior sulcus tumor or Pancoast tumor, involving vital structures in the thoracic inlet and spine. A combined posterior and anterior approach will be necessary for complete resection (see description in text). The patient will be placed prone for the spine resection and stabilization. Once that is completed, the patient will be rotated into the lateral decubitus position and a posterolateral thoracotomy performed to complete the lobectomy and chest wall resection and reconstruction.

References

1. Pancoast HK. Importance of careful roentgen-ray investigations of apical chest tumors. J Am Med Assoc. 1924;83:1407–11.
2. Pancoast HK. Superior pulmonary sulcus tumor. J Am Med Assoc. 1932;99:1391–6.
3. Nesbitt JC, Wind GG, Rusch VW, Walsh GL. Superior sulcus tumor resection. In: Nesbitt JC, Wind GG, Deslauriers J, Faber LP, Ginsberg RJ, Moores DWO, et al., editors. Thoracic surgical oncology. Philadelphia: Lippincott Williams & Wilkins; 2003. p. 162–93.
4. Arcasoy SM, Jett JR. Superior pulmonary sulcus tumors and Pancoast's syndrome. N Engl J Med. 1997;337:1370–6.
5. Detterbeck FC. Changes in the treatment of Pancoast tumors. Ann Thorac Surg. 2003;75:1990–7.
6. Rusch VW, Parekh KR, Leon L, et al. Factors determining outcome after surgical resection of T3 and T4 lung cancers of the superior sulcus. J Thorac Cardiovasc Surg. 2000;119:1147–53.
7. Chardack WM, MacCallum JD. Pancoast tumor (five year survival without recurrence or metastases following radical resection and postoperative irradiation). J Thorac Surg. 1956;31:535–42.
8. Shaw RR, Paulson DL, Kee JL Jr. Treatment of the superior sulcus tumor by irradiation followed by resection. Ann Surg. 1961;154:29–40.
9. Ginsberg RJ, Martini N, Zaman M, et al. Influence of surgical resection and brachytherapy in the management of superior sulcus tumor. Ann Thorac Surg. 1994;57:1440–5.
10. Albain KS, Rusch VW, Crowley JJ, et al. Concurrent cisplatin/etoposide plus chest radiotherapy followed by surgery for stages IIIA (N2) and IIIB non-small cell lung cancer: mature results of Southwest Oncology Group Phase II study 8805. J Clin Oncol. 1995;13:1880–92.
11. Rusch VW, Giroux DJ, Kraut MJ, et al. Induction chemoradiation and surgical resection for superior sulcus non-small cell lung carcinomas: long-term results of Southwest Oncology Group trial 9416 (Intergroup trial 0160). J Clin Oncol. 2007;25:313–8.
12. Marra A, Eberhardt W, Pöttgen C, et al. Induction chemotherapy, concurrent chemoradiation and surgery for Pancoast tumour. Eur Respir J. 2007;29:117–27.
13. Fischer S, Darling G, Pierre AF, et al. Induction chemoradiation therapy followed by surgical resection for non-small cell lung cancer (NSCLC) invading the thoracic inlet. Eur J Cardiothorac Surg. 2008;33:1129–34.
14. Kunitoh H, Kato H, Tsuboi M, et al. Phase II trial of preoperative chemoradiotherapy followed by surgical resection in patients with superior sulcus non-small cell lung cancers: report of Japan Clinical Oncology Group Trial 9806. J Clin Oncol. 2008;26:644–9.
15. Kappers I, van Sandick JW, Burgers JA, et al. Results of combined modality treatment in patients with non-small cell lung cancer of the superior sulcus and the rationale for surgical resection. Eur J Cardiothorac Surg. 2009;36:741–6.
16. Antonoff MB, Hofstetter WL, Correa AM, et al. Clinical prediction of pathologic complete response in superior sulcus non-small cell lung cancer. Ann Thorac Surg. 2016;101:211–7.
17. Bilsky MH, Vitaz TW, Boland PJ, Bains MS, Rajaraman V, Rusch VW. Surgical treatment of superior sulcus tumors with spinal and brachial plexus involvement. J Neurosurg. 2002;97(3 Suppl):301–9.
18. Gandhi S, Walsh GL, Komaki R, et al. A multidisciplinary surgical approach to superior sulcus tumors with vertebral invasion. Ann Thorac Surg. 1999;68:1778–85.
19. Bolton WD, Rice DC, Goodyear A, et al. Superior sulcus tumors with vertebral body involvement: a multimodality approach. J Thorac Cardiovasc Surg. 2009;137(6):1379–87.
20. Masaoka A, Ito Y, Yasumitsu T. Anterior approach for tumor of the superior sulcus. J Thorac Cardiovasc Surg. 1979;78:413–5.
21. Niwa H, Masaoka A, Yamakawa Y, Fukai I, Kiriyama M. Surgical therapy for apical invasive lung cancer: different approaches according to tumor location. Lung Cancer. 1993;10:63–71.
22. Nazari S. Transcervical approach (Dartevelle technique) for resection of lung tumors invading the thoracic inlet, sparing the clavicle. J Thorac Cardiovasc Surg. 1996;112:558.
23. Marshall MB, Kucharczuk JC, Shrager JB, Kaiser LR. Anterior surgical approaches to the thoracic outlet. J Thorac Cardiovasc Surg. 2006;131(6):1255–60.
24. Grunenwald D, Spaggiari L, Girard P, Baldeyrou P. Transmanubrial approach to the thoracic inlet. J Thorac Cardiovasc Surg. 1997;113:958.
25. Klima U, Lichtenberg A, Haverich A. Transmanubrial approach reproposed: reply. Ann Thorac Surg. 1999;68:1888.
26. Dartevelle PG, Chapelier AR, Macchiarini P, et al. Anterior transcervical-thoracic approach for radical resection of lung tumors invading the thoracic inlet. J Thorac Cardiovasc Surg. 1993;105:1025–34.
27. Macchiarini P. Resection of superior sulcus carcinomas (anterior approach). Thorac Surg Clin. 2004;14:229–40.
28. Fadel E, Missenard G, Chapelier A, et al. En bloc resection of non-small cell lung cancer invading the thoracic inlet and intervertebral foramina. J Thorac Cardiovasc Surg. 2002;123:676–85.
29. Keyhani K, Miller CC III, Estrera AL, Wegryn T, Sheinbaum R, Safi HJ. Analysis of motor and somatosensory evoked potentials during thoracic and thoracoabdominal aortic aneurysm repair. J Vasc Surg. 2009;49(1):36–41.
30. Higgs M, Hackworth RJ, John K, Riffenburgh R, Tomlin J, Wamsley B. The intraoperative effect of methadone on somatosensory evoked potentials. J Neurosurg Anesthesiol. 2017;29(2):168–74.
31. Lee JH, Jeon Y, Bahk JH, et al. Pulse pressure variation as a predictor of fluid responsiveness during one-lung ventilation for lung surgery using thoracotomy: randomised controlled study. Eur J Anaesthesiol. 2011;28(1):39–44.
32. Bala E, Sessler DI, Nair DR, McLain R, Dalton JE, Farag E. Motor and somatosensory evoked potentials are well maintained in patients given dexmedetomidine during spine surgery. Anesthesiology. 2008;109(3):417–25.
33. Schubert A, Licina MG, Glaze GM, Paranandi L. Systemic lidocaine and human somatosensory-evoked potentials during sufentanil-isoflurane anaesthesia. Can J Anaesth. 1992;39(6):569–75.

Anesthesia for Esophageal Surgery

38

Randal S. Blank, Stephen R. Collins, Julie L. Huffmyer,
and J. Michael Jaeger

Key Points
- Patients presenting for esophageal surgery frequently have comorbidities including cardiopulmonary disease which should be evaluated per published ACC/AHA guidelines. Particular attention should be paid to symptoms and signs of esophageal obstruction, GERD, and malnutrition which may affect the risk of perioperative complications.
- Postoperative pain control strategies are dictated by the surgical approach to the esophagus. Use of thoracic epidural analgesia in patients undergoing transthoracic esophageal surgery provides optimal pain control, permits early patient extubation and mobilization, and may improve outcomes.
- Patients presenting for esophageal surgery commonly have pathology which increases their risk of regurgitation and aspiration. This is particularly true for patients with achalasia and other motor disorders of the esophagus, high-grade esophageal obstruction, esophageal diverticula, and severe GERD. Consideration should be given to awake intubation or rapid sequence induction with the patient in a head-up position and appropriate postoperative care, including gastric drainage.

- Excessive perioperative intravenous fluid administration may lead to exaggerated fluid shifts toward the interstitial space causing increased complications such as poor wound healing, slower return of GI function, abdominal compartment syndrome, impaired anastomotic healing, increased cardiac demand, pneumonia, and respiratory failure. The ideal fluid regimen for major esophageal surgery should be individualized, optimizing cardiac output and oxygen delivery while avoiding excessive fluid administration.
- Patients presenting for emergent repair of esophageal disruption, rupture, or perforation may present with hypovolemia, sepsis, and shock. Anesthetic management strategies should be based on the severity of these presenting conditions and the nature of the planned procedure.
- Esophageal anastomotic leak is a frequent complication associated with high morbidity and mortality and is likely to be a function of numerous surgical, systemic, and possibly anesthetic factors. Since anastomotic integrity is dependent upon adequate blood flow and oxygen delivery, the development of anastomotic leak may be related to intraoperative management variables, particularly systemic blood pressure, cardiac output, and oxygen delivery and may thus be modifiable by anesthetic management. In the euvolemic patient, the use of pressors does not appear to compromise conduit or anastomotic perfusion.

R. S. Blank (✉) · S. R. Collins
J. L. Huffmyer · J. M. Jaeger
Department of Anesthesiology, University of Virginia Health
System, Charlottesville, VA, USA
e-mail: rsb8p@virginia.edu; SRC2F@hscmail.mcc.virginia.edu;
JH3WD@hscmail.mcc.virginia.edu; JMJ4W@hscmail.mcc.
virginia.edu

Abbreviations

ALI	Acute lung injury
ARDS	Acute respiratory distress syndrome
COPD	Chronic obstructive pulmonary disease

© Springer Nature Switzerland AG 2019
P. Slinger (ed.), *Principles and Practice of Anesthesia for Thoracic Surgery*, https://doi.org/10.1007/978-3-030-00859-8_38

CT	Computerized tomography
CXR	Chest X-ray (radiograph)
DLT	Double-lumen endotracheal tube(s)
ECG	Electrocardiogram
EGD	Esophagogastroduodenoscopy
ERAS	Enhanced recovery after surgery
EUS	Endoscopic ultrasound
GDFT	Goal-directed fluid therapy
GERD	Gastroesophageal reflux disease
GI	Gastrointestinal
LEA	Lumbar epidural analgesia
LES	Lower esophageal sphincter
LVEDVI	Left ventricular end-diastolic volume index
MIE	Minimally invasive esophagectomy
MRI	Magnetic resonance imaging
NGT	Nasogastric tube
OLV	One-lung ventilation
PCA	Patient-controlled analgesia
PEEP	Positive end-expiratory pressure
PET	Positron emission tomography
PH	Paraesophageal hernia(s)
PONV	Postoperative nausea and vomiting
PVB	Paravertebral block
SLT	Single-lumen endotracheal tube(s)
SVV	Stroke volume variation
TEA	Thoracic epidural analgesia
TEF	Tracheoesophageal fistula
THE	Transhiatal esophagectomy
TTE	Transthoracic esophagectomy
UES	Upper esophageal sphincter

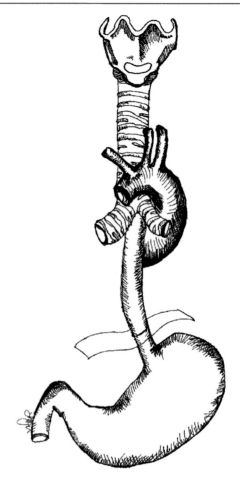

Fig. 38.1 Anatomic relationships between the esophagus, airway, aorta, diaphragm, and stomach

Anatomy and Physiology of the Esophagus

The adult esophagus is a muscular tube, 18–26 cm in length, which acts as a conduit for the passage of food from the oral cavity into the stomach (Fig. 38.1). The esophagus begins at the level of the oropharynx; it then enters the superior mediastinum behind the trachea and left recurrent laryngeal nerve and passes into the posterior mediastinum behind the left mainstem bronchus. It continues caudad passing posteriorly to the left atrium but anterior to the descending thoracic aorta. At the level of T10, the esophagus joins the stomach at the cardia after passing through the hiatus in the right diaphragm.

The upper esophagus is supplied by arterial branches of the superior and inferior thyroid arteries, whereas the mid-esophagus receives its blood supply from the bronchial and right intercostal arteries as well as branches of the descending aorta. Distally, the esophagus is supplied by branches of the left gastric, left inferior phrenic, and splenic arteries. Venous drainage from the upper segment is to the inferior thyroid veins, from the mid-segment to the azygous veins and from the lower esophageal segment to the gastric veins. The azygous and gastric veins form an anastomotic network between the portal and systemic venous systems and are thus the site of esophageal varices in patients with high portal pressure.

The esophagus receives innervation from both parasympathetic and sympathetic nerves. The parasympathetic input affects peristalsis via the vagus nerve, originating in the medulla, whereas both parasympathetic and sympathetic afferent nerves transmit information to the central nervous system via the spinal cord. Esophageal neuroanatomic pathways are shared by both the cardiac and respiratory systems; thus it may be difficult to ascertain which organ is responsible for chest pain syndromes.

Structurally, the esophagus is made up of four layers: the mucosa, submucosa, muscularis propria, and adventitia. The muscularis propria carries out most of the motor function of the esophagus. In the upper third of the esophagus, this muscularis propria is skeletal muscle, but in the distal third, it is smooth muscle, and the mid-section is mixed skeletal and smooth muscle. The upper esophageal sphincter (UES) is at the proximal origin of the esophagus where the inferior pharyngeal constrictor joins the cricopharyngeus muscle. UES tone is contracted at rest thus preventing aspiration of air during normal breathing. The lower esophageal sphincter (LES) is a 2–4 cm length of asymmetric circular smooth muscle within the diaphragmatic hiatus. At rest, the LES is contracted, preventing regurgitation of gastric contents. Swallowing elicits a wave of peristalsis which is under vagal control and carries a bolus of food from the pharynx to the stomach in 5–10 s. The coordinated relaxation of the LES allows the food bolus to enter the stomach.

A number of medications affect LES tone. Drugs known to decrease LES pressure include anticholinergics, sodium nitroprusside, dopamine, beta-adrenergic agonists, tricyclic antidepressant medications, and opioids. Drugs that have been found to increase LES tone include anticholinesterases, metoclopramide, prochlorperazine, and metoprolol.

Nonmalignant Disorders of the Esophagus and Surgical Therapies

Hiatal Hernia, Gastroesophageal Reflux Disease (GERD), and Esophageal Stricture

Gastroesophageal reflux and hiatal hernia may be present independently or may coexist. Esophageal strictures may be caused by a number of insults but are frequently related to gastroesophageal reflux. Gastroesophageal reflux is a common disorder and, depending on diet and lifestyle, may affect up to 80% of the population. The term gastroesophageal reflux disease (GERD) applies when symptoms are more frequent or severe than the population norm. Pharmacotherapies including histamine blockers and proton pump inhibitors are widely used and may dramatically ameliorate symptoms and reduce the need for surgical therapy. Indications for surgery in patients with GERD include symptoms that are refractory to optimized medical therapy, esophageal stricture, pulmonary symptoms such as asthma and chronic cough, and severe erosive esophagitis. Fundoplication surgery is generally associated with superior symptom control and higher patient satisfaction when compared to medical management [1], but considerable uncertainty remains regarding the long-term benefits and potential harm of surgical therapy for GERD [2].

GERD frequently coexists with hiatal hernia, but many patients with a hiatal hernia remain asymptomatic. Hiatal hernias include the sliding hiatal hernia (type I) and paraesophageal hernias (types II, III, IV) (see Fig. 38.2a and b). Sliding hiatal hernias are most common and occur when the gastroesophageal junction and part of the fundus of the stomach herniate axially through the diaphragm into the thoracic cavity. Hiatal hernia is associated with a decrease in LES pressure [3] reducing barrier pressure between the esophagus and stomach, which in turn promotes reflux.

a   b

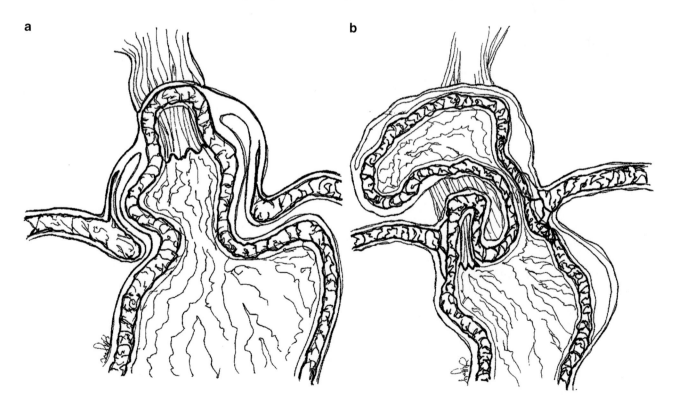

Fig. 38.2 (a) Type I hiatal hernia (sliding hernia). Note widening of the muscular hiatal orifice that allows cephalad herniation of the gastric cardia. (b) Type II hiatal hernia (paraesophageal hernia). The leading part of the herniating stomach is the fundus

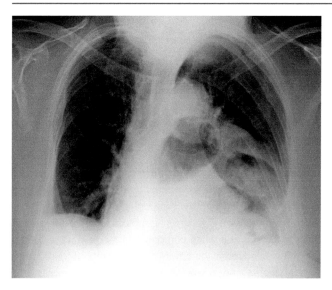

Fig. 38.3 Chest radiograph demonstrating a large left-sided type 4 paraesophageal hernia

Paraesophageal hernias (PH) occur when a portion of the stomach, typically the fundus, herniates into the thorax anterolateral to the distal esophagus (see Figs. 38.2b and 38.3). PH are much less common than type I hiatal hernias and comprise approximately 5–15% of hiatal hernias [4]. PH are at risk of incarceration, and the presence of a PH is thus considered an indication for surgical repair [5].

Surgical therapies for GERD and hiatal hernia can be achieved via a number of surgical approaches, but most are performed via laparoscopy. Although the laparoscopic Nissen fundoplication (utilizing a 360° wrap) is a mainstay of surgical GERD therapy, the Toupet fundoplication (270° wrap) may be equally effective with a superior postoperative symptom profile [6]. Other surgical alternatives include endoluminal, robotic-assisted laparoscopic, and transthoracic approaches. The recently developed transoral incisionless fundoplication (TIF) is an entirely endoluminal procedure which can be performed by gastroenterologists or surgeons. Although additional studies are required, TIF appears to be a safe and relatively effective alternative to more invasive surgical procedures, producing lasting reduction in medication requirements in approximately 75% of patients [7]. Robotic-assisted laparoscopic fundoplications produce outcomes comparable to that of standard laparoscopic procedures [8, 9] but at an appreciably higher cost [8]. Relative to laparotomy or transthoracic approaches, laparoscopic surgeries may produce considerably less pain, eliminate the need for a tube thoracostomy, utilize smaller incisions which decrease the risk of postoperative incisional hernias, and provide visualization for the diagnosis of other intra-abdominal pathology. A transthoracic approach may be preferred for patients with severe peptic strictures, patients requiring reoperation, and for those with other intrathoracic pathologies.

Table 38.1 Common transthoracic esophageal procedures and anesthetic considerations

Surgical procedure	Surgical incision(s)/ approach	Anesthetic considerations
Transthoracic total fundoplication (Nissen)	Left thoracotomy	Pain control One-lung ventilation Aspiration risk
Transthoracic partial fundoplication (Belsey)		
Collis gastroplasty		
Thoracoscopic esophagomyotomy	Left thoracoscopy (4–5 ports)	Pain control One-lung ventilation High aspiration risk
Heller myotomy and modified Heller myotomy	Left thoracotomy	Intraoperative esophagoscopy
Transhiatal esophagectomy	Midline laparotomy	Aspiration risk
	Left cervical incision	Risk of tracheobronchial injury, bleeding, cardiac compression, and dysrhythmias
Transthoracic esophagectomy (Ivor Lewis)	Midline laparotomy	Aspiration risk
	Right thoracotomy	One-lung ventilation Protective ventilation
Three-hole esophagectomy (McKewin)	Right thoracotomy	Fluid and hemodynamic management to optimize oxygen delivery
	Midline laparotomy	Pain control
	Left cervical incision	Early extubation
Minimally invasive esophagectomy	Right thoracoscopy (4 ports)	Aspiration risk
	Laparoscopy (5 ports)	Protective ventilation
	Left cervical incision (variable)	Procedure duration
Robotic-assisted esophagectomy	Multiple abdominal and thoracic ports	Aspiration risk Procedure duration Positioning requirements and risks Hypercarbia Cardiovascular compromise Conversion to open

The transthoracic total fundoplication (Nissen) is performed through a left lateral thoracotomy (see Table 38.1 for a summary of thoracic esophageal procedures and anesthetic considerations). The distal esophagus and the esophagogastric junction are mobilized with preservation of the vagus nerve and exposure of the crura and left hepatic lobe. At the surgeon's request, the anesthesiologist places an esophageal dilator orally and advances it through the gastroesophageal junction. The proximal stomach is brought into the chest and a 2 cm fundoplication wrap is created with the fundus of the stomach. The dilator is removed and the fundoplication wrap placed below the diaphragm without tension. A nasogastric tube (NGT) and a chest drain are left in place postoperatively. Nissen fundoplication yields a high patient satisfaction rate (90–95%) when the procedure is performed by experienced surgeons [10, 11]. The transthoracic partial fundoplication (Belsey) is similar to the Nissen fundoplication, but the esophageal wrap extends only 240–270° and is thus a partial fundoplication. The Belsey fundoplication yields a reduction in GERD symptoms comparable to that of the Nissen and may cause fewer postoperative obstructive symptoms.

Chronic GERD can cause esophageal ulceration which leads to inflammation and may cause axial esophageal shortening and stricture formation. Medical therapy is inadequate for symptomatic stricture, though most can be internally dilated using any one of a number of dilating techniques. After dilation, surgical therapy aims to reduce reflux and prevent recurrence. The Collis gastroplasty, classically performed via a transthoracic approach, aims to lengthen the esophagus to facilitate a subsequent tension-free fundoplication. This procedure creates a tube of esophageal diameter from the lesser gastric curvature tissues via surgical stapling so that subsequent intra-abdominal fundoplication can be performed around the "neoesophagus." In the context of advanced GERD with esophageal shortening, Collis gastroplasty combined with either a Belsey [12] or Nissen fundoplication [13] can provide excellent relief of GERD symptoms in the majority of treated patients. Esophageal strictures that are not amenable to dilation may require esophagoplasty or esophagectomy.

PH can be repaired through a midline laparotomy, a laparoscopic approach, or via thoracotomy. Through a left thoracotomy incision, the esophagus can be easily isolated and encircled, the hernia sac opened, its contents reduced to the abdomen, and the hiatus narrowed. Esophageal lengthening and fundoplication procedures are also frequently performed as part of the same procedure. Both transthoracic and laparoscopic approaches to the repair of PH are associated with good results, though recurrence rates remain a concern for both procedures [14–16].

Esophageal Perforation and Rupture

Esophageal perforation typically occurs in the hospital and is often iatrogenic. Multiple etiologies of perforation exist including upper gastrointestinal endoscopy and the traumatic placement of esophageal dilators, nasogastric tubes, and misplaced endotracheal tubes. Perforation or disruption of the esophagus may also occur from external trauma, typically gunshot wounds or less commonly, from blunt trauma, and from a foreign body or chemical ingestion but may also follow misadventures in airway management, resulting from the use of a Combitube [17] or esophageal obturator airway [18]. Hospital mortality and 3-year survival in patients with esophageal perforation are 17.5% and 67%, respectively [19].

In contrast, esophageal rupture typically results from a sudden increase in intra-abdominal pressure with a relaxed LES and an obstructed esophageal orifice with vomiting, straining, weight lifting, childbirth, defecation, or blunt crush traumatic injuries to the abdomen and chest. Spontaneous rupture of the esophagus during vomiting is known as Boerhaave's syndrome. This rupture of the distal esophagus occurs under high pressure which forces gastric contents into the mediastinum and pleura [20].

Clinical presentation may be related to the mode of injury but is often nonspecific. Pain is the most common symptom [21], though fever, dyspnea, and crepitus may also be present. Mackler's triad, often associated with spontaneous esophageal rupture includes chest pain, vomiting, and subcutaneous emphysema. Soilage of the mediastinum elicits an inflammatory response that results in mediastinitis. Abdominal perforation may result in peritonitis. These patients may present with septic shock and are likely to deteriorate rapidly, particularly without aggressive resuscitation and definitive therapy.

Evaluation for esophageal perforation or rupture includes a plain film chest X-ray (CXR) which may reveal mediastinal or free peritoneal air, pleural effusion, pneumothorax, widened mediastinum, and subcutaneous emphysema [22]. Computerized tomography (CT) scan will also confirm the rupture as evidenced by esophageal edema and thickening, possible abscess formation, as well as air and/or fluid in the pleural space. A water-soluble esophagogram will help to confirm the location and extent of the tear by allowing visualization of the extravasation of contrast.

Treatment of esophageal rupture or perforation depends mainly on the extent and location of the injury and the disease state of the esophagus. Factors affecting patient outcome include the location, association with malignancy, sepsis, respiratory failure, and other comorbidities [23] as well as the interval between diagnosis and treatment [24, 25]. Perforation of the cervical esophagus may be treated solely by drainage; surgical repair is typically preferred for thoracic or abdominal esophageal perforations. In a stable patient without severe esophageal pathology, primary closure of a thoracic or abdominal esophageal perforation can be attempted. If the area of injury is diseased, an esophagectomy may be required. In one study, emergent esophagectomy for perforation was associated with a short-term survival equivalent to that of elective esophagectomy. However, survival at 1 year and 5 years was markedly diminished [26]. Early aggressive surgical treatment of Boerhaave's syndrome is favored; left untreated this condition is virtually always fatal [20]. Conservative non-operative therapies emphasizing aggressive drainage of fluid collections and appropriate antibiotic therapy are preferred by some clinicians for stable patients with contained esophageal leaks [24, 27] and may be associated with acceptably low morbidity and mortality [24, 27, 28]. Numerous case series have also demonstrated the efficacy of treating esophageal perforation and esophageal anastomotic leaks with self-expandable plastic and metallic stents [29–32]. Additional recently developed endoscopic modalities used with some success in managing esophageal perforation include endoscopic clipping and vacuum therapy [33].

Achalasia and Motility Disorders

Achalasia is a disease of impaired esophageal motility, most often affecting the distal esophagus. It affects approximately 1 in 100,000 persons per year, with an equal gender distribution [34]. The etiology of achalasia is unknown, but characteristic features include increased LES pressure, incomplete relaxation of the LES with swallowing, and loss of peristalsis which causes impaired esophageal emptying. Primary achalasia is due to a complete loss or relative absence of ganglion cells in the myenteric plexus. This causes an imbalance between excitatory and inhibitory neurons which results in impaired relaxation of the LES [35]. Other primary motor disorders of the esophagus include nutcracker esophagus and diffuse esophageal spasm. Secondary achalasia is most often caused by Chagas' disease, a systemic disease due to infection with Trypanosoma cruzi [36]. Other secondary motor disorders are associated with systemic disease processes such as scleroderma, diabetes, amyloidosis, Parkinson's disease, and neuromuscular diseases of skeletal muscle.

Achalasia progresses slowly, and thus when patients finally present for treatment, they are often at advanced stages of the disease. Symptoms of achalasia include dysphagia, first for solids and then liquids. As the esophagus dilates, reflux becomes a more frequent problem. Patients may describe chest pain due to esophageal spasm. Weight loss, symptoms of GERD, and history suggestive for aspiration such as pneumonia and chronic cough are also consistent with achalasia [37, 38].

Radiographic findings in advanced achalasia include absence of gastric bubble, esophageal dilation, and fluid filling [39]. Barium swallow reveals the esophageal air-fluid level and a characteristic bird's beak narrowing caused by the impaired relaxation of the LES [39] (see Fig. 38.4). Esophageal manometry is a sensitive diagnostic test for achalasia, and manifestations include elevated LES resting pressure and incomplete relaxation of the LES, aperistalsis

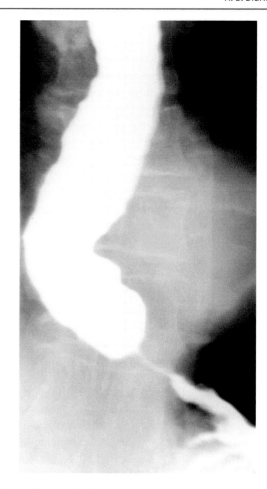

Fig. 38.4 This thoracic level barium swallow esophagogram illustrates a classic radiologic feature of achalasia – bird-beak appearance of the esophagus

of the esophageal body, and elevated lower esophageal baseline pressure [37]. At this time, achalasia cannot be cured. Treatment goals for achalasia include elimination of the esophageal outflow obstruction due to the tight LES, alleviating dysphagia and minimizing gastroesophageal reflux [37]. Medical treatments include calcium channel blockers and nitrates, but because of their adverse effects and unpredictable absorption in these patients, medical therapy is typically reserved for patients who are not candidates for surgical or endoscopic therapies. Botulinum toxin injection of the LES produces relaxation of this sphincter and can improve dysphagia temporarily [40], but relapse is common, and most patients required repeated therapy. Pneumatic dilatation of the LES is associated with a low risk of perforation [41]. While surgical myotomy with fundoplication produces a greater response than a single dilation [42], the strategy of serial dilation may be similarly efficacious [43].

Laparoscopic esophagomyotomy is typically performed with the patient in reverse Trendelenburg position and includes an anterior longitudinal myotomy of the distal esophagus, esophagogastric junction, and proximal stomach.

Thoracoscopic esophagomyotomy is performed through a thoracoscope via the left chest which allows for optimal visualization of the lower esophagus and cardioesophageal junction [44, 45]. The thoracic Heller and modified Heller myotomy procedures are performed via a left thoracotomy incision and differ in the extent of the myotomy incision and the inclusion of a fundoplication to minimize reflux. The Heller procedure utilizes a shorter myotomy incision extended only 1 cm or less onto the stomach. The modified Heller myotomy includes a 10 cm myotomy incision and a partial anterior gastric fundoplication to decrease the risk of reflux postoperatively [45].

Minimally invasive laparoscopic and thoracoscopic Heller and modified Heller myotomy procedures have been shown to be safe, effective, and durable treatments for achalasia [46–59]. Patient outcomes after minimally invasive myotomy surgery for achalasia generally favor the laparoscopic approaches, however. Multiple investigators have found that patients experience superior dysphagia relief and less postoperative reflux with the laparoscopic approach as compared to the thoracoscopic approach [46, 49, 53, 54]. This difference may result from the limitations in extending the myotomy incision into the stomach and creating a fundoplication wrap from the thoracoscopic approach.

Per-oral endoscopic myotomy (POEM) represents the newest therapy for achalasia. POEM is an entirely endoscopic procedure; a small mid-esophageal incision is made in the mucosa and a submucosal tract is created and tunneled to the gastric cardia. Electrocautery is then used to create a myotomy of the circular muscle fibers. POEM is a relatively new development, and although initial results suggest that this technique is safe, effective, and well tolerated [7, 60–64], randomized trials are needed.

Tracheoesophageal Fistula (TEF)

Acquired TEF or bronchoesophageal fistula in the adult patient is typically the result of malignancy, prolonged endotracheal intubation, esophageal surgery including esophagectomy, trauma, stent erosion, and infection [65–71]. Though less common, TEF of congenital origin has also been reported [72–74]. Rarely, the diagnosis of TEF may be made intraoperatively [75], in the perioperative period [72, 76] or in chronically intubated patients [69–71].

Treatment of TEF varies depending upon the etiology and location of the fistula and the nature and severity of associated symptoms and clinical sequelae. The mainstay of therapy for malignant TEF involves placement of self-expandable coated stents with the esophagus or trachea or both, whereas surgical therapy is rarely indicated and associated with high risk for morbidity and mortality [66]. Surgical therapy is preferred for most patients with nonmalignant TEF, and retro-

spective studies of clinical cohorts confirm a high rate of successful closures with low incidence of TEF recurrence [65, 77]. In critically ill patients dependent on mechanical ventilation, the use of esophageal stents to provide temporary closure of benign TEF has been demonstrated to be safe and effective for palliation [78].

Esophageal Diverticula

Esophageal diverticula are classified according to their anatomic location (cervical or thoracic) and pathophysiology (pseudo- or traction diverticula). Most diverticula are acquired and occur in an elderly patient population. Pulsion or pseudodiverticula are the most common form and consist of a localized outpouching which lacks a muscular covering; that is, the wall consists of only mucosa and submucosa herniating through the muscle layer. Most pseudodiverticula are of Zenker's variety, located in the hypopharynx. Epiphrenic diverticula are located within the thoracic esophagus, typically in the distal esophagus [79]. True or traction diverticula occur within the middle one third of the thoracic esophagus as a result of paraesophageal granulomatous mediastinal lymphadenitis usually due to tuberculosis or histoplasmosis and are characterized by full-thickness involvement of the esophageal wall. These diverticula are typically small and most are asymptomatic. Complications are uncommon but may include TEF formation.

Clinical presentation of Zenker's diverticulum usually includes dysphagia for solid food and regurgitation of undigested food substances. Patients may also complain of halitosis, gurgling associated with swallowing, and symptoms associated with aspiration such as nighttime cough, hoarseness of voice, bronchospasm, and chronic respiratory infection. Diagnostic confirmation is accomplished with barium contrast study which clearly demonstrates the diverticulum.

Surgical correction of Zenker's diverticulum is usually accomplished via a left cervical incision and includes a cricopharyngeal myotomy. While the myotomy may be sufficient therapy for small diverticula, larger sacs require diverticulectomy or diverticulopexy [79, 80]. Minimally invasive techniques used to treat Zenker's diverticulum have included endoscopic stapling diverticulostomy, fiberoptic endoscopic electrocautery, and laser coagulation techniques [79–82]. In general, minimally invasive treatments for Zenker's diverticulum have yielded satisfactory results in the majority of patients [82, 83], and most can be performed in an endoscopy unit with a brief general anesthetic or in an awake patient. A recent large systematic review of treatments for Zenker's diverticulum reported a failure rate for open and endoscopic approaches of 4.2% and 18.4%, respectively [84]. Mortality was low in both groups, but open procedures were associated with a higher complication rate [84].

Thus, endoscopic techniques may be preferable for frail patients who are less likely to tolerate a general anesthetic.

Thoracic esophageal diverticula are usually epiphrenic, and most are found to be associated with an esophageal motor disorder such as achalasia. While many patients do not have symptoms specifically referable to the diverticulum, if present these may be difficult to distinguish from those of the associated motor disorder. Patients who are asymptomatic or present with mild symptoms are not surgical candidates. Presenting symptoms may include dysphagia, chest pain, regurgitation of ingested foods, and symptoms of aspiration. Patients with epiphrenic diverticula are advised to undergo both barium swallow examination (see Fig. 38.5 for barium esophagogram of a mid-esophageal diverticulum) and esophageal manometry to delineate any associated pathology such as motility disorder, malignancy, or stricture. Patients with incapacitating symptom profiles are referred for surgery.

Surgical goals include resection of the diverticulum, typically with a myotomy to treat the accompanying motor disorder, and may be performed with or without an anti-reflux procedure. The classical surgical approach has been through

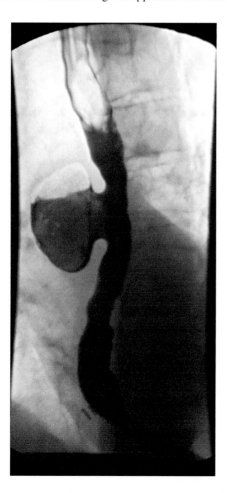

Fig. 38.5 A thoracic level barium swallow esophagogram which demonstrates a large mid-esophageal diverticulum filled with contrast

a left thoracotomy incision, through which the diverticulum is dissected and excised; a myotomy and a fundoplication may also be performed. Results of surgical therapy are favorable, completely eliminating symptoms in 74% of patients [85]. Thoracoscopic and laparoscopic approaches, as well as combined approaches, have been reported [86–88] and appear to be feasible. The laparoscopic approach has been associated with a lower postoperative morbidity rate relative to that of the thoracotomy [89]. Definitive conclusions regarding the ideal surgical approach(es) to epiphrenic diverticula await larger studies, which are in turn limited by the relative rarity of these lesions.

Malignant Disease of the Esophagus and Esophagectomy

Esophageal Cancer

Malignant esophageal tumors can be classified on the basis of histologic types – squamous cell carcinoma and adenocarcinoma – which differ with respect to affected populations, incidence, etiology, and risk factors. While squamous cell carcinoma still accounts for the vast majority of esophageal cancers worldwide, the incidence of adenocarcinoma has risen sharply throughout the Western world, now accounting for nearly half of esophageal cancers in many countries [90–92]. Potential etiologic and predisposing factors identified through epidemiologic study include tobacco use and excessive alcohol ingestion, gastroesophageal reflux, obesity, achalasia, and low socioeconomic status [90, 92].

Clinical presentation of patients with esophageal cancer is variable; patients may present with symptoms of dysphagia, odynophagia, and progressive weight loss. Patient evaluation should include a thorough history and physical examination with attention to local tumor effects, possible sites of metastasis, and general health. Clinical investigations include the barium contrast swallow study to define esophageal anatomy and esophagogastroscopy to permit biopsy and definitive identification of tumor type. Both CT scans and magnetic resonance imaging (MRI) are used clinically for noninvasive staging of esophageal cancer. Endoscopic ultrasound (EUS) has been used for imaging of local/regional esophageal disease and may be considered complementary to CT scanning (see Fig. 38.6 for CT image of thickened esophagus in a patient with esophageal cancer). Positron emission tomography (PET) is being used with greater frequency for the purpose of staging esophageal cancer and for assessing the response to induction chemotherapy.

In an effort to avoid the morbidity, mortality, and expense associated with esophagectomy, many centers are employing relatively new approaches to esophageal preservation in

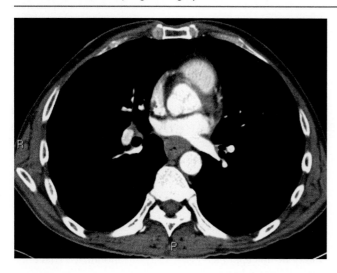

Fig. 38.6 A CT scan demonstrating thickened esophagus in a patient with esophageal cancer and dysphagia

patients with malignant and premalignant esophageal lesions. The close surveillance of many patients with premalignant disease of the esophagus has led to the early identification of many cases of high-grade dysplasia and superficial adenocarcinoma. Advances in the use of minimally invasive endoscopic techniques permit the staging of superficial esophageal cancers by endoscopic biopsy [93, 94] and, where appropriate, endoscopic resection of adenocarcinoma limited to the esophageal mucosa [95, 96].

Unfortunately, patients often present with advanced local/regional and metastatic disease. The failure of surgery to cure most advanced local and regional disease and the early systemic dissemination of esophageal cancers has led to significant interest in improving chemotherapeutic regimens and developing more focused therapies. Chemotherapeutic goals are to reduce tumor burden prior to surgical resection and to reduce tumor spread and micrometastasis. Chemotherapies are used in the context of esophageal cancer both for palliation of locally advanced and metastatic disease and increasingly as an adjunct to surgical resection. 5-Fluorouracil and cisplatin are widely used in combination preoperative therapy for both adenocarcinoma and squamous cell carcinoma of the esophagus [97, 98]. Induction chemotherapy with radiation before esophagectomy is recommended for patients undergoing esophagectomy for both locally advanced squamous cell and adenocarcinoma [99].

Esophagectomy

Esophagectomy is indicated for the resection of esophageal cancer without local invasion or metastasis [100], curative resection of high-grade dysplasia [101], and severe nonmalignant disorders including esophageal injury, non-dilatable stricture, severe recurrent GERD, and achalasia [102, 103]. Esophagectomy surgery can be performed via a transhiatal approach by laparotomy, a two-incision surgery utilizing both laparotomy and right thoracotomy (Ivor Lewis), a three-incision approach (McKewin) which also requires a cervical incision for anastomosis, a left thoracoabdominal approach, and minimally invasive approaches utilizing laparoscopy and/or thoracoscopy with or without robotic assistance (see Table 38.1). Consideration for the transhiatal, transthoracic, minimally invasive esophagectomy and robotic esophagectomy will be discussed below.

Transhiatal esophagectomy (THE) is performed for tumors throughout the esophagus but is often preferred for lower tumors. The primary advantage of this resection is that it avoids a thoracotomy and the possibility of an intrathoracic anastomotic leak. This procedure is accomplished via a large upper abdominal incision which is used to mobilize the stomach and through which transhiatal esophageal dissection is carried out and a cervical incision through which the conduit is introduced and the anastomosis is made. The transhiatal approach to esophagectomy requires the manual dissection of the esophagus from the mediastinum blindly via the abdominal hiatus.

There continues to be considerable debate regarding the relative risk of THE relative to the transthoracic esophagectomy (TTE), from both surgical and oncologic standpoints. While the morbidity and mortality associated with THE have declined over the past several decades [104], the advantage of THE over TTE remains controversial with both early morbidity and mortality advantages demonstrated [105, 106] and refuted [107]. In a recent Society of Thoracic Surgeons Database study, combined perioperative morbidity and mortality were similar between open transhiatal and open Ivor Lewis esophagectomy [108]. Similar results were reported in a NSQIP study; there was no significant difference between the two approaches with regard to mortality or morbidity [109]. Similarly, a recent meta-analysis reported no difference in 5-year survival between the two surgical approaches [110]. It should be understood that the finding of equivalence with regard to oncologic, and perhaps other outcomes, may not necessarily be indicative of equivalent efficacy, as the transthoracic groups may have more advanced cancer [110]. Overall, transhiatal esophagectomy is associated with a higher rate of anastomotic leak, stricture, and recurrent laryngeal nerve injury [110, 111], whereas transthoracic esophagectomy is associated with a longer length of stay and higher rates of respiratory complications and wound infections [110]. It should also be noted that various transthoracic approaches to esophagectomy may not be equivalent with regard to outcome risk. The open three-hole (or McKeown) esophagectomy may represent a higher-risk approach than the Ivor Lewis esophagectomy given the recent finding that this approach is associated with an increased risk of morbidity and mortality in a risk adjustment model (OR 1.59; 1.20–2.10) [108].

The transthoracic approach to esophagectomy is performed for malignant, premalignant, or nonmalignant disease of the esophagus and employs an abdominal incision for mobilization of the stomach and formation of a gastric tube or other esophageal conduit and a right thoracotomy through which the diseased esophageal portion is resected and the anastomosis is made. The transthoracic esophagectomy is often preferred when the resection extends to other mediastinal structures, mediastinal fibrosis is known or suspected, tumor may involve the airway or vascular structures, or an intrathoracic anastomosis is required.

The term "minimally invasive esophagectomy" (MIE) encompasses a variety of surgical approaches to esophagectomy that attempt to minimize the degree of surgical trespass in one or more body cavities. True minimally invasive esophagectomy using laparoscopy and thoracoscopy is performed in a limited number of centers. Analogous to open procedures, several variants are possible, including the minimally invasive equivalents of the Ivor Lewis, three-hole, and transhiatal esophagectomies.

Avoiding large thoracotomy and/or laparotomy incisions in the context of MIE has significant potential to reduce major morbidity after esophagectomy, particularly pulmonary morbidity. Feasibility and safety of MIE has been widely demonstrated [112–115], but, although numerous randomized trials are planned, very little objective data comparing these approaches are currently available. A small randomized trial comparing MIE to open esophagectomy for patients with esophageal cancer demonstrated significant reduction in pulmonary infections in the MIE group [116]. Follow-up at 1 year revealed better quality of life and pain in the MIE group at 1 year [117] and equivalent disease-free survival at 3 years [118]. Most retrospective, non-randomized studies and meta-analyses also report equivalent or better clinical outcomes [114, 119–122] with similar or improved oncologic outcomes [123].

Robotic-assisted minimally invasive esophagectomy procedures utilize the proprietary da Vinci surgical system to aid in the minimally invasive approach to the laparoscopic and thoracoscopic components of esophagectomy surgery. This system provides a number of theoretical and practical surgical advantages – a three-dimensional magnified operating field view, normal hand-eye coordination, tremor filtering, and motion scaling. Although robotic esophagectomy surgery is a nascent and evolving field, several reports of clinical series have demonstrated the feasibility and relative safety of this approach [124, 125]. A randomized trial comparing robotic assisted to open transthoracic esophagectomy is currently underway [126] and should further delineate benefits with regard to short- and long-term outcomes, if any.

Esophageal Conduits

Although a variety of conduits have been used after esophageal resection, the stomach is usually preferred because of its excellent blood supply, because it can be readily mobilized to reach the thorax or neck, and because only one anastomosis is required (see Fig. 38.7a and b). However, the stomach may not be a suitable conduit in the case of prior gastric surgery or tumor involvement. In such cases, an alternative conduit must be used. The pedicled colonic interposition utilizes a segment of colon with an attached vascular pedicle as an esophageal replacement conduit. While the pedicled colon graft has adequate mobility, its use is associated with numerous complications including conduit redundancy and symp-

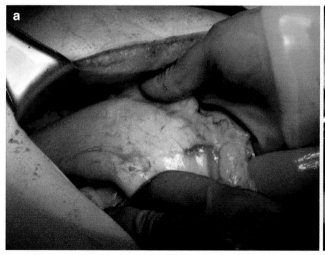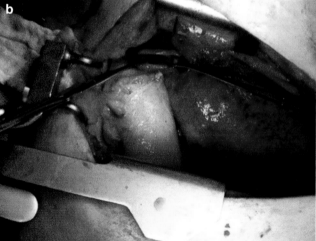

Fig. 38.7 (**a**) Gastric conduit prior to anastomosis. (**b**) Gastric conduit and proximal esophagus via thoracotomy prior to anastomosis during Ivor Lewis esophagectomy

toms related to inadequate food transit [127–131] which may impact quality of life [128] and long-term outcomes [132]. Additionally, atherosclerotic disease may affect vascular supply to the colon which may in turn increase the risk of colonic ischemia and necrosis, a major cause of morbidity and mortality [133–135].

Jejunum has a number of theoretical advantages over that of colon for use as an esophageal replacement. First, its diameter more closely approximates that of the esophagus. Secondly, it is generally disease-free. Additionally its intrinsic peristaltic activity may improve food transit and reduce symptoms postoperatively [136–140]. Use of the jejunum for interposition has previously been limited by the vascular anatomy of the jejunum. The jejunal mesentery lacks the collateral arcades of the colon which permit them to reach interposition sites in the thorax and neck. Ischemia of the interposition graft is the likely cause of jejunal loop gangrene which plagued early attempts and led to an interest in vascular augmentation of the interposition graft, now known as "supercharging," or vascular enhancement.

Recent advances in microvascular surgery have enabled specialized centers to expand the indications for jejunal interposition beyond short-segment esophageal replacement. Esophagectomy with "supercharging" jejunal interposition graft is undertaken as a one-stage procedure which includes esophageal resection, construction of the interposition graft with esophageal and jejunal reconstruction. The superior jejunal vascular arcade is "supercharged" by reimplantation into cervical or internal mammary arteries. The inferior arcade retains its native supply from the superior mesenteric artery. Clinical series have demonstrated the feasibility and relative safety of this approach [141–143]. Use of the supercharging technique for construction of jejunal interposition grafts for esophageal reconstruction led to a 92% success rate for discharge with an intact flap, and 95% of patients were discharged on a regular diet and without reflux symptoms [142, 143]. A recent study comparing conduit function in patients who previously received either supercharged pedicled jejunal interposition grafts or conventional gastric revealed similar levels of conduit function with regard to reflux, dumping, dysphagia, stricture, and conduit emptying [144]. Despite these successes, this technique remains the purview of highly specialized centers with multidisciplinary teams and is considered only in the absence of a suitable gastric conduit.

Anesthetic Management of Esophageal Surgery Patients

Preoperative Evaluation and Preparation

A thorough history and physical examination should be performed prior to anesthetizing a patient for esophageal sur- gery. Comorbid conditions should be evaluated and optimized prior to surgery. Preanesthetic assessment for thoracic surgery is discussed in Chap. 2. Particular attention should be given to signs and symptoms of esophageal obstruction, GERD, and silent aspiration. Symptoms of obstruction, particularly dysphagia and odynophagia, may lead to reduced oral intake and malnutrition which can lead to increased morbidity and mortality [145, 146]. Symptoms of severe GERD with aspiration may include water brash (hypersalivation in response to reflux), coughing when supine, globus sensation (feeling of lump in throat), laryngitis, and asthmatype symptoms.

The presence of significant cardiovascular disease has important implications for patients undergoing major surgical procedures involving the esophagus. Patients may be evaluated for cardiovascular risk with attention to the ACC/AHA guidelines for perioperative cardiovascular evaluation [147, 148]. The risk of cardiovascular complications during major surgical procedures of the esophagus may be increased by a number of factors inherent to surgery and anesthesia care, including the degree of planned physiologic trespass, hypoxemia, hemorrhage, dysrhythmias, and pain. One-lung ventilation (OLV) is often required for surgery of the esophagus. Oxygenation, ventilation, and weaning from mechanical ventilation may be more difficult in the patient with pulmonary disease. The minimum preoperative evaluation of the cardiopulmonary system should include a 12-lead electrocardiogram (ECG) and CXR. A preoperative ECG serves as a screening test for myocardial ischemia and arrhythmias and provides a baseline for comparison in the event of perioperative cardiac complications. Preoperative CXR may reveal evidence of aspiration as well as coexisting pulmonary and cardiac disease. Patients with a history of morbid obesity or chronic lung disease should also undergo preoperative pulmonary function testing if the procedure involves a thoracotomy approach.

Patients with severe GERD or those otherwise at risk for aspiration pneumonitis may benefit from prophylactic medication to increase gastric pH and decrease gastric volume. Though definitive evidence of risk reduction is lacking, appropriate pharmacologic prophylaxis with H_2 receptor antagonists or proton pump inhibitors is known to reduce gastric volume and acidity [149–154] and is thus likely to reduce the incidence and severity of pneumonitis should aspiration occur.

Patients may present for esophagectomy surgery after having received neoadjuvant chemotherapy and/or radiotherapy, either of which may improve survival compared to surgical therapy alone [97, 155–157]. The chemotherapeutic agents used to treat esophageal cancer cause bone marrow suppression, and patients often present with some degree of anemia and thrombocytopenia. The need for optimizing patient status prior to major surgery should be balanced with the risk of delaying the resection of malignant tumors. Occasionally, severe thrombocytopenia may preclude the preoperative placement of an epidural catheter in which case alternative plans for analgesia should be made.

Intraoperative Monitoring

In general, intraoperative monitoring for esophageal surgery cases should be commensurate with the degree of physiological trespass inherent in the planned procedure and the nature and severity of patient comorbidity (see Chap. 20 for discussion of intraoperative monitoring). Routine monitoring should include pulse oximetry, noninvasive blood pressure monitoring, and electrocardiography. Since many patients presenting for esophageal surgery have comorbid disease of the cardiovascular and respiratory systems, consideration should be given to invasive monitors where appropriate. With the exception of patients with advanced cardiovascular or pulmonary disease, routine intraoperative monitors will generally suffice for those patients presenting for endoscopic and minimally invasive procedures limited to the abdominal cavity. Transthoracic approaches to the esophagus generally mandate a more aggressive approach to monitoring. An indwelling arterial catheter for continuous measurement of systemic arterial blood pressure is the standard of care for these procedures. Surgical manipulation of thoracic and mediastinal structures can profoundly affect determinants of cardiac performance including venous return and cardiac filling and may contribute to the development of dysrhythmias, all of which can compromise cardiac output and hemodynamic status. In addition, many of these procedures require lung isolation and OLV, a ventilation strategy which substantially limits arterial oxygenation and may increase the risk of lung injury. Surgical dissection can lead to unexpected bleeding, occasionally massive in nature. Point of care testing of arterial blood samples can aid in the assessment and maintenance of adequate arterial oxygenation, acid base status, as well as hemoglobin and electrolyte concentrations.

In the patient with normal cardiovascular reserve, central venous access is not generally necessary and does not provide useful information for volume management. Nonetheless, central access may be required in patients with very limited peripheral venous access, especially obese patients in whom it may be difficult to re-establish lost venous access intraoperatively, patients requiring emergency surgery for esophageal trauma or perforation as septic complications can rapidly ensue, and those patients who are likely to require vasopressor or inotropic support. Patients undergoing esophageal surgery should also undergo bladder catheterization for decompression and for the monitoring of urine output. Temperature monitoring is easily accomplished via a probe in the oropharynx, axilla, or bladder catheter.

Euthermia can be achieved by use of commercially available forced warm air heating blankets and fluid warmers.

Pain Control

Pain control after esophageal surgery is dictated largely by the surgical approach to the esophagus (see Chaps. 59–61 for detailed discussion of pain management). Most patients undergoing endoscopic surgery of the esophagus have little pain postoperatively and thus do not require an aggressive plan for analgesia. Similarly a laparoscopic approach is generally not associated with high analgesic requirement postoperatively. However, the thoracotomy incision utilized in most transthoracic esophageal surgeries, is one of the most painful surgical incisions in common use. As such, anesthetic techniques for postoperative pain control play an extremely important role in optimizing outcomes after transthoracic esophageal procedures. Although a variety of pain control approaches have been utilized, most centers favor the use of thoracic epidural analgesia (TEA) for its excellent analgesia [158, 159], favorable safety profile, cost savings [160, 161], its potential role in mitigating the perioperative inflammatory response [162, 163], and improving outcomes after transthoracic esophageal surgery [161, 163–168] and as a component of multimodal strategies to expedite patient mobilization and recovery after esophagectomy [169–176]. In comparison to parenteral opioid pain therapy alone, TEA provides superior analgesia after esophagectomy [158, 159, 162] and is considered by most anesthesiologists and surgeons to represent the "gold standard" with regard to postoperative pain control after transthoracic esophagectomy. However, for technical and safety reasons, not all patients are suitable candidates for the placement of thoracic epidural catheters. For patients in whom TEA is not possible but epidural analgesia per se is not contraindicated, lumbar epidural analgesia (LEA) may represent a compromise approach for analgesia after thoracoabdominal esophagectomy though pain control postoperatively is inferior to that obtained by TEA [177].

A variety of non-neuraxial techniques have been studied and recommended for post-thoracotomy pain control; the most promising of these include intrapleural, intercostal, and paravertebral approaches. Intercostal nerve catheters in combination with patient-controlled analgesia (PCA) have been compared to TEA with mixed results [178, 179]. Intrapleural and thoracotomy wound catheters have also been utilized, though rigorous comparison to standard therapies are lacking [180, 181]. Paravertebral blockade has shown promise as an alternative therapy [182] with analgesic efficacy for thoracotomy comparable to that of TEA by randomized trial [183] and meta-analysis [184–186] and with a favorable side effect profile [184] and has been advocated as a superior modality by several authors [187, 188]. A recent Cochrane review comparing PVB and TEA for thoracotomy confirmed comparable analgesic efficacy for PVB with reduced risks of minor complications. However, there were no differences between the two modalities with regard to mortality, length of stay, or major complications [185]. An obvious limitation of PVB for analgesia for open thoracoabdominal esophagectomy is the wide range of spinal/dermatomal levels to be blocked in order to provide adequate analgesia for both a midline laparotomy and a high posterolateral thoracotomy. These challenges have limited enthusiasm for PVB in open thoracoabdominal esophagectomy, though reasonable efficacy has been demonstrated for a combined approach utilizing intravenous sufentanil and bilateral PVB in minimally invasive esophagectomy [189]. Subcostal transversus abdominis plane (TAP) block combined with PVB [190] and TAP block [191] alone have shown some efficacy in minimally invasive esophagectomy and hybrid Ivor Lewis esophagectomy, respectively, and warrant further study. Whether paravertebral analgesia will replace TEA for post-thoracotomy pain will likely depend on both the ability to adapt this technique to the specific analgesic challenges associated with esophagectomy and on the identification of outcome advantages that have thus far been ascribed only to TEA.

Specific epidural management strategies should ideally consider the dermatomal range of incision(s), the impact of incisional pain on respiratory function, the likelihood and impact of respiratory depression, and the intraoperative impact of an epidural-induced sympathectomy on hemodynamic status. Since the thoracoabdominal esophagectomy requires both thoracotomy and laparotomy incisions, any plan for postoperative pain control should address this fact. A variety of management strategies have been reported, but most centers which perform transthoracic and thoracoabdominal esophageal surgeries utilize a multimodal approach to pain management including preoperative placement of a thoracic epidural catheter unless contraindicated, intra- or postoperative bolus, and infusion of a dilute local anesthetic such as ropivacaine or bupivacaine along with fentanyl or hydromorphone. A dual epidural catheter technique has also been reported and may improve analgesia for Ivor Lewis esophagectomy [192], though this is likely to further increase the complexity of management. An epidural bolus of preservative-free morphine may provide a wider neuraxial spread and may provide synergism with the infused local anesthetics but requires postoperative respiratory monitoring because of the possibility of delayed respiratory depression. Whether to bolus or infuse epidural local anesthetics pre- or intraoperatively has been a subject of debate among anesthesiologists. Arguments that a preemptive initiation of analgesia might provide better acute and chronic pain control have been based largely on theoretical considerations. Results

thus far are inconclusive but suggest that preoperative dosing of epidural catheters may produce better acute pain control [193–195]. However, while epidural analgesia may reduce the incidence of chronic post-thoracotomy pain [196], preemptive dosing does not improve chronic post-thoracotomy pain [194, 196].

Induction and Airway Management

Induction of general anesthesia and airway management in patients undergoing esophageal surgery is dictated largely by patient factors including cardiopulmonary status, hemodynamic and nutritional status at the time of induction, mediastinal mass effect if any, perceived risk of aspiration pneumonitis, and procedural factors including anticipated length of and nature of the procedure (i.e., if OLV is required for an intrathoracic procedure). Patients presenting for emergency procedures of the esophagus and stomach may lack the desired preoperative evaluation of cardiopulmonary status and can present with unstable hemodynamic or pulmonary status from a variety of factors including underlying cardiopulmonary disease, aspiration, sepsis, acute respiratory distress syndrome (ARDS), or hemorrhage. Most practitioners favor intravenous induction agents such as propofol, thiopental, etomidate, or ketamine in conjunction with a rapidly acting neuromuscular blocking agent such as succinylcholine or rocuronium to facilitate smooth induction of anesthesia and rapid tracheal intubation.

Patients presenting for elective esophageal procedures will be stable at induction, but complications arising from the presence of a mediastinal mass may accompany the induction of anesthesia, positive-pressure ventilation, and muscle relaxation. Tracheobronchial compression or obstruction and cardiovascular collapse associated with anesthetic induction in patients with mediastinal masses has been well described and is discussed in Chap. 14. Airway compromise has also been reported spontaneously or during the conduct of anesthesia in patients with posterior [197–201] and superior [202–204] mediastinal masses. Posterior mediastinal masses, including those of esophageal origin [197–199], may impinge on the airway and cause obstruction. Patients with achalasia are at particular risk as the dilated esophagus may cause respiratory compromise by direct compression of the upper airway [205], tracheobronchial tree [206–208], or lung parenchyma [209].

The trachea is most easily compressed posteriorly because of the lack of cartilaginous support, and thus, posterior compression can result in near complete expiratory obstruction [201]. The identification of patients with mediastinal masses who are at risk for cardiopulmonary complications is imprecise, but specific factors associated with increased risk have been reported [210] and may aid in management.

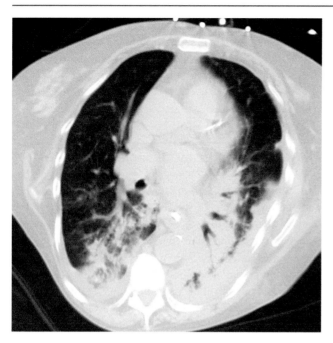

Fig. 38.8 CT scan of the thorax which demonstrates multifocal bibasilar consolidations consistent with aspiration pneumonitis

Anesthetic management of patients for esophageal surgery presents an additional challenge with regard to the perceived risk of aspiration. Patients in need of esophageal surgery are widely considered to be at elevated risk of aspiration and its sequelae [211–214] (Fig. 38.8), and the use of rapid sequence induction techniques is widely used and advocated [212, 213, 215]. A retrospective analysis of perioperative aspiration at a university hospital demonstrated that, among a variety of surgical service lines, those patients undergoing thoracic esophageal surgery exhibited the highest incidence of pulmonary aspiration [216].

Patients with severe gastroesophageal pathology, particularly those with obstructive disease, dysmotility syndromes, paraesophageal hernias, and esophageal diverticula, may represent high-risk subgroups, but clear risk stratification is lacking. Achalasia in particular has been associated with spontaneous aspiration pneumonitis [217, 218], and these patients may benefit from longer periods of NPO status. Practice guidelines for preoperative fasting have been published [219], and effects of fasting regimens have been reviewed [220, 221] but apply to healthy patients and elective surgical procedures. Optimal periods of NPO status in patients with severe gastroesophageal pathology are not known.

Rapid sequence induction and intubation has been widely advocated in patients thought to be at elevated risk of regurgitation and aspiration. This technique has classically referred to the rapid intravenous administration of induction agent and muscle relaxant, accompanied by the application of cricoid pressure (Sellick maneuver) and immediate laryngoscopy and tracheal intubation without intervening positive-pressure ventilation. The rationale underlying this approach is (1) that the cricoid cartilage is positioned anterior to the esophagus, (2) that downward pressure on the cricoid cartilage on a patient in the supine position would be transmitted to the esophagus occluding the esophageal lumen by compressing it against the adjacent vertebral body, and (3) that this compression would result in a clinically significant effect on passive regurgitation and thus aspiration in the anesthetized patient. Arguably, rapid sequence induction with cricoid pressure has represented the standard of care for patients at risk for pulmonary aspiration in many centers. There is currently, however, considerable controversy regarding the efficacy and safety of this maneuver [222–225]; this topic has been recently and extensively reviewed [225]. There is also an awareness that the assumptions underlying the use of cricoid pressure and the efficacy of cricoid pressure in preventing regurgitation and aspiration remain unproven [226]. A recent randomized pilot trial compared cricoid pressure versus no cricoid pressure in patients at risk for microaspiration. Despite the use of sensitive biomarkers for microaspiration, no statistically significant differences were seen between the two groups [227].

Pressure applied to the cricoid cartilage may increase the lateral displacement of the esophagus [228] without reliably compressing it [229]. Cricoid pressure does appear to compress the hypopharynx, decreasing its diameter by 35% [230] and may obliterate the esophageal entrance [231]. The appropriate amount of force needed to prevent aspiration has also been a subject of considerable debate. However, a recent clinical study has quantified the force needed to occlude the esophageal entrance. Not surprisingly, a considerable amount of inter-patient variability was seen. The median cricoid force needed to completely occlude the esophageal entrance in 50% of men and women was 30.8 and 18.7 N, respectively [232]. Since excessive force may complicate airway management (see below) and insufficient force may fail to accomplish the desired clinical effect, modalities which enable the practitioner to monitor the degree of occlusion would seem desirable. Real-time ultrasound of the esophagus shows some early promise in this regard and has been advocated to confirm adequate esophageal compression and occlusion during RSI with cricoid pressure [233], but its utility in this regard remains unproven.

It should be understood by the practitioner that the application of cricoid pressure has the potential to displace and compress the airway [228], potentially increasing the difficulty associated with airway management [224, 234–237], and is contraindicated in the context of known or suspected cricoid or tracheal injury and unstable cervical spine and during active vomiting. Additionally, cricoid pressure has been associated with fracture of the cartilage [238] and a variety of other risks [234, 235, 239]. It is also worth noting that cricoid pressure is associated with a decrease in lower esophageal sphincter pressure and esophageal barrier pressure [240] which could increase the risk of passive regurgitation in the anesthetized patient. This is consistent with the well-described phenomenon of regurgitation and aspiration during the application of cricoid pressure [211, 241, 242]. Since our current understanding of aspiration and the protective effects of cricoid pressure, if any, are incomplete, the decision to apply cricoid pressure in the context of a rapid sequence induction should be individualized and based on an understanding of the relevant anatomic and physiologic principles and the specific clinical context.

Though there is little definitive evidence with regard to practical aspects of aspiration risk reduction to guide the practitioner, we suggest the following approach. If there is any anatomic or historical evidence to suggest a difficult intubation, serious consideration should be given to intubation in the awake patient, particularly for patients at highest risk of aspiration – those presenting with achalasia, high-grade esophageal obstruction, and those requiring emergency procedures. The awake placement of a large-bore gastric tube and awake intubation have been proposed for patients with severe achalasia [243]. For those patients with airways judged to be easily manageable, the use of a rapid sequence induction is prudent. Minimizing the time between loss of consciousness, muscle relaxation, and tracheal intubation with a lubricated cuffed tube may reduce risk. It is also worth considering the possible effect of patient position on aspiration risk. We routinely utilize the head-up, or reverse Trendelenburg position, as this is likely to reduce the passive reflux of gastric contents and aspiration risk [244–246]. Additionally, this position improves pulmonary mechanics, particularly in the obese patient, and has been previously advocated [211, 244]. It should be noted that, while a head-up position may reduce passive reflux, there is also a rationale for a head down tilt – placing the mouth in a more inferior position than that of the laryngeal inlet and trachea [224, 247], particularly in the patient at risk for vomiting during induction.

The suggestion that aspiration of gastric contents may be a contributing factor in the development of pulmonary complications in thoracic surgery patients is derived, in part, from evidence of intraoperative tracheal aspiration in intubated patients undergoing thoracotomy [248]. In this study, premedication with ranitidine decreased the incidence of measured gastric acid regurgitation, but effects on reduction of tracheal acid aspiration were not statistically significant. Clearly, acid aspiration in patients intubated with double-lumen endotracheal tubes is possible [248] though dye studies suggest that gel lubrication of the tube cuff may reduce leakage and aspiration [249, 250]. Other strategies to minimize the risk of tracheal aspiration in patients undergoing esophageal surgery include the placement of a large-bore gastric tube for highest-risk patients and preoperative suctioning of an in situ gastric tube [243] and of the gastric tube and oropharynx prior to tracheal extubation. A low level of continuous suctioning of the nasogastric tube after major esophageal surgery may also help reduce the incidence of subacute and chronic aspiration postoperatively [251].

Intraoperative Management

After the induction of general anesthesia and tracheal intubation, the maintenance of anesthesia can be accomplished by a variety of approaches, though many authors prefer a balanced anesthetic technique with the use of a volatile inhalational agent such as isoflurane, sevoflurane, or desflurane, a nondepolarizing paralytic agent, intravenous opioids, and opioids and/or local anesthetic agents via an epidural catheter if present [170, 172]. As volatile anesthetic agents are known to precondition the myocardium against subsequent ischemic insult, there is a theoretical advantage in the use of these agents. Given the overlap of risk factors for coronary disease and esophageal disease, patients presenting with surgical esophageal disease may also be at risk for myocardial ischemia and thus may benefit from such protection, though clinical evidence of benefit in this population is lacking. A total intravenous anesthetic with propofol infusion is also a viable option, though this technique lacks the theoretical advantage of myocardial preconditioning and may be significantly more expensive, particularly for longer surgeries.

Anesthetics have been shown to modulate the systemic and pulmonary inflammatory responses associated with major surgeries, mechanical ventilation, and OLV in particular. Since the inflammatory response associated with major esophageal surgeries can be severe [252] and since both systemic [253] and pulmonary inflammation [254] predict postoperative pulmonary complications, there has been considerable research interest in defining these modulatory effects. However, studies comparing primarily volatile anesthetic-based regimens to those based on propofol have produced somewhat discordant results. In a porcine model, sevoflurane elicited an immune lymphocytic response when compared with propofol and appeared to trigger apoptosis in lung tissue [255], though sevoflurane more effectively attenuates the pulmonary inflammatory response and oxygen impairment associated with ARDS [256] and ALI [257] in two different animal models. In randomized trials in patients undergoing thoracic surgery, however, anti-inflammatory effects have been attributed to both propofol and volatile agents. In a small trial of propofol vs sevoflurane in esophagectomy patients, propofol more effectively decreased the intrapulmonary concentration of inflammatory cytokines [258]. In contrast, sevoflurane dramatically attenuated the systemic [259, 260] and pulmonary [261] inflammatory responses to major thoracic surgery. Thus far, however, neither intravenous- nor volatile-based anesthetic strategies have been demonstrated to be unambiguously superior with regard to meaningful clinical outcomes and recent large clinical trial comparing propofol with desflurane demonstrated no differences in major morbidity between the two anesthetic regimens [262].

Lung Isolation and One-Lung Ventilation

Surgical approaches to the thoracic esophagus have been greatly facilitated by the development of techniques for lung isolation and OLV (see Chap. 6 for discussion of OLV and Chaps. 16–18 for details regarding lung isolation). In most major centers, lung isolation and one-lung ventilation are considered the standard of care for transthoracic approaches to the esophagus and are essential for thoracoscopic esophageal surgery. The most commonly utilized modalities are double-lumen endotracheal tubes (DLT) and endobronchial blockers. The left-sided DLT is most commonly employed for transthoracic esophageal surgery; it has the advantage of being easily placed by experienced practitioners, providing excellent lung isolation and operating conditions while providing access to both lungs for bronchoscopy, suctioning, ventilation, and oxygen insufflation. Additionally, because the left mainstem bronchus is longer than that of the right, positioning is more easily accomplished without compromising left upper lobe ventilation.

However, the use of a DLT may be relatively or absolutely contraindicated in some patients or may be difficult to achieve, necessitating another approach. First, endotracheal intubation with a DLT may require more time than with a single-lumen tube [263]. This may increase the risk of aspiration in the high-risk patient, especially in the context of a difficult airway. The use of adjunctive airway devices such as the endotracheal tube introducer may be more difficult with a DLT [264], though difficult endotracheal intubation with a DLT can be aided by the use of adjunctive devices such as the GlideScope video laryngoscope [265, 266], the McGrath video laryngoscope [267], the Airway Scope [268], and the Airtraq laryngoscope [269, 270]. Videolaryngoscopy improves visualization of the larynx during DLT intubation and has been recommended [271].

Some patients may present with anatomic abnormalities of the airway such as subglottic stenosis or extrinsic compression of the trachea or either mainstem bronchus. Passage of a DLT may be difficult or even dangerous in this context. If it is likely that the patient will require postoperative mechanical ventilation or if extubation is delayed for another reason, exchanging the DLT for a single-lumen tube at the end of surgery places the patient at additional risk for loss of airway and aspiration. The above limitations of DLT have

prompted interest in the use of endobronchial blockers for esophageal surgeries. A detailed discussion of endobronchial blockers and their applications can be found in Chaps. 16–18. Endobronchial blockers are placed through (coaxially) or occasionally alongside single-lumen endotracheal tubes (SLT) and can be used in patients with tracheostomies or nasal airway access. The use of endobronchial blockers is well described for thoracic procedures, including esophageal surgery [272], and is preferred by some authors [264] because of the perceived reduction in aspiration risk with the use of the SLT and rapid sequence induction, the improved ease of managing difficult airways, and lung collapse scores equivalent to [273] or better [274] than that of DLTs.

Fluid Management

Fluid requirements vary widely among patients and procedures and ultimately represent the sum of preoperative deficits, maintenance requirements, and ongoing losses (see Chap. 21 for a discussion of fluid management in thoracic surgery). Preoperative fluid deficits in patients with severe esophageal disease may be substantial, though they have not been well defined. Fluid requirements in patients undergoing esophageal procedures may be complicated by the fact that patients may be relatively hypovolemic after long preoperative fasts, particularly if esophageal obstruction or dysphagia limit fluid intake. Perioperative losses occur via a number of mechanisms including urinary, gastrointestinal, and evaporative losses, bleeding, and interstitial fluid shifting. This shift of fluid from the vascular compartment into the interstitial space accompanies surgical trauma and is likely to reflect vascular injury and loss of endothelial integrity. So-called "third-space" losses describe fluid loss into non-interstitial extracellular spaces which are not in equilibrium with the vascular compartment and thus considered to be a "nonfunctional" extracellular fluid compartment. This space has not been well characterized and its existence is unlikely [275–277].

In general, minor procedures and those involving minimally invasive surgical procedures tend to be associated with low fluid requirements. Patients undergoing longer and more complex procedures involving open abdominal and/or thoracic incisions may require more intraoperative fluid to maintain homeostasis. While evidence-based guidelines on fluid management for thoracic surgery do not yet exist, a consensus of best practice is beginning to evolve. Principles of perioperative fluid management principles for esophagectomy [278] and pathophysiology of fluid shifting in the perioperative setting have been extensively reviewed [275, 279]. Recent advances in understanding of glycocalyx function, the pathophysiologic implications of excessive fluid administration, and the application of advanced monitoring modalities to drive rational goal-directed fluid therapies (GDFT) justify several conclusions.

First, excessive perioperative intravenous fluid administration, particularly crystalloid, contributes to an exaggerated fluid shifting toward the interstitial space, potentially increasing complications associated with poor wound healing, slower return of GI function, abdominal compartment syndrome, impaired anastomotic healing, increased cardiac demand, pneumonia, and respiratory failure [280]. The adverse consequences of excessive fluid administration may be particularly problematic in esophagectomy patients, since edema in the conduit and at the anastomotic site may lead to inflammatory infiltration [281] and reduced tissue oxygenation [215], potentially placing the anastomosis at greater risk for necrosis and leak.

Prospective trials examining "liberal" versus "restrictive" fluid regimens in patients undergoing major surgical procedures generally favor greater fluid restriction [282–284] as do retrospective studies of patients undergoing pulmonary resection surgery [285–287] and esophagectomy [288, 289]. Interpretation of these prospective trials is limited, however, by a lack of standard definition of the terms "restrictive" and "liberal." What is liberal in one study may be restrictive in another. Retrospective analyses are limited in this regard by the potential for uncontrolled bias. Most studies of both types, however, are consistent with the idea that fluid overload is indeed related to adverse outcomes. This concept is supported by a large meta-analysis of trials comparing liberal versus restrictive fluid management in elective surgeries which reported a large reduction in perioperative complications in the restrictive group [290]. Perioperative fluid administration appears to be an independent risk predictor of morbidity after esophagectomy for cancer [291], and a positive fluid balance predicts pulmonary complications after esophagectomy [292].

However, inadequate fluid resuscitation in patients with significant perioperative fluid losses may also be detrimental, causing hypovolemia and a decrement in stroke volume, cardiac output, and tissue oxygen delivery which could compromise renal function, wound healing, anastomotic integrity, and even cardiovascular stability. Fluid requirements for major esophageal surgery appear to be lower than previously thought and expert recommendations have been published [278]. Concerns regarding the implications for acute kidney injury in major thoracic surgical patients subjected to fluid restriction may be exaggerated, given recent findings that fluid restriction (<3 mL/kg/h) was not a risk factor for kidney injury in major thoracic surgery [293].

Optimizing fluid regimens is likely to be dependent upon adequately measuring fluid requirements or surrogates thereof in individual patients rather than relying upon formulas for "restrictive" or "liberal" regimens. While fluid requirements have not been well characterized in patients undergoing esophageal surgery specifically, recent evaluation of crystalloid requirements to maintain the left ventricular end-diastolic volume index (LVEDVI) in patients undergoing colorectal surgery has been made. The rate of crystalloid infusion required to maintain LVEDVI in patients undergoing open and laparoscopic colorectal surgery was 5.9 mL/kg/h and 3.4 mL/kg/h, respectively [294]. However, inter-individual variability was high, consistent with the need for an individualized approach. It would seem intuitive that an ideal fluid regimen for major surgeries including esophageal surgeries is individualized and optimizes cardiac output and oxygen delivery while avoiding excessive fluid administration. There is an emerging body of evidence that fluid therapies which are designed to achieve individualized and specific flow-related hemodynamic endpoints such as stroke volume, cardiac output, or measures of fluid responsiveness such as stroke volume variation (collectively referred to as goal-directed fluid therapy (GDFT)) may provide a superior alternative to fixed regimens or those based on static measures of cardiac filling such as central venous pressure which does not predict fluid responsiveness or correlate with circulating blood volume in hospitalized patients [295] or after transthoracic esophagectomy [296]. GDFT in the setting of major surgery has been shown to reduce hospital length of stay [297–304], promote earlier return of bowel function [297], and reduce postoperative nausea and vomiting (PONV) [297], morbidity [299–301, 305], and vasopressor use [306]. A review of nine studies utilizing GDFT revealed that of these, seven reported reduced hospital length of stay, three reported reduced PONV and ileus, and four reported a reduction in complications [307]. Several large meta-analyses have also supported the use of defined protocols including fluid management and inotropic therapies to optimize hemodynamics and/or tissue perfusion [308–310]. Indeed, a goal-directed approach to fluid management in the context of an enhanced recovery program for colorectal surgery has been recommended in a joint consensus statement by the American Society for Enhance Recovery and the Perioperative Quality Initiative [311].

The role of GDFT for outcome improvement in thoracic surgery is less clear and most available studies are small and have investigated primarily patients undergoing cardiac surgery. In addition to the pulmonary artery catheter-derived cardiac output measurements, which are not typically used for most general thoracic surgeries, and the transesophageal echocardiographic and esophageal Doppler modalities, which are inappropriate for esophageal surgery, a number of minimally invasive modalities compatible with transthoracic esophageal surgery are available. These include primarily devices that use proprietary algorithms to estimate stroke volume index, cardiac index, and/or stroke volume variation (SVV) [312–315]. Most of the available minimally invasive technologies used to guide GDFT depend upon respiratory variation and cardiorespiratory interaction to predict fluid responsiveness. Since these interactions are likely to be sub-

Chest radiography and arterial blood gas analysis should be performed immediately in any patient with acute respiratory decompensation after thoracic surgery.

Anesthetic Considerations for Specific Esophageal Procedures and Disorders

Esophagoscopy

Esophagoscopy may be performed with either a rigid or flexible endoscope and is used for a number of specific diagnostic and therapeutic purposes. In general, most diagnostic esophagoscopies are performed using flexible endoscopes, often in awake/sedated patients and frequently in a gastroenterology suite without the care of an anesthesiologist. Conscious sedation performed by a nurse or other assistant under the direction of an endoscopist, usually a gastroenterologist, is most often accomplished with the use of a benzodiazepine such as diazepam or midazolam with or without the addition of an opioid such as meperidine or fentanyl. Often, a local anesthetic such as lidocaine or benzocaine is applied topically to facilitate patient acceptance and reduce gagging during the procedure. Using a traditional approach, patient acceptance of the procedure without sedation, even with ultrathin esophagoscopes, is quite limited [341]. However, more recent clinical experience with a transnasal approach to flexible esophagoscopy confirms that this procedure is well tolerated under local anesthesia without sedation when performed by otolaryngologists [342, 343]. If local anesthetic is used, the total acceptable dose should be carefully considered as methemoglobinemia has been associated with topical use of benzocaine for surgical procedures [344], including esophagogastroduodenoscopy (EGD) [345]. Flexible esophagoscopy is also routinely performed by thoracic surgeons immediately prior to esophageal surgery to assess the location and extent of esophageal lesions and the degree of esophageal obstruction. Most of these patients have known esophageal disease and are presenting for curative or palliative esophageal surgery. These patients are usually at elevated risk for regurgitation and aspiration and should be treated appropriately. The airway should be secured prior to instrumentation of the esophagus under general anesthesia.

More complex endoscopic procedures often require deeper levels of sedation or general anesthesia. Maintaining a patient airway, optimizing oxygenation, and preventing aspiration are the primary concerns during these procedures, particularly in obese patients, longer procedures, and with prone positioning. While some degree of desaturation is common during extended esophagoscopic procedures in patients not endotracheally intubated, the presence of an in situ endoscope may help stent open the airway at the pharyngeal level [346]. Nonetheless, a high degree of vigilance is required to detect airway obstruction and impending hypoxemia in these cases. If standard maneuvers fail to relieve airway obstruction, extraction of the esophagoscope may be required for definitive airway management. A number of commercially available devices have been designed to accommodate an endoscope while permitting oxygen insufflation and/or ventilation. These include face masks, a gastrolaryngeal tube [346], and the recently available LMA Gastro Airway – a supraglottic device designed to create an oropharyngeal seal while providing a large channel for endoscope passage.

Rigid esophagoscopy is most frequently employed for the extraction of esophageal foreign bodies, often in children, as well as for the removal of retained food items. As with laryngoscopy, this is a very stimulating procedure and not likely to be well tolerated without general anesthesia. These patients should also be considered high risk for aspiration and managed accordingly, with the rapid placement of a cuffed endotracheal tube before or immediately after induction of anesthesia. In selected patients who are felt to be at lower risk for aspiration with this procedure and who meet NPO guidelines, it may be appropriate to consider deeper levels of sedation. Monitored anesthesia care with sedation using dexmedetomidine infusion for rigid esophagoscopy and dilation of the UES with botulinum toxin injection for dysphagia has been described [347]. Propofol-based monitored anesthesia care is also commonly used for patients who do not require endotracheal intubation and may be particularly useful for longer or more difficult cases, including submucosal dissections for esophagogastric cancer [348]. Anesthetic management considerations for rigid esophagoscopy include the extreme neck extension desired by surgeons for alignment of the oral-esophageal axis, the risk of aspirating objects once extracted from the esophagus [349], and the need for a relaxed patient to minimize movement during the procedure. The latter need can be achieved with deep levels of inhalational anesthetic or with short-acting muscle relaxants.

Additional therapeutic uses of esophagoscopy include esophageal stent placement for tracheoesophageal fistula (TEF), benign and malignant strictures [350, 351], and perforation [29, 352] and nonsurgical treatment of achalasia, including esophageal dilatation and intraesophageal delivery of botulinum toxin [353], as well as the per-oral endoscopic myotomy (POEM) procedure [354] – an endoscopic alternative to the classical Heller myotomy. Endoscopic techniques are also used in the staging of superficial esophageal tumors and complete resection and ablation of mucosal adenocarcinoma [93–96, 355].

Tracheoesophageal Fistula (TEF)

Anesthetic management of the patient with TEF is uniquely challenging for several reasons. First, positive-pressure ventilation inevitably results in ventilatory gas entering the esophagus and stomach. Second, the inevitable large airway leak may render pulmonary ventilation difficult or impossible. Third, ventilation of the gastrointestinal tract may result in worsening pulmonary compliance because of abdominal distention which may also increase the risk of further aspiration and other complications [72, 356, 357]. For these reasons, maintenance of spontaneous ventilation is often preferred and can be accomplished with either an inhalational induction or an awake intubation, though baseline decrements in pulmonary function and compliance on the affected side are likely to increase difficulties associated with oxygenation and adequate ventilation after induction of anesthesia. The preoperative placement of a gastrostomy tube will aid in venting the stomach in the event that positive-pressure ventilation becomes necessary but is contraindicated if the stomach is to be used as a conduit. Additionally, chronic aspiration and its sequelae of pneumonia, sepsis, and hypoxemia may complicate the anesthetic management of these patients, particularly during OLV. Positive-pressure ventilation can be safely performed once lung isolation has been accomplished. Lung isolation is essential to prevent ventilation of the fistula, to provide adequate pulmonary ventilation, and to prevent further soilage of the lung.

The anesthetic plan for airway management and ventilation in adult patients with TEF should reflect the anatomic position of the fistula in the respiratory tract. Typically, the identification and localization of the fistula is made before presentation to the operating theater. On rare occasions, a previously undiagnosed TEF may manifest itself after otherwise uncomplicated airway management [76]. Occasionally, the exact level of the fistula is not known. Though not always successful, bronchoscopic examination of the airway may identify the level of airway involvement and can be performed preoperatively. Bronchoscopy can also be performed after tracheal intubation with either a DLT [358] or SLT [359] and used to guide placement after localization of the TEF. Rarely, esophagoscopy may also be used to identify SLT position relative to the fistula [360].

The DLT is preferred in most cases of TEF since it can be placed into the mainstem bronchus contralateral to the fistula, providing lung isolation, OLV, and protection from soilage of the ventilated lung. Thus, the right-sided DLT should be used for left-sided lesions and vice versa. Alternatively, an SLT (ideally one designed for endobronchial placement) can be placed in the contralateral bronchus. Occasionally, for a tracheal TEF well above the carina, a SLT may be used if the cuff can be inflated below the fistula. If this is not possible, a right DLT is preferable for distal tracheal fistulae or if the fistula site is not identified preoperatively. In patients with severe pulmonary disease, OLV may be incompatible with adequate oxygenation and ventilation. Rarely, alternative approaches for oxygenation and ventilation that minimize

gas flow into the esophagus may be required. The use of a left DLT for lung isolation with high-frequency oscillation ventilation on the right side has been described for optimizing gas exchange in a patient with a low tracheal TEF and ARDS [361]. An alternative approach in critically ill ventilated patients with benign TEF utilizes temporary stenting to functionally separate the airway and esophagus, minimizing air leak and improving CO_2 removal [78]. This procedure was easily performed and well tolerated and could presumably serve as a bridge to definitive surgical correction following improvement in the patient's status.

Postoperative goals include optimizing pulmonary function to facilitate a return to spontaneous ventilation with adequate gas exchange. The continuation of positive-pressure ventilation may lead to disruption of the esophageal closure and could thus cause a ventilatory leak. Achieving this goal requires adequate pain control and may also require aggressive pulmonary toilet with bronchoscopy prior to emergence.

Transthoracic Nissen and Belsey Fundoplication, Collis Gastroplasty, and Paraesophageal Hernia Repair

Transthoracic anti-reflux procedures require monitoring arterial and venous access commensurate with a thoracotomy. Most patients presenting with hiatal hernias, particularly those with paraesophageal hernia and/or symptomatic GERD, are considered to be at elevated risk for perioperative aspiration of gastric contents, although clear risk stratification is lacking. For this reason, rapid sequence induction is preferred by many practitioners for patients with reassuring airway anatomy.

Lung isolation and OLV are required for transthoracic approaches to the esophagus. Bronchial blockers are ideal in these cases for the following reasons: (1) blocker placement can follow definitive airway management via rapid sequence induction with SLT in the protected (intubated) airway, (2) rapid sequence induction is performed more rapidly and arguably, more easily and safely, when a SLT rather than DLT is used, (3) as discussed above, performance of modern bronchial blockers with regard to lung isolation and operating conditions are equivalent to that of DLTs, and (4) since most of these procedures utilize a left thoracotomy approach, left bronchial blockade is easily achieved due to the longer left main bronchus.

An aggressive plan for postoperative pain control is also required – typically TEA. Following induction, intubation, and placement of vascular cannulae, the patient is placed in the right lateral decubitus position. After withdrawing an indwelling gastric tube, a large bougie/dilator is advanced into the esophagus at the surgeon's request to facilitate the fundoplication. The dilator should be well lubricated with a water-soluble lubricant and passed atraumatically into the upper esophagus with manual guidance or with the use of a laryngoscope to aid engagement with the esophageal orifice. Caution should be exercised during advancement, and communication with the surgeon is important, particularly if resistance is encountered as esophageal disruption can occur. It is then passed slowly through the esophagogastric junction and left in this position until the fundoplication sutures are secured at which time it can be withdrawn.

Unless complications are encountered intraoperatively, most patients can be allowed to emerge from anesthesia at the conclusion of surgery and extubated at emergence. The stomach should be drained with a nasogastric tube postoperatively. Oral feeding is begun after return of normal bowel activity which may require several days after open repair. Dysphagia to solid foods can be experienced by some patients for several weeks after surgery and is more common with transthoracic procedures and total fundoplications but typically resolves spontaneously.

Esophagectomy

Transhiatal Esophagectomy (THE)

Patients presenting for this procedure require standard monitoring, a urinary catheter and an arterial catheter for continuous arterial blood pressure monitoring. Patients will also benefit from the preoperative placement of an epidural catheter for postoperative pain control. After preoxygenation and induction of general anesthesia, the trachea is intubated with a single-lumen endotracheal tube and both arterial and adequate intravenous access are obtained – generally two peripheral venous cannulae and an arterial catheter. A nasogastric tube is placed and secured in its position after the esophageal anastomosis is made.

The transhiatal approach to esophagectomy requires the manual dissection of the esophagus from the mediastinum blindly via the abdominal hiatus. The manual compression of the heart and great veins commonly causes hypotension, usually transiently. Optimizing volume status prior to this step may partially mitigate the decrement in blood pressure and cardiac output. Close communication between surgeon and anesthesiologist is critical during this stage, as it may become necessary for the surgeon to temporarily discontinue the dissection to permit hemodynamic recovery, particularly in the elderly or fragile patient. The duration of hypotension during dissection may be related to a patient history of cardiac disease and the presence of a mid-esophageal tumor [362]. The transhiatal dissection may also precipitate atrial and/or ventricular ectopy which could contribute to hypotension and reduced cardiac output during this phase. Atrial arrhythmias are commonly associated with transhiatal dissection [363] and are more likely in patients with cardiac

disease [362]. In a small study of transhiatal esophagectomies, arrhythmias occurred during transhiatal manipulation in 65% of cases, but were transient, did not require treatment, and were not correlated with hypotension [363]. Other potential intraoperative complications include pneumothorax, mediastinal bleeding from injuries to the aorta or azygous vein, and injury of the membranous trachea. Pneumothorax is easily managed surgically with the placement of a tube thoracostomy from the operative field. Massive hemorrhage is rare but is likely to require emergent thoracotomy and repair with aggressive transfusion and resuscitation. Tracheal injury also requires definitive repair, and the anesthesiologist may be required to advance the endotracheal tube beyond the site of injury to facilitate ventilation during the repair. For this reason, only full-length uncut endotracheal tubes should be used for THE.

Following completion of the cervical anastomosis and wound closure, the nasogastric tube is secured in position. If in situ, the epidural catheter should be appropriately dosed prior to emergence. Tracheal extubation is performed at emergence with return of protective airway reflexes, and the patient is transferred to a unit where appropriate monitoring and pain control can be accomplished. The head of the bed should be elevated between 30° and 45° to optimize respiratory mechanics and to minimize the potential for reflux and aspiration. Postoperative therapy includes antibiotics and thromboprophylaxis. Postoperative complications attributable to the THE include recurrent laryngeal nerve injury which results in hoarseness and an increased risk of aspiration pneumonitis, chylothorax, and anastomotic leak.

Transthoracic Esophagectomy (Ivor Lewis; TTE)

Unless contraindicated, a thoracic epidural catheter should be placed preoperatively. Induction and maintenance of general anesthesia can be accomplished with standard agents. For the reasons enumerated above, a rapid sequence induction is recommended, and endotracheal intubation should ideally be accomplished with attention to the risks of aspiration. Lung isolation is not required for laparotomy, and thus, some practitioners intubate initially with a SLT, replacing it with a DLT prior to the thoracotomy incision and after suctioning of the stomach. It is also reasonable to place a DLT at induction unless difficult placement is predicted in a patient with elevated risk of aspiration, such as high-grade obstruction, gastroparesis, or emergency surgery. In such cases, the practitioner should first rapidly secure the airway with a SLT, evacuate stomach contents intraoperatively, and then either place a DLT prior to thoracotomy or simply use an endobronchial blocker.

After induction, a nasogastric tube is placed with consideration to possible partial or complete esophageal obstruction that may necessitate surgical assistance for positioning distally. Decompression of the stomach and esophageal conduit is of paramount importance; thus the tube should be secured intraoperatively to prevent its removal by the patient or inadvertent removal during patient movement and transport. Muscle relaxation with nondepolarizing muscle relaxants provides optimal operating conditions. An arterial catheter and large-bore peripheral or central venous access should be obtained after induction.

Intraoperative hypotension may occur during transthoracic esophagectomy surgery and typically results from hypovolemia and/or TEA-related sympathectomy. Hypotension may precipitate myocardial or cerebral ischemia and may also contribute to gastric tube ischemia. Thus, potential causes should be immediately sought and treated. The mobilized gastric tube has a limited blood supply, usually from the right gastroepiploic artery, and blood flow at the distal segment is decreased. Factors such as hypotension may further compromise perfusion of the gastric tube and may thus increase the risk of anastomotic leak [364]. Since anastomotic integrity is dependent upon adequate blood flow and oxygen delivery [365–369], the development of anastomotic leak may be related to intraoperative management variables, particularly systemic blood pressure [364] and cardiac output and may thus be modifiable by anesthetic management.

Some esophageal surgeons eschew the use of vasoconstricting agents for fear of the theoretical adverse effects on gastric tube blood flow. However, the available data do not support this reasoning. The effect of vasoconstrictors on gastric tube blood flow is likely to reflect volume status and other variables, but the clinical and experimental evidence supports the following concepts: (1) dysregulated blood flow in the newly formed conduit is blood pressure-dependent, (2) hypotension impairs conduit blood flow, (3) a supranormal blood pressure does not improve conduit blood flow above that of normotension, and (4) in the euvolemic patient, the use of vasopressors to treat hypotension, rather than compromising conduit blood flow, actually has the potential to substantially improve perfusion. Al-Rawi and colleagues demonstrated that a TEA-induced sympathectomy decreased gastric tube blood flow during esophagectomy and that the intravenous infusion of epinephrine restored blood flow [370]. The use of norepinephrine to maintain arterial blood pressure during esophagectomy as part of a multimodal anesthetic regimen has been associated with reduced respiratory morbidity without increasing the incidence of anastomotic complications [172]. These findings are consistent with those of an elegant porcine gastric tube model in which the use of norepinephrine to attain supranormal blood pressures did not improve gastric tube blood flow but likewise did not adversely affect this variable [371]. Clinically useful conclusions can also be derived from the study by Pathak et al. [372] who demonstrated that hypotension induced by a local anesthetic bolus via an in situ thoracic epidural catheter

adversely affected conduit blood flow and that a phenylephrine infusion restored both mean blood pressure and conduit perfusion. Given the established relationship between gastric tube blood flow and anastomotic leak, maintenance of normal hemodynamics should be a priority in the intraoperative management of these patients. Toward this end it may be prudent to modify or postpone dosing of an indwelling epidural catheter in a hypotensive patient and to consider the use of inotropic agents with or without vasopressor activity.

Following uneventful transthoracic esophagectomy, most patients can be extubated in the operating room provided that they are normothermic, metabolically and hemodynamically stable, well oxygenated, and appropriate pain control modalities have been employed. Although an older randomized trial comparing early versus late extubation after esophagectomy reported a higher mortality in the early extubation group, this difference was not statistically significant [373] and has not been observed subsequently. Early extubation after esophagectomy has been well studied and is supported by a number of retrospective and observational analyses [169, 374, 375] as well as reports of standardized management approaches [170] and fast-track clinical pathways [169, 171, 376]. Factors which may predict failure or complications associated with early extubation include a history of smoking and chronic obstructive pulmonary disease (COPD) [377]. Epidural analgesia has been demonstrated to facilitate successful early extubation [169, 375, 377].

Considerable interest in enhanced recovery (enhanced recovery after surgery (ERAS)) protocols in a variety of surgical service lines follows from initial successes in colorectal surgery [378]. Although considerable heterogeneity exists between institutions, most ERAS programs employ efforts to optimize pain control while minimizing opioid use, prevent iatrogenic fluid overload, and improve pre- and postoperative rehabilitation. Specific elements of ERAS care for esophagectomy patients have included preoperative education, prehabilitation including inspiratory muscle training, preoperative carbohydrate nutrition, epidural analgesia, early mobilization and rehabilitation, avoidance of or early discontinuation of nasogastric and other drains, early feeding, and discharge education. While ERAS for esophagectomy is still in its infancy relative to that of other surgical service lines, considerable evidence has accrued to support a protocolized pathway for perioperative care in the esophagectomy patient. Thus far, a number of outcome advantages have been ascribed to ERAS-like protocols in esophagectomy; these include a reduction in postoperative complications [175, 379, 380], pain [175], hospital length of stay [174, 175], hospital costs (or charges) [176, 379, 380], and time to return to normal activity [175], without an increase in readmission rate [174, 379, 380]. Optimizing perioperative care in this way also appears to reduce the systemic inflammatory response associated with esophagectomy [176] which may account for improvements in certain outcomes. A recent meta-analysis of ERAS programs [381] for esophagectomy confirms a large degree of variation in program design and the limitations associated with uncontrolled potential confounding variables. However, within these constraints, the efficacy of ERAS is generally supported – leading to a reduction in anastomotic and pulmonary complications and hospital length of stay without any change in the readmission rate (ERAS in thoracic surgery is discussed in Chap. 52).

At emergence, patients should be seated 30° above supine and extubated upon return of protective airway reflexes. Supplemental oxygen may be delivered via face tent or nasal cannulae. If postoperative ventilatory support is required or extubation must be delayed for other reasons, tube exchange can be performed with laryngoscopy, adjunctive airway devices, or via a tube exchange catheter.

Minimally Invasive Esophagectomy (MIE)

Minimally invasive esophagectomy (MIE) is a blanket term which has been used to describe a variety of less invasive approaches to esophagectomy. MIE may refer to a laparoscopic approach to transhiatal esophagectomy, fully minimally invasive equivalents of the Ivor Lewis esophagectomy (laparoscopy and thoracoscopy), or a number of hybrid approaches. At this time, there is little specific data available to guide anesthetic management of the patient undergoing minimally invasive esophagectomy, but principles of management in the patient undergoing open esophagectomy are likely to apply. OLV is considered essential for any thoracoscopic procedure, including MIE, and thus, lung isolation is required. The use of DLT and bronchial blockers for esophageal surgery has been discussed above and applies here as well.

It is not clear that patients undergoing MIE require aggressive pain control modalities such as TEA for optimal postoperative pain control. However, the TEA remains the standard of care in centers which perform these surgeries largely because of the theoretical and demonstrated advantages of TEA in the context of open esophagectomy and thoracic surgery in general.

Robotic Esophagectomy

From an anesthesiologist's perspective, use of the da Vinci robotic surgical system to aid in the performance of esophagectomy has the potential to significantly affect patient care and safety during the operative procedure. It is thus incumbent upon the practitioner to understand the implications of robot use particularly with regard to patient access and specific risks. The da Vinci robotic system utilizes a console for the surgeon, a side cart with four robotic arms which interact with the patient, and an additional cart which houses optical devices for the camera system. Typically, the patient axis is turned at least 90° away from the anesthesiologist and anesthesia machine. After port placement and robot docking, access to the patient is very limited. Position of the robot chassis above the patient's head limits access to the airway. The anesthesiologist should be aware of the risks associated with positioning for robotic surgery – including the known risk of brachial plexus injury from extreme arm positioning and the possibility of robotic arm collision with the patient's body. Likewise, access to the patient's body is also quite restrictive. It is essential for the anesthesiologist to confirm ideal position of the DLT or bronchial blocker prior to final robot positioning. All vascular access must also be secured and line patency confirmed. Extension tubing for arterial and venous lines is often required. The recently developed lung isolation products (Viva Sight, ET View) incorporate a small high-resolution imaging camera in the DLT or single-lumen tube to provide for continuous and real-time imaging of the distal airway. These devices allow the anesthesiologist to continuously monitor the DLT or blocker position, potentially providing both confirmation of correct positioning and an early warning when a malposition is imminent.

Additional concerns for the anesthesiologist during robotic surgery arise from the use of carbon dioxide insufflation to improve surgical exposure. Pressurized insufflation of carbon dioxide can contribute to hypercarbia, gas embolism, and bradycardia. Hemithoracic gas insufflation can be associated with hemodynamic compromise to the extent that it creates a state similar to that of a tension pneumothorax. In general low-pressure insufflation (<5 mmHg) is well tolerated in stable patients [382] and most patients can tolerate moderate pressures (8–10 mmHg). However, higher pressures may cause hemodynamic compromise, and efforts should be made to minimize insufflation pressures. If higher pressures are needed, a slow increase in insufflation pressure (up to 14 mmHg) may minimize hemodynamic effects [383]. Additionally, surgical violation of the contralateral pleura may cause respiratory or hemodynamic compromise. Finally, the anesthesiologist should be prepared for open thoracotomy in the event the robotic approach fails (see Chap. 39 for a detailed discussion of anesthesia for robotic thoracic surgery).

Postoperative Care of the Esophagectomy Patient

With appropriate pain control regimens, most patients are extubated in the operating room. Early ambulation and chest physiotherapy are used to reduce respiratory complications.

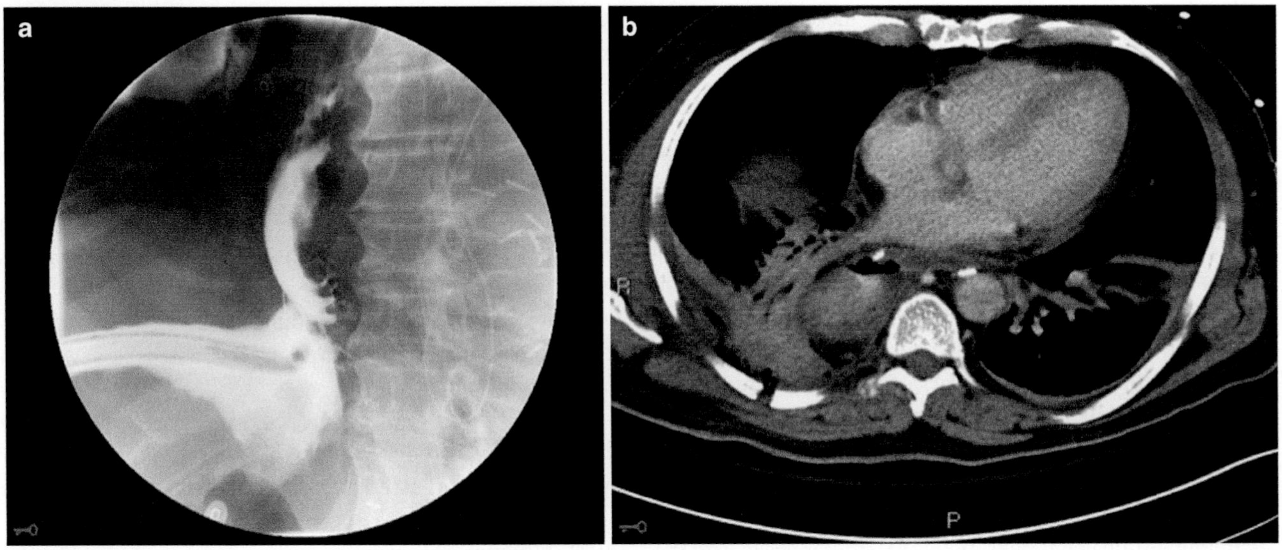

Fig. 38.9 (a) Fluoroscopic image of anastomotic leak after esophagectomy. Note contrast material leak into right hemithorax. (b) Chest CT scan revealing contrast medium leaking into right hemithorax from anastomotic leak after esophagectomy

Pleural drains are removed as soon as drainage is minimal and absence of air leak is confirmed, though mediastinal drains may be left until confirmation of intrathoracic anastomotic integrity is confirmed. The indwelling epidural catheter is generally used and left in situ until pleural drains are removed, at which time pain control can be adequately accomplished with parenteral or enteral medications. Feeding via a jejunostomy tube is typically initiated after 24 h postoperatively and advanced over a period of several days. A contrast study of the esophagus is usually performed on or about the fifth postoperative day, and if normal, a clear diet by mouth is begun at that time. As noted in the discussion above, there is substantial interest in, and some evidence supporting, immediate oral nutrition following esophagectomy, though widespread adoption is likely to await the completion of, and favorable outcomes from, a randomized trial. At discharge, the patient should be eating solid food and the jejunostomy tube is clamped. At surgical follow-up in several weeks, the feeding tube is removed.

Adverse Outcomes After Esophagectomy

Adverse outcomes after esophagectomy surgery have historically been divided into surgical and anesthetic complications. At first glance, this division is logical and appealing, but recent insight into the pathophysiology of complications after major thoracic and thoracoabdominal surgeries is beginning to blur this distinction.

Esophageal Anastomotic Leaks

As mentioned above, the development of an esophageal anastomotic leak is a frequent and serious complication of esophagectomy (see Fig. 38.9a and b). In a recent large retrospective review of data from the Society of Thoracic Surgeons database, the incidence of anastomotic leak was 12.9% [108]. This complication is particularly worrisome when the leak is mediastinal in location. Mortality rates from intrathoracic leaks range from 3.3% to 71% [384]. Preoperative, operative, and postoperative factors that may predispose to the development of anastomotic leak have been well described in the literature [384] and include comorbidities such as diabetes, pulmonary disease, and cardiovascular disease, a variety of surgical and technical factors, and postoperative factors including gastric distension, prolonged ventilatory support, and hypoxia. Though still considered a surgical complication, accumulating evidence suggests that intraoperative management may have an impact on the incidence of this complication. Because of the tenuous blood supply to the mobilized gastric tube, fluid status, hemodynamics, and oxygenation may affect anastomotic integrity through effects on oxygen delivery [365, 366] and blood flow [365]. Though the optimization of tissue oxygen delivery through appropriate management of hemodynamics, fluid status, and oxygenation is a priority for all perioperative patients, this truism may be particularly critical for patients undergoing esophageal anastomoses.

Cardiovascular Complications

Cardiovascular complications account for significant morbidity and mortality after esophagectomy. The most common cardiac complication is arrhythmia, typically atrial tachyarrhythmias such as atrial fibrillation, atrial flutter, and paroxysmal supraventricular tachycardia. While generally considered benign after cardiac surgery, these diagnoses may be more ominous after general thoracic surgery including esophagectomy. There is considerable evidence that atrial tachyarrhythmias after esophagectomy are associated with a higher rate of ICU admission, greater length of hospital stay, and a higher mortality [385–387]. These findings are consistent with those for general non-cardiac thoracic surgery patients in whom atrial fibrillation was a marker for increased morbidity and mortality [388]. Atrial fibrillation after esophagectomy is also associated with a higher rate of pulmonary complications, anastomotic leakage, and sepsis [386]. Risk factors for the development of atrial dysrhythmias after esophagectomy include transthoracic approach [389], older age, perioperative theophylline use, a low diffusion capacity [385, 390], COPD, male sex, and history of cardiac disease [390]. Larger studies of general thoracic surgery patients including esophagectomies point to similar risks for the development of atrial fibrillation – male sex, older age, history of congestive heart failure, arrhythmia, peripheral vascular disease and resection of mediastinal tumor, pulmonary resection, esophagectomy, and intraoperative blood transfusion [388].

The prophylaxis of atrial tachyarrhythmias in general thoracic surgery has been the subject of numerous clinical trials and observational studies, but no clinical standard for prophylaxis exists. A review of trials of pharmacologic prophylaxis for postoperative atrial arrhythmias reported that calcium channel blockers and beta-blockers reduced the risk of tachyarrhythmias, though the latter increased the risk of pulmonary edema [391]. The routine prophylactic use of digoxin, flecainide, and amiodarone is not supported by the available evidence [391]. A randomized trial in patients undergoing transthoracic esophagectomy demonstrated a relative risk reduction of 62.5% for postoperative atrial fibrillation in patients randomized to receive amiodarone [392]. The available evidence supports prophylaxis in patients at higher risk of atrial tachyarrhythmias. Such prophylaxis should be individualized and may include amiodarone, calcium channel blockers, or beta-blockers, with attention to the potential for adverse effects of the latter.

Pulmonary Complications

Respiratory morbidity occurs frequently after thoracic surgery in general and after esophagectomy in particular [167, 393]. Pulmonary complications of thoracic surgery are variably defined in the literature but include pneumonia, aspiration pneumonitis, ARDS, bronchopleural fistula, atelectasis, and pulmonary embolism. Any individual or cluster of these complications can result in respiratory insufficiency or respiratory failure, which may require specific therapies including the continuation or reinstitution of mechanical ventilation. The overall incidence of serious respiratory morbidity is highly variable but is between 10% and 30% in most large series [108, 394–398]. Factors predictive of pulmonary complications after esophagectomy include age [394, 395, 398], smoking [398], alcohol use [398], COPD [398], proximal location of esophageal tumor, and duration of surgery [394, 398], as well as forced expiratory volume in 1 s (FEV_1) [395] which predicts pulmonary complications in patients with COPD [399]. Additionally, preoperative airway bacterial colonization predicts an increase in postoperative pulmonary complications and is associated with an increased mortality [400].

ALI and ARDS are among the most severe pulmonary complications associated with esophagectomy, and their incidence in a large series was 23.8% and 14.5%, respectively [401]. ARDS is associated with a 50% mortality rate [401], a higher risk of non-respiratory organ failure, and a longer ICU and hospital stay [402]. Risk factors included low body mass index, tobacco history, surgeon experience, duration of surgery and OLV, anastomotic leak, and cardiorespiratory instability. The pathophysiology of ALI and ARDS are complex and thought to result from direct or indirect pulmonary injury. Though injury can occur from a variety of mechanisms, the final pathway appears to involve inflammatory mediators including cytokines and cellular mediators. Still a very active area of investigation, it has become clear that surgical stress itself elicits an already well-characterized and profound inflammatory response that includes cytokines such as IL-1, IL-8, TNF-alpha, IL-6, selectins, neutrophil elastase, and thrombomodulin [252, 403–406]. In particular, IL-8 has been implicated in the development of ARDS [407] and is likely to provide a strong signal for the chemotactic migration of neutrophils [408, 409], the alveolar infiltration of which is characteristic of the disease process. The degranulation of neutrophils and an increase in pulmonary capillary permeability has been demonstrated after esophagectomy and has been proposed as a human model of lung injury [406]. Causative involvement of IL-8 is suggested by studies of IL-8 antagonists in animal models [408], the presence of high concentrations in both ventilated and non-ventilated lungs [410] and the relationship between IL-8 concentrations in lavage fluid, and the subsequent development of pulmonary complications after esophagectomy [411].

Improving Outcomes After Esophagectomy

Since esophagectomy patients are at increased risk for malnutrition and since malnutrition places them at substantially elevated risk for morbidity and possibly mortality, improving preoperative and postoperative nutritional status has become a major focus for perioperative physicians caring for these patients. Patients presenting for esophagectomy may be malnourished for a number of reasons – including decreased nutrient intake, increased catabolism and nutrient requirements, and impaired absorption. Preoperative sarcopenia [412] and low body mass index [413] are associated with poorer prognosis following esophagectomy. Malnutrition in this patient population has been shown to predict reoperation, respiratory morbidity, and a decrement in both overall and cancer-specific survival [414]. Preoperative nutritional status appears to be an independent risk factor for morbidity after esophagectomy and may improve risk prediction using existing prognostic scoring methodologies [415]. Moreover, nutritional disturbances appear to persist through the first postoperative year [416] and may never normalize in some patients [417]. Nutritional intervention appears to have significant potential to improve outcomes, though most studies address only postoperative nutrition. In a randomized trial, the parenteral administration of amino acids before and during the esophagectomy procedure resulted in an increase in core temperature and a decrease in the incidence of surgical infectious complications [418]. Postoperatively, enteral nutrition is superior to other routes, reducing weight loss and reducing the incidence of pneumonia [419], and may attenuate the cytokine response to surgery [420]. Further improvements in postoperative outcomes, including wound infection and length of stay, have been attributed to immunonutrition (containing specific immune system-enhancing nutrients) in upper gastrointestinal surgery [421] and to immediate resumption of oral nutrition following esophagectomy [422]. This latter approach to enteral nutrition (oral route) remains controversial because of concerns regarding possible aspiration and leak. A multicenter randomized trial to directly compare oral versus jejunostomy feeding after esophagectomy has been planned [423].

The high incidence of pulmonary complications following esophagectomy has prompted significant interest in efforts to improve preoperative cardiorespiratory function through inspiratory muscle training, an approach which has some preliminary support in the context of other thoracic surgical procedures. A prospective study comparing the effects of chest physical therapy in both thoracoscopic and open transthoracic esophagectomy demonstrated an improvement in pulmonary mechanical function in both groups [424], suggesting the utility of this approach for both surgical approaches.

Whether pulmonary prehabilitation results in improvements in clinical outcomes remains controversial. Retrospective review of esophagectomy patients suggests an association between physical therapy for reducing respiratory complications [425].

Prospective trials comparing high-intensity and endurance inspiratory muscle training demonstrated the feasibility of both protocols and the effectiveness of the high-intensity training for improvement of respiratory muscle function but

differ with regard to the ability of such therapy for reducing postoperative pulmonary complications [426, 427].

The use of TEA for postoperative analgesia has been reviewed above, but its potential value in improving outcomes after esophagectomy merits additional mention. Improved outcomes associated with the use of TEA after transthoracic esophageal surgery [161, 164–167] may be related to improved postoperative pulmonary function and resultant decrease in pulmonary complications [164] and an improvement in gastric tube blood flow [428, 429]. The use of TEA has been associated with a decreased risk of anastomotic leak in a retrospective study of esophagectomy patients [166]. A causative role is implied by animal experiments in which the use of TEA improved microcirculation and motility in the gastric tube [429] and a clinical study with similar findings [428]. For these reasons and the overwhelming evidence of superior pain control, TEA represents the standard of care for TTE in most institutions.

Though lung injury in this context is multifactorial, there is a growing awareness that anesthetic and perioperative factors are involved (see Chap. 10 for discussion of perioperative lung injury). These include atelectasis, which is obligate in the non-ventilated lung during OLV, direct injurious effect of volutrauma or barotrauma in the contralateral lung during OLV, oxygen stress and toxicity in the ventilated lung, and ischemia reperfusion injury in the ipsilateral lung after reventilation. Current knowledge of these mechanisms has been extensively reviewed [430]. Strategies to protect the lung and optimize outcomes after major thoracic surgery are most likely to be successful if they minimize these injurious stimuli. Guidance in the absence of definitive outcome data in the perioperative thoracic surgery setting is based largely on results from studies of animal models, surrogate markers of lung injury, patients with established lung injury, and more recently patients undergoing a variety of surgical procedures. Expert recommendations have been published [431], and several randomized trials [432–435], including one trial in minimally invasive esophagectomy [436], have revealed strategies which may improve clinical outcomes.

Ventilation strategies, particularly during OLV, should be tailored to patient physiology. That OLV itself may be a factor in the inflammatory response accompanying thoracic esophageal surgery is suggested by studies of cytokine and complement levels during and after OLV [252, 434, 437]. Thus, ventilation should be as physiologic as possible in an effort to minimize the likelihood of volutrauma. So-called "protective ventilation" strategies represent a physiologic approach to tidal ventilation and are likely to improve outcomes in this patient population by minimizing the risk of alveolar overdistension as well as cyclic collapse of alveoli (atelectrauma) and atelectasis. Specifically, protective ventilation in the context of thoracic surgery and OLV has referred to lower tidal volumes (4–6 mL/kg ideal body weight) with added positive end-expiratory pressure (PEEP) [431]. This ventilatory strategy in patients undergoing transthoracic esophagectomy has been shown to minimize surrogate markers of systemic inflammation (IL-1beta, IL-6, IL-8) [252, 438] while improving oxygenation intra- and postoperatively and decreasing the duration of mechanical ventilation [252]. Since oxygen toxicity and oxidative stress may also contribute to the development of adverse outcomes, it may be prudent to minimize FIO_2, though the large obligate right to left shunt in the non-ventilated lung during OLV limits the extent to which this maneuver is practicable.

Observations that the intense inflammatory responses accompanying esophagectomy may predict postoperative outcomes have led to a considerable effort to use pharmacologic therapies to attenuate inflammation. Numerous studies have documented the effects of corticosteroid administration on outcomes after esophagectomy, and, although there is a suggestion of possible benefit [439, 440], definitive conclusions await the results of an appropriately powered randomized trial [439–441]. Additional anti-inflammatory therapies tested in esophagectomy patients include simvastatin [442] and the neutrophil elastase inhibitor – sivelestat [443].

Surgery for Esophageal Rupture and Perforation

Patients presenting for emergent repair of esophageal disruption, rupture, or perforation may present with pain, hypovolemia, sepsis, and shock. Anesthetic management should be based on the severity of these presenting conditions and the nature of the planned procedure which may include endoscopic closure, primary surgical closure with mediastinal drainage, or esophagectomy. To the extent possible, fluid deficits should be corrected preoperatively and may be guided by standard and invasive monitoring as appropriate. Because of the likelihood of further fluid losses and hemodynamic decompensation, an arterial catheter for continuous blood pressure monitoring and arterial blood gas sampling is indicated.

The principles of anesthetic management are based on correcting preoperative fluid deficits, minimizing hemodynamic derangements, avoiding increases in abdominal pressure which may exacerbate leakage of gastroesophageal contents, and minimizing the risk of aspiration, particularly during induction. In general, a rapid sequence induction is indicated with the choice and dose of induction and neuromuscular blocking agents tailored to the patient's hemodynamic status. If a thoracotomy is planned or likely, surgical exposure will benefit from the use of a DLT, but this advantage should be considered in light of airway anatomy, anticipated ease of intubation, and the potentially elevated risk of aspiration should placement of the DLT require additional time.

Intraoperative management is likely to be dominated by the need for continuous fluid resuscitation. Arterial blood gas analysis and pulmonary artery catheter data may be used to guide fluid management and plasma volume expansion as well as the likely need for blood products. This factor combined with the probability of ongoing fluid shifts, pulmonary edema, and the need for inotropic and vasopressor support often mandate postoperative ventilatory support.

Surgery for Achalasia

Esophagomyotomy is most commonly performed to relieve esophageal obstruction at the sphincter level as well as for the relief of pain from esophageal spasm. Esophagomyotomy can be performed endoscopically, laparoscopically, thoracoscopically, or via thoracotomy, with or without the addition of an anti-reflux procedure. Arguably, the most important anesthetic consideration is the possibility of aspiration on induction of anesthesia with loss of protective airway reflexes. Because achalasia results in a dilated esophagus with impaired motility, the likelihood of retained food material in the esophagus is dramatically increased. It may also be desirable to restrict oral intake to only clear liquids for 2 days prior to surgery in an effort to reduce food retention. Approaches to minimize the risk of regurgitation and aspiration have been discussed previously and are especially important in these patients.

Additional anesthetic considerations for esophagomyotomy procedures include pain control (non-endoscopic surgeries) and lung isolation (transthoracic approaches). The use of thoracoscopy to perform a transthoracic myotomy undoubtedly reduces pain intensity relative to that of a thoracotomy and may not require TEA, though many practitioners still prefer it. After induction and intubation with a DLT or SLT with blocker and placement of a gastric tube, the patient is turned in the lateral decubitus position, usually right lateral decubitus, and the transthoracic myotomy is performed. Most patients can be extubated in the operating room after return of protective airway reflexes. The gastric tube is usually removed and feedings initiated and advanced after return of normal peristaltic activity.

Anesthetic management for POEM has been described recently. Clinical series report the use of a balanced general anesthetic in endotracheally intubated patients with [444] and without [445] the preoperative use of an esophagoscope to clear esophageal contents. Aspiration risk is minimized by an extended NPO period (24–48 hours) and an extended period (3–5 days) of diet restricted to clear liquids in patients judged to be at higher risk based on esophageal food retention during prior EGD. Since carbon dioxide insufflation is utilized for POEM procedures, the anesthesiologist is advised to monitor closely for potential problems and complications including hypercarbia, elevated ventilator pressures, and subcutaneous emphysema.

Surgery for Esophageal Diverticula

Zenker's Diverticulum

While Zenker's diverticulum is not a disorder of the thoracic esophagus, its repair is often undertaken by thoracic surgeons, and so it will be briefly discussed. Anesthetic management of patients with Zenker's diverticulum should be focused on the prevention of aspiration. Patients should be restricted to clear liquids for at least 24 h preoperatively and encouraged to manually express and empty the diverticulum prior to anesthetic induction if this is possible. Other efforts to avoid aspiration of diverticular contents include a head-up position (30°) during induction and a rapid sequence induction without cricoid pressure. In the patient with difficult airway anatomy, it may be preferable to intubate the trachea prior to induction of anesthesia. Caution should be exercised during placement of a gastric drain tube or esophageal bougie as these may enter the diverticulum and cause perforation.

Thoracic Diverticula

Patients presenting with thoracic esophageal diverticula may represent a subclass of patients at the highest risk for aspiration in the perioperative period. The reasons for this are twofold. First, these diverticula may be large and potentially contain significant quantities of food material. Second, these diverticula cannot be emptied by manual expression, though drainage may be possible with the careful placement of a large-bore drain tube. Additionally, most thoracic diverticula are associated with an esophageal motility disorder such as achalasia which is itself a high-risk condition with regard to aspiration. Thus, all reasonable precautions should be taken, including a head-up position if appropriate and either a rapid sequence induction or an awake intubation depending on the anticipated ease of airway management.

Transthoracic repair of esophageal diverticula is usually accomplished via a left thoracotomy incision. Surgical exposure is facilitated by lung isolation and OLV. During dissection, the anesthesiologist may assist by passing a large esophageal bougie with surgical guidance until it passes the diverticular aperture. If not already in situ, a nasogastric tube should be placed prior to emergence and should remain in place until esophageal integrity has been demonstrated by a contrast esophagram several days postoperatively. Most patients presenting for elective transthoracic resection of esophageal diverticula can be extubated following the procedure provided that a suitable plan for pain control has been initiated.

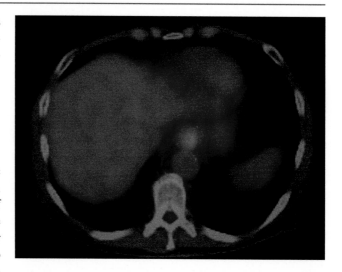

Fig. 38.10 PET scan reveals focal soft tissue thickening with increased uptake of FDG in the distal esophagus at the gastroesophageal junction consistent with esophageal carcinoma

Esophageal Surgery Clinical Case Discussion

Case: A 61-year-old male presents with a 14-month history of episodic dysphagia to solids that is progressively worsening. He notes no pain or weight loss. His evaluation included an EGD and biopsy showing high-grade dysplasia with features highly suspicious for invasive esophageal adenocarcinoma. Further evaluation in preparation for surgery included a whole-body PET-CT scan following injection of 14.014 mCi of F-18-FDG intravenously. Figure 38.10 shows the distal esophageal lesion illuminated by the marker. His past medical history is significant for CAD (MI 12 years prior treated with angioplasty). He has not had a recent cardiac catheterization. He also has intermittent supraventricular tachycardia (PSVT) controlled with diltiazem. He denies ever having a electrophysiologic study performed. He also suffers from HTN (enalapril), hypercholesterolemia (simvastatin), and asthma (albuterol as needed and Claritin). His only prior surgeries are a C4–7 discectomy and fusion and a L4–S1 laminectomy. He is scheduled for an Ivor Lewis esophagectomy.

Questions

- What further preoperative evaluation might be considered reasonable?
- What are the anesthetic considerations for this esophageal surgery?
- What specific intraoperative preparation of this patient might be prudent?
- What are postoperative considerations for this patient?

Focused   preoperative   history,   physical,   and investigations:

- Patient reports a daily requirement for his MDI and has recovered recently from a viral pharyngitis (physical exam, preoperative MDI use; see Chap. 8).
- Cardiac evaluation: baseline ECG to evaluate impulse initiation site, AV node conduction, and QTc in the context of PSVT history and diltiazem use. Stress echocardiogram to evaluate audible murmur and function (see Chap. 2).
- Careful airway evaluation with particular attention to cervical extension after cervical fusion.
- Focused neurologic exam to identify any preoperative deficits given the risk of position-related neurologic injury in left lateral decubitus position (see Chap. 19).

What intraoperative management considerations will optimize the patient's surgery?

- Thoracic epidural to provide postoperative analgesia for a right thoracotomy and upper midline laparotomy (see Chaps. 38 and 59).
- Avoidance of beta-blockade because of a significant history of reactive airway disease and chronic calcium channel blockade use. Intraoperative application of external electrodes for emergency cardioversion, pacing, or defibrillation. Calcium channel blockers indicated for treating hemodynamically stable PSVT (see Chap. 8).
- Fluid management strategy which seeks to optimize overall oxygen delivery, with particular attention to the high-risk esophageal anastomosis. A variety of methods can be used to guide fluid therapy (base deficit, serum lactate, mixed venous O_2 saturation). Optimal fluid management will seek to optimize cardiac output and oxygen delivery while avoiding excessive fluid administration (see Chaps. 21 and 38).
- High postoperative risk of atrial arrhythmias, in particular, atrial fibrillation. Treatment usually includes rate control with a beta-blocker especially in the patient with CAD, but preoperative use of a calcium channel blocker and history of asthma may preclude its use. Amiodarone can be used if atrial fibrillation is sustained and resistant to rate control with calcium channel blockers (see Chaps. 53 and 56).

References

1. Rickenbacher N, Kotter T, Kochen MM, Scherer M, Blozik E. Fundoplication versus medical management of gastroesophageal reflux disease: systematic review and meta-analysis. Surg Endosc. 2014;28(1):143–55.
2. Garg SK, Gurusamy KS. Laparoscopic fundoplication surgery versus medical management for gastro-oesophageal reflux disease (GORD) in adults. Cochrane Database Syst Rev. 2015;(11):CD003243.
3. Fein M, Ritter MP, DeMeester TR, et al. Role of the lower esophageal sphincter and hiatal hernia in the pathogenesis of gastroesophageal reflux disease. J Gastrointest Surg. 1999;3(4):405–10.
4. Skinner DB. Hernias (hiatal, traumatic, and congenital). 4th ed. Philadelphia: W.B. Saunders; 1985.
5. Halpin VJ, Soper NJ. Paraesophageal hernia. Curr Treat Options Gastroenterol. 2001;4(1):83–8.
6. Tian ZC, Wang B, Shan CX, Zhang W, Jiang DZ, Qiu M. A meta-analysis of randomized controlled trials to compare long-term outcomes of Nissen and Toupet fundoplication for gastroesophageal reflux disease. PLoS One. 2015;10(6):e0127627.
7. Testoni PA, Mazzoleni G, Testoni SG. Transoral incisionless fundoplication for gastro-esophageal reflux disease: techniques and outcomes. World J Gastrointest Pharmacol Ther. 2016;7(2):179–89.
8. Owen B, Simorov A, Siref A, Shostrom V, Oleynikov D. How does robotic anti-reflux surgery compare with traditional open and laparoscopic techniques: a cost and outcomes analysis. Surg Endosc. 2014;28(5):1686–90.
9. Yao G, Liu K, Fan Y. Robotic Nissen fundoplication for gastro-esophageal reflux disease: a meta-analysis of prospective randomized controlled trials. Surg Today. 2014;44(8):1415–23.
10. Dassinger MS, Torquati A, Houston HL, Holzman MD, Sharp KW, Richards WO. Laparoscopic fundoplication: 5-year follow-up. Am Surg. 2004;70(8):691–4; discussion 694–5
11. Cowgill SM, Arnaoutakis D, Villadolid D, et al. Results after laparoscopic fundoplication: does age matter? Am Surg. 2006;72(9):778–83; discussion 783–4
12. Ritter MP, Peters JH, DeMeester TR, et al. Treatment of advanced gastroesophageal reflux disease with Collis gastroplasty and Belsey partial fundoplication. Arch Surg. 1998;133(5):523–8; discussion 528–9
13. Lugaresi M, Mattioli B, Perrone O, Daddi N, Di Simone MP, Mattioli S. Results of left thoracoscopic Collis gastroplasty with laparoscopic Nissen fundoplication for the surgical treatment of true short oesophagus in gastro-oesophageal reflux disease and type III–IV hiatal hernia. Eur J Cardiothorac Surg. 2016;49(1):e22–30.
14. Patel HJ, Tan BB, Yee J, Orringer MB, Iannettoni MD. A 25-year experience with open primary transthoracic repair of paraesophageal hiatal hernia. J Thorac Cardiovasc Surg. 2004;127(3):843–9.
15. Gangopadhyay N, Perrone JM, Soper NJ, et al. Outcomes of laparoscopic paraesophageal hernia repair in elderly and high-risk patients. Surgery. 2006;140(4):491–8; discussion 498–9
16. Targarona EM, Grisales S, Uyanik O, Balague C, Pernas JC, Trias M. Long-term outcome and quality of life after laparoscopic treatment of large paraesophageal hernia. World J Surg. 2013;37(8):1878–82.
17. Bagheri SC, Stockmaster N, Delgado G, et al. Esophageal rupture with the use of the Combitube: report of a case and review of the literature. J Oral Maxillofac Surg. 2008;66(5):1041–4.
18. Harrison EE, Nord HJ, Beeman RW. Esophageal perforation following use of the esophageal obturator airway. Ann Emerg Med. 1980;9(1):21–5.
19. Biancari F, Saarnio J, Mennander A, et al. Outcome of patients with esophageal perforations: a multicenter study. World J Surg. 2014;38(4):902–9.
20. Khan AZ, Strauss D, Mason RC. Boerhaave's syndrome: diagnosis and surgical management. Surgeon. 2007;5(1):39–44.
21. Nesbitt JC, Sawyers JL. Surgical management of esophageal perforation. Am Surg. 1987;53(4):183–91.
22. Han SY, McElvein RB, Aldrete JS, Tishler JM. Perforation of the esophagus: correlation of site and cause with plain film findings. AJR Am J Roentgenol. 1985;145(3):537–40.
23. Bhatia P, Fortin D, Inculet RI, Malthaner RA. Current concepts in the management of esophageal perforations: a twenty-seven year Canadian experience. Ann Thorac Surg. 2011;92(1):209–15.

24. Minnich DJ, Yu P, Bryant AS, Jarrar D, Cerfolio RJ. Management of thoracic esophageal perforations. Eur J Cardiothorac Surg. 2011;40(4):931–7.

25. Shaker H, Elsayed H, Whittle I, Hussein S, Shackcloth M. The influence of the "golden 24-h rule" on the prognosis of oesophageal perforation in the modern era. Eur J Cardiothorac Surg. 2010;38(2):216–22.

26. Seo YD, Lin J, Chang AC, Orringer MB, Lynch WR, Reddy RM. Emergent esophagectomy for esophageal perforations: a safe option. Ann Thorac Surg. 2015;100(3):905–9.

27. Abbas G, Schuchert MJ, Pettiford BL, et al. Contemporaneous management of esophageal perforation. Surgery. 2009;146(4):749–55; discussion 755–6

28. Vogel SB, Rout WR, Martin TD, Abbitt PL. Esophageal perforation in adults: aggressive, conservative treatment lowers morbidity and mortality. Ann Surg. 2005;241(6):1016–21;discussion 1021–3

29. Fischer A, Thomusch O, Benz S, von Dobschuetz E, Baier P, Hopt UT. Nonoperative treatment of 15 benign esophageal perforations with self-expandable covered metal stents. Ann Thorac Surg. 2006;81(2):467–72.

30. Gelbmann CM, Ratiu NL, Rath HC, et al. Use of self-expandable plastic stents for the treatment of esophageal perforations and symptomatic anastomotic leaks. Endoscopy. 2004;36(8):695–9.

31. Siersema PD, Homs MY, Haringsma J, Tilanus HW, Kuipers EJ. Use of large-diameter metallic stents to seal traumatic nonmalignant perforations of the esophagus. Gastrointest Endosc. 2003;58(3):356–61.

32. Dasari BV, Neely D, Kennedy A, et al. The role of esophageal stents in the management of esophageal anastomotic leaks and benign esophageal perforations. Ann Surg. 2014;259(5):852–60.

33. Gomez-Esquivel R, Raju GS. Endoscopic closure of acute esophageal perforations. Curr Gastroenterol Rep. 2013;15(5):321.

34. Podas T, Eaden J, Mayberry M, Mayberry J. Achalasia: a critical review of epidemiological studies. Am J Gastroenterol. 1998;93(12):2345–7.

35. Kraichely RE, Farrugia G. Achalasia: physiology and etiopathogenesis. Dis Esophagus. 2006;19(4):213–23.

36. de Oliveira RB, Rezende Filho J, Dantas RO, Iazigi N. The spectrum of esophageal motor disorders in Chagas' disease. Am J Gastroenterol. 1995;90(7):1119–24.

37. Williams VA, Peters JH. Achalasia of the esophagus: a surgical disease. J Am Coll Surg. 2009;208(1):151–62.

38. Pandolfino JE, Gawron AJ. Achalasia: a systematic review. JAMA. 2015;313(18):1841–52.

39. Ott DJ, Richter JE, Chen YM, Wu WC, Gelfand DW, Castell DO. Esophageal radiography and manometry: correlation in 172 patients with dysphagia. AJR Am J Roentgenol. 1987;149(2):307–11.

40. Pasricha PJ, Rai R, Ravich WJ, Hendrix TR, Kalloo AN. Botulinum toxin for achalasia: long-term outcome and predictors of response. Gastroenterology. 1996;110(5):1410–5.

41. Lynch KL, Pandolfino JE, Howden CW, Kahrilas PJ. Major complications of pneumatic dilation and Heller myotomy for achalasia: single-center experience and systematic review of the literature. Am J Gastroenterol. 2012;107(12):1817–25.

42. Campos GM, Vittinghoff E, Rabl C, et al. Endoscopic and surgical treatments for achalasia: a systematic review and meta-analysis. Ann Surg. 2009;249(1):45–57.

43. Boeckxstaens GE, Annese V, des Varannes SB, et al. Pneumatic dilation versus laparoscopic Heller's myotomy for idiopathic achalasia. New Engl J Med. 2011;364(19):1807–16.

44. Finley RJ. Achalasia: thoracoscopic and laparoscopic myotomy. 2nd ed. Philadelphia: Churchill Livingstone; 2002.

45. Heitmiller RF, Buzdon MM. Surgery for achalasia and other motility disorders. 2nd ed. Philadelphia: Lippincott, Williams, and Wilkins; 2007.

46. Stewart KC, Finley RJ, Clifton JC, Graham AJ, Storseth C, Inculet R. Thoracoscopic versus laparoscopic modified Heller Myotomy for achalasia: efficacy and safety in 87 patients. J Am Coll Surg. 1999;189(2):164–9; discussion 169–70

47. Maher JW. Thoracoscopic esophagomyotomy for achalasia: maximum gain, minimal pain. Surgery. 1997;122(4):836–40; discussion 840–1

48. Maher JW, Conklin J, Heitshusen DS. Thoracoscopic esophagomyotomy for achalasia: preoperative patterns of acid reflux and long-term follow-up. Surgery. 2001;130(4):570–6; discussion 576–7

49. Champion JK, Delisle N, Hunt T. Comparison of thoracoscopic and laparoscopic esophagomyotomy with fundoplication for primary motility disorders. Eur J Cardiothorac Surg. 1999;16(Suppl 1):S34–6.

50. Rosemurgy A, Villadolid D, Thometz D, et al. Laparoscopic Heller myotomy provides durable relief from achalasia and salvages failures after botox or dilation. Ann Surg. 2005;241(5):725–33; discussion 733–5

51. Costantini M, Zaninotto G, Guirroli E, et al. The laparoscopic Heller-Dor operation remains an effective treatment for esophageal achalasia at a minimum 6-year follow-up. Surg Endosc. 2005;19(3):345–51.

52. Gholoum S, Feldman LS, Andrew CG, et al. Relationship between subjective and objective outcome measures after Heller myotomy and Dor fundoplication for achalasia. Surg Endosc. 2006;20(2):214–9.

53. Patti MG, Arcerito M, De Pinto M, et al. Comparison of thoracoscopic and laparoscopic Heller myotomy for achalasia. J Gastrointest Surg. 1998;2(6):561–6.

54. Patti MG, Pellegrini CA, Horgan S, et al. Minimally invasive surgery for achalasia: an 8-year experience with 168 patients. Ann Surg. 1999;230(4):587–93; discussion 593–4

55. Schuchert MJ, Luketich JD, Landreneau RJ, et al. Minimally-invasive esophagomyotomy in 200 consecutive patients: factors influencing postoperative outcomes. Ann Thorac Surg. 2008;85(5):1729–34.

56. Mehra M, Bahar RJ, Ament ME, et al. Laparoscopic and thoracoscopic esophagomyotomy for children with achalasia. J Pediatr Gastroenterol Nutr. 2001;33(4):466–71.

57. Rebecchi F, Giaccone C, Farinella E, Campaci R, Morino M. Randomized controlled trial of laparoscopic Heller myotomy plus Dor fundoplication versus Nissen fundoplication for achalasia: long-term results. Ann Surg. 2008;248(6):1023–30.

58. Jeansonne LO, White BC, Pilger KE, et al. Ten-year follow-up of laparoscopic Heller myotomy for achalasia shows durability. Surg Endosc. 2007;21(9):1498–502.

59. Persson J, Johnsson E, Kostic S, Lundell L, Smedh U. Treatment of achalasia with laparoscopic myotomy or pneumatic dilatation: long-term results of a prospective, randomized study. World J Surg. 2015;39(3):713–20.

60. Jain D, Singhal S. Transoral incisionless fundoplication for refractory gastroesophageal reflux disease: where do we stand? Clin Endosc. 2016;49(2):147–56.

61. Brar TS, Draganov PV, Yang D. Endoluminal therapy for gastroesophageal reflux disease: in between the pill and the knife? Dig Dis Sci. 2017;62(1):16–25.

62. Crespin OM, Liu LW, Parmar A, et al. Safety and efficacy of POEM for treatment of achalasia: a systematic review of the literature. Surg Endosc. 2017;31(5):2187–201.

63. Schneider AM, Louie BE, Warren HF, Farivar AS, Schembre DB, Aye RW. A matched comparison of per oral endoscopic myotomy to laparoscopic Heller myotomy in the treatment of achalasia. J Gastrointest Surg. 2016;20(11):1789–96.

64. Marano L, Pallabazzer G, Solito B, et al. Surgery or peroral esophageal myotomy for achalasia: a systematic review and meta-analysis. Medicine (Baltimore). 2016;95(10):e3001.

65. Shen KR, Allen MS, Cassivi SD, et al. Surgical management of acquired nonmalignant tracheoesophageal and bronchoesophageal fistulae. Ann Thorac Surg. 2010;90(3):914–8; discussion 919

66. Hurtgen M, Herber SC. Treatment of malignant tracheoesophageal fistula. Thorac Surg Clin. 2014;24(1):117–27.

67. Reed WJ, Doyle SE, Aprahamian C. Tracheoesophageal fistula after blunt chest trauma. Ann Thorac Surg. 1995;59(5):1251–6.

68. Drage SM, Pac Soo C, Dexter T. Delayed presentation of tracheo-oesophageal fistula following percutaneous dilatational tracheostomy. Anaesthesia. 2002;57(9):932–3.

69. Chang CY, Chang YT, Lee PL, Lin JT. Tracheoesophageal fistula. Gastrointest Endosc. 2004;59(7):870.

70. Collier KP, Zubarik RS, Lewis JH. Tracheoesophageal fistula from an indwelling endotracheal tube balloon: a report of two cases and review. Gastrointest Endosc. 2000;51(2):231–4.

71. Mooty RC, Rath P, Self M, Dunn E, Mangram A. Review of tracheo-esophageal fistula associated with endotracheal intubation. J Surg Educ. 2007;64(4):237–40.

72. Grant DM, Thompson GE. Diagnosis of congenital tracheo-esophageal fistula in the adolescent and adult. Anesthesiology. 1978;49(2):139–40.

73. Lancaster JL, Hanafi Z, Jackson SR. Adult presentation of a tracheoesophageal fistula with co-existing laryngeal cleft. J Laryngol Otol. 1999;113(5):469–72.

74. Zacharias J, Genc O, Goldstraw P. Congenital tracheoesophageal fistulas presenting in adults: presentation of two cases and a synopsis of the literature. J Thorac Cardiovasc Surg. 2004;128(2):316–8.

75. Finkelstein RG. The intraoperative diagnosis of a tracheoesophageal fistula in an adult. Anesthesiology. 1999;91(6):1946–7.

76. Smith HM, Bacon DR, Sprung J. Difficulty assessing endotracheal tube placement in a patient with undiagnosed iatrogenic tracheoesophageal fistula. J Cardiothorac Vasc Anesth. 2006;20(2):223–4.

77. Muniappan A, Wain JC, Wright CD, et al. Surgical treatment of nonmalignant tracheoesophageal fistula: a thirty-five year experience. Ann Thorac Surg. 2013;95(4):1141–6.

78. Eleftheriadis E, Kotzampassi K. Temporary stenting of acquired benign tracheoesophageal fistulas in critically ill ventilated patients. Surg Endosc. 2005;19(6):811–5.

79. Cassivi SD, Deschamps C, Nichols FC 3rd, Allen MS, Pairolero PC. Diverticula of the esophagus. Surg Clin North Am. 2005;85(3):495–503; ix

80. Rascoe PA, Smythe WR. Excision of esophageal diverticula. 2nd ed. Philadelphia: Lippincott, Williams, and Wilkins; 2007.

81. van Overbeek JJ. Pathogenesis and methods of treatment of Zenker's diverticulum. Ann Otol Rhinol Laryngol. 2003;112(7):583–93.

82. Costantini M, Zaninotto G, Rizzetto C, Narne S, Ancona E. Oesophageal diverticula. Best Pract Res Clin Gastroenterol. 2004;18(1):3–17.

83. Visosky AM, Parke RB, Donovan DT. Endoscopic management of Zenker's diverticulum: factors predictive of success or failure. Ann Otol Rhinol Laryngol. 2008;117(7):531–7.

84. Verdonck J, Morton RP. Systematic review on treatment of Zenker's diverticulum. Eur Arch Otorhinolaryngol. 2015;272(11):3095–107.

85. Varghese TK Jr, Marshall B, Chang AC, Pickens A, Lau CL, Orringer MB. Surgical treatment of epiphrenic diverticula: a 30-year experience. Ann Thorac Surg. 2007;84(6):1801–9; discussion 1801–9

86. Achim V, Aye RW, Farivar AS, Vallieres E, Louie BE. A combined thoracoscopic and laparoscopic approach for high epiphrenic diverticula and the importance of complete myotomy. Surg Endosc. 2017;31(2):788–94.

87. Hirano Y, Takeuchi H, Oyama T, et al. Minimally invasive surgery for esophageal epiphrenic diverticulum: the results of 133 patients in 25 published series and our experience. Surg Today. 2013;43(1):1–7.

88. Andolfi C, Wiesel O, Fisichella PM. Surgical treatment of epiphrenic diverticulum: technique and controversies. J Laparoendosc Adv Surg Tech A. 2016;26(11):905–10.

89. Onwugbufor MT, Obirieze AC, Ortega G, Allen D, Cornwell EE 3rd, Fullum TM. Surgical management of esophageal diverticulum: a review of the nationwide inpatient sample database. J Surg Res. 2013;184(1):120–5.

90. Kamangar F, Chow WH, Abnet CC, Dawsey SM. Environmental causes of esophageal cancer. Gastroenterol Clin N Am. 2009;38(1):27–57, vii

91. Liu W, Zhang X, Sun W. Developments in treatment of esophageal/gastric cancer. Curr Treat Options in Oncol. 2008;9(4–6):375–87.

92. Napier KJ, Scheerer M, Misra S. Esophageal cancer: a review of epidemiology, pathogenesis, staging workup and treatment modalities. World J Gastrointest Oncol. 2014;6(5):112–20.

93. Maish MS, DeMeester SR. Endoscopic mucosal resection as a staging technique to determine the depth of invasion of esophageal adenocarcinoma. Ann Thorac Surg. 2004;78(5):1777–82.

94. Prasad GA, Buttar NS, Wongkeesong LM, et al. Significance of neoplastic involvement of margins obtained by endoscopic mucosal resection in Barrett's esophagus. Am J Gastroenterol. 2007;102(11):2380–6.

95. Ell C, May A, Pech O, et al. Curative endoscopic resection of early esophageal adenocarcinomas (Barrett's cancer). Gastrointest Endosc. 2007;65(1):3–10.

96. Pech O, Behrens A, May A, et al. Long-term results and risk factor analysis for recurrence after curative endoscopic therapy in 349 patients with high-grade intraepithelial neoplasia and mucosal adenocarcinoma in Barrett's oesophagus. Gut. 2008;57(9):1200–6.

97. Ilson DH. Esophageal cancer chemotherapy: recent advances. Gastrointest Cancer Res. 2008;2(2):85–92.

98. Le Bras GF, Farooq MH, Falk GW, Andl CD. Esophageal cancer: the latest on chemoprevention and state of the art therapies. Pharmacol Res. 2016;113(Pt A):236–44.

99. Berry MF. The role of induction therapy for esophageal cancer. Thorac Surg Clin. 2016;26(3):295–304.

100. Veuillez V, Rougier P, Seitz JF. The multidisciplinary management of gastrointestinal cancer. Multimodal treatment of oesophageal cancer. Best Pract Res Clin Gastroenterol. 2007;21(6):947–63.

101. Fernando HC, Murthy SC, Hofstetter W, et al. The Society of Thoracic Surgeons practice guideline series: guidelines for the management of Barrett's esophagus with high-grade dysplasia. Ann Thorac Surg. 2009;87(6):1993–2002.

102. Orringer MB, Marshall B, Stirling MC. Transhiatal esophagectomy for benign and malignant disease. J Thorac Cardiovasc Surg. 1993;105(2):265–76; discussion 276–7

103. Ferraro P, Duranceau A. Esophagectomy for benign disease. In: Pearson FG, Cooper JD, Deslauriers J, et al., editors. Esophageal surgery. 2nd ed. New York: Churchill Livingstone; 2002. p. 453–64.

104. Orringer MB, Marshall B, Chang AC, Lee J, Pickens A, Lau CL. Two thousand transhiatal esophagectomies: changing trends, lessons learned. Ann Surg. 2007;246(3):363–72; discussion 372–4

105. Hulscher JB, Tijssen JG, Obertop H, van Lanschot JJ. Transthoracic versus transhiatal resection for carcinoma of the esophagus: a meta-analysis. Ann Thorac Surg. 2001;72(1):306–13.

106. Hulscher JB, van Sandick JW, de Boer AG, et al. Extended transthoracic resection compared with limited transhiatal resection for adenocarcinoma of the esophagus. N Engl J Med. 2002;347(21):1662–9.

107. Rentz J, Bull D, Harpole D, et al. Transthoracic versus transhiatal esophagectomy: a prospective study of 945 patients. J Thorac Cardiovasc Surg. 2003;125(5):1114–20.

108. Raymond DP, Seder CW, Wright CD, et al. Predictors of major morbidity or mortality after resection for esophageal cancer: a society of thoracic surgeons general thoracic surgery database risk adjustment model. Ann Thorac Surg. 2016;102(1):207–14.

109. Papenfuss WA, Kukar M, Attwood K, et al. Transhiatal versus transthoracic esophagectomy for esophageal cancer: a 2005-2011 NSQIP comparison of modern multicenter results. J Surg Oncol. 2014;110(3):298–301.

110. Boshier PR, Anderson O, Hanna GB. Transthoracic versus transhiatal esophagectomy for the treatment of esophagogastric cancer: a meta-analysis. Ann Surg. 2011;254(6):894–906.

111. Ryan CE, Paniccia A, Meguid RA, McCarter MD. Transthoracic anastomotic leak after esophagectomy: current trends. Ann Surg Oncol. 2017;24(1):281–90.

112. Luketich JD, Alvelo-Rivera M, Buenaventura PO, et al. Minimally invasive esophagectomy: outcomes in 222 patients. Ann Surg. 2003;238(4):486–94; discussion 494–5

113. Luketich JD, Pennathur A, Franchetti Y, et al. Minimally invasive esophagectomy: results of a prospective phase II multicenter trial-the eastern cooperative oncology group (E2202) study. Ann Surg. 2015;261(4):702–7.

114. Sihag S, Kosinski AS, Gaissert HA, Wright CD, Schipper PH. Minimally invasive versus open esophagectomy for esophageal cancer: a comparison of early surgical outcomes from the society of thoracic surgeons national database. Ann Thorac Surg. 2016;101(4):1281–8; discussion 1288–9

115. Wang W, Zhou Y, Feng J, Mei Y. Oncological and surgical outcomes of minimally invasive versus open esophagectomy for esophageal squamous cell carcinoma: a matched-pair comparative study. Int J Clin Exp Med. 2015;8(9):15983–90.

116. Biere SS, van Berge Henegouwen MI, Maas KW, et al. Minimally invasive versus open oesophagectomy for patients with oesophageal cancer: a multicentre, open-label, randomised controlled trial. Lancet. 2012;379(9829):1887–92.

117. Maas KW, Cuesta MA, van Berge Henegouwen MI, et al. Quality of life and late complications after minimally invasive compared to open esophagectomy: results of a randomized trial. World J Surg. 2015;39(8):1986–93.

118. Straatman J, van der Wielen N, Cuesta MA, et al. Minimally invasive versus open esophageal resection: three-year follow-up of the previously reported randomized controlled trial: the TIME trial. Ann Surg. 2017;266(2):232–6.

119. Yerokun BA, Sun Z, Yang CJ, et al. Minimally invasive versus open esophagectomy for esophageal cancer: a population-based analysis. Ann Thorac Surg. 2016;102(2):416–23.

120. Tapias LF, Mathisen DJ, Wright CD, et al. Outcomes with open and minimally invasive Ivor Lewis esophagectomy after neoadjuvant therapy. Ann Thorac Surg. 2016;101(3):1097–103.

121. Zhou C, Zhang L, Wang H, et al. Superiority of minimally invasive oesophagectomy in reducing in-hospital mortality of patients with resectable oesophageal cancer: a meta-analysis. PLoS One. 2015;10(7):e0132889.

122. Rodham P, Batty JA, McElnay PJ, Immanuel A. Does minimally invasive oesophagectomy provide a benefit in hospital length of stay when compared with open oesophagectomy? Interact Cardiovasc Thorac Surg. 2016;22(3):360–7.

123. Guo W, Ma X, Yang S, et al. Combined thoracoscopic-laparoscopic esophagectomy versus open esophagectomy: a meta-analysis of outcomes. Surg Endosc. 2016;30(9):3873–81.

124. Cerfolio RJ, Wei B, Hawn MT, Minnich DJ. Robotic esophagectomy for cancer: early results and lessons learned. Semin Thorac Cardiovasc Surg. 2016;28(1):160–9.

125. Sarkaria IS, Rizk NP, Grosser R, et al. Attaining proficiency in robotic-assisted minimally invasive esophagectomy while maximizing safety during procedure development. Innovations (Phila). 2016;11(4):268–73.

126. van der Sluis PC, Ruurda JP, van der Horst S, et al. Robot-assisted minimally invasive thoraco-laparoscopic esophagectomy versus open transthoracic esophagectomy for resectable esophageal cancer, a randomized controlled trial (ROBOT trial). Trials. 2012;13:230.

127. Urschel JD. Late dysphagia after presternal colon interposition. Dysphagia. 1996;11(1):75–7.

128. Cense HA, Visser MR, van Sandick JW, et al. Quality of life after colon interposition by necessity for esophageal cancer replacement. J Surg Oncol. 2004;88(1):32–8.

129. Domreis JS, Jobe BA, Aye RW, Deveney KE, Sheppard BC, Deveney CW. Management of long-term failure after colon interposition for benign disease. Am J Surg. 2002;183(5):544–6.

130. Jeyasingham K, Lerut T, Belsey RH. Revisional surgery after colon interposition for benign oesophageal disease. Dis Esophagus. 1999;12(1):7–9.

131. de Delva PE, Morse CR, Austen WG Jr, et al. Surgical management of failed colon interposition. Eur J Cardiothorac Surg. 2008;34(2):432–7; discussion 437

132. Doki Y, Okada K, Miyata H, et al. Long-term and short-term evaluation of esophageal reconstruction using the colon or the jejunum in esophageal cancer patients after gastrectomy. Dis Esophagus. 2008;21(2):132–8.

133. Cerfolio RJ, Allen MS, Deschamps C, Trastek VF, Pairolero PC. Esophageal replacement by colon interposition. Ann Thorac Surg. 1995;59(6):1382–4.

134. Briel JW, Tamhankar AP, Hagen JA, et al. Prevalence and risk factors for ischemia, leak, and stricture of esophageal anastomosis: gastric pull-up versus colon interposition. J Am Coll Surg. 2004;198(4):536–41; discussion 541–2

135. Wain JC, Wright CD, Kuo EY, et al. Long-segment colon interposition for acquired esophageal disease. Ann Thorac Surg. 1999;67(2):313–7; discussion 317–8

136. Ring WS, Varco RL, L'Heureux PR, Foker JE. Esophageal replacement with jejunum in children: an 18 to 33 year follow-up. J Thorac Cardiovasc Surg. 1982;83(6):918–27.

137. Smith RW, Garvey CJ, Dawson PM, Davies DM. Jejunum versus colon for free oesophageal reconstruction: an experimental radiological assessment. Br J Plast Surg. 1987;40(2):181–7.

138. Meyers WC, Seigler HF, Hanks JB, et al. Postoperative function of "free" jejunal transplants for replacement of the cervical esophagus. Ann Surg. 1980;192(4):439–50.

139. Wright C, Cuschieri A. Jejunal interposition for benign esophageal disease. Technical considerations and long-term results. Ann Surg. 1987;205(1):54–60.

140. Moreno-Osset E, Tomas-Ridocci M, Paris F, et al. Motor activity of esophageal substitute (stomach, jejunal, and colon segments). Ann Thorac Surg. 1986;41(5):515–9.

141. Baker CR, Forshaw MJ, Gossage JA, Ng R, Mason RC. Long-term outcome and quality of life after supercharged jejunal interposition for oesophageal replacement. Surgeon. 2015;13(4):187–93.

142. Swisher SG, Hofstetter WL, Miller MJ. The supercharged microvascular jejunal interposition. Semin Thorac Cardiovasc Surg. 2007;19(1):56–65.

143. Ascioti AJ, Hofstetter WL, Miller MJ, et al. Long-segment, supercharged, pedicled jejunal flap for total esophageal reconstruction. J Thorac Cardiovasc Surg. 2005;130(5):1391–8.

144. Stephens EH, Gaur P, Hotze KO, Correa AM, Kim MP, Blackmon SH. Super-charged pedicled jejunal interposition performance compares favorably with a gastric conduit after esophagectomy. Ann Thorac Surg. 2015;100(2):407–13.

145. Sungurtekin H, Sungurtekin U, Balci C, Zencir M, Erdem E. The influence of nutritional status on complications after major intraabdominal surgery. J Am Coll Nutr. 2004;23(3):227–32.

146. Windsor JA, Hill GL. Weight loss with physiologic impairment. A basic indicator of surgical risk. Ann Surg. 1988;207(3):290–6.

147. Fleisher LA, Fleischmann KE, Auerbach AD, et al. 2014 ACC/AHA guideline on perioperative cardiovascular evaluation and management of patients undergoing noncardiac surgery: a report of the American College of Cardiology/American Heart Association Task Force on practice guidelines. J Am Coll Cardiol. 2014;64(22):e77–137.

148. Fleisher LA, Fleischmann KE, Auerbach AD, et al. 2014 ACC/AHA guideline on perioperative cardiovascular evaluation and management of patients undergoing noncardiac surgery: a report of the American College of Cardiology/American Heart Association Task Force on Practice Guidelines. Circulation. 2014;130(24):e278–333.

149. Yamanaka Y, Mammoto T, Kita T, Kishi Y. A study of 13 patients with gastric tube in place after esophageal resection: use of omeprazole to decrease gastric acidity and volume. J Clin Anesth. 2001;13(5):370–3.

150. Pisegna JR, Karlstadt RG, Norton JA, et al. Effect of preoperative intravenous pantoprazole in elective-surgery patients: a pilot study. Dig Dis Sci. 2009;54(5):1041–9.

151. Nishina K, Mikawa K, Takao Y, Shiga M, Maekawa N, Obara H. A comparison of rabeprazole, lansoprazole, and ranitidine for improving preoperative gastric fluid property in adults undergoing elective surgery. Anesth Analg. 2000;90(3):717–21.

152. Jeske HC, Borovicka J, von Goedecke A, et al. Preoperative administration of esomeprazole has no influence on frequency of refluxes. J Clin Anesth. 2008;20(3):191–5.

153. Ng A, Smith G. Gastroesophageal reflux and aspiration of gastric contents in anesthetic practice. Anesth Analg. 2001;93(2):494–513.

154. Pisegna JR, Martindale RG. Acid suppression in the perioperative period. J Clin Gastroenterol. 2005;39(1):10–6.

155. Wijnhoven BP, van Lanschot JJ, Tilanus HW, Steyerberg EW, van der Gaast A. Neoadjuvant chemoradiotherapy for esophageal cancer: a review of meta-analyses. World J Surg. 2009;33(12):2606–14.

156. Ardalan B, Spector SA, Livingstone AS, et al. Neoadjuvant, surgery and adjuvant chemotherapy without radiation for esophageal cancer. Jpn J Clin Oncol. 2007;37(8):590–6.

157. Oppedijk V, van der Gaast A, van Lanschot JJ, et al. Patterns of recurrence after surgery alone versus preoperative chemoradiotherapy and surgery in the CROSS trials. J Clin Oncol. 2014;32(5):385–91.

158. Rudin A, Flisberg P, Johansson J, Walther B, Lundberg CJ. Thoracic epidural analgesia or intravenous morphine analgesia after thoracoabdominal esophagectomy: a prospective follow-up of 201 patients. J Cardiothorac Vasc Anesth. 2005;19(3):350–7.

159. Flisberg P, Tornebrandt K, Walther B, Lundberg J. Pain relief after esophagectomy: thoracic epidural analgesia is better than parenteral opioids. J Cardiothorac Vasc Anesth. 2001;15(3):282–7.

160. Smedstad KG, Beattie WS, Blair WS, Buckley DN. Postoperative pain relief and hospital stay after total esophagectomy. Clin J Pain. 1992;8(2):149–53.

161. Tsui SL, Law S, Fok M, et al. Postoperative analgesia reduces mortality and morbidity after esophagectomy. Am J Surg. 1997;173(6):472–8.

162. Fares KM, Mohamed SA, Hamza HM, Sayed DM, Hetta DF. Effect of thoracic epidural analgesia on pro-inflammatory cytokines in patients subjected to protective lung ventilation during Ivor Lewis esophagectomy. Pain Physician. 2014;17(4):305–15.

163. Li W, Li Y, Huang Q, Ye S, Rong T. Short and long-term outcomes of epidural or intravenous analgesia after esophagectomy: a propensity-matched cohort study. PLoS One. 2016;11(4):e0154380.

164. Ballantyne JC, Carr DB, deFerranti S, et al. The comparative effects of postoperative analgesic therapies on pulmonary outcome: cumulative meta-analyses of randomized, controlled trials. Anesth Analg. 1998;86(3):598–612.

165. Cense HA, Lagarde SM, de Jong K, et al. Association of no epidural analgesia with postoperative morbidity and mortality after transthoracic esophageal cancer resection. J Am Coll Surg. 2006;202(3):395–400.

166. Michelet P, D'Journo XB, Roch A, et al. Perioperative risk factors for anastomotic leakage after esophagectomy: influence of thoracic epidural analgesia. Chest. 2005;128(5):3461–6.

167. Whooley BP, Law S, Murthy SC, Alexandrou A, Wong J. Analysis of reduced death and complication rates after esophageal resection. Ann Surg. 2001;233(3):338–44.

168. Heinrich S, Janitz K, Merkel S, Klein P, Schmidt J. Short- and long term effects of epidural analgesia on morbidity and mortality of esophageal cancer surgery. Langenbecks Arch Surg. 2015;400(1):19–26.

169. Yap FH, Lau JY, Joynt GM, Chui PT, Chan AC, Chung SS. Early extubation after transthoracic oesophagectomy. Hong Kong Med J. 2003;9(2):98–102.

170. Neal JM, Wilcox RT, Allen HW, Low DE. Near-total esophagectomy: the influence of standardized multimodal management and intraoperative fluid restriction. Reg Anesth Pain Med. 2003;28(4):328–34.

171. Low DE, Kunz S, Schembre D, et al. Esophagectomy – it's not just about mortality anymore: standardized perioperative clinical pathways improve outcomes in patients with esophageal cancer. J Gastrointest Surg. 2007;11(11):1395–402; discussion 1402

172. Buise M, Van Bommel J, Mehra M, Tilanus HW, Van Zundert A, Gommers D. Pulmonary morbidity following esophagectomy is decreased after introduction of a multimodal anesthetic regimen. Acta Anaesthesiol Belg. 2008;59(4):257–61.

173. Gemmill EH, Humes DJ, Catton JA. Systematic review of enhanced recovery after gastro-oesophageal cancer surgery. Ann R Coll Surg Engl. 2015;97(3):173–9.

174. Porteous GH, Neal JM, Slee A, Schmidt H, Low DE. A standardized anesthetic and surgical clinical pathway for esophageal resection: impact on length of stay and major outcomes. Reg Anesth Pain Med. 2015;40(2):139–49.

175. Cao S, Zhao G, Cui J, et al. Fast-track rehabilitation program and conventional care after esophagectomy: a retrospective controlled cohort study. Support Care Cancer. 2013;21(3):707–14.

176. Chen L, Sun L, Lang Y, et al. Fast-track surgery improves postoperative clinical recovery and cellular and humoral immunity after esophagectomy for esophageal cancer. BMC Cancer. 2016; 16:449.

177. Kahn L, Baxter FJ, Dauphin A, et al. A comparison of thoracic and lumbar epidural techniques for post-thoracoabdominal esophagectomy analgesia. Can J Anaesth. 1999;46(5 Pt 1):415–22.

178. Luketich JD, Land SR, Sullivan EA, et al. Thoracic epidural versus intercostal nerve catheter plus patient-controlled analgesia: a randomized study. Ann Thorac Surg. 2005;79(6):1845–9; discussion 1849–50

179. Debreceni G, Molnar Z, Szelig L, Molnar TF. Continuous epidural or intercostal analgesia following thoracotomy: a prospective randomized double-blind clinical trial. Acta Anaesthesiol Scand. 2003;47(9):1091–5.

180. Francois T, Blanloeil Y, Pillet F, et al. Effect of interpleural administration of bupivacaine or lidocaine on pain and morphine requirement after esophagectomy with thoracotomy: a randomized, double-blind and controlled study. Anesth Analg. 1995;80(4):718–23.

181. Wheatley GH 3rd, Rosenbaum DH, Paul MC, et al. Improved pain management outcomes with continuous infusion of a local anesthetic after thoracotomy. J Thorac Cardiovasc Surg. 2005;130(2):464–8.

182. Marret E, Bazelly B, Taylor G, et al. Paravertebral block with ropivacaine 0.5% versus systemic analgesia for pain relief after thoracotomy. Ann Thorac Surg. 2005;79(6):2109–13.

183. Casati A, Alessandrini P, Nuzzi M, et al. A prospective, randomized, blinded comparison between continuous thoracic paravertebral and epidural infusion of 0.2% ropivacaine after lung resection surgery. Eur J Anaesthesiol. 2006;23(12):999–1004.

184. Davies RG, Myles PS, Graham JM. A comparison of the analgesic efficacy and side-effects of paravertebral vs epidural blockade for thoracotomy – a systematic review and meta-analysis of randomized trials. Br J Anaesth. 2006;96(4):418–26.

185. Yeung JH, Gates S, Naidu BV, Wilson MJ, Gao Smith F. Paravertebral block versus thoracic epidural for patients undergoing thoracotomy. Cochrane Database Syst Rev. 2016;2:CD009121.

186. Scarfe AJ, Schuhmann-Hingel S, Duncan JK, Ma N, Atukorale YN, Cameron AL. Continuous paravertebral block for post-cardiothoracic surgery analgesia: a systematic review and meta-analysis. Eur J Cardiothorac Surg. 2016;50(6):1010–8.

187. Conlon NP, Shaw AD, Grichnik KP. Postthoracotomy paravertebral analgesia: will it replace epidural analgesia? Anesthesiol Clin. 2008;26(2):369–80, viii

188. Daly DJ, Myles PS. Update on the role of paravertebral blocks for thoracic surgery: are they worth it? Curr Opin Anaesthesiol. 2009;22(1):38–43.

189. Zhang W, Fang C, Li J, et al. Single-dose, bilateral paravertebral block plus intravenous sufentanil analgesia in patients with esophageal cancer undergoing combined thoracoscopic-laparoscopic esophagectomy: a safe and effective alternative. J Cardiothorac Vasc Anesth. 2014;28(4):966–72.

190. Li NL, Liu CC, Cheng SH, et al. Feasibility of combined paravertebral block and subcostal transversus abdominis plane block in postoperative pain control after minimally invasive esophagectomy. Acta Anaesthesiol Taiwanica. 2013;51(3):103–7.

191. Barbera C, Milito P, Punturieri M, Asti E, Bonavina L. Serratus anterior plane block for hybrid transthoracic esophagectomy: a pilot study. J Pain Res. 2017;10:73–7.

192. Brown MJ, Kor DJ, Allen MS, et al. Dual-epidural catheter technique and perioperative outcomes after Ivor-Lewis esophagectomy. Reg Anesth Pain Med. 2013;38(1):3–8.

193. Yegin A, Erdogan A, Kayacan N, Karsli B. Early postoperative pain management after thoracic surgery; pre- and postoperative versus postoperative epidural analgesia: a randomised study. Eur J Cardiothorac Surg. 2003;24(3):420–4.

194. Bong CL, Samuel M, Ng JM, Ip-Yam C. Effects of preemptive epidural analgesia on post-thoracotomy pain. J Cardiothorac Vasc Anesth. 2005;19(6):786–93.

195. Salengros JC, Huybrechts I, Ducart A, et al. Different anesthetic techniques associated with different incidences of chronic post-thoracotomy pain: low-dose remifentanil plus presurgical epidural analgesia is preferable to high-dose remifentanil with postsurgical epidural analgesia. J Cardiothorac Vasc Anesth. 2010;24(4):608–16.

196. Rodriguez-Aldrete D, Candiotti KA, Janakiraman R, Rodriguez-Blanco YF. Trends and new evidence in the management of acute and chronic post-thoracotomy pain-an overview of the literature from 2005 to 2015. J Cardiothorac Vasc Anesth. 2016;30(3):762–72.

197. Chen HC, Huang HJ, Wu CY, Lin TS, Fang HY. Esophageal schwannoma with tracheal compression. Thorac Cardiovasc Surg. 2006;54(8):555–8.

198. Mizuguchi S, Inoue K, Imagawa A, et al. Benign esophageal schwannoma compressing the trachea in pregnancy. Ann Thorac Surg. 2008;85(2):660–2.

199. Sasano H, Sasano N, Ito S, et al. Continuous positive airway pressure applied through a bronchial blocker as a treatment for hypoxemia due to stenosis of the left main bronchus. Anesthesiology. 2009;110(5):1199–200.

200. Andronikou S, Wieselthaler N, Kilborn T. Significant airway compromise in a child with a posterior mediastinal mass due to tuberculous spondylitis. Pediatr Radiol. 2005;35(11):1159–60.

201. Blank RS, Waldrop CS, Balestrieri PJ. Pseudomeningocele: an unusual cause of intraoperative tracheal compression and expiratory obstruction. Anesth Analg. 2008;107(1):226–8.

202. ul Huda A, Siddiqui KM, Khan FH. Emergency airway management of a patient with mediastinal mass. J Pak Med Assoc. 2007;57(3):152–4.

203. Tokunaga T, Takeda S, Sumimura J, Maeda H. Esophageal schwannoma: report of a case. Surg Today. 2007;37(6):500–2.

204. Hasan N, Mandhan P. Respiratory obstruction caused by lipoma of the esophagus. J Pediatr Surg. 1994;29(12):1565–6.

205. Walton AR. Acute upper airway obstruction due to oesophageal achalasia. Anaesthesia. 2009;64(2):222–3.

206. Kaths JM, Foltys DB, Scheuermann U, et al. Achalasia with megaesophagus and tracheal compression in a young patient: a case report. Int J Surg Case Rep. 2015;14:16–8.

207. Westbrook JL. Oesophageal achalasia causing respiratory obstruction. Anaesthesia. 1992;47(1):38–40.

208. Arcos E, Medina C, Mearin F, Larish J, Guarner L, Malagelada JR. Achalasia presenting as acute airway obstruction. Dig Dis Sci. 2000;45(10):2079–83.

209. Layton J, Ward PW, Miller DW, Roan RM. Acute respiratory failure secondary to esophageal dilation from undiagnosed achalasia. A A Case Rep. 2014;3(5):65–7.

210. Bechard P, Letourneau L, Lacasse Y, Cote D, Bussieres JS. Perioperative cardiorespiratory complications in adults with mediastinal mass: incidence and risk factors. Anesthesiology. 2004;100(4):826–34; discussion 825A

211. Black DR, Thangathurai D, Senthilkumar N, Roffey P, Mikhail M. High risk of aspiration and difficult intubation in post-esophagectomy patients. Acta Anaesthesiol Scand. 1999;43(6):687.

212. Pennefather SH. Anaesthesia for oesophagectomy. Curr Opin Anaesthesiol. 2007;20(1):15–20.

213. Ng JM. Perioperative anesthetic management for esophagectomy. Anesthesiol Clin. 2008;26(2):293–304, vi

214. de Souza DG, Gaughen CL. Aspiration risk after esophagectomy. Anesth Analg. 2009;109(4):1352.

215. Bartels K, Fiegel M, Stevens Q, Ahlgren B, Weitzel N. Approaches to perioperative care for esophagectomy. J Cardiothorac Vasc Anesth. 2015;29(2):472–80.

216. Sakai T, Planinsic RM, Quinlan JJ, Handley LJ, Kim TY, Hilmi IA. The incidence and outcome of perioperative pulmonary aspiration in a university hospital: a 4-year retrospective analysis. Anesth Analg. 2006;103(4):941–7.

217. Robinson GV, Kanji H, Davies RJ, Gleeson FV. Selective pulmonary fat aspiration complicating oesophageal achalasia. Thorax. 2004;59(2):180.

218. Akritidis N, Gousis C, Dimos G, Paparounas K. Fever, cough, and bilateral lung infiltrates. Achalasia associated with aspiration pneumonia. Chest. 2003;123(2):608–12.

219. Practice Guidelines for Preoperative Fasting and the Use of Pharmacologic Agents to Reduce the Risk of Pulmonary Aspiration: Application to Healthy Patients Undergoing Elective Procedures: An Updated Report by the American Society of Anesthesiologists Task Force on Preoperative Fasting and the Use of Pharmacologic Agents to Reduce the Risk of Pulmonary Aspiration. Anesthesiology. 2017;126(3):376–93.

220. Brady M, Kinn S, Stuart P. Preoperative fasting for adults to prevent perioperative complications. Cochrane Database Syst Rev. 2003;(4):CD004423.

221. Brady M, Kinn S, Ness V, O'Rourke K, Randhawa N, Stuart P. Preoperative fasting for preventing perioperative complications in children. Cochrane Database Syst Rev. 2009;(4):CD005285.

222. Ovassapian A, Salem MR. Sellick's maneuver: to do or not do. Anesth Analg. 2009;109(5):1360–2.

223. Lerman J. On cricoid pressure: "may the force be with you". Anesth Analg. 2009;109(5):1363–6.

224. El-Orbany M, Connolly LA. Rapid sequence induction and intubation: current controversy. Anesth Analg. 2010;110(5):1318–25.

225. Salem MR, Khorasani A, Zeidan A, Crystal GJ. Cricoid pressure controversies: narrative review. Anesthesiology. 2017;126(4):738–52.

226. Algie CM, Mahar RK, Tan HB, Wilson G, Mahar PD, Wasiak J. Effectiveness and risks of cricoid pressure during rapid sequence induction for endotracheal intubation. Cochrane Database Syst Rev. 2015;(11):CD011656.

227. Bohman JK, Kashyap R, Lee A, et al. A pilot randomized clinical trial assessing the effect of cricoid pressure on risk of aspiration. Clin Respir J. 2018;12(1):175–82.

228. Smith KJ, Dobranowski J, Yip G, Dauphin A, Choi PT. Cricoid pressure displaces the esophagus: an observational study using magnetic resonance imaging. Anesthesiology. 2003;99(1):60–4.

229. Boet S, Duttchen K, Chan J, et al. Cricoid pressure provides incomplete esophageal occlusion associated with lateral deviation: a magnetic resonance imaging study. J Emerg Med. 2012;42(5):606–11.

230. Rice MJ, Mancuso AA, Gibbs C, Morey TE, Gravenstein N, Deitte LA. Cricoid pressure results in compression of the postcricoid hypopharynx: the esophageal position is irrelevant. Anesth Analg. 2009;109(5):1546–52.

231. Zeidan AM, Salem MR, Mazoit JX, Abdullah MA, Ghattas T, Crystal GJ. The effectiveness of cricoid pressure for occluding the esophageal entrance in anesthetized and paralyzed patients: an experimental and observational glidescope study. Anesth Analg. 2014;118(3):580–6.

232. Zeidan AM, Salem MR, Bamadhaj M, et al. The cricoid force necessary to occlude the esophageal entrance: is there a gender difference? Anesth Analg. 2017;124(4):1168–73.

233. Byas-Smith M, Prinsell JR Jr. Ultrasound-guided esophageal occlusion during rapid sequence induction. Can J Anaesth. 2013;60(3):327–8.

234. Brimacombe JR, Berry AM. Cricoid pressure. Can J Anaesth. 1997;44(4):414–25.

235. Ellis DY, Harris T, Zideman D. Cricoid pressure in emergency department rapid sequence tracheal intubations: a risk-benefit analysis. Ann Emerg Med. 2007;50(6):653–65.

236. Asai T, Barclay K, Power I, Vaughan RS. Cricoid pressure impedes placement of the laryngeal mask airway. Br J Anaesth. 1995;74(5):521–5.

237. Aoyama K, Takenaka I, Sata T, Shigematsu A. Cricoid pressure impedes positioning and ventilation through the laryngeal mask airway. Can J Anaesth. 1996;43(10):1035–40.

238. Heath KJ, Palmer M, Fletcher SJ. Fracture of the cricoid cartilage after Sellick's manoeuvre. Br J Anaesth. 1996;76(6):877–8.

239. Landsman I. Cricoid pressure: indications and complications. Paediatr Anaesth. 2004;14(1):43–7.

240. Garrard A, Campbell AE, Turley A, Hall JE. The effect of mechanically-induced cricoid force on lower oesophageal sphincter pressure in anaesthetised patients. Anaesthesia. 2004;59(5):435–9.

241. Whittington RM, Robinson JS, Thompson JM. Prevention of fatal aspiration syndrome. Lancet. 1979;2(8143):630–1.

242. Williamson R. Cricoid pressure. Can J Anaesth. 1989;36(5):601.

243. Salem MR, Khorasani A, Saatee S, Crystal GJ, El-Orbany M. Gastric tubes and airway management in patients at risk of aspiration: history, current concepts, and proposal of an algorithm. Anesth Analg. 2014;118(3):569–79.

244. Gobindram A, Clarke S. Cricoid pressure: should we lay off the pressure? Anaesthesia. 2008;63(11):1258–9.

245. Snow RG, Nunn JF. Induction of anaesthesia in the foot-down position for patients with a full stomach. Br J Anaesth. 1959;31:493–7.

246. Hodges RJ, Bennett JR, Tunstall ME, Knight RF. General anaesthesia for operative obstetrics: with special reference to the use of thiopentone and suxamethonium. Br J Anaesth. 1959;31(4):152–63.

247. Takenaka I, Aoyama K, Iwagaki T. Combining head-neck position and head-down tilt to prevent pulmonary aspiration of gastric contents during induction of anaesthesia: a volunteer and manikin study. Eur J Anaesthesiol. 2012;29(8):380–5.

248. Agnew NM, Kendall JB, Akrofi M, et al. Gastroesophageal reflux and tracheal aspiration in the thoracotomy position: should ranitidine premedication be routine? Anesth Analg. 2002;95(6):1645–9, table of contents

249. Blunt MC, Young PJ, Patil A, Haddock A. Gel lubrication of the tracheal tube cuff reduces pulmonary aspiration. Anesthesiology. 2001;95(2):377–81.

250. Sanjay PS, Miller SA, Corry PR, Russell GN, Pennefather SH. The effect of gel lubrication on cuff leakage of double lumen tubes during thoracic surgery. Anaesthesia. 2006;61(2):133–7.

251. Shackcloth MJ, McCarron E, Kendall J, et al. Randomized clinical trial to determine the effect of nasogastric drainage on tracheal acid aspiration following oesophagectomy. Br J Surg. 2006;93(5):547–52.

252. Michelet P, D'Journo XB, Roch A, et al. Protective ventilation influences systemic inflammation after esophagectomy: a randomized controlled study. Anesthesiology. 2006;105(5):911–9.

253. Tsujimoto H, Takahata R, Nomura S, et al. Predictive value of pleural and serum interleukin-6 levels for pneumonia and hypooxygenations after esophagectomy. J Surg Res. 2013;182(2):e61–7.

254. D'Journo XB, Michelet P, Marin V, et al. An early inflammatory response to oesophagectomy predicts the occurrence of pulmonary complications. Eur J Cardiothorac Surg. 2010;37(5):1144–51.

255. Kalimeris K, Christodoulaki K, Karakitsos P, et al. Influence of propofol and volatile anaesthetics on the inflammatory response in the ventilated lung. Acta Anaesthesiol Scand. 2011;55(6):740–8.

256. Ferrando C, Aguilar G, Piqueras L, Soro M, Moreno J, Belda FJ. Sevoflurane, but not propofol, reduces the lung inflammatory response and improves oxygenation in an acute respiratory distress syndrome model: a randomised laboratory study. Eur J Anaesthesiol. 2013;30(8):455–63.

257. Kellner P, Muller M, Piegeler T, et al. Sevoflurane abolishes oxygenation impairment in a long-term rat model of acute lung injury. Anesth Analg. 2017;124(1):194–203.

258. Wakabayashi S, Yamaguchi K, Kumakura S, et al. Effects of anesthesia with sevoflurane and propofol on the cytokine/chemokine production at the airway epithelium during esophagectomy. Int J Mol Med. 2014;34(1):137–44.

259. Lee JJ, Kim GH, Kim JA, et al. Comparison of pulmonary morbidity using sevoflurane or propofol-remifentanil anesthesia in an Ivor Lewis operation. J Cardiothorac Vasc Anesth. 2012;26(5):857–62.

260. Potocnik I, Novak Jankovic V, Sostaric M, et al. Antiinflammatory effect of sevoflurane in open lung surgery with one-lung ventilation. Croat Med J. 2014;55(6):628–37.

261. Schilling T, Kozian A, Senturk M, et al. Effects of volatile and intravenous anesthesia on the alveolar and systemic inflammatory response in thoracic surgical patients. Anesthesiology. 2011;115(1):65–74.

262. Beck-Schimmer B, Bonvini JM, Braun J, et al. Which anesthesia regimen is best to reduce morbidity and mortality in lung surgery?: a multicenter randomized controlled trial. Anesthesiology. 2016;125(2):313–21.

263. Benumof JL. Difficult tubes and difficult airways. J Cardiothorac Vasc Anesth. 1998;12(2):131–2.

264. Vanner R. Arndt endobronchial blocker during oesophagectomy. Anaesthesia. 2005;60(3):295–6.

265. Chen A, Lai HY, Lin PC, Chen TY, Shyr MH. GlideScope-assisted double-lumen endobronchial tube placement in a patient with an unanticipated difficult airway. J Cardiothorac Vasc Anesth. 2008;22(1):170–2.

266. Russell T, Slinger P, Roscoe A, McRae K, Van Rensburg A. A randomised controlled trial comparing the GlideScope((R)) and the Macintosh laryngoscope for double-lumen endobronchial intubation. Anaesthesia. 2013;68(12):1253–8.

267. Yao WL, Wan L, Xu H, et al. A comparison of the McGrath(R) series 5 videolaryngoscope and Macintosh laryngoscope for double-lumen tracheal tube placement in patients with a good glottic view at direct laryngoscopy. Anaesthesia. 2015;70(7): 810–7.

268. Yamazaki T, Ohsumi H. The airway scope is a practical intubation device for a double-lumen tube during rapid-sequence induction. J Cardiothorac Vasc Anesth. 2009;23(6):926.

269. Wasem S, Lazarus M, Hain J, et al. Comparison of the Airtraq and the Macintosh laryngoscope for double-lumen tube intubation: a randomised clinical trial. Eur J Anaesthesiol. 2013;30(4):180–6.

270. Hirabayashi Y, Seo N. The Airtraq laryngoscope for placement of double-lumen endobronchial tube. Can J Anaesth. 2007;54(11):955–7.

271. Purugganan RV, Jackson TA, Heir JS, Wang H, Cata JP. Video laryngoscopy versus direct laryngoscopy for double-lumen endotracheal tube intubation: a retrospective analysis. J Cardiothorac Vasc Anesth. 2012;26(5):845–8.

272. Angie Ho CY, Chen CY, Yang MW, Liu HP. Use of the Arndt wire-guided endobronchial blocker via nasal for one-lung ventilation in patient with anticipated restricted mouth opening for esophagectomy. Eur J Cardiothorac Surg. 2005;28(1):174–5.

273. Narayanaswamy M, McRae K, Slinger P, et al. Choosing a lung isolation device for thoracic surgery: a randomized trial of three bronchial blockers versus double-lumen tubes. Anesth Analg. 2009;108(4):1097–101.

274. Bussieres JS, Somma J, Del Castillo JL, et al. Bronchial blocker versus left double-lumen endotracheal tube in video-assisted thoracoscopic surgery: a randomized-controlled trial examining time and quality of lung deflation. Can J Anaesth. 2016;63(7):818–27.

275. Chappell D, Jacob M, Hofmann-Kiefer K, Conzen P, Rehm M. A rational approach to perioperative fluid management. Anesthesiology. 2008;109(4):723–40.

276. Brandstrup B, Svensen C, Engquist A. Hemorrhage and operation cause a contraction of the extracellular space needing replacement – evidence and implications? A systematic review. Surgery. 2006;139(3):419–32.

277. Jacob M, Chappell D, Rehm M. The "third space" – fact or fiction? Best Pract Res Clin Anaesthesiol. 2009;23(2):145–57.

278. Chau EH, Slinger P. Perioperative fluid management for pulmonary resection surgery and esophagectomy. Semin Cardiothorac Vasc Anesth. 2014;18(1):36–44.

279. Collins SR, Blank RS, Deatherage LS, Dull RO. Special article: the endothelial glycocalyx: emerging concepts in pulmonary edema and acute lung injury. Anesth Analg. 2013;117(3):664–74.

280. Holte K, Sharrock NE, Kehlet H. Pathophysiology and clinical implications of perioperative fluid excess. Br J Anaesth. 2002;89(4):622–32.

281. Kulemann B, Timme S, Seifert G, et al. Intraoperative crystalloid overload leads to substantial inflammatory infiltration of intestinal anastomoses-a histomorphological analysis. Surgery. 2013;154(3):596–603.

282. Brandstrup B, Tonnesen H, Beier-Holgersen R, et al. Effects of intravenous fluid restriction on postoperative complications: comparison of two perioperative fluid regimens: a randomized assessor-blinded multicenter trial. Ann Surg. 2003;238(5):641–8.

283. Lobo DN, Bostock KA, Neal KR, Perkins AC, Rowlands BJ, Allison SP. Effect of salt and water balance on recovery of gastro-intestinal function after elective colonic resection: a randomised controlled trial. Lancet. 2002;359(9320):1812–8.

284. Nisanevich V, Felsenstein I, Almogy G, Weissman C, Einav S, Matot I. Effect of intraoperative fluid management on outcome after intraabdominal surgery. Anesthesiology. 2005;103(1): 25–32.

285. Bernard A, Deschamps C, Allen MS, et al. Pneumonectomy for malignant disease: factors affecting early morbidity and mortality. J Thorac Cardiovasc Surg. 2001;121(6):1076–82.

286. Licker M, de Perrot M, Spiliopoulos A, et al. Risk factors for acute lung injury after thoracic surgery for lung cancer. Anesth Analg. 2003;97(6):1558–65.

287. Fernandez-Perez ER, Keegan MT, Brown DR, Hubmayr RD, Gajic O. Intraoperative tidal volume as a risk factor for respiratory failure after pneumonectomy. Anesthesiology. 2006;105(1): 14–8.

288. Wei S, Tian J, Song X, Chen Y. Association of perioperative fluid balance and adverse surgical outcomes in esophageal cancer and esophagogastric junction cancer. Ann Thorac Surg. 2008;86(1):266–72.

289. Kita T, Mammoto T, Kishi Y. Fluid management and postoperative respiratory disturbances in patients with transthoracic esophagectomy for carcinoma. J Clin Anesth. 2002;14(4):252–6.

290. Schol PB, Terink IM, Lance MD, Scheepers HC. Liberal or restrictive fluid management during elective surgery: a systematic review and meta-analysis. J Clin Anesth. 2016;35:26–39.

291. Glatz T, Kulemann B, Marjanovic G, Bregenzer S, Makowiec F, Hoeppner J. Postoperative fluid overload is a risk factor for adverse surgical outcome in patients undergoing esophagectomy for esophageal cancer: a retrospective study in 335 patients. BMC Surg. 2017;17(1):6.

292. Xing X, Gao Y, Wang H, et al. Correlation of fluid balance and postoperative pulmonary complications in patients after esophagectomy for cancer. J Thorac Dis. 2015;7(11):1986–93.

293. Ahn HJ, Kim JA, Lee AR, Yang M, Jung HJ, Heo B. The risk of acute kidney injury from fluid restriction and hydroxyethyl starch in thoracic surgery. Anesth Analg. 2016;122(1):186–93.

294. Concha MR, Mertz VF, Cortinez LI, et al. The volume of lactated Ringer's solution required to maintain preload and cardiac index during open and laparoscopic surgery. Anesth Analg. 2009;108(2):616–22.

295. Marik PE, Baram M, Vahid B. Does central venous pressure predict fluid responsiveness? A systematic review of the literature and the tale of seven mares. Chest. 2008;134(1):172–8.

296. Oohashi S, Endoh H. Does central venous pressure or pulmonary capillary wedge pressure reflect the status of circulating blood volume in patients after extended transthoracic esophagectomy? J Anesth. 2005;19(1):21–5.

297. Gan TJ, Soppitt A, Maroof M, et al. Goal-directed intraoperative fluid administration reduces length of hospital stay after major surgery. Anesthesiology. 2002;97(4):820–6.

298. Pearse R, Dawson D, Fawcett J, Rhodes A, Grounds RM, Bennett ED. Early goal-directed therapy after major surgery reduces complications and duration of hospital stay. A randomised, controlled trial [ISRCTN38797445]. Crit Care. 2005;9(6):R687–93.

299. Donati A, Loggi S, Preiser JC, et al. Goal-directed intraoperative therapy reduces morbidity and length of hospital stay in high-risk surgical patients. Chest. 2007;132(6):1817–24.

300. Lopes MR, Oliveira MA, Pereira VO, Lemos IP, Auler JO Jr, Michard F. Goal-directed fluid management based on pulse pressure variation monitoring during high-risk surgery: a pilot randomized controlled trial. Crit Care. 2007;11(5):R100.

301. Noblett SE, Snowden CP, Shenton BK, Horgan AF. Randomized clinical trial assessing the effect of Doppler-optimized fluid management on outcome after elective colorectal resection. Br J Surg. 2006;93(9):1069–76.

302. Mythen MG, Webb AR. Perioperative plasma volume expansion reduces the incidence of gut mucosal hypoperfusion during cardiac surgery. Arch Surg. 1995;130(4):423–9.

303. Sinclair S, James S, Singer M. Intraoperative intravascular volume optimisation and length of hospital stay after repair of proximal femoral fracture: randomised controlled trial. BMJ. 1997;315(7113):909–12.

304. McKendry M, McGloin H, Saberi D, Caudwell L, Brady AR, Singer M. Randomised controlled trial assessing the impact of a nurse delivered, flow monitored protocol for optimisation of circulatory status after cardiac surgery. BMJ. 2004;329(7460):258.

305. Wakeling HG, McFall MR, Jenkins CS, et al. Intraoperative oesophageal Doppler guided fluid management shortens postoperative hospital stay after major bowel surgery. Br J Anaesth. 2005;95(5):634–42.

306. Goepfert MS, Reuter DA, Akyol D, Lamm P, Kilger E, Goetz AE. Goal-directed fluid management reduces vasopressor and catecholamine use in cardiac surgery patients. Intensive Care Med. 2007;33(1):96–103.

307. Bundgaard-Nielsen M, Holte K, Secher NH, Kehlet H. Monitoring of peri-operative fluid administration by individualized goal-directed therapy. Acta Anaesthesiol Scand. 2007;51(3):331–40.

308. Gurgel ST, do Nascimento P Jr. Maintaining tissue perfusion in high-risk surgical patients: a systematic review of randomized clinical trials. Anesth Analg. 2011;112(6):1384–91.

309. Hamilton MA, Cecconi M, Rhodes A. A systematic review and meta-analysis on the use of preemptive hemodynamic intervention to improve postoperative outcomes in moderate and high-risk surgical patients. Anesth Analg. 2011;112(6):1392–402.

310. Pearse RM, Harrison DA, MacDonald N, et al. Effect of a perioperative, cardiac output-guided hemodynamic therapy algorithm on outcomes following major gastrointestinal surgery: a randomized clinical trial and systematic review. JAMA. 2014;311(21):2181–90.

311. Thiele RH, Raghunathan K, Brudney CS, et al. American Society for Enhanced Recovery (ASER) and Perioperative Quality Initiative (POQI) joint consensus statement on perioperative fluid management within an enhanced recovery pathway for colorectal surgery. Perioper Med (Lond). 2016;5:24.

312. Manecke GR. Edwards FloTrac sensor and Vigileo monitor: easy, accurate, reliable cardiac output assessment using the arterial pulse wave. Expert Rev Med Devices. 2005;2(5):523–7.

313. Cannesson M, Musard H, Desebbe O, et al. The ability of stroke volume variations obtained with Vigileo/FloTrac system to monitor fluid responsiveness in mechanically ventilated patients. Anesth Analg. 2009;108(2):513–7.

314. Manecke GR Jr, Auger WR. Cardiac output determination from the arterial pressure wave: clinical testing of a novel algorithm that does not require calibration. J Cardiothorac Vasc Anesth. 2007;21(1):3–7.

315. Godje O, Hoke K, Goetz AE, et al. Reliability of a new algorithm for continuous cardiac output determination by pulse-contour analysis during hemodynamic instability. Crit Care Med. 2002;30(1):52–8.

316. Haas S, Eichhorn V, Hasbach T, et al. Goal-directed fluid therapy using stroke volume variation does not result in pulmonary fluid overload in thoracic surgery requiring one-lung ventilation. Crit Care Res Pract. 2012;2012:687018.

317. Lee JH, Jeon Y, Bahk JH, et al. Pulse pressure variation as a predictor of fluid responsiveness during one-lung ventilation for lung surgery using thoracotomy: randomised controlled study. Eur J Anaesthesiol. 2011;28(1):39–44.

318. Fu Q, Duan M, Zhao F, Mi W. Evaluation of stroke volume variation and pulse pressure variation as predictors of fluid responsiveness in patients undergoing protective one-lung ventilation. Drug Discov Ther. 2015;9(4):296–302.

319. Suehiro K, Okutani R. Stroke volume variation as a predictor of fluid responsiveness in patients undergoing one-lung ventilation. J Cardiothorac Vasc Anesth. 2010;24(5):772–5.

320. Suehiro K, Okutani R. Influence of tidal volume for stroke volume variation to predict fluid responsiveness in patients undergoing one-lung ventilation. J Anesth. 2011;25(5):777–80.

321. Ishihara H, Hashiba E, Okawa H, Saito J, Kasai T, Tsubo T. Neither dynamic, static, nor volumetric variables can accurately predict fluid responsiveness early after abdominothoracic esophagectomy. Perioper Med (Lond). 2013;2(1):3.

322. Kobayashi M, Koh M, Irinoda T, Meguro E, Hayakawa Y, Takagane A. Stroke volume variation as a predictor of intravascular volume depression and possible hypotension during the early postoperative period after esophagectomy. Ann Surg Oncol. 2009;16(5):1371–7.

323. Veelo DP, van Berge Henegouwen MI, Ouwehand KS, et al. Effect of goal-directed therapy on outcome after esophageal surgery: a quality improvement study. PLoS One. 2017;12(3): e0172806.

324. Kimberger O, Arnberger M, Brandt S, et al. Goal-directed colloid administration improves the microcirculation of healthy and peri-anastomotic colon. Anesthesiology. 2009;110(3):496–504.

325. Moretti EW, Robertson KM, El-Moalem H, Gan TJ. Intraoperative colloid administration reduces postoperative nausea and vomiting and improves postoperative outcomes compared with crystalloid administration. Anesth Analg. 2003;96(2):611–7, table of contents

326. Jungheinrich C, Scharpf R, Wargenau M, Bepperling F, Baron JF. The pharmacokinetics and tolerability of an intravenous infusion of the new hydroxyethyl starch 130/0.4 (6%, 500 mL) in mild-to-severe renal impairment. Anesth Analg. 2002;95(3):544–51, table of contents

327. Boldt J, Brosch C, Ducke M, Papsdorf M, Lehmann A. Influence of volume therapy with a modern hydroxyethyl starch preparation on kidney function in cardiac surgery patients with compromised renal function: a comparison with human albumin. Crit Care Med. 2007;35(12):2740–6.

328. Mukhtar A, Aboulfetouh F, Obayah G, et al. The safety of modern hydroxyethyl starch in living donor liver transplantation: a comparison with human albumin. Anesth Analg. 2009;109(3):924–30.

329. Gandhi SD, Weiskopf RB, Jungheinrich C, et al. Volume replacement therapy during major orthopedic surgery using Voluven (hydroxyethyl starch 130/0.4) or hetastarch. Anesthesiology. 2007;106(6):1120–7.

330. Gallandat Huet RC, Siemons AW, Baus D, et al. A novel hydroxyethyl starch (Voluven) for effective perioperative plasma volume substitution in cardiac surgery. Can J Anaesth. 2000;47(12):1207–15.

331. Nohe B, Johannes T, Reutershan J, et al. Synthetic colloids attenuate leukocyte-endothelial interactions by inhibition of integrin function. Anesthesiology. 2005;103(4):759–67.

332. Ozturk T, Onur E, Cerrahoglu M, Calgan M, Nizamoglu F, Civi M. Immune and inflammatory role of hydroxyethyl starch 130/0.4 and fluid gelatin in patients undergoing coronary surgery. Cytokine. 2015;74(1):69–75.

333. Perner A, Haase N, Guttormsen AB, et al. Hydroxyethyl starch 130/0.42 versus Ringer's acetate in severe sepsis. New Engl J Med. 2012;367(2):124–34.

334. Myburgh JA, Finfer S, Bellomo R, et al. Hydroxyethyl starch or saline for fluid resuscitation in intensive care. New Engl J Med. 2012;367(20):1901–11.

335. Raghunathan K, Miller TE, Shaw AD. Intravenous starches: is suspension the best solution? Anesth Analg. 2014;119(3):731–6.

336. Annane D, Siami S, Jaber S, et al. Effects of fluid resuscitation with colloids vs crystalloids on mortality in critically ill patients presenting with hypovolemic shock: the CRISTAL randomized trial. JAMA. 2013;310(17):1809–17.

337. Jacob M, Fellahi JL, Chappell D, Kurz A. The impact of hydroxy-ethyl starches in cardiac surgery: a meta-analysis. Crit Care. 2014;18(6):656.

338. Chappell D, Jacob M. Hydroxyethyl starch – the importance of being earnest. Scand J Trauma Resusc Emerg Med. 2013;21:61.

339. Jorgenson A, Jaeger JM, de Souza DG, Blank RS. Acute intra-operative pulmonary embolism: an unusual cause of hypoxemia during one-lung ventilation. J Cardiothorac Vasc Anesth. 2011;25(6):1113–5.

340. Bechtold ML, Nguyen DL, Palmer LB, Kiraly LN, Martindale RG, McClave SA. Nasal bridles for securing nasoenteric tubes: a meta-analysis. Nutr Clin Pract. 2014;29(5):667–71.

341. Faulx AL, Catanzaro A, Zyzanski S, et al. Patient tolerance and acceptance of unsedated ultrathin esophagoscopy. Gastrointest Endosc. 2002;55(6):620–3.

342. Bush CM, Postma GN. Transnasal esophagoscopy. Otolaryngol Clin N Am. 2013;46(1):41–52.

343. Streckfuss A, Bosch N, Plinkert PK, Baumann I. Transnasal flexible esophagoscopy (TNE): an evaluation of the patient's experience and time management. Eur Arch Otorhinolaryngol. 2014;271(2):323–8.

344. Nguyen ST, Cabrales RE, Bashour CA, et al. Benzocaine-induced methemoglobinemia. Anesth Analg. 2000;90(2):369–71.

345. Gunaratnam NT, Vazquez-Sequeiros E, Gostout CJ, Alexander GL. Methemoglobinemia related to topical benzocaine use: is it time to reconsider the empiric use of topical anesthesia before sedated EGD? Gastrointest Endosc. 2000;52(5):692–3.

346. Goudra B, Singh PM. Airway management during upper GI endoscopic procedures: state of the art review. Dig Dis Sci. 2017;62(1):45–53.

347. Busick T, Kussman M, Scheidt T, Tobias JD. Preliminary experience with dexmedetomidine for monitored anesthesia care during ENT surgical procedures. Am J Ther. 2008;15(6):520–7.

348. Nonaka S, Kawaguchi Y, Oda I, et al. Safety and effectiveness of propofol-based monitored anesthesia care without intubation during endoscopic submucosal dissection for early gastric and esophageal cancers. Dig Endosc. 2015;27(6):665–73.

349. Gitzelmann CA, Gysin C, Weiss M. Dorsal flexion of head and neck for rigid oesophagoscopy – a caution for hidden foreign bodies dropped into the epipharynx. Acta Anaesthesiol Scand. 2003;47(9):1178–9.

350. Lee SH. The role of oesophageal stenting in the non-surgical management of oesophageal strictures. Br J Radiol. 2001;74(886):891–900.

351. Verschuur EM, Kuipers EJ, Siersema PD. Esophageal stents for malignant strictures close to the upper esophageal sphincter. Gastrointest Endosc. 2007;66(6):1082–90.

352. Freeman RK, Van Woerkom JM, Ascioti AJ. Esophageal stent placement for the treatment of iatrogenic intrathoracic esophageal perforation. Ann Thorac Surg. 2007;83(6):2003–7; discussion 2007–8

353. Annese V, Bassotti G. Non-surgical treatment of esophageal achalasia. World J Gastroenterol. 2006;12(36):5763–6.

354. Uppal DS, Wang AY. Update on the endoscopic treatments for achalasia. World J Gastroenterol. 2016;22(39):8670–83.

355. Worrell S, DeMeester SR. Endoscopic resection and ablation for early-stage esophageal cancer. Thorac Surg Clin. 2016;26(2):173–6.

356. Calverley RK, Johnston AE. The anaesthetic management of tracheo-oesophageal fistula: a review of ten years' experience. Can Anaesth Soc J. 1972;19(3):270–82.

357. Baraka A, Slim M. Cardiac arrest during IPPV in a newborn with tracheoesophageal fistula. Anesthesiology. 1970;32(6):564–5.

358. Horishita T, Ogata J, Minami K. Unique anesthetic management of a patient with a large tracheoesophageal fistula using fiberoptic bronchoscopy. Anesth Analg. 2003;97(6):1856.

359. Chan CS. Anaesthetic management during repair of tracheo-oesophageal fistula. Anaesthesia. 1984;39(2):158–60.

360. Truong A. Esophagoscopy to confirm tracheal tube position in a patient with a large tracheoesophageal fistula. Anesth Analg. 2011;113(5):1284–5.

361. Ichinose M, Sakai H, Miyazaki I, et al. Independent lung ventilation combined with HFOV for a patient suffering from tracheo-gastric roll fistula. J Anesth. 2008;22(3):282–5.

362. Patti MG, Wiener-Kronish JP, Way LW, Pellegrini CA. Impact of transhiatal esophagectomy on cardiac and respiratory function. Am J Surg. 1991;162(6):563–6; discussion 566–7

363. Malhotra SK, Kaur RP, Gupta NM, Grover A, Ramprabu K, Nakra D. Incidence and types of arrhythmias after mediastinal manipulation during transhiatal esophagectomy. Ann Thorac Surg. 2006;82(1):298–302.

364. Fumagalli U, Melis A, Balazova J, Lascari V, Morenghi E, Rosati R. Intra-operative hypotensive episodes may be associated with post-operative esophageal anastomotic leak. Updates Surg. 2016;68(2):185–90.

365. Ikeda Y, Niimi M, Kan S, Shatari T, Takami H, Kodaira S. Clinical significance of tissue blood flow during esophagectomy by laser Doppler flowmetry. J Thorac Cardiovasc Surg. 2001;122(6):1101–6.

366. Kusano C, Baba M, Takao S, et al. Oxygen delivery as a factor in the development of fatal postoperative complications after oesophagectomy. Br J Surg. 1997;84(2):252–7.

367. Urschel JD. Esophagogastrostomy anastomotic leaks complicating esophagectomy: a review. Am J Surg. 1995;169(6):634–40.

368. Koyanagi K, Ozawa S, Oguma J, et al. Blood flow speed of the gastric conduit assessed by indocyanine green fluorescence: new predictive evaluation of anastomotic leakage after esophagectomy. Medicine (Baltimore). 2016;95(30):e4386.

369. Pham TH, Perry KA, Enestvedt CK, et al. Decreased conduit perfusion measured by spectroscopy is associated with anastomotic complications. Ann Thorac Surg. 2011;91(2):380–5.

370. Al-Rawi OY, Pennefather SH, Page RD, Dave I, Russell GN. The effect of thoracic epidural bupivacaine and an intravenous adrenaline infusion on gastric tube blood flow during esophagectomy. Anesth Analg. 2008;106(3):884–7, table of contents

371. Klijn E, Niehof S, de Jonge J, Gommers D, Ince C, van Bommel J. The effect of perfusion pressure on gastric tissue blood flow in an experimental gastric tube model. Anesth Analg. 2010;110(2):541–6.

372. Pathak D, Pennefather SH, Russell GN, et al. Phenylephrine infusion improves blood flow to the stomach during oesophagectomy in the presence of a thoracic epidural analgesia. Eur J Cardiothorac Surg. 2013;44(1):130–3.

373. Bartels H, Stein HJ, Siewert JR. Early extubation vs. late extubation after esophagus resection: a randomized, prospective study. Langenbecks Arch Chir Suppl Kongressbd. 1998;115:1074–6.

374. Caldwell MT, Murphy PG, Page R, Walsh TN, Hennessy TP. Timing of extubation after oesophagectomy. Br J Surg. 1993;80(12):1537–9.

375. Lanuti M, de Delva PE, Maher A, et al. Feasibility and outcomes of an early extubation policy after esophagectomy. Ann Thorac Surg. 2006;82(6):2037–41.

376. Jiang K, Cheng L, Wang JJ, Li JS, Nie J. Fast track clinical pathway implications in esophagogastrectomy. World J Gastroenterol. 2009;15(4):496–501.

377. Chandrashekar MV, Irving M, Wayman J, Raimes SA, Linsley A. Immediate extubation and epidural analgesia allow safe management in a high-dependency unit after two-stage oesophagectomy. Results of eight years of experience in a specialized upper gastrointestinal unit in a district general hospital. Br J Anaesth. 2003;90(4):474–9.

378. Greco M, Capretti G, Beretta L, Gemma M, Pecorelli N, Braga M. Enhanced recovery program in colorectal surgery: a meta-analysis of randomized controlled trials. World J Surg. 2014;38(6):1531–41.

379. Cooke DT, Calhoun RF, Kuderer V, David EA. A defined esophagectomy perioperative clinical care process can improve outcomes and costs. Am Surg. 2017;83(1):103–11.

380. Schmidt HM, El Lakis MA, Markar SR, Hubka M, Low DE. Accelerated recovery within standardized recovery pathways after esophagectomy: a prospective cohort study assessing the effects of early discharge on outcomes, readmissions, patient satisfaction, and costs. Ann Thorac Surg. 2016;102(3):931–9.

381. Markar SR, Karthikesalingam A, Low DE. Enhanced recovery pathways lead to an improvement in postoperative outcomes following esophagectomy: systematic review and pooled analysis. Dis Esophagus. 2015;28(5):468–75.

382. Brock H, Rieger R, Gabriel C, Polz W, Moosbauer W, Necek S. Haemodynamic changes during thoracoscopic surgery the effects of one-lung ventilation compared with carbon dioxide insufflation. Anaesthesia. 2000;55(1):10–6.

383. Wolfer RS, Krasna MJ, Hasnain JU, McLaughlin JS. Hemodynamic effects of carbon dioxide insufflation during thoracoscopy. Ann Thorac Surg. 1994;58(2):404–7; discussion 407–8

384. Martin LW, Hofstetter W, Swisher SG, Roth JA. Management of intrathoracic leaks following esophagectomy. Adv Surg. 2006;40:173–90.

385. Amar D, Burt ME, Bains MS, Leung DH. Symptomatic tachydysrhythmias after esophagectomy: incidence and outcome measures. Ann Thorac Surg. 1996;61(5):1506–9.

386. Murthy SC, Law S, Whooley BP, Alexandrou A, Chu KM, Wong J. Atrial fibrillation after esophagectomy is a marker for postoperative morbidity and mortality. J Thorac Cardiovasc Surg. 2003;126(4):1162–7.

387. Chin JH, Moon YJ, Jo JY, et al. Association between postoperatively developed atrial fibrillation and long-term mortality after esophagectomy in esophageal cancer patients: an observational study. PLoS One. 2016;11(5):e0154931.

388. Vaporciyan AA, Correa AM, Rice DC, et al. Risk factors associated with atrial fibrillation after noncardiac thoracic surgery: analysis of 2588 patients. J Thorac Cardiovasc Surg. 2004;127(3):779–86.

389. Lohani KR, Nandipati KC, Rollins SE, et al. Transthoracic approach is associated with increased incidence of atrial fibrillation after esophageal resection. Surg Endosc. 2015;29(7):2039–45.

390. Ma JY, Wang Y, Zhao YF, et al. Atrial fibrillation after surgery for esophageal carcinoma: clinical and prognostic significance. World J Gastroenterol. 2006;12(3):449–52.

391. Sedrakyan A, Treasure T, Browne J, Krumholz H, Sharpin C, van der Meulen J. Pharmacologic prophylaxis for postoperative atrial tachyarrhythmia in general thoracic surgery: evidence from randomized clinical trials. J Thorac Cardiovasc Surg. 2005;129(5):997–1005.

392. Tisdale JE, Wroblewski HA, Wall DS, et al. A randomized, controlled study of amiodarone for prevention of atrial fibrillation after transthoracic esophagectomy. J Thorac Cardiovasc Surg. 2010;140(1):45–51.

393. Law SY, Fok M, Wong J. Risk analysis in resection of squamous cell carcinoma of the esophagus. World J Surg. 1994;18(3):339–46.

394. Law S, Wong KH, Kwok KF, Chu KM, Wong J. Predictive factors for postoperative pulmonary complications and mortality after esophagectomy for cancer. Ann Surg. 2004;240(5):791–800.

395. Ferguson MK, Durkin AE. Preoperative prediction of the risk of pulmonary complications after esophagectomy for cancer. J Thorac Cardiovasc Surg. 2002;123(4):661–9.

396. Bailey SH, Bull DA, Harpole DH, et al. Outcomes after esophagectomy: a ten-year prospective cohort. Ann Thorac Surg. 2003;75(1):217–22; discussion 222

397. Muller JM, Erasmi H, Stelzner M, Zieren U, Pichlmaier H. Surgical therapy of oesophageal carcinoma. Br J Surg. 1990;77(8):845–57.

398. Molena D, Mungo B, Stem M, Lidor AO. Incidence and risk factors for respiratory complications in patients undergoing esophagectomy for malignancy: a NSQIP analysis. Semin Thorac Cardiovasc Surg. 2014;26(4):287–94.

399. Jiao WJ, Wang TY, Gong M, Pan H, Liu YB, Liu ZH. Pulmonary complications in patients with chronic obstructive pulmonary disease following transthoracic esophagectomy. World J Gastroenterol. 2006;12(16):2505–9.

400. Bludau M, Holscher AH, Bollschweiler E, et al. Preoperative airway colonization prior to transthoracic esophagectomy predicts postoperative pulmonary complications. Langenbecks Arch Surg. 2015;400(6):707–14.

401. Tandon S, Batchelor A, Bullock R, et al. Peri-operative risk factors for acute lung injury after elective oesophagectomy. Br J Anaesth. 2001;86(5):633–8.

402. Howells P, Thickett D, Knox C, et al. The impact of the acute respiratory distress syndrome on outcome after oesophagectomy. Br J Anaesth. 2016;117(3):375–81.

403. Nakanishi K, Takeda S, Terajima K, Takano T, Ogawa R. Myocardial dysfunction associated with proinflammatory cytokines after esophageal resection. Anesth Analg. 2000;91(2):270–5.

404. Kooguchi K, Kobayashi A, Kitamura Y, et al. Elevated expression of inducible nitric oxide synthase and inflammatory cytokines in the alveolar macrophages after esophagectomy. Crit Care Med. 2002;30(1):71–6.

405. Reid PT, Donnelly SC, MacGregor IR, et al. Pulmonary endothelial permeability and circulating neutrophil-endothelial markers in patients undergoing esophagogastrectomy. Crit Care Med. 2000;28(9):3161–5.

406. Rocker GM, Wiseman MS, Pearson D, Shale DJ. Neutrophil degranulation and increased pulmonary capillary permeability following oesophagectomy: a model of early lung injury in man. Br J Surg. 1988;75(9):883–6.

407. Donnelly SC, Strieter RM, Kunkel SL, et al. Interleukin-8 and development of adult respiratory distress syndrome in at-risk patient groups. Lancet. 1993;341(8846):643–7.

408. Hay DW, Sarau HM. Interleukin-8 receptor antagonists in pulmonary diseases. Curr Opin Pharmacol. 2001;1(3):242–7.

409. Zeilhofer HU, Schorr W. Role of interleukin-8 in neutrophil signaling. Curr Opin Hematol. 2000;7(3):178–82.

410. Cree RT, Warnell I, Staunton M, et al. Alveolar and plasma concentrations of interleukin-8 and vascular endothelial growth factor following oesophagectomy. Anaesthesia. 2004;59(9):867–71.

411. Tsukada K, Hasegawa T, Miyazaki T, et al. Predictive value of interleukin-8 and granulocyte elastase in pulmonary complication after esophagectomy. Am J Surg. 2001;181(2):167–71.

412. Harada K, Ida S, Baba Y, et al. Prognostic and clinical impact of sarcopenia in esophageal squamous cell carcinoma. Dis Esophagus. 2016;29(6):627–33.

413. Watanabe M, Ishimoto T, Baba Y, et al. Prognostic impact of body mass index in patients with squamous cell carcinoma of the esophagus. Ann Surg Oncol. 2013;20(12):3984–91.

414. Yoshida N, Harada K, Baba Y, et al. Preoperative controlling nutritional status (CONUT) is useful to estimate the prognosis after esophagectomy for esophageal cancer. Langenbecks Arch Surg. 2017;402(2):333–41.

415. Filip B, Scarpa M, Cavallin F, et al. Postoperative outcome after oesophagectomy for cancer: nutritional status is the missing ring in the current prognostic scores. Eur J Surg Oncol. 2015;41(6):787–94.

416. Haverkort EB, Binnekade JM, Busch OR, van Berge Henegouwen MI, de Haan RJ, Gouma DJ. Presence and persistence of nutrition-related symptoms during the first year following esophagectomy

with gastric tube reconstruction in clinically disease-free patients. World J Surg. 2010;34(12):2844–52.

417. Baker M, Halliday V, Williams RN, Bowrey DJ. A systematic review of the nutritional consequences of esophagectomy. Clin Nutr. 2016;35(5):987–94.

418. Fujita T, Okada N, Kanamori J, et al. Thermogenesis induced by amino acid administration prevents intraoperative hypothermia and reduces postoperative infectious complications after thoracoscopic esophagectomy. Dis Esophagus. 2017;30(1):1–7.

419. Takesue T, Takeuchi H, Ogura M, et al. A prospective randomized trial of enteral nutrition after thoracoscopic esophagectomy for esophageal cancer. Ann Surg Oncol. 2015;22(Suppl 3):S802–9.

420. Okamura A, Takeuchi H, Matsuda S, et al. Factors affecting cytokine change after esophagectomy for esophageal cancer. Ann Surg Oncol. 2015;22(9):3130–5.

421. Wong CS, Aly EH. The effects of enteral immunonutrition in upper gastrointestinal surgery: a systematic review and meta-analysis. Int J Surg. 2016;29:137–50.

422. Weijs TJ, Berkelmans GH, Nieuwenhuijzen GA, et al. Immediate postoperative oral nutrition following esophagectomy: a multicenter clinical trial. Ann Thorac Surg. 2016;102(4):1141–8.

423. Berkelmans GH, Wilts BJ, Kouwenhoven EA, et al. Nutritional route in oesophageal resection trial II (NUTRIENT II): study protocol for a multicentre open-label randomised controlled trial. BMJ Open. 2016;6(8):e011979.

424. Nakatsuchi T, Otani M, Osugi H, Ito Y, Koike T. The necessity of chest physical therapy for thoracoscopic oesophagectomy. J Int Med Res. 2005;33(4):434–41.

425. Lunardi AC, Cecconello I, Carvalho CR. Postoperative chest physical therapy prevents respiratory complications in patients undergoing esophagectomy. Rev Bras Fisioter. 2011;15(2):160–5.

426. van Adrichem EJ, Meulenbroek RL, Plukker JT, Groen H, van Weert E. Comparison of two preoperative inspiratory muscle training programs to prevent pulmonary complications in patients undergoing esophagectomy: a randomized controlled pilot study. Ann Surg Oncol. 2014;21(7):2353–60.

427. Dettling DS, van der Schaaf M, Blom RL, Nollet F, Busch OR, van Berge Henegouwen MI. Feasibility and effectiveness of pre-operative inspiratory muscle training in patients undergoing oesophagectomy: a pilot study. Physiother Res Int. 2013;18(1):16–26.

428. Michelet P, Roch A, D'Journo XB, et al. Effect of thoracic epidural analgesia on gastric blood flow after oesophagectomy. Acta Anaesthesiol Scand. 2007;51(5):587–94.

429. Lazar G, Kaszaki J, Abraham S, et al. Thoracic epidural anesthesia improves the gastric microcirculation during experimental gastric tube formation. Surgery. 2003;134(5):799–805.

430. Lohser J, Slinger P. Lung injury after one-lung ventilation: a review of the pathophysiologic mechanisms affecting the ventilated and the collapsed lung. Anesth Analg. 2015;121(2):302–18.

431. Brassard CL, Lohser J, Donati F, Bussieres JS. Step-by-step clinical management of one-lung ventilation: continuing professional development. Can J Anaesth. 2014;61(12):1103–21.

432. Severgnini P, Selmo G, Lanza C, et al. Protective mechanical ventilation during general anesthesia for open abdominal surgery improves postoperative pulmonary function. Anesthesiology. 2013;118(6):1307–21.

433. Futier E, Constantin JM, Paugam-Burtz C, et al. A trial of intraoperative low-tidal-volume ventilation in abdominal surgery. New Engl J Med. 2013;369(5):428–37.

434. Shen Y, Zhong M, Wu W, et al. The impact of tidal volume on pulmonary complications following minimally invasive esophagectomy: a randomized and controlled study. J Thorac Cardiovasc Surg. 2013;146(5):1267–73; discussion 1273–4

435. Yang M, Ahn HJ, Kim K, et al. Does a protective ventilation strategy reduce the risk of pulmonary complications after lung cancer surgery?: a randomized controlled trial. Chest. 2011;139(3):530–7.

436. Serpa Neto A, Hemmes SN, Barbas CS, et al. Incidence of mortality and morbidity related to postoperative lung injury in patients who have undergone abdominal or thoracic surgery: a systematic review and meta-analysis. Lancet Respir Med. 2014;2(12):1007–15.

437. Tsai JA, Lund M, Lundell L, Nilsson-Ekdahl K. One-lung ventilation during thoracoabdominal esophagectomy elicits complement activation. J Surg Res. 2009;152(2):331–7.

438. Terragni PP, Del Sorbo L, Mascia L, et al. Tidal volume lower than 6 ml/kg enhances lung protection: role of extracorporeal carbon dioxide removal. Anesthesiology. 2009;111(4):826–35.

439. Engelman E, Maeyens C. Effect of preoperative single-dose corticosteroid administration on postoperative morbidity following esophagectomy. J Gastrointest Surg. 2010;14(5):788–804.

440. Gao Q, Mok HP, Wang WP, Xiao F, Chen LQ. Effect of perioperative glucocorticoid administration on postoperative complications following esophagectomy: a meta-analysis. Oncol Lett. 2014;7(2):349–56.

441. Weijs TJ, Dieleman JM, Ruurda JP, Kroese AC, Knape HJ, van Hillegersberg R. The effect of perioperative administration of glucocorticoids on pulmonary complications after transthoracic oesophagectomy: a systematic review and meta-analysis. Eur J Anaesthesiol. 2014;31(12):685–94.

442. Shyamsundar M, McAuley DF, Shields MO, et al. Effect of simvastatin on physiological and biological outcomes in patients undergoing esophagectomy: a randomized placebo-controlled trial. Ann Surg. 2014;259(1):26–31.

443. Wang ZQ, Chen LQ, Yuan Y, et al. Effects of neutrophil elastase inhibitor in patients undergoing esophagectomy: a systematic review and meta-analysis. World J Gastroenterol. 2015;21(12):3720–30.

444. Tanaka E, Murata H, Minami H, Sumikawa K. Anesthetic management of peroral endoscopic myotomy for esophageal achalasia: a retrospective case series. J Anesth. 2014;28(3):456–9.

445. Yang D, Pannu D, Zhang Q, White JD, Draganov PV. Evaluation of anesthesia management, feasibility and efficacy of peroral endoscopic myotomy (POEM) for achalasia performed in the endoscopy unit. Endosc Int Open. 2015;3(4):E289–95.

Anesthesia for Robotic Thoracic Surgery

39

Javier Campos

Key Points

- The management of the robotic thoracic surgical patient requires the knowledge of minimally invasive surgery techniques involving the chest.
- Familiarity with the da Vinci® robot surgical system by the anesthesiologist is mandatory.
- Management of one-lung ventilation techniques with a left-sided double-lumen endotracheal tube or an independent bronchial blocker is required, along with flexible fiber-optic bronchoscopy techniques.
- Patient positioning and prevention of complications such as nerve or crashing injuries, while the robotic system is used.
- Recognition of the hemodynamic effects of carbon dioxide (CO_2) during insufflation in the chest is required.
- Potential for conversion to open thoracotomy or open procedure in the abdomen.

Introduction

Minimally invasive surgery approaches have become increasingly popular in cardiac, thoracic, and esophageal surgery [1–5]. With the introduction of robotic systems, specifically the da Vinci® robot surgical system, more than 10 years ago, a wide variety of surgical operations have been performed with some provocative results and limited defined advantages. This chapter provides an overview of the anesthetic implications and the use of the robotic system in patients undergoing mediastinal mass resection, pulmonary resections, and esophageal surgery.

J. Campos (✉)
Department of Anesthesia, University of Iowa Health Care, Roy and Lucille Carver College of Medicine, Iowa City, IA, USA
e-mail: javier-campos@uiowa.edu

The da Vinci® Robot Surgical System

The da Vinci® robot surgical system provides three-dimensional (3D) video imaging plus a set of telemanipulated flexible effector instruments [6]. The system consists of three major components, a console for the operating surgeon, a patient-side cart with four interactive robotic arms, and a vision cart including optical devices for the robotic camera [7]. Figure 39.1 displays the da Vinci® robot surgical system.

In brief the surgeon operates while seated at a console and views a 3D image of the surgical fields through the vision system. The patient-side cart (the actual robot) consists of three or four robotic arms, two or three instrument arms, and one endoscope arm which houses the camera. A full range of EndoWrists (Intuitive Surgical) instruments are used to assist with the surgery. These EndoWrists provide seven degrees of motion which exceeds the capacity of a surgeon's hand in open surgery and two degrees of axial rotation to replicate human wrist-like movements. In clinical practice, the first two arms,

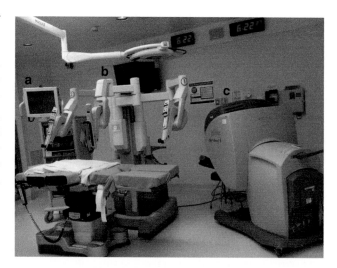

Fig. 39.1 Displays (**a**) Video Monitor (**b**) a three-arm da Vinci® robot surgical system and (**c**) the console

P. Slinger (ed.), *Principles and Practice of Anesthesia for Thoracic Surgery*, https://doi.org/10.1007/978-3-030-00859-8_39

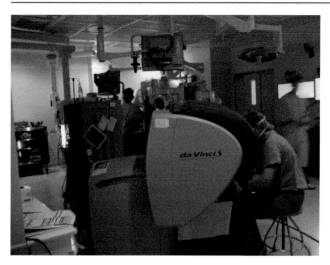

Fig. 39.2 Displays the console and a surgeon seated and performing robotic surgery

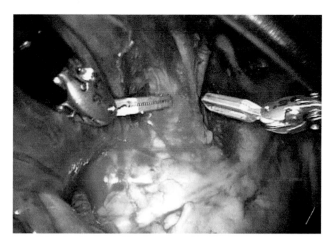

Fig. 39.3 Displays the EndoWrist instruments during a thoracic surgical case

Table 39.1 Advantages and disadvantages of robotic thoracic surgery

Advantages of robotic thoracic surgery
Shorter hospital length of stay
Less pain
Less blood loss and need for transfusion
Minimal scarring
Faster recovery
Faster return to normal activities
Disadvantages
Increasing surgical times
Increased number of operating room personnel needed
Potential for conversion to open procedure
Cost and outcomes (need to be compared with other techniques)

Table 39.2 Surgical procedures performed in thoracic surgery with the da Vinci® robot surgical system

Thymectomy
Mediastinal mass resection
Nissen fundoplications
Esophageal dissections
Esophagectomy
Pulmonary lobectomy

geon, who introduces the trocars and connects them with the robotic arms and changes the robotic instruments through the other ports if needed. The size of the robotic trocar is 10 mm for the binocular robotic camera and 8 mm for the instruments. Some of the potential advantages of using a robotic surgical system in thoracic surgery include shorter hospital length of stay, less pain, less blood loss and transfusion, minimal scarring, faster recovery, and probably a faster return to normal activities [8, 9]. Table 39.1 displays the advantages and disadvantages of robotic thoracic surgery. Table 39.2 displays the surgical procedures performed in thoracic surgery with the da Vinci® robot surgical system.

representing the surgeon's left and right hands, hold the EndoWrist instruments; a third arm positions the endoscope; and the optional fourth arm, which represents the latest design in the da Vinci® robot surgical system, adds surgical capabilities by enabling the surgeon to add a third EndoWrist instrument. The surgical instruments are introduced via special ports and attached to the arms of the robot. The surgeon sitting at the console triggers highly sensitive motion sensors that transfer the surgeon's movement to the tip of the instruments. In addition, the da Vinci robot surgical system has developed the da Vinci skills simulator; therefore surgeons and surgical teams can participate with the system skill exercise within their specialty. Figure 39.2 displays the console and a surgeon seated and performing robotic surgery. Figure 39.3 displays the EndoWrist instruments during a thoracic surgical case.

Robotic surgical procedures are usually performed by two surgeons, the surgeon at the console and the table-side sur-

Anesthetic Implications in Robotic Thoracic Surgery

The basic principles applied to minimally invasive surgery of the chest (i.e., thoracoscopic surgery; see also Chap. 24) also apply to robotic-assisted thoracic surgery. The combination of patient position, management of one-lung ventilation (OLV) techniques, and surgical manipulations alters ventilation and perfusion from the dependant and nondependant or collapsed lung. The preferred method for lung isolation during robotic-assisted thoracic surgery is the use of a left-sided double-lumen endotracheal tube (DLT) because of the greater margin of safety and faster and more reliable lung collapse. Also, it provides ready access for bronchoscopic evaluation of the airway during surgical resection.

In general, careful attention must be given to airway devices because changes in body position may cause tube migration. OLV anesthetic management is more challenging during robotic thoracic surgery due to the presence of the robot chassis that is stationed over the patient. The patient's airway is also usually located far from the anesthesia field. In some instances, access to the airway, if needed, is not optimal because of the presence of the robotic arms nearby. In addition, visualization during robotic thoracic surgery may be enhanced by continuous intrathoracic carbon dioxide (CO_2) insufflation, which may increase airway pressures. When CO_2 is used, it should not exceed intrathoracic pressures of 10–15 mmHg. Increasing the intrathoracic pressure (i.e., >25 mmHg) can compromise venous return and cardiac compliance; also the dependant lung develops higher airway pressures, and ventilation can become difficult. During the surgical procedure, the FiO_2 should be maintained at 100%, and the peak inspiratory pressure should be kept <30 cm H_2O. The ventilatory parameters should be adjusted to maintain a $PaCO_2$ at approximately 40 mmHg.

Robotic-Assisted Surgery and Anesthesia for Mediastinal Masses

Among the thoracic surgical procedures performed to date with the use of the da Vinci® robot surgical system is thymectomy [10]. Of the patients scheduled for robotic-assisted thymectomy, some have the diagnosis of myasthenia gravis because of the presence of a thymoma. Preparation of the patient for surgery includes neurological evaluation to assess the patient's neurological status and optimization of neurological conditions; continuation of anticholinesterase therapy and plasmapheresis may be indicated in some cases [11, 12] (see also Chap. 15). Precautions regarding anesthetic management include the proper dosing of muscle relaxants and the potential consequences of a large mediastinal mass on oxygenation and ventilation.

Positioning the patient for a thymectomy with the use of the robot system requires an optimal surgical position. In these cases, the patients are placed in an incomplete side-up position at a 30° angle right or a left lateral decubitus position with the use of a beanbag. The arm of the elevated side is positioned at the patient's side as far back as possible so the surgeon can gain enough space for the robotic arms (Fig. 39.4). While the robot is in use, it is imperative to consider strategies to protect all pressure points and to avoid unnecessary stretching of the elevated arm because this can cause damage to the brachial plexus. Also, because the arm of the robot is in the chest cavity, a complete lung collapse must be maintained throughout the procedure. Robotic surgery with the da Vinci® robot surgical system does not allow for changes in patient position on the operating room table once the robot has been docked. Robotic thymectomy requires that the operating room table be rotated 90° away

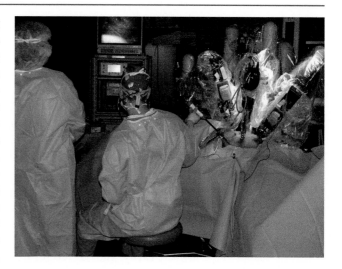

Fig. 39.4 Mediastinal mass resection

from the anesthesiologist's field. For this reason access to the airway to make adjustments to the DLT during the surgery can be challenging. In some cases, a bilateral approach may be required. In these cases, the operation is performed in two stages and requires rotating the table 180° to provide the surgeon access to the contralateral chest for the second stage of the operation. The anesthesiologist must be cautious during these changes to avoid problems with the airway and to ensure that the lines and monitor wires have enough slack to accommodate changes in position. The anesthesiologist must be aware during these cases about possible injury to the contralateral pleura, especially if CO_2 capnothorax is being used, as the elevated intrathoracic pressure in the contralateral hemithorax can make ventilation difficult and cause cardiovascular collapse or tension pneumothorax because of malfunction of the chest tube. Special attention must be given to the patient's elevated arm and head to prevent crushing injuries with the robotic arms. A recent case report [13] showed a brachial plexus injury in an 18-year-old male after robot-assisted thoracoscopic thymectomy. In this report, the left upper limb was in slight hyperabduction. It is important to keep in mind that hyperabduction of the elevated arm to give optimal space to the operating arm of the robot can lead to a neurologic injury. Close communication between surgeon and anesthesiologist in relation to the positioning and function of the robot is mandatory, and all proper measures must be taken, including the use of soft padding and measures to avoid hyperabduction of the arm. The elevated arm should be protected by using a sling resting device. Operating room staff should always be vigilant of telescope light sources because direct contact of these devices with surgical drapes and the patient's skin can quickly cause serious burns, while telescopes and cameras are being changed.

An early report by Bodner et al. [14] involving 13 patients with mediastinal masses resected with the da Vinci® robot surgical system showed no intraoperative complications or surgical mortality. In this series of patients, a complete thymectomy with en bloc removal of all mediastinal fat around the tumor was performed. In this report, cases were restricted to patients with a tumor size less than 10 cm in diameter.

In a report by Savitt et al. [4] involving 14 patients undergoing robot-assisted thymectomy, all patients received a DLT for selective lung ventilation; in addition, patients were managed with arterial and central venous pressure catheters. Complete thymectomy was performed on all 14 patients. Right-lung deflation was accomplished with selective lung ventilation and CO_2 insufflation to a pressure of 10–15 mmHg to maintain the lung away from the operative area. It is important that the anesthesiologist recognizes the effects of CO_2 insufflation in the thoracic cavity. The outcome of this report included no conversion to open thoracotomy nor any intraoperative complications or deaths; the median hospital stay was 2 days with a range of 1–4 days.

In another report, Rückert et al. [9] had zero mortality and an overall postoperative morbidity rate of 2% in 106 consecutive robot-assisted thymectomies. Therefore, robotic thymectomy is a promising technique for minimally invasive surgery. Length of stay was shorter with robotic thymectomy when compared to the conventional approach via sternotomy. Figure 39.5 displays a case of mediastinal mass resection.

A recent systematic review and meta-analysis comparing robotic-assisted minimally invasive surgery versus open thymectomy [15] clearly showed that the patients undergoing robotic thymectomy have a reduced hospital length of stay, less intraoperative blood loss, fewer chest-in-tube days, and less postoperative complications when compared to open thymectomy.

In contrast another meta-analysis study [16] comparing robotic-assisted minimally invasive thymectomy versus video-assisted thoracic surgery thymectomy showed no statistically significant differences in surgery outcomes among the two groups (no significant difference on conversion rates, surgical times or average days, or length of stay).

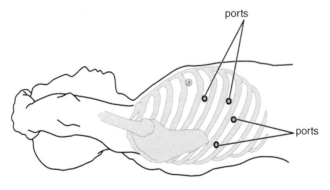

Fig. 39.5 Positioning during robotic thoracic approach

In addition the indications for the use of the robotic surgery have been extended for cases with posterior mediastinal tumor where the access can be challenging and it reported good outcomes [17, 18].

Robotic-Assisted Pulmonary Lobectomy

With the introduction of the da Vinci® robot surgical system, there has been widespread interest in its use in minimally invasive surgery involving the chest [19–21]. Lobectomy with lymph node dissection remains the cornerstone of radical resection of early-stage cancer [22]. However due to the use of low-dose computed tomography, CT scans are increasing the number of patients diagnosed with early-stage disease each year; these patients can be treated via lobectomy or segmentectomy. In order to offer more minimally invasive resection options to patients with lung disease, video-assisted lobectomy/segmentectomy and subsequently robotic-assisted lobectomy/segmentectomy approaches have been developed [23].

The robotic-assisted lobectomy/segmentectomy has attracted interest of thoracic surgeons since its introduction in 2002. The advantages of robotic lobectomy/segmentectomy include smaller incisions, decreased postoperative pain, faster recovery time, and superior survival when compared to conventional open thoracotomy [19].

A report by Park et al. [24] showed robot-assisted thoracic surgical lobectomy to be feasible and safe. In the report, the operation was accomplished with the robotic system in 30 out of 34 scheduled patients. The remaining four patients required conversion to open thoracotomy. Anderson et al. [25] reported a series of 21 patients that underwent robotic lung resection for lung cancer. In this report, the 30-day mortality and conversion rate was 0%. The median operating room time and blood loss were 3.6 h and 100 mL. The complication rate was 27% and included atrial fibrillation and pneumonia. Gharagozloo et al. [26] reported a series of 100 consecutive robotic-assisted lobectomies for lung cancer and concluded that robotic surgery is feasible for mediastinal, hilar, and pulmonary vascular dissection during video-assisted thoracoscopy lobectomy.

Positioning the patient for a robotic lobectomy includes placing the patient over a beanbag in a maximally flexed lateral decubitus position with the elevated arm slightly extended so that the thoracic cavity can be accessed and no damage to the arm occurs during manipulation of the robotic arms. Patients undergoing robotic lobectomy must have a lung isolation device to achieve OLV. In the vast majority of these cases, a left-sided DLT is used, and optimal position is achieved with the flexible fiber optic bronchoscope [27]. In a few cases in which the airway is deemed to be difficult, an independent bronchial blocker could be used and optimal position achieved with the use of a fiber optic bronchoscope [28]. Initial thoracic exploration is performed with conventional thoracoscopy to verify tumor location. During robot-assisted lobectomy, it is mandatory that lung collapse is achieved effectively to allow the surgeon the best field of vision and to avoid unnecessary damage to vessels or lung parenchyma.

All patients undergoing robot-assisted thoracic lobectomy should have an arterial line. The anesthesiologist must be ready for potential conversion to an open thoracotomy. In the Park report [24], three out of four cases that needed to be converted had minor bleeding; in addition, in one case lung isolation was lost, requiring an open thoracotomy. It is mandatory that the anesthesiologist involved in these cases has experience in placing a DLT [29] and can guarantee optimal position with the aid of flexible fiber optic bronchoscope. Using intraoperative fiber optic bronchoscopy to make adjustments to the DLT during surgery is challenging because the table is rotated 180° away from the anesthesiologist's field. The chassis of the robot is often positioned over the patients' head leaving a very small area for the anesthesiologist to access the airway.

A report by Gharagozloo et al. [26] involving 100 patients who underwent lobectomy and complete mediastinal nodal dissection for early-stage lung cancer (stages I and II) with the robotic system reported 1 nonemergent conversion to open thoracotomy. In this report, postoperative analgesia was managed with the infusion of a local anesthetic (0.5% bupivacaine, 4 mL/h) through catheters placed in a subpleural tunnel encompassing intercostal spaces 2 through 8. All patients were extubated in the operating room. Mean operating room time was 216 min (range 173–369). Overall mortality within 30 days was 4.9%, and median length of stay was 4 days. Postoperative complications included atrial fibrillation in four cases, prolonged air leak in two cases, and pleural effusion requiring drainage in two cases – complications that are not different from those occurring with video-assisted thoracoscopic surgery.

A meta-analysis report [30] in 2015 has evaluated the perioperative outcomes of robotic-assisted thoracoscopic surgery for early-stage lung cancer. This meta-analysis report showed that the morbidity and perioperative 30-day mortality were similar in both groups. In contrast a recent meta-analysis study [23] comparing robotic- versus video-assisted lobectomy/segmentectomy for lung cancer showed that robotic lobectomy is a feasible and safe alternative to a video-assisted thoracoscopic surgery with a low 30-day mortality and similar morbidity; also this study reported lower open thoracotomy conversion rate, but longer operative time which increases the cost of surgery. Robotic cases surgical times must be shorter with a reduced cost and improve morbidity to become an alternative to other surgical techniques.

Acute and chronic pain after open thoracotomy continues to be a problem [31]. Minimally invasive thoracic surgery approach results in less tissue trauma, shorter recovery, and improved cosmesis [32, 33]. A recent study [34] evaluating the outcomes of the acute and chronic pain after robotic, video-assisted thoracoscopic surgery or open anatomic pulmonary resection showed that robotic- and video-assisted thoracoscopic surgery (VATS) approach resulted in less acute pain and chronic numbness when compared to open thoracotomy. However, there was no significant difference between robotic- and video-assisted thoracic surgery. This report indicates that in terms to pain control, there are no difference regardless what minimally invasive surgery the surgical team chooses and no advantage of one versus the other technique (robotic vs VATS).

Carbon Dioxide Insufflation During Robotic Surgery

Continuous low-flow insufflation of CO_2 has been demonstrated as an aid for surgical exposure during minimally invasive thoracic procedures. It has been used as the only means of providing surgical exposure to the thoracic cavity (during two-lung ventilation for VATS) or more frequently in conjunction with a DLT or an independent bronchial blocker and OLV. The compression of the lung parenchyma by CO_2 acts as a retractor [35].

A study by Ohtsuka et al. [36] involving 38 patients undergoing minimally invasive internal mammary harvest during cardiac surgery found significant increases in mean central venous pressure, pulmonary artery pressure, and the pulmonary artery wedge pressure. They also found that with insufflation of the right hemithorax, but not the left side, slight decreases were noted in the mean arterial blood pressure and cardiac index. They concluded that the hemodynamic effect from continuous insufflation of CO_2 at 8–10 mmHg for 30–40 min is mild in both hemithoraces, although the impact is greater on the right. This information was supported by another study [37]. This study involving 20 patients undergoing thoracoscopic sympathectomy and concluded that compared to the left side hemithorax, the impact of CO_2 insufflation on the vena cava and the right atrium during right-sided procedures was associated with reduction of venous return and low cardiac index and stroke volume. The impact of CO_2 insufflation on the respiratory system has also been studied. El-Dawlatly et al. [38] reported a significant pressure-dependent increase in peak airway pressure and a decrease in dynamic lung compliance but no difference in tidal volume or minute ventilation during volume-controlled ventilation.

Insufflation of CO_2 should only be started after initial thoracoscopic evaluation has ruled out that the port of insufflation has not compromised a vascular structure or the lung parenchyma. Communication between the surgeon, anesthesiologist, and operating room personnel is crucial at this point. Insufflation is ideally started at low pressures of 4–5 mmHg and is gradually increased while monitoring the patient's vital signs. The anesthesiologist should always be aware of the possibility of gas embolization during these cases. In the case of sudden cardiac collapse, the CO_2 flow should be discontinued immediately. Ventilation during CO_2 insufflation should be titrated to keep adequate oxygenation and a normal $PaCO_2$ and pH. Also, damage to the contralateral pleura may occur resulting in CO_2 flow to the contralateral chest, making ventilation difficult and also causing hemodynamic compromise, along with the potential development of subcutaneous emphysema. In addition, venous return compromise or progressive arterial desaturation can occur [39, 40].

Robotic-Assisted Esophageal Surgery and Anesthetic Implications

Transthoracic esophagectomy with extended lymph node dissection is associated with higher morbidity rates than transhiatal esophagectomy. Esophagectomy is a palliative and potentially curative treatment for esophageal cancer. Minimally invasive esophagectomy has been performed to lessen the biological impact of surgery and potentially reduce pain. The initial esophagectomy experience with the da Vinci® robot surgical system involved a patient who had a thoracic esophagectomy with wide celiac axis lymphadenectomy. The case was reported by Kernstine et al. [41] and had promising results. Thereafter another report using the da Vinci® robot surgical system has been published of six patients undergoing esophagectomy without intraoperative complications [42]. The surgical approach in this report was performed from the right side of the chest. A left-sided DLT was used to selectively collapse the right lung, while, at the same time, ventilation was maintained in the left lung.

In a report by Hillegersberg et al. [43] involving 21 consecutive patients with esophageal cancer who underwent robot-assisted thoracoscopic esophagolymphadenectomy, 18 were completed thoracoscopically, and 3 required open procedures (because adhesions or intraoperative hemorrhage). In this case series report, all patients received a left-sided DLT and a thoracic epidural catheter as part of their anesthetic management. Positioning of these patients was in a left lateral decubitus position, and the patient was tilted 45° toward the prone position. Once the robotic thoracoscopic phase was completed, the patient was then put in supine position, and a midline laparotomy was performed. A cervical esophagogastrostomy was performed in the neck for the completion of surgery.

Of interest in this series is the fact that pulmonary complications occurred in the first ten cases (60%), caused primarily by left-sided pneumonia and associated acute respiratory distress syndrome in three patients (33%). These complications were probably related to barotrauma to the left lung (ventilated lung) attributed to high tidal volumes and high peak inspiratory pressures. In the 11 patients that followed, the same authors modified their ventilatory setting to administer continuous positive airway pressure ventilation 5 cm H_2O during single-lung ventilation, and pressure-controlled ventilation was used; with this approach the respiratory complication rate was reduced to 32%.

A recent report by Kim et al. [44] described 21 patients who underwent robotic-assisted thoracoscopic esophagectomy performed in a prone position with the use of a Univent® bronchial blocker tube (Fuji Systems Corp, Tokyo Japan). All thoracoscopic procedures were completed with robotic-assisted techniques followed by a cervical esophagogastrostomy. In Kim's report, major complications included anastomotic leakage in four patients, vocal cord paralysis in six patients, and intra-abdominal bleeding in one patient. The prone position led to an increase in central venous pressure and mean pulmonary arterial pressure and a decrease in static lung compliance. The overall conclusion from this report is that robotic-assisted esophagectomy in the prone position is technically feasible and safe. Others have reported a robotic-assisted transhiatal esophagectomy technique feasible and safe as well [45].

Another study [5] involved 14 patients who underwent esophagectomy using the da Vinci® robot surgical system in different surgical stages. It showed that for a complete robotic esophagectomy including laparoscopic gastric conduct, the operating room time was an average of 11 h with a console time by the surgeon of 5 h and an estimated mean blood loss of 400 ± 300 mL. In this report after the robotic thoracoscopic part of the surgery was accomplished with the patient in the lateral decubitus position, patients were then placed in supine position and reintubated, and the DLT was replaced with a single-lumen endotracheal tube. The head of each patient was turned upward and to the right, exposing the left neck for the cervical part of the operation. Among the pulmonary complications in the postoperative period, arterial fibrillation occurred in 5 out of 14 patients.

In Kernstine's report [5] among the recommendations to improve efficiency in these cases is the "use of an experienced anesthesiologist who can efficiently intubate and manage single-lung ventilation and hemodynamically support the patient during the procedure." This follows what Nifong and Chitwood [29] have reported in their editorial views regarding anesthesia and robotics: that a team approach with expertise in these procedures involving nurses, anesthesiologists, and surgeons with an interest in robotic procedures is required.

The data on robotic-assisted esophagectomy suggest that the procedure is safe, feasible, and associated with preoperative outcomes similar to open and minimally invasive esophagectomy. No data, however, demonstrate improved outcomes in terms of operative morbidity, pain, operative time, or total costs [46]. Table 39.3 displays the complications of robotic-assisted thoracic surgery involving the mediastinum lung and esophagus.

Although the outcome of robotic-assisted minimally invasive esophagectomy compared to thoracic minimally invasive esophagectomy is comparable, one of the advantages of using robotic technique is the reduced incidence of vocal cord paralysis. Three-dimensional images enhance identification of recurrent laryngeal nerve; therefore it could reduce the chance of damaging the nerve. One study [47] reported a reduced incidence of vocal cord paralysis around 50% when robotic-assisted technique was used (6/38 versus 15/20); other reported complications include anastomotic leakage, bleeding, dysrhythmia, and acute lung injury [48–50].

Summary

The use of the da Vinci® robot surgical system in thoracic and esophageal surgery continues to gain acceptance. Although its use has reduced surgical scarring and decreased length of stay, specific indications for use in these areas need to be determined. All reports to date describe the use of lung isolation devices, most often a left-sided DLT, as part of the intraoperative management of thoracic surgery patients to facilitate surgical exposure. In addition, because the surgical approach varies depending on the thoracic procedure, optimal positioning is not standard and varies among the specific surgical procedures. Vigilance is required with patients' elevated arms to avoid nerve injuries or crush injuries from the robotic arms. Continuous low-flow insufflation of CO_2 has been used as an aid for surgical exposure during minimally invasive thoracic procedures. The potential to convert to an open thoracotomy requires preparation by the surgical team and anesthesiologist. The use of the da Vinci® robot surgical

Table 39.3 Complications of robotic-assisted thoracic surgery

References	$n =$ cases	Operation	Intraoperative complications	Postoperative complications
Rea et al. [3]	33	Thymectomy	0	Chylothorax $n = 1$ Hemothorax $n = 1$
Savitt et al. [4]	15	Mediastinal mass resection	0	Atrial fibrillation $n = 1$
Kernstine et al. [5]	14	Esophagectomy	Conversion to open procedure $n = 1$	Thoracic duct leak $n = 3$ Vocal cord paralysis $n = 3$ Atrial fibrillation $n = 5$
Rückert et al. [9]	106	Thymectomy	Bleeding $n = 1$	Phrenic nerve injury $n = 1$
Pandey et al. [13]	1	Thymectomy	–	Brachial plexus injury
Bodner et al. [14]	14	Mediastinal mass resection	0	Postoperative hoarseness due to lesion to left laryngeal recurrent nerve
Cerfolio et al. [18]	153	Anterior mediastinal Inferior/posterior pathology	0	Conversion to thoracotomy $n =1$ Esophageal leak $n =1$ Atrial fibrillation $n =4$ Pneumothorax $n =2$ Prolonged air leak $n =1$
Park et al. [24]	34	Lobectomy	Conversion to open thoracotomy $n = 3$ Lack lung isolation $n = 1$	Supraventricular arrhythmia $n = 6$ Bleeding $n = 1$ Air leak $n = 1$
Gharagozloo et al. [26]	100	Lobectomy	0	Atrial fibrillation $n = 4$ Air leak $n = 2$ Bleeding $n = 1$ Pleural effusion $n = 2$
Van Hillegersberg et al. [43]	21	Esophagectomy	Conversion to open procedure $n = 3$	Pulmonary complication 60% first 10 cases Pulmonary complication 32%, 11 patients
Kim et al. [44]	21	Esophagectomy	Bleeding $n = 1$	Anastomotic leakage $n = 4$ Vocal cord paralysis $n = 6$
Suda et al. [47]	16	Esophagectomy		Vocal cord paralysis $n=6$ Anastomotic leakage $n = 6$ Pneumonia $n = 1$
Dunn et al. [48]	40	Esophagectomy		Anastomotic leakage $n = 10$ Recent laryngeal nerve injury $n = 14$
Cerfolio et al. [49]	22	Esophagectomy	Conversion from laparoscopy to laparotomy $n = 1$	Anastomotic leakage $n = 1$ Atrial Fibrillation $n = 1$

system is expected to grow in the years to come [51, 52]. Prospective studies are needed to define the specific advantages of this robotic system.

References

1. Tatooles AJ, Pappas PS, Gordon PJ, Slaughter MS. Minimally invasive mitral valve repair using the da Vinci robotic system. Ann Thorac Surg. 2004;77:1978–82.
2. Nifong LW, Chitwood WR, Pappas PS, Smith CR, Argenziano M, Starnes VA, et al. Robotic mitral valve surgery: a United States multicenter trial. J Thorac Cardiovasc Surg. 2005;129:1395–404.
3. Rea F, Marulli G, Bortolotti L, Feltracco P, Zuin A, Sartori F. Experience with the "da Vinci" robotic system for thymectomy in patients with myasthenia gravis. Ann Thorac Surg. 2006;8:455–9.
4. Savitt MA, Gao G, Furnary AP, Swanson J, Gately HL, Handy JR. Application of robotic-assisted techniques to the surgical evaluation and treatment of the anterior mediastinum. Ann Thorac Surg. 2005;79:450–5.
5. Kernstine KH, DeArmond DT, Shamoun DM, Campos JH. The first series of completely robotic esophagectomies with three-field lymphadenectomy: initial experience. Surg Endosc. 2007;21:2285–92.
6. Mack MJ. Minimally invasive and robotic surgery. JAMA. 2001;285:568–72.
7. Campos JH. An update on robotic thoracic surgery and anesthesia. Curr Opin Anaesthesiol. 2010;23:1–6.
8. Bodner J, Wykypiel H, Wetscher G, Schmid T. First experiences with the da Vinci operating robot in thoracic surgery. Eur J Cardiothorac Surg. 2004;25:844–51.
9. Rückert JC, Ismail M, Swierzy M, Sobel H, Rogalla P, Meisel A, et al. Thoracoscopic thymectomy with the da Vinci robotic system for myasthenia gravis. Ann N Y Acad Sci. 2008;1132:329–35.
10. Campos JH. Anaesthesia for robotic surgery: mediastinal mass resection and pulmonary resections. Anaesth Int. 2011:19–22.
11. Baraka A. Onset of neuromuscular block in myasthenic patients. Br J Anaesth. 1992;69:227–8.
12. Abel M, Eisenkraft JB. Anesthetic implications of myasthenia gravis. Mt Sinai J Med. 2002;69:31–7.
13. Pandey R, Elakkumanan LB, Garg R, Jyoti B, Mukund C, Chandralekha, et al. Brachial plexus injury after robotic-assisted thoracoscopic thymectomy. J Cardiothorac Vasc Anesth. 2009;23:584–6.
14. Bodner J, Wykypiel H, Greiner A, Kirchmayr W, Freund MC, Margreiter R, et al. Early experience with robot-assisted surgery for mediastinal masses. Ann Thorac Surg. 2004;78:259–65.
15. Buentzel J, Straube C, Heinz RC, Beham A, Emmert A, et al. Thymectomy via open surgery or robotic video assisted thoracic surgery: can a recommendation already be made? Medicine (Baltimore). 2017;96(24):e7161.
16. Buentzel J, Heinz J, Hinterthaner M, Schöndube FA, Straube C, Roever C, et al. Robotic versus thoracoscopic thymectomy: the current evidence. Int J Med Robot. 2017; 13.
17. Kajiwara N, Kakihana M, Usuda J, Ohira T, Kawate N, Ikeda N. Extended indications for robotic surgery for posterior mediastinal tumors. Asian Cardiovasc Thorac Ann. 2012;20:308–13.
18. Cerfolio RJ, Bryant AS, Minnich DJ. Operative techniques in robotic thoracic surgery for inferior or posterior mediastinal pathology. J Thorac Cardiovasc Surg. 2012;143:1138–43.
19. Zhang L, Gao S. Robot-assisted thoracic surgery versus open thoracic surgery for lung cancer: a system review and meta-analysis. Int J Clin Exp Med. 2015;8:17804–10.
20. Lee BE, Korst RJ, Kletsman E, Rutledge JR. Transitioning from video-assisted thoracic surgical lobectomy to robotics for lung cancer: are there outcomes advantages? J Thorac Cardiovasc Surg. 2014;147:724–9.
21. Yang HX, Woo KM, Sima CS, Bains MS, Adusumilli PS, Huang J, et al. Long-term survival based on the surgical approach to lobectomy for clinical stage I nonsmall cell lung Cancer: comparison of robotic, video-assisted thoracic surgery, and thoracotomy lobectomy. Ann Surg. 2017;265:431–7.
22. Ginsberg RJ, Rubinstein LV. Randomized trial of lobectomy versus limited resection for T1 N0 non-small cell lung cancer. Lung Cancer Study Group. Ann Thorac Surg. 1995;60:615–22.
23. Liang H, Liang W, Zhao L, Chen D, Zhang J, Zhang Y, et al. Robotic versus video-assisted lobectomy/Segmentectomy for lung Cancer: a meta-analysis. Ann Surg. 2017 (in press).
24. Park BJ, Flores RM, Rusch VW. Robotic assistance for video-assisted thoracic surgical lobectomy: technique and initial results. J Thorac Cardiovasc Surg. 2006;131:54–9.
25. Anderson CA, Filsoufi F, Aklog L, Farivar RS, Byrne JG, Adams DH. Robotic-assisted lung resection for malignant disease. Innovations. 2007;2:254–8.
26. Gharagozloo F, Margolis M, Tempesta B, Strother E, Najam F. Robot-assisted lobectomy for early-stage lung cancer: report of 100 consecutive cases. Ann Thorac Surg. 2009;88:380–4.
27. Campos JH. Update on tracheobronchial anatomy and flexible fiberoptic bronchoscopy in thoracic anesthesia. Curr Opin Anaesthesiol. 2009;22:4–10.
28. Campos JH. Progress in lung separation. Thorac Surg Clin. 2005;15:71–83.
29. Nifong LW, Chitwood WR Jr. Challenges for the anesthesiologist: robotics? Anesth Analg. 2003;96:1–2.
30. Ye X, Xie L, Chen G, Tang JM, Ben XS. Robotic thoracic surgery versus video-assisted thoracic surgery for lung cancer: a meta-analysis. Interact Cardiovasc Thorac Surg. 2015;21:409–14.
31. Kampe S, Lohmer J, Weinreich G, Hahn M, Stamatis G, Welter S. Epidural analgesia is not superior to systemic postoperative analgesia with regard to preventing chronic or neuropathic pain after thoracotomy. J Cardiothorac Surg. 2013;8:127.
32. Nagahiro I, Andou A, Aoe M, Sano Y, Date H, Shimizu N. Pulmonary function, postoperative pain, and serum cytokine level after lobectomy: a comparison of VATS and conventional procedure. Ann Thorac Surg. 2001;72:362–5.
33. Grogan EL, Jones DR. VATS lobectomy is better than open thoracotomy: what is the evidence for short-term outcomes. Thorac Surg Clin. 2008;18:249–58.
34. Kwon ST, Zhao L, Reddy RM, Chang AC, Orringer MB, Brummett CM, et al. Evaluation of acute and chronic pain outcomes after robotic, video-assisted thoracoscopic surgery, or open anatomic pulmonary resection. J Thorac Cardiovasc Surg. 2017;154:652–9.
35. Wolfer RS, Krasna MJ, Hasnain JU, McLaughlin JS. Hemodynamic effects of carbon dioxide insufflation during thoracoscopy. Ann Thorac Surg. 1994;58:404–7.
36. Ohtsuka T, Nakajima J, Kotsuka Y, Takamoto S. Hemodynamic response to intrapleural insufflation with hemipulmonary collapse. Surg Endosc. 2001;15:1327–30.
37. El-Dawlatly AA, Al-Dohayan A, Samarkandi A, Algahdam F, Atef A. Right vs left side thoracoscopic sympathectomy: effects of carbon dioxide insufflation on haemodynamics. Ann Chir Gynaecol. 2001;90:206–8.
38. El-Dawlatly AA, Al-Dohayan A, Abdel-Meguid ME, Turkistani A, Alotaiby WM, Abdelaziz EM. Variations in dynamic lung compliance during endoscopic thoracic sympathectomy with carbon dioxide insufflation. Clin Auton Res. 2003;13(Suppl 1):I94–7.
39. Steenwyk B, Lyerly R. Advancements in robotic-assisted thoracic surgery. Anesthesiol Clin. 2012;30:699–708.

40. Campos JH, Ueda K. Update on anesthetic complications of robotic thoracic surgery. Minerva Anestesiol. 2014;80:83–8.

41. Kernstine KH, DeArmond DT, Karimi M, Van Natta TL, Campos JH, Yoder MR, et al. The robotic, 2-stage, 3-field esophagolymphadenectomy. J Thorac Cardiovasc Surg. 2004;127:1847–9.

42. Bodner JC, Zitt M, Ott H, Wetscher GJ, et al. Robotic-assisted thoracoscopic surgery (RATS) for benign and malignant esophageal tumors. Ann Thorac Surg. 2005;80:1202–6.

43. van Hillegersberg R, Boone J, Draaisma WA, Broeders IA, et al. First experience with robot-assisted thoracoscopic esophagolymphadenectomy for esophageal cancer. Surg Endosc. 2006;20: 1435–9.

44. Kim DJ, Hyung WJ, Lee CY, Lee JG, Haam SJ, Park IK, et al. Thoracoscopic esophagectomy for esophageal cancer: feasibility and safety of robotic assistance in the prone position. J Thorac Cardiovasc Surg. 2010;139:53–9.

45. Gutt CN, Bintintan VV, Köninger J, Müller-Stich BP, Reiter M, Büchler MW. Robotic-assisted transhiatal esophagectomy. Langenbeck's Arch Surg. 2006;391:428–34.

46. Watson TJ. Robotic esophagectomy: is it an advance and what is the future? Ann Thorac Surg. 2008;85:757–9.

47. Suda K, Ishida Y, Kawamura Y, Inaba K, Kanaya S, Teramukai S, et al. Robot-assisted thoracoscopic lymphadenectomy along the left recurrent laryngeal nerve for esophageal squamous cell carcinoma in the prone position: technical report and short-term outcomes. World J Surg. 2012;36:1608–16.

48. Dunn DH, Johnson EM, Morphew JA, Dilworth HP, Krueger JL, Banerji N. Robot-assisted transhiatal esophagectomy: a 3-year single-center experience. Dis Esophagus. 2013;26:159–66.

49. Cerfolio RJ, Bryant AS, Hawn MT. Technical aspects and early results of robotic esophagectomy with chest anastomosis. J Thorac Cardiovasc Surg. 2013;145:90–6.

50. Choi YS, Shim JK, Na S, Hong SB, Hong YW, Oh YJ. Pressure-controlled versus volume-controlled ventilation during one-lung ventilation in the prone position for robot-assisted esophagectomy. Surg Endosc. 2009;23:2286–91.

51. Czibik G, D'Ancona G, Donias HW, Karamanoukian HL. Robotic cardiac surgery: present and future applications. J Cardiothorac Vasc Anesth. 2002;16:495–501.

52. Hubens G, Ruppert M, Balliu L, Vaneerdeweg W. What have we learnt after two years working with the da Vinci robot system in digestive surgery? Acta Chir Belg. 2004;104:609–14.

Anaesthesia for Combined Cardiac and Thoracic Procedures

40

Marcin Wąsowicz

Key Points

- From a physiologic point of view, alveolar-capillary membrane is the most important part of the respiratory system. It always undergoes micro-injury during cardiac surgery with the use of cardiopulmonary bypass. Therefore, a second insult, such as loss of part of the pulmonary parenchyma, can lead to acute lung injury and unfavourable outcomes from combined thoracic and cardiac procedures.
- Additional insult to the respiratory system can be caused by phrenic nerve injury subsequent diaphragmatic dysfunction and disturbances in chest wall mechanics caused by sternotomy or thoracotomy.
- Clinicians should be very selective in choosing to combine pulmonary resection and heart surgery. Concomitant pulmonary resection and cardiac surgery entail substantial additional risk, especially pulmonary complications and bleeding problems. These procedures should be performed in tertiary care centres with expertise in cardiac and thoracic surgery including use of extracorporeal life support systems.
- Anaesthetic management must be individualized and based on preoperative assessment, extent of surgery and need to use cardiopulmonary bypass. Anaesthesiologists managing these cases should have extensive training in both cardiac and thoracic anaesthesia. An expertise in transesophageal echocardiography is strongly recommended.

Introduction

Combined cardiac and thoracic procedures are rare; however thanks to progress of surgical techniques and recent advances in use of extracorporeal life support (ECLS) techniques the number of these procedures is increasing.

Anaesthesia and optimal perioperative management for these complex, high-risk surgical interventions requires an expertise in both cardiac and pulmonary physiologies, lung isolation techniques, the multiorgan impact of cardiopulmonary bypass (CPB) and additional monitoring techniques (e.g. transesophageal echocardiography-TEE). Combined procedures may include excision of invasive tumours, pulmonary endarterectomy, cardiac revascularization combined with lung resection and cardiac procedures combined with lung transplantation (e.g. PFO closure). Optimal management of these procedures remains controversial and is not well described; in fact it is mainly limited to case reports [1, 2]. Proponents of single-stage operations will argue in favour of the avoidance of a second surgery and anaesthetic and reduced hospital stay [2, 3]. The opponents will argue for divided, two-stage procedures on the basis of limiting surgical trauma, blood loss, multiorgan impact of cardiopulmonary bypass and high intensive care morbidity and thus may potentially confer a better long-term survival [3, 4].

The following chapter will briefly describe the anaesthetic management for various combined thoracic and cardiac procedures. For a better understanding of why CPB is detrimental for lung function, the author will briefly describe the structure and function of the air-blood barrier and pathophysiology of its injury during procedures with the use of CPB.

M. Wąsowicz (✉)
Department of Anesthesia and Pain Management, Toronto General Hospital, University Health Network and Department of Anesthesia University of Toronto, Toronto, ON, Canada

Cardiovascular Intensive Care Unit, Toronto General Hospital, Toronto, ON, Canada
e-mail: marcin.wasowicz@uhn.ca

Structure of the Alveolar-Capillary Barrier

The human lung consists of 300,000,000 alveoli. Each of them has a dense network of capillaries, which form air-blood barriers (alveolar-capillary membranes). From a phys-

© Springer Nature Switzerland AG 2019
P. Slinger (ed.), *Principles and Practice of Anesthesia for Thoracic Surgery*, https://doi.org/10.1007/978-3-030-00859-8_40

iological point of view, the air-blood barrier is the most important part of the respiratory system. It is the site of gas exchange. Additionally, the alveolar-capillary barrier separates the external environment from the pulmonary circulation, regulates transport of fluid and molecules from alveoli to capillaries and is a vital part of the natural defence mechanism of the human body (see also Chap. 7) [5].

Structure The alveolar-capillary barrier has three components: thin processes of type I pneumocytes (epithelial cells), endothelial cells and their common basement membranes (Fig. 40.1). Typically, endothelial and epithelial cells have separate basement membranes; but the pulmonary alveolus is a unique site where the basement membranes are fused together. This creates an extremely thin barrier (0.2–0.4 μm) enabling efficient exchange of oxygen and carbon dioxide [6, 7]. The processes of type I pneumocytes are very thin and

Fig. 40.1 (**a**) Picture presents a scheme of an air-blood barrier, which consists of endothelial cell, epithelial cell (type I pneumocyte) and their common basement membrane. Large cuboidal cell is type II pneumocyte producing surfactant contained within its cytoplasm as lamellar bodies (onion-like structures), which are exocytosed into the alveolar lumen and then transform into tubular myelin and finally monolayed of the surfactant covering the surface of type I pneumocytes. Left-hand side inset shows details of thin alveolar-capillary membrane; right-hand side inset shows a scheme on surfactant monolayer. (**b**) Electron microscope photograph which is showing an air-blood barrier

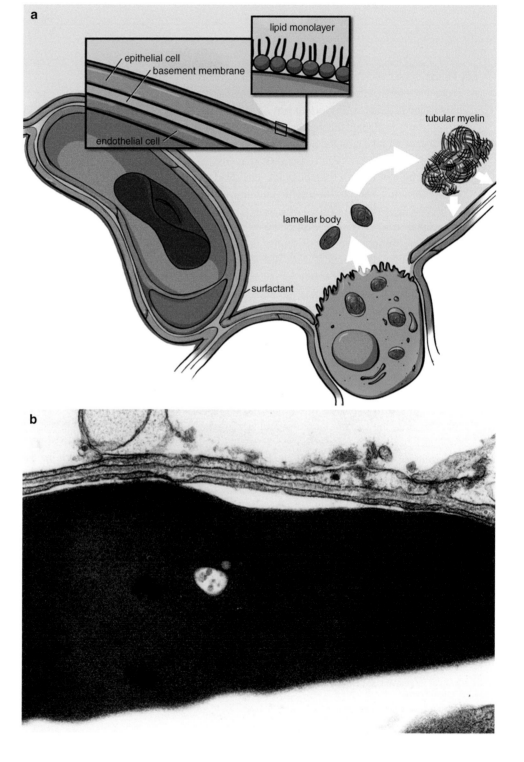

cover 95% of the alveolar surface. The remaining 5% is covered by type II pneumocytes, which produce surfactant. Type II pneumocytes (also called granular cells) reside within the "corners" of the alveoli because their large cellular structure makes them inefficient for gas exchange (Fig. 40.1). Type II pneumocytes eventually divide into type I pneumocytes (progenitor cells). During injury of the alveolar surface, the damaged type I pneumocytes are replaced by large, cubical, quickly dividing, type II pneumocytes. These large cuboidal cells create a thicker alveolar-capillary barrier leading to inefficient gas exchange.

Tight intercellular junctions between epithelial cells (pneumocytes) are impermeable to fluid, which contrasts with endothelial cell junctions which are highly permeable to fluids and allow the continuous exchange of plasma components between capillaries and the pulmonary interstitium. The common basement membrane consists of laminin, glycosaminoglycans, collagen type IV and fibronectin [6–8]. Glycosaminoglycans are concentrated on one side of basement membrane regulating its permeability. Among all the components of the alveolar-capillary barrier, this is the most critical part, and its injury leads to permanent damage of the blood-gas interface [9, 10]. There are three stabilizing elements of the alveolar-capillary barrier: surfactant, the pulmonary circulation and the connective tissue of the intra-alveolar septa [7, 11].

Surfactant Surfactant is composed from lipids (90%) and proteins (10%). The lipid component mainly consists of phosphatidylcholine (bipolar lipid) and phosphatidylglycerol [12]. Both lipids have a hydrophilic "head" and "lipophilic" tail (see Fig. 40.1a, right-hand inset]. Surfactant forms a monolayer lining the alveolar surface with the hydrophilic part directed towards the epithelial cells. The biochemical structure of the pulmonary surfactant resembles a detergent, surface-active layer, which aims to lower the surface tension and stabilizes the alveolar shape and structure. Surfactant protects the alveolus from collapse and prevents overdistension [13]. Moreover, surfactant acts as an anti-pulmonary oedema substance.

The protein component consists of four, distinct surfactant proteins – A, B, C and D (SP-A surfactant protein A, SP-B, SP-C and SP-D). These molecules play an important role in local defence mechanisms, surfactant metabolism, recirculation and spreading on the alveolar surface. Additionally they participate in local defence mechanisms. SP-A is a 28,000–36,000 kD protein and participates in monolayer formation and in recirculation of pulmonary surfactant. It has hydrophilic character. SP-D is the biggest surfactant protein (42,000 kD) and has also hydrophilic character, and its main role is to regulate local defence mech-

anisms. SP-B and SP-C are relatively small proteins (9.000 and 4.000 kD, respectively) with lipophilic character, and they are essential for monolayer formation [14]. Surfactant is produced in type II pneumocytes and is seen as so-called lamellar bodies (onion-like structures) (Fig. 40.2). Lamellar bodies are excreted into the alveolar lumen, transform into tubular myelin (Fig. 40.3) and then spread as a monolayer on the surface of type I pneumocytes (Fig. 40.1). The metabolism of surfactant is unique; it is recycled. Molecules of surface-active material are endocytosed back into type II pneumocytes and without any breakdown incorporated back into the lamellar bodies. Small amounts of surfactant (7–8%) are digested by alveolar macrophages. In the normal physiological situation, surfactant is not present within the pulmonary circulation (except for newborns when the lung is drying out after delivery). If surfactant is present within the pulmonary circulation, its amount reflects the extent of damage to the alveolar-capillary barrier [15, 16].

Pulmonary Circulation Flow through the pulmonary circulation equals the systemic flow enabling effective gas exchange. The pulmonary circulation also plays an important role in metabolic and filtrating functions of the lung. The pulmonary circulation is a low-pressure system, which is influenced by gravitation forces creating West's zones. The alveolar capillaries make contact with multiple alveoli,

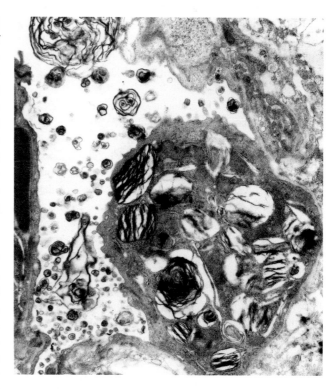

Fig. 40.2 Electron microscope photograph showing a type II pneumocyte filled with lamellar bodies (onion-like structures), some of them exocytosed into the lumen of the alveolar space

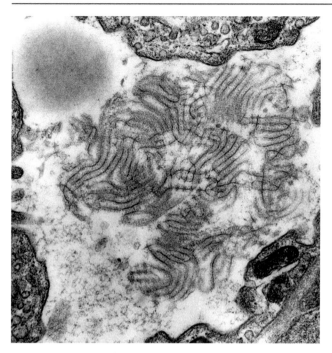

Fig. 40.3 Electron microscope picture, which presents structure of the tubular myelin

which increases the efficiency of gas exchange. The alveolar vessels are stabilized by a delicate network of collagen and elastic fibres, which form a continuum connected to basement membranes of the air-blood barriers. The location and structure of the alveolar capillaries make them susceptible to pressure changes occurring within the alveolar space. Rising intra-alveolar pressure will decrease the volume of the alveolar capillaries and increase their resistance.

Connective Tissue The connective tissue (mesenchyma) of the inter-alveolar septae is responsible for both their elasticity and mechanical resistance [11, 17]. The mesenchyma consists of the cellular and extracellular components. The cellular part is largely composed from fibroblasts, which are responsible for producing extracellular elements of the connective tissue, for example, collagen fibres, elastic fibres, fibronectin, entactin, glycosaminoglycans and components of the basement membranes [7]. The extracellular connective tissue forms a continuum extending from the hilum to each alveolus [18]. Thus any structural change within the lung tissue will have a transmitted effect upon every alveolus. This means that any change of shape within the lung affects every alveolus. Collagen fibres form the main mechanical support and restrictive force. This is counterbalanced by the presence of elastic fibres, which are responsible for the elastic recoil of lung parenchyma and its compliance. Collagen fibres are interwoven with elastic fibres, and both elements aid in stabilization of the alveolar-capillary membranes. During injury, the elastic fibres are more susceptible to damage,

which creates an imbalance in the resistive-elastic forces of the lung in favour of a stiffer lung with low compliance.

Lung Injury During Surgery with Use of Cardiopulmonary Bypass

Combined cardiac and thoracic surgical procedures with the use of CPB are controversial. If a cardiac procedure is performed with the use of CPB and is combined with thoracic surgery, which involves resection of lung parenchyma (lobectomy or pneumonectomy), respiratory complications may reach an incidence as high as 49% [19, 20]. It is postulated that CPB is the main causative factor of the aforementioned complications; therefore the most common injuries of the respiratory system caused by CPB will be briefly described in the following paragraphs [21–23].

Respiratory complications occurring after cardiac surgery with use of CPB are relatively common, but the vast majority are mild and self-limiting [24–26]. It is important to emphasize that the cause of lung failure after operations involving CPB is multifactorial [27, 28]; patient factors combine with the direct detrimental effects of CPB to compromise pulmonary function in the early postoperative period. A second insult to the respiratory system, such as loss of part of the pulmonary parenchyma, can be detrimental and lead to acute lung injury and unfavourable outcomes.

Prolonged mechanical ventilation after cardiac surgery occurs in about 6–7% of patients, and strongest predictors of this complication are previous cardiac surgery, lower left ventricular ejection fraction, shock, surgery involving repair of congenital heart disease and cardiopulmonary bypass time [26]. The most severe form of injury to the respiratory system – acute respiratory distress syndrome (ARDS) – occurs in 1–2% of cardiac cases with a very high mortality (40%) [10, 24].

Histological Injury Most patients who undergo cardiac surgery with the use of CPB present some degree of histological lung injury [30]. Microscopic observations reveal a range of injuries detected within the structures of the air-blood barriers [7, 8, 30, 31]. Mild injury presents as oedema of endothelial (type I pneumocytes) and epithelial cells. More severe forms cause denuding of the basement membranes with loss of epithelial lining (Fig. 40.4). In the most severe cases, basement membranes of alveolar-capillary membranes lose their continuity, which means they are permanently damaged. The alveoli with damaged basement membrane fill with fluid and lamellar bodies (surfactant) are not able to spread on the surface of epithelial cells. Beyond the damage visualized within the alveolar-capillary membranes, authors have observed congestion within alveolar capillaries and the accumulation of polynuclear leukocytes (neutrophils), many

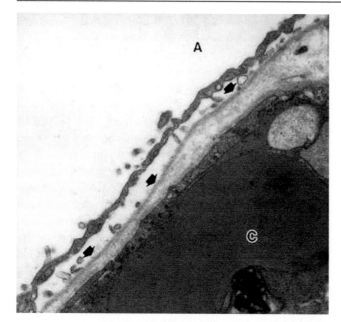

Fig. 40.4 Electron microscope photograph presenting a portion of alveolar-capillary barrier with partially "denuded" basement membrane (arrows). A, alveolar lumen; C, capillary lumen. (Permission for publication obtained from Taylor & Francis, from Ref. [29])

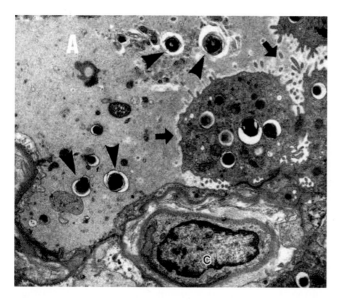

Fig. 40.5 Electron microscope photograph showing severe microscopic injury of air-blood barrier occurring post-CPB. Alveolar lumen is filled with oedema fluid, and surfactant structures (lamellar bodies-arrows' heads) are not able to spread. Arrows are indicating type II pneumocyte. (Permission for publication obtained from Taylor & Francis, From Ref. [29])

of which are extravasated (Fig. 40.5). Upon migrating from the intravascular space to the interstitium or alveolar space, neutrophils are able to survive for 6 h. Subsequent breakdown of neutrophils will exacerbate alveolar damage by releasing an abundance of proteolytic enzymes, reactive oxygen species and free radicals [29, 32]. In summary, in all

patients undergoing surgery utilizing CPB, some injury will occur within the pulmonary parenchyma [8, 30, 31].

Systemic Inflammatory Response Syndrome CPB causes a systemic inflammatory response syndrome (SIRS) [29, 32–35]. This leads to the activation of neutrophils, macrophages and multiple cytokines including complement and is commonly associated with free radical formation [32–37]. Complement proteins, mainly C3a and C5a, promote neutrophil activation, which can subsequently adhere to the endothelial cells and migrate into the interstitium promoting local damage and inflammation [36, 35]. The lung acts as a "filter" to activated neutrophils and therefore is often more vulnerable to CPB-related injury compared to other organs [24, 25]. In addition to the release of pro-inflammatory mediators and enzymes, activated neutrophils express surface receptors, CD11a and CD 18b, which facilitate further leukocyte-endothelial adhesion and chemotaxis. Those activated neutrophils, which remain within the lumen of the alveolar capillaries, tend to accumulate in congested blood vessels and release their contents causing "leakage" from alveolar capillaries to the extracellular spaces and alveolar lumen [29–31]. Neutrophils are not the only cells which are activated by an extracorporeal circuit. Macrophages also belong to the first line of cells which are stimulated by CPB [37]. They release multiple cytokines. The main cytokines involved in the inflammatory process and lung injury are interleukin 6 and 8. At the end of CPB, their concentration within the alveolar lining is much higher than within plasma [32, 33, 35].

Lipid Peroxidation Another line of activation caused by CPB is lipid peroxidation and release of free radicals [38]. They are mainly freed as a consequence of ischemia-reperfusion injury. It should be stressed that during aortic cross-clamp, the lung has no blood supply, except for a small amount of flow coming from the bronchial arteries. During reperfusion, large amounts of free radicals are flushed from ischemic lung tissue (as a result of xanthine oxidase activation) [16]. Free radicals have a high affinity for cellular membranes causing oxidation of lipid components (so-called peroxidation) [39, 40]. Free radicals also activate leukocytes [24].

Surgical Factors CPB is not the only cause of respiratory system dysfunction after cardiac surgery. Other common factors include:

- Changes in lung mechanics related to sternotomy, internal mammary artery harvesting and other surgical manipulations. These present as an increased elastance of the pulmonary tissue (decreased compliance). Decreased compliance is also caused by the injury caused by CPB, i.e. increased pulmonary vasculature permeability, positive fluid balance and accumulation of neutrophils [41].

- Atelectasis is a common postoperative complication after any major, prolonged surgery performed under general anaesthesia. Atelectasis occurs in up to 70% of patients undergoing cardiac surgery with or without the use of CPB [27, 41]. After cardiac surgery, atelectasis is observed most frequently in the left lower lobe and is considered the most common cause of an increased alveolar-arterial PO2 gradient [42, 43]. Atelectasis is also thought to be one of the main factors leading to further inflammatory injury leading to further deterioration in pulmonary function during the recovery phase after cardiac surgery. During the postoperative period, atelectasis is aggravated by pleural effusion(s) or pneumothorax, which may develop as a result of mechanical ventilation, central line cannulation or air leaks from surgical manipulations [9, 24, 27].
- Phrenic nerve injury leading to poor diaphragmatic function. The most common cause of phrenic nerve injury is the use of cold saline flush or ice slush as a method of additional cardiac preservation. Fortunately, most of the centres have abandoned this method of cardioprotection.
- Postoperative infections – pneumonia. All the aforementioned factors impairing pulmonary mechanics and ciliary clearance increase the risk of postoperative infections. Moreover, if a patient remains intubated for a prolonged period of time after any cardiac procedure, the risk of ventilator-associated pneumonia (VAP) increases to 44% (after 7 days of intubation) [41, 43]. Other significant risk factors for postoperative pulmonary infectious complications include cigarette smoking (a very common habit in patients undergoing combined cardiac and thoracic surgery) and the use of H_2 blockers [44].
- Massive transfusions of red blood cells and other blood products also contribute to respiratory dysfunction postoperatively [45, 46].

Prevention of Lung Injury After Cardiac Procedures

Although severe lung injury after CPB (ARDS) is uncommon (1–2%), other pulmonary complications remain a significant cause of mortality and morbidity after cardiac surgery [9, 25]. There are many patient-related risk factors, which contribute to postoperative pulmonary dysfunction, and some of them are modifiable. Among most important ones are smoking, obesity, COPD (see Chap. 2) and the use of proton-pump inhibitors [41, 43, 44]. Recently, we were also able to identify the intraoperative risk factors for prolonged mechanical surgery after surgery with the use of CPB [26]. At the same time prolonged mechanical ventilation might be detrimental to lung function aggravating injury to the remaining lung parenchyma.

There is little doubt that CPB is considered a "main culprit" of the pulmonary dysfunction occurring after cardiac surgery; however other factors also play an important role in their pathogenesis. Since the pathophysiology of respiratory complications following cardiac surgery has been extensively studied for the last 40 years, clinicians have developed multiple strategies to prevent them [24]. One of the most common approaches is the avoidance of CPB, which can be applied to coronary artery bypass surgeries [46]. On the other hand, currently available results are still inconclusive as to the true benefits of the off-pump CABG. Certainly, the new types of oxygenators (hollow fibre) and use of centrifugal pumps instead of roller pumps decrease activation of neutrophils and subsequent pulmonary dysfunction. The addition of leukoreduction filters which filter out activated polynuclear leucocytes has also been proven to have a beneficial effect [25, 27]. Similarly, a beneficial effect is observed with the use of heparin-coated circuits. Alternatively, some authors propose the use of the patient's lungs as a natural oxygenator (so-called Drew-Anderson technique) [47]. Even though it improves the function of the respiratory system after surgery, it increases the complexity of the surgical technique (additional cannulation sites) and makes it impractical for combined cardiothoracic procedures. It seems that a much easier approach would be to continue ventilation with small tidal volumes, PEEP and the use of air during the surgical procedure and use of the vital capacity manoeuvre just prior to discontinuation of CPB [48]. One of the oldest methods used in the cardiac surgery aiming to attenuate of detrimental effects of CPB (including pulmonary dysfunction) is use of corticosteroids [49]. Even though use of methylprednisolone decreased the release of inflammatory interleukins (IL-6 and IL-8) and complement activation, it has been frequently proven to work as a double-edged sword. While preventing pulmonary complications, it can be attributed to other significant postoperative problems (sternal wound infection, insulin resistance and abdominal complications).

Among the many methods aimed at prevention of respiratory complications, we should also mention strategies used during the postoperative period. They include use of low-tidal volume ventilation, active preventions of VAP (detailed discussion is beyond the scope of this chapter), early extubation whenever possible and aggressive physiotherapy and incentive spirometry. One of the keys to achieve the above-mentioned aims is to maintain effective pain control during the postoperative period.

In summary, the incidence of postoperative pulmonary complications occurring after cardiac surgery is high, and the incidence of prolonged mechanical ventilation is 6–7% [26, 43]. Most likely the incidence of prolonged mechanical ventilation is even higher after combined cardiothoracic procedures; however there is no data in the literature. Progress in their prevention and advance in surgical and anaesthetic techniques make most of them temporary. On the other hand, given that many patients currently undergoing cardiac surgery are older and suffering from many co-morbidities, this is probably the main reason for reluctance to perform combined cardiac and thoracic procedures. The main argument against combined procedures is that most of the patients suffer some degree of lung injury related to the use of CPB, and an additional insult to lung tissue caused by surgical resection might significantly increase mortality and morbidity [50, 51].

Surgical Considerations

Many thoracic surgeons are familiar with techniques of extracorporeal circulation. There are some thoracic procedures, which are routinely performed with use of CPB. Among the most common are lung transplantation and pulmonary endarterectomy; however recently most of the centres prefer the use of VA-ECMO over CPB. Since anaesthetic management during these procedures is discussed in different chapters of this textbook, they will not be further reviewed here (see Chaps. 47 and 49). The scope of the discussion in this section will concentrate on the perioperative management of patients with intrathoracic malignancies invading cardiac or major vascular structures and patients undergoing thoracic surgery who are suffering from coexisting coronary artery disease. Many surgeons are reluctant to perform one-stage cardiac-thoracic operation because of the concerns mentioned above [50–52]. Moreover, surgical access to the lung structures might be difficult if surgical incision and subsequent CPB cannulation are performed via median sternotomy. Additionally, there is anxiety regarding heparin use and the possibility of excessive bleeding. Apart from the injury to the respiratory system, a frightening consideration is the possibility of dissemination of pulmonary malignancy through the use of CPB [19, 52–54]. On the other hand, a one-stage combined procedure avoids the need for a second major thoracic surgery [3, 53, 54]. In the case of coexisting pulmonary malignancy and coronary artery disease, the answer seems to be straightforward [21, 50, 54, 55]. Preoperative revascularizations performed by interventional cardiologists (PCI – primary coronary intervention) may cause significant time delays for subsequent cancer surgery [56]. Thus, combined surgical coronary revascularization and resection of the lung cancer may be the optimal management. In most cases, revascularization can be performed without the use of CPB (off-pump coronary artery bypass grafting – OPCABG); therefore the detrimental effects of CPB can be avoided [21, 50, 54]. The results of these combined tho-

racic and cardiac surgeries are encouraging; however published results usually involve small number of patients [20, 21, 57–59].

When considering proper management of thoracic malignancies invading heart structures, it should be mentioned that surgical resection remains the only curative option for most intrathoracic malignancies [52, 53, 59, 60, 61]. Sometimes conventional thoracic surgical techniques do not allow complete resection of a pulmonary tumour which is invading the heart or large vessels; therefore radical surgical removal may necessitate the use of CPB [52]. The most common examples are tumours involving the left atrium and pulmonary artery or infiltrating the descending portion of the aorta [53, 58, 59].

Most of the procedures involving resection or opening of the heart structures are performed via median sternotomy. Surgical exposure to some of the hilar structures is more difficult when compared to a lateral thoracotomy approach. Left lower lobectomy and mediastinal lymph nodes dissection are especially technically challenging when performed via median sternotomy. Probably in most of the cases, mediastinoscopy or EBUS are is indicated initially to rule out mediastinal spread of the disease. All these concerns raise a question as to whether aggressive treatment including surgical resection of lung parenchyma and cardiac or major vascular structures should be a routine management. The answer is clearly no. This mode of treatment should be only performed in departments that are prepared for the complexity of those cases and can offer expertise in both cardiac and thoracic surgery, and anaesthesia, and postoperative ICU care for these patients. Moreover, the functional status of the patient prepared for this type of surgery should be excellent to allow them to survive a potential prolonged stay within an intensive care setting.

Anaesthetic Management for Combined Cardiac and Thoracic Procedures

The literature describing the anaesthetic management of the patient undergoing combined thoracic and cardiac procedures is very scarce and includes mainly case reports [1, 2, 62]. Subsequent paragraphs will try to summarize current information described as individual cases and the experience of the institution where the author practices cardiac and thoracic anaesthesia. The anaesthesiologist who is looking after the patient who is scheduled to undergo combined thoracic and cardiac surgery should possess an expertise in both cardiac and thoracic anaesthesia. Quite often these procedures are complex and require management by two consultants. For most of the cases, we also require the presence of perfusionist, who will be either actively involved with management of the case requiring the use of

CPB and ECLS or prepare the machine for extracorporeal circulation in a "standby" mode.

Preoperative Assessment

Apart from standard preoperative evaluations before surgery, the anaesthesiologist preparing the patient for combined cardiac and thoracic procedure must perform a detailed assessment of the respiratory and cardiovascular systems. An extensive description of respiratory system evaluation is described elsewhere in this monograph (see Chap. 2). Briefly, the anaesthesiologist who is assessing the pulmonary function should concentrate on lung mechanics, pulmonary parenchymal function and cardiorespiratory reserve. The most popular test performed to assess lung mechanics is spirometry. The value most commonly used by anaesthesiologists is the forced expiratory volume in 1 s (FEV1). FEV1 is also used to calculate the predicted postoperative FEV1 (ppo-FEV1) once part of the pulmonary parenchyma is resected. Values below 30–35% for ppo-FEV1 are considered as predictors of increased risk of respiratory complications and prolonged weaning from mechanical ventilation. Maximal oxygen consumption is used to assess cardiopulmonary reserve, and diffusing capacity of carbon monoxide is measured to estimate the gas exchange function of lung parenchyma. Any patient being prepared for a combined procedure requires a very careful airway evaluation. Intrathoracic malignancies necessitating these types of procedures often result in airway involvement, causing deviation or invasion of large airways. Moreover, they can infiltrate or compress large vascular structures. Apart from clinical symptoms, the anaesthesiologist must examine the results of computed tomography (CT) scans, which show precisely the extent of the disease and possible vascular involvement. A preoperative echocardiogram will be complimentary to the radiological examination and should routinely be performed before any cardiac surgical procedure. In the context of pulmonary resection, we should pay particular attention to the function of the right ventricle and value of right ventricular systolic pressure reflecting on pressure in pulmonary circulation.

The "second leg" of preoperative evaluation focuses on the status of the cardiovascular system. The mortality and morbidity of cardiac surgical patients are strongly influenced by their preoperative severity of the illness. The important factors included in most preoperative risk assessment scores include age, sex, left ventricular function, type of surgery, urgency of the surgery, redo cardiac surgery, unstable angina, congestive heart failure, history of peripheral vascular disease and cerebral vascular disease, renal insufficiency and history of diabetes. In most cases, this information can be obtained from the medical history, physical examination and simple laboratory findings including electro- and echocardiogram. Additionally, results of echocardiography provide a detailed description of valve structure and pathology, contractility of the left and right ventricle and morphology of most of the large vessels. In the case of poor ventricular function (ejection fraction <30%), it is recommended to consider an alternative therapeutic approach rather than combined cardiac-thoracic surgery. If the patient suffers from coronary artery disease, the degree of coronary stenosis (es) is assessed preoperatively by cardiac catheterization (coronary angiogram). This information is important for the anaesthesiologist who will be intraoperatively assessing the contractility of the particular segments of the myocardium with the use of transesophageal echocardiography (TEE).

Patients who are scheduled to undergo combined cardiac-thoracic surgery frequently suffer from multiple co-morbidities. Among the most significant, we should mention peripheral vascular disease, diabetes mellitus and kidney dysfunction. Most of these co-morbidities are aggravated during the perioperative period, and this in turn is what significantly increases mortality and morbidity. The anaesthesiologist must collect a detailed list of which medications the patient is currently taking.

Anaesthetic Management

The anaesthesiologist providing care during combined cardiac-thoracic procedures faces multiple challenges. Quite often she/he must simultaneously manage haemodynamic instability, hypoxemia, problems with ventilation and excessive bleeding. It is beyond the scope of this chapter to fully discuss all of the challenges of cardiac anaesthesia, and most of the topics related to thoracic anaesthesia are presented elsewhere in this textbook. Therefore, the author will discuss only the most important problems occurring during combined thoracic and cardiac procedures.

1. Airway management. If pulmonary resection is performed before or after CPB, the patient will require lung isolation. Detailed techniques and methods of choice are discussed in Chap. 16. The position of a double lumen tube or bronchial blocker should be always verified with a fibre-optic bronchoscope. If resection of pulmonary parenchyma is to be performed during CPB, the patient can be intubated with standard, single-lumen tube.
2. Management of hypoxemia during one lung ventilation is discussed in Chap. 6.
3. Transesophageal echocardiography (see Chap. 20). The use of TEE is one of the key components of intraoperative anaesthetic management of patients undergoing com-

bined cardiac and thoracic procedures. The important information obtained from intraoperative TEE during combined cardiac and thoracic procedures includes assessment of left and right ventricular function (especially important after pneumonectomy), diagnosis of new wall-motion abnormalities (coronary artery bypass surgery), evaluation of effects of valve repair/replacement and extension of the disease (e.g. lung tumour invading left atrium or pulmonary vein).

4. Pulmonary artery catheter (PAC). TEE is an excellent diagnostic tool, but at current stage, its use is limited to this role. It does not allow for continuous monitoring of haemodynamic status particularly RV function and afterload for RV. Therefore, PAC is very useful in management of combined cardiac and thoracic procedures particularly during postoperative period. It allows to monitor cardiac output (read function of RV), pulmonary pressures and their changes as response to therapy and certain physiological phenomena and provides warning of RV dysfunction (high CVP, low PAD pressures or presence of square root sign in case we have RV channel in our PA line). During surgery anesthesiologist must remember to ask surgeon to palpate catheter before PA or its branch is being clamped in case pulmonary resection is being performed. If necessary PA must be pulled back prior to resection.

5. The anaesthesiologist and extracorporeal techniques (cardiopulmonary bypass, CPB, and extracorporeal lung support, ECLS). CPB has three main functions during cardiac procedures: (1) replacing function of the heart (circulation of the blood), (2) replacing function of the lungs (oxygenation and CO_2 removal) and (3) diversion of the blood from the operating field to create optimal surgical conditions. To achieve these purposes, superior and inferior vena cavae are cannulated, and the blood is passively drained into the CPB venous reservoir. The blood is then oxygenated and returned back to the patient via an aortic cannula usually placed in the distal part of the ascending aorta. In the case of combined thoracic-vascular surgery including the resection of the tumour invading the descending aorta, one can use partial bypass, which diverts some of the blood from the left atrium and returns it back to one of the femoral arteries. Since the primary function of CPB is to oxygenate blood and perfuse the vital organs, an important question for the anaesthesiologist is what perfusion/oxygenation is optimal? Even though it has been over 50 years since the first human use of extracorporeal circulation, there is no definite answer. Blood is exposed multiple times to the foreign surface of the extracorporeal circuit causing SIRS and microembolization, which can affect every organ of the human body. Apart from lung injury, CPB can contribute to cognitive

dysfunction, renal injury or failure, pancreatitis or, in the worst-case scenario, multiorgan dysfunction. It is the anaesthesiologist's role to prevent or minimize these complications. Due to advancement in development of extracorporeal techniques and better availability of ECLS perfusion in some cases, venoarterial ECMO might be used instead of full CPB. It allows for using relatively small doses of heparin (typically ACT is between 140–200 s), and subsequently it leads to less significant disturbances in coagulation. On the other hand, ECLS can still cause systemic inflammatory reaction and subsequent vasoplegia. When ECLS is used, we must remember that it is entirely a closed system, which does not allow perfusionist to add any volume. When used in venoarterial configuration, it allows to offload the heart; however it does not allow full circulatory arrest.

6. The anaesthetic approach to combined procedures performed without the use of CPB. Off-pump coronary artery grafting (OPCABG) is the preferred surgical management of coronary artery disease in patients who require pulmonary resection at the same time as coronary revascularization [21, 54, 56]. Revascularization is usually performed as the first part of the procedure followed by the resection of the pulmonary pathology. The most important principles of anaesthetic management for OPCABG include aggressive maintenance of normothermia to prevent bleeding and/or acidosis and preservation of haemodynamic stability during surgical manipulation of the heart. The first aim is achieved by use of warm blankets, body warmers, fluid warmers and adjustment of the room temperature in the operating theatre. Maintaining haemodynamic stability is crucial for ultimate success of the procedure; thus it requires ideal communication and cooperation between the surgeon and the anaesthesiologist. It is accomplished by a combination of inotropic support, proper volume therapy (quite often achieved by "deep" Trendelenburg position) and antiarrhythmic prophylaxis. The surgeon should use gentle manipulations (e.g. incision of right pleura to avoid compression of the heart) and devices (e.g. Starfish™, Medtronic International Ltd., Minneapolis, MN or intracoronary shunts) in order to preserve the geometry of the heart ventricles and their contractility, and prevent mitral regurgitation.

7. Haemodynamic support, right ventricular failure. Cardiothoracic anaesthesiologist must be familiar with all forms of circulatory support to provide haemodynamic stability during and after surgery. It can be achieved by optimization of pre- and after load, maintaining or improving contractility and preservation of a stable sinus rhythm. The most worrisome haemodynamic problem complicating combined cardiac-thoracic procedures is

right ventricular dysfunction or failure. It is commonly caused by a rapid increase in the afterload (pressure) for the right side of the heart, especially after major resection of the pulmonary parenchyma (e.g. pneumonectomy). The warning symptoms include right ventricular distension visualized directly by the surgeon and the anaesthesiologist, a low cardiac output state and a central venous pressure (CVP) higher than the pulmonary diastolic pressure (PAD). If we are monitoring RV pressure, the analysis of pressure tracing might show characteristic square root sign warning anaesthesiologist about RV dysfunction.

The treatment includes:

- Reduction of RV preload (e.g. promotion of diuresis with diuretics) or early introduction of renal replacement therapy if there is no response to diuretics.
- Manoeuvres to decrease the pressure in the pulmonary circulation – hyperventilation, hyperoxia and pharmacological support. Among the intravenous agents, which decrease afterload for the RV and improve its contractility, the first choices are dobutamine and milrinone. Inhalational pulmonary vasodilators (nitric oxide or prostacyclin) are used when a lack of response to intravenous agents occurs.
- Preservation of good perfusion pressure to the right ventricle and ventricular interdependence (norepinephrine or vasopressin) and/or the use of an intra-aortic balloon pump.
- Since stroke volume is usually fixed in RV dysfunction or failure and in order to increase the cardiac output, it is recommended to increase heart rate (e.g. A-V pacing).

8. Treatment of coagulopathy. Combined cardiothoracic procedures performed with the use of CPB are frequently complicated by excessive bleeding, which can have two possible causes: surgical (extensive surgery) and coagulopathy related to prolonged CPB. In cases of surgical resection of pulmonary parenchyma combined with a cardiac procedure, CPB duration often exceeds 2 h. Duration of CPB directly correlates with the magnitude of coagulopathy. There are multiple mechanisms of excessive, non-surgical bleeding caused by extracorporeal circulation; among the most important are the dilutional effect, SIRS, platelet consumption, depleted amount of clotting factors, secondary fibrinolysis, low haemoglobin and hypothermia. Treatment is based on the results of laboratory tests (INR, aPTT, fibrinogen level and platelet count) or use of point-of-care devices. Currently many tertiary care centres use them routinely; its application delivers quick assessment of coagulation status based on results obtained from a whole-blood sample. Among the most popular ones are thromboelas-

tography (TEG) and thromboelastometry (ROTEM). In the context of high likelihood of massive bleeding and coagulopathy in our institution, for most of the combined cardiac-thoracic cases, we secure at least two, large-bore venous catheters to be able to transfuse large volumes of blood products in a relatively short period of time. In most of these cases, we use routinely infusion of tranexamic acid as an antifibrinolytic agent. We follow protocol proposed by Dowd and Karski; however infusion rate should be modified (decreased) in patients with kidney dysfunction or failure [63–65].

Summary

There is no complete agreement about the optimal surgical management of patients who are suffering from both cardiac and thoracic diseases requiring surgery [1, 2, 52, 62]. The arguments for one-stage procedures are avoidance of a second surgery/anaesthetic and reduced hospital stay and cost. However, two-stage procedures may be associated with less surgical trauma and blood loss and may offer better long-term survival because the consequences of cardiopulmonary bypass (CPB) are minimized.

Combined cardiac-thoracic procedures should be performed only for selected cases in specialized centres, which pose an expertise in both cardiac and thoracic anaesthesia and surgeries. This chapter briefly describes the important perioperative considerations and management. Since there is minimal literature describing the anaesthetic management for combined cardiac-thoracic procedures, the a forementioned recommendations are based on the experience and clinical practice developed in the institution where author works.

Case Presentation

Case A 21-year-old patient admitted for redo cardiac surgery for resection of recurrent left atrial angiosarcoma invading pulmonary tissue which was demonstrated on a recent follow-up chest X-ray and CT scan (see Figs. 40.6 and 40.7). The proposed procedure will also involve resection of pulmonary parenchyma. His previous surgery was performed 3 years ago without complications and followed by multiple courses of chemotherapy. He has no other significant co-morbidities. Anaesthesiologist is asked to decide whether patient is going to tolerate combined cardiac-thoracic procedure and what additional test he would like to perform.

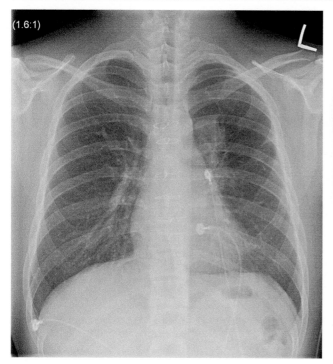

Fig. 40.6 Chest X-ray taken before surgery

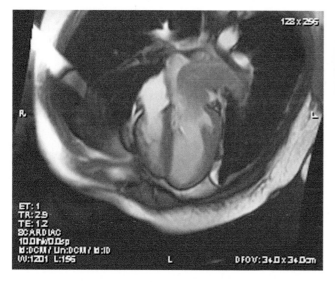

Fig. 40.7 Computed tomogram showing invasion of the tumour obtained before surgery

Questions

- What additional tests would you order?
- Will the patient tolerate procedure? What kind of thoracic procedure will the patient require to achieve complete eradication of his tumour?

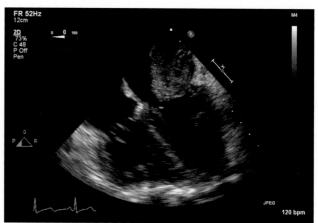

Fig. 40.8 Picture obtained during intraoperative, transesophageal examination. Mid-esophageal, four-chamber view

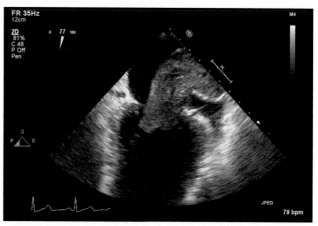

Fig. 40.9 Picture obtained during intraoperative, transesophageal examination. Mid-esophageal, two-chamber view

- What is your anaesthetic plan?
- Do you have any specific concerns related to intraoperative management?
- What kind of postoperative complications can you expect?

Picture presents intraoperative transesophageal echo findings (Figs. 40.8 and 40.9).

Questions

- What cardiac procedure should be performed?
- Which pulmonary veins are invaded?
- What postoperative complications would you expect?

References

1. Marseu K, Minkovich L, Zubrinic M, Keshavjee S. Anesthetic considerations for pneumonectomy with left atrial resection on cardiopulmonary bypass in a patient with lung Cancer: a case report. A A Case Rep. 2017;8:61–3.

2. Slinger PD, Chang DCH, David TE, editors. Perioperative Care in Cardiac Anesthesia and Surgery. Philadelphia/Baltimore/New York/London/Buenos Aires/Homg Kong/Sydney/Tokyo: Lippincott, Williams&Wilkins; 2006. p. 43–8.

3. Rao V, Todd TRJ, Weisel RD, et al. Results of combined pulmonary resection and cardiac operation. Ann Thorac Surg. 1996;62:342–7.

4. Ciracio P, Carretta A, Calori G, Mazzone P, Zannini P. Lung resection for cancer in patients with coronary artery disease: analysis of short term results. Eur J Cardiothorac Surg. 2002;22:35–40.

5. Wąsowicz M, Biczysko W, Marszałek A, Yokoyama S, Nakayama I. Ultrastructural studies on selected elements of the extra cellular matrix in the developing rat lung alveolus. Folia Histochem Cytobiol. 1998;36:3–13.

6. Wąsowicz M, Kashima K, Yokoyama S, Nakayama I. Pulmonary surfactant migrates into the alveolar capillaries of newborn rats an immunoelectron microscopic study. Acta Anat. 1996;156:11–21.

7. Wąsowicz M. Biczysko W. In: Andres J, Wąsowicz M, editors. Selected problems of anesthesia and critical care in cardiovascular surgery. Kraków: Danbert; 2002. p. 174–89.

8. Wąsowicz M, Drwiła R, Biczysko W, Marszałek A, Florek E, Andres J. Effects of exogenous surfactant on alveolar barrier. An experimental study. Anaesth Inten Ther. 2002;34:76–80.

9. Wąsowicz M, Sobczyński P, Szulc R, Biczysko W. Ultrastructural changes in the lung alveoli after cardiac surgical operations with the use of cardiopulmonary bypass (CPB). Pol J Pathol. 1999;50:189–96.

10. Ng CSH, Wan S, Yim APC, Arifi AA. Pulmonary dysfunction after cardiac surgery. Chest. 2002;121:1269–77.

11. Biczysko W, Wąsowicz M, Marszałek A. Stromal compartment in the developing lung's alveoli- an electron microscopic study. Clin Perinat Gynaecol. 1994;6:107–19.

12. Wąsowicz M, Biczysko W, Sobczyński P. Structure and activity of pulmonary surfactant and their implications for intensive therapy. Inten Care Emerg Med. 1998;1:35–44.

13. Biczysko W, Wąsowicz M, Metzner J, Marszałek A. In: Drobnik L, Jurczyk W, editors. Problems of anesthesiology and intensive therapy. Warszawa: Wydawnictwo Lekarskie PZWL; 1998. p. 96–109.

14. Biczysko W, Marszałek A, Wąsowicz M. Maturation of lung epithelia in transmission electron microscopic study. Clin Perinat Gynaecol. 1993;3:3–23.

15. Doyle I, Nicholas TE, Bernste AD. Serum surfactant protein a levels in patients with acute cardiogenic pulmonary edema and adult respiratory distress syndrome. Am J Respir Crit Care Med. 1995;152:307–17.

16. Sobczyński P, Wąsowicz M. In: Zapalski S, Checinski P, editors. Clinical aspects of lung reperfusion. Clinical aspects of ischemia and reperfusion. Bielsko Biała: Alfa Medica Press; 1997. p. 79–89.

17. Wąsowicz M, Yokoyama S, Kashima K, Nakayama I. The connective tissue compartment in the terminal region of the developing rat lung. Acta Anat. 1996;156:268–82.

18. Biczysko W, Wąsowicz M, Marszałek A, Florek E. Why do the lungs of premature newborns function improperly? A morphological study of the connective tissue and vascular compartments in the developing lung. Arch Perinat Med. 1999;5:19–26.

19. Danton MHD, Anikin VA, McManus KG, McGuigan JA, Campalani G. Simultaneous cardiac surgery with pulmonary resection: presentation of series and review of literature. Eur J Cardiothorac Surg. 1998;13:667–72.

20. Wiebe K, Baraki H, Macchiarini M, Haverich A. Extended pulmonary resections of advanced thoracic malignancies with support of cardiopulmonary bypass. Eur J Cardiothorac Surg. 2006;29:571–8.

21. Dyszkiewicz W, Jemielity M, Piwkowski C, et al. The early and late results of combined off-pump coronary artery bypass grafting and pulmonary resection in patients with concomitant lung cancer and unstable coronary heart disease. Eur J Cardiothorac Surg. 2008;34:531–5.

22. Spaggiari L, D'Aiuto M, Veronesi G, et al. Extended pneumonectomy with partial resection of the left atrium, without cardiopulmonary bypass for lung cancer. Ann Thorac Surg. 2005;79:234–40.

23. Voets AJ, Sheik Joesoef K, van Teeffelen MEJM. Synchronously occurring lung cancer (stages I-II) and coronary artery disease: concomitant versus staged surgical approach. Eur J Cardiothorac Surg. 1997;12:713–7.

24. Wąsowicz M. In: Andres J, Wąsowicz M, editors. Selected problems of anesthesia and critical care in cardiovascular surgery. Kraków: Danbert; 2002. p. 191–207.

25. Clark SC. Lung injury after cardiopulmonary bypass. Perfusion. 2006;21:225–8.

26. Sharma V, Rao V, Manlhiot C, Boruvka A, Fremes S, Wąsowicz M. A derived and validated score to predict prolonged mechanical ventilation in patients undergoing cardiac surgery. J Thorac Cardiovasc Surg. 2017;153:108–15.

27. Weissman C. Pulmonary complications after cardiac surgery. Semin Cardiothorac Vasc Anesth. 2004;8:185–211.

28. Picone AL, Lutz CJ, Finck C, et al. Multiple sequential insults cause post-pump syndrome. Ann Thorac Surg. 1999;67:978–85.

29. Tonz M, Milhajevic T, Von Segesser LK. Acute lung injury during cardiopulmonary bypass. Are the neutrophils responsible? Chest. 1995;198:1551–6.

30. Wąsowicz M, Drwiła R, Sobczyński P, Przybyłowski P, Dziatkowiak A. Lung alveolar damage during coronary artery bypass grafting with use of cardiopulmonary-bypass: and old nemesis? Br J Anaesth. 2000;84(supp 1):18.

31. Wąsowicz M, Sobczyński P, Drwiła R, Biczysko W, Marszałek A, Andres J. Air-blood barrier injury during cardiac operations with the use of cardiopulmonary bypass (CPB). An old story? Scand Cardiovasc J. 2003;37:216–21.

32. Kotani N, Hashimoto H, Sessler DI, et al. Neutrophil number and interleukin-8 and elastase concentration in bronchoalveolar lavage fluid correlate with decreased arterial oxygenation after cardiopulmonary bypass. Anesth Analg. 2000;90:1046–51.

33. Kotani N, Hashimoto H, Sessler DI, et al. Cardiopulmonary bypass produces greater pulmonary than systemic proinflammatory cytokines. Anesth Analg. 2000;90:1039–45.

34. Sinclair DG, Haslam PL, Quinlan GL, Pepper JR, Evans TW. The effects of cardiopulmonary bypass on interstitial and pulmonary endothelial permeability. Chest. 1995;108:718–24.

35. Kawamura T, Wakusawa R, Okada K, Inada S. Elevation of cytokines during open heart surgery with cardiopulmonary bypass: participation of interleukin 8 and 6 in reperfusion injury. Can J Anesth. 1993;40:1016–21.

36. Chenoweth DE, Cooper SW, Hugli TE, et al. Complement activation during cardiopulmonary bypass. Evidence for generation C3a and C5a anaphylatoxins. N Engl J Med. 1981;304:497–503.

37. Warner AE. Pulmonary intravascular macrophages. Role in acute lung injury. Clin Cest Med. 1996;17:125–35.

38. Royston D, Fleming JS, Desai JB, et al. Increased production of peroxidation products associated with cardiac operations. Evidence for free radical generation. J Thorac Cardiovasc Surg. 1986;91:75–766.

39. Wąsowicz M, Drwiła R, Jeleń H, Przybyłowski P, Andres J, Dziatkowiak A. Lipid peroxidation (LO) during cardiac operations with use of cardiopulmonary bypass measured by headspace chromatography. Eur J Anaesthesiol. 2001;18(supp. 22):19.

40. Wąsowicz M, Drwiła R, Jeleń H, Przybyłowski P, Andres J, Dziatkowiak A. Lipid peroxidation (LO) during cardiac operations with use of cardiopulmonary bypass measured by headspace chromatography. Eur J Anaesthesiol. 2001;18(supp. 22):19.

41. Rady MY, Ryan T, Star NY. Early onset of acute pulmonary dysfunction after cardiovascular surgery; risk factors and clinical outcomes. Crit Care Med. 1997;25:1831–9.

42. Magnusson L, Zemgulis V, Wicky ZS, Tyden H, Thelin S, et al. Atelectasis is a major cause of hypoxemia and shunt after cardiopulmonary bypass. Anethesiology. 1997;87:1153–63.

43. Bouza E, Perez A, Munoz P, et al. Ventilator-associated pneumonia after heart surgery: a prospective analysis and the value of surveillance. Crit Care Med. 2003;31:1964–70.

44. Gaynes R, Bizek B, Movry-Hanley J, et al. Risk factors for nosocomial pneumonia after coronary artery bypass operations. Ann Thorac Surg. 1991;51:215–8.

45. Karkouti K, Wijeysundera DN, Yau TM, et al. The independent association of massive blood loss with mortality in cardiac surgery. Transfusion. 2004;44:1453–62.

46. Taggard DP. Respiratory dysfunction after cardiac surgery: effect of avoiding cardiopulmonary bypass and the use of bilateral internal mammary artery. Eur J Cardiovasc Surg. 2000;18:31–7.

47. Richter JA, Meisner H, Tassani P, et al. Drew-Anderson technique attenuates systemic inflammatory response syndrome and improves respiratory function after coronary artery bypass grafting. Ann Thorac Surg. 2000;69:7783.

48. Minkovich L, Djaiani G, Katznelson R, et al. Effects of alveolar recruitment on arterial oxygenation in patients after cardiac surgery: a prospective, randomized, controlled clinical trial. J Cardiothorac Vasc Anesth. 2007;21:375–8.

49. Tassani P, Richter P, Barankay A, et al. Does high-dose methylprednisolone in aprotinin-treated patients attenuates the systemic inflammatory response during coronary artery bypass grafting procedures? J Cardiothorac Vasc Anesth. 1999;13:165–72.

50. Saxena P, Tam RKW. Combined off-pump coronary artery bypass surgery and pulmonary resection. Ann Thorac Surg. 2004;78:498–501.

51. Ng CSH, Arifi AA, Wan S, Wai S, Lee TW, Yim APC. Cardiac operation with associated pulmonary resection: a word of caution. Asian Cardiovasc Thorac J. 2002;10:362–4.

52. Klepetko W. Surgical intervention for T4 lung cancer with infiltration of the thoracic aorta: are we back to the archetype of surgical thinking? J Thorac Cardiovasc Surg. 2005;129:727–9.

53. De Perrot M, Fadel ZE, Mussot S, de Palma A, Chapelier A, Dartevelle P. Resection of locally advanced (T4) non-small cell lung cancer with cardiopulmonary bypass. Ann Thorac Surg. 2005;79:1691–7.

54. Dyszkiewicz W, Jemielity MM, Piwkowski CT, Perek B, Kasprzyk M. Simultaneous lung resection for cancer and myocardial revascularization without cardiopulmonary bypass (off-pump coronary artery bypass grafting). Ann Thorac Surg. 2004;77:1023–7.

55. Mariani M, vn Boven W, Duurkens VAM, et al. Combined off-pump coronary surgery and right lung resections through midline sternotomy. Ann Thorac Surg. 2001;71:1342–4.

56. Marcucci C, Chassot P-G, Gardaz J-P, Magnusson L, et al. Fatal myocardial infarction after lung resection in a patient with prophylactic preoperative coronary stenting. Br J Anaesth. 2004;92:743–7.

57. Shudo Y, Takahashi T, Ohta M, et al. Radical operation for invasive thymoma with intracaval, intracardiac and lung invasion. J Card Surg. 2007;22:330–2.

58. Nakajima J, Morota T, Matsumoto J, et al. Pulmonary intimal sarcoma treated by a left pneumonectomy with pulmonary arterioplasty under cardiopulmonary bypass: report of case. Surg Today. 2007;37:496–9.

59. Venuta F, Ciccone AM, Anile M, et al. Reconstruction of the pulmonary artery for lung cancer: long-term results. J Thorac Cardiovasc Surg. 2009;138:1185–91.

60. Ratto GB, Costa R, Vassallo G, et al. Twelve-year experience with left atrial resection in the treatment of non-small cell lung cancer. Ann Thorac Surg. 2004;78:234–7.

61. Francesca L, Frazier OH, Radovancevic B, De Caro LF, Reul GJ, Cooley DA. Concomitant cardiac and pulmonary operations for lung cancer. Tex Heart Inst J. 1995;22:296–300.

62. Lennon PF, Hartigan PM, Friedberg JS. Clinical management of patients undergoing concurrent cardiac surgery and pulmonary resection. J Cardiothorac Vac Anesth. 1998;12:587–90.

63. Dowd NP, Karski JM, Cheng DC, Carroll JA, Lin Y, James RL, Butterworth J. Pharmacokinetics of tranexamic acid during cardiopulmonary bypass. Anesthesiology. 2002;97(2):390–9.

64. Sharma V, Fan J, Jerath A, Pang KS, Bojko B, Pawliszyn J, Karski JM, Yau T, McCluskey S, Wąsowicz M. Pharmacokinetics of tranexamic acid in patients undergoing cardiac surgery with use of cardiopulmonary bypass. Anaesthesia. 2012 Nov 1;67(11):1242–50.

65. Jearth A, Yang JQ, Pang KS, Lobby N, Vasicic T, Reyes N, Bojko B, PAwliszyn J, Wijeysundera D, Beattie WS, Wąsowicz M. Tranexamic acid dosing for cardiac surgical patients with chronic renal dysfunction: a new dosing regimen. Anesth Analg. 2018.; published ahead of print

Open Thoracoabdominal Aortic Aneurysm Repair

41

Helen A. Lindsay, Coimbatore Srinivas, and Maral Ouzounian

Key Points

- Open thoracoabdominal aortic surgery is high risk, with placement of an aortic cross-clamp resulting in significant physiological derangements. The main complications include respiratory failure, renal failure, paraplegia, stroke, and major cardiac complications.
- The anesthetic technique is demanding and requires a high level of expertise, including proficiencies in managing one-lung ventilation, massive blood loss, coagulopathy, and cerebrospinal fluid drains.
- To prevent spinal cord ischemia, different techniques may be used to achieve the same physiological goal of maintaining spinal cord perfusion pressure. Techniques to prevent and minimize spinal cord ischemia primarily focus on maximizing collateral flow by supporting mean arterial pressure and reducing cerebrospinal fluid pressure while prolonging ischemic tolerance and reducing reperfusion injury with hypothermia and pharmacotherapy.
- The mainstay interventions to prevent renal injury include avoidance of nephrotoxic insults and selective cold renal perfusion.
- There is an increasing shift to recognize the importance of consensus definitions, standards for reporting outcomes, and coordinated multicentered trials in order to improve the quality of evidence necessary for guideline development.

H. A. Lindsay
Department of Anesthesia & Perioperative Medicine, Auckland City Hospital, Auckland, New Zealand

C. Srinivas (✉)
Department of Anesthesia, Toronto General Hospital, Toronto, ON, Canada
e-mail: coimbatore.srinivas@uhn.ca

M. Ouzounian
Division of Cardiovascular Surgery, Department of Surgery, Toronto General Hospital, Toronto, ON, Canada

Introduction

The aorta and arterial system is an essential component of the cardiovascular system, providing oxygen and other essential elements to tissues and cells for aerobic metabolism. This is critical to preserving end-organ function and preventing ischemic injury. Repair of a thoracoabdominal aortic aneurysm (TAAA) is among the most challenging cases for an anesthesiologist. A demanding anesthetic plan comprises of many elements to contend with the significant physiological derangements that occur during the case. Additionally, despite improvements in surgical technique, the potential for significant morbidity and mortality remains [1]. A high level of expertise and an exacting level of care from all members of the perioperative team have been shown to have a significant impact on outcomes [2, 3].

Diseases of the aorta are many and varied [4, 5]: from acute aortic syndromes including aortic dissection or traumatic injuries that are an immediate threat to life requiring emergent repair to progressive, often asymptomatic aneurysmal disease that prompts elective repair to prevent progression to acute rupture. Disease not only develops in the elderly due to degenerative and atherosclerotic disease related to smoking and hypertension risk factors but also the young with various genetic aortopathies such as Marfan syndrome. Clearly the associated comorbidities anticipated in these different subgroups are unique and the management plan should reflect this variability. A full discussion of the diagnostic guidelines and indications for surgical correction of various types of aortic disease is beyond the scope of this chapter. Additionally, this chapter outlines the management for elective TAAA surgery. While many details discussed are equally relevant to the emergent case, the feasibility of implementation will need to be considered.

Clinicians have recognized the risk of spinal cord injury (SCI) since the inception of surgical repair of TAAAs in the 1950s [6]. Lower extremity neurological deficit may be temporary or permanent and range from minor deficits to

© Springer Nature Switzerland AG 2019
P. Slinger (ed.), *Principles and Practice of Anesthesia for Thoracic Surgery*, https://doi.org/10.1007/978-3-030-00859-8_41

paralysis. The reported incidence of SCI after open TAAA procedures varies widely from 0% to 44% [7, 8]. A general decline in rates to 6–8% has been described since the turn of the century [5], potentially because of more routine employment of protective adjuncts [7, 9]. More recently, a permanent paraplegia and paraparesis rate of 2.9% and 2.4%, respectively, was reported in the largest published single-center experience of open TAAA repair [10]. All the same, when permanent paralysis does occur, it has a devastating impact on a patient's quality of life [11] and long-term prognosis, with a higher complication and mortality rate and longer intensive care and hospital stay [12–18]. As with all major thoracic and vascular surgery, the risk of other complications is also significant and is associated with a substantial potential for morbidity and mortality. The risk of myocardial infarction, heart failure, ventricular arrhythmia, infectious complications, and reoperation for bleeding is quoted in the range of 1–5%, neurocognitive deficits and renal failure requiring hemodialysis up to 10%, and respiratory failure, the most common postoperative complication, between 5% and 15% [4].

Robust clinical evidence validating optimal anesthetic management to achieve improved clinical outcomes in TAAA is lacking. This is largely due to a dependence on single-center observational studies, with substantial heterogeneity in technical details, a lack of universal definitions, and inconsistent standards in reporting outcomes. While research groups and national and international registries are beginning to address these issues in aortic arch and other types of cardiothoracic and vascular surgery [19–22], further

work is to be done before substantive evidence-based guidelines may be produced. The purpose of this chapter is to review the current literature and provide a rationale for a structured approach for the patient presenting for thoracoabdominal aortic surgery. Some content is complemented by other chapters in this textbook, so particular attention is paid to the requirements unique to TAAA surgery, particularly spinal cord and renal protection measures [23].

Anatomy and Physiology

Crawford Classification of TAAA Repair

TAAAs are commonly categorized by the classification devised by Crawford and colleagues, which divides TAAAs into four anatomic categories based on the extent of the repair required [24] (see Fig. 41.1). *Type I* extends from proximal to the sixth rib, typically at the origin of the left subclavian artery, to the suprarenal abdominal aorta and typically includes a beveled distal anastomosis at the visceral segment. *Type II* is the most extensive and extends from the left subclavian artery to the aortoiliac bifurcation. *Type III* extends from the thoracic aorta distal to the sixth rib to the aortoiliac bifurcation. *Type IV* extends from below the diaphragm and involves the entire visceral aortic segment and typically most of the abdominal aorta.

In addition to providing a uniform description of the anatomic extent of repair, the Crawford classification also allows the clinical team to estimate the operative risk. In particular,

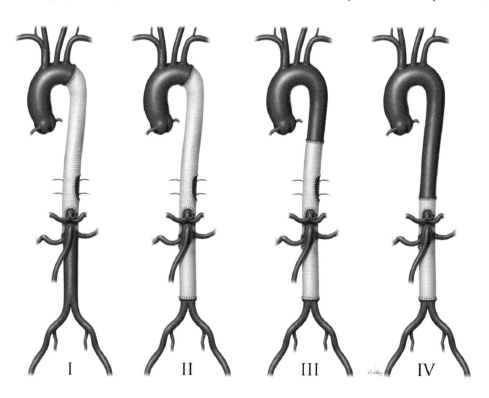

Fig. 41.1 Crawford classification of thoracoabdominal aortic aneurysms. (Courtesy of Baylor College of Medicine)

I   II   III   IV

type II TAAA repairs have the greatest potential for morbidity and mortality, specifically the highest incidence of spinal cord ischemia and renal dysfunction.

Pathophysiology of Aortic Clamp

The application and release of a thoracic aortic clamp has major mechanical, humoral, inflammatory, and metabolic effects. Our understanding of these effects is incomplete, largely limited to historical animal studies that have not lead to any therapeutic interventions with proven clinical benefit to date. This is largely due to the complexity of the physiology involved, with an interplay of multiple factors that vary depending on the type of pre-existing disease, location, and duration of the aortic cross-clamp and that not only affect multiple end targets with unique sequential effects but macro- as well as microvascular structures in a dynamic system that is simultaneously responding to the effects of bleeding, anesthetic medications, and fluid treatment [23].

After application of a thoracic aortic clamp, systemic vascular resistance suddenly increases, arterial blood pressure proximal to the clamp increasing up to 40%, with limited changes in heart rate. Distal to the aortic clamp, end-organ perfusion pressures are reduced to 10–20% of baseline. Pre-existing occlusive disease that has stimulated collateral blood vessel development or more distal placement of the clamp reduces the severity of these changes with greater potential for collateral runoff. Animal models have substantiated that the increase in preload and blood pressure proximal to the aortic clamp is due to a shift in blood flow from the splanchnic vasculature into the vena cava, by various potential mechanical and/or humoral mechanisms [25, 26]. On assessment with transesophageal echocardiogram, the left ventricle filling pressures can increase by 40%, the end-diastolic area by 28%, and end-systolic areas by 70% [27]. The ability to compensate for the left ventricular dilation secondary to a significant increase in afterload and to a lesser extent preload is largely dependent on the reserve ionotropic function of the heart. This can be severely limited in the context of coronary artery disease and subendocardial ischemia or with prolonged clamp placement and increasing concentrations of humoral and inflammatory products.

Upon removal of the aortic clamp, the arterial blood pressure suddenly drops with a sudden reduction in systemic vascular resistance due to both mechanical and complex ischemic dilating humoral/metabolic mechanisms. Cardiac output should increase in response but is variable depending on the patient's cardiac reserve and the effect of returning cold, hyperkalemic, acidotic, ischemic metabolites, as well as other dynamic factors such as the degree of acute bleeding.

Pathophysiology of Spinal Cord Injury

In the last 10 years, significant advances in our understanding of spinal cord blood supply have emphasized the need for a broader, more physiological approach to SCI [28].

Blood Supply of the Spinal Cord

Adamkiewicz and Kady provided the first accurate description of spinal cord blood supply in 1881 [29]. Their *classical model* was based on two posterolateral and one anterior spinal artery (ASA), the ASA being reinforced at multiple levels by segmental arteries originating from the aorta via the intercostal and lumbar arteries. Significant inter-individual variation within this anatomical model is recognized. During fetal development, an original 31 bilateral segmental arteries variably regress to 6 on average, with a broad range of 2 to 14 [29]. The largest segmental artery ("the artery of Adamkiewicz") arises most commonly from a left intercostal artery, between T9 and T12 in 75% of patients but as high as T5–T8 in 15% or as low as L1–L2 in 10% [30, 31]. Functional studies using motor-evoked potentials (MEP) also indicate acquired aneurysmal and atherosclerotic disease of the aorta results in significant anatomical variability [32].

In the last decade, evidence of a *spinal collateral arterial network* (SCAN) has supplanted the classical model of an anatomically defined single important blood supply, whereby a substantial arterial plexus along the entire length of the spinal cord supports its blood supply [9]. The intercostal and lumbar segmental arteries have multiple degrees of connection longitudinally and transversely to arterial networks in the spinal canal (consisting of the ASA and epidural arcades), paravertebral tissues, and multiple paraspinous muscles, the latter being the largest and most extensive of the three [9, 29] (see Fig. 41.2). The importance of additional inflow vessels is emphasized in this model, including the subclavian artery through the vertebral artery, the thyrocervical and costocervical trunks, the internal thoracic arteries through the intercostal arteries, and the hypogastric arteries through the lateral sacral and iliolumbar arteries [9, 29, 33]. There is also evidence of significant inter-individual variation with remodeling potential in porcine studies [9, 34].

Considering the potential for inter-individual variation in both conceptual models, advances in imaging the spinal cord blood supply offer potential benefits in defining and modifying an individual's risk [29]. However, options are currently limited. Invasive intra-arterial catheter angiography provides the best image quality when successful; however, its reported sensitivity is variable, with a risk of renal impairment or iatrogenic paraplegia. Magnetic resonance angiogram (MRA) technology has advanced significantly to reliably image the artery of Adamkiewicz and other larger segmental arteries but is still limited when it comes to the smaller caliber collateral vessels. When collateral arteries are distal to the

Fig. 41.2 Schematic diagram of the blood supply of the spinal cord. (Courtesy of Etz et al. [9])

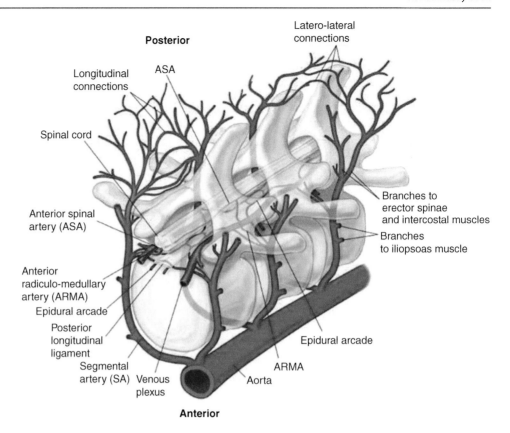

A Physiological Approach to SCI

While anatomical knowledge has advanced, understanding of circulatory physiology at the level of SCAN remains limited and is central to why the development and management of SCI remains poorly understood.

Simplistically, ischemia occurs when the supply of nutrients required for cellular metabolism does not met the demands for tissue viability. Absolute interruption of spinal cord blood supply for a sufficient period of time will cause irreversible ischemic necrosis. On the basis of early studies using a "clamp and sew" technique, this risk is significantly increased after 30 min of aortic cross-clamp and almost certain after 60 min [36, 37]. Alternatively, perfusion may be permanently marginal and become inadequate for viable cord function at a certain "tipping point" [38], explaining how cases of delayed SCI can present up to 27 days after intervention [39]. Added complexity lies in how variable this can be between individuals, for instance, chronic hypertension appears to shift the tipping point [34], while therapeutic interventions can improve ischemic tolerance. This concept is highlighted in studies where complete segmental arterial supply sacrifice consistently reduced spinal cord perfusion pressure (SCPP), but only lead to SCI in approximately half

planned aortic clamp on MRA, intraoperative decline of MEPs has a high negative (97%) but poor positive predictive value (37%) [35].

the cases [40]. Furthermore, while staging the arterial sacrifice minimized the drop in SCPP and improved functional outcomes overall, the cohort that could have tolerated the drop in SCPP without staging was unpredictable [34]. This is important to consider when interpreting the variability in published results.

Additionally, SCPP may be compromised by multiple mechanisms [33, 39, 41]. Spinal cord blood flow is reduced by direct arterial occlusion with placement of an aortic clamp or replacing aortic tissue with a graft. The primary aortic disease process (atherosclerosis, dissection) and embolic phenomena can also compromise the anastomotic capacity of the SCAN [29, 42]. Increased cerebrospinal fluid (CSF) pressure as occurs with placement of an aortic cross-clamp or edema secondary to an ischemic-reperfusion injury can create a "compartment syndrome" effect [43–45]. Systemic hypotension or steal phenomenon will further exacerbate suboptimal perfusion [39]. The potential interconnectedness of these various factors adds further complexity, where ischemia can exacerbate edema that further exacerbates ischemia in a spiral-like effect [8, 29, 42, 46].

Ultimately, the adequacy of SCPP is determined by an interplay of multiple factors that not only affects an individual's SCPP but also determines the SCPP required to prevent SCI (see Fig. 41.3). This creates a unique risk balance in each individual patient and demands a multimodal approach to prevent SCI following TAA intervention.

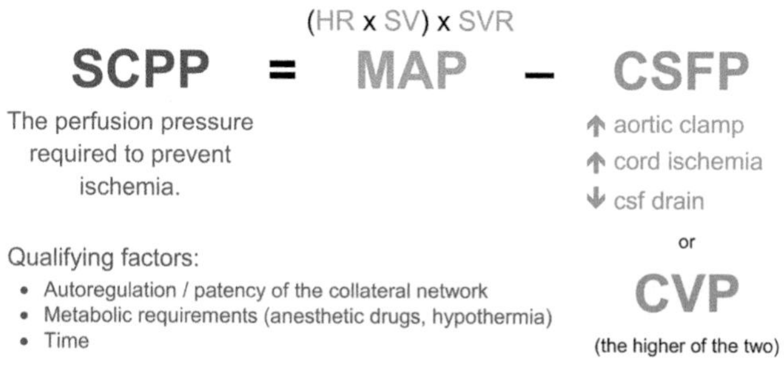

$$\text{SCPP} = \text{MAP} - \text{CSFP}$$

$$\frac{(\text{HR} \times \text{SV}) \times \text{SVR}}{}$$

The perfusion pressure required to prevent ischemia.

↑ aortic clamp
↑ cord ischemia
↓ csf drain

or

CVP

(the higher of the two)

Qualifying factors:
- Autoregulation / patency of the collateral network
- Metabolic requirements (anesthetic drugs, hypothermia)
- Time

Fig. 41.3 Multiple factors determine an individual's spinal cord perfusion pressure (SCPP), and the SCPP required to prevent spinal cord injury (SCI). MAP mean arterial pressure, HR heart rate, SV stroke volume, SVR systemic vascular resistance, CSFP cerebrospinal fluid pressure, CVP central venous pressure

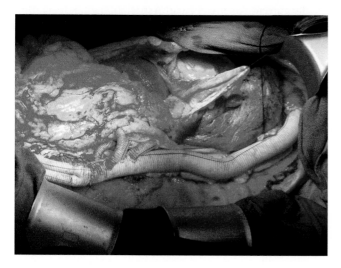

Fig. 41.4 Completed extent II thoracoabdominal repair with multi-branched graft and bifurcated distal aortic graft. (Courtesy of Baylor College of Medicine)

Surgical Technique

In order to surgically repair aortic disease, a clamp is placed above and below the lesion, the aorta opened, and the diseased segment replaced with a graft (see Fig. 41.4). The thoracic aorta is accessed via a left thoracotomy, which is extended to a paramedian laparotomy when access to the abdominal aorta is also required.

Established surgical methods for TAAA surgery include the "clamp and sew" technique, left heart bypass [47], partial cardiopulmonary bypass [48], and deep hypothermic arrest [49]. There are no established criteria to justify one technique over another and current guidelines recognizing that institutional experience is an important factor in technique selection [4]. The simple "clamp and sew" *technique* is no longer used in most institutions and is not advisable when the cross-clamp duration is expected to exceed 30 min because of the sig-

nificant risk of postoperative neurological deficit and mesenteric and renal ischemia.

Left heart bypass provides distal aortic perfusion during aortic clamping by means of a centrifugal pump, with the potential for additional selective perfusion of mesenteric visceral and renal arteries. Proximal decompression is provided by draining oxygenated blood through a left pulmonary vein cannula. The left atrial appendage may alternatively be used, but the positioning is often more awkward with a greater risk of air embolism. Blood is returned to provide distal perfusion through a distal aorta or femoral artery cannula. Close communication between the anesthesiologist and perfusionist is required to ensure that the balance of preload and the pump speed are optimal. *Partial bypass* is similar in that it ensures distal perfusion by cannulation of the femoral artery and vein while maintaining enough preload in the heart to support the cardiac and cerebral circulations but contrastingly achieves this by the use of full extracorporeal cardiopulmonary bypass. This can achieve higher flow rates that are advantageous in patients with poor left ventricular function or during a prolonged aortic cross-clamp time; however, it requires full heparinization, which increases the risk of increased blood loss and coagulopathy.

Deep hypothermic circulatory arrest (DHCA) is indicated when a proximal aortic clamp site is unable to be safely secured, often when the arch is dissected and/or aneurysmal. The benefits of use are in its simplicity, with a bloodless field and no need for additional cannula or aortic manipulation. Its main limitation is time on cardiopulmonary bypass. On the basis of advanced physiological and clinical testing, the upper safe limit of profound to deep HCA (12–20 °C) is 25–30 min [50, 51]. In a landmark clinical study by Svensson et al., >40 min of profound HCA increased the risk of neurological injury, and >65 min increased the risk in mortality [52]. In a more recent study of 490 patients, safe use of DHCA (18–20 °C) was reported for up to 50 min in terms of stroke risk, but only 61 patients had arrest times >40 min [53]. While it is established that organ metabolism is reduced proportionally to the degree of hypothermia, there is increasing recognition of the potential harm associated with profound and deep hypothermia (<14–20 °C). Various experimental studies raise concerns about the risks of coagulopathy, a proinflammatory response, and end-organ dysfunction, but these concerns are yet to be substantiated in clinical studies [19, 54]. Inconsistent standards in the reporting of outcomes related to end-organ ischemia significantly limits assessment of safe temperature and time parameters for these techniques [19, 54]. Additionally, the impact of relevant patient or interventional modifiers on these parameters is poorly understood [55–57].

Selective cerebral perfusion is not commonly used and more difficult to implement for TAA surgery. The specifics of this are covered in more detail in a previous review [58].

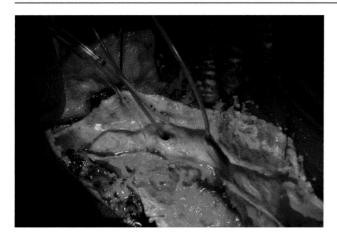

Fig. 41.5 Visceral perfusion. Isothermic blood is delivered from the return line of the left heart bypass circuit to the celiac artery and the superior mesenteric artery. Cold crystalloid solution is delivered intermittently to the left and right renal arteries. (Courtesy of Baylor College of Medicine)

If renal ischemia exceeds 30 min, some guidelines recommend selective cold crystalloid renal perfusion, as discussed later in section "Renal Protection" [5] (see Fig. 41.5).

Preoperative Evaluation

As already recognized, the variability in presentation of aortic disease is extensive and will have a major impact in guiding appropriate preoperative assessment and planning. A detailed description of these nuances is beyond the scope of this chapter, and we recommend review of current guidelines as appropriate [4, 5]. From an anesthetic perspective, recognizing certain distinctions is important to assess for likely associated disease, the required urgency, and risk benefits of surgical management.

In addition to a complete anesthetic, medical history and examination, a systematic approach should be taken in considering the need for additional investigations. Review of the content in Chap. 2 related to the preoperative assessment and optimization of the thoracotomy patient is relevant to TAAA surgery. Considering TAAA surgery qualifies as major surgery by entering both the thoracic and abdominal cavities, specific considerations include:

- Blood assays. Electrolytes and creatinine to assess renal and endocrine function, for side effects of pharmacotherapy, and potential avenues for optimization in the event of arrhythmia. Complete blood count to assess for myelo-suppression and anemia. In the event of anemia, iron studies, CRP, vitamin B12, folate, and thyroid function studies should be reviewed to assess for reversible causes. Coagulation studies to assess for bleeding dyscrasias. Liver function studies should be completed if there is sug-

gestion or risk factors for liver disease. Albumin is also a potential marker of nutritional status and frailty.
- A 12-lead electrocardiogram to provide a baseline measure and assess for evidence of arrhythmic or structural cardiac disease. 24 hour Holter monitoring may be considered for those with a history of intermittent symptoms of palpitations or pre-syncope.
- A resting echocardiogram if there are any risk factors or evidence of cardiac disease, including age > 40 years in some guidelines [4].
- A BNP level is recommended by the current Canadian Cardiovascular Society guidelines [59]. Dynamic cardiac testing (including a dobutamine stress echocardiogram or myocardial perfusion scan) is indicated according to the current American Heart Association guidelines if the patient's functional capacity is poor or cannot be assessed [60]. Current expert opinion is that patients with unstable coronary syndromes and significant coronary artery disease (i.e., left main stenosis or three-vessel disease) should undergo revascularization prior to or at the time of thoracic surgery, while the benefits for those with clinically stable flow-limiting coronary disease remain unclear [4].
- Neurocognitive testing, a carotid artery duplex scan, brachiocephalic angiography, and brain imaging should be considered if there are risk factors or evidence of cerebrovascular disease. While they are considered reasonable investigations in some guidelines to help assess a patient's risk profile [4], they are not routine, and their utility is uncertain.
- A recent chest x-ray or computed tomography (CT) is required to assess for cardiopulmonary disease including distortion of the trachea or left main bronchus by the aortic disease and to assist in sizing the double-lumen tube (DLT).
- The utility of an arterial blood gas on air, spirometry, pulmonary function testing, and cardiopulmonary testing are discussed at length in Chap. 2.

To complement this assessment, communication with the multidisciplinary team is important to insure optimal patient care. The surgical team will provide important insights into the indications for surgical management and the specific requirements of the surgical plan, including planned clamp positions, the need for additional shunt, bypass support, or selective organ perfusion techniques. Liaison with intensive care services is important to ensure suitability for a period of postoperative support. In the patient with significant comorbidity, referral for assessment or liaison with their treating medical subspecialist may be required. This can be to insure maximal optimization and/or provide an opinion as to the patient's long-term survival prognosis with respect to their comorbidity.

Putting all of this together, the anesthesiologist needs to provide the patient and surgeon with an individualized summative assessment of the risks of not proceeding with surgery, weighed against the perioperative risk. A perioperative plan should make provision for preoperative optimization of all elements of the patient's health.

Current international guidelines provide the best evidential support to optimize medical management of cardiac risk [59, 60]. In addition to specifically withhold angiotensin-converting enzyme inhibitors/angiotensin receptor blockers for 24 h prior to surgery to prevent the risk of death and vascular complications [61], other sources recommend withholding all antihypertensive agents the morning of surgery to help support compromised distal perfusion pressures [13, 34]. Counselling to support smoking cessation should be provided. In those with a reversible airways disease component, inhaler therapy should be optimized. Reversible causes of anemia and kidney injury should be treated if the urgency of surgery allows. The intra- and postoperative plan should outline the monitoring and interventions needed to minimize the risk of complication, in particular protective strategies to reduce the risk of spinal cord and renal injury, as discussed later in sections "Spinal Cord Protection Strategies" and "Renal Protection Strategies."

Although guidelines suggest identifying the "high risk" for implementation of spinal cord protection techniques, there are no recognized criteria to define "high risk" in this population [4]. The extent of the intended aortic repair has long been recognized as an important determinant since Crawford's classification of TAAA disease [24]; however, many institutions classify all open TAAA repairs as high risk. Although many other patient and procedural factors have been proposed as risk factors for postoperative SCI, none have been consistently validated. The rationale for instituting spinal cord protective strategies is determined on a surgeon and patient-case basis. The following is a summary of independent predictors of SCI with open repair identified by logistic regression modelling that could be considered:

- Extent of disease, including type II only [62, 63], I and II [15], and I, II, and III [64] Crawford TAA aneurysm classification.
- Previous thoracic or TAA surgery [65]. In another study thoracic aneurysm repair was protective [62].
- Presence of aortic rupture [15].
- Total aortic clamp time [15]. In a later study by the same group distal aortic perfusion eliminated this as a risk factor on repeat analysis [63].
- Diabetes [62].
- History of preoperative renal dysfunction [15], renal dysfunction (Cr >2.0 mg/dL, a previous history of renal failure or insufficiency or being on active dialysis) [63].

In the most recent and largest publication of a single-center experience to date, Coselli et al. identified that the independent risk factors for permanent paraplegia varied depending on the extent of TAAA. For extent II repairs, coronary artery disease and chronic aortic symptoms increased risk, while having a genetically triggered disorder was protective. For extent III repairs, cerebrovascular disease, emergency repair, and selective visceral perfusion increased risk of SCI [10].

Intraoperative Management

Monitoring

In addition to ASA standard monitoring [66], extra monitoring of cardiac and neurological function is required for the early detection and minimization of complications. Again, much of what is discussed with regard to monitoring in Chap. 20 should be reviewed.

Five-Lead Electrocardiogram (ECG) and Defibrillation Pads

While lead V provides assessment of the left ventricle lateral wall and provides the greatest sensitivity for detecting intraoperative ischemia, the lead position is directly in the surgical field. Defibrillation pads should also be anteroposteriorly placed prior to induction.

Invasive Blood Pressure

Right radial or brachial arterial line placement provides information about pressures proximal to the aortic clamp, including the cerebral circulation even if the left subclavian arterial flow is compromised by the clamp. If distal perfusion techniques are used, a right femoral artery line may be placed, reserving the left femoral artery for bypass cannulation. If distal perfusion pressure monitoring is not required, we recommend using a second line in the left radial or brachial artery. This is dedicated to blood sampling in order to prevent interruption in pressure monitoring or compromise of the right line from frequent blood sampling.

Pulmonary Artery Catheter (PAC)

While recognizing there is no support for improved clinical outcomes [67], we routinely place a sheath and PAC in the right internal jugular for these cases. Recognizing the standard limitations in its use, including the likely overestimation of the left ventricular end-diastolic pressure with isolated right-lung ventilation, we find the additional information about left ventricular function in terms of filling pressures and cardiac output useful in optimizing hemodynamic management.

Fig. 41.6 An ergonomic
anesthetic space

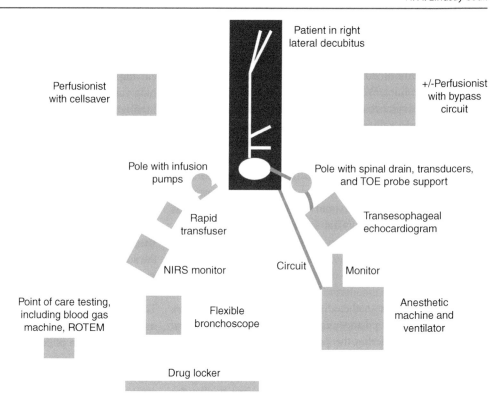

Hemodynamic Management

A key priority for major vascular surgery of this nature is tight hemodynamic control throughout the perioperative period. Minimizing acute extremes in blood pressure and heart rate is important in order to limit changes in wall shear stress across the diseased aorta. In the context of using aortic clamps and massive bleeding, this can be demanding. There are many ways of achieving this same outcome, and the treating anesthesiologist should consider agents with the appropriate pharmacological properties that they are familiar with in order to achieve the best results.

With placement of the proximal aortic clamp, it is important to avoid an excessively high left ventricular filling pressure and heart rate that will increase myocardial oxygen consumption while reducing coronary perfusion. In patients with a degree of coronary artery disease this will result in subendocardial ischemia. Equally, at least a "normal" (i.e., relative to the patient's awake baseline blood pressure) proximal aortic pressure will need to be maintained if end-organ perfusion distal to the aortic clamp is dependent on collateral flow. While euvolemia should be maintained preoperatively to avoid pre-renal injury, excessive fluid resuscitation should be avoided prior to aortic clamp placement. There is a small body of evidence to support nitroglycerin as more effective that nitroprusside for reducing preload and filling pressures once the clamp is placed, with superior preservation of collateral coronary, renal, and spinal blood flow [86–88]. Using β-blockers such as labetalol with its alpha- and beta-effects

or esmolol with its short-acting, β1-selective effects could be considered as second-line agents, but the negative inotropy will need to be monitored closely. Nicardipine is a dihydropyridine calcium channel antagonist with a relatively rapid onset and offset of effect that predominately relates to arterial dilation. Its use may be more favorable to β-blockers in the context of bradycardia or reactive airways disease.

Acute hypotension following release of the aortic clamp should be limited by preemptively bolusing fluid and instituting vasopressor/inotropic support approximately 10 min prior. In the event of refractory or severe hypotension, reapplication of the aortic clamp may be required for 1–2 min. Again, while supporting adequate organ perfusion postclamp release, excess blood pressure that will stress the suture lines of the graft and increase the risk of bleeding must be avoided.

Fluid Management with Massive Blood Loss

A full discussion of the management of massive transfusion and coagulopathy is beyond the scope of this chapter. Rather we would refer to current international guidelines [89, 90]. Close communication with blood bank and operating room staff such as the nurses, anesthetic assistants, and attendants can help meet the high level of resource intensity potentially required.

Targeted transfusion using point-of-care viscoelastic assay (e.g., thromboelastography (TEG) or rotational thromboelastometry (ROTEM))-guided algorithms have been shown to reduce blood transfusion requirements [90]. No single algorithm can be recommended at this time; rather this should be developed at an institutional level with multi-departmental input and regular audit. Figure 41.7 provides an example of the validated algorithm used for cardiac surgery with bypass support at our institution [91]. If available, a massive transfusion protocol may need to be used as a strategy to optimize the delivery of blood products to massively bleeding patients.

Prophylactic use of antifibrinolytic therapy, in particular tranexamic acid, has been shown to reduce perioperative blood loss and reduce transfusion requirements. The evidence is most substantive for use in cardiac surgery and is appropriate for TAAA surgery in light of the risk for excessive bleeding. In multiple randomized trials, including the largest and most recent ATACAS trial, there is no evidence of

an increased risk of thrombotic complications; however, there is a recognized dose-dependent risk of postoperative seizures [90, 92].

Spinal Cord Protection Strategies

To prevent spinal ischemia, different techniques can be used to achieve the same outcomes, as long as the physiological principles of maintaining perfusion pressure to prevent paraplegia are accounted for. Techniques to prevent and minimize SCI primarily focus on maximizing collateral flow by supporting mean arterial pressure and reducing CSF pressure while prolonging ischemic tolerance and reducing reperfusion injury with hypothermia and pharmacotherapy. Despite a wealth of options, interpretation of the large volume of conflicting literature allows for few conclusive

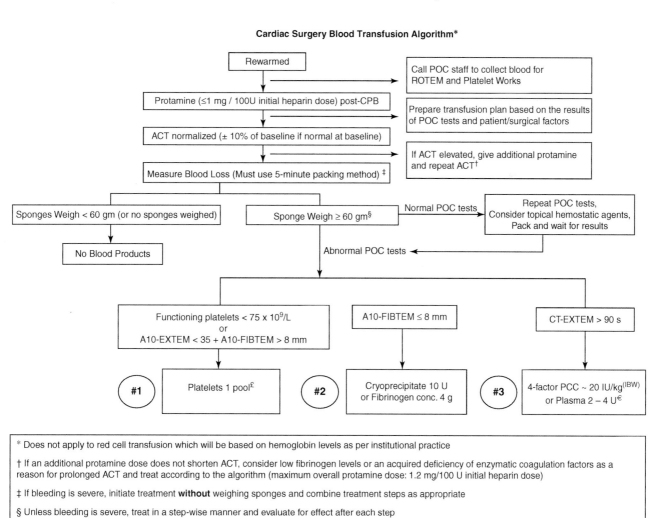

Fig. 41.7 ROTEM-guided algorithm for targeted transfusion. (Courtesy of Karkouti et al. [91])

recommendations. Except for one randomized controlled trial on cerebrospinal fluid drainage (CSFD), the vast majority of evidence is level B with single-center cohort studies of a few hundred patients [4, 5]. Besides the inherent variability in pathophysiology, comparability of results between studies is limited by the heterogeneity in definitions, inclusion/exclusion criteria, and therapy combinations [8, 31]. The risk of generalizing results from single centers of excellence must also be considered [2, 4], as a surgeon's experience, treatment volume of an institution [2], and implementation of a protocoled care package [41] have been shown to have a significant effect on outcomes.

Cerebrospinal Fluid Drainage (CSFD)

Evidence from animal studies in the 1960s showing that reduced CSF pressures improved SCPP provided the initial justification for trialing CSFD [8, 30, 31]. Cases of CSFD reversing SCI symptoms [8, 93] and Coselli et al.'s landmark randomized controlled trial [94] validate their potential benefit in humans. Conversely there are cases of SCI developing despite prophylactic CSFD and recovering without it [95], with conflicting findings in the literature as highlighted in the systematic [8] and Cochrane review [31]. While recognizing the weaknesses in the current data, both of these reviews concluded there is sufficient evidence to support the role of CSFD in high-risk patients as part of a multimodal proactive approach [8, 31]. The 2010 ACCF and 2014 ESC guidelines made similar recommendations for use as a protective strategy in high-risk open thoracic aortic repair procedures [4, 5]. However, the clarity of this statement is misleading, with no criteria to identify the "high-risk" patient. While the authors of the Cochrane review caution against extrapolating benefit beyond the selection criteria in the Coselli trial (i.e., open repair of Crawford type I–II TAA in a center of excellence) [31], the other systematic review specified "high risk" as open repair of Crawford types I–III with and without dissection [8]. Given that the risk of SCI is unpredictable, many centers use CSFD in all patients, including those undergoing extent IV repair.

Increasingly the risks of CSFD are recognized, although in a large portion of the literature systemic evaluation of the rate and risks of CSFD complications are poorly reported [96]. Intracranial hemorrhage is the most significant in terms of the potential morbidity and mortality, with an incidence 0.45–7.8%, of whom 10–50% develop significant neurological deficit or die [68, 97–103]. CSF leak with post-dural puncture headache (incidence 0.74–9.7% [12, 98, 99, 102, 103]), neuraxial hematoma (incidence 0–3% [68, 98, 103–105]), catheter fracture, meningitis, para-lumbar infection, and abducens nerve palsy (incidence <1% [68, 103, 106]) is also reported in the literature.

Even more importantly, there is a paucity of literature to substantiate important management standards for CSFD to minimize complications with use. This includes specifics about pressure thresholds and drainage limits, duration of use, and infrastructure requirements. Drainage of larger volumes of CSF is the most consistent independent predictor of hemorrhagic complication [97, 102], with high CVP at the time of cross-clamping also being noted by one group [102]. Maintenance of CSFP >7–10 mmHg with continuous monitoring, limiting drainage to <15–25 mL/h, maintenance of a recumbent position (<30 degrees reverse Trendelenburg), early removal within 48–72 h postoperatively, capping the drain 24 h prior to removal to allow CSFP to normalize, and cautious use of anticoagulation therapy even after drain removal are the most common expert recommendations for safe CSFD in the literature [95, 97, 98, 102, 106], with various "care bundles" described in the literature [98, 107–110]. However, this is far from universal, with one group advocating a more flexible approach, limiting drainage volumes to the upper limits of CSF circulating volume (140–165 mL) intra- and postoperatively [102], while others individualize the baseline pressure target based on the preoperative "opening pressure" at the time of drain placement [42]. While drainage of bloody CSF is only associated with radiological evidence of intracranial hemorrhage in 50% of cases, it is widely recognized as a sensitive indicator of increased risk for ICH requiring the immediate attention to limit significant morbidity and mortality [97, 98, 102], as covered in section "Technical Specifics of Cerebrospinal Fluid Drainage." Irrespective of the value of each component, a recent study that protocoled CSFD management achieved a substantial reduction in their institution's complication rate (from 24.1% to 5.7%, $p = 0.067$) [68].

Supporting SCPP

Increasingly the importance of supporting systemic blood pressure (with mean arterial pressures 80–100 mmHg) and cardiac output to maintain SCPP is recognized for at least 48 h postoperatively until SCAN has sufficiently remodeled to compensate for the loss of segmental arterial supply [41, 42, 68, 106]. While direct measurement of SCPP [40, 111], functional MEP testing [44, 109], and risk factor analysis [99, 112, 113] have supported this, the role of blood pressure augmentation in reversing symptomatic SCI is most compelling [95, 114]. Consideration of the patient's preoperative baseline arterial pressure and withholding antihypertensive preoperatively is recommended [13, 34]. Optimization of oxygen delivery with aggressive blood transfusion targets also features in recent institutional protocols [41, 68].

Intraoperatively the established benefits of distal aortic perfusion by cardiopulmonary bypass (CPB) or left heart bypass are recognized for open repair of type I–II TAAA in centers with significant experience [63, 115]. Guidelines recommend a proximal mean arterial pressure of 90–100 mmHg and distal arterial pressure of 60 mmHg to ensure adequate spinal cord perfusion [4]. There is also evidence that non-pulsatile perfusion is inferior to pulsatile perfusion at the same mean pressure [34]. Further technical aspects of these techniques are covered above in section "Surgical Technique."

Other surgical techniques to optimize collateral blood flow to the spinal are largely controversial. Historically, re-implantation of segmental arterial supply via the intercostal and lumbar arteries has been a dominant protective strategy in surgical TAAA repair. However, by prolonging the aortic cross-clamp time, this intervention is not without risk. Techniques may be indiscriminate or selective based on clinical assessment of back-bleeding, intraoperative MEP, or preoperative imaging [8, 116]. Some retrospective analyses have shown a tenfold increase in SCI risk when critical zone (T9-L1) intercostal vessels were oversewn in type I/II open repair [117, 118], and selective re-implantation has been associated with a significant protective effect when used as part of a multimodal strategy [46, 116, 119, 120]. However, the work of Griepp et al. ($n = 95$) and later Etz et al. ($n = 100$) challenged this doctrine by extensively sacrificing segmental arteries under EP monitoring without SCI [121, 122]. While recognizing the limitations of these observational studies, the authors contested re-implantation was not only unnecessary when other means are used to support the SCAN, but it is potentially harmful by prolonging surgery and causing steal phenomenon. In reality, both arguments are likely to hold merit, and while not necessary in the majority, it may be critical in a few, justifying a balanced approach with selective re-implantation in current guidelines [4, 42, 46].

The importance of patency and revascularization of independent arterial beds contributing to the SCAN is equally controversial. While some studies have identified left subclavian artery coverage as a risk factor for SCI [13, 123], it is not a consistent finding [124–127]. Additionally, prophylactic revascularization may be justified in order to reduce the risk of stroke or left arm ischemia [128, 129].

Staged repair is a relatively new concept based on supporting collateral flow through SCAN remodeling. While the physical effects of staging on SCPP are compelling [34], the complexity of how these impact clinical outcomes, especially for an individual patient, is yet to be fully understood. This is not limited to open repair, with various hybrid and endovascular staging methods described that are beyond the scope of this chapter, and we refer to a previous review for further detail on this [58].

Hypothermia

The protective benefits of hypothermia have been long recognized [130]. Various methods including local epidural cooling [117, 131], profound (<20–22 °C) hypothermia with CPB with or without circulatory arrest [132, 133], moderate (30–34 °C) hypothermia with partial bypass (aortofemoral or atriofemoral) [134, 135], and mild permissive hypothermia [136] have been advocated, with a protective effect in high-risk cases when used in institutions with significant experience.

However, as already noted above in section "Surgical Technique," the association between hypothermia (<34.5 °C) and an increase in postoperative organ dysfunction and mortality in patients having aortic surgery [137] cautions against routine use, with specific concerns about an increased risk of coagulopathy, pulmonary dysfunction [132, 138], and arrhythmias [134] in open TAAA repair studies. Currently moderate systemic hypothermia is considered a reasonable strategy to protect the spinal cord during open surgical repair of the descending thoracic aorta, and epidural irrigation with a hypothermic solution may be considered [4].

Drugs

While the desire for a pharmacologically protective agent has been exhaustive, the evidence base remains weak [106]. While intravenous naloxone [139, 140] and intrathecal papaverine [135, 141] have been shown to have protective benefit in human trials, the benefits of thiopentone [142], systemic steroids [143], lidocaine [144], intrathecal methylprednisolone [145], deferoxamine [146], superoxide dismutase [146, 147], minocycline [148] and erythropoietin [149], testosterone [150], and dexmedetomidine [151] are limited to animal studies.

The 2010 ACCF guidelines recommend that use of high-dose systemic glucocorticoids, mannitol for osmotic diuresis, intrathecal papaverine, and various anesthetic agents to suppress metabolic suppression may be considered [4].

Hyperbaric Oxygen

In our institution we have had positive experience with early institution of hyperbaric oxygen therapy in three patients, all of whom recovered full neurological function. While the evidence base is currently limited to case reports, this is an emerging field of research.

Technical Specifics of Cerebrospinal Fluid Drainage

Use and familiarly with the manufacture's recommendations of a dedicated lumbar drainage kit that includes a 14ga introducer needle, specialized multi-orificed silastic drainage catheter, and external drainage and monitoring system is required. Once identifying that a CSFD is indicated, important contraindications should be considered. Current coagulation guidelines for neuraxial techniques should be followed [152]. The presence of intracranial disease that could predispose to neuraxial or intracranial bleeding complications in the context of iatrogenic intracranial hypotension should be considered in liaison with the surgeon, including cerebral aneurysms, arteriovenous malformations, cerebral atrophy, cranial vault abnormalities, chronic subdural hematomas, or a history of recent head trauma [153]. An assessment of risk for infectious complications should also be made as per current guidelines for neuraxial techniques, and while a bacteremia or epidural abscess would be grounds to delay surgery altogether, the drain should also not be placed over a localized area of infection [154]. Other preparations in terms of fully informed consent, strict asepsis, and monitoring are also as per local/national requirements for any neuraxial technique [155, 156].

CSFDs are usually inserted the day prior to surgery in our institution, in an awake patient, in the lateral position, and in a low lumbar intervertebral space [107]; however, variations on this with good clinical outcomes are described [98]. Placement the day prior to surgery allows for contingency planning in the event of a traumatic/bloody tap, including delaying surgery and systemic anticoagulation for 24 h [4, 152]. However, this can be resource intensive with the need to observe the patient in the CVICU overnight to insure the drain doesn't become blocked due to kinking or clot formation. Placing the patient in the lateral position is intended to decrease the hydrostatic pressure of the column of CSF and limit the volume of CSF uncontrollably drained during insertion of the drain. Puncture of the dura below the level of the conus medullaris is theoretically less likely to transfix the filum terminale. With the patient awake, redirection of the needle and drain in the event of paresthesia may also limit the potential for nerve injury.

Published techniques variably describe feeding 8–20 cm of catheter into the subarachnoid space beyond the epidural tip [107]. While ensuring that a sufficient length is inserted to avoid the accidental displacement of the catheter with patient movement, the length of catheter that can be inserted is often limited by mechanical difficulties feeding the catheter, a desire to limit uncontrolled drainage of CSF, or patient complaints of paresthesia. If adjustment of the catheter position is required, particular care should be taken when withdrawing the catheter back through the needle due to the risk of shearing it against the needle tip. If any slight resistance is felt, the whole needle and catheter must be withdrawn as one unit and the procedure started again.

Once the drain is inserted and the introducer needle removed, the drain should be secured with care to minimize the risk of kinking and connected to the pressure transducer and drainage bag while maintaining strict sterility (see Fig. 41.8). The level of the transducer should be set and zeroed at the level of the right atrium and ideally fixed to the patient and/or bed. When the drain is open, the level of the transducer and drain should be closely monitored and the patient kept at less than 30 degrees reverse Trendelenburg, with a high level of vigilance to avoid accidental excess CSF

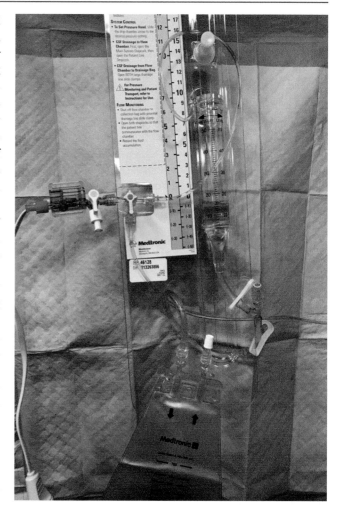

Fig. 41.8 Setting up electronic pressure transduction of the cerebrospinal fluid pressure. Note that with using this set-up the pressurized flush function on the transducer must be removed

drainage. Development of an automated device for pressure- or volume-controlled CSF drainage with simultaneous measurement is described in the literature (LiquoGuard®, Moller Medical GmbH, Fulda, Germany), and while potentially having safety benefits over standard dripping chambers, this is yet to be substantiated [157].

If placed the day before surgery, the drain should be left off overnight and opened once an hour to drain 1–2 drops to ensure patency. Once the patient is in the operating room and positioned for surgery, the transducer should be carefully checked and the drain opened to drain to a CSF pressure of 10 mmHg prior to aortic clamp placement, limited to 10–20 ml/h (or as per the agreed institutional practice, the rationale for which was explored in section "Spinal Cord Protection Strategies" above). At least hourly review and documentation of the drainage pressure (absolute number and waveform), drainage volumes, and the presence of any blood are crucial for safe use. Similarly, at the end of the case, the drain should be clamped before repositioning the patient and only resumed once the patient is finally positioned on their CVICU bed and close monitoring is possible.

In the context of intra- or postoperative evidence of neurological deficit, spinal cord perfusion should be optimized with an increase in mean arterial pressure targets, review of hemoglobin targets, and consideration to further decrease CSF pressure and increase drainage targets. In the postoperative period, the need for imaging (ideally magnetic resonance imaging (MRI) but not always feasible) to assess whether spinal ischemia or an epidural hematoma is the precipitant cause of deficit and the role of hyperbaric therapy can also be considered following optimization of CSF hemodynamics. In the event of frankly bloody CSF drainage, a cessation or reduction in the drainage volume limit should be considered, coagulation function optimized, with imaging to assess for intracranial hemorrhage as soon as the patient is stable enough, with neurosurgical consultation as appropriate.

The CSFD should be removed as soon as possible to reduce infectious complications. Some guidelines recommend drainage for at least 48 h and up to 72 h postoperatively to prevent delayed onset paraplegia [5, 31]. Alternatively, once the patient is neurologically accessible with normal lower limb findings and hemodynamically stable, the CSFD can be clamped and removed if the neurological status remains stable for a further 24 h. Coagulation status should be reviewed before removal of the drain, as described prior to drain insertion. In the event a patient develops sepsis in the postoperative period, the risk-benefit balance of removing the CSFD should be carefully considered, the CSFD not only being a potential source of infection but also a receptacle for colonization. In the event of delayed neurological deterioration after removal of the CSFD that does not improve with blood pressure support, the need to reinsert the CFSD will need to be considered.

While there is limited evidence to validate the optimal technique for CSFD placement and management, evidence substantiates that there should be an agreed standard operating procedure developed at an institutional level [68]. All staff involved in the care of patient's having TAAA surgery should be orientated to this, and any deviations from care be discussed at a multidisciplinary level.

Renal Protection Strategies

Renal dysfunction is a common complication after TAAA surgery, and while a much smaller proportion proceed to require permanent dialysis, it is a consistent independent predictor of major morbidity and mortality [158, 159]. The ability to assess the incidence, risk factors, and effective therapeutic interventions to prevent renal dysfunction continues to be hampered by the lack of consistency in the crite-

ria to define acute kidney failure [159, 160]. Additionally, the mechanisms for renal injury are diverse, and the contribution variable between patients, including [85, 161, 162]:

- Nephrotoxic insult, namely, with contrast media preoperatively
- Ischemia related to the aortic cross-clamp, hypotension, and anemia
- Atheroembolic phenomenon
- Reperfusion tubular injury, mediated by various chemical immunomodulating agents

Preoperative renal dysfunction (creatinine >1.5 mg/dL) is consistently found to be an important predictor of postoperative renal dysfunction [85, 158, 159, 161, 162]. Complex surgery with prolonged ischemic times (clamp time > 100 min), greater intraoperative hemodynamic instability, increased bleeding, and the need to return to operating room is understandably associated with worse renal outcomes [158, 159].

In the absence of any effective interventions to treat renal failure, prevention of injury is critical. Despite an extensive body of research, there is limited evidence to support any pharmacological agents as being renoprotective [163]. Furosemide, mannitol, and dopamine [164–167] have been shown to be ineffective and potentially even harmful [4, 168–170], while the utility of corticosteroids, fenoldopam, and dopexamine remains unproven [85, 158].

Considering the potential for preoperative optimization is important if possible. Identifying the "at-risk" patient provides an opportunity to institute additional intraoperative support. Contrast-induced nephropathy should be allowed to resolve with hydration support and N-acetylcysteine [171, 172] or avoid contrast altogether by using alternative imaging techniques such as magnetic resonance angiography [162]. Limited evidence from animal studies also support the concept of post-conditioning, where a gradual increase in blood flow on unclamping reduces the degree of reperfusion injury [173].

In addition to maintaining euvolemia and supporting an adequate cardiac output and blood pressure perioperatively, renal perfusion can be selectively supported. This involves inserting perfusion catheters into the renal ostia and infusing a rapid 250–300 ml bolus, followed by ~20 ml/min or ~1000 ml/h of a cold crystalloid perfusion solution into each kidney. Although technically simple, the specific indications for use and techniques are controversial. Randomized data supports the use of cold (4 °C) crystalloid (Ringer's lactate) as superior to normothermic or cold blood [174, 175]; however, the specifics of the type of crystalloid or the utility of adding mannitol or steroids to the perfusate is unclear. American guidelines recommend considering cold (4 °C) crystalloid or blood perfusion [4], while the European guidelines specify utility of cold renal perfusion when the ischemia time is greater than 30 min [5].

Postoperative Care

Part XII of this textbook comprehensively covers the postoperative requirements and potential complications following thoracic surgery. Chapters 46 and 47 specifically cover strategies for managing significant postoperative pain and preventing chronic post-thoracotomy pain.

Specific to TAAA surgery, preservation of spinal cord and end-organ function continues to be the primary concern in the immediate postoperative period. As in the intraoperative period, tight hemodynamic control, euvolemia, normal coagulation function, close protocolized CSFD management, and one hourly neurological assessment are crucial to optimal long-term recovery outcomes.

In our institute patients are transferred to the intensive care sedated and ventilation. Once the patient is hemodynamically stable, the sedation is temporarily held to assess neurological function by regular clinical examination. Sedation is weaned, and the patient is usually extubated in the first 12–24 h postoperatively. Our routine postoperative analgesia regimen comprises of a continuous local anesthetic infusion (ropivacaine 0.2% 5 cc/h) through surgically placed paravertebral catheters started on arrival to the ICU and opioid (hydromorphone/morphine) patient-controlled analgesia (PCA) boluses once the patient is conscious.

Summary

Cambria said it best – "absolutes in TAAA surgery are usually proven to be wrong" [176]. This not only recognizes the many limitations in the quality of current literature but the multifaceted complexity of the pathology, with no individual case being predictable.

Despite the limitations in knowledge and specifics in practice standards, fundamentals in improving outcomes are being established, including the development of protocols/packages of care, establishing institutional familiarity and experience, proactive measures to protect sensitive neural and renal tissue from ischemia, and the early identification of compromise in order to minimize the severity of long-term injury.

Clinical Case Discussion

A 40-year-old lady with Marfan syndrome has a Crawford type II TAAA which measures 6.4 cm. She is an ex-smoker with no other significant comorbidities.

Question 1. What are the major perioperative concerns?

Question 2: There is a suitable proximal clamp site just distal to the left subclavian artery. What are the options for perfusion management for this case?

Question 3: The patient develops weakness in both legs in ICU on the first postoperative day. How would you manage this situation?

Answer 1: For a complete discussion of these issues, see the section "Intraoperative Management" (from page 14)
  (a) Massive bleeding and coagulopathy
  (b) Spinal cord injury
  (c) Acute kidney injury
  (d) Acute lung injury due to prolonged OLV, surgical manipulation, and massive transfusion

Answer 2: For a complete discussion, see section "Surgical Technique" (from page 6)
  (a) Left heart bypass – preferred
  (b) Partial cardiopulmonary bypass
  (c) Deep hypothermic circulatory arrest

Answer 3: For a complete discussion, see sections "Spinal Cord Protection Strategies" and "Technical Specifics of Cerebrospinal Fluid Drainage" (specifically page 21)
  (a) Increase MAP to 90–100 mmHg
  (b) Increase CSF drainage to maintain ICP less than 10 mmHg
  (c) Raise the hemoglobin to over 90–100 g/dl
  (d) MRI/CT scan to rule out epidural hematoma

References

1. Acher C, Wynn M. Outcomes in open repair of the thoracic and thoracoabdominal aorta. J Vasc Surg. 2010;52(4 Suppl):3S–9S.
2. Cowan JA Jr, Dimick JB, Henke PK, Huber TS, Stanley JC, Upchurch GR Jr. Surgical treatment of intact thoracoabdominal aortic aneurysms in the United States: hospital and surgeon volume-related outcomes. J Vasc Surg. 2003;37(6):1169–74.
3. Schermerhorn ML, Giles KA, Hamdan AD, Dalhberg SE, Hagberg R, Pomposelli F. Population-based outcomes of open descending thoracic aortic aneurysm repair. J Vasc Surg. 2008;48(4):821–7.
4. Hiratzka LF, Bakris GL, Beckman JA, Bersin RM, Carr VF, Casey DE Jr, et al. 2010 ACCF/AHA/AATS/ACR/ASA/SCA/SCAI/SIR/STS/SVM Guidelines for the diagnosis and management of patients with thoracic aortic disease: executive summary: a report of the American College of Cardiology Foundation/American Heart Association Task Force on Practice Guidelines, American Association for Thoracic Surgery, American College of Radiology, American Stroke Association, Society of Cardiovascular Anesthesiologists, Society for Cardiovascular Angiography and Interventions, Society of Interventional Radiology, Society of Thoracic Surgeons, and Society for Vascular Medicine. Anesth Analg. 2010;111(2):279–315.
5. Erbel R, Aboyans V, Boileau C, Bossone E, Bartolomeo RD, Eggebrecht H, et al. 2014 ESC guidelines on the diagnosis and treatment of aortic diseases: document covering acute and chronic aortic diseases of the thoracic and abdominal aorta of the adult. The task force for the diagnosis and treatment of aortic diseases of the European Society of Cardiology (ESC). Eur Heart J. 2014;35(41):2873–926.

6. Adams HD, Van Geertruyden HH. Neurologic complications of aortic surgery. Ann Surg. 1956;144(4):574–610.

7. Panthee N, Ono M. Spinal cord injury following thoracic and thoracoabdominal aortic repairs. Asian Cardiovasc Thorac Ann. 2015;23(2):235–46.

8. Cina CS, Abouzahr L, Arena GO, Lagana A, Devereaux PJ, Farrokhyar F. Cerebrospinal fluid drainage to prevent paraplegia during thoracic and thoracoabdominal aortic aneurysm surgery: a systematic review and meta-analysis. J Vasc Surg. 2004;40(1):36–44.

9. Etz CD, Kari FA, Mueller CS, Silovitz D, Brenner RM, Lin HM, et al. The collateral network concept: a reassessment of the anatomy of spinal cord perfusion. J Thorac Cardiovasc Surg. 2011;141(4):1020–8.

10. Coselli JS, LeMaire SA, Preventza O, de la Cruz KI, Cooley DA, Price MD, et al. Outcomes of 3309 thoracoabdominal aortic aneurysm repairs. J Thorac Cardiovasc Surg. 2016;151(5):1323–37.

11. Mehmedagic I, Jorgensen S, Acosta S. Mid-term follow-up of patients with permanent sequel due to spinal cord ischemia after advanced endovascular therapy for extensive aortic disease. Spinal Cord. 2015;53(3):232.

12. Bisdas T, Panuccio G, Sugimoto M, Torsello G, Austermann M. Risk factors for spinal cord ischemia after endovascular repair of thoracoabdominal aortic aneurysms. J Vasc Surg. 2015;61(6):1408–16.

13. Buth J, Harris PL, Hobo R, van Eps R, Cuypers P, Duijm L, et al. Neurologic complications associated with endovascular repair of thoracic aortic pathology: incidence and risk factors. A study from the European Collaborators on Stent/Graft Techniques for Aortic Aneurysm Repair (EUROSTAR) registry. J Vasc Surg. 2007;46(6):1103–10. discussion 10-1.

14. Conrad MF, Ye JY, Chung TK, Davison JK, Cambria RP. Spinal cord complications after thoracic aortic surgery: long-term survival and functional status varies with deficit severity. J Vasc Surg. 2008;48(1):47–53.

15. Svensson LG, Crawford ES, Hess KR, Coselli JS, Safi HJ. Experience with 1509 patients undergoing thoracoabdominal aortic operations. J Vasc Surg. 1993;17(2):357–68. discussion 68-70

16. Eagleton MJ, Shah S, Petkosevek D, Mastracci TM, Greenberg RK. Hypogastric and subclavian artery patency affects onset and recovery of spinal cord ischemia associated with aortic endografting. J Vasc Surg. 2014;59(1):89–94.

17. Becker DA, McGarvey ML, Rojvirat C, Bavaria JE, Messe SR. Predictors of outcome in patients with spinal cord ischemia after open aortic repair. Neurocrit Care. 2013;18(1):70–4.

18. Keith CJ Jr, Passman MA, Carignan MJ, Parmar GM, Nagre SB, Patterson MA, et al. Protocol implementation of selective postoperative lumbar spinal drainage after thoracic aortic endograft. J Vasc Surg. 2012;55(1):1–8. discussion 8.

19. Yan TD, Tian DH, LeMaire SA, Misfeld M, Elefteriades JA, Chen EP, et al. The ARCH projects: design and rationale (IAASSG 001). Eur J Cardiothorac Surg. 2014;45(1):10–6.

20. The Society of Thoracic Surgeons. STS National Database, Data Managers 2017. Available from: http://www.sts.org/sts-national-database/data-managers.

21. Boening A, Karck M, Conzelmann LO, Easo J, Krüger T, Rylski B, et al. German registry for acute aortic dissection type A: structure, results, and future perspectives. Thorac Cardiovasc Surg. 2017;65(2):77–84.

22. Beck AW, Sedrakyan A, Mao J, Venermo M, Faizer R, Debus S, et al. Variations in abdominal aortic aneurysm care: a report from the international consortium of vascular registries. Circulation. 2016;134(24):1948–58.

23. Zammert M, Gelman S. The pathophysiology of aortic cross-clamping. Best Pract Res Clin Anaesthesiol. 2016;30(3):257–69.

24. Crawford ES, Crawford JL, Safi HJ, Coselli JS, Hess KR, Brooks B, et al. Thoracoabdominal aortic aneurysms: preoperative and intraoperative factors determining immediate and long-term results of operations in 605 patients. J Vasc Surg. 1986;3(3):389–404.

25. Gelman S, Khazaeli MB, Orr R, Henderson T. Blood volume redistribution during cross-clamping of the descending aorta. Anesth Analg. 1994;78(2):219–24.

26. Stokland O, Miller MM, Ilebekk A, Kiil F. Mechanism of hemodynamic responses to occlusion of the descending thoracic aorta. Am J Phys. 1980;238(4):H423–9.

27. Roizen MF, Beaupre PN, Alpert RA, Kremer P, Cahalan MK, Shiller N, et al. Monitoring with two-dimensional transesophageal echocardiography. Comparison of myocardial function in patients undergoing supraceliac, suprarenal-infraceliac, or infrarenal aortic occlusion. J Vasc Surg. 1984;1(2):300–5.

28. Acher CW, Wynn M. A modern theory of paraplegia in the treatment of aneurysms of the thoracoabdominal aorta: an analysis of technique specific observed/expected ratios for paralysis. J Vasc Surg. 2009;49(5):1117–24. discussion 24.

29. Melissano G, Bertoglio L, Rinaldi E, Leopardi M, Chiesa R. An anatomical review of spinal cord blood supply. J Cardiovasc Surg. 2015;56(5):699–706.

30. Connolly JE. Hume memorial lecture. Prevention of spinal cord complications in aortic surgery. Am J Surg. 1998;176(2):92–101.

31. Khan SN, Stansby G. Cerebrospinal fluid drainage for thoracic and thoracoabdominal aortic aneurysm surgery. Cochrane Database Syst Rev. 2012;10:CD003635.

32. Jacobs MJ, de Mol BA, Elenbaas T, Mess WH, Kalkman CJ, Schurink GW, et al. Spinal cord blood supply in patients with thoracoabdominal aortic aneurysms. J Vasc Surg. 2002;35(1):30–7.

33. Griepp RB, Griepp EB. Spinal cord protection in surgical and endovascular repair of thoracoabdominal aortic disease. J Thorac Cardiovasc Surg. 2015;149(2 Suppl):S86–90.

34. Etz CD, Zoli S, Bischoff MS, Bodian C, Di Luozzo G, Griepp RB. Measuring the collateral network pressure to minimize paraplegia risk in thoracoabdominal aneurysm resection. J Thorac Cardiovasc Surg. 2010;140(6 Suppl):S125–30. discussion S42-S46.

35. Backes WH, Nijenhuis RJ, Mess WH, Wilmink FA, Schurink GW, Jacobs MJ. Magnetic resonance angiography of collateral blood supply to spinal cord in thoracic and thoracoabdominal aortic aneurysm patients. J Vasc Surg. 2008;48(2):261–71.

36. Svensson LG, Crawford ES. Cardiovascular and vascular disease of the aorta. Philadelphia: W.B. Saunders Company; 1997.

37. Katz NM, Blackstone EH, Kirklin JW, Karp RB. Incremental risk factors for spinal cord injury following operation for acute traumatic aortic transection. J Thorac Cardiovasc Surg. 1981;81(5):669–74.

38. O'Callaghan A, Mastracci TM, Eagleton MJ. Staged endovascular repair of thoracoabdominal aortic aneurysms limits incidence and severity of spinal cord ischemia. J Vasc Surg. 2015;61(2):347–54. e1.

39. Davidovic L, Ilic N, Koncar I. Differences between immediate and late onset of spinal cord ischemia after open and endovascular aortic interventions. J Cardiovasc Surg. 2015;56(5):737–44.

40. Etz CD, Homann TM, Plestis KA, Zhang N, Luehr M, Weisz DJ, et al. Spinal cord perfusion after extensive segmental artery sacrifice: can paraplegia be prevented? Eur J Cardiothorac Surg. 2007;31(4):643–8.

41. Maurel B, Delclaux N, Sobocinski J, Hertault A, Martin-Gonzalez T, Moussa M, et al. The impact of early pelvic and lower limb reperfusion and attentive peri-operative management on the incidence of spinal cord ischemia during thoracoabdominal aortic aneurysm endovascular repair. Eur J Vasc Endovasc Surg. 2015;49(3):248–54.

42. Etz CD, Weigang E, Hartert M, Lonn L, Mestres CA, Di Bartolomeo R, et al. Contemporary spinal cord protection during thoracic and thoracoabdominal aortic surgery and endovascular aortic repair: a position paper of the vascular domain of the

European Association for Cardio-Thoracic Surgery dagger. Eur J Cardiothorac Surg. 2015;47(6):943–57.

43. Marini CP, Levison J, Caliendo F, Nathan IM, Cohen JR. Control of proximal hypertension during aortic cross-clamping: its effect on cerebrospinal fluid dynamics and spinal cord perfusion pressure. Semin Thorac Cardiovasc Surg. 1998;10(1):51–6.

44. Jacobs MJ, Mess W, Mochtar B, Nijenhuis RJ, Statius van Eps RG, Schurink GW. The value of motor evoked potentials in reducing paraplegia during thoracoabdominal aneurysm repair. J Vasc Surg. 2006;43(2):239–46.

45. Safi HJ, Miller CC 3rd, Azizzadeh A, Iliopoulos DC. Observations on delayed neurologic deficit after thoracoabdominal aortic aneurysm repair. J Vasc Surg. 1997;26(4):616–22.

46. Acher CW, Wynn MM, Mell MW, Tefera G, Hoch JR. A quantitative assessment of the impact of intercostal artery reimplantation on paralysis risk in thoracoabdominal aortic aneurysm repair. Ann Surg. 2008;248(4):529–40.

47. Estrera AL, Miller CC, Chen EP, Meada R, Torres RH, Porat EE, et al. Descending thoracic aortic aneurysm repair: 12-year experience using distal aortic perfusion and cerebrospinal fluid drainage. Ann Thorac Surg. 2005;80(4):1290–6. discussion 6.

48. Minatoya K, Ogino H, Matsuda H, Sasaki H, Yagihara T, Kitamura S. Replacement of the descending aorta: recent outcomes of open surgery performed with partial cardiopulmonary bypass. J Thorac Cardiovasc Surg. 2008;136(2):431–5.

49. Kulik A, Castner CF, Kouchoukos NT. Replacement of the descending thoracic aorta: contemporary outcomes using hypothermic circulatory arrest. J Thorac Cardiovasc Surg. 2010;139(2):249–55.

50. Di Luozzo G, Griepp RB. Experimental basis and clinical studies of brain protection in aortic arch surgery. In: Bosner RS, Pagano D, Haverich A, editors. Brain protection in cardiac surgery. London: Springer; 2011. p. 219–28.

51. Di Mauro M, Iaco AL, Di Lorenzo C, Gagliardi M, Varone E, Al Amri H, et al. Cold reperfusion before rewarming reduces neurological events after deep hypothermic circulatory arrest. Eur J Cardiothorac Surg. 2013;43(1):168–73.

52. Svensson LG, Crawford ES, Hess KR, Coselli JS, Raskin S, Shenaq SA, et al. Deep hypothermia with circulatory arrest. Determinants of stroke and early mortality in 656 patients. J Thorac Cardiovasc Surg. 1993;106(1):19–28; discussion -31.

53. Ziganshin BA, Rajbanshi BG, Tranquilli M, Fang H, Rizzo JA, Elefteriades JA. Straight deep hypothermic circulatory arrest for cerebral protection during aortic arch surgery: safe and effective. J Thorac Cardiovasc Surg. 2014;148(3):888–98; discussion 98-900.

54. Tian DH, Wan B, Bannon PG, Misfeld M, LeMaire SA, Kazui T, et al. A meta-analysis of deep hypothermic circulatory arrest versus moderate hypothermic circulatory arrest with selective antegrade cerebral perfusion. Ann Cardiothorac Surg. 2013;2(2):148–58.

55. De Paulis R, Czerny M, Weltert L, Bavaria J, Borger MA, Carrel TP, et al. Current trends in cannulation and neuroprotection during surgery of the aortic arch in Europe. Eur J Cardiothorac Surg. 2015;47(5):917–23.

56. Kamiya H, Hagl C, Kropivnitskaya I, Bothig D, Kallenbach K, Khaladj N, et al. The safety of moderate hypothermic lower body circulatory arrest with selective cerebral perfusion: a propensity score analysis. J Thorac Cardiovasc Surg. 2007;133(2):501–9.

57. Zierer A, El-Sayed Ahmad A, Papadopoulos N, Moritz A, Diegeler A, Urbanski PP. Selective antegrade cerebral perfusion and mild (28–30 °C) systemic hypothermic circulatory arrest for aortic arch replacement: results from 1002 patients. J Thorac Cardiovasc Surg. 2012;144(5):1042–9.

58. Lindsay H, Srinivas C, Djaiani G. Neuroprotection during aortic surgery. Best Pract Res Clin Anaesthesiol. 2016;30(3):283–303.

59. Duceppe E, Parlow J, MacDonald P, Lyons K, McMullen M, Srinathan S, et al. Canadian cardiovascular society guidelines on perioperative cardiac risk assessment and management

for patients who undergo noncardiac surgery. Can J Cardiol. 2017;33(1):17–32.

60. Fleisher LA, Fleischmann KE, Auerbach AD, Barnason SA, Beckman JA, Bozkurt B, et al. 2014 ACC/AHA guideline on perioperative cardiovascular evaluation and management of patients undergoing noncardiac surgery: executive summary: a report of the American College of Cardiology/American Heart Association task force on practice guidelines. Circulation. 2014;130(24):2215–45.

61. Roshanov PS, Rochwerg B, Patel A, Salehian O, Duceppe E, Belley-Côté EP, et al. Withholding versus continuing angiotensin-converting enzyme inhibitors or angiotensin II receptor blockers before noncardiac surgery: an analysis of the vascular events in noncardiac surgery patIents cOhort evaluatioN prospective cohort. Anesthesiology. 2017;126(1):16–27.

62. Coselli JS, LeMaire SA, Miller CC 3rd, Schmittling ZC, Koksoy C, Pagan J, et al. Mortality and paraplegia after thoracoabdominal aortic aneurysm repair: a risk factor analysis. Ann Thorac Surg. 2000;69(2):409–14.

63. Safi HJ, Estrera AL, Miller CC, Huynh TT, Porat EE, Azizzadeh A, et al. Evolution of risk for neurologic deficit after descending and thoracoabdominal aortic repair. Ann Thorac Surg. 2005;80(6):2173–9; discussion 9

64. Greenberg RK, Lu Q, Roselli EE, Svensson LG, Moon MC, Hernandez AV, et al. Contemporary analysis of descending thoracic and thoracoabdominal aneurysm repair: a comparison of endovascular and open techniques. Circulation. 2008;118(8):808–17.

65. Schlosser FJ, Mojibian H, Verhagen HJ, Moll FL, Muhs BE. Open thoracic or thoracoabdominal aortic aneurysm repair after previous abdominal aortic aneurysm surgery. J Vasc Surg. 2008;48(3):761–8.

66. American Society of Anesthesiologists. 10.28.15 Standards for Basic Anesthetic Monitoring Amended 2010, Affirmed 2015.

67. Sandham JD, Hull RD, Brant RF, Knox L, Pineo GF, Doig CJ, et al. A randomized, controlled trial of the use of pulmonary-artery catheters in high-risk surgical patients. N Engl J Med. 2003;348(1):5–14.

68. Dias NV, Sonesson B, Kristmundsson T, Holm H, Resch T. Short-term outcome of spinal cord ischemia after endovascular repair of thoracoabdominal aortic aneurysms. Eur J Vasc Endovasc Surg. 2015;49(4):403–9.

69. Meylaerts SA, Jacobs MJ, van Iterson V, De Haan P, Kalkman CJ. Comparison of transcranial motor evoked potentials and somatosensory evoked potentials during thoracoabdominal aortic aneurysm repair. Ann Surg. 1999;230(6):742–9.

70. Coselli JS, Tsai PI. Motor evoked potentials in thoracoabdominal aortic surgery: CON. Cardiol Clin. 2010;28(2):361–8.

71. Etz CD, von Aspern K, Gudehus S, Luehr M, Girrbach FF, Ender J, et al. Near-infrared spectroscopy monitoring of the collateral network prior to, during, and after thoracoabdominal aortic repair: a pilot study. Eur J Vasc Endovasc Surg. 2013;46(6):651–6.

72. Boezeman RP, van Dongen EP, Morshuis WJ, Sonker U, Boezeman EH, Waanders FG, et al. Spinal near-infrared spectroscopy measurements during and after thoracoabdominal aortic aneurysm repair: a pilot study. Ann Thorac Surg. 2015;99(4):1267–74.

73. Urbanski PP, Lenos A, Kolowca M, Bougioukakis P, Keller G, Zacher M, et al. Near-infrared spectroscopy for neuromonitoring of unilateral cerebral perfusion. Eur J Cardiothorac Surg. 2013;43(6):1140–4.

74. Zheng F, Sheinberg R, Yee MS, Ono M, Zheng Y, Hogue CW. Cerebral near-infrared spectroscopy monitoring and neurologic outcomes in adult cardiac surgery patients: a systematic review. Anesth Analg. 2013;116(3):663–76.

75. Arrowsmith JE, Ganugapenta MSSR. Intraoperative brain monitoring in cardiac surgery. In: Bosner RS, Pagano D, Haverich A,

editors. Brain protection in cardiac surgery. London: Spinger; 2011. p. 83–111.

76. Douds MT, Straub EJ, Kent AC, Bistrick CH, Sistino JJ. A systematic review of cerebral oxygenation-monitoring devices in cardiac surgery. Perfusion. 2014;29(6):545–52.

77. Fedorow C, Grocott HP. Cerebral monitoring to optimize outcomes after cardiac surgery. Curr Opin Anaesthesiol. 2010;23(1):89–94.

78. Mohandas BS, Jagadeesh AM, Vikram SB. Impact of monitoring cerebral oxygen saturation on the outcome of patients undergoing open heart surgery. Ann Cardiac Anesth. 2013;16(2):102–6.

79. Deschamps A, Hall R, Grocott H, Mazer CD, Choi PT, Turgeon AF, et al. Cerebral oximetry monitoring to maintain Normal Cerebral Oxygen Saturation during high-risk cardiac surgery: a randomized controlled feasibility trial. Anesthesiology. 2016;124(4):826–36.

80. Khoyratty SI, Gajendragadkar PR, Polisetty K, Ward S, Skinner T. Flow rates through intravenous access devices: an in vitro study. J Clin Anesth. 2016;31:101–5.

81. van der Zee EN, Egal M, Gommers D, Groeneveld AB. Targeting urine output and 30-day mortality in goal-directed therapy: a systematic review with meta-analysis and meta-regression. BMC Anesthesiol. 2017;17(1):22.

82. Egal M, de Geus HR, van Bommel J, Groeneveld AB. Targeting oliguria reversal in perioperative restrictive fluid management does not influence the occurrence of renal dysfunction: a systematic review and meta-analysis. Eur J Anaesthesiol. 2016;33(6):425–35.

83. Alpert RA, Roizen MF, Hamilton WK, Stoney RJ, Ehrenfeld WK, Poler SM, et al. Intraoperative urinary output does not predict postoperative renal function in patients undergoing abdominal aortic revascularization. Surgery. 1984;95(6):707–11.

84. Kheterpal S, Tremper KK, Englesbe MJ, O'Reilly M, Shanks AM, Fetterman DM, et al. Predictors of postoperative acute renal failure after noncardiac surgery in patients with previously normal renal function. Anesthesiology. 2007;107(6):892–902.

85. Sear JW. Kidney dysfunction in the postoperative period. Br J Anaesth. 2005;95(1):20–32.

86. Shine T, Nugent M. Sodium nitroprusside decreases spinal cord perfusion pressure during descending thoracic aortic cross-clamping in the dog. J Cardiothorac Anesth. 1990;4(2):185–93.

87. Flaherty JT, Magee PA, Gardner TL, Potter A, MacAllister NP. Comparison of intravenous nitroglycerin and sodium nitroprusside for treatment of acute hypertension developing after coronary artery bypass surgery. Circulation. 1982;65(6):1072–7.

88. Gelman S, Reves JG, Fowler K, Samuelson PN, Lell WA, Smith LR. Regional blood flow during cross-clamping of the thoracic aorta and infusion of sodium nitroprusside. J Thorac Cardiovasc Surg. 1983;85(2):287–91.

89. National Blood Authority. Patient Blood Management Guidelines: Module 1- Critical Bleeding/Massive Transfusion. Canberra, Australia 2011.

90. Management ASoATFoPB. Practice guidelines for perioperative blood management: an updated report by the American Society of Anesthesiologists Task Force on Perioperative Blood Management*. Anesthesiology. 2015;122(2):241–75.

91. Karkouti K, Callum J, Wijeysundera DN, Rao V, Crowther M, Grocott HP, et al. Point-of-care hemostatic testing in cardiac surgery: a stepped-wedge clustered randomized controlled trial. Circulation. 2016;134(16):1152–62.

92. Myles PS, Smith JA, Forbes A, Silbert B, Jayarajah M, Painter T, et al. Tranexamic acid in patients undergoing coronary-artery surgery. N Engl J Med. 2017;376(2):136–48.

93. Cheung AT, Weiss SJ, McGarvey ML, Stecker MM, Hogan MS, Escherich A, et al. Interventions for reversing delayed-onset postoperative paraplegia after thoracic aortic reconstruction. Ann Thorac Surg. 2002;74(2):413–9; discussion 20-1.

94. Coselli JS, LeMaire SA, Koksoy C, Schmittling ZC, Curling PE. Cerebrospinal fluid drainage reduces paraplegia after tho-

racoabdominal aortic aneurysm repair: results of a randomized clinical trial. J Vasc Surg. 2002;35(4):631–9.

95. Ullery BW, Cheung AT, Fairman RM, Jackson BM, Woo EY, Bavaria J, et al. Risk factors, outcomes, and clinical manifestations of spinal cord ischemia following thoracic endovascular aortic repair. J Vasc Surg. 2011;54(3):677–84.

96. Wong CS, Healy D, Canning C, Coffey JC, Boyle JR, Walsh SR. A systematic review of spinal cord injury and cerebrospinal fluid drainage after thoracic aortic endografting. J Vasc Surg. 2012;56(5):1438–47.

97. Dardik A, Perler BA, Roseborough GS, Williams GM. Subdural hematoma after thoracoabdominal aortic aneurysm repair: an underreported complication of spinal fluid drainage? J Vasc Surg. 2002;36(1):47–50.

98. Estrera AL, Sheinbaum R, Miller CC, Azizzadeh A, Walkes JC, Lee TY, et al. Cerebrospinal fluid drainage during thoracic aortic repair: safety and current management. Ann Thorac Surg. 2009;88(1):9–15; discussion 15.

99. Hanna JM, Andersen ND, Aziz H, Shah AA, McCann RL, Hughes GC. Results with selective preoperative lumbar drain placement for thoracic endovascular aortic repair. Ann Thorac Surg. 2013;95(6):1968–74; discussion 74-5.

100. McHardy FE, Bayly PJ, Wyatt MG. Fatal subdural hemorrhage following lumbar spinal drainage during repair of thoracoabdominal aneurysm. Anaesthesia. 2001;56(2):168–70.

101. Verhoeven EL, Katsargyris A, Bekkema F, Oikonomou K, Zeebregts CJ, Ritter W, et al. Editor's choice-ten-year experience with endovascular repair of thoracoabdominal aortic aneurysms: results from 166 consecutive patients. Eur J Vasc Endovasc Surg. 2015;49(5):524–31.

102. Wynn MM, Sebranek J, Marks E, Engelbert T, Acher CW. Complications of spinal fluid drainage in thoracic and thoracoabdominal aortic aneurysm surgery in 724 patients treated from 1987 to 2013. J Cardiothorac Vasc Anesth. 2015;29(2):342–50.

103. Youngblood SC, Tolpin DA, LeMaire SA, Coselli JS, Lee VV, Cooper JR Jr. Complications of cerebrospinal fluid drainage after thoracic aortic surgery: a review of 504 patients over 5 years. J Thorac Cardiovasc Surg. 2013;146(1):166–71.

104. Weaver KD, Wiseman DB, Farber M, Ewend MG, Marston W, Keagy BA. Complications of lumbar drainage after thoracoabdominal aortic aneurysm repair. J Vasc Surg. 2001;34(4):623–7.

105. Bobadilla JL, Wynn M, Tefera G, Acher CW. Low incidence of paraplegia after thoracic endovascular aneurysm repair with proactive spinal cord protective protocols. J Vasc Surg. 2013;57(6):1537–42.

106. Augoustides JG, Stone ME, Drenger B. Novel approaches to spinal cord protection during thoracoabdominal aortic interventions. Curr Opin Anaesthesiol. 2014;27(1):98–105.

107. Fedorow CA, Moon MC, Mutch WA, Grocott HP. Lumbar cerebrospinal fluid drainage for thoracoabdominal aortic surgery: rationale and practical considerations for management. Anesth Analg. 2010;111(1):46–58.

108. Field M, Doolan J, Safar M, Kuduvalli M, Oo A, Mills K, et al. The safe use of spinal drains in thoracic aortic surgery. Interact Cardiovasc Thorac Surg. 2011;13(6):557–65.

109. Cheung AT, Pochettino A, McGarvey ML, Appoo JJ, Fairman RM, Carpenter JP, et al. Strategies to manage paraplegia risk after endovascular stent repair of descending thoracic aortic aneurysms. Ann Thorac Surg. 2005;80(4):1280–8; discussion 8-9.

110. Rizvi AZ, Sullivan TM. Incidence, prevention, and management in spinal cord protection during TEVAR. J Vasc Surg. 2010;52(4 Suppl):86s–90s.

111. Kise Y, Kuniyoshi Y, Inafuku H, Nagano T, Hirayasu T, Yamashiro S. Directly measuring spinal cord blood flow and spinal cord perfusion pressure via the collateral network: correlations with

changes in systemic blood pressure. J Thorac Cardiovasc Surg. 2015;149(1):360–6.

112. Chiesa R, Melissano G, Marrocco-Trischitta MM, Civilini E, Setacci F. Spinal cord ischemia after elective stent-graft repair of the thoracic aorta. J Vasc Surg. 2005;42(1):11–7.

113. Crawford ES, Svensson LG, Hess KR, Shenaq SS, Coselli JS, Safi HJ, et al. A prospective randomized study of cerebrospinal fluid drainage to prevent paraplegia after high-risk surgery on the thoracoabdominal aorta. J Vasc Surg. 1991;13(1):36–45; discussion -6.

114. Chang CK, Chuter TA, Reilly LM, Ota MK, Furtado A, Bucci M, et al. Spinal arterial anatomy and risk factors for lower extremity weakness following endovascular thoracoabdominal aortic aneurysm repair with branched stent-grafts. J Endovasc Ther. 2008;15(3):356–62.

115. Coselli JS, LeMaire SA. Left heart bypass reduces paraplegia rates after thoracoabdominal aortic aneurysm repair. Ann Thorac Surg. 1999;67(6):1931–4; discussion 53–8.

116. Nijenhuis RJ, Jacobs MJ, Schurink GW, Kessels AG, van Engelshoven JM, Backes WH. Magnetic resonance angiography and neuromonitoring to assess spinal cord blood supply in thoracic and thoracoabdominal aortic aneurysm surgery. J Vasc Surg. 2007;45(1):71–7; discussion 7–8

117. Cambria RP, Clouse WD, Davison JK, Dunn PF, Corey M, Dorer D. Thoracoabdominal aneurysm repair: results with 337 operations performed over a 15-year interval. Ann Surg. 2002;236(4):471–9; discussion 9.

118. Cambria RP, Davison JK, Carter C, Brewster DC, Chang Y, Clark KA, et al. Epidural cooling for spinal cord protection during thoracoabdominal aneurysm repair: a five-year experience. J Vasc Surg. 2000;31(6):1093–102.

119. Svensson LG, Hess KR, Coselli JS, Safi HJ. Influence of segmental arteries, extent, and atriofemoral bypass on postoperative paraplegia after thoracoabdominal aortic operations. J Vasc Surg. 1994;20(2):255–62.

120. Safi HJ, Miller CC 3rd, Carr C, Iliopoulos DC, Dorsay DA, Baldwin JC. Importance of intercostal artery reattachment during thoracoabdominal aortic aneurysm repair. J Vasc Surg. 1998;27(1):58–66; discussion -8.

121. Etz CD, Halstead JC, Spielvogel D, Shahani R, Lazala R, Homann TM, et al. Thoracic and thoracoabdominal aneurysm repair: is reimplantation of spinal cord arteries a waste of time? Ann Thorac Surg. 2006;82(5):1670–7.

122. Griepp RB, Ergin MA, Galla JD, Lansman S, Khan N, Quintana C, et al. Looking for the artery of Adamkiewicz: a quest to minimize paraplegia after operations for aneurysms of the descending thoracic and thoracoabdominal aorta. J Thorac Cardiovasc Surg. 1996;112(5):1202–13; discussion 13–5.

123. Czerny M, Eggebrecht H, Sodeck G, Verzini F, Cao P, Maritati G, et al. Mechanisms of symptomatic spinal cord ischemia after TEVAR: insights from the European Registry of Endovascular Aortic Repair Complications (EuREC). J Endovasc Ther. 2012;19(1):37–43.

124. Amabile P, Grisoli D, Giorgi R, Bartoli JM, Piquet P. Incidence and determinants of spinal cord ischemia in stent-graft repair of the thoracic aorta. Eur J Vasc Endovasc Surg. 2008;35(4):455–61.

125. Drinkwater SL, Goebells A, Haydar A, Bourke P, Brown L, Hamady M, et al. The incidence of spinal cord ischemia following thoracic and thoracoabdominal aortic endovascular intervention. Eur J Vasc Endovasc Surg. 2010;40(6):729–35.

126. Rizvi AZ, Murad MH, Fairman RM, Erwin PJ, Montori VM. The effect of left subclavian artery coverage on morbidity and mortality in patients undergoing endovascular thoracic aortic interventions: a systematic review and meta-analysis. J Vasc Surg. 2009;50(5):1159–69.

127. Patterson BO, Holt PJ, Nienaber C, Fairman RM, Heijmen RH, Thompson MM. Management of the left subclavian artery and neurologic complications after thoracic endovascular aortic repair. J Vasc Surg. 2014;60(6):1491–7.e1.

128. Sepehripour AH, Ahmed K, Vecht JA, Anagnostakou V, Suliman A, Ashrafian H, et al. Management of the left subclavian artery during endovascular stent grafting for traumatic aortic injury - a systematic review. Eur J Vasc Endovasc Surg. 2011;41(6):758–69.

129. Weigang E, Parker JA, Czerny M, Lonn L, Bonser RS, Carrel TP, et al. Should intentional endovascular stent-graft coverage of the left subclavian artery be preceded by prophylactic revascularization? Eur J Cardiothorac Surg. 2011;40(4):858–68.

130. De Bakey ME, Cooley DA, Creech O Jr. Resection of the aorta for aneurysms and occlusive disease with particular reference to the use of hypothermia; analysis of 240 cases. Trans Am Coll Cardiol. 1955;5:153–7.

131. Conrad MF, Crawford RS, Davison JK, Cambria RP. Thoracoabdominal aneurysm repair: a 20-year perspective. The Annals of thoracic surgery. 2007;83(2):S856–61; discussion S90–2.

132. Kouchoukos NT, Masetti P, Murphy SF. Hypothermic cardiopulmonary bypass and circulatory arrest in the management of extensive thoracic and thoracoabdominal aortic aneurysms. Semin Thorac Cardiovasc Surg. 2003;15(4):333–9.

133. Kulik A, Castner CF, Kouchoukos NT. Outcomes after thoracoabdominal aortic aneurysm repair with hypothermic circulatory arrest. J Thorac Cardiovasc Surg. 2011;141(4):953–60.

134. Frank SM, Parker SD, Rock P, Gorman RB, Kelly S, Beattie C, et al. Moderate hypothermia, with partial bypass and segmental sequential repair for thoracoabdominal aortic aneurysm. J Vasc Surg. 1994;19(4):687–97.

135. Svensson LG, Hess KR, D'Agostino RS, Entrup MH, Hreib K, Kimmel WA, et al. Reduction of neurologic injury after high-risk thoracoabdominal aortic operation. Ann Thorac Surg. 1998;66(1):132–8.

136. Griepp RB, Di Luozzo G. Hypothermia for aortic surgery. J Thorac Cardiovasc Surg. 2013;145(3 Suppl):S56–8.

137. Bush HL Jr, Hydo LJ, Fischer E, Fantini GA, Silane MF, Barie PS. Hypothermia during elective abdominal aortic aneurysm repair: the high price of avoidable morbidity. J Vasc Surg. 1995;21(3):392–400; discussion -2.

138. Safi HJ, Miller CC 3rd, Subramaniam MH, Campbell MP, Iliopoulos DC, O'Donnell JJ, et al. Thoracic and thoracoabdominal aortic aneurysm repair using cardiopulmonary bypass, profound hypothermia, and circulatory arrest via left side of the chest incision. J Vasc Surg. 1998;28(4):591–8.

139. Acher CW, Wynn MM, Hoch JR, Popic P, Archibald J, Turnipseed WD. Combined use of cerebral spinal fluid drainage and naloxone reduces the risk of paraplegia in thoracoabdominal aneurysm repair. J Vasc Surg. 1994;19(2):236–46; discussion 47–8.

140. Kunihara T, Matsuzaki K, Shiiya N, Saijo Y, Yasuda K. Naloxone lowers cerebrospinal fluid levels of excitatory amino acids after thoracoabdominal aortic surgery. J Vasc Surg. 2004;40(4): 681–90.

141. Lima B, Nowicki ER, Blackstone EH, Williams SJ, Roselli EE, Sabik JF 3rd, et al. Spinal cord protective strategies during descending and thoracoabdominal aortic aneurysm repair in the modern era: the role of intrathecal papaverine. J Thorac Cardiovasc Surg. 2012;143(4):945–52.e1.

142. Nylander WA Jr, Plunkett RJ, Hammon JW Jr, Oldfield EH, Meacham WF. Thiopental modification of ischemic spinal cord injury in the dog. Ann Thorac Surg. 1982;33(1):64–8.

143. Fowl RJ, Patterson RB, Gewirtz RJ, Anderson DK. Protection against postischemic spinal cord injury using a new 21-aminosteroid. J Surg Res. 1990;48(6):597–600.

144. Apaydin AZ, Buket S. Regional lidocaine infusion reduces postischemic spinal cord injury in rabbits. Tex Heart Inst J. 2001;28(3):172–6.

145. Wu GJ, Chen WF, Sung CS, Jean YH, Shih CM, Shyu CY, et al. Preventive effects of intrathecal methylprednisolone administration on spinal cord ischemia in rats: the role of excitatory amino acid metabolizing systems. Neuroscience. 2007;147(2):294–303.

146. Qayumi AK, Janusz MT, Jamieson WR, Lyster DM. Pharmacologic interventions for prevention of spinal cord injury caused by aortic crossclamping. J Thorac Cardiovasc Surg. 1992;104(2):256–61.

147. Lim KH, Connolly M, Rose D, Siegman F, Jacobowitz I, Acinapura A, et al. Prevention of reperfusion injury of the ischemic spinal cord: use of recombinant superoxide dismutase. Ann Thorac Surg. 1986;42(3):282–6.

148. Smith PD, Bell MT, Puskas F, Meng X, Cleveland JC Jr, Weyant MJ, et al. Preservation of motor function after spinal cord ischemia and reperfusion injury through microglial inhibition. Ann Thorac Surg. 2013;95(5):1647–53.

149. Mares JM, Foley LS, Bell MT, Bennett DT, Freeman KA, Meng X, et al. Erythropoietin activates the phosporylated cAMP [adenosine 3'5' cyclic monophosphate] response element-binding protein pathway and attenuates delayed paraplegia after ischemia-reperfusion injury. J Thorac Cardiovasc Surg. 2015;149(3):920–4.

150. Gurer B, Kertmen H, Kasim E, Yilmaz ER, Kanat BH, Sargon MF, et al. Neuroprotective effects of testosterone on ischemia/reperfusion injury of the rabbit spinal cord. Injury. 2015;46(2):240–8.

151. Freeman KA, Fullerton DA, Foley LS, Bell MT, Cleveland JC Jr, Weyant MJ, et al. Spinal cord protection via alpha-2 agonist-mediated increase in glial cell-line-derived neurotrophic factor. J Thorac Cardiovasc Surg. 2015;149(2):578–84; discussion 84–6.

152. Horlocker TT, Wedel DJ, Rowlingson JC, Enneking FK, Kopp SL, Benzon HT, et al. Regional anesthesia in the patient receiving antithrombotic or thrombolytic therapy: American Society of Regional Anesthesia and Pain Medicine evidence-based guidelines (third edition). Reg Anesth Pain Med. 2010;35(1):64–101.

153. Wynn MM, Mell MW, Tefera G, Hoch JR, Acher CW. Complications of spinal fluid drainage in thoracoabdominal aortic aneurysm repair: a report of 486 patients treated from 1987 to 2008. J Vasc Surg. 2009;49(1):29–34; discussion -5.

154. American Society of Anesthesiologists. Practice advisory for the prevention, diagnosis, and management of infectious complications associated with neuraxial techniques: an updated report by the American Society of Anesthesiologists Task Force on infectious complications associated with neuraxial techniques and the American Society of Regional Anesthesia and Pain Medicine. Anesthesiology. 2017;126(4):585–601.

155. Australia New Zealand College of Anaesthetists Guidelines for the Management of Major Regional Analgesia. Australia New Zealand College of Anaesthetists; 2011. p. 6.

156. Obstetric Anaesthetists' Association, Campbell JP, Plaat F, Checketts MR, Bogod D, Tighe S, et al. Safety guideline: skin antisepsis for central neuraxial blockade. Anaesthesia. 2014;69(11):1279–86.

157. Tshomba Y, Leopardi M, Mascia D, Kahlberg A, Carozzo A, Magrin S, et al. Automated pressure-controlled cerebrospinal fluid drainage during open thoracoabdominal aortic aneurysm repair. J Vasc Surg. 2017;66:37.

158. Wynn MM, Acher C, Marks E, Engelbert T, Acher CW. Postoperative renal failure in thoracoabdominal aortic aneurysm repair with simple cross-clamp technique and 4°C renal perfusion. J Vasc Surg. 2015;61(3):611–22.

159. Kashyap VS, Cambria RP, Davison JK, L'Italien GJ. Renal failure after thoracoabdominal aortic surgery. J Vasc Surg. 1997;26(6):949–55; discussion 55–7.

160. Dariane C, Coscas R, Boulitrop C, Javerliat I, Vilaine E, Goeau-Brissonniere O, et al. Acute kidney injury after open repair of intact abdominal aortic aneurysms. Ann Vasc Surg. 2017;39:294–300.

161. Yeung KK, Groeneveld M, Lu JJ, van Diemen P, Jongkind V, Wisselink W. Organ protection during aortic cross-clamping. Best Pract Res Clin Anaesthesiol. 2016;30(3):305–15.

162. Swaminathan M, Stafford-Smith M. Renal dysfunction after vascular surgery. Curr Opin Anaesthesiol. 2003;16(1):45–51.

163. Zacharias M, Mugawar M, Herbison GP, Walker RJ, Hovhannisyan K, Sivalingam P, et al. Interventions for protecting renal function in the perioperative period. Cochrane Database Syst Rev. 2013;9:CD003590.

164. Marik PE. Low-dose dopamine: a systematic review. Intensive Care Med. 2002;28(7):877–83.

165. Bellomo R, Chapman M, Finfer S, Hickling K, Myburgh J. Low-dose dopamine in patients with early renal dysfunction: a placebo-controlled randomized trial. Australian and New Zealand Intensive Care Society (ANZICS) Clinical Trials Group. Lancet. 2000;356(9248):2139–43.

166. Kellum JA, M Decker J. Use of dopamine in acute renal failure: a meta-analysis. Crit Care Med. 2001;29(8):1526–31.

167. Friedrich JO, Adhikari N, Herridge MS, Beyene J. Meta-analysis: low-dose dopamine increases urine output but does not prevent renal dysfunction or death. Ann Intern Med. 2005;142(7):510–24.

168. Doi K, Ogawa N, Suzuki E, Noiri E, Fujita T. Mannitol-induced acute renal failure. Am J Med. 2003;115(7):593–4.

169. Perdue PW, Balser JR, Lipsett PA, Breslow MJ. "Renal dose" dopamine in surgical patients: dogma or science? Ann Surg. 1998;227(4):470–3.

170. Visweswaran P, Massin EK, Dubose TD. Mannitol-induced acute renal failure. J Am Soc Nephrol. 1997;8(6):1028–33.

171. Subramaniam RM, Suarez-Cuervo C, Wilson RF, Turban S, Zhang A, Sherrod C, et al. Effectiveness of prevention strategies for contrast-induced nephropathy: a systematic review and meta-analysis. Ann Intern Med. 2016;164(6):406–16.

172. Xu R, Tao A, Bai Y, Deng Y, Chen G. Effectiveness of N-Acetylcysteine for the prevention of contrast-induced nephropathy: a systematic review and meta-analysis of randomized controlled trials. J Am Heart Assoc. 2016;5(9):e003968.

173. Durrani NK, Yavuzer R, Mittal V, Bradford MM, Lobocki C, Silberberg B. The effect of gradually increased blood flow on ischemia-reperfusion injury in rat kidney. Am J Surg. 2006;191(3):334–7.

174. Köksoy C, LeMaire SA, Curling PE, Raskin SA, Schmittling ZC, Conklin LD, et al. Renal perfusion during thoracoabdominal aortic operations: cold crystalloid is superior to normothermic blood. Ann Thorac Surg. 2002;73(3):730–8.

175. Lemaire SA, Jones MM, Conklin LD, Carter SA, Criddell MD, Wang XL, et al. Randomized comparison of cold blood and cold crystalloid renal perfusion for renal protection during thoracoabdominal aortic aneurysm repair. J Vasc Surg. 2009;49(1):11–9; discussion 9.

176. Cambria R. Commentary. Thoracic and thoracoabdominal aneurysm repair: is reimplantation of spinal cord arteries a waste of time? Perspect Vasc Surg Endovasc Ther. 2008;20(2):221–3.

Thoracic Anesthesia in the Developing World

42

Swapnil Yeshwant Parab and Sheila Nainan Myatra

Key Points

- Surgical and anesthesia practices are often modified to strike a balance between available resources and improving outcome of the patients.
- Patients presenting for thoracic surgeries are often suffering from pyogenic infections, TB, and helminthiasis. In addition to being sick and infectious, they also suffer from chronic malnourishment and anemia.
- Respiratory physiotherapy, including muscle-strengthening exercises, helps to improve the cardiorespiratory conditioning of the patient. The quantity of time spent performing physiotherapy exercises is an important determinant of improvement in respiratory functions.
- In developing countries, the choice of lung isolation device depends largely on the availability of the device and fiber-optic bronchoscopes. In absence of a pediatric fiber-optic bronchoscope, DLTs are preferred over bronchial blockers as DLTs can be inserted blindly and their position can be confirmed by clinical methods like inspection of chest expansion and auscultation.
- Thoracic surgery for infectious processes is more likely to develop intraoperative bleeding.
- With improvements in anesthesia and surgical methods, thoracic surgery for complications of pulmonary tuberculosis is less morbid than previously. As a result, the need for surgery is increasing.
- Some patients who present for surgery due to empyema will have an underlying bronchopleural fistula. A history of position-related productive cough should be carefully sought.

Introduction

The last five decades have witnessed a significant decline in total perioperative mortality (from 10,603 per million before the 1970s to 1176 per million in the 1990s–2000s) [1]. Reduction in anesthesia-related perioperative mortality has been one of the reasons for improvement in perioperative care. This improvement has been largely due to vast research and development in fields of anesthesia and perioperative medicine leading to better understanding of physiology; application of evidence-based safe anesthesia practices, drugs, and techniques; and vigilant perioperative monitoring. However, the improvement is not uniform across the globe and has occurred mainly in developed countries. Perioperative mortality risk is still two to three times higher in low-income countries as compared to high-income countries [1]. Degrees of development in the field of anesthesia and perioperative medicine vary from country to country and also within each country. In developing countries, there are few centers which maintain similar standard of care as that in developed countries and struggle to meet the demands of heavy patient load, within the limits of available resources [2]. In these countries where primary healthcare needs are unmet, specialty fields like thoracic anesthesia have a long way to go.

Challenges Faced by Thoracic Anesthesiologist in the Developing World

(a) Spectrum of disease:
   Respiratory diseases are among the leading causes of death worldwide. Lung infections (mostly pneumonia and tuberculosis), lung cancer, and chronic obstructive pulmonary disease (COPD) together accounted for 9.5 million deaths worldwide during 2008 (one-sixth of the global total) [3]. Among these diseases, lung infection is

S. Y. Parab · S. N. Myatra (✉)
Department of Anesthesiology, Critical Care and Pain,
Tata Memorial Hospital, Mumbai, Maharashtra, India

© Springer Nature Switzerland AG 2019
P. Slinger (ed.), *Principles and Practice of Anesthesia for Thoracic Surgery*, https://doi.org/10.1007/978-3-030-00859-8_42

the leading overall cause of mortality in developing countries [4]. Low immunization rates, overcrowding, poor nutrition, and HIV infection are among the common causes for acute lung infections. On the other hand, industrialization, air pollution, indoor smoke, and cigarette smoking are common causes for growing incidence of chronic respiratory conditions like COPD, asbestosis, pneumoconiosis, and asthma. Growing civilization has increased the numbers of road traffic accidents and chest trauma. Thoracic surgeries are conducted largely for the management of infection-related diseases like bronchiectasis, empyema, lung abscess, pulmonary hydatid cysts, and complicated tuberculosis (TB). These patients are often sick and infectious. Many patients are chronically malnourished and anemic. They often present late for the treatment due to ignorance and poverty.

(b) Human resources:

In the developing world, especially in the rural and the underprivileged areas, safe anesthesia services are lacking [5]. Some tertiary care centers and private institutes offer subspecialty services like thoracic anesthesia, but they are few in numbers and unable to meet the huge patient load. Often patients have to travel a long distance to reach these centers. Majority of trained doctors prefer to work in major cities for better opportunities, income, and lifestyle, leading to uneven distribution of skilled manpower. A study on anesthesia services in Haiti, a developing country, showed that non-physicians conduct majority of anesthesia procedures [6]. Another survey showed severe shortage of manpower and other resources was present even at the university teaching hospital in Zambia [7]. Dubowitz et al. highlighted that number of anesthesia providers per capita of population in developing countries was significantly less in comparison to developed world [8].

Apart from anesthesiologists and thoracic surgeons, a thoracic surgery unit involves the active participation of well-trained nursing staff, chest physicians, and physiotherapists. In many developing countries, there is neither a nurse anesthetist nor a technician. The anesthesiologist has the sole responsibility to deliver safe anesthesia. Lack of structured educational programs for nurses and other paramedical staff and meagre salaries are often the reasons for shortage of skilled support staff.

(c) Technical and infrastructural resources:

Apart from a trained anesthesiologist, safety of anesthesia services depends upon availability of monitors, drugs, anesthesia workstations, and other equipment. In addition, adequate laboratory, blood bank, and radiodiagnostic facilities are essential. In developing countries, uniform availability of such technical and infrastructural resources is lacking. Even in the twenty-first century, in developing country like Uganda, 74% of anesthesiolo-

gists reported lack of pulse oximetry in the operation theaters, the most commonly used volatile anesthetic was ether (68%), and drugs like non-depolarizing muscle relaxants were not available to 69% of anesthesiologists [9]. Specific to thoracic anesthesia, pediatric fiber-optic bronchoscopes, fluoroscopy machines, ultrasound machines, small sizes of bronchial blockers and double-lumen tubes (DLT), and multichannel monitors are unavailable in many centers. In some centers, pulmonary functions are often assessed by bedside tests, and objective spirometry examination is not available. Cardiopulmonary exercise testing (CPET) and lung perfusion scans are available only at few centers across the country. Common reasons for the unavailability of these resources are financial burden and lack of trained staff to maintain these services. As a result, the thoracic anesthesiologist often has to adapt to the needs and situation and make proper utilization of available resources to deliver safe anesthesia. This has led to development of many "adaptive modifications" in the practices of thoracic anesthesia. These have been discussed in separate section later in the chapter.

(d) Education and research:

In developing countries, there is a lack of uniformity in delivering proper education in anesthesia. Tertiary care centers are few in numbers, and in these centers, there is often a shortage of teaching staff. Many trained professionals do not take up teaching jobs, due to meagre salaries paid in teaching institutes. As a result, training to medical students, residents, and nurses cannot be imparted properly. In many developing countries, language barrier is a major hurdle in imparting education in anesthesia. Even within a country, a uniform national language is not followed, and local languages are often used for communications. Hence, it becomes a great difficulty for faculties from developed countries to impart education in conferences.

Underreporting, poorly maintained medical records, lack of electronic database, failure to conduct proper audits, and quality improvement drills are some of the obstacles in fields of medical research. If publication in journals is considered as crude indicator of research standards, then a bibliometric analysis of highly cited anesthesia journals showed a meagre (0.3%) contribution from low-income countries [10].

Conduct of Thoracic Anesthesia in Developing World: Meeting the Challenge

Surgical and anesthesia practices are often modified to strike a balance between available resources and improving outcome of the patients. Principles of anesthesia management for patients undergoing thoracic surgeries in developing world share some common aspects during preoperative, intraoperative, and postoperative periods. At the same time, certain aspects are disease specific and need modifications in anesthesia management. Following are the common aspects of anesthesia management for thoracic surgeries in developing countries.

Preoperative Care: Assessment and Optimization

- *Malnutrition*: Patients presenting for thoracic surgeries are often suffering from pyogenic infections, TB, and helminthiasis. In addition to being sick and infectious, they also suffer from chronic malnourishment and anemia. With ongoing catabolism and inadequate oral intake, patients tend to lose weight and muscle mass, developing a state of protein-energy malnutrition (defined as a negative balance of 100 g of nitrogen and 10,000 kcal within a few days) [11]. Resultant physiological and psychological changes lead to "deconditioning" of the patient [12]. It requires a team of nutritionist, respiratory physiotherapist, and psychologist to optimize the general health of the patient. In the developing world, shortage of skilled support staff results in the responsibility for optimization of patient being shared by primary physician, anesthesiologist, and family members of the patient, sometimes with additional help from medical social workers. All the efforts to improve nutritional status of the patients are required to be started as early as possible. Nutritional demands vary from patient to patient, but care needs to be taken to meet the requirements for protein, energy, and micronutrients. Enteral nutrition is preferred over parenteral route. Patients with esophageal diseases suffer from severe dysphagia. Such patients should undergo endoscopy-guided nasogastric tube insertion. Neoadjuvant chemotherapy in case of esophageal cancers relieves dysphagia in many patients. Usually, a week of nutritional support is required to halt the catabolic state of the patient, and a month is required to regain nutritional status. However, often due to late presentation, there is hardly any time available for nutritional optimization. Nonavailability of good value nutritional products, poor financial status of the patient, and illiteracy leads to inadequate nutritional optimization of patient.
- *Anemia*: Anemia is a major public health problem in developing world. In developing countries, anemia affects 42% of children less than 5 years of age and 53% children between 5 and 14 years of age [13]. Women of childbearing age form another vulnerable population suffering from anemia. Nearly 7.5–33% patients suffering from COPD are also affected by anemia, the most common cause being anemia of chronic disease [14]. Anemia is often due to iron deficiency, following anorexia, faulty food habits, diet deficient in iron supplements, and worm infestations. Deworming agents like oral albendazole as a single dose should be considered especially in children. Hematinic and multivitamin supplements should be started from the first visit. If patient is intolerant to oral iron supplements or unable to swallow, then intravenous iron replacement or packed cell transfusions should be given prior to surgery. Recently, available intravenous iron supplementations are safe, effective, and quick in increasing hemoglobin level prior to surgery and can avoid transfusion-related risks.
- *Respiratory optimization*: Infections of the respiratory tract are the leading cause of mortality in the developing world. Chronic respiratory diseases are also prevalent in developing countries. They include restrictive lung diseases like pneumoconiosis, asbestosis, byssinosis, etc. and obstructive airway diseases like asthma and forms of COPD – emphysema, peripheral airway diseases, and chronic bronchitis. Patients undergo preoperative radiological imaging and pulmonary function tests to know the severity of the disease. Respiratory optimization includes administration of bronchodilators, good hydration, frequent nebulization, postural drainage of the secretions, and treatment of infections. Respiratory physiotherapy, including muscle-strengthening exercises, helps to improve the cardiorespiratory conditioning of the patient. The quantity of time spent performing physiotherapy exercises is an important determinant of improvement in respiratory functions. Patients with excessive sputum production (e.g., chronic bronchitis) are most benefited by chest physiotherapy. Hence, chest physiotherapy should begin as early as possible. Proper education and counselling of the patient are required to improve the compliance of the patient to perform physiotherapy exercises.

Intraoperative Care

During the intraoperative period, the aim of the thoracic anesthesiologist is to maintain the safety of the patient, amidst the deficiencies of technical resources and skilled manpower. The inadequately optimized general condition of the patient often adds to the challenges. Following is a discussion about certain areas of special attention when administering anesthesia for thoracic surgery in developing world.

- *Use of antibiotics*: Patients with respiratory infections are usually on preoperative antibiotics. The anesthesiologist needs to ensure that adequate doses have been given preoperatively and necessary intraoperative doses are repeated in time. Some of the antibiotics like vancomycin can cause severe allergic reactions and hypotension intra-operatively. Drug interactions need to be considered, especially when a patient is on antitubercular treatment. (Separately covered in another section of the chapter).

- *Low serum albumin and choice of intravascular fluids*: Malnourished patients with low serum albumin levels fail to maintain intravascular volume due to decreased colloid osmotic pressure. Low serum albumin level is also identified as independent preoperative indicator of acute kidney injury in patients undergoing esophageal cancer surgeries [15]. Intraoperatively, intravascular volume replacement is done with semisynthetic colloid solutions like succinylated gelatin and hydroxyethyl starch. Intravenous albumin is often not available and is also expensive. In absence of colloids, blood products are also used for volume replacement.

- *Blood loss*: Patients with acute and chronic inflammatory lung diseases tend to have higher blood loss during thoracic surgeries. In cases of preoperative anemia, packed cell transfusions are required even with minimal blood loss, thus increasing blood transfusion-related infection and anaphylactic and immunological risks in the perioperative period. Some institutes do not have in-hospital transfusion medicine departments. In such cases, delay may occur in receiving blood products in the operating theater, and anesthesiologists prefer to call for one unit of packed cell or whole blood well in advance.

- *Positioning*: Most thoracic surgeries are carried out in lateral decubitus positions, except when median sternotomy is required. It is the shared responsibility of the anesthesiologist and surgeon to correctly position the patient. Care needs to be taken to prevent neurovascular injuries due to faulty positioning. Chronically malnourished and dehydrated patients tend to develop hypotension after turning from supine to lateral position. Such patients also carry a higher chance of developing decubitus ulcers or pressure sores at bony prominences. Anesthesiologists need to be extra vigilant to provide adequate padding under bony prominences to prevent pressure sores.

- *Lung isolation*: In developing countries, lung isolation techniques are required primarily to facilitate surgical exposure during thoracoscopic surgeries and to prevent contamination of non-infected areas of lungs. Lung isolation devices of adequate sizes, pediatric flexible bronchoscopes, fluoroscopic backup, and facilities for advanced hemodynamic monitoring are often unavailable in many institutes in developing countries. In many centers, surgeries are carried out with an open thoracotomy approach, and both lungs are ventilated with low tidal volumes. In such centers, if lung isolation is mandatory, then patients are referred to centers where advanced facilities are available. Some centers have advanced surgical technologies (e.g., thoracoscopes, robotic surgery unit, etc.), but anes-

thesia equipment (flexible bronchoscopes, bronchial blockers, etc.) required for lung isolation are not available. In such conditions, the anesthesiologist needs to be adaptable and innovative to use the available resources to provide good quality lung isolation without compromising with safety of the patient. Many such adaptations remain underreported in medical journals. It must be remembered that these are not standard practices and limited evidence is available to recommend the use of these methods. Standard equipment and techniques should be preferred whenever available. Following is the discussion about few such adaptations which have been reported in the literature.

Selection of Lung Isolation Devices

In developing countries, the choice of lung isolation device depends largely on the availability of the device and fiber-optic bronchoscopes. In absence of a pediatric fiber-optic bronchoscope, DLTs are preferred over bronchial blockers as DLTs can be inserted blindly and their position can be confirmed by clinical methods like inspection of chest expansion and auscultation, followed by fine adjustments in their position. DLTs of smaller sizes (26 F, 28 F, and 32 F) and bronchial blockers of pediatric sizes are often not available. Hence lung isolation in children and adults of short stature becomes difficult. In such conditions, adaptations like endobronchial intubation and the use of Fogarty catheters are commonly followed in developing countries.

In places where DLTs are not available or in young children (less than 8 years old), a single-lumen endotracheal tube is advanced into the main bronchus on the opposite side of surgery. If in the right main bronchus, the Murphy's eye would ventilate the right upper lobe. Bronchial diameter and distance from the tip of tube to the upper margin of cuff are taken into account while deciding the size of endotracheal tube. The major problems with endobronchial intubation are dislodgment of the tube and inability to apply suction to the opposite bronchus. These problems can be overcome by use of largest possible size of the single-lumen tube, a steep head-down tilt of the table, and frequent suctioning through an extra-luminal suction catheter placed in trachea. This technique is commonly followed in pediatric cases in developing countries.

Fogarty arterial embolectomy catheters (Edwards Lifesciences, Irvine, CA, USA) are not created for use in airways; however use of Fogarty catheters is prevalent in developing countries for the purpose of lung isolation in small children, as pediatric size bronchial blockers and DLTs are not available. These catheters can be passed intraluminally or extra-luminally, and their position is confirmed by flexible bronchoscope, if available. Two major difficulties faced in placement of Fogarty catheters are to direct the catheter tip into target bronchus and to identify the transparent balloon by FOB. The catheter tip is bent to 45° by using wire stylet to facilitate guidance into desired bronchus. The balloon can be filled with saline containing methylene blue to facilitate identification by a flexible bronchoscope.

Methods to Aid Insertion of Lung Isolation Devices

In absence of a pediatric flexible bronchoscope, blind insertion of the DLT followed by auscultation to confirm placement of the DLT is the most commonly followed practice in developing countries. However, there are certain techniques that may help inserting a lung isolation device when a pediatric flexible bronchoscope is not available. These techniques are discussed below.

- *Pre-intubation measurements of trachea and bronchus*:
  In absence of a pediatric flexible bronchoscope, an adult flexible bronchoscope, which is commonly available, can be used to measure the distance from central incisor to carina, and from carina to secondary carina, before placement of any lung isolation device. These measurements are then used to guide a DLT or bronchial blocker through the exact distance from central incisor. A study showed that the success rate of optimal positioning of the DLT was significantly higher in the group where DLTs were placed as per distances measured by flexible bronchoscope as compared to the group where DLTs were placed blindly [16].
  Measurement of tracheal diameter at cricoid level, and bronchial diameter, using CT scan or chest radiograph, helps to choose correct size of DLTs. This is especially important in the Asian population in whom height-based criteria for choosing DLTs are not helpful. In Asian patients who are shorter than 150 cm, anesthesiologists often encounter difficulty in passing a 35 F DLT through the subglottic portion of trachea. In a retrospective analysis of Japanese women shorter than 150 cm, the primary reason for failure of first attempt of intubation was narrow tracheal diameter at cricoid level [17]. The use of another lung isolation device leads to additional cost to the patient, apart from to hemodynamic stress of a second intubation. Hence, it may be useful to measure the tracheal diameter at cricoid level prior to choosing a DLT size, especially in Asian patients shorter than 150 cm in height. It is also common practice to use one size smaller DLTs in these patients rather than using larger one.
- *Extra-luminal use of bronchial blockers*:
  Bronchial blockers are meant to be deployed through the lumen of an endotracheal tube into the desired bronchus with the help of a pediatric flexible bronchoscope. However, there are conditions where bronchial blockers and a pediatric flexible bronchoscope are difficult to pass together through an endotracheal tube, especially in small

children and patients with a tracheostomy. In such conditions, or when a pediatric flexible bronchoscope is not available, bronchial blockers are passed extra-luminally and are guided into position using an adult or pediatric bronchoscope passed through the lumen of the endotracheal tube. There are case reports of the use of pediatric 5 F Arndt blockers (Cook Medical Ltd) extra-luminally in children less than 2 years of age [18, 19]. A study by Templeton et al. compared intraluminal versus extra-luminal use of 9 F Arndt blocker in adult patients and found that the extra-luminal placement of a bronchial blocker is faster, as compared to intraluminal placement, without any difference in the quality of lung isolation or postoperative sore throat [20].

Methods to Monitor the Position of the Lung Isolation Device

- *Use of basic clinical skills and auscultation*:
  In developing countries, the position of a DLT is most commonly confirmed by inspection of chest expansion and auscultation. In conditions where minimum basic monitoring devices are not available, it is a safe practice to fix the chest piece of the stethoscope to the patient's chest on non-operative side and monitor regional ventilation through auscultation. This practice enables the anesthesiologist to detect problems like intraoperative bronchospasm, dislodgment of lung isolation device, pulmonary edema, atelectasis of the lung, etc. Modern anesthesia workstations give accurate outputs in the form of compliance, peak inspiratory pressure, end-tidal carbon dioxide curve, exhaled tidal volumes, etc. and provide continuous monitoring of ventilation. However, in many centers in developing countries, anesthesia workstations are not available, and patients are ventilated manually. In these situations, the reservoir bag in the hand of the anesthesiologist is sometimes the only means to monitor the lung mechanics of the patient. Clinical methods like a hand on the pulse are useful in assessing hemodynamic status of the patient. Such basic ways of monitoring help the anesthesiologist to continue safe delivery of anesthesia when advanced monitoring devices are not available.
- *Fluoroscopy and chest radiography*:
  Fluoroscopy can be used to positon lung isolation devices in the desired bronchus. Fluoroscopy machines are often available in institutes where orthopedic and interventional radiological procedures are carried out. Placement of a DLT, bronchial blocker (BB), or endobronchial intubation with a single-lumen tube can be confirmed using fluoroscopy [19, 21, 22]. This method is used when a pediatric flexible bronchoscope is not available. Chest radiography has also been used for the same purposes. These methods,

however, increase radiation exposure risk to the patient and healthcare workers in operating room.

- *Use of lung ultrasonography*:

The flexible bronchoscope confirms the position of the double-lumen tube (DLT) in trachea and bronchus, but it cannot confirm good quality of lung collapse. Whether the lung to be isolated has collapsed, and whether the other lung is getting properly ventilated, is determined by assessment of regional ventilation. Traditionally, this is confirmed by auscultation. However, auscultation has low accuracy to confirm correct placement of lung isolation device [23]. Lung ultrasonography can differentiate ventilated lung from non-ventilated lung using lung sliding and lung pulse signs. Application of a linear transducer to the chest wall detects hypoechoic shadows of ribs with hyperechoic bright pleural line (see Chap. 28). During ventilation of the lung, movement at parietal-visceral pleural interface is detected by a sliding movement of the pleural line. This sign is called lung sliding. When the lung is not ventilated, then there is no such movement, and lung sliding is not visible. In an atelectatic lung, the pleural line moves with heartbeats, and this sign is called the lung pulse sign. Lung pulse is 93% sensitive and 100% specific for the diagnosis of atelectasis [24]. These signs can be used to determine regional distribution of ventilation following placement of lung isolation devices. This is a bedside, noninvasive, cost-effective, and real-time monitor of regional ventilation. This method has been used to determine position of DLTs and has been proved to be more efficacious than auscultation [25–27]. In centers where flexible pediatric bronchoscopes are not available, or in situations where bronchoscopes cannot be used, lung ultrasonography can be a better method than auscultation to determine position of DLTs.

Ultrasonography has number of applications in perioperative medicine right from echocardiography to securing of vascular access. Though an ultrasonography machine is a costly instrument, a wide range of its applications and low maintenance cost make it a cost-effective option. A limitation of this technique is that ultrasonography is subjective and interindividual variations in findings can be possible. Anesthesiologists need to acquire the additional skill of ultrasonography. Intraoperatively, it cannot be performed on draped areas. With these limitations in mind, lung ultrasound can still be useful for thoracic anesthesiologist in the developing world to determine regional ventilation after placement of DLTs.

- *Bronchial cuff pressure monitoring*:

Lung isolation devices can get dislodged intraoperatively which may lead to a loss of lung isolation and contamination of the other lung. The pediatric flexible bronchoscope is used to confirm and rectify any malposition of the lung isolation device. However, if a pediatric flexible bronchoscope is not available, the anesthesiologist has to rely upon clinical acumen to diagnose and correct the malposition. Araki et al. monitored bronchial cuff pressure using aneroid manometer and found out that continuous bronchial cuff pressure monitoring is a sensitive technique for detection of DLT displacement. When the DLT gets displaced, bronchial cuff pressure decreases even before any changes are detected in pressure volume or end-tidal carbon dioxide curves [28]. Bronchial cuff pressure can also be used to guide blind insertion of DLT when a pediatric flexible bronchoscope is unavailable. In a study of 79 patients, the DLT was introduced into the trachea using laryngoscopy, and further advancement into bronchus was done blindly by rotation of the tube to the ipsilateral side. The DLT was advanced until resistance was felt for any further movement. At this time, the bronchial cuff was inflated with 1–2 cc of air, and the DLT was withdrawn slowly while monitoring the bronchial cuff pressure manually. When a drop in bronchial cuff pressure was felt, further withdrawal of DLT was stopped, and after deflation of bronchial cuff, DLT was advanced by 1 cm (1.5 cm in case of 39 F DLT). Later, upon bronchoscopic confirmation, DLTs were found to be in the optimum position in 50 cases and within margin of safety in 27 patients [29, 30]. Thus, in case of unavailability of flexible bronchoscope, this method can help to place DLT blindly.

Postoperative Care and Analgesia for Thoracic Patients

Postoperatively, patients are transferred to a recovery room area, which is often understaffed. Often there is no designated post-anesthesia care unit. A high patient to nurse ratio means that one nurse has to look after more than two to three patients. Multichannel monitors are often not available, and vital signs are monitored manually, mostly by a junior nurse. This leads to infrequent and suboptimal monitoring of patient by the available nursing staff. Doctors managing recovery room areas are often not trained in intensive care medicine. Machines for arterial blood gas analysis, portable chest radiography, and ultrasonography are often not available. Lack of these machines may delay the diagnosis and treatment of any complications of the patients. It often leads to transfer of patients out of recovery rooms for diagnostic purposes, costing manpower and time. It also increases risk of transferring patient to the areas where monitoring is suboptimal. Support staff, like physiotherapist and nutritionist, are fewer in number as compared to the patient population and cannot spend adequate time with each patient. Family members of the patient play an important role, looking after the physiotherapy, feeding, ambulation, cleaning, and also providing psychological support to the patient.

Postoperative pain relief is poorly addressed partly due to ignorance, the fear of respiratory depression, the non-availability of drugs or equipment such as infusion pumps, and inadequate nursing care. Post-thoracotomy pain is severe and incapacitating, leading to inadequate chest physiotherapy exercises, poor clearance of sputum, delayed ambulation, and chronic post-thoracotomy pain syndrome, which, if untreated, can lead to increased morbidity and mortality. Optimal pain management is of paramount importance. The pain score, which is considered the fifth vital sign, is often neither evaluated nor documented by the nursing staff. There is no preoperative counselling of the patient regarding various options available for control of pain. Many patients are uneducated and unaware of the options available for the pain control and often believe that pain is expected with surgery or that taking too many pain medications will lead to side effects. A designated acute postoperative pain management service is present in very few centers.

Opioids form the important component of postoperative analgesia being of low cost and effective as well. However, opioids are not available at many centers in developing world. As per a report, nearly 85% of world's morphine is consumed by 15% of world's population across ten developed countries, whereas 85% of remaining population consumes only 13% of morphine [31]. Fear of addiction, stringent rules and regulations for prescribing morphine, and high cost of importing morphine are some of the barriers for effective use of morphine in developing world. Even if they are available, there is significant fear among the treating physicians regarding the use of opioids for pain control, commonly referred as "opiophobia" [32]. Also, inadequate nursing staff and monitoring equipment make it unsafe to prescribe opioids in postoperative wards. Nonsteroidal anti-inflammatory drugs (NSAIDs) and paracetamol are the most commonly used drugs for postoperative pain management. Regional analgesia techniques like epidural analgesia, paravertebral blocks, or intercostal nerve blocks which play important role for postoperative pain management are often underutilized due to shortage of equipment (e.g., infusion pumps, patient-controlled analgesia systems, etc.), drugs (e.g., liposomal bupivacaine, additives like clonidine), and lack of clinical expertise. Drugs like ketamine, which have postoperative analgesic potential, are commonly used in the pediatric population. A study on prescription patterns and adequacy of analgesia in postoperative patients in University College in Nigeria showed that nearly 68% patient complained of unbearable pain postoperatively. Weak opioids were prescribed, and intramuscular injection was the most common route of administration of analgesics [33]. Thus, postoperative pain management has a long way to go in developing world.

Anesthesia for Thoracic Surgeries in Patients with Infective Lung Diseases

Respiratory infections form the major burden of lung diseases in the developing world. Though these infections are primarily treated by medical management, thoracic surgery may be required to manage the complications arising from infectious process. Pulmonary TB along with pyogenic and parasitic infections of pleura and parenchyma forms a majority of the lower respiratory tract infections, which may require surgical treatment. These include bronchiectasis, empyema, lung abscess, and pulmonary helminthiasis. Management of these patients requires special precautions in preoperative, intraoperative, and postoperative periods. Following is a discussion about commonly prevalent infectious conditions in developing world and their anesthetic management.

Tuberculosis

Incidence and Prevalence

Tuberculosis (TB) is a leading cause of morbidity and mortality worldwide, more so in low- and middle-income countries. In 2015, approximately 10.4 million new TB cases and 1.4 million TB deaths were reported worldwide. Six countries, which accounted for 60% of the new cases, were India, Indonesia, China, Nigeria, Pakistan, and South Africa, in the descending order of the number of cases. Approximately 1.2 million patients (i.e., 11% of all new TB cases) were co-infected with human immunodeficiency virus (HIV) [34]. Apart from HIV, smoking, diabetes mellitus, anti-TNFα drugs, and new immunosuppressive treatments are important risk factors for TB [35, 36].

The World Health Organization End TB Strategy was approved by the World Health Assembly in 2014. It targets a 90% reduction in TB deaths and an 80% reduction in the TB incidence rate by 2030, compared with 2015. Incidence of TB has declined significantly in high-income countries, mainly due to improved socioeconomic conditions and better use of anti-TB drugs [37]. After the introduction of rifampicin and isoniazid, chemotherapy has been the mainstay of treatment of TB, while surgical treatment has been used for complicated cases only. Currently followed chemotherapy regimens with directly observed treatment short course (DOTS) approach have achieved cure rates in excess of 85%; however, it is not so effective in countries where multidrug-resistant strains are prevalent. In 2015, there were an estimated 480,000 new cases of multidrug-resistant TB (MDR-TB), where the mycobacterium TB strains were resistant to at least rifampicin and isoniazid. An additional 100,000 people with rifampicin-resistant TB (RR-TB) were also eligible for MDR-TB treatment. Three countries, namely, India, China, and the Russian Federation, accounted for 45% of the combined total of 580,000 cases [34]. There is growing concern over rapid emergence of "extensively drug-resistant TB" (XDR-TB), which is defined as resistance to rifampicin, isoniazid, fluoroquinolones, and at least one of the following injectable anti-TB drugs – capreomycin, kanamycin, or amikacin [38, 39]. A combination of 5–7s line drugs has been suggested by WHO for the management of MDR-TB. A few new drugs (bedaquiline, delamanid) and some repurposed drugs (carbapenems, linezolid, mefloquine, etc.) are also being investigated for the treatment of MDR-TB.

Pathophysiology

Spread of mycobacterium tuberculosis occurs via the transmission of small airborne droplets (0.5–5 μm). Although the lung is the most commonly affected organ, TB can affect any organ of the body. Affection of lung parenchyma and lymphadenitis forms the primary complex of TB (Ghon focus), usually in the middle third of the lung. The primary site of infection can also be subpleural. In most cases, these lesions heal spontaneously. However, in immunocompromised hosts, primary TB progresses rapidly from exudative pneumonia to necrosis and cavitation in the lungs (see Fig. 42.1a, b). Caseation necrosis also occurs in hilar lymph nodes and leads to hematoge-

nous spread to other organs. Affection of bronchi or endobronchial TB occurs due to direct extension of infection from primary parenchymal focus and affected lymph nodes or by hematogenous spread. Right upper lobe bronchus and right main bronchus are the most commonly affected bronchi. Infiltration of bronchial mucosa by lymphocytes leads to congestion and edema. Further inflammation leads to the development of caseation necrosis and granuloma formation. Fibrotic changes following inflammation lead to narrowing of bronchial lumen, which is called as bronchostenosis [40]. Compression of bronchi by the enlarged lymph nodes or bronchostenosis leads to obstructive atelectasis.

Bacteria within the granuloma can become dormant, resulting in latent infection. At this stage, the patient is often asymptomatic but may show a positive response to a tuberculin skin test. Endogenous reactivation of latent infection results in postprimary or secondary TB. The most common site of affection is the apical or apical-posterior segment of an upper lobe due to relatively high oxygen tension, which favors growth of mycobacteria. Diffuse pulmonary involvement leads to military TB (see Fig. 42.2a, b). Productive cough with variable quantities of sputum and/or hemoptysis in a debilitated patient is a hallmark of pulmonary TB. Other pulmonary complications include pneumothorax, pleural effusion, empyema, BPF, massive hemoptysis, fibrosis with loss of parenchymal volume, and distortion of the tracheobronchial tree including bronchial stenosis.

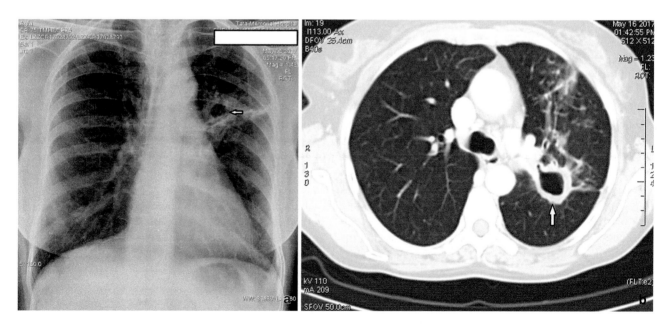

Fig. 42.1 (**a**) Chest radiograph showing cavitary lesion (marked by an arrow) with adjacent plate atelectasis in left mid-zone. (**b**) Computed tomography scan of chest showing a thick-walled, heterogeneously enhancing cavitary lesion (marked by an arrow) in left upper lobe, with surrounding spiculations and a speck of eccentric calcification. Also seen are subjacent areas of collapse/consolidation with multiple ill-defined nodules in left upper lobe. Interseptal thickening and areas of traction bronchiectasis are also seen

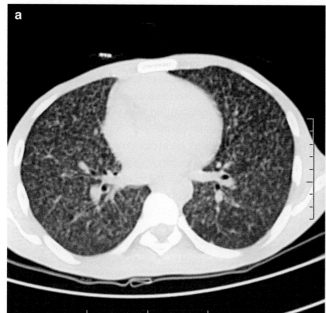 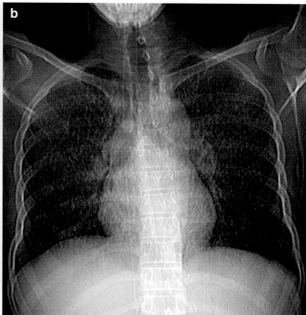

Fig. 42.2 (**a**) A positron emission tomography scan of the chest showing innumerable small pulmonary nodules distributed uniformly in both lungs suggestive of military TB. (**b**) Anteroposterior image of positron emission tomography scan of the chest showing widespread distribution of discrete nodules throughout both the lungs, suggestive of military TB

Surgery and TB

Historically the first thoracic surgery procedure was open drainage of a TB pleural empyema, performed by Hippocrates. During first half of the twentieth century, a number of surgical procedures were carried out to deprive the mycobacterium TB of oxygen. These included thoracoplasty, induced pneumothorax, plombage, and phrenic nerve crushing [41]. Similar to open surgery, thoracoscopy was also first used for pleural biopsy and adhesiolysis in TB patients [42]. Following introduction of rifampicin in 1960, chemotherapy became first-line treatment of TB, and surgery remained the option for complications arising from TB.

In the last two decades, there has been resurgence in the role of surgery in the management of TB, primarily due to global incidence and emergence of MDR-TB. With improvements in anesthesia and surgical methods, thoracic surgery is less morbid procedure. As a result, the need for surgery is increasing.

Indications for thoracic surgery in patients with pulmonary TB are:

1. Management of pulmonary complications of TB like hemoptysis, empyema, tuberculomas, "destroyed lung" due to fibrosis, etc.
2. Treatment of patients who present with inadequate clinical or radiological or microbiological improvement despite appropriate chemotherapy regimen

Patients with persistently positive sputum even after at least 6–8 months of appropriate anti-TB therapy benefit from surgical resection of pulmonary lesions. A meta-analysis evaluating role of pulmonary resection in cases with MDR-TB reported success rate of 84%, with only 6% failure rate, 3% relapse, and 5% mortality [43]. Parenchymal-sparing pulmonary resections are performed, lobectomies being more common than pneumonectomies [44]. Pneumonectomies are performed in patients with multiple cavitary lesions. In case of bilateral lesions, unilateral dominant lesions are removed surgically, and small lesions on opposite side are treated with medical management. However, sometimes these small lesions require surgery in the future [45].

Thus, lung resection should be considered when the following criteria are fulfilled [46]:

1. Adequate (i.e., 6–8 months) anti-TB treatment has failed to cure the patient.
2. Disease is localized to allow anatomical lung resection.
3. Patient has adequate cardiopulmonary reserve and acceptable surgical risk to tolerate the resection.

A "Destroyed lung" is a sequel of pulmonary TB, which is characterized by fibrotic cavities and caseous lymphadenitis and further complicated by sub-lobar atelectasis or bronchiectasis. Patient presents with history of prolonged and multiple anti-TB treatment, drug resistance, and progressive deterioration in pulmonary functions. Surgery is performed to decrease the infectious load and to prevent life-threatening complications [47]. Similarly tuberculomas also present as pulmonary nodules of varying sizes and are resected to reduce the infectiousness. Recurrent hemoptysis is a common presentation in advanced pulmonary TB. Emergency surgery may be required in patients where massive hemoptysis occurs and embolization cannot be performed or is unavailable [48]. Surgical decortications are recommended for management of tuberculous empyema when there is major residual pleural thickening leading to non-expansion of underlying lung [49].

TB and Anesthesia Implications

In the patient with pulmonary TB undergoing thoracic surgery, there are three major implications for the anesthetist:

1. The general condition of patient and the effect of TB on functions of affected organs
2. The potential for drug interactions between anti-TB treatment and anesthetic drugs
3. The risk of transmission of TB to staff and other patients

The following care should be taken when anesthetizing a patient with pulmonary TB for thoracic surgery:

- A detailed history, examination, and relevant investigations are required to determine the extent of organ dysfunction. Patients with pulmonary TB are often chronically ill, malnourished, and frequently anemic. Chronic longstanding TB leads to parenchymal fibrosis and bronchiectasis causing progressive decrease in lung functions. Severe adrenocortical insufficiency may occur perioperatively in patients suffering from TB of adrenal glands. In patients with TB of the cervical spine, special precautions should be taken during airway manipulation especially while giving neck extension for procedures like mediastinoscopy to avoid injury to the cervical spine.
- Elective surgical procedures should be postponed until patients are no longer considered infectious. Patients are considered noninfectious if they have received anti-TB chemotherapy for 2–3 weeks, are improving clinically, and have had three consecutive negative sputum smears [50].
- The anesthesiologist should review liver function tests because anti-TB medications (isoniazid, pyrazinamide, rifampicin) are hepatotoxic. Combining anti-TB treatment with antiretroviral therapy leads to a mild elevation in liver enzymes. However, symptomatic hepatitis is a potentially dangerous complication and carries a mortality of almost 5% [51]. In such condition, anti-TB drugs should be immediately stopped and alternate medications

considered. After improvement of hepatic function, they may be restarted carefully, under specialist care. An elective surgery should be avoided during this period.
- Rifampicin can cause thrombocytopenia when used in high doses. INH can cause sensory neuropathy, which should be checked and documented before performing regional nerve blocks. Administration of pyridoxine helps in treatment of neuropathy.
- Anti-TB agents may be ordered on the day of surgery to keep blood levels constant.
- Drug interactions occur due to pharmacokinetic changes following the induction of liver enzymes. Rifampicin is a potent inducer of the cytochrome P450 system, especially isoenzyme 3A4. It leads to increased metabolism, causing subtherapeutic effects of anesthetic drugs and/or increased production of toxic metabolites. INH is a CYP450 inhibitor. Drug interactions are further complicated when patient is receiving concurrent antiretroviral treatment, specifically protease inhibitors. Induction agents, when used as intravenous infusions, are metabolized rapidly. This can lead to potential chances of awareness during TIVA. Infusion rates need to be increased to avoid this phenomenon. With use of halothane, chances of hepatitis are increased. Hence newer volatile agents are preferred. Increased metabolism affects duration of action of non-depolarizing muscle relaxants like vecuronium and rocuronium. Neuromuscular monitoring is required to titrate the doses of these drugs. Increased metabolism also affects opioids, and more frequent dosing may be required.

Preventing Transmission of TB to Other Patients and Healthcare Workers (HCW)

Operating room (OR), hospital staff, and other personnel in close contact with a TB patients are at risk of getting infected with TB. Characteristics that exist in a patient with TB disease and increase the risk of infectiousness are given in Table 42.1.

Table 42.1 Characteristics in a TB patient that increase risk of infectivity

1	Presence of cough
2	Cavitation on chest radiograph
3	Sputum smear positive for acid-fast bacilli
4	Respiratory tract disease with involvement of the larynx (substantially infectious)
5	Respiratory tract disease with involvement of the lung or pleura (exclusively pleural involvement is less infectious)
6	Untreated, inappropriate, or short duration of anti-TB treatment
7	Undergoing cough-inducing or aerosol-generating procedures (e.g., bronchoscopy, sputum induction, and administration of aerosolized medications)

According to the American Society of Anesthesiologist guidelines regarding perioperative management of TB patients [50], the following recommendations are made to prevent transmission of TB to healthcare workers:

- Elective surgery should not be done until patient is noninfectious (a TB patient is considered as noninfectious when, for 2–3 weeks, he/she is clinically getting better and has had three negative sputum samples on different days).
- Procedures should be scheduled for patients with suspected or confirmed TB disease when a minimum number of healthcare workers and other patients are present in the surgical suite and at the end of the day to maximize the time available for removal of airborne contamination.
- Surgical staff, particularly those close to the surgical field, should use respiratory protection (e.g., a valveless N95 disposable respirator) to protect themselves and the patient undergoing surgery.
- If a surgical suite has an anteroom, the anteroom should be either (1) positive pressure compared with both the corridor and the suite or (2) negative pressure compared with both the corridor and the suite. In the usual design in which an OR has no anteroom, doors to the OR should be closed, and traffic into and out of the room should be minimized.
- A bacterial filter (ability to filter particles 0.3 μm in size in both the unloaded and loaded states with a filter efficiency of ≥95% at the maximum design flow rates of the ventilator for the service life of the filter) should be placed on the patient's endotracheal tube (or at the expiratory side of the breathing circuit of a ventilator or anesthesia machine, if used).

Postoperative Care

The patient with TB should be nursed in isolation room with airborne infection isolation (AII) precautions. This isolation area should receive ≥12 air changes per hour (ACH) and should be under negative pressure. Room should direct exhaust of air from the room to the outside of the building or recirculation of air through a HEPA filter.

Postoperative care includes antibiotics, analgesics, chest physiotherapy, breathing exercises, blood replacement whenever needed, and good care of chest tubes. One should routinely monitor drain outputs and general condition of the patient, and chest radiographs should be performed as required. Early and late post-thoracotomy complications can develop like air leak, bronchopleural fistula, residual pleural space, empyema, consolidations, etc., which should be appropriately managed.

Table 42.2 Duration of postoperative anti-TB treatment

Culture-negative patients at the time of surgery:
With susceptible TB, at least 4 months after surgery
With M/XDR-TB, 6–8 months after surgery (depending on postoperative recovery)
Culture-positive patients at the time of surgery:
With susceptible TB – 4–6 months after culture conversion
With MDR-TB, at least 18 months after culture conversion
With XDR-TB, at least 24 months after culture conversion

Preoperative anti-TB chemotherapy should be resumed as soon as patient tolerates enteral feeding. Surgical material should be analyzed for bacteriological culture. Guidelines on durations of postoperative anti-TB chemotherapy are summarized in Table 42.2 [46].

Bronchiectasis

Bronchiectasis is defined as an abnormal and permanent dilatation of bronchi. It may be focal, where bronchi in the limited region of pulmonary parenchyma are dilated, or diffuse, where airways are affected with widespread distribution. Focal or localized forms of bronchiectasis usually follow an inadequately treated pulmonary infection and are associated with good prognosis. On the other hand, a diffuse form of bronchiectasis is seen in patients suffering from congenital ciliary defects and immunoglobulin deficiencies. The diffuse form of bronchiectasis is associated with bilateral presentation and rapid decline in respiratory function.

Pathophysiology and Causes

Bronchiectasis results as a consequence of inflammatory destruction of structural components of bronchial wall. Inflammation is triggered by infection or exposure to toxic substances or by immunological reaction. Dilated airways, lack of ciliary motility, and airway obstruction lead to stagnation of pulmonary secretions and further infections. This sets up a vicious cycle of progressive inflammation and recurrent infections (see Fig. 42.3 and 42.4a, b).

Common causes of bronchiectasis are enumerated in Table 42.3.

The use of effective antibiotics, immunization policies, and improved hygiene has led to a decreased incidence of bronchiectasis in developed countries. However, in developing countries where pulmonary infections are prevalent, bronchiectasis is a major respiratory illness.

Patients suffer from chronic cough, excessive sputum production, hemoptysis, and progressive decline in respiratory function. Cough is often related to change in position. Hemoptysis can be life-threatening as well. History and

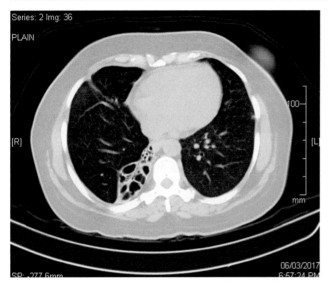

Fig. 42.3 Computed tomography scan of the chest showing cystic bronchiectasis changes with resultant collapse of the lung in postero-basal segment of right lower lobe, suggestive of acute or chronic infective etiology

examination in addition to radiological imaging confirm the diagnosis.

Most patients can be treated with medical management. It involves:

1. Antibiotics to treat causative infection
2. Bronchodilators to improve reversible obstruction of airways
3. Mucolytic therapy and physiotherapy to facilitate loosening and clearance of secretions

Surgical management is considered for the patients who:

- Fail or do not tolerate medical management
- Show signs of disease progression
- Present with life-threatening hemoptysis or recurrent pneumonia
- Have a localized disease amenable to anatomical lung resection

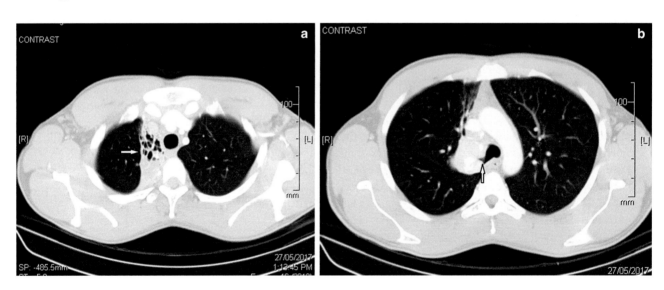

Fig. 42.4 (**a**, **b**) Computed tomography scan of the chest showing a homogenously enhancing mass in right hilum with endobronchial extension into right main bronchus (marked by an arrow). Post-obstructive bronchiectasis is seen in right upper lobe

Table 42.3 Causes of bronchiectasis

A. Acquired:	B. Host factors:
Infection:	Immunoglobulin deficiency
Viral (e.g., adenovirus, influenza virus)	Primary ciliary motility disorders
Bacterial (necrotizing organisms like *Staphylococcus* spp., *Klebsiella*, anaerobes, etc.)	Cystic fibrosis
Pulmonary TB – direct destruction of parenchyma by necrotizing inflammation and indirect way of airway obstruction due to bronchostenosis and extrinsic compression of airways by enlarged lymph nodes	Ulcerative colitis, rheumatoid arthritis, Sjogren's syndrome
Chronic obstruction of airways due to endobronchial tumors and foreign bodies	Alpha-1 antitrypsin deficiency
Exposure to toxic substance like ammonia or acidic gastric contents	Yellow nail syndrome
Immunological – allergic bronchopulmonary aspergillosis	

Surgery involves careful resection of involved segments of the lung. For widespread disease presenting with hemoptysis, bronchial artery embolization is preferred. For diffuse bronchiectasis showing progressive worsening despite optimum medical treatment, lung transplantation is a therapeutic option.

Anesthetic Considerations

Some principles of anesthesia management are common during perioperative care of patient with infectious lung diseases. These are summarized in Table 42.4 and have been discussed in detail in early part of the chapter. Certain salient aspects, pertaining to bronchiectasis, during perioperative care, are discussed here:

- A bronchoscopic aspiration of sputum should be done in preoperative period. It not only provides a sample for culture, but it also clears the sputum and improves regional ventilation. In case of hemoptysis, bronchoscopy can aid in localizing source of bleeding in tracheobronchial tree. Endobronchial tumors or foreign bodies can be identified, and surgical treatment can be planned accordingly.
- Appropriate antibiotic therapy should be started prior to surgery based on culture reports. In case of immunodeficiency disorders, intravenous or subcutaneous immunoglobulin G is administered in preoperative periods. Inhaled corticosteroids can be considered in case of noninfective inflammatory causes.
- A primary concern of the anesthesiologist is to prevent contamination of the non-operative lung. During induction of anesthesia, in absence of lung isolation, secretions can spill from affected segment to other lobes of lungs. Hence, the patient should be positioned in such a way that

the affected segment is in a dependent position, e.g., left lateral and semi-sitting position in case of left lower lobe bronchiectasis.
- If there are copious secretions in spite of all efforts, then awake, bronchoscope-guided intubation can be performed, followed by bronchoscopic suctioning of sputum and placement of bronchial blocker to achieve selective lobar blockade to avoid contamination of the non-affected lung.
- DLTs are always preferred over bronchial blockers, as bronchial blockers have higher chance of intraoperative displacement and have a narrow working channel which does not facilitate suctioning of affected segment.
- The left or right upper lobes can be deliberately obstructed by a left-sided double lumen placed in the ipsilateral main stem bronchus with fiber-optic bronchoscopic guidance. Saline-soaked gauze can be used to block lower or right middle lobe bronchi, using rigid bronchoscope at induction. During surgery once the bronchus is opened, the gauze is removed.
- The presence of inflammation increases the risk of intraoperative hemorrhage. A wide-bore intravenous cannula and preoperative confirmation of availability of cross-matched blood are always necessary.
- The use of neuraxial anesthetic techniques, specifically thoracic epidural analgesia in bronchiectasis and other infectious diseases, carries a risk of epidural abscess in the patient with an infectious process. An individual risk/benefit assessment should be performed and discussed with the patient and/or family in advance. In most cases, in a patient who is not septic and has significant pulmonary disability, the risks are acceptable due to the superior analgesia of thoracic epidural techniques.

Table 42.4 Principles for anesthesia management for patients with infectious lung disease

Preoperative nutritional supplementation, correction of anemia, cessation of smoking, chest physiotherapy, postural drainage, and preoperative antibiotics if necessary
Careful positioning of patient during anesthesia induction to minimize contamination of healthy areas of lungs
Use of lung isolation device especially DLT prior to re-positioning of patient, to prevent contamination
Anticipation, monitoring, and replacement of blood loss intraoperatively
Repetition of antibiotic doses to continue perioperative antibiotic coverage
Careful titration of anesthesia drugs, keeping in mind the interactions with the ongoing antibiotics
Use of precautions to prevent transmission of infection from patient to healthcare workers and other patients
Nutritional support, chest physiotherapy, adequate analgesia, and antibiotics postoperatively

Empyema

Empyema is collection of infected fluid between parietal and visceral layers of pleura. It occurs most commonly secondary to pneumonia but can also occur after thoracic surgery, trauma, or esophageal leaks. Empyema following surgical lung resections occurs in 2–16% of cases and is associated with 40% increase in perioperative mortality [52]. Empyema is commonly seen in pediatric and elderly populations and is associated with high morbidity and mortality. Due to underreporting, data from developing countries is lacking, but in developed countries like the UK and the USA combined, the approximate annual incidence of pleural infections is up to 80,000 cases. In the UK, 20% of patients with empyema die, and 20% need surgery within 12 months of their infection [53, 54].

Bacteriology

Community-acquired pleural infections are most commonly due to gram-positive aerobic organisms (*Streptococcus* spp., *Staphylococcus aureus*), whereas hospital-acquired pleural infections are frequently due to *Staphylococcus aureus*, methicillin-resistant *S. aureus* (MRSA) being the commonest. Infections with gram-negative organisms (Enterobacteriaceae, *E. coli*, *H. influenzae*) and anaerobes (*Fusobacterium* spp., *Bacteroides* spp.) are seen in patients with decreased immunity and comorbidities [54].

Pathophysiology

Development of empyema following pneumonia progresses through three stages:

1. Simple exudate
2. Fibrinopurulent stage
3. Organizing stage with pleural peel formation

In the first stage, fluid in pleural cavity is free flowing with low white cell count, with LDH level less than half of that in serum level, and with normal pH and often sterile. Treatment with antibiotics is adequate, and most often chest tube drainage is not required (see Fig. 42.5).

If untreated in first stage, then the infection progresses to fibrinopurulent stage where bacteria invade across the damaged endothelium. It leads to active immune response with increased procoagulant and decreased fibrinolytic activity. Biochemical examination of fluid at this stage shows rise in WBC count and LDH levels and fall in pH. Chest tube drainage is alone insufficient, and patient requires use of fibrinolytic agents or thoracoscopic surgery to facilitate adhesiolysis and removal of pus. Though fibrinolytic agents have been found to improve pleural fluid drainage, the use of these agents is not associated with reduced mortality, frequency of surgery, length of hospital stay, or long-term radiological outcome.

In the third stage, there is marked thickening of pleura with formation of solid pleural peel, preventing lung expansion. Most patients are referred to tertiary care centers at this stage and are treated with surgical decortication.

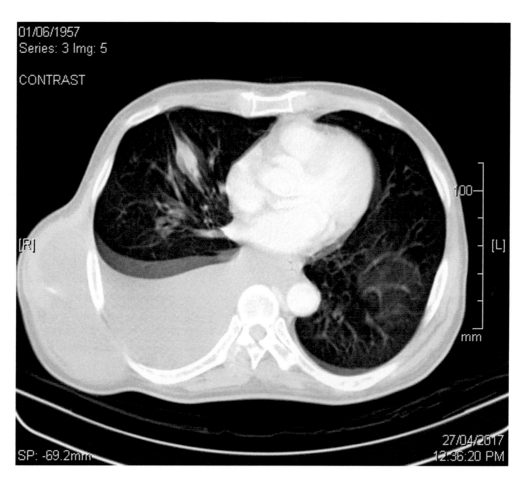

Fig. 42.5 Computed tomography scan of the chest and abdomen showing a moderate effusion on right side and a minimal effusion on left side. Effusion on right side is in communication with a collection in right lateral chest wall. Empyema necessitans was suspected. Patient underwent subsequent USG-guided tapping of collection and based on culture received 4-week course of antibiotics

Surgery for Empyema

Surgical options are required when patient has persistent pleural collection and associated sepsis despite chest tube drainage and antibiotics. For chronic hemothoraces, decortication is required when there is 50% compression of the lung, and there is no appreciable pulmonary expansion for 4–6 weeks following aspiration [55]. Goals of surgery are thorough surgical debridement of pleural peel, excision of necrotic tissues, adhesiolysis, and careful closure of all major air leaks. Surgery can be performed by open thoracotomy or a video-assisted thoracoscopic surgical (VATS) approach depending on the severity of the empyema. Surgery carries the best results when performed at the earliest stages.

The following are the anesthesia implications in management of patient with empyema:

- Some patients will present with an underlying bronchopleural fistula (BPF). A history of position-related productive cough should be carefully sought. History regarding chronicity of infection, past complications, and requirement of chest tube drainage can give hints about the presence of BPF. If there is uncertainty regarding the presence of a BPF based on history and examination, then it is a safest to assume the presence of an underlying BPF and plan anesthesia accordingly.
- Empyema and formation of pleural peel, being an inflammatory process, result in increased vascularity. Debridement of pleural peel results in significant blood loss. Major blood loss should be anticipated and necessary arrangements made in advance. Re-expansion of chronically collapsed lung should be done gradually to prevent re-expansion pulmonary edema.
- Adhesiolysis can result in air leaks from the pulmonary parenchyma. Lung isolation may be required if there are significant air leaks. Amount of air leak should be checked intraoperatively, and postoperative plans should be discussed with the surgeon accordingly.
- In case of BPF or lung abscess communicating with airways, lung isolation should be perfect to avoid loss of tidal volumes or contamination of the opposite lung. DLTs are preferred over bronchial blockers in such cases.

Lung Abscess

Lung abscess is an infection of lung parenchyma, leading to liquefactive necrosis of parenchyma with formation of well-circumscribed debris containing cavities. In the pre-antibiotic era, lung abscess had a high mortality. Causes of lung abscess are divided into primary and secondary.

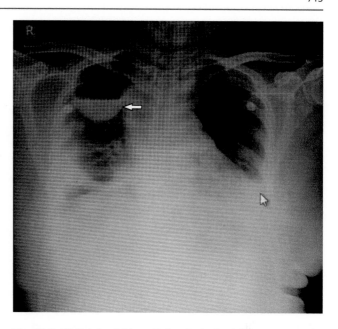

Fig. 42.6 Well-defined thin-walled cavity in the right upper zone with air fluid level within (marked by an arrow), suggestive of lung abscess of infective etiology. The right middle and lower zones show patchy areas of consolidation with blunting of the right costophrenic angle

Primary causes include infection of lung parenchyma due to aspiration of infected oropharyngeal secretions or a sequel of necrotizing pneumonia in immunocompromised host (see Fig. 42.6). On the other hand, secondary causes include hematogenous spread of infection from a distant focus. Elderly, alcoholic, comatose, diabetic, and those on immunosuppression treatments carry a high risk for developing lung abscess. Patients present with fever with chills, chest pain, night sweats, productive cough, progressive dyspnea, and weight loss. Obstruction of a bronchus causing distal stagnation of secretions can lead to lung abscess. Such an abscess may be incidentally detected during resection of bronchus and can lead to contamination of non-infected areas of lungs. Hence, the anesthesiologist should review preoperative imaging of the patient to find out if there is a lung abscess distal to an obstructed bronchus. Microbiologically, causative organisms are predominantly anaerobic (*Bacteroides*, *Fusobacterium* spp., *Peptostreptococcus*) or polymicrobial including aerobic organisms like *Staphylococcus aureus*, *Streptococcus pneumoniae*, *Klebsiella pneumoniae*, *Pseudomonas aeruginosa*, *Haemophilus influenzae*, etc. [56]. Open thoracotomy and drainage of abscess used to be the treatment of choice. However, currently medical management with antibiotics for 4–6 weeks or CT-guided percutaneous drainage forms the mainstay of the treatment, and surgery is rarely required.

Surgical management is reserved for the patients who show no improvement despite appropriate antibiotics administered for 6–8 weeks. Also complications arising from lung abscess like empyema and bronchopleural fistula warrant surgical management. Percutaneous drainage of the abscess guided by computed tomography (CT) scan is a safe and effective alternative to open thoracotomy and drainage especially in critically ill patients with ongoing sepsis and progressively enlarging abscess or those not amenable for extensive thoracic surgery [57].

Spillage from the abscess into non-infected areas of the lung is the chief concern during surgical management of patients. Anesthesia management principles are essentially the same as those involved in management of bronchiectasis or empyema (discussed in the earlier section of chapter).

Pneumatoceles

Pneumatoceles are thin-walled cyst-like air-filled cavities that occur following trauma or pneumonia (see Fig. 42.7). These are often the sequel of pneumonia (usually within first week of pneumonia) or trauma, and they resolve spontaneously within 6 weeks. Secondary infection and progressive enlargement of cavities remain the major complications. Cavities may rupture and develop tension pneumothorax. Tension pneumatocele is an unusual phenomenon that results from a one-way valve mechanism in patients on positive-pressure ventilation [58]. Large pneumatocele (occupying 50% of hemithorax) may be complicated by lung atelectasis, bronchopleural fistula, and non-resolving secondary infection, which requires surgical resection [59]. Surgical decompression can be performed by percutaneous needle aspiration and catheter or chest tube drainage under guidance of CT scan or fluoroscopy.

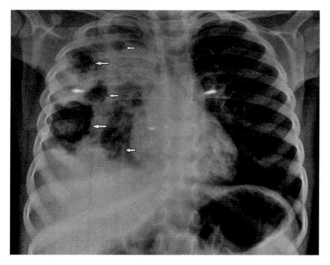

Fig. 42.7 Patchy areas of opacity involving the right lung with thin-walled cystic spaces (marked by arrows) having smooth inner margins without any air fluid level – suggestive of pneumatoceles

Hydatid Disease of the Lung or Pulmonary Echinococcosis

Pulmonary hydatid cysts are watery, parasitic cysts, containing larvae of the dog tapeworm, *Echinococcus granulosus* [60]. Echinococcosis is endemic in Australia, New Zealand, South America, Arctic North America, Africa, and parts of Asia.

Cyst Composition

The fully matured cysts are composed of three layers. The outer layer, or pericyst, is composed of inflamed fibrous tissue of lung parenchyma; the exocyst is a middle acellular lamina and the innermost endocyst which is a germinative layer, producing brood capsules or secondary cysts. An intact cyst may be filled with liters of fluid which is antigenic in nature. It contains debris consisting of hooklets and scolices referred to as "hydatid sand." The liver and lungs are the most commonly affected organs. Pulmonary hydatid cysts in children occur more commonly on the right side (~60%), 30% of patients have multiple pulmonary cysts, and 60% of cysts are found in the lower lobes [61]. Diameter of pulmonary cysts increases progressively at the rate of approximately 1–5 cm per year.

Whereas small cysts remain asymptomatic, large cysts can produce symptoms due to mass effect, causing compression of adjacent structures like bronchus, esophagus, and pulmonary vessels. Spontaneous or traumatic rupture may occur, disbursing fluid, parasites, and debris into surrounding lung parenchyma or bronchus, pleura, or even in the circulation. Spillage into blood vessels leads to systemic embolization of debris and parasites. Hypersensitivity reactions can present with urticarial or even life-threatening bronchospasm and anaphylaxis. Bursting of cyst into bronchi leads to sudden violent cough, respiratory distress, or feeling of asphyxiation. Rupture into the pleural space results in a hydropneumothorax. Rupture becomes more dangerous and more likely as cysts become larger or the patient has been treated with anti-helminthic. It is recommended that any cyst larger than 7 cm should be removed [62]. Ruptured cysts may become infected with bacteria or saprophytic or invasive fungi [63]. Diagnosis is by chest radiograph or CT scan.

Surgical Options

Surgical goals are complete resection of the intact cyst with maximal preservation of lung parenchyma. Anatomical lobar resection is required when single or multiple cysts occupy most of the lobe. An alternative surgical technique is to inject a scolicidal agent (hypertonic saline, cetrimide, povidone-iodine, formalin, ethanol, or hydrogen peroxide) into the intact cyst to sterilize it and then aspiration of the contents and removal of the evacuated cyst.

Anesthesia Considerations

- Postural drainage and antibiotics are started preoperatively in patients with suppurative cysts. Anti-helminthic drugs weaken the cyst wall and increase the likelihood of cyst rupture [64]. However, in case of spillage of cyst contents, either mebendazole or albendazole is administered to decrease the risk of secondary hydatidosis. Prophylactic medical therapy is started 4 days prior to surgery and is continued for 1–3 months.

- During dissection of the cyst, lung isolation or decreasing tidal volumes help in preventing early herniation of the cyst. Increased airway pressure with manual inspiratory hold helps in delivery of the cyst. The operative field is protected with hypertonic saline or 1% formaldehyde solution.

- After removal of cyst, parenchymal and bronchial leaks are checked with flooding the operative field with saline and ventilating the lungs to look for air bubbles (leak tests). Attempts are made to suture and close as many leaks as possible.

- Capitonnage (i.e., quilting or suturing of the anterior to posterior cyst walls) is recommended to close the cavity completely. A deliberately created broncho-atmospheric fistula (BAF) has been described in cases where there are large bronchial openings and there is fear of leaving a BPF or compromising airflow distally, if sutured. Ventilation is best managed spontaneously after creation of the BAF [65].

Acknowledgment We thank Dr. Anila Malde, Professor, Department of Anesthesia, Lokmanya Tilak Municipal Medical College and Hospital, Mumbai, India, for her valuable inputs.

We thank Dr. Sandeep Tandon, Dr. Maheema Bhaskar, and Dr. Aparna Iyer, Chest Physicians, Pulmonary Medicine Unit, Tata Memorial Hospital, India, for providing the images.

We thank Dr. Amit Janu, Consultant Radiologist, Department of Radiodiagnosis, Tata Memorial Hospital, Mumbai, India, for reporting the images.

Financial Support Nil

Conflicts of Interest None

References

1. Bainbridge D, Martin J, Arango M, et al., Evidence-based Peri-operative Clinical Outcomes Research (EPiCOR) Group. Perioperative and anesthetic-related mortality in developed and developing countries: a systematic review and meta-analysis. Lancet. 2012; 380:1075–81.

2. Jacob R. Challenges in the practice of thoracic anesthesia in developing countries. In: Slinger P, editor. Progress in thoracic anesthesia. Baltimore: Lippincott Williams and Wilkins; 2004. p. 267–85.

3. European Lung White Book. The burden of lung disease. Available from: http://www.erswhitebook.org/chapters/the-burden-of-lung-disease. Last accessed on 11 May 2017.

4. Ferkol T, Schraufnagel D. The global burden of respiratory disease. Ann Am Thorac Soc. 2014;11(3):404–6.

5. Hodges SC, Mijumbi C, Okello M, et al. Anesthesia services in developing countries: defining the problems. Anesthesia. 2007;62:4–11.

6. Rosseel P, Trelles M, Guilavogui S, et al. Ten years of experience training non-physician anesthesia providers in Haiti. World J Surg. 2010;34:453–8.

7. Jochberger S, Ismailova F, Banda D, et al. A survey of the status of education and research in anesthesia and intensive care medicine at the University Teaching Hospital in Lusaka, Zambia. Arch Iran Med. 2010;13:5–12.

8. Dubowitz G, Detlefs S, McQueen KA. Global anesthesia workforce crisis: a preliminary survey revealing shortages contributing to undesirable outcomes and unsafe practices. World J Surg. 2010;34:438–44.

9. Edwards J. Taking the pulse of pulse oximetry in Africa. CMAJ. 2012;184:E244–5.

10. Bould MD, Boet S, Riem N, et al. National representation in the anesthesia literature: a bibliometric analysis of highly cited anesthesia journals. Anaesthesia. 2010;65:799–804.

11. Babineau TJ, Borlase BC, Blackburn GL. Applied total parental nutrition in the critically ill. In: Rippe JM, Irwin RS, Alpert JS, Fink MP, editors. Intensive Care Medicine. Boston: Little, Brown and Co; 1991. p. 1675.

12. Gillis A, MacDonald B. Deconditioning in the hospitalized elderly. Can Nurse. 2005;101(6):16–20.

13. Administrative Committee on Coordination/Standing Committee on Nutrition, ACC/SCN. Fourth report on the world nutrition situation. New York: United Nations; 2000.

14. Sarkar M, Rajta PN, Khatana J. Anemia in chronic obstructive pulmonary disease: prevalence, pathogenesis, and potential impact. Lung India. 2015;32(2):142–51.

15. Lee EH, Kim HR, Baek SH, et al. Risk factors of postoperative acute kidney injury in patients undergoing esophageal cancer surgery. J Cardiothorac Vasc Anesth. 2014;28(4):936–42.

16. Amin N, Tarwade P, Shetmahajan M, et al. A randomized trial to assess the utility of preintubation adult fiberoptic bronchoscope assessment in patients for thoracic surgery requiring one-lung ventilation. Ann Card Anaesth. 2016;19(2):251–5.

17. Sato M, Kayashima K. Difficulty in inserting left double-lumen endobronchial tubes at the cricoid level in small-statured women: a retrospective study. Indian J Anesthesia. 2017;61(5):393–7.

18. Bastien JL, O'Brien JG, Frantz FW. Extraluminal use of the Arndt pediatric endobronchial blocker in an infant: a case report. Can J Anaesth. 2006;53(2):159–61.

19. Marciniak B, Fayoux P, Hébrard A, et al. Fluoroscopic guidance of Arndt endobronchial blocker placement for single-lung ventilation in small children. Acta Anaesthesiol Scand. 2008;52(7):1003–5.

20. Templeton TW, Downard MG, Simpson CR, et al. Bending the rules: a novel approach to placement and retrospective experience with the 5 French Arndt endobronchial blocker in children <2 years. Paediatr Anaesth. 2016;26(5):512–20.

21. Maheshwari A, Sharma N, Mathur P. Successful placement of double lumen endotracheal tube using fluoroscopy. J Anaesthesiol Clin Pharmacol. 2013;29(1):130–1.

22. Cohen DE, McCloskey JJ, Motas D, et al. Fluoroscopic-assisted endobronchial intubation for single-lung ventilation in infants. Paediatr Anaesth. 2011;21:681–4.

23. Alliaume B, Coddens J, Deloof T. Reliability of auscultation in positioning of double-lumen endobronchial tubes. Can J Anaesth. 1992;39(7):687–90.

24. Lichtenstein DA, Lascols N, Prin S, et al. The "lung pulse": an early ultrasound sign of complete atelectasis. Intensive Care Med. 2003;29(12):2187–92.

25. Parab SY, Divatia JV, Chogle A. A prospective comparative study to evaluate the utility of lung ultrasonography to improve the accuracy of traditional clinical methods to confirm position of left sided DLT in elective thoracic surgeries. Indian J Anaesth. 2015;59(8):476–81.

26. Saporito A, Lo Piccolo A, Franceschini D, et al. Thoracic ultrasound confirmation of correct lung exclusion before one-lung ventilation during thoracic surgery. J Ultrasound. 2013;16(4):195–9.

27. Ponsonnard S, Karoutsos S, Gardet E, et al. Value of lung sonography to control right-sided double lumen endotracheal tube location. J Anesth Clin Res. 2014;5:453.

28. Araki K, Nomura R, Urushibara R, et al. Displacement of the double-lumen endobronchial tube can be detected by bronchial cuff pressure change. Anesth Analg. 1997;84(6):1349–53.

29. Bahk JH, Oh YS. A new and simple maneuver to position the left-sided double-lumen tube without the aid of fiberoptic bronchoscopy. Anesth Analg. 1998;86(6):1271–5.

30. Zong ZJ, Shen QY, Lu Y, et al. A simple blind placement of the left-sided double-lumen tubes. Medicine (Baltimore). 2016;95(45):e5376.

31. Pain & Policy Studies Group. Availability of opioid analgesics in Asia: consumption trends, resources, recommendations. Madison: University of Wisconsin Pain and Policy Studies Group/WHO Collaborating Center for Policy and Communications in Cancer Care. Prepared for 17th Study Programme for Overseas Experts on Drug Abuse and Narcotics Control; Tokyo, Japan, 26 June, 2002 (Monograph).

32. Bennett DS, Carr DB. Opiophobia as a barrier to the treatment of pain. J Pain Palliat Care Pharmacother. 2002;16(1):105–9.

33. Faponle AF, Soyannwo OA, Ajayi IO. Postoperative pain therapy: a survey of prescribing patterns and adequacy of analgesia in Ibadan, Nigeria. Cent Afr J Med. 2001;47:70–4.

34. Global tuberculosis report 2016. Geneva: World Health Organisation (WHO); 2016.

35. Ferrara G, Murray M, Winthrop K, et al. Risk factors associated with pulmonary tuberculosis: smoking, diabetes and anti-TNFα drugs. Curr Opin Pulm Med. 2012;18:233–40.

36. Sotgiu G, Matteelli A, Migliori GB, et al. Diabetes and tuberculosis: what else beyond? Int J Tuberc Lung Dis. 2015;19:1127–8.

37. Hermans S, Horsburgh CR Jr, Wood RA. Century of tuberculosis epidemiology in the northern and southern hemisphere: the differential impact of control interventions. PLoS One. 2015;10:e0135179.

38. CDC. Emergence of mycobacterium tuberculosis with extensive resistance to second-line drugs – worldwide, 2000–2004. MMWR Morb Mortal Wkly Rep. 2006;55:301–5.

39. CDC. Notice to readers: revised definition of extensively drug-resistant tuberculosis. MMWR Morb Mortal Wkly Rep. 2006;55:1176.

40. Albert RK, Petty TL. Endobronchial tuberculosis progressing to bronchial stenosis; fiberoptic bronchoscopic manifestations. Chest. 1976;70(4):537–9.

41. Pomerantz M. Surgery for the management of mycobacterium tuberculosis and nontuberculous mycobacterial infections of the lung. In: Shields TW, Lo Cicero J, Ponn RB, et al., editors. General thoracic surgery. 6th ed. Philadelphia: Lippincott Williams & Wilkins; 2005. p. 1251–61.

42. Jacobaeus HC. The cauterization of adhesions in artificial pneumothorax treatment of pulmonary tuberculosis under thoracoscopic control. Proc R Soc Med. 1923;16:45–62.

43. Xu HB, Jiang RH, Li L. Pulmonary resection for patients with multidrug-resistant tuberculosis: systematic review and meta-analysis. J Antimicrob Chemother. 2011;66:1687–95.

44. Somocurcio JG, Sotomayor A, Shin S, et al. Surgery for patients with drug-resistant tuberculosis: report of 121 cases receiving community-based treatment in Lima, Peru. Thorax. 2007;62:416–21.

45. Shiraishi Y, Nakajima Y, Katsuragi N, et al. Resectional surgery combined with chemotherapy remains the treatment of choice for multidrug-resistant tuberculosis. J Thorac Cardiovasc Surg. 2004;128:523–8.

46. Masoud Dara. The role of surgery in the treatment of pulmonary TB and multidrug- and extensively drug resistant TB. Available from: http://www.euro.who.int/__data/assets/pdf_file/0005/259691/The-role-of-surgery-in-the-treatment-of-pulmonary-TB-and-multidrug-and-extensively-drug-resistant-TB.pdf?ua=1. Last accessed on 27 May 2017.

47. Bai L, Hong Z, Gong C, et al. Surgical treatment efficacy in 172 cases of tuberculosis-destroyed lungs. Eur J Cardiothorac Surg. 2012;41:335–40.

48. Ozgül MA, Turna A, Yildiz P, et al. Risk factors and recurrence patterns in 203 patients with hemoptysis. Tuberk Toraks. 2006;54:243–8.

49. Kerti CA, Miron I, Cozma GV, et al. The role of surgery in the management of pleuropulmonary tuberculosis– seven years' experience at a single institution. Interact Cardiovasc Thorac Surg. 2009;8:334–7.

50. Jensen PA, Lambert LA, Iademarco MF, et al. Guidelines for preventing the transmission of mycobacterium tuberculosis in healthcare settings. Centers for Disease Control and Prevention. 2005. c2012. Available from: https://www.cdc.gov/mmwr/preview/mmwrhtml/rr5417a1.htm. Last accessed on 26 May 2017.

51. Forget EJ, Menzies D. Adverse reactions to first-line antituberculous drugs. Expert Opin Drug Saf. 2006;5(2):231–49.

52. Pairolero PC, Deschamps C, Allen MS, et al. Postoperative empyema. Chest Surg Clin North Am. 1992;2:813–20.

53. Ferguson AD, Prescott RJ, Selkon JB, et al. The clinical course and management of thoracic empyema. Q J Med. 1996;89:285–9.

54. Maskell NA, Batt S, Hedley EL, et al. The bacteriology of pleural infection by genetic and standard methods and its mortality significance. Am J Respir Crit Care Med. 2006;174:817–23.

55. Rocco G, Descamps C, Deslariers J. Fibrothorax and decortication. In: Patterson GA, editor. Pearson's thoracic and esophageal surgery. 3rd ed. Philadelphia: Churchill Livingston; 2008. p. 1170–85.

56. Kuhajda I, Zarogoulidis K, Tsirgogianni K, et al. Lung abscess-etiology, diagnostic and treatment options. Ann Transl Med. 2015;3(13):183.

57. Herth F, Ernst A, Becker HD. Endoscopic drainage of lung abscesses: technique and outcome. Chest. 2005;127(4):1378–81.

58. Shen H, Lu FL, Wu H, et al. Management of tension pneumatocele with high-frequency oscillatory ventilation. Chest. 2002;121:284–7.

59. Fujii AM, Moulton S. VATS management of an enlarging multicysticpneumatocele. J Perinatol. 2008;28(6):445–7.

60. Morar R, Feldman C. Pulmonary echinococcus. Eur Respir J. 2003;21:1069–77.

61. Thumler J, Munoz A. Pulmonary and hepatic echinococcus in children. Pediatr Radiol. 1978;7:164–71.

62. Aletras H, Symbas PN. Hydatid disease of the lung. In: Shields TW, LoCicero J, Ponn RB, editors. General thoracic surgery. 5th ed. Philadelphia: Lippincott Williams and Wilkins; 2000. p. 1113.

63. Date A, Zachariaih N. Saprophytic mycosis with pulmonary echinococcosis. J Trop Med Hyg. 1995;98:404–6.

64. Kuzucu A, Soysal O, Ozgel M, et al. Complicated hydatic cysts of the lung: clinical and therapeutic issues. Ann Thorac Surg. 2004;77:1200–4.

65. Jacob R, Sen S. The anesthetic management of a deliberately created bronchoatmospheric fistula in bilateral pulmonary hydatids. Paediatr Anaesth. 2001;11:733–6.

Bronchopleural Fistulae

43

Andrew Ian Levin

Summary

Bronchopleural fistulae (BPFs) are air leaks that occur via connections between airways and the pleural space. They may be divided into two broad categories, alveolar-parenchymal-pleural and bronchopleural fistulae when they originate from lung parenchyma or tracheobronchial tree, respectively [1, 2]. Prior to anesthesia induction, anesthesiologists must evaluate not only the absolute size of the fistula but also the "effective" size of the fistula. The effective size of the fistula considers both the physical size of the fistula and the effect of lung mechanics on the distribution of ventilation and fistula gas flow during positive pressure ventilation (IPPV). If IPPV results in preferential gas flow via the fistula, difficult or impossible alveolar ventilation could result. As total functional residual capacity may be reduced in the presence of a large BPF, severe hypoxia and difficulty in ventilation can result after anesthesia induction and initiation of IPPV. The safest approach is to determine effective fistula size before anesthesia induction and let that decision guide the safest for anesthesia induction technique. Small "effective size" fistulae can be managed with conventional induction of anesthesia followed by lung isolation if needed. Fistulae that have a large effective size need a more conservative approach, with maintenance of spontaneous respiration during induction and until fistula isolation. This latter goal can be achieved with volatile induction and placement of a double-lumen endotracheal tube; alternatively, awake single-lumen tube intubation may be performed followed by lung isolation prior to commencement of IPPV. Bronchopleural fistulae are increasingly being managed by interventional pulmonologists using minimally invasive techniques, endobronchial valves placement having proved successful on many occasions. The management of BPFs in the ICU is a complex issue, the primary aim being treatment of the underlying lung disease and optimizing IPPV and arterial oxygenation, with management of the air leak using lung isolation or other techniques usually being of secondary importance.

Pathophysiology and Pathogenesis of Bronchopleural Fistulae

Lung mechanics dictate that a balance be maintained between two opposing forces, the lung's elastic recoil which promotes

A. I. Levin (✉)
Department of Anaesthesiology and Critical Care, University of Stellenbosch, Tygerberg Hospital, Cape Town, WC, South Africa
e-mail: ail@sun.ac.za

© Springer Nature Switzerland AG 2019
P. Slinger (ed.), *Principles and Practice of Anesthesia for Thoracic Surgery*, https://doi.org/10.1007/978-3-030-00859-8_43

lung collapse and the tendency of the chest wall to expand [3]. These opposing forces create the negative intrapleural pressure.

Following disruption of the hermetic pleural seal, pulmonary elastic recoil promotes lung collapse. Gas (usually air) fills the pleural space (pneumothorax). If such a disruption is caused by a chest wall penetrating injury that does not affect the lung itself, a simple pneumothorax will ensue. A simple pneumothorax is easily drained using a thoracostomy (chest) tube attached to an underwater seal drain or one-way flapper-type valve. Once the simple pneumothorax is drained, the air leak will not persist. The lung should expand following restoration of the negative intrapleural pressure.

A different picture will result if the injury causes a bronchus or other airways to be disrupted and simultaneously sets up a connection to the pleural space. Under such circumstances, bronchial gas will enter the pleural cavity by either being sucked in during spontaneous respiration or forced in during intermittent positive pressure ventilation. The negative intrapleural pressure is eliminated, and lung elastic recoil will promote its collapse. Percutaneous chest tube insertion and attachment to an underwater seal drain will reveal continuous air leak. The lung will only partially inflate or not re-inflate at all. This is termed a bronchopleural-cutaneous fistula. With bronchopleural or even a simple pleural-cutaneous fistula, if gas continues to enter the pleural space, is not able to escape and intrapleural pressure becomes positive, a tension pneumothorax ensues. A tension pneumothorax may occur during either positive pressure or spontaneous ventilation, if the fistula functions as a one-way valve. The consequences of a tension pneumothorax are progressive cardiovascular and respiratory compromise. In this respect, a critical assumption and prerequisite when dealing with a patient with a bronchopleural fistula is the presence of a functioning, correctly positioned chest tube and underwater seal or flapper drain.

The pathophysiology can be divided into or bronchopleural and alveolar-pleural fistulae. The pathogenesis of these two pathophysiological entities is different, although the two could coexist (Table 43.1).

Table 43.1 A simple approach to causes of bronchopleural fistula

1. Bronchopleural fistula:
   1. Penetrating trauma:
      1. Iatrogenic injury following instrumentation from inside the airway
      2. Iatrogenic injury following tissue disruption from outside the airway or pleura
      3. Non-iatrogenic penetrating trauma such as gunshots, stab wounds, or impalement
      4. Blunt trauma, crush injuries such as being crushed by a falling heavy objet, and acceleration-deceleration injuries as in motor vehicle accidents
      5. *Medical disorders* radiotherapy and chemotherapy
2. Alveolar-parenchymal-pleural fistulae:
   1. Ventilation trauma is commonly associated with this type of fistula

A bronchopleural fistula may follow either *penetrating or blunt traumatic injury*, which causes bronchus disruption and creates a bronchopleural connection.

Penetrating non-iatrogenic trauma may follow knife or gunshot injuries, impalement, or other forms of trauma. They typically present with non-resolving pneumothoraxes or immediate large air leaks.

Penetrating iatrogenic trauma may follow medical-surgical instrumentation from inside the airway (endotracheal tube introducer or bougie, airway exchange catheters, endobronchial biopsy, misplaced nasogastric tubes endobronchial biopsy, etc.) or from outside the lung (thoracostomy tube insertion, percutaneous lung biopsy, central vein cannulation). Bronchopleural fistulae are very common post-thoracic surgical complications, occurring after 1.5–28% of all pulmonary surgeries (e.g., pneumonectomy, lobectomy, bullectomy, etc.) [4–7]. Post-lung resection BPFs are most often located in the residual lobe's bronchial stump [8]. Other associations include pneumonectomy rather than lobectomy; right-sided pulmonary resections; concurrent infections such as tuberculosis, lung abscess, and empyema; resection for malignancy; residual bronchial tumor; preoperative radiotherapy and/or chemotherapy; and poor wound healing conditions such as diabetes, malnutrition, anemia, and steroid administration. Bronchial stump disruption has been associated with postoperative intermittent positive pressure ventilation or bronchoscopy for secretion removal [9–16]. Because of the high incidence, much emphasis has been placed on surgical strategies to prevent this complication. These include avoidance of excessively tight bronchial sutures, avoidance of a long residual bronchial stump, avoidance of excessive peribronchial and paratracheal dissection, staple line buttressing, and protocol-driven chest tube management [17].

Blunt trauma may cause bronchopleural fistulae by one of the three mechanisms:

1. *A crush injury* with chest compression in the presence of a closed glottis can cause the membranous portion of the tracheobronchial tree to rupture [18–20]. Tracheobronchial injuries mostly [76%] occurr within 2 cm of the carina. The greater prevalence of right-sided injuries is due to the longer and more pliable left main bronchus being protected by the aorta and mediastinal structures, while the shorter right bronchus is attached to the heavier lung.
2. Abrupt anterior-posterior thoracic compression can cause lateral widening of the chest and lungs with distraction of the carina [18, 21].
3. Acceleration-deceleration injury can cause the weight of the lungs to apply traction to the relatively fixed carina. This may cause tracheobronchial rupture.

Ventilation trauma is a common cause of alveolar-parenchymal-pleural fistulae. Macklin and colleagues clarified the mechanism of how intermittent positive pressure ventilation causes bronchopleural fistulae. The "Macklin effect" is made up of three steps (Fig. 43.1):

1. During mechanical ventilation, volutrauma causes rupture of alveoli and terminal bronchioles. It is important to appreciate that alveoli do not usually rupture through the dense pleural membrane into the pleural cavity unless there has been penetrating trauma [22, 23].

2. Gas escaping from the alveoli and terminal bronchioles dissects along the bronchovascular sheaths to reach the mediastinum [23–28]. This process manifests as pulmonary interstitial emphysema.

3. The pneumomediastinum then dissects along fascial sheaths to create a cervical or thoracic subcutaneous emphysema and/or pneumothorax with typical character-

Fig. 43.1 The "Macklin effect". (Reprinted with permission from Visser et al. [23])

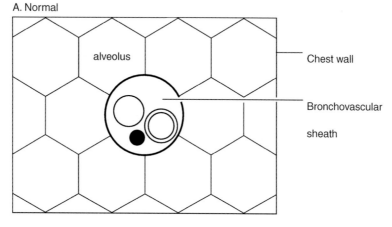

A. Normal

alveolus

Chest wall

Bronchovascular

sheath

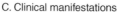

B. Interstitial emphysema

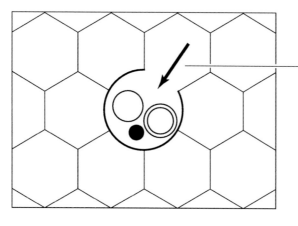

Alveolus ruptures into bronchovascular

sheath (no support from neighboring

alveoli)

C. Clinical manifestations

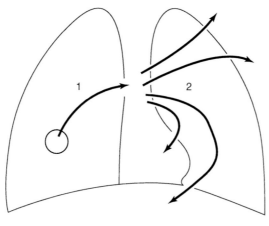

Air moves from bronchovascular sheath

to mediastinum and from there migrates

to become clinically apparent as one or

more of the following:

    a)   Surgical emphysema

    b)   Pneumothorax

    c)   Pneumopericardium

    d)   Air under the diaphragm

istics of a bronchopleural fistula. These "peripheral" air leaks are referred to as a alveolar-pleural or parenchymal-pleural fistulae [29, 30]. Other possible complications of pneumomediastinum and fascial sheath dissection are pneumopericardium or pneumoperitoneum [22].

Medical disorders and treatment can cause BPFs. Primary (no known underlying lung disease) or secondary spontaneous pneumothorax may result in persistent air leaks [31]. Close investigation suggests many (90%) of these patients have underlying chronic pulmonary obstructive disease with subpleural blebs or bullae [32–34]. Larger bullae can rupture into the pleural space and cause a BPF. Occasionally, infections (lung abscesses, tuberculosis), primary lung or pleural tumors, or metastatic tumors erode bronchi and create bronchopleural connections. Iatrogenic BPFs have been caused by radiotherapy and chemotherapy [10, 35–45].

The Pathophysiological Consequences of Large Air Leaks

In the presence of an air leak, a proportion of the tidal volume is lost via the bronchopleural fistula. The gas lost into the pleural space forms wasted (dead space) ventilation, with reduction of alveolar ventilation.

The affected lung will collapse in the presence of a large unilateral air leak. Pulmonary blood flow will be diverted from the affected to the "normal" lung by the increase in pulmonary vascular resistance induced by both hypoxic pulmonary vasoconstriction and the decrease in lung volume. This will limit the size of the shunt and the amount of low ventilation-perfusion units in the affected lung. Hypoxia is therefore not a prominent feature of uncomplicated bronchopleural fistula.

The dead space lesion will cause a respiratory acidosis. The respiratory center will then stimulate minute ventilation, which will aggravate the sensation of air hunger. During intermittent positive pressure ventilation, the gas leaked via the bronchopleural fistula contributes somewhat to carbon dioxide elimination [46].

In the presence of a large unilateral bronchopleural fistula, the mechanics of breathing become ineffective. The diaphragm and intercostal muscle action cannot generate the usual negative intrapleural pressure needed to increase the transpulmonary pressure gradient and expand the lungs. This ineffective mechanism, combined with the increased minute ventilation due to the respiratory acidosis, will lead to dyspnea, respiratory distress, air hunger, and tachypnea. This may be aggravated by any underlying infection with an increase in carbon dioxide production or contralateral lung parenchymal (restrictive) disease processes. It may be diffi-

cult to separate the effects of a bronchopleural fistula from the patient's underlying lung disease [47].

Other complications and consequences of a BPF include the inability to maintain PEEP and de-recruitment of the unaffected lung during intermittent positive pressure ventilation [2]. Large bilateral BPFs may rapidly lead to death. Bronchopleural fistulae can allow airway organisms to reach the normally sterile pleural space, leading to clinical infection and further impeding closure of the leak [2]. Lung function tests are unreliable in the presence of a bronchopleural fistula.

Bronchopleural Fistula, Intermittent Positive Pressure Ventilation, and Effective Fistula Size

Positive pressure ventilation may cause preferential gas flow via the BPF and chest tube and compromise effective alveolar ventilation. To appreciate how this works, the interaction of the physical factors governing fistula flow and the mechanics of alveolar ventilation need to be considered. Fistula gas flow is inversely proportional to the resistance and directly proportional to the pressure gradient over the fistula. During IPPV, the proximal fistula driving pressure is effectively peak (or if distally located, mean) airway pressure.

The worst-case scenario is represented by the combination of a large fistula and non-compliant lungs. Non-compliant lungs (restrictive disease such as pulmonary fibrosis, cystic fibrosis, acute lung injury, small lung volumes, pleural or chest wall disease) will require a higher transpulmonary pressure gradient with higher airway pressures to generate effective tidal volumes. This higher airway pressure will favor fistula gas flow. Furthermore, in the presence of a very large fistula, it may not be able to achieve high enough airway and transpulmonary pressures to effect adequate tidal volumes . In this scenario, intermittent positive pressure ventilation will result in preferential fistula flow and ineffective alveolar ventilation.

The best-case scenario is the combination of a small BPF with two normal or emphysematous, highly compliant lungs. The presence of normal or high pulmonary compliance requires low transpulmonary pressures to effect adequate tidal volumes. The low airway pressures and small fistula size result in limited BPF gas flow and adequate alveolar ventilation. This scenario typically occurs with a patient with a spontaneous pneumothorax with bullous COAD, or post-pneumonectomy with a small, persistent bronchial stump fistula with a relatively unscathed, or healthy non-resected lung.

The above emphasizes that it is not only the absolute physical size and physical characteristics of the fistula that matters. Lung mechanics affect how fistulae function. These concepts are summarized by the term "effective fistula size" which is essentially a clinical estimate of the balance between BPF flow and the effective tidal volume that will likely be generated during intermittent positive pressure ventilation. With a large effective fistula size, the majority of the tidal volume delivered during intermittent positive pressure ventilation will escape via the fistula with concomitant poor alveolar ventilation.

Anesthesia and BPF

Prior to starting anesthesia induction, it is essential to ensure correct pleural cavity positioning of the thoracostomy tube. Furthermore, the thoracostomy tube and the underwater drain seal or one-way flapper valve system must function properly. Thoracostomy tubes may become blocked with infective material or clotted blood, or the drainage system tubing may be deliberately clamped or become accidentally kinked during patient transport. The combination of a non-functional thoracostomy tube and the initiation of intermittent positive pressure ventilation can produce a tension pneumothorax with associated (hemodynamic) consequences. The only exception to the presence of a functional thoracostomy tube is if the bronchopleural fistula is small and restrictive, as may occur after lung surgery.

The chest tube should be of adequate diameter and low enough resistance to effectively evacuate the pleural space so tension pneumothorax does not develop during intermittent positive pressure ventilation [48]. Gas flow via a chest tube is summed up by the Fanning equation, $V = \prod^2 r^5 [P1 - P2]/fL$ where V is flow rate, $[P1-P2]$ is the pressure gradient over the chest tube, "f" is the Fanning friction factor, "L" is the length of the tube, and "r" is the radius of the tube. The Fanning equation effectively says that shorter, wider chest tubes support the highest pleural cavity gas evacuation rates [2, 48].

If the thoracostomy tube was subject to negative pressure suction in the ward, it is advisable to keep this operational during anesthesia induction while considering that this may cause or aggravate anesthesia gas and vapor evacuation during induction.

The physiological tolerance to both apnea and the ability to tolerate intermittent positive pressure ventilation are critical elements to consider when deciding on how to best manage induction (Table 43.2). Apnea at induction may follow opioid and/or induction agent administration and will occur after neuromuscular blocker administration. It is critical that the anesthesia providers consider whether initiation of positive pressure ventilation may result in preferential gas flow via the fistula. This could result in difficult or impossible alveolar ventilation. A cannot ventilate-cannot oxygenate scenario could possibly ensue.

A further inconvenient physiological consideration is the potential for rapid onset of hypoxia with apnea and/or ineffective lung ventilation. On the fistula affected side, pulmo-

Table 43.2 Considerations for anesthesia management of bronchopleural fistula

(i) *Safety before starting:* Is the thoracostomy tube in the pleural cavity and correctly positioned, of appropriate size, and functioning correctly?

(ii) *Safety with induction:* Before induction of anesthesia, carefully estimate the effective fistula size and the distribution of ventilation on initiation of intermittent positive pressure ventilation?

(iii) *Safety with respect to distribution of ventilation ± lung isolation:* What is the best method of isolating the lung? Is there a risk of tearing the fistula with airway instrumentation, and if so, how is this best avoided? Is there a risk of contamination of the "healthy lung," usually from an empyema or lung abscess, and how is that best avoided?

(iv) *Consider* what is the surgeon and/or pulmonologist going to do?

(v) In the light of the previous three statements, what is the best method of inducing anesthesia? If the fistula size is small, consider conventional general anesthesia. If the effective fistula size is large, consider volatile induction with spontaneous respiration and of a double-lumen tube placement guided preferably by a fiber-optic scope to avoid fistula damage. Alternatively, with a large fistula, perform an awake single-lumen intubation and then isolate the lung by advancing the endotracheal tube into an appropriate bronchus; alternatively place a bronchial blocker considering that it is not the most secure isolation device

(vi) *Postoperative concerns:* Can postoperative ventilation be avoided to prevent causing or re-opening the fistula? What is the best method of providing postoperative analgesia? Is epidural analgesia possible, or is there local infection?

nary elastic recoil will result in varying degrees of lung collapse. This diminishes the patient's functional residual capacity and oxygen reservoir. Furthermore, oxygen consumption may be increased by the greater work of breathing and/or the presence of infection. After anesthesia induction, the occurrence of apnea, hypoventilation, or difficult alveolar ventilation can therefore result in the rapid onset of hypoxia in the presence of a bronchopleural fistula [49].

When presented with a scenario of difficult ventilation with a rapidly desaturating patient, the anesthesiologist may hastily attempt lung isolation and control of ventilation. Incorrect double- or single-lumen tube position can lead to failure to control either the air leak or effect adequate alveolar ventilation. Another risk is that the tube enters or tears the fistula and aggravates the situation.

This is therefore a potentially difficult [lower] airway scenario, and, as with all potentially difficult airways, it is critical to plan thoroughly beforehand. The plan must consider how anesthetic induction and lung isolation are best conducted. It is also not always possible to know or predict the precise size of the fistula. Indeed, there is a paucity of high-quality scientific evidence on which to base the treatment of BPFs, most literature being small case series or dramatic case reports.

Before induction of anesthesia, this author looks for clues regarding the physical size of the fistula and underlying lung mechanics to evaluate the "effective fistula size" (see above), which is a clinical evaluation of the balance between BPF flow and tidal volume that will likely be generated during intermittent positive pressure ventilation. Determining "effective fistula size" is not an exact science but is useful to decide how to best manage anesthetic induction. With a large effective fistula size, the majority of the tidal volume delivered during intermittent positive pressure ventilation will likely escape via the fistula and is accompanied by poor alveolar ventilation. Under such circumstances, IPPV is best avoided during induction and before distribution of ventilation has been controlled. Control of the distribution of ventilation is usually achieved by employing lung isolation techniques.

Estimating the physical size of the fistula can be assumed from a variety of sources of information. Determining the pathogenesis of the BPF may be useful. For example, it may be obvious that a large fistula resulted from a penetrating or blunt injury, or it is a small, post-lung resection fistula. Inspection of the imaging, particularly the chest computerized tomograms, often indicates the physical size and exact location of the fistula (Fig. 43.2). Fiber-optic bronchoscopy can also be used to evaluate the position and size of the lesion.

Pulmonary mechanics significantly affects how BPFs function. Evaluating the mechanics of both lungs is useful to evaluate whether the peak airway pressures needed for effective alveolar ventilation will be high or low. The transpulmonary pressure gradient needed for adequate alveolar ventilation is largely determined by the ventilated lung compliance and resistance. A high and a low peak airway pressures will aggravate and ameliorate fistula flow, respectively. Gaining a clinical appreciation of the underlying pathophysiology helps evaluate pulmonary compliance. This may be obvious from the patient's history or the context, such as a long smoking history with severe obstructive airways dis-

ease, a history of restrictive pulmonary disease, or a patient in ICU with acute lung injury. Furthermore, chest wall and pleural conditions as well as factors affecting lung volumes such as intra-abdominal pressures and obesity all affect the transpulmonary pressure gradient. These important determinants of pulmonary mechanics will influence fistula functioning. The lung imaging may offer useful information on the underlying lung parenchymal or pleural diseases and lung volumes.

The mechanics and particularly the compliance of the affected lung having the BPF also matter when evaluating the "effective fistula size." When evaluating the transpulmonary pressure gradient likely needed to effect an adequate tidal volume, the extent of ipsilateral lung collapse on imaging is potentially useful. Complete ipsilateral lung collapse despite both tube thoracostomy and negative pressure suction suggests that the fistula is large and/or the lung compliance is low. This suggests a large effective fistula size and heralds that problems can be expected with intermittent positive pressure ventilation. However, a fully expanded lung on the affected side with only tube thoracostomy indicates the presence of a small BPF and/or a very compliant lung. This suggests that the effective fistula size is small, and problems with intermittent positive pressure ventilation are unlikely. The amount of respiratory distress also relates to the effective size of the fistula.

The amount of underwater drain bubbling (i.e., the effective volume of gas going through the fistula) may offer clues to the effective size of the fistula. Fistula size is typically classified into small, medium, or large according to the magnitude of the air leak and whether the bubbling is during inspiration or during expiration and whether it is continuous during both inspiration and expiration or if it only occurs during coughing:

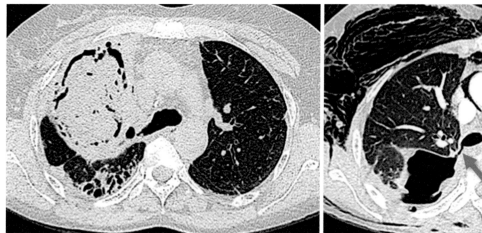
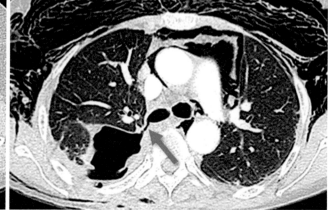

Fig. 43.2 The chest CT scan of a patient with previous pulmonary tuberculosis and a right upper lobe mycetoma. The left-hand image is prior to resection, and the arrow in the right-hand image points to a residual bronchopleural fistula 2 weeks after resection. This was closed surgically

1. Small, trivial: Air leak present only with Valsalva maneuver or coughing.
2. Medium: Air leak present with expiration only.
3. Large: Air leak present during both inspiration and expiration.

The volume of gas escaping via the fistula may be quantified with a spirometer or pneumotachograph placed between the thoracostomy tube and the underwater seal or flapper valve drainage device [29, 50–52]. Kempainen and Pierson suggest that a difference of more than 100 ml between the inspired and expired tidal volumes in a ventilated patient is indicative of a large leak [29]. In clinic medicine, this is not practical and seldom performed [2]. Despite being suggested as being a reliable indicator of effective fistula size, the "degree" of bubbling depends heavily on the patency of the underwater drain, drains being easily blocked by pus or clotted blood. Furthermore, while the resistance offered by the chest tube and drainage system is assumed minimal, this may not be so when using "waterless, pleural drainage units containing a flapper, one-way, Heimlich-type valve". Such systems are not all equivalently designed or constructed and may have inherent resistance which prevents the evaluation of airflow as described above in the classic, older water seal type systems [53].

The anesthesiologist faced with a bronchopleural fistula must therefore try to predict the effective fistula size, i.e., the distribution of gas flow via the BPF compared to how effective alveolar ventilation will likely be during intermittent positive pressure ventilation. With a large effective size fistulae, intermittent positive pressure ventilation will be problematic, most of the delivered tidal volume escaping via the BPF rather than being directed to effective alveolar ventilation. This prediction of "effective fistula size" requires "clinical judgment," the astute clinician weighing up multiple factors. This prediction is not an exact science, and the evaluation can prove wrong. A note of caution is that BPFs may be damaged and/or enlarged by airway instrumentation. Furthermore, if loose material partially obstructs the orifice, this material can be dislodged by airway instrumentation or coughing. Therefore, the initial physical appearance of the hole or the "effective fistula size" may not always represent the actual or potential size of the opening.

Having decided on the effective fistula size, a decision how to induce anesthesia and isolate the lungs needs to be made (Table 43.2). Despite being discussed "separately," a suitable method of both induction and lung isolation [and alternatives if the chosen method is ineffective]need to be decided upon beforehand. Practical preparations then need to be made to facilitate the chosen technique prior to commencement of the anaesthetic. If the effective fistula size is judged to be small, it is invariably safe to perform a "conventional" anesthesia induction sequence using opioids, induction agent, and a non-depolarizing or depolarizing neuromuscular blocker, followed by facemask intermittent positive pressure ventilation. Flexible or rigid bronchoscopic airway inspection is then frequently performed to better define the anatomy.

If the effective fistula size is evaluated as being large, it is crucial to avoid intermittent positive pressure ventilation until lung isolation has occurred. Under such circumstances, the anesthesiologist must use a "non-conventional" induction technique to ensure that the patient continues to breathe spontaneously until lung isolation and the distribution of ventilation is controlled. These goals can be achieved using volatile anesthesia induction or an awake intubation followed by lung isolation. Volatile anesthesia induction using sevoflurane accompanied by high oxygen concentrations is usually safe and efficient. After volatile induction of general anesthesia, placement of a double-lumen tube and lung isolation is usually easily performed to control the distribution of ventilation during intermittent positive pressure ventilation. Alternatively, a single-lumen tube can be used to effect lung isolation. Anesthetists practicing thoracic surgery must be proficient and practiced with a spontaneous breathing, gas induction technique to facilitate double lumen tube placemement, the authors preferred technique described in Table 43.3. Alternatively, placement of a single-lumen endotracheal tube into the upper airway, proximal to where the fistula is expected to be found, can be performed. This single-lumen tube is then used to establish control of the distribution of ventilation either using a bronchial blocker or using the single lumen tube to efffect lung isolation. This can be performed awake or after spontaneous respiration, gas induction of anaesthesia. Anesthetists need to be proficient at awake (single-lumen) endotracheal intubation without distressing the patient, the staff, or themselves. Being proficient also reduces reluctance to perform awake intubation [54, 55]. A technique often touted for control of ventilation is awake placement of a double-lumen tube. It is suggested that this be railroaded over a tracheally placed fiber-optic scope or an (appropriately sized, stiff enough, long enough) airway exchange catheter. This approach is technically challenging, and this author seldom if ever uses it . [54, 55].

In the presence of a large bronchopleural fistula, *unconventional ways of ventilation and oxygenation* have included high-frequency oscillation in combination with spontaneous ventilation, ECMO, or avoiding general anesthesia and airway instrumentation altogether and utilizing epidural or regional anesthesia [56–58]. Dependent positioning of the affected lung has reduced BPF flow [59].

The question often arises how best to manage the patient when it is difficult to decide whether the effective fistula size is small or large and/or it is truly a "medium"-sized fistula? Is the case best managed using the unconventional "complicated" spontaneous breathing volatile induction method, or does the anesthetist risk using a conventional induction with a non-depolarizing neuromuscular blocker followed by

Table 43.3 A suggested technique for volatile spontaneous induction of anesthesia:

(i) *Step 1:* Prepare airway equipment including a Saunders injector, rigid and fiber-optic bronchoscopes, airway exchange catheters, and suction catheters, and the surgeon present

(ii) *Step 2: Preoxygenation:* Preoxygenate using high fresh gas flow and 100% oxygen. During all upper airway instrumentation maneuvers, high-flow nasal oxygen may be useful to maintain oxygenation provided it does not cause excessive PEEP and damage the fistula

(iii) *Step 3: Volatile induction while maintaining spontaneous respiration:*

   1. Perform sevoflurane volatile anesthesia induction using in 100% oxygen while maintaining spontaneous respiration

   2. Consider administering a *small* dose of midazolam (1–2 mg/80–100 kg) when induction commences

   3. Gentle pressure support may be useful during gas induction. Note that spontaneous respiration under volatile anesthesia occurs at a carbon dioxide partial pressure of approximately 0.5 kPa above the apnea point. Excessive assistance may render the patient apneic

(iv) Step *4: Options to obtund airway reflexes prior to laryngoscopy and double-lumen tube placement. The advantages and disadvantages of each maneuver below must be carefully considered.*

   1. *The one possibility is to topicalize the airway.* This may be performed using rigid laryngoscopy to instill 10–15 ml of 2% lidocaine down the tracheobronchial tree, when the patient is "deeply enough anesthetized." The author invariably uses this method. After topicalization, reapply the anesthesia mask and administer sevoflurane in 100% oxygen until the patient is "deep enough" again

   2. Laryngeal spasm following local anesthetic instillation could be very problematic, this seldom occurring if the patient was deep enough. Alternatively, transtracheal local anesthetic injection in the awake patient may be used to topicalize the airway, a method that seldom induces laryngeal spasm

   3. Anticholinergic pretreatment is usually not needed but may be considered

   4. *An alternative to airway topicalization is to administer an ultra-short-acting opioid,* either a bolus of alfentanil 10–15 mg/kg or start a remifentanil infusion ≥ 0,1 ug/kg/minute or TCI targeting 1 to 2 ng/ml 1 minute prior to airway instrumentation. The disadvantage of opioids is they will inevitably cause apnea, and the time to begin spontaneous respiration again when combined with general anaesthesthetics is somewhat uncertain!

   5. Despite airway topicalization, this author invariably administers *Propofol 0.5 mg/kg* during spontaneous respiration with sevoflurane just prior to airway instrumentation. Again, apnea can ensue!

Airway instrumentation:

   1. Perform laryngoscopy and advance the desired airway device (double- or single-lumen endotracheal tube) only into the upper part of the trachea, proximal to the suspected location of the BPF. DLT placement is usually easy under volatile anesthesia if the patient does not have a difficultly airway

   2. After upper airway location of the airway device, airway toilet is often useful to facilitate fiber-optic inspection of the airway. This may be performed using a suction catheter or via a fiber-optic scope. To avoid physical disruption of the bronchopleural fistula, guide the double-lumen tube or airway device into its more distal position using a fiber-optic scope

IPPV? A technique often suggested as an alternative is to preoxygenate, induce anesthesia, and administer suxamethonium. The airway and distribution of ventilation will be easily controlled with the chosen lung isolation technique, which will not take long. The assumption is that the period of apnea before the airway is secured or before spontaneous respiration resumes will be short, as suxamethonium is "short-acting." With the widespread introduction of sugammadex, the use of rocuronium will eventually be touted as alternative to suxamethonium. However, with compromise of the functional residual capacity, severe hypoxia may ensue before the distribution of ventilation can be controlled or spontaneous respiration resumes. Furthermore, in a race against time prior to desaturation, hasty airway instrumentation may damage the fistula. It is far preferable to make a definitive decision before induction of anesthesia, declare it a small or large fistula, and use a conventional or nonconventional anesthesia induction sequence, as appropriate. Such an approach also makes anesthetists use, practice, and teach their "non-conventional" techniques more often which may promote patient safety.

After induction of anesthesia using conventional or inhalation techniques, double-lumen tubes are commonly used to control airflow in the presence of a BPF. A left-sided DLT is commonly used with a right-sided fistula and vice versa.

After anesthetized or awake placement of a single-lumen endotracheal tube, control of the distribution of ventilation is usually achieved using unilateral bronchial intubation or using a bronchial blocker. Unilateral bronchial intubation by advancing an appropriately sized single-lumen tube into a bronchus under bronchoscopic guidance is usually simple to perform. The simplicity of the technique means it is potentially useful in acute life-threatening situations. Selective left main bronchus intubation is better suited to this technique as it allows ventilation of the entire left lung. Disadvantages of this technique are that toilet of the contralateral bronchus cannot be performed and that selective right main or bronchus intermedius intubation usually allows only two-lobe ventilation and a high risk of hypoxia. After single-lumen tube placement, a bronchial blocker can be placed via the endotracheal tube and located proximally to the fistula. Alternatively, the bronchial blocker may be placed outside the endotracheal tube and then advanced into position under fiber-optic guidance. This latter "outside the tube" approach is better suited to the anaesthetised patient.

There is some controversy about the use of bronchial blockers in the presence of bronchopleural fistulae. Double-lumen tubes are considered more reliable in ensuring lung isolation and control of the distribution of ventilation [60, 61]. Because of poorer reliability, particularly when placed in the short right main bronchus, bronchial blockers have been considered less suitable devices. However, this concern must be balanced against the considerations that awake intubation with a double-lumen tube can be very difficult, whereas awake single-lumen tube tracheal intubation followed by bronchial blocker placement through the tube is much easier. These considerations may apply even more in the patient who has a difficult upper airway. Bronchial blocker placement may also be considerably easier in the patient already intubated with a single-lumen tube, for example, in the ICU.

When lower airway instrumentation is performed in patients with bronchopleural fistulae, it is very important this be performed under bronchoscopic vision to avoid compromising fistula integrity. Airway devices can enter and damage or enlarge the fistula. Despite being small, the tissue surrounding the fistula may be very friable and tenuous. Airway devices such as endotracheal, double-lumen tubes or blockers can snag on bronchial sutures and directly enter and further disrupt the fistula. It is therefore critical to avoid blind advancement of any airway device and advance airway devices gently, only under direct vision facilitated by a flexible bronchoscope. This may require meticulous prior airway toilet to clear pus and secretions. Airway instrumentation is unlikely to aggravate alveolar-parenchymal fistula damage.

The affected pleural cavity may contain copious amounts of pus or infected material. This often occurs in the presence of post-thoracic surgery infection. If the pus is thin and/or the fistula is large, there is a risk of contaminating the dependent lung after turning the patient into the lateral decubitus position. During induction but before lung isolation has been achieved, gravity can be used to prevent or limit spillage to the normal lung. The affected side should be placed below the normal side by appropriate tilting of the operating table or patient during the induction sequence. Furthermore, the double-lumen tube or bronchial blocker should effect a watertight seal and also must not dislodge when turning the patient into the lateral decubitus position. The anesthesiologists must carefully consider the advisability of adhering to the conventional directive to deflate the bronchial cuff during turning. Suitable suction catheters and effective suction should be present. If the fistula is very small, classic lung isolation may not be needed to control the distribution of ventilation. Nonetheless, even with a small fistula, the risk of soiling of the "normal" lung still exists particularly if thin pus is present in the affected pleural cavity.

Postoperative ventilation may put strain on a sutured bronchus or repaired fistula and has been associated with fistula formation or re-occurrence. It is prudent to avoid postoperative IPPV in these circumstances. Noninvasive ventilatory support may be more suitable after such surgery.

In the presence of systemic and local infection, and pus draining from a chest drain, it may be inadvisable to use epidural analgesia.

Interventional Pulmonology Management of Bronchopleural Fistula

Interventional pulmonology techniques have been used to treat BPFs [32]. These techniques were previously reserved for high-risk surgical patients but are becoming more commonly used as the primary intervention [9, 32, 62, 63]. The anesthesiologist needs to appreciate what the surgeon is planning and incorporate it into the anesthesia technique. The interested reader is referred to Slade's clear review of the pulmonary interventional techniques available to treat BPFs [32].

The precise bronchial source of the air leak can be identified using computed tomography scanning or may be visible on bronchoscopy. Sometimes, the "feeding" bronchi cannot be identified as they are too distal or there is haste. In these cases, the offending bronchi may be identified using a sequential Fogarty catheter bronchial occlusion technique [32, 64, 65].

Once identified, the offending bronchi can be occluded with a variety of techniques. Mechanical occlusion has been achieved by deploying Watanabe silicone spigots, vascular occlusion coils, and tracheobronchial silicone or self-expanding metal stents [66–75]. A novel, successful approach to larger lesions has been the use of Amplatzer intracardiac and vascular occlusion devices placed over the BPF [76–82]. Bronchial instillation of cyanoacrylate or fibrin glue has been successful with smaller less than 5 mm diameter fistulae but risk damage to expensive bronchoscopes [83–87]. Bronchial occlusion has also been achieved following submucosal sclerosing agent injection or endobronchial coagulation using Nd:YAG laser or argon plasma coagulation [32, 88].

While most interventional pulmonology approaches rely on case reports or case series, the strongest evidence base comes from the use of unidirectional endobronchial valves [32, 62, 89–104]. These devices were originally designed for lung volume reduction procedures. After endobronchial placement, they limit or prevent gas passage out of the particular bronchus and promote distal parenchymal atelectasis. The available evidence suggests great success in treating BPFs of various etiologies including spontaneous pneumothorax; postsurgical, traumatic, and iatrogenic BPFs; and in cystic fibrosis [62, 64, 93, 105, 106]. Endobronchial valves have also been used urgently in critically ill patients that have developed BPFs. Their use has allowed weaning from ECMO and mechanical ventilation and facilitated chest tube removal [107, 108]. Interventional pulmonology approaches become logistically difficult or impossible as the number and/or size of the air leaks increases; thus, in situations of massive air leaks, ventilator strategies are preferable [29, 50].

A bronchopleural fistula (BPF) is usually a manifestation of the underlying lung disease, particularly in adult respiratory distress syndrome (ARDS). Therefore, measures to reduce the air leak are generally unsuccessful until the patient's underlying lung disease has improved. Even if the severity of the air leak is successfully reduced, there tends to be little effect on gas exchange, as measured by arterial blood gases [29, 50, 109].

Management of Bronchopleural Fistula in Ventilated Patients

Anesthesiologists will encounter bronchopleural fistulae that develop in the ICU. Ventilated patients usually develop alveolar-parenchymal fistulae rather than central connections with the bronchi. Their occurrence invariably indicates the severity of the underlying lung disease or ventilation trauma and is associated with a poor prognosis [47, 48, 110–112]. Anesthesiologists may be involved in both the medical and ventilatory management and also the definitive interventional pulmonology or surgical attempts to close the fistula. While a detailed discussion being beyond the scope of this chapter, brief notes on this topic may be useful.

The primary therapeutic aim should be optimal medical treatment and ventilatory management of the underlying lung disease, often, acute lung injury [29, 113]. Small fistulae invariably resolve as the underlying lung condition improves. Bronchospasm and infection need aggressive treatment. Healing may be facilitated by improved nutritional status. A secondary therapeutic aim is ventilator optimization to minimize the air leak, promote BPF closure, and improve gas exchange [47, 48, 51, 114]. Fistula airflow is increased by higher peak and mean airway pressures. Ventilatory strategies essentially aim at minimizing airway pressures by any means possible [50, 51, 114]. This should employ judicious amounts of PEEP, lowest tidal volumes and transpulmonary pressures possible, and allow permissive hypercapnia.

Conventional ventilation strategies to achieve this aim have included reducing tidal volume, reducing inspiratory time, minimizing PEEP, and using different ventilatory modes (pressure support, pressure control, synchronized intermittent mandatory positive pressure ventilation) and (partially) weaning the patient from ventilation [2, 48, 115–118]. When pressure support ventilation is utilized, the practitioner must consider that inspiratory support is terminated when inspiratory flow is reduced to below a particular value, which may

not occur in the presence of a large air leak [29]. Kempainen and colleagues suggest adopting a ventilatory strategy comprising of "appropriate inaction". This strategy incorporates tolerating larger air leaks, employing higher inspired oxygen concentrations, and tolerating permissive hypercapnia. Nonetheless, while having substantial wisdom, the effect of these strategies on outcome is uncertain [29, 50, 109, 118].

Non-conventional ventilation methods have been advocated. High-frequency jet ventilation has been associated with lower peak airway pressures and is apparently useful in airway disruption with normal lung parenchyma [29, 48, 110, 111, 119–123]. However, change from conventional to high-frequency jet ventilation has been associated with worsening hypoxemia with alveolar-parenchymal disease-related fistulae [114, 124, 125]. Alveolar-parenchymal fistula flow is reduced only if high-frequency ventilation decreases peak and mean airway pressures [48, 51, 52, 119, 124, 126–133]. High-frequency ventilation's propensity to produce PEEP may possibly be the reason for its failure in alveolar-parenchymal disease and utility in tracheo-bronchial disruption [121, 133, 134]. High-frequency oscillation may be an option in acute lung injury complicated with BPF [135].

Another non-conventional "ICU" technique within the anesthesiologist's expertise is placement of a double-lumen endotracheal tube. This can be used for control of the distribution of ventilation and will buy time to develop a definitive therapeutic strategy. Moreover, a double-lumen tube also facilitates differential, independent lung ventilation, particularly if the lungs have different pathologies [2, 29, 48, 129, 136–161]. Independent lung ventilation does not have to use only one ventilator or be of the same mode; for example, one lung can be ventilated with synchronized intermittent mandatory ventilation, while the BPF affected lung is administered continuous positive airway pressure or high-frequency ventilation [129, 136, 138, 139, 143, 147, 162, 163]. Independent lung ventilation can employ ventilation techniques to "rest" (minimize transpulmonary pressures) the BPF affected lung and allow spontaneous healing of small fistulae [113, 118, 129, 137, 164, 165]. By facilitating better non-affected lung management, independent lung ventilation may effect better alveolar ventilation, facilitate gas exchange, and prevent further ventilation trauma. Independent lung ventilation has few deleterious hemodynamic effects and does not require synchronization [148, 166, 167]. Nonetheless, ventilator electronic linking and synchronization have been used.

The use of double-lumen endotracheal tubes DLTs in the ICU is fraught with potential technical problems, particularly displacement, airway toilet, and blockage by secretions. These problems may occur even if the patient is deeply sedated and had recieved non-depolarizing muscle relaxants, and meticulous suctioning . For these reasons, when a DLT is used in the ICU, it is imperative that a suitable bronchoscope and skilled anesthesiologists are immediately available, a significant human resource problem. The high-pressure DLT bronchial and tracheal cuffs can compromise mucosal blood flow. Weaning from the double-lumen to a single-lumen tube to conventional ventilation may be considered when the air leak is resolved; the between-lung tidal volume and compliance difference are less than 100 mL and 20%, respectively [136, 159]. An alternative successfully used approach to differential lung ventilation is selective lobar blockade using a Fogarty catheter or bronchial blocker [168].

Definitive closure may be considered. Open surgery or video-assisted thoracoscopy may be used to visualize and facilitate fistula closure, pleurectomy, and/or pleurodesis. Any of the minimally invasive techniques discussed above, particularly the use of endobronchial valves, can and have been used to effect definitive fistula closure. ECMO has been employed after lung transplantation as a bridge for both successful surgical repairs of BPF and postoperatively to allow bronchial healing with less ventilatory support [57].

When using conventional and non-conventional ventilatory techniques in the ICU, it is assumed that a functional thoracostomy tube is in situ. This may be difficult in the presence of pleural infection, adhesion, and multiple leakage sites. These issues may necessitate careful placement of more than one chest tube [29]. Chest tube manipulations, particularly thoracostomy tube suction, are frequently advocated to induce better pleural space drainage and lung expansion, thereby facilitating fistula closure. Pierson prudently suggests maintaining only the minimum amount of negative thoracostomy tube suction to just keep the affected lung inflated [113]. Excessive thoracostomy suction may cause respiratory alkalosis, not improve or even worsen gas exchange, and initiate ventilator autotriggering [117, 132, 169]. The application of positive intrapleural pressure equal to PEEP may improve oxygenation [115, 116]. Intermittent inspiratory chest tube occlusion has been touted, albeit, it is a technique neither widely available nor feasible with multiple chest tubes [29, 170–173].

References

1. Musani AI, Dutau H. Management of alveolar-pleural fistula: a complex medical and surgical problem. Chest. 2015;147(3):590–2.
2. Shekar K, Foot C, Fraser J, Ziegenfuss M, Hopkins P, Windsor M. Bronchopleural fistula: an update for intensivists. J Crit Care. 2010;25(1):47–55.
3. West JB. Respiratory physiology-the essentials. 9th ed. Philadelphia, PA: Wolters Kluwer; 2012.
4. Yano M, Yokoi K, Numanami H, Kondo R, Ohde Y, Sugaya M, et al. Complications of bronchial stapling in thoracic surgery. World J Surg. 2014;38(2):341–6.
5. Watanabe S, Watanabe T, Urayama H. Endobronchial occlusion method of bronchopleural fistula with metallic coils and glue. Thorac Cardiovasc Surg. 2003;51(2):106–8.
6. Darling GE, Abdurahman A, Yi QL, Johnston M, Waddell TK, Pierre A, et al. Risk of a right pneumonectomy: role of bronchopleural fistula. Ann Thorac Surg. 2005;79(2):433–7.
7. Asamura H, Naruke T, Tsuchiya R, Goya T, Kondo H, Suemasu K. Bronchopleural fistulas associated with lung cancer operations. Univariate and multivariate analysis of risk factors, management, and outcome. J Thorac Cardiovasc Surg. 1992;104(5):1456–64.
8. Sato M, Saito Y, Nagamoto N, Endo C, Usuda K, Takahashi S, et al. An improved method of bronchial stump closure for prevention of bronchopleural fistula in pulmonary resection. Tohoku J Exp Med. 1992;168(3):507–13.
9. Lois M, Noppen M. Bronchopleural fistulas: an overview of the problem with special focus on endoscopic management. Chest. 2005;128(6):3955–65.
10. Frytak S, Lee RE, Pairolero PC, Arnold PG, Shaw JN. Necrotic lung and bronchopleural fistula as complications of therapy in lung cancer. Cancer Investig. 1988;6(2):139–43.
11. McManigle JE, Fletcher GL, Tenholder MF. Bronchoscopy in the management of bronchopleural fistula. Chest. 1990;97(5):1235–8.
12. Sirbu H, Busch T, Aleksic I, Schreiner W, Oster O, Dalichau H. Bronchopleural fistula in the surgery of non-small cell lung cancer: incidence, risk factors, and management. Ann Thorac Cardiovasc Surg. 2001;7(6):330–6.
13. Turk AE, Karanas YL, Cannon W, Chang J. Staged closure of complicated bronchopleural fistulas. Ann Plast Surg. 2000;45(5):560–4.
14. al-Kattan K, Cattelani L, Goldstraw P. Bronchopleural fistula after pneumonectomy for lung cancer. Eur J Cardiothorac Surg. 1995;9(9):479–82.
15. Conlan AA, Lukanich JM, Shutz J, Hurwitz SS. Elective pneumonectomy for benign lung disease: modern-day mortality and morbidity. J Thorac Cardiovasc Surg. 1995;110(4 Pt 1):1118–24.
16. Cerfolio RJ. The incidence, etiology, and prevention of postresectional bronchopleural fistula. Semin Thorac Cardiovasc Surg. 2001;13(1):3–7.
17. Drahush N, Miller AD, Smith JS, Royer AM, Spiva M, Headrick JR Jr. Standardized approach to prolonged air leak reduction after pulmonary resection. Ann Thorac Surg. 2016;101(6):2097–101.
18. Kiser AC, O'Brien SM, Detterbeck FC. Blunt tracheobronchial injuries: treatment and outcomes. Ann Thorac Surg. 2001;71(6):2059–65.
19. Eastridge CE, Hughes FA Jr, Pate JW, Cole F, Richardson R. Tracheobronchial injury caused by blunt trauma. Am Rev Respir Dis. 1970;101(2):230–7.
20. Martin de Nicolas JL, Gamez AP, Cruz F, Diaz-Hellin V, Marron M, Martinez JI, et al. Long tracheobronchial and esophageal rupture after blunt chest trauma: injury by airway bursting. Ann Thorac Surg. 1996;62(1):269–72.
21. Chesterman JT, Satsangi PN. Rupture of the trachea and bronchi by closed injury. Thorax. 1966;21(1):21–7.
22. Wintermark M, Schnyder P. The Macklin effect: a frequent etiology for pneumomediastinum in severe blunt chest trauma. Chest. 2001;120(2):543–7.
23. Visser F, Heine AM, Levin AI, Coetzee A. Pneumopericardium: two case reports and a review. S African J Anaesth Analg. 2008;14(2):5.
24. Levin AI, Visser F, Mattheyse F, Coetzee A. Tension pneumopericardium during positive-pressure ventilation leading to cardiac arrest. J Cardiothorac Vasc Anesth. 2008;22(6):879–82.
25. Macklin CC. Pneumothorax with massive collapse from experimental local over-inflation of the lung substance. Can Med Assoc J. 1937;36(4):414–20.
26. Baydur A, Gottlieb LS. Pneumopericardium and pneumothorax complicating bronchogenic carcinoma. West J Med. 1976;124(2):144–6.
27. Hadjis T, Palisaitis D, Dontigny L, Allard M. Benign pneumopericardium and tamponade. Can J Cardiol. 1995;11(3):232–4.

28. Kim HY, Song KS, Goo JM, Lee JS, Lee KS, Lim TH. Thoracic sequelae and complications of tuberculosis. Radiographics. 2001;21(4):839–58. discussion 59-60

29. Kempainen RR, Pierson DJ. Persistent air leaks in patients receiving mechanical ventilation. Semin Respir Crit Care Med. 2001;22(6):675–84.

30. Stern EJ, Sun H, Haramati LB. Peripheral bronchopleural fistulas: CT imaging features. AJR Am J Roentgenol. 1996;167(1):117–20.

31. Mathur NN, Kumar S, Bothra R, Dhawan R. Multi-lobulated cervical pneumatocoele communicating with pyopneumothorax and bronchopleural fistula. Int J Pediatr Otorhinolaryngol. 2004;68(12):1525–7.

32. Slade M. Management of pneumothorax and prolonged air leak. Semin Respir Crit Care Med. 2014;35(6):706–14.

33. Donahue DM, Wright CD, Viale G, Mathisen DJ. Resection of pulmonary blebs and pleurodesis for spontaneous pneumothorax. Chest. 1993;104(6):1767–9.

34. Lesur O, Delorme N, Fromaget JM, Bernadac P, Polu JM. Computed tomography in the etiologic assessment of idiopathic spontaneous pneumothorax. Chest. 1990;98(2):341–7.

35. Stein ME, Haim N, Drumea K, Ben-Itzhak O, Kuten A. Spontaneous pneumothorax complicating chemotherapy for metastatic seminoma. A case report and a review of the literature. Cancer. 1995;75(11):2710–3.

36. Torre M, Chiesa G, Ravini M, Vercelloni M, Belloni PA. Endoscopic gluing of bronchopleural fistula. Ann Thorac Surg. 1987;43(3):295–7.

37. Stamatis G, Eberhard W, Pottgen C. Surgery after multimodality treatment for non-small-cell lung cancer. Lung Cancer. 2004;45(Suppl 2):S107–12.

38. Sonett JR, Suntharalingam M, Edelman MJ, Patel AB, Gamliel Z, Doyle A, et al. Pulmonary resection after curative intent radiotherapy (>59 Gy) and concurrent chemotherapy in non-small-cell lung cancer. Ann Thorac Surg. 2004;78(4):1200–5. discussion 6

39. Mansour Z, Kochetkova EA, Ducrocq X, Vasilescu MD, Maxant G, Buggenhout A, et al. Induction chemotherapy does not increase the operative risk of pneumonectomy! Eur J Cardiothorac Surg. 2007;31(2):181–5.

40. Fehr M, von Moos R, Furrer M, Cathomas R. Spontaneous pneumothorax during chemotherapy: a case report. Onkologie. 2010;33(10):527–30.

41. Bonomi P, Faber LP, Warren W, Lincoln S, LaFollette S, Sharma M, et al. Postoperative bronchopulmonary complications in stage III lung cancer patients treated with preoperative paclitaxel-containing chemotherapy and concurrent radiation. Semin Oncol. 1997;24(4 Suppl 12):S12-123–S12-9.

42. Li S, Fan J, Liu J, Zhou J, Ren Y, Shen C, et al. Neoadjuvant therapy and risk of bronchopleural fistula after lung cancer surgery: a systematic meta-analysis of 14 912 patients. Jpn J Clin Oncol. 2016;46(6):534–46.

43. Li S, Fan J, Zhou J, Ren Y, Shen C, Che G. Residual disease at the bronchial stump is positively associated with the risk of bronchopleural fistula in patients undergoing lung cancer surgery: a meta-analysis. Interact Cardiovasc Thorac Surg. 2016;22(3):327–35.

44. Li SJ, Fan J, Zhou J, Ren YT, Shen C, Che GW. Diabetes mellitus and risk of bronchopleural fistula after pulmonary resections: a meta-analysis. Ann Thorac Surg. 2016;102(1):328–39.

45. Toyooka S, Soh J, Shien K, Sugimoto S, Yamane M, Oto T, et al. Sacrificing the pulmonary arterial branch to the spared lobe is a risk factor of bronchopleural fistula in sleeve lobectomy after chemoradiotherapy. Eur J Cardiothorac Surg. 2013;43(3):568–72.

46. Bishop MJ, Benson MS, Pierson DJ. Carbon dioxide excretion via bronchopleural fistulas in adult respiratory distress syndrome. Chest. 1987;91(3):400–2.

47. Pierson DJ, Horton CA, Bates PW. Persistent bronchopleural air leak during mechanical ventilation. A review of 39 cases. Chest. 1986;90(3):321–3.

48. Baumann MH, Sahn SA. Medical management and therapy of bronchopleural fistulas in the mechanically ventilated patient. Chest. 1990;97(3):721–8.

49. Benumof JL, Dagg R, Benumof R. Critical hemoglobin desaturation will occur before return to an unparalyzed state following 1 mg/kg intravenous succinylcholine. Anesthesiology. 1997;87(4):979–82.

50. Luks AM. Management of bronchopleural fistula in patients on mechanical ventilation 2017.

51. Albelda SM, Hansen-Flaschen JH, Taylor E, Lanken PN, Wollman H. Evaluation of high-frequency jet ventilation in patients with bronchopleural fistulas by quantitation of the airleak. Anesthesiology. 1985;63(5):551–4.

52. Ritz R, Benson M, Bishop MJ. Measuring gas leakage from bronchopleural fistulas during high-frequency jet ventilation. Crit Care Med. 1984;12(9):836–7.

53. Rusch VW, Capps JS, Tyler ML, Pierson DL. The performance of four pleural drainage systems in an animal model of bronchopleural fistula. Chest. 1988;93(4):859–63.

54. Allan AG. Reluctance of anaesthetists to perform awake intubation. Anaesthesia. 2004;59(4):413.

55. Basi SK, Cooper M, Ahmed FB, Clarke SG, Mitchell V. Reluctance of anaesthetists to perform awake intubation. Anaesthesia. 2004;59(9):918.

56. Poulin V, Vaillancourt R, Somma J, Gagne N, Bussieres JS. High frequency ventilation combined with spontaneous breathing during bronchopleural fistula repair: a case report. Can J Anaesth. 2009;56(1):52–6.

57. Khan NU, Al-Aloul M, Khasati N, Machaal A, Leonard CT, Yonan N. Extracorporeal membrane oxygenator as a bridge to successful surgical repair of bronchopleural fistula following bilateral sequential lung transplantation: a case report and review of literature. J Cardiothorac Surg. 2007;2:28.

58. Saleemi MS, McLaren C, Sharma BK, Muthialu N, Roebuck D, Ng C. Bronchopleural fistula in a newborn undergoing ECMO-transbronchial closure. J Perinatol. 2013;33(8):659–60.

59. Lau KY. Postural management of bronchopleural fistula. Chest. 1988;94(5):1122.

60. Campos JH. Which device should be considered the best for lung isolation: double-lumen endotracheal tube versus bronchial blockers. Curr Opin Anaesthesiol. 2007;20(1):27–31.

61. Cohen E. Pro: the new bronchial blockers are preferable to double-lumen tubes for lung isolation. J Cardiothorac Vasc Anesth. 2008;22(6):920–4.

62. Travaline JM, McKenna RJ Jr, De Giacomo T, Venuta F, Hazelrigg SR, Boomer M, et al. Treatment of persistent pulmonary air leaks using endobronchial valves. Chest. 2009;136(2):355–60.

63. Wood DE, Cerfolio RJ, Gonzalez X, Springmeyer SC. Bronchoscopic management of prolonged air leak. Clin Chest Med. 2010;31(1):127–33. Table of Contents

64. Firlinger I, Stubenberger E, Muller MR, Burghuber OC, Valipour A. Endoscopic one-way valve implantation in patients with prolonged air leak and the use of digital air leak monitoring. Ann Thorac Surg. 2013;95(4):1243–9.

65. Ratliff JL, Hill JD, Tucker H, Fallat R. Endobronchial control of bronchopleural fistulae. Chest. 1977;71(1):98–9.

66. Dalar L, Kosar F, Eryuksel E, Karasulu L, Altin S. Endobronchial Watanabe spigot embolisation in the treatment of bronchopleural fistula due to tuberculous empyema in intensive care unit. Ann Thorac Cardiovasc Surg. 2013;19(2):140–3.

67. Jindal A, Agarwal R. Novel treatment of a persistent bronchopleural fistula using a customized spigot. J Bronchology Interv Pulmonol. 2014;21(2):173–6.

68. Ueda Y, Huang CL, Itotani R, Fukui M. Endobronchial Watanabe Spigot placement for a secondary pneumothorax. J Bronchology Interv Pulmonol. 2015;22(3):278–80.

69. Uchida T, Wada M, Sakamoto J, Arai Y. Treatment for empyema with bronchopleural fistulas using endobronchial occlusion coils: report of a case. Surg Today. 1999;29(2):186–9.

70. Ozgul MA, Cetinkaya E, Cortuk M, Tanriverdi E, Yildirim BZ, Balci MK, et al. Oki stent application in different indications: Six cases. Clin Respir J. 2016;12(1):234–40

71. Cao M, Zhu Q, Wang W, Zhang TX, Jiang MZ, Zang Q. Clinical application of fully covered self-expandable metal stents in the treatment of bronchial fistula. Thorac Cardiovasc Surg. 2016;64(6):533–9.

72. Wu G, Li ZM, Han XW, Wang ZG, Lu HB, Zhu M, et al. Right bronchopleural fistula treated with a novel, Y-shaped, single-plugged, covered, metallic airway stent. Acta Radiol. 2013;54(6):656–60.

73. Bille A, Giovannetti R, Calarco G, Pastorino U. Tailored stent for bronchial stump fistula closure and omentoplasty for infection control: a combined approach with low morbidity. Tumori. 2014;100(4):157e–9e.

74. Amaral B, Feijo S. Fistula of the stump: a novel approach with a "stapled" stent. J Bronchology Interv Pulmonol. 2015;22(4):365–6.

75. Cusumano G, Terminella A, Vasta I, Riscica Lizzio C, Bellofiore S, Saita S. Endoscopic stenting for double bronco-pleural fistula after lobectomy. Asian Cardiovasc Thorac Ann. 2015;23(8):995–7.

76. Kramer MR, Peled N, Shitrit D, Atar E, Saute M, Shlomi D, et al. Use of Amplatzer device for endobronchial closure of bronchopleural fistulas. Chest. 2008;133(6):1481–4.

77. Gulkarov I, Paul S, Altorki NK, Lee PC. Use of Amplatzer device for endobronchial closure of bronchopleural fistulas. Interact Cardiovasc Thorac Surg. 2009;9(5):901–2.

78. Fruchter O, Bruckheimer E, Raviv Y, Rosengarten D, Saute M, Kramer MR. Endobronchial closure of bronchopleural fistulas with Amplatzer vascular plug. Eur J Cardiothorac Surg. 2012;41(1):46–9.

79. Krumpolcova M, Durand M, Rossi-Blancher M, Heylbroeck C, Vanzetto G, Albaladejo P, et al. Endobronchial closure of bronchopleural fistula with Amplatzer PFO device. Thorac Cardiovasc Surg. 2012;60(5):366–8.

80. Papiashvilli M, Bar I, Sasson L, Priel IE. Endobronchial closure of recurrent bronchopleural and tracheopleural fistulae by two amplatzer devices. Heart Lung Circ. 2013;22(11):959–61.

81. Fruchter O, El Raouf BA, Abdel-Rahman N, Saute M, Bruckheimer E, Kramer MR. Efficacy of bronchoscopic closure of a bronchopleural fistula with amplatzer devices: long-term follow-up. Respiration. 2014;87(3):227–33.

82. Klotz LV, Gesierich W, Schott-Hildebrand S, Hatz RA, Lindner M. Endobronchial closure of bronchopleural fistula using Amplatzer device. J Thorac Dis. 2015;7(8):1478–82.

83. Inaspettato G, Rodella L, Laterza E, Prattico F, Kind R, Lombardo F, et al. Endoscopic treatment of bronchopleural fistulas using N-butyl-2-cyanoacrylate. Surg Laparosc Endosc. 1994;4(1):62–4.

84. Clemson LA, Walser E, Gill A, Lynch JE, Zwischenberger JB. Transthoracic closure of a postpneumonectomy bronchopleural fistula with coils and cyanoacrylate. Ann Thorac Surg. 2006;82(5):1924–6.

85. Petter-Puchner AH, Simunek M, Redl H, Puchner KU, Van Griensven M. A comparison of a cyanoacrylate [corrected] glue (Glubran) vs. fibrin sealant (Tisseel) in experimental models of partial pulmonary resection and lung incision [corrected] in rabbits. J Investig Surg. 2010;23(1):40–7.

86. York EL, Lewall DB, Hirji M, Gelfand ET, Modry DL. Endoscopic diagnosis and treatment of postoperative bronchopleural fistula. Chest. 1990;97(6):1390–2.

87. York JA. Treating bronchopleural fistulae percutaneously with N-butyl cyanoacrylate glue. J Vasc Interv Radiol. 2013;24(10):1581–3.

88. Kiriyama M, Fujii Y, Yamakawa Y, Fukai I, Yano M, Kaji M, et al. Endobronchial neodymium:yttrium-aluminum garnet laser for noninvasive closure of small proximal bronchopleural fistula after lung resection. Ann Thorac Surg. 2002;73(3):945–8. discussion 8-9

89. Gkegkes ID, Mourtarakos S, Gakidis I. Endobronchial valves in treatment of persistent air leaks: a systematic review of clinical evidence. Med Sci Monit. 2015;21:432–8.

90. Feller-Kopman D, Bechara R, Garland R, Ernst A, Ashiku S. Use of a removable endobronchial valve for the treatment of bronchopleural fistula. Chest. 2006;130(1):273–5.

91. Gilbert CR, Casal RF, Lee HJ, Feller-Kopman D, Frimpong B, Dincer HE, et al. Use of one-way Intrabronchial valves in air leak management after tube Thoracostomy drainage. Ann Thorac Surg. 2016;101(5):1891–6.

92. Mitchell KM, Boley TM, Hazelrigg SR. Endobronchial valves for treatment of bronchopleural fistula. Ann Thorac Surg. 2006;81(3):1129–31.

93. Gillespie CT, Sterman DH, Cerfolio RJ, Nader D, Mulligan MS, Mularski RA, et al. Endobronchial valve treatment for prolonged air leaks of the lung: a case series. Ann Thorac Surg. 2011;91(1):270–3.

94. Jenkins M, Vaughan P, Place D, Kornaszewska M. Endobronchial valve migration. Eur J Cardiothorac Surg. 2011;40(5):1258–60.

95. Schweigert M, Kraus D, Ficker JH, Stein HJ. Closure of persisting air leaks in patients with severe pleural empyema--use of endoscopic one-way endobronchial valve. Eur J Cardiothorac Surg. 2011;39(3):401–3.

96. Alexander ES, Healey TT, Martin DW, Dupuy DE. Use of endobronchial valves for the treatment of bronchopleural fistulas after thermal ablation of lung neoplasms. J Vasc Interv Radiol. 2012;23(9):1236–40.

97. El-Sameed Y, Waness A, Al Shamsi I, Mehta AC. Endobronchial valves in the management of broncho-pleural and alveolo-pleural fistulae. Lung. 2012;190(3):347–51.

98. Gudbjartsson T, Helgadottir S, Ek L. One-way endobronchial valve for bronchopleural fistula after necrotizing pneumonia. Asian Cardiovasc Thorac Ann. 2013;21(4):498–9.

99. Venkatappa N, Fadul R, Raymond D, Cicenia J, Gildea TR. Endobronchial valves for treatment of bronchopleural fistula in granulomatous polyangitis: a longitudinal case report. J Bronchology Interv Pulmonol. 2013;20(2):186–8.

100. Cundiff WB, McCormack FX, Wikenheiser-Brokamp K, Starnes S, Kotloff R, Benzaquen S. Successful management of a chronic, refractory bronchopleural fistula with endobronchial valves followed by talc pleurodesis. Am J Respir Crit Care Med. 2014;189(4):490–1.

101. Giddings O, Kuhn J, Akulian J. Endobronchial valve placement for the treatment of bronchopleural fistula: a review of the current literature. Curr Opin Pulm Med. 2014;20(4):347–51.

102. Hance JM, Martin JT, Mullett TW. Endobronchial valves in the treatment of persistent air leaks. Ann Thorac Surg. 2015;100(5):1780–5. discussion 5-6

103. Reed MF, Gilbert CR, Taylor MD, Toth JW. Endobronchial valves for challenging air leaks. Ann Thorac Surg. 2015;100(4):1181–6.

104. Bakhos C, Doelken P, Pupovac S, Ata A, Fabian T. Management of Prolonged Pulmonary Air Leaks With Endobronchial Valve Placement. JSLS. 2016;20(3):e2016.00055.

105. Dooms CA, Decaluwe H, Yserbyt J, De Leyn P, Van Raemdonck D, Ninane V. Bronchial valve treatment for pulmonary air leak after anatomical lung resection for cancer. Eur Respir J. 2014;43(4):1142–8.

106. Fischer W, Feller-Kopman D, Shah A, Orens J, Illei P, Yarmus L. Endobronchial valve therapy for pneumothorax as a bridge to lung transplantation. J Heart Lung Transplant. 2012;31(3):334–6.

107. Mahajan AK, Verhoef P, Patel SB, Carr G, Kyle HD. Intrabronchial valves: a case series describing a minimally invasive approach to bronchopleural fistulas in medical intensive care unit patients. J Bronchology Interv Pulmonol. 2012;19(2):137–41.

108. Brichon PY, Poquet C, Arvieux C, Pison C. Successful treatment of a life-threatening air leakage, complicating severe abdominal sepsis, with a one-way endobronchial valve. Interact Cardiovasc Thorac Surg. 2012;15(4):779–80.

109. Luks AM, Pierson DJ. Barotrauma and bronchopleural fistula. In: Tobin MJ, editor. Principles and Practice of Mechanical Ventilation. 23rd ed. New York: McGrawHill; 2012.

110. Turnbull AD, Carlon G, Howland WS, Beattie EJ Jr. High-frequency jet ventilation in major airway or pulmonary disruption. Ann Thorac Surg. 1981;32(5):468–74.

111. Carlon GC, Ray C Jr, Pierri MK, Croeger J, Howland WS. High-frequency jet ventilation: theoretical considerations and clinical observations. Chest. 1982;81(3):350–4.

112. Steiger Z, Wilson RF. Management of bronchopleural fistulas. Surg Gynecol Obstet. 1984;158(3):267–71.

113. Pierson DJ. Management of bronchopleural fistula in the adult respiratory distress syndrome. New Horiz. 1993;1(4):512–21.

114. Albelda SM, Gefter WB, Epstein DM, Miller WT. Bronchopleural fistula complicating invasive pulmonary aspergillosis. Am Rev Respir Dis. 1982;126(1):163–5.

115. Downs JB, Chapman RL Jr. Treatment of bronchopleural fistula during continuous positive pressure ventilation. Chest. 1976;69(3):363–6.

116. Phillips YY, Lonigan RM, Joyner LR. A simple technique for managing a bronchopleural fistula while maintaining positive pressure ventilation. Crit Care Med. 1979;7(8):351–3.

117. Zimmerman JE, Colgan DL, Mills M. Management of bronchopleural fistula complicating therapy with positive end expiratory pressure (PEEP). Chest. 1973;64(4):526–9.

118. Litmanovitch M, Joynt GM, Cooper PJ, Kraus P. Persistent bronchopleural fistula in a patient with adult respiratory distress syndrome. Treatment with pressure-controlled ventilation. Chest. 1993;104(6):1901–2.

119. Carlon GC, Ray C Jr, Klain M, McCormack PM. High-frequency positive-pressure ventilation in management of a patient with bronchopleural fistula. Anesthesiology. 1980;52(2):160–2.

120. Fernandez NA, Lynch RD. High frequency jet ventilation in tracheopleural fistula: case report. Tex Med. 1985;81(3):61–2.

121. Dennis JW, Eigen H, Ballantine TV, Grosfeld JL. The relationship between peak inspiratory pressure and positive end expiratory pressure on the volume of air lost through a bronchopleural fistula. J Pediatr Surg. 1980;15(6):971–6.

122. Sjostrand UH, Smith RB, Hoff BH, Bunegin L, Wilson E. Conventional and high-frequency ventilation in dogs with bronchopleural fistula. Crit Care Med. 1985;13(3):191–3.

123. Orlando R 3rd, Gluck EH, Cohen M, Mesologites CG. Ultra-high-frequency jet ventilation in a bronchopleural fistula model. Arch Surg. 1988;123(5):591–3.

124. Schuster DP, Klain M, Snyder JV. Comparison of high frequency jet ventilation to conventional ventilation during severe acute respiratory failure in humans. Crit Care Med. 1982;10(10):625–30.

125. Beamer WC, Prough DS, Royster RL, Johnston WE, Johnson JC. High-frequency jet ventilation produces auto-PEEP. Crit Care Med. 1984;12(9):734–7.

126. Holzapfel L, Robert D, Perrin F, Gaussorgues P, Giudicelli DP. Comparison of high-frequency jet ventilation to conventional ventilation in adults with respiratory distress syndrome. Intensive Care Med. 1987;13(2):100–5.

127. Campbell D, Steinmann M, Porayko L. Nitric oxide and high frequency jet ventilation in a patient with bilateral bronchopleural fistulae and ARDS. Can J Anaesth. 2000;47(1):53–7.

128. Derderian SS, Rajagopal KR, Abbrecht PH, Bennett LL, Doblar DD, Hunt KK Jr. High frequency positive pressure jet ventilation in bilateral bronchopleural fistulae. Crit Care Med. 1982;10(2):119–21.

129. Mortimer AJ, Laurie PS, Garrett H, Kerr JH. Unilateral high frequency jet ventilation. Reduction of leak in bronchopleural fistula. Intensive Care Med. 1984;10(1):39–41.

130. Rubio JJ, Algora-Weber A, Dominguez-de Villota E, Chamorro C, Mosquera JM. Prolonged high-frequency jet ventilation in a patient with bronchopleural fistula. An alternative mode of ventilation. Intensive Care Med. 1986;12(3):161–3.

131. Bishop MJ, Benson MS, Sato P, Pierson DJ. Comparison of high-frequency jet ventilation with conventional mechanical ventilation for bronchopleural fistula. Anesth Analg. 1987;66(9):833–8.

132. Roth MD, Wright JW, Bellamy PE. Gas flow through a bronchopleural fistula. Measuring the effects of high-frequency jet ventilation and chest-tube suction. Chest. 1988;93(1):210–3.

133. Spinale FG, Linker RW, Crawford FA, Reines HD. Conventional versus high frequency jet ventilation with a bronchopleural fistula. J Surg Res. 1989;46(2):147–51.

134. Ray C Jr, Miodownik S, Carlon G, Groeger J, Howland WS. Pneumatic-to-electrical analog for high-frequency jet ventilation of disrupted airways. Crit Care Med. 1984;12(9):711–2.

135. Ha DV, Johnson D. High frequency oscillatory ventilation in the management of a high output bronchopleural fistula: a case report. Can J Anaesth. 2004;51(1):78–83.

136. Minhas JS, Halligan K, Dargin JM. Independent lung ventilation in the management of ARDS and bronchopleural fistula. Heart Lung. 2016;45(3):258–60.

137. Cheatham ML, Promes JT. Independent lung ventilation in the management of traumatic bronchopleural fistula. Am Surg. 2006;72(6):530–3.

138. Wendt M, Hachenberg T, Winde G, Lawin P. Differential ventilation with low-flow CPAP and CPPV in the treatment of unilateral chest trauma. Intensive Care Med. 1989;15(3):209–11.

139. Crimi G, Candiani A, Conti G, Mattia C, Gasparetto A. Clinical applications of independent lung ventilation with unilateral high-frequency jet ventilation (ILV-UHFJV). Intensive Care Med. 1986;12(2):90–4.

140. McGuive GP. Lung ventilation and bronchopleural fistula. Can J Anaesth. 1996;43(12):1275–6.

141. Ost D, Corbridge T. Independent lung ventilation. Clin Chest Med. 1996;17(3):591–601.

142. Parish JM, Gracey DR, Southorn PA, Pairolero PA, Wheeler JT. Differential mechanical ventilation in respiratory failure due to severe unilateral lung disease. Mayo Clin Proc. 1984;59(12):822–8.

143. Sawulski S, Nestorowicz A, Wosko J, Dabrowski W, Kowalczyk M, Fijalkowska A. Independent lung ventilation for treatment of post-traumatic ARDS. Anaesthesiol Intensive Ther. 2012;44(2):84–8.

144. Hedenstierna G. Differential ventilation in bilateral lung disease. Eur J Anaesthesiol. 1985;2(1):1–10.

145. Hedenstierna G, Baehrendtz S, Frostell C, Mebius C. Differential ventilation in acute respiratory failure. Indications and outcome. Bull Eur Physiopathol Respir. 1985;21(3):281–5.

146. Powner DJ. Differential lung ventilation during adult donor care. Prog Transplant (Aliso Viejo, Calif). 2010;20(3):262–7. quiz 8

147. Hillman KM, Barber JD. Asynchronous independent lung ventilation (AILV). Crit Care Med. 1980;8(7):390–5.

148. Baehrendtz S, Hedenstierna G. Differential ventilation and selective positive end-expiratory pressure: effects on patients with acute bilateral lung disease. Anesthesiology. 1984;61(5):511–7.

149. Baehrendtz S, Klingstedt C. Differential ventilation and selective PEEP during anaesthesia in the lateral decubitus posture. Acta Anaesthesiol Scand. 1984;28(3):252–9.

150. Anantham D, Jagadesan R, Tiew PE. Clinical review: independent lung ventilation in critical care. Crit Care. 2005;9(6):594–600.

151. Diaz O, Iglesia R, Ferrer M, Zavala E, Santos C, Wagner PD, et al. Effects of noninvasive ventilation on pulmonary gas exchange

and hemodynamics during acute hypercapnic exacerbations of chronic obstructive pulmonary disease. Am J Respir Crit Care Med. 1997;156(6):1840–5.

152. Siegel JH, Stoklosa JC, Borg U, Wiles CE 3rd, Sganga G, Geisler FH, et al. Quantification of asymmetric lung pathophysiology as a guide to the use of simultaneous independent lung ventilation in posttraumatic and septic adult respiratory distress syndrome. Ann Surg. 1985;202(4):425–39.

153. Thomas AR, Bryce TL. Ventilation in the patient with unilateral lung disease. Crit Care Clin. 1998;14(4):743–73.

154. Dodds CP, Hillman KM. Management of massive air leak with asynchronous independent lung ventilation. Intensive Care Med. 1982;8(6):287–90.

155. Carvalho P, Thompson WH, Riggs R, Carvalho C, Charan NB. Management of bronchopleural fistula with a variable-resistance valve and a single ventilator. Chest. 1997;111(5):1452–4.

156. Charan NB, Carvalho CG, Hawk P, Crowley JJ, Carvalho P. Independent lung ventilation with a single ventilator using a variable resistance valve. Chest. 1995;107(1):256–60.

157. Feeley TW, Keating D, Nishimura T. Independent lung ventilation using high-frequency ventilation in the management of a bronchopleural fistula. Anesthesiology. 1988;69(3):420–2.

158. Shekar K, Foot CL, Fraser JF. Independent lung ventilation in the intensive care unit: desperate measure or viable treatment option? Crit Care Resusc. 2008;10(2):144–8.

159. Cinnella G, Dambrosio M, Brienza N, Giuliani R, Bruno F, Fiore T, et al. Independent lung ventilation in patients with unilateral pulmonary contusion. Monitoring with compliance and EtCO(2). Intensive Care Med. 2001;27(12):1860–7.

160. Gavazzeni V, Iapichino G, Mascheroni D, Langer M, Bordone G, Zannini P, et al. Prolonged independent lung respiratory treatment after single lung transplantation in pulmonary emphysema. Chest. 1993;103(1):96–100.

161. Adoumie R, Shennib H, Brown R, Slinger P, Chiu RC. Differential lung ventilation. Applications beyond the operating room. J Thorac Cardiovasc Surg. 1993;105(2):229–33.

162. Marraro G. Simultaneous independent lung ventilation in pediatric patients. Crit Care Clin. 1992;8(1):131–45.

163. Marraro G, Marinari M, Rataggi M. The clinical application of synchronized independent lung ventilation (S.I.L.V.) in pulmonary disease with unilateral prevalence in pediatrics. Int J Clin Monit Comput. 1987;4(2):123–9.

164. Konstantinov IE, Saxena P. Independent lung ventilation in the postoperative management of large bronchopleural fistula. J Thorac Cardiovasc Surg. 2010;139(2):e21–2.

165. Garlick J, Maxson T, Imamura M, Green J, Prodhan P. Differential lung ventilation and venovenous extracorporeal membrane oxygenation for traumatic bronchopleural fistula. Ann Thorac Surg. 2013;96(5):1859–60.

166. Katsaragakis S, Stamou KM, Androulakis G. Independent lung ventilation for asymmetrical chest trauma: effect on ventilatory and haemodynamic parameters. Injury. 2005;36(4):501–4.

167. Officer TM, Wheeler DR, Frost AE, Rodarte JR. Respiratory control during independent lung ventilation. Chest. 2001;120(2):678–81.

168. Neustein SM. The use of bronchial blockers for providing one-lung ventilation. J Cardiothorac Vasc Anesth. 2009;23(6):860–8.

169. Sager JS, Eiger G, Fuchs BD. Ventilator auto-triggering in a patient with tuberculous bronchopleural fistula. Respir Care. 2003;48(5):519–21.

170. Gallagher TJ, Smith RA, Kirby RR, Civetta JM. Intermittent inspiratory chest tube occlusion to limit bronchopleural cutaneous airleaks. Crit Care Med. 1976;4(6):328–32.

171. Blanch PB, Koens JC Jr, Layon AJ. A new device that allows synchronous intermittent inspiratory chest tube occlusion with any mechanical ventilator. Chest. 1990;97(6):1426–30.

172. Gramm HJ, Frucht U, Simgen WL, Dennhardt R. Respiratory controlled intermittent inspiratory pleural drainage--a method for handling life threatening bronchopleural fistulas. Anaesthesist. 1984;33(10):507–10.

173. Toneloto MG, Moreira MM, Bustorff-Silva JM, Souza GF, Martins LC, Dragosavac D, et al. Adjustable inspiratory occlusion valve in experimental bronchopleural fistula. A new therapeutic perspective. Acta Cir Bras. 2015;30(8):561–7.

Massive Hemoptysis

44

Jean S. Bussières and Marili Frenette

Key Points

- With massive hemoptysis, death is usually caused by asphyxiation rather than by exsanguination.
- Urgent management focuses on the prevention of asphyxia while the source of bleeding is addressed.
- Endobronchial and/or angiographic control are usually possible.
- Bronchial artery embolization (BAE) is now the treatment of choice.
- There is now less indication for surgery, and surgical results are better in stabilized, "elective," non-bleeding patient.
- Pulmonary artery injury is rare but associated with high mortality and is curable with BAE.

Introduction

Massive hemoptysis (MH) is a medical emergency that places the patient at risk of asphyxiation and death. Because of the explosive clinical presentation of MH, it is essential to respond quickly and appropriately. This is a potential lethal condition that deserves to be investigated thoroughly and brought under control promptly [1].

The definition of MH may vary depending of the publications. It is usually based on the volume of blood expectorated. In the literature, we can find large variations between the definitions. They range from 100 to 1000 mL/24 h [2–4]. By consensus (Table 44.1 and Fig. 44.1), MH is defined as a rate of bleeding exceeding 600 mL/24 h, meaning 25 mL/h. Only 1.5–5% of hemoptysis are really massive [1]. Exsanguinating hemoptysis is defined as a bleeding rate exceeding 150 mL/h or blood loss over 1000 mL/24 h or over 300 mL during one expectoration [5].

Quantification of MH may be difficult, and from a clinical point of view, such criteria are not useful. Based on the fact that the anatomic dead space of the major tracheobronchial tree is about 200 mL in most adults [6], other definitions relying on the magnitude of the clinical effects have been proposed. MH can be defined as the volume of expectorated blood that is life-threatening mainly by virtue of airway obstruction and rarely by blood loss.

J. S. Bussières (✉)
Department of Anesthesiology, Institut Universitaire de Cardiologie et de Pneumologie de Quebec – Université Laval, Quebec City, QC, Canada
e-mail: jbuss@criucpq.ulaval.ca

M. Frenette
Department of Anesthesiology and Critical Care, Université Laval, Quebec City, QC, Canada

Table 44.1 Definition of hemoptysis

Hemoptysis	Massive	Exsanguinating
One expectoration (mL)		>300
mL by hour	>25	>150
mL by 24 h	>600	>1000

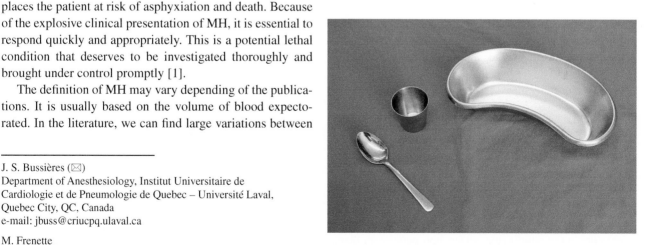

Fig. 44.1 Evaluation of the severity of hemoptysis. From left to right: a tespoon = 5 cc, a medicine cup = 60 cc, a kidney basin = 650 cc

Massive hemoptysis compared to moderate or minor hemoptysis represents a higher risk of mortality for the patient. Published series on patients presenting massive hemoptysis showed a mortality rate with medical management varying from 12% to 50%. Mortality rate was greater than 50% in patients not treated adequately [1].

Decision-making is a multidisciplinary process involving a critical care physician, pulmonary medicine bronchoscopist, interventional radiologist, thoracic surgeon, and anesthesiologist.

Historical Considerations

MH treatment was at first exclusively surgical. From the 1940s to the 1960s, different surgical approaches have been used to control and treat MH. In 1973, Remy and colleagues [7] changed management forever with the first report of bronchial artery embolization. Hiebert in 1974 [8] described the first successful use of a Fogarty balloon catheter through a rigid bronchoscope to tamponade bleeding in a moribund patient with massive bronchial hemorrhage. Subsequently, the use of the bronchoscope progressively changed from a rigid device to the flexible fiber-optic bronchoscopy (FOB). More recently, the role of early bronchoscopy, mainly with a FOB, is questioned since bronchial artery embolectomy (BAE) is easy to perform and so effective.

Since the introduction of radiological embolization, there are less frequent interventions by anesthesiologists for massive hemoptysis. With the rapid use of BAE, potentially massive hemoptysis is rapidly controlled, and there is less and less need for surgical interventions (emergent, semi-emergent, or elective post treatment), and therefore there is less anesthesia management. Consequently, anesthesiologists are nowadays only occasionally required to help with airway management, lung protection, and assistance during radiological intervention.

The literature usually refers to old publications, and there are only retrospective series or anecdotic reports that support recommendations for investigation and a treatment plan for MH. It is easy to understand that it is very difficult to design a prospective, randomized, controlled trial in this type of population.

Etiologies

Hemoptysis is defined by coughing of blood that originates from the tracheobronchial tree or pulmonary parenchyma. There are many potential causes of massive hemoptysis. It is very important to rapidly rule out any non-pulmonary bleeding since it can originate from the nasopharynx or from the upper gastrointestinal tract.

The lungs have a dual blood supply, the pulmonary circulation and the bronchial arteries. The bronchial circulation is a high-pressure system providing only 1% of the arterial supplies to the lungs, but the bronchial tree is implicated in MH in more than 90% of cases. Bronchial arterial bleeding is distinctively brisk and bright red. Bronchial arteries originate from the aorta that brings nutrients to the lung parenchyma and major airways. Seventy percent of the bronchial arteries typically arise from the descending thoracic aorta in regard to the fifth and the sixth vertebrae. The 30% remaining arise from other locations such as the subclavian arteries [9]. The same vessels that supply the bronchial arteries may also supply the esophagus, the mediastinal nodes, and, more importantly, the spinal cord, through a complex anastomotic network [10].

Pulmonary arterial circulation is responsible for gas exchanges and is involved in less than 5–10% of massive hemoptysis. The pulmonary bed is a high-compliance and usually a low-pressure system (15–20 mmHg systolic and 5–10 mmHg diastolic). However, if there is pulmonary artery hypertension, this low-pressure system may be modified to a high-pressure system, reaching sometimes the systemic level. Dark blood is more consistent with pulmonary artery bleeding since the blood is not sufficiently oxygenated.

Hemoptysis originates from systemic, namely, bronchial, or from pulmonary vessels. The most frequent causes of bronchial tree hemoptysis are inflammatory lung disease (bronchiectasis and tuberculosis) and neoplasia (Table 44.2). The most common causes of hemoptysis from pulmonary circulation are arteriovenous malformation (AVM) and Rasmussen's aneurysms (due to tuberculosis). Iatrogenic

Table 44.2 Possible causes of massive hemoptysis

Infectious
Bronchiectasis (including cystic fibrosis)
Chronic bronchitis
Tuberculosis
Non-tuberculous mycobacteria
Lung abscess
Necrotizing pneumonia
Mycetoma
Cardiovascular
Arteriovenous malformation
Pulmonary embolism or infarct
Mitral stenosis
Aortic aneurysm or bronchovascular fistula
Vasculitis, Wegener's granulomatosis
Neoplastic
Lung cancer
Bronchial adenoma
Pulmonary metastases
Miscellaneous
Aspirated foreign body
Pulmonary contusion, trauma
Idiopathic pulmonary hemosiderosis
Iatrogenic (transthoracic or transbronchial biopsy, pulmonary artery catheter)

pulmonary artery rupture from pulmonary catheter (Swan-Ganz) occurs rarely, but since anesthesiologists are frequently implicated in its causality, this subject will be discussed more deeply in another section of this chapter.

Clinical Manifestation

In the acute phase of hemoptysis, there is an accumulation of blood in the dependent parts of the lungs. Through the cough reflex, blood is expelled, producing the hemoptysis. During that time, blood can be dispersed bilaterally into the bronchial tree, and the evaluation can mislead to lateralization.

The degree of bleeding may be easily underrated because the volume of blood engulfing the involved lobes or lungs is not quantified and may be significant [1]. Many patients with hemoptysis have a medical history of compromised lung function, and even small quantities of blood into the bronchial tree can lead to significant respiratory distress. Expectorated blood is often swallowed and cannot be measured. Asphyxia is the most life-threatening manifestation of MH, well before hemodynamic instability appears, and is the usual cause of death associated with MH.

Initial Management of MH

There is little consensus regarding the optimal management of patients presenting with MH. Moreover, from the beginning of the twenty-first century, there are few recent large series of patients studied [11]. In this section, conclusions of these studies, some consensus from the literature, and also various controversies will be presented.

Initial management of massive hemoptysis needs to achieve a few objectives quickly and simultaneously. The initial step in management of hemoptysis is to differentiate between minor and massive hemoptysis. The approach to the patient presenting MH can be generally done in three steps [12]: airway protection, localization, and treatment. The initial approach to the patient should be dictated by the clinical presentation. Patients with rapid bleeding or severe functional decompensation need protection of the airway first, meaning that every effort should be made to protect the non-affected lung against blood spillage and to maintain adequate gas exchange to prevent asphyxia [13]. Hypoxia secondary to lung spillage or blood clots is the main cause leading to death. Secondly, it is essential to localize the source of bleeding, meaning finding as precisely as possible its origin or at least the side of the MH. Thirdly, the administration of a specific therapy is mandatory. Definitive treatment options include conservative medical therapy, endobronchial therapy, arterial embolization, or surgery.

All patients presenting MH should be admitted to an intensive care unit for further investigation and treatment or transferred to the radiological suite for CT or angiogram examination or, less frequently, directly to the operating room. While undergoing diagnostic procedures, the patient should be kept upright, and 100% oxygen should be administered. Appropriate venous access should be put in place, and blood should be available from the blood bank. A coagulation profile should be obtained to show any coagulopathy, including platelet dysfunction from drugs such as acetylsalicylic acid (Aspirin®), clopidogrel (Plavix®), and other antiplatelets and new anticoagulants. Every effort should be made to reverse anticoagulation, when possible. Invasive therapeutic measures are not indicated for the control of hemoptysis caused by anticoagulant therapy, blood dyscrasia, or Goodpasture's syndrome [1]. Blood loss is rarely massive enough to cause a great threat to hemodynamics. Slight hypotension can occur and may be treated with volume replacement.

Light sedation with anxiolytic drugs or cough suppression drugs is rarely useful in the acute phase of MH [13]. Once the immediate danger has passed and bleeding is settling, these drugs may be used to depress the excessive coughing that can aggravate or stimulate hemoptysis [6]. Bronchodilators cannot be administered since they can have a vasodilation effect and may precipitate renewed bleeding [14].

Life-Threatening Intervention

When facing MH, many strategies to prevent airway contamination should be available. If lung isolation is delayed or not available, the patient intubated or not should be placed in the lateral decubitus position with the bleeding lung on the dependent (inferior) side to prevent spillage to the unaffected lung (nondependent, superior side).

Lung isolation may be used to avoid spillage to the unaffected lung by blood from the bleeding lung. Lung isolation can be performed with different techniques including a selective endobronchial intubation with a standard endotracheal tube, the use of a bronchial blocker (BB), or the insertion of a double-lumen tube (DLT). The two last lung isolation techniques are not specific to hemoptysis as they are regularly used during anesthesia for thoracic surgery [15] (see Chap. 16).

Main stem bronchial selective intubation with a large uncut endotracheal tube is facilitated using FOB, if the visualization is good enough to allow the guidance of the tube. Unfortunately, blood and clots can obstruct the view from FOB. Blood highly absorbs the light of the FOB and consequently alters its capacity to identify the tracheal bifurcation and the guidance of the endobronchial tube. Blind endobronchial insertion may be attempted and verified by auscultation.

However, the presence of large amount of blood in the main airway may confuse the sound perceived unilaterally.

Bronchial blockers (BBs) may be used for lung isolation or act as a therapeutic avenue when facing MH. It can be a temporary measure in life-threatening situations until a more specific treatment is applied. Bronchial blockers may be inserted into a bleeding bronchus under the control of a FOB to induce an endobronchial tamponade. Bronchial blocking device is useful for lung separation when the DLT is not immediately available or when there is some difficulty in inserting the DLT (e.g., percutaneous tracheotomy) [16]. As for any other lung isolation devices, the use of FOB is mandatory, but the airway visualization may be difficult because of the presence blood and blood clots. BB can be used in a non-intubated (through nostrils) or intubated patient. It can be positioned and stabilized alongside or inside the lumen of the endotracheal tube or DLT. In some situations, the BB may be introduced through a DLT. At that time, the use of very small FOB (2.8 mm) may be necessary, mainly with a smaller-sized DLT (35–37 Fr). The Uniblocker BB (Fuji Systems Corporation, Tokyo, Japan) is easy to use compared to other models, and it is now the golden standard for that procedure.

It is an excellent method to achieve control of the bleeding and to protect the contralateral lung and potentially the ipsilateral non-bleeding lobes or segments. The technique of endobronchial tamponade for bleeding control in MH was first introduced by Hiebert in 1974 [8]. The author occluded a bleeding bronchus with a balloon catheter inserted through a rigid bronchoscope. Different catheters have been used for this application, Foley catheter, Fogarty catheter, Swan-Ganz catheter, specific double balloon catheter, and more recently bronchial blockers. In addition to the tamponade effect, the administration of vasoactive drugs is possible through the inner channel [17]. This gives time to proceed with a therapeutic and more definitive intervention. If possible, the BB should be replaced by a DLT or a simple lumen tube to allow further evaluation and suctioning of the bleeding lung. The bronchial blocker should always be deflated under FOB vision. In 2006, Giannoni et al. [18] described a bilateral concurrent massive hemoptysis successfully controlled with the placement of more than one balloon catheter. In 2017, Caddell reported a case of an emergency surgical pulmonary embolectomy complicated by an acute massive hemoptysis [19, 20]. The authors used a double bronchial blocker system with a sequential inflate and deflate technique to localize the hemorrhage and provide lung isolation and ventilation.

A third alternative for the management of the airway during MH is the placement of a double-lumen tube (DLT) or endobronchial tube. These DLTs are specially designed for selective intubation of the right or left main stem bronchi [21]. For MH, selective intubation of the left lung is preferable. The left-sided tube is easier to position than the right-sided tube which carries the risk obstructing the right upper lobe bronchus. Double-lumen tubes have a bad reputation in the literature when used in the context of MH. Nevertheless, some of these observations were published before [22] the introduction of the polyvinyl DLTs whose positioning can be verified with the FOB. Other publications [1] refer to the use of DLTs for other conditions than MH, and their conclusions cannot be used to determine the safety of DLTs during MH [23]. However, it has been demonstrated that anesthesiologists with limited experience in thoracic anesthesia frequently fail to successfully place lung isolation devices, DLT, or bronchial blockers [24].

It is the authors' opinion that inserting a left-sided double-lumen tube is a good strategy. Many problems with DLT were described with older nondisposable model of DLT or with older models of FOB. When confronted with massive hemoptysis, the use of polyvinyl DLT and new FOB with larger suction channel can be helpful. The lumen inserted into the non-bleeding lung is used to ventilate the patient. The other lumen, connected to the bleeding lung, allows the insertion of a specific FOB. These FOBs, with a diameter less than 4.2 mm, have a working channel allowing suction of blood and blood clots from the bleeding site. The lumen directed to the bleeding lung may be used to carry out a relatively "blind" and very careful catheter aspiration. With attentive care, the lumen may be cleared of blood or clots. The application of CPAP or mechanical ventilation with PEEP on the bleeding lung may help to decrease the bleeding and/or to improve the patient's gas exchange.

Nevertheless, insertion of a DLT may be difficult, even for an experienced anesthesiologist, because large amounts of blood can make the visibility poor with FOBs. Also, a well-positioned DLT may be easily displaced during the frequent transfers of the patient from ICU to radiologic suites or frequent patient's repositioning in bed. The authors prefer to use left-sided DLT with a carinal hook to stabilize the DLT onto the carina and fix it to the maxillary bone to minimize its displacement. Sometime, when facing a massive hemoptysis, the use of a carinal hook helps to "blindly" position a DLT. It is important to note that BBs are at higher risk of dislodgement with movement or transfer of the patient than DLTs. Consequently, patients with a DLT or a BB usually should not be moved unless in absolute necessity, and sometime these patients should be with muscle relaxants to prevent coughing until the hemoptysis has been treated [25, 26].

Once adequate lung isolation is achieved, the patient can be placed in the lateral decubitus position with the bleeding lung on the nondependent (superior) side. The dependent non-bleeding lung will thus receive most of the pulmonary blood flow, and this will help to control the hemorrhage, as it decreases the perfusion in the upper lung. This position will also improve ventilation/perfusion (V/Q) ratio. The patient should be ventilated with 100% oxygen, and PEEP should be applied on the inferior lung to improve gas exchange. PEEP or CPAP may also be used on the upper bleeding lung acting as a hemostatic effect and help gas exchange.

Diagnostic Tools and Therapeutic Approaches

There is a controversy regarding the sequence of bronchoscopic and radiological interventions. Initial computed tomographic scan (CT) is thought to shorten examination time in critical patients, but in a patient with massive hemoptysis, etiologic diagnosis is less important than immediate interruption of the bleeding process [27].

Chest radiography is readily available and is an important diagnostic tool in finding the cause of the bleeding and localizing pulmonary pathology. High-definition computed tomographic (HDCT) scanning angiography is also an excellent diagnostic tool. Except for life-threatening situations, CT scan should be performed before the bronchoscopic exploration. It has superior diagnostic capacity over bronchoscopy and chest radiography for demonstrating underlying pathology and the site of bleeding in hemoptysis, especially in bronchiectasis, bronchogenic carcinoma, and aspergilloma cases. Vascular pathologies such as arteriovenous malformation or aneurysm, which are rare causes of hemoptysis, are also depicted very clearly in contrast-enhanced CT scan examinations [13]. With recent developments in multidetector CT scan technique, it is now possible to scan the whole thorax into very thin slices (1.25 mm) in a very short time (12–15 s) [14, 15]. Both the lesion causing hemoptysis and bronchial or nonbronchial systemic feeding arteries are detected during the same study using 80–100 mL of contrast medium. In angiography-controlled studies, 86–87% of the pathologic vessels detected by angiography were discovered with CT angiography (CTA) [14, 15].

Bronchoscopy

For a patient presenting MH, the medical team may choose to proceed with early or late bronchoscopy. This bronchoscopy may be rigid or flexible, and its primary goal is to localize the site or at least lateralize the side of the bleeding source. The secondary goal is to clear the airway of gross blood. Finally, the third goal may be to use a therapeutic agent to control the bleeding. If the situation is not critical, a quick trial of fiber-optic bronchoscopy (FOB) can be performed to determine the origin or at least the side of the bleeding. If the patient's oxygenation is significantly compromised or the bleeding continues at a brisk pace, elective oral intubation with an endotracheal tube (8.0 mm or larger)

should be performed; this may be done simultaneously with the bronchoscopy [28].

Timing

Although most authorities advocate bronchoscopy to help localize bleeding during MH, the moment when to use the bronchoscopy is still controversial [12]. In the literature, it is frequently mentioned that patients with MH require urgent bronchoscopy. The argument for this assertion is that bleeding will increase with time, making visualization difficult. It is reported that bronchoscopy helps to detect the bleeding site in a lung or lobe in patients with diffuse pulmonary disease [10].

More recently a new option emerged. Patients presenting with MH are immediately directed to the angiographic suite to get a diagnostic angiogram and bronchial artery embolization (BAE) at the same time. Patients at risk of asphyxia prior to the BAE benefit from lung isolation techniques. The FOB is then carried out a few days later. The main argument for this sequence is that during the acute phase of severe MH, airways are filled with large volumes of blood restricting the use of bronchoscopy and consequently invalidating endobronchial treatment [7, 29]. Sometimes, endoscopic examination may aggravate bleeding and delay more effective treatment. Hsiao et al. reported in 2001 [30] that bronchoscopy was not a prerequisite in the treatment process considering risk of airway compromised from sedation, delay in definitive treatment, hypoxemia, and high cost [11]. In this study, bronchoscopy findings were taken into consideration whenever they were available. Not having to perform a bronchoscopy did not affect the progress of endovascular treatment. Bronchoscopy findings have not altered the course of angiography and endovascular treatment in any of their patients. In this observational retrospective study of 28 patients, there was no need for emergency bronchoscopy during active and abundant bleeding.

In a retrospective study of 28 patients with massive hemoptysis, flexible bronchoscopy successfully localized the site of bleeding in 26 patients [2]. In comparison, chest radiographs localized the bleeding site in 23 patients. This suggests that flexible bronchoscopy is effective at identifying the site of bleeding in patients with massive hemoptysis, but localizing a radiographic abnormality is sufficiently accurate to warrant proceeding to bronchial artery embolization without bronchoscopy [28].

Despite the "lack of proof" showing that early bronchoscopy is beneficial, the general expert consensus favors an early bronchoscopy, especially for patients with massive hemoptysis [3]. The early procedure provides clinicians with the maximal amount of information upon which to base future decisions, particularly in patients who develop sudden recurrence or acceleration of their bleeding. Nevertheless, early bronchoscopy has not been strictly proven to improve outcome [28].

Practically speaking, early bronchoscopy should be done within the first 12–18 h for the patient who is clinically stable or for whom bleeding has become quiescent. Alternatively, bronchoscopy is performed as early as it is safely feasible on the unstable, decompensating patient [28]. In some institutions, in patients with MH who are unstable, diagnostic angiography is the imaging method of choice to localize the bleeding site because it allows for immediate treatment [31].

Type of Bronchoscopy

Depending on each institution's local practice, rigid or flexible bronchoscopes are used to evaluate and to stabilize any patient presenting MH. The selection is likely to reflect the institution's or the user's experience [12]. No study addressed this issue.

Rigid

Rigid bronchoscopy has been, until recently, the procedure of choice after initial chest radiography. Many surgeons and much of the older literature strongly advocate the use of the rigid bronchoscope. Rigid bronchoscopy is preferred because of its ability to suction large quantities of liquid and clotted blood, to use a great variety of therapies during bronchoscopy, such as direct cauterization or packing of bronchial lesions, and to continuously provide ventilation. Obviously, operating room setting and general anesthesia are required. By contrast, the visual range of inspection is significantly reduced compared to the fiber-optic bronchoscopy.

Changing over time, the technique of rigid bronchoscopy is being less and less used and, as a result, is not available in many institutions [13]. Consequently, a rigid bronchoscope is usually used for patients with ongoing massive hemoptysis after an unsuccessful bedside fiber-optic bronchoscopy. The flexible bronchoscope can also be used in conjunction with the rigid bronchoscope by passing it through its lumen. This allows a better examination of the more distal and upper lobe airways [28].

A survey in 1998 noted that 79% of physicians treating massive hemoptysis favored the flexible optic bronchoscope (FOB) as the initial technique compared to 48% in a similar survey performed in 1988 [32, 33].

Flexible

FOB has become more acceptable as an initial procedure for intubated or not intubated patients. The main limitation of FOB compared to the rigid bronchoscope is its limited ability to produce adequate suction through its smaller port. Also, with massive hemoptysis, the presence of blood in the inferior airway may absorb the light transmitted by the FOB and consequently decrease the capacity of visualization [13]. As described above, FOB can be used through the rigid bronchoscope for further examination.

For maximal safety, most patients should be intubated when bronchoscopy is indicated in presence of massive hemoptysis. If bleeding increases or recurs during the procedure, the bronchoscope can be removed, and suction can be applied while controlling the airway. The perception obtained through the bronchoscope is commonly obscured by clots on the tip of the scope; thus, it is important to be able to safely remove the scope, clean the tip, and suction the channel to continue the examination [28]. The disadvantages of bronchoscopy in an acute bleeding situation include poor visibility due to endobronchial blood and frequent ineffective therapeutic options [1].

Endobronchial Therapy

Laser photocoagulation or resection, electrocauterization, and cryotherapy are useful tools for minor or moderate hemoptysis. Unfortunately, these techniques are rarely efficient against massive hemoptysis [13]. If bronchoscopy allows visualization of a localized bleeding mucosal lesion, laser therapy or electrocauterization may be considered, if available. Both techniques can be used through a flexible or rigid bronchoscope. Since excellent visualization of the bleeding site is required, the rigid bronchoscope may be preferred because of its better suction capability [11].

Pharmacologic Adjuncts

Some pharmacologic adjuncts may be used through the FOB. Topical agents such as warm saline may initially help to break down gross clots and identify the bleeding site [13]. After identification of the bleeding side, initial control may be obtained by using 50 mL sequential aliquots of up to 500 mL ice-saline lavage [12]. Topical epinephrine (1:20,000) is also used to act locally as a vessel's vasoconstrictor to stop bleeding. Thrombin, fibrinogen-thrombin, or fibrin precursor solutions, such as hemostatic agents, can be injected via intrabronchial infusion through a catheter inserted into a FOB wedged against the bleeding bronchus [34, 35].

Mechanical Therapy

When a lesion is not treatable by embolization, as there is no feeding vessel and if surgical resection is not thought to be a viable option, the protection of the contralateral lung can be achieved by the insertion of a lung isolation device. But this measure may offer only a temporary relief. At that time, the use of self-expanding airway stent to cover the bleeding segmental bronchial orifice may act as both tamponade and isolation of the bleeding source [36].

Systemic Therapy

Intravenous vasopressin has been used to treat massive hemoptysis, in a similar way as its use in gastrointestinal hemorrhage [37]. Therefore, its administration may prevent successful BAE [38–40]. Other therapies that may promote coagulation and that have been used successfully for massive hemoptysis include intravenous estrogens (Premarin®), desmopressin (DDAVP®), ADH (vasopressin), tranexamic acid (Cyklokapron®) [41–44], and recombinant activated coagulation factor VII [45].

Bronchial Artery Embolization (BAE)

First reported by Remy et al. in 1973 [7], the use of BAE for management of MH has become widespread. It has become the main option for the treatment of MH, either at first presentation or in case of recurrence. Development of BAE has been a huge advance in treatment of patients with MH, both as a temporizing measure and as a definitive treatment for some patients [46]. After several improvements, BAE is now considered the procedure of choice in cases of both massive and recurring hemoptysis and should be undertaken promptly [29]. It is also now considered the most effective nonsurgical treatment in MH [1]. This approach reduces the systemic arterial perfusion pressure from the fragile bronchial arteries within the diseased lung parenchyma [47]. In the hands of experienced angiographers, embolization successfully stops bleeding more than 85% of the time, especially if the bronchial circulation and the systemic arterial supply are carefully defined [11, 48].

Multiple imaging modalities are used to confirm the diagnosis and to locate the bleeding site in stable patients. These include plain chest radiography, chest computed tomography, and bronchoscopy. But in patients with MH who are unstable, diagnostic angiography is the preferred imaging method for localizing the bleeding site because it allows for immediate treatment [31].

The initial step for transcatheter embolization is performing a thoracic angiogram to visualize and localize all the main systemic arteries to the lung(s). Once the feeding arteries are localized, selective bronchial arteriography is performed to characterize the bleeding vessel. When the bleeding vessel is identified, an embolic agent is used. There are numerous options regarding material used for BAE. They all have different characteristics as being particles or coils or having irregular or spherical form or different sizes [49].

Postembolization, bronchial arteriogram, and thoracic aortogram are performed to ensure the complete block of all the feeding arteries with no further bleeding from vessels. Immediate recurrent hemoptysis often occurs due to missed feeding arteries that went untreated, whereas later recurrence may take place as a result of collateralization or recanalization of either the feeding artery or new bleeding vessels [31].

Multiple publications (10 series including 609 patients, from 1983 to 2007) have demonstrated an immediate suc-

cessful rate of controlled bleeding varying from 70% to 95% with a recurrence rate ranging between 13% and 43%. These studies also report a minimal immediate complication rate of less than 1% [31]. The most serious complication of BAE is the accidental embolization of the anterior spinal artery (Adamkiewicz) either by contrast material or the embolizing particles causing ischemic injuries [1]. The anterior spinal artery originates from a bronchial artery in about 5% of patients. The reported prevalence of this complication has been described as 1% [50]. This risk has been decreased by superselective embolization techniques using smaller catheters that can be placed distally [51]. Renal dysfunction resulting from the contrast load is a concern, especially in patients who are hemodynamically unstable due to blood loss [6].

Correct clinical evaluation and ventilation stabilization of the patient are mandatory before BAE in massive hemoptysis [27]. Intubating a patient with a single- or double-lumen tube helps to monitor, with the help of a FOB, the interruption of bleeding through a radiologic intervention and to clean the inferior airways from any residual blood and blood clots.

Surgery

Historically, pulmonary resection has been the most effective method to control and prevent recurrent bleeding [6]. Comparing the results with those of medical or surgical management is difficult for several reasons. The criteria of eligibility for surgery differ among institutions and seem to be subject to surgical or institutional bias [1]. The primary problem in selection bias is that patients who are more likely to die are less likely to be operated on [6].

Patients with lateralized, ideally well-localized, uncontrollable bleeding should be assessed early for possible surgery in case the bleeding remains brisk and unresponsive to other measures. Surgery is reserved as an absolute last resort for operative candidates not salvageable by BAE [6].

Patients presenting MH are too ill for physiologic testing; historical data are therefore used to estimate the patient's ability to undergo lung resection. Relative contraindications to surgery include severe underlying pulmonary disease, active TB, diffuse underlying lung disease (cystic fibrosis, multiple arteriovenous malformations, multifocal bronchiectasis), and diffuse alveolar hemorrhage [11].

Morbidity and mortality are significantly greater with emergent surgery for persistent massive bleeding compared to elective surgery in non-bleeding patients. In most series of emergent therapy, surgical mortality for treatment of massive hemoptysis is approximately 20%, ranging from 10% to 38% for series published between 2000 and 2003 [52–54], with morbidity occurring in an additional 25–50% of patients; however, most of these series are more than 20 years old.

The reasons for such high mortality and morbidity may be related to the ongoing bleeding in unstable hemodynamic conditions, together with soiling of the remaining healthy bronchopulmonary segments before and during the operation. Contamination of the contralateral lung before, during, and after surgery is the main cause of postoperative respiratory failure leading to prolonged ventilation, nosocomial pneumonia, and death [6]. One solution is to delay the surgery with BAE, to obtain hemodynamic stability preoperatively, and to perform bronchial toilet pre- and postoperatively. Before the critical decision to perform surgery is taken, the surgeons should make sure that available interventional modalities such as balloon bronchial blockers, rigid bronchoscopy, or BAE can be used in an optimal manner to buy time to delay surgery for a better surgical outcome.

Iatrogenic Pulmonary Artery Rupture (IPAR)

The use of a pulmonary artery catheter (PAC) is becoming less frequent in the operating room since the general use of transesophageal echocardiography. Nevertheless, PAC remains a useful tool for diagnosis and management of many patients with cardiac or lung diseases. Sicker patients may need the insertion of a PAC, and these sicker patients are usually the patients most at risk for catheter-induced pulmonary artery rupture. Prevention is the first approach to develop when confronted with an iatrogenic complication. The first step of prevention is the judicious selection of patients. Risk factors for catheter-induced pulmonary artery rupture include female gender, age over 60 years old, improper catheter placement, and pre-existing pulmonary hypertension. The second is the appropriate use and management of the PAC. Nevertheless, when a catheter-induced pulmonary artery rupture occurs, the physician needs to have a clear scheme of intervention to deal with this severe complication.

The incidence of rupture is not very high, with an average of 0.01–0.47%. In a large retrospective study of patients with a Swan-Ganz catheter, Kearney et al. [55] found an incidence of pulmonary artery rupture (PAR) of 0.031% and a mortality of 70% [55]. The mortality rate of pulmonary artery rupture averages 50% but can be as high as 75% in anticoagulated patients. Death occurs most often secondary to asphyxia. If a delay before the appropriate management is instituted, it will contribute to a higher mortality rate.

The initial presentation may be as obvious as massive pulmonary hemorrhage or as subtle as a minor hemoptysis associated with cough, or it may be totally asymptomatic [56]. Moreover, any hemoptysis in the presence of a PAC should be investigated because of the high suspicion of PAR or false aneurysm formation. Hemothorax may be the mode of presentation when blood enters the pleural space instead of the airway.

The proposed mechanisms for catheter-induced PAR include catheter tip lodged in the vessel wall when the PAC is advanced while the balloon is not inflated or when eccentric balloon inflation exposes the catheter tip and guides it into the arterial wall or migration of catheter in a smaller arteriole with subsequent rupture caused by balloon inflation. Primary management of catheter-induced pulmonary artery rupture focuses on the prevention of asphyxia. Asphyxia secondary to lung spillage or blood clots is the main factor leading to death. Prevention of contamination of the unaffected lung is essential. As for other types of MH, blood loss is rarely massive enough to cause a great threat in hemodynamics, and slight hypotension may be treated with volume replacement.

The management of IPAR is a three-pronged approach, with targeted therapy derived from the basic "ABC" principles of resuscitation, airway, breathing, and circulation. The goals are (A) lung isolation, (B) maintaining appropriate gas exchange and oxygen delivery, and (C) volume resuscitation. The decision to leave the PAC in place may be critical at that time for the next steps in the radiologic management of this complication. It is essential not to inflate the balloon without radiologic imaging support (see later discussion). Management differs depending on the clinical presentation, mainly in which setting it is presenting, intensive care unit, operating room, or radiology suite.

Intensive Care Unit Setting

When a pulmonary artery catheter is inserted and there is hemoptysis, whether it is massive or negligible, a chest radiograph is usually obtained and will show infiltration around the catheter tip or pleural effusion. The side of a PAC can serve as a guide to determine from which side the hemorrhage may come from. Since most PACs are located in the right lung (90%), mainly the right lower lobe, it can be assumed that hemorrhage comes from the right side if the situation is critical [20, 57].

While diagnostic procedures are performed, 100% oxygen should be administered to the patient. If the lungs are not isolated, the patient should be placed with the bleeding lung on the dependent (inferior) side to prevent spillage to the unaffected side. If the situation is not critical, a short fiber-optic bronchoscopy can be performed to determine the origin of bleeding.

The patient must undergo selective intubation to obtain lung isolation. Lung isolation can be performed with various techniques, including selective intubation with a standard endotracheal tube, bronchial blocker, or DLT. As mentioned earlier, it is our opinion that the best strategy is to place a DLT, but a bronchial blocker can be used for lung separation if a DLT is not immediately available or is difficult to insert.

After lung isolation, fiber-optic bronchoscopy can be useful to confirm the good positioning of the device used for the lung isolation and to identify the bleeding site. It is frequently difficult to get a good view of the structures because the blood in the tracheobronchial tree highly absorbs the light of the fiber-optic bronchoscope.

It has been suggested that the PAC could be deflated, withdrawn of a few centimeters, and left in the pulmonary artery. The balloon may be inflated to compress the bleeding vessels or to temporarily obstruct the feeding artery [58, 59]. We recommend that this technique should be used only under fluoroscopy and angiographic control to finely adjust the position of the balloon, in order to avoid malpositioning of the balloon. Improper positioning could augment the bleeding by increasing the vascular laceration or by diverting the pulmonary blood flow to the injured vessel.

Pulmonary angiogram generated through a PAC may be difficult to realize because of the very small inner lumen of the Swan-Ganz catheter. With a stable patient or if the diagnosis remains unclear, a contrast-enhanced CT scan may be performed and is a valuable diagnostic tool. It can confirm the possibility of a pulmonary artery false aneurysm (PAFA) but also exclude any other causes of hemoptysis. CT scan-

ning is usually followed by an angiography with embolization, if indicated and feasible (Table 44.3).

Operating Room Setting

Most cases of life-threatening hemoptysis described during cardiac surgery result from a catheter-induced pulmonary artery perforation [1]. If a hemoptysis happens during surgery, lung isolation can be rapidly achieved, and the diagnostic and therapeutic procedures started, while the patient is still under anesthesia. If the hemoptysis happens before the scheduled surgery, elective surgery must be postponed until the PAR is investigated and stabilized. During cardiac surgery, when a hemorrhage happens after cardiopulmonary bypass (CPB) but before heparin reversal, CPB should be restarted to bypass the lung circulation and stop the bleeding, giving time to the anesthesia team to identify the side of the bleeding, to isolate the lungs, and to maximize oxygenation (see Fig. 44.2). If the hemoptysis begins after protamine administration, the best conduct is to finish the surgery as quickly as possible, isolate the lung, and proceed to a definite investigation and treatment of the pulmonary artery rupture.

Iatrogenic pulmonary artery rupture can be localized at the proximal trunk of the pulmonary artery (PA). As this perforation occurred outside the lung parenchyma, it explains the absence of hemoptysis [60]. Surgical repair is then indicated.

After ruling out the implication of PAC as the cause of MH during cardiac surgery, other causes, including surgical trauma, traumatic intubation, or concomitant disease (neoplasia, pulmonary edema) amplified by heparin and anticoagulation, should be considered. When no pre-existing disease and no lesion can be identified by bronchoscopy or by the surgeons to explain unilateral bleeding and that the patient is too instable to be transferred to the angiographic

Table 44.3 Management of pulmonary artery catheter-induced pulmonary hemorrhage

1. Initially place the patient with the non-isolated, bleeding lung in the inferior position
2. Endotracheal intubation, oxygenation, airway toilet
3. Lung isolation: endobronchial double- or single-lumen tube or bronchial blocker
4. Withdraw the pulmonary artery catheter several centimeters, leaving it in the main pulmonary artery. Do not inflate the balloon (except with fluoroscopic guidance).
5. Position the patient with the isolated bleeding lung nondependent. PEEP to the bleeding lung if possible
6. Transport to medical imaging for diagnosis and embolization if feasible

Fig. 44.2 Flow diagram of management of massive hemoptysis during weaning from cardiopulmonary bypass. *CPB* cardiopulmonary bypass, *FOB* fiber-optic bronchoscopy, *ETT* endotracheal tube, *PA* pulmonary artery, *Parenc.* lung parenchyma

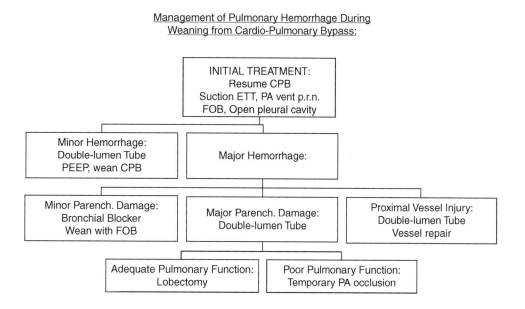

Management of Pulmonary Hemorrhage During Weaning from Cardio-Pulmonary Bypass:

room, temporary pulmonary vascular exclusion by thoracotomy is an effective alternative to radiologic embolization for managing unilateral hemoptysis during heart surgery [61].

Radiological Setting

During cardiac catheterization, the PAC can be used to evaluate pulmonary vascular resistance and the wedge pressure. When catheter-induced pulmonary artery rupture happens in this setting, it is relatively easy to pull back the PAC of a few cm and to reinflate the balloon under direct visualization [59, 62]. Thus, it may be possible to stop the bleeding pending further radiological intervention. However, this measure does not always enable physician to contain the hemorrhage [63]. This is the reason why the authors recommend using fluoroscopy and contrast injection to confirm that the PAC is still proximal to the injured vessel and that balloon inflation impedes flow through the lacerated vessel. Diagnostic angiography and embolization can be easily performed at that point. This may help to avoid intubation, lung isolation, and post-procedure ventilation in some circumstances [59]. Since the use of a FOB to initially position a DLT or BB in a patient with MH can be difficult due to obstruction of the view by blood, one option in the radiology suite is to use fluoroscopy to help guide the lung isolation device (see Fig. 44.3) [62].

Pulmonary Artery False Aneurysm (PAFA)

PAFA formation is secondary to the accumulation of blood in an aneurismal sac compressed by the lung parenchyma. While there is no intact vessel wall lining containing the bleeding, the lung parenchyma may prevent further extrava-

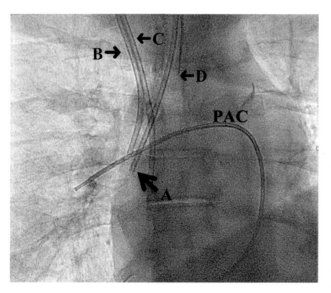

Fig. 44.3 An Arndt bronchial blocker (arrow A) has been positioned under fluoroscopic guidance into the right main stem bronchus of a patient who developed massive hemoptysis during right heart catheterization. The bronchial blocker can be seen between the central venous catheter (arrow B), proximal pulmonary artery catheter (arrow C), distal end of the endotracheal tube (arrow D). *PAC* distal pulmonary artery catheter (Modified with permission from Addante et al. [62])

sation. The presence of a PAFA requires intervention, because one can never be certain that spontaneous healing will occur. Delayed pulmonary hemorrhage occurs in 30–40% of cases of a PAFA caused by a previous catheter-induced pulmonary artery rupture. Rebleeding can occur as late as 2 weeks to 7 months after the initial event [64].

With the development of interventional cardiology and different vascular devices, novel therapeutic approaches to IPAR have been recently developed. For instance, vascular plug (Amplatzer® AGA Medical Corp., North Plymouth, MN) has been used with success [65, 66].

If there is suspicion of a PAFA on the CT scan, an angiogram should be done. When the clinical suspicion of pulmonary artery rupture is high or when the patient is unstable, angiography remains the procedure of choice because it allows both diagnostic and therapeutic intervention (see Fig. 44.4) [67]. If diagnosis of a PAFA is confirmed, selective embolization helps to reduce morbidity and mortality. Embolization is successful in 75% of cases, with a rebleeding rate of about 20%. Sometimes, it can be deleterious to embolize the PAFA regarding global lung function. In these cases, conservative treatment can be tried. Follow-up of this type of patients with repeat contrast CT scan is required.

Other Causes

Some other causes or presentations of IPAR have been described. Its occurrence is extremely rare during insertion of a thoracic percutaneous drainage tubes but may be devastating due to the large-bore chest tube typically used and sometimes may be rapidly fatal [68]. An idiopathic bilateral bronchial hemorrhage during cardiac surgery has been reported in the literature. Despite a very aggressive treatment, the patient died on day 6 [19].

Management Post Hemoptysis

Following massive hemoptysis, treated either by endoscopy, radiological intervention or surgery, it is important to perform a bronchoscopy to clean the tracheobronchial tree and to remove any blood and clots in the distal airway. This action will help promote better and faster patient recuperation.

Tracheostomy Hemorrhage

Another clinically challenging scenario involving massive airway bleeding is tracheostomy hemorrhage. Hemorrhage in the immediate postoperative period following a tracheostomy is usually from local vessels in the incision such as the anterior jugular or inferior thyroid veins. Massive hemorrhage 1–6 weeks postoperatively is most common due to tracheo-innominate artery fistula [69]. A small sentinel bleed occurs in most patients before a massive bleed.

Fig. 44.4 (a) Radiographic contrast dye injection showing a false aneurysm of the pulmonary artery of the right lower lobe following massive hemoptysis induced by pulmonary artery catheter rupture. (b) A coil has been placed by interventional radiology in the false aneurysm of the right lower pulmonary artery in the same patient. Dye injection shows that the aneurysm has embolized with no further leakage

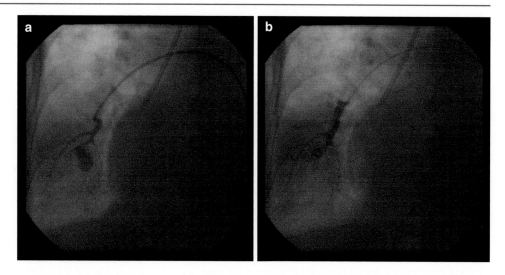

Table 44.4 Management of tracheo-innominate artery fistula hemorrhage

1. Overinflate the tracheostomy cuff to tamponade the hemorrhage. If this fails:
2. Replace the tracheostomy tube with an oral endotracheal tube. Position the cuff with FOB guidance just above the carina
3. Digital compression of the innominate artery against the posterior sternum using a finger passed through the tracheostomy stoma. If this fails:
4. Slow withdrawal of the ETT and overinflation of the cuff to tamponade
5. Then proceed with definitive therapy: sternotomy and ligation of the innominate artery

The management protocol for tracheo-innominate artery fistula is outlined in Table 44.4.

Conclusion

Endobronchial control measures and artery embolization have radically changed the management of massive hemoptysis. In experienced hands, BAE is an effective therapeutic tool and plays a pivotal role in the management of life-threatening massive hemoptysis. With control of hemorrhage, nonsurgical patients can be identified and surgical candidates accurately assessed to allow an elective operation, with lower morbidity and mortality, if conservative measures are unsuccessful [6].

Based on the above information, the following approach is a reasonable way to manage a patient with massive hemoptysis. First, stabilize the patient's oxygenation, ventilation, and hemodynamic status. Early correction of coagulopathy and consultation with critical care physician, pulmonary medicine (bronchoscopist), interventional radiologist, thoracic surgery, and anesthesiologist are essential. Perform early bronchoscopy along with other appropriate diagnostic evaluations. If the patient

continues to bleed aggressively, arteriography is most reasonable for localization and therapy. If bleeding persists despite embolization or if the patient is too ill to undergo an angiography, blockade therapy or insertion of a double-lumen tube should be considered in preparation for rigid bronchoscopy in the operating room with possible lung resection if warranted. While surgery remains the only truly definitive therapy, it should not be used in the acute emergent setting unless it cannot be avoided [11]. Surgery, including pulmonary artery ligature, segmentectomy, lobectomy, or pneumonectomy, is reserved for extreme cases since it is technically challenging and associated to high morbidity [64].

Clinical Case Discussion

A 26-year-old woman is well known in the authors' institution for Eisenmenger's syndrome secondary to a complex congenital heart disease. She had a patent ductus arteriosus for which no surgical option was available when diagnosed at 4 years old. She was referred to our center 4 years ago for pulmonary hypertension. At that time, it was observed that the right pulmonary artery originates directly from the aorta. She has been treated with epoprostenol (Flolan) for 3 years.

A few months ago, she presented some episodes of moderate hemoptysis treated with BAE. Someday, she presented a new moderate hemoptysis necessitating BAE. She was admitted to the intensive care unit for 5 days, and no bleeding was observed. She was then transferred to the bronchoscopy suite to search for a blood occluding the right inferior lobe bronchus. With the aid of sedation and local anesthesia, the area was easily reached. The blood clot was partially dislodged without any problem. While trying to dislodge the remaining of the clot, coughing was provoked, and it induced a massive bleeding from the inferior lobe.

Questions

Which immediate procedure should be undertaken?

1. Nasal oxygen was already in place for the FOB exam.
2. Right lateral decubitus position to protect the left lung from blood spillage.
3. Irrigation of the origin of bleeding with cold saline.

Bleeding continues and becomes a MH. What is the next step?

4. Left-side endobronchial intubation with single-lumen tube with the assistance of the FOB.
5. Left lateral decubitus position to improve left lung gas exchange and minimize bleeding from the right lung.
6. Exchange the endobronchial simple lumen tube for a double-lumen tube.

The patient was directed, with anesthesia assistance, to the radiological suite for angiography and BAE as needed. Following diagnostic angiography and therapeutic embolization, the radiologist wanted to know about the bleeding in the right lung. What we can do to help her?

7. Fiber-Optic Bronchoscopy Examination

Following this procedure, the right-side bronchial tree was suctioned. At that time, active bleeding was identified originating from the right inferior super dorsal bronchus. Following a new BAE, the bleeding ceased, and the cleaning of the bilateral bronchial tree was completed without finding any other bleeding site.

The patient was transferred to the ICU with the DLT in place. She was sedated and ventilated until the next morning when she was extubated. She did not present any recurrence, and she was transferred to another center for evaluation for lung transplantation.

References

1. Jean-Baptiste E. Clinical assessment and management of massive hemoptysis. Crit Care Med. 2000;28(5):1642–7.
2. Amirana M, Frater R, Tirschwell P, Janis M, Bloomberg A, State D. An aggressive surgical approach to significant hemoptysis in patients with pulmonary tuberculosis. Am Rev Respir Dis. 1968;97(2):187–92.
3. Bobrowitz ID, Ramakrishna S, Shim YS. Comparison of medical v surgical treatment of major hemoptysis. Arch Intern Med. 1983;143(7):1343–6.
4. Corey R, Hla KM. Major and massive hemoptysis: reassessment of conservative management. Am J Med Sci. 1987;294(5):301–9.
5. Garzon AA, Cerruti MM, Golding ME. Exsanguinating hemoptysis. J Thorac Cardiovasc Surg. 1982;84(6):829–33.
6. Wigle DA, Waddell TK. Chapter 38: Investigation and management of massive hemoptysis. In: Pearson's thoracic & esophageal surgery. J, D., Meyerson, S. L., A, P. (Ed.), & JD, C. (Ed.). Pearson's Thoracic and Esophageal Surgery 3rd edition. Philadelphia: Churchill Livingstone. 2008
7. Remy J, Voisin C, Ribet M, Dupuis C, Beguery P, Tonnel AB, et al. Treatment, by embolization, of severe or repeated hemoptysis associated with systemic hypervascularization. Nouv Press Med. 2060;2(31):1973.
8. Hiebert CA. Balloon catheter control of life-threatening hemoptysis. Chest. 1974;66(3):308–9.
9. Cauldwell EW, Siekert RG, et al. The bronchial arteries; an anatomic study of 150 human cadavers. Surg Gynecol Obstet. 1948;86(4):395–412.
10. Fraser KL, Grosman H, Hyland RH, Tullis DE. Transverse myelitis: a reversible complication of bronchial artery embolisation in cystic fibrosis. Thorax. 1997;52(1):99–101.
11. Ingbar DH. Causes and management of massive hemoptysis in adults. Post TW, ed. UpToDate. Waltham, MA: UpToDate Inc. http://www.uptodate.com; 2009.
12. Dweik RA, Stoller JK. Role of bronchoscopy in massive hemoptysis. Clin Chest Med. 1999;20(1):89–105.
13. Karmy-Jones R, Cuschieri J, Vallieres E. Role of bronchoscopy in massive hemoptysis. Chest Surg Clin N Am. 2001;11(4):873–906.
14. Wedzicha JA, Pearson MC. Management of massive haemoptysis. Respir Med. 1990;84(1):9–12.
15. Campos JH. Progress in lung separation. Thorac Surg Clin. 2005;15(1):71–83.
16. Spicek-Macan J, Hodoba N, Nikolic I, Stancic-Rokotov D, Kolaric N, Popovic-Grle S. Exsanguinating tuberculosis-related hemoptysis: bronchial blocker introduced through percutaneous tracheostomy. Minerva Anestesiol. 2009;75(6):405–8.
17. Freitag L, Tekolf E, Stamatis G, Montag M, Greschuchna D. Three years experience with a new balloon catheter for the management of haemoptysis. Eur Respir J. 1994;7(11):2033–7.
18. Giannoni S, Buti G, Allori O, Conti D, Ferri L. Bilateral concurrent massive hemoptysis successfully controlled with double endobronchial tamponade. A case report. Minerva Anestesiol. 2006;72(7–8):665–74.
19. Uzuka T, Nakamura M, Nakajima T, Kusudoh S, Usubuchi H, Tanaka A, et al. Idiopathic bronchial hemorrhage: a rare but catastrophic complication in cardiac surgery. J Cardiothorac Surg. 2016;11(1):78.
20. Caddell B, Yelverton B, Tippett JC, Ravi Y, Sai-Sudhakar CB, Culp WC Jr. Management of massive hemoptysis after pulmonary thromboembolectomy using a double bronchial blocker system. J Cardiothorac Vasc Anesth. 2017;31(2):633–6.
21. Jardin M, Remy J. Control of hemoptysis: systemic angiography and anastomoses of the internal mammary artery. Radiology. 1988;168(2):377–83.
22. Gourin A, Garzon AA. Operative treatment of massive hemoptysis. Ann Thorac Surg. 1974;18(1):52–60.
23. Klein U, Karzai W, Bloos F, Wohlfarth M, Gottschall R, Fritz H, et al. Role of fiberoptic bronchoscopy in conjunction with the use of double-lumen tubes for thoracic anesthesia: a prospective study. Anesthesiology. 1998;88(2):346–50.
24. Campos JH, Hallam EA, Van Natta T, Kernstine KH. Devices for lung isolation used by anesthesiologists with limited thoracic experience: comparison of double-lumen endotracheal tube, Univent torque control blocker, and Arndt wire-guided endobronchial blocker. Anesthesiology. 2006;104(2):261–6, discussion 5A
25. Campos JH. Which device should be considered the best for lung isolation: double-lumen endotracheal tube versus bronchial blockers. Curr Opin Anaesthesiol. 2007;20(1):27–31.
26. Narayanaswamy M, McRae K, Slinger P, Dugas G, Kanellakos GW, Roscoe A, et al. Choosing a lung isolation device for thoracic surgery: a randomized trial of three bronchial blockers versus double-lumen tubes. Anesth Analg. 2009;108(4):1097–101.
27. de Gregorio MA, Medrano J, Laborda A, Higuera T. Hemoptysis workup before embolization: single-center experience with a 15-year period follow-up. Tech Vasc Interv Radiol. 2007;10(4):270–3.

28. Ingbar DH. Diagnostic approach to massive hemoptysis in adults. Post TW, ed. UpToDate. Waltham, MA: UpToDate Inc. http://www.uptodate.com; 2009

29. Poyanli A, Acunas B, Rozanes I, Guven K, Yilmaz S, Salmaslioglu A, et al. Endovascular therapy in the management of moderate and massive haemoptysis. Br J Radiol. 2007;80(953):331–6.

30. Hsiao EI, Kirsch CM, Kagawa FT, Wehner JH, Jensen WA, Baxter RB. Utility of fiberoptic bronchoscopy before bronchial artery embolization for massive hemoptysis. AJR Am J Roentgenol. 2001;177(4):861–7.

31. Lee EW, Grant JD, Loh CT, Kee ST. Bronchial and pulmonary arterial and venous interventions. Semin Respir Crit Care Med. 2008;29(4):395–404.

32. Haponik EF, Chin R. Hemoptysis: clinicians' perspectives. Chest. 1990;97(2):469–75.

33. Lippmann ML, Walkenstein MD, Goldberg SK. Bronchoscopy in hemoptysis. Chest. 1990;98(6):1538.

34. Tsukamoto T, Sasaki H, Nakamura H. Treatment of hemoptysis patients by thrombin and fibrinogen-thrombin infusion therapy using a fiberoptic bronchoscope. Chest. 1989;96(3):473–6.

35. Bense L. Intrabronchial selective coagulative treatment of hemoptysis. Report of three cases. Chest. 1990;97(4):990–6.

36. Brandes JC, Schmidt E, Yung R. Occlusive endobronchial stent placement as a novel management approach to massive hemoptysis from lung cancer. J Thorac Oncol. 2008;3(9):1071–2.

37. Magee G, Williams MH Jr. Treatment of massive hemoptysis with intravenous pitressin. Lung. 1982;160(3):165–9.

38. Mal H, Rullon I, Mellot F, Brugiere O, Sleiman C, Menu Y, et al. Immediate and long-term results of bronchial artery embolization for life-threatening hemoptysis. Chest. 1999;115(4):996–1001.

39. Remy J, Arnaud A, Fardou H, Giraud R, Voisin C. Treatment of hemoptysis by embolization of bronchial arteries. Radiology. 1977;122(1):33–7.

40. Stoller J. Diagnosis and management of massive hemoptysis: a review. Respir Care. 1992;37:564–81.

41. Bilton D, Webb AK, Foster H, Mulvenna P, Dodd M. Life threatening haemoptysis in cystic fibrosis: an alternative therapeutic approach. Thorax. 1990;45(12):975–6.

42. Chang AB, Ditchfield M, Robinson PJ, Robertson CF. Major hemoptysis in a child with cystic fibrosis from multiple aberrant bronchial arteries treated with tranexamic acid. Pediatr Pulmonol. 1996;22(6):416–20.

43. Graff GR. Treatment of recurrent severe hemoptysis in cystic fibrosis with tranexamic acid. Respiration. 2001;68(1):91–4.

44. Popper J. The use of premarin IV in hemoptysis. Dis Chest. 1960;37:659–60.

45. Tien HC, Gough MR, Farrell R, Macdonald J. Successful use of recombinant activated coagulation factor VII in a patient with massive hemoptysis from a penetrating thoracic injury. Ann Thorac Surg. 2007;84(4):1373–4.

46. Johnson JL. Manifestations of hemoptysis. How to manage minor, moderate, and massive bleeding. Postgrad Med. 2002;112(4):101–6, 8–9, 13

47. Marshall TJ, Jackson JE. Vascular intervention in the thorax: bronchial artery embolization for haemoptysis. Eur Radiol. 1997;7(8):1221–7.

48. Yoon W, Kim JK, Kim YH, Chung TW, Kang HK. Bronchial and nonbronchial systemic artery embolization for life-threatening hemoptysis: a comprehensive review. Radiographics. 2002;22(6):1395–409.

49. Ittrich H, Klose H, Adam G. Radiologic management of haemoptysis: diagnostic and interventional bronchial arterial embolisation. RoFo. 2015;187(4):248–59.

50. Zhang JS, Cui ZP, Wang MQ, Yang L. Bronchial arteriography and transcatheter embolization in the management of hemoptysis. Cardiovasc Intervent Radiol. 1994;17(5):276–9.

51. Tanaka N, Yamakado K, Murashima S, Takeda K, Matsumura K, Nakagawa T, et al. Superselective bronchial artery embolization for hemoptysis with a coaxial microcatheter system. J Vasc Interv Radiol. 1997;8(1 Pt 1):65–70.

52. Lee TW, Wan S, Choy DK, Chan M, Arifi A, Yim AP. Management of massive hemoptysis: a single institution experience. Ann Thorac Cardiovasc Surg. 2000;6(4):232–5.

53. Knott-Craig CJ, Oostuizen JG, Rossouw G, Joubert JR, Barnard PM. Management and prognosis of massive hemoptysis. Recent experience with 120 patients. J Thorac Cardiovasc Surg. 1993;105(3):394–7.

54. Endo S, Otani S, Saito N, Hasegawa T, Kanai Y, Sato Y, et al. Management of massive hemoptysis in a thoracic surgical unit. Eur J Cardiothorac Surg. 2003;23(4):467–72.

55. Kearney TJ, Shabot MM. Pulmonary artery rupture associated with the Swan-Ganz catheter. Chest. 1995;108(5):1349–52.

56. Poplausky MR, Rozenblit G, Rundback JH, Crea G, Maddineni S, Leonardo R. Swan-Ganz catheter-induced pulmonary artery pseudoaneurysm formation: three case reports and a review of the literature. Chest. 2001;120(6):2105–11.

57. Stratmann G, Benumof JL. Endobronchial hemorrhage due to pulmonary circulation tear: separating the lungs and the air from the blood. Anesth Analg. 2004;99(5):1276–9.

58. Dopfmer UR, Braun JP, Grosse J, Hotz H, Duveneck K, Schneider MB. Treatment of severe pulmonary hemorrhage after cardiopulmonary bypass by selective, temporary balloon occlusion. Anesth Analg. 2004;99(5):1280–2; table of contents

59. Fortin M, Turcotte R, Gleeton O, Bussieres JS. Catheter-induced pulmonary artery rupture: using occlusion balloon to avoid lung isolation. J Cardiothorac Vasc Anesth. 2006;20(3):376–8.

60. Booth KL, Mercer-Smith G, McConkey C, Parissis H. Catheter-induced pulmonary artery rupture: haemodynamic compromise necessitates surgical repair. Interact Cardiovasc Thorac Surg. 2012;15(3):531–3.

61. Fortin J, Vaillancourt R, Vigneault L, Laflamme M, Simon M, Bussières JS. Unusual cause of life-threatening hemoptysis during cardiac operation: surgical management revisited. Ann Thorac Surg. 2017;104:e251.

62. Addante RA, Chen J, Goswami S. Successful management of a patient with pulmonary artery rupture in a catheterization suite. J Cardiothorac Vasc Anesth. 2016;30(6):1618–20.

63. Gottwalles Y, Wunschel-Joseph ME, Hanssen M. Coil embolization treatment in pulmonary artery branch rupture during Swan-Ganz catheterization. Cardiovasc Intervent Radiol. 2000;23(6):477–9.

64. Mullerworth MH, Angelopoulos P, Couyant MA, Horton AM, Robinson SM, Petring OU, et al. Recognition and management of catheter-induced pulmonary artery rupture. Ann Thorac Surg. 1998;66(4):1242–5.

65. Kalra A, Heitner S, Topalian S. Iatrogenic pulmonary artery rupture during Swan-Ganz catheter placement--a novel therapeutic approach. Catheter Cardiovasc Interv. 2013;81(1):57–9.

66. Rudzinski PN, Henzel J, Dzielinska Z, Lubiszewska BM, Michalowska I, Szymanski P, et al. Pulmonary artery rupture as a complication of Swan-Ganz catheter application. Diagnosis and endovascular treatment: a single centre's experience. Postepy Kardiol Interwencyjnej. 2016;12(2):135–9.

67. Utsumi T, Kido T, Ohata T, Yasukawa M, Takano H, Sakakibara T. Swan-Ganz catheter-induced pseudoaneurysm of the pulmonary artery. Jpn J Thorac Cardiovasc Surg. 2002;50(8):347–9.

68. Bozzani A, Arici V, Bellinzona G, Pirrelli S, Forni E, Odero A. Iatrogenic pulmonary artery rupture due to chest-tube insertion. Tex Heart Inst J. 2010;37(6):732–3.

69. Grant CA, Dempsey G, Harrison J, Jones T. Tracheo-innominate artery fistula after percutaneous tracheostomy: three case reports and a clinical review. Br J Anaesth. 2006;96:127–30.

Whole Lung Lavage

45

Jean S. Bussières and Etienne J. Couture

Key Points
- Patients with pulmonary alveolar proteinosis have a restrictive disease and are hypoxic.
- Lavage of one lung with large quantities of saline requires careful lung isolation.
- For more than 10 years, bilateral lung lavage has been performed during the same anesthetic period.
- GM-CSF is now a complementary treatment to whole lung lavage when needed.

Introduction

This chapter reviews the historical considerations of whole lung lavage (WLL), when its performance is appropriate, details of the technique, complications, and finally benefits of this unusual treatment modality. It is important to differentiate WLL from bronchoalveolar lavage (BAL). BAL is a diagnostic tool performed with the aid of a fiberoptic bronchoscope (FOB) under local anesthesia, which uses only 300 mL of liquid in one segment of the lung. WLL is a treatment modality that requires over 10 L of normal saline instilled through a double-lumen tube in one whole lung while the patient is under general anesthesia.

Historical Consideration

WLL was first described in 1928 [1]. In the early 1960s, the first application of this technique was used to treat pulmonary alveolar proteinosis (PAP) [2–5]. At that time, the procedure consisted in repeated segmental flooding through a percutaneous transtracheal catheter positioned blindly into the bronchial tree. This technique was performed in an awake patient and was repeated four times a day for 2–3 weeks, using physical positioning to direct the saline sequentially into different lung segments. The 1980–2000 period **led** to the development of a modern technique of unilateral WLL, which is carried out under general anesthesia and lung separation [6, 7]. Since the beginning of this century, performing bilateral WLL during the same anesthesia period is the gold standard. In parallel with this evolution, the pathogenesis of WLL has been better defined since the discovery of the role of granulocyte-macrophage colony-stimulating factor (GM-CSF) in surfactant catabolism.

Indications

WLL is the most effective proven treatment modality for symptomatic pulmonary alveolar proteinosis [1, 2]. Various pathologic states have been also treated by WLL including cystic fibrosis, asthma, chronic obstructive lung disease, radioactive dust inhalation, alveolar microlithiasis, lipoid pneumonitis or exogenous lipoid pneumonia, and silicosis with variable success [8].

Pulmonary Alveolar Proteinosis

Primary pulmonary alveolar proteinosis (PAP) is a rare disorder of unknown cause and variable natural history. This lung disease is caused by alveolar accumulation of a lipoproteic material that has the aspect of surfactant. This accumulation of material creates a true alveolo-capillary blockade,

J. S. Bussières (✉)
Department of Anesthesiology, Institut Universitaire de Cardiologie et de Pneumologie de Québec – Université Laval, Québec City, QC, Canada
e-mail: jbuss@criucpq.ulaval.ca

E. J. Couture
Department of Medicine, Critical Care Division, University of Montreal, Montreal, QC, Canada
e-mail: Etienne.Couture.3@ULaval.ca

© Springer Nature Switzerland AG 2019
P. Slinger (ed.), *Principles and Practice of Anesthesia for Thoracic Surgery*, https://doi.org/10.1007/978-3-030-00859-8_45

and the patient presents with dyspnea and hypoxemia, aggravated by exercise.

Pathogenesis and Classification

Until recently, the pathogenesis of PAP was unknown. Most investigators have postulated a decreased clearance of surfactant from the alveolar space. Over the last decade, rapid progresses were made toward the elucidation of the molecular mechanisms of PAP. Recent data suggest that GM-CSF has a pivotal role in PAP pathogenesis, as it is required for normal surfactant homeostasis. The disease is associated with neutralizing autoantibodies against GM-CSF. This new information allows the development of a new classification for this orphan lung disease and the use of new therapies. Some studies have been conducted with inhaled and subcutaneous GM-CSF. The latter form shows improvement in oxygenation and quality of life in 48% of patients [9]. The main conclusion is that GM-CSF treatment appears to benefit a subset of patients with adult PAP and may represent a novel alternative to the repeated whole lung lavages.

Three forms of PAP are now recognized: primary, secondary, and congenital [10]. The primary (idiopathic) form of PAP is the most common disease presentation, representing more than 90% of all cases. Its onset occurs in adulthood, and it has an autoimmune origin. It is associated with a high prevalence of circulating anti-GM-CSF antibodies. Reduction of localized GM-CSF activity in the lung, secondary to the presence of neutralizing anti-GM-CSF antibodies, causes alveolar macrophage dysfunction, resulting in surfactant excess and accumulation [11]. There is no other associated underlying illness or exposure.

The secondary form also develops in adulthood, occurs with other conditions, and can be separated into two broad subgroups. These are systemic inflammatory diseases or malignancy and specific exogenous exposure. Exposure to a high level of inorganic dusts (e.g., silica, aluminum, titanium, cement, wood) or fumes (chlorine, gas, gasoline, plastics) has been incriminated. Secondary PAP is likely related to a relative deficiency of GM-CSF and related macrophage dysfunction.

The congenital form is often present in the neonatal period and results from a very rare gene mutation. This mutation is related to the surfactant receptor gene or to the GM-CSF gene. This form is rare but is usually very severe. Neonatal respiratory distress syndrome is a presentation form of congenital PAP.

Clinical Manifestations

Among adults, the typical age of apparition of the illness is 30–50 years. There is a male to female ratio of 2:1. The major symptom of PAP is a progressive dyspnea and hypoxemia on exertion, spread over months and sometimes years. Dyspnea, the most common presenting symptom, is reported by approximately 55–80% of patients; however, approximately one-third of affected patients are asymptomatic, despite the infiltration of the alveolar air space. Nonproductive cough, fatigue, weight loss, and low-grade fever have also been described.

Spontaneous remission can occur, but the therapeutic decision in PAP depends on the progression of the illness and the extent of the physiological impairment. The prognosis of PAP has greatly improved since the introduction of WLL by Ramirez in 1965. The usual objective of WLL is the improvement in the clinical, physiological, and radiological condition of the patient.

Radiographic Findings

Chest radiography is the most useful screening test, although very nonspecific [12, 13]. On chest radiography, bilateral symmetric alveolar opacities located centrally in mid- and lower or upper lung zones are typical, yielding a "butterfly" distribution. High-resolution CT scanning (HRCT) reveals ground-glass opacification, predominantly in a homogeneous distribution. Thickened intralobular structures and interlobular septa in typical polygonal shapes may also be observed, referred to as "crazy paving." Crazy paving is characteristic but not specific to PAP and can also be observed in patients with an acute respiratory distress syndrome, lipoid pneumonia, acute interstitial pneumonia, drug-related hypersensitivity reactions, and diffuse alveolar damage superimposed on usual interstitial pneumonitis [14].

Physiological Testing

Pulmonary function tests show a restrictive ventilatory defect with reduction in the total lung capacity and vital capacity. When present, the decrement in diffusing capacity for carbon dioxide (DLCO) is often out of proportion to the degree of the restrictive defect. Arterial blood gas analysis shows mild to moderate hypoxemia, with an elevated alveolar-arterial gradient and elevation in shunt fraction while breathing 100% O_2 [15].

Laboratory Investigation

Bronchoalveolar lavage (BAL) may help in establishing the diagnosis in clinically suspected cases. BAL fluid is opaque and presents a "milky" appearance, with large amounts of granular, acellular eosinophilic lipoproteinaceous material which is periodic acid-Schiff (PAS). Electron microscopic exam of BAL fluid can confirm the diagnosis [16, 17]. When allowed to stand, the fluid spontaneously separates into pale yellow, almost translucent supernatant, and thick sediment.

Obtaining tissue for histopathology by open lung biopsy has been the gold standard for a long time. This biopsy performed by VATS is now unnecessary in the majority of cases of PAP. The combination of the clinical presentation, imaging findings, and BAL results are generally sufficient to make the diagnosis. Transbronchial biopsies may be occasionally used when needed. Surgical lung biopsy is rarely necessary to make the diagnosis [18–20].

Furthermore, anti-GM-CSF antibodies are increasingly used as a diagnostic tool in PAP. The quantitative assessment of anti-GM-CSF antibodies in reference laboratories constitutes an important diagnostic and therapy-guiding measurement [21]. GM-CSF antibodies are present in all serum and BAL fluid samples from primary, idiopathic, PAP patients. BAL fluid levels of anti-GM-CSF antibodies correlate better with the severity of PAP compared to serum titers [22]. Serial measurements of BAL or serum anti-GM-CSF antibodies may be useful in monitoring disease activity and response to treatment.

Therapy

The treatment depends on the form of PAP. When dealing with idiopathic PAP, the use of WLL, GM-CSF, rituximab (Rituxan®), or plasmapheresis (see later) can be considered. For secondary PAP, treatment of the underlying condition or removal of the offending agent should be the first step to consider. When confronted with congenital PAP, WLL, supportive therapy, or lung transplantation is the ultimate treatment.

Whole Lung Lavage

Treatment of idiopathic PAP has evolved from the use of a variety of nonspecific and largely ineffective agents to the physical removal of the lipoproteinaceous material from the lungs (WLL) and to the development of specific therapy targeting the underlying pathogenesis of the disorder. WLL has, for a long time, been considered the definitive therapy for PAP. The idea that the accumulated material could be physically removed from the lungs of PAP patients was first advanced in the early 1960s.

Specific indications for lung lavage include a definitive histological diagnosis and one of the following: resting PaO_2 < 65 mmHg, alveolar-arterial O_2 gradient ≥40 mmHg, measured shunt fraction >10–12%, severe dyspnea, and hypoxemia at rest or on exercise. It is critical not to perform WLL when a patient has active bacterial pneumonia, since this can result in generalized sepsis and shock [11].

Physical removal of the lipoproteinaceous material through repeated dilutions with saline solution is believed to be the mechanism from which WLL shows benefits; additional mechanisms including the bulk removal of anti-GM-CSF antibody, as well as other possible immunologic effects on the effector cells, such as the alveolar macrophage or the type II epithelial cell, are possible [23].

Although fairly well tolerated, WLL sometimes only provides temporary symptomatic benefit and has then to be repeated several times. The lavage requires prolonged general anesthesia, is complex to perform, and is associated with potential morbidity. All these considerations make repeated WLL a less-than-desirable treatment. Hence, the search for alternative modalities of therapy is still crucial.

GM-CSF

Discovery of the alveolar macrophage involvement and anti-GM-CSF neutralizing antibodies led to multiple trials examining the usefulness of GM-CSF therapy. Preliminary data suggest that about 48% of patients treated with subcutaneous GM-CSF experienced improvement in pulmonary symptoms and function; however, the number of respondents appears to be less than with whole lung lavage. Given the experimental nature of GM-CSF therapy, the use of lung lavage is still the primary therapy for PAP.

Inhalation of nebulized GM-CSF has also been reported to improve lung function and facilitate clearance of the GM-CSF-antibody complexes from the lung. Additionally, a recent study using a two-pronged approach showed a decrease in GM-CSF requirements by performing WLL followed by nebulization of GM-CSF. It also appears that high amounts of exogenous GM-CSF can overcome the endogenous neutralizing antibodies, especially if GM-CSF is directly administered to the lung. This result would seem to be explained by the lipoproteinaceous material cleared by WLL, and consequently the inhaled GM-CSF could more readily reach the alveoli [11].

Although the positive effect of GM-CSF has been shown in idiopathic PAP, many important questions remain, including the optimal dose of GM-CSF, the optimal duration of treatment, the relation to the anti-GM-CSF titers, and the optimal route of GM-CSF administration.

Other Therapies

Rituximab (Rituxan®) is a monoclonal antibody directed against B lymphocytes. Since 1997, rituximab has been demonstrated to be effective in various autoantibody-mediated diseases like PAP [24]. Treatment with plasmapheresis to decrease the level of GM-CSF antibodies has yielded mixed results [25, 26]. Lung transplantation has been performed in patients whose health has deteriorated despite multimodal therapy, but recurrence in the allograft has been reported [27].

Whole-Lung Lavage Technique

In the author's quaternary center, the team is composed of trained and experienced staff consisting of two respiratory therapists, one nurse, two physiotherapists, and one anesthesiologist in charge of the anesthesia and of the lung lavage [7] (Table 45.1).

Monitoring

Whole lung lavage is realized under general anesthesia with basic monitoring, supplement respiratory monitoring, and sometimes invasive monitoring. In addition to the standard monitoring devices, an arterial cannulation is used for

Table 45.1 Whole lung lavage – proceeding

Stages	Whole lung lavage – proceeding
1	*Induction of anesthesia* Insertion of the left DLT with carinal hook
2	*Pre-lavage evaluation* (FiO$_2$ 1) Conventional ventilation for 5 min → arterial blood gas (ABG) Left OLV for 5 min → ABG Right OLV for 5 min → ABG
3	*First lung lavage* Lung lavage on the lung with the worst PaO$_2$ on OLV Multiple lavage/drainage cycles Fifth cycle done in lateral decubitus position * Contamination risk on the dependent lung Following fifth cycle: manual ventilation halfway through drainage phase End of cycles when the drainage fluid returns clear Aspiration with soft suction and FOB
4	*Recovery/lung rest* Protective 2 lung ventilation TV 6–8 mL/ kg, PEEP 7–12 cmH$_2$O, FiO$_2$ < 0.6 if well tolerated Fluid balance and diuretics if needed Cover the patient with heating blanket Length: 30–45 min
5	*Preparation for second lung lavage* (FiO$_2$ 1) OLV on the fresh lavaged lung for 5 min → ABG If PaO$_2$ > 70 mmHg If PaO$_2$ < 70 mmHg Proceed with the 2nd lung Consider adjuvants (iNO, PAC) Report proceeding with the 2nd lung
6	*Second lung lavage* Idem as the first lavage
7	*Landing phase* Replace the DLT by a single-lumen tube Aspiration with soft suction and FOB
8	*Emerging phase* Protective ventilation (2–4 h) in a monitored unit Post-anesthesia care unit Intensive care unit ABG and chest X-ray Awakening and extubation
9	*Observation phase* 24 h in a monitored unit ABG and chest X-ray evaluation *Noninvasive positive-pressure ventilation as needed*

beat-to-beat measurement of blood pressure and for blood gases analysis. Some authors also suggest the use of pulmonary artery catheter, continuous monitoring of mixed venous oxygen saturation [28, 29], and transesophageal echocardiography (TEE) [30, 31]. The pulmonary artery catheter may be used more as a therapeutic aid than a monitoring device by diverging blood flow away from the lavaged lung. TEE is sometimes useful to evaluate the cardiac function, mainly the right ventricle, in the presence of pulmonary hypertension.

The ventilator monitor found on most new anesthesia machines provides essential information during the

WLL. The observation of the airway pressure/volume loop (spirometry) on a breath-to-breath basis is useful to detect any loss of lung isolation and to prevent flooding of the ventilate lung [7, 32].

General Anesthesia

Only light premedication with anxiolytic drugs is used. Efficient preoxygenation is mandatory. General anesthesia is induced and maintained with intravenous agents, such as narcotics, benzodiazepine, intravenous anesthetic, and muscle relaxants. Inhaled anesthetic is rarely used. Minimal intravenous hydration is administrated since many liters of fluids originating from the alveolar space will be reabsorbed into the vascular space. Usually, the procedure for unilateral lavage lasts between 3–4 h and 5–6 h for a bilateral lavage. The use of a warming blanket over the legs helps to minimize heat loss as the thorax is completely denuded for the procedure.

Lung Separation

Lung separation is obtained by using a disposable left double-lumen tube (DLT). For the purpose of WLL, a left DLT with a carinal hook is used. The carinal hook offers a better stability of the tube given the numerous manipulations that occur during lung lavage. Adequate positioning of the DLT is achieved by the use of FOB, and air tightness is confirmed by a well-closed pressure-volume loop. Gas exchanges are obtained from both lungs simultaneously and then from each lung separately before and after the procedure to measure the effects of the WLL objectively.

Lung Lavage

The patient is kept in the supine position. To improve the effectiveness of the lavage, ventilation with FiO$_2$ 1.0 is initiated for a few minutes to denitrogenate both lungs. Pre-lavage evaluation confirms which lung is the most impaired, mainly through imaging evaluations and blood gas exchange during bilateral sequential one-lung ventilation (OLV). The most impaired lung is the first to be lavaged.

OLV is instituted in the non-lavaged lung, and confirmation of perfect lung isolation is obtained from the spirometry loop. A homemade disposable irrigation and drainage system (Fig. 45.1) is used to instill approximately 1 L of warm normal saline (37 °C). The irrigating liquid is suspended 30 cm above the patient's mid-chest level, and the instillation takes about 2–5 min.

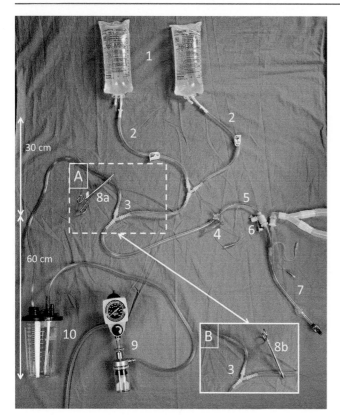

Fig. 45.1 Irrigation and drainage system. (1) Normal saline bag, (2) large bore tubular set for bladder irrigation, (3) Y-adaptor, (4) three-way for enteral feeding, (5) 5.0 mm single-lumen endotracheal tube, (6) swivel adaptor, (7) double-lumen endotracheal tube, (8a) clamp on the drainage side tubing during instillation phase, (8b) clamp on the instillation side tubing during drainage phase, (9) suction unit, (10) suction bottle. (Reproduced with permission of Libbey [52])

Approximately 2 min after the lung is completely filled with saline, it is rapidly drained over a 5–10 min period into a container positioned 60 cm below the patient's mid-chest level, with the assistance of a low suction pressure level (<20 cm H_2O). This process is repeated ten times or more, as necessary, to obtain a clear effluent lavage fluid.

Mechanical maneuvers are used to increase the efficacy of the WLL. These techniques consist of manual chest physiotherapy, mainly percussions, vibrations, and pressure applied during the filling and the drainage phase [33, 34]. A flannel cloth is used to protect the patient's skin from irritation provoked by repetitive manipulations. Positional modifications are very useful to irrigate and to drain all the different segments of the lung. The full lateral position is used at least once during the procedure, usually at the fifth cycle. When the lavaged lung is up, extreme care must be taken to avoid the risk of leakage from this nondependent lavaged lung into the dependent and ventilated one. After six or seven cycles of lavage and drainage, manual ventilation of the lavaged lung is frequently used halfway during the drainage phase to help the evacuation of the alveolar material

[35]. When the effluent lavage fluid is clear, the procedure is completed.

Bilateral WLL

For more than 15 years, bilateral WLL is done during the same anesthetic period and is performed with good results. Before bilateral WLL was performed in the same anesthetic episode, it was initially performed on the sickest lung; then at least a week later, the WLL of the contralateral lung was completed. At that time, oxygenation was usually not a problem because the treated and now near-normal lung was used to support gas exchange during the second procedure. We realized, with the experience of the bilateral WLL, that the lung recuperates rapidly enough to allow the contralateral WLL in less than an hour after the initial one.

When the effluent lavage fluid is clear on the first lavaged lung, careful aspiration is done, blindly with a suction catheter and also under direct vision with the use of a FOB. In order to safely proceed with WLL on the contralateral lung, a recuperation period has to be respected for the recently lavaged lung. Both lungs are ventilated with normal tidal volume (8–10 mL /kg) with addition of PEEP at a level varying from 7 to 12 cmH_2O for a period of 30–45 min. Furosemide can be administered (10 mg) to induce diuresis during this period, and patient's body is entirely covered with a warming blanket to keep its temperature close to normal.

Following determination of the ability of the recently lavaged lung to support the OLV necessary for the lavage of the contralateral lung, another WLL is done as previously described. Our goal is to obtain a PaO_2 greater than 70 mmHg with a FiO_2 1.0, with or without PEEP prior to begin WLL. When a satisfactory oxygenation cannot be achieved, inhaled nitric oxide is used at 20 ppm, and/or a pulmonary artery catheter is inserted under fluoroscopy in order to diverge blood flow from the lavaged lung to the ventilated lung [36]. When the adequacy of oxygenation is demonstrated, the WLL on the second lung is performed similarly to the first one.

Associated Bronchoalveolar Lavage (BAL)

In some specific cases, when the distribution of the alveolar infiltration is not homogeneous and is more localized into some specific lobes, the author adds to the standard WLL a series of BAL, well directed to the main involved lobes. BAL is performed after the WLL, following the exchange from DLT to a large, over 8 mm, single-lumen endotracheal tube. A regular FOB is used to obtain a bigger suctioning channel. BAL is performed at the segmental level. A maximum of 150 mL aliquots of normal saline is injected, followed by a drainage period assisted by the same system as the one used during regular WLL. BALs are repeated as needed, that is, until the return of clear liquid from the treated lobe. Every involved lobe is lavaged with the same technique.

Complications

The main complication is a decrease in arterial oxygen saturation, mainly during the drainage phase. Some liquid spillage from the lavaged lung to the non-lavaged lung may also occur. Other complications such as pneumothorax and hydrothorax are rare but may need to be drained, resulting in a postponed procedure. Post-procedure complications are pneumonia, sepsis, and, rarely, acute respiratory distress syndrome.

Desaturation

Increase in the blood flow in the non-ventilated lung occurs during the drainage phase (Fig. 45.2). This causes a decrease in arterial oxygen saturation. The use of PEEP on the ventilated lung helps to improve oxygenation during the filling phase but may worsen the PaO_2 during the drainage phase [37]. At that time, if needed (low $SatO_2$, i.e., <80% and/or for a prolonged period), a temporary partial unilateral pulmonary artery balloon occlusion with a pulmonary artery catheter, positioned under fluoroscopy in the artery of the lavaged lung, may be used. The occlusion diverts blood flow from the lavaged lung to the ventilated lung to improve oxygenation [36]. The use of nitric oxide with or without almitrine infusion has been described [38]. Others have performed the whole lung lavage under hyperbaric conditions [39]. Sometimes the patient presents severe impairment in gas exchange not allowing OLV. At that time, the use of vevovenous or venoarterial extracorporeal membrane oxygen-

ation (ECMO) or cardiopulmonary bypass (CPB) is useful to avoid severe hypoxemia during OLV [40]. The use of an extracorporeal membrane oxygenator has been also described to perform bilateral simultaneous whole lung lavage [41–43]. The use of a hyperoxygenated solution has been investigated. Its use improved oxygen supply in comparison to normal saline, as lavage solution, without obvious side effects [44].

Leakage

Spirometry must be used continuously to monitor and diagnose any liquid spillage from the lavaged lung. The mechanism of liquid spillage differs depending on which side the lavaged lung is lying (Fig. 45.3). When the whole lung lavage is performed in the right lung with a left-sided DLT in place, overpressure comes from the trachea over the bronchial balloon. When leaking occurs, there is flooding of the left ventilated lung. When it is happening during lavage of the left lung, leaking is caused by an overpressure in the left lung over the bronchial balloon or from a proximal displacement of the DLT. It creates leakage from the left lung to the trachea and finally to the right ventilated lung.

If there is a modification of the aspect of the spirometry loops, it is important to suspect flooding of the ventilated lung. At that time, it is essential to stop the irrigation or to increase the drainage, depending on timing. Confirmation by FOB and treatment by vigorous suctioning and inflation of the involved lung should be performed. It is essential to assess the non-lavaged lung function before continuing the lavage to ensure that the flooded lung can provide adequate oxygenation during subsequent one-lung ventilation. In the context of unilateral WLL, when flooding of the non-lavaged lung occurs, it frequently requires prolongation of ventilation during the post-procedure period to allow recovery. The best treatment for this complication is prevention, which can be done with a secure fixation of the double-lumen tube, the use of a double-lumen tube with a carinal hook, and by being

Fig. 45.2 Desaturation. (**a**) During the filling phase (circle), there is reduction of blood flow to the non-ventilated lung, by compression of the pulmonary blood vessels (arrow). (**b**) During the drainage phase (circle), there is reperfusion of the non-ventilated lung (arrow), creating a shunt and leading to desaturation. (Reproduced with permission of *Anesthesiology Clinics of North America* [7] (September 2001))

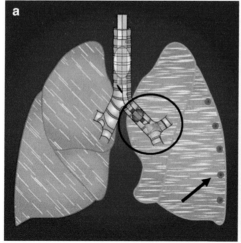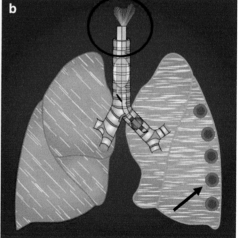

Fig. 45.3 Leakage from the lavaged lung to the non-lavaged lung. (**a**) During right lung lavage, overpressure in the trachea provokes flooding in the left ventilated lung. (**b**) During left lung lavage, overpressure in the left lung or displacement of the DLT provokes flooding of the right ventilated lung. (Reproduced with permission of *Anesthesiology Clinics of North America* [7] (September 2001))

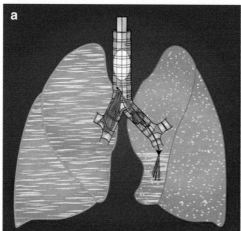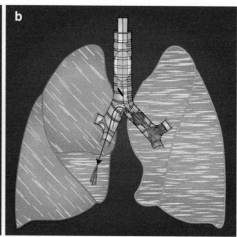

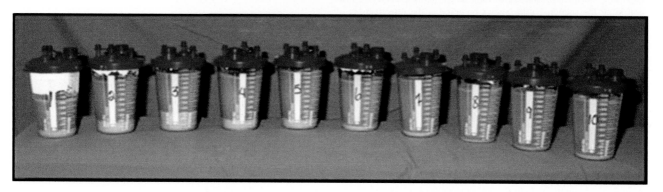

Fig. 45.4 Fluids collected from whole lung lavage. Fluids collected from WLL in pulmonary alveolar proteinosis seem milky. When fluid lavages are allowed to stand for a few hours, thick sediment appears in the bottom of the collecting bottle. It is more abundant in the first bottles going to near zero in the last ones. (Reproduced with permission of *Anesthesiology Clinics of North America* [7] (September 2001))

careful not to dislodge the double-lumen tube during patient and head manipulations.

Ending

The end point that is clinically used to cease a lung lavage is when the effluent lavage fluid is clear. Usually, between 10 and 15 L of saline are instilled into each lung (up to 50 L), and more than 90% of this volume is recovered, leaving a recuperation deficit of less than 10%. At the end of the procedure, the lavaged lung is thoroughly suctioned, and the volume of the residual liquid aspirated is calculated in a strict "in and out" balance of lavage liquid.

The effluent liquid of the whole lung lavage looks different depending on the pathology being treated. The sediment may seem milky following WLL for PAP (Fig. 45.4), while it may appear sandy if lung lavage is performed for silicosis. Over the past few years, the author has evaluated the amount of sediment recuperated during WLL for each lung separately (Fig. 45.5). The sediment amount is determined after fluid lavages are allowed to stand for at least

2–3 h. Then, the fluid spontaneously separates into a translucent supernatant and a thick sediment. The total height of sedimentary deposition in all the suction bottles allows quantifying the effectiveness of WLL in each lung individually. The accumulation may vary from 50 to 150 mm for each lung, meaning up to 300 mm following bilateral WLL.

After reintubation with a single-lumen endotracheal tube, a fiberoptic bronchoscopy control inspection is performed to look for the occurrence of undetected leakage throughout the procedure. During the FOB inspection, the author regularly observes local irritation of the distal tracheal mucosa, secondary to the movement of the double-lumen tube during WLL. The use of a double-lumen tube with a carinal hook has noticeably decreased the incidence of this irritation.

Conventional ventilation with PEEP is continued, usually for less than 2–4 h, to restore lung function, until the patient awakens in the recovery room. Alveolar infiltrates seen on the chest X-ray immediately after WLL normally clear within 24–36 h (Fig. 45.6). Observation in the ICU for 24 h is part of routine procedure.

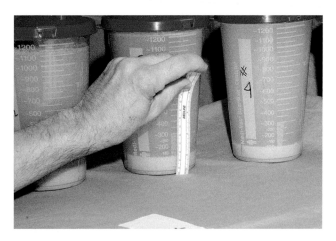

Fig. 45.5 Sediment measurment. Total height of sedimentary deposition in all the suction bottles allows quantifying the effectiveness of whole lung lavage in each lung individually

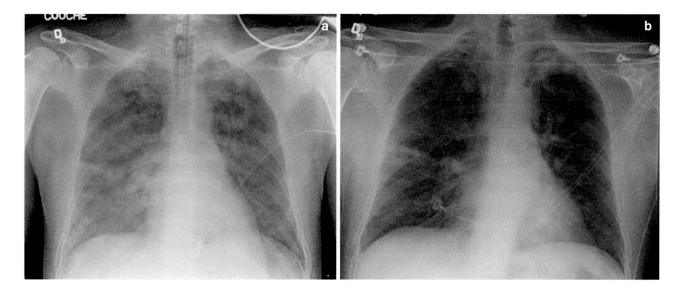

Fig. 45.6 Radiological imaging. (**a**) Immediately after left whole lung lavage, note the important alveolar edema resulting from the procedure. (**b**) The day after the right-side whole lung lavage, note the important amelioration of the two lungs. (Reproduced with permission of Springer)

Post Whole-Lung Lavage Evolution

The impact of WLL on the natural history of idiopathic PAP is difficult to ascertain, given the absence of randomized prospective trials or large, long-standing registries. However, practitioners of this procedure widely believe that patients with PAP improve symptomatically due to better gas exchanges. After whole lung lavage, patients usually have marked subjective improvement that correlates with increases in PaO_2 (at rest and exercise), vital capacity, diffusing capacity, and clearing of the chest roentgenogram (Fig. 45.6) or CT-scan (Fig. 45.7). Some patients require lavage every few months, whereas others remain in remis-

sion for several years. The disease may eventually show late recurrence. In PAP, WLL is proven to be successful because the lavage removes enormous accumulations of alveolar lipoproteinaceous material but also probably because it interrupts the pathogenic loop, decreasing the level of anti GM-GSF at the alveolar site, and temporarily restores the activity and function of the macrophages. It should be noted that congenital PAP appears to be particularly unlikely to respond to WLL [18].

An excellent retrospective review of all published articles, describing over 400 individual cases of PAP, was published in 2002 by Seymour and Presneill [18]. They reported that 41 patients with pre-lavage and post-lavage paired gas exchange results have seen their PaO_2 improved by

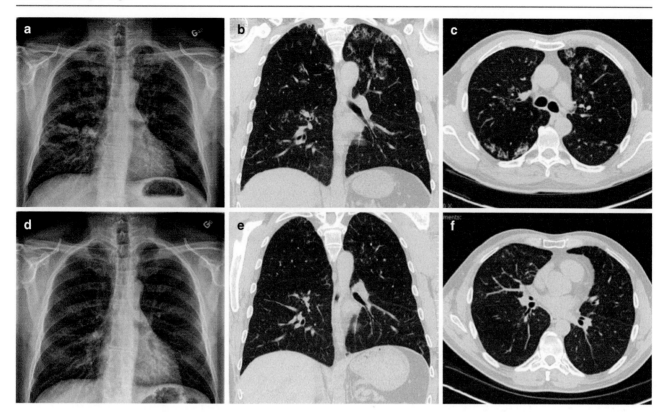

Fig. 45.7 Radiological imaging before (**a**–**c**) and following (**d**–**f**) whole lung lavage and GM-CSF by inhalation. (**a**) Anteroposterior view demonstrating the heterogeneous radiological infiltrations. They are mainly localized in the left superior lobe and the supero-dorsal segment of the bilateral inferior lobes. (**b**) High-definition computed tomography scan, coronal plane, showing the same involvement. (**c**) High-definition computed tomography scan, axial plane, showing crazy paving imaging in the left upper lobe. (**d**) Anteroposterior view demonstrating the disappearance of radiological infiltrations. (**e**) High-definition computed tomography scan, coronal plane, showing the same improvement. (**f**) High-definition computed tomography scan, axial plane, showing that the alveolar material has cleared out compared to **c**. (Reproduced with permission of Springer [53])

20 mmHg following WLL. The improvements in other pulmonary function parameters or diffusing capacity were less impressive. Their results also indicate that the median total number of lavages performed was two and that the median symptom-free period after one session of WLL was 15 months.

With regard to survival, in their analysis of the literature, Seymour and Presneill indicated that the overall survival at 5 years from the time of diagnosis is higher for patients who underwent therapeutic lung lavage during the course of their disease (94% vs. 85%, for those not lavaged). This was based on a series of 146 patients who were lavaged and 85 patients who were not [18].

Pediatric Whole Lung Lavage

Whole lung lavage has been used in the pediatric and neonatal population with some success. Whole lung lavage is technically difficult in infants and small children because of the incapacity to ventilate part of the lung or one lung safely and adequately during lavage of other areas or the other lung.

Small double-lumen tube (Bronchopart ®, size 26, 28, and 32, Willy Rusch AG, 71394 Kernen, Germany or Broncho-Cath ® size 28 and 32, Mallinckrodt Medical, Athlone, Ireland) is now available for use in children aged over 8–10 years old or weighing over 30 kg. Small FOB are also available to verify and adjust the final position of the DLT. When the airway of a child accepts a DLT, the WLL technique is similar to the one performed in adults.

If the airway is too small to insert a DLT, WLL is technically more challenging. Different methods to isolate both lungs have been described [45, 46]. The use of two alongside cuffed tubes (one tracheal 3.0 mm and one bronchial 3.5 mm) in a 11 kg child for unilateral WLL has been described [47]. Airway isolation has been obtained even for an infant as small as 2 kg [48]. When the perfect isolation of both lungs is obtained, WLL is performed similarly as when a DLT is placed but with much more attention to the stability of the airway devices.

When the techniques described above cannot be applied, mainly in patients weighing less than 10 kg, ECMO can be used to oxygenate the patient while bilateral simultaneous WLL is performed. Different approaches for the vascular cannulation have been described [49, 50]. Finally, one case report described the use of partial liquid ventilation with per-flubron (LiquidVent ®; Alliance Pharmaceuticals Corp. and Hoechst Marion Roussel) for 4 days following WLL done under ECMO in a 3.4 kg infant aged 6 weeks [51].

Conclusion

After more than 50 years of evolution, whole lung lavage is an efficient and safe technique. This procedure can be adapted to a large variety of patients and diseases. When WLL does not lead to a substantial effect, there are now new modalities that can be combined to WLL.

Clinical Case Discussion

A 47-year-old woman was referred to our team for WLL 10 years ago (2008). At that time, she presented some symptoms, mainly increasing dyspnea, for 6 months. An open lung biopsy had been performed at her hospital to establish the diagnosis of PAP. Pulmonary function tests performed in our center showed a light restrictive syndrome, a DLCO at 58%, and a PaO_2 of 68 mmHg. Radiological investigation revealed a homogeneous distribution with the involvement of bilateral superior lobes, middle lobe, and bilateral supero-dorsal segment of the inferior lobe. BAL confirmed the diagnosis of PAP.

A first bilateral WLL was performed, and moderately effective results were obtained. During the next 2.5-year period, the patient underwent six bilateral WLL, at intervals varying between 4 and 12 months, without good improvement in the clinical status, laboratory results, and radiological imaging. During the last WLL, BAL was performed as the radiological infiltrations were localized mainly in the left superior lobe and the supero-dorsal segment of the bilateral inferior lobes.

Nine months later, the patient complained about the same symptoms without marked improvement following any of the performed WLL. The dosage of GM-CSF was measured, and the dosage result, 203 µg/mL (N < 3 µg/ml), confirmed the diagnosis of primary PAP. In the following months, the patient received GM-CSF, but this treatment was ended because no improvement occurred and many secondary effects were observed. A few months later, the patient was placed on rituximab (Rituxan®), but the treatment was also ended after a few cycles since there was clinical and radiological deterioration.

Given this situation, we performed a new WLL, associated with specific BAL. The sediment recuperation was increased following the BAL. In the following days after the recovery from the WLL, we began GM-CSF by inhalation, once daily. At 1- and 3-month follow-up, the patient presented a significant improvement of her clinical status, for the first time since the first WLL. The radiologic images were completely cleared with this associated therapy, but the laboratory investigation remained stable.

We followed her to evaluate the long-term effect of this therapy. Up to 4 years after the last WLL, she received GM-CSF by inhalation following the yearly CT scan imaging, since the images reported small infiltrations. The last follow-up was done 8 years following the last WLL, and she was still asymptomatic. The annual CT scan was clean, as for the last four ones, and she did not take any GM-CSF inhalation.

This case report promotes the usefulness of a multimodal therapy that should be carried out to efficiently treat patients suffering from PAP.

References

1. Vincente G. Le lavage des poumons. Presse Med. 28:1266–8.
2. Ramirez-Riviera J. The strange beginnings of diagnostic and therapeutic bronchoalveolar lavage. PRHS. 1992;11(1):27.
3. Ramirez-Riviera J, Kieffer RF, Ball WC Jr. Bronchopulmonary lavage in man. Ann Intern Med. 1965;63(5):819–28.
4. Ramirez J. Bronchopulmonary lavage. New techniques and observations. Dis Chest. 1966;50(6):581–8.
5. Ramirez-Riviera J, Schultz RB, Dutton RE. Pulmonary alveolar proteinosis: a new technique and rationale for treatment. Arch Intern Med. 1963;112:419–31.
6. Spragg RG, Benumof JL, Alfery DD. New methods for the performance of unilateral lung lavage. Anesthesiology. 1982;57(6):535–8.
7. Bussieres JS. Whole lung lavage. Anesthesiol Clin North Am. 2001;19(3):543–58.
8. Wilt JL, Banks DE, Weissman DN, Parker JE, Vallyathan V, Castranova V, et al. Reduction of lung dust burden in pneumoconiosis by whole-lung lavage. J Occup Environ Med. 1996;38(6):619–24.
9. Venkateshiah SB, Yan TD, Bonfield TL, Thomassen MJ, Meziane M, Czich C, et al. An open-label trial of granulocyte macrophage colony stimulating factor therapy for moderate symptomatic pulmonary alveolar proteinosis. Chest. 2006;130(1):227–37.
10. Trapnell BC, Whitsett JA, Nakata K. Pulmonary alveolar proteinosis. N Engl J Med. 2003;349(26):2527–39.
11. Huizar I, Kavuru MS. Alveolar proteinosis syndrome: pathogenesis, diagnosis, and management. Curr Opin Pulm Med. 2009;15(5):491–8.
12. Lee K, Levin D, Webb W, Chen D, Storto M, Golden J. Pulmonary alveolar proteinosis: high-resolution CT, chest radiographic, and functional correlations. Chest. 1997;111:989–95.
13. Arcasoy SM, Lanken PN. Images in clinical medicine. Pulmonary alveolar proteinosis. N Engl J Med. 2002;347(26):2133.
14. Wong CA, Wilsher ML. Treatment of exogenous lipoid pneumonia by whole lung lavage. Aust NZ J Med. 1994;24(6):734–5.
15. Martin RJ, Rogers RM, Myers NM. PUlmonary alveolar proteinosis: shunt fraction and lactic acid dehydrogenase concentration as aids to diagnosis. Am Rev Respir Dis. 1978;117(6):1059–62.

16. Costello JF, Moriarty DC, Branthwaite MA, Turner-Warwick M, Corrin B. Diagnosis and management of alveolar proteinosis: the role of electron microscopy. Thorax. 1975;30(2):121–32.

17. Gilmore LB, Talley FA, Hook GE. Classification and morphometric quantitation of insoluble materials from the lungs of patients with alveolar proteinosis. Am J Pathol. 1988;133(2):252–64.

18. Seymour JF, Presneill JJ. Pulmonary alveolar proteinosis: progress in the first 44 years. Am J Respir Crit Care Med. 2002;166(2):215–35.

19. Goldstein LS, Kavuru MS, Curtis-McCarthy P, Christie HA, Farver C, Stoller JK. Pulmonary alveolar proteinosis: clinical features and outcomes. Chest. 1998;114(5):1357–62.

20. Rubinstein I, Mullen JB, Hoffstein V. Morphologic diagnosis of idiopathic pulmonary alveolar lipoproteinosis-revisited. Arch Intern Med. 1988;148(4):813–6.

21. Bonfield TL, Kavuru MS, Thomassen MJ. Anti-GM-CSF titer predicts response to GM-CSF therapy in pulmonary alveolar proteinosis. Clin Immunol. 2002;105(3):342–50.

22. Lin FC, Chang GD, Chern MS, Chen YC, Chang SC. Clinical significance of anti-GM-CSF antibodies in idiopathic pulmonary alveolar proteinosis. Thorax. 2006;61(6):528–34.

23. Kavuru MS, Popovich M. Therapeutic whole lung lavage: a stop-gap therapy for alveolar proteinosis. Chest. 2002;122(4):1123–4.

24. Borie R, Debray MP, Laine C, Aubier M, Crestani B. Rituximab therapy in autoimmune pulmonary alveolar proteinosis. Eur Respir J. 2009;33(6):1503–6.

25. Luisetti M, Rodi G, Perotti C, Campo I, Mariani F, Pozzi E, et al. Plasmapheresis for treatment of pulmonary alveolar proteinosis. Eur Respir J. 2009;33(5):1220–2.

26. Garber B, Albores J, Wang T, Neville TH. A plasmapheresis protocol for refractory pulmonary alveolar proteinosis. Lung. 2015;193(2):209–11.

27. Parker LA, Novotny D. Recurrent alveolar proteinosis following double lung transplantation. Chest. 1997;111:1457.

28. Loubser PG. Validity of pulmonary artery catheter-derived hemodynamic information during bronchopulmonary lavage. J Cardiothorac Vasc Anesth. 1997;11(7):885–8.

29. Cohen E, Eisenkraft JB. Bronchopulmonary lavage: effects on oxygenation and hemodynamics. J Cardiothorac Anesth. 1990;4(5):609–15.

30. McMahon CC, Irvine T, Conacher ID. Transoesophageal echocardiography in the management of whole lung lavage. Br J Anaesth. 1998;81(2):262–4.

31. Swenson JD, Astle KL, Bailey PL. Reduction in left ventricular filling during bronchopulmonary lavage demonstrated by transesophageal echocardiography. Anesth Analg. 1995;81(3):634–7.

32. Bardoczky GI, Engelman E, d'Hollander A. Continuous spirometry: an aid to monitoring ventilation during operation. Br J Anaesth. 1993;71(5):747–51.

33. Hammon WE, McCaffree DR, Cucchiara AJ. A comparison of manual to mechanical chest percussion for clearance of alveolar material in patients with pulmonary alveolar proteinosis (phospholipidosis). Chest. 1993;103(5):1409–12.

34. Bracci L. Role of physical therapy in management of pulmonary alveolar proteinosis. A case report. Phys Ther. 1988;68(5):686–9.

35. Bingisser R, Kaplan V, Zollinger A, Russi EW. Whole-lung lavage in alveolar proteinosis by a modified lavage technique. Chest. 1998;113(6):1718–9.

36. Nadeau MJ, Cote D, Bussieres JS. The combination of inhaled nitric oxide and pulmonary artery balloon inflation improves oxygenation during whole-lung lavage. Anesth Analg. 2004;99(3):676–9. table of contents.

37. Julien T, Caudine M, Barlet H, Wintrebert P, Aubas P, du Cailar J. Effect of positive end expiratory pressure on arterial oxygenation during bronchoalveolar lavage for proteinosis. Annales francaises d'anesthesie et de reanimation. 1986;5(2):173–6.

38. Moutafis M, Dalibon N, Colchen A, Fischler M. Improving oxygenation during bronchopulmonary lavage using nitric oxide inhalation and almitrine infusion. Anesth Analg. 1999;89(2):302–4.

39. Biervliet J, Peper J, Roos C, et al. Whole-lung lavage under hyperbaric conditions. In: Erdmann W, editor. Oxygen transport to tissue XIV. New York: Plenum Press; 1992.

40. Vymazal T, Krecmerova M. Respiratory strategies and airway management in patients with pulmonary alveolar proteinosis: a review. Biomed Res Int. 2015;2015:639543.

41. Cohen ES, Elpern E, Silver MR. Pulmonary alveolar proteinosis causing severe hypoxemic respiratory failure treated with sequential whole-lung lavage utilizing venovenous extracorporeal membrane oxygenation: a case report and review. Chest. 2001;120(3):1024–6.

42. Chauhan S, Sharma KP, Bisoi AK, Pangeni R, Madan K, Chauhan YS. Management of pulmonary alveolar proteinosis with whole lung lavage using extracorporeal membrane oxygenation support in a postrenal transplant patient with graft failure. Ann Card Anaesth. 2016;19(2):379–82.

43. Hasan N, Bagga S, Monteagudo J, Hirose H, Cavarocchi NC, Hehn BT, et al. Extracorporeal membrane oxygenation to support whole-lung lavage in pulmonary alveolar proteinosis: salvage of the drowned lungs. J Bronchology Interv Pulmonol. 2013;20(1):41–4.

44. Zhou B, Zhou HY, Xu PH, Wang HM, Lin XM, Wang XD. Hyperoxygenated solution for improved oxygen supply in patients undergoing lung lavage for pulmonary alveolar proteinosis. Chin Med J. 2009;122(15):1780–3.

45. Ciravegna B, Sacco O, Moroni C, Silvestri M, Pallecchi A, Loy A, et al. Mineral oil lipoid pneumonia in a child with anoxic encephalopathy: treatment by whole lung lavage. Pediatr Pulmonol. 1997;23(3):233–7.

46. McKenzie B, Wood RE, Bailey A. Airway management for unilateral lung lavage in children. Anesthesiology. 1989;70(3):550–3.

47. Paquet C, Karsli C. Technique of lung isolation for whole lung lavage in a child with pulmonary alveolar proteinosis. Anesthesiology. 2009;110(1):190–2.

48. Moazam F, Schmidt JH, Chesrown SE, Graves SA, Sauder RA, Drummond J, et al. Total lung lavage for pulmonary alveolar proteinosis in an infant without the use of cardiopulmonary bypass. J Pediatr Surg. 1985;20(4):398–401.

49. Hiratzka LF, Swan DM, Rose EF, Ahrens RC. Bilateral simultaneous lung lavage utilizing membrane oxygenator for pulmonary alveolar proteinosis in an 8-month-old infant. Ann Thorac Surg. 1983;35(3):313–7.

50. Lippmann M, Mok MS, Wasserman K. Anaesthetic management for children with alveolar proteinosis using extracorporeal circulation. Report of two cases. Br J Anaesth. 1977;49(2):173–7.

51. Tsai WC, Lewis D, Nasr SZ, Hirschl RB. Liquid ventilation in an infant with pulmonary alveolar proteinosis. Pediatr Pulmonol. 1998;26(4):283–6.

52. Libbey J. Anesthésie-Réanimation en Chirurgie Thoracique. In: Bussières JS, Léone M. Anesthésie-Réanimation en Chirurgie Thoracique. Paris: Arnette-Collection verte, John Libbey; 2017

53. Slinger PD. Principles and practice of anesthesia for thoracic surgery. 1st ed. New York/London: Springer; 2011.

Lung Volume Reduction

Erin A. Sullivan

Key Points
- Lung volume reduction surgery (LVRS) is a viable option for a select group of emphysema patients.
- Effective preoperative pulmonary rehabilitation and careful patient selection criteria promote favorable outcomes.
- Effective perioperative pain management and early extubation are significant factors that minimize postoperative complications and lead to better outcome.
- LVRS improves dyspnea and exercise tolerance and increases potential for patient survival in appropriately selected patients.

Introduction

Approximately 13.5 million persons in the United States are afflicted with COPD, and 3.1 million of these patients have emphysema [1]. Airflow obstruction associated with chronic bronchitis or emphysema occurs due to a loss of the elastic recoil properties of the lung and chest wall and the collapse of small airways, creating a permanent state of hyperinflation. The anterior–posterior diameter of the chest wall is markedly expanded, and the diaphragm is flattened leading to progressive dyspnea and a gradual increase in the work of breathing. As the disease progresses, patients become increasingly debilitated, require supplemental oxygen, and display poor exercise tolerance. Lung volume reduction surgery (LVRS) offers a select group of patients the possibility of improved exercise tolerance, reduction in dyspnea, improved quality of life, and an extended life span. It has

been suggested that LVRS may provide these patients with a benefit that otherwise cannot be achieved by any means other than lung transplantation.

More recently, less invasive bronchoscopic procedures have been used to achieve the same goals as LVRS. Bronchial blockers, bronchial valves, and biologic glue have been used in an attempt to provide lung reduction with an acceptable risk profile in patients with advanced heterogenous emphysema. This technique could provide palliation to patients who are currently not considered for LVRS.

History of Lung Volume Reduction Surgery (LVRS)

In 1957, Otto Brantigan, M.D., described a surgical technique for patients with end-stage emphysema that was designed to alleviate symptoms of severe dyspnea and exercise intolerance [2]. It was Brantigan's intent to remove functionally useless areas of the lung in order to restore pulmonary elastic recoil, thus increasing the outward traction on small airways and subsequently improve airflow. Brantigan believed that this technique could restore diaphragmatic and thoracic contours that would improve respiratory excursion. Additionally, he reasoned that by excising the nonfunctional lung tissue, the compressive effects exerted on normal lung tissue could be relieved and result in improved V/Q matching. Unfortunately, the operative mortality was significant, and no objective measures of benefit could be documented. Thus, early LVRS was abandoned as a viable therapy for patients with end-stage emphysema until 1993.

In 1996, Joel Cooper, M.D., authored an editorial advocating the technique of LVRS as a "logical, physiologically sound procedure of demonstrable benefit for a selected group of patients with no alternative therapy" [3]. He further stated that the successful application of LVRS was "made possible through an improved understanding of pulmonary physiology, improved anesthetic and surgical techniques, and lessons

E. A. Sullivan (✉)
Department of Anesthesiology, UPMC Presbyterian Hospital,
University of Pittsburgh Medical Center, Pittsburgh, PA, USA
e-mail: sullivanea@upmc.edu

© Springer Nature Switzerland AG 2019
P. Slinger (ed.), *Principles and Practice of Anesthesia for Thoracic Surgery*, https://doi.org/10.1007/978-3-030-00859-8_46

learned from experience with lung transplantation." Although Dr. Cooper touted the benefits of LVRS for certain patients, he did not minimize the surgical risk and suggested that this was not a procedure to be performed in all healthcare centers across the country. He made the following proposal: (1) healthcare providers should restrict the application of this (LVRS) procedure to a limited number of centers of excellence; (2) such centers should be required to document and report specified information regarding morbidity, mortality, and objective measures of outcome; and (3) these data should be periodically reviewed and evaluated by a scientific panel before approval to continue performing the procedure is approved. Additionally, he advocated that the patients who would otherwise qualify for lung transplantation should be simultaneously evaluated for LVRS so that they would receive the procedure proving to be most appropriate. LVRS was considered to be a palliative procedure to reduce dyspnea, improve exercise tolerance and the quality of daily life. Most of Dr. Cooper's patients achieved these goals as well as an improvement in airflow, a reduction of lung hyperinflation, and an improved alveolar gas exchange.

Shortly after Dr. Cooper's report regarding the success of LVRS was published, there was a widespread application of the technique. Analysis of the outcome data for Medicare patients revealed a 23% mortality rate at 12 months following LVRS prompting the discontinuation of funding for this procedure in 1996 due to the associated high risks and costs [4]. Subsequently, the National Heart, Blood, and Lung Institute designed a prospective, randomized clinical trial, the National Emphysema Treatment Trial (NETT), that evaluated the efficacy and safety of LVRS plus medical therapy vs. medical therapy alone [5].

Clinical Features of Emphysema

Emphysema is usually the end result of cigarette smoking, but can also be caused by alpha-1-antitrypsin deficiency [6, 7]. It is a chronic progressive disorder that ultimately leads to disability and early death. The cardinal physiologic defect in emphysema is a decrease in elastic recoil of the lung tissue that results in the principal physiologic abnormalities of decreased maximum expiratory airflow, leading to air trapping and hyperinflation and severely limited exercise capacity [7, 8].

Areas of severely emphysematous lung constitute dead space and result in compression of the adjacent lung tissue rendering it less capable of exerting the better-preserved elastic recoil on its adjoining airways. This leads to an increase in airway resistance and a reduction of expiratory airflow due to decreases in the driving and transmural pressures that maintain the patency of intraparenchymal airways.

The distribution of emphysema in the lung parenchyma adversely affects alveolar gas exchange compounded by an increase in ventilatory drive, premature initiation of inspiration, hyperinflation, and positive alveolar pressure at end expiration (auto-PEEP). As the disease progresses, inspiration becomes more difficult as a more negative inspiratory pressure is required to counteract auto-PEEP. Hyperinflation of the lungs leads to remodeling of the chest wall via progressive flattening of the diaphragm and alterations in the anterior–posterior diameter of the rib cage. These changes contribute directly to the increased work of breathing associated with emphysema [9].

Preoperative Medical Management of Emphysema Patients

The American Thoracic Society established guidelines for the diagnosis and management of emphysema [10]. Patients who are evaluated and considered for LVRS may remain symptomatic despite optimal medical management. Prior to LVRS, a structured pulmonary rehabilitation program is instituted with the goals of halting the progressive decline in lung function, preventing exacerbations of the disease, improving exercise capacity and quality of life, and prolonging survival. This is achieved through exercise training, optimization of medical therapy, patient education, psychosocial evaluation, and nutritional counseling and management.

The only treatment that has been shown to alter the rate of progression of COPD is cessation of smoking [11]. The majority of programs will require cessation of smoking for at least 6 months prior to considering the patient as a surgical candidate for LVRS.

Patients with severe emphysema are usually severely dyspneic even during minimal physical activity, and as a result, they become sedentary leading to progressive exercise deconditioning. For this reason, exercise training is an essential component for the preoperative preparation of the patient undergoing LVRS. The optimal training program is supervised by a specialized nurse and physician and lasts for at least 6 weeks prior surgery. Training consists of walking for a distance on a flat surface, bicycle ergometer training, and weight lifting. These exercises are combined with a special diet. There are several advantages of an exercise program prior to surgery: (a) the patient's willingness to cooperate can be assessed; (b) endurance and exercise tolerance is increased, which will be helpful for early mobilization after surgery [12]; and (c) maximal oxygen consumption can be increased in many subjects [13].

Influenza immunization and pneumococcal vaccination are recommended for the prevention of life-threatening infection [10]. Exacerbations of bronchospasm and infection are treated with steroids and antibiotics, respectively [14, 15].

Furthermore, beta-adrenergic agonists such as theophylline and anticholinergics are recommended for treatment of COPD and asthma [10]. Although these interventions are believed to shorten the duration of individual episodes and to minimize symptoms, there is little evidence that they either alter the natural history of the disease or reduce mortality. Bronchodilators improve lung function, exercise capacity, and quality of life in patients with COPD but are of limited benefit to patients without reversible airway disease [10].

Long-term home oxygen therapy in chronically hypoxemic patients is the only treatment for COPD that has been documented to decrease mortality rates [16, 17]. Adjunctive forms of therapy, such as the use of mucolytics to control respiratory secretions or narcotics to reduce the sensation of dyspnea, have been used in selected COPD patients [10]. In end-stage COPD patients, single or double-lung transplantation has been used as a last resort, but this option is limited by financial resources and the number of donor organs.

Patients presenting for LVRS are frequently very anxious secondary to the dyspnea and asthmatic crises they experienced in the past. Psychological factors can induce an asthma attack that is a dangerous complication during the perioperative period. Anxiety is associated with an increase in respiratory frequency leading to an increase in dynamic pulmonary hyperinflation and dyspnea [18]. Therefore, it is important that the anesthesiologist is able to establish a good relationship with the patient before surgery. The optimal psychological preconditions are likely to be achieved when the preoperative preparation, preoperative visit, insertion of a thoracic epidural catheter, administration of general anesthesia, and early postoperative therapy are conducted by the same physician or a team well known to the patient. Anxiolytic therapy may be necessary during the preoperative and perioperative period.

Evaluation of Patients for LVRS and Selection Criteria

General Evaluation

General criteria for patient selection and recommendations for screening procedures are described by Weinmann and Hyatt [19]. These selection criteria may vary between institutions. Distinct selection criteria for LVRS candidates were published by Daniel et al. [20] and are shown in Table 46.1.

Whether patients with significant hypercapnia should undergo LVRS is controversial [19, 21]. Furthermore, some institutions report significant coronary artery disease (coronary artery stenosis >70%) diagnosed in 15% of their asymptomatic LVRS candidates, and thus, they recommend left and right heart cardiac catheterization preoperatively [22]. This invasive cardiac screening seems justified by several case

Table 46.1 General inclusion criteria for LVRS

Diagnosis of COPD
Patient history, physical examination, lung function test, chest X-ray, etc.
Smoking cessation for greater than 1 month
Age < 75 years
FEV_1 between 15% and 35% of predicted
P_aCO_2 < 55 mmHg
Prednisone requirement <20 mg/day
PAP_{sys} < 50 mmHg
No previous thoracotomy or pleurodesis
Absence of symptomatic coronary artery disease
Absence of chronic asthma or bronchitis
Commitment to pre-op and post-op supervised pulmonary rehabilitation for 6 weeks

Reprinted from Daniel et al. [20] with permission from Wolters Kluwer Health
COPD chronic obstructive pulmonary disease, *FEV₁* forced expiratory volume in 1 s, *PaCO₂* arterial carbon dioxide pressure in mmHg, *PAPsys* systolic pulmonary arterial pressure in mmHg

reports of myocardial infarction during and after LVRS. Other institutions recommend limiting cardiac screening to transthoracic echocardiography [19]. In general, it is reasonable for centers with less experience to employ strict criteria for patient selection to minimize patient morbidity and mortality.

Anatomic/Radiologic Evaluation

The chest X-ray should provide evidence of hyperinflated lungs, large intercostal spaces, retrosternal airspace, flattened diaphragm, and high transparency of the lungs (see Fig. 46.1a). For a precise morphologic evaluation, a high-resolution computer tomography (HRCT) of the chest is essential for identification of nonhomogeneous areas within the lungs. HRCT locates the target areas for resection. An ideal anatomical precondition for LVRS is marked inhomogeneity of the lung structure, where normal lung tissue and severely destroyed, overdistended tissue are present in the same lung (see Fig. 46.2a). Homogeneous distribution of the disease proved to be an unfavorable precondition (see Fig. 46.2b).

Several authors have demonstrated that patients presenting with severe inhomogeneity are very likely to benefit from LVRS [23–25]. Two reasons might account for this: (1) compressed, normal lung tissue is released after removing adjoining hyperinflated, nonfunctional, destroyed tissue, and thus, the pulmonary mechanics of the remaining tissue are improved; and (2) surgery is easier to perform if the target areas are clearly visible. In many centers, lung perfusion scintography is still routinely performed for screening LVRS candidates primarily to rule out ventilation–perfusion mismatch. However, chest computed tomography has been

Fig. 46.3 (**a**) Depicts the Zephyr® EBV (registered trademark of PulmonX, Inc.). (**b**) Depicts the IBV (Spiration Inc.). Both devices have been used to provide bronchoscopic LVRS for patients with heterogenous forms of emphysema. (**c**) Depicts the Chartis system (PulmonX) that is used to detect collateral flow and determine the suitability of patients for the Zephyr® EBV. A hollow balloon-tipped catheter is used to obstruct a lobar or segmental bronchus. Collateral flow to the obstructed region can be detected by measuring continued expired gas flow distal to the balloon. (Reprinted with permission from © 2010 PulmonX, Inc. all rights reserved)

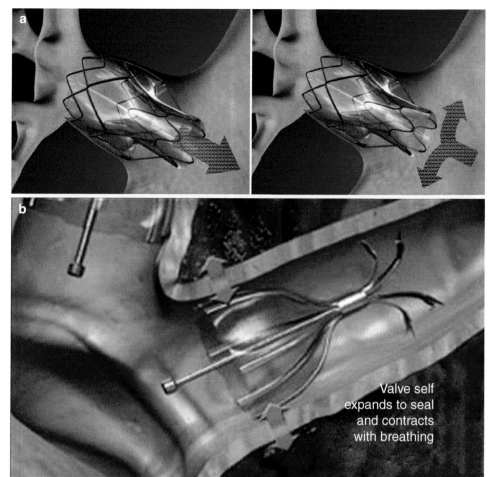

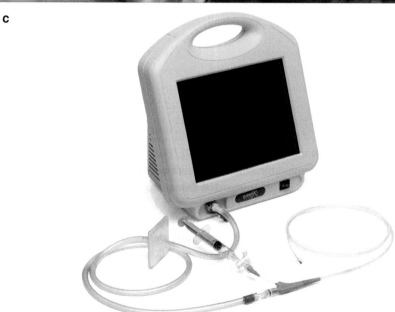

will respond well to Zephyr® valve therapy. Chartis collateral flow screening must be performed under moderate sedation with the patient breathing normally in order to obtain an accurate assessment.

Another alternative to combat less optimal results in bronchoscopic lung volume reduction for heterogenous emphysema was developed by Ingenito et al. He and his colleagues developed a transbronchoscopic technique to create and maintain

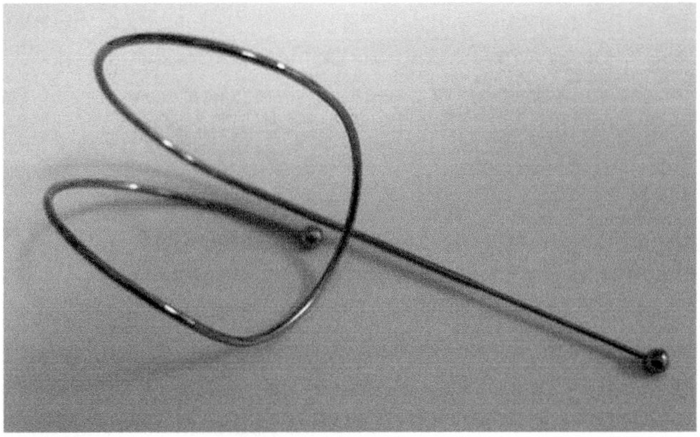

Fig. 46.4 The RePneu™ lung volume reduction device (PneumRx, Mountain View, CA) is designed to reduce lung volume for both heterogenous and homologous forms of emphysema. It is effective even when collateral ventilation due to compromises in the fissures between lung lobes exists. The preformed coil is delivered into a segmental or subsegmental bronchus in a straight configuration via a fiber-optic bronchoscope. After deployment, the device resumes its coil shape gathering and compressing emphysematous lung tissue

volume loss using a washout solution and fibrin-based glue to collapse, seal, and scar target regions of abnormal lung. Initial results show that in short-term follow-up there was improved mean vital capacity, reduced mean residual volume, reduced mean residual volume/total lung capacity ratio, longer mean 6-min walk distance, and improved mean dyspnea score [41].

There is a device designed to reduce lung volume for patients with heterogenous or homologous emphysema, and it is effective even when there are compromises in the fissures between lung lobes. The RePneu™ LVRC (see Fig. 46.4) is constructed of Nitinol that is preformed in a coil shape and that can be deployed into a target lobe via a bronchoscope and using either moderate sedation or general anesthesia. Multiple implants are used to obtain optimal results. This device is completely removable, and preclinical studies have indicated that lung volume reduction of up to 50% has been achieved in human lungs.

At present there does not seem to be a consensus on interventional therapy for severe emphysema. There has not been an appropriate randomized study. Individual centers tend to favor either lung volume reduction surgery or bronchoscopic procedures. Centers that favor interventional bronchoscopy tend to favor mainly valves or coils [42].

Anesthetic Management

Preoperative Assessment

Pharmacologic Preparation
Most of the patients presenting for LVRS require long-term bronchodilator therapy (beta adrenergic agonists), steroid therapy (inhalation or systemic), and mucolytic therapy. Additionally, these patients frequently require antibiotics. Most centers recommend continuation of bronchodilator and mucolytic therapy before LVRS, including the day of surgery. The patient must be free from respiratory infections for at least 3 weeks prior to LVRS and require no antibiotic therapy preoperatively. In terms of steroid therapy, the goal is to gradually reduce the dose of systemic steroids prior to LVRS.

Many patients have received chronic theophylline therapy before LVRS, and some patients experience toxic symptoms while theophylline blood levels are in the therapeutic range [43]. The main side effects are nervousness, tremor, and tachycardia. Theophylline therapy should be discontinued before LVRS if the patient shows significant side effects or if the serum levels are >20 ng/mL.

Pain Management

Thoracic Epidural Analgesia
By now it is a generally accepted concept that thoracic epidural analgesia (TEA) is mandatory for optimal postoperative pain management following LVRS. A thoracic epidural catheter is inserted at the T3–T4 or T4–T5 vertebral level in the awake patient immediately prior to surgery. The spread of anesthesia and analgesia should be assessed carefully before induction of general anesthesia in order to avoid inadequate pain management that may cause ventilatory depression during the immediate postoperative period. A local anesthetic such as bupivacaine or ropivacaine can be used for TEA preferably in combination with an opioid. Since emphysema patients tend to be volume depleted, it is important that they are adequately volume loaded (1–2 mL/kg) before fully activating the TEA so as to avoid severe hypotension. A potent vasopressor such as norepinephrine or phenylephrine should be available before activating the TEA. Ropivacaine is frequently preferred over bupivacaine as the local anesthetic since it causes less circulatory depression and helps to reduce the incidence of hypotension.

Most anesthesiologists providing care to patients for LVRS are convinced that TEA is crucial to reduce perioperative patient morbidity and mortality. Unfortunately, there are no controlled studies available to validate this theory. Some anesthesiologists might consider such a study unethical since patients would potentially be denied optimal pain management. In patients with normal lung function undergoing lung resection, there is evidence that sufficient postoperative analgesia with TEA can reduce morbidity and mortality [44]; however, other authors emphasize that the influence of TEA on outcome after lung resection has not been proven [45]. Nevertheless, the use of TEA is the worldwide established means for intraoperative and postoperative analgesia for patients undergoing LVRS. In order to guarantee optimal analgesia, TEA should be maintained until all chest drains are removed.

Paravertebral Nerve Block

Paravertebral nerve blocks are multiple-level intercostal nerve blocks that have replaced the direct and multiple applications of local anesthetics to intercostal nerves, cryotherapy, and interpleural local anesthetics [46]. Paravertebral nerve blocks may be performed either by multiple injections or by inserting a catheter into the paravertebral space for use with a continuous infusion of local anesthetic [47, 48]. The levels of analgesia and restoration of pulmonary function seen with TEA can also be achieved with paravertebral nerve block when a multimodal analgesic regimen including the use of intravenous opioids and nonsteroidal anti-inflammatory agents (NSAIDS) are added. Outcome studies of the effect of paravertebral nerve blocks on morbidity and mortality rates following thoracic surgery, in particular LVRS, have yet to be determined. It is widely accepted that the use of multimodal analgesia in conjunction with paravertebral nerve block is an excellent alternative to TEA. Paravertebral catheters may be inserted either percutaneously or under direct vision during thoracotomy. This technique is particularly useful for patients in whom placement of TEA is difficult or contraindicated.

Intraoperative Management

Monitors

Monitors for LVRS should include a six-lead ECG, pulse oximetry, invasive blood pressure monitoring, a temperature probe for continuous core temperature measurement, and a central venous catheter to assess central venous pressure. The routine use of a pulmonary artery catheter is controversial; however, continuous monitoring of pulmonary artery pressure (PAP) may be helpful since PAP can increase substantially during single-lung ventilation, thus causing acute right ventricular failure. Transesophageal echocardiography may also be useful for intraoperative cardiac monitoring.

General Anesthesia

During endotracheal intubation with a double-lumen tube, the intravenous analgesic requirement can be substantially reduced if the pharynx and larynx are carefully anesthetized with a topical anesthetic spray (e.g., 2% lidocaine) [49]. Following intubation, analgesia should be maintained with TEA. It is important to mention that intubation of a poorly anesthetized emphysema patient can precipitate life-threatening bronchospasm [50].

Only short-acting drugs should be used for sedation and neuromuscular blockade during general anesthesia for LVRS in order to facilitate tracheal extubation as early as possible after the procedure in order to avoid prolonged air leakage associated with prolonged positive pressure ventilation. Propofol is therefore a suitable choice for sedation. If the patient is susceptible to bronchospasm, a volatile inhalation anesthetic such as sevoflurane or isoflurane may be preferred over an intravenous agent. Neuromuscular blocking agents with short duration and absence of histamine liberation (e.g., vecuronium or cisatracurium) are frequently chosen.

Sufficient patient warming can be achieved using warming blankets, heating mats, and warm intravenous fluid infusions. Core body temperature and the peripheral temperature of the patient should be maintained within the normal range. A decrease in the body heat content of the patient will ultimately lead to shivering after extubation along with increased carbon dioxide production and oxygen consumption. It is frequently impossible for the end-stage emphysema patient to meet the increased ventilatory demands caused by shivering. Shivering is an undesirable complication that may lead to reintubation in the postoperative period.

Mechanical Ventilation

Optimal mechanical ventilation for LVRS must provide sufficient arterial oxygenation while strictly avoiding air trapping [18], which can potentiate the threat of pneumothorax. Air trapping can be minimized by using moderate tidal volumes (≤ 9 mL/kg during ventilation of both lungs and ≤ 5 mL/kg during single-lung ventilation), low respiratory frequencies (≤ 12 breaths/min during ventilation of both lungs and ≤ 16 breaths/min during single-lung ventilation), and a prolonged expiratory time (I/E = 1:3 during double- and single-lung ventilation). If the preoperative HRCT exhibits a substantial difference in the quality of lung tissue between the right and left lung, it may be more desirable to resect the less functional lung first.

It is important to limit airway pressure generated (≤ 35 cmH$_2$O) by the ventilator in order to avoid barotraumas resulting in a pneumothorax or tension pneumothorax. The anesthesiologist should pay constant attention to the inspired and expired volumes during mechanical ventilation. For this purpose it is necessary to monitor the configuration of the end-tidal CO_2 waves closely. In most patients undergoing LVRS, the anesthesiologist will have to accept elevated values of end-tidal and P_aCO_2 (arterial carbon dioxide tension) during single-lung ventilation. This permissive hypercapnia is the price for the prevention of barotrauma during mechanical ventilation for LVRS. P_aCO_2 values will return to the normal range soon after the procedure when both lungs can be ventilated again.

Early Extubation

It is difficult to avoid air leakage entirely despite the use of new surgical techniques that use staplers buttressed with bovine pericardium. Air leakage can be exacerbated by positive pres-

Table 46.2 Extubation criteria after LVRS

1. Patient awake and cooperative
2. Patient breathing sufficiently, i.e., rapid shallow breathing index (respiratory frequency per min/tidal volume in L) is below 70
3. Sufficient arterial oxygenation: $S_aO_2 \geq 92$ while patient is breathing spontaneously ($F_iO_2 \leq 0.35$)
4. Adequate pain management achieved
5. Patient core temperature >35.5 °C
6. No shivering
7. Stable hemodynamic conditions

sure ventilation, whereas the negative intrapleural pressure generated during spontaneous breathing minimizes air leakage. Therefore, early extubation after LVRS is of prime importance. Several criteria must be satisfied before the patient can be extubated (Table 46.2). Should the patient fail to meet all of these criteria, it is reasonable to stabilize the patient in a quiet environment such as an intensive care unit or the postanesthesia care unit before extubation. Successful extubation will usually be possible within 1–2 h and is not harmful to the patient. This is preferable to premature extubation in the operating room followed by prolonged episodes of arterial hypoxemia.

Postoperative Management

More than 50% of patients who undergo LVRS experience a complication during the postoperative period. They include (1) oversedation, (2) accumulation of airway secretions, (3) pneumothorax, (4) bronchospasm, (5) pulmonary embolism, (6) pneumonia, (7) persistent air leaks, (8) arrhythmias, (9) myocardial infarction, and (10) pulmonary embolism. Reintubation and mechanical ventilation are associated with a high morbidity and mortality.

The majority of patients are extubated in the operating room and rarely require reintubation during the initial 48 h. However, significant hypercarbia and acidosis may be present for several hours owing to the residual effects of the anesthesia or incomplete analgesia. Unlike other patients undergoing pulmonary resection, the chest tubes in these patients are attached to water-seal drainage without suction. The loss of elastic recoil and the obstructive physiology of the remaining lung make it resistant to the usual loss of volume associated with a postoperative pneumothorax. The fragile nature of the lungs renders them more susceptible to the adverse effects of increased transpulmonary pressure and overdistention that would be caused by chest tube suction. This has a tendency to increase the magnitude and prolong the duration of air leaks in these patients. Postoperative management is directed to minimize these adverse side effects: (1) judicious pulmonary toilet, (2) bronchodilator therapy, (3) effective perioperative analgesia with TEA or paravertebral/multimodal analgesia, and (4) avoidance of systemic corticosteroids.

Summary

LVRS is a viable option for a select group of emphysema patients, and endobronchial valves and blockers that are undergoing clinical trials in the United States hold much promise as a treatment alternative for all emphysema patients. Regardless of the selection of treatment modality, the goals are the same: improvements in dyspnea, exercise tolerance, quality of life, and prolonged patient survival.

Patient selection is of crucial importance for a successful outcome after LVRS. The anesthesiologist must be actively involved in patient selection since he or she will be responsible for the patient's immediate perioperative management. Patient history and preoperative status as well as the results obtained from the evaluation of chest X-rays, HRCT scans, and catheterization of the right heart should be carefully weighed during the patient selection process. The careful selection and preoperative preparation of patients is essential to minimize perioperative complications and obtain a successful outcome. Furthermore, it has to be emphasized that the role of the anesthesiologist is of crucial importance for the successful conduct of LVRS.

Clinical Case Discussion

Case: A 58-year-old female patient with end-stage emphysema is scheduled for bilateral LVRS using a video-assisted thoracoscopic approach (VATS). She has a past medical history that is significant for smoking (60 pack years; quit for the past 2 years), hypertension, and atrial fibrillation that is controlled with metoprolol. Her other medication includes an 81-mg aspirin that she takes once per day. She successfully completed a preoperative exercise program 8 weeks ago. The patient is very anxious and wishes to speak with the anesthesiologist who will provide her care prior to the date of surgery.

Questions

- What additional preoperative preparation is necessary from a pulmonary standpoint?
- How will you treat the patient's anxiety?
- What will you recommend for perioperative pain management?
- What are your specific concerns regarding postoperative management?

Preoperative Pulmonary Preparation

- Successful completion of a preoperative exercise program including a 6-min walk on a flat surface, bicycle ergometer, and weight lifting (see section "Preoperative Medical Management of Emphysema Patients").

- Continue supplemental oxygen use, bronchodilators, and mucolytics up to and including the day of surgery (see section "Pharmacologic Preparation").
- Gradually reduce the dose of steroids prior to surgery if they are being administered.
- If the patient is receiving theophylline therapy and exhibiting symptoms of toxicity (nervousness, tremor, tachycardia) or if serum levels exceed 20 ng/mL, discontinue the drug.
- Ensure that the patient is free from infection and does not require antibiotics for at least a 3-week period prior to surgery.

Treatment of Anxiety

- Untreated anxiety may precipitate an episode of acute bronchospasm, an increase in dynamic pulmonary hyperinflation, and dyspnea (see section "Preoperative Medical Management of Emphysema Patients").
- An effective way to allay a patient's anxiety is for the anesthesiologist to establish a good relationship with the patient prior to the date of surgery by scheduling a meeting in the anesthesia preoperative evaluation clinic.
- Anxiolytic therapy may be necessary during the preoperative and perioperative period.

Perioperative Analgesia

- The patient is at high risk for perioperative pulmonary complications if analgesia is insufficient or ineffective.
- The risk of pulmonary complications may be improved with the use of thoracic epidural or paravertebral analgesia (see sections "Thoracic Epidural Analgesia" and "Paravertebral Nerve Block").
- TEA or paravertebral nerve block catheters should be maintained until the chest drains are removed and the patient is tolerating oral pain medications.

Postoperative Management (see sections "Early Extubation" and "Postoperative Management")

- Air leakage can be exacerbated by positive pressure ventilation. Therefore, the patient should be extubated as soon as it is safe to do so, preferably in the operating room. It is safe, however, to maintain mechanical ventilation for 1–2 h following surgery, and this is preferable to premature extubation and the subsequent development of arterial hypoxemia.
- Fifty percent of LVRS patients develop a postoperative complication.
- Reintubation and mechanical ventilation in the postoperative period are associated with a high morbidity and mortality.

- Postoperative complications can be minimized by implementing judicious pulmonary toilet, bronchodilator therapy, effective pain management with thoracic epidural or paravertebral analgesia, and avoidance of systemic corticosteroids.

References

1. Prevalence and incidence of chronic obstructive pulmonary disease. 2010. http://www.cureresearch.com/c/copd/prevalence.html. Accessed 24 Jan 2010.
2. Brantigan OC, Mueller E, Kress MB. A surgical approach to pulmonary emphysema. Am Rev Respir Dis. 1959;80(1 Pt. 2): 194–206.
3. Cooper JD, Lefrak SS. Is volume reduction surgery appropriate in the treatment of emphysema? Yes. Am J Respir Crit Care Med. 1996;153:1201–4.
4. McKenna RJ Jr, Benditt JO, DeCamp M, et al. Safety and efficacy of median sternotomy versus video-assisted thoracic surgery for lung volume reduction surgery. J Thorac Cardiovasc Surg. 2004;127:1350–60.
5. National Emphysema Treatment Trial Group. Rationale and design of the national emphysema treatment trial (NETT): a prospective randomized trial of lung volume reduction surgery. J Thorac Cardiovasc Surg. 1999;118:518–28.
6. Carrell RW, Jeppsson JO, Laurell CB, et al. Structure and variation of the human alpha-1-antitrypsin. Nature. 1982;298:329–34.
7. Janus ED, Phillips NT, Carrell RW. Smoking, lung function and alpha-1-antitrypsin deficiency. Lancet. 1985;1:152–4.
8. Potter WA, Olafsson S, Hyatt RE. Ventilatory mechanics and expiratory flow limitation during exercise in patients with obstructive lung disease. J Clin Invest. 1971;50:910–9.
9. Stubbing DC, Pengelly LD, Morse JLC, et al. Pulmonary mechanics during exercise in subjects with chronic airflow obstruction. J Appl Physiol. 1980;49:511–5.
10. American Thoracic Society. Standards for the diagnosis and care of patients with chronic obstructive pulmonary disease (COPD) and asthma. Am Rev Respir Dis. 1987;136:225–44.
11. Buist AS, Sexton GJ, Nagy JM, Ross BB. The effect of smoking cessation and modification on lung function. Am Rev Respir Dis. 1976;114:115–22.
12. Cooper JD, Trulock EP, Triantafillou AN, et al. Bilateral pneumectomy volume reduction for chronic obstructive pulmonary disease. J Thorac Cardiovasc Surg. 1995;109:106–19.
13. Hughes RL, Davison R. Limitations of exercise reconditioning in COPD. Chest. 1983;83:241–9.
14. Sahn SA. Corticosteroid therapy in chronic obstructive pulmonary disease. Pract Cardiol. 1985;11(8):150–6.
15. Tager I, Speizer FE. Role of infection in chronic bronchitis. N Engl J Med. 1975;292:563–71.
16. Anthonisen NR. Long-term oxygen therapy. Ann Intern Med. 1983;99:519–27.
17. Nocturnal Oxygen Therapy Trail Group. Continuous or nocturnal oxygen therapy in hypoxemia chronic obstructive lung disease: a clinical trial. Ann Intern Med. 1980;91:391–8.
18. Tuxen DV, Lane S. The effects of ventilatory pattern on hyperinflation, airway pressures, and circulation in mechanical ventilation of patients with severe air-flow obstruction. Am Rev Respir Dis. 1987;136:872–9.
19. Weinmann GG, Hyatt R. Evaluation and research in lung volume reduction surgery. Am J Respir Crit Care Med. 1996;154:1913–8.

20. Daniel TM, Barry BK, Chan MD, et al. Lung volume reduction surgery: case selection, operative technique, and clinical results. Ann Surg. 1996;223(5):526–33.

21. Wisser W, Klepetko W, Senbaklavaci O, et al. Chronic hypercapnia should not exclude patients from lung volume reduction surgery. Eur J Cardiothorac Surg. 1998;14:107–12.

22. Thurnheer R, Muntwyler J, Stammberger U, et al. Coronary artery disease in patients undergoing lung volume reduction surgery for emphysema. Chest. 1997;112(1):122–8.

23. Hamacher J, Block KE, Stammberger U, et al. Two years' outcome of lung volume reduction surgery in different morphologic emphysema types. Ann Thorac Surg. 1999;68:1792–8.

24. Rogers RM, Coxson HO, Sciurba FC, et al. Preoperative severity of emphysema predictive of improvement after lung volume reduction surgery – use of CT morphometry. Chest. 2000;118:1240–7.

25. Salzman SH. Can CT measurement of emphysema severity aid patient selection for lung volume reduction surgery? Chest. 2000;118:1231–2.

26. Thurnheer R, Engel H, Weder W, et al. Role of lung perfusion scintigraphy in relation to chest computed tomography and pulmonary function in the evaluation of candidates for lung volume reduction surgery. Am J Respir Crit Care Med. 1999;159(1):301–10.

27. National Emphysema Treatment Trial Research Group. Patients at high risk of death after lung-volume-reduction surgery. N Engl J Med. 2001;345(15):1075–83.

28. Dueck R, Cooper S, Kapelanski D, Colt H, Clauser J. A pilot study of expiratory flow limitation and lung volume reduction surgery. Chest. 1999;116:1762–71.

29. Gelb AF, Zamel N, McKenna RJ, Brenner M. Mechanism of short-term improvement in lung function after emphysema resection. Am J Respir Crit Care Med. 1996;154:945–51.

30. Marchand E, Gayan-Ramirez G, De Leyn P, Decramer M. Physiological basis of improvement after lung volume reduction surgery for severe emphysema: where are we? Eur Respir J. 1999;13(3):686–96.

31. Sciurba FC, Rogers RM, Keenan RJ, Slivka WA, Gorcsan J, Ferson PF, Holbert JM, Brown ML, Landreneau RJ. Improvement in pulmonary function and elastic recoil after lung-reduction surgery for diffuse emphysema. N Engl J Med. 1996;334:1095–9.

32. Tschernko EM, Wisser W, Hofer S, et al. Influence of lung volume reduction on ventilatory mechanics in patients suffering from severe COPD. Anesth Analg. 1996;83:996–1001.

33. Ingenito EP, Evans RB, Loring SH, et al. Relation between preoperative inspiratory lung resistance and the outcome of lung-volume-reduction surgery for emphysema. N Engl J Med. 1998;338:1181–5.

34. Tschernko EM, Kritzinger M, Gruber EM, et al. Lung volume reduction surgery: preoperative functional predictors for postoperative outcome. Anesth Analg. 1999;88:28–33.

35. Tutic M, Lardinois D, Imfeld S, et al. Lung – volume reduction surgery as an alternative or bridging procedure to lung transplantation. Ann Thorac Surg. 2006;82:208–13.

36. The National Emphysema Treatment Trial Research Group. Effects of lung volume reduction surgery versus medical therapy: results from the National Emphysema Treatment Trial. N Engl J Med. 2003;324:2059–73.

37. Naunheim KS, Wood DE, Mohnsenifar Z, et al. Long-term follow-up of patients receiving lung-volume reduction surgery versus medical therapy for severe emphysema by the National Emphysema Treatment Trial Research Group. Ann Thorac Surg. 2006;82:431–3.

38. Toma TP, Hopkinson NS, Hillier J, et al. Bronchoscopic volume reduction with valve implants in patients with severe emphysema. Lancet. 2003;361:931–3.

39. Yim AP, Hwong TM, Lee TW, et al. Early results of endoscopic lung volume reduction for emphysema. J Thorac Cardiovasc Surg. 2004;127:1564–73.

40. Salanitri J, Kalff V, Kelly M, et al. 133Xenon ventilation scintigraphy applied to bronchoscopic lung volume reduction techniques for emphysema: relevance of interlobar collaterals. Int Med J. 2005;35:97–103.

41. Reilly J, Washko G, Pinto-Plata V, et al. Biological lung volume reduction: a new bronchoscopic therapy for advanced emphysema. Chest. 2007;131:1108–13.

42. Shah PL, van Geffen WH, Desiee G, Slebos D-J. Lung volume reduction for emphysema. Lancet Respir Med. 2017;5:147–56.

43. Weinberg M, Hendeles L. Methylxanthines. In: Weiss EB, Segal MS, Stein M, editors. Bronchial asthma. Mechanisms and therapeutics. 2nd ed. Boston: Little Brown and Company; 1985.

44. Ballantyne JC, Carr DB, deFerranti S, et al. The comparative effects of postoperative analgesic therapies on pulmonary outcome: cumulative meta-analyses of randomized, controlled trials. Anesth Analg. 1998;86(3):598–612.

45. Warner DO. Preventing postoperative pulmonary complications. Anesthesiology. 2000;92:1467–72.

46. Keenan DJM, Cave K, Langdon L, et al. Comparative trial of rectal indomethacin and cryoanalgesia for control of early postthoracotomy pain. Br Med J. 1983;287:1335.

47. Karmakar MJ. Thoracic paravertebral block. Anesthesiology. 2001;95:771–80.

48. Hill SE, Keller RA, Stafford-Smith M, et al. Efficacy of single-dose, multilevel paravertebral nerve blockade for analgesia after thoracoscopic procedures. Anesthesiology. 2006;104:1047–53.

49. Loehning RW, Waltemath CL, Bergman NA. Lidocaine and increased respiratory resistance produced by ultrasonic aerosols. Anesthesiology. 1976;44:306–10.

50. Brandus V, Joffe S, Benoit CV, et al. Bronchial spasm during general anesthesia. Can Anesth Soc J. 1970;17:269–74.

Lung Transplantation

47

Andrew Roscoe and Rebecca Y. Klinger

Key Points
- Preoperative assessment is paramount for planning intraoperative strategies.
- Careful induction of anesthesia is essential to avoid cardiovascular collapse.
- Transesophageal echocardiography is an invaluable intraoperative tool.
- Perioperative extracorporeal membrane oxygenation support is beneficial for patients but provides new challenges for the anesthesiologist.
- Reduction in early postoperative complications confers a long-term survival benefit.

Introduction

Lung transplantation (LT) is the treatment of choice for some patients with end-stage lung disease or pulmonary vascular disease [1]. The term "lung transplantation" encompasses a group of operations, comprised of lobar transplant, single-lung transplant (SLT), double-lung transplant, bilateral sequential lung transplant (BSLT), and heart-lung transplant (HLT). The first reported human LT was undertaken in 1963 [2], but outcomes were poor until the introduction of ciclosporin (also spelled cyclosporin) and the development of newer surgical techniques in the 1980s. The first reported successful LT was performed in 1983 at Toronto General Hospital [3]. The number of LT has increased significantly over the last 30 years (Fig. 47.1) and outcomes have gradually improved; median survival for LT is now approximately 6 years (Fig. 47.2) [1].

A. Roscoe (✉)
Department of Anesthesia, Papworth Hospital, Cambridge, UK
e-mail: andyroscoe@doctors.org.uk

R. Y. Klinger
Department of Anesthesiology, Duke University Medical Center, Durham, NC, USA

Donor Organ Management

The potential donor patient is often cared for in a nontransplant critical care unit [4]. After the diagnosis of brain stem death (BSD), the pathophysiological sequelae must be appropriately managed to effectuate organ preservation [5–9]. This includes intravenous fluid administration and vasoactive drug therapy to achieve a mean arterial pressure (MAP) above 70 mmHg, heart rate 60–120 beats per minutes, and a central venous pressure (CVP) or pulmonary artery wedge pressure (PAWP) between 6 and 10 mmHg [10, 11]. Intravenous fluid restriction and judicious use of diuretics help to reduce fluid accumulation in the lungs. The use of "hormonal" therapy, comprised of thyroxine, methylprednisolone, and vasopressin, has been shown to increase the number of transplantable organs. Ventilatory settings are altered to protect the potential donor lungs. This includes the use of pressure-controlled ventilation with appropriate positive end-expiratory pressure (PEEP) to give tidal volumes of 6–8 mL/kg. Bronchoscopic pulmonary toilet is used to clear retained secretions. Basic critical care therapies, including normothermia, antimicrobial use, nutrition, correction of electrolyte imbalance, and treatment of diabetes insipidus are essential [12–15].

During procurement, the donor receives systematic heparinization, and the pulmonary artery is flushed with a cold preservation solution. Prostaglandin is infused into the donor pulmonary circulation to inhibit the vasoconstrictive response to the cold pneumoplegia solution and to inhibit platelet aggregation. The donor lungs are ventilated throughout the flush and are inflated to a pressure of 10–20 cmH$_2$O prior to dividing the airways. The harvested allograft is then stored at 4 °C for transfer to the recipient center [16–18].

Less than 20% of donors of other solid organs have lungs that are suitable for transplantation. This may be related to the etiology of BSD or secondary to pulmonary aspiration of gastric contents at the time of brain injury [12, 19]. Due to the imbalance between the number of candidates awaiting transplantation and the availability of suitable donor organs, the

© Springer Nature Switzerland AG 2019
P. Slinger (ed.), *Principles and Practice of Anesthesia for Thoracic Surgery*, https://doi.org/10.1007/978-3-030-00859-8_47

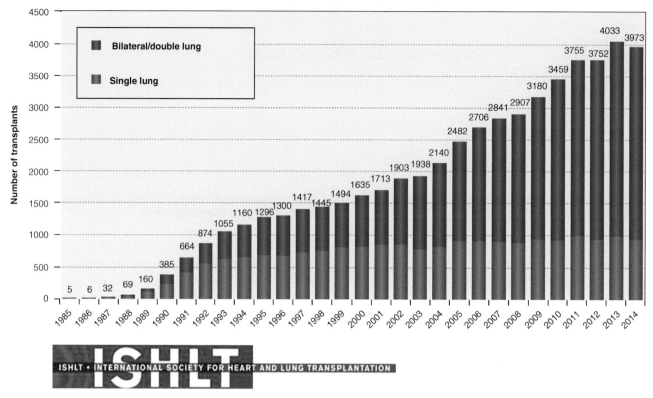

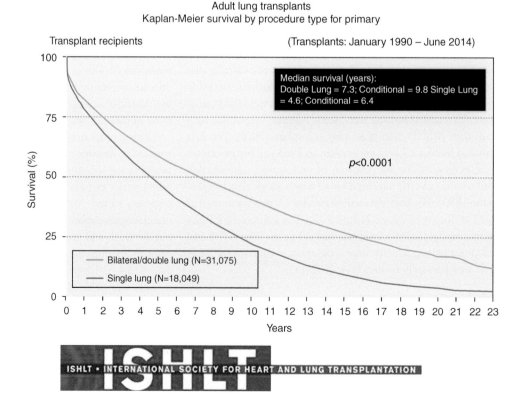

Fig. 47.1 Number of lung transplants reported by year. (From the International Society for Heart and Lung Transplantation, with permission)

Fig. 47.2 Survival for adult lung transplantation. The median survival is the estimated time point at which 50% of all of the recipients have died. The conditional median survival is the estimated time point at which 50% of the recipients who survive to at least 1 year have died. Because the decline in survival is greatest during the first year following transplantation, the conditional survival provides a more realistic expectation of survival time for recipients who survive the early post-transplant period. (From the International Society for Heart and Lung Transplantation, with permission)

Table 47.1 Donor lung criteria

	Standard donor	Marginal donor
ABO compatibility	Yes	Yes
Age (years)	<55	>55
pO$_2$/FiO$_2$ (mmHg)	>300	<300
Smoking history (pack years)	<20	>20
Chest X-ray	Clear	Pulmonary edema
Microbiology	Gram stain negative	Antimicrobial therapy
Bronchoscopy	Non-purulent	Purulent/inflamed
Chest trauma	Absence	Minor

FiO$_2$ fraction of inspired oxygen

"standard" criteria for donor lung acceptance have been extended to include "marginal" donors (Table 47.1). The survival of recipients from these "marginal" donors may be decreased to those from standard donors, and a higher incidence of primary graft dysfunction (PGD) has been reported [20–23]. Several strategies have been developed in an attempt to increase the donor organ pool. This includes the use of patients in Maastricht category III: donation after cardiac death (DCD). Donors are typically patients in a critical care environment, who are expected to die within 60–90 min of withdrawal of active treatment. Ethical considerations mandate the use of two separate teams: one for therapy withdrawal and the second for organ harvesting. Lung preservation interventions are withheld until cardiac death has been certified [10, 24–26]. The lungs are unique in their ability to tolerate a warm ischemia time of at least 1 h [27]. Outcomes of recipients from DCD are comparable to those from BSD donors [26, 28]. Ex vivo lung perfusion (EVLP) and reconditioning are techniques that allow assessment and optimization of potential donor lungs outside of the donor. After organ harvesting, the lungs are perfused on an external circuit and ventilated (Fig. 47.3). The lungs can then be optimized and assessed for adequate function prior to transplantation [29–31]. Patient outcomes are similar to those with conventional transplants [32, 33]. The role of EVLP is now being extended: assessment of lungs from uncontrolled circulatory death; standard donor organs can be evaluated ex vivo to allow for exclusion of functionally impaired lungs; and the extension of graft perfusion time may facilitate better timing of transplant operations [34–36].

Recipient Candidates

Transplantation is indicated for patients with end-stage lung disease who are failing medical therapy, with the goal to provide a survival benefit. Due to the relative shortage of donor organs, it is necessary to list only patients with realistic beneficial outcomes. Listing for transplantation should occur when life expectancy after transplant exceeds life expectancy without the procedure. Donors and recipients are matched

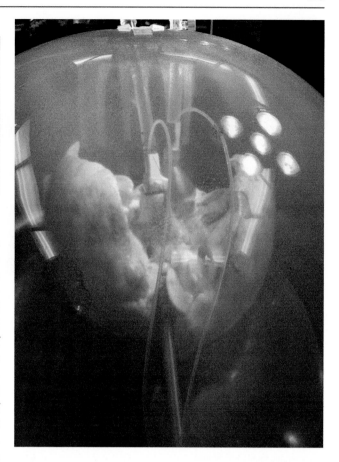

Fig. 47.3 Donor lungs inside a sterile plastic dome undergoing ex vivo perfusion. During ventilation via an endotracheal tube in the donor trachea, the lungs are perfused with a crystalloid solution. The yellow cannula is in the main pulmonary artery and the green cannula in the cuff of the donor left atrium

according to blood group and size [37–39]. The common underlying pathologies responsible for LT referral include chronic obstructive pulmonary disease (COPD), alpha-1 antitrypsin deficiency (AATD), cystic fibrosis (CF), pulmonary hypertension (PHT), and interstitial lung disease (ILD), incorporating usual interstitial pneumonitis (UIP), fibrosing non-specific interstitial pneumonitis (NSIP), and non-idiopathic interstitial pneumonitis (non-IIP) (Fig. 47.4). Contraindications to LT are listed in Table 47.2.

Disease-specific indications for referral and listing for transplantation are summarized in Table 47.3 [39]. Patients suffering from emphysematous diseases are assessed using the BODE index, which involves scoring body mass index, airflow obstruction, degree of dyspnea, and exercise capacity on a scale from 0 to 10. A BODE index ≥7 is associated with lower survival than would be expected after transplantation. Three or more severe exacerbations within 1 year are associated with increased mortality, and an episode of acute hypercapnic respiratory failure carries a 43% 1-year mortality [39, 40]. Lung volume reduction surgery may provide an alternative or a bridge-to-transplant in some emphysema patients [41, 42]. Cystic fibrosis patients are

Fig. 47.4 Indications for lung transplantation. AATD alpha-1 antitrypsin deficiency, CF cystic fibrosis, COPD chronic obstructive pulmonary disease, ILD interstitial lung disease, PHT pulmonary hypertension, Re-Tx re-transplantation. (Based on data form the International Society of Heart and Lung Transplantation <https://www.ishlt.org> accessed May 2017)

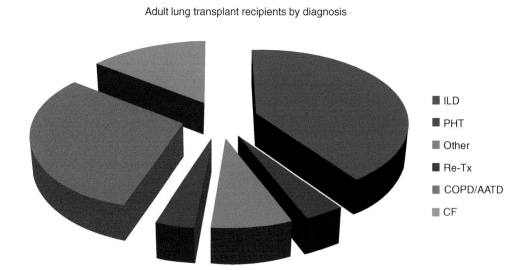

Adult lung transplant recipients by diagnosis

- ■ ILD
- ■ PHT
- ■ Other
- ■ Re-Tx
- ■ COPD/AATD
- ■ CF

Table 47.2 Contraindications to lung transplantation [39]

Absolute
Malignancy within 2 years/hematological malignancy within 5 years
Untreatable major organ dysfunction, not amenable to combined transplant
Significant coronary artery disease, not amenable to revascularization
Chronic infection with resistant organisms
Active *Mycobacterium tuberculosis* infection
Significant chest wall deformity
Body mass index >35 kg/m²
Psychiatric conditions associated with nonadherence to medical therapy
Substance abuse/dependence
Absence of adequate social support structure
Relative
Age > 65 years
Body mass index >30 kg/m²
Previous extensive thoracic surgery
Colonization with highly resistant organisms
Infection with HIV, Hepatitis, *Burkholderia cepacia*, or *Mycobacterium abscessus*
Severe malnutrition
Severe symptomatic osteoporosis

HIV Human immunodeficiency virus

Table 47.3 Disease-specific criteria for lung transplantation listing [39]

COPD/AATD	BODE index ≥7
	FEV_1 < 20% predicted
	Three severe exacerbations in 1 year
	Development of pulmonary hypertension
Cystic fibrosis	Chronic respiratory failure: pO_2 < 60 mmHg/pCO_2 > 50 mmHg
	FEV_1 < 30% with rapidly declining function
	WHO functional class IV
	Development of pulmonary hypertension
Interstitial lung disease	FVC < 80% predicted and decrease in FVC > 10% over 6 months
	D_{LCO} < 40% predicted and decrease D_{LCO} > 15% over 6 months
	6-MWT: distance <250 m or desaturation <88%
	Development of pulmonary hypertension
Pulmonary Hypertension	6-MWT: distance < 350 m
	Cardiac index < 2 L/min/m²
	Right atrial pressure > 15 mmHg
	WHO functional class III or IV

6-MWT 6-min walk test, *AATD* alpha-1 antitrypsin deficiency, *COPD* chronic obstructive pulmonary disease, D_{LCO} diffusing capacity for carbon monoxide, FEV_1 forced expiratory volume in 1 s, *FVC* forced vital capacity, *WHO* World Health Organization

prone to colonization with resistant pathogens. Infection with *Burkholderia cenocepacia* and non-tuberculous *Mycobacterium* is associated with increased morbidity and mortality and confers a contraindication in some centers [39, 43]. Patients with ILD have the worst prognosis of those referred for LT. The introduction of the lung allocation score (LAS) system, designed to prioritize patients with the highest mortality on the waiting list, has increased the number of ILD candidates receiving transplantation [44, 45]. Significant developments in targeted medical therapy for pulmonary hypertension had led to improvements in management and a postponement in referral for LT listing in this population [39]. Patients with PHT secondary to pulmonary veno-occlusive disease should be referred for LT assessment at the time of diagnosis, as there is no established medical therapy,

and the prognosis is poor [46]. The incidence of re-transplantation has increased since the introduction of the LAS system. The same criteria for initial LT listing are used. Whether SLT or BSLT is planned, removal of the failed allograft is recommended to reduce infection risk and ongoing stimulation of the immune system. Patients requiring re-transplant after 2 years of their original procedure have better outcomes than those who are re-transplanted within 30 days [39, 47–49]. Previously, patients in a critical condition, supported with mechanical ventilation or extracorporeal life support (ECLS) were deemed unsuitable candidates [50]. However, improvements in technology and expanded experience in the management of ECLS have allowed for such patients to be bridged to transplantation with ECLS, with acceptable outcomes [51–53].

Anesthesia for Lung Transplantation

Preoperative Assessment

Due to the nature of LT, the anesthesiologist usually has limited time for preoperative assessment [54]. In some centers the listed candidates are reviewed in an assessment clinic by an anesthesiologist to highlight pertinent anesthetic considerations. Patients are typically debilitated, with poor cardiorespiratory reserve. Latent ischemic heart disease and right ventricular (RV) dysfunction are not uncommon, especially in elderly patients, although the presence of noncritical coronary artery disease does not appear to influence postoperative outcomes [55–58]. After admission to hospital for surgery, there is limited time to optimize the patient: chest physiotherapy to clear secretions, bronchodilator therapy, and drainage of significant pleural effusions or pneumothoraces. In addition to a standard preoperative evaluation, anesthetic assessment should focus on [59]:

- Underlying diagnosis: obstructive, restrictive, or suppurative pathology. This facilitates selection of appropriate ventilator settings.
- Pulmonary artery (PA) pressure: this will dictate the likelihood of undertaking the procedure without the use of ECLS.
- Ventilation/perfusion (V/Q) scan: the differential perfusion to each lung (in BSLT) will determine which lung initially will better tolerate PA clamping and pneumonectomy.
- Arterial blood gases (ABGs): baseline pO_2/pCO_2 helps define acceptable intraoperative limits.
- Echocardiography: knowledge of RV and left ventricular (LV) function will influence the requirement for ECLS.

Standard premedication involves immunosuppressant drugs, bronchodilator therapy, and supplemental oxygen. The routine use of anxiolytic medication is not recommended, and any sedative agents should be administered with caution, as they can exacerbate hypoxemia and hypercapnia, leading to worsening PHT and RV failure.

Monitoring

Routine monitoring includes electrocardiography (ECG), pulse oximetry, invasive arterial and central venous pressure (CVP) measurements, pulmonary artery catheterization (PAC), temperature measurement, capnography, and inhalational agent monitoring. Minimally invasive cardiac output monitoring has been used extensively in the nontransplant perioperative setting and in nonpulmonary transplantation with mixed conclusions [60–63]. Mixed venous

oximetry has been used successfully intraoperatively, and cerebral oximetry has been shown to improve outcomes in cardiac surgery [64–67]. The use of depth of anesthesia monitoring may reduce the incidence of awareness, and when used in combination with a closed-loop anesthesia, delivery system provides better titration of drugs, giving the anesthesiologist more time to focus on intraoperative hemodynamic and surgical events [68, 69]. Early detection and prevention of intraoperative hypothermia is important to prevent cardiac dysrhythmias, coagulopathy, and altered drug metabolism and to reduce the risk of postoperative infection [70, 71].

Transesophageal Echocardiography

The value of intraoperative transesophageal echocardiography (TEE) in LT surgery is well established [72–75]. TEE is more accurate at determining preload and volemic status compared to PAC [76]. It facilitates rapid diagnosis of hemodynamic instability, including evaluation of RV function after PA clamping, LV dysfunction, detection of gaseous emboli, and assessment of surgical anastomotic sites [75, 77–79]. Significant stenosis of pulmonary vein anastomoses is more commonly seen on the left (Fig. 47.5) and can result in pulmonary venous congestion and graft failure. However, TEE can overestimate pulmonary vein Doppler peak velocities, and caution is required when interpreting findings [80, 81]. The presence of an interatrial septal defect or patent foramen ovale can lead to a significant right-to-left shunt during periods of increased pulmonary vascular resistance (PVR) or when increased PEEP is employed. Prompt detection by TEE can aid in diagnosing this cause of worsening hypoxemia

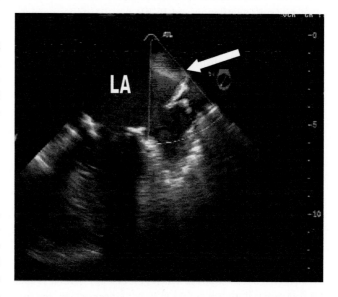

Fig. 47.5 Transesophageal echocardiography showing turbulence on color flow Doppler imaging (arrow) in a stenotic left pulmonary vein anastomosis. LA left atrium

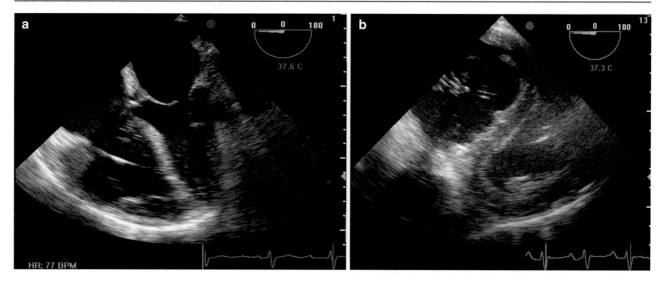

Fig. 47.6 Transesophageal echocardiography midesophageal (**a**) and transgastric (**b**) views showing right ventricular dilatation and flattening of the interventricular septum with leftward shift. LV left ventricle, RV right ventricle

[82]. With the expansion of intraoperative extracorporeal membrane oxygenation (ECMO) support in LT surgery, TEE is also beneficial in assisting in positioning of cannulae and differentiating between hypovolemia and cannula obstruction when low ECMO flows are encountered (Fig. 47.6) [83, 84].

Induction of Anesthesia

Thorough preoxygenation of the patient is prudent. Induction of anesthesia may precipitate cardiovascular collapse due to a combination of factors: systemic vasodilation and negative inotropic effects of anesthetic drugs, reduced venous return due to an increase in intrathoracic pressure secondary to positive pressure ventilation and PEEP, and RV failure caused by an increase in PVR due to hypoventilation and subsequent hypercapnia [85–87].

In patients with obstructive lung pathologies, it is important to allow sufficient time for the expiratory phase to occur and to avoid PEEP, in order to reduce the risk of dynamic hyperinflation. Overenthusiastic manual ventilation after induction of anesthesia can lead to severe gas trapping in emphysematous lungs, resulting in reduced venous return and direct cardiac compression: "pulmonary tamponade" [88, 89]. Profound hypotension ensues, and correct management is to disconnect the patient from the breathing circuit to allow sufficient time for expiration of trapped gases [90].

Patients with restrictive lung disease typically require higher ventilatory pressures to deliver an adequate tidal volume and often benefit from the application of increased levels of PEEP. Adoption of a ventilation strategy similar to that used in acute lung injury (ALI) is more appropriate for this group of patients [91, 92].

Recipients with suppurative pathologies may have mixed obstructive/restrictive respiratory defects, so appropriate ventilation should be individualized. Thorough bronchial lavage after intubation of the patient may reduce intraoperative sputum plugging and assist in maintaining adequate ventilation throughout the procedure.

In patients with pulmonary vascular disease, smooth induction of anesthesia is critical to prevent systemic hypotension, PA hypertensive crises, myocardial depression, hypoxemia, and hypercapnia. It may be useful to obtain central venous access before induction of anesthesia for administration of vasopressors. Anesthetic goals include [93]:

- Avoid acute increases in RV preload: RV dilatation increases RV wall tension, increasing oxygen demand; elevates RV end-diastolic pressure (RVEDP), reducing oxygen delivery; and worsens tricuspid regurgitation (TR), exacerbating volume overload.
- Maintain RV perfusion: avoid systemic hypotension and increases in RVEDP.
- Maintain sinus rhythm and positive chronotropy.
- Augment RV contractility with inotropic support when necessary.
- Decrease PVR: avoid hypoxemia, hypercapnia, and acidemia.

Ketamine may be a more appropriate induction agent in severe cases, with vasoactive infusions commenced prior to induction. The use of inhaled pulmonary vasodilators and preinduction ECLS has been described [94, 95]. The anesthesiologist should be prepared for emergency institution of cardiopulmonary bypass (CPB) after induction.

Table 47.4 Disease-specific intraoperative considerations

Pathology	Intraoperative complications
COPD/AATD	Elderly with concomitant coronary artery disease
	Dynamic hyperinflation, gas-trapping and auto-PEEP with positive pressure ventilation, causing "pulmonary tamponade"
Cystic fibrosis	Thick, tenacious secretions, plugging the DLT lumens
	Difficult to maintain normocapnia
	Difficult surgery: small chest cavity, multiple adhesions
Interstitial lung disease	High ventilatory pressures, reducing venous return
	Secondary pulmonary hypertension
	Associated pathologies: scleroderma, rheumatoid arthritis
Pulmonary hypertension	Cardiovascular collapse at induction of anesthesia
	Right ventricular failure

AATD alpha-1 antitrypsin deficiency, *COPD* chronic obstructive pulmonary disease, *DLT* double-lumen tube, *PEEP* positive end-expiratory pressure

Disease-specific intraoperative anesthetic considerations are summarized in Table 47.4.

Following induction, the airway is secured with either a single-lumen or double-lumen tube (DLT). A single-lumen tube in combination with an endobronchial blocker provides an alternative technique to DLT [96, 97]. In BSLT, the blocker will need repositioning under bronchoscopic guidance to allow surgery on the opposite side. A left-sided DLT is preferred to a right-sided DLT, which may interfere with the right-sided bronchial anastomosis. In patients with significant suppurative pathologies (e.g., cystic fibrosis), it is common to initially insert a single-lumen tube in order to facilitate bronchoscopic toilet and suctioning of thick secretions, prior to exchanging for a DLT. Bronchoscopic lavage samples can be sent for microbiological analysis to direct postoperative antimicrobial therapy. Prophylactic antibiotic regimens are institution-related but must provide adequate gram-positive and gram-negative cover. Patients with CF often require alternative antimicrobials, depending on their history of allergies, microbe colonization, and presence of drug-resistant organisms [98, 99].

Maintenance of Anesthesia

Maintenance of anesthesia is achieved with either inhalational or intravenous agents [100, 101]. Nitrous oxide should be avoided as it may increase PVR [102]. SLT can be performed through a standard posterolateral thoracotomy, with the patient in the lateral position, or via an anterior thoracotomy, in the supine position. This latter approach provides easier surgical cannulation access if urgent ECLS is needed. BSLT may be performed either via a midline sternotomy, bilateral thoracotomies, or "clamshell" incision [103].

Initiation of one-lung ventilation (OLV) will initially cause an increase in shunt with worsening hypoxemia until surgical stapling of the PA. During OLV pressure-controlled ventilation may proffer some benefits over volume-controlled ventilation, by reducing peak airway pressures [104, 105]. Patients unable to tolerate OLV will require CPB or ECMO support [106].

Optimal fluid management is paramount during the intraoperative period. Patient hemodynamics are influenced by volemic status and preload optimization is essential. However, the lung allograft is prone to low-pressure pulmonary edema, secondary to re-expansion injury, ischemia-reperfusion microvascular leak, and the absence of lymphatic drainage. A restrictive fluid regimen is recommended, with surgical blood loss replaced by boluses of colloid or blood products as indicated [107, 108].

Management of RV Dysfunction

Surgical clamping of the PA during OLV will reduce shunt and improve oxygenation but will result in an acute increase in PA pressures. In patients with pre-existing PHT, it is prudent for the surgeon to apply temporary PA clamping to determine the effect on PA pressures and RV function [109]. Early diagnosis of RV failure by TEE allows for prompt management and potential avoidance of ECLS [78]. Recipients with severe PHT rarely tolerate PA clamping, and the elective use of ECLS is employed [110].

An acute elevation in PVR causes a combination of detrimental effects, which may ultimately result in RV failure. The increase in RV afterload will initially reduce RV stroke volume, leading to a rise in RVEDV. RV dilatation can worsen the severity of TR, exacerbating volume overload, further raising RVEDV and consequently RVEDP. There is a leftward shift of the interventricular septum, inhibiting LV diastolic filling and decreasing LV stroke volume. The subsequent fall in cardiac output leads to systemic hypotension and, coupled with an increase in RVEDP, a reduction in RV perfusion pressure. RV ischemia follows, with further RV decompensation and failure [93].

The use of selective pulmonary vasodilators, inhaled nitric oxide (iNO), and prostacyclin therapy reduces PVR, improves oxygenation, and can reverse RV failure [111–114]. Catecholamines and phosphodiesterase inhibitors (PDE-I) will provide positive inotropy and improve RV contractility. PDE-I may reduce PVR but also have the less desirable side effect of systemic vasodilatation and hypotension, often necessitating the addition of vasopressor support to maintain coronary perfusion [115–118]. Levosimendan restores RV-PA coupling by decreasing PVR and increasing RV contractility but is also associated with systemic vasodilatation [119].

Norepinephrine is the initial vasoconstrictor of choice: it improves ventricular systolic interaction and coronary perfusion and may also improve RV-PA coupling. Vasopressin can be added in cases of refractory hypotension [118].

Extracorporeal Support

There is institutional and surgical variation in preference for utilization of CPB. Elective use of ECLS, either full CPB or ECMO, is indicated in recipients with severe PHT and in HLT [120]. SLT is typically performed "off-pump" via a thoracotomy. When BSLT is performed "off-pump," the lung receiving less perfusion (from the preoperative V/Q scan) should be replaced first. For BSLT with CPB, the heart remains warm and beating. After implantation of the first allograft, the heart is allowed to eject a little, and the lung is gently ventilated.

In recent years, the use of full CPB has been replaced by other forms of ECLS: veno-venous (VV) and venoarterial (VA) ECMO support [121–123]. VA-ECMO, like full CPB, provides both cardiac and respiratory support but requires less heparinization. Central cannulation sites, right atrium (RA) and ascending aorta, are generally preferred, as higher ECMO flows can be achieved, necessitating less anticoagulation. Peripheral cannulation, usually femoral vein (FV) to femoral artery, allows for continued ECLS support into the postoperative period in cases of severe PGD, and the chest can be closed [124, 125]. However, the anesthesiologist must remain vigilant during the intraoperative period, as lower ECMO flows permit more blood flow through the heart and lungs, which may be significantly deoxygenated: ECMO Harlequin syndrome may occur, resulting in cerebral hypoxia with peripheral VA cannulation. Pulse oximetry and arterial pressure monitoring should be placed on the right upper limb to ensure adequate oxygenation, and cerebral oximetry is advantageous [126, 127]. VV-ECMO provides only respiratory support, but the correction of hypoxemia and hypercapnia can markedly enhance RV function, leading to improved hemodynamics. Cannulation is typically peripheral and can be achieved with either a single dual-lumen cannula or by two cannulae [128, 129]. Fluid management is more challenging during ECMO support: ECMO flows are highly dependent on patient venous pressures, so sufficient fluid must be administered to maintain adequate ECMO flows without causing fluid overload and "wet" lungs. The utilization of ECMO support instead of CPB has led to better patient outcomes [130–134]. If postoperative VV-ECMO is probable, it may be useful to avoid using the right internal jugular vein for central access during surgery.

Organ Reperfusion

Reperfusion of the allograft should occur gradually, over a period of 5–10 min, as it may result in significant hypotension due to release of stored pneumoplegia, inflammatory mediators, and gas emboli into the systemic circulation [135]. Simultaneously, gentle alveolar recruitment and ventilation are commenced with limited peak airway pressures, moderate PEEP (5–10 cmH$_2$O), and initially with a fraction of inspired oxygen (FiO$_2$) less than 40% [136–139]. In BSLT the residual native lung can be ventilated with a high FiO$_2$ to maintain arterial oxygenation, while the new allograft is reperfusing with protective ventilation. After this initial period of reperfusion, the FiO$_2$ to the allograft is increased as necessary, while ventilation to the native lung is stopped to enable surgical explantation. Ischemia-reperfusion injury (IRI) presents as hypoxemia despite increasing FiO$_2$, reduced lung compliance, PHT, and, in severe cases, pulmonary edema. PGD due to IRI is associated with an increased mortality [140]. The administration of iNO is effective in improving oxygenation in cases of IRI, but its routine use to prevent IRI is of less benefit [141–143]. Severe PGD can be managed with ECLS, usually VV-ECMO, with acceptable outcomes [144, 145].

Analgesia

In the postoperative period, insufficient pain control hinders spontaneous deep breathing, adequate coughing, and sputum clearance. Analgesic options comprise paracetamol, intravenous opiates, and regional techniques, including epidural and paravertebral analgesia. Opioid-sparing regimens are encouraged to reduce respiratory depression. Epidural insertion can be performed prior to surgery, to facilitate earlier postoperative extubation, or postoperatively, after coagulopathy has been excluded [146, 147]. Paravertebral catheters can be placed by the surgeon at the end of a SLT as an alternative to epidural analgesia [148]. There may be a role for low-dose intravenous ketamine as an adjunct to reduce postoperative opiate requirements [149, 150]. Nonsteroidal anti-inflammatory drugs are avoided due to the increased risk of renal dysfunction in patients receiving calcineurin inhibitors for immunosuppression [151].

Postoperative care

Early extubation in the operating room is feasible, especially after SLT [152, 153]. The advantages include avoidance of positive pressure ventilation, with potential barotrauma, reduced extravascular lung water, decreased PA pressures, lower requirements for vasoactive drugs, and early mobilization with physiotherapy. This is facilitated by the use of short-acting anesthetic agents, epidural analgesia, and the absence of intraoperative complications [153, 154]. For patients returning to the intensive care unit for postoperative ventilation, the DLT is changed to a single-lumen tube, and a nasogastric tube is passed to permit early administration of enteral immunosuppression.

Ventilatory support involves a lung protective strategy and potential differential lung ventilation in patients with SLT for emphysema. Tracheostomy is considered if prolonged ventilation is anticipated [155–158].

Early complications include PGD, hemorrhage, iatrogenic surgical anastomotic anomalies, infection, cardiac dysrhythmias, renal failure, and venous thromboembolism [159–165]. Early complications have a negative impact on long-term survival [166]. Prevention of acute rejection is managed with a combination of steroids, calcineurin inhibitors, antiproliferatives, and mammalian target of rapamycin (mTOR) inhibitors. The routine use of induction therapy with monoclonal or polyclonal antibodies is controversial but may confer some survival benefit in BSLT [167]. Late complications include chronic rejection, presenting as bronchiolitis obliterans, infection, renal dysfunction, diabetes mellitus, and malignancy [1, 168].

Clinical Case Discussion

Case Presentation

A 52-year-old male with mixed interstitial lung disease/COPD presents for right single-lung transplantation via right thoracotomy and left hemidiaphragm plication. He requires supplemental oxygen at 3 lpm at rest and 10 lpm with exertion. He has a 40-pack-year smoking history and quit 5 years ago. His history is notable for five-vessel coronary artery bypass graft 8 years ago and endovascular repair of an abdominal aortic aneurysm 5 years ago. As a teenager, he suffered a traumatic injury to his left neck, resulting in left vocal cord and hemidiaphragm paralysis.

His preoperative medication list includes albuterol, atorvastatin, azithromycin, gabapentin, metoprolol, omeprazole, sertraline, and sildenafil. He has no medication allergies.

The patient's preoperative workup reveals the following information:

Weight: 87 kg, Height: 176 cm, Heart rate: 80 bpm, Blood pressure: 108/70 mmHg Temperature: 37.0 °C, SpO$_2$: 97% on 3 L nasal cannulae

ECG: normal sinus rhythm with occasional premature ventricular contractions, left ventricular hypertrophy

Hemoglobin: 13.7 g/dL, hematocrit: 42.3%, white blood cell count: 10 x109/L, platelets 229 × 109/L

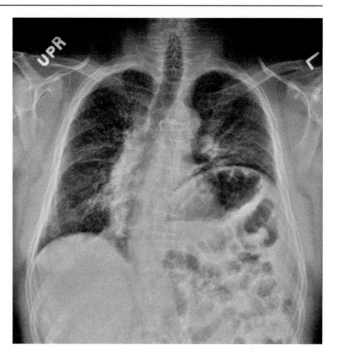

Fig. 47.7 Preoperative upright posterior-anterior chest X-ray. Notable findings include left hemidiaphragm elevation, changes consistent with post median sternotomy and CABG, and aortic stent graft within the abdomen

Na+: 138 mmol/L, K+: 4.1 mmol/L, Cl-: 103 mmol/L, CO$_2$: 28 mmol/L, BUN 20 mg/dL, Cr 0.8 mg/dL, Glucose 103 mg/dL, INR 1.0

Arterial blood gas on room air: pH 7.37, pCO$_2$ 49 mmHg, pO$_2$ 59 mmHg, bicarbonate 28 mmol/L, base excess 2 mmol/L

FEV1 51% predicted, FVC 59% predicted, FEV1/FVC 86

Ventilation/perfusion scan: differential perfusion is 46% to left lung, 54% to right lung

Transthoracic echocardiogram: left ventricular ejection fraction 50% with inferior hypokinesis, normal right ventricular systolic function, trivial tricuspid regurgitation

Left heart catheterization: significant native vessel coronary artery disease, all grafts patent

Right heart catheterization: pulmonary artery (PA) pressure 52/14 mmHg (mean 28), pulmonary vascular resistance 2.4 Wood units, cardiac index 2.6 L/min-m^2, pulmonary capillary wedge pressure 9 mmHg

Preoperative imaging studies are shown in Figs. 47.7 and 47.8.

Questions

1. Would you insert a central line and/or pulmonary artery catheter prior to the induction of anesthesia? Does the laterality of central line insertion matter?
2. How would you induce anesthesia in this patient?
3. How would you secure the airway?

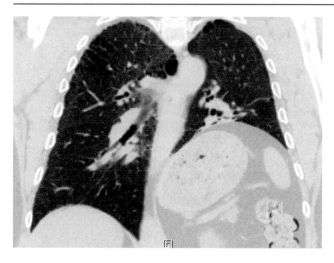

Fig. 47.8 Coronal slice from preoperative computed tomography (CT) scan of the chest. Notable findings are left hemidiaphragm elevation with volume loss in the left hemithorax, right lung hyperinflation, and paraseptal emphysema in the bilateral lung apices

4. How would your anesthetic considerations differ if the patient had:
   (a) Cystic fibrosis?
   (b) COPD?
   (c) Primary pulmonary hypertension?
5. Can this transplant be done without cardiopulmonary bypass (CPB) or extracorporeal membrane oxygenation (ECMO)?

Case Continuation

After the induction of anesthesia, intubation with a left-sided double-lumen tube, and insertion of all invasive monitors and a TEE probe, lung isolation is achieved, and one-lung ventilation (OLV) is established. After 30 min of dissection and OLV, the patient remains hemodynamically stable, but the SpO$_2$ has decreased to 85% on 100% inspired oxygen, and the arterial blood gas now reads pH 7.21, pCO$_2$ 68 mmHg, pO$_2$ 51 mmHg, bicarbonate 22 mmol/L, and base excess −2 mmol/L.

Questions

6. How will you manage OLV?
7. How will you address the hypoxemia that has developed during OLV? What degree of hypoxemia and/or hypercarbia will you tolerate?

Case Continuation

In preparation for explant of the native right lung, the surgeon clamps the right PA. After clamping, the vitals are heart

rate 90 bpm, blood pressure 129/74 mmHg, central venous pressure 10 mmHg, PA pressure 46/17 (mean 29) mmHg, and SpO$_2$ 99%.

The right lung is explanted. Then the right donor lung is implanted and reperfused, during which time there is severe hemodynamic instability.

Questions

8. How would you expect pulmonary arterial pressures to change with clamping of the left PA?
9. What has caused the hemodynamic instability?

Case Continuation

The donor (right) lung is now ventilated. Soon after, frank pulmonary edema is seen coming from the tracheal (right) lumen of the double-lumen tube.

Questions

10. How would you ventilate the donor lung?
11. Transesophageal echocardiography pulse-wave Doppler evaluation of the right pulmonary veins reveals a peak velocity of 110 cm/s. How would you advise the surgeon?
12. What is the reason for the development of pulmonary edema?

Discussion

Question 1: Would you insert a central line and/or pulmonary artery catheter prior to the induction of anesthesia? Does the laterality of central line insertion matter?

This patient does not have significant pulmonary hypertension; thus, the preinduction insertion of a pulmonary artery catheter (PAC) is not required. However, in a patient with significant pulmonary hypertension, the preinduction insertion of a PAC allows for precise hemodynamic management during induction of anesthesia. Central access also offers the advantage of allowing for the use of inotrope infusions (e.g., epinephrine) to support the right ventricle, although this central access is not necessarily required for temporary infusions. Of note, many lung transplant patients will not be able to tolerate preinduction central line/PAC insertion because they may not tolerate Trendelenburg or even supine positioning. Importantly, extreme caution must be taken in administering sedation to lung transplant recipients who often have tenuous respiratory status. The potential exacerbation of baseline hypercapnia or hypoxemia with sedation may precipitate an acute increase in pulmonary vascular resistance and subsequent right ventricular dysfunction/failure with cardiovascular collapse.

If the patient's pulmonary arterial pressures are approaching or even supra-systemic, it may be prudent to consider preinduction cannulation of the femoral vessels under local anesthesia for either preemptive or emergent institution of ECMO/CPB. Our practice is to typically place the central line and PAC via the left internal jugular vein under ultrasound guidance; this leaves the right internal jugular vein accessible should circulatory support (e.g., ECMO) be required during or after the transplant procedure. In this patient, vascular access in the left neck may be complicated by his previous injury.

Question 2: How would you induce anesthesia in this patient?

The induction of anesthesia in lung transplant recipients should focus on extreme attention to hemodynamic stability and management of pulmonary hypertension as well as rapid securement of the airway. With regard to the management of pulmonary hypertension, it is paramount to avoid significant decreases in systemic vascular resistance that will reduce right ventricular perfusion, thus compromising RV function. One must also limit any increase in pulmonary vascular resistance by avoiding hypoxemia, hypercarbia, acidosis, and "light" anesthesia during laryngoscopy and intubation. A preinduction arterial catheter is mandatory for beat-to-beat blood pressure monitoring, and a cardiac-style induction relying primarily on narcotics and benzodiazepines often provides the desired hemodynamic stability. Although rapid securement of the airway is desirable, conventional rapid sequence induction techniques may not be tolerated in patients with RV dysfunction. Despite the potential for adrenocortical suppression, some practitioners select etomidate as part of a rapid sequence induction in combination with succinylcholine. Regardless of the drugs selected for induction, vasoconstrictors and inotropes should be readily available for hemodynamic support and resuscitation. Inotropes without systemic vasodilatory effects are preferred. Careful preoperative assessment of the airway and contingency planning for difficult airway access are prudent, as these patients may not tolerate prolonged periods of apnea. Given the left hemidiaphragm paralysis in this patient, with resultant low lung volumes on the left, this patient may experience more rapid desaturation during induction than might be predicted from his lung disease. Furthermore, this patient is only undergoing single-lung transplantation; therefore, precautions against aspiration, which could compromise the remaining native lung, should be taken.

Question 3: How would you secure the airway?

In the vast majority of lung transplant patients, a left-sided double-lumen endotracheal tube (ETT) placed with bronchoscopic guidance is typically used. Patients with a suppurative pathology (e.g., cystic fibrosis) will benefit from initial insertion of a single-lumen ETT to allow for pulmonary toilet via bronchoscopy. This will mostly likely improve oxygenation during one-lung ventilation.

Bronchial blockers to achieve lung isolation are more prone to movement within the airway during manipulation of the hilum and do not allow for effective suctioning, the application of continuous positive airway pressure (CPAP) to the non-ventilated lung, or differential ventilation of the two lungs.

Question 4: How would your anesthetic considerations differ
if the patient had:
  (a) Cystic fibrosis?
  (b) COPD?
  (c) Primary pulmonary hypertension?

The leading indications for lung transplantation today are pulmonary fibrosis, COPD, and cystic fibrosis. The underlying pathology impacts the surgical procedure as well as the anesthetic considerations. For example, patients with fibrosis often receive single-lung transplants, while patients with cystic fibrosis always require a double-lung transplant.

Induction techniques are similar for all pathologies and reflect consideration of pulmonary artery pressures and underlying right ventricular function, as described above.

Ventilation strategies, on the other hand, should be tailored to the underlying pulmonary pathology. Patients with pulmonary fibrosis have low lung compliance and are at risk for barotrauma associated with mechanical ventilation. Pressure control ventilation may be preferable to volume control ventilation to decrease the airway pressure transmitted to the lungs. Patients with obstructive lung disease, such as COPD or cystic fibrosis, are prone to air trapping and dynamic hyperinflation (see question 6).

Patients such as this one who receive single-lung transplants may have a significant imbalance in pulmonary compliance between the native lung and the transplanted lung, requiring differential lung ventilation via a double-lumen ETT.

Question 5: Can this transplant be done without cardiopulmonary bypass (CPB) or extracorporeal membrane oxygenation (ECMO)?

Cardiopulmonary bypass (CPB) offers the advantage of improved hemodynamic stability and systemic oxygenation during lung transplantation. However, CPB has many disadvantages, including bleeding related to full heparinization and coagulopathy, increased use of blood products, increased crystalloid administration, inflammation, and possible damage to other organs. Nonetheless, patients with intractable hypoxemia during one-lung ventilation or RV dysfunction causing hemodynamic compromise may require ECMO or CPB to safely complete the procedure. ECMO is often preferred over CPB because it allows for less heparinization and can be easily extended into the postoperative period if required.

Question 6: How will you manage OLV?

Concerns during OLV before transplant include hypoxemia, hypercarbia, dynamic hyperinflation (in cases of obstructive lung disease), and excessively high airway pressures (which may precipitate RV failure). To address dynamic hyperinflation, ventilation should focus on permissive hypercapnia with reduced tidal volume, lower respiratory rate, elimination of positive end-expiratory pressure (PEEP), and adjustments to inspiratory/expiratory (I:E) ratio to favor exhalation. Elevated airway pressures can be ameliorated through reduced tidal volumes, higher respiratory rate, and adjustment of the ventilator I:E ratio.

Question 7: How will you address the hypoxemia that has developed during OLV? What degree of hypoxemia and/or hypercarbia will you tolerate?

Hypoxemia during one-lung ventilation (OLV) can be treated with either continuous positive airway pressure (5–10 cmH$_2$O) to the non-ventilated lung to oxygenate the shunt fraction or with PEEP (5–10 cmH$_2$O) to the ventilated lung to minimize atelectasis. Of note, PEEP can potentially reduce venous return to the heart, impair hypoxic pulmonary vasoconstriction, and elevate pulmonary vascular resistance. Definitive treatment of hypoxemia due to shunt during OLV is achieved with surgical clamping of the PA to the non-ventilated lung. Hypoxic pulmonary vasoconstriction may be improved by reducing inhaled volatile anesthetic concentration or utilizing TIVA only and by avoiding IV vasodilators (e.g., nitroglycerin). If intractable hypoxemia occurs despite the above maneuvers and utilization of 100% inspired oxygen, ECMO or CPB may be required.

Management of arterial blood gas values should target the patient's baseline values prior to induction of anesthesia. While some degree of permissive hypercarbia may be necessary to achieve adequate oxygenation, severe hypercarbia, hypoxemia, or acidosis that produce hemodynamic instability are indications for ECMO or CBP.

Question 8: How would you expect pulmonary arterial pressures to change with clamping of the left PA?

It is reasonable to expect a rise in the PA pressure after surgical clamping of either pulmonary artery because the entire cardiac output is now passing through the contralateral lung. This PA pressure increase may be variable depending on the degree of baseline perfusion through the native lung (reference the preoperative ventilation/perfusion lung scan). While a lack of increase in PA pressure with PA clamping may seem reassuring, the anesthesiologist should always be vigilant about the possibility of worsening of RV function.

Question 9: What has caused the hemodynamic instability?

Possible causes of hemodynamic instability in this scenario include worsening of RV function, worsening of LV function due to ischemia in this patient with significant coronary disease, and air embolism occurring during reperfusion of the transplanted lung. The best tool for monitoring cardiac function and for diagnosing the cause of intraoperative hemodynamic instability is transesophageal echocardiography (TEE). TEE will be able to differentiate between these scenarios and allow for determination of the cause of hemodynamic instability.

Question 10: How would you ventilate the donor lung?

Goals for the management of any newly transplanted lung include the avoidance of atelectasis, hyperoxia, and barotrauma, which can rapidly cause pulmonary edema. During double-lung transplantation, a particularly vulnerable period occurs between the first and second implant when the newly reperfused first lung must tolerate twice the normal blood flow (i.e., the full cardiac output). Single-lung transplants are vulnerable to differences in compliance between the newly implanted lung and the remaining native lung. Institutional perioperative standardized practices for ventilation of the newly transplanted lung are common for goal PEEP (e.g., 8 mmHg), preferred oxygen levels (e.g., room air or the lowest inspired oxygen concentration to maintain SpO$_2$ above 90%), and peak inspiratory pressure (e.g., less than 30 mmHg). At our institution, inhaled nitric oxide (iNO) or inhaled epoprostenol are routinely administered to reduce pulmonary artery pressure and support RV function, although the benefits in lung transplantation are controversial.

Question 11: TEE pulse-wave Doppler evaluation of the R pulmonary veins reveals a peak velocity of 110 cm/s. How would you advise the surgeon?

Pre-procedure and post-procedure TEE evaluation provides invaluable information to assist with anesthetic management and to aide in diagnosing surgical complications. Pre-procedure evaluation should focus on RV and LV function, the identification and quantification of any valvular lesions or intracardiac shunts (e.g., PFO), and an assessment of baseline pulmonary vein velocities and pulmonary artery size.

Post-transplant TEE should again evaluate RV and LV function. Most importantly, following reperfusion there should be a careful assessment of the right and left pulmonary arteries and all four pulmonary veins (if possible), including:

- Assessment of the diameter of pulmonary artery and pulmonary vein anastomoses, if visible
- Color flow Doppler evaluation of pulmonary artery anastomoses, if visible
- Color flow Doppler evaluation of pulmonary vein flows and pulsed-wave Doppler determination of pulmonary vein velocities

In general, anastomoses >0.5 cm in diameter and pulmonary vein pulse-wave Doppler peak systolic velocities ≤100 cm/s are acceptable. Although few specific guidelines exist, peak systolic velocities >100–170 cm/s are worrisome for obstruction (kinked or narrow anastomoses) and should prompt discussion with the surgical team before chest closure.

Question 12: What is the reason for the development of pulmonary edema?

Reperfusion injury typically presents with poor oxygenation, high PA pressures, and pulmonary edema. It is important to exclude a mechanical cause, such as pulmonary vein or arterial anastomotic stenosis or kinking (best evaluated via TEE, as described above). Otherwise, protective lung ventilation strategies should be employed. Inhaled pulmonary vasodilators can help to reduce the inspired oxygen concentration in patients with high oxygen requirements. Ultimately, significant reperfusion injury or primary graft dysfunction may necessitate the use of ECMO.

References

1. Yusen RD, Edwards LB, Dipchand AI, et al. The registry of the International Society for Heart and Lung Transplantation: thirty-third adult lung and heart-lung transplant report-2016. J Heart Lung Transplant. 2016;35:1170–84.
2. Hardy JD, Webb WR, Dalton ML Jr. Lung homotransplantations in man: report of the initial case. JAMA. 1963;18:1065–74.
3. Toronto Lung Transplant Group. Unilateral lung transplantation for pulmonary fibrosis. N Engl J Med. 1986;314:1140–5.
4. Liao WC, Hwang SL, Ko WJ, et al. Analysis of heart donation for cardiac transplantation at the National Taiwan university Hospital: fifteen-year cases review. Transplant Proc. 2004;36:2365–8.
5. Cameron EJ, Bellini A, Damian MS, et al. Confirmation of brain-stem death. Pract Neurol. 2016;16:129–35.
6. Smith M. Physiologic changes during brain stem death – lessons for management of the organ donor. J Heart Lung Transplant. 2004;23:S217–22.
7. Dictus C, Vienenkoetter B, Esmaeilzadeh M, et al. Critical care management of potential organ donors: our current standard. Clin Transpl. 2009;23:2–9.
8. Faropoulos K, Apostolakis E. Brain death and its influence on the lungs of the donor: how is it prevented? Transplant Proc. 2009;41:4114–9.
9. Shutter L. Pathophysiology of brain death: what does the brain do and what is lost in brain death? J Crit Care. 2014;29:683–6.
10. Shemie SD, Ross H, Pagliarello J, et al. Organ donor management in Canada: recommendations of the forum on medical management to optimize donor organ potential. CMAJ. 2006;174:S13–32.
11. Grissom TE, Richards JE, Herr DL. Critical care management of the potential organ donor. Int Anesthesiol Clin. 2017;55:18–41.
12. Angel LF, Levine DJ, Restrepo MI, et al. Impact of a lung transplantation donor-management protocol on lung donation and recipient outcomes. Am J Respir Crit Care Med. 2006;174:710–6.
13. Mascia L, Pasero D, Slutsky AS, et al. Effect of a lung protective strategy for organ donors on eligibility and availability of lungs for transplantation: a randomized controlled trial. JAMA. 2010;304:2620–7.
14. Novitzky D, Mi Z, Videla LA, et al. Hormone resuscitation therapy for brain-dead donors: is insulin beneficial or detrimental? Clin Transpl. 2016;30:754–9.
15. Anderson TA, Bekker P, Vagefi PA. Anesthetic considerations in organ procurement surgery: a narrative review. Can J Anaesth. 2015;62:529–39.
16. Oto T, Griffiths AP, Rosenfeldt F, et al. Early outcomes comparing Perfadex, Euro-Collins and Papworth solutions in lung transplantation. Ann Thorac Surg. 2006;82:1842–8.
17. Latchana N, Peck JR, Whitson B, et al. Preservation solutions for cardiac and pulmonary donor grafts: a review of the current literature. J Thorac Dis. 2014;6:1143–9.
18. Van Raemdonck DE, Jannis NC, Rega FR, et al. Extended preservation of ischemic pulmonary graft function by postmortem alveolar expansion. Ann Thorac Surg. 1997;64:801–8.
19. Orens JB, Boehler A, de Perrot M, et al. A review of lung transplant donor acceptability criteria. J Heart Lung Transplant. 2003;22:1183–200.
20. Van Raemdonck D, Neyrinck A, Verleden GM, et al. Lung donor selection and management. Proc Am Thorac Soc. 2009;15:28–38.
21. Bittle GJ, Sanchez PG, Kon ZN, et al. The use of lung donors older than 55 years: a review of the UNOS database. J Heart Lung Transplant. 2013;32:760–8.
22. Mulligan MJ, Sanchez PG, Evans CF, et al. The use of extended criteria donors decreases one-year survival in high-risk lung recipients: a review of the UNOS database. J Thorac Cardiovasc Surg. 2016;152:891–8.
23. Botha P, Trivedi D, Weir CJ. Extended donor criteria in lung transplantation: impact on organ allocation. J Thorac Cardiovasc Surg. 2006;131:1154–60.
24. Van Raemdonck D, Rega FR, Neyrinck A, et al. Non-heart beating donors. Semin Cardiovasc Surg. 2004;16:309–21.
25. Oto T, Levvey B, McEgan R, et al. A practical approach to clinical lung transplantation from a Maastricht category III donor with cardiac death. J Heart Lung Transplant. 2007;26:196–9.
26. Wigfield C. Donation after cardiac death for lung transplantation: a review of current clinical practice. Curr Opin Organ Transplant. 2014;19:455–9.
27. Egan TM. Non-heart-beating donors in thoracic transplantation. J Heart Lung Transplant. 2004;23:3–10.
28. De Vleeschauwer SI, Wauters S, Dupont LJ, et al. Medium-term outcome after lung transplantation is comparable between brain-dead and cardiac-dead donors. J Heart Lung Transplant. 2011;30:975–81.

29. Steen S, Ingemansson R, Eriksson L, et al. First human transplantation of a nonacceptable donor lung after reconditioning ex vivo. Ann Thorac Surg. 2007;83:2191–4.

30. Sanchez PG, Bittle GJ, Burdorf L, et al. State of the art: clinical ex-vivo lung perfusion: rationale, current status, and future directions. J Heart Lung Transplant. 2012;31:339–48.

31. Van Raemdonck D, Neyrinck A, Cypel M, et al. Ex-vivo lung perfusion. Transplant Int. 2015;28:643–56.

32. Cypel M, Yeung JC, Machuca T, et al. Experience with the first 50 ex vivo lung perfusions in clinical transplantation. J Thorac Cardiovasc Surg. 2012;144:1200–6.

33. Wallinder A, Riise GC, Ricksen SE, et al. Transplantation after ex vivo lung perfusion: a midterm follow-up. J Heart Lung Transplant. 2016;35:1303–10.

34. Valenza F, Citerio G, Palleschi A, et al. Successful transplantation of lungs from an uncontrolled donor after circulatory death preserved in situ by alveolar recruitment maneuvers and assessed by ex vivo lung perfusion. Am J Transplant. 2016;16:1312–8.

35. Slama A, Schillab L, Barta M, et al. Standard donor lung procurement with normothermic ex vivo lung perfusion: a prospective randomized clinical trial. J Heart Lung Transplant. 2017;36:744–53.

36. Yeung JC, Krueger T, Yasufuku K, et al. Outcomes after transplantation of lungs preserved for more than 12h: a retrospective study. Lancet Respir Med. 2017;5:119–24.

37. Orens JB, Estenne M, Arcasoy S, et al. International guidelines for the selection of lung transplant candidates: 2006 update – a consensus report from the Pulmonary Scientific Council of the International Society for Heart and Lung Transplantation. J Heart Lung Transplant. 2006;25:745–55.

38. Shah PD, Orens JB. Guidelines for the selection of lung-transplant candidates. Curr Opin Organ Transplant. 2012;17:467–73.

39. Weill D, Benden C, Corris PA, et al. A consensus document for the selection of lung transplant candidates: 2104 – an update from the Pulmonary Transplantation Council of the International Society for Heart and Lung Transplantation. J Heart Lung Transplant. 2015;34:1–15.

40. Celli BR, Cote CG, Marin JM, et al. The body-mass index, airflow obstruction, dyspnea, and exercise capacity index in chronic obstructive pulmonary disease. N Engl J Med. 2004;350:1005–12.

41. Van Agteren JE, Carson KV, Tiong LU, et al. Lung volume reduction surgery for diffuse emphysema. Cochrane Database Syst Rev. 2016;(10):CD001001.

42. Tutic M, Lardinois D, Imfeld S, et al. Lung-volume reduction surgery as an alternative or bridging procedure to lung transplantation. Ann Thorac Surg. 2006;82:208–13.

43. Morrell MR, Pilewski JM. Lung transplantation for cystic fibrosis. Clin Chest Med. 2016;37:127–38.

44. Egan TM, Murray S, Bustami RT, et al. Development of the lung allocation system in the United States. Am J Transplant. 2006;6:1212–27.

45. Egan TM, Edwards LB. Effect of the lung allocation score on lung transplantation in the United States. J Heart Lung Transplant. 2016;35:433–9.

46. Task Force for the Diagnosis and Treatment of Pulmonary Hypertension of the European Society of Cardiology and the European Respiratory Society. Guidelines for the diagnosis and treatment of pulmonary hypertension. Eur Heart J. 2009;30:2493–537.

47. Aigner C, Jaksch P, Taghavi S, et al. Pulmonary retransplantation: is it worth the effort? A long-term analysis of 46 cases. J Heart Lung Transplant. 2008;27:60–5.

48. Schumer EM, Rice JD, Kistler AM, et al. Single versus double lung retransplantation does not affect survival based on previous transplant type. Ann Thorac Surg. 2017;103:236–40.

49. Aigner C. Retransplantation. Curr Opin Organ Transplant. 2015;20:521–6.

50. Maurer JR, Frost AE, Estenne M, et al. International guidelines for the selection of lung transplant candidates. Transplantation. 1998;66:951–6.

51. Chiumello D, Coppola S, Froio S, et al. Extracorporeal life support as a bridge to lung transplantation: a systematic review. Crit Care. 2015;19:19.

52. Rajagopal K, Hoeper MM. State of the art: bridging to lung transplantation using artificial organ support technologies. J Heart Lung Transplant. 2016;35:1385–98.

53. Lehr CJ, Zaas DW, Cheifetz IM. Ambulatory extracorporeal membrane oxygenation as a bridge to lung transplantation: walking while waiting. Chest. 2015;147:1213–8.

54. Myles PS. Aspects of anesthesia for lung transplantation. Semin Cardiothorac Vasc Anesth. 1998;2:140–54.

55. Jones RM, Enfield KB, Mehrad B, et al. Prevalence of obstructive coronary artery disease in patients undergoing lung transplantation: case series and review of the literature. Catheter Cardiovasc Interv. 2014;84:1–6.

56. Vizza CD, Lynch JP, Ochoa LL, et al. Right and left ventricular dysfunction in patients with severe pulmonary disease. Chest. 1998;113:576–83.

57. Koprivanac M, Budev MM, Yun JJ, et al. How important is coronary artery disease when considering lung transplant candidates? J Heart Lung Transplant. 2016;35:1453–61.

58. Choong CK, Meyers BF, Guthrie TJ, et al. Does the presence of preoperative mild or moderate coronary artery disease affect the outcomes of lung transplantation? Ann Thorac Surg. 2006;82:1038–42.

59. Hoechter DJ, von Dossow V. Lung transplantation: from the procedure to managing patients with lung transplantation. Curr Opin Anesthesiol. 2016;29:8–13.

60. Funk DJ, Moretti EW, Gan TJ. Minimally invasive cardiac output monitoring in the perioperative setting. Anesth Analg. 2009;108:887–97.

61. Missant C, Rex S, Wouters PF. Accuracy of cardiac output measurements with pulse contour analysis (PulseCO) and Doppler echocardiography during off-pump coronary artery bypass grafting. Eur J Anaesthesiol. 2008;25:243–8.

62. Sangkum L, Liu GL, Yu L, et al. Minimally invasive or noninvasive cardiac output measurement: an update. J Anesth. 2016;30:461–80.

63. Rudnick MR, Marchi LD, Plotkin JS. Hemodynamic monitoring during liver transplantation: a state of the art review. World J Hepatol. 2015;7:1302–11.

64. Conacher ID, Paes ML. Mixed venous oxygen saturation during lung transplantation. J Cardiothorac Vasc Anesth. 1994;8:671–4.

65. Shepherd SJ, Pearse RM. Role of central and mixed venous oxygen saturation measurement in perioperative care. Anesthesiology. 2009;111:649–56.

66. Murkin JM, Adams SJ, Novick RJ, et al. Monitoring brain oxygen saturation during coronary bypass surgery: a randomized, prospective study. Anesth Analg. 2007;104:51–8.

67. Harilall Y, Adam JK, Biccard BM, et al. The effect of optimising cerebral tissue oxygen saturation on markers of neurological injury during coronary artery bypass graft surgery. Heart Lung Circ. 2014;23:68–74.

68. Myles PS, Leslie K, McNeil J, et al. Bispectral index monitoring to prevent awareness during anaesthesia: the B-Aware randomised controlled trial. Lancet. 2004;363:1757–63.

69. De Smet T, Struys MM, Neckebroek MM, et al. The accuracy and clinical feasibility of a new bayesian-based closed-loop control system for propofol administration using the bispectral index as a controlled variable. Anesth Analg. 2008;107:1200–10.

70. NICE clinical guideline 65: inadvertent perioperative hypothermia. https://www.nice.org.uk/guidance/cg65. Accessed 14 April 2017.

71. Sessler DI. Perioperative thermoregulation and heat balance. Lancet. 2016;387:2655–64.

72. Flachskampf FA, Badano L, Daniel WG, et al. Recommendations for transoesophageal echocardiography: update 2010. Eur J Echocardiogr. 2010;11:557–76.

73. American Society of Anesthesiologists and Society of Cardiovascular Anesthesiologists Task Force on Transesophageal Echocardiography. Practice guidelines for perioperative transesophageal echocardiography. Anesthesiology. 2010;112:1084–96.

74. Sullivan B, Puskas F, Fernandez-Bustamante A. Transesophageal echocardiography in noncardiac thoracic surgery. Anesthesiol Clin. 2012;30:657–69.

75. Evans A, Dwarakanath S, Hogue C, et al. Intraoperative echocardiography for patients undergoing lung transplantation. Anesth Analg. 2014;118:725–30.

76. Della Rocca G, Brondani A, Costa MG. Intraoperative hemodynamic monitoring during organ transplantation: what is new? Curr Opin Organ Transplant. 2009;14:291–6.

77. Tan TC, Dudzinski DM, Hung J, et al. Peri-operative assessment of right heart function: role of echocardiography. Eur J Clin Investig. 2015;45:755–66.

78. Ashes C, Roscoe A. Transesophageal echocardiography in thoracic anesthesia: pulmonary hypertension and right ventricular function. Curr Opin Anaesthesiol. 2015;28:38–44.

79. Miyaji K, Nakamura K, Maruo T, et al. Effect of a kink in unilateral pulmonary artery anastomosis on velocities of blood flow through bilateral pulmonary vein anastomoses in living-donor lobar lung transplantation. J Am Soc Echocardiogr. 2004;17:998–9.

80. Cartwright BL, Jackson A, Cooper J. Intraoperative pulmonary vein examination by transesophageal echocardiography: an anatomic update and review of utility. J Cardiothorac Vasc Anesth. 2013;27:111–20.

81. Felton ML, Michel-Cherqui M, Sage E, et al. Transesophageal and contact ultrasound echographic assessments of pulmonary vessels in bilateral lung transplantation. Ann Thorac Surg. 2012;93:1094–100.

82. Shaikh N, Saif AS, Nayeemuddin M, et al. Patent foramen ovale: its significance in anesthesia and intensive care: an illustrated case. Anesth Essays Res. 2012;6:94–7.

83. Subramaniam K, Esper SA. Role of transesophageal echocardiography in perioperative patient management of lung transplantation surgery. J Perioper Echocardiogr. 2013;1:48–56.

84. Doufle G, Roscoe A, Billia F, et al. Echocardiography for adult patients supported with extracorporeal membrane oxygenation. Crit Care. 2015;19:326.

85. Hohn L, Schweizer A, Morel DR, et al. Circulatory failure after anesthesia induction in a patient with severe primary pulmonary hypertension. Anesthesiology. 1999;91:1943–5.

86. Manthous CA. Avoiding circulatory complications during endotracheal intubation and initiation of positive pressure ventilation. J Emerg Med. 2009;38(5):622–31.

87. Schisler T, Marquez JM, Hilmi I, et al. Pulmonary hypertensive crisis on induction of anesthesia. Sem Cardiothorac Vasc Anesth. 2017;21:105–13.

88. Conacher ID. Anaesthesia for the surgery of emphysema. Br J Anaesth. 1997;79:530–8.

89. Quinlan JJ, Buffington CW. Deliberate hypoventilation in a patient with air trapping during lung transplantation. Anesthesiology. 1993;78:1177–81.

90. Myles PS, Ryder IG, Weeks AM, et al. Diagnosis and management of dynamic hyperinflation during lung transplantation. J Cardiothorac Vasc Anesth. 1997;11:100–4.

91. Petrucci N, De Feo C. Lung protective ventilation strategy for the acute respiratory distress syndrome. Cochrane Database Syst Rev. 2013;(2):CD003844.

92. Papiris SA, Manali ED, Kolilekas L, et al. Clinical review: idiopathic pulmonary fibrosis acute exacerbations – unravelling Ariadne's thread. Crit Care. 2010;14:246.

93. Hosseinian L. Pulmonary hypertension and noncardiac surgery: implications for the anesthesiologist. J Cardiothorac Vasc Anesth. 2014;28:1064–74.

94. Snell GI, Salamonsen RF, Bergin P, et al. Inhaled nitric oxide as a bridge to heart-lung transplantation in a patient with end-stage pulmonary hypertension. Am J Respir Crit Care Med. 1995;151:1263–6.

95. de Boer WJ, Waterbolk TW, Brugemann J, et al. Extracorporeal membrane oxygenation before induction of anesthesia in critically ill thoracic transplant patients. Ann Thorac Surg. 2001;72:1407–8.

96. Scheller MS, Kriett JM, Smith CM, et al. Airway management during anesthesia for double-lung transplantation using a single-lumen endotracheal tube with an enclosed bronchial blocker. J Cardiovasc Thorac Anesth. 1992;6:204–7.

97. Campos JH. Which device should be considered the best for lung isolation: double-lumen endotracheal tube versus bronchial blockers. Curr Opin Anaesthesiol. 2007;20:27–31.

98. Conway SP, Brownlee KG, Denton M, et al. Antibiotic treatment of multidrug-resistant organisms in cystic fibrosis. Am J Respir Med. 2003;2:321–32.

99. Haja Mydin H, Corris PA, Nicholson A, et al. Targeted antibiotic prophylaxis for lung transplantation in cystic fibrosis patients colonized with Pseudomonas aeruginosa using multiple combination bactericidal testing. J Transp Secur. 2012;2012:135738.

100. Pruszkowski O, Dalibon N, Moutafis M, et al. Effects of propofol vs sevoflurane on arterial oxygenation during one-lung ventilation. Br J Anaesth. 2007;98:539–44.

101. Módolo NS, Módolo MP, Marton MA, et al. Intravenous versus inhalation anaesthesia for one-lung ventilation. Cochrane Database Syst Rev. 2013;(7):CD006313.

102. Schulte-Sasse U, Hess W, Tarnow J. Pulmonary vascular responses to nitrous oxide in patients with normal and high pulmonary vascular resistance. Anesthesiology. 1982;57:9–13.

103. Awori Hayanga JW, D'Cunha J. The surgical technique of bilateral sequential lung transplantation. J Thorac Dis. 2014;6:1063–9.

104. Kim KN, Kim DW, Jeong MA. Comparison of pressure-controlled ventilation with volume-controlled ventilation during one-lung ventilation: a systematic review and meta-analysis. BMC Anesthesiol. 2016;16:72.

105. Pardos PC, Garutti I, Pineiro P, et al. Effects of ventilatory mode during one-lung ventilation on intraoperative and postoperative arterial oxygenation in thoracic surgery. J Cardiothorac Vasc Anesth. 2009;23:770–4.

106. Bittner HB, Binner C, Lehmann S, et al. Replacing cardiopulmonary bypass with extracorporeal membrane oxygenation in lung transplantation operations. Eur J Cardiothorac Surg. 2007;31:462–7.

107. McIlroy DR, Pilcher DV, Snell GI. Does anaesthetic management affect early outcomes after lung transplant? An exploratory analysis. Br J Anaesth. 2009;102:506–14.

108. Geube MA, Perez-Protto SE, McGrath TL, et al. Increased intraoperative fluid administration is associated with severe primary graft dysfunction after lung transplantation. Anesth Analg. 2016;122:1081–8.

109. Feltracco P, Serra E, Barbieri F, et al. Anesthetic considerations in lung transplantation for severe pulmonary hypertension. Transplant Proc. 2007;39:1976–80.

110. Triantafillou AN, Pasque MK, Huddleston CB, et al. Predictors, frequency and indications for cardiopulmonary bypass during lung transplantation in adults. Ann Thorac Surg. 1994;57:1248–51.

111. Wright BJ. Inhaled pulmonary vasodilators in refractory hypoxemia. Clin Exp Emerg Med. 2015;2:184–7.

112. Rocca GD, Passariello M, Coccia C, et al. Inhaled nitric oxide administration during one-lung ventilation in patients undergoing thoracic surgery. J Cardiothorac Vasc Anesth. 2001;15:218–23.

113. Muzaffar S, Shukla N, Angelini GD, et al. Inhaled prostacyclin is safe, effective and affordable in patients with pulmonary hypertension, right-heart dysfunction, and refractory hypoxemia after cardiothoracic surgery. J Thorac Cardiovasc Surg. 2004;128:949–50.

114. Ventetuolo CE, Klinger JR. Management of acute right ventricular failure in the intensive care unit. Ann Am Thorac Soc. 2014;11:811–22.

115. Forrest P. Anaesthesia and right ventricular failure. Anaesth Intensive Care. 2009;37:370–85.

116. Vachiery JL, Huez S, Gillies H, et al. Safety, tolerability and pharmacokinetics of an intravenous bolus of sildenafil in patients with pulmonary arterial hypertension. Br J Pharmacol. 2011;71:289–92.

117. Price LC, Wort SJ, Finney SJ, et al. Pulmonary vascular and right ventricular dysfunction in adult critical care: current and emerging options for management: a systematic literature review. Crit Care. 2010;14:R169.

118. Harjola VP, Mebazaa A, Celutkiene J, et al. Contemporary management of acute right ventricular failure: a statement from the Heart Failure Association and the Working Group on Pulmonary Circulation and Right Ventricular Function of the European Society of Cardiology. Eur J Heart Fail. 2016;18:226–41.

119. Kerbaul F, Gariboldi V, Giorgi R, et al. Effects of levosimendan on acute pulmonary embolism-induced right ventricular failure. Crit Care Med. 2007;35:1948–54.

120. Nagendran M, Maruthappu M, Sugand K. Should double lung transplant be performed with or without cardiopulmonary bypass? Interact Cardiovasc Thorac Surg. 2011;12:799–804.

121. Yu WS, Paik HC, Haam SJ, et al. Transition to routine use of venoarterial extracorporeal oxygenation during lung transplantation could improve early outcomes. J Thorac Dis. 2016;8:1712–20.

122. Ius F, Sommer W, Tudorache I, et al. Five-year experience with intraoperative extracorporeal membrane oxygenation in lung transplantation: indications and midterm results. J Heart Lung Transplant. 2016;35:49–58.

123. Odell DD, D'Cunha J, Shigemura N, et al. Intraoperative extracorporeal membrane oxygenation as an alternative to cardiopulmonary bypass in lung transplantation. J Heart Lung Transplant. 2013;32:S167–8.

124. Pavlushkov E, Berman M, Valchanov K. Cannulation techniques for extracorporeal life support. Ann Transl Med. 2017;5:70.

125. Salman J, Ius F, Sommer W, et al. Mid-term results of bilateral lung transplant with postoperatively extended intraoperative extracorporeal membrane oxygenation for severe pulmonary hypertension. Eur J Cardiothorac Surg. 2017;52:163–70.

126. Chung M, Shiloh AL, Carlese A. Monitoring of the adult patient on venoarterial extracorporeal membrane oxygenation. ScientificWorldJournal. 2014;2014:393258.

127. Rupprecht L, Lunz D, Philipp A, et al. Pitfalls in percutaneous ECMO cannulation. Heart Lung Vessel. 2015;7:320–6.

128. Sidebotham D, Allen SJ, McGeorge A, et al. Venovenous extracorporeal membrane oxygenation in adults: practical aspects of circuits, cannulae, and procedures. J Cardiothorac Vasc Anesth. 2012;26:893–909.

129. Reis Miranda D, van Thiel R, Brodie D, et al. Right ventricular unloading after initiation of venovenous extracorporeal membrane oxygenation. Am J Respir Crit Care Med. 2015;191:346–8.

130. Mohite PN, Sabashnikov A, Patil NP, et al. The role of cardiopulmonary bypass in lung transplantation. Clin Transpl. 2016;30:202–9.

131. Machuca TN, Collaud S, Mercier O, et al. Outcomes of intraoperative extracorporeal membrane oxygenation versus cardiopulmonary bypass for lung transplantation. J Thorac Cardiovasc Surg. 2015;149:1152–7.

132. Bermudez CA, Shiose A, Esper SA, et al. Outcomes of intraoperative venoarterial extracorporeal membrane oxygenation versus cardiopulmonary bypass during lung transplantation. Ann Thorac Surg. 2014;98:1936–42.

133. Diamond JM, Lee JC, Kawut SM, et al. Clinical risk factors for primary graft dysfunction after lung transplantation. Am J Respir Crit Care Med. 2013;187:527–34.

134. Hoechter DJ, Shen YM, Kammerer T, et al. Extracorporeal circulation during lung transplantation procedures: a meta-analysis. ASAIO J. 2017;63:551–61.

135. Castillo M. Anesthetic management for lung transplantation. Curr Opin Anaesthesiol. 2011;24:32–6.

136. Shaver CM, Ware LB. Primary graft dysfunction: pathophysiology to guide new preventive therapies. Expert Rev Respir Med. 2017;11:119–28.

137. Silva CA, Carvalho RS, Cagido VR, et al. Influence of lung mechanical properties and alveolar architecture on the pathogenesis of ischemia-reperfusion injury. Interact Cardiovasc Thorac Surg. 2010;11:46–51.

138. DeCampos KN, Keshavjee S, Slutsky AS, et al. Alveolar recruitment prevents rapid-reperfusion-induced injury of lung transplants. J Heart Lung Transplant. 1999;18:1096–102.

139. Singh RR, Laubach VE, Ellman PI, et al. Attenuation of lung reperfusion injury by modified ventilation and reperfusion techniques. J Heart Lung Transplant. 2006;25:1467–73.

140. Porteous MK, Diamond JM, Christie JD. Primary graft dysfunction: lessons leaned about the first 72h after lung transplantation. Curr Opin Organ Transplant. 2015;20:506–14.

141. Della Rocca G, Pierconti F, Costa MG, et al. Severe reperfusion lung injury after lung transplantation. Crit Care. 2002;6:240–4.

142. Tavare AN, Tsakok T. Does prophylactic inhaled nitric oxide reduce morbidity and mortality after lung transplantation? Interact Cardiovasc Thorac Surg. 2011;13:516–20.

143. Pasero D, Martin EL, Davi A, et al. The effects of inhaled nitric oxide after lung transplantation. Minerva Anestesiol. 2010;76:353–61.

144. Hsu HH, Ko WJ, Chen JS, et al. Extracorporeal membrane oxygenation in pulmonary crisis and primary graft dysfunction. J Heart Lung Transplant. 2008;27:233–7.

145. Fischer S, Bohn D, Rycus P, et al. Extracorporeal membrane oxygenation for primary graft dysfunction after lung transplantation: analysis of the Extracorporeal Life Support Organization (ELSO) registry. J Heart Lung Transplant. 2007;26:472–7.

146. Pottecher J, Falcoz PE, Massard G, et al. Does thoracic epidural analgesia improve outcome after lung transplantation? Interact Cardiovasc Thorac Surg. 2011;12:51–3.

147. Feltracco P, Barbieri S, Milevoj M, et al. Thoracic epidural analgesia in lung transplantation. Transplant Proc. 2010;42:1265–9.

148. Yeung JH, Gates S, Naidu BV, et al. Paravertebral block versus thoracic epidural for patients undergoing thoracotomy. Cochrane Database Syst Rev. 2016;(2):CD009121.

149. Jouguelet-Lacoste J, La Colla L, Schilling D, et al. The use of intravenous infusion or single dose of low-dose ketamine for postoperative analgesia: a review of the current literature. Pain Med. 2015;16:383–403.

150. Laskowski K, Stirling A, McKay WP, et al. A systematic review of intravenous ketamine for postoperative analgesia. Can J Anaesth. 2011;58:911–23.

151. Scheffert JL, Raza K. Immunosuppression in lung transplantation. J Thorac Dis. 2014;6:1039–53.

152. Augoustides JG, Watcha SM, Pochettino A, et al. Early tracheal extubation in adults undergoing single-lung transplantation for chronic obstructive pulmonary disease: pilot evaluation of perioperative outcome. Interact Cardiovasc Thorac Surg. 2008;7:755–8.

153. Felten ML, Moyer JD, Dreyfus JF, et al. Immediate postoperative extubation in bilateral lung transplantation: predictive factors and outcome. Br J Anaesth. 2016;116:847–54.

154. Rocca GD, Coccia C, Costa GM, et al. Is very early extubation after lung transplantation feasible? J Cardiothorac Vasc Anesth. 2003;17:29–35.

155. Thakuria L, Davey R, Romano R, et al. Mechanical ventilation after lung transplantation. J Crit Care. 2016 Feb;31(1):110–8.

156. Mitchell JB, Shaw AD, Donald S, et al. Differential lung ventilation after single-lung transplantation for emphysema. J Cardiothorac Vasc Anesth. 2002;16:459–62.

157. Fuehner T, Kuehn C, Welte T, et al. ICU care before and after lung transplantation. Chest. 2016;150:442–50.

158. Pilarczyk K, Carstens H, Heckmann J, et al. Safety and efficiency of percutaneous dilatational tracheostomy with direct bronchoscopic guidance for thoracic transplant recipients. Respir Care. 2016;61:235–42.

159. Najafizadeh K, Daneshvar A, Dezfouli AA, et al. Pulmonary artery stenosis shortly after lung transplantation: successful balloon dilation and stent insertion in one case. Ann Transplant. 2009;14:52–5.

160. Yserbyt J, Dooms C, Vos R, et al. Anastomotic airway complications after lung transplantation: risk factors, treatment modalities and outcome – a single-centre experience. Eur J Cardiothorac Surg. 2016;49:e1–8.

161. Yun JH, Lee SO, Jo KW, et al. Infections after lung transplantation: time of occurrence, sites, and microbiologic etiologies. Korean J Intern Med. 2015;30:506–14.

162. Parada MT, Alba A, Sepúlveda C. Early and late infections in lung transplantation patients. Transplant Proc. 2010;42:333–5.

163. Raghavan D, Gao A. Ahn C, et al Contemporary analysis of incidence of post-operative atrial fibrillation, its predictors, and association with clinical outcomes in lung transplantation. J Heart Lung Transplant. 2015;34:563–70.

164. Jacques F, El-Hamamsy I, Fortier A, et al. Acute renal failure following lung transplantation: risk factors, mortality and long-term consequences. Eur J Cardiothorac Surg. 2012;41:193–9.

165. Evans CF, Iacono AT, Sanchez PG, et al. Venous thromboembolic complications of lung transplantation: a contemporary single-institution review. Ann Thorac Surg. 2015;100: 2033–9.

166. Chan EG, Bianco V III, Richards T, et al. The ripple effect of a complication in lung transplantation: evidence for increased long-term survival. J Thorac Cardiovasc Surg. 2016;151: 1171–80.

167. Sweet SC. Induction therapy in lung transplantation. Transpl Int. 2013;26:696–703.

168. Tabarelli W, Bonatti H, Tabarelli D, et al. Long term complications following 54 consecutive lung transplants. J Thorac Dis. 2016;8:1234–44.

Anesthesia for the Patient with a Previous Lung Transplant

48

Maureen Cheng

Key Points
- Post lung transplantation, patients have an altered physiology which predisposes them to adverse respiratory events during the perioperative period.
- Anesthetic concerns include allograft function and airway complications, consequences of immuno-suppression, impact of surgery on airway management, and interference with lung function.
- For patients who have undergone single lung transplants, the effects of the differing compliances in the native and transplanted lung must be taken into account during positive-pressure ventilation.

Introduction

Lung transplantation is an established mode of treatment for patients with end-stage lung disease, and an increasing number of procedures are being performed annually [1]. Patients have a longer life expectancy due to current medical advances, with the median survival rate for a patient post double lung transplant (LT) being 7.3 years [1]. As such, there is an increasing likelihood of encountering these patients who may return for the management of transplant-related complications, surveillance procedures, or for the treatment of other surgical conditions. The physiological changes that occur post LT, implications of the primary pathology that necessitated transplantation, and interactions with immunosuppressive agents will have to be taken into consideration when formulating a perioperative management strategy.

M. Cheng (✉)
Department of Anesthesia and Intensive Care, Papworth Hospital, Papworth Everard, Cambridge, UK
e-mail: Maureen.cheng@nhs.net

Common Procedures After Lung Transplantation

Common surgical procedures can be broadly divided into those that are in the immediate postoperative period, related to transplant surveillance or surgical intervention for other non-transplant-related conditions.

Bleeding complications such as drainage of pericardial effusions or hemothoraces and those related to stenosis of pulmonary venous and arterial anastomoses [2] may necessitate a return to the operating room in the early postoperative period. As part of their follow-up, patients often require surveillance bronchoscopies for assessment of anastomotic healing or transbronchial biopsies to rule out infection and graft rejection.

Gastrointestinal issues that commonly present in the post transplant population include gastrointestinal reflux disease (GERD) (22.9%), infectious colitis (15.1%), gastroparesis (10.7%), peptic ulcer disease (8.8%), and cholecystitis (8.3%), necessitating surgery in over 20% of patients [3]. In addition, patients with cystic fibrosis have a predilection for complications such as pancreatitis and distal intestinal obstruction syndrome. Osteoporosis from the use of immunosuppressive agents may result in fractures or avascular necrosis of the hip requiring orthopedic fixation [4]. Lung volume reduction surgery on the native lung for single LT patients or pulmonary resections for carcinoma may also be performed.

Pulmonary Physiology Post Lung Transplantation

Pulmonary function rapidly improves in the first year following transplantation, though the degree of approximation to the recipient's ideal predicted spirometry values and diffusion capacity are dependent on whether a single or double LT is performed. In a study by Pochettino et al. [5], peak forced expiratory volume in 1 s (FEV1) values achieved by patients

© Springer Nature Switzerland AG 2019
P. Slinger (ed.), *Principles and Practice of Anesthesia for Thoracic Surgery*, https://doi.org/10.1007/978-3-030-00859-8_48

who underwent bilateral LT for chronic obstructive pulmonary disease (COPD) were 80% as opposed to 50% for single LT. Declines in the FEV1/forced vital capacity (FVC) ratio can reflect deteriorating graft function due to infection, rejection, or airway complications such as bronchial anastomotic stenosis. In the absence of other confounding conditions, a persistent decrease in the FEV1 ≤ 80% may represent the development of bronchiolitis obliterans syndrome (BOS) which is caused by progressive obliteration of small airways and reduction of the air passages to stenotic scar tissue [6].

Disruption of the sensory fibers of the vagus nerve results in a loss of the afferent signals for the cough reflex in the airways distal to the bronchial anastomosis and impairment of mucociliary clearance, though on follow-up Duarte et al. reported that the sensory innervation for the cough reflex may be restored in 6–12 months [7]. LT recipients have also been shown to have a high prevalence of GERD, which further increases following transplantation [4]. This results in an increased susceptibility to aspiration and the development of chest infections. Bronchial hyperreactivity is another common feature, with 24% of patients having a positive methacholine challenge test at 6 months post LT [8]. The pulmonary hypoxic vasoconstriction reflex is preserved [9]; however, the response to hypercarbia has been reported to be variable [10]. During the transection of the bronchi, there is also disruption of lymphatic drainage, and it has not been established whether there is eventual regeneration as demonstrated in animal studies [11], though LT patients are known to have a high incidence of pleural collections [12]. Preclinical studies have also shown that there is increased extravascular lung water prior to reestablishment of lymphatic drainage in canine models [13].

More than 90% of single LTs are performed for restrictive or obstructive causes [1]. Post implantation, the distribution of ventilation and perfusion is predominantly shifted toward the pulmonary allograft, and this effect is more marked in patients who have COPD than patients who have pulmonary fibrosis [14]. The effects of the differing compliances in the native and transplanted lung must be taken into account as this will affect the distribution of ventilation during positive-pressure ventilation via a single-lumen tube. Single LT patients with COPD have been reported to have a ratio of compliance in the native lung that is more than 2.6 times that of the transplanted lung [15], resulting in a larger proportion of the ventilatory flow being directed toward the native lung which can potentially cause hyperinflation and mediastinal shift.

Anesthetic Considerations

Preoperative assessment should focus on (1) allograft function and airway complications (2), consequences of immunosuppression, and (3) impact of surgery on airway management and interference with lung function.

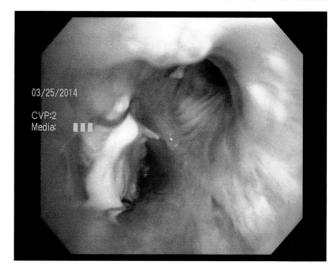

Fig. 48.1 Bronchus intermedius stenosis post LT. (Reproduced with permission [16])

A multidisciplinary approach should be taken in the perioperative care of LT patients, and it is important to liaise with the transplant team who is involved in the routine follow-up of the patient. A review of the patient's prior spirometry and diffusion capacity tests should be carried out to identify patients who have low pulmonary reserve. BOS accounts for a considerable proportion of deterioration in lung function and affects more than half of the recipients that survive beyond 5 years [6]. It is the main cause of mortality in patients who survive more than a year [1]. Airway complications such as bronchial stenosis which presents most commonly in the bronchus intermedius (Fig. 48.1), tracheobronchomalacia, and infectious complications resulting in necrosis, dehiscence, or fistula formation [17] should be highlighted particularly if lung isolation will be required. Recent episodes of chest infection may also require targeted antibiotic therapy.

It is important to ascertain if the patient has had any recent episodes of allograft rejection requiring pulsed steroid therapy or alterations to their immunosuppressive regimen as these may result in drug interactions and complications affecting various other organ systems. Common immunosuppressive regimens will include a glucocorticoid (prednisolone), a calcineurin inhibitor (cyclosporine or tacrolimus), and a nucleotide blocking agent (mycophenolate or azathioprine). Inhibitors of the mammalian target of rapamycin such as sirolimus or everolimus may be used in patients who have allograft rejection that is unresponsive to nucleotide blocking agents or are intolerant of the side effects of these medications. Therapeutic drug monitoring should be carried out in the perioperative period, and note should be taken of drug interactions such as an increase in drug levels of calcineurin inhibitors with the concurrent use of antifungals or macrolide antibiotics. Patients should continue their

Table 48.1 Adverse effects of commonly used immunosuppressive agents

Immunosuppressant	Adverse effect
Corticosteroids	
Prednisolone	Cushing's syndrome, hypertension, sodium and water retention Glucose intolerance Peptic ulcer disease Osteoporosis, avascular necrosis of femoral head
Calcineurin inhibitors	
Cyclosporine	Renal and hepatic dysfunction
Tacrolimus (FK-506)	Hypertension, hyperlipidemia Hyperkalemia, hypomagnesaemia, hyperuricemia Neurotoxicity (headache, visual disturbances, seizures) Glucose intolerance
Antimetabolites	
Mycophenolate mofetil (MMF)	Hyper-/hypotension, peripheral edema Hyperglycemia Hypokalemia, hypomagnesemia, and hypocalcemia Renal and hepatic dysfunction Hematological disorders (pancytopenia)
Azathioprine	Hepatotoxicity Leukopenia and thrombocytopenia

current immunosuppressive regime, and if unable to take orally, consultation should be made with the transplant team regarding conversion to intravenous formulations. The side effects of commonly used immunosuppressive agents are listed in Table 48.1. Within 5 years, the incidence of renal dysfunction is 53.6%, with 3.3% requiring chronic dialysis [1]. Standard preoperative management should be performed for the frequently encountered side effects of glucocorticoid and calcineurin inhibitor use such as diabetes mellitus (80.3%) and hypertension (37.4%) [1].

The choice of anesthetic technique should take into consideration the surgical procedure and the intraoperative effects on ventilation and pulmonary function. Orthopedic fixation procedures may be complicated by bone cement implantation syndrome that increases pulmonary vascular resistance and the risk of right ventricular failure [18]. Upper abdominal surgery results in diaphragmatic splinting which worsens chest wall mechanics.

If peripheral surgery is being performed, regional techniques provide the advantages of avoiding manipulation of the airway and the respiratory depressant effects of opiates. Peripheral nerve blocks can be performed for surgery on extremities; however, as phrenic nerve palsy occurs in approximately 3% of patients post LT [19], the use of techniques such as interscalene blocks that are known to affect the phrenic nerve may result in increased respiratory distress in patients who have preexisting impairment of diaphragmatic function. Central neuraxial techniques can be employed for orthopedic procedures such as hip replacements or as an

adjuvant analgesic technique for major abdominal or thoracic surgeries. Caution should be taken to avoid excessive fluid preloading, and patients should be carefully monitored for worsening respiratory parameters caused by impairment of intercostal muscle function.

Intraoperative Airway and Ventilation Management

In procedures which do not require tracheal intubation or muscle paralysis, a supraglottic device such as a laryngeal mask airway can be used with spontaneous ventilation, though severe mucositis from immunosuppressant use should first be excluded. Due to the high incidence of GERD in this patient population, a rapid sequence induction with tracheal intubation may be more appropriate for patients who have reflux disease.

Placement of a lung isolation device such as a double-lumen tube (DLT) may be indicated either to facilitate surgical exposure in thoracic surgery such as pulmonary resections or bullectomies or in patients who have had a single LT requiring controlled mechanical ventilation. The differential distribution of ventilation due to unequal compliances in the native and transplanted lung may result in over distention of the more compliant lung and can lead to serious complications such as mediastinal shift (Fig. 48.2) and barotrauma and tension pneumothoraces. Note should be taken of any preexisting airway complications, the most common being granulation tissue resulting in stenosis of bronchial anastomoses which may have been stented. During intubation, care should be taken with the use of airway adjuncts such as gum elastic bougies to avoid disruption of the bronchial anasto-

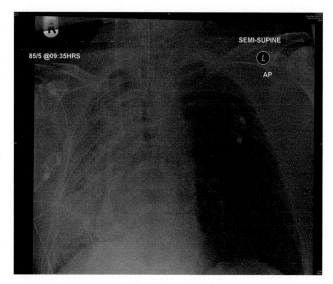

Fig. 48.2 Chest X-ray of a post right single lung transplant patient (COPD) with hyperinflation of the native lung causing mediastinal shift

moses or stents. The use of fiber-optic bronchoscopy is recommended to guide the placement of lung isolation devices. Ventilation strategies for patients post single LT will need to be tailored to accommodate the underlying primary pathology (obstructive vs restrictive). In single LT patients who require positive-pressure ventilation and whose primary pathology is obstructive, after the placement of a DLT, the ventilation settings for the allografted lung may be adjusted as per routine one-lung ventilation, and the native lung should receive only oxygen insufflation or low-pressure ventilation with a prolonged expiratory phase.

Intraoperative Management

The aims of a general anesthetic should be to maintain hemodynamic stability with the use of short-acting agents to facilitate an early extubation. It has been postulated that cyclosporine may enhance the neuromuscular blockade with some agents such as atracurium and vecuronium [20] though the mechanism remains unclear. At present, there have not been any studies which have conclusively demonstrated adverse drug interactions with other induction agents or neuromuscular blockers. Given the high incidence of renal dysfunction in LT patients, it would be prudent to avoid agents with a long duration of action and to perform depth of neuromuscular blockade monitoring to guide dosing. Drugs that may potentiate acute kidney injury such as nonsteroidal anti-inflammatory drugs should also be avoided.

The effects of absent lymphatic drainage have not been clearly demonstrated, and given that there is a significant incidence of renal dysfunction in this group of patients, the perioperative fluid balance should be carefully titrated. The use of a central venous catheter and close monitoring of the urinary output and fluid balance may be warranted depending on the clinical situation.

Patients who are on steroids as part of their immunosuppressive regime should receive their baseline steroid requirement. The perioperative supplementation of stress-dose steroids is controversial [21] but can be administered in patients who are undergoing major surgery to compensate for the suppression of the hypothalamic pituitary axis.

Postoperative Care

As this group of patients has compromised airway reflexes and is at risk of aspiration, care should be taken to ensure return of adequate airway control, and a careful assessment of respiratory function and residual neuromuscular blockade should be made prior to extubation. Depending on the patient's underlying residual lung function and scope and duration of the surgical procedure, an admission to the intensive care unit may be required for postoperative ventilation.

Clinical Case Discussion

Case: A 54-year-old male presents for elective laparoscopic cholecystectomy. He underwent right single lung transplantation for emphysema previously. He has no other major comorbidities. His preoperative pulmonary function tests show an FEV1 of 1.6 L (69% predicted), FVC 2.5 L (78% predicted), and DLCO of 84% predicted.

Questions

- What other transplant-related history is important?
- What are your intraoperative concerns, and how would you ventilate this patient for the surgical procedure?
- What are the postoperative analgesic options?

Transplant-Related History

It is important to ascertain if the patient has had any recent episodes of allograft rejection requiring pulsed high-dose steroid therapy or changes to his immunosuppressive medications as drug dose manipulations may have important interactions and effects on renal function. The perioperative dosing of immunosuppressant drugs should be discussed with the primary transplant team. Recent infective episodes requiring changes to his antimicrobial regimen should also be noted.

Intraoperative Concerns

A rapid sequence induction can be considered if he has a significant history of GERD. As the patient's native lung is highly compliant and prone to gas trapping, differential lung ventilation should be employed for this procedure. Positive-pressure ventilation through a single-lumen tube would result in preferential distribution of ventilation to the native lung resulting in hyperinflation, direct cardiac compression, and profound hypotension. A DLT should be positioned using fiber-optic bronchoscopic guidance to avoid disrupting the bronchial anastomoses. The ventilation settings for the allografted lung may be adjusted as per routine one-lung ventilation, and the native lung should receive only oxygen insufflation or low-pressure ventilation with a prolonged expiratory phase. The perioperative fluid balance should be carefully monitored and titrated to avoid fluid overload. Adequate reversal of neuromuscular blockade should be demonstrated, and care should be taken to ensure recovery of airway reflexes prior to extubation.

Postoperative Analgesia

Multimodal analgesia should be employed including paracetamol, opiates, and local anesthetic infiltration. If the procedure is converted from a laparoscopic to an open procedure, an epidural should be considered to avoid large doses of opiates. Nonsteroidal anti-inflammatory drugs should be avoided due to their potential nephrotoxicity when given in combination with calcineurin inhibitors.

References

1. Yusen RD, Edwards LB, Dipchand AI, Goldfarb SB, Kucheryavaya AY, Levvey BJ, et al. The registry of the International Society for Heart and Lung Transplantation: thirty-third adult lung and heart-lung transplant report-2016; focus theme: primary diagnostic indications for transplant. J Heart Lung Transplant. 2016;35(10):1170–84.
2. Siddique A, Bose AK, Ozalp F, Butt TA, Muse H, Morley KE, et al. Vascular anastomotic complications in lung transplantation: a single institution's experience. Interact Cardiovasc Thorac Surg. 2013;17(4):625–31.
3. Grass F, Schafer M, Cristaudi A, Berutto C, Aubert JD, Gonzalez M, et al. Incidence and risk factors of abdominal complications after lung transplantation. World J Surg. 2015;39(9):2274–81.
4. Lyu DM, Zamora MR. Medical complications of lung transplantation. Proc Am Thorac Soc. 2009;6(1):101–7.
5. Pochettino A, Kotloff RM, Rosengard BR, Arcasoy SM, Blumenthal NP, Kaiser LR, et al. Bilateral versus single lung transplantation for chronic obstructive pulmonary disease: intermediate-term results. Ann Thorac Surg. 2000;70(6):1813–8; discussion 8–9.
6. Meyer KC, Raghu G, Verleden GM, Corris PA, Aurora P, Wilson KC, et al. An international ISHLT/ATS/ERS clinical practice guideline: diagnosis and management of bronchiolitis obliterans syndrome. Eur Respir J. 2014;44(6):1479–503.
7. Duarte AG, Myers AC. Cough reflex in lung transplant recipients. Lung. 2012;190(1):23–7.
8. Stanbrook MB, Kesten S. Bronchial hyperreactivity after lung transplantation predicts early bronchiolitis obliterans. Am J Respir Crit Care Med. 1999;160(6):2034–9.
9. Robin ED, Theodore J, Burke CM, Oesterle SN, Fowler MB, Jamieson SW, et al. Hypoxic pulmonary vasoconstriction persists in the human transplanted lung. Clin Sci (Lond). 1987;72(3):283–7.
10. Frost AE, Zamel N, McClean P, Grossman R, Patterson GA, Maurer JR. Hypercapnic ventilatory response in recipients of double-lung transplants. Am Rev Respir Dis. 1992;146(6):1610–2.
11. Ruggiero R, Muz J, Fietsam R Jr, Thomas GA, Welsh RJ, Miller JE, et al. Reestablishment of lymphatic drainage after canine lung transplantation. J Thorac Cardiovasc Surg. 1993;106(1):167–71.
12. Arndt A, Boffa DJ. Pleural space complications associated with lung transplantation. Thorac Surg Clin. 2015;25(1):87–95.
13. Cowan GM Jr, Staub NC, Edmunds LH,J. Changes in the fluid compartments and dry weights of reimplanted dog lungs. J Appl Physiol. 1976;40(6):962–70.
14. Chacon RA, Corris PA, Dark JH, Gibson GJ. Comparison of the functional results of single lung transplantation for pulmonary fibrosis and chronic airway obstruction. Thorax. 1998;53(1):43–9.
15. Mitchell JB, Shaw AD, Donald S, Farrimond JG. Differential lung ventilation after single-lung transplantation for emphysema. J Cardiothorac Vasc Anesth. 2002;16(4):459–62.
16. Rosenblatt W, Popescu W. Master techniques in upper and lower airway management. 1st ed: Wolters Kluwer; 2015.
17. Santacruz JF, Mehta AC. Airway complications and management after lung transplantation: ischemia, dehiscence, and stenosis. Proc Am Thorac Soc. 2009;6(1):79–93.
18. Donaldson AJ, Thomson HE, Harper NJ, Kenny NW. Bone cement implantation syndrome. Br J Anaesth. 2009;102(1):12–22.
19. Maziak DE, Maurer JR, Kesten S. Diaphragmatic paralysis: a complication of lung transplantation. Ann Thorac Surg. 1996;61(1):170–3.
20. Sidi A, Kaplan RF, Davis RF. Prolonged neuromuscular blockade and ventilatory failure after renal transplantation and cyclosporine. Can J Anaesth. 1990;37(5):543–8.
21. Marik PE, Varon J. Requirement of perioperative stress doses of corticosteroids: a systematic review of the literature. Philadelphia, United States. Arch Surg. 2008;143(12):1222–6.

Anesthesia for Pulmonary Thromboendarterectomy

Timothy M. Maus and Dalia Banks

Key Points
- Chronic thromboembolic pulmonary hypertension (CTEPH) results from recurrent or residual intraluminal organized fibrotic clot leading to increased pulmonary vascular resistance (PVR), severe PH, and eventually right heart failure (RHF).
- Incidence of thromboembolic disease is difficult to estimate because of the nonspecific nature of the presenting symptoms and the lack of public awareness of the disorder.
- Pulmonary thromboendarterectomy is an endarterectomy of the proximal pulmonary vascular tree and is the preferred treatment for chronic thromboembolic pulmonary hypertension.
- The most common presenting symptom of chronic thromboembolic pulmonary hypertension is exertional dyspnea. The diagnosis is confirmed with echocardiography, right-sided cardiac catheterization, and pulmonary angiogram.
- Most common complications of PTE procedure are reperfusion pulmonary edema (RPE), pulmonary hemorrhage, and persistent pulmonary hypertension

- Riociguat is the first FDA-approved medication for treating certain patient subgroups with chronic thromboembolic pulmonary hypertension (CTEPH).
- Balloon pulmonary angioplasty is an alternative approach to thromboendarterectomy surgery in patients with surgically inaccessible chronic thromboembolic disease.

Introduction

Pulmonary thromboendarterectomy (PTE), a complete endarterectomy of the pulmonary vascular tree, is the definitive treatment for chronic thromboembolic pulmonary hypertension (CTEPH). Pulmonary embolism (PE) is a relatively common cardiovascular event, and in a small percentage of cases, it leads to a chronic condition in which repeated microemboli as well as ongoing inflammatory response lead to accumulation of connective and elastic tissue on the endovascular surface of the pulmonary vessels [1, 2].

Pulmonary thromboembolism is a significant cause of morbidity and mortality worldwide. Acute PE has been estimated to occur in approximately 63 per 100,000 patients per year in the United States with in-hospital mortality occurring in 11.1% [3–5]. These statistics probably represent underestimates; however, since in 70–80% of patients in whom the primary cause of death was PE, the diagnosis was unsuspected premortem [6].

If left untreated, the prognosis for patients with CTEPH is poor. In fact, once the mean pulmonary pressure in patients with CTEPH reaches 50 mmHg or more, the 3-year mortality approaches 90% [7]. Although medical management can provide temporary symptomatic relief, it is noncurative and generally ineffective. The only potentially curative options are lung transplantation and PTE, with PTE preferred because of its favorable long-term morbidity and mortality profile.

Electronic Supplementary Material The online version of this chapter (https://doi.org/10.1007/978-3-030-00859-8_49) contains supplementary material, which is available to authorized users.

T. M. Maus (✉) · D. Banks
Department of Anesthesiology, University of California San Diego Health, La Jolla, CA, USA
e-mail: tmaus@ucsd.edu

This chapter, based in large part on the experience at UCSD, provides a review of the natural history of CTEPH, a description of PTE, a discussion of anesthetic factors unique to PTE and CTEPH, and a case discussion on managing massive pulmonary hemorrhage, one of the feared complications of the operation.

Classification of Pulmonary Hypertension

Pulmonary hypertension (PH) is classified by the World Health Organization into five types known as the Evian classification [8]: (1) pulmonary arterial hypertension (PAH); (2) pulmonary venous hypertension typically from left heart disease; (3) PH due to respiratory disease such as chronic bronchitis, emphysema, and hypoxemia; (4) pulmonary hypertension due to embolic disease (CTEPH); and (5) PH caused by diseases affecting the pulmonary vasculature.

Further classification of pulmonary hypertension by Galie et al. [9, 10] is defined by the presence of precapillary and postcapillary PH. Precapillary PH as assessed by right heart catheterization is characterized by mean pulmonary artery pressure (mPAP) >25 mmHg; normal pulmonary capillary wedge pressure (PCWP), i.e., <15 mmHg; and an elevated pulmonary vascular resistance (PVR) more than 300 dynes·s·cm^{-5}. Postcapillary PH, often due to left heart disease, is the most frequent form of PH and is characterized by mPAP >25 mmHg, PCWP >15 mmHg, and normal PVR [11].

Chronic Thromboembolic Pulmonary Hypertension (CTEPH)

Most cases of acute PE resolve within weeks and the patient recovers to their previous level of function. However, for unknown reasons, embolic resolution is sometimes incomplete. If the acute emboli are not lysed in 1–2 weeks, the embolic material becomes attached to the pulmonary arterial and arteriolar walls [12]. With time, the embolic material progressively becomes converted to connective and elastic tissue [13]. This chronic obstructive disease may lead to a small vessel arteriolar vasculopathy characterized by excessive smooth muscle cell proliferation in pulmonary arterioles. This vasculopathy is seen in the remaining open vessels, which are subjected to long exposure to high flow and pressure. Pulmonary hypertension results from both mechanical obstruction and from small vessel vasculopathy. Once pulmonary hypertension has developed, patients require expeditious treatment. CTEPH patients generally do not respond well to medical management, which is reserved for patients who are not surgical candidates

[14–16]. The only curative option is to proceed with surgical removal of the thromboembolic material by means of endarterectomy.

Incidence

The incidence of pulmonary hypertension caused by PE remains unknown. It has been estimated that there are more than 500,000 survivors of symptomatic episodes of acute PE per year [17]. One recent prospective study indicates that thromboembolic disease develops in as many as 3.8% of patients with acute PE [18]. Thus, a conservative estimate is that 19,000 individuals progress to CTEPH in the United States each year. Considering that only 200–300 PTEs are performed annually worldwide, it is clear that acute PE and CTEPH are under-diagnosed, and PTE is underutilized.

Etiologic Factors

No clear etiology has been defined for the development of CTEPH, although hypercoagulability is certainly a risk. Lupus anticoagulant may be detected in approximately 10% of chronic thromboembolic patients, and 20% carry anticardiolipin antibodies, lupus anticoagulant, or both [19]. A recent study has demonstrated that the plasma level of factor VIII, a protein that is associated with both primary and recurrent venous thromboembolism, is elevated in 39% of patients with CTEPH. Analyses of plasma proteins in patients with chronic thromboembolic disease have shown that fibrin from these patients is resistant to thrombolysis in vitro. In this study, the fibrin β chain N-terminus was particularly resistant to thrombolysis, suggesting that it could be responsible for thrombus nonresolution [20].

Case reports and anecdotal experience have suggested links between chronic thromboembolism and previous splenectomy, permanent intravenous catheters, and ventriculoatrial shunts for the treatment of hydrocephalus or chronic inflammatory conditions. In addition to these observations, associations with sickle cell disease, hereditary stomatocytosis, and the Klippel-Trenaunay syndrome have been described [21]. However, the vast majority of cases of CTEPH cannot be traced to a specific known coagulation defect or underlying medical condition.

Pathology and Pathogenesis

Although most individuals with CTEPH are unaware of a past thromboembolic or deep venous thrombosis, CTEPH likely stems from acute embolic episodes that do not completely resolve. Why some patients fail to resolve their emboli is unclear, but a variety of factors may play a role. The volume of acute embolic material may simply overwhelm the lytic mechanisms. The total occlusion of a major arterial branch may prevent lytic material from reaching, and therefore dissolving, the embolus completely. The emboli may be made of substances that cannot be lysed by normal mechanisms. These may include organized fibrous thrombus, fat, or tumor emboli, from stomach, breast, kidney, and right atrial (myxoma) origin. The lytic mechanisms themselves may be abnormal, or some patients may have a hypercoaguable state. Hypercoagulability may result in spontaneous thrombosis within the pulmonary vascular bed, embolization, or lead to proximal propagation of embolic material. With time, the increased pressure and flow of redirected pulmonary blood flow in the previously normal pulmonary vascular bed can create a vasculopathy in the arterioles, similar to that of the Eisenmenger syndrome. This, as well as resulting right-sided heart failure, can lead to an inoperable, lethal situation, so early surgical intervention is recommended.

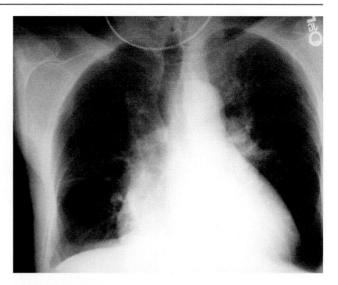

Fig. 49.1 Chest radiograph of a patient with advanced chronic thromboembolic pulmonary hypertension. Cardiomegaly, hilar fullness, and decrease in vascularity of the lung fields are apparent

Clinical Presentation

The most common symptom of CTEPH, as with pulmonary hypertension in general, is exertional dyspnea. This dyspnea is out of proportion to abnormalities found on clinical examination. Syncope is another common symptom of pulmonary hypertension, particularly in patients with advanced disease. Other common findings include chest tightness, hemoptysis, peripheral edema, and early satiety.

The physical signs of pulmonary hypertension are the same regardless of the underlying pathophysiology. Jugular venous distension is common, with prominent V waves. The right ventricle is usually palpable near the lower left sternal border, and pulmonary valve closure may be audible in the second intercostal space. Patients with advanced disease may be cyanotic. A systolic murmur characteristic of tricuspid regurgitation is common, and murmurs over the lung fields resulting from turbulent flow in the pulmonary vessels may also be appreciated.

Workup may include chest radiograph (CXR), pulmonary function testing, right heart catheterization with pulmonary angiography, high-resolution magnetic resonance imaging, arterial blood gas analysis, ventilation/perfusion scanning, and echocardiography. CXR may show lung opacities suggestive of previous scarring, hyperlucent areas suggestive of regional decreased blood flow, right-sided cardiomegaly, and dilatation of the pulmonary vessels (Fig. 49.1). Diffusing capacity (DLCO) is often reduced and may be the only abnormality on pulmonary function testing. Pulmonary arterial pressure is elevated, sometimes being supra-systemic. Resting cardiac output is often low, with reduced pulmonary

arterial oxygen saturation. Many patients exhibit hypoxia, particularly with exercise; room air arterial oxygen tension ranges between 50 and 83 torr, the average being 65 torr [22]. CO_2 tension is often slightly reduced, although dead space ventilation is increased. Ventilation-perfusion studies show moderate mismatch but correlate poorly with the degree of pulmonary vascular obstruction [23].

Transthoracic echocardiography is often the first study to provide clear evidence of pulmonary hypertension. An estimate of pulmonary artery systolic pressure is often provided by Doppler of the tricuspid regurgitant envelope. Echocardiographic findings vary depending on the stage of the disease and include right ventricular enlargement, leftward displacement of the interventricular septum, and encroachment of the enlarged right ventricle on the left ventricular cavity with abnormal systolic and diastolic function of the left ventricle. Thankfully, many of these abnormalities resolve after successful PTE [24]. Contrast echocardiography may demonstrate a persistent foramen ovale, the result of high right atrial pressures opening the previously closed intra-atrial communication.

Pulmonary angiography is the gold standard for defining pulmonary vascular anatomy and is performed to confirm the diagnosis and to determine the location and surgical accessibility of thromboembolic disease. In angiographic imaging, thrombi appear as unusual filling defects, pouches, webs, or bands, or completely thrombosed vessels that may resemble congenital absence of a vessel (Fig. 49.2). More recently, high-resolution computed tomography scanning [25], SPECT-CT fusion imaging [26], and magnetic resonance angiography [27] have been used successfully to screen patients with suspected thromboembolic disease.

Fig. 49.2 Pulmonary angiogram showing perfusion defects (*arrows*) and large hyperlucent areas result from pulmonary vascular obstruction

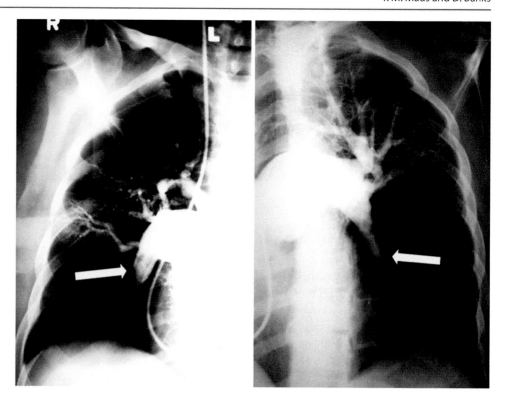

In approximately 10% of cases, the differential diagnosis between primary pulmonary hypertension and distal and small vessel pulmonary thromboembolic disease remains unclear and difficult to establish. In these patients, pulmonary angioscopy is often helpful. The pulmonary angioscope is a fiberoptic scope that is placed through a central line into the pulmonary artery. The tip contains a balloon that is then filled with saline and pushed against the vessel wall. A bloodless field can thus be obtained to view the pulmonary artery wall. The classic appearance of chronic pulmonary thromboembolic disease by angioscopy consists of intimal thickening, with intimal irregularity and scarring, and webs across small vessels. The presence of embolic disease, occlusion of vessels, or the presence of thrombotic material is diagnostic.

Many CTEPH patients have longstanding pulmonary hypertension; as many as 37% of them receive medical pulmonary vasodilator therapy [28]. This therapy may consist of phosphodiesterase 5 inhibition (e.g., sildenafil) [29], endothelin-1 inhibition (e.g., bosentan) [30, 31], and prostacyclin analogs (e.g., iloprost, flolan, remodulin) [32–34]. It is prudent to continue these medications preoperatively and to consider their use postoperatively if the surgical result is suboptimal. Abrupt cessation of a prostacyclin analog can result in potentially catastrophic rebound pulmonary hypertension [35]. If a patient presents with an epoprostenol (Flolan™) infusion, one approach is to continue this infusion throughout the pre-CPB period, discontinue it during CPB, and restart it after CPB if the surgical result is suboptimal. If the surgical result is good, keep it available to be restarted if pulmonary hypertension develops postoperatively.

The Surgical Procedure

Surgical Approach and Technique

PTE, being an endarterectomy of the proximal pulmonary vascular tree, is performed through a midline sternotomy and requires cardiopulmonary bypass (CPB) with deep hypothermic circulatory arrest (DHCA). Although used in the past, lateral thoracotomy is suboptimal [36]. Median sternotomy allows treatment of both pulmonary arteries, which is necessary in almost all cases [36, 37]. The use of CPB with periods of complete circulatory arrest provides the bloodless operative field necessary for complete meticulous lobar and segmental dissections [38].

The procedure follows four basic but important principles. (1) The endarterectomy must be bilateral; therefore the approach is through a median sternotomy. (2) Identification of the correct dissection plane is crucial, and at times the plane of dissection has to be identified in each of the segmental and subsegmental branches. (3) Perfect visualization is essential, and a thorough distal endarterectomy cannot be performed without the use of circulatory arrest. Circulatory arrest is usually limited to 20 min at a time, and supported by cooling to 18 °C. (4) A complete endarterectomy all the way to the distal ends of the smallest vessels is essential.

Following median sternotomy, CPB is established with cannulation of the ascending aorta and the inferior and superior vena cava. Cooling is instituted immediately. A gradient of not more than 10 °C is maintained between the arterial blood and the bladder/rectal temperature. This allows an even distribution of cooling and warming, as well as helping to prevent release of gas bubbles into the circulation upon rewarming. Pulmonary artery and pulmonary venous vents are inserted. During the cooling phase venous oxygen saturation increases, with a saturation of 80% typical at 25 °C, and 90% at 20 °C. Hemodilution to a hematocrit of 18–25% is utilized to decrease blood viscosity, optimize capillary blood flow, and promote uniform cooling. Complete cooling typically requires 45–60 min, depending on the size and perfusion characteristics of the patient.

As core temperature approaches 20 °C and tympanic membrane temperature approaches 16–18 °C, the aorta is cross-clamped. Immediately after aortic cross-clamping, cardioplegia solution is administered into the aortic root. Additional myocardial protection is afforded by a circulating cold water cooling jacket around the heart. An incision is made in the right pulmonary artery with the surgeon standing on the patient's left. The right pulmonary artery endarterectomy plane is established and dissection continues until bronchial artery flow impairs good visualization. At this point circulatory arrest is imperative. Bronchial flow in these patients is frequently substantial and without circulatory arrest complete endarterectomy cannot be accomplished.

Circulatory arrest is limited to 20-min epochs. An experienced surgeon can usually accomplish the entire unilateral endarterectomy within this time period. If additional arrest time is necessary, reperfusion is carried out at 18 °C core temperature for a minimum of 10 min. At the completion of the endarterectomy, perfusion is reestablished, while the pulmonary artery incision is closed.

Following a 10-min period of hypothermic perfusion, the left pulmonary artery is incised, and an endarterectomy is performed. Following completion of the left endarterectomy, a patent foramen ovale (PFO), if present, is repaired. Any additional procedures such as coronary artery bypass grafting or valve replacement can be performed during the rewarming period.

Surgical Subtypes

There are five categories of pulmonary occlusive disease related to disease extent that can be appreciated. The UCSD classification system describes these different levels based on the thromboembolic specimen and corresponds to the degree of difficulty of the endarterectomy [39] (Table 49.1).

Level 0 represents no evidence of chronic thromboembolic disease present; in other words, there has been a misdiagnosis, or perhaps one lung is completely unaffected by

Table 49.1 UCSD CTE classification

Level I Level I C	Chronic thromboembolic disease in the main pulmonary arteries Complete occlusion of one main pulmonary artery with chronic thromboembolic disease
Level II	Chronic thromboembolic disease starting at the level of lobar arteries or in the main descending pulmonary arteries
Level III	Chronic thromboembolic disease starting at the level of the segmental arteries
Level IV	Chronic thromboembolic disease starting at the level of the subsegmental arteries
Level 0	No evidence of chronic thromboembolic disease in either lung

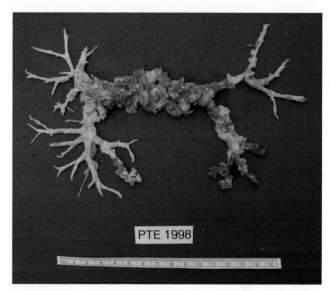

Fig. 49.3 Endarterectomy specimen of Type I thromboembolic disease. Thrombus and fibrous connective tissue were removed from much of the pulmonary vascular tree

thromboembolic disease, both of which are rare. In this entity there is intrinsic small vessel disease, although secondary thrombus may occur as a result of stasis. Small vessel disease may be unrelated to thromboembolic events ("primary" pulmonary hypertension) or occurs in relation to thromboembolic hypertension as a result of a high-flow or high-pressure state in previously unaffected vessels similar to the generation of Eisenmenger's syndrome. We believe that there may also be sympathetic "cross-talk" from an affected contralateral side or stenotic areas in the same lung. Level I (Fig. 49.3) disease refers to the situation in which thromboembolic material is present and is readily visible on the opening of the main left and right pulmonary arteries. A subset of level I disease, level Ic, is complete occlusion of either the left or right pulmonary artery and non-perfusion of that lung. Complete occlusion may present an entirely different disease, especially when it is unilateral and on the left side. In level II (Fig. 49.4), the disease starts at the lobar or

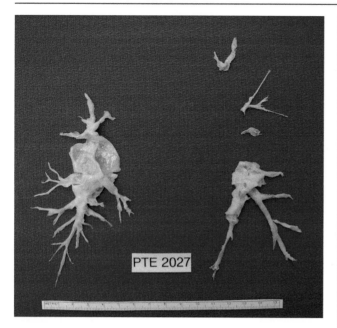

Fig. 49.4 Endarterectomy specimen of Type 2 thromboembolic disease. Fibrous connective tissue was removed from much of the pulmonary vascular tree

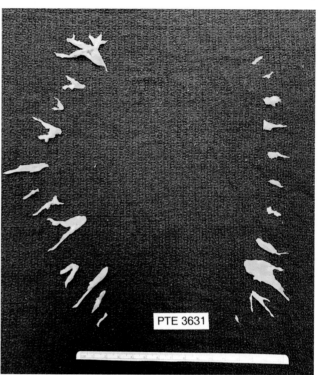

Fig. 49.6 Endarterectomy specimen of Type 4 thromboembolic disease. Only subsegmental fibrous connective tissue was found at surgery

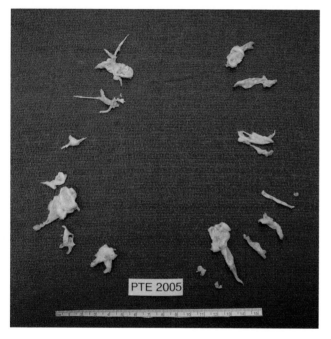

Fig. 49.5 Endarterectomy specimen of Type 3 thromboembolic disease. Only distal fibrous connective tissue was found at surgery

Anesthetic Management

Setup and Preparation

A typical "setup" for a pulmonary endarterectomy includes preparation for transesophageal echocardiography (TEE), pulmonary artery catheterization, hemodynamic support, cerebral function monitoring, and a cooling device for head cooling. On the day of surgery, a large bore peripheral intravenous catheter and a radial arterial catheter are inserted. The patient may then be given light sedation (with caution) and brought to the operating room. Even small amounts of sedation may cause respiratory depression, leading to a catastrophic rise in pulmonary vascular resistance. Supplemental oxygen should be considered in the preoperative area, particularly if sedation is administered.

Anesthetic Induction and Pre-CPB Management

After thorough preoxygenation and ventilation encouragement, anesthetic induction can be accomplished with midazolam, fentanyl, and a muscle relaxant. Myocardial depressants such as propofol should be used with extreme caution, if at all. In cases of tenuous hemodynamics,

intermediate level arteries and the main pulmonary arteries are unaffected. Level III (Fig. 49.5) disease is limited to thromboembolic disease originating in the segmental vessels only. Level IV (Fig. 49.6) is disease of the subsegmental vessels, with no other disease appreciated at more proximal levels. Level III and level IV disease present the most challenging surgical situation. The disease is very distal and confined to the segmental and subsegmental branches.

etomidate may be useful because of its relative lack of cardiovascular depression. A pulmonary artery catheter is generally placed after induction rather than before, since the hemodynamic status and goals are usually known by the time the patient reaches the operating room. Also, lying awake in the supine or Trendelenburg position may be stressful for patients with advanced disease, occasionally leading to cardiorespiratory instability. If preoperative transthoracic echocardiography shows evidence of right atrial or right ventricular thrombi, TEE is performed immediately after induction, prior to placement of a pulmonary artery catheter.

Although some patients with CTEPH presenting for pulmonary endarterectomy have associated left ventricular pathology, most do not. Hemodynamic management is thus centered on right ventricular function. The right ventricle is usually hypertrophic and dilated, as is the right atrium. Because of the high right-sided pressures, the coronary blood supply to right ventricle is at risk. Maintenance of adequate systemic vascular resistance (SVR), inotropic state, and normal sinus rhythm serve to preserve systemic hemodynamics as well as right ventricular coronary perfusion. The preoperative cardiac catheterization data, including cardiac output, pulmonary vascular resistance (PVR), patency of coronary arteries, and right ventricular end-diastolic pressure (RVEDP) are useful in planning the induction sequence. Elevated RVEDP (>14 mmHg), severe tricuspid regurgitation, and preoperative PVR > 1000 dyne-s-cm^{-5} are signs of impending decompensation. In such cases inotropic support (e.g., dopamine or epinephrine), as well as vasopressor support (e.g., phenylephrine or vasopressin), should be considered for the induction and pre-CPB period. Generally, patients with CTEPH have fixed PVR because of mechanical obstruction. However, high PVR can still be exacerbated by factors that increase PVR (e.g., hypoxia, hypercarbia, acidosis, pain, and anxiety). Thus, these stressors should be minimized during induction and immediate pre-CPB period. Attempts to lower the PVR pharmacologically (e.g., nitroglycerin, nitroprusside) should be avoided as they have minimal efficacy in treating CTEPH and can dangerously jeopardize the coronary perfusion pressure to the right ventricular myocardium. This can rapidly lead to hypotension and cardiovascular collapse. Direct pulmonary vasodilators such as nitric oxide and prostaglandins, which may be useful in the medical management of patients with other types of pulmonary hypertension, generally show limited benefit for pulmonary endarterectomy patients in the perioperative period. The effects of phenylephrine on right ventricular performance in pulmonary hypertension has been studied by Rich et al. [40] They documented improved right ventricular performance (increased MAP, coronary artery perfusion pressure, maintained cardiac output) with phenylephrine administration. Since hemodynamic collapse can occur very rapidly in these patients, it is particularly important to treat

decreases in blood pressure and heart rate rapidly and aggressively. The muscle relaxant is chosen according to airway issues and desired hemodynamic response. Pancuronium, rocuronium, and vecuronium have all been used successfully in these patients.

If the superior vena cava is patent, an internal jugular introducer and pulmonary artery catheter are inserted. Placement of the pulmonary artery catheter may be difficult because of right atrial and right ventricular dilatation, as well as tricuspid regurgitation and pulmonary artery pathology. Transesophageal echocardiography has been shown to be helpful in the live guidance of pulmonary arterial catheter placement in CTEPH patients [41].

Next, a femoral arterial catheter is placed. This is because, in cases involving prolonged hypothermic CPB, the systemic arterial pressure is significantly underestimated by the radial artery catheter in the post-CPB period [42]. This phenomenon has been noticed by others [43] and appears to be accentuated by prolonged periods of profound hypothermia. It is not uncommon for a mean arterial pressure (MAP) gradient of as much as 20 mmHg to develop after CPB. The mechanism is unclear; causes involving peripheral vasoconstriction and vasodilatation have been proposed [44]. Although the time course for recovery of the radial arterial wave is variable, typically the radial and femoral pressure measurements show reasonable agreement by the morning following surgery [42].

TEE is valuable in monitoring and assessing cardiac function and filling during PTE. The most useful views include the transgastric mid-papillary short-axis view to assess left ventricular size and septal motion (Fig. 49.7; Video 49.1); the midesophageal four-chamber view for relative chamber sizes, intracardiac thrombus, and tricuspid valve assessment (Fig. 49.8; Video 49.2); the midesophageal bicaval view (interatrial septal integrity, thrombosis of the great veins); and the midesophageal ascending aortic short-axis view for

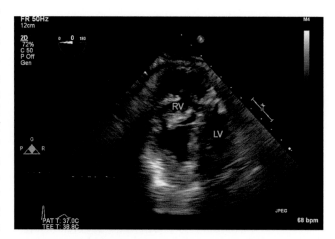

Fig. 49.7 Transgastric mid-papillary short-axis view in a PTE patient with a massive enlarged right ventricle and a shifted interventricular septum. RV right ventricle, LV left ventricle

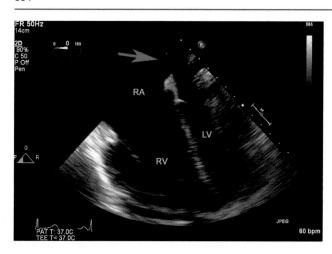

Fig. 49.8 Midesophageal four-chamber view in a PTE patient with a severely dilated right atrium and right ventricle. Note the shifted interventricular septum and interatrial septum (*red arrow*) as well as the underfilled left heart. RA right atrium, RV right ventricle, LV left ventricle

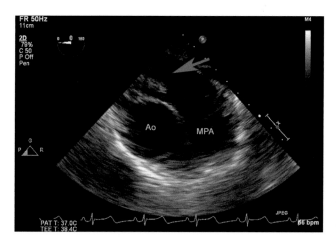

Fig. 49.9 Midesophageal ascending aortic short-axis view demonstrating thromboembolic material at the origin of the right pulmonary artery (*red arrow*). Ao ascending aorta, MPA main pulmonary artery

size of the pulmonary artery (PA) and detecting PA thrombus. It is not uncommon to find substantial dilatation of the PA, as well as thromboembolic material (Fig. 49.9; Video 49.3). The integrity of the interatrial septum is investigated with the use of an agitated saline test. PFO is present in 25–35% of PTE patients [45]. If a PFO is present, it is repaired, since, postoperatively some patients may experience high right-sided pressures. Such pressures, in the presence of a PFO, could lead to right-to-left shunt and hypoxemia.

Processed electroencephalogram (EEG) is monitored throughout the procedure. This allows confirmation of minimal oxygen utilization of the brain prior to circulatory arrest (isoelectric EEG), as well as monitoring of level of consciousness during normothermia. In our institution the

SedLine monitor (Masimo, Irvine, CA), a four-channel processed electroencephalograph monitor, provides monitoring of the isoelectric electroencephalogram and confirmation of minimal oxygen utilization of the brain before circulatory arrest. Temperature monitoring is accomplished with a urinary catheter with temperature monitoring capabilities, a rectal probe, and tympanic membrane probe, which provides an estimation of brain temperature [46]. The rectal and bladder probes estimate core temperature, and the PA catheter measures blood temperature, allowing quantification of thermal gradients.

During the precardiopulmonary bypass period, the head is wrapped in a circulating cold water blanket. The water, maintained at 4 °C, is circulated through the blanket by an electric pump. This system (Polar Care, Breg, Inc., Vista, CA), originally designed as a "knee wrap" for orthopedic and physical medicine purposes, is easily applied to the head. It contains a thermometer within the fluid circulation system for confirmation of adequate blanket cooling, as well as a flow control dial. This head wrap is used in all PTEs at UCSD, with no complications. It is our belief that the blanket provides better cooling to the surface of the cranium, particularly posterior regions, than application of ice bags, and is easier to apply.

If the hematocrit and hemodynamics permit, 1–2 units of autologous blood are harvested for reinfusion after CPB. Another consideration is prior exposure and response to heparin. Because of prior exposure, some patients develop heparin-induced antiplatelet antibodies, causing a propensity to heparin-induced thrombocytopenia. Anticoagulation for these patients has been managed with preheparin administration of iloprost (a prostacyclin analog), heparinoid [37, 38], hirudin, and bivalirudin [47, 48]. Most recently, we have had success using the platelet-inhibitor tirofiban [49, 50].

Management of Deep Hypothermic Circulatory Arrest (DHCA)

Prior to DHCA mannitol (12.5 g), methylprednisolone sodium succinate (30 mg/kg; maximum dose of 3 g), and phenytoin sodium (15 mg/kg) are administered. Mannitol is used to promote an osmotic diuresis, minimize cellular edema, and for free radical scavenging. Methylprednisolone theoretically functions as a cell-membrane stabilizer and anti-inflammatory agent. Phenytoin may provide some protection against postoperative seizures. Historically sodium thiopental (6 mg/kg) was administered as a cerebral protection agent. Due to sodium thiopental's lack of commercial availability, propofol (2.5 mg/kg) is utilized to ensure complete isoelectricity immediately prior to instituting deep hypothermic circulatory arrest. While there is no clear clinical evidence supporting added benefit of propofol or barbiturate administration for DHCA, we give propofol for three reasons: (1) brain cooling may be uneven or incomplete, (2) cerebral emboli may occur during rewarming (pulmonary endarterectomy is an "open-chamber" procedure), and (3) even at 18 °C we often notice sparse EEG activity which is then abolished with administration of propofol.

After assurance of an isoelectric EEG, tympanic membrane temperature 18 °C or less, and a bladder or rectal temperature of 20 °C or less, circulatory arrest is instituted. At this time, all monitoring lines are turned off to the patient, decreasing the risk of entraining air into the vasculature during exsanguination. The duration of DHCA is limited to 20 min epochs, typically one epoch per left and right pulmonary endarterectomy, respectively. If additional time is needed on either side, hypothermic circulation is reestablished for 10 min prior to additional periods of DHCA.

Monitoring jugular venous bulb oxygen saturation may be useful in detecting adverse cerebral effects of rapid warming [51] or for prognosticating postoperative neurologic function [52]. However, since our warming rate is slow, and our neurologic results are good, we choose not to expose our patients to the added risks of jugular venous bulb catheterization. Surface cerebral oximetry is a noninvasive technique applying near-infrared spectroscopy to measure hemoglobin oxygen saturation in the brain underlying the sensor. The number reported by the monitor is rSO_2, which is a measure of the mixed arterial and venous blood in the brain. Since venous blood volume accounts for 70–90% of total cerebral blood volume, rSO_2 reflects oxygen saturation of venous blood and thus the relationship between cerebral oxygen metabolism (demand) and cerebral blood flow (supply). In healthy volunteers, rSO_2 has been found to correlate with jugular venous saturation [53, 54], although, during cardiac surgery, the correlation between the two monitors is not always close [55]. Ongoing research in this area and additional neuropsychiatric outcome studies may prove this monitor useful during the conduct of DHCA.

Post-DHCA Rewarming

A 10° gradient between blood and bladder/rectal temperature is not exceeded during rewarming, and the perfusate temperature is never greater than 37.5°. Warming too quickly promotes systemic gas bubble formation, cerebral oxygen desaturation, and uneven warming. Rewarming times are variably related to the patient's weight and systemic perfusion; 90–120 min is usually required to achieve a core temperature of 36.5 °C. Adequate and even rewarming aims to prevent "after-drop", whereby uneven rewarming redistributes post-CPB leading to a drop in temperature with the attendant risks of hypothermia.

Separation from CPB

With the following few exceptions, the process of separation from CPB is similar to other surgeries involving CPB. End-tidal carbon dioxide ($ETCO_2$) is a poor measure of ventilation adequacy in these patients both pre- and post-CPB, since dead space ventilation is an integral part of the disease process. After successful surgery, the arterial-$ETCO_2$ gradient may be decreased compared to preoperative values, but the time course for this improvement is variable often with weeks to months for complete resolution. Aggressive hyperventilation is utilized due to the metabolic acidosis that may occur from cardiopulmonary bypass, hypothermia, and deep hypothermic circulatory arrest. The anesthesiologist checks the endotracheal tube for frothy sputum or bleeding because reperfusion pulmonary edema and airway bleeding, two of the most dreaded complications of the procedure, may manifest at this time [56]. Suction of the endotracheal tube during rewarming (while the surgical PA vent remains in place) allows the early identification of bleeding prior to pressurization of the pulmonary arterial circuit. While still on CPB, the TEE is used to detect intracavitary air as well as to evaluate left and right ventricular function.

For separation from CPB, modest inotropic support (e.g., dopamine, 3–7 μg/kg/min) is often necessary because of the long hypothermic period and long aortic cross-clamp time. In patients with particularly poor ventricular function epinephrine 0.04–0.15 μg/kg/min is added. Discussion with the surgical team regarding CTEPH classification and the success of the endarterectomy should occur prior to separation. If the surgery has only been partially successful because of small vessel disease, pulmonary vasodilators such as milrinone, intravenous prostacyclin, and nitric oxide are considered. If the surgery has been successful, the TEE reveals immediate improvements in the left- and right-sided geometry [57, 58]. The distention of the right atrium and right ventricle is greatly decreased, resulting in improvement of function of both ventricles (Fig. 49.10a, b; Videos 49.4 and 49.5). Tricuspid regurgitation, if it was present before the endarterectomy, has greatly decreased or resolved. Significant improvement in hemodynamic status is usually noted, including a doubling of the cardiac index, dramatic decrease in PA pressures, and a drop in the PVR to 25% of the preoperative value [4].

Post-CPB Management

After heparin reversal, bleeding diathesis is rare, and transfusion requirements are usually minimal [4]. Antifibrinolytic agents such as ε-amino-caproic acid are not routinely used for pulmonary endarterectomy in our institution. Two procedure-related complications may potentially present

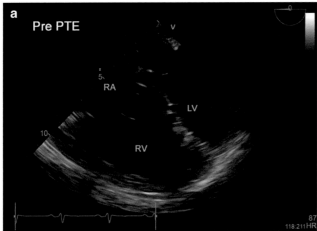
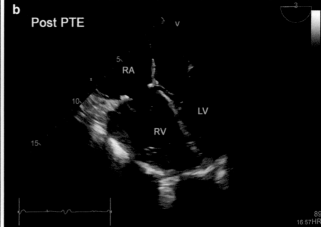

Fig. 49.10 (a) Midesophageal four-chamber view in a patient with CTEPH prior to pulmonary thromboendarterectomy. Note the dilated right heart, deviated septums, and underfilled left heart. RA right atrium, RV right ventricle, LV left ventricle. (**b**) Midesophageal four-chamber view of the same patient status post-pulmonary thromboendarterectomy and tricuspid valve repair. Note the decompression of the RA and RV with increased left heart size. RA right atrium, RV right ventricle, LV left ventricle

themselves immediately upon separation from CPB. Pink frothy sputum, if present, likely indicates the onset of reperfusion pulmonary edema. In this case, the endotracheal tube is suctioned, and increasing amounts of positive end-expiratory pressure (PEEP) are applied beginning with 5 cmH$_2$O escalating to 8 and 10 cmH$_2$O. The volume of pulmonary edema can be profound requiring frequent anesthesia circuit changes and maintenance of high levels of PEEP. If oxygenation and ventilation are significantly impaired, the resultant hypoxia and hypercarbia can lead to worsening RV dysfunction. Venovenous extracorporeal membrane oxygenation may be considered to improve the hypoxia and hypercarbia.

Secondly, if frank blood is emanating from the endotracheal tube, disruption of the blood-airway barrier has likely occurred secondary to surgical injury. The approach to this clinical scenario often begins with the surgeon's high index of suspicion of adventitial disruption. Prior to pressurizing the pulmonary arterial circuit via reduction of the PA vent, the anesthesiologist should pass an airway suction catheter. Identification of blood in the endotracheal tube warrants a fiberoptic bronchoscopy. If identification of pulmonary hemorrhage occurs after pressurization of the pulmonary arteries during cardiac ejection, localization of the culprit segment may be difficult. With the assistance of the surgical team and perfusionist, a slow reinstitution of cardiac ejection while concurrently visualizing via bronchoscopy can identify the specific lesion location. Management subsequently includes lung or lobar isolation via bronchial blocker placement, PEEP, separation from CPB, reversing anticoagulation, and treatment of coagulopathy. Assuming adequate oxygenation, ventilation, and coagulation, bronchial blocker balloon deflation may occur under direct fiberoptic visualization [59].

Significant pulmonary hemorrhage may lead to inadequate oxygenation, ventilation, and potential subsequent cardiac dysfunction prompting the use of various methods of extracorporeal life support. The choice of support depends upon the clinical scenario as outlined in the algorithm in Fig. 49.11. With preserved cardiac function, oxygenation and ventilation may be assisted via venovenous extracorporeal membrane oxygenation (ECMO). Utilization of the Avalon Elite Bicaval Dual-Lumen Catheter (Maquet, Rastatt, Germany) via the right internal jugular vein allows the institution of venovenous ECMO with minimal or no anticoagulation, an advantage in the setting of massive pulmonary hemorrhage [59]. As RV dysfunction develops, ECMO may be employed with right atrial inflow and pulmonary arterial outflow. Lastly if biventricular failure ensues, venoarterial ECMO may be employed.

Postoperative Management

Intensive care unit management is similar to other post-cardiac surgical patients with a few exceptions. Two major postoperative complications unique to PTE that can present in the ICU are reperfusion pulmonary edema and pulmonary arterial steal. Reperfusion pulmonary edema is a localized form of high-permeability (noncardiogenic) lung injury, a form of adult respiratory distress syndrome, localized to the area of lung having received the endarterectomy. It usually occurs within the first 24 h but may appear up to 72 h following PTE [60]. In most cases it is mild; reperfusion edema resulting in clinically significant morbidity occurs in only 10% of cases. In its most severe form, it begins immediately post-CPB, in the operating room as described above.

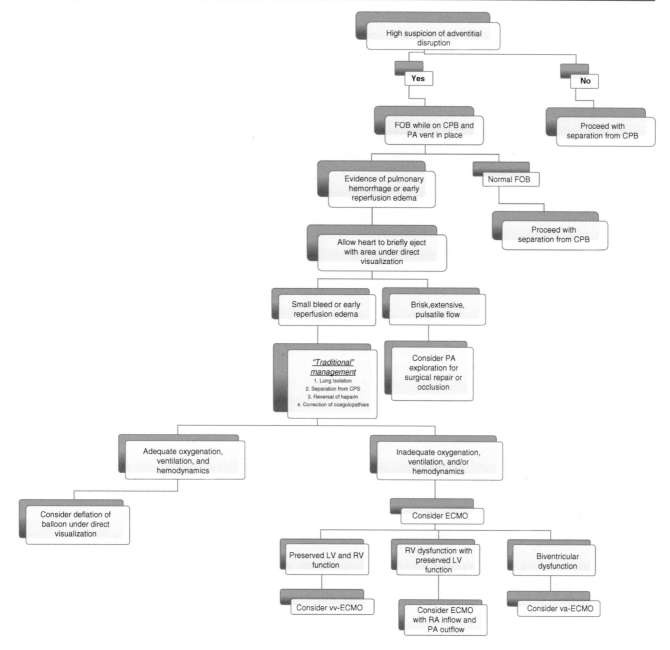

Fig. 49.11 Algorithm for the management of post-pulmonary thromboendarterectomy pulmonary hemorrhage. *CPB* cardiopulmonary bypass, *FOB* fiberoptic bronchoscopy, *ECMO* extracorporeal membrane oxygenation, *LV* left ventricular, *PA* pulmonary artery, *RA* right atrial, *RV* right ventricular, *va* venoarterial, *vv* venovenous. (Reprinted with permission from Cronin et al. [59])

These patients are often extremely ill, requiring aggressive intensive care and ventilator management. Pressure control, PEEP, and inverse ratio ventilation are used judicially in an effort to improve *V/Q* matching and minimize further pulmonary injury. Occasionally extracorporeal support is required [61, 62]. Pulmonary arterial steal represents a postoperative redistribution of pulmonary arterial blood away from the previously well-perfused segments into the newly endarterectomized segments [63]. Whether the cause is failure of autoregulation in the newly endarterectomized segments or

secondary small vessel, changes in the previously open segments have not been clarified. However, long-term follow-up has documented a decrease in pulmonary vascular steal in the majority of patients, suggesting a remodeling process in the pulmonary vascular bed [64].

Other postoperative complications are rare but can include pulmonary hemorrhage (0.4%), neurologic sequelae (0.4%), mediastinal bleeding (3.5%), GI bleeding (1.6%), atrial fibrillation (2.6%), renal failure requiring renal replacement therapy (1%), and sepsis (1.2%) [65].

PTE patients usually awaken within 1–2 h after surgery, and a brief neurologic examination is performed. The patient is then sedated with a propofol infusion and analgesics. They remain intubated overnight, since the onset of reperfusion pulmonary edema may be delayed. If pulmonary, cardiac, and neurologic function is good, and there is no bleeding diathesis, extubation occurs the following morning. Discharge from the intensive care unit typically occurs on the second or third postoperative day, and the patients are usually discharged from the hospital 1 week after the operation.

Outcome After PTE

There has been steady improvement in mortality rate at UCSD since 1980, with current perioperative mortality rate being less than 3% (Fig. 49.12). We believe these result from improvements in preoperative preparation, surgical technique, anesthetic care, perfusion technique, and postoperative management. The positive effect of experience, in the form of case volume, on outcome has been well documented for other types of complicated surgery, such as liver transplantation [66]. In addition, we have developed close collaboration between the Pulmonary Medicine, Cardiac Surgery, and Anesthesiology departments. This "team approach," we believe, is absolutely essential to a successful PTE program.

With this operation, a reduction in pulmonary pressures and resistance to normal levels and corresponding improvement in pulmonary blood flow and cardiac output are generally immediate and sustained [65, 67, 68]. Mortality rate and improvements in hemodynamics depend heavily on surgical subtype, with CTEPH Type 1 and 2 fairing better than Types 3 and 4. Type 0, not being CTEPH but rather small vessel disease, is associated with poor outcome [65]. There is a trend of patients presenting with more segmental and subsegmental disease as identified by Madani et al [69]. Despite a trend of patients presenting with more distal disease with its attendant increased surgical complexity, our experience

Table 49.2 Preoperative/postoperative hemodynamic results and operating times

Variable	Group 1 (n = 1000)	Group 2 (n = 500)	p value
PVR (dynes/sec/cm^{-5})			
Preoperative	861.2 ± 446.2	719.0 ± 383.2	< 0.001[a]
Postoperative	294.8 ± 204.2	253.4 ± 148.6	< 0.001[a]
Cardiac output (L/min)			
Preoperative	3.9 ± 1.3	4.3 ± 1.4	< 0.001[a]
Postoperative	5.4 ± 1.5	5.6 ± 1.4	< 0.001[a]
Systolic pulmonary artery pressure (mm Hg)			
Preoperative	75.7 ± 18.8	75.5 ± 19.1	0.8932
Postoperative	46.8 ± 17.3	41.7 ± 14.1	< 0.001[a]
Mean pulmonary artery pressure (mm Hg)			
Preoperative	46.1 ± 11.4	45.5 ± 11.6	0.3854
Postoperative	28.7 ± 10.1	26.0 ± 8.4	< 0.001[a]
Tricuspid regurgitant velocity (m/s)			
Preoperative	4.2 ± 0.7	4.0 ± 0.8	0.0263[a]
Postoperative	3.0 ± 0.6	2.9 ± 0.6	0.0075[a]
Operating times			
Total operating room time (min)	488.6 ± 80.1	534.6 ± 64.3	< 0.001[a]
Surgical time (min)	388.5 ± 73.4	430.5 ± 58.8	<0.001[a]
CPB time (min)	231.5 ± 45.6	265.4 ± 37.9	< 0.001[a]
Cross-clamp time (min)	95.7 ± 26.5	105.7 ± 25.4	< 0.001[a]
Circulatory arrest time (min)	35.2 ± 12.5	36.3 ± 12.5	0.1309

Data are shown as mean + standard deviation or number (percentages). Top numbers are preoperative values and bottom numbers are postoperative values
CPB cardiopulmonary bypass, *PVR* pulmonary vascular resistance
[a]Statistically significant with p value <0.05
Group 1 included 1000 patients operated on between March 1999 and October 2006, and group 2 included 500 patients operated on between October 2006 and December 2010
Adapted with permission from Madani et al. [69]

continues to demonstrate a dramatic reduction in pulmonary arterial pressures and pulmonary vascular resistance (Table 49.2). Patients who have undergone a successful PTE enjoy long-term benefit. Typically patients preoperatively present as New York Heart Association (NYHA) class III or IV and often maintain NYHA I and II function indefinitely following the operation [70].

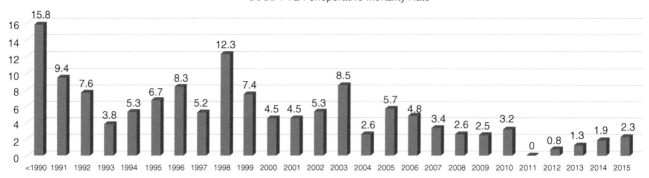

Fig. 49.12 Bar graph showing progressive improvement in perioperative mortality at UCSD. Years are on the *X*-axis, percentage mortality on the *Y*-axis

Future

While surgical management of CTEPH continues to be the proven mainstay of treatment, there are continued advances both in medical management and percutaneous treatments of these patients. Adempas® (Riociguat) is an FDA-approved drug which acts via guanylate cyclase and nitric oxide; the drug is a pulmonary vasodilator specifically indicated for the treatment of residual or recurrent pulmonary hypertension after PTE or those with inoperable CTEPH. Its role and the role of other pulmonary vasodilators (i.e., phosphodiesterase inhibitors, endothelin antagonists, prostaglandins, etc.) in the treatment are continuing to be elucidated. The exact role of medical management prior to surgical PTE still remains unknown.

The experience with percutaneous balloon pulmonary angioplasty (BPA) has continued to grow either as an alternative to those patients with surgically inaccessible CTEPH or those with high perioperative risk due to comorbidities. Reperfusion pulmonary edema and pulmonary vascular injury remain concerns with this percutaneous technique as well. The exact role of BPA in the management of CTEPH patients requires further study.

Research to determine the etiology of CTEPH, as well as the mechanisms and factors leading to reperfusion pulmonary edema, vascular steal, and ischemic neurologic injury continues. Understanding these processes will most likely lead to improved prophylaxis and treatment. Anesthesiologists, in particular, will be an integral part of future research on the immediate perioperative period. This will include efforts to improve the management of residual "small vessel disease," right ventricular failure, cerebral function and oxygenation monitoring, postoperative pulmonary edema, pulmonary bleeding, and organ protection.

Clinical Case Discussion

Case: A 68-year-old woman with CTEPH underwent a PTE and has just been separated from CPB. The surgeon tells you that the endarterectomy was difficult because it was Type 3 disease and the thromboembolic material was particularly "sticky." You suspected such because the surgeon required two circulatory arrests on the right side, and he usually requires only one on each side. Large amounts of dark blood appear in the endotracheal tube as you begin ventilating.

Questions

- What is the most likely cause of this bleeding?
- What diagnostic maneuvers can be performed to determine the cause and location of the bleeding?
- What are the therapeutic options, and how will they be chosen?

The most likely cause is surgical trauma, puncture of the distal pulmonary arteries resulting from aggressive endarterectomy. Other possibilities include nonsurgical PA rupture (high pressure, PA catheter trauma). Initial maneuvers include reinstitution of CPB including decompression of the pulmonary arterial tree with a PA vent, thereby temporarily reducing the amount of airway bleeding. Fiberoptic bronchoscopy can assist in localizing the site of the bleeding. Smaller bleeds may be managed with lung isolation, separation from CPB, reversal of heparin, as well as correction of coagulopathies. Lung isolation techniques include double-lumen tubes and bronchial blockers. A preferred technique is to exchange the endotracheal tube for a larger size (i.e., 9.0 mm ETT) to allow a bronchial blocker and a larger adult-sized bronchoscope simultaneously. The use of a pediatric size scope yields a smaller suction channel. Attempts to place the bronchial blocker in a subsegment if possible should be sought to maximize the amount of salvaged lung and prevent spillage of blood into the remaining segments. Larger pulmonary hemorrhage events or those associated with worsening hypoxia and hypercarbia may require ECMO. The decision for the method of ECMO rests on the hemodynamic status of the patient with TEE evidence of ventricular dysfunction playing a key role. Assuming biventricular function is intact, venovenous ECMO may be instituted via a single cannula placed percutaneously through the right internal jugular vein. This approach allows for ECMO support with minimal anticoagulation [59]. An algorithm for management of post-CPB hemorrhage is presented in Fig. 49.11.

References

1. Moser KM, Houk VN, Jones RC, Hufnagel CC. Chronic, massive thrombotic obstruction of the pulmonary arteries: analysis of four operated cases. Circulation. 1965;32(3):377–85.
2. McLaughlin VV, Langer A, Tan M, et al. Contemporary trends in the diagnosis and management of pulmonary arterial hypertension. Chest. 2013;143(2):324–32.
3. Moser KM, Auger WR, Fedullo PF. Chronic major-vessel thromboembolic pulmonary hypertension. Circulation. 1990;81(6):1735–43.
4. Jamieson SW, Kapelanski DP. Pulmonary endarterectomy. Curr Probl Surg. 2000;37(3):165–252.
5. DeMonaco NA, Dang Q, Kapoor WN, Ragni MV. Pulmonary embolism incidence is increasing with use of spiral computed tomography. Am J Med. 2008;121(7):611–7.
6. Lindblad B, Eriksson A, Bergqvist D. Autopsy-verified pulmonary embolism in a surgical department: analysis of the period from 1951 to 1988. Br J Surg. 1991;78(7):849–52.
7. Riedel M, Stanek V, Widimsky J, Prerovsky I. Longterm follow-up of patients with pulmonary thromboembolism. Chest. 1982;81(2):151–8.
8. Rich S Rubin L, Abenhail L, et al. Executive summary from the World Symposium on Primary Pulmonary Hypertension. Paper presented at: World Symposium on Primary Pulmonary Pulmonary Hypertension; September 6–10, 1998, Evian; 1998.
9. Galie N, Hoeper MM, Humbert M, et al. Guidelines for the diagnosis and treatment of pulmonary hypertension. Eur Respir J. 2009;34(6):1219–63.

10. Dadfarmay S, Berkowitz R, Kim B, Manchikalapudi RB. Differentiating pulmonary arterial and pulmonary venous hypertension and the implications for therapy. Congest Heart Fail. 2010;16(6):287–91.

11. Bossone E, D'Andrea A, D'Alto M, et al. Echocardiography in pulmonary arterial hypertension: from diagnosis to prognosis. J Am Soc Echocardiogr. 2013;26(1):1–14.

12. Bernard J, Yi ES. Pulmonary thromboendarterectomy: a clinicopathologic study of 200 consecutive pulmonary thromboendarterectomy cases in one institution. Hum Pathol. 2007;38(6):871–7.

13. Guillinta P, Peterson KL, Ben-Yehuda O. Cardiac catheterization techniques in pulmonary hypertension. Cardiol Clin. 2004;22(3):401–15.

14. Post MC, Plokker HWM, Kelder JC, Snijder RJ. Long-term efficacy of bosentan in inoperable chronic thromboembolic pulmonary hypertension. Neth Hear J. 2009;17(9):329–33.

15. Vassallo FG, Kodric M, Scarduelli C, et al. Bosentan for patients with chronic thromboembolic pulmonary hypertension. Eur J Intern Med. 2009;20(1):24–9.

16. Jaïs X, D'Armini AM, Jansa P, et al. Bosentan for treatment of inoperable chronic thromboembolic pulmonary hypertension. J Am Coll Cardiol. 2008;52(25):2127–34.

17. Dalen JE, Alpert JS. Natural history of pulmonary embolism. Prog Cardiovasc Dis. 1975;17(4):259–70.

18. Pengo V, Lensing AWA, Prins MH, et al. Incidence of chronic thromboembolic pulmonary hypertension after pulmonary embolism. N Engl J Med. 2004;350(22):2257–64.

19. Fedullo PF, Auger WR, Kerr KM, Rubin LJ. Chronic thromboembolic pulmonary hypertension. N Engl J Med. 2001;345(20):1465–72.

20. Bonderman D, Turecek PL, Jakowitsch J, et al. High prevalence of elevated clotting factor VIII in chronic thromboembolic pulmonary hypertension. Thromb Haemost. 2003;90:372–6.

21. Lang IM. Chronic thromboembolic pulmonary hypertension — not so rare after all. N Engl J Med. 2004;350(22):2236–8.

22. Kapitän KS, Buchbinder M, Wagner PD, Moser KM. Mechanisms of hypoxemia in chronic thromboembolic pulmonary hypertension. Am Rev Respir Dis. 1989;139(5):1149–54.

23. Moser KM. Thromboendarterectomy for chronic, major-vessel thromboembolic pulmonary hypertension. Ann Intern Med. 1987;107(4):560.

24. D'Armini AM, Zanotti G, Ghio S, et al. Reverse right ventricular remodeling after pulmonary endarterectomy. J Thorac Cardiovasc Surg. 2007;133(1):162–8.

25. Reichelt A, Hoeper MM, Galanski M, Keberle M. Chronic thromboembolic pulmonary hypertension: evaluation with 64-detector row CT versus digital substraction angiography. Eur J Radiol. 2009;71(1):49–54.

26. Suga K, Kawakami Y, Iwanaga H, Hayashi N, Seto A, Matsunaga N. Comprehensive assessment of lung CT attenuation alteration at perfusion defects of acute pulmonary thromboembolism with breath-hold SPECT-CT fusion images. J Comput Assist Tomogr. 2006;30(1):83–91.

27. Nikolaou K, Schoenberg SO, Attenberger U, et al. Pulmonary arterial hypertension: diagnosis with fast perfusion MR imaging and high-spatial-resolution MR angiography—preliminary experience. Radiology. 2005;236(2):694–703.

28. Jensen KW, Kerr KM, Fedullo PF, et al. Pulmonary hypertensive medical therapy in chronic thromboembolic pulmonary hypertension before pulmonary thromboendarterectomy. Circulation. 2009;120(13):1248–54.

29. Archer SL, Michelakis ED. Phosphodiesterase type 5 inhibitors for pulmonary arterial hypertension. N Engl J Med. 2009;361(19):1864–71.

30. Rubin LJ, Badesch DB, Barst RJ. Bosentan therapy for pulmonary arterial hypertension. ACC Curr J Rev. 2002;11(5):30.

31. Confalonieri M, Kodric M, Longo C, Vassallo FG. Bosentan for chronic thromboembolic pulmonary hypertension. Expert Rev Cardiovasc Ther. 2009;7(12):1503–12.

32. Nagaya N, Sasaki N, Ando M, et al. Prostacyclin therapy before pulmonary thromboendarterectomy in patients with chronic thromboembolic pulmonary hypertension*. Chest. 2003;123(2):338–43.

33. Ono F, Nagaya N, Okumura H, et al. Effect of orally active prostacyclin analogue on survival in patients with chronic thromboembolic pulmonary hypertension without major vessel obstruction. Chest. 2003;123(5):1583–8.

34. Vizza CD, Badagliacca R, Sciomer S, et al. Mid-term efficacy of Beraprost, an Oral prostacyclin analog, in the treatment of distal CTEPH: a case control study. Cardiology. 2006;106(3):168–73.

35. Augoustides JG, Culp K, Smith S. Rebound pulmonary hypertension and cardiogenic shock after withdrawal of inhaled prostacyclin. Anesthesiology. 2004;100(4):1023–5.

36. Jamieson SW. Pulmonary thromboendarterectomy. Heart. 1998;79(2):118–20.

37. Fedullo PF, Auger WR, Channick RN, Moser KM, Jamieson SW. Chronic thromboembolic pulmonary hypertension. Clin Chest Med. 1995;16(2):353–74.

38. Jamieson SW, Auger WR, Fedullo PF, et al. Experience and results with 150 pulmonary thromboendarterectomy operations over a 29-month period. J Thorac Cardiovasc Surg. 1993;106(1):116–26; discussion 126–7.

39. Madani M. Surgical Treatment of Chronic Thromboembolic Pulmonary Hypertension: Pulmonary Thromboendarterectomy. Methodist Debakey Cardiovasc J. 2016; 12(4): 213–218.

40. Rich S, Gubin S, Hart K. The effects of phenylephrine on right ventricular performance in patients with pulmonary hypertension. Chest. 1990;98(5):1102–6.

41. Cronin B, Robbins R, Maus T. Pulmonary artery catheter placement using transesophageal echocardiography. J Cardiothorac Vasc Anesth. 2017;31(1):178–83.

42. Manecke GR, Parimucha M, Stratmann G, et al. Deep hypothermic circulatory arrest and the femoral-to-radial arterial pressure gradient. J Cardiothorac Vasc Anesth. 2004;18(2):175–9.

43. Mohr R, Lavee J, Goor D. Inaccuracy of radial artery pressure measurement after cardiac operations. Surv Anesthesiol. 1988;32(1):1.

44. Urzua J. Aortic-to-radial arterial pressure gradient after bypass. Anesthesiology. 1990;73(1):191.

45. Dittrich HC, McConn HA, Wilson WC. Identification of interatrial communication in patients with elevated right atrial pressure using surface and transesophageal contrast echocardiography. J Am Coll Cardiol. 1993;21(Suppl):135A.

46. Schuhmann MU, Suhr DF, v Gösseln HH, Bräuer A, Jantzen J-P, Samii M. Local brain surface temperature compared to temperatures measured at standard extracranial monitoring sites during. J Neurosurg Anesthesiol. 1999;11(2):90–5.

47. Riess F-C, Löwer C, Seelig C, et al. Recombinant hirudin as a new anticoagulant during cardiac operations instead of heparin: successful for aortic valve replacement in man. J Thorac Cardiovasc Surg. 1995;110(1):265–7.

48. Pötzsch B, Hund S, Madlener K, Unkrig C, Müller-Berghaus G. Monitoring of recombinant hirudin: assessment of a plasma-based ecarin clotting time assay. Thromb Res. 1997;86(5):373–83.

49. von Segesser LK, Mueller X, Marty B, Horisberger J, Corno A. Alternatives to unfractionated heparin for anticoagulation in cardiopulmonary bypass. Perfusion. 2001;16(5):411–6.

50. Warkentin TE, Greinacher A. Heparin-induced thrombocytopenia and cardiac surgery. Ann Thorac Surg. 2003;76(2):638–48.

51. Vanderlinden J, Ekroth R, Lincoln C, Pugsley W, Scallan M, Tyden H. Is cerebral blood flow/metabolic mismatch during rewarming a risk factor after profound hypothermic procedures in small children? Eur J Cardiothorac Surg. 1989;3(3):209–15.

52. Yoshitani K, Kawaguchi M, Sugiyama N, et al. The association of high jugular bulb venous oxygen saturation with cognitive decline after hypothermic cardiopulmonary bypass. Anesth Analg. 2001;92:1370–6.

53. Henson LC, Calalang C, Temp JA, Ward DS. Accuracy of a cerebral oximeter in healthy volunteers under conditions of Isocapnic hypoxia. Anesthesiology. 1998;88(1):58–65.

54. Daubeney PEF, Pilkington SN, Janke E, Charlton GA, Smith DC, Webber SA. Cerebral oxygenation measured by near-infrared spectroscopy: comparison with jugular bulb oximetry. Ann Thorac Surg. 1996;61(3):930–4.

55. Chen CSLN, Liu K. Detection of cerebral desaturation during cardiopulmonary bypass by cerebral oximetry. Acta Anaesthesiol Sin. 1997;35(1):59.

56. Manecke GR, Kotzur A, Atkins G, et al. Massive pulmonary hemorrhage after pulmonary thromboendarterectomy. Anesth Analg. 2004;99(3):672–5.

57. Dittrich HC, Nicod PH, Chow LC, Chappuis FP, Moser KM, Peterson KL. Early changes of right heart geometry after pulmonary thromboendarterectomy. J Am Coll Cardiol. 1988;11(5):937–43.

58. Dittrich HC, Chow LC, Nicod PH. Early improvement in left ventricular diastolic function after relief of chronic right ventricular pressure overload. Circulation. 1989;80(4):823–30.

59. Cronin B, Maus T, Pretorius V, et al. Case 13 – 2014: management of pulmonary hemorrhage after pulmonary endarterectomy with venovenous extracorporeal membrane oxygenation without systemic anticoagulation. J Cardiothorac Vasc Anesth. 2014;28(6):1667–76.

60. Levinson RM, Shure D, Moser KM. Reperfusion pulmonary edema after pulmonary artery thromboendarterectomy. Am Rev Respir Dis. 1986;134(6):1241–5.

61. Thistlethwaite PA, Madani MM, Kemp AD, Hartley M, Auger WR, Jamieson SW. Venovenous extracorporeal life support after pulmonary endarterectomy: indications, techniques, and outcomes. Ann Thorac Surg. 2006;82(6):2139–45.

62. Berman M, Tsui S, Vuylsteke A, et al. Successful extracorporeal membrane oxygenation support after pulmonary thromboendarterectomy. Ann Thorac Surg. 2008;86(4):1261–7.

63. Olman MA, Auger WR, Fedullo PF, Moser KM. Pulmonary vascular steal in chronic thromboembolic pulmonary hypertension. Chest. 1990;98(6):1430–4.

64. Moser KM, Metersky ML, Auger WR, Fedullo PF. Resolution of vascular steal after pulmonary Thromboendarterectomy. Chest. 1993;104(5):1441–4.

65. Thistlethwaite PA, Kaneko K, Madani MM, Jamieson SW. Technique and outcomes of pulmonary endarterectomy surgery. Ann Thorac Cardiovasc Surg. 2008;14(5):274–82.

66. Edwards EB, Roberts JP, McBride MA, Schulak JA, Hunsicker LG. The effect of the volume of procedures at transplantation centers on mortality after liver transplantation. N Engl J Med. 1999;341(27):2049–53.

67. Menzel T, Kramm T, Mohr-Kahaly S, Mayer E, Oelert H, Meyer J. Assessment of cardiac performance using Tei indices in patients undergoing pulmonary thromboendarterectomy. Ann Thorac Surg. 2002;73(3):762–6.

68. Thistlethwaite PA, Madani M, Jamieson SW. Outcomes of pulmonary endarterectomy surgery. Semin Thorac Cardiovasc Surg. 2006;18(3):257–64.

69. Madani MM, Auger WR, Pretorius V, et al. Pulmonary endarterectomy: recent changes in a single institution's experience of more than 2,700 patients. Ann Thorac Surg. 2012;94(1):97–103. discussion 103

70. Corsico AG, D'Armini AM, Cerveri I, et al. Long-term outcome after pulmonary endarterectomy. Am J Respir Crit Care Med. 2008;178(4):419–24.

Anesthesia for Pediatric Thoracic Surgery

50

Robert Schwartz and Cengiz Karsli

Key Points

- Pediatric patients present in varying stages of development, from the premature neonate to full-grown teenager. Appreciation of the unique physiologic states associated with the different stages of development will direct anesthetic management.
- Preoperative evaluation of the small child should include the neonatal history as this may indicate comorbid pulmonary and cardiac disease and linked syndromes which must be investigated.
- Lung isolation is not always necessary in pediatric thoracic surgery. Appropriate lung isolation techniques will depend on the age and size of the patient as there is no single technique that is suitable for all pediatric patients.
- Physiologic manifestation of one-lung ventilation may be more pronounced in children than in adults. The compliant rib cage, compressible lung parenchyma, reduced FRC under anesthesia, and higher oxygen consumption in the child contribute to aggravate hypoxemia during lung isolation.
- Adult thoracic surgery is often related to tumor excision, whereas pediatric thoracic disease encompasses a greater variety of pathology. Each specific disease state has its own particular anesthetic considerations and management strategy.
- Pain management in the pediatric population has evolved to include a greater use of regional and neuraxial techniques, even in the smallest of infants.
- Postoperative disposition will depend on the type and length of surgery, extent of resection or manipulation, and nature of the underlying condition. Many pediatric patients will require postoperative ventilation or close cardiorespiratory monitoring following the procedure.

Introduction

Pediatric and neonatal thoracic anesthesia begins with an understanding of the physiologic and anatomic differences that occur in this patient population. Pediatric patients will present in varying sizes and weights from less than 1 kg to greater than 100 kg and in varying stages of development from the extremely premature to the older teenage child. It is therefore the requirement of the pediatric anesthesiologist to understand the physiologic differences associated with these extremes and how they influence anesthetic management.

The determinants of these physiologic restraints and the practicality of securing ventilation and oxygenation will often dictate both the anesthetic management and the surgical approach. Unlike the adult population where one-lung isolation can almost universally be applied, in much of the neonatal population, this can be at best a harrowing challenge or even an impossibility. As well, securing invasive monitors such as arterial or central venous lines may be problematic in the pediatric population. This means that the pediatric anesthesiologist must appreciate the compromise that arises due to the nature of the patient and procedure and yet be flexible and knowledgeable enough to safely carry out the anesthetic management. Postoperative pain management

R. Schwartz
Department of Anesthesia, Children's Hospital of Eastern Ontario, Ottawa, ON, Canada

C. Karsli (✉)
Department of Anesthesiology, The Hospital for Sick Children, Toronto, ON, Canada
e-mail: Cengiz.karsli@sickkids.ca

© Springer Nature Switzerland AG 2019
P. Slinger (ed.), *Principles and Practice of Anesthesia for Thoracic Surgery*, https://doi.org/10.1007/978-3-030-00859-8_50

and monitored postoperative disposition may differ significantly from that of the adult population and depend largely on the disease process, surgical intervention, and the physiologic maturity of the patient. Thoracoscopic procedures continue to be applied to smaller and younger patients with their own set of unique challenges and hazards.

The purpose of this chapter is to provide the anesthesiologist with the basic physiologic and anatomic characteristics associated with this patient population and how these differences are practically managed. A general discussion on the cardiopulmonary development of the pediatric patient will be presented; however, specialty texts should be sought for in-depth coverage of this topic. Case presentation and examples will be used where possible to provide the reader with a practical approach to common pediatric thoracic procedures. The understanding and practice of these techniques should then enable the pediatric anesthesiologist to apply this knowledge to more complicated and challenging cases.

Pediatric Growth and Development

Normal embryonic development begins at the time of conception and continues throughout the first 8 weeks of life. During this period of time, fetal cells will divide and begin the process of organogenesis. By the fourth week of embryonic development, the primitive heart and lungs appear. At this point neurulation also begins, a process that will see the eventual creation of the brain and spinal cord.

From this early lung, the trachea and bronchial tree will emerge, and by the eighth week of life, the segmental bronchi and diaphragm are complete. In the following months, the airways will canalize, and surfactant will be produced. Although lung maturation will continue post delivery, it is generally accepted that by the 27th week of gestation, fetal lung maturity is sufficient to sustain ex uterine life.

Similarly the heart tube which began to beat at approximately day 22 will undergo a series of foldings and septate formation such that the four-chambered heart will be complete at the eighth week of gestation. Shortly thereafter, the valves separating these chambers will also form. Once the process of organogenesis is complete, the remainder of fetal development is devoted to an increase in cell numbers and the maturation of these organs. Intestinal rotation will proceed as well as a significant increase in overall size and weight. Interruption of this normal developmental pathway can have significant impact on the fetus. Teratogens acting at the time of organogenesis can impact organ formation. Abnormal morphogenesis may lead to cleft palate and congenital diaphragmatic hernia (CDH) among others. Chromosomal abnormalities, those that are not lethal, may have a cluster of symptoms that when grouped together form the basis of pediatric syndromes. As well the problems associated with premature infants (born <37 week GA) are almost entirely due to the immature nature of the fetal organ systems.

Lung and airway maturation continues until approximately the eighth year of life, during which time the number and size of alveoli steadily increase. Transition from intrauterine to the extrauterine environment will see the replacement of the previously fluid-filled alveoli with air as the first breaths are taken. The oxygen-Hb dissociation curve will begin to transition rightward as the alveolar oxygen partial pressure increases from that of intrauterine life.

The anatomic changes that the airway undergoes from that of the neonate to infant and onward to adulthood have been well described. The glottic opening is typically located at the level of the third cervical vertebra as opposed to C4–C5 in adults. In addition, the tongue is relatively large, and the epiglottis is long and floppy in infants up to 1 year in age. As a result the entire tongue of the neonate and infant is located in the oral cavity, whereas only the anterior two thirds of the tongue in older children and adults occupy the oral cavity. This accounts for the propensity to upper airway obstruction in neonates and infants who are sedated, have decreased level of consciousness, or during anesthetic induction. Until 7 or 8 years of age, the tracheal diameter at the level of the cricoid cartilage is narrower than that at the vocal cords, resulting in a conical larynx. A tracheal tube that passes through the vocal cords may not necessarily then pass through the cricoid ring. A relatively large head, short neck, and trachea mean that tracheal intubation, although not typically difficult, requires a subtly different technique than that used in the adult patient.

As the lungs fill with air during the first moments of extrauterine life, pulmonary vascular resistance (PVR) will fall and cause a dramatic increase in pulmonary blood flow. As PaO_2 rises, the ductus arteriosus will constrict and usually fully closes by the end of the first week of life. Left-sided cardiac pressures will rise and close the foramen ovale. The myocardium of the neonate is relatively noncompliant and cannot adjust contractility in response to changes in filling pressures. The cardiac output in the neonate is thus dependent on HR, and the normal heart rate is typically between 100 and 150 bpm.

Relative body composition changes also occur during the first year of life. The highest percent body fat is at 1 year of age (approximately 30%) and typically decreases throughout adult life. Total body water (as a percentage of body weight) is highest at birth (75%) and drops to adult (60%) levels by 1 year of age. The estimated blood volume (as a percent of body weight) also decreases. Term infants typically have an estimated blood volume of 95 mL/kg, whereas by 1 year of age, it has decreased to 65 mL/kg. In addition to this, the fluid, electrolyte composition, energy requirements, hematologic system, and vital signs all change significantly throughout the various stages of growth. The pediatric anesthesiologist's understanding of these changes will necessarily guide the management of the patient as drug dosages, ventilation parameters, and equipment must be adjusted for the age and maturation of the patient.

Special Considerations

Prematurity

Premature infants have several unique features that will briefly be addressed here. In-depth coverage of this topic can be found in any neonatal or pediatric specific anesthesia text.

Fetal surfactant is produced by type II pneumocytes at approximately the 22nd week of gestation. Half of this production is usually complete by the 28th week, with the remainder by the 37th week. Steroid administration to the mother can speed up this process. Deficiency in surfactant production may result in respiratory distress syndrome (RDS) [1]. The constellation of tachypnea, indrawing, and oxygen desaturation results from collapse of alveoli caused by insufficient surfactant levels. This leads to decreased lung compliance, higher opening pressures, decreased FRC, and increased work of breathing. Arterial blood gas analysis will often reveal hypoxemia, hypercarbia, and acidosis.

The early management of RDS consists of oxygenation and assisted ventilation in the form of noninvasive CPAP/BIPAP [2–4]. Exposure to high oxygen concentrations may lead to retinopathy of prematurity (ROP) and other complications in these patients, although the role of anesthetic agents in causing ROP remains undefined. Balancing the need to avoid tissue hypoxemia and avoiding the toxic effects of oxygen can be challenging. Prudence would seem to suggest that using the lowest possible FiO_2 to maintain adequate tissue oxygenation is advisable. Oxygen therapy is often adjusted to achieve an oxygen saturation of 90–95% [5]; however, if there is evidence of hypoxia-induced hemodynamic instability or other end-organ failures, oxygen therapy should not be sacrificed in order to prevent ROP. Continued oxygen desaturation (below 90%) or persistent acidosis may require endotracheal intubation and mechanical ventilation be instituted. The goal of ventilation is to minimize baro- and volu-trauma while maintaining oxygen saturation between 90 and 95%. To this end, relative hypercapnia ($PaCO_2$ 45–60 mmHg) is often permitted. Much like the management of ARDS, the FiO_2 and PEEP ratio should be carefully adjusted to minimize both while achieving the above stated goals.

Exogenous surfactant can also be administered to these infants both at the time of birth and at regular intervals thereafter [6]. Surfactant acts to decrease alveolar surface tension and has been shown to decrease RDS-related morbidity and mortality [1, 7]. The long-term sequela from RDS is typically bronchopulmonary dysplasia (BPD). These children may continue to have respiratory difficulty secondary to decreased lung compliance and increased airway resistance with increased dead space.

Pulmonary Hypertension

Pulmonary hypertension is classically defined as mean pulmonary arterial pressure (PAP) >25 mmHg at rest or > 30 mmHg with activity [8]. In neonates, echocardiographic evidence of PVR greater than the half the systemic vascular resistance is commonly considered as evidence of pulmonary hypertension [9]. This state arises when PVR fails to decrease after the transition to extrauterine life occurs. Severely elevated pulmonary pressures will cause a decrease in blood flow through the lungs and encourage right-to-left shunting, resulting in cyanosis and hypoxemia. The causes of persistent pulmonary hypertension in the newborn are described in Table 50.1.

Management of pulmonary hypertension involves treating the underlying cause and reducing pulmonary vascular tone. To this end supplemental oxygen administration is employed as well as control of ventilation to avoid hypercapnia and acidosis. Pharmacologic pulmonary vasodilators such as intravenous prostacyclin, phosphodiesterase III inhibitors (e.g., milrinone), and/or inhaled nitric oxide may be administered if necessary [10]. Sildenafil has shown promise and is increasingly being used to treat responsive pulmonary hypertension in this patient population [11, 12]. Individual or combination therapies have

Table 50.1 Causes of persistent pulmonary hypertension in the newborn

Acute pulmonary vasoconstriction due to perinatal events
Meconium aspiration
Respiratory distress syndrome
Pneumonia
Hypoventilation/asphyxia
Hypothermia
Hypoglycemia
Sepsis
Idiopathic
Maternal NSAID or SSRI use
Pulmonary vascular hypoplasia
Congenital diaphragmatic hernia
Oligohydramnios
Congenital cystic adenomatoid malformation (CCAM)
Pulmonary sequestration
Cardiac lesions
Pulmonary atresia with intact ventricular septum
Transposition of the great arteries (TGA)
Total anomalous pulmonary venous drainage (TAPVD)
Tricuspid atresia

been used in neonatal and infant populations with some success [13–15]. Nitric oxide offers the theoretical advantage of improving V/Q matching by preferentially increasing blood flow to ventilated alveoli. Alternatively, extracorporeal membrane oxygenation (ECMO) has been utilized to temporize pulmonary hypertension or as a bridge to lung transplantation [9, 16, 17].

Cardiac Disease

Patent ductus arteriosus (PDA) is a common finding in the premature infant. Blood flow through the PDA is typically left to right, although this can reverse if pulmonary hypertension exists. Preoperative echocardiography should be performed to evaluate this. Depending on the reason for prematurity, these infants may also have other forms of congenital heart disease (CHD) that should be evaluated prior to undergoing any anesthetic. Although pharmacologic or surgical closure of the PDA is often indicated, if other cyanotic CHD exists, the closure of the PDA is delayed until the lesion is repaired or palliated via another form of surgical shunt. The anesthetic management of thoracic procedures in patients with unrepaired or palliated shunts is particularly challenging. Increased positive-pressure ventilation and compromised oxygenation may lead to worsening of right-to-left shunts.

Immature organ function and depleted metabolic reserves predispose the premature infant to several other age-related disorders. Lack of glycogen stores in the premature neonatal liver places these patients at risk for hypoglycemia. The implications of untreated hypoglycemia can be quite severe and include seizures and developmental delay. The normal stress response of surgery is to increase plasma glucose levels secondary to catecholamine and cortisol production. This may not occur, however, in the very sick child. Five or ten percent dextrose solution should be used as maintenance fluid in the pediatric population, although at what age this practice should cease is not clear [18]. To avoid hyperglycemia a balanced salt solution should be used for fluid bolus administration [19].

Apnea of prematurity is common, and its incidence is inversely proportional to the gestational age and weight of the child. Apnea (airflow cessation lasting more than 15 s) may be accompanied by bradycardia and hypoxia. The presumptive mechanism is due to immature neuronal control at the level of the brainstem and peripheral chemoreceptors [20]. An obstructive component to the apnea is often present as well. Other risk factors include a hemoglobin <100 or Hct < 30. Management may include minimizing narcotic use, stimulation and airway support, and pharmacology (e.g., caffeine). Postoperative observation and monitoring for apnea are mandatory in premature and ex-premature infants less than 50–60 weeks postconceptual age.

Preoperative Evaluation

As in adults the preoperative evaluation of the pediatric patient focuses on the history, physical exam, and laboratory investigations, although an age-appropriate evaluation is necessary. The pediatric practitioner must be aware that certain congenital anomalies do not occur in isolation. For example, tracheoesophageal fistula may be associated with other significant anomalies as part of the VACTERL syndrome (vertebral, anal, cardiac, TE fistula, renal, radial, and limb anomalies). The presence and severity of the associated anomalies should be identified as they may affect anesthetic management.

The evaluation of the neonate or infant typically begins with a history of the pregnancy, labor, and delivery. Apgar scores and resuscitation efforts at delivery are important as they may provide diagnostic clues. For example, prolonged tracheal intubation early in life may predict the presence of subglottic stenosis. RDS leading to BPD may affect children many years after their NICU discharge. Both these examples may lead the anesthesiologist to modify his approach to airway management or ventilation strategy.

As this may be the first anesthetic the child is to receive, the biological parents must be questioned with regard to prior familial anesthetic complications. Malignant hyperthermia and pseudocholinesterase deficiency (among others) have a genetic transmission and may present with the first anesthetic. If a prior anesthetic record is available, it should be reviewed. As in adults particular attention should be focused on the ease of bag-mask ventilation and intubation. In the pediatric population, one must also look for evidence of difficulty with intravenous access and the disposition of the child prior to induction. Endotracheal tube (ETT) size and the presence of a leak around the tracheal tube should also be noted.

Functional capacity should be assessed keeping in mind the patient's age. An infant's inability to take full feeds, sweating, and/or cyanosis during feeds may be an indicator of heart failure. In toddlers and older children, activity level or ability to run or play is a better measure of cardiothoracic functional capacity. A helpful indicator is whether the child is able to keep up with his peers when at play. A child who takes more frequent naps or must stop and sit while his peers continue to play is a clear indication of decreased functional capacity. Height- and weight-based growth analysis will also provide evidence of failure to thrive which can be caused by or exacerbate a decreased functional capacity.

The physical exam can be challenging in the pediatric patient. Noncompliance and occasionally combativeness will prevent thorough examination. Most adult markers for difficult bag-mask ventilation and intubation are not appropriate for infants and children. Assessing Mallampati score in a newborn may be impossible and futile. In its place many pediatric anesthesiologists assess the craniofacial silhouette or profile, focusing on evidence of retro- or micrognathia. A gloved finger can also be used to feel for the presence of a high arched and/or cleft palate, which may be associated with difficult laryngoscopy.

Respiratory compromise or distress will manifest not only as tachypnea but perhaps also as indrawing, nasal flaring, grunting, accessory muscle use, or paradoxical breathing. All are easily identifiable in children. Peripheral cyanosis and evidence of decreased perfusion should be sought. Assessment of intravascular volume status in the pediatric patient may be challenging. Orthostatic vital signs are generally not done in neonates, and the JVP cannot be easily seen. Skin turgor, capillary refill, fontanelle fullness, level of consciousness, and urine output, however, are easily assessed, as is total fluid intake. A newborn that consistently is gaining weight is very unlikely to be hypovolemic.

Vital signs change with age and should therefore be compared to the statistical norms for the patients' cohort. Blood pressure measurements in an irritable or uncooperative child can be unreliable or impossible to attain. Auscultation for normal heart sounds and murmurs of concern is important to document. Evidence of heart failure, pulmonary edema, and wheezing on respiratory exam should also raise concerns.

Laboratory investigations in the pediatric population should be based on the presenting illness and the surgery proposed. Often children that are booked for thoracic procedures will have at minimum a CXR that can be evaluated for pulmonary pathology, edema, and evidence of scoliosis and engorgement of the vascular structures. If available the computed tomography (CT) scan or MRI should also be viewed. This will prove a valuable aide in determining the feasibility of lung isolation and the extent of the pathology. Particular attention should be noted if the disease is in communication with the bronchi (e.g., congenital cystic adenomatoid malformation, CCAM) as this will potentially alter the ventilation strategy. Anterior mediastinal masses may compress the great vessels, the trachea, or the heart itself. Evidence of cardiovascular compromise, whether on history or physical exam, warrants further investigation with transthoracic echocardiography. Often an understanding of the disease pathophysiology and associated cardiac anomalies will warrant this investigation. An ECG can be very helpful in these circumstances.

Since most thoracic procedures have the potential for blood loss, a CBC should be obtained preoperatively. This test may also indicate the degree of hypoxia if the hematocrit is significantly elevated. Often electrolytes and renal function indicators will be ordered. In an otherwise healthy child, no blood work may be needed. Baseline arterial blood gases may be useful but may not be practical in the frightened young child. Capillary or venous gases are more easily obtained in pediatrics and provide almost as much useful information as arterial gases. Unlike the adult patient that presents for thoracic surgery, it is often impossible to obtain reliable pulmonary function tests or spirometry. This, however, should not be an impediment to proceeding with the planned surgery. Any further testing should be based on those areas of concern elucidated during the preoperative evaluation.

Lastly, the preoperative evaluation should be used to explain to the child and/or parents the anesthetic plan and the eventual disposition of the patient. Risks and complications should be addressed and assent or consent obtained. Decisions regarding preoperative sedation and parental presence at induction can also be made at this time. The postoperative pain management strategy should be outlined and questions or concerns addressed.

Strategies for Lung Isolation

The indications for lung isolation in children include prevention of contamination by blood or pus, treatment of a large bronchopleural fistula or severe unilateral bronchiectasis, as well as facilitating surgical exposure during thoracic procedures. Although thoracoscopic procedures may be performed without lung isolation in very small infants (the induced pneumothorax is often enough to compress the lung tissue and provide surgical exposure; see Fig. 50.1), one must be prepared to isolate the lungs in the event surgical exposure is inadequate. The techniques and approach to lung isolation in the pediatric population may differ from that of adults since infant and small child-sized bronchial

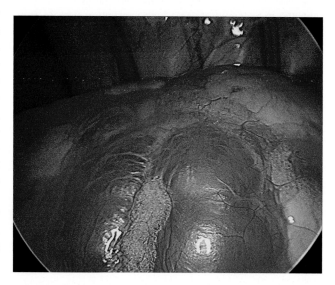

Fig. 50.1 Thoracoscopic view of a 6-month-old infant's right hemithorax in whom adequate surgical lung exposure was achieved with the induced capnothorax and without the need for lung isolation. The right lower lobe almost entirely consists of congenital cystic adenomatoid malformation (CCAM)

tubes are not available. Despite this, the basic principles of lung isolation in the child are similar to those for the adult. There are three fundamental techniques of lung isolation: single-lumen endobronchial intubation, bronchial blockers, and double-lumen bronchial tubes [21].

Historically, the use of single-lumen tubes for selective endobronchial intubation was the only method to isolate the lungs in small children. Although it is now rarely the preferred method of lung isolation, it has the advantage of being readily available, requiring little technical expertise, and can be performed on any patient, regardless of size. Right mainstem bronchus intubation is easily accomplished and has been performed (inadvertently or otherwise) by virtually every anesthesiologist. Left mainstem bronchus intubation, if done blindly, simply requires the ETT be rotated 180° with the patient's head turned to the right. This maneuver turns the bevel of the tracheal tube to favor left mainstem bronchus intubation with advancement. Alternatively, flexible fiberoptic bronchoscopy can be used to place the tracheal tube in the appropriate mainstem bronchus under indirect vision. Regardless of which technique is used, fiberoptic verification of proper tube placement is recommended [22, 23].

Other advantages of this technique include very rapid isolation that can be applied in emergency situations such as pulmonary hemorrhage. Limited technical experience is required, and specialized equipment is not necessary. Because single-lumen tubes are available in a wide variety of sizes, there is no patient that cannot be managed by this method. Note, however, that since airway diameter narrows further down the trachea and bronchi, one should consider placing a slightly smaller ETT than otherwise indicated.

Disadvantages of this technique are numerous. Firstly, conversion to temporary two-lung ventilation (i.e., to reexpand the nondependent lung) may be cumbersome. This requires withdrawing the secured ETT from the bronchus to the trachea. Reisolating the lung with the patient in lateral decubitus position and under surgical drapes can be problematic. As well, an incomplete seal at the bronchus will allow gases to escape and inflate the nondependent lung. Leak gas will also contaminate the room; however, more importantly debris, blood, and secretions from the operative side may soil the poorly isolated lung. If intubating the right mainstem bronchus, obstruction of the right upper lobe is possible, especially if a cuffed ETT is used. Finally, if hypoxemia arises, it is impossible to apply CPAP to the nondependent lung. If adjusting PEEP to the dependent lung does not improve the hypoxemia, repositioning the ETT above the carina and reverting to two-lung ventilation will be the only solution.

Bronchial blockers play an important role in pediatric lung isolation, particularly in patients 3 months to 9 years of age. There are currently three main devices available: Fogarty arterial embolectomy catheters (Edwards Lifesciences,

Irvine, CA, USA), Univent® tube (Vitaid, Lewinston, NY, USA), and the Arndt endobronchial blocker (Cook® Critical Care, Bloomington, IN, USA). The use of the Fogarty catheter for lung isolation is well described and has been used for all types of thoracic procedures [24–27]. The catheter can be placed either alongside the standard ETT or within it. If it is to be placed outside the ETT, the catheter is advanced under direct laryngoscopy through the vocal cords. The blocker catheter tip (which if larger than 3F can be slightly flexed; see Fig. 50.2) is then rotated 90° toward the desired lung and advanced into the mainstem bronchus. The ETT is then placed in the trachea. With fiberoptic visualization, the position of the catheter can be verified prior to inflation of the balloon tip. The entire apparatus is then secured to the patient.

If the Fogarty catheter is to be placed within the lumen of the ETT, the method of placement is as follows. As described earlier for selective endobronchial intubation, the ETT is advanced into the desired bronchus. The 15 mm adapter is removed from the tracheal tube, and the Fogarty catheter is placed through the lumen of the ETT into the bronchus. The ETT is withdrawn to a position above the carina while maintaining the endobronchial position of the catheter. Again verification and inflation of the Fogarty should be performed under flexible fiberoptic visualization. The ETT adapter will then have to be securely fastened such that the Fogarty is trapped between the adapter and ETT itself (see Fig. 50.3). A disadvantage of placing the Fogarty within the lumen of the ETT is that it may significantly decrease the internal diameter. This can interfere with ventilation if using a very small ETT, but more commonly it will make passage of the fiberoptic scope difficult. The fit of all scopes and airway devices must be prepared and tested prior to anesthetic induction.

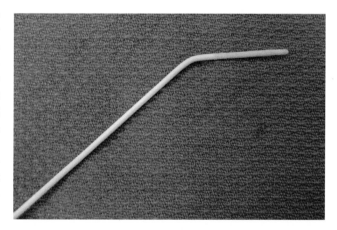

Fig. 50.2 Tip of a size 4F Fogarty embolectomy catheter (Edwards Lifesciences, Irvine, CA, USA) which has been shaped to facilitate maneuverability and insertion into a mainstem bronchus. All Fogarty embolectomy catheters except the size 2F and 3F contain a removable guide wire that can be used to shape the tip in this fashion

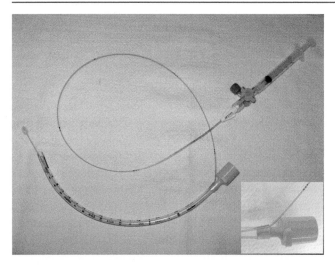

Fig. 50.3 Embolectomy catheter and tracheal tube assembly used for lung isolation in the small child. A size 3F Fogarty embolectomy catheter (Edwards Lifesciences, Irvine, CA, USA) inserted through a 4.5 mm ID tracheal tube (Sheridan) and placed in a mainstem bronchus. The embolectomy catheter is secured in place and sealed between the tracheal tube inner lumen and the 15 mm adapter (inset). Alternatively, the embolectomy catheter may be placed outside the tracheal tube in the mainstem bronchus

Table 50.2 Bronchial blocker sizes used for lung isolation in children

Age	ETT size (ID, mm)	Bronchial blocker size (F)[a]	Max balloon gas capacity (cc)	Inflated balloon diameter (mm)
<2 months	3.0–3.5	3	0.6	5
2–6 months	3.5–4.0	4	1.7	9
6 months–1 year	4.0	4	1.7	9
1–2 years	4.0–4.5	5	3.0	11
2–4 years	4.5–5.0	5	3.0	11
4–6 years	5.0–5.5	5	3.0	11
6–8 years	5.0–5.5 cuffed	6	4.5	13
8–10 years	5.5–6.0 cuffed	6	4.5	13

Abbreviations: ETT endotracheal tube, *ID* internal diameter
[a]Fogarty arterial embolectomy catheters (Edwards Lifesciences, Irvine, CA, USA)

The main advantage of the Fogarty catheter is that it can be used in very small infants as well as older children. Table 50.2 outlines the various embolectomy catheter sizes as well as the corresponding appropriate tracheal tube sizes used in pediatric practice. In general, the smaller the patient, the more challenging proper catheter placement becomes. Deflation of the balloon tip will enable easy and rapid reexpansion of the operative lung without requiring manipulation of the ETT.

A drawback to the Fogarty catheter is that the balloon is a low-volume, high-pressure device. For this reason, balloon inflation should be done under direct visualization and only the minimum of pressure be applied to provide bronchial sealing. Table 50.2 illustrates the maximum inflation volumes of the various embolectomy catheters. Since migration of the blocker by even a few millimeters can cause the balloon to slip into the lumen of the trachea and obstruct both lungs, one must be vigilant and prepared to immediately intervene by deflating the catheter cuff.

The Univent® tube has been designed with a channel that contains a bronchial blocker. Conventional laryngoscopy places the single-lumen tube into the trachea, and fiberoptic guidance of the balloon-tip catheter into the operative lung can then be performed. When seated appropriately, the Univent will isolate the lung and allow for easy conversion to conventional two-lung ventilation by simply deflating the bronchial cuff.

Pediatric sizes are available as small as 3.5 mm internal diameter. However, this device has an 8 mm external diameter and as such should not be used in patients less than 6 years old. In these smaller tube sizes, the bronchial blocker and its channel will also encroach into the lumen of the ETT and proportionally increase the airflow resistance as well as necessitate the use of a smaller fiberoptic scope. Univent® tubes below 6.5 mm ID do not have a central lumen in the bronchial blockers. Therefore, oxygen and CPAP cannot be applied with the smaller Univent® tubes [28–30].

The Arndt endobronchial blocker is a more recent addition to the armamentarium available to the pediatric anesthesiologist [31–33]. It consists of a conventional blocker with balloon tip and four-way adapter. The balloon is designed as a high-volume low-pressure system. Pediatric sizes include a 5F and 7F size blocker which can be used in a 4.5 and 6.5 mm ID tracheal tube, respectively (Table 50.3). Preparation and use of the Arndt endobronchial blocker are identical to that for adults (see Chap. 16).

A unique challenge of using the pediatric-sized Arndt blocker is adequate ventilation while the blocker and FOB both occupy the lumen of the ETT. The smallest-sized FOB must be used that allows placement of the endobronchial blocker. If such a small (i.e., 2.2 mm OD) fiberoptic bronchoscope is not available, the blocker can be positioned outside the ETT much like an embolectomy catheter. The tip of the FOB is passed through the nylon loop of the blocker, and the assembly is inserted in the operative bronchus. The FOB

Table 50.3 Pediatric Arndt endobronchial blocker sizes[a]

Blocker size (F)	ETT size (ID, mm)	FOB size (OD, mm)	Balloon inflation volume (cc)
5.0	≥4.5	≤2.8	0.5–2.0
7.0	≥6.5	≤3.5	2.0–6.0

Abbreviations: ETT endotracheal tube, *ID* internal diameter, *OD* outer diameter
[a]Cook® Critical Care, Bloomington, IN, USA

is then removed and the tracheal tube placed using direct laryngoscopy. Alternatively, if the patient remains adequately oxygenated and ventilated with the FOB-blocker apparatus in the operative bronchus, the FOB may be withdrawn to a position above the blocker, and inflation of the blocker cuff can be observed prior to removing the FOB. Once in position the nylon guide can be removed from the bronchial blocker (it cannot later be reinserted), and the central channel can be used for suctioning, providing supplemental oxygen, and CPAP. Fuji Systems (Tokyo, Japan) has recently released a 5F pediatric size of its independent bronchial blocker, the Uni-Blocker®.

The double-lumen endobronchial tube (DLT, Bronchopart®; Rüsch Inc., Duluth, GA, USA) differs significantly from the above designs in that selective intubation of either mainstem bronchus can be achieved with a second lumen located within the trachea. In this way, ventilation can be applied through either lumen individually or collectively. Unfortunately, pediatric sizes are limited due to the necessarily larger outer diameter of such a design. The 26F is currently the smallest available size and has an outer diameter of 9.3 mm, equivalent to a 6.5 mm ID ETT [34]. It is suitable for children approximately 8–10 years of age or approximately 30 kg in weight. Below this, one of the aforementioned isolation techniques is more appropriate. Double-lumen tube sizing will depend on the child's height as well as age. In general, a 28F DLT is suitable for a 12-year-old child, a 32F is appropriate for a 14-year old, and a size 35F is suitable for a 16-year old.

The DLT is straightforward in its application. Conventional laryngoscopy places the device into the trachea where it can be advanced into position by rotation to the appropriate side in a manner identical to that for adult patients. Fiberoptic bronchoscopy is recommended to ensure proper positioning [35]. Most often a left-sided DLT is used as it is easier to insert and eliminates the risk of right upper lobe obstruction. Correct positioning will mean the bronchial lumen is within the appropriate mainstem bronchus and the tracheal lumen above the carina. Inflation of the bronchial cuff can be observed with the FOB placed within the tracheal lumen. Once inflated the specialized circuit adapter can be manipulated such that ventilation to that lumen is obstructed while egress of gases from the lung is permitted.

Advantages of the DLT include easy access to either lung for suctioning or ventilation, application of supplemental oxygen, and CPAP. Conversion to two-lung ventilation is rapid and simple. Disadvantages of the DLT are mainly due to its awkward size and shape. Iatrogenic injury has been reported, and placement in patients with a difficult airway may be particularly challenging [36, 37]. The DLT should be replaced with a conventional ETT if postoperative ventilation is required.

Anesthetic Management of Specific Procedures and Diseases

Bronchoscopy

Evaluation of the airway by bronchoscopy, either rigid or flexible, has both diagnostic and therapeutic indications [38]. It is one of the few pediatric thoracic procedures that can be performed outside of the operating room under sedation or general anesthesia. In fact, depending on the age of the patient and indication for bronchoscopy, the anesthesiologist may not be involved at all, as some pediatric pulmonologists will provide airway topicalization and intravenous sedation in an ambulatory setting. This approach should be reserved for older, cooperative children who do not have severe respiratory compromise. Those patients that do require operative bronchoscopy must be evaluated with particular focus on the reason for bronchoscopy and the level of respiratory derangement. The type of procedure will often determine the means by which the airway is maintained, the type of anesthetic to be given, and whether paralysis is warranted. Rigid bronchoscopy for foreign body removal will require that a general anesthetic be given. Diagnostic evaluation of the trachea and bronchi for other etiologies can generally be performed via flexible bronchoscopy. Communication between the bronchoscopist and anesthesiologist is essential in any such shared airway case. An appropriately sized ETT or supraglottic airway should be selected for the specific fiberoptic bronchoscope in order to ensure ventilation can be maintained during bronchoscopy.

Older children who are able to understand and cooperate with the anesthesiologist and bronchoscopist can be successfully managed with airway topicalization and intravenous sedation. This can include an infusion of one or a combination of propofol, remifentanil, or ketamine, with or without midazolam [39–43]. More recently, an infusion of dexmedetomidine and propofol has been used in this setting [44]. Although ideally this should be carried out in the OR setting, such procedures are now frequently performed outside the operating room to contain costs and increase efficiency. Children tend to need a deeper level of sedation than adults in order to tolerate the bronchoscope, and titrating the sedation/anesthesia to achieve acceptable procedural conditions while maintaining spontaneous respiration can be challenging. Monitoring and preparation for possible conversion to a general anesthetic are essential. A second physician for patient monitoring and airway management should be at hand.

For those patients that are not suitable for sedation and airway topicalization, several options for airway management exist. These include but are not limited to mask ventilation, laryngeal mask, endotracheal intubation, and ventilation through the side port of a rigid bronchoscope [45]. Face mask ventilation has an advantage over the other methods listed as it allows for fiberoptic inspection of the oropharynx and/or nasopharynx and can be managed by one of two methods. The simplest is intermittent bag-mask ventilation or support with bronchoscopy conducted while the mask is temporarily removed from the patient. This requires coordination between the anesthesiologist and bronchoscopist and may involve periods of hypoventilation or apnea. If an inhalation agent is chosen as the means of anesthesia, then both awareness and waste gas pollution are a concern as the patient will be exhaling the agent into the room during the procedure. Careful titration of TIVA may therefore be the preferred approach for this option [46]. In addition, the diagnostic value of the procedure may be impaired as the bronchoscopist must enter and exit the airway repeatedly. To overcome these limitations, face masks with angled side ports have been developed that allow for continuous application of the mask to the patient and ventilation through the adapter, while the bronchoscopist uses an inline diaphragm that minimizes gas leakage (Fig. 50.4).

Although the laryngeal mask does not allow for inspection of the upper airway, it has nevertheless become the most commonly used conduit for diagnostic and therapeutic bronchoscopy in the pediatric patient outside the critical care unit [47]. The availability of smaller sizes and its ease of use make it ideally suited for this procedure. It is better tolerated than a tracheal tube and accommodates both spontaneous ventilation and positive-pressure ventilation as required. It has been shown in several studies to be well suited for bronchoscopy, even in small infants [48–50]. An angled adapter with an inline diaphragm for the bronchoscope is required. If the LMA has aperture bars, they may need to be removed as

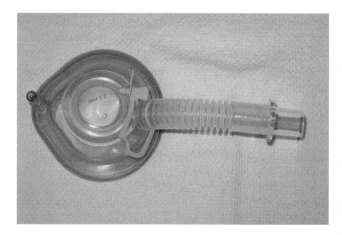

Fig. 50.4 Pediatric endoscopy mask (VBM Medizintechnik GmbH, Sulz, Germany) designed to allow simultaneous ventilation and endoscopy of the child. The assembly may be used for flexible fiberoptic intubation or airway endoscopy

they can impair the scope from passing through. In most cases, the bronchoscope will align itself with the glottic opening and not require any further manipulation of the LMA once seated.

Endotracheal intubation provides the most secure, stable, and controlled means of airway management for bronchoscopy. The majority of children in the critical care unit undergoing bronchoscopy will have an ETT in situ and undergo bronchoscopy to assess bronchial patency or pathology, tracheomalacia, and for sputum sampling. Outside the critical care unit, elective tracheal intubation for bronchoscopy may be preferred for infants and small children as well as patients with significant respiratory compromise. A period of postoperative ventilation may also be required for high-risk patients. Disadvantages of bronchoscopy through an ETT include the inability to examine the upper airway as well as bronchoscope size limitations. An appropriately sized scope must be chosen that allows adequate ventilation around itself in the remaining lumen of the ETT.

Rigid bronchoscopy offers the advantage of allowing dynamic examination of the airway from the oropharynx to the subsegmental bronchi. Most pediatric rigid bronchoscopes contain a 15 mm side port that allows for gas insufflation and even positive-pressure ventilation. It is the instrument of choice for pediatric foreign body removal. Disadvantages of rigid bronchoscopy include the fact that deep anesthesia is required to tolerate the bronchoscope and, if volatile anesthetic agents are used, room air contamination is a concern. In that case, suction or gas scavenging can be positioned at the base of the bronchoscope to minimize contamination. The practice of many pediatric anesthesiologists is to therefore use a propofol-based TIVA technique with local anesthetic applied to the vocal cords and carina. To this end a low-dose remifentanil (0.05 μg/kg/min) or dexmedetomidine (0.5–2.0 μg/kg/hr) infusion may be a useful adjunct. Typical goals are to maintain spontaneous ventilation without the use of muscle relaxants. However, positive-pressure ventilation can be applied via the side port of the rigid bronchoscope which may be facilitated by muscle relaxation.

Fever is not an uncommon sequela of flexible bronchoscopy, and it is not necessary to treat all such patients with antibiotics. Case reports of fever associated with sepsis following bronchoscopy have been reported; however, these are generally in immunocompromised patients in whom antibiotic therapy is warranted [51, 52]. Similarly rigid bronchoscopy has been shown to induce transient bacteremia, but again antibiotic treatment is generally unnecessary. Complication rates for bronchoscopy are low. The most common adverse event is transient desaturation; however, laryngospasm and bronchospasm can also occur [53, 54].

Thoracotomy and Video-Assisted Thoracoscopic Surgery (VATS)

Traditionally, all thoracic procedures in children were performed via a thoracotomy or median sternotomy. Mechanical retraction of the ribs and lung tissue would often be applied to provide the required surgical exposure. Because of technological advances and greater surgical experience gained from the adult population, video-assisted thoracoscopic surgery (VATS) is now used more readily in the pediatric population, even at the extremes of age and weight (Fig. 39.5) [55–58]. The reported advantages of VATS in the adult population, including less postoperative pain and shorter length of stay, accelerated the use of this technique in children. Although very few outcome studies have been conducted in children, VATS is utilized for an increasing number of conditions including empyema, lung biopsy and resection, mediastinal mass, trauma, pulmonary sequestration, and CCAM (Fig. 50.1) [59]. Even PDA closure is being performed thoracoscopically in very small infants [60]. Trocars for pediatric use are available in 5 and 3 mm diameters (Fig. 50.5).

Whereas thoracotomy does not always require the lungs be isolated in children, VATS is quite challenging without proper lung isolation and collapse of the surgical lung. An exception is in small infants, whose lungs can be collapsed with the induced capnothorax.

Single-lung ventilation in the pediatric population incurs many of the same physiologic derangements as in the adult population (see Chap. 6). Collapse of the nondependent lung preferentially directs ventilation to the dependent (nonsurgical) lung. Hypoxic pulmonary vasoconstriction (HPV) in the nondependent lung increases perfusion to the dependent lung and therefore attempts to correct the shunt. In adults

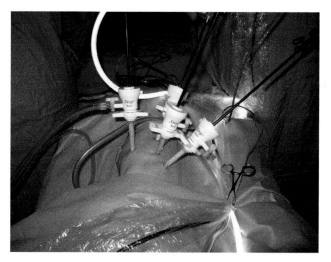

Fig. 50.5 Thoracoscopic trocars inserted in an infant for VATS. Surgical trocars used in children are available in 5 mm (shown) and 3 mm diameters

with the diseased lung in a nondependent position, this arrangement may actually improve oxygenation. Unfortunately in infants and neonates, this is often not the case. A compliant rib cage and compressible lung parenchyma allows for mediastinal excursion into the dependent lung thus reducing ventilation of that lung. Poor positioning and increased insufflating pressures will further contribute to this. Decreased hydrostatic pressure gradients between the two hemithoraces translate into relatively little improvement in V/Q matching even when HPV is intact. Moreover, alveolar collapse occurs more readily in infants as FRC approaches residual volume. The higher ratio of oxygen consumption to FRC, as compared to adults, will further exacerbate deoxygenation.

Many of the same complications of VATS occur in the pediatric population as in adults. Trocar misplacement (into the spleen or liver) may cause significant morbidity. High thoracoscopic insufflating pressures will decrease cardiac output and blood pressure by reducing preload and afterload. Patient positioning is even more important in pediatric procedures as an inappropriately located bolster will easily compress the compliant rib cage and reduce lung volumes in the dependent lung. Abdominal compression in the lateral decubitus position, from padding or "bean bags," will force the abdominal contents into the chest. As with any procedure that involves CO_2 insufflation under pressure, CO_2 gas embolism, though rare, must be considered in the event of sudden severe hemodynamic derangement.

As in adults maneuvers to preserve and treat hypoxemia with single-lung ventilation apply equally in the pediatric setting. Initial routine use of 100% oxygen upon lung isolation offers an increased safety margin and decreases HPV of the dependent lung. Once the procedure is underway and hemodynamic stability confirmed, the FiO_2 may be decreased as tolerated. Pressure-controlled ventilation may be used provided it delivers volumes in the range of 5–10 mL/kg. To this end mild hypercapnia is permitted, to avoid barotrauma. The application of PEEP to the dependent lung may improve oxygenation and if kept to <10 mmHg usually has minimal effects on PVR and does not divert blood flow away from the ventilated lung. Application of CPAP to the nondependent lung is not as practically applicable in the small child and often interferes with surgical exposure.

To conclude, the decision to proceed with a thoracotomy vs. VATS procedure must be discussed ahead of time by surgeon and anesthesiologist. A thorough understanding of the risks and benefits must be assessed by both teams and then explained to the parents/patient. A discussion between the anesthesiologist and surgeon must include a time line with respect to how long the VATS technique will be employed. If surgical goals are not met during this time line, then conversion to thoracotomy should be considered. Most importantly, emergency management of intraoperative bleeding must be discussed and a plan formulated for emergent conversion to thoracotomy. Pediatric patients, especially small infants and neonates, will very rapidly hemorrhage into the chest cavity. By the time thoracotomy is performed and surgical control of bleeding is established, significant morbidity may have occurred. Resuscitation, even with rapid/immediate transfusion, is extremely difficult in such cases. A low threshold is recommended for release of capnothorax and possible immediate conversion to thoracotomy if significant hemodynamic instability arises.

Empyema

Pediatric pleural effusions are most often infectious in nature with 50–70% being parapneumonic [61]. Other less common causes of pleural effusions, including those associated with renal disease, malignancy, and congenital heart disease, will not be discussed in this section.

There are three generally accepted stages of empyema formation. Stage one is *exudative* with a small volume of sterile fluid accumulation and neutrophil recruitment. Stage two involves bacterial translocation across the now damaged pleural endothelium followed by further neutrophil activation. This *bacterial invasive stage* is characterized by fibrin and collagen fluid loculations. The pleural chemistry will now be acidic as glucose is metabolized and carbon dioxide and lactic acid levels increase. The final stage of *organized empyema* formation results in a thick purulent fluid, filled with cellular debris and deposition of a pleural "peel" along the membrane.

Aside from clinical examination, the most common investigational techniques will involve two-view chest X-rays and ultrasonography (US). US has the advantage of being able to quantify the fluid, indicate loculations, and locate ideal insertion sites for drainage tubes. Computed tomography can also provide detailed assessment of the pleural space but is not usually indicated.

Medical management is still the mainstay of management of parapneumonic effusions in most institutions [62], although early surgical intervention with VATS is associated with shorter hospitalization and equivalent clinical outcomes [63].

Empiric antibiotic therapy is initiated based on the common bacterial pathogens as determined by patient demographics and known community pathogens. Common pathogens include *Streptococcus pneumonia, Streptococcus pyogenes, Staphylococcus aureus, and Haemophilus influenza* [64]. Retrospective case analysis shows that approximately one-quarter of cases will be successfully managed with antibiotic therapy alone [65]. Fine needle thoracentesis and/or small-bore chest tube drainage is required in the remaining cases.

Clinical pathways for pleural effusion drainage are typically institutionally driven and based on the most recent literature. Several different groups have proposed indications for chest drainage [66]. Any effusion greater than 1 cm or 25% of the width of the hemithorax on US or CXR or ongoing respiratory distress despite adequate antimicrobial coverage may warrant small-bore drainage tube insertion. This is typically achieved in the interventional radiology suite with IV sedation and local anesthetic infiltration at the insertion site. Most commonly the use of midazolam, ketamine, dexmedetomidine, and/or fentanyl in titrated doses is sufficient, although sedating doses of propofol will be tolerated by most patients. Nasal prong oxygen and standard monitoring are employed.

If the effusion persists despite drainage tube insertion, it is typically a result of loculation and fibrin deposition. The initial approach is to instill a thrombolytic agent (e.g., streptokinase, urokinase, tPA) through the chest tube into the pleural space. This will ideally break down the adhesions and facilitate further drainage [67]. Approximately 15% of patients will require multiple fibrinolysis treatments [65].

Failure of clinical improvement or progression of fluid accumulation will necessitate discussion regarding surgical decortication. Three percent of patients may require such surgical intervention following conservative medical management [68]. Surgery can be accomplished by open thoracotomy or more commonly video-assisted thoracoscopic surgery (VATS). At this stage the empyema has likely developed a thick fibrous plaque that prevents collapse of the affected pleural space. As such lung isolation is not routinely applied. Trocar insertion into the pleural space is performed without the need for lung isolation as the empyema fluid and thickened pleura have created a fluid-filled space with the affected lung collapsed away from the chest wall.

Anesthetic monitoring of these patients includes conventional noninvasive monitors with the addition of an arterial line if clinically warranted. As blood transfusion may occasionally be required, adequate venous access is essential. Induction of anesthesia is usually not complicated, although these patients may have significant respiratory distress.

In most cases, tracheal extubation and transfer to a monitored ward bed are sufficient; however, these patients may require postoperative ventilation. Intravenous antibiotic therapy should be continued. Most children will recover uneventfully with full resolution of symptoms and no ongoing sequelae.

Patent Ductus Arteriosus (PDA)

Surgical PDA repair is perhaps the most common cardiac procedure to be managed by the noncardiac specialized pediatric anesthesiologist. As technology and surgical technique have evolved, so too has the surgical management of this disease. The historic use of a large lateral thoracotomy has today been replaced by smaller muscle-sparing "mini" thoracotomies. Moreover, many centers have established good success rates with the VATS technique [60, 69]. Percutaneous coiling of the PDA via interventional angiography is also widely available but will not be discussed herein [70, 71].

The ductus arteriosus is an essential conduit directing blood flow away from the high-pressure pulmonary circulation toward the systemic circulation during fetal development. It most often arises at the anterior surface of the main PA and attaches to the descending aorta near the left subclavian artery. In response to the increased PaO_2 after birth, the musculature of the ductus constricts and effectively closes the structure. Smaller birth weight infants and premature infants are more likely to have persistently PDA. If left untreated the left-to-right shunt created by the PDA will result in pulmonary overcirculation, pulmonary edema, and respiratory insufficiency. RV failure may also develop, especially if pulmonary pressures increase. Rarely, this may result in shunt reversal. In children who have a hemodynamically stable PDA, closure is still required as the risk of bacterial endocarditis is quite high [72].

If significant pulmonary overcirculation exists, the patient may require tracheal intubation in NICU to help support ventilation prior to surgery. These patients may often be fluid restricted and given diuretics in order to help alleviate the resultant pulmonary valvular insufficiency. To this end, inotropic support will also occasionally be required. Surgical stress will further strain the already compromised preexisting respiratory and hemodynamic status. Likewise, any preexisting medical condition or syndrome should be evaluated prior to induction of anesthesia. Whether performed via mini thoracotomy or VATS, surgical closure of a PDA is usually of short duration (<1 h typically) and involves minimal blood loss. In order to assess the blood flow in both the ascending (preductal) and descending (postductal) aorta, a noninvasive blood pressure cuff may be placed on a lower limb with an oxygen saturation probe applied to both the right hand and the left foot. Invasive arterial measurement is no longer routinely required. When identification of the PDA is difficult, the surgeon may place temporary clips across the vascular structure and observe the effects on the patient. Correct positioning across the PDA will result in a rise in diastolic pressures, whereas occlusion of the main PA will result in decreased oxygen saturation and $ETCO_2$. Temporary occlusion of the descending aorta will result in a sudden loss of lower extremity saturation tracing and blood pressure while simultaneously preserving the preductal saturation.

Induction of anesthesia is dependent on the preexisting condition of the patient. Those that present with respiratory or hemodynamic compromise may typically receive a high-dose narcotic (e.g., fentanyl 10–20 μg/kg IV) at induction with muscle paralysis. Minimal volatile anesthetics should be used in these cases, and supplemental narcotic dosing may be given as required. Alternatively, a remifentanil infusion along with low volatile anesthetic concentration may be used in those patients suitable for postoperative tracheal extubation. In addition to the standard intravenous used for induction, a larger peripheral intravenous catheter should be inserted after induction. Blood should be available in the operating theater for fluid resuscitation in the event of surgical misadventure. Open thoracotomy for PDA closure does not require lung isolation or single-lung ventilation. Simple retraction is sufficient to provide surgical exposure. Recent studies, however, have shown the efficacy of the VATS approach to PDA repair [73–76]. Ventilatory strategies for this include lung isolation (by any technique described earlier) or placement of a single-lumen ETT and allowing the pneumothorax to dictate surgical exposure. Muraldihar et al. [77] evaluated right mainstem bronchial intubation vs. low tidal volume high-frequency ventilation of both lungs and showed more profound desaturation in the mainstem intubated patients. Miyagi et al. [78] reported on the successful use of the Fogarty catheter as a bronchial blocker for a series of PDA closures performed via VATS. Despite the potential for hemorrhage, many studies have shown the safety and efficacy of this surgical approach for the repair of PDA [79]. Risk factors, regardless of approach, continue to be hemorrhage, residual patency, and recurrent laryngeal nerve injury. Odegard et al. [80] describe a simple yet effective means to identify the recurrent laryngeal nerve and thus prevent injury during VATS procedures by using a thin Teflon nerve-stimulating probe and recording the evoked electromyograms.

Tracheoesophageal Fistula (TEF)

The incidence of TEF is approximately 1 in 3000, and although it may occur in isolation, about 50% of cases will present in association with other congenital anomalies [81]. The VACTERL association (vertebral, anal, and cardiovascular defects, TEF, renal and radial limb defects) has been well described [82, 83]. The most commonly associated cardiac defects are atrial septal defect, PDA, and tetralogy of Fallot [84]. Investigation of these defects is essential prior to any surgical intervention. The trachea and esophagus are derived from the primitive foregut during the fourth and fifth weeks of life. The trachea emerges ventrally from the primitive foregut, and a septum between the esophagus and trachea is created by fusion of the tracheoesophageal folds. Failure of incomplete separation of these two structures can result in isolated esophageal atresia (rare) or more commonly TEF. The Gross classification describes six of the most common forms of TEF [85]. Type C, accounting for 85% of all cases of TEF, consists of a fistula located slightly above the carina with proximal esophageal atresia. It is suggested shortly after birth with copious salivation associated with choking, coughing, and cyanosis coincident with the onset of feeding. Diagnosis is confirmed by the inability to pass a suction catheter into the stomach, and a gastric air bubble is often visible on radiograph. In most patients, surgical intervention will be planned for within the first week of life. During this time, these patients should be kept in a head-up or lateral decubitus position with a nasoesophageal suction catheter inserted to help prevent aspiration. Early tracheal intubation is rarely required. In otherwise healthy newborn infants, there is almost 100% survivability. Survival declines rapidly if TEF is associated with low birth weight, prematurity, cardiac anomalies, or pulmonary complications [71, 86].

Primary repair consists of fistula ligation and esophageal anastomosis. Occasionally, a staged repair will be required in patients that are unstable and premature or have very low birth weight. This consists of placement of a balloon-tip catheter into the distal esophagus via percutaneous gastrostomy under local anesthesia [87]. This temporizing measure helps prevent reflux and will enable more efficient ventilation, particularly if high airway pressures are required. When the patient becomes more stable, the definitive repair can be performed. This has traditionally been undertaken through a thoracotomy on the side opposite the aortic arch. Fistula ligation is followed by esophageal anastomosis. If the two ends of the esophagus are separated by too great a distance, the fistula is ligated, and a section of the colon can be interposed at a later date. Thoracoscopic repair has been described, and in some centers it has become the preferred surgical approach [88, 89].

Anesthetic management begins with the understanding that positive-pressure ventilation should be minimized on induction. If the fistula is large, pressurized gas flow will follow the path of least resistance through the fistula and into the stomach. This will cause gastric dilatation leading to further impairment of ventilation and possible reflux of gastric contents into the lungs. Profound respiratory failure and cardiac arrest have been reported. The goal of induction is to place the ETT distal to the fistula and proximal to the carina. This is often accomplished by blind mainstem intubation and subsequent retraction of the ETT until bilateral breath sounds are auscultated. Many centers now advocate initial rigid bronchoscopy with the patient breathing spontaneously under volatile or intravenous anesthesia in order to identify the size and location of the fistula prior to tracheal intubation. Flexible fiberoptic bronchoscopy may also be used to verify tube positioning following tracheal intubation. Prior to induction the patient should have thorough suctioning of the esophageal catheter and be well preoxygenated. Pretreatment with atropine is recommended. Traditionally,

an awake tracheal intubation would have been performed on these patients. More recently, pediatric anesthesiologists prefer to induce anesthesia with inhaled volatile anesthetic while maintaining spontaneous respiration or alternatively, perform a rapid sequence induction. Once the ETT is carefully positioned to ensure lung ventilation without fistula insufflation, muscle relaxation and gentle positive pressure can be provided. Some anesthesiologists will prefer not to paralyze or provide positive-pressure ventilation until the fistula is ligated. For thoracoscopic TEF repair, lung isolation is generally not attempted. Anesthetic induction and tracheal tube placement are as for open repair; however, maintaining spontaneous respiration until the fistula is ligated is impractical. The induced pneumothorax/capnothorax often produces adequate surgical exposure.

Intraoperative monitoring consists of the usual noninvasive monitors and possibly an arterial line. A large peripheral intravenous for fluid resuscitation should be obtained. A precordial stethoscope placed in the left axilla will help identify movement of the ETT into the right mainstem bronchus. The flexible fiberoptic bronchoscope should be available as it may be required to confirm intraoperative tube placement. Tracheal suction catheters should be on hand as surgical manipulation of the nondependent lung may cause debris or secretions to obstruct the ETT.

Intraoperative complications usually consist of ventilation difficulties, leading to hypoxemia and/or hypercapnia. Increasing FiO$_2$, adjusting ventilatory settings, and providing muscle relaxation may help improve this. Occasionally, and more commonly during thoracoscopic procedures, a degree of hypercapnia and desaturation must be tolerated. Although some of the most robust patients may be suitable for postoperative tracheal extubation, most will benefit from a short period of elective ventilation. The tracheal tube is carefully withdrawn to a position proximal to the fistula, and the nondependent lung is gently reexpanded under direct vision. The hemithorax is simultaneously filled with warmed saline to ensure there is no air leak from the repaired fistula site. Early postoperative complications include atelectasis, increased airway secretions causing small airway collapse, and electrolyte disturbances associated with increased fluid requirements. Later complications include esophageal anastomotic leak, formation of bronchoesophageal fistula, and esophageal stricture formation [90].

Mediastinal Mass

Management of the pediatric patient with a mediastinal mass presents unique and serious challenges to the anesthesiologist. A common misconception is that a mediastinal mass is more likely to cause symptoms in children compared to adults [91]. In fact children are less likely to be symptomatic compared to an adult [92–94]. The presence of symptoms may be predictive of malignancy in the adult; however, this does not seem to hold true for children [95]. A finding of orthopnea (supine dyspnea) in the child may be predictive of significant tracheal narrowing [96, 97], and its presence should alert the clinician to the possibility of airway obstruction upon induction of anesthesia. The presence and degree of orthopnea should be assessed in every patient. The older child with mild symptoms can lie supine with some cough or pressure sensation. The patient with moderate symptoms will only be able to lie supine for short periods, and the severely symptomatic patient will not tolerate the supine position [98]. Characterizing the degree of orthopnea in the infant or small child is more challenging. The infant without symptoms will not seem stressed when supine, whereas the mildly symptomatic infant may look frightened or upset when supine. It is difficult and of little clinical use to attempt to distinguish between moderate or severe symptoms in the small child or infant. In either case, the infant will look severely distressed, may be gasping, or even cyanotic when supine.

Despite the predictive value of orthopnea in older children with a mediastinal mass, life-threatening complications may occur in the absence of symptoms, particularly in infants and small children [99].

The other major complication is cardiovascular collapse secondary to compression of the heart or major vessels. The presence of a pericardial effusion is associated with an increased risk of cardiovascular complications during anesthesia [100]. Death upon induction of general anesthesia in patients with an anterior mediastinal mass is always a risk. Anesthetic deaths have mainly been reported in children [101]. This may be due to the fact that:

1. Children have a more compressible cartilaginous airway structure.
2. The presenting signs and symptoms correlate poorly with tumor size.
3. Children are less able to give a reliable history.
4. Children more often receive a general anesthetic for tissue biopsy.

Diagnosis and Risk Stratification

The most important diagnostic test in the patient with a mediastinal mass is CT of the trachea and chest. Although a chest X-ray is often helpful in detecting a mediastinal mass, the CT scan provides useful information such as the size and compressive effects of the mass. For proper tumor staging, however, a CT scan of the chest, abdomen, and pelvis is required. Fortunately, this can be accomplished with an average scan time of under 20 s with the more modern, faster CT scanners. In addition, the patient's head and chest can be elevated to 30° without affecting scan quality. Alternatively, the scan can be done with the patient in lateral or even prone position, if necessary.

It is essential to determine the patient's most comfortable position prior to starting the CT scan. Most patients, including the otherwise uncooperative child, will often assume that position while confined to the hospital bed. Furthermore, many major pediatric centers have adopted the resourceful practice of performing the scan at a time that coincides with that child's natural sleep. Distraction (with music or video) has been used with success in older children. For practical purposes, this means that the scan can be done with the patient in his/her most comfortable position during natural sleep, thus minimizing the need for sedation. The anesthesiologist should never feel compelled to have the severely symptomatic patient lay flat and supine, be deeply sedated, or anesthetized for a CT scan. In such a situation, if the above measures are unsuccessful or impractical, serious consideration should be given to steroid administration or selective irradiation prior to CT in order to reduce the tumor mass.

For those patients that are uncooperative but do not have severe symptoms, sedation may be administered, provided a cautious approach is adopted. Although nothing is absolute, careful titration of a single agent may be safer or preferable to polypharmacy, particularly for small children. A 6-year review of over 16,000 sedations performed on children revealed that the odds of having an adverse event were nearly 5 times higher when multiple agents were used (odds ratio [OR] 4.9, 95% CI 2.9–8.4) [102]. As a single agent, nitrous oxide 50% in oxygen is often all that is needed in small children to provide analgesia and sedation. Alternatively, midazolam or etomidate 0.1 mg/kg, ketamine or propofol 0.25 mg/kg IV boluses, or continuous infusion may be carefully titrated to effect. Although many agree that the risk of airway obstruction and hypoxemia increases when a combination of benzodiazepines and opioids is used [103], sedation even with a single agent may not be tolerated in the high-risk patient [104]. Of equal importance is appropriate monitoring of the patient, early recognition and treatment of complications, and attention to patient positioning during the procedure. The flat, supine position is never mandatory.

Obstruction of the superior vena cava (SVC) causing venous hypertension and engorgement of venous collaterals leading to cyanosis and edema of the head, neck, and upper extremities is known as the SVC syndrome [105]. The most common cause of SVC syndrome in children is primary lymphoma or lymphoblastic leukemia [106]. SVC syndrome is often present without associated airway compromise in the adult with a mediastinal mass. In children with such a mass, however, the SVC syndrome is closely associated with and may predict the development of acute airway compromise. Tracheal intubation may be more difficult due to laryngeal edema that results from SVC obstruction. This obstruction may also cause pulmonary artery or myocardial compression or affect right ventricular output, causing right heart failure [107]. Anesthetic-induced myocardial depression will aggravate these effects, with potentially disastrous consequences. Cerebral venous drainage and cerebral perfusion pressure may also be reduced in the patient with significant SVC obstruction. As such, any patient presenting with SVC syndrome should be considered high risk. Patients with cardiovascular symptoms and SVC syndrome or those patients unable to give an adequate history should therefore have transthoracic echocardiography to assess for cardiac, systemic, or pulmonary vascular compression.

Historically, children with tracheobronchial compression greater than 50% on CT have been considered high risk for general anesthesia [108]. More recent reviews have found the presence of orthopnea or SVC syndrome may be predictive of anesthesia-related complications [104, 107], but the extent of symptoms do not correlate well with the degree of tracheal narrowing on CT scan [96]. Based on these studies and the authors' clinical experience, the following risk stratification guideline regarding safety for general anesthesia is suggested. The patient with minimal to no orthopnea and near-normal tracheobronchial area on CT scan will likely tolerate general anesthesia. In contrast, the child with moderate to severe orthopnea and tracheobronchial area < 50% of normal on CT scan or the patient with evidence of SVC syndrome or a pericardial effusion should be considered high risk. Unfortunately, there are several patient groups whose risk for general anesthesia remains uncertain. They include the child with mild orthopnea whose tracheobronchial diameter is unknown and older child who is unable to give a history.

Direct examination of mediastinal mass tissue has been the traditional and preferable approach to making the diagnosis. In high-risk or symptomatic patients, however, the risk of general anesthesia and thoracotomy, mediastinoscopy, or VATS may be considerable. Excisional biopsy of extrathoracic lymph nodes has often been sufficient to confirm the diagnosis and allow for appropriate therapy. Increasingly, cytometric and immunocytochemical studies of pleural fluid have also been used with success to secure a diagnosis, obviating the need to deliver deep sedation or general anesthesia. Thoracentesis is particularly useful in lymphoblastic lymphoma, which is associated with a high incidence of pleural effusion [109, 110].

In the high-risk patient without extrathoracic lymphadenopathy or a pleural effusion, percutaneous needle biopsy of the tumor under ultrasound or CT guidance may be a safe alternative [111, 112]. In centers equipped with interventional radiology expertise, core needle biopsies can be obtained under ultrasound guidance with the patient in a semi-upright or lateral position [113, 114]. This can be achieved under local anesthesia and mild sedation as required. The most obvious disadvantage to needle biopsy is the inherent "failure to diagnose" rate due to insufficient tissue for complete histological and molecular classification, although a failure rate exists also for open biopsy [115].

The use of prebiopsy corticosteroid treatment to reduce tumor size has generally been avoided if possible due to the extreme and rapid responsiveness to this (and radiation) therapy. There is widespread belief that prebiopsy steroid therapy will impair accurate histological diagnosis and result in suboptimal treatment or recurrence with a less favorable prognosis. A 10-year review of children presenting with an anterior mediastinal tumor sheds light on and refutes this myth [116]. Twenty-three of the 86 patients in that series received prebiopsy hydrocortisone because of clinical evidence of respiratory compromise. Prebiopsy steroid treatment was felt to have had an adverse effect on the pathological diagnosis in 5 of the 23 children; however, survival in those 5 patients was unaffected, and the authors concluded that prebiopsy steroid administration is defensible in symptomatic patients. In a more recent series, one third of children with a mediastinal mass were treated with corticosteroids prior to diagnosis because they were considered high risk. A clear diagnosis was made in 95% of these patients despite steroid therapy [99]. In these cases, close and ongoing consultation with the oncologist is essential. Prebiopsy steroid therapy may be justifiable (and arguably necessary) if the patient has symptoms and CT evidence of significant airway or cardiovascular compression and is too young or uncooperative to tolerate local anesthetic alone. A typical regimen consists of 20 mg prednisone equivalents per meter square of body surface area, administered three times daily. Coordination between the oncologist, surgeon, and anesthesiologist is essential as biopsy tissue should be obtained between 12 and 24 h after starting steroid therapy. These patients should be monitored and treated in anticipation of developing tumor lysis syndrome, a constellation of metabolic abnormalities which can include hyperkalemia, hyperuricemia, hyperphosphatemia, secondary hypocalcemia, and acute renal failure [117].

Another alternative to preoperative steroids in the high-risk patient includes irradiating the tumor while leaving a small area covered with lead for subsequent biopsy. This is not a viable option for the majority of pediatric patients presenting with a mediastinal mass as it requires the patient be cooperative and able to lie still for the duration of the treatment.

Flow-volume loops are commonly ordered as part of the preoperative assessment for patients with an anterior mediastinal mass. Specifically, the development of an increased expiratory plateau when changing from the upright to the supine position is thought to be pathognomonic for a variable intrathoracic airway obstruction and an indicator of patients who are at risk for airway collapse during induction of anesthesia.

However, a careful examination of the literature reveals that this emphasis on flow-volume loops derives from a single case report [118]. Apart from isolated case reports, studies of flow-volume loops have shown a poor correlation with the degree of airway obstruction [119–121]. The use of flow-volume loops in the assessment of patients with anterior mediastinal masses is well described in standard anesthesia texts and frequently asked on anesthesia specialty exams. However in clinical practice, it is difficult to see how flow-volume loops add any useful information beyond that which is obtained from the history and chest imaging. Certainly flow-volume loops may show some correlation with airway obstruction in selected patients. However, modern chest imaging will tell the clinician not only if there is an obstruction but also its location, severity, and extent. This is the truly vital information in deciding how to manage the airway of a patient with an anterior mediastinal mass.

Although deep general anesthesia and muscle relaxation can be avoided in most patients with symptomatic lesions, invariably the anesthesiologist will be faced with the uncooperative child with a compressive mediastinal mass requiring general anesthesia for a diagnostic or therapeutic procedure. Management of these patients is guided by their symptoms and the CT scan. A stepwise induction of anesthesia with continuous monitoring of gas exchange and hemodynamics is recommended. This may be achieved by inhalation of a volatile agent such as sevoflurane or IV titration of propofol, ketamine, and/or dexmedetomidine which maintains spontaneous ventilation until either the airway is definitively secured or the procedure is completed [122]. Awake intubation of the trachea before induction is a possibility only in older, mature pediatric patients if the CT scan shows a distal area of noncompressed trachea to which the ETT can be advanced before induction. If muscle relaxation is required, ventilation should first be gradually taken over manually to assure that positive-pressure ventilation is possible and only then can a muscle relaxant be administered. In some centers, muscle relaxation is avoided throughout the entire procedure if at all possible, as there have been cases of cardiorespiratory collapse that were likely caused by the resultant loss of muscle tone [123].

Airway or vascular compression can develop at any stage of the procedure and should be anticipated. In the preoperative assessment, the patient will often report that there is one side or position that causes less symptoms of compression. This, along with the findings on chest imaging, should be communicated to the entire operative team prior to anesthetic induction. In the event of intraoperative life-threatening airway or cardiovascular collapse, the patient should immediately be placed in that predetermined position, which will often result in a dramatic clinical improvement. The prone position has also been lifesaving in this setting [124]. Rigid bronchoscopy and ventilation distal to the obstruction may be necessary. As such, an experienced bronchoscopist and rigid bronchoscopy equipment must always be immediately available. In emergent situations, it is often not possible to push a standard ETT distally through the collapsed trachea. Ventilation and oxygenation can be reestablished temporarily with either a ventilating rigid bronchoscope or with jet ventilation via a rigid scope. Ultimately a reinforced ETT should be placed distal to the obstruction to stent the airway. This can be done by passing an airway exchange catheter or bougie distally under direct vision through the rigid bronchoscope, then withdrawing the bronchoscope, and using the airway catheter as a guide for the ETT [125]. In fact it may be reasonable to use an armored tube in all patients with a mediastinal mass; however, a stylet will still be needed to advance the tube distal to the compressed portion of the airway. Depending on the response to the above emergency measures, the patient may have to be awakened as rapidly as possible and other options for surgery explored.

Heliox may be used in the event of subtotal airway collapse to decrease the work of breathing. Heliox is a mixture of helium and oxygen (most commonly 70:30) and decreases the turbulent airflow resistance through a narrowed airway due to the decreased density of helium.

Femorofemoral cardiopulmonary bypass (CPB) before induction of anesthesia is a possibility for older and more cooperative children who are considered "unsafe" for general anesthesia. Although emergency percutaneous CPB has been used successfully in an adult patient with impending complete airway obstruction [126], this is not a practical option in the young, frightened child. In addition, even the smallest femoral bypass cannulae are too large in diameter to be used in the patient weighing less than 15–20 kg. In such a case, preoperative steroid therapy should be considered.

The concept of CPB "standby" during attempted induction of anesthesia is fraught with danger because there is not enough time after sudden airway collapse to establish CPB before hypoxic cerebral injury occurs. It is not a practical option in the pediatric patient with a large anterior mediastinal mass. For patients who present with primarily cardiovascular rather than airway compression, rigid bronchoscopy will not be a useful resuscitation maneuver in the event of cardiovascular collapse. Resuscitation intraoperatively may require emergent sternotomy and lifting the tumor off the heart and great vessels [127]. For this reason, whenever possible, patients with cardiovascular compression should be prepped and draped for surgery prior to induction of anesthesia.

Congenital Diaphragmatic Hernia (CDH)

Congenital herniation of the abdominal contents into the thoracic cavity occurs in approximately 1 in every 2500 live births [128]. The majority of cases will present prenatally if the mother has undergone standard ultrasonography [129, 130]. Occasionally, the diagnosis will be made in the early postnatal period. Intrusion of abdominal viscera into the thorax during fetal lung development leads to pulmonary hypoplasia and pulmonary vascular hypertension. This may promote persistence of fetal circulation (i.e., patent foramen ovale and PDA) after birth. Most cases of CDH occur on the left side at the foramen of Bochdalek, accounting for 80% of unilateral herniations. Less common is herniation at the foramen of Morgagni or at the esophageal hiatus itself. Mortality is related to the size of the defect and the association of cardiovascular anomalies. Approximately 10–30% of patients with CDH will have other congenital anomalies. These include congenital cardiac disease, chromosomal abnormalities (e.g., trisomy 18 and 21), CNS (e.g., spina bifida, hydrocephalus), and gastrointestinal anomalies (e.g., TEF, malrotation, atresia) [131]. Right-sided hernias are more often associated with these other defects. Large diaphragmatic hernias not diagnosed prenatally will present at delivery with severe respiratory distress and cyanosis. Physical findings include decreased breath sounds unilaterally or bilaterally. Indrawing, nasal flaring, and accessory muscle use indicate impending respiratory failure. Palpation of the trachea often reveals deviation away from the affected side. Peristaltic (bowel) sounds may be heard over the affected hemithorax. Chest X-ray will reveal mediastinal shift away from the affected hemithorax as well as air-filled bowel loops in the chest. The position of a nasogastric tube will be above the diaphragm.

As a result of compression and interference with normal lung development, the affected lung is reduced in volume and hypoplastic. Pulmonary surfactant deficiency contributes to poor lung compliance. This results in poor gas exchange and worsening of hypoxia, hypercapnia, and acidosis. PVR may remain elevated with persistent fetal circulation. High airway pressures and hemodynamic instability can further drive pulmonary hypertension. With elevated PVR and a PDA, right-to-left shunting will occur. Other sites of shunting may also exist depending on the associated cardiac pathology. Systemic hypoxia will continue because of this shunting, and disease progression will accelerate. Without appropriate preoperative support, this cascade of hypoxia, acidosis, increasing PVR, and right-to-left shunt will lead to cardiac dysfunction and patient demise. Routine preoperative echocardiogram is mandated to screen for the aforementioned defects, PVR and ventricular function.

Management strategies for CDH have changed over the last few decades [80, 132]. Currently, preoperative stabilization followed by surgical repair is recommended. That being said the optimal timing of repair is currently debated. Much of the recent work has focused on optimizing hemodynamic and ventilatory support in this patient population [133]. At present no one best strategy has been universally agreed

upon. Historically, resuscitative efforts were aimed at achieving alkalosis through active hyperventilation with the goal of minimizing pulmonary vascular hypertension. Contemporary "gentle" ventilation guidelines aim to minimize barotrauma by limiting maximal inspiratory pressures (<25 cmH$_2$O) and tidal volumes. Much like in the management of adult RSD, a degree of hypoxia and hypercapnia is accepted. Survivability has actually been shown to improve in these patients managed in this way provided PaO$_2$ is kept at 60 mmHg and PaCO$_2$ approaches 65 mmHg [134–136]. Until invasive arterial vascular access can be gained, one may aim for a preductal oxygen saturation of 85% with postductal saturation of 60%. Failure to achieve these goals with conventional ventilation may be an indication for conversion to high-frequency oscillatory (HFO) or jet ventilation. To facilitate this method of ventilation, judicious use of sedatives, narcotics, and muscle relaxants will be required. Alternatively, progressive hypercapnia and acidosis with an A-a gradient >500 mmHg are indications for ECMO [137, 138].

Pharmacologic adjuncts for the management of pulmonary hypertension have included inhaled nitric oxide, sildenafil, prostaglandins, and prostacyclins [139]. In this case, inotropic support is often required. With improvements in preoperative management, the overall survival rate has been reported as >75% [140].

The anesthesiologist may first become involved during resuscitative efforts at the time of birth. Early insertion of a nasogastric tube will be necessary to decompress the stomach. The reduced volume of air in the stomach will aid ventilatory mechanics. Likewise bag-mask ventilation should be kept to a minimum to avoid further gastric distension. If oxygen saturation continues to decrease despite NG tube insertion and high-flow oxygen, then tracheal intubation is appropriate. Sedatives, narcotics, and muscle relaxants are often administered to facilitate tracheal intubation and positive-pressure ventilation.

Intraoperatively the anesthesiologist must attempt to maintain ventilation and oxygenation as discussed earlier. Conversion from HFO to conventional ventilation should be attempted prior to surgery, although CDH repair is possible with the patient on HFO ventilation [141, 142]. Peak airway pressures should be limited to avoid barotrauma and worsening PVR. A sudden rise in airway pressures or decrease in lung compliance can indicate a contralateral pneumothorax which must be diagnosed and treated promptly as it may be associated with a worse outcome. Anesthetic management typically includes a narcotic and muscle relaxant technique. In addition to basic monitoring, an arterial line (preferably right radial) as well as pre- and postductal oxygen saturation monitors should be placed. Decreasing postductal saturation may indicate worsening right-to-left shunt and increasing PVR. Closure of the diaphragmatic hernia may compromise venous return from the lower extremities, and therefore intravenous access in the upper limbs is preferred. Insertion of an internal jugular venous line is not essential and risks causing a pneumothorax but if already present can be a useful adjunct for monitoring right-sided pressures and venous oxygen saturation.

Surgery usually consists of an abdominal incision with the herniated contents being reduced into the abdomen. Small defects can then be closed primarily, while larger ones may require the use of a synthetic patch. Closure of the abdomen may also necessitate the use of a patch to avoid cardiopulmonary compromise in the event of elevated abdominal pressures. With reduction complete, the hypoplastic lung should not be aggressively ventilated as this will increase the risk of barotrauma and contralateral pneumothorax and is typically of little or no therapeutic value.

Minimally invasive repair of CDH has been documented in the pediatric population [143]. Unfortunately the literature in favor of this technique likely suffers from patient selection bias (most stable patients selected for this technique). Current consensus statements do not recommend the routine use of minimally invasive repair [143, 144].

Lung Biopsy

Optimum management of solid lung masses almost always requires correct pathological diagnosis via biopsy of the affected tissue. Obtaining such samples, however, can be challenging, especially when dealing with pediatric patients. The traditional method for acquiring these samples has been open lung biopsy, which is associated with morbidity and considerable pain. Increasingly, less invasive procedures such as endobronchial biopsy and image-guided percutaneous biopsy have been used in children [145]. Concerns regarding endobronchial biopsy include bleeding and the histologic adequacy of the sample obtained. Minor mucosal bleeding is common and not of great concern as experience with airway foreign body removal would indicate that minor bleeding of the mucosa is not associated with a worse outcome [146]. Although not all lung masses are accessible via transbronchial biopsy, it is useful as a diagnostic measure in patients with poorly controlled asthma [147], cystic fibrosis (CF) [148, 149], and postlung transplant monitoring [150]. Salva et al. [54] prospectively studied 170 children between the ages of 2.5 and 16 years who underwent flexible endobronchial biopsy for a variety of chronic respiratory conditions. At least three biopsy samples were taken from each patient. These children received a general anesthetic in an ambulatory setting with the use of an LMA (as described earlier). The results were encouraging as no patient required intervention for mucosal bleeding and there were no cases of pneumothorax, hemoptysis, or pneumonia.

Image-guided percutaneous lung biopsy can be performed with CT or ultrasound guidance depending on the location and accessibility of the tumor. Deep sedation with local anesthetic infiltration [151] or general anesthesia can be performed depending on age, cooperation, and medical status of the patient. Disadvantages compared to general anesthesia include the inability to suspend respiration to aide biopsy localization. In a series of CT-guided percutaneous lung biopsies performed in children between the ages of 0.6 and 20 years, most cases were performed successfully with deep sedation. Adequate tissue samples were obtained in 85% of the cases [152]. Perioperative complications that did not require intervention included subclinical pneumothorax (17%), pleural effusion (3%), subcutaneous hemorrhage (12%), and postprocedural hemoptysis (3%). There was one case of tension pneumothorax requiring chest tube insertion. There was no association between adverse events and the number of biopsy attempts. All children received a chest X-ray approximately 6 h after the procedure or sooner as clinically indicated. Despite an overall complication rate of 28%, percutaneous biopsy fares favorably when compared to historic data on surgical open biopsy. Procedure length, overall hospital stay, and procedural costs also tend to favor percutaneous biopsy.

For those patients in whom percutaneous biopsy has failed to yield a diagnosis and those in whom the lung pathology is not amenable to such a technique, surgical lung biopsy is required. This can be performed with open thoracotomy or VATS. Although postoperative morbidity is increased in comparison to percutaneous biopsy, surgical biopsy is still considered by many the gold standard diagnostic tool. Gluer et al. [153] prospectively evaluated the feasibility, efficacy, and safety of the VATS technique for lung biopsy in patients with diffuse parenchymal lung disease. This was performed with general anesthesia using a single-lumen tube without lung isolation. The average age of the 21 patients was 3 years (range 12 days to 15 years). Only two cases required conversion from VATS to mini-thoracotomy, and no other intraoperative complications were noted. Studies comparing thoracoscopic and open lung resection in children have shown comparable success rates, safety parameters, and clinical outcomes [154, 155]. As experience with pediatric VATS procedures increases, we are seeing an increase in the number of biopsy procedures performed using this technique.

Cystic Fibrosis (CF)

Thick inspissated secretions causing airway obstruction, atelectasis, and superimposed pneumonia are some of the pulmonary sequelae of this multiorgan disease. Respiratory dysfunction can be quite pronounced with patients becoming extremely ill. Progression of the disease can lead to cor pulmonale, pneumothorax, antibiotic-resistant infections, and bronchiectasis. Intestinal malabsorption and pancreatic and liver dysfunction are the most frequent extrapulmonary effects. Measures such as chest physiotherapy, bronchodilators, antimicrobial treatments, and medications to break down secretions (i.e., Pulmozyme), have significantly improved outcome and quality of life for many patients. Despite this, eventual respiratory failure is the rule, and, for many, lung transplant may be the only alternative. Children with CF may present for surgery at various stages of life. The neonate may present with meconium ileus or for central line placement for nutritional supplementation. Older children may present with pneumothorax requiring chest tube insertion and bronchoscopy for lavage of inspissated secretions, and microbrial diagnosis of infections can happen at any stage of life.

Anesthetic management is predicated on optimizing preoperative respiratory function. Consultation with the pulmonologist is indicated for all patients with CF. Medical management including appropriate antibiotic treatment, optimizing bronchodilator use, and initiating Pulmozyme therapy often requires the patient be admitted to hospital prior to the scheduled procedure. Preoperative laboratory investigations should include arterial blood gas, electrolyte panel, liver function tests, and blood glucose. Reviewing the most recent spirometry or PFTs and available chest imaging will also help in determining the degree of respiratory dysfunction. Chest physiotherapy for secretion clearance should be ordered preoperatively and early in the postoperative period. Controversy exists as to the most favorable perioperative fluid management strategy. Although aggressive fluid supplementation may decrease the viscosity of pulmonary secretions, some anesthesiologists prefer to limit fluid administration to decrease the volume of secretions. To date no one best strategy has been found. Whichever approach is taken, it is advisable to have the patient euvolemic at the start of the procedure. Bronchoscopy, bronchoalveolar lavage, and transbronchial biopsies may be performed through an LMA with the patient breathing spontaneously; however, anesthetic depth must be sufficient to prevent coughing and laryngospasm. Increasingly, muscle relaxation and gentle positive-pressure ventilation through the LMA have simplified anesthesia for bronchoscopic procedures in children with CF. If a tracheal tube is to be used, it must be adequately large to allow for ventilation around the fiberoptic scope as well as tracheobronchial suctioning. Routine noninvasive monitoring is acceptable for straightforward procedures; however, an arterial line may be helpful in more involved cases to assess oxygenation, ventilation, and blood glucose monitoring.

Inhalational induction may be slow in patients with severe respiratory dysfunction, and therefore intravenous induction is often preferred in this patient group. Intraoperative complications to be aware of include mucus plugging, pneumothorax, bronchospasm, and atelectasis. Inspired gases should be humidified, and tracheobronchial suctioning should be performed at regular intervals throughout the procedure. Some clinicians advocate against the use of ketamine in children with CF as this drug can increase airway secretions. Regional techniques for pain management have the theoretical advantage of minimizing respiratory depression associated with systemic narcotic use and should be considered. In the mature child or teenager with CF undergoing peripheral surgery, regional anesthesia with or without mild sedation may be a reasonable option. A plan for postoperative ventilatory support must be discussed among the surgical team, anesthesia, intensivist, and the patient/family. Respiratory compromise due to surgery, postoperative sedation, narcotic analgesia, and a weakened cough will increase the likelihood of needing postoperative ventilator support.

Pulmonary Alveolar Proteinosis

PAP is a rare disease in which accumulation of phospholipoproteinaceous material in the alveoli causes pulmonary impairment [156]. A deficiency in granulocyte-macrophage colony-stimulating factor (GM-CSF) activity results in defective macrophages and reduced clearance of surfactant from the lungs [157]. Regular administration of GM-CSF as well as bronchoalveolar or whole-lung lavage is an important part of treatment for this disease and often results in temporary improvement of symptoms and radiographic appearance (see also Chap. 45).

The small child with PAP requiring whole-lung lavage presents a particular challenge to the anesthesiologist. In adolescents and adults, double-lumen bronchial tubes are often used to isolate the lungs for lavage; however, such tubes do not currently exist for use in smaller children. Several techniques have been described to isolate the lungs in smaller children in order to allow for lavage. No single method has been shown to be ideal, and each has its risks and limitations. Extracorporeal circulation has been used which allows for thorough bilateral whole-lung lavage; however, it is invasive and may be associated with significant morbidity [158]. Lavage through a flexible bronchoscope adjacent to a cuffed ETT allows for improved lung isolation [159]; however, this can be a lengthy process and also carries a risk of causing trauma to bronchial mucosa. Lavage through a pulmonary artery catheter has also been performed either through a rigid bronchoscope [160] or through an ETT [161]. This method also allows for lung isolation; however, the diameter of a pulmonary artery catheter port is small, and drainage may be inadequate. The most commonly used method of lung lavage in children is individual or multilobar lavage through a flexible fiberoptic bronchoscope. This may be performed through an ETT or an LMA. It is more time-consuming than whole-lung lavage, however, may be associated with lower lavage returns, and does not isolate the lung.

For whole-lung lavage in a child under the age of 9 years, true lung isolation may be achieved by using an assembly that mimics commercially available double-lumen tubes. Two cuffed tracheal tubes are passed through the glottis, one seated endobronchially to isolate the lung to be lavaged and the second seated in the trachea. These tubes are then connected to the angled and Y-connectors from a standard double-lumen bronchial tube set (Fig. 50.6) [162]. Although this approach may allow for proper lung lavage, one-lung ventilation, and obviate the need for postprocedural ventilation, the nature of the underlying illness may nevertheless dictate the need for monitoring in a high-acuity setting. Because of the nature of the procedure and the airway assembly, total intravenous anesthesia is likely preferable if this technique is to be used. This type of airway assembly

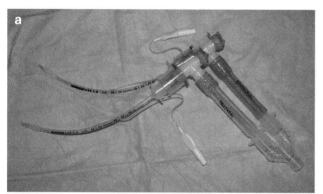
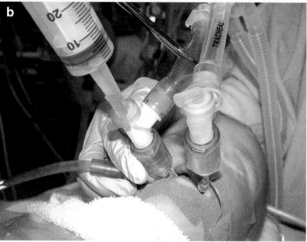

Fig. 50.6 (**a**) Airway assembly for use in the small child that mimics commercially available double-lumen bronchial tubes. Two cuffed tracheal tubes are passed through the glottis, one seated endobronchially to isolate the lung to be lavaged and the second seated in the trachea. These tubes are then connected to the angled and Y-connectors from a standard double-lumen bronchial tube set. (**b**) Whole-lung lavage being performed in a 3-year-old child via the bronchial tube of the airway assembly, while positive-pressure ventilation is applied via the tracheal tube

can be used in the small child requiring differential lung ventilation and/or strict lung isolation for a variety of procedures other than lung lavage. Disadvantages include the necessarily smaller sizes of the two tracheal tubes needed to simultaneously pass through the vocal cords. Dexamethasone 0.1 mg/kg IV may be given prior to the procedure to reduce the risk of mucosal edema at the level of the cricoid cartilage.

Trauma, Pneumothorax, and Hemothorax

Due to the unique and changing physiology and psychology of children, the management of the pediatric trauma patient may be quite different from that of the adult. Although isolated chest injuries are rare in children (5–15% of traumas), when associated with other injuries, the mortality rate can be as high as 25% [163–165]. Between 60% and 80% of all pediatric trauma is blunt impact, usually from motor vehicle collision [105]. Incomplete ossification of the ribs in children means that the rib cage is more likely to deflect under traumatic assault as opposed to fracture. Therefore, pulmonary contusions are more likely in children as compared to adults even in the absence of overlying rib fractures [166]. Conversely, a child that presents with rib fractures has likely suffered a severe, high force trauma to the chest. Insertion of a thoracic epidural catheter should be considered in the analgesic management of the child with multiple rib fractures [167]. Penetrating chest injuries due to gun violence and knife stabbings are less common in children. The presence of rib fractures in the infant should raise suspicion of child abuse [168, 169].

Pulmonary contusion is perhaps the most common traumatic thoracic injury in the pediatric population [170, 171]. Within the lung parenchyma, this manifests as alveolar edema and consolidation, sometimes associated with hemorrhage. Because of the child's higher metabolic oxygen consumption, lung injury may be accompanied by significant hypoxemia. Mechanical ventilation may be required although most pulmonary contusions can be treated by less invasive measures [172]. This includes BiPAP, supplemental oxygen, pain control, fluid restriction, and incentive spirometry when appropriate. Preventing and treating atelectasis are essential as this will reduce the risk of pneumonia and further respiratory compromise.

Pneumothorax may occur spontaneously in susceptible patients but is more often encountered at the conclusion of surgical thoracic procedures or in the setting of trauma. An open pneumothorax, one in which the pleura communicates with atmosphere, is treated with the insertion of a chest tube that allows for drainage without further entrainment of air upon inspiration. The chest tube apparatus is usually placed under water seal or to a suction device. Toward the end of most major thoracic procedures, the surgeon will choose to electively place such a device. For minor intrathoracic procedures, some surgeons will elect not to place a chest tube. In these cases, air is removed as the chest wall is closed, while the anesthesiologist provides positive pressure to the lung. These maneuvers should minimize any residual pneumothorax. A postoperative chest X-ray is required with careful monitoring of the patient for signs of increasing pneumothorax. Most small (i.e., <10%) pneumothoraces are insignificant and will resolve over a period of a few days.

Tension pneumothorax occurs when air accumulates in the pleural space without communicating with atmosphere. As the pressure builds within the pleural space, the ipsilateral lung will further collapse with increasing mediastinal shift. Clinical deterioration of the patient will become apparent. Hypotension, hypoxia, and decreased cardiac output will require emergent management. Diagnosis is confirmed by decreased breath sounds on the ipsilateral side, tracheal deviation away from the affected lung, and shift of the maximal cardiac impulse. Radiographic diagnosis should not delay the emergent placement of a chest tube or needle decompression followed by chest tube insertion.

Bleeding into the pleural cavity can occur intraoperatively or postoperatively following any thoracic procedure. The amount of blood loss due to hemothorax in this setting should be minimal if hemostasis was achieved prior to closure. In the case of thoracic trauma, however, the amount of blood loss can quickly become life-threatening. Disruption of intercostal arteries or veins is the most common culprit in this setting. As with tension pneumothorax, the accumulation of blood will compromise ventilation and cardiac output. If this blood is not promptly drained, it may reorganize into a fibrous scar thus causing chronic atelectasis and V/Q mismatch. In addition to this, the blood may become a medium for bacterial growth with ensuing sepsis and empyema formation. Operative exploration of a hemothorax must be considered when there is ongoing drainage from the chest tube and/or the patient remains hemodynamically unstable. Some clinicians advocate a quantitative approach that would require surgical exploration if greater than 15 mL/kg of blood is recovered upon chest tube insertion or if ongoing drainage exceeds 4 mL/kg/h [173].

Major airway disruption is rare in pediatric trauma but may occur in the setting of penetrating injury or rapid acceleration or deceleration. When present these injuries can be immediately life-threatening. In 80% of cases, the disruption is located at the distal trachea or main bronchus [174, 175]. Airway injury should be suspected in the setting of pneumomediastinum, subcutaneous emphysema, large persistent air leak within the chest tube, and frank respiratory collapse.

Diagnosis is usually confirmed by bronchoscopy, either rigid or flexible. When airway injury is suspected, intubation should be performed fiberoptically and the ETT placed distal to the disruption to avoid further trauma or creation of a false passage. Immediate operative repair of major airway injuries may be required although minor injuries can be observed with delayed surgical repair as required. Distal injuries can be treated with simple resection, while more proximal injuries may require quite extensive repairs. Postoperative complications may include dehiscence, airway stenosis, atelectasis, and pneumonia. A severe blow to the chest while the vocal cords are adducted can lead to a rare injury pattern that is unique to pediatrics. Traumatic asphyxia presents with neck and facial swelling and ecchymosis, subcutaneous emphysema, and pneumomediastinum [176]. The sudden increase in intrathoracic pressure causes a small tear in the upper trachea and forces air into the tissues of the neck, face, and around the mediastinum. Management is often supportive and nonsurgical.

Lung Transplantation

Pediatric lung transplantation continues to account for a small fraction of all lung transplant operations performed. Despite this, the number of transplants performed on children is increasing, and the minimum age of transplantation is decreasing. Many large pediatric transplant centers have established living donor programs and life-sustaining temporizing measures such as the Novalung® have been introduced for use in children awaiting a donor lung (Toronto Lung Transplant Program, Hospital for Sick Children Statistics, 2009, personal communication). The vast majority of pediatric lung transplant procedures are carried out in children between 10 and 17 years of age. CF accounts for over 64% of cases in children, followed by primary pulmonary hypertension (14%), pulmonary interstitial disease (7%), and retransplant (7%) [177]. Actuarial survival rates tend to be favorable for pediatric lung transplantation as compared to those for older adults.

A multidisciplinary team and approach are crucial to meet the surgical, medical, psychological, physical, and dietary challenges that will be faced. At the time or writing, children smaller than 10 years of age (i.e., those too small to accept a double-lumen bronchial tube) usually undergo lung transplantation under cardiopulmonary bypass. Other indications for the use of bypass during lung pediatric transplantation include primary pulmonary hypertension and severe right ventricular dysfunction. There also continues to be a significant rate of conversion from off-bypass double sequential lung transplant to urgent bypass in children due to worsening pulmonary hypertension or relentless hypoxemia. The advantage of off-bypass sequential lung transplantation is the avoidance of systemic anticoagulation needed for cardiopulmonary bypass. A short period of postoperative ventilation is provided to monitor for early complications such as ischemic-reperfusion injury, infection, acute rejection, bleeding, and anastomotic leaks.

Postoperative and Pain Management

The postoperative disposition of a child who has undergone a thoracic procedure will depend on many criteria including the type and length of surgery, extent of resection or manipulation, and nature of the underlying condition. In general, infants and small children will be more frequently managed with a short period of postoperative ventilation when compared to adult patients. Regardless of the type of surgery or reason for intervention, the pediatric patient should be monitored for respiratory status and adequate pain control in a suitable environment. Constant care or high-acuity nursing and monitoring should be considered even if the patient's trachea was extubated in the operating room.

Because many procedures are now being done with the less invasive video-assisted thoracoscopic technique, postoperative pain management has become somewhat easier. These patients can often be managed with nonopioid analgesics, a simple narcotic infusion, or patient-controlled analgesia. Table 50.4 outlines commonly used analgesics in pediatric practice. Local anesthetic can also be infiltrated

prior to the placement of trocars, and multimodal analgesia should be considered in all patients. Pain control for the pediatric patient has recently regained a renaissance with the more aggressive use of regional anesthesia techniques. These techniques are being applied to a wider range of the pediatric population with good success and minimal complications. The proper management of postoperative pain can avoid some of the negative physiologic outcomes associated with poorly treated pain. These include heightened sympathetic drive, increased metabolism, decreased immune function, and, specifically for thoracic procedures, poor respiratory function [177]. A simple option for regional analgesia includes intercostal nerve blocks performed prior to skin incision or just before surgical closure under direct visualization. Local anesthetic dosages should be reduced as plasma uptake at this site is rapid [178]. The overlap of thoracic dermatomes requires that the nerves above and below the surgical site also be blocked. Indwelling intercostal catheters can also be placed by the surgeon and managed as a constant infusion postoperatively [179].

The epidural space in the child can be assessed in a similar fashion to that of adults. Ideally the epidural catheter tip should be placed at the dermatome level corresponding to the surgical site. Specific pediatric-sized Touhy needles should be used to minimize complications and provide for better control. Unlike in adults, thoracic epidural catheters are almost always placed when the child has already been anesthetized. Therefore, greater care must be exercised when advancing the needle as the patient will not be able to articulate the presence of radicular pain. Despite this drawback, there is no evidence to suggest the incidence of complications is higher in children compared to adults [180].

In smaller infants, the caudal epidural space can be easily accessed and a catheter advanced to the required thoracic level, using an ultrasound-guided approach [181]. As in adults many different local anesthetic solutions and adjuncts have been used in the pediatric population. The most commonly used local anesthetics continue to be bupivacaine and ropivacaine for either "single shot" or continuous infusion epidurals [182]. Suggested neuraxial blocks and dosing guidelines suitable for pediatric thoracic procedures can be found in Table 50.5. Epidural narcotics are commonly coadministered as they reduce the dosage requirement for local anesthetics and improve the block quality. Epidural morphine, fentanyl, and hydromorphone are the most commonly prescribed narcotics for this use [183, 184]. The purpose of optimizing pain management strategies is not only to keep the child comfortable but also to avoid pulmonary dysfunction by enabling deep breathing and coughing. This can aide in the prevention of atelectasis and postoperative pneumonia. Early ambulation is also encouraged to further accelerate the recovery of the patient and prevent those diseases associated with prolonged immobilization and hospitalization.

Table 50.4 Commonly used analgesics in pediatric practice[a]

Analgesic	Dose[b]	Infusion dose	PCA dosing (µg/kg q 6–10 min) or comment
Morphine	50 µg/kg	10–40 µg/kg/hr	10–30
Fentanyl	0.5 µg/kg	0.5–2 µg/kg/hr	0.2–0.5
Hydromorphone	0.15 µg/kg	3–5 µg/kg/hr	3–5
Remifentanil	0.5 µg/kg	0.05–2 µg/kg/min	Intraoperative use only
Ketamine	0.15 µg/kg	1–4 µg/kg/min	Narcotic-sparing effect; may be useful if opioid side effects considerable
Acetaminophen	75 mg/kg/day po	N/A	q4h dosing for oral, q6h for rectal
Ibuprofen	5–10 mg/kg po q6h	N/A	For children >6 months of age
Ketorolac	0.5 mg/kg (maximum 15 mg) q6h	N/A	For children >6 months of age. Limit to 48 h, and then switch to po ibuprofen

Abbreviations: PCA patient-controlled analgesia, *po* per os
[a]Adapted from Sick Kids Acute Pain Handbook, 2010. The Hospital for Sick Children, Toronto, Canada
[b]Doses are intravenous unless otherwise specified

Table 50.5 Neuraxial blocks and dosing guidelines suitable for pediatric thoracic procedures[a]

Type of block	Solution	Infusion rate (mL/kg/h)
Thoracic epidural[b]	0.125% bupivacaine + epi 1:400,000 ± fentanyl 1–2 µg/mL	0.1–0.16 maximum 10 mL/h
Thoracic epidural[b]	0.1% bupivacaine + epi 1:500,000 ± fentanyl 1–2 µg/mL	0.1–0.16 maximum 12 mL/h
Thoracic epidural[b]	0.0625% bupivacaine + epi 1:800,000 ± fentanyl 1–2 µg/mL	0.1–0.16 maximum 14 mL/h
Paravertebral[c]	0.125% bupivacaine + epi 1:400,000	0.2 maximum 15 mL/h
Intercostal[d]	0.125% bupivacaine + epi 1:400,000	0.016–0.032 per rib maximum 1 mL/h/rib
Intrapleural[e]	0.125% bupivacaine + epi 1:400,000	0.2–0.3 maximum 20 mL/h

[a]Adapted from Sick Kids Acute Pain Handbook, 2010. The Hospital for Sick Children, Toronto, Canada
[b]Alternatively, caudal or lumbar approach with epidural catheter threaded to thoracic level. Suggested loading dose of 0.2–0.25 mL/kg of 0.25% bupivacaine + epi 1:200,000 up to maximum 10 mL
[c]Suggested loading dose of 0.3–0.5 mL/kg of 0.25% bupivacaine + epi 1:200,000 up to maximum 15 mL
[d]Suggested loading dose of 0.05 mL/kg (maximum 2 mL) of 0.25% bupivacaine + epi 1:200,000 per intercostal space
[e]Suggested loading dose of 0.2–0.3 mL/kg (maximum 20 mL) of 0.25% bupivacaine + epi 1:200,000

Clinical Case Discussion

A 3-year-old child with a newly diagnosed left lung mass presents for tissue diagnosis followed 1 week later by thoracotomy and tumor resection.

The initial workup of the child will focus on the functional status and size of lung mass. Imaging will be essential to identify the size and location of tumor and to rule out a mediastinal mass. A CT scan will be required which may be done without sedation if the child is cooperative. Otherwise a stepwise approach of cautious sedation may be required. Any sedation should be delayed to verify the absence of a significant mediastinal mass. Tissue samples may be obtained through a mini-thoracotomy; however, in tertiary pediatric centers, image-guided needle core biopsy is preferred and associated with lower morbidity. Most 3-year olds will require deep sedation or general anesthesia. Spontaneous respiration can be maintained during the biopsies, which might be CT or ultrasound guided. Often tracheal intubation is not required, and the patient's airway can be managed by face mask, bag-mask support, or insertion of an LMA. Sedation/anesthesia may be achieved by TIVA (propofol or ketamine, alone or in combination with a short-acting opioid or benzodiazepine) and/or inhalation. Occasionally, a brief period of apnea will be requested to

facilitate biopsy. This may be achieved temporarily deepening the anesthetic and providing positive-pressure ventilation. Postbiopsy X-ray should be performed to ensure there is no significant residual pneumothorax. Chest tube insertion is rarely required.

Tumor resection may be performed via VATS or open thoracotomy. In either case the anesthesiologist should be prepared to isolate the lung. Options in a 3-year old include (1) selective right mainstem bronchus intubation with a 4.5 or 5.0 mm ID tracheal tube, (2) insertion of a size 5F embolectomy catheter in the left mainstem bronchus inside or (more practically) outside a 4.5 mm ID tracheal tube, or (3) a 5F Arndt endobronchial blocker inserted in a 5.0 mm ID tracheal tube and placed in the left mainstem bronchus. Regardless of the option chosen, fiberoptic verification of proper tube or blocker positioning is crucial. A 2.2 or 2.8 mm OD pediatric fiberoptic bronchoscope should be used to ensure adequate ventilation may be provided while the scope occupies the lumen of the tracheal tube. The author prefers not to perform selective right mainstem bronchus intubations as quite often the tube slips distal to the right upper lobe takeoff, resulting in atelectasis of that lobe and worsening hypoxemia. Monitoring should include an invasive arterial blood pressure line in addition to standard monitors. Pain control will depend partly on whether VATS or open thoracotomy is performed. As a general guideline, central neuraxial blockade is offered in the event of open thoracotomy, and systemic analgesics are administered if VATS is performed. Postoperative monitoring in a high-acuity setting (step-down or critical care unit) is warranted for the first 12–24 h.

References

1. Sweet DG, Halliday HL. The use of surfactants in 2009. Arch Dis Child Educ Pract Ed. 2009;94(3):78–83.
2. Sekar KC, Corff KE. To tube or not to tube babies with respiratory distress syndrome. J Perinatol. 2009;29(Suppl 2):S68–72.
3. Verder H, Bohlin K, Kamper J, Lindwall R, Jonsson B. Nasal CPAP and surfactant for treatment of respiratory distress syndrome and prevention of bronchopulmonary dysplasia. Acta Paediatr. 2009;98(9):1400–8. Epub 2009 Jul 1.
4. Lista G, et al. Nasal continuous positive airway pressure (CPAP) versus bi-level nasal CPAP in preterm babies with respiratory distress syndrome: a randomised control trial. Arch Dis Child Fetal Neonatal Ed. 2010;95(2):F85–9.
5. Askie LM, et al. Effects of targeting lower versus higher arterial oxygen saturations on death or disability in preterm infants. Cochrane Database Syst Rev. 2017;(4):CD011190.
6. Cogo PE, et al. Dosing of porcine surfactant: effect on kinetics and gas exchange in respiratory distress syndrome. Pediatrics. 2009;124(5):e950–7. Epub 2009 Oct 12.
7. Suresh GK, Soll RF. Overview of surfactant replacement trials. J Perinatol. 2005;25(Suppl 2):S40–4.
8. Blaise G, et al. Pulmonary arterial hypertension pathophysiology and anesthetic approach. Anesthesiology. 2003;99:1415–32.

9. Hawkins A, Tulloh R. Treatment of pediatric pulmonary hypertension. Vasc Health Risk Manag. 2009;5(2):509–24. Epub 2009 Jun 7.

10. Konduri GG, Kim UO. Advances in the diagnosis and management of persistent pulmonary hypertension of the newborn. Pediatr Clin N Am. 2009;56(3):579–600. Table of Contents.

11. Knoderer CA, Morris JL, Ebenroth ES. Sildenafil for the treatment of pulmonary hypertension in pediatric patients. Pediatr Cardiol. 2009;30(7):871–82. Epub 2009 Aug 25.

12. Krishnan U, Krishnan S, Gewitz M. Treatment of pulmonary hypertension in children with chronic lung disease with newer oral therapies. Pediatr Cardiol. 2008;29(6):1082–6. Epub 2008 Jul 2.

13. MacKnight B, Martinez EA, Simon BA. Anesthetic management of patients with pulmonary hypertension. Semin Cardiothorac Vasc Anesth. 2008;12(2):91–6.

14. Galante D. Intraoperative management of pulmonary arterial hypertension in infants and children. Curr Opin Anaesthesiol. 2009;22(3):378–82.

15. Rosenzweig EB, Barst RJ. Pulmonary arterial hypertension in children: a medical update. Indian J Pediatr. 2009;76(1):77–81. Epub 2009 Apr 18.

16. Friesen RH, Williams GD. Anesthetic management of children with pulmonary arterial hypertension. Paediatr Anaesth. 2008;18(3):208–16.

17. Taylor K, Holtby H. Emergency interventional lung assist for pulmonary hypertension. Anesth Analg. 2009;109(2):382–5.

18. Ayers J, Graves SA. Perioperative management of total parenteral nutrition, glucose containing solutions, and intraoperative glucose monitoring in paediatric patients: a survey of clinical practice. Paediatr Anaesth. 2001;11(1):41–4.

19. Fösel TH, Uth M, Wilhelm W, Grüness V. Comparison of two solutions with different glucose concentrations for infusion therapy during laparotomies in infants. Infusionsther Transfusionsmed. 1996;23(2):80–4.

20. Gauda EB, McLemore GL, Tolosa J, Marston-Nelson J, Kwak D. Maturation of peripheral arterial chemoreceptors in relation to neonatal apnoea. Semin Neonatol. 2004;9(3):181–94.

21. Choudhry DK. Single-lung ventilation in pediatric anesthesia. Anesthesiol Clin N Am. 2005;23:693–708.

22. Rowe R, Andropoulos D, Heard M, et al. Anesthestic management of pediatric patients undergoing thoracoscopy. J Cardiothorac Vasc Anesth. 1994;8:563–6.

23. Kubota H, Kubota Y, Toyoda Y, et al. Selective blind endobronchial intubation in children and adults. Anesthesiology. 1987;67:587–9.

24. Rehman M, Sherlekar S, Schwartz R, et al. One lung anesthesia for video assisted thoracoscopic lung biopsy in a paediatric patient. Paediatr Anaesth. 1999;9:85–7.

25. Hammer GB, Harrison TK, Vricella LA, Black MD, Krane EJ. Single lung ventilation in children using a new paediatric bronchial blocker. Paediatr Anaesth. 2002;12(1):69–72.

26. Takahashi M, Yamada M, Honda I, Kato M, Yamamuro M, Hashimoto Y. Selective lobar – bronchial blocking for pediatric video-assisted thoracic surgery. Anesthesiology. 2001;94(1):170–2.

27. Chengod S, Chandrasekharan AP, Manoj P. Selective left bronchial intubation and left-lung isolation in infants and toddlers: analysis of a new technique. J Cardiothorac Vasc Anesth. 2005;19(5):636–41.

28. Gayes JM. Pro: one-lung ventilation is best accomplished with the Univent endotracheal tube. J Cardiothorac Vasc Anesth. 1993;7:103–7.

29. Kamaya H, Krishna PR. New endotracheal tube (univent tube) for selective blockade of one lung. Anesthesiology. 1985;63:342–3.

30. Hammer GB, Brodsky JB, Redpath JH, Cannon WB. The Univent tube for single-lung ventilation in paediatric patients. Paediatr Anaesth. 1998;8(1):55–7.

31. Arndt GA, DeLessio ST, Kranner PW, Orzepowski W, Ceranski B, Valtysson B. One-lung ventilation when intubation is difficult – presentation of a new endobronchial blocker. Acta Anaesthesiol Scand. 1999;43(3):356–8.

32. Yun ES, Saulys A, Popic PM, Arndt GA. Single-lung ventilation in a pediatric patient using a pediatric fibreoptically-directed wire-guided endobronchial blocker. Can J Anaesth. 2002;49(3):256–61.

33. Li PY, Gu HH, Liang WM. Sequential one-lung ventilation using one Arndt endobronchial blocker in a pediatric patient undergoing bilateral, video-assisted thoracoscopic surgery (VATS). J Clin Anesth. 2009;21(6):464.

34. Hammer GB, Fitzmaurice BG, Brodsky JB. Methods for single-lung ventilation in pediatric patients. Anesth Analg. 1999;89:1426–9.

35. Klein U, Karzai W, Bloos F, Wohlfarth M, Gottschall R, Fritz H, et al. Role of fiberoptic bronchoscopy in conjunction with the use of double-lumen tubes for thoracic anesthesia: a prospective study. Anesthesiology. 1998;88(2):346–50.

36. Fitzmaurice BG, Brodsky JB. Airway rupture from double-lumen tubes. J Cardiothorac Vasc Anesth. 1999;13:322–9.

37. Tezel C, Okur E, Baysungur V. Iatrogenic tracheal rupture during intubation with a double-lumen tube. Thorac Cardiovasc Surg. 2010;58(1):54–6.

38. Nicolai T. Pediatric bronchoscopy. Pediatr Pulmonol. 2001;31(2):150–64.

39. Slonim AD, Ognibene FP. Amnestic agents in pediatric bronchoscopy. Chest. 1999;116(6):1802–8.

40. Berkenbosch JW, Graff GR, Stark JM, Ner Z, Tobias JD. Use of a remifentanil-propofol mixture for pediatric flexible fiberoptic bronchoscopy sedation. Paediatr Anaesth. 2004;14(11):941–6.

41. Larsen R, Galloway D, Wadera S, Kjar D, Hardy D, Mirkes C, Wick L, Pohl JF. Safety of propofol sedation for pediatric outpatient procedures. Clin Pediatr (Phila). 2009;48(8):819–23. Epub 2009 May 29.

42. Tobias JD. Sedation and anesthesia for pediatric bronchoscopy. Curr Opin Pediatr. 1997;9(3):198–206.

43. Dilos BM. Anesthesia for pediatric airway endoscopy and upper gastrointestinal endoscopy. Int Anesthesiol Clin. 2009;47:55–62.

44. Seybold JL. The use of dexmedetomidine during laryngoscopy, bronchoscopy, and tracheal extubation following tracheal reconstruction. Pediatr Anesth. 2007;17:1212–4.

45. Niggemann B, Haack M, Machotta A. How to enter the pediatric airway for bronchoscopy. Pediatr Int. 2004;46(2):117–21.

46. Zestos MM, Bhattacharya D, Rajan S, Kemper S, Haupert M. Propofol decreases waste anesthetic gas exposure during pediatric bronchoscopy. Laryngoscope. 2004;114(2):212–5.

47. Nussbaum E, Zagnoev M. Pediatric fiberoptic bronchoscopy with a laryngeal mask airway. Chest. 2001;120(2):614–6.

48. Bandla HP, Smith DE, Kiernan MP. Laryngeal mask airway facilitated fibreoptic bronchoscopy in infants. Can J Anaesth. 1997;44(12):1242–7.

49. Naguib ML, Streetman DS, Clifton S, Nasr SZ. Use of laryngeal mask airway in flexible bronchoscopy in infants and children. Pediatr Pulmonol. 2005;39(1):56–63.

50. Somri M, Barna Teszler C, Tome R, Kugelman A, Vaida S, Gaitini L. Flexible fiberoptic bronchoscopy through the laryngeal mask airway in a small, premature neonate. Am J Otolaryngol. 2005;26(4):268–71.

51. Picard E, Schwartz S, Goldberg S, Glick T, Villa Y, Kerem E. A prospective study of fever and bacteremia after flexible fiberoptic bronchoscopy in children. Chest. 2000;117(2):573–7.

52. Picard E, Goldberg S, Virgilis D, Schwartz S, Raveh D, Kerem E. A single dose of dexamethasone to prevent postbronchoscopy fever in children: a randomized placebo-controlled trial. Chest. 2007;131(1):201–5.

53. Nussbaum E. Pediatric fiberoptic bronchoscopy: clinical experience with 2,836 bronchoscopies. Pediatr Crit Care Med. 2002;3(2):171–6.

54. Salva PS, Theroux C, Schwartz D. Safety of endobronchial biopsy in 170 children with chronic respiratory symptoms. Thorax. 2003;58(12):1058–60.

55. Shah R, Reddy AS, Dhende NP. Video assisted thoracic surgery in children. J Minim Access Surg. 2007;3(4):161–7.

56. Oak SN, Parelkar SV, Satishkumar KV, Pathak R, Ramesh BH, Sudhir S, et al. Review of video-assisted thoracoscopy in children. J Minim Access Surg. 2009;5(3):57–62.

57. de Campos JR, Andrade Filho LO, Werebe EC, Minamoto H, Quim AO, Filomeno LT, et al. Thoracoscopy in children and adolescents. Chest. 1997;111(2):494–7.

58. Tobias JD. Thoracic surgery in children. Curr Opin Anaesthesiol. 2001;14(1):77–85.

59. Sundararajan L, Parikh DH. Evolving experience with video-assisted thoracic surgery in congenital cystic lung lesions in a British pediatric center. J Pediatr Surg. 2007;42(7): 1243–50.

60. Dutta S, Mihailovic A, Benson L, Kantor PF, Fitzgerald PG, Walton JM, Langer JC, Cameron BH. Thoracoscopic ligation versus coil occlusion for patent ductus arteriosus: a matched cohort study of outcomes and cost. Surg Endosc. 2008;22(7):1643–8. Epub 2007 Nov 20.

61. Efrati O, Barak A. Pleural effusions in the pediatric population. Pediatr Rev. 2002;23:417–26.

62. Praskakis E, et al. Current evidence for the management of paediatric parapneumonic effusions. Curr Med Res Opin. 2012;28(7):1179–92.

63. Gates RL, et al. Drainage, fibrinolytics, or surgery: a comparison of treatment options in pediatric empyema. J Pediatr Surg. 2004;39(3):381–6.

64. Hawkins JA, et al. Current treatment of pediatric empyema. Semin Thorac Cardiovasc Surg. 2004;16:196–200.

65. Long A-M, et al. 'Less may be best'-Pediatric parapneumonic effusion and empyema management: lessons from a UK center. J Pediatr Surg. 2016;51:588–91.

66. Hendaus MA, Janahi IA. Parapneumonic effusion in children: an up-to-date review. Clin Pediatr. 2016;55(1):10–8.

67. Israel EN, Blackmer AB. Tissue plasminogen activator for the treatment of parapneumonic effusions in pediatric patients. Pharmacotherapy. 2014;34(5):521–32.

68. Krenke K, et al. Clinical characteristics of 323 children with parapneumonic pleural effusion and pleural empyema due to community acquired pneumonia. J Infect Chemother. 2016;22: 292–7.

69. Nezafati MH, Soltani G, Vedadian A. Video-assisted ductal closure with new modifications: minimally invasive, maximally effective, 1,300 cases. Ann Thorac Surg. 2007;84(4):1343–8.

70. Mavroudis C. Forty-six years of patient ductus arteriosus division at Children's Memorial Hospital of Chicago. Standards for comparison. Ann Surg. 1994;220(3):402–10.

71. Wang JK, Hwang JJ, Chiang FT, Wu MH, Lin MT, Lee WL, Lue HC. A strategic approach to transcatheter closure of patent ductus: gianturco coils for small-to-moderate ductus and Amplatzer duct occluder for large ductus. Int J Cardiol. 2006;106(1):10–5. Epub 2005 Sep 15.

72. Daher AH. Infective endocarditis in neonates. Clin Pediatr (Phila). 1995;34(4):198–206.

73. Vanamo K. Video-assisted thoracoscopic versus open surgery for persistent ductus arteriosus. J Pediatr Surg. 2006;41(7):1226–9.

74. Villa E. Video-assisted thoracoscopic clipping of patent ductus arteriosus: close to the gold standard and minimally invasive competitor of percutaneous techniques. J Cardiovasc Med (Hagerstown). 2006;7(3):210–5.

75. Villa E. Paediatric video-assisted thoracoscopic clipping of patent ductus arteriosus: experience in more than 700 cases. Eur J Cardiothorac Surg. 2004;25(3):387–93.

76. Burke RP. Video-assisted thoracoscopic surgery for patent ductus arteriosus in low birth weight neonates and infants. Pediatrics. 1999;104(2 Pt 1):227–30.

77. Muralidhar KS, Shetty DP. Ventilation strategy for video-assisted thoracoscopic clipping of patent ductus arteriosus in children. Paediatr Anaesth. 2001;11(1):45–8.

78. Miyagi K. One-lung ventilation for video-assisted thoracoscopic interruption of patent ductus arteriosus. Surg Today. 2004;34(12):1006–9.

79. Stankowski, et al. Minimally invasive thoracoscopic closure versus thoracotomy in children with patent ductus arteriosus. J Surg Res. 2017;208:1–9.

80. Odegard KC. Intraoperative recurrent laryngeal nerve monitoring during video-assisted throracoscopic surgery for patent ductus arteriosus. J Cardiothorac Vasc Anesth. 2000;14(5):562–4.

81. Clark DC. Esophageal atresia and tracheoesophageal fistula. Am Fam Physician. 1999;59(4):910–6; 919–20.

82. Keckler SJ, St Peter SD, Valusek PA, Tsao K, Snyder CL, Holcomb GW 3rd, Ostlie DJ. VACTERL anomalies in patients with esophageal atresia: an updated delineation of the spectrum and review of the literature. Pediatr Surg Int. 2007;23(4):309–13. Epub 2007 Feb 15.

83. Geneviève D, de Pontual L, Amiel J, Sarnacki S, Lyonnet S. An overview of isolated and syndromic oesophageal atresia. Clin Genet. 2007;71(5):392–9.

84. Spitz L. Oesophageal atresia. Orphanet J Rare Dis. 2007;2:24.

85. Gross RE. The surgery of infancy and childhood. Philadelphia: WB Saunders; 1953.

86. Okamoto T, Takamizawa S, Arai H, Bitoh Y, Nakao M, Yokoi A, Nishijima E. Esophageal atresia: prognostic classification revisited. Surgery. 2009;145(6):675–81. Epub 2009 Apr 11.

87. Aziz D, Chait P, Kreichman F, Langer JC. Image-guided percutaneous gastrostomy in neonates with esophageal atresia. J Pediatr Surg. 2004;39(11):1648–50.

88. Krosnar S, Baxter A. Thoracoscopic repair of esophageal atresia with tracheoesophageal fistula: anesthetic and intensive care management of a series of eight neonates. Paediatr Anaesth. 2005;15(7):541–6.

89. Lugo B, Malhotra A, Guner Y, Nguyen T, Ford H, Nguyen NX. Thoracoscopic versus open repair of tracheoesophageal fistula and esophageal atresia. J Laparoendosc Adv Surg Tech A. 2008;18(5):753–6.

90. Orford J. Advances in the treatment of oesophageal atresia over three decades: the 1970s and the 1990s. Pediatr Surg Int. 2004;20(6):402–7. Epub 2004 May 18.

91. Narang S, Harte BH, Body SC. Anesthesia for patients with a mediastinal mass. Anesthesiol Clin N Am. 2001;19: 559–79.

92. Takeda SI, Miyoshi S, Akashi A, Ohta M, Minami M, Okumura M, et al. Clinical spectrum of primary mediastinal tumors: a comparison of adult and pediatric populations at a single Japanese institution. J Surg Oncol. 2003;83:24–30.

93. Davis RD, Oldham NH, Sabiston DC. Primary cysts and neoplasms of the mediastinum: recent changes in clinical presentation, methods of diagnosis, management and results. Ann Thorac Surg. 1987;44:229–37.

94. Sairanen H, Leijala M, Louhimo I. Primary mediastinal tumors in children. Eur J Cardiothorac Surg. 1987;1:148–51.

95. Azarow KS, Pearl RH, Zurcher R, Edwards FH, Cohen AJ. Primary mediastinal masses: a comparison of adult and pediatric populations. J Thorac Cardiovasc Surg. 1993;106:67–72.

96. Shamberger RC, Holzman RS, Griscom NT, Tarbell NJ, Weinstein HJ. CT quantification of tracheal cross sectional area as a guide to

the surgical and anesthetic management of children with anterior mediastinal mass. J Pediatr Surg. 1991;26:138–42.

97. Sakakeeny-Zaal K. Pediatric orthopnea and total airway obstruction. Am J Nurs. 2007;107:40–3.

98. Slinger P, Karsli C. Management of the patient with a large anterior mediastinal mass: recurring myths (Editorial). Curr Opin Anaesthesiol. 2007;20:1–3.

99. Hack HA, Wright NB, Wynn RF. The anaesthetic management of children with anterior mediastinal masses. Anaesthesia. 2008;63(8):837–46.

100. Bechard P, Letourneau L, Lacasse Y, Cote D, Bussieres JS. Perioperative cardiorespiratory complications in adults with mediastinal mass: incidence and risk factors. Anesthesiology. 2004;100:826–34.

101. Victory RA, Casey W, Doherty P, Breatnach F. Cardiac and respiratory complications of mediastinal lymphomas. Anaesth Intensive Care. 1993;21:366–9.

102. Sanborn PA, Michna E, Zurokowski D, Burrows PE, Fontaine PJ, Connor L, et al. Adverse cardiovascular and respiratory events during sedation of pediatric patients for imaging examinations. Radiology. 2005;237:288–94.

103. Bailey PL, Pace NL, Ashburn MA, Moll JW, East KA, Stanley TH. Frequent hypoxemia and apnea after sedation with midazolam and fentanyl. Anesthesiology. 1990;73:826–30.

104. Anghelescu DL, Burgoyne LL, Liu T, Li CS, Pui CH, Hudson MM, et al. Clinical and diagnostic imaging findings predict anesthetic complications in children presenting with malignant mediastinal masses. Paediatr Anaesth. 2007;17:1090–8.

105. Rice TW, Rodriguez RM, Light RW. The superior vena cava syndrome: clinical characteristics and evolving etiology. Medicine. 2006;85:37–42.

106. Arya LS, Narain S, Tomar S, Thavaraj V, Dawar R, Bhargawa M. Superior vena cava syndrome. Indian J Pediatr. 2002;69: 293–7.

107. Lam JCM, Chui CH, Jacobsen AS, Tan AM, Joseph VT. When is a mediastinal mass critical in a child? An analysis of 29 children. Pediatr Surg Int. 2004;20:180–4.

108. Azizkhan RG, Dudgeon DL, Buck JR, Colombani PM, Yaster M, Nichols D, et al. Life-threatening airway obstruction as a complication to the management of mediastinal masses in children. J Pediatr Surg. 1985;20(6):816–22.

109. Chaignaud BE, Bonsack TA, Kozakewich HP, Shamberger RC. Pleural effusions in lymphoblastic lymphoma: a diagnostic alternative. J Pediatr Surg. 1998;33:1355–7.

110. Das DK. Serous effusions in malignant lymphomas: a review. Diagn Cytopathol. 2006;3:335–47.

111. Güllüoğlu MG, Kiliçaslan Z, Toker A, Kayalci G, Yilmazbayhan D. The diagnostic value of image guided percutaneous fine needle aspiration biopsy in equivocal mediastinal masses. Langenbeck's Arch Surg. 2006;39:222–7.

112. Chait P, Rico L, Amaral J, Connolly B, John P, Temple M. Ultrasound-guided core biopsy of mediastinal masses in children. Pediatr Radiol. 2005;35:S76.

113. Lachar W, Shahab I, Saad A. Accuracy and cost-effectiveness of core needle biopsy in the evaluation of suspected lymphoma: a study of 101 cases. Arch Pathol Lab Med. 2007;131:1033–9.

114. Annessi V, Paci M, Ferrari G, Sgarbi G. Ultrasonically guided biopsy of mediastinal masses. Interact Cardiovasc Thorac Surg. 2003;2:319–21.

115. Gupta A, Kumar A, Walters S, Chait P, Irwin MS, Gerstle JT. Analysis of needle versus open biopsy for the diagnosis of advanced stage pediatric neuroblastoma. Pediatr Blood Cancer. 2006;47:875–9.

116. Borenstein SH, Gerstle T, Malkin D, Thorner P, Filler RM. The effects of prebiopsy corticosteroid treatment on the diagnosis of mediastinal lymphoma. J Pediatr Surg. 2000;35:973–6.

117. Rampello E, Fricia T, Malaguarnera M. The management of tumor lysis syndrome. Nat Clin Pract Oncol. 2006;3:438–47.

118. Neuman GG, Weingarten AE, Abramowitz RM, Kushins LG, Abramson AL, Ladner W. The anesthetic management of a patient with an anterior mediastinal mass. Anesthesiology. 1984;60:144–7.

119. Torchio R, Gulotta C, Perbondi A, Ciacco C, Guglielmo M, Orlandi F, et al. Orthopnea and tidal expiratory flow limitation in patients with euthyroid goiter. Chest. 2003;124:133–40.

120. Hnatiuk OW, Corcoran PC, Sierra P. Spirometry in surgery for anterior mediastinal masses. Chest. 2001;120:1152–6.

121. Vander Els NJ, Sorhage F, Bach AM, Straus DJ, White DA. Abnormal flow volume loops in patients with intrathoracic Hodgkin's disease. Chest. 2000;117:1256–61.

122. Frawley G, Low J, Brown TCK. Anaesthesia for an anterior mediastinal mass with ketamine and midazolam infusion. Anaesth Intensive Care. 1995;23:610–2.

123. Bergman NA. Reduction in resting end-expiratory position of the respiratory system with induction of anesthesia and neuromuscular paralysis. Anesthesiology. 1982;57:14–7.

124. Lin SH, Su NY, Hseu SS, Ting CK, Yien HW, Cheng HC, et al. Anesthetic management of patients with giant mediastinal tumors – a report of two cases. Acta Anaesthesiol Sin. 1999;37:133–9.

125. Riley RH, Raper GD, Newman MAJ. Helium-oxygen and cardiopulmonary bypass standby in anesthesia for tracheal stenosis. Anaesth Intensive Care. 1994;22:710–3.

126. Asai T. Emergency cardiopulmonary bypass in a patient with a mediastinal mass. Anaesthesia. 2007;62:859–60.

127. Takeda S, Miyoshi S, Omori K, Okumura M, Matsuda H. Surgical rescue for life-threatening hypoxemia caused by a mediastinal tumor. Ann Thorac Surg. 1999;68:2324–6.

128. Langham MR Jr, Kays DW, Ledbetter DJ, Frentzen B, Sanford LL, Richards DS. Congenital diaphragmatic hernia. Epidemiology and outcome. Clin Perinatol. 1996;23(4):671–88.

129. Deeprest J. Current consequences of prenatal diagnosis of congenital diaphragmatic hernia. J Pediatr Surg. 2006;41(2):423–30.

130. Suita S, et al. Fetal stabilization for antenatally diagnosed diaphragmatic hernia. J Pediatr Surg. 1999;34(11):1652–7.

131. Bosenberg AT, Brown RA. Management of congenital diaphragmatic hernia. Curr Opin Anaesthesiol. 2008;21(3):323–31.

132. Bohn D. Congenital diaphragmatic hernia. Am J Respir Crit Care Med. 2002;166:911–5.

133. Vitali SH, Arnold JH. Bench-to-bedside review: ventilator strategies to reduce lung injury – lessons from pediatric and neonatal intensive care. Crit Care. 2005;9(2):177–83. Epub 2004 Nov 4.

134. Wung JT. Congenital diaphragmatic hernia: survival treated with very delayed surgery, spontaneous respiration, and no chest tube. J Pediatr Surg. 1995;30(3):406–9.

135. Boloker J. Congenital diaphragmatic hernia in 120 infants treated consecutively with permissive hypercapnea/spontaneous respiration/elective repair. J Pediatr Surg. 2002;37:357–66.

136. Kays DW. Detrimental effects of standard medical therapy in congenital diaphragmatic hernia. Ann Surg. 1999;230(3):340–51.

137. Bryner BS, et al. Congenital diaphragmatic hernia requiring extracorporeal membrane oxygenation: does timing of repair matter? J Pediatr Surg. 2009;44(6):1165–71.

138. Guner YS, et al. Outcome analysis of neonates with congenital diaphragmatic hernia treated with venovenous vs. venoarterial extracorporeal membrane oxygenation. J Pediatr Surg. 2009;44(9):1691–701.

139. van den Hout L. Can we improve outcome of congenital diaphragmatic hernia? Pediatr Surg Int. 2009;25:733–43.

140. Butler E, et al. The Canadian Pediatric Surgery Network (CAPSNet): lessons learned from a national registry devoted to the study of congenital diaphragmatic hernia and gastroschisis. Eur J Pediatr Surg. 2015;25(6):474–80.

141. Liem NT, Dien TM, Ung NQ. Thoracoscopic repair in the neonatal intensive care unit for congenital diaphragmatic hernia during high-frequency oscillatory ventilation. J Laparoendosc Adv Surg Tech A. 2010;20(1):111–4.

142. Hsu HT, et al. Total intravenous anesthesia for repair of congenital diaphragmatic hernia: a case report. Kaohsiung J Med Sci. 2004;20(9):465–9.

143. Terui K, et al. Surgical approaches for neonatal congenital diaphragmatic hernia: a systematic review and meta-analysis. Pediatr Surg Int. 2015;31:891–7.

144. Tsao K. Minimally invasive repair of congenital diaphragmatic hernia. J Pediatr Surg. 2011;46(6):1158–64.

145. Hussain HK, et al. Imaging-guided core biopsy for the diagnosis of malignant tumors in pediatric patients. AJR Am J Roentgenol. 2001;176(1):43–7.

146. Elston WJ, et al. Safety of research bronchoscopy, biopsy and bronchoalveolar lavage in asthma. Eur Respir J. 2004;24(3):375–7.

147. Lex C, et al. Airway eosinophilia in children with severe asthma: predictive values of noninvasive tests. Am J Respir Crit Care Med. 2006;174(12):1286–91.

148. Regamey N, et al. Quality, size, and composition of pediatric endobronchial biopsies in cystic fibrosis. Chest. 2007;131(6):1710–7.

149. Molina-Teran A, et al. Safety of endobronchial biopsy in children with cystic fibrosis. Pediatr Pulmonol. 2006;41(11):1021–4.

150. Dishop MK, Mallory GB, White FV. Pediatric lung transplantation: perspectives for the pathologist. Pediatr Dev Pathol. 2008;11(2):85–105.

151. Mahmoud M, et al. Dexmedetomidine and ketamine for large anterior mediastinal mass biopsy. Paediatr Anaesth. 2008;18(10):1011–3.

152. Cahill AM, et al. CT-guided percutaneous lung biopsy in children. J Vasc Interv Radiol. 2004;15(9):955–60.

153. Gluer S, et al. Thoracoscopic biopsy in children with diffuse parenchymal lung disease. Pediatr Pulmonol. 2008;43(10):992–6.

154. Kulayat AN, et al. Comparing 30-day outcomes between thoracoscopic and open approaches for resection of pediatric congenital lung malformations: evidence from NSQIP. J Pediatr Surg. 2015;50(1):1716–26.

155. Kunisaki SM, et al. Thoracoscopic vs open lobectomy in infants and young children with congenital lung malformations. J Am Coll Surg. 2014;218(2):261–70.

156. Shah PL, Hansell D, Lawson PR, Reid KBM, Morgan C. Pulmonary alveolar proteinosis: clinical aspects and current concepts on pathogenesis. Thorax. 2000;55:67–771.

157. Trapnell BC, Whitsett JA, Nakata K. Mechanisms of disease: pulmonary alveolar proteinosis. N Engl J Med. 2003;349:2527–39.

158. Lippmann M, Mok MS, Wasserman K. Anaesthetic management for children with alveolar proteinosis using extracorporeal circulation. Report of two cases. Br J Anaesth. 1977;49:173–7.

159. Mahut B, de Blic J, Le Bourgeois M, Beringer A, Chevalier JY, Scheinmann P. Partial and massive lung lavages in an infant with severe pulmonary alveolar proteinosis. Pediatr Pulmonol. 1992;13:50–3.

160. Moazam F, Schmidt JH, Chesrown SE, Graves SA, Sauder RA, Drummond J, et al. Total lung lavage for pulmonary alveolar proteinosis in an infant without the use of cardiopulmonary bypass. J Pediatr Surg. 1985;20:398–401.

161. Paschen C, Reiter K, Stanzel F, Teschler H, Griese M. Therapeutic lung lavages in children and adults. Respir Res. 2005;6:138.

162. Paquet C, Karsli C. Technique of lung isolation for whole lung lavage in a child with pulmonary alveolar proteinosis. Anesthesiology. 2009;110:190–2.

163. Bliss D, Silen M. Pediatric thoracic trauma. Crit Care Med. 2002;30(11 Suppl):S409–15.

164. Holmes JF, Sokolove PE, Brant WE, Kuppermann N. A clinical decision rule for identifying children with thoracic injuries after blunt torso trauma. Ann Emerg Med. 2002;39(5):492–9.

165. Peclet MH, et al. Thoracic trauma in children: an indicator of increased mortality. J Pediatr Surg. 1990;25(9):961–5.

166. Bonadio WA, Hellmich T. Post-traumatic pulmonary contusion in children. Ann Emerg Med. 1989;18(10):1050–2.

167. Karamakar MK, Ho A. Acute pain management of patients with multiple fractured ribs. J Trauma. 2003;54:615–25.

168. Cadzow SP, Armstrong KL. Rib fractures in infants: red alert. J Paediatr Child Health. 2000;36:322–6.

169. Bulloch B, et al. Cause and clinical characteristics of rib fractures in infants. Pediatrics. 2000;105(4):E48.

170. Roux P, Fisher RM. Chest injuries in children: an analysis of 100 cases of blunt chest trauma from motor vehicle accidents. J Pediatr Surg. 1992;27(5):551–5.

171. Haxhija EQ, Nöres H, Schober P, Höllwarth ME. Lung contusion-lacerations after blunt thoracic trauma in children. Pediatr Surg Int. 2004;20(6):412–4. Epub 2004 Apr 30.

172. Taira BR, et al. Ventilator-associated pneumonia in pediatric trauma patients. Pediatr Crit Care Med. 2009;10(4): 491–4.

173. Cullen ML. Pulmonary and respiratory complications of pediatric trauma. Respir Care Clin N Am. 2001;7(1):59–77.

174. Hancock BJ, Wiseman NE. Tracheobronchial injuries in children. J Pediatr Surg. 1991;26(11):1316–9.

175. Grant WJ, Meyers RL, Jaffe RL, Johnson DG. Tracheobronchial injuries after blunt chest trauma in children – hidden pathology. J Pediatr Surg. 1998;33(11):1707–11.

176. Eichelberger MR, Randolph JG. Thoracic trauma in children. Surg Clin N Am. 1981;61(5):1181–97.

177. Golianu B, Hammer GB. Pain management for pediatric thoracic surgery. Curr Opin Anaesthesiol. 2005;18:13–21.

178. Nunn JF, Slavin G. Posterior intercostal nerve blocks for pain relief after cholecystectomy. Anatomical basis and efficacy. Br J Anaesth. 1980;52:253–60.

179. Gibson MP, Vetter T, Crow JP. Use of continuous retropleural bupivacaine in postoperative pain management for pediatric thoracotomy. J Pediatr Surg. 1999;34(1):199–201.

180. Krane EJ, Dalens BJ, Murat I, Murrell D. The safety of epidurals placed during general anesthesia. Reg Anesth Pain Med. 1998;23:433–8.

181. Tsui BC. Innovative approaches to neuraxial blockade in children: the introduction of epidural nerve root stimulation and ultrasound guidance for epidural catheter placement. Pain Res Manag. 2006;11(3):173–80.

182. Ingelmo P, et al. The optimum initial pediatric epidural bolus: a comparison of four local anesthetic solutions. Paediatr Anaesth. 2007;17(12):1166–75.

183. Goodarzi M. Comparison of epidural morphine, hydromorphone and fentanyl for postoperative pain control in children undergoing orthopaedic surgery. Paediatr Anaesth. 1999;9(5):419–22.

184. Serlin S. Single-dose caudal epidural morphine in children: safe, effective, and easy. J Clin Anesth. 1991;3(5):386–90.

Anesthetic Management of Thoracic Trauma

51

Stephen V. Panaro and Tzonghuei Herb Chen

Key Points

- The initial assessment and stabilization of the thoracic trauma patient is critical for successful outcomes. An understanding of the relevant anatomy and familiarization with the signs and symptoms of injury to the vital structures will minimize the chance of missed injury which could be catastrophic.
- Transesophageal echocardiography is a valuable tool in the care of the hemodynamically unstable thoracic trauma patient, reliably diagnosing and guiding the management of blunt cardiac injury, aortic injury, and hypovolemia.
- Airway management and lung isolation provide challenges to the anesthesiologist. Identification of the location of a tracheobronchial injury preoperatively will dictate the method of isolation beyond the injury. Lung isolation techniques are more challenging to novice anesthesiologists. Anesthesiologists who may be asked to manage thoracic trauma patients should familiarize themselves with these techniques.
- There is no level I evidence for the management of pulmonary contusion. There are similarities between the contused lung and ARDS and patients who present with pulmonary contusion should be ventilated with lung protective strategies.

- Management of cardiac trauma requires an understanding of the type of injury and prompt diagnosis is of paramount importance. Signs of cardiac tamponade must be identified quickly and the pericardium decompressed urgently. Echocardiography is a useful tool in evaluating injury and guiding therapy in unstable patients if available.
- Injury to the thoracic aorta is increasingly being managed with endovascular techniques, but not all patients are candidates. An understanding of the physiology of the thoracic aortic clamp and its implications for hemodynamic management remains important. Similarly, strategies for spinal cord protection during open repair must be considered. Expectant management of minimal aortic injury may become more common.
- Anesthesiologists play an integral role in the management of pain in the patient with chest wall injury. There is potential for improved outcomes with epidural analgesia, but many patients will not be candidates for neuraxial analgesia. In the patients who will meet exclusion criteria, other techniques including paravertebral blocks should be considered.

Introduction

Thoracic trauma is a morbid business. The American College of Surgeons estimates it is associated with a 10% mortality [1] with 16,000 deaths annually. That represents 25% of all trauma deaths. Considering that injury is the leading cause of death from ages 1 to 45 (more than half of all deaths ages 13–32 and 80% in teenage years) [2] and the leading cause of years of life lost before 75, its impact is enormous [3]. In one analysis, if injury is taken into account, the life expectancy in

Electronic Supplementary Material The online version of this chapter (https://doi.org/10.1007/978-3-030-00859-8_51) contains supplementary material, which is available to authorized users.

S. V. Panaro (✉)
Department of Anesthesia, Hartford Hospital, Hartford, CT, USA

T. H. Chen
Department of Anesthesiology, Warren Alpert Medical School of Brown University, Rhode Island Hospital, Providence, RI, USA

© Springer Nature Switzerland AG 2019
P. Slinger (ed.), *Principles and Practice of Anesthesia for Thoracic Surgery*, https://doi.org/10.1007/978-3-030-00859-8_51

845

the United States rockets from 19th in the developed world to first [4]. Since the vital structures in the chest are so well protected by the bony thorax, a great deal of force is required to disrupt them, and they are uncommonly injured in isolation in blunt trauma. Indeed, 70% of the time, insults to the chest are associated with multisystem injury.

This chapter will attempt to describe thoracic trauma in terms of the underlying injury and its treatment. This approach is not new and dates (at least) to the ancient Egyptian Edwin Smith Papyrus in the seventeenth century B.C. While our tools and management have changed (we no longer treat hemorrhage with the binding of fresh meat on the first day), the organization of the chapter will follow theirs – structured to some degree by injury type.

While the presentation of a patient with traumatic injury to the thorax can seem daunting, the principles in managing these patients are the familiar backbone of our specialty. A rational stepwise approach to the evaluation and management of these patients will not only yield the best results, but make it clear that there is nothing mystical about them. That process begins, as always, with an understanding of the relevant physiology, anatomy, and the tools we use to assess them.

Anatomy

The chest is by definition the upper part of the trunk between the neck and the abdomen formed by the 12 thoracic vertebrae and the corresponding ribs. Thoracic trauma may include injury to the chest wall, pleura, airways, heart, great vessels, diaphragm, and esophagus. The implications of injury vary by structure and its mechanism of insult. The most lethal injuries are those involving the mediastinal structures. The mediastinum itself is divided into four parts. The anterior mediastinum lies between the sternum and the pericardium and contains little other than fat, lymph nodes, the internal thoracic (mammary) vessels, and the thymus. The middle mediastinum contains the pericardium, heart, lower half of the superior vena cava, ascending aorta, tracheal bifurcation, as well as the pulmonary arteries and veins. The posterior mediastinum is the space between the tracheal bifurcation and vertebral column and contains the descending aorta, azygous, esophagus, and thoracic duct. Lastly, the superior mediastinum is bound by the manubrium and the first four vertebrae. It holds the aortic arch, brachiocephalic veins, upper half of the SVC, the left common carotid, and subclavian arteries as well as the brachiocephalic trunk. Stab injuries to the heart are thru the classic precordium (so-called box of death) bound by the sternal notch superiorly, nipples laterally, and inferiorly by the anterior ribs 80% of the time. Because the entry site for gunshot injuries to the heart are thru the precordium only a

minority (46%) of the time, any entrance wound to the torso should raise concern of injury to the heart.

Initial Approach to the Patient with Thoracic Trauma

Many thoracic injuries are highly lethal. In fact, only two-thirds of patients will actually reach the hospital alive. Of those that do, the immediate identification and treatment of the six most lethal injuries is paramount, and the assessment of the thoracic trauma patient should follow the protocol detailed in ATLS®. Despite these statistics, most patients (90% of blunt injury and 70–85% of penetrating thoracic injury) who reach the hospital will not need operative intervention, and most can be treated by simple procedures commonly taught in the ATLS course including airway control and chest decompression (tube thoracotomy or needle decompression) [5]. The assessment of the thoracic trauma patient does not differ from the assessment of any trauma patient, and it begins with the primary survey focusing where the six most immediately lethal injuries to the chest are sought. These include airway obstruction, tension pneumothorax, cardiac tamponade, open pneumothorax, massive hemothorax, and flail chest. Each of these major problems is addressed as they are identified since each can be immediately lethal. Once the primary survey is completed and the patient is stabilized, the secondary survey is undertaken. The injuries typically found on secondary survey are not easily recognized on physical exam and can be missed. Still, each can be potentially lethal. The ATLS student manual focuses on eight potentially lethal diagnoses including simple pneumothorax, hemothorax, pulmonary contusion, tracheobronchial injury, blunt cardiac injury, traumatic aortic disruption, traumatic diaphragmatic injury, and blunt esophageal rupture. We will begin with the most lethal six.

The diagnosis of airway obstruction should be clear to any anesthesiologist. The physical findings of apnea, cyanosis, stridor, subcutaneous emphysema, and the appearance of a patient with air hunger should be familiar to us. The etiology may be from avulsed teeth, secretions, expanding neck hematomas, laryngeal trauma, or tracheal tears or transection. As always immediate intubation is indicated in any patient with airway compromise. Special considerations for patients with airway disruption will be discussed later in the chapter as will the management of the airway in the trauma patient.

Tension pneumothorax occurs when air enters the pleural space and cannot exit. This results in shift of the mediastinum, kinking of the superior and inferior vena cava, and a profound decrease in cardiac output. Patients present with respiratory distress, unilateral breath sounds, neck vein distention, tracheal deviation (rarely), and cyanosis (very late finding). If this constellation of symptoms occurs just after intubation, one must become immediately suspicious. An old surgical adage holds that one should never have a chest X-ray (CXR) of a tension pneumothorax. This constellation of findings should be immediately treated with needle decompression (the classic teaching calls for the insertion of a 14-gauge catheter in the second intercostal space, midclavicular line) followed by tube thoracostomy, although a midaxillary approach for needle decompression is also acceptable (see below).

Cardiac tamponade is most often the result of penetrating trauma but can be seen in blunt trauma. The normal pericardial sac is tough and fibrous, and – when fluid builds quickly – only 75–100 ccs will cause tamponade physiology. The classic Beck's triad (JVD, hypotension, and muffled heart sounds) is only present in a third of patients. While Kussmaul's sign (rise in central venous pressure with inspiration) is reliable, it is not practical in the trauma setting since few patients have a central line in place before the diagnosis must be made. The equalization of pressures (should one happen to have a Swan-Ganz catheter in place) or systolic to diastolic gradient of less than 30 mm Hg may also suggest tamponade. Most commonly in trauma, the diagnosis will be suggested by ongoing hypotension without obvious blood loss. FAST (Focused Assessment with Sonography for Trauma) examination is highly accurate [6]. The patient can be temporized with pericardiocentesis occasionally, but this procedure is technically less challenging in the patient with chronic pericardial effusions than in traumatic tamponade because of the small amount of fluid necessary to cause the physiology and because clotted blood can be difficult to aspirate. In reality, trauma patients in extremis should be treated with ED thoracotomy. Those more stable should be evaluated with FAST, TEE if the expertise is available, or even a subxiphoid pericardial window depending on local experience, resources, and clinical scenario. The latter can be performed in the operating room but can be considered in the emergency department if necessary [7]. Once the diagnosis is made, the patient should be treated aggressively with fluids until they can be taken for definitive treatment. If a penetrating injury to the myocardium has occurred, it may be possible to treat without cardiopulmonary bypass [8]. This is fortuitous, because the administration of large volumes of heparin is often contraindicated in the trauma patient. Adenosine may provide the surgeon with 15 or 20 s of asystole and has been described to facilitate repair [9].

The other three of the lethal six are usually not difficult to diagnose. Massive hemothorax (>1500 cc of blood or more than 200 cc/h for 4 h) should be suspected in any trauma patient with shock and absent or distant breath sounds on one side. While patient physiology should be the primary driver of urgent surgical management, any patient with an output of greater than 1500 cc of blood in a 24 h period should prompt

consideration of surgical exploration [10]. A CXR will show the fluid in the chest but should not be necessary in all cases. Extended FAST (E-FAST) in experienced hands provides a rapid and sensitive evaluation for hemothorax and will be discussed in the section on echocardiography for thoracic trauma. The last two of the six (open pneumothorax and flail chest) should be easily recognizable. We will discuss the treatment of the latter in later sections.

Echocardiography in Thoracic Trauma

Echocardiography has become an incredibly useful tool in the assessment of the trauma patient and this begins with the FAST exam, a rapid bedside ultrasound examination which functions as a screening tool for pericardial effusion and hemoperitoneum after trauma. In particular, FAST has proven extremely reliable in the assessment of the pericardium and can be completed in less than a minute and a half with sensitivity as high as 100% for patients with suspected pericardial tamponade. The extended FAST (or eFAST) adds bilateral anterior thoracic ultrasound to FAST, which allows for the detection of pneumothorax.

Though not currently recommended as a primary screening tool for blunt cardiac injury (BCI) in the hemodynamically stable patient [11], formal echocardiography–transthoracic echocardiography (TTE) and transesophageal echocardiography (TEE) – expands on the power of FAST and eFAST and plays a critical role in the care of the thoracic trauma patient, rapidly diagnosing intrathoracic pathologies causing severe hemodynamic instability and/or cardiopulmonary arrest. Expeditious diagnosis and treatment with TTE and/or TEE can stabilize the patient and help prevent end-organ ischemia and subsequent morbidity and mortality. Both modalities are portable and, unlike other radiographic imaging modalities such as computerized tomography (CT) and angiography, can be performed anywhere an echocardiography machine and probe can be brought. With an experienced operator, it also provides easy and rapid return of data which is updated in real time.

TEE appears to be superior, however, in the trauma population. A prospective study comparing TTE and TEE in 105 blunt thoracic trauma patients found that TTE yielded poor image quality in 19% of the patients who required TEE instead, which was superior in diagnosing myocardial contusion, 30% of which were missed by TTE, and aortic injury. The problem with TTE probably lies in its limitations in patients with chest wall trauma [12]. Another prospective study comparing the two modalities reported similar findings, with the transthoracic approach significantly limited by mechanical ventilation, subcutaneous emphysema, the presence of chest or abdominal tubes, and possible interference with other ongoing procedures [13].

TEE was first used in cardiac surgery in the early 1980s [14]. In the decades since then, its use has expanded to the point where TEE is now used in 91% of US teaching hospitals [15]. Specifically, it is used in nearly every cardiac operating room, routinely revealing new pathology and occasionally altering surgical management [16], and is frequently seen in non-cardiac surgery, typically in the form of "rescue echocardiography" in unstable patients to help identify the cause of the hemodynamic derangements, often with great success [17]. It has a distinct advantage over other invasive hemodynamic monitors because it directly assesses intracardiac volume and biventricular systolic function.

Though generally safe when available guidelines for TEE probe insertion and manipulation are followed, serious complications have been reported including esophageal perforation, esophageal injury, hematoma, laryngeal palsy, dysphagia, dental injury, and death. Mortality associated with TEE has been reported to be <1 in 10,000 while morbidity is 2–5/1000 [18, 19]. While there is insufficient literature to define contraindications to TEE, most experts agree that prior esophagectomy or esophagogastrectomy, esophageal stricture, tracheoesophageal fistula, and esophageal trauma are absolute contraindications. Outside of these recommendations, there is little consensus regarding the safety of TEE in patients with esophageal varices, prior radiation therapy, previous bariatric surgery, Zenker diverticulum, and colonic interposition. However, as long as the expected benefit outweighs potential risk, the experts agree that the use of TEE is justified [20]. Specific to the trauma patient, extreme caution should be taken in a patient with a suspected or known esophageal or cervical spine injury [19, 21].

In the absence of contraindications, current guidelines recommend using TEE in all open adult heart and thoracic aortic surgical procedures and considering its use in coronary artery bypass surgeries and transcatheter intracardiac procedures to confirm preoperative diagnoses, detect new pathology, guide the anesthetic and surgical plan, and assess surgical results. In the non-cardiac realm, use of TEE is recommended "when the nature of the planned surgery or the patient's known or suspected cardiovascular pathology might result in severe hemodynamic, pulmonary, or neurologic compromise" and "when unexplained life-threatening circulatory instability persists despite corrective therapy." The guidelines specifically mention the use of TEE in patients who have suffered major thoracic trauma [20].

In the hemodynamic unstable thoracic trauma patient needing immediate surgical intervention, TEE is able to diagnose the most common pathologies in this patient population, reliably detecting various blunt cardiac injuries (myocardial contusion, acute valvular insufficiency, pericardial tamponade), aortic injury, and hypovolemia. It is also an ideal tool to guide and alter perioperative management of hypotensive patient who is undergoing resuscitation with fluid, blood, vasopressors, and inotropes. In a prospective study assessing the impact of TEE on trauma patients initially screened using clinical exam, ECG, CK-MB, and chest radiography, TEE was able to detect unexpected myocardial contusions, valve injuries, pericardial effusions, aortic lesions, and hypovolemia. In total, 30 new diagnoses were made while 32 previous diagnoses were invalidated. In 20% of patients, the use of TEE "made a new clinically relevant diagnosis leading to an emergency treatment" [22]. A retrospective study demonstrated that TEE was able to make a wide variety of diagnoses without complications in 16 cardiothoracic trauma patients, 10 penetrating and 6 blunt ranging from right ventricular infarction and aortic injury to valvular insufficiency, aorto-right ventricular fistulas, and intracardiac foreign bodies, positively influencing treatment in every case [23]. More recently, in a case series of 37 perioperative rescue echocardiograms of trauma patients in shock, management changes were prompted by echocardiographic findings in 49% of the patients. Hypovolemia was the most common finding, followed by left ventricular (LV) and right ventricular (RV) failure, dynamic left ventricular outflow tract obstruction (LVOTO), pericardial tamponade, valvular dysfunction, type B aortic dissection, and mediastinal air. The diagnoses of LVOTO and RV failure made the most impact on patient management [24]. Another article reviewing 364 perioperative rescue echocardiograms similarly found that echo findings influenced management in 59% of patients [25].

Image Acquisition

A comprehensive TEE exam has been described in the literature by the American Society of Echocardiography (ASE) and the Society of Cardiovascular Anesthesiologists (SCA) [14, 19], with recommendations on the maintenance, cleaning, and decontamination of the TEE probe, safe insertion and manipulation of the probe within the esophagus, and acquisition and optimization of images required for a complete examination. An experienced echocardiographer can complete the comprehensive exam which is comprised of 20 standard views in less than 10 min, but this may not be feasible in the hemodynamically unstable thoracic trauma patient. A focused TEE exam can be performed instead, with many examples described in the literature [25–27]. Ultimately, the images obtained and the order of acquisition will be driven by provider preference and specific areas of interest for the individual patient, but at a minimum, the echocardiographer obtains the views shown in Table 51.1 and answers the following:

1. Volume status: is there hypovolemia?
2. Myocardial function: Are the LV and RV contracting adequately? Are there any wall motion abnormalities?
3. Are there any valve abnormalities?
4. Is there a pericardial effusion or pericardial tamponade?
5. Is the aorta intact?

Table 51.1 Suggested TEE exam for the trauma patient

Views	Omniplane angle	Key structures visualized	Pathology diagnosed
TG mid-papillary SAX	0	LV, RV	BCI, hypovolemia
ME 4 chamber +/− CFD	0	LV, RV, LA, RA, MV, TV, IAS, IVS	BCI
ME 2 chamber +/− CFD	90	LV, LA, MV	BCI
ME RV inflow-outflow +/− CFD	60	RA, RV, TV, PV	BCI
ME AV SAX, LAX +/− CFD	40, 130	AV, ascending aorta	BCI, TAI
ME Asc Ao SAX, LAX	0, 90	Ascending aorta	TAI
UE to LE Desc Ao SAX, LAX	0, 90	Descending aorta	TAI
UE aortic arch SAX, LAX	0, 90	Aortic arch	TAI

Abbreviations: *TG* transgastric, *SAX* short axis, *LV* left ventricle, *RV* right ventricle, *ME* mid-esophageal, *CFD* color flow Doppler, *LA* left atrium, *RA* right atrium, *MV* mitral valve, *TV* tricuspid valve, *IAS* intra-atrial septum, *IVS* intraventricular septum, *AV* aortic valve, *LAX* long axis, *Asc Ao* ascending aorta, *Desc Ao* descending aorta, *UE* upper esophageal, *BCI* blunt cardiac injury, *TAI* traumatic aortic injury

A diagnosis of blunt cardiac injury, hypovolemia, or traumatic aortic injury should then be made and treatment should be tailored appropriately.

Blunt Cardiac Injury (Myocardial Contusion, Valvular Insufficiency, Pericardial Effusion, and Tamponade)

There exist a number of ways of evaluating blunt cardiac injury. Cardiac isoenzyme testing, in particular for troponin I (cTnI) which is very specific for myocardial damage, is often performed but is not terribly sensitive. The value of the cTnI increases when combined with the electrocardiogram (ECG), which is recommended in all patients suspected of having a BCI. On its own, ECG is not an ideal diagnostic tool as abnormalities are often nonspecific and can occur as a result of other conditions often associated with trauma [28, 29]. Moreover, the ECG primarily evaluates the left ventricle and can therefore miss a right ventricular contusion, the most common BCI [30]. However, an abnormal ECG combined with abnormal cardiac isoenzymes appears to correlate with clinically significant cardiac complications [31]. On the contrary, it has been established that a normal ECG combined with two serial negative troponin I tests all but excludes BCI with a negative predictive value of 100%. There are many manifestations of BCI, and while these tests can predict the presence or absence of BCI, they are unable to elucidate the exact pathology or physiology. Echocardiography has proven useful and superior to other imaging modalities in the evaluation of BCI [32–34]. It can directly visualize the presence of

both right and left ventricular contusions [35, 36] and pinpoint segmental wall motion abnormalities [37]. TEE can also readily detect and facilitate treatment for unanticipated valve injury, a less common lesion usually affecting the tricuspid valve where early or late rupture of supporting structures such as papillary muscles or chordae tendineae causes valvular regurgitation [32, 36, 38–42]. Pericardial effusions are also effectively evaluated with TEE [36] and there are reports describing the use of echocardiography to diagnose such injuries as atrial septal rupture [34], an inferior vena cava (IVC) tear [43], right atrial free wall rupture [44], pulmonary vein rupture [33], and an aorta-left atrial fistula [45].

A complete evaluation of blunt cardiac injury will require the acquisition of several images. The most common BCI is RV contusion which is best assessed in the ME 4C view (see Fig. 51.1, Video 51.1). Visual estimation of reduced RV contractility and RV dilatation, relative dilatation compared to the LV, and tricuspid annular plane systolic excursion (TAPSE) <16 mm are all signs of RV injury [46]. TAPSE, a very specific sign of RV dysfunction, is best measured with M-mode, with the cursor directed through the lateral annulus of the tricuspid valve, measuring the longitudinal distance of systolic annular motion [26].

Global and regional LV function is best viewed in the transgastric LV short-axis (TG LV SAX) view, the mid-esophageal four-chamber (ME 4C) view, and the mid-esophageal two-chamber (ME 2C) view, though in the hemodynamically unstable patient, the TG LV SAX view is probably most useful. Global function can be evaluated quantitatively but most basic echocardiographers rely on a qualitative estimate of systolic function [19]. A thorough assessment of regional wall motion is described in the ASE guidelines based on ME views [47], but an abbreviated assessment based on the TG LV SAX view at the mid-papillary level may also suffice [48].

Potential valvular injuries should be evaluated in multiple ME views (see Table 51.1) with both two-dimensional (2D)

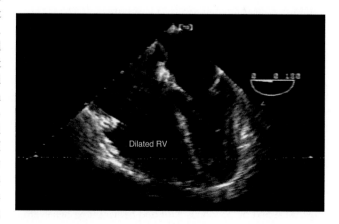

Fig. 51.1 A mid-esophageal four-chamber view showing a right ventricular contusion

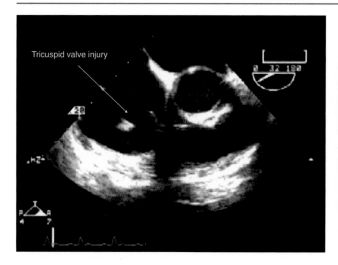

Fig. 51.2 A mid-esophageal right ventricular inflow-outflow view showing a tricuspid valve injury

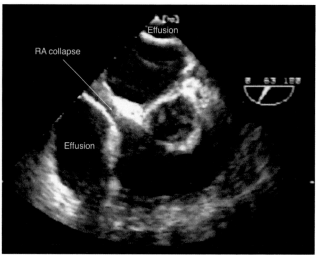

Fig. 51.4 A large traumatic pericardial effusion with evidence of right atrial systolic collapse, suggesting pericardial tamponade

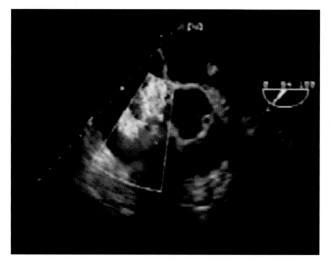

Fig. 51.3 A mid-esophageal right ventricular inflow-outflow view demonstrating severe tricuspid regurgitation associated with a traumatic tricuspid valve injury

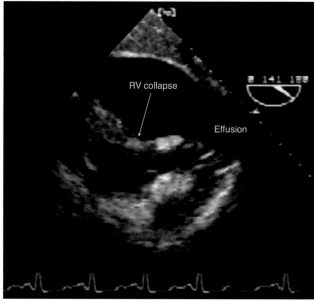

Fig. 51.5 A large traumatic pericardial effusion with evidence of right ventricular diastolic collapse, suggesting pericardial tamponade

echo to check for gross valve abnormalities and color flow Doppler (CFD) to determine the presence or absence of a significant regurgitant lesion. The severity of valvular regurgitation can be determined by visual inspection of the regurgitant jet area in the receiving chamber (the right atrium in the case of a tricuspid valve injury; see Figs. 51.2 and 51.3, Videos 51.2 and 51.3) and by vena contracta width. It is important to use caution when assessing eccentric jets, however, as degree of pathology is often underestimated [19].

Pericardial effusions are easily seen by TEE as a fluid-filled hypoechoic space extending circumferentially around the heart, occasionally containing floating echodense materials (see Figs. 51.4 and 51.5, Videos 51.4 and 51.5). Large acute effusions frequently develop into pericardial tamponade, which can be diagnosed by systolic right atrial collapse lasting for more

than a third of systole, right ventricular diastolic collapse, interventricular dependence, IVC plethora, and exaggerated respiratory changes in mitral and tricuspid inflow. Emergent pericardiocentesis is indicated in this scenario and can be guided by TTE to minimize injury to nearby structures [26, 27, 49].

Aortic Injury

TEE has become a major contributor in the evaluation of the aorta due to its safety, portability, and diagnostic accuracy. It provides superior visualization of the entire aortic isthmus, where most traumatic aortic injuries (TAI) occur [49]. It can be performed during an emergency operation, does not interfere with ongoing resuscitation, can be interpreted immediately, does not require contrast media, and is able to detect concomitant BCI. It is considered to be at least equal to helical computerized tomography (CT) [50] and aortography in the diagnosis of traumatic aortic injuries (TAI), with a reported sensitivity of 94–100% and a specificity of 77–100% [51] and comparable to helical CT and MRI specifically for the diagnosis of type A dissections, with a sensitivity of 98% and a specificity of 95% [52]. The main limitation of TEE in the evaluation of the thoracic aorta is that it is unable to assess the proximal aortic arch or the distal ascending aorta due to the presence of the tracheobronchial bifurcation, where 20% of injuries occur in aortic trauma [53]. It has also been shown to be highly operator-dependent [54]. For these reasons, it should not be the only imaging modality used when TAI is suspected.

Evaluation of the aorta involves direct echocardiographic examination of the entire visible thoracic aorta. The ascending aorta is visible in the upper esophageal (UE) view and the descending aorta in mid-esophageal aortic views and should be examined with 2D echo in the short axis and longitudinal views and with CFD. The presence of a thin, mobile, linear echodensity on the inner surface of the aortic wall suggests a traumatic intimal tear while a thin, less mobile intimal flap dividing the aorta into true and false lumens with or without thrombus formation indicates the presence of a traumatic aortic dissection (see Fig. 51.6, Video 51.6). A more mobile "thick flap" or "medial flap" consisting of intima and media with a potentially ruptured pseudoaneurysm points to a subadventitial traumatic aortic disruption (see Figs. 51.7 and 51.8, Video 51.7). The appearance of the flap and the pattern of blood flow as seen on CFD can distinguish between a partial, subtotal, and complete aortic disruption [49]. The presence of a mediastinal hematoma is a sensitive and specific indirect indicator of a traumatic aortic

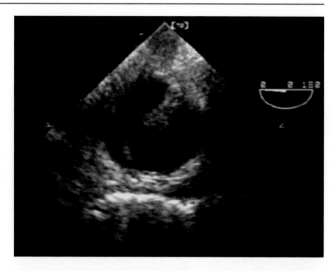

Fig. 51.7 A view of the descending thoracic aorta with a "medial flap" demonstrating traumatic aortic disruption

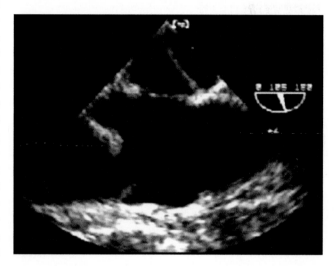

Fig. 51.8 A view of the ascending aorta with a "medial flap" demonstrating traumatic aortic disruption

disruption and can be especially useful in diagnosing injuries of the aorta not visible with TEE [55]. One study suggested that a distance of more than 5.5 mm between the esophageal probe and the posterolateral aortic wall or 6.6 mm between the anteromedial aortic wall and left visceral pleura was predictive of injury to the descending aorta or its branches [56].

Hypovolemia

Hypovolemia secondary to hemorrhage is very prevalent in trauma patients [24]. There are many ways of assessing intravascular volume status, but TEE is the only modality which can provide us with direct measurements of static intracardiac volume and dynamic fluid responsiveness. While the various ME views can yield valuable information, the most basic and most commonly used view for the diagnosis of hypovolemia is

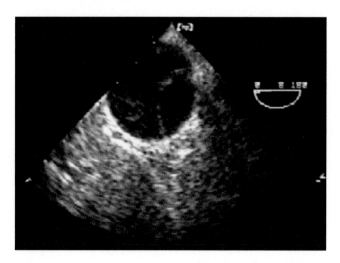

Fig. 51.6 A view of the descending thoracic aorta demonstrating a traumatic aortic dissection with a thin intimal flap dividing the aorta into true and false lumens

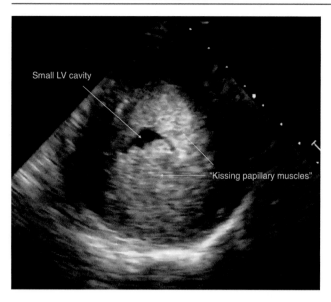

Fig. 51.9 A transgastric left ventricular short axis view showing severe hypovolemia

the TG mid-papillary LV SAX view, where LV end-diastolic diameter and LV end-diastolic area are measured [19]. In the severely hypovolemic patient, the appearance of "kissing papillary muscles" has been described [21] (see Fig. 51.9, Video 51.8). IVC size and collapsibility is another index of volume status but has been described only for TTE in the spontaneously breathing patient and is not applicable to TEE in the mechanically ventilated patient [26, 46, 51]. Stroke volume measurements can be useful. The cross-sectional area of a site (usually the LVOT) is determined using 2D echo and then multiplied by the stroke distance or velocity-time integral (VTI) of blood through that site, determined with pulse-wave (PW) Doppler in the deep TG AV LAX view [26]. A low stroke volume in the setting of normal contractility suggests hypovolemia, while significant stroke volume respiratory variation is a dynamic indication of fluid responsiveness [24].

Training and Certification

Echocardiography is invaluable in hemodynamically unstable trauma patients to elucidate volume status, evaluate global and regional biventricular and valvular function, and detect the presence of pericardial or aortic pathology. The expanding role of TEE in these critically ill patients highlights the need for standardized echocardiographic training. TEE is a powerful tool but it is an invasive procedure with rare but potentially life-threatening complications. Many have tried to define the knowledge needed to safely and effectively perform and interpret exams, while several societies, including the European Association of Cardiovascular Imaging, Society of Critical Care Medicine, and the ASE, have published education guidelines [57–59]. While the echocardiographer with basic TEE proficiency should be

able to obtain and interpret most echocardiographic findings to help guide therapy for the thoracic trauma patient, advanced skills are required for thorough evaluation of valvular injury and interpretation of quantitative parameters [19]. The National Board of Echocardiography (www.echoboards.org), in collaboration with the ASE and SCA, now offers certification in basic and advanced perioperative transesophageal (PTE) echocardiography, which can be achieved by passing a written examination and performing and interpreting a certain number of studies, and courses are available to help interested providers (anesthesiologists, cardiologists, intensivists) achieve and maintain certification in PTE echocardiography.

Traumatic Airway Management

Few topics seem to generate more discussion among anesthesiologists than the presentation of a trauma patient in need of an emergent airway. There are questions of whether manual in-line stabilization is always helpful or can be harmful in restricting the view at laryngoscopy [60, 61]. There are questions of whether Sellick and his 26 patients should have had the influence they have over the last half century [62–66], and there are a myriad of devices to aid us. The discussion is not without merit, since the consequences of failure are dire. The fact that 2% of blunt trauma patients have a cervical spine injury adds to the angst. Furthermore, every method of airway intervention causes motion of the cervical spine including a jaw thrust and placement of an LMA. The basic tenants of airway management remain in place, however, and the ASA difficult airway algorithm (modified for trauma) remains a valuable tool [67] (Fig. 51.10). The modifications for trauma recognize, among other things, that stopping and returning another day is not feasible and that a surgical airway may often be the best option. As such, anesthesiologists who treat trauma patients should be familiar with the techniques and equipment necessary for percutaneous or open cricothyrotomy or tracheostomy. An outstanding recent review of the literature on the topic of airway management in the trauma patient (beyond the scope of this chapter) also provides perspective [68]. What should never be lost amid all the controversy is that the cornerstone of emergent airway management remains direct laryngoscopy. There is strong historical data suggesting that direct laryngoscopy is both highly successful and associated with few credible reports of neurologic deterioration even in the face of known cervical spine injury [68, 69]. A recent review at a major trauma center, in fact, looked at over 6000 patients who were intubated within 1 h of their arrival, and of the 31 patients who required a surgical airway in the first 24 hours, 87% survived to discharge [70]. Only four patients died and none of these were judged to be airway related. This study did not include the

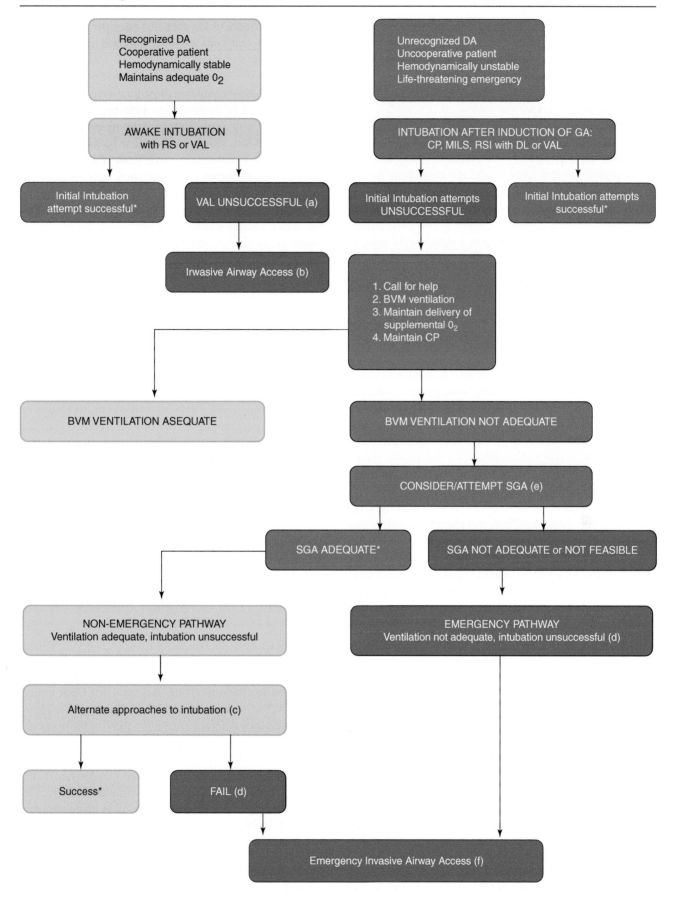

Fig. 51.10 Difficult airway Management in Trauma Updated by COTEP. Originally published by ASA Newsletter. C Hagberg, O Kaslow [67] reprinted with permission

number of patients that were intubated fiberoptically. Their high success rate compared to other series may have been a result of an attending anesthesiologist's presence as part of their protocol. While their protocol calls for in-line stabilization and cricoid pressure, they wisely will relax one or both of these if there is a sense that intubation is being hampered by either technique.

This is not to minimize the role of awake (or asleep) fiberoptic intubation in patients with a difficult airway or known or suspected cervical spine injury. For those with the skill set, bronchoscopic intubation is an excellent rescue as well as primary technique. This is by far the author's preference for known difficult airways in stable cooperative patients with cervical spine injuries and as a rescue technique. No technology has yet replaced it. Still, the reality is that awake fiberoptic intubation requires a cooperative patient and can be difficult with blood in the airway. Many of the limitations to fiberoptic intubation can be overcome, however, with the use of an adult bronchoscope (5.5 mm in diameter or greater) with a modern powerful light source. Anesthesiologists often use smaller bronchoscopes for use in double-lumen endobronchial tubes, but these are less ideal than full size scopes for intubation. The use of an adult bronchoscope adds stiffness which aids in directing the bronchoscope, and the larger port on an adult-sized bronchoscope can be used to either suction or blow oxygen to free the view of secretions or blood. Lastly, a 6.0 endotracheal tube fits snugly around 5.5 mm bronchoscopes, while a 7.0 tube will fit tightly around the largest bronchoscope, minimizing the chance the tube will catch on the arytenoids or epiglottis after the scope has passed into the trachea. Still, it is always best to be familiar with the other emergency airway devices available in one's practice such as the bougie, light wand, GlideScope®, Airtraq®, and McGrath® video laryngoscope or kits for retrograde intubation. This is especially true since awake, cooperative patients are in the minority in the trauma population. In one 7-year review, 83% of the patients were legally intoxicated on presentation [69].

Lung Isolation

One of the more challenging aspects of the management of patients with thoracic injury is lung isolation, which may be required for injury to the thorax. Techniques include right mainstem intubation, Univent® tubes, a variety of commercially available bronchial blockers, and right- and left-sided double-lumen tubes. Since right mainstem intubation will most often result in ventilation of the right middle and lower lobes, it would be expected to result in the highest shunt fraction and higher rates of hypoxia. Each of the other devices requires some expertise, however, and they each have an equivalent high failure rate of 39% in faculty with limited

thoracic experience of less than two cases per month [71]. In this study all malpositions were corrected easily by more experienced thoracic staff. The choice of isolation technique must be based on other factors. Traditionally, double-lumen tubes (DLTs) are the standard of performance for lung isolation. In experienced hands isolation can be achieved quickly and definitively in most cases. In institutions with extensive experience, in fact, right-sided tubes can be used with as few complications (desaturation, high peak airway pressures, etc.) as left-sided tubes [72]. Still, there may be disadvantages to DLTs especially in the trauma population. They may be associated with more airway trauma (especially if an airway injury already exists) with placement. Further, if the patient is to remain intubated following the procedure, double-lumen endobronchial tubes should be changed to single-lumen endotracheal tubes for many reasons. Most obviously, pulmonary toilet is much more difficult with standard length suction devices in the ICU. Their bulk may lead to torsion and injury to the airway over the long term in a patient who is awake and moving. They also have a much larger outer diameter and higher work of breathing given their added length. Recently, three commercially available bronchial blockers have been shown to perform well when compared to left-sided DLTs in their ability to isolate the lung. These designs are continuing to evolve. They did require a longer time to place and had to be repositioned frequently, however [73]. They may be a better option for thoracic trauma patients, although anesthesiologists' familiarity should also play a role in selecting a lung isolation device.

Tracheobronchial Injury

Like so many injuries to the thorax, tracheobronchial injuries are highly lethal. In an older autopsy series of trauma patients, 81% of patients died before reaching a hospital [74]. In a much more recent review of a single institution's 15-year experience including over 12,000 trauma patients, 0.9% of patients reaching the hospital had a tracheobronchial injury (TBI). The numbers were very different for blunt and penetrating mechanisms (0.4% incidence for blunt trauma victims, 4.5% for penetrating) [75]. This review considered all traumatic airway injuries including those of the upper airway and thoracic trachea. In the larger of the North American series, around 60% of these injuries treated will be the result of penetrating trauma [76]. These patients tend to have better outcomes, possibly because of fewer associated injuries [75, 76]. Patients who do appear after a delay in diagnosis often will present when granulation tissue appears in their airway causing a narrowing and post-obstructive pneumonia or recurrent pneumothoraces.

There are classic signs of TBI, but they can be misleading or absent, and a high index of suspicion is required.

Surprisingly, in a comprehensive review of all TBIs reported in the literature up until 1996, the median time to diagnosis was 9 days [77]. In more recent single-institution review, long delays in diagnosis were not reported [75, 76]. When present the classic signs of subcutaneous or mediastinal emphysema, hemoptysis, pneumothorax (especially with a large air leak or with a failure to expand the lung after tube thoracostomy), tension pneumothorax, as well as unexplained dyspnea should all raise suspicion of an airway injury. Blunt TBIs may be associated with fractures of the first rib, clavicle, sternum, and chest wall and lung contusions. The location of injury to the tracheobronchial tree has been consistent over several series [76, 77]. By far, most injuries seem to be within 2 cm of the carina with a predilection for the right side. The latter may be a result of a heavier right lung with a shorter right mainstem bronchus in deceleration injuries. The most likely theory explaining the consistent data showing injury close to the bifurcation is that a rapid deceleration of relatively mobile lungs in the pleura against a fixed carina causes a tear. Bronchial rupture may also be from compression of the chest against a closed glottis. This has been shown in a canine model.

Whatever the mechanism, securing the airway in patients with TBIs can be a daunting task. Indeed, some very heroic measures have been described including thoracotomy [78], jet ventilation via intrabronchial catheters [79], and ECMO [80]. The ASA does have an airway disruption algorithm which emphasizes above all else spontaneous ventilation if possible. The critical tool for both assessing the injury as well as controlling the airway is fiberoptic bronchoscopy. The goal in most cases should be to place the cuff of the endotracheal tube beyond the injury or at least to protect the injury from positive pressure ventilation in some fashion. This is complicated by the fact that most blunt injuries to the trachea are within 2 cm of the carina [76, 77]. In this instance, placement of a side-specific double-lumen endotracheal tube is often most appropriate, although caution must be exercised in placing these bulky rigid tubes past an already injured airway. Passing the cuff of a single-lumen tube beyond the injury and using a bronchial blocker for lung isolation in more proximal injuries seems more prudent. This also has the added advantage of avoiding the changing of the endotracheal tube at the end of the procedure should the patient need to remain intubated. A scenario of cross field ventilation can also be envisioned but should be rare. In every case knowledge of the location of injury is paramount in providing the best airway.

One cannot overemphasize the importance of maintaining spontaneous ventilation in patients with severe tracheal injury. There have been reports of patients arriving with essentially transected airways who maintain spontaneous ventilation through a "neo-trachea" via mediastinal tissues. Attempts at blind instrumentation can be disastrous [81]. It is

the author's strong presence when TBI is suspected for a fiberoptic intubation to be performed. This allows not only a diagnosis and characterization of any pathology, but placement of a single-lumen tube beyond the injury under direct visualization when feasible and proper planning (both surgical and from an airway management perspective) if the injury is more distal. Unfortunately, making the diagnosis can be difficult prior to the need for intubation although clues may be present in a lateral c-spine film. Suspicion should be heightened in a patient with difficulty breathing and any of the classic signs of TBI including subcutaneous emphysema. Fortuitously complete transaction of the airways in patients surviving to reach the hospital is quite rare. The liberal use of bronchoscopy should help lower the incidence of missed injury, help define injury when present, and help secure the airway [76]. In the Toronto series, 29% of patients with TBI required interventions more complex than direct laryngoscopy. These included around 10% each of FOB, surgical airway, and temporary airway through the wound [75].

There is literature evolving for conservative management of tracheobronchial injuries. Most have focused on iatrogenic injury to the membranous portion of the trachea. Unfortunately these injuries are becoming more common and represented half the injuries in a recent series [82]. They may be as common as 1 in 20,000 intubations or 0.12% of DLT placements [83]. Patients may present removed from the trauma with either a delay in their diagnosis or a delay in their treatment. These patients allow for surgical planning and controlled airway management and have a lower mortality [77].

Aortic Injury

In 1958 Parmley reviewed 296 cases of aortic injury from the Armed Forces Institute of Pathology and found 80% mortality prior to arrival at a hospital [84]. It is unlikely that we have made much progress on that front in the intervening five decades [85]. Since this is thought to be largely a deceleration injury, it may be that restraints have had little impact. We have, however, made progress on the patients who do reach the hospital and may be seeing a major advancement over the last few years as thoracic stent grafts become increasingly common.

Because most aortic injuries occur following a rapid deceleration and are most often at the isthmus, traditional discussions of the pathophysiology of the tear have focused on the interaction between the fixed descending aorta and relatively mobile heart and great vessels. Still, injuries have been described in the ascending aorta, more distal thoracic aorta, and abdominal aorta suggesting that other mechanisms may play a role as well [86]. Other mechanisms described include a pinching of the aorta against the vertebral column and a "water hammer effect" describing a sudden occlusion of the aorta and increase in aortic pressure. These have recently been summarized elsewhere [87].

The prompt diagnosis of this injury is essential. As is often quoted, 30–50% of the patients who reach the hospital will die within the first 24 h [84, 88]. Imaging is crucial since there can be few external signs of aortic injury. While the classic findings on CXR such as widening of the mediastinum, blurring of the aortic knob, deviation of the NG tube, and shift of the right bronchus all suggest the diagnosis, they are not diagnostic. Helical computed tomography has become the dominant modality for this purpose. It is fast, allows the quick evaluation of concomitant injuries elsewhere in the body, and has a sensitivity approaching 100% [89]. TEE, MRI, and intravascular ultrasound have also all been described, although it is unclear if any are as accurate as helical CT.

The treatment of aortic injury once a diagnosis is made is almost always prompt. It should be noted for completeness that there is a small subgroup of patients presenting with hemodynamic stability that have been treated expectantly with tight blood pressure and heart rate control either because their severe comorbid conditions precluded operative repair or because their injury was considered minimal [90, 91]. Although small in number, these patients have done quite well. Still, defining minimal aortic injury is an ongoing process and most patients will present to the operating room. This has been especially true in the last decade as thoracic endovascular repair has become commonplace. A period of nonoperative management may be indicated for patients who are unstable from associated injuries, those with traumatic brain injury, severe pulmonary contusion unable to tolerate one-lung ventilation, etc., but again the endovascular approach is making this far less common. While surgery may be successfully delayed while associated injuries are evaluated and stabilized with the use of beta-blockers and antihypertensive agents, the care of these complex patients will eventually fall to the anesthesiologist.

Despite our advances, a prospective look at 50 trauma centers in North America over a 2.5-year period suggested an overall mortality of 31% [88]. All patients who arrived in extremis or who ruptured prior to definitive therapy died. Mortality in patients who were operated on was 14% with an 8.7% paraplegia rate. This study was published before endovascular grafts were increasing in use, and all patients who were operated on had an open repair.

Open surgical repair in general begins with a high left posterolateral thoracotomy and some form of lung isolation – most typically a double-lumen endobronchial tube (DLT). Hypoxia may be a formidable challenge in patients with associated pulmonary contusion. The pros and cons of various methods of lung isolation were reviewed earlier in the chapter. The anesthesiologist must be prepared for the massive hemodynamic swings that accompany proximal thoracic aortic cross clamping (sometimes above the left subclavian artery) as well as attending to all the issues of blood loss and the concomitant injuries the patient brings to the operating theater. There are three main methods of surgical repair, all aimed at preserving spinal cord function. The first is speed in a traditional clamp and sew technique. The advantage of this technique is its simplicity and avoidance of the large doses of systemic heparin used for cardiopulmonary bypass. Bypass from the left atrium (or pulmonary vein) to the distal aorta involves the use of a relatively simple centrifugal pump system and also minimizes the use of heparin. Bypass from the femoral vein cannulation site to the femoral artery requires an oxygenator in the circuit and may require high-dose anticoagulation, although heparin-coated tubing may minimize the dose [87]. There may be advantages in having an oxygenator in the circuit, however, if the patient has lung injury where one-lung ventilation may not be optimal [87]. Clearly it would seem that any technique that limits the need for anticoagulation in the multi-injured trauma patient is advantageous, although concerns of short-term anticoagulation may be exaggerated in patients without head injury [88]. The pros and cons of these techniques are beyond the scope of this text, but the anesthesiologist must be familiar with the norms of the institution and be prepared to manage the techniques preferred by their surgeons. Although lumbar cerebrospinal fluid (CSF) drainage has not been proven in blunt aortic injury, its use was shown prospectively to be of benefit in patients undergoing thoracic aortic aneurysm repair and should be considered in the stable, cooperative patient [92]. Even under the best circumstances, open repair can negatively affect the patients underlying pulmonary, cardiac, and neurologic status [93].

Recently, attention has focused on endovascular treatment of thoracic aortic injuries [94]. There are many theoretical advantages of this approach. For patients with closed head injury, it can be done without significant heparinization and large hemodynamic swings complicating the management of intracranial hypertension and can even be done in reverse Trendelenburg if needed. It can be done in patients in traction for long bone injuries, does not require lung isolation, and avoids position changes for patients with pelvic injury that may exacerbate pelvic hematoma. These facts broaden the patient population who can be treated and avoids delays in treating others. Published series show improved mortality, fewer perioperative complications compared to open repair, and a low or zero rate of paraplegia [33, 93, 95, 96]. The low rate of paraplegia may relate to the short segment of thoracic aorta that needs coverage in the typical injury [95]. Concerns remain, however. Many are technical and some revolve around the specifics of a device developed for aneurysmal disease being placed in a normal, smaller thoracic aorta. There can also be difficulties with the proximity to the left subclavian artery, and there can be challenges in dealing with the curvature of the aorta. Still, there has been a dramatic shift away from open repair to endovascular treatments. Open repair has fallen from 100% of repairs in 1997 to 35% in the second American Association for the Surgery of Trauma study in 2008 [97, 98]. These numbers of course reflect the behavior of 18 select trauma centers. The percentage of stent grafts placed in the country as a whole is probably smaller. Still, in these two studies, there has been a dramatic fall in procedure-related mortality and paraplegia (8.7–1.6% overall from first study to the second). Device issues (early endoleak, left subclavian artery compromise, left carotid artery occlusion (resulting in CVA), etc.) remain a concern. There also remains a lack of long-term follow-up of these devices, and how they will perform as a young trauma patient ages is as of yet unknown. These patients will also need long-term, perhaps lifelong follow-up to assure endoleaks do not develop. Lastly, it is unclear if some of these devices were placed in patients who had minimal aortic injury and may not have required treatment at all as pointed out in the discussion that accompanies this chapter [97].

Despite these caveats and the absence of randomized controlled trials, nonrandomized controlled trials are pushing us in the direction of TEVAR, and the Society for Vascular Surgery has issued guidelines suggesting that blunt traumatic aortic injury be managed with endovascular repair preferentially. While it is acknowledged that randomized trials are lacking, it is also acknowledged that such trials may never be completed and while imperfect, available evidence points to the less invasive and expedient approach in these often profoundly injured patients [99–101].

Pulmonary Contusion

Pulmonary contusion is a clinical entity that complicates as many as 65% of blunt chest trauma patients who present for surgery [102]. In a sobering look at the long-term sequela, a recent review suggested that 70% of patients will have deficits in pulmonary function 6 months after injury and will report a loss of physical function [103]. Signs on presentation are as one would expect, namely, tachypnea, hypoxia, hypercarbia, wheezing, and sometimes hemoptysis. CXR and even CT findings can lag behind the clinical picture by hours. Chest ultrasound may aid in the rapid diagnosis especially as the extended focused assessment with ultrasonography for trauma (EFAST) evolves [104, 105]. The gross pathology results from the loss of vessel integrity at the alveolar capillary membrane leading to intraparenchymal and alveolar hemorrhage and edema. Surfactant production decreases and shunt ensues. As in ARDS the lung becomes functionally smaller as alveoli fill with blood and edema. Pain then leads to splinting and progressive atelectasis. Worse, pulmonary contusion can lead to

true ARDS. Evidence continues to mount that lung injury is itself inflammatory, and the localized inflammatory response may be what leads to ARDS [106–109]. Further, the immediate inflammatory response in the lung may lead to delayed immunosuppression that increases patients' susceptibility to an infectious challenge later [110, 111]. Despite its inflammatory nature, steroids cannot be recommended [112].

Making specific, evidence-based recommendations based on the available literature is difficult. This is underscored by the absence of a single level I evidence-based recommendation in the Eastern Association for the Surgery of Trauma (EAST) guidelines for pulmonary contusion [112]. Level II recommendations describe supportive care such as optimal pain management (with epidurals when possible), avoiding obligatory ventilation and overly aggressive resuscitation. The anesthesiologists' primary role in lung contusion outside the operating room will be to assist in the management of pain. This will be discussed in more detail later. In the operating theater, issues will center around fluid and ventilatory management. Adapting lung protective strategies developed for and accepted in ARDS patients seems prudent. Because alveolar over distention and alveolar opening and collapse can only exacerbate the inflammatory process, part of this should be recruitment maneuvers and PEEP [112, 113]. The initial resuscitation should not be compromised, but the administration of fluids afterward should be meticulous in an effort not to augment extravascular lung water. The best method for monitoring fluid management is open to question although dynamic assessments to predict fluid responsiveness (improvement in cardiac output) seem to be better than static measurements of CVP and PCWP in a myriad of recent clinical trials. There is also a suggestion that Hextend® may have a role [114, 115].

Blunt Cardiac Injury

The term blunt cardiac injury (BCI) covers a wide range of injuries whose clinical significance is related to both the type and severity of the injury. The pathophysiology results from either direct transfer of energy during the impact of the myocardium against the thorax; the rapid decelertaion of the heart, or from compression of the heart between the sternum and spine [30]. The pattern and pathophysiology of injury will reflect the details of the impact and position of the heart in the cardiac cycle. The ventricles, for example, are most vulnerable at end diastole and the valves most vulnerable when closed. Even modest impacts can lead to sudden cardiac death, most commonly from ventricular arrhythmias. Commotion cordis, for example, results from an impact during the vulnerable moment of repolarization just prior to T wave peak [116, 117]. Most deaths due to blunt cardiac injury require more force, however. Almost every injury one can imagine can occur and has been described. The heart can be contused, torn, or ruptured (freely or septal). Coronary arteries can be torn or become thrombosed. The pericardium can become distended with blood and cause tamponade. Finally, the heart is a muscle, and when it is contused, local hemorrhage, edema, and often necrosis cause poor performance. As the contused portion begins to swell, perfusion to that portion of myocardium may be compromised causing ventricular dysfunction to be exacerbated. Further, this may make the patient susceptible to arrhythmias possibly from a reentry mechanism [118]. Of concern, these arrhythmias can present very late (up to 6 days in one case report) after an initial 24 h arrhythmia free period [119]. Lastly, the practitioner must remember that myocardial performance may be drastically compromised even without direct injury to the heart. This is most commonly and sometimes dramatically seen in patients with traumatic brain injury. The most common mechanism of cardiac injury remains motor vehicle crashes in the most recent series. In patients who died of blunt trauma, 66% had either a cardiac or thoracic aortic injury (or both). Injuries to the right atrium and to the right ventricle predominate [120].

The approach to the patient is determined by their clinical presentation. Taking a history from the patient who is able to provide one will give valuable clues not only by detailing symptoms, but by documenting prior cardiac issues that may help avoid confusion of acute and chronic conditions. The physical exam should focus not only on the heart, but on associated chest wall injuries that will raise the index of suspicion for associated BCI. These include chest tenderness, crepitus, seatbelt marks, etc. Beck's triad of hypotension, muffled heart sounds, and distended neck veins or pulsus paradoxus suggest tamponade and urgent surgical attention.

Echocardiography has become an incredibly useful tool in the assessment of the BCI patient, and this begins with the FAST assessment. FAST has proven extremely reliable in the assessment of the pericardium and can be completed in less than a minute and a half with sensitivity as high as 100% [121, 122] for patients with suspected pericardial tamponade. Formal echocardiography (transthoracic or transesophageal when transthoracic is inadequate) is the primary tool for assessing hemodynamic instability in patients with BCI. Hemodynamic instability can result from etiologies that require very different treatments, and defining whether failure is due to acute valvular insufficiency, septal rupture leading to left to right shunt, cardiac rupture, wall motion abnormalities from contusion, LAD thrombosis from crush injury, or any other pathology is essential. Despite its usefulness as a tool in the sickest patients, it is not a cost-effective screening tool. The EAST practice guidelines reflect most authors' opinion and the bulk of the literature when they state that formal echocardiography adds little to the hemodynamically stable patient and should be reserved for patients with instability or with a clinical question that cannot be explained [123, 124]. Part of the rationale for this statement is that even in patients diag-

nosed with BCI by echocardiography, in hemodynamically stable patients, there was no sequela of the injury that required treatment even at 1-year follow-up [125]. One of the difficulties in BCI, in fact, is evaluating and triaging patients with significant chest trauma and risk for BCI (e.g., patients with fractured ribs, sternum, and pulmonary contusion) who have no initial symptoms of BCI. The negative predictive value of two serial negative troponin I tests and a normal ECG was 100% in one study suggesting that these patients need no further observation or treatment [126]. While an abnormal ECG does correlate with the risk of developing a complication requiring treatment in BCI [31], the findings are often nonspecific and may not help define the pathology or physiology that is crucial to aiding in treatment.

Specific generalizations for the anesthesiologists managing the patient with blunt cardiac injury are few since the individual patient's injury pattern and physiology must dictate specific treatments. As we have stated, defining any abnormality of the function of the ventricle is generally accomplished with echocardiography. Clinical suspicion of the possibility of tamponade and an understanding of the signs will aid in the prompt diagnosis of this problem. In truth, all three signs of Beck's triad may not be present in trauma patients with tamponade who are profoundly hypovolemic. The most common etiology is rupture of the right atrial appendage followed by rupture of the right ventricle [31, 120, 127]. This is true in autopsy and clinical series although the percentage of right-sided rupture is higher in clinical series presumably because of the high lethality of left ventricular rupture. Pericardiocentesis as a diagnostic tool is used less frequently than in the past because of a higher number of complications and lower sensitivity/specificity compared to FAST. For unstable patients either subxiphoid window or anterolateral thoracotomy is preferred as discussed in the section on pericardial tamponade.

Cardiac failure can occur from several different etiologies in blunt trauma. As stated above, contusions can cause inflammation, hemorrhage within the myocardium, and cellular necrosis all of which change the compliance of the ventricle and its contractility. Complicating this may be small vessel thrombosis worsening ischemia [128]. Coronary artery occlusion, laceration, and thrombosis have all been described as well [2, 127]. Acute valvular incompetence may also precipitate failure. Care is supportive and consists of appropriate fluid resuscitation based on the injury and the use of vasopressors and inotropes. There are case reports of intra-aortic balloon counter pulsation (IABP). Since most cardiac contusion involves the right ventricle, avoiding common causes for increased pulmonary vascular resistance (e.g., hypoxia, hypercarbia) would be prudent. When pulmonary contusion is present, the increased afterload may worsen right ventricular function. Increasing mean intrathoracic pressures further with large tidal volumes should be avoided.

While vasopressors may be unavoidable, vasopressin specifically may improve systemic hemodynamics without increasing pulmonary vascular resistance, although this is hardly proven [129]. While heightened vigilance for arrhythmias seems prudent, no prophylactic treatment is warranted and management is as dictated by ACLS. Arrhythmias are in fact the most common finding in patients with BCI. If one includes sinus tachycardia and bradycardia in the definition, they are present in the majority of patients [127]. Arrhythmias requiring treatment, conversely, will be rare. In a large meta-analysis, only around 2% of patients out of over 2200 in their population suffered arrhythmias requiring treatment, and some of these were frequent PVCs that may no longer be considered worthy of pharmacologic intervention [31].

Chest Wall Injury

The rationale for optimal pain control for the population with blunt thoracic injury is not complex and lies in the high rate of morbidity and mortality in these patients and the now accepted tenants of its treatment. Rib fractures are present in roughly 10% of trauma admissions and they are a marker of more severe injuries [130]. Ninety percent of patients will have associated injuries and 12% will die of their injuries [73]. More pertinently, 35% will have a pulmonary complication [130]. Flail chest in isolation carries a 16% mortality [131]. Thirty percent of patients with seven or more rib fractures will die [73]. Elderly patients may be particularly vulnerable with a 36% rate of pulmonary complications and 8% mortality for isolated rib fractures reported [132]. A combination of age and number of ribs fractured dramatically increased morbidity and mortality with each additional rib fracture in patients over 65 causing a 27% increase risk of pneumonia and a 19% increase in the risk of death [133]. The management of blunt thoracic trauma has evolved from stabilization of the bony injury (either physical or "pneumatic" via positive pressure ventilation) to a reliance on pain control and adequate chest physiotherapy [134]. Indeed, most patients with rib fractures will be treated primarily with one or a combination of the modalities discussed in the next section. Still, it must be noted that there is a resurgence of interest in operative fixation of rib fractures after blunt trauma. There is a recent guideline, in fact, from the Eastern Association for the Surgery of Trauma (EAST) that conditionally recommends rib open reduction internal fixation (ORIF) for the subset of patients with flail chest while acknowledging the poor quality of the evidence that their recommendation is based on [135].

Flail Chest

A flail segment exists when a portion of the chest wall loses its mechanical continuity with the remainder of the chest wall [136]. For this to occur, at least two ribs must be fractured in two places (anteriorly and posteriorly). The conse- quence is that the flail segment responds to changes in pleural pressure and therefore moves inward with inhalation rather than outward. The reverse happens with exhalation. Together this results in a paradoxical movement of the segment. The resulting pathophysiology is not only from the paradoxical motion, but from the inevitable lung injury that results from the impact. The gravity of this injury can lead to a mortality as high as 35% in these patients. They also often have other injuries associated with the impact including pulmonary contusion, lung laceration leading to pneumothorax and hemothorax, as well as injury to other thoracic and extrathoracic structures. The extent that it is the flail segment itself that needs to be addressed is not an academic point since one must decide whether the treatment should be focused primarily at the flail segment per se (positive pressure ventilation, surgical fixation), pain-associated splinting, or the underlying physiology or a combination of all three. Inefficient ventilation, pulmonary contusion, and atelectasis from hypoventilation all play a role in the pathophysiology [136]. The result is V/Q mismatch. The treatment for these patients is therefore as complex as the injury itself. In other sections of this chapter, we will address pulmonary contusion, hemothorax, and analgesia for blunt thoracic trauma leaving the treatment of the mechanics of the flail segment left to be discussed here.

The initial treatment of the flail segment may ultimately be dictated by other underlying injuries. For example, the severity of other injuries to the patient may necessitate tracheal intubation and positive pressure ventilation. This will solve (for the time being) the mechanically discordant movement of the chest wall caused by the flail segment itself. Noninvasive ventilation is also increasingly being utilized for respiratory failure of a variety of etiologies. It has the theoretical advantage of resolving the sequela of paradoxical movement and the resulting V/Q mismatches without the complications of intubation, and there is data emerging to support this approach in selected patients [137].

The notion of surgical fixation of rib fractures is not a new one (the first successful description was in the 1950s [138]) and has a noble goal. Inadequate ventilation and cough because of pain lead to atelectasis. Atelectasis also may occur from the paradoxical chest wall movement itself. In both cases the result is hypoxemia. Further, inadequate analgesia may lead to poor pulmonary toilet and the clearance of secretions. The result is often pneumonia leading to prolonged mechanical ventilation and ICU stays. If surgical fixation could improve pain and therefore clearance of secretions as well as the mechanical handicap, it would be well worth pursuing. Assessing the value of surgical intervention critically has been difficult. Studies have been hampered by small size and cover a variety of surgical techniques. Similarly, standardization of nonoperative management has varied widely with differences in intubation and tracheostomy thresholds, analgesic strategies, pulmonary toilet regimens, fluid administration, etc. [135]. Still, based on available evidence, EAST has conditionally recommended operative ORIF for patients with flail segments with the caution that the level of evidence is poor. The goal is to decrease mortality, shorten time on the ventilator, and shorten ICU length of stay and hospital length of stay, and there is some evidence for each of these outcomes, although most was retrospective in nature and there were concerns of imprecision given the high heterogeneity and by wide confidence intervals. There was no evidence that rib fixation improved pain. They were not able to make any recommendation for patients with non-flail rib fractures based on the available evidence. In our experience, most of these fixations have recently been done with rib plating. Given that, there is usually no need for lung isolation in the operating room, and the main goal of the anesthesiologist is to ventilate the patient with the lung protective strategies dictated by the underlying lung pathology and current best practice.

Pleural Space

The pleural space is normally a potential space between the visceral (covers each lung) and parietal (covers the chest wall) pleural filled with nothing more than a thin film of serous fluid. In trauma, air can enter this space either from the outside world (open pneumothorax) or more commonly from a disruption in the visceral pleura causing air to escape from the lung or the tracheobronchial tree. Air in the pleural space that is not under pressure can lead to a varied clinical presentation from asymptomatic to severe pleuritic chest pain, dyspnea, and tachypnea. The diagnosis is typically made on CXR. Small asymptomatic collections may be managed by observation only, but most in the trauma patient are practically managed by tube thoracostomy. Although this procedure is generally straightforward when performed by experienced providers, a variety of complications can occur including cardiac injury, intercostal artery injury, lung parenchymal injury, extrapleural placement, and even sub-diaphragmatic placement leading to intraabdominal injury and bleeding (spleen, liver). Anesthesiologists should also be aware that a conservatively treated pneumothorax (or one previously undiagnosed) can convert to a tension pneumothorax – air in the pleural space under pressure – when positive pressure ventilation applied. This diagnosis should be kept in mind as part of a differential when a patient with chest trauma has a significant hemodynamic deterioration following intubation. Indeed, the need to go to the operating room should be factored into the decision-making process before a simple pneumothorax is treated with only observation, although studies supporting or refuting the need for thoracostomy tube prior to positive pressure ventilation are conflicting and suffer from very small numbers [139, 140]. At the very

least, clear communication of the presence of a pneumothorax to the anesthesia personnel should occur prior to taking a patient to the operating room with a known or suspected pneumothorax thus treated. A tension pneumothorax occurs when a one-way mechanism allows air into the pleural space with no means of egress. The potential for this exists with injury to the lung parenchyma, tracheobronchial injury, or injury to the chest wall itself. As noted above, positive pressure air in the pleural space leads physiologically to lung collapse, mediastinal shift, and crimping of the IVC and SVC. The result is a sharp decrease in cardiac output. Signs include tracheal deviation, jugular venous distention, unilateral breath sounds, and cyanosis (late finding). Also as noted above, the goal of treatment is immediate relief of the pressure in the pleural space. Needle decompression followed by tube thoracostomy is indicated when suspected. Classically this is accomplished with a 14-gauge needle in the second intercostal space in the midclavicular line. This approach does risk injury to the great vessels and, because of the thickness of the chest wall in this location, can cause an angiocatheter to fail to reach the pleural space. Some (including the author) have advocated an approach via the fifth intercostal space in the midaxillary line where the largest vessel that can be injured is an intercostal artery [141].

Aside from air, blood can invade the pleural space in trauma. When ongoing or with an initial massive output along with hemodynamic instability, thoracotomy is undertaken as described in the section of the lethal six. The injuries leading to this grave situation are usually large lacerations to the pulmonary parenchyma or injury to an intercostal, mammary artery or great vessel, if not the heart itself. Less dramatically, the smaller and more common hemothorax can present with a wide variety of symptoms similar to a pneumothorax including pleuritic chest pain and dyspnea. Physical findings include decreased breath sounds and dullness to percussion. Imaging modalities now include not only chest radiograph, but E-FAST and chest computed tomography depending on the clinical situation [10]. The main drawback of the upright CXR is the volume of blood needed to demonstrate hemothorax, which can be as much as 400–500 cc. Twice that may be necessary with portable supine film. Ultrasound has the advantage of speed and portability with an excellent sensitivity for hemothorax, but it lacks the more comprehensive evaluation of the thorax that computed tomography offers [10]. Mediastinal and bony injuries are not well visualized with ultrasound. Computed tomography provides an excellent diagnostic study in the trauma patient with pleural-based pathology. Its one drawback may be that it is overly sensitive and it is not yet clear what should be done with the very small hemothorax found on initial chest computed tomography (CT). Chest CT may also help define persistent opacities on CXR after thoracostomy placement or be helpful later in the course of chest trauma. The initial treatment of most hemothoraces is tube thoracostomy. EAST qualifies this recommendation with the caveat that it is based on level 3 evidence. More certain (level 1 evidence) is that persistent opacities after initial tube thoracostomy are treated with VATS within the first 3–7 days of injury to reduce the risk of empyema [10].

As a general statement, the diagnosis and optimal management strategies for posttraumatic retained hemothorax remain problematic. The goal of an aggressive approach to the problem is to prevent not only empyema, but fibrothorax (trapped lung) [142]. Still, the natural history of retained hemothorax has not been well elucidated, and individual therapy must be tailored to the risks associated with operative management in each patient. In the American Association for the Surgery of Trauma (AAST) study, nearly one third of patients were treated with observation after the initial chest tube that proved successful 83% of the time. Smaller collections (less than or equal to 300 cc) also predicted success with observation. Overall, VATS success as the primary therapy approached that of thoracotomy (70% versus 79%) with less theoretical morbidity. Caution should be used when comparing the success rate with observation alone given the observational nature of the AAST study [142]. Taken together, the EAST guidelines and the AAST study suggest we will continue to see frequent and early management of patients with retained hemothorax for VATS.

Pain Management for Blunt Thoracic Trauma

It seems intuitive that providing analgesia to a patient with painful injuries to the thorax would be of great importance and, in an ideal world, lead to improved outcomes. What is less obvious is how to provide optimal pain management. The ideal regimen would provide long-lasting analgesia and allow the patient to comfortably participate in chest physiotherapy. It would improve dynamic measurements of respiratory function. It would be easy to administer, have a favorable side effect profile, and be cost-effective. We have no such technique or pharmaceutical. What we do have is a variety of tools that can each be useful in a given circumstance. Each has pros and cons and they should be viewed as complementary in many cases. As clinicians, we often feel one technique is superior to another. Free of bias, we can see that many of these modalities have their uses and can and should be used in combination depending on the clinical picture. Until the perfect solution is created, we must recognize that while some of our tools are more valuable than others, many of them will be needed in busy trauma centers to optimize patient management. We will review the modalities, their strengths and weakness, and the relevant literature.

Systemic narcotics remain the most prevalent modality for pain management in patients with blunt chest trauma. They are easy to prescribe and can be administered orally, transderfmally or intravenously. There are no procedural-related complications and they are inexpensive. They improve visual analog scales and may improve vital capacity [143]. When compared to epidural analgesia, however patients retain more CO_2, have a lower PaO_2, and do not improve maximum inspiratory pressure. They also cause respiratory depression, suppress cough, and increase sedation [143].

Intrapleural anesthesia involves infiltration of local anesthetic into the pleural space either via an indwelling thoracostomy tube or placement of a dedicated intrapleural catheter [144, 145]. The procedure is a unilateral modality that has few hemodynamic penalties. The theoretical and real disadvantages are considerable, however. Instillation of local anesthetic thru a chest tube requires its clamping to retain the drug in the intrapleural space risking tension pneumothorax [134]. Hemothorax may impair absorption across the pleura [146]. Concerns have also been raised about high plasma levels from intrapleural infusions of local anesthetic. Phrenic nerve paralysis and Horner's syndrome have been described [147–149]. Furthermore, a complication of placement of an intrapleural catheter in a patient without a thoracostomy tube is pneumothorax. Position of the catheter in relation to the fractured ribs, the number and location of the fractured ribs, and patient position may all affect the technique's efficacy. When compared in a randomized fashion (albeit in small numbers) to epidural analgesia, the intrapleural catheter provided less pain relief and more narcotic use. However, the use of epidural analgesia improved negative inspiratory pressure and tidal volume. The authors concluded that continuous epidural block was superior to intrapleural block [145]. Although some have used the technique with success, an admittedly small study more recently showed no benefit compared even to systemic narcotics [146, 150]. In the end, the large number of variables that affect this technique, the short duration of effect, the lack of consistent data showing efficacy, and the potential complications severely limit its use in our practice.

Intercostal nerve blocks have a long history of use and success in patients with blunt chest trauma [151]. They involve injections of the intercostal nerve proximal to the point of injury and at a level above and below the injured rib. While some authors advocate the block be performed proximal to the midaxillary line to ensure blockade of the lateral and anterior cutaneous branches of the intercostal nerve, this should only be necessary when analgesia of the skin is required [151, 152]. The block will be unilateral and should have few hemodynamic consequences. Intercostal nerve block has been shown to improve peak expiratory flow rate as well as arterial oxygen and carbon dioxide tensions, but these effects last only hours [153–155]. Despite this, Shanti observed that the vast majority of trauma patients need only one or two injections [156]. The blocks are not sedating. Still there are limitations to the technique. Palpating fractured ribs can be painful, and there can be technical difficulties with the block in higher ribs because of the scapula. Of more concern is that the rate of pneumothorax is 1.4% for each individual intercostal nerve blocked leading to an overall rate of 8.7% per patient in Shanti's study [91]. With patients who have several ribs fractured, there would be a need for multiple injections raising the risk not only of pneumothorax but of local anesthetic toxicity and increased pain of the procedure. Intercostal catheters have been described in small numbers, but the anatomic endpoint of placement can be nebulous and maintaining the proper position of the catheter a challenge [134, 157, 158]. In the end they are simple to perform and can remain a viable alternative in patients who have contraindications or unsuccessful placement of either an epidural catheter or paravertebral block – especially in patients who have a tube thoracostomy in place.

Paravertebral blocks using both a single shot and continuous infusion of local anesthetic are gaining momentum. This seems to be true both in the thoracic trauma and the thoracic surgery literature. Although expertise in the technique may be more limited than it is for epidural placement, the theoretical advantages may soon change that [159, 160]. There seems to be mounting enthusiasm for this technique first described over 100 years ago, and the discussion has begun on the possibility that it will replace epidural analgesia in the world of thoracic surgery and thoracic trauma [161, 162]. Because the technique involves the block of the intercostal nerve, its dorsal ramus, and the sympathetic chain, it produces a dense sensory and sympathetic block [161]. Because the block is unilateral (although unintentional epidural injection is a potential complication), there is less hypotension when compared to epidural analgesia [162, 163]. The block is reported as being simple to perform and perhaps easier to place than a thoracic epidural, although trouble threading the catheter into the paravertebral space has been reported more than once [160, 164]. There are other advantages as well. When compared to epidural analgesia, there seems to be less urinary retention, and there are theoretic reasons to expect less respiratory depression and pruritis since there is no neuraxial opioids as there commonly are with an epidural. It also may be safer to place in patients who are sedated or even ventilated [134, 151]. Placement of a paravertebral block could in theory relax strict restrictions on the placement of epidural catheters in the face of mild coagulopathy or DVT prophylaxis with low molecular weight heparins. Further, many trials of epidurals in blunt thoracic trauma patients have used any injury to the spine as an exclusion criterion [165]. The presence of a spine fracture was in fact the most frequent exclusion criteria accounting for more than twice as many as any other in a frequently quoted study [165].

The exclusion of patients with spine injuries may not be necessary for placement of a paravertebral catheter. It would, for example, be hard to imagine that a lumbar transverse process fracture would be a contraindication for a paravertebral block or catheter. There are also now being described ultrasound-guided techniques of placement that may make this technique safer and easier [166–168]. Lastly, the paravertebral approach does seem to be effective. It has been shown to improve pain, bedside spirometry, and blood gasses [164]. In one small study (15 patients, each arm), it was as effective as epidural analgesia. Unfortunately, these are the only patients comparing the techniques in trauma patients. If one were to extrapolate data from thoracotomy patients, paravertebral catheters still seem to do as well, but again the data is very limited and that extrapolation may or may not be valid [161].

Still there remain some challenges for paravertebral blocks. The most obvious may be familiarity with the technique among current practitioners. Secondly, the technique is not complication free. In Karmakar's series of 15 patients having a continuous paravertebral catheter placed for unilateral rib fractures, for example, there was one inadvertent placement of the catheter in the epidural space that was not appreciated until a large volume of local anesthetic was given. That patient became hypotensive. Twenty percent of the patients in that same series had bilateral analgesia. It is unclear whether that was from epidural spread or spread to the contralateral paravertebral space, but these facts taken together along with the known incidence of pneumothorax and pleural placement make the position of the catheter to be less than certain [164, 169]. The failure rate is also as high as 10% and vascular puncture is 3.8% [169]. Dural puncture and subarachnoid injection have also been described [170, 171]. One of the 15 patients that received a paravertebral infusion in Mohta's recent trial suffered a seizure presumably from local anesthetic toxicity [162]. Certainly strict attention to dose is necessary especially if bilateral catheters would be contemplated for patients with bilateral rib fractures.

In the end, the application of paravertebral blocks in blunt trauma may gain wider acceptance as familiarity with the technique spreads. There are numerous theoretical advantages and some of these have been realized in small trials. Ultrasound guidance may add to the safety of the technique. While data in trauma patients remains limited for now, this technique will undoubtedly become more commonplace. Its utility at present is limited both by widespread technical expertise and its greater utility in patients with unilateral rib fractures [172].

Epidural analgesia remains the standard by which all other pain management modalities are compared. Its theoretical advantages are myriad. It provides nearly immediate bilateral pain relief. It is less sedating than systemic narcotics so patients can participate in pulmonary toilet [173]. It has been shown to increase functional residual capacity, vital capacity, tidal volume, and compliance and decrease the movement of flail segments as well as to increase PaO_2 [151, 174, 175]. There have been two randomized prospective trials comparing systemic narcotics and epidural analgesia [165, 174]. In the study by Bulger, there was an impressive decrease in the rate of nosocomial pneumonia and duration of mechanical ventilation [165]. In the Ullman study, there were fewer ventilator days, a shorter ICU stay, and a shorter hospitalization. They also had fewer tracheostomies and a larger tidal volume [174]. These results were achieved without what the author would propose is the most effective manor to use an epidural suggesting that the technique could be even more effective. The Ullman study used only epidural narcotics, while the Bulger study had no standardization of their epidural regimen. Neither study used patient-controlled epidural analgesia (PCEA) or programmed intermittent epidural bolus (PIEB) which should result in improved pain control in the trauma patient as it has in the obstetric patient [176, 177]. There is also evidence in the thoracic surgery literature that a combination of local anesthetic and opioids is more effective than either alone [178]. Epidurals may even modulate the immune response in thoracic trauma patients [134, 179].

Despite all of this data and 30 years of experience, there remains as stated above only two randomized controlled trials showing improved outcomes with epidural pain management compared to systemic narcotics, and both of these trials were very small (46 enrolled was the larger of the two) [180]. The size of the studies actually points to some of the concerns of epidural analgesia. In the Bulger study, for example, 408 patients were identified over 3.5 years, and yet 282 met exclusion criteria and 80 could not be consented leaving only 46 [165]. By their own admission, they were fairly conservative in their enrollment (all patients with any spine fracture were excluded). The point remains that many patients who would benefit from epidural placement will not be able to receive one, even if the criteria for exclusion in that study were relaxed. For example, a patient with a lumbar transverse process fracture may be expected to have an epidural placed without significant additional risk [165]. Still other exclusion criteria will remain firm (hemodynamic instability, coagulopathy, altered mental status). Epidurals can cause hypotension especially in the hypovolemic patient or after large volume bolus with local anesthetic. Epidural infections have also been documented [173]. Epidural catheters can be challenging to place especially in patients in pain. Lastly, epidural combinations of local anesthetic and opioids can cause pruritus, nausea, urinary retention, and respiratory depression.

The aim of pain management for the blunt thoracic trauma patient is twofold. First and most obviously pain control is an end onto itself. Patient satisfaction and comfort should be the anesthesiologist's goal under any circumstance. It is improving their respiratory mechanics thru that pain relief that will alter outcome. If we can break the cycle of shallow breathing and poor cough leading to atelectasis, sputum retention, decreased functional residual capacity (FRC), and worsening hypoxia from V/Q mismatch, we can hopefully intubate fewer patients and avoid all the complications that come with it. These include the need for sedation, ventilator-associated pneumonia, DVT, the possibility of nutritional deficiency, etc. The elderly are particularly hard hit by this process as detailed before [133]. Epidural catheters and paravertebral blocks seem to offer the best pain control, although the role of each continues to be a topic of debate and our understanding continues to evolve [181]. Each has its strengths and weakness, and therapy must be individualized. A patient who is able to achieve a vital capacity of 12–15 cc/kg without significant sedation from systemic narcotics, for example, may require no invasive procedures. The presence of a protocol in each institution to standardize therapy may be helpful. It should be noted that the use of other systemic agents for the use of pain control have not been mentioned. Interestingly, there is a paucity of data for the use of NSAIDs or acetaminophen in thoracic injury. Still they are frequently used for the outpatient management of rib fractures, and as a tenant of multimodality therapy, it is reasonable to include them in the management of patients without contraindication. Figure 51.11 represents a modified version of the protocol at our institution. It may serve as a model for departments wishing to address the issue of optimum pain control for their hospital. Even with a protocol in place, the clinician must be aware that patients vary in their clinical presentation and analgesic requirements. This protocol should not serve as a substitute for acumen, but as a guide and source of discussion in the management of pain which must be, in the end, individualized.

With no perfect analgesic agent and with the acknowledgment that surgical fixation may have a role – but is clearly no panacea – and with the realization of the obvious fact that blunt trauma is a heterogeneous entity in a heterogeneous population, it may be that the best way to improve the care of these patients is with a systems approach. The literature in this arena is in its infancy [182]. At our institution a protocol has been implemented that created a standard approach in the care of these patients. It defined standard criteria for ICU admission with an emphasis on pain control and pulmonary toilet. All patients over 45 with four or more rib fractures and over 65 with two or more rib fractured are admitted to the ICU. When pain was not well

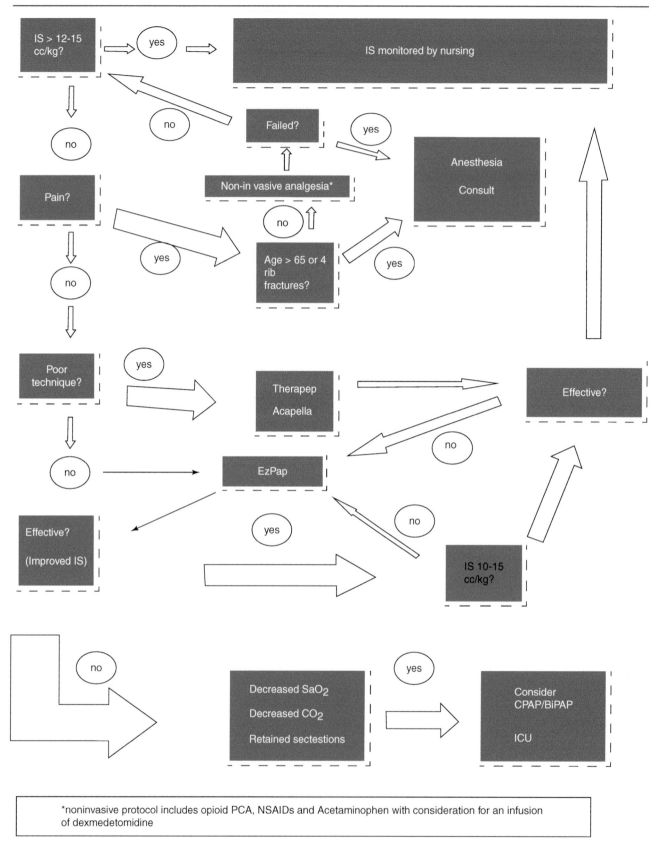

Fig. 51.11 An example protocol for the treatment of pain in patients with blunt chest trauma. Anesthesia consult may trigger additional modalities of pharmacologic management or a variety of nerve blocked in eluding serrates anterior plane block, paravertebral block, or epidural

controlled with PCA and ketorolac leading to poor cough and incentive spirometry performance, early consultation with the anesthesia service is obtained for epidural placement. In a retrospective review, this led to a dramatic reduction in mortality in the elderly patient (9% versus 24%) without a dramatic increase in cost [183]. As is the trend in our specialty, continued examination of evolving evidence will point the way to a standardized approach to this difficult clinical dilemma.

Clinical Case Discussion

Case Pt is a 27-year-old male who was stabbed at the base of the neck and thrown off the top of a three-story building. He arrives in the emergency room intoxicated but awake and alert. He is hemodynamically stable. His past medical history is noncontributory. He is extremely tachypnic, anxious, and complaining of shortness of breath. He is coughing up a small amount of blood. He is wearing a cervical collar. On secondary survey he is found to have subcutaneous emphysema.

Questions

1. What are the anesthesiologists concerns?
2. Should any further imaging be obtained prior to intubation?
3. What airway device should be placed?
4. What technique should be used to intubate the patient?

Given the mechanism of injury and the presence of subcutaneous emphysema and hemoptysis, the anesthesiologist should be concerned that there is an injury to the airway. While under ideal conditions an awake fiberoptic intubation would be preferred, the scenario presented describes a patient who is in respiratory distress and could not be expected to participate in an awake fiberoptic intubation. No further imaging should be necessary in this patient who clearly needs urgent control of the airway. Rapid sequence intubation with in-line stabilization remains the standard of care and should be performed without delay. Strict attention should be made to the patient's hemodynamics after intubation, since converting a presumed pneumothorax to a tension pneumothorax is possible in this scenario. Every attempt must be made to place the endotracheal tube with great care in an effort not to disrupt a potential injury to the trachea.

Scenario continues: The patient is successfully intubated, and a chest tube is placed for decreased breath sounds over

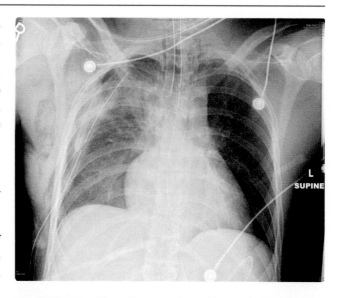

Fig. 51.12 Chest X-ray shows a patient with a persistent right pneumothorax despite a well-positioned thoracotomy tube and an endotracheal tube above the carina

the right chest. A large air leak is found. The following CXR is obtained.

Figure 51.12 CXR shows a patient with a persistent right pneumothorax despite well-positioned thoracostomy tube and an endotracheal tube just above the carina

Questions

1. What would be the next step in the evaluation of this patient?
2. How can the anesthesiologist manage the air leak?
3. The patient is being taken to the operating room for surgical repair. What form of lung isolation should be used?

The patient should undergo fiberoptic bronchoscopy to define the tracheal injury and if possible to move the cuff of the endotracheal tube beyond the tear. This patient also underwent computed tomography which revealed a posterior tear in the trachea. The CT also demonstrated continued pneumothorax on the right as well as subcutaneous air. Lastly the CT demonstrated five posterior rib fractures on the right (Fig. 51.13).

The first choice for lung isolation in this case would be a bronchial blocker thru the original endotracheal tube. This would prevent any further tracheal injury by passing a larger stiffer device thru the injury. In addition, the patient has not had injury to the cervical spine ruled out, and this will minimize movement of the neck. He is taken to the operating room for repair of this injury shown in Fig. 51.14.

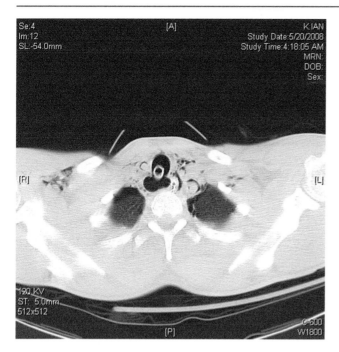

Fig. 51.13 Computed tomography scan demonstrating posterior tracheal tear, subcutaneous emphysema and persistent right pneumothorax. Subcutaneous emphysema is also demonstrated

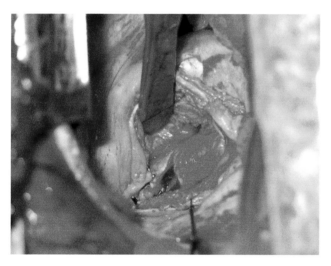

Fig. 51.14 Intraoperative view of posterior tracheal injury seen through a right thoracotomy. (Photo courtesy of Thomas NG, MD, thoracic surgery, Rhode Island Hospital)

Questions

Would you extubate this patient at the end of the case? How would you control his pain from the rib fractures?

These are both difficult questions. In general, every effort to extubate the patient as soon as possible should be made given his tracheal repair. Managing the pain of his rib fractures may be difficult. If he is awake and cooperative post extubation, an epidural can be considered. If not, paraverte-

bral blocks or a catheter may be an option since the rib fractures are unilateral.

References

1. American College of Surgeons Committee on Trauma. Thoracic trauma. In: ATLS® program for doctors student course manual. 6th ed. Chicago: American College of Surgeons; 1997. p. 127–41.
2. Bergen G, Chen LH, Warner M, Fingerhut LA. Injury in the United States: 2007 Chartbook. Hyattsville: National Center for Health Statistics; 2008.
3. Fingerhaut LA, Warner M. Injury Chartbook. Health, United States, 1996–7. Hyattsville: National Center for Health Statistics; 1998.
4. Ohsfeldt RL, Schneider JE. The business of health. The role of competition, markets, and regulation. 1st ed. Washington DC: AEI Press; 2006.
5. American College of Surgeons Committee on Trauma. Thoracic trauma. In:ATLS® program for doctors student course manual. 9th ed. Chicago: American College of Surgeons; 2012. p. 94–112.
6. Rozycki GS, Feliciano DV, Ochsner MG, et al. The role of ultrasound in patients with possible penetrating cardiac wounds: a prospective multicenter study. J Trauma Acute Care Surg. 1999;46:543–51.
7. Kirkpatrick AW, Ball CG, D'Armours SK, Zygun D. Acute resuscitation of the unstable adult trauma patient: bedside diagnosis and therapy. Can J Surg. 2008;5(1):57–69.
8. Hakuba T, Minato N, Minematsu T, Kamohara K. Surgical management and treatment of traumatic right atrial rupture. Gen Thorac Cardiovasc Surg. 2008;56(11):551–4.
9. Lim R, Gill IS, Temes RT, Smith CE. The use of adenosine for repair of penetrating cardiac injuries: a novel method. Ann Thoracic Surg. 2001;71:1714–5.
10. Mowery NT, Gunter OL, Collier BR, Jose'J D Jr, Haut E, Hildreth A, Holevar M, Mayberry J, Streib E. Practice management guidelines for management of hemothorax and occult Pneumothorax. J Trauma Acute Care Surg. 2011;70(2):510–8.
11. Clancy K, Velopulos C, Bilaniuk JW, et al. Screening for blunt cardiac injury. J Trauma Acute Care Surg. 2012;73(5):S301–6.
12. Karalis D, Victor M, Davis G, McAllister M, Covalesky V, Ross J, Foley R, Kerstein M, Chandrasekaran K. The role of echocardiography in blunt chest trauma. J Trauma. 1994;36(1):53–8.
13. Chirillo F, Totis O, Cavarzerani A, et al. Usefulness of transthoracic and transoesophageal echocardiography in recognition and management of cardiovascular injuries after blunt chest trauma. Heart. 1996;75(3):301–6.
14. Shanewise JS, Cheung AT, Aronson S, et al. ASE/SCA guidelines for performing a comprehensive intraoperative multiplane transesophageal echocardiography examination: recommendations of the American Society of Echocardiography Council for Intraoperative Echocardiography and the Society of Cardiovasc. Anesth Analg. 1999;89:870–84.
15. Poterack KA. Who uses transesophageal echocardiography in the operating room? Anesth Analg. 1995;80(3):454–8.
16. Minhaj M, Patel K, Muzic D, et al. The effect of routine intraoperative transesophageal echocardiography on surgical management. J Cardiothorac Vasc Anesth. 2007;21(6):800–4.
17. Memtsoudis SG, Rosenberger P, Loffler M, et al. The usefulness of transesophageal echocardiography during intraoperative cardiac arrest in noncardiac surgery. Anesth Analg. 2006;102(6):1653–7.
18. Kallmeyer IJ, Collard CD, Fox JA, Body SC, Shernan SK. The safety of intraoperative transesophageal echocardiography: a case series of 7200 cardiac surgical patients. Anesth Analg. 2001;92(5):1126–30.

19. Reeves ST, Finley AC, Skubas NJ, et al. Basic perioperative transesophageal echocardiography examination: a consensus statement of the American Society of Echocardiography and the Society of Cardiovascular Anesthesiologists. J Am Soc Echocardiogr. 2013;26:443–56.

20. Thys DM, Abel MD, Brooker RF, Cahalan MK, Connis RT, Duke PG, Nickinovich DG, Reeves ST, Rozner MA, Russell IA, Streckenbach SC. Practice guidelines for perioperative transesophageal echocardiography. Anesthesiology. 2010;112(5):1084–96.

21. Leichtle SW, Singleton A, Singh M, Griffee MJ, Tobin JM. Transesophageal echocardiography in the evaluation of the trauma patient: a trauma resuscitation transesophageal echocardiography exam. J Crit Care. 2017;40:202–6.

22. Catoire P, Orliaguet G, Liu N, et al. Systemic transoesophageal echocardiography for detection of mediastinal lesions in patients with multiple injuries. J Trauma. 1995;38(1):96–8.

23. Mollod M, Felner JM. Transesophageal echocardiography in the evaluation of cardiothoracic trauma. Am Heart J. 1996;132(4):841–9.

24. Griffee MJ, Singleton A, Zimmerman JM, Morgan DE. The effect of perioperative rescue transesophageal echocardiography on the management of trauma patients. Anesth Analg. 2016;6(12):387–90.

25. Markin NW, Gmelch BS, Griffee MJ, Holmberg TJ, Morgan DE, Zimmerman JM. A review of 364 perioperative rescue echocardiograms: findings of an anesthesiologist-staffed perioperative echocardiography service. J Cardiothorac Vasc Anesth. 2015;29(1):82–8.

26. Porter TR, Shillcutt SK, Adams MS, et al. Guidelines for the use of echocardiography as a monitor for therapeutic intervention in adults: a report from the American Society of Echocardiography. J Am Soc Echocardiogr. 2015;28(1):40–56.

27. Shillcutt SK, Markin NW, Montzingo CR, Brakke TR. Use of rapid "rescue" perioperative echocardiography to improve outcomes after hemodynamic instability in noncardiac surgical patients. J Cardiothorac Vasc Anesth. 2012;26(3):362–70.

28. Kaye P, O'Sullivan I. Myocardial contusion: emergency investigation and diagnosis. Emerg Med J. 2002;19(1):8–10.

29. Sousa RC, Garcia-Fernandez MA, Moreno M, Quero F, Torrecilla E, San Roman D, Delcan JL. Value of transesophageal echocardiography in the assessment of blunt chest trauma: correlation with electrocardiogram, heart enzymes, and transthoracic echocardiogram. Rev Port Cardiol. 1994;13(11):833–43. 807-8.

30. Orliaguet G, Ferjani M, Riou B. The heart in blunt trauma. Anesthesiology. 2001;95:544–8.

31. Maenza RL, Seaberg D, D'Amico F. A meta-analysis of blunt cardiac trauma: ending myocardial confusion. Am J Emerg Med. 1996;14(3):237–41.

32. Yousef R, Carr JA. Blunt cardiac trauma: a review of the current knowledge and management. Ann Thorac Surg. 2014;98(3):1134–40.

33. Ouda A, Kappert U, Ghazy T, et al. Isolated rupture of the right upper pulmonary vein: a blunt cardiac trauma case. Ann Thorac Surg. 2011;91(4):1267–9.

34. Rowe SK, Porter CB. Atrial septal hematoma: two-dimensional echocardiographic findings after blunt chest trauma. Am Heart J. 1987;114(3):650–2.

35. Fegheli NT, Prisant LM. Blunt myocardial injury. Chest. 1995;108:1673–7.

36. Shapiro M, Yanofski S, Trapp J, et al. Cardiovascular evaluation in blunt thoracic trauma using Transesophageal Echocardiography (TEE). J Trauma. 1991;31(6):835–40.

37. Brooks SW, Young JC, Cmolik B, et al. The use of transesophageal echocardiography in the evaluation of chest trauma. J Trauma. 1992;32(6):761–6.

38. Zakynthinos EG, Vassilakopoulos T, Routsi C, Roussos C, Zakynthinos S. Early- and late-onset atrioventricular valve rupture after blunt chest trauma: the usefulness of transesophageal echocardiography. J Trauma. 2002;52(5):990–6.

39. Varahan SL, Farah GM, Caldeira CC, Hoit BD, Askari AT. The double jeopardy of blunt chest trauma: a case report and review. Echocardiography. 2006;23(3):235–9.

40. Bruschi G, Agati S, Iorio F, Vitali E. Papillary muscle rupture and pericardial injuries after blunt chest trauma. Eur J Cardiothorac Surg. 2001;20(1):200–2.

41. Nelson M, Wells G. A case of traumatic tricuspid valve regurgitation caused by blunt chest trauma. J Am Soc Echocardiogr. 2007;20(2):198.e4–5.

42. Ellis JE, Bender EM. Intraoperative transesophageal echocardiography in blunt thoracic trauma. J Cardiothorac Vasc Anesth. 1991;5(4):373–6.

43. Kennedy N, Ireland M, McConaghy P. Transoesophageal echocardiographic examination of a patient with venacaval and pericardial tears after blunt chest trauma. Br J Anaesth. 1995;75:495–7.

44. De Maria E, Gaddi O, Navazio A, Monducci I, Tirabassi G, Guiducci U. Right atrial free wall rupture after blunt chest trauma. J Cardiovasc Med (Hagerstown). 2007;8(11):946–9.

45. Nandate K, Krishnamoorthy V, McIntyre LK, Verrier ED, Mackensen GB. Gunshot-induced aorto-left atrial fistula diagnosed by intraoperative transesophageal echocardiography. Ann Thorac Surg. 2016;101(2):771–3.

46. Rudski LG, Lai WW, Afilalo J, et al. Guidelines for the echocardiographic assessment of the right heart in adults: a report from the American Society of Echocardiography. J Am Soc Echocardiogr. 2010;23(7):685–713.

47. Lang RM, Bierig M, Devereux RB, et al. Recommendations for chamber quantification: a report from the American Society of Echocardiography's guidelines and standards committee and the chamber quantification writing group, developed in conjunction with the European Association of Echocardiography, a branch of the European Society of Cardiology. J Am Soc Echocardiogr. 2005;18(12):1440–63.

48. Reichert CLA, Visser CA, van den Brink RBA, et al. Prognostic value of biventricular function in hypotensive patients after cardiac surgery as assessed by transesophageal echocardiography. J Cardiothorac Vasc Anesth. 1992;6(4):429–32.

49. Vignon P, Gueret P, Vedrinne JM, Lagrange P, Cornu E, Abrieu O, Gastinne H, Bensaid J, Lang R. Role of transesophageal echocardiography in the diagnosis and management of traumatic aortic disruption. Circulation. 1995;92(10):2959–68.

50. Vignon P, Boncoeur MP, François B, Rambaud G, Maubon A, Gastinne H. Comparison of multiplane transesophageal echocardiography and contrast-enhanced helical CT in the diagnosis of blunt traumatic cardiovascular injuries. Anesthesiology. 2001;94(4):615–22.

51. Saranteas T, Mavrogenis AF, Mandila C, Poularas J, Panou F. Ultrasound in cardiac trauma. J Crit Care. 2017;38:144–51.

52. Lanigan MJ, Chaney MA, Gologorsky E, Chavanon O, Augoustides JG. CASE 2 – 2014: aortic dissection: real or artifact? J Cardiothorac Vasc Anesth. 2014;28(2):398–407.

53. Ahrar K, Smith DC, Bansal RC, Razzouk A, Catalano RD. Angiography in blunt thoracic aortic injury. J Trauma. 1997;42(4):665–9.

54. Bansal V, Lee J, Coimbra R. Current diagnosis and management of blunt traumatic rupture of the thoracic aorta. J Vasc Bras. 2007;6(1):64–73.

55. Le Bret F, Ruel P, Rosier H, Goarin JP, Riou B, Viars P. Diagnosis of traumatic mediastinal hematoma with transesophageal echocardiography. Chest. 1994;105(2):373–6.

56. Vignon P, Rambaud G, François B, Preux P-M, Lang RM, Gastinne H. Quantification of traumatic hemomediastinum using transesophageal echocardiography. Chest. 1998;113(6):1475–80.

57. Hahn RT, Abraham T, Adams MS, et al. Guidelines for performing a comprehensive transesophageal echocardiographic examination: recommendations from the American Society of Echocardiography and the Society of Cardiovascular Anesthesiologists. Anesth Analg. 2014;118(1):21–68.

58. Neskovic AN, Hagendorff A, Lancellotti P, et al. Emergency echocardiography: the European Association of Cardiovascular Imaging recommendations. Eur Heart J Cardiovasc Imaging. 2013;14(1):1–11.

59. Levitov A, Frankel HL, Blaivas M, et al. Guidelines for the appropriate use of bedside general and cardiac ultrasonography in the evaluation of critically ill patients—part II. Crit Care Med. 2016;44(6):1206–27.

60. Santoni BG, Hindman BJ, Puttit CM, Weeks JB, Johnson N, Maktabi MA, Todd MM. Manuel in-line stabilization increases pressures applied by the laryngoscope blade during direct laryngoscopy and orotracheal intubation. Anesthesiology. 2009;110:24–31.

61. Manoach S, Paladino L. Laryngoscopy force, visualization and intubation failure in acute trauma. Anesthesiology. 2009;110:6–7.

62. Rice MJ, Mancuso AA, Gibbs C, Morey TE, Gravenstein N, Deitte LA. Cricoid pressure results in compression of the postcricoid hypopharynx: the esophageal position is irrelevant. Anesth Analg. 2009;109:1546–52.

63. Ovassapian A, Salem MR. Sellick's maneuver: to do or not to do. Anesth Analg. 2009;109:1360–2.

64. Lerman J. On cricoid pressure: "may the force be with you". Anesth Analg. 2009;109:1363–6.

65. Priebe HJ. Cricoid pressure: an alternative view. Semin Anesth. 2005;24(2):120–6.

66. Birenbaum A, Hajage D, Roche S, et al. Effect of cricoid pressure compared with a sham procedure in the rapid sequence induction of anesthesia: the IRIS randomized clinical trial. JAMA Surg. 2018; https://doi.org/10.1001/jamasurg.2018.3577.

67. Hagberg CA, Kaslow O. Difficult airway management in trauma updated by COTEP. ASA Monitor. 2014;78(9):56–60.

68. Crosby ET. Airway management in adults after cervical spine trauma. Anesthesiology. 2006;104:1293–318.

69. Shatney CH, Brunner RD, Nguyen TQ. The safety of orotracheal intubation in patients with unstable cervical spine fracture or high spinal cord injury. Am J Surg. 1995;170:676–80.

70. Stephens CT, Kahntroff S, Dutton RP. The success of emergency endotracheal intubation in trauma patients: a 10-year experience at a major adult trauma referral center. Anesth Analg. 2009;109:866–72.

71. Campos JH, Hallam EA, Van Natta T, Kernstine KH. Devices for lung isolation used by anesthesiologists with limited thoracic experience. Anesthesiology. 2006;104:261–6.

72. Narayanaswamy M, McRae K, Slinger P, Dugas G, Kanellakos GW, Roscoe A, Lacroix M. Choosing a lung isolation device for thoracic surgery: a randomized trial of three bronchial blockers and double lumen tubes. Anesth Analg. 2009;108:1097–01.

73. Ehrenfeld JM, Walsh JL, Sandberg WA. Right- and left-sided Mallinckrodt double-lumen tubes have identical clinical performance. Anesth Analg. 2008;106:1847–52.

74. Kemmerer WT, Eckert WG, Gathright JB, Reemtsma k CO. Patterns of thoracic injuries in fatal traffic accidents. J Trauma. 1961;1:595–9.

75. Kummer C, Netto FS, Rizoli S, Yee D. A review of traumatic airway injuries: potential implications for airway assessment and management. Injury Int J Care Injured. 2007;38:27–33.

76. Rossbach MM, Johnson SB, Gomez MA, Sako EY, Miller L, Calhoon JH. Management of tracheobronchial injuries: a 28-year experience. Ann Thorac Surg. 1998;65:182–6.

77. Kisser AC, Obrien SM, Detterbeck FC. Blunt tracheobronchial injuries: treatment and outcomes. Ann Thorac Surg. 2001;71:2059–65.

78. Shah AS, Forbess JM, Skaryak LA, Lilly RE, Vaslef SN, D'Amico TA. Emergent thoracotomy for airway control after intrathoracic tracheal injury. J Trauma. 2000;48(6):1163–4.

79. Naghibi K, Hashemi SL, Sajedi P. Anesthetic management of tracheobronchial rupture following blunt chest trauma. Acta Anaesthesiol Scand. 2003;47:901–3.

80. Symbas PN, Justicz AG, Ricketts RR. Rupture of the airways from blunt trauma: treatment of complex injuries. Ann Thorac Surg. 1992;54:177–83.

81. Shweikh AM, Nadkarni AB. Laryngotracheal separation with pneumopericardium after a blunt trauma to the neck. Emerg Med J. 2001;18:410–1.

82. Gómez-Caro A, Ausín P, et al. Role of conservative medical management of tracheobronchial injuries. J Trauma. 2006;61: 1426–35.

83. Borasio P, Arissone F, Chiampo G. Post-intubation tracheal rupture. A report on ten cases. Eur J Cardiothorac Surg. 1997;12:98–100.

84. Parmley LF, Mattingly TW, Manion WC, Jahnke EJ Jr. Nonpenetrating traumatic injury of the aorta. Circulation. 1958;17:1086–101.

85. Schulman CI, Carvajal D, Lopez PP, Soffer D, Habib F, Augenstein J. Incidence and crash mechanisms of aortic injury during the past decade. J Trauma. 2007;62:664–7.

86. Bruno VD, Batchelor TJP. Late aortic injury: a rare complication of a posterior rib fracture. Ann Thorac Surg. 2009;87:301–3.

87. Neschis DG, Scalea TM, Flinn WR, Griffith BP. Blunt aortic injury. N Engl J Med. 2008;359:1708–16.

88. Fabian TC, Richardson JD, Croce MA, Smith JS Jr, Rodman G Jr, Kearney PA, et al. Prospective study of blunt aortic injury: multicenter trial of the American Association for the surgery of trauma. J Trauma. 1997;42:374–80.

89. Fabian TC, Davis KA, Gavant ML, et al. Prospective study of blunt aortic injury; helical CT is diagnostic and antihypertensive therapy reduces rupture. Ann Surg. 1998;227:666–76.

90. Malhotra AK, Fabian TC, Croce MA, Weinman DS, Gavant ML, Pate JW. Minimal aortic injury: a lesion associated with advancing diagnostic techniques. J Trauma. 2001;51:1042–8.

91. Hirose H, Gill IS, Malangoni MA. Nonoperative management of traumatic aortic injury. J Trauma. 2006;60:597–601.

92. Coselli JS, LeMaire SA, Köksoy C, Schmittling ZC, Curling PE. Cerebrospinal fluid drainage reduces paraplegia after thoracoabdominal aortic aneurysm repair: results of a randomized clinical trial. J Vasc Surg. 2002;35:631–9.

93. Feezor RJ, Hess PJ, Martin TD, Klodell CT, Beaver TM, Lottenberg L, Martin LC, Lee WA. Endovascular treatment of traumatic aortic injuries. J Am Coll Surg. 2009;208:510–6.

94. Lettinga-van de Poll T, Schurink GWH, DeHaan MW, Verbruggen JPAM, Jacobs MJ. Endovascular treatment of traumatic rupture of the thoracic aorta. Br J Surg. 2007;94:525–33.

95. Ehrlich MP, Rosseau H, Heijman R, Piquet P, Beregi JP, Nienaber CA, Sodeck G, Fattori R. Early outcome of endovascular repair of acute traumatic aortic injuries: the talent thoracic retrospective registry. Ann Thorac Surg. 2009;88:1258–66.

96. Reed AB, Thompson JK, Grafton CJ, Delvecchio C, Giglia JS. Timing of endovascular repair of blunt traumatic thoracic transections. J Vasc Surg. 2006;43:684–8.

97. Demetriades D, Velmahos GC, Scalea TM, et al. Operative repair or endovascular stent graft in blunt traumatic thoracic aortic injuries: results of an American association for the surgery of trauma multicenter study. J Trauma. 2008;64:561–70.

98. Demetriades D, Velmahos GC, Scalea TM, et al. Diagnosis and treatment of blunt thoracic aortic injuries: changing perspectives. J Trauma. 2008;64:1415–8.

99. Pang D, Hildebrand D, Bachoo P. Thoracic Endovascular Repair (TEVAR) versus open surgery for blunt traumatic thoracic aortic injury. Cochrane Database Syst Rev. 2015;(9):CD006642.

100. Lee AW, Matsumura JS, Mitchell RS, Farber MA, Greenberg RK, Azizzadeh A, Murad MH, Fairman RM. Endovascular repair of traumatic thoracic aortic injury: clinical practice guidelines of the Society for Vascular Surgery. J Vast Surg. 2011;53:187–92.

101. DuBose JJ, Leake SS, Brennar M, Pasley J, O'Callaghan T, Luo-Owen X, et al. Contemporary management and outcomes of blunt thoracic aortic injury: a multi center retrospective study. J Trauma Acute Care Surg. 2015;78(2):360–9.

102. Devitt JH, McLean RF, Koch JP. Anaesthetic management of acute blunt thoracic trauma. Can J Anaesth. 1991;308:506–10.

103. Leone M, Brégeon F, Antonini F, et al. Long term outcome in chest trauma. Anesthesiology. 2008;109:864–71.

104. Soldati G, Testa A, Silva FR, et al. Chest ultrasonography in lung contusion. Chest. 2006;130:533–8.

105. Ball CG, Ranson MK, Rodriguez-Galvez M, Lall R, Kirkpatrick AW. Sonographic depiction of posttraumatic alveolar-interstitial disease: the hand held diagnosis of a pulmonary contusion. J Trauma. 2009;66:962.

106. Hoth JJ, Stitzel JD, Gayzik S, Brownlee NA, Miller PR, Yoza BK, McCall CE, Meredith JW, Payne RM. The pathogenesis of pulmonary contusion: an open chest model in the rat. J Trauma. 2006;61:32–45.

107. Keel M, Ecknauer E, Stocker R, et al. Different pattern of local and systemic release of proinflammatory and anti-inflammatory mediators in severely injured patients with chest trauma. J Trauma. 1996;40:907–12.

108. Keel M, Trentz O. Pathophysiology of polytrauma. Injury. 2005;36:691–709.

109. Muehlstedt SG, Richardson CJ, Lyte M, Rodriguez JL. Systemic and pulmonary effector cell function after injury. Crit Care Med. 2002;30:1322–6.

110. Perl M, Gebhard F, Brückner UB, Ayala A, Braumüller C, Kinzl L, Knöferl MW. Pulmonary contusion causes impairment of macrophage and lymphocyte immune function and increases mortality associated with a subsequent septic challenge. Crit Care Med. 2005;33(6):1351–8.

111. Knöferl MW, Liener UC, Perl M, et al. Blunt chest trauma induces delayed splenic immunosupression. Shock. 2004;22:51–6.

112. Simon B, Ebert J, Bokhari F, Capella J, Emhoff T, et al. EAST practice management workgroup for pulmonary contusion-flail chest. Eastern Association for the Surgery of Trauma. 2006. www.east.org/tpg/pulmcontflailchest.pdf.

113. Schreiter D, Reske A, Stichert B, Seiwerts M, et al. Alveolar recruitment in combination with sufficient positive end-expiratory pressure increases oxygenation and lung aeration in patients with severe chest trauma. Crit Care Med. 2004;32(4):968–75.

114. Kelly ME, Miller PR, Greenshaw JJ, Fabian TC, Proctor KG. Novel resuscitation strategy for pulmonary contusion after severe chest trauma. J Trauma. 2003;55:94–105.

115. Jacobs JV, Hooft NM, Robinson BR, et al. The use of extracorporeal membrane oxygenation in blunt thoracic trauma: a study of the extracorporeal life support organization database. J Trauma Acute Care Surg. 2015;79(6):1049–54.

116. Maron BJ, Gohman TE, Kyle SB, Estes NA, Link MS. Clinical profile and spectrum of commotion cordis. JAMA. 2002;287:1142–6.

117. Link MS, Wang PJ, Pandian NG, et al. An experimental model of sudden death due to low-energy chest-wall impact (commotion cordis). N Engl J Med. 1998;338:1805–11.

118. Robert E, de la Coussaye JE, Aya AGM, Bertinchant JP, Polge A, Fabbro-Péray P, Pignodel C, Eledjam JJ. Mechanisms of ventricular arrhythmias induced by myocardial contusion. Anesthesiology. 2000;92:1132–43.

119. Sakka SG, Huettermann E, Giebe W, Reinhart K. Late cardiac arrhythmias after blunt chest trauma. Intensive Care Med. 2000;26:792–5.

120. Teixeria PG, Georgiou C, Inaba K, et al. Blunt cardiac trauma: lessons learned from the medical examiner. J Trauma. 2009;67:1259–64.

121. Sisley AC, Rozycki GS, Ballard RN, et al. Rapid detection of traumatic effusion using surgeon performed ultrasonography. J Trauma. 1998;44(2):291–6.

122. Rozycki GS, Feliciano DV, Oschner MG, et al. The role of surgeon performed ultrasound in patients with possible cardiac wounds. Ann Surg. 1996;223(6):737–44.

123. Pasquale MD, Nagy K, Clark J. Practice management guidelines for the screening of blunt cardiac injury. Eastern Association for the Surgery of Trauma. 1998. Available on URL www.east.org/tpg/chap2.pdf. Accessed 1/1/2010.

124. Christensen MA, Sutton KR. Myocardial contusion: new concepts in diagnosis and management. Am J Crit Care. 1993;2(1):28–34.

125. Lindstaedt M, Germing A, Lawo T, et al. Acute and long-term clinical significance of myocardial contusion following blunt thoracic trauma: results of a prospective study. J Trauma. 2002;52:479–85.

126. Velmahos GC, Karaiskakis M, Salim A, Toutouzas KG, Murray J, Asensio J, Demetriades D. Normal electrocardiography and serum troponin I levels preclude the presence if clinically significant cardiac injury. J Trauma. 2003;54:45–51.

127. Schultz JM, Trunkey DD. Blunt cardiac injury. Crit Care Clin. 2004;20(1):57–70.

128. Parmley LF, Manion WC, Mattingly TW. Nonpenetrating traumatic injury of the heart. Circulation. 1958;18(3):371–96.

129. Jeon Y, Ryu JH, Lim YJK, Kim CSB, Bahk JH, Yoon SZ, Choi JY. Comparative effects of vasopressin and norepinephrine after milrinone-induced hypotension in off-pump coronary artery bypass surgical patients. Eur J Cardiothoracic Surg. 2006;29(6):952–6.

130. Ziegler DW, Agarwal NN. The morbidity and mortality of rib fractures. J Trauma. 1994;37(6):975–9.

131. Clark GC, Schecter WP, Trunkey DD. Variables affecting outcome in blunt chest trauma: flail chest vs. pulmonary contusion. J Trauma. 1988;28:298–304.

132. Barnea Y, Kashtan H, shornick Y, Werbin N. Isolated rib fractures in elderly patients; mortality and morbidity. Can J Surg. 2002;45:43–6.

133. Bulger EM, Arenson MA, Mock CN, Jurkovich GJ. Rib fractures in the elderly. J Trauma. 2000;48(6):1040–7.

134. Simon BJ, Cushman J, Barraco R, et al. For the EAST practice management guidelines work group. Pain management guidelines for blunt thoracic trauma. J Trauma. 2005;59:1256–67.

135. Kasotakis G, Hasenboehler EA, Streib EW, Patel N, Patel MB, Alarcon L, Bosarge PL, Love J, Haut ER, Como JJ. Operative fixation of rib fractures after blunt trauma: a practice management guideline from the Eastern Association for the Surgery of Trauma. J Trauma Acute Care Surg. 2017;82(3):618–26.

136. Davignon K, Kwo J, Bigatello LM. Pathophysiology and management of the flail chest. Minerva Anestesiol. 2004;70:193–9.

137. Roberts S, Skinner D, Biccard B, Rodseth RN. The role of non-invasive ventilation in blunt chest trauma: systemic review and meta-analysis. Eur J Trauma Emerg Surg. 2014;40:553–9.

138. Proctor H, London PS. The stove-in chest with paradoxical respiration. Br J Surg. 1955;42(176):622–33.

139. Enderson BL, Abdalla R, Frame SB, Casey MT, Gould H, Maull KI. Tube thoracotomy for occult pneumothorax; a prospective randomized study of its use. J Trauma. 1993;35:726–9.

140. Brasel KJ, Stafford RE, Wiegelt JA, Tenquist JE, Borgstrom DC. Treatment of occult pneumothoraces from blunt trauma. J Trauma. 1999;46:987–90.

141. Harcke HT, Mabry RL, Mazuchowski EL. Needle thoracentesis decompression: observations from postmortem computed tomography and autopsy. J Spec Oper Med. 2013;13:53–6.

142. DuBose J, Inaba K, Demetriades D, Scalea TM, O'Connor J, Menaker J, Morales C, Konstantinidis A, Shiflett A, Copwood B, AAST retained hemoythroax study group. Management of post-traumatic retained hemothorax: a prospective, observational, multicenter AAST study. J Trauma Acute Care Surg. 2011;72(1):11–24.

143. Mackersie RC, Karagianes TG, Hoyt DB, Davis JW. Prospective evaluation of epidural and intravenous administration of fentanyl

for pain control and restoration of ventilator function following multiple rib fractures. J Trauma. 1991;31(4):443–51.

144. Knottenbelt JD, James MF, Bloomfield M. Intrapleural bupivacaine analgesia in chest trauma: a randomized double-blind controlled trial. Injury. 1991;22(2):114–6.

145. Lunchette FA, Radafshar SM, Kaiser R, Flynn W, Hassett JM. Prospective evaluation of epidural versus intrapleural catheters for analgesia in chest wall trauma. J Trauma. 1994;36(6):865–70.

146. Short K, Scheeres D, Mlakar J, et al. Evaluation of intrapleural analgesia in the management of blunt traumatic chest wall pain: a clinical trial. Am Surg. 1996;62:488–93.

147. el-Baz N, Faber LP, Ivankovich AD. Intrapleural infusion of local anesthetic: a word of caution. Anesthesiology. 1988;68:809–10.

148. Lauder GR. Interpleural analgesia and phrenic nerve palsy. Anaesthesia. 1993;48:315–6.

149. Parkinson SK, Mueller JB, Rich TJ, Little WL. Unilateral Horner's syndrome associated with interpleural catheter injection of local anesthetic. Anesth Analg. 1989;68:61–2.

150. Shinohara K, Iwama H, Akama Y, Tase C. Interpleural block for patients with multiple rib fractures: comparison with epidural block. J Emerg Med. 1994;12:441–6.

151. Karmakar MK, Ho AM. Acute pain management of patients with multiple fractured ribs. J Trauma. 2003;54:615–25.

152. Moore KL, Dalley AF. Thorax. In: Kelly PJ, editor. Clincially oriented anatomy. 4th ed. Philadelphia: Lippincott Williams & Wilkins; 1999. p. 59–173.

153. Pedersen VM, Schulze S, Hoier-Madsen K, Halkier E. Air flow meter assessment of the effect of intercostals nerve blockade on respiratory function in rib fractures. Acta Chir Scand. 1983;149:119–20.

154. Toledo-Pereyra LH, DeMeester TR. Prospective randomized evaluation of intrathoracic nerve block with bupivacaine on postoperative ventilator function. Ann Thor Surg. 1979;27:203–5.

155. Kaplan JA, Miller ED, Gallagher EG. Postoperative analgesia of thoracotomy patients. Anesth Analg. 1975;54:773–7.

156. Shanti CM, Carlin AM, Tyburski JG. Incidence of pneumothorax from intercostals nerve blocks for analgesia in rib fractures. J Trauma. 2001;51:536–9.

157. Baxter AD, Flynn JF, Jennings FO. Continuous intercostal nerve blockade. Br J Anaesth. 1984;56:665–6.

158. Mowbray A, Wong KK, Murray JM. Intercostal catheterization; an alternative approach to the paravertebral space. Anaesthesia. 1987;42:959–61.

159. Slinger P. Informal poll taken at thoracic conference. MD Anderson Cancer center, Houston, Nov 2008.

160. Gerner P. Postthoracotomy pain management problems. Anesthesiol Clin. 2008;26:355–67.

161. Conlon NP, Shaw AD, Grichnik KP. Postthoracotomy paravertebral analgesia: will it replace epidural analgesia? Anesthesiol Clin. 2008;26:369–80.

162. Mohta M, Verma P, Saxena AK, Sethi AK, Tyagi A, Girotra G. Prospective, randomized comparison of continuous thoracic epidural and thoracic paravertebral infusion in patients with unilateral multiple fractured ribs- a pilot study. J Trauma. 2009;66:1096–101.

163. Davies RG, Myles PS, Graham JM. A comparison of the analgesic efficacy and side-effects of paravertebral vs epidural blockade for thoracotomy- a systematic review and meta-analysis of randomized trials. Br J Anaesth. 2006;96:418–26.

164. Karmakar MK, Critchley LAH, Ho AMH, Gin T, Lee TW, Yin APC. Continuous thoracic paravertebral infusion of bupivacaine for pain management in patients with multiple fractured ribs. Chest. 2003;123:424–31.

165. Bulger EM, Edwards T, Klotz P, Jurkovich GJ. Epidural analgesia improves outcome after multiple rib fractures. Surgery. 2004;136:426.

166. Shibata Y, Nishiwaki K. Ultrasound-guided intercostals approach to thoracic paravertebral block. Anesth Analg. 2009;109(3):996–7.

167. Ben-Ari A, Moreno M, Chelly JE, Bigeleisen PE. Ultrasound-guided paravertebral block using an intercostals approach. Anesth Analg. 2009;109(5):1691–4.

168. Hara K, Sakura S, Nomura T, Saito Y. Ultrasound guided thoracic paravertebral block in breast surgery. Anaesthesia. 2009;64(2):223–5.

169. Lönnqvist PA, MacKenzie J, Soni AK, Conacher ID. Paravertebral blockade. Failure rate and complications. Anaesthesia. 1995;50(9):813–5.

170. Evans PJ, Lloyd JW, Wood GJ. Accidental intrathecal injection of bupivacaine and dextran. Anaesthesia. 1981;36:685–7.

171. Sharrock NE. Postural headache following thoracic somatic paravertebral block. Anesthesiology. 1980;52:360–2.

172. Khalil AE, Abdallah NM, Bashandy GM, Kaddah TA. Ultrasound-guided serratus anterior plane block versus thoracic epidural analgesia for thoracotomy pain. J Cardiothorac Vasc Anesth. 2017;31(1):152–8.

173. Worthley LI. Thoracic epidural management of chest trauma. Intensive Care Med. 1985;11:312–5.

174. Ullman DA, Wimpy RE, Fortune JB, Kennedy TM, Greenhouse BB. The treatment of patients with multiple rib fractures using continuous thoracic epidural narcotic infusion. Regional Anesth. 1989;14:43–7.

175. Dittman M, Keller R, Wolff G. A rationale for epidural analgesia in the treatment of multiple rib fractures. Intensive Care Med. 1978;4:193–7.

176. Ueda K, Ueda W, Manabe M. A comparative study of sequential epidural bolus technique and continuous epidural infusion. Anesthesiology. 2005;103:126–9.

177. Halpern SH, Carvalho B. Patient-controlled epidural analgesia for labor. Anesth Analg. 2009;108:921–8.

178. Joshy GP, Bonnet F, Shah R, Wilkinson RC, Camu F, et al. A systematic review of randomized trials evaluating regional techniques for postthoracotomy analgesia. Anesth Analg. 2008;107:1026–40.

179. Moon MR, Luchette FA, Gibson SW, et al. Prospective, randomized comparison of epidural versus parenteral opioid analgesia in thoracic trauma. Ann Surg. 1999;229:684–91.

180. Galvagno SM, Smith CE, Varon AJ, et al. Pain management for blunt thoracic trauma: a joint practice management guideline from the Eastern Association for the Surgery of Trauma and Trauma Anesthesiology Society. J Trauma Acute Care Surg. 2016;81(5):936–51.

181. Malekpour M, Hashmi A, Dove J, Torres D, Wild J. Analgesic choice in management of rib fractures: paravertebral block or epidural analgesia? Anesth Analg. 2017;124:1906–11.

182. Unsworth A, Curtis K, Asha SE. Treatments for blunt chest trauma and their impact on patient outcomes and health service delivery. Scand J Trauma Resusc Emerg Med. 2015;23:17.

183. Monaghan SF, Adams CA, Connolly MD, Stephen AH, Lueckel SN, Harrington DT, Cioffi WG, Heffernan DS. A geriatric specific rib fracture protocol significantly improves mortality. Oral presentation as part of the 73rd annual meeting of the American Association for the Surgery of Trauma and Clinical Congress of Acute Care Surgery, Philadelphia, 10–13 Sept 2014.

Part XIV

Post-operative Management

Enhanced Recovery After Surgery (ERAS) for Thoracic Surgery

Emily G. Teeter, Gabriel E. Mena, Javier D. Lasala, and Lavinia M. Kolarczyk

Key Points

- Enhanced recovery after surgery (ERAS) describes a multidisciplinary approach to reducing the perioperative stress response, decreasing potential complications, and enabling a faster return to baseline functional status.
- The core tenets of ERAS span the entire perioperative period.
- Pre-operative components of ERAS include patient education, "prehabilitation," and optimization of underlying medical conditions such as COPD and anemia.
- Intraoperatively, multimodal opioid-sparing analgesia, minimally invasive surgical techniques, avoidance of salt and crystalloid excess, protective ventilatory strategies, and limited use of tubes and drains should be considered.
- In the post-operative period, early mobilization, early enteral nutrition, and early removal of tubes and drains are encouraged.
- While ERAS is well-established in some fields, ERAS for thoracic surgery is still relatively new.
- In order to be successful, an ERAS program must have buy-in from all members of the team, including personnel in the pre-operative, intraoperative, and post-operative settings. Anesthesiologists play a major role in the success of ERAS programs, and patients are active participants in their care.

Background

The concept of enhanced recovery after surgery (ERAS) was introduced in the late 1990s by Kehlet. This model of care provides a multidisciplinary, comprehensive approach aimed at reducing the perioperative stress response, decreasing potential complications, and enabling a faster return to baseline functional status [1]. From a systems perspective, ERAS programs are associated with reduced length of hospital stay, increased patient satisfaction, and lower costs [2]. In the oncologic population, faster recovery means an earlier return to planned adjuvant chemotherapy or radiation therapy, a so-called return to intended oncologic therapy (RIOT) score [3]. ERAS programs challenge traditional clinical practice and emphasize application of evidence-based best practices throughout the perioperative spectrum [4–6].

Healthcare systems in the United States and abroad have implemented ERAS protocols in a variety of surgical patient populations. Given the changes in healthcare reimbursement from fee-for-service to value-based models, there is a growing emphasis on delivering quality, improving outcomes, and decreasing cost [7]. ERAS programs serve as a vehicle to deliver value-based care, as ERAS principles promote early physiologic recovery, improved pain management, and early hospital discharge.

Fast-track and thoracic ERAS protocols have evolved over the past two decades in parallel with cardiac fast-track protocols, likely due to the clinical overlap between cardiac and thoracic surgery practitioners. Fast-track cardiac surgery protocols gained popularity in the 1990s as a way to facilitate early extubation after surgery and in turn decrease intensive care unit cost. Early extubation after cardiac surgery helped to mitigate the well-described deleterious effects of prolonged mechanical ventilation. Some fast-track cardiac protocols included extubation in the operating room at the end of the procedure [8–15]. The success of these cardiac surgery protocols led to the evolution of pathways in other cardiothoracic procedures, including pulmonary resection and esophageal surgery [16–19].

E. G. Teeter (✉) · L. M. Kolarczyk
Department of Anesthesiology, University of North Carolina at Chapel Hill, Chapel Hill, NC, USA
e-mail: eteeter@aims.unc.edu

G. E. Mena · J. D. Lasala
Department of Anesthesiology and Perioperative Medicine, The University of Texas MD Anderson Cancer Center, Houston, TX, USA

© Springer Nature Switzerland AG 2019
P. Slinger (ed.), *Principles and Practice of Anesthesia for Thoracic Surgery*, https://doi.org/10.1007/978-3-030-00859-8_52

In 2008, Muehling et al. [20] performed a prospective, randomized, controlled study investigating fast-track versus conservative care in thoracic surgery. The conservative patient group fasted for 6 h and had an intraoperative intercostal nerve block followed by IV patient-controlled analgesia (PCA). Enteral feeding and ambulation started on the day after surgery. The fast-track group fasted for 2 h and received patient-controlled epidural analgesia. In this group, enteral feeding and ambulation started on the evening of the operation. The primary end points of the study were the presence of post-operative pulmonary complications, namely, atelectasis, pneumonia, prolonged air leak, and pleural effusion. The researchers found that the overall rates of post-operative pulmonary complications were 36% in the conservative group and 7% in the fast-track group ($P = 0\ 0.009$). In this study, researchers found no significant difference in overall morbidity or mortality.

In 2009, Das-Neves-Pereira et al. [21] published their 5-year experience with patients undergoing open, muscle-sparing lobectomy who were provided care in a fast-track rehabilitation program. Comparison of their post-operative complications and hospital length of stay showed that non-fast-tracked patients experienced more frequent post-operative complications and a longer average hospital stay. Of particular importance, early patient ambulation was the only predictive (i.e., protective) independent variable of post-operative complications.

In esophageal surgery, fast-track surgery protocols have demonstrated an improvement in biochemical markers of inflammation. Chen et al. [16] demonstrated that fast-track surgery improves post-operative clinical recovery and effectively inhibited the release of inflammatory factors via the immune system after esophagectomy for esophageal cancer.

As compared to thoracotomy, minimally invasive thoracic surgery is associated with lower cytokine release, less effect on white cell function, and less impact on the immune system [22]. The translation to clinical outcomes, however, has not yet been demonstrated. Findlay et al. provided the first systematic review of enhanced recovery protocols for esophagectomy [17, 18]. The findings of this review support that ERAS pathways for esophagectomy are safe, feasible, and likely beneficial for this high-risk group, although more studies are needed.

ERAS General Overview

The Enhanced Recovery After Surgery (ERAS(R)) Society and American Society of Enhanced Recovery (ASER) has described core components for ERAS pathways across a variety of surgical specialties (Fig. 52.1). These core concepts include pre-operative patient education, pre-operative carbohydrate fluids up to 2 h before surgery, multimodal opioid-sparing analgesia, minimally invasive surgery when possible, avoidance of salt and crystalloid excess, early mobilization, early enteral nutrition, and limited use of and early removal of tubes and drains. Additionally, avoidance of bowel preps is strongly advised. The ERAS Society has published specific guidelines for a variety of surgical patient populations, including bariatric surgery, colorectal surgery, gynecologic surgery, pancreatic surgery, urologic surgery, liver surgery, and head and neck surgery [23, 24]. Thoracic ERAS pathways are still in their infancy, and currently there is significant variability in institutional practices with limited evidence [25, 26].

PREOPERATIVE	INTRAOPERATIVE	POSTOPERATIVE
Patient education	Defined blood pressure goals	Multimodal analgesia, avoidance of systemic Opioids
Consumption of carbohydrate drink	Antibiotic prophylaxis (per SCIP guidelines)	Early and frequent mobilization
Multimodal analgesia	Standardized anesthetic approach	Early removal of nasogastric tube
VTE Prophylaxis	Multimodal analgesia, avoidance of systemic opiates	Early removal of urinary (Foley) catheter
Avoidance of bowel preps	Avoidance of IV crystalloid and salt excess	Early discontinuation of IV fluds
		Early PO intake

Fig. 52.1 Core components of an enhanced recovery after surgery pathway

ERAS for Thoracic Surgery: Rationale

Application of ERAS principles to thoracic surgery seems prudent, as this patient population represents an at-risk group for increased perioperative complications. Thoracic surgical patients tend to be older with multiple comorbidities including chronic obstructive pulmonary disease (COPD), hypertension, and coronary artery disease. Thoracic surgery patients are also more likely to be current or former tobacco smokers [27]. These patient factors contribute to prolonged length of hospital stay and increased risk of perioperative morbidity and mortality [28].

While ERAS for thoracic surgery is a novel concept, there is emerging literature demonstrating proof of concept in lobectomy, video-assisted thoracoscopy (VATS), and esophagectomy [29–31]. Pre-operative components of an ERAS clinical pathway for thoracic surgery focus on risk reduction and optimization, which may include tobacco cessation, nutrition, and improving functional capacity [30]. Intraoperative components of an ERAS clinical pathway may include multimodal opioid-sparing analgesia and interventions to prevent post-operative pulmonary complications. Post-operative components serve to prevent common complications including oxygen dependency, delirium, and suboptimal pain control [30].

ERAS Thoracic Surgery: Pre-operative Components

Surgical stress is associated with a sharp decline in functional status, typically followed by a slow recovery (Fig. 52.2). "Prehabilitation" is a term used to describe the pre-operative physical conditioning and optimization of patient functional status in order to facilitate tolerance to surgical stress and enable a smooth perioperative course [32–34]. The core components of prehabilitation include exercise, nutritional counseling, and stress reduction. Specific to thoracic surgery, pre-operative interventions should focus on encouraging tobacco cessation, correcting anemia, optimizing comorbid conditions, and improving pulmonary and nutritional status. In addition, the importance of patient education, clear communication of expectations, and involving patients as active participants in their own care cannot be overstated.

Much like training for an endurance race, prehabilitation aims to optimize physiologic reserve in light of the impending physical and psychological insult of surgery. While prehabilitation makes intuitive sense, the literature is mixed, particularly when the primary outcomes are morbidity, mortality, and hospital length of stay. A review of 12 randomized controlled trials of patients undergoing

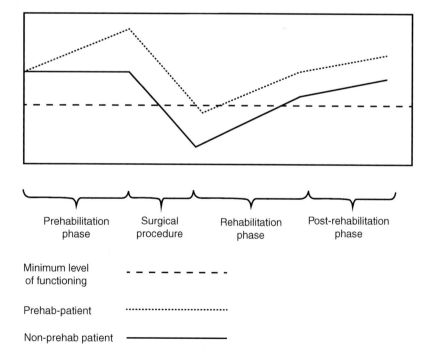

Fig. 52.2 Functional ability through the perioperative period with and without pre-operative physical conditioning ("prehabilitation"). (Carli and Zavorsky [125] with permission. https://journals.lww.com/co-clinicalnutrition/Abstract/2005/01000/Optimizing_functional_exercise_capacity_in_the.5.aspx)

orthopedic, cardiac, and abdominal surgery reported decreased length of hospital stay and fewer post-operative pulmonary complications in those who had participated in pre-operative exercise programs [35]. A similar systematic review of pre-operative exercise therapy in thoracic surgery patients found beneficial effects of exercise on physical fitness, exercise capacity, as well as post-operative complications and hospital length of stay. Conversely, a review of eight randomized controlled trials by Lemanu found only one study demonstrating physiologic benefit of prehabilitation. Interestingly, the group that did show benefit (less decline in respiratory parameters as compared to controls) was a group of patients undergoing coronary artery bypass grafting (CABG) surgery [36].

Traditionally, rehabilitation begins after surgery, and while anecdotally prehabilitation has benefit, the specific benefit of beginning this in the pre-operative setting rather than post-operatively is unclear. A prospective, randomized controlled trial comparing pre-operative rehabilitation with standard post-operative rehabilitation in patients undergoing colon resection was performed by Gillis et al. Both groups participated in aerobic and resistance exercise, nutritional counseling, and relaxation exercises. The prehabilitation group experienced a significant improvement in functional exercise capacity both pre-operatively and post-operatively, although no difference in outcomes was demonstrated [37]. While data specifically looking at thoracic surgery is sparse, a study following 82 patients who began pulmonary prehabilitation during induction chemotherapy and were followed through the perioperative period found an overall improvement in forced expiratory volume in one second (FEV1) and forced vital capacity (FVC) post-operatively, and the improvement was most marked in high-risk patients (smokers and those with the poorest baseline pulmonary function tests) [38]. However, this was an observational study, which by definition has no control group, so they were unable to demonstrate any comparative benefit. To date, no randomized controlled trials in the thoracic population demonstrate decreased pulmonary complications, length of stay, or morbidity/mortality in patients who complete pre-operative rehabilitation programs [39]. Further studies exploring the impact of prehabilitation in thoracic surgery are needed in order to establish the benefit of including prehabilitation in enhanced recovery protocols.

Optimization of Comorbid Conditions

Thoracic surgery patients are among the most medically complex, partly due to concomitant respiratory pathology and high rates of long-term tobacco abuse. Often, patients are scheduled for lung resection surgery soon after a cancer diagnosis, which does not leave much time for optimization of comorbid conditions. Specifically, COPD is a common finding in patients who present for thoracic surgery and is an independent risk factor for post-operative pulmonary complications [40]. A long-acting bronchodilator and/or inhaled steroid should be considered for patients whose COPD is untreated or not optimally controlled [41–43]. As discussed above, perioperative respiratory physiotherapy programs may improve FEV1 and FVC such that some patients who may not be proper surgical candidates could be reconsidered for a surgical procedure [44]. Other comorbid conditions, such as hypertension and diabetes, should be addressed as aggressively as possible without delaying surgery. The pre-operative assessment clinic is invaluable in providing a comprehensive assessment and recommendations for management of thoracic surgery patients in the pre-operative period.

Nutrition

Malnutrition has deleterious consequences in the perioperative period; namely, delayed wound healing, as well as muscle weakness leading to respiratory complications, increased morbidity, and prolonged recovery [40, 45–47]. Patients with cancer are prone to malnutrition, and among these, patients with esophageal cancer are at especially high risk due to accompanying dysphagia and obstructive gastrointestinal symptoms. Recent emerging guidelines, such as the European Society for Nutrition and Metabolism Guidelines, recommend that patients be screened for malnutrition in the pre-operative period [48]. Multiple risk stratification tools exist, including the subjective global assessment (SGA) and Nutritional Risk Screening 2002. Patients at high risk should undergo nutritional counseling and supplementation. Up to 28% of patients undergoing lung resection surgery fall into the high-risk category, as defined by weight loss >10–15% within 6 months, BMI < 18.5 kg/m^2, SGA Grade C, or serum albumin <30 g/L [49]. Not surprisingly, most esophagectomy patients should be considered high-risk and would benefit from aggressive nutritional support pre-operatively [17]. While no studies to date have specifically examined the impact of pre-operative correction of malnutrition in patients undergoing lung resection or esophagectomy, such interventions are still recommended [17]. Small trials have investigated the impact of pre-operative immunonutrient and micronutrient supplementation (such as a-ketoglutaric acid and 5-hydroxymethylfurfural) in patients with non-esophageal gastrointestinal or non-small cell lung cancer and found a reduction in infectious complications and ICU and hospital length of stay [50, 51]. However, randomized control trials specifically focusing on micronutrient supplementation in patients with esophageal cancer found no benefit [52, 53].

Anemia Screening

Anemia, defined as a hemoglobin concentration <12 g/dL in females and <13 g/dL in males, is a common pre-operative finding which has been associated with increased morbidity and mortality [54, 55]. Transfusion is typically avoided unless absolutely necessary, as it carries the risks of transfusion reaction, infection, immunosuppression, and cancer recurrence [56]. Other strategies to correct anemia pre-operatively include iron supplementation and erythropoietin administration; however, typically their use is limited by the short time interval between cancer diagnosis and surgery [40]. Regardless, anemia should be investigated and corrected as much as possible prior to thoracic surgery.

Tobacco

An estimated 20% of the US population smokes [57], and this number is even higher in the thoracic surgery patient population [58]. Smokers are at significantly higher risk of post-operative complications than non-smokers. Smoking increases the odds of 30-day mortality, post-operative pulmonary complications, major adverse cardiac events, and wound infection [57]. Pre-operative smoking cessation reduces morbidity and mortality, although the optimal timing has been a source of debate. Currently, the literature does not support the formerly held notion that tobacco cessation within 2 months of surgery is associated with a paradoxical increase in post-operative pulmonary complications [59]. According to the NICE guidelines, patients should be counseled to stop smoking before surgery, regardless of the timeline [60]. Among smoking cessation methods, no randomized control trials have shown one method to be most successful [61].

ERAS Thoracic Surgery: Intraoperative Components

Analgesia

Multimodal analgesia involves the use of non-opioid analgesics with different mechanisms of action, which work synergistically to provide pain relief with reduced analgesic-related adverse effects. The analgesic modalities available for postoperative pain management after thoracic surgery include regional or local analgesia techniques, such as thoracic epidural analgesia (TEA), paravertebral block (PVB), intercostal nerve blocks (ICNB), and wound infiltration. In addition, acetaminophen, non-steroidal anti-inflammatory drugs (NSAIDs), or cyclo-oxygenase-2 (COX-2) specific inhibitors and analgesic adjuncts, such as steroids, ketamine, alpha-2 agonists, and gabapentinoids (e.g., gabapentin and pregabalin), have been evaluated [62]. An ideal analgesic combination would reduce the intensity of movement-evoked pain (e.g., during coughing and ambulation), while avoiding analgesic-related adverse effects, and improve post-operative outcome.

Gabapentinoids, namely, gabapentin and pregabalin, have both been shown to be effective in the prevention of post-thoracotomy pain syndromes [63, 64]. COX-2 inhibitors and NSAIDs have demonstrated clinical effectiveness in treating ipsilateral shoulder pain after thoracic surgery [65]. The alpha-2 agonist dexmedetomidine has been shown to decrease opioid use in thoracic surgical patients [66, 67].

Neuraxial and regional anesthesia techniques to minimize perioperative opioid use include thoracic epidural analgesia, paravertebral blocks, intercostal blocks, and serratus anterior nerve blocks. Historically, the gold standard for thoracotomy pain management has been thoracic epidural analgesia [68, 69]. The dense analgesic block provided by an epidural has been shown to decrease post-operative pulmonary complications [70] and prevent long-term chronic post-thoracotomy pain syndromes [71]. However, the risks associated with TEA remain an ongoing concern. These risks include hypotension, urinary retention, epidural abscess, and epidural hematoma. As such, there has been a growing interest in the use of regional anesthetic techniques for thoracic surgery, which theoretically have fewer systemic side effects.

The thoracic PVB continues to show promise as a safe and equally efficacious analgesic method for thoracic surgery [72]. A recent Cochrane review compared TEA to PVB for elective thoracotomy with respect to analgesic efficacy, the incidence of major and minor complications, length of hospital stay, and cost-effectiveness [25]. The conclusion from this review was that PVB was equally as effective as TEA for acute thoracotomy pain and that PVB reduced the risks of minor complications commonly associated with TEA. There was not enough evidence to evaluate length of hospital stay and cost-effectiveness [73].

There has been a renewed interest in the use of intercostal nerve blockade (ICB) for thoracic surgical analgesia with the introduction of liposomal bupivacaine (Exparel®, Pacira Pharmaceuticals, Parsippany, NJ) and the growing popularity of ERAS pathways for thoracic surgery [25]. The advantages of ICB include ease of block placement, placement of block under direct visualization by the surgeon, low risk of hemodynamic issues, and good safety profile. Liposomal bupivacaine adds yet another advantage in that it does not require placement or management of an indwelling catheter while providing up to 96 h of analgesia. The use of liposomal bupivacaine for peripheral nerve blockade is not yet FDA-approved, but several studies using liposomal bupivacaine for ICB in thoracic surgery have demonstrated a promising safety profile. A retrospective study of 108 patients compared TEA ($n = 54$) to ICB with Exparel® ($n = 54$) for lung resection surgery [26]. The authors found no differences in mean or maximal pain scores or in opioid consumption between ICB with Exparel® and TEA. The authors were able to conclude that a posterior intercostal block performed under direct vision via a thoracoscopic view and using long-acting encapsulated bupivacaine (Exparel®) is safe and provides effective analgesia for patients undergoing thoracic surgery. It may be considered as a suitable alternative to TEA. Of note, there was significant heterogeneity in surgical approach, as the study included patients who had video-assisted thoracoscopic (VATS), robotic, and open thoracotomy approaches. A second retrospective study of 85 patients compared TEA to ICB with Exparel® specifically for thoracotomy patients [74]. Patients in the Exparel® ICB group had lower pain scores on post-operative days 1 and 3, and there was no difference in pain scores on post-operative day 2. The authors found no difference in supplemental opioid use between groups. While these results are promising, these studies are small retrospective reviews.

The serratus anterior block (SAB) has been recently introduced as a novel regional technique for thoracic surgical analgesia. The SAB targets the lateral cutaneous branches of the intercostal nerve as they pass through this fascial plane before these nerves divide into anterior and posterior branches to innervate the chest wall. The block is performed by injecting local anesthetic either superficially or deep to the serratus muscle under ultrasound guidance [75]. A recent prospective randomized controlled trial evaluated TEA versus serratus anterior nerve block (SAB) infusion for thoracotomy patients [76]. The authors found no difference in pain scores or morphine consumption between groups for the first 24 h after surgery. The SAB group had fewer episodes of hypotension. While this study is promising, larger studies that follow patients for longer periods of time are needed to demonstrate the effectiveness and safety profile of the SAB.

Mechanical Ventilation Strategy

In thoracic surgery, pulmonary complications outnumber cardiovascular complications and are the most common cause of post-operative death in esophageal cancer patients [77, 78]. Injury from OLV can manifest as re-expansion pulmonary edema (REPE), acute lung injury (ALI), or acute respiratory distress syndrome (ARDS). While bronchopneumonia or aspiration can contribute to delayed ALI, the risk of early ALI is increased by high intraoperative ventilation pressures, increased surgery duration, and excessive intravenous volume replacement [79–82]. Thus, protective ventilatory strategies and judicious fluid use may decrease the incidence of ALI [80].

Historical ventilator schemes focused on prevention of atelectasis, and tidal volumes as high as 10–12 mL/kg were advocated. Tidal volumes <8 mL/kg were thought to result in decreased functional residual capacity (FRC) and worsening atelectasis. OLV was achieved with parameters similar to two-lung ventilation. This ventilator strategy proved to be detrimental because it led to a cascade of inflammatory mediators due to the stimulation of stretch-activated cation channels, oxygen-derived free radicals, activated neutrophils, and cytokine upregulation contributing to increased microvascular-alveolar permeability [83]. The current strategy to minimize OLV-associated lung injury advocates lung protective ventilation to decrease inflammatory mediators, which contribute to ventilator-induced lung injury (VILI) [84]. Reduction of tidal volumes during OLV to 5 ml/kg was shown to reduce alveolar concentration of TNF-α and sICAM-1 [85]. The addition of 5 cm H2O PEEP was associated with better oxygenation and earlier extubation [86]. Current lung protective ventilation consists of tidal volume of 5–6 mL/kg, maintaining low fraction of inspired O2 (FiO2) to avoid absorption atelectasis and worsening shunt [87], PEEP above the lower inflection point on the static pressure-volume curve, plateau pressures of less than 20 cm H2O above the PEEP value, peak inspiratory pressures less than 35 cm H2O, and preferential use of pressure-limited ventilatory modes [82].

Lung protective ventilation primarily refers to the dependent lung, which shows a more pronounced inflammatory response than the non-ventilated lung [88, 89]. However, the nondependent lung may experience ischemia-reperfusion injury, and it is likely that physiologic and pathologic insults to both lungs contribute to post-operative complications.

Maintenance of Anesthesia

The influence of anesthetic type on the inflammatory response and post-operative clinical outcomes is unknown. Studies comparing propofol to volatile anesthetics such as sevoflurane and desflurane have yielded conflicting results [90]. Overall, differences in surgical time, duration of OLV, and laboratory techniques in existing studies have complicated interpretation of the data [82]. Volatile agents are thought to have immune-modulating effects. While previous work showed anti-inflammatory effects of propofol, recent studies have demonstrated decreased inflammatory markers in both the operative and non-operative lung with volatile anesthesia [90–92]. Sugasawa and colleagues found that sevoflurane use was significantly associated with a suppressed inflammatory response compared to propofol [92]. Thus, the choice of anesthetic agent and other drugs such as ropivacaine, ketamine, thiopental, and dexmedetomidine may have anti-inflammatory effects that may be protective during lung surgery with OLV. Further study is needed to elucidate the role of these agents [93].

Fluid Management

Appropriate perioperative fluid management during thoracic surgery and specifically lung resection including VATS is a subject of a long-standing debate between thoracic surgeons and anesthesiologists. The controversy centers around the fact that restrictive fluid management may induce hypovolemia leading to a negative impact on organ perfusion and increased perioperative morbidity (e.g., renal impairment [94], myocardial ischemia) as well as prolonged length of stay (LOS), whereas fluid overload leads to increased perioperative morbidity (GI complications, i.e., anastomosis leak, ileus, infections) [95–98].

In the operative setting, surgical insults may cause an inflammatory response characterized by alterations in microvascular integrity. Specifically, the protective glycocalyx may be compromised, thus allowing abnormal transmicrovascular fluid flux. Due to this increase in permeability, interstitial edema may develop, which decreases O2 diffusion and results in hypoxic cell injury. This injury propagates a vicious cycle involving further cell death and the subsequent release of inflammatory cytokines.

Goal-directed therapy (GDT) describes the administration of intravenous fluids, vasopressors, and inotropes guided by flow-based dynamic parameters such as stroke volume variation (SVV), cardiac index (CI), and stroke volume (SV) in order to achieve individualized hemodynamic and fluid optimization. Cecconi et al. reviewed 32 randomized controlled trials including 2808 patients and concluded that GDT decreases morbidity and mortality in high-risk surgical patients (those who had predicted mortality >20%) undergoing elective surgery [99]. However, the use of these monitors, which include Vigileo FloTrac™, PiCCOplus™, and LiDCO™, is limited in thoracic surgery by open-chest physiology, one-lung ventilation, and lateral positioning. In patients undergoing thoracic surgery with one-lung ventilation (OLV), these commercially available hemodynamic monitoring tools may be used to follow perioperative hemodynamic trends, but the anesthesiologist should recognize their limitations.

Slinger describes a rational approach to fluid administration for thoracic surgery patients [100]. The thorax is not assumed to be a third space. Total positive fluid balance in the first 24 h post-operatively should not exceed 20 ml/kg or approximately 3 L of crystalloid. Unless the patient is at high risk of developing renal insufficiency, urine output of greater than 0.5 mL/kg/h is probably unnecessary. In the case of reduced tissue perfusion, as in the case of epidural-induced sympathectomy, it is preferable to invasively monitor and use GDT. The use of inotropes may be preferable to aggressive fluid overload.

ERAS Thoracic Surgery: Post-operative Components

In order for an enhanced recovery pathway for thoracic surgery to succeed, the post-operative care must be a multidisciplinary continuation of the components begun in the pre-operative period. Namely, multimodal analgesia, mobilization, chest physiotherapy, and nutritional optimization are

paramount. Additionally, early removal of chest tubes, lines, and urinary catheters should be performed.

Removal of Lines and Drains

The "early" removal of lines, tubes, and drains challenges traditional surgical dogma. Nonetheless, indwelling urinary catheters limit mobility and are associated with an increased incidence of urinary tract infection, which can lead to post-operative delirium, sepsis, increased length of stay, and mortality [17]. Therefore, even in the presence of a thoracic epidural, the Foley catheter should be removed as early as possible. While the need for catheter replacement in the setting of urinary retention remains a concern, randomized controlled trials in thoracic and abdominal surgery patients demonstrate that in patients with normal urinary function, the rate of recatheterization remains extremely low and the risk of urinary tract infection was overall reduced [17].

Unless placed for esophagectomy, nasogastric tubes ought to be removed by post-operative day 1 or not placed at all if possible. In our institution, both the urinary catheter and nasogastric tube are labeled with a fluorescent "ERAS" sticker as a visual reminder for the surgical team to consider early removal.

Chest Drains

Indwelling chest drains cause pain and impair mobilization, thus slowing recovery [101]. Significant heterogeneity exists in the practice patterns for chest drain management, even in matters so simple as whether or not to apply suction [102, 103]. Some argue that suction decreases air leaks by encouraging the two layers of pleura to appose, while others argue that suction maintains or even encourages air leaks. The threshold for chest drain removal remains unstandardized, although absence of an air leak and output of less than 150 mL per day are common [104]. Unfortunately, for many patients, discharge is delayed due solely to persistent air leak or chest drain output. Thus, several studies have examined a lower threshold for drain removal and concluded that removal at a higher threshold (200 mL or even higher) is indeed safe [104, 105], and patients can be discharged sooner, particularly if the patients can be discharged with portable suction or a similar device. When possible, placing only one chest drain may improve pain and expedite discharge without increasing morbidity as compared to two or more drains [106–109]. Surgical sealants have been developed to decrease post-operative air leak, and while some evidence supports their efficacy in this regard, they do not contribute to a shorter length of stay and cannot be recommended [110].

Early Mobilization

Although post-operative convalescence has been traditionally thought to aid recovery by decreasing metabolic demands, bed rest has several undesirable consequences. Specifically, muscle atrophy due to catabolism takes place in a matter of days, even in healthy adults, with an estimated loss of 10–20% of muscle mass per week, and pulmonary function rapidly declines [40, 111]. Therefore, early mobilization ought to be a priority in the post-operative period as soon as it is safely possible. Patients who were mobilized as soon as 4 h after lung resection required less supplemental oxygen and made a smoother psychological recovery in one prospective cohort study [112].

Incentive Spirometry

Pulmonary complications, such as atelectasis, pneumonia, prolonged ventilation, and exacerbation of chronic obstructive pulmonary disease (COPD), remain a major source of morbidity and mortality in thoracic patients [113]. Altered respiratory mechanics, atelectasis, and shallow breathing due to pain can contribute to post-operative pulmonary complications [114]. To date, several studies have examined the role of post-operative chest physiotherapy and incentive spirometry in preventing post-operative pulmonary complications in thoracic surgery patients. Methods of chest physiotherapy vary but include airway clearance techniques (percussion, effective coughing), deep breathing exercises, and mobilization. Incentive spirometry is a low-cost technique utilizing a device that provides visual feedback of the patient's inspiratory efforts (Fig. 52.3). The goal of incentive spirometry is to encourage lung re-expansion and mitigate atelectasis by encouraging deep breathing with an inspiratory hold [115].

The benefit of pulmonary rehabilitation for patients undergoing thoracic surgery is well established [116]. Intensive chest physiotherapy reduces the risk of pulmonary complications and hospital length of stay [117]. The use of incentive spirometry, however, remains controversial. Weiner et al. performed a randomized controlled trial on patients with COPD who were undergoing lung resection and found that patients who used incentive spirometry in the pre-operative and post-operative period had higher post-operative FEV1 and FVC as compared to controls who did not receive training in incentive spirometry [118]. A similar study by Agostini failed to demonstrate an improvement in post-operative pulmonary complications for post-thoracotomy and lung resection patients who added incentive spirometry to a standardized post-operative lung expansion program. A systematic review by Carvalho revealed inconclusive results regarding the benefit of incentive spirometry in thoracic sur-

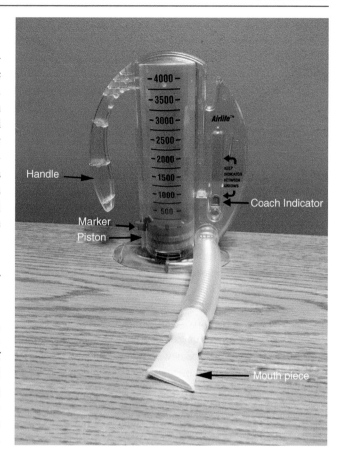

Fig. 52.3 Incentive spirometer

gery patients, further stating that no study supports the post-operative use of IS [119]. Overall, there is little evidence supporting the use of chest physiotherapy or incentive spirometry after thoracic surgery [115]. However, incentive spirometry remains a low-cost and noninvasive option to encourage lung expansion in the perioperative period [120]. Although support from the literature is weak, in our institutional experience, patients who begin incentive IS in the pre-operative period fare better post-operatively, likely due in part to an increased level of ownership and investment in their health and outcome.

Multimodal Analgesia

The majority of thoracic enhanced recovery pathways incorporate a multimodal approach to analgesia as previously discussed. It is imperative that these efforts continue into the post-operative period in order to provide adequate analgesia and decrease dependence on opioid pain medications. While a single pre-operative dose of gabapentin does not decrease pain or morphine consumption, 2 days or more of use can provide superior pain control as compared to morphine PCA alone [121]. A 60-day post-operative regimen of gabapentin provides significant improvement in pain control with minimal side effects and cost [63]. Acetaminophen is another low-cost, low-risk addition to the post-operative multimodal regimen.

Barriers to Implementation and Sustainability

A common barrier to implementation of ERAS pathways is lack of buy-in by surgeons, anesthesiologists, and nurses [122, 123]. ERAS programs often represent disruptive change in traditional practices, otherwise known as culture change [124]. Changing culture within a healthcare organization takes time: time to get all members to agree to standardized, evidence-based practice, time to educate perioperative teams, time to obtain feedback, and time to collect and share data on quality metrics. Buy-in from all members of the perioperative team comes with time and persistence, fueled by a dedicated core group of individuals engaged in the quality improvement process. In order to sustain an ERAS program, it is imperative to evaluate individual pathway components for effectiveness and make changes based on data.

Current State, Future Directions, and Applicability

While ERAS has shown great promise in other surgical subspecialties, thoracic ERAS is still in its infancy and requires further investigation. In the future, enhanced recovery principles and practices will become integrated as standard of care for thoracic surgery as well as other specialties, particularly in light of the changes in healthcare and the growing opioid epidemic in the United States.

In conclusion, enhanced recovery after surgery represents a multidisciplinary approach to perioperative care with a goal of early return to baseline function through the core tenets described in this chapter. The key components span the pre-operative, intraoperative, and post-operative period and require the participation of all members of the perioperative team and, most importantly, the patients themselves.

References

1. Kehlet H. Multimodal approach to control postoperative pathophysiology and rehabilitation. Br J Anaesth. 1997;78:606–17.
2. Nelson G, Kalogera E, Dowdy SC. Enhanced recovery pathways in gynecologic oncology. Gynecol Oncol. 2014;135:586–94. https://doi.org/10.1016/j.ygyno.2014.10.006.
3. Aloia TA, et al. Return to intended oncologic treatment (RIOT): a novel metric for evaluating the quality of oncosurgical therapy for malignancy. J Surg Oncol. 2014;110:107–14. https://doi.org/10.1002/jso.23626.
4. Kehlet H. Enhanced Recovery After Surgery (ERAS): good for now, but what about the future? Can J Anesth (Journal canadien d'anesthésie). 2015;62:99–104. https://doi.org/10.1007/s12630-014-0261-3.
5. Nelson G, et al. Guidelines for pre- and intra-operative care in gynecologic/oncology surgery: Enhanced Recovery After Surgery (ERAS®) Society recommendations — Part I. Gynecol Oncol. 2016;140:313–22. https://doi.org/10.1016/j.ygyno.2015.11.015.
6. Nelson G, et al. Guidelines for postoperative care in gynecologic/oncology surgery: Enhanced Recovery After Surgery (ERAS®) Society recommendations — Part II. Gynecol Oncol. 2016;140:323–32. https://doi.org/10.1016/j.ygyno.2015.12.019.
7. Teisberg EO, Wallace S. Creating a high-value delivery system for health care. Semin Thorac Cardiovasc Surg. 2009;21:35–42. https://doi.org/10.1053/j.semtcvs.2009.03.003.
8. Borracci RA, et al. Routine operation theatre extubation after cardiac surgery in the elderly. Interact Cardiovasc Thorac Surg. 2016;22:627–32. https://doi.org/10.1093/icvts/ivv409.
9. Cheng DC, et al. Randomized assessment of resource use in fast-track cardiac surgery 1-year after hospital discharge. Anesthesiology. 2003;98:651–7.
10. Djaiani GN, et al. Ultra-fast-track anesthetic technique facilitates operating room extubation in patients undergoing off-pump coronary revascularization surgery. J Cardiothorac Vasc Anesth. 2001;15:152–7. https://doi.org/10.1053/jcan.2001.21936.
11. Kianfar AA, et al. Ultra fast-track extubation in heart transplant surgery patients. Int J Crit Illn Inj Sci. 2015;5:89–92. https://doi.org/10.4103/2229-5151.158394.
12. Meissner U, Scharf J, Dotsch J, Schroth M. Very early extubation after open-heart surgery in children does not influence cardiac function. Pediatr Cardiol. 2008;29:317–20. https://doi.org/10.1007/s00246-007-9023-0.
13. Plumer H, Markewitz A, Marohl K, Bernutz C, Weinhold C. Early extubation after cardiac surgery: a prospective clinical trial including patients at risk. Thorac Cardiovasc Surg. 1998;46:275–80. https://doi.org/10.1055/s-2007-1010238.
14. Svircevic V, et al. Fast-track anesthesia and cardiac surgery: a retrospective cohort study of 7989 patients. Anesth Analg. 2009;108:727–33. https://doi.org/10.1213/ane.0b013e318193c423.
15. Zhu F, Lee A, Chee YE. Fast-track cardiac care for adult cardiac surgical patients. Cochrane Database Syst Rev. 2012;10:CD003587. https://doi.org/10.1002/14651858.CD003587.pub2.
16. Chen L, et al. Fast-track surgery improves postoperative clinical recovery and cellular and humoral immunity after esophagectomy for esophageal cancer. BMC Cancer. 2016;16:449. https://doi.org/10.1186/s12885-016-2506-8.
17. Findlay JM, et al. Enhanced recovery for esophagectomy: a systematic review and evidence-based guidelines. Ann Surg. 2014;259:413–31. https://doi.org/10.1097/SLA.0000000000000349.
18. Findlay JM, et al. The effect of formalizing enhanced recovery after esophagectomy with a protocol. Dis Esophagus. 2015;28:567–73. https://doi.org/10.1111/dote.12234.
19. Zayat R, et al. Benefits of ultra-fast-track anesthesia in left ventricular assist device implantation: a retrospective, propensity score matched cohort study of a four-year single center experience. J Cardiothorac Surg. 2017;12:10. https://doi.org/10.1186/s13019-017-0573-9.
20. Muehling BM, et al. Reduction of postoperative pulmonary complications after lung surgery using a fast track clinical pathway. Eur J Cardiothorac Surg. 2008;34:174–80. https://doi.org/10.1016/j.ejcts.2008.04.009.
21. Das-Neves-Pereira JC, et al. Fast-track rehabilitation for lung cancer lobectomy: a five-year experience. Eur J Cardiothorac Surg.

2009;36:383–91; discussion 391–382. https://doi.org/10.1016/j.ejcts.2009.02.020.

22. Nagahiro I, et al. Pulmonary function, postoperative pain, and serum cytokine level after lobectomy: a comparison of VATS and conventional procedure. Ann Thorac Surg. 2001;72:362–5.

23. Wolk S, et al. Use of activity tracking in major visceral surgery-the Enhanced Perioperative Mobilization (EPM) trial: study protocol for a randomized controlled trial. Trials. 2017;18:77. https://doi.org/10.1186/s13063-017-1782-1.

24. Miralpeix E, et al. A call for new standard of care in perioperative gynecologic oncology practice: Impact of enhanced recovery after surgery (ERAS) programs. Gynecol Oncol. 2016;141:371–8. https://doi.org/10.1016/j.ygyno.2016.02.019.

25. Mehran RJ, Martin LW, Baker CM, Mena GE, Rice DC. Pain management in an enhanced recovery pathway after thoracic surgical procedures. Ann Thorac Surg. 2016;102:e595–6. https://doi.org/10.1016/j.athoracsur.2016.05.050.

26. Rice DC, et al. Posterior intercostal nerve block with liposomal bupivacaine: an alternative to thoracic epidural analgesia. Ann Thorac Surg. 2015;99:1953–60. https://doi.org/10.1016/j.athoracsur.2015.02.074.

27. Meguid RA, et al. Long-term survival outcomes by smoking status in surgical and nonsurgical patients with non-small cell lung cancer: comparing never smokers and current smokers. Chest. 2010;138:500–9. https://doi.org/10.1378/chest.08-2991.

28. Fernandez FG, et al. The Society of Thoracic Surgeons lung cancer resection risk model: higher quality data and superior outcomes. Ann Thorac Surg. 2016;102:370–7. https://doi.org/10.1016/j.athoracsur.2016.02.098.

29. Madani A, et al. An enhanced recovery pathway reduces duration of stay and complications after open pulmonary lobectomy. Surgery. 2015;158:899–908; discussion 908–810. https://doi.org/10.1016/j.surg.2015.04.046.

30. Gimenez-Mila M, Klein AA, Martinez G. Design and implementation of an enhanced recovery program in thoracic surgery. J Thorac Dis. 2016;8:S37–45. https://doi.org/10.3978/j.issn.2072-1439.2015.10.71.

31. Li C, et al. An enhanced recovery pathway decreases duration of stay after esophagectomy. Surgery. 2012;152:606–14; discussion 614–606. https://doi.org/10.1016/j.surg.2012.07.021.

32. Carli F, et al. Randomized clinical trial of prehabilitation in colorectal surgery. Br J Surg. 2010;97:1187–97. https://doi.org/10.1002/bjs.7102.

33. Santa Mina D, et al. Effect of total-body prehabilitation on postoperative outcomes: a systematic review and meta-analysis. Physiotherapy. 2014;100:196–207. https://doi.org/10.1016/j.physio.2013.08.008.

34. Furze G, et al. "Prehabilitation" prior to CABG surgery improves physical functioning and depression. Int J Cardiol. 2009;132:51–8. https://doi.org/10.1016/j.ijcard.2008.06.001.

35. Valkenet K, et al. The effects of preoperative exercise therapy on postoperative outcome: a systematic review. Clin Rehabil. 2011;25:99–111. https://doi.org/10.1177/0269215510380830.

36. Weiner P, et al. Prophylactic inspiratory muscle training in patients undergoing coronary artery bypass graft. World J Surg. 1998;22:427–31.

37. Gillis C, et al. Prehabilitation versus rehabilitation: a randomized control trial in patients undergoing colorectal resection for cancer. Anesthesiology. 2014;121:937–47. https://doi.org/10.1097/ALN.0000000000000393.

38. Tarumi S, et al. Pulmonary rehabilitation during induction chemoradiotherapy for lung cancer improves pulmonary function. J Thorac Cardiovasc Surg. 2015;149:569–73. https://doi.org/10.1016/j.jtcvs.2014.09.123.

39. Nagarajan K, Bennett A, Agostini P, Naidu B. Is preoperative physiotherapy/pulmonary rehabilitation beneficial in lung resection

patients? Interact Cardiovasc Thorac Surg. 2011;13:300–2. https://doi.org/10.1510/icvts.2010.264507.

40. Jones NL, Edmonds L, Ghosh S, Klein AA. A review of enhanced recovery for thoracic anaesthesia and surgery. Anaesthesia. 2013;68:179–89. https://doi.org/10.1111/anae.12067.

41. Ueda K, Tanaka T, Hayashi M, Hamano K. Role of inhaled tiotropium on the perioperative outcomes of patients with lung cancer and chronic obstructive pulmonary disease. Thorac Cardiovasc Surg. 2010;58:38–42. https://doi.org/10.1055/s-0029-1186269.

42. Bolukbas S, Eberlein M, Eckhoff J, Schirren J. Short-term effects of inhalative tiotropium/formoterol/budenoside versus tiotropium/formoterol in patients with newly diagnosed chronic obstructive pulmonary disease requiring surgery for lung cancer: a prospective randomized trial. Eur J Cardiothorac Surg. 2011;39:995–1000. https://doi.org/10.1016/j.ejcts.2010.09.025.

43. Gruffydd-Jones K, Loveridge C. The 2010 NICE COPD Guidelines: how do they compare with the GOLD guidelines? Prim Care Respir J. 2011;20:199–204. https://doi.org/10.4104/pcrj.2011.00011.

44. Gomez Sebastian G, et al. Impact of a rescue program on the operability of patients with bronchogenic carcinoma and chronic obstructive pulmonary disease. Arch Bronconeumol. 2007;43:262–6.

45. Kunisaki C, et al. Immunonutrition risk factors of respiratory complications after esophagectomy. Nutrition. 2004;20:364–7. https://doi.org/10.1016/j.nut.2003.12.008.

46. Han-Geurts IJ, Hop WC, Tran TC, Tilanus HW. Nutritional status as a risk factor in esophageal surgery. Dig Surg. 2006;23:159–63. https://doi.org/10.1159/000093756.

47. Nozoe T, et al. Correlation of pre-operative nutritional condition with post-operative complications in surgical treatment for oesophageal carcinoma. Eur J Surg Oncol. 2002;28:396–400.

48. Weimann A, et al. ESPEN Guidelines on Enteral Nutrition: Surgery including organ transplantation. Clin Nutr. 2006;25:224–44. https://doi.org/10.1016/j.clnu.2006.01.015.

49. Win T, Ritchie AJ, Wells FC, Laroche CM. The incidence and impact of low body mass index on patients with operable lung cancer. Clin Nutr. 2007;26:440–3. https://doi.org/10.1016/j.clnu.2007.01.009.

50. Matzi V, et al. The impact of preoperative micronutrient supplementation in lung surgery. A prospective randomized trial of oral supplementation of combined alpha-ketoglutaric acid and 5-hydroxymethylfurfural. Eur J Cardiothorac Surg. 2007;32:776–82. https://doi.org/10.1016/j.ejcts.2007.07.016.

51. Zhang Y, Gu Y, Guo T, Li Y, Cai H. Perioperative immunonutrition for gastrointestinal cancer: a systematic review of randomized controlled trials. Surg Oncol. 2012;21:e87–95. https://doi.org/10.1016/j.suronc.2012.01.002.

52. Lobo DN, et al. Early postoperative jejunostomy feeding with an immune modulating diet in patients undergoing resectional surgery for upper gastrointestinal cancer: a prospective, randomized, controlled, double-blind study. Clin Nutr. 2006;25:716–26. https://doi.org/10.1016/j.clnu.2006.04.007.

53. Sultan J, et al. Randomized clinical trial of omega-3 fatty acid-supplemented enteral nutrition versus standard enteral nutrition in patients undergoing oesophagogastric cancer surgery. Br J Surg. 2012;99:346–55. https://doi.org/10.1002/bjs.7799.

54. Halabi WJ, et al. Blood transfusions in colorectal cancer surgery: incidence, outcomes, and predictive factors: an American College of Surgeons National Surgical Quality Improvement Program analysis. Am J Surg. 2013;206:1024–32; discussion 1032–1023. https://doi.org/10.1016/j.amjsurg.2013.10.001.

55. Acheson AG, Brookes MJ, Spahn DR. Effects of allogeneic red blood cell transfusions on clinical outcomes in patients undergoing colorectal cancer surgery: a systematic review and meta-analysis. Ann Surg. 2012;256:235–44. https://doi.org/10.1097/SLA.0b013e31825b35d5.

56. Churchhouse AM, Mathews TJ, McBride OM, Dunning J. Does blood transfusion increase the chance of recurrence in patients

undergoing surgery for lung cancer? Interact Cardiovasc Thorac Surg. 2012;14:85–90. https://doi.org/10.1093/icvts/ivr025.

57. Turan A, et al. Smoking and perioperative outcomes. Anesthesiology. 2011;114:837–46. https://doi.org/10.1097/ALN.0b013e318210f560.

58. Alberg AJ, Brock MV, Ford JG, Samet JM, Spivack SD. Epidemiology of lung cancer: diagnosis and management of lung cancer, 3rd ed: American College of Chest Physicians evidence-based clinical practice guidelines. Chest. 2013;143:e1S–29S. https://doi.org/10.1378/chest.12-2345.

59. Mason DP, et al. Impact of smoking cessation before resection of lung cancer: a Society of Thoracic Surgeons General Thoracic Surgery Database study. Ann Thorac Surg. 2009;88:362–70; discussion 370–361. https://doi.org/10.1016/j.athoracsur.2009.04.035.

60. Killoran A, Crombie H, White P, Jones D, Morgan A. NICE public health guidance update. J Public Health (Oxf). 2010;32:451–3. https://doi.org/10.1093/pubmed/fdq057.

61. Zeng L, Yu X, Yu T, Xiao J, Huang Y. Interventions for smoking cessation in people diagnosed with lung cancer. Cochrane Database Syst Rev. 2015:CD011751. https://doi.org/10.1002/14651858.CD011751.pub2.

62. De Cosmo G, Aceto P, Gualtieri E, Congedo E. Analgesia in thoracic surgery: review. Minerva Anestesiol. 2009;75:393–400.

63. Solak O, et al. Effectiveness of gabapentin in the treatment of chronic post-thoracotomy pain. Eur J Cardiothorac Surg. 2007;32:9–12. https://doi.org/10.1016/j.ejcts.2007.03.022.

64. Yoshimura N, et al. Effect of postoperative administration of pregabalin for post-thoracotomy pain: a randomized study. J Cardiothorac Vasc Anesth. 2015;29:1567–72. https://doi.org/10.1053/j.jvca.2015.05.117.

65. Mac TB, et al. Acetaminophen decreases early post-thoracotomy ipsilateral shoulder pain in patients with thoracic epidural analgesia: a double-blind placebo-controlled study. J Cardiothorac Vasc Anesth. 2005;19:475–8. https://doi.org/10.1053/j.jvca.2004.11.041.

66. Wahlander S, et al. A prospective, double-blind, randomized, placebo-controlled study of dexmedetomidine as an adjunct to epidural analgesia after thoracic surgery. J Cardiothorac Vasc Anesth. 2005;19:630–5. https://doi.org/10.1053/j.jvca.2005.07.006.

67. Lee SH, et al. Intraoperative dexmedetomidine improves the quality of recovery and postoperative pulmonary function in patients undergoing video-assisted thoracoscopic surgery: a CONSORT-prospective, randomized, controlled trial. Medicine (Baltimore). 2016;95:e2854. https://doi.org/10.1097/MD.0000000000002854.

68. Joshi GP, et al. A systematic review of randomized trials evaluating regional techniques for postthoracotomy analgesia. Anesth Analg. 2008;107:1026–40. https://doi.org/10.1213/01.ane.0000333274.63501.ff.

69. Teeter EG, Kumar PA. Pro: thoracic epidural block is superior to paravertebral blocks for open thoracic surgery. J Cardiothorac Vasc Anesth. 2015;29:1717–9. https://doi.org/10.1053/j.jvca.2015.06.015.

70. Bauer C, et al. Lung function after lobectomy: a randomized, double-blinded trial comparing thoracic epidural ropivacaine/sufentanil and intravenous morphine for patient-controlled analgesia. Anesth Analg. 2007;105:238–44. https://doi.org/10.1213/01.ane.0000266441.58308.42.

71. Katz J, Jackson M, Kavanagh BP, Sandler AN. Acute pain after thoracic surgery predicts long-term post-thoracotomy pain. Clin J Pain. 1996;12:50–5.

72. El-Tahan MR Role of thoracic epidural analgesia for thoracic surgery and its perioperative effects. J Cardiothorac Vasc Anesth. 2016. https://doi.org/10.1053/j.jvca.2016.09.010.

73. Yeung JH, Gates S, Naidu BV, Wilson MJ, Gao Smith F. Paravertebral block versus thoracic epidural for patients undergoing thoracotomy. Cochrane Database Syst Rev. 2016;2:CD009121. https://doi.org/10.1002/14651858.CD009121.pub2.

74. Khalil KG, et al. Operative intercostal nerve blocks with long-acting bupivacaine liposome for pain control after thoracotomy. Ann Thorac Surg. 2015;100:2013–8. https://doi.org/10.1016/j.athoracsur.2015.08.017.

75. Blanco R, Parras T, McDonnell JG, Prats-Galino A. Serratus plane block: a novel ultrasound-guided thoracic wall nerve block. Anaesthesia. 2013;68:1107–13. https://doi.org/10.1111/anae.12344.

76. Khalil AE, Abdallah NM, Bashandy GM, Kaddah TA. Ultrasound-guided serratus anterior plane block versus thoracic epidural analgesia for thoracotomy pain. J Cardiothorac Vasc Anesth. 2017;31:152–8. https://doi.org/10.1053/j.jvca.2016.08.023.

77. Fleischmann KE, Goldman L, Young B, Lee TH. Association between cardiac and noncardiac complications in patients undergoing noncardiac surgery: outcomes and effects on length of stay. Am J Med. 2003;115:515–20.

78. Law S, Wong KH, Kwok KF, Chu KM, Wong J. Predictive factors for postoperative pulmonary complications and mortality after esophagectomy for cancer. Ann Surg. 2004;240:791–800.

79. Kooguchi K, et al. Elevated expression of inducible nitric oxide synthase and inflammatory cytokines in the alveolar macrophages after esophagectomy. Crit Care Med. 2002;30:71–6.

80. Licker M, et al. Risk factors for acute lung injury after thoracic surgery for lung cancer. Anesth Analg. 2003;97:1558–65.

81. Misthos P, et al. Postresectional pulmonary oxidative stress in lung cancer patients. The role of one-lung ventilation. Eur J Cardiothorac Surg. 2005;27:379–82; discussion 382–373. https://doi.org/10.1016/j.ejcts.2004.12.023.

82. Ng JM. Update on anesthetic management for esophagectomy. Curr Opin Anaesthesiol. 2011;24:37–43. https://doi.org/10.1097/ACO.0b013e32834141f7.

83. Amato MB, et al. Effect of a protective-ventilation strategy on mortality in the acute respiratory distress syndrome. N Engl J Med. 1998;338:347–54. https://doi.org/10.1056/NEJM199802053380602.

84. Lionetti V, Recchia FA, Ranieri VM. Overview of ventilator-induced lung injury mechanisms. Curr Opin Crit Care. 2005;11:82–6.

85. Schilling T, et al. The pulmonary immune effects of mechanical ventilation in patients undergoing thoracic surgery. Anesth Analg. 2005;101:957–65, table of contents,. https://doi.org/10.1213/01.ane.0000172112.02902.77.

86. Michelet P, et al. Protective ventilation influences systemic inflammation after esophagectomy: a randomized controlled study. Anesthesiology. 2006;105:911–9.

87. Mols G, Priebe HJ, Guttmann J. Alveolar recruitment in acute lung injury. Br J Anaesth. 2006;96:156–66. https://doi.org/10.1093/bja/aei299.

88. Sugasawa Y, et al. The effect of one-lung ventilation upon pulmonary inflammatory responses during lung resection. J Anesth. 2011;25:170–7. https://doi.org/10.1007/s00540-011-1100-0.

89. Zingg U, et al. Inflammatory response in ventilated left and collapsed right lungs, serum and pleural fluid, in transthoracic esophagectomy for cancer. Eur Cytokine Netw. 2010;21:50–7. https://doi.org/10.1684/ecn.2009.0180.

90. De Conno E, et al. Anesthetic-induced improvement of the inflammatory response to one-lung ventilation. Anesthesiology. 2009;110:1316–26. https://doi.org/10.1097/ALN.0b013e3181a10731.

91. Schilling T, et al. Effects of propofol and desflurane anaesthesia on the alveolar inflammatory response to one-lung ventilation. Br J Anaesth. 2007;99:368–75. https://doi.org/10.1093/bja/aem184.

92. Sugasawa Y, et al. Effects of sevoflurane and propofol on pulmonary inflammatory responses during lung resection. J Anesth. 2012;26:62–9. https://doi.org/10.1007/s00540-011-1244-y.

93. Blumenthal S, et al. Ropivacaine decreases inflammation in experimental endotoxin-induced lung injury. Anesthesiology. 2006;104:961–9.

94. Brienza N, Giglio MT, Marucci M, Fiore T. Does perioperative hemodynamic optimization protect renal function in surgical patients? A meta-analytic study. Crit Care Med. 2009;37:2079–90. https://doi.org/10.1097/CCM.0b013e3181a00a43.

95. Ishikawa S, Griesdale DE, Lohser J. Acute kidney injury after lung resection surgery: incidence and perioperative risk factors. Anesth Analg. 2012;114:1256–62. https://doi.org/10.1213/ANE.0b013e31824e2d20.

96. Ahn HJ, et al. The risk of acute kidney injury from fluid restriction and hydroxyethyl starch in thoracic surgery. Anesth Analg. 2016;122:186–93. https://doi.org/10.1213/ane.0000000000000974.

97. Giglio MT, Marucci M, Testini M, Brienza N. Goal-directed haemodynamic therapy and gastrointestinal complications in major surgery: a meta-analysis of randomized controlled trials. Br J Anaesth. 2009;103:637–46. https://doi.org/10.1093/bja/aep279.

98. Dalfino L, Giglio MT, Puntillo F, Marucci M, Brienza N. Haemodynamic goal-directed therapy and postoperative infections: earlier is better. A systematic review and meta-analysis. Crit Care (London, England). 2011;15:R154. https://doi.org/10.1186/cc10284.

99. Cecconi M, et al. Clinical review: Goal-directed therapy-what is the evidence in surgical patients? The effect on different risk groups. Crit Care. 2013;17:209. https://doi.org/10.1186/cc11823.

100. Slinger PD. Perioperative fluid management for thoracic surgery: the puzzle of postpneumonectomy pulmonary edema. J Cardiothorac Vasc Anesth. 1995;9:442–51.

101. Nomori H, Horio H, Suemasu K. Early removal of chest drainage tubes and oxygen support after a lobectomy for lung cancer facilitates earlier recovery of the 6-minute walking distance. Surg Today. 2001;31:395–9. https://doi.org/10.1007/s005950170128.

102. Deng B, Tan QY, Zhao YP, Wang RW, Jiang YG. Suction or non-suction to the underwater seal drains following pulmonary operation: meta-analysis of randomised controlled trials. Eur J Cardiothorac Surg. 2010;38:210–5. https://doi.org/10.1016/j.ejcts.2010.01.050.

103. Lagarde SM, et al. Predictive factors associated with prolonged chest drain production after esophagectomy. Dis Esophagus. 2007;20:24–8. https://doi.org/10.1111/j.1442-2050.2007.00639.x.

104. Hessami MA, Najafi F, Hatami S. Volume threshold for chest tube removal: a randomized controlled trial. J Inj Violence Res. 2009;1:33–6. https://doi.org/10.5249/jivr.v1i1.5.

105. Younes RN, Gross JL, Aguiar S, Haddad FJ, Deheinzelin D. When to remove a chest tube? A randomized study with subsequent prospective consecutive validation. J Am Coll Surg. 2002;195:658–62.

106. Gomez-Caro A, et al. Successful use of a single chest drain postlobectomy instead of two classical drains: a randomized study. Eur J Cardiothorac Surg. 2006;29:562–6. https://doi.org/10.1016/j.ejcts.2006.01.019.

107. Pawelczyk K, Marciniak M, Kacprzak G, Kolodziej J. One or two drains after lobectomy? A comparison of both methods in the immediate postoperative period. Thorac Cardiovasc Surg. 2007;55:313–6. https://doi.org/10.1055/s-2007-964930.

108. Alex J, et al. Comparison of the immediate postoperative outcome of using the conventional two drains versus a single drain after lobectomy. Ann Thorac Surg. 2003;76:1046–9.

109. Dawson AG, Hosmane S. Should you place one or two chest drains in patients undergoing lobectomy? Interact Cardiovasc Thorac Surg. 2010;11:178–81. https://doi.org/10.1510/icvts.2010.235853.

110. Belda-Sanchis J, Serra-Mitjans M, Iglesias Sentis M, Rami R. Surgical sealant for preventing air leaks after pulmonary resections in patients with lung cancer. Cochrane Database Syst Rev. 2010:CD003051. https://doi.org/10.1002/14651858.CD003051.pub3.

111. Kortebein P, et al. Functional impact of 10 days of bed rest in healthy older adults. J Gerontol A Biol Sci Med Sci. 2008;63:1076–81.

112. Kaneda H, et al. Early postoperative mobilization with walking at 4 hours after lobectomy in lung cancer patients. Gen Thorac Cardiovasc Surg. 2007;55:493–8. https://doi.org/10.1007/s11748-007-0169-8.

113. Garcia-Miguel FJ, Serrano-Aguilar PG, Lopez-Bastida J. Preoperative assessment. Lancet. 2003;362:1749–57.

114. Lumb AB, Nunn JF. Nunn's applied respiratory physiology. 6th ed. Edinburgh: Elsevier/Butterworth Heinemann; 2005.

115. Agostini P, Singh S. Incentive spirometry following thoracic surgery: what should we be doing? Physiotherapy. 2009;95:76–82. https://doi.org/10.1016/j.physio.2008.11.003.

116. Glattki GP, et al. Pulmonary rehabilitation in non-small cell lung cancer patients after completion of treatment. Am J Clin Oncol. 2012;35:120–5. https://doi.org/10.1097/COC.0b013e318209ced7.

117. Varela G, Ballesteros E, Jimenez MF, Novoa N, Aranda JL. Cost-effectiveness analysis of prophylactic respiratory physiotherapy in pulmonary lobectomy. Eur J Cardiothorac Surg. 2006;29:216–20. https://doi.org/10.1016/j.ejcts.2005.11.002.

118. Weiner P, et al. The effect of incentive spirometry and inspiratory muscle training on pulmonary function after lung resection. J Thorac Cardiovasc Surg. 1997;113:552–7. https://doi.org/10.1016/S0022-5223(97)70370-2.

119. Carvalho CR, Paisani DM, Lunardi AC. Incentive spirometry in major surgeries: a systematic review. Rev Bras Fisioter. 2011;15:343–50.

120. Lawrence VA, Cornell JE, Smetana GW, American College of, P. Strategies to reduce postoperative pulmonary complications after noncardiothoracic surgery: systematic review for the American College of Physicians. Ann Intern Med. 2006;144:596–608.

121. Zakkar M, Frazer S, Hunt I. Is there a role for gabapentin in preventing or treating pain following thoracic surgery? Interact Cardiovasc Thorac Surg. 2013;17:716–9. https://doi.org/10.1093/icvts/ivt301.

122. Alawadi ZM, et al. Facilitators and barriers of implementing enhanced recovery in colorectal surgery at a safety net hospital: a provider and patient perspective. Surgery. 2016;159:700–12. https://doi.org/10.1016/j.surg.2015.08.025.

123. Gotlib Conn L, McKenzie M, Pearsall EA, McLeod RS. Successful implementation of an enhanced recovery after surgery programme for elective colorectal surgery: a process evaluation of champions' experiences. Implement Sci. 2015;10:99. https://doi.org/10.1186/s13012-015-0289-y.

124. Lyon A, Solomon MJ, Harrison JD. A qualitative study assessing the barriers to implementation of enhanced recovery after surgery. World J Surg. 2014;38:1374–80. https://doi.org/10.1007/s00268-013-2441-7.

125. Carli F, Zavorsky GS. Optimizing functional exercise capacity in the elderly surgical population. Curr Opin Clin Nutr Metab Care. 2005;8(1):25.

Anesthetic Management of Post-thoracotomy Complications

53

Michael A. Hall and Jesse M. Raiten

Key Points

- The immediate postoperative period following thoracic surgery is a dynamic time characterized by rapidly changing physiology. Anesthetic and surgical complications may become evident and may require immediate intervention.
- Although most patients undergoing thoracic surgery are extubated immediately following surgery, preexisting lung disease may necessitate postoperative mechanical ventilation. Patients remaining intubated postoperatively should be weaned to ventilator modes that promote spontaneous ventilation and low airway pressures, and they should be assessed frequently for extubation criteria.
- Airway-related complications are not uncommon and may be due to anesthetic or surgical technique. The large caliber of double-lumen endotracheal tubes may increase the risk of airway injury. Glottic injury and airway bleeding may also occur.
- Intrathoracic complications range from relatively minor air leaks to life-threatening bronchopleural fistulas. Preoperative prophylaxis against deep vein thrombosis helps prevent pulmonary embolism. Other complications such as phrenic nerve injury may become evident immediately postoperatively or after a prolonged period of mechanical ventilation in the ICU.

- Atrial fibrillation is a very common complication following thoracic surgery. Its management depends on the patient's hemodynamic status. New-onset postoperative atrial fibrillation should prompt a thorough review of the patient's overall well-being. Other cardiac complications are less common, including cardiac herniation and interatrial shunting.

Introduction

The immediate postoperative period following thoracotomy is characterized by rapidly changing physiology, during which careful management and attention to possible surgical or anesthetic complications is necessary. The normal physiological changes associated with emergence from anesthesia and mechanical ventilation may be less predictable in a patient having just undergone thoracic surgery. Patients undergoing thoracic procedures often have multiple comorbidities and poor baseline lung function. The surgeries can be long, may be associated with significant blood loss, and risk damage to intrathoracic structures including the lungs, airway, great vessels, and peripheral nervous system. Thoracic surgery may also cause significant stress on the cardiovascular system. Many factors may preclude the patient's immediate liberation from mechanical ventilation, and anesthetic or surgical complications may become evident in the operating room or shortly after arrival in the recovery room or intensive care unit (ICU). In this chapter, we will explore some of the common management challenges and potential complications that may be encountered in the immediate postoperative period following thoracotomy.

M. A. Hall
Anesthesia Services, P.A., Department of Anesthesiology,
Christiana Care Health System,
Newark, DE, USA

J. M. Raiten (✉)
Department of Anesthesiology and Critical Care,
Perelman School of Medicine at the University of Pennsylvania,
Philadelphia, PA, USA
jesse.raiten@uphs.upenn.edu

© Springer Nature Switzerland AG 2019
P. Slinger (ed.), *Principles and Practice of Anesthesia for Thoracic Surgery*, https://doi.org/10.1007/978-3-030-00859-8_53

Mechanical Ventilation and Extubation

Classification of Respiratory Failure

The decision regarding tracheal extubation of a patient following surgery must take into account many variables. Patients requiring mechanical ventilation all have respiratory failure that falls into one (or more) of the following four categories [1].

1. *Type I* (hypoxemic respiratory failure) is characterized by $PaO_2 < 60$ mmHg at sea level.
2. *Type II* (hypercapnic respiratory failure) is characterized by $PaCO_2 > 45$ mmHg.
3. *Type III* (perioperative respiratory failure) is due to increased atelectasis and low functional residual capacity (FRC). This may occur in the setting of abnormal respiratory muscle mechanics, and may precipitate Types I or II failure.
4. *Type IV* (respiratory failure secondary to shock) may be present when mechanical ventilation is utilized to decrease oxygen consumption and increase oxygen delivery in the setting of resuscitation and shock.

Criteria for Extubation

Patients immediately post-thoracotomy may experience any of these types of respiratory failure, although Types I, II, and III are more likely than Type IV. All patients emerging from anesthesia who require continued mechanical ventilation suffer, to some extent, from Type III failure. Even patients with healthy lungs experience hypoxemia secondary to airway closure and atelectasis [2]. Indeed, collapsed lung tissue is observed in 90% of patients under anesthesia [3]. Residual anesthetics and neuromuscular blocking agents may also contribute to hypoventilation and subsequent hypoxemia and hypercarbia. In patients requiring one-lung ventilation for thoracic surgery, changes in ventilation and perfusion may be even more pronounced on account of the delayed offset of hypoxic pulmonary vasoconstriction in the operative lung, placing patients at higher risk of hypoxia [4]. While recruitment maneuvers on the ventilator may be useful to expand portions of collapsed lung tissue [3], patients with poor baseline lung function may not tolerate extubation at the conclusion of surgery because of hypoxia attributable to a combination of Types I and III respiratory failure. These patients may require continued mechanical ventilation postoperatively until adequate gas exchange can be reestablished.

Patients may also fail extubation due to impaired CO_2 removal. In the case of thoracic surgery, pain from a thoracotomy incision may prevent deep breathing and adequate CO_2 elimination. Epidural analgesia is very effective at controlling post-thoracotomy pain and minimizing postoperative hypercarbia [5]. In cases where thoracotomy is unplanned, epidural placement at the end of surgery, or shortly after extubation, may help reduce the need for reintubation [6].

Complications of Prolonged Intubation and Mechanical Ventilation

In 2001, a task force (represented by the American College of Chest Physicians, the American Association for Respiratory Care, and the American College of Critical Care Medicine) established guidelines for the assessment and implementation of discontinuation of patients from mechanical ventilation [7]. These guidelines call for evidence of the resolution of the underlying cause of respiratory failure, adequate oxygenation ($PaO_2/FiO_2 > 150$–200, PEEP ≤ 5–8 cmH$_2$O, FiO$_2 \leq 0.4$–0.5), adequate pH (≥ 7.25), hemodynamic stability, and the capability to initiate spontaneous ventilation. Patients meeting these criteria may then undergo a formal spontaneous breathing trial (SBT) for 30–120 min. More recently published guidelines of ventilator liberation in critically ill adults suggest utilizing a ventilator liberation protocol, checking for an endotracheal tube (ETT) cuff leak in patients at risk for stridor, and considering systemic steroids in patients who fail a cuff leak test but are otherwise stable for extubation [8].

Those who successfully pass an SBT have a high likelihood of tolerating extubation, and assessment of the patient's ability to protect the airway, mental status, and likelihood of airway obstruction should be performed prior to removal of the endotracheal tube [9]. Although not a guarantee, an intact gag reflex and alert state of mind suggest the patient will be able to protect the airway against aspiration. This may not be true in the case of vocal cord injury, however [10]. Aspiration risk may be better assessed after extubation via a flexible endoscopic evaluation of swallowing with sensory testing (FEESST) examination [11].

While extubation in the immediate postoperative period requires fulfilling many of the abovementioned criteria, emergence from anesthesia is a rapid and dynamic process, and assessment of these variables may be made on a minute-to-minute basis. Additional physiologic parameters are also assessed, including tidal volume (desire 5–10 cc/kg), respiratory rate (≤ 20 breaths/min), body temperature, electrolytes, and volume status.

When comparing predictors of a successful extubation, two useful tests are the rapid shallow breathing index (RSBI, respiratory rate/tidal volume) and the negative inspiratory force (NIF). While an NIF >20 cmH$_2$O does not guarantee a successful extubation, a poor performance in this test usually predicts failure [12]. In a review of studies of factors associated with ventilator weaning, a RSBI <105 breaths/min/L had a sensitivity up to 96% and specificity up to 73% for prediction of a successful extubation [13].

In patients immediately after lung resection, a prompt transition from positive pressure ventilation to spontaneous breathing is usually desirable in light of new suture lines or staples within the tracheobronchial tree. In practice, the majority of patients undergoing thoracic surgery are extubated in the operating room.

In a retrospective study of 214 patients undergoing lung transplantation, the need for mechanical ventilation for greater than 72 h was identified as an independent risk factor for airway complications [14], and early postoperative extubation may help reduce this risk [15]. Following esophagectomy, early extubation has been shown to be safe and lead to short ICU lengths of stay [16, 17]. Similarly, immediate extubation following tracheal surgery has yielded good results. In a retrospective review of 60 patients undergoing tracheal resection and reconstruction, all but one patient was successfully extubated in the operating room [18]. Likewise, extubation in the operating room immediately following lung resection has been shown to be safe, reduce the risk of postoperative complications, decrease time in the ICU, and reduce hospital costs [19].

Adverse effects associated with intubation and mechanical ventilation include ventilator-associated pneumonia (VAP), laryngeal and tracheal injury, hemodynamic changes, patient discomfort and the need for sedation, and difficulty obtaining an accurate neurologic examination [20].

Independent Lung Ventilation

While severe unilateral lung disease in the postoperative setting is uncommon, it may occur following single lung transplantation or pneumonectomy (Fig. 53.1). In the case of lung transplantation, independent lung ventilation in the ICU may be necessary to allow different ventilation strategies to each lung. Independent lung ventilation requires a double-lumen endotracheal tube (DLT). DLTs are rarely utilized outside of the OR as they are technically more difficult to manage and require constant attention to ensure proper position, and their larger size makes laryngeal and tracheal trauma more likely compared to single-lumen tubes. The narrower lumen can make it more difficult to perform bronchoscopy and endotracheal suctioning. Nevertheless, in cases of severe unilateral acute respiratory distress syndrome (ARDS), as may occur after lung transplantation, the ability to provide different tidal volumes and oxygen concentrations to each lung may be critical to patient management.

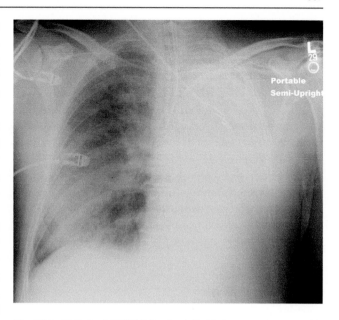

Fig. 53.1 Unilateral ARDS following left-sided pneumonectomy

Airway Complications

Endotracheal Intubation and Airway Injury

Airway complications following thoracic surgery may be related to anesthetic or surgical technique. The larger external diameter and more invasive positioning of DLTs may increase the likelihood of airway trauma compared to a single-lumen ETT. Anesthetic-related airway complications that may become apparent immediately postoperatively include injury to dentition, sore throat, laryngeal trauma, bronchial erythema and edema, vocal cord injury, and tracheobronchial rupture (TBR). Risk factors associated with vocal cord injury include intubating conditions, type of surgery, and endotracheal tube size, among others [21].

In a study comparing DLT to bronchial blockers in patients undergoing pulmonary resection, the overall incidence of bronchial and vocal cord injury was 25% and 30%, respectively [21]. In both cases, the most common injuries were erythema and edema. Severe complications such as TBR are unusual, with an estimated incidence between 0.05% and 0.37% for all intubations at a single institution [22], and this risk is increased with the use of a DLT versus a SLT [23]. Symptoms of TBR include neck emphysema and hemoptysis, and may be identified as an increase in fresh gas flow requirements intraoperatively. Surgical factors are also important when assessing the risk of TBR, as tracheal perforation has a reported incidence of 0.4% during transhiatal esophagectomy at high-volume centers [23].

Airway Bleeding and Secretions

The nature of the surgical procedures and proximity to structures vital to proper respiratory function make patients undergoing thoracic surgeries particularly prone to airway injuries and complications. The blood and secretions may accumulate in the upper or lower airways in patients undergoing lung resection surgery. Removal of the blood by endotracheal suctioning may be difficult in a patient with a DLT, and a pediatric-sized bronchoscope may be necessary to pass through the tube's narrow lumen. If significant secretions and debris are present within the airways, changing the DLT to a larger diameter single-lumen ETT may better facilitate pulmonary toilet prior to emergence and extubation.

Vocal Cord Injuries

Vocal cord palsies may occur in patients undergoing mediastinoscopy or esophagectomy, with an incidence between 1–6% and 5–22%, respectively [24]. Damage to the recurrent laryngeal nerve may occur intraoperatively from traction in the anterior mediastinum [24], or from direct trauma to the nerve. Unilateral vocal cord paralysis may result in voice changes, but usually does not result in airway obstruction. While bilateral vocal cord injury is rare except in the case of neck surgery, it has been reported following lung resection under video-assisted thoracic surgery (VATS) [25]. In this case report, vocal cord injury may have resulted from the DLT. Bilateral vocal cord injury may lead to dyspnea and stridor. Unilateral and bilateral injuries will increase the risk of aspiration [10].

Vocal cord injuries may also be attributed to the act of orotracheal intubation or the subsequent presence of the ETT, especially after prolonged intubation. Vocal cord hematoma or edema can cause dyspnea, stridor, and partial or complete airway obstruction. Luxation of the arytenoid cartilage during passage of the ETT through the glottis can result in unilateral vocal cord immobility without neurologic injury [26]. Tapia's syndrome, or unilateral vocal cord palsy, can present after short-term intubation, most likely secondary to compression of the recurrent laryngeal nerve between the ETT and the thyroid cartilage [27].

Prompt recognition of vocal cord injury in the extubated patient is critical to prevent potentially life-threatening airway obstruction. While a hoarse voice is relatively common after endotracheal intubation, the presence of stridor or respiratory distress is abnormal, and a sign indicating a more serious process may be occurring. Prompt intubation may be the safest approach to the patient in acute, severe respiratory distress, particularly if it presents in the immediate postoperative period. However, it is difficult to examine the vocal cords in an intubated patient.

If symptoms are mild and the patient remains stable, it is reasonable to treat the patient conservatively with oxygen by mask, steroids, and racemic epinephrine. The vocal cords may then be examined by flexible fiber-optic laryngoscopy in cases with a high clinical suspicion of vocal cord injury or palsy. Heliox is a mixture of helium and oxygen (usually 70% helium and 30% oxygen) that has a lower density than air with a similar viscosity. Work of breathing is affected by the resistance to flow within the airway and the pressure gradient that must be generated to produce flow. Narrowing of the airway, such as at the glottis after vocal cord paralysis or swelling, will increase resistance to flow in itself, and it will also increase the tendency of inspired gas to generate turbulent flow. Turbulent flow generates higher resistance than laminar flow within the same airway, further increasing work of breathing. The lower density of heliox will lower the Reynolds number of the gas flow in the airway, increasing the likelihood of laminar flow. Other parameters of fluid mechanics, including the formula for calculation of orifice flow and the application of Bernoulli's principle, support the assertion that the decreased density of heliox relative to mixtures of oxygen and nitrogen will lead to increased flow, decreased resistance, and decreased pressure requirements to generate gas flow through a partially obstructed glottis [28]. Its effects may be seen very rapidly. Most studies of heliox are in the pediatric population. One additional complication for thoracic surgery patients is that underlying lung parenchymal disease may reveal the obligate 0.30 FiO_2 of heliox to be inadequate to maintain oxygenation, thus requiring airway intubation to bypass the obstructed glottis and deliver higher concentrations of oxygen.

Intrathoracic Complications

Patients requiring thoracic surgery are among the sickest patients in the hospital – many are diabetic, have chronic obstructive pulmonary disease (COPD), and coronary artery disease (CAD). Despite optimal preoperative evaluation and intraoperative technique, the high acuity of this patient population contributes to the significant rate of postoperative surgical complications. Common complications include persistent air leak, pneumothorax, and atrial fibrillation. Other complications include bronchopleural fistula (BPF), pulmonary embolism, postpneumonectomy syndrome, phrenic nerve injury, cardiac herniation, massive hemorrhage, mediastinal emphysema, and intracardiac shunting.

Air Leak, Pneumothorax, and Bronchopleural Fistula

Postoperative air leaks are common after thoracic surgery and can be easily recognized by the presence of bubbles in the water seal chamber of the drainage system. The presence of an air leak with a properly positioned chest tube indicates that air is passing from the pleural space into the drainage system. If the chest tube has been placed for a pneumothorax, an air leak signifies the pneumothorax is being successfully evacuated, and the leak should resolve as the pneumothorax improves.

Any surgery in which the pleural space is entered leads to the creation of a pneumothorax. A pneumothorax that remains in communication with atmospheric pressure is rarely dangerous. If it is not in communication with the atmosphere, a tension pneumothorax may develop. A tension pneumothorax may rapidly expand in a patient receiving positive pressure ventilation, leading to hemodynamic collapse.

When the lung parenchyma is cut, as in the case of a lobectomy, an air leak may be caused by small fistulas between the distal airways and the pleural space. This should resolve as the lung tissue heals and becomes apposed to the parietal pleura. In patients with COPD, a new air leak may be caused by rupture of a pulmonary bleb. An inadequate seal at the site of chest tube exit from the skin may also allow air to track back to the pleural space and communicate with the drainage system.

In the immediate postoperative period small air leaks rarely cause problems. In patients having undergone pneumonectomy, however, a large new air leak can indicate rupture of the bronchial stump and creation of a bronchopleural fistula (BPF). There may be significant mediastinal shift toward the remaining lung, as well as subcutaneous emphysema. This is a surgical emergency that requires immediate attention. In a retrospective study of patients undergoing pneumonectomy, 1.9% developed BPF [29]. Two-thirds of these patients died. The diameter of the bronchial stump has also been associated with postpneumonectomy BPF [30], and right-sided pneumonectomy has a higher incidence of developing a BPF than left-sided pneumonectomy [31]. Other risk factors include malnutrition, history of chemotherapy or radiation treatment, active smoking, and untreated pulmonary infection. Chest radiograph of a postpneumonectomy patient who develops a BPF will demonstrate a decrease in the air-fluid level on the operative side, usually with the meniscus at the level of the bronchial stump.

While many pneumonectomy patients are extubated immediately after surgery in the operating room, it is not uncommon to remain intubated postoperatively in the ICU. A prompt extubation and transition from positive pressure to spontaneous ventilation is important to help reduce intrathoracic pressure. If a BPF does occur, and is associated with hemodynamic and respiratory instability, intubation with either a DLT or single-lumen ETT placed into the main stem bronchus is a reasonable approach to secure the airway. The latter approach is easier on the left side due to the greater distance between the carina and branching of the left upper and lower lobes. Again, spontaneous ventilation, or the use of very low inspiratory pressures, is desirable.

Mediastinal Emphysema

Mediastinal emphysema occurs when air accumulates in the mediastinal space. It may occur with airway, alveolar, or esophageal rupture, or following intrathoracic surgery. Patients may present with dyspnea or subcutaneous emphysema, and the diagnosis can be readily obtained with chest radiography or CT scan. Often, no treatment is necessary, although a chest tube may be placed if a pneumothorax is present. In the case of esophageal rupture, immediate surgical repair or esophageal stenting may be necessary.

Deep Vein Thrombosis and Pulmonary Embolism

Deep vein thrombosis (DVT) and pulmonary embolism (PE) are potentially fatal complications that may follow thoracic surgery. In a review of 690 patients undergoing chest surgery for malignant lung disease, there were 12 (1.7%) venous thromboembolic complications, of which 9 (1.3%) were PE [32]. All events occurred in patients who were receiving DVT prophylaxis with heparin. Prolonged surgical times and malignancy are risk factors for the development of DVT that are common to many patients undergoing thoracic surgery. Antithrombotic prophylaxis with heparin (either low molecular weight or unfractionated) has become common practice in the perioperative period.

A high index of suspicion is necessary to ensure detection of DVT and PE, as many PE are subclinical and only detected at autopsy. The initial chest radiograph is often normal in patients with PE. Pulmonary angiography represents the gold standard diagnostic technique. However, computed tomography angiography (CT angiogram) is easier to perform and is the most commonly employed technique for PE diagnosis. Ventilation-perfusion scans are less widely used as the results may be difficult to interpret. In the presence of a large PE with hemodynamic compromise, right ventricular dilatation and strain may be seen on echocardiogram.

When a clinically significant PE does occur, a variety of therapies may be employed including operative embolectomy [33], catheter embolectomy, systemic anticoagulation, or thrombolytic administration. The decision of how to proceed depends on a variety of factors including the size of the embolus, the location within the pulmonary vasculature, and the hemodynamic status of the patient.

Postpneumonectomy Syndrome

Postpneumonectomy syndrome is an uncommon condition that may be observed following left- or right-sided pneumonectomy [34]. It is characterized by a mediastinal shift toward the side of the resected lung, with associated herniation of the overinflated remaining lung in the same direction. Subsequent compression of the distal trachea or main stem bronchus against the vertebral column or aorta may cause airway compression and obstruction [35].

Patients may present with progressive dyspnea, stridor, or heartburn and dysphagia if esophageal compression develops [34]. Symptoms develop months to years after a pneumonectomy. A high index of suspicion is necessary to make the diagnosis, which may be confirmed with a variety of techniques including awake bronchoscopy, pulmonary function tests, and CT scan. Treatment often involves mediastinal repositioning with expandable saline prostheses [36]. A recent case series reported nine out of ten patients had symptomatic improvement after placement of tissue expanders within the operative hemithorax and were discharged home without supplemental oxygen therapy [37].

Post Lung Resection Pulmonary Edema

Post lung resection pulmonary edema is a serious complication that carries a mortality rate greater than 50% [38]. In a series of 146 patients who underwent pneumonectomy, mild to moderate noncardiogenic pulmonary edema was observed in 15% of patients and was strongly associated with previous radiotherapy and excess intraoperative volume administration [39]. The incidence of pulmonary edema is higher following right pneumonectomy compared to left, with clinical symptoms typically appearing between postoperative day (POD) 2–4. While an association with excess fluid administration exists, pulmonary artery occlusion pressure (PAOP) is often low, suggesting a multifactorial etiology [38]. Pulmonary edema may also follow lobectomy, although this is less common.

Post lung resection pulmonary edema is a diagnosis of exclusion, and all other etiologies of pulmonary congestion must be ruled out (heart failure, pulmonary aspiration, sepsis, pulmonary embolism, transfusion reaction). As with cardiac herniation, a high level of suspicion is necessary to make the diagnosis. Once identified, treatment is largely supportive and may include high-dose corticosteroids and the use of pulmonary artery vasodilators [40] or extracorporeal ventilatory support.

Phrenic Nerve Injury

Phrenic nerve injury may occur in patients undergoing thoracic surgery. Both hypothermia (associated with pericardial cooling in cardiac surgery) and mechanical trauma may be contributing factors [41]. Injury to the phrenic nerve is associated with diaphragmatic dysfunction. Unilateral diaphragmatic paralysis is often well tolerated by patients without significant underlying pulmonary disease [42]. However,

thoracic surgery patients often have poor baseline lung function, and difficulty weaning from the ventilator may be the first sign that phrenic nerve injury has occurred. An elevated hemidiaphragm may also be observed on chest radiography, and the diagnosis can be confirmed by electromyography. In severe cases, techniques such as diaphragmatic pacing may be useful [42]. Abnormal diaphragmatic motion postoperatively has been associated with diminished lung volumes and reduced exercise capacity [43].

Cardiac Complications

Cardiac Failure and Arrhythmias

Thoracic surgery places a considerable stress on the cardiovascular system and postoperative cardiac complications are not uncommon. Patients often have preexisting cardiac disease and may be at risk for perioperative myocardial infarction (MI) and heart failure. Adequate preoperative evaluation and optimization of cardiac function may decrease these risks. In a patient with risk factors, postoperative hemodynamic instability should trigger an evaluation of cardiac status.

Arrhythmias are a common cardiac complication following thoracic surgery, with atrial fibrillation (AF) being the most prevalent. The incidence of AF may reach 20% after lobectomy and as high as 40% following pneumonectomy [44]. It is unclear whether postoperative supraventricular tachycardias (SVT) worsen patient outcome. In an observational study of 82 patients undergoing elective thoracotomy, there was no association between SVT and myocardial ischemia or adverse outcome [45].

AF complicating lung cancer resection has been associated with increased hospital length of stay, costs, and in-hospital mortality [46]. While AF is often relatively asymptomatic and easy to treat, its onset must not be ignored. Roselli and colleagues identified a temporal association between the onset of AF and other complications, particularly respiratory and infectious in etiology [46]. New-onset postoperative AF in the immediate postoperative period should prompt a thorough review of the patient's overall condition.

Management of postoperative AF is well described in the literature and largely dictated by the patient's hemodynamic status (Fig. 53.2). There is some controversy regarding what should be the initial therapy (rate or rhythm control) for new-onset postoperative AF in patients who are hemodynamically stable. A large randomized trial recently conducted in patients with new-onset postoperative AF after cardiac surgery found that the two strategies were largely equivocal [47]. In hemodynamically unstable patients, rhythm control is preferred. The use of amiodarone in

Fig. 53.2 Treatment
algorithm for new-onset
postoperative atrial fibrillation

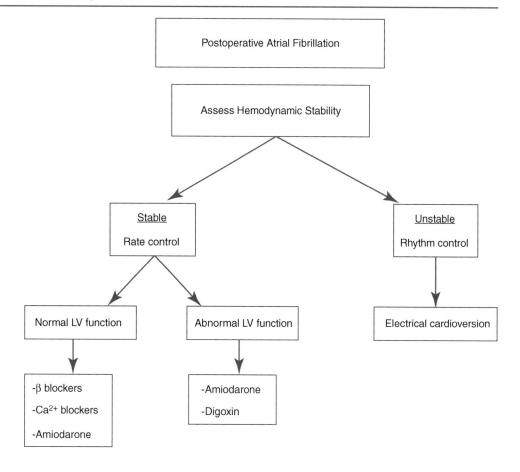

patients having undergone lung transplant is relatively common despite its potential pulmonary toxicity. Amiodarone-induced pulmonary toxicity correlates with total dose administered and is more common after 2 months of therapy [48]. Judicious use in the perioperative period may be justified in the appropriate clinical situation.

Cardiac Herniation

Cardiac herniation is a rare and potentially lethal complication of thoracic procedures, most commonly occurring within 24 h following intrapericardial pneumonectomy [49]. Sudden hypotension and tachycardia should trigger the physician to consider the diagnosis. In the case of right-sided herniation, central venous pressure (CVP) may be elevated, and cyanosis of the face and neck is common and related to impaired venous drainage by the superior vena cava (SVC) [50]. This impaired drainage may reduce cardiac filling and lead to obstructive shock. Left-sided herniation can lead to myocardial ischemia and arrhythmias due to ventricular strangulation by the pericardial edges [51].

Herniation may be triggered by multiple factors. Positive intrathoracic pressure (due to coughing or mechanical ventilation), suction on a chest tube, or even patient reposi-

tioning may be contributing factors [51]. A prompt diagnosis is critical and may be obtained by chest radiography (easier to diagnose right-sided herniation than left), or echocardiogram. Immediate surgical repositioning of the heart and closure of the pericardial defect is necessary.

It should be noted that while cardiac herniation typically presents with rapidly deteriorating hemodynamics, this is not universally the case. Buniva and colleagues describe a patient in which cardiac herniation and torsion developed following right-sided pneumonectomy and partial pericardiectomy [52]. In this case, the patient remained hemodynamically stable, and herniation was detected 2 h later on routine chest radiography. Herniation has also been reported 6 months following pneumonectomy [53]; however, this is exceedingly uncommon. Adhesions between the heart and pericardium help prevent delayed herniation [51]. Along with the risk of bronchial stump rupture, the risk of cardiac herniation underscores the importance of a prompt transition to spontaneous ventilation in patients following pneumonectomy.

Interatrial Shunting

Interatrial shunting (right to left) is a rare cause of hypoxemia in patients having undergone pneumonectomy. The exact pathophysiology is poorly understood but may involve the development of a right- to left-sided pressure gradient or decreased compliance of the right ventricle relative to the left [54]. Shunting across an atrial septal defect (ASD) occurs primarily during diastole, and right to left blood flow may be accentuated by a stiffer right ventricle [54]. Case reports of shunting after pneumonectomy highlight three common features: a positional nature of the shunt, whereby it is worsened when the patient is upright (platypnea), an asymptomatic interval following surgery, and an increased shunt fraction with hypovolemia [55]. Diagnosis of interatrial shunting can be readily made by echocardiogram.

Clinical Case Discussion

A 67-year-old man is in the ICU 4 h following left-sided pneumonectomy for lung cancer. His medical history is significant for a 50-pack-year smoking history and ischemic cardiomyopathy with a left ventricular ejection fraction of 30%. At the end of the surgery, he was oxygenating poorly with a PaO_2 55 mmHg on 100% inspired oxygen and is currently receiving mechanical ventilation in the ICU. His EKG changes from sinus rhythm to rapid atrial fibrillation with a heart rate of 144 bpm, and his blood pressure falls to 60/40. You are called emergently to the bedside.

Questions

- What type of respiratory failure is this patient suffering from?
- Why is it important to extubate this patient and reestablish spontaneous ventilation in a timely fashion?
- How would you assess and treat this patient when you are called to the bedside?

Respiratory failure, extubation, and assessment of atrial fibrillation:

- Type III respiratory failure (perioperative), likely due to atelectasis from anesthesia and positive pressure ventilation, hypoxia, and hypercarbia from baseline lung disease (see section "Classification of Respiratory Failure").
- Improved hemodynamics, decreased ventilator-associated pneumonia, lower risk of surgical suture line damage, and development of a bronchopleural fistula (see sections "Complications of Prolonged Intubation and Mechanical Ventilation," and "Intrathoracic Complications").
- Assess patient's overall condition and search for possible etiology of new-onset postoperative atrial fibrillation. Hemodynamically unstable atrial fibrillation should be

treated with electrical cardioversion (see section "Cardiac Complications" and Fig. 53.2).

Weaning from mechanical ventilation:

- When postoperative patients require mechanical ventilation, it is usually temporary and they should be frequently assessed for extubation.
- Evaluate respiratory rate, tidal volume, oxygen and positive end expiratory pressure (PEEP) requirements, level of consciousness, hemodynamic stability, volume status, pH and CO_2 levels, ability to cough and clear secretions, analgesia, temperature, and electrolyte status (see section "Classification of Respiratory Failure").
- The rapid shallow breathing index and negative inspiratory force may help predict whether a patient will tolerate extubation. When a patient meets extubation criteria, a spontaneous breathing trial should be attempted (see section "Criteria for Extubation").

Considerations with new-onset postoperative atrial fibrillation:

- New-onset postoperative atrial fibrillation is common after pneumonectomy.
- Patients should undergo a complete evaluation of their overall well-being, including a search for underlying infection, volume status, hypoxia and hypercarbia, and electrolyte abnormalities, particularly hypokalemia and hypomagnesemia (see section "Cardiac Complications").
- Patients who are hemodynamically stable may be managed medically with rate or rhythm control, while hemodynamically unstable patients should be electrically cardioverted (Fig. 53.2).

References

1. Naureckas E, Wood L. The pathophysiology and differential diagnosis of acute respiratory failure. In: Hall J, Schmidt G, Kress J, editors. Principles of critical care. 4th ed. New York, NY: McGraw-Hill; 2014. p. 370–6.
2. Rothen HU, Sporre B, Engberg G, Wegenius G, Hedenstierna G. Airway closure, atelectasis and gas exchange during general anaesthesia. Br J Anaesth. 1998;81(5):681–6.
3. Hedenstierna G, Rothen HU. Atelectasis formation during anesthesia: causes and measures to prevent it. J Clin Monit Comput. 2000;16(5–6):329–35.
4. Lohser J, Slinger P. Lung injury after one-lung ventilation: a review of the pathophysiologic mechanisms affecting the ventilated and the collapsed lung. Anesth Analg. 2015;121(2):302–18. https://doi.org/10.1213/ANE.0000000000000808.
5. Slinger P, Shennib H, Wilson S. Postthoracotomy pulmonary function: a comparison of epidural versus intravenous meperidine infusions. J Cardiothorac Vasc Anesth. 1995;9(2):128–34. https://doi.org/10.1016/S1053-0770(05)80182-X.

6. Cense HA, Lagarde SM, de Jong K, et al. Association of no epidural analgesia with postoperative morbidity and mortality after transthoracic esophageal cancer resection. J Am Coll Surg. 2006;202(3):395–400. https://doi.org/10.1016/j.jamcollsurg.2005.11.023.

7. MacIntyre NR, Cook DJ, Ely EWJ, et al. Evidence-based guidelines for weaning and discontinuing ventilatory support: a collective task force facilitated by the American College of Chest Physicians; the American Association for Respiratory Care; and the American College of Critical Care Medicine. Chest. 2001;120(6 Suppl):375S–95S.

8. Girard TD, Alhazzani W, Kress JP, et al. An Official American Thoracic Society/American College of Chest Physicians Clinical Practice Guideline: Liberation from Mechanical Ventilation in Critically Ill Adults. Rehabilitation Protocols, Ventilator Liberation Protocols, and Cuff Leak Tests. Am J Respir Crit Care Med. 2017;195(1):120–33. https://doi.org/10.1164/rccm.201610-2075ST.

9. MacIntyre N. Discontinuing mechanical ventilatory support. Chest. 2007;132(3):1049–56. https://doi.org/10.1378/chest.06-2862.

10. Bhattacharyya N, Kotz T, Shapiro J. Dysphagia and aspiration with unilateral vocal cord immobility: incidence, characterization, and response to surgical treatment. Ann Otol Rhinol Laryngol. 2002;111(8):672–9. https://doi.org/10.1177/000348940211100803.

11. Aviv JE, Kim T, Sacco RL, et al. FEESST: a new bedside endoscopic test of the motor and sensory components of swallowing. Ann Otol Rhinol Laryngol. 1998;107(5 Pt 1):378–87. https://doi.org/10.1177/000348949810700503.

12. Yang KL, Tobin MJ. A prospective study of indexes predicting the outcome of trials of weaning from mechanical ventilation. N Engl J Med. 1991;324(21):1445–50. https://doi.org/10.1056/NEJM199105233242101.

13. Meade M, Guyatt G, Cook D, et al. Predicting success in weaning from mechanical ventilation. Chest. 2001;120(6 Suppl):400S–24S.

14. Moreno P, Alvarez A, Algar FJ, et al. Incidence, management and clinical outcomes of patients with airway complications following lung transplantation. Eur J Cardiothorac Surg. 2008;34(6):1198–205. https://doi.org/10.1016/j.ejcts.2008.08.006.

15. Alvarez A, Algar J, Santos F, et al. Airway complications after lung transplantation: a review of 151 anastomoses. Eur J Cardiothorac Surg. 2001;19(4):381–7.

16. Yap FHY, Lau JYW, Joynt GM, Chui PT, Chan ACW, Chung SSC. Early extubation after transthoracic oesophagectomy. Hong Kong Med J. 2003;9(2):98–102.

17. Lanuti M, de Delva PE, Maher A, et al. Feasibility and outcomes of an early extubation policy after esophagectomy. Ann Thorac Surg. 2006;82(6):2037–41. https://doi.org/10.1016/j.athoracsur.2006.07.024.

18. Cordos I, Bolca C, Paleru C, Posea R, Stoica R. Sixty tracheal resections--single center experience. Interact Cardiovasc Thorac Surg. 2009;8(1):62–5.; discussion 65. https://doi.org/10.1510/icvts.2008.184747.

19. Almada CP d S, Martins FAN d C, Tardelli MA, JLG A. Time of extubation and postoperative outcome after thoracotomy. Rev Assoc Med Bras. 2007;53(3):209–12.

20. Raiten J, Thiele R, Nemergut E. Anesthesia and intensive care management of patients with brain tumors. In: Kaye AH, Laws ER, editors. Brain tumors. 3rd ed. Philadelphia: Elsevier; 2011. p. 249–81.

21. Knoll H, Ziegeler S, Schreiber J-U, et al. Airway injuries after one-lung ventilation: a comparison between double-lumen tube and endobronchial blocker: a randomized, prospective, controlled trial. Anesthesiology. 2006;105(3):471–7.

22. Minambres E, Gonzalez-Castro A, Buron J, Suberviola B, Ballesteros MA, Ortiz-Melon F. Management of postintubation tracheobronchial rupture: our experience and a review of the literature. Eur J Emerg Med. 2007;14(3):177–9. https://doi.org/10.1097/MEJ.0b013e3280bef8f0.

23. Lui N, Wright C. Intraoperative tracheal injury. Thorac Surg Clin. 2015;25(3):249–54. https://doi.org/10.1016/j.thorsurg.2015.04.008.

24. Roberts JR, Wadsworth J. Recurrent laryngeal nerve monitoring during mediastinoscopy: predictors of injury. Ann Thorac Surg. 2007;83(2):382–8. https://doi.org/10.1016/j.athoracsur.2006.03.124.

25. Sagawa M, Donjo T, Isobe T, et al. Bilateral vocal cord paralysis after lung cancer surgery with a double-lumen endotracheal tube: a life-threatening complication. J Cardiothorac Vasc Anesth. 2006;20(2):225–6. https://doi.org/10.1053/j.jvca.2005.01.037.

26. Lee DH, Yoon TM, Lee JK, Lim SC. Clinical characteristics of arytenoid dislocation after endotracheal intubation. J Craniofac Surg. 2015;26(4):1358–60. https://doi.org/10.1097/SCS.0000000000001749.

27. Tesei F, Poveda LM, Strali W, Tosi L, Magnani G, Farneti G. Unilateral laryngeal and hypoglossal paralysis (Tapia's syndrome) following rhinoplasty in general anaesthesia: case report and review of the literature. Acta Otorhinolaryngol Ital. 2006;26(4):219–21.

28. Hess DR, Fink JB, Venkataraman ST, Kim IK, Myers TR, Tano BD. The history and physics of heliox. Respir Care. 2006;51(6):608–12.

29. Javadpour H, Sidhu P, Luke DA. Bronchopleural fistula after pneumonectomy. Ir J Med Sci. 2003;172(1):13–5.

30. Hollaus PH, Setinek U, Lax F, Pridun NS. Risk factors for bronchopleural fistula after pneumonectomy: stump size does matter. Thorac Cardiovasc Surg. 2003;51(3):162–6. https://doi.org/10.1055/s-2003-40321.

31. Zanotti G, Mitchell JD. Bronchopleural fistula and empyema after anatomic lung resection. Thorac Surg Clin. 2015;25(4):421–7. https://doi.org/10.1016/j.thorsurg.2015.07.006.

32. Dentali F, Malato A, Ageno W, et al. Incidence of venous thromboembolism in patients undergoing thoracotomy for lung cancer. J Thorac Cardiovasc Surg. 2008;135(3):705–6. https://doi.org/10.1016/j.jtcvs.2007.10.036.

33. Chen Q, Tang AT, Tsang GM. Acute pulmonary thromboembolism complicating pneumonectomy: successful operative management. Eur J Cardiothorac Surg. 2001;19(2):223–5.

34. Soll C, Hahnloser D, Frauenfelder T, Russi EW, Weder W, Kestenholz PB. The postpneumonectomy syndrome: clinical presentation and treatment. Eur J Cardiothorac Surg. 2009;35(2):319–24. https://doi.org/10.1016/j.ejcts.2008.07.070.

35. Shen KR, Wain JC, Wright CD, Grillo HC, Mathisen DJ. Postpneumonectomy syndrome: surgical management and long-term results. J Thorac Cardiovasc Surg. 2008;135(6):1210–9. https://doi.org/10.1016/j.jtcvs.2007.11.022.

36. Ng T, Ryder BA, Maziak DE, Shamji FM. Thoracoscopic approach for the treatment of postpneumonectomy syndrome. Ann Thorac Surg. 2009;88(3):1015–8. https://doi.org/10.1016/j.athoracsur.2009.02.021.

37. Jung JJ, Cho JH, Kim HK, et al. Management of postpneumonectomy syndrome using tissue expanders. Thorac Cancer. 2016;7(1):88–93. https://doi.org/10.1111/1759-7714.12282.

38. Slinger P. Post-pneumonectomy pulmonary edema: is anesthesia to blame? Curr Opin Anaesthesiol. 1999;12(1):49–54.

39. Parquin F, Marchal M, Mehiri S, Herve P, Lescot B. Post-pneumonectomy pulmonary edema: analysis and risk factors. Eur J Cardiothorac Surg. 1996;10(11):929–32. discussion 933

40. Alvarez JM, Bairstow BM, Tang C, Newman MA. Post-lung resection pulmonary edema: a case for aggressive management. J Cardiothorac Vasc Anesth. 1998;12(2):199–205.

41. Mogayzel PJJ, Colombani PM, Crawford TO, Yang SC. Bilateral diaphragm paralysis following lung transplantation and cardiac surgery in a 17-year-old. J Heart Lung Transplant. 2002;21(6):710–2.

42. Qureshi A. Diaphragm paralysis. Semin Respir Crit Care Med. 2009;30(3):315–20. https://doi.org/10.1055/s-0029-1222445.

43. Ugalde P, Miro S, Provencher S, et al. Ipsilateral diaphragmatic motion and lung function in long-term pneumonectomy patients. Ann Thorac Surg. 2008;86(6):1742–5. https://doi.org/10.1016/j.athoracsur.2008.05.081.

44. De Decker K, Jorens PG, Van Schil P. Cardiac complications after noncardiac thoracic surgery: an evidence-based current review. Ann Thorac Surg. 2003;75(4):1340–8.

45. Groves J, Edwards ND, Carr B, Sherry KM. Perioperative myocardial ischaemia, heart rate and arrhythmia in patients undergoing thoracotomy: an observational study. Br J Anaesth. 1999;83(6):850–4.

46. Roselli EE, Murthy SC, Rice TW, et al. Atrial fibrillation complicating lung cancer resection. J Thorac Cardiovasc Surg. 2005;130(2):438–44. https://doi.org/10.1016/j.jtcvs.2005.02.010.

47. Gillinov AM, Bagiella E, Moskowitz AJ, et al. Rate control versus rhythm control for atrial fibrillation after cardiac surgery. N Engl J Med. 2016;374(20):1911–21. https://doi.org/10.1056/NEJMoa1602002.

48. Diaz-Guzman E, Mireles-Cabodevila E, Arrossi A, Kanne JP, Budev M. Amiodarone pulmonary toxicity after lung transplantation. J Heart Lung Transplant. 2008;27(9):1059–63. https://doi.org/10.1016/j.healun.2008.05.023.

49. Baaijens PF, Hasenbos MA, Lacquet LK, Dekhuijzen PN. Cardiac herniation after pneumonectomy. Acta Anaesthesiol Scand. 1992;36(8):842–5.

50. Deiraniya AK. Cardiac herniation following intrapericardial pneumonectomy. Thorax. 1974;29(5):545–52.

51. Shimizu J, Ishida Y, Hirano Y, et al. Cardiac herniation following intrapericardial pneumonectomy with partial pericardiectomy for advanced lung cancer. Ann Thorac Cardiovasc Surg. 2003;9(1):68–72.

52. Buniva P, Aluffi A, Rescigno G, Rademacher J, Nazari S. Cardiac herniation and torsion after partial pericardiectomy during right pneumonectomy. Texas Hear Inst J. 2001;28(1):73.

53. Zandberg FT, Verbeke SJME, Snijder RJ, Dalinghaus WH, Roeffel SM, Van Swieten HA. Sudden cardiac herniation 6 months after right pneumonectomy. Ann Thorac Surg. 2004;78(3):1095–7. https://doi.org/10.1016/S0003-4975(03)01404-8.

54. Bakris NC, Siddiqi AJ, Fraser CDJ, Mehta AC. Right-to-left interatrial shunt after pneumonectomy. Ann Thorac Surg. 1997;63(1):198–201.

55. Zueger O, Soler M, Stulz P, Jacob A, Perruchoud AP. Dyspnea after pneumonectomy: the result of an atrial septal defect. Ann Thorac Surg. 1997;63(5):1451–2.

Postoperative Respiratory Failure and Treatment

54

Wendy Smith, Alan Finley, and James Ramsay

Key Points

- Although pure hypoxemic or pure hypercapnic respiratory failure may occur after thoracic surgery, most patients exhibit a mixed picture.
- The single most important preoperative patient-related risk factor for respiratory failure after thoracic surgery is the presence of severe COPD.
- High-flow nasal cannula oxygen and noninvasive ventilation (NIV) can be safely administered in the post-thoracic surgery patient, both to reduce respiratory complications and to prevent the need for re-intubation.
- Mechanical ventilation after thoracic surgery should follow a "lung-protective" strategy of appropriate combinations of PEEP and low tidal volume, in association with increased respiratory rate as needed.
- Ventilator-associated pneumonia (VAP) is associated with a high mortality, so prevention is a priority. The "VAP "bundle" is a variety of care processes either known or believed to reduce the risk of acquiring VAP.
- A daily spontaneous breathing trial is the most effective way to identify patients ready for withdrawal of ventilator support.
- Tracheotomy should be considered if mechanical ventilation is expected to be required for more than a total of 7–10 days.

Respiratory failure following thoracic surgery is a significant cause of morbidity and mortality in this high-risk patient population. The incidence of major post-thoracotomy pulmonary complications such as pneumonia, lobar atelectasis, or need for mechanical ventilation for more than 24 h ranges from 22% to 25%, while the incidence of respiratory failure (requiring mechanical ventilation for more than 48 h after surgery) ranges from about 3 to 10% [1–5]. In most reports respiratory failure accounts for approximately half of the 30-day mortality. The reported incidence of respiratory failure and overall mortality for several thoracic procedures is given in Table 54.1. Respiratory failure and mortality are greater after right-sided as compared to left-sided pneumonectomy and after extra vs. intrapleural pneumonectomy [6]. The addition of chest wall resection to intrathoracic surgery also adds to the incidence of respiratory failure and mortality [2]. Preexisting pulmonary disease and other concomitant disease processes increase the risk of postoperative

Table 54.1 Respiratory failure[a] and 30-day mortality after open[b] thoracic surgery procedures

	Respiratory failure	Overall mortality
Lung resection		
Wedge resection	(Not reported)	0.8–1.4% [1, 2]
Lobectomy	3.2–6.6% [3–5]	1.2–4% [1–5]
Pneumonectomy	6.9–9.3% [3–5]	3.2–11.5% [1–5]
Esophagogastrectomy	16% [57]	2.1–9.8% [54–57]
Lung volume reduction surgery	13.6% [48]	2.3–16% [47–50]

In two reports lobectomy was not separated from pneumonectomy: in one the incidence of tracheostomy was 14% [1]; in the other the incidence of respiratory failure was 6% [2]

[a]Defined as the need for mechanical ventilation for more than 48 h after surgery

[b]Limited data for thoracoscopic procedures suggests reduced overall complications but not mortality VS open procedures [48]. Preliminary data for robotic-assisted surgeries suggests reductions in morbidity and mortality that is at least comparable to VATS and in some instances superior to both VATS and open procedures [25]

W. Smith
Department of Anesthesiology and Perioperative Care, University of California at San Francisco, San Francisco, CA, USA

A. Finley
Department of Anesthesia and Perioperative Medicine, Medical University of South Carolina, Charleston, SC, USA

J. Ramsay (✉)
Department of Anesthesia and Preoperative Care, University of California San Francisco, San Francisco, CA, USA
e-mail: James.Ramsay@ucsf.edu

© Springer Nature Switzerland AG 2019
P. Slinger (ed.), *Principles and Practice of Anesthesia for Thoracic Surgery*, https://doi.org/10.1007/978-3-030-00859-8_54

respiratory insufficiency and failure. Anticipation and early recognition are essential to provide the best possible outcome for the patient in respiratory failure.

Definition

Respiratory failure is the inability of the respiratory system to provide sufficient gas exchange to prevent life-threatening hypoxemia and/or hypercapnia. The clinical picture suggests the diagnosis, and the arterial blood gas analysis is confirmatory (Table 54.2). Respiratory failure may be purely hypoxemic, in which arterial partial pressure of oxygen in the blood is inadequate, but partial pressure of carbon dioxide is low or normal. Physiologic causes of hypoxemic respiratory failure include hypoventilation, ventilation-perfusion mismatch, right-to-left intrapulmonary or intracardiac shunts,

Table 54.2 Diagnosis of acute respiratory failure

Clinical	Central nervous system	Agitation, restlessness, diaphoresis from distress
		Headache, confusion from hypercarbia or hypoxemia
		Dizziness, focal twitching from hypercarbia
		Insomnia, personality change from hypoxemia
		Stupor, confusion, coma from severe hypercarbia or severe hypoxemia
		Seizures from severe hypoxemia
	Cardiovascular system	Tachyarrhythmias from hypoxemia or hypercarbia
		Bradyarrhythmias from severe hypoxemia
		Systemic hypertension from hypoxemia or hypercarbia
		Pulmonary hypertension from hypoxemia or hypercarbia
		Hypotension/cardiac failure from severe hypoxemia or hypercarbia
	Respiratory system	Intact respiratory drive: Tachypnea Labored respirations, dyspnea Intercostal retractions
		Impaired respiratory drive: Bradypnea or apnea
		Cheyne-stokes respirations
Laboratory	Oxygenation[a]	Arterial pO_2 < 50–60 mmHg
		Peripheral arterial saturation (pulse oximetry) <90%
	Carbon dioxide[b]	Arterial pCO_2 > 50–60 mmHg associated with acidosis

[a]Respiratory "failure" due to hypoxemia may not require mechanical ventilatory support if it is responsive to supplemental oxygen therapy
[b]Chronic elevations in arterial pCO_2 are accompanied by retention of bicarbonate and relatively normal arterial pH and do not necessarily indicate respiratory "failure." Hypercarbia associated with acidosis always indicates respiratory failure and usually requires mechanical ventilatory support

abnormalities in alveolar oxygen diffusion, and low fraction of inspired oxygen [7]. Failure to oxygenate the blood after thoracic surgery is usually the result of severe mismatch of ventilation and perfusion ("V:Q mismatch") such that pulmonary blood flows through poorly ventilated or edematous lung and there is inadequate time or alveolar exposure for absorption of O_2. Increased pulmonary water from direct surgical injury, capillary leak, or fluid overload may cause V:Q mismatch, as may focal areas of consolidation from collections (air, blood), infection, inflammation, or atelectasis. The most severe form of V:Q mismatch is true shunting of pulmonary blood without any absorption of O_2, as might occur with a completely atelectatic or consolidated segment or lobe.

Hypoventilation alone may result in hypoxemia. The simplified form of the alveolar gas equation estimates the partial pressure of oxygen in the alveoli based on the inspired partial pressure of oxygen and the partial pressure of arterial carbon dioxide:

$$P_A O_2 = P_I O_2 - P_a CO_2 / R$$

$P_A O_2$ is the alveolar partial pressure of oxygen, $P_I O_2$ is the partial pressure of inspired oxygen, and $P_a CO_2$ is the arterial partial pressure of carbon dioxide (R represents the respiratory exchange ratio). Severe hypoventilation, with a resultant rise in $P_a CO_2$, would therefore be expected to result in some degree of hypoxemia. The degree of hypoxemia caused by pure hypoventilation can usually be overcome by supplemental oxygen [8].

Intracardiac shunt with right- to left-sided blood flow causes arterial desaturation independent of pulmonary pathology. The condition where this most commonly occurs in the adult is a patent foramen ovale (PFO), which is present – at least in a probe-patent form – in approximately 25% of the population [9]. In short actual closure of the shunt, the treatment requires reducing the gradient for blood flow from right to left, either reducing the right atrial pressure or increasing the left atrial pressure. In the presence of a PFO, application of increasing levels of positive intrathoracic pressure (positive end-expiratory pressure or PEEP) can worsen arterial oxygenation [10]. Positive intrathoracic pressure can increase impedance to ejection by the right ventricle, resulting in an elevation in the central venous pressure (CVP). This may increase blood flow across the atrial septum from right to left.

Hypercapnic respiratory failure occurs when ventilation of the lungs is insufficient to maintain an adequate arterial partial pressure of carbon dioxide. Hypercapnic respiratory failure may occur with structural or functional abnormalities of the chest wall and muscles of respiration. Decreased function of the muscles of respiration may be seen with residual neuromuscular blockade and with surgical disruption.

Structural or mechanical problems with the chest wall induced by surgery can lead to hypoventilation by affecting the normal decrease in intrathoracic pressure seen during inspiration. These include pneumothorax, pulmonary contusion leading to decreased distensibility of the lung tissue, and flail chest. These types of hypercapnic failure are associated with respiratory distress and usually tachypnea: the patient is trying to achieve a normal arterial pCO_2 but cannot. Decreased central respiratory drive results in hypoventilation. Decreased central drive may be seen with residual anesthesia, postoperative sedation, or central nervous system disease (e.g., perioperative stroke). Conditions associated with chronic carbon dioxide retention (e.g., obstructive airways disease, obesity-hypoventilation syndrome) may be exacerbated by depressant medications or structural changes induced by surgery.

Although pure hypoxemic or pure hypercapnic respiratory failure may be seen, most surgical patients with postoperative respiratory failure exhibit a mixed picture. Chest wall and parenchymal injury, edema, retained secretions or blood, and atelectasis interfere with gas exchange and increase the work of breathing. Surgical injury to the chest wall and pain also interfere with normal mechanical function, thus decreasing the effectiveness of the respiratory effort and increasing the work of breathing.

Preoperative Predictors of Postoperative Respiratory Failure

Conflicting results in the available literature make establishing precise criteria for determining those patients most at risk for postoperative respiratory failure difficult. The history, physical examination, and specific investigations enable the surgeon and anesthesiologist to estimate risk and identify processes that can be treated or optimized prior to surgery. Preoperative assessment for pulmonary resection is discussed in Chap. 2. Preoperative factors associated with an increased incidence of postoperative respiratory failure are summarized in Table 54.3.

History

Preexisting conditions which have been associated with increased risk of respiratory dysfunction and failure in the general surgery patient population include advanced age (greater than 70 years), chronic pulmonary disease, smoking, cardiac dysfunction, and neuromuscular diseases affecting the muscles of respiration or glutition [11]. Arozullah et al. published a multifactorial index for predicting postoperative respiratory failure which includes chronic obstructive pulmonary disease (COPD), increased age, dependent func-

Table 54.3 Preoperative factors associated with increased risk of postoperative respiratory failure

History
Age > 70 years
Smoking history with chronic obstructive pulmonary disease
Cardiac dysfunction
Neuromuscular disease
Dyspnea at rest or with light exertion
Inability to climb 1 flight of stairs
Physical findings
Increased baseline work of breathing
Preoperative wheezing (not controlled by bronchodilators)
Lower extremity edema/jugular venous distension (suggestive of right heart dysfunction)
Cachexia
Laboratory
PCO₂ > 45 mmHg
PO₂ < 50 mmHg on room air
ppoFEV1 < 40% predicted
ppoDLCO < 40% predicted
RV/TLC > 30%
VO₂max < 15 ml/kg/min
Increased serum creatinine

ppo predicted postoperative, *DLCO* diffusion capacity for carbon monoxide, *FEV1* forced expiratory volume in one second, *RV* residual volume, *TLC* total lung capacity, *VO₂max* maximum oxygen consumption

tional status, and surgical site as independent risk factors for patients in the general surgical population [12]. Patients who report dyspnea at rest, with light exercise (walking on a level surface 100 yards), or with activities of daily living (dressing, talking) have an approximate twofold increase in respiratory complications following thoracotomy [13]. In a review from the Cleveland Clinic, preoperative predictors of postoperative ventilator support after thoracotomy for lung resection included elevated creatinine and low preoperative forced expiratory volume in one second (FEV_1) [14].

There is some data to suggest an elevated BNP level, on postoperative day 1, may also be predictive of cardiopulmonary complications [15]. The single most important preoperative patient-related risk factor is the presence of COPD, and the incidence of postoperative pulmonary complications associated with COPD increases with the severity of the disease. The relative risk of pulmonary complications in patients with COPD is three- to fourfold [16]. These patients should have management of their airway obstruction optimized prior to surgery with a multimodal approach consisting of bronchodilators, smoking cessation, antibiotics, and corticosteroids.

Asymptomatic asthma is not associated with any increase in the incidence of pulmonary complications or need for postoperative mechanical ventilation after thoracotomy. If the patient is free of wheezing in the immediate preoperative period and the FEV_1 is greater than 80% predicted, there is no increased risk of bronchospasm or other pulmonary complications [17].

On the other hand, an asthmatic patient with recent episodes of bronchospasm and wheezing should be treated cautiously. These patients may benefit from prophylactic corticosteroid use before anesthesia and surgery. Inhaled corticosteroids are recommended for virtually all patients with persistent asthma [18]. Steroids may be administered orally or by inhalation with inhaled steroids leading to less systemic side effects. Patients who have recently had significant asthma symptoms and received systemic glucocorticosteroids within the past 6 months should have systemic coverage during the perioperative period. All asthmatic patients should remain on their routine bronchodilator and anti-inflammatory medications in the perioperative period.

Procedure and Extent of Resection

Thoracotomy for Lung Resection

The extent of resection during thoracotomy for lung cancer is a risk factor for the need for postoperative mechanical ventilation, pulmonary complications, and 30-day mortality (Table 54.1) [14]. In addition, Busch et al. reported an 82% incidence of postoperative pulmonary complications in patients requiring extensive resection, including the chest wall. This compared to an overall incidence of 39% in their study of patients undergoing thoracotomy [2]. On the other hand, a review of the muscle-sparing thoracotomy approach (where the latissimus dorsi and serratus anterior muscles are not severed) vs. standard thoracotomy found no morbidity or mortality benefit [19]. Not surprisingly, increasing age is a major risk factor for the development of serious pulmonary complications, including respiratory failure and mortality [4, 5, 20].

Video-Assisted Thoracic Surgery for Lung Resection

Minimally invasive lung surgery has gained popularity because of the smaller incision, potentially shorter hospital stay, and quicker recovery (see also Chap. 23). Video-assisted thoracic surgery (VATS) is performed through several small ports rather than a single long incision, resulting in less interference with pulmonary mechanics, decreased postoperative pain, and possibly less morbidity and mortality. Imperatori et al. reported a reduced incidence of prolonged air leak and pneumonia; other postoperative pulmonary complications were not reported [21]. Although some studies support better outcomes compared to thoracotomy, limited evidence supports the theory that VATS for lobectomy improves long-term outcomes [22, 23]. Also, concern still exists that the extent of the resection may be inadequate in certain patient populations [22]. The reality is that many surgeons are performing VATS, and many patients are requesting it.

Robot Video-Assisted Thoracic Surgery for Lung Resection

Robotic surgery provides all the benefits of VATS while providing better surgical control through the use of a three-dimensional field and wristed instrumentation. Thus, the experienced surgeon is able to perform a meticulous dissection in a nearly bloodless field [24]. Though robotic lung resections are in their infancy, preliminary data suggest a reduction in morbidity and mortality that is at least comparable to that of VATS compared to open procedures. In some instances, outcomes were superior to both VATS and traditional thoracotomy [25].

Lung Volume Reduction Surgery

Lung volume reduction is a surgical strategy to improve ventilation-perfusion matching in patients with severe emphysema (see also Chap. 46). Prospective candidates usually have a FEV_1 of less than 30% predicted and poor exercise tolerance secondary to dyspnea. During lung volume reduction surgery, nonfunctional portions of lung are removed (up to 30% of lung volume in some patients). The goal is improvement of chest wall mechanics and elastic recoil of lung by removing poorly ventilated and perfused apical segments [26]. Surgery in these very high-risk patients does carry a significant risk of postoperative respiratory complications. In one report the incidence of postoperative acute respiratory failure was 29.8%, with 43% of mortality related to a respiratory etiology [27]. Overall, the reported mortality following lung volume reduction surgery ranges from a low of 2.3% to up to 16% [28, 29].

Trans-sternal Thymectomy

Thymectomy is performed in patients with myasthenia gravis who have worsening symptoms despite maximal medical therapy with anticholinesterase medications and/or corticosteroids and has been shown to improve symptoms in up to 75% of patients (see also Chap. 15) [30]. In the perioperative period, the myasthenic patient may show exquisite sensitivity to non-depolarizing neuromuscular blocking medications and may have increased sensitivity to medications with respiratory depression side effects. In the past these patients remained intubated after surgery and were only extubated after careful assessment and reinstitution of preoperative anticholinesterase medications. As medical management has improved, many of these patients now present for surgery with their disease well controlled and with careful anesthetic management can be extubated immediately after the procedure. Historically, preoperative predictors of the need for postoperative ventilatory support include duration of the disease greater than 6 years, chronic lung disease, a daily dose of pyridostigmine greater than 750 mg (or its equivalent), and a preoperative vital capacity less than 2.9 liters [31]. In a series of 71 patients undergoing thymoma resection, the incidence of postoperative respiratory complications was 13%, with only one death due to respiratory failure [32]. An increasing use of thoracoscopic techniques for this procedure may reduce the incidence of postoperative respiratory complications.

Esophagogastrectomy

The incidence of adenocarcinoma of the distal esophagus has increased over the last several decades, with risk factors including a history of tobacco use and alcohol consumption [33]. Esophagogastrectomy offers the only hope of cure.

Esophagogastrectomy for carcinoma at or near the gastroesophageal junction may be performed via a transhiatal approach or via a transthoracic approach (see also Chap. 38). Pulmonary complications occur in 15–25% of patients, with pneumonia and/or respiratory failure comprising about half of this incidence. The in-hospital mortality rate following transthoracic esophagogastrectomy ranges from 2.1% to 9.8% [34–36]. Two of three postesophagectomy mortalities are related to pulmonary complications; aspiration pneumonia secondary to postoperative swallowing disorders is the most common etiology [37].

Lung Transplantation

Lung transplantation is increasingly performed for end-stage lung disease secondary to many etiologies, limited to a large degree by donor availability. Following reperfusion of the donor lung, more than half of the patients exhibit some degree of non-cardiogenic pulmonary edema, and postoperative mechanical ventilation for at least 24 h is normal. This is discussed below under "pulmonary edema."

Thoracoabdominal Aortic Aneurysm (TAAA) Repair

The most common complications after open thoracoabdominal aortic aneurysm repair are pulmonary. These procedures require extensive incisions, prolonged periods of one lung ventilation, and large volume fluid resuscitation (see also Chap. 41). Reporting on 100 consecutive thoracoabdominal aortic aneurysm repairs, Money et al. found the mean duration of intubation to be 5.8 days, with a 21% incidence of respiratory failure [38]. An earlier report from Crawford's group suggested an incidence of respiratory failure in patients with chronic pulmonary disease of 58% and a mortality of 43% in this group [39]. Etz et al. reported an incidence of prolonged respiratory failure of 27% [40].

Specific Etiologies of Respiratory Failure: Their Prevention and Treatment

Table 54.4 summarizes the common conditions leading to acute postoperative respiratory failure. Similar to the diagno-

Table 54.4 Acute causes of respiratory failure following thoracic surgery

| Atelectasis/retained secretions |
| Pneumonia |
| Pulmonary embolus |
| Pulmonary edema |
| Postpneumonectomy pulmonary edema |
| Pulmonary reimplantation response |
| Acute respiratory distress syndrome |
| Pneumothorax |
| Bronchopulmonary fistula |
| Torsion of residual lobe |
| Neurologic injuries |
| Phrenic nerve |
| Recurrent laryngeal nerves |

sis itself, the cause is seldom single or simple; more often it represents the combination of postoperative factors with predisposing physiology or underlying conditions.

Atelectasis

Surgery on the thorax and the upper abdomen leads to some degree of postoperative pulmonary dysfunction and atelectasis, which may persist for days or weeks. Inhibition of surfactant, gas resorption, and compression of lung tissue all are potential mechanisms by which atelectasis occurs. Although general anesthesia has been shown to depress the function of surfactant, inhibition of surfactant is not believed to play a major role in the formation of atelectasis [41, 42]. Resorption atelectasis refers to the continued gas uptake in alveoli after airway occlusion and ultimately leads to collapse of the gas pocket [43]. Resorption atelectasis increases with increasing inspired oxygen concentration [44]. Lastly, loss of intercostal muscle tone and cephalad displacement of the diaphragm and abdominal contents leads to an increase in pleural pressures and compression atelectasis [45].

The relationship between functional residual capacity (FRC) and closing capacity (CC) must also be considered. FRC is defined as the amount of air remaining in the lung at end-expiration of a normal tidal volume. CC is the volume of gas that must be in the lungs to prevent small airway collapse. In healthy lungs, FRC exceeds CC, and no atelectasis occurs. If CC exceeds FRC and the tidal volume lies within the CC, then small airways will open and close with each tidal volume. This will result in areas of low ventilation/perfusion ratio or shunt. If CC far exceeds FRC, then small airways never open during the respiratory cycle resulting in atelectasis (Fig. 54.1). Thus, factors that decrease FRC like general anesthesia, obesity, and supine position will subject patients to atelectasis.

While some degree of atelectasis occurs in almost all post-thoracotomy patients, the severity and clinical

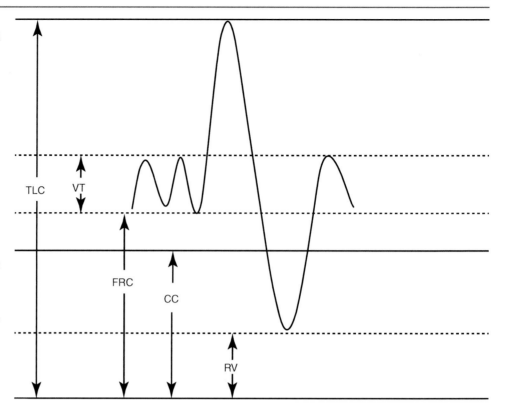

Fig. 54.1 Lung volumes in a normal young adult showing tidal volume (VT), total lung capacity reached on a maximum inspiration (TLC), functional residual capacity which is the volume in the lung at the end of normal expiration (FRC), closing capacity which is the lung volume below which small airways begin to close (CC), and residual volume, the volume of the lung remaining after maximum expiration (RV). With increasing age the CC increases bringing the normal tidal ventilation into a lung volume where small airways are closing, leading to shunt and predisposing to atelectasis. In addition, with obesity, supine posture, or Trendelenburg position, FRC decreases, while the CC does not, also leading to small airway closure and atelectasis

implications vary widely. Mild atelectasis usually requires little treatment other than supplemental oxygen administration in the postanesthesia care unit and will resolve as the patient awakens and increases depth of breathing. Decreased compliance, impaired oxygenation, increased pulmonary vascular resistance, and development of lung injury represent the more severe pathophysiologic effects of atelectasis. The most severe form of post-lobectomy atelectasis, lobar atelectasis, occurs in approximately 5% of patients after pulmonary resection. Lobar atelectasis is defined radiographically by complete lobar collapse and mediastinal shift. Risk factors include male gender, advanced age, and reduced preoperative FEV_1 [45]. This extreme form of atelectasis usually requires bronchoscopy, may require mechanical ventilatory support, and can lead to longer ICU and hospital lengths of stay. Lastly, atelectasis has been shown to promote bacterial overgrowth and increase lung permeability [46].

Prevention and treatment of atelectasis has traditionally consisted of cough and deep breathing exercises (Table 54.5). While coughing and deep breathing help clear secretions and potentially reopen atelectatic areas of lung, the ability of surgical patients to cough is significantly impaired after thoracic surgery. The maximal intrapleural pressures produced during voluntary coughing are reduced to as low as 29% of preoperative values and may remain as low as 50% of the preoperative value at 3 weeks postsurgery [47]. The cough effort may be improved with the

Table 54.5 Adjuvants to routine postoperative respiratory care

Inhaled bronchodilators and mucolytics
Incentive spirometry
Positive expiratory pressure valves
Flutter valves
Chest physiotherapy
Percussion/vibration
Nasotracheal suctioning
Fiber-optic bronchoscopy
Therapeutic
Diagnostic
Minitracheostomy

patient in the sitting position and with manually assisted compression of the chest wall. Simply mobilizing patients from sitting in bed to sitting in a chair improved FRC at an average of 17% [48].

Incentive spirometry (IS) is a simple and inexpensive method of helping patients obtain maximal inspiratory effort [49]. IS encourages patients to maintain inspiration for a prolonged period while using slow and deep breaths. Figure 54.2 shows a typical single-patient use incentive spirometry device. Incentive spirometry can also be followed as a bedside test for evaluation of postoperative pulmonary function after lung surgery. The performance on IS correlates well with inspiratory reserve volume and forced vital capacity [50]. A decline in a patient's ability to perform IS can be an early indicator of an acute worsening of the

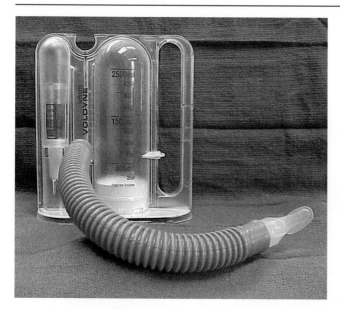

Fig. 54.2 Incentive spirometer (Hudson RCI, Teleflex Medical). The patient makes a sustained inhalation effort through the mouthpiece, guided by an effort indicator on the right side of the device. This causes the "floating" marker inside the graduated cylinder to be drawn up to a set target indicated to the left of the cylinder

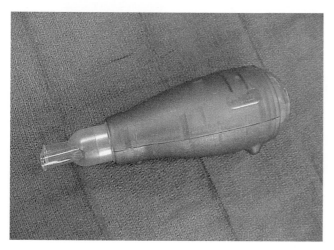

Fig. 54.3 Positive expiratory pressure vibratory device ("Acapella" device, Smiths Medical ASD, Inc.). Exhalation through this device is intermittently occluded at a high frequency which "vibrates" the airways facilitating clearance of secretions and possibly opening closed airways

patient's pulmonary status. While IS is widely accepted as a tool to help prevent atelectasis, this has not been clearly established in clinical studies. Several reviews of the literature have failed to find supporting evidence for the routine use of IS following cardiac, thoracic, or upper abdominal surgery [51–56].

An alternative approach to IS is to focus on maintaining airway patency during expiration. This is termed "positive expiratory pressure therapy ("PEP") and has been shown to

improve clearance of secretions [57] (Fig. 54.3). The patient uses this device for several breaths and then makes coughing or "huffing" efforts. A third type of device is the "flutter valve" which causes "fluttering" of the expiratory airway pressure, aiding the mobilization of secretions.

Positive-pressure breathing (i.e., positive inspiratory pressure) through a mouthpiece or face mask or continuous positive airway pressure (CPAP; see description in "ventilatory modes") delivered by nasal or face mask may be beneficial in maintaining and recruiting atelectatic lung [58]. Biphasic, or bi-level, positive airway pressure (BiPAP) has also been used to support hypoxemic patients in the postanesthesia care unit [59]. Figure 54.4a illustrates the mask used for BiPAP or CPAP. More recently, the use of high-flow nasal cannula (HFNC) oxygen (up to 60 L/min) has been described in the same setting. A typical HFNC setup is depicted in Fig. 54.4b. The application of these noninvasive ventilator modes, to assist in the prevention and/or treatment of acute respiratory failure, is discussed below.

Pain is a major factor contributing to the reduction in cough effort and deep breathing in patients following thoracotomy. Adequate control of postoperative pain, including use of epidural analgesia, improves maximal cough pressures in post-thoracotomy patients, and lack of a thoracic epidural catheter was found to be a risk factor for the need for postoperative mechanical ventilation after lung resection [14, 60]. While the use of opoid infusions through either lumbar-level or thoracic-level epidural catheters can provide adequate post-thoracotomy analgesia, only analgesia provided by thoracic-level catheters was demonstrated to decrease mortality in a meta-analysis of postoperative outcomes [61]. Various infusions may be used including an opoid alone or, for a thoracic level catheter, an opoid and local anesthetic combination. The combination of an opoid and local anesthetic has been shown to be synergistic and allows for a lower dose of each than if either is used alone [62]. A technique gaining popularity for thoracic patients is a continuous paravertebral catheter. This technique offers the advantages of fewer side effects compared to a thoracic epidural and is not contraindicated in anticoagulated patients. A literature review by Davies indicates that continuous paravertebral catheters are just as efficacious in pain control as thoracic epidurals [63]. Other modalities of regional anesthesia to provide post-thoracotomy analgesia include intrapleural administration of local anesthetic and intercostal nerve blocks. Intercostal nerve blocks may be performed by the anesthesiologist pre- or postoperatively or by the surgeon during the procedure. The blocks may be performed with plain local anesthetic with or without epinephrine or, for a more protracted duration of analgesia, liposomal bupivacaine [64]. Intraoperative cryoablation of intercostal nerves has also been used to provide an extended period of analgesia.

Fig. 54.4 (**a**) Full face mask used to provide CPAP or BIPAP (Respironics/Philips). An air-filled sealing rim provides an occlusive seal around the mouth and nose, with head straps to keep the mask in place as well as provide adequate pressure for the level of CPAP/BIPAP applied. Nasal masks are also available. (**b**) HFNC – right: typical high-flow nasal cannula (HFNC) setup consisting of flow meter, oxygen blender (not shown), active humidifier, and heated inspiratory circuit. Though mobile, HFNC, given the rates of oxygen delivery, is best delivered by attaching to a wall circuit. Left: HFNC is delivered through a heated humidified circuit, which at the patient end does not seem significantly different from a standard nasal cannula. As stated in the text, patients can receive the benefits of noninvasive ventilation without the discomfort of a mask, and practitioners have the benefit of an unencumbered view of the patient's face

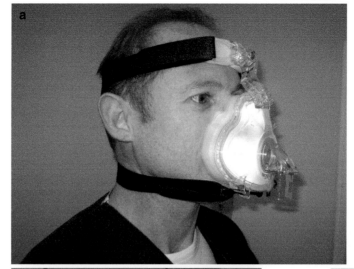

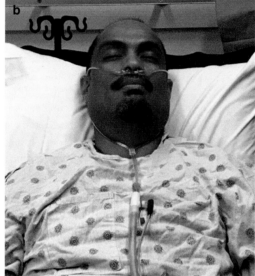

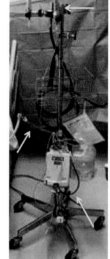

Flow meter

Heated
inspiratory
circuit

Active
Humidifier

Bronchospasm

In patients with known bronchospastic disease or in patients with chronic obstructive pulmonary disease shown to have improvement after bronchodilators during preoperative spirometry, postoperative airway constriction may contribute to respiratory failure. Increased airway resistance contributes to increased work of breathing and also can create the "auto-PEEP" effect. This occurs when terminal bronchioles/alveoli do not fully empty through narrowed airways during expiration, resulting in a positive rather than zero pressure at end-expiration distal to the obstruction. In order to generate flow into these alveoli during inspiration, this positive pressure must first be overcome, creating a further increase in the work of breathing [65].

Inhaled bronchodilating agents should be considered in all patients exhibiting respiratory distress after thoracic sur-

gery. Inhaled beta-adrenergic agonists enhance smooth muscle relaxation by increasing intracellular levels of cyclic AMP and ultimately result in bronchodilation [66]. Inhaled albuterol is the beta-adrenergic agonist most often prescribed in the postoperative period due to its short onset time and ability to act as a rescue medication. The half-life of albuterol is short and requires dosing every 4 h. Salmeterol and formoterol are longer-acting beta-adrenergic agonists and are mainly used as maintenance therapy [67]. Racemic epinephrine also has beta-adrenergic properties and may reduce respiratory mucosal edema through its alpha-adrenergic effects on mucosal vasculature. A concern with these agents, especially epinephrine, is absorption and systemic side effects.

Anticholinergic medications are also effective bronchodilators. These medications induce smooth muscle relaxation by antagonism of acetylcholine at the M3 receptor and decrease intracellular levels of cyclic-GMP. Ipratropium is a short onset and short duration anticholinergic medication commonly used in combination with albuterol for bronchospastic disease. Like albuterol, it needs to be dosed approximately every 4 h. Tiotropium is a longer-acting anticholinergic medication that can be used for maintenance. These medications are poorly absorbed and have limited systemic side effects.

Combination therapy with a beta-adrenergic agonist and anticholinergic medication provides greater improvement in symptoms. By having different mechanism of action and durations, these medications work synergistically to improve bronchodilation [68]. A combination of the short acting beta-adrenergic agonist albuterol and short-acting anticholinergic ipratropium is available in the United States.

Lastly, steroidal compounds are also available for inhalational administration and serve a useful role in prevention of inflammatory-mediated bronchospasm. These medications are mainly used in maintenance therapy and are not indicated for acute bronchospasm.

Retained Secretions

Inability to clear secretions contributes to atelectasis and pulmonary infections.

Dehydration of the tracheobronchial mucosa occurs with use of non-humidified oxygen. This leads to mucociliary dysfunction and drying of secretions. The ensuing decrease in ability to mobilize and clear secretions can contribute to the formation of atelectasis; humidification of oxygen is therefore recommended. Patients with tenacious secretions may benefit from inhaled agents that decrease the viscosity of secretions such as N-acetylcysteine or dornase alfa (Pulmozyme ®, Genetech, Inc.). Dornase is a recombinant human DNAse, which has been demonstrated to decrease viscosity of respiratory secretions in cystic fibrosis patients and help re-expand atelectatic lobes in this population [69]. Efficacy in patients with chronic bronchitis has not been demonstrated for long-term use but has been suggested in acute exacerbations.

For the patient who fails to respond to deep breathing exercises, IS, and PEP therapy, along with inhaled bronchodilators and/or mucolytics, there are several adjuvant therapies that may be utilized to improve the patient's status (Table 54.5). Modalities of chest physiotherapy include postural drainage, percussion and vibration over the affected lung segments, and incentive to cough. Postural drainage is performed by positioning the patient, so the lung segments to be drained are in a superior position. Drainage is most effective when combined with percussion and vibration, but proper positioning may be limited by the patient's condition. Percussion is performed throughout the respiratory cycle and is followed by vibration during the exhalation phase.

Tracheal suctioning can be used to mechanically remove secretions from the trachea and to induce deep breathing and coughing. In the non-intubated patient, tracheal suctioning is usually performed by a blind nasal technique. Suctioning should be performed after preoxygenating the patient with a high FIO_2 and may be better tolerated through a nasal airway or "trumpet." The catheter should be advanced without suction and removed from the trachea with intermittent suction. Blind nasotracheal suctioning is a very unpleasant experience for most patients; while it may induce better coughing, it may also induce gagging and vomiting, and frequent or aggressive suctioning can cause mucosal damage and may induce bronchospasm, laryngospasm, and cardiac rhythm disturbances.

An alternative to blind nasotracheal suctioning is placement of a minitracheostomy (a small, uncuffed endotracheal tube through an incision in the cricothyroid membrane) to facilitate suctioning of secretions. This procedure is safe and effective in decreasing the need for other interventions such as chest physiotherapy. This procedure also may decrease postoperative respiratory complications [70–72]. Potential complications are rare, including bleeding into the trachea, infection, and tracheal occlusion by granuloma formation [73]. Minitracheostomy is not intended to provide a means for positive-pressure ventilation and is not a replacement for endotracheal intubation when indicated.

Fiber-optic bronchoscopy (FOB) may be used for more aggressive clearance of secretions or blood in the tracheobronchial tree or as a diagnostic study in the patient with an acute worsening of respiratory function. Under direct visualization, tenacious secretions can be suctioned from affected airways. A review of the practice of FOB in a large teaching hospital confirmed the safety of the procedure with a major complication rate of 0.5% and a minor complication rate of 0.8% [74]. Complications include laryngospasm, bronchospasm, pneumothorax, and pulmonary hemorrhage. In the awake, non-intubated patient, fiber-optic bronchoscopy requires topical anesthesia of the upper airway and often requires moderate sedation.

Pneumonia

Decreased mucociliary clearance and persistent atelectasis place the thoracic surgical patient at increased risk for postoperative nosocomial pneumonia. Following thoracotomy, patients also have altered systemic and lung host defenses which increase susceptibility to postoperative pneumonia [75]. The occurrence of pneumonia, especially after lung resection, significantly increases the patient's risk for respiratory insufficiency and need for mechanical ventilation. Nosocomial pneumonia is the single most important risk factor for mortality in the post-thoracotomy patient [4]. In a prospective trial, Nan found the rate of postoperative respiratory infections after lung surgery (pneumonia, empyema) to be ~19% [76]. Overall, mortality rates for nosocomial pneumonia range from 20% to 80% with Gram-negative bacilli and *Staphylococcus aureus* being the most common pathogens [77]. Ventilator-associated pneumonia is discussed below.

Initiation of therapy should not be delayed for the results of initial cultures. Mortality is reduced with appropriate empiric antibiotic therapy versus delaying until BAL is performed [78]. For suspected pneumonia occurring early in the postoperative period in a patient who was not in the hospital preoperatively, community-acquired organisms such as *Streptococcus pneumonia* and *Haemophilus influenzae* should be targeted. For a patient who has been in the hospital preoperatively or in whom pneumonia is suspected more than 48 h after surgery, empiric antibiotic therapy should target hospital-acquired organisms such as *Pseudomonas aeruginosa*, *Acinetobacter* and *Klebsiella* species, and methicillin-resistant *Staphylococcus aureus*. The importance of initial appropriate empiric antibiotic therapy cannot be understated and should be targeted to institution or community-specific pathogens. Inappropriate antibiotic therapy, even if corrected within 48 h when the results of culture become available, has been associated with higher mortality, a longer ICU stay, and a trend toward longer mechanical ventilation. Inappropriate initial antibiotic therapy has been reported to be as high as 50% [79]. Ventilator-associated pneumonia is discussed below.

Pulmonary Embolism

In a study of 77 patients undergoing thoracotomy before the use of subcutaneous heparin prophylaxis, the incidence of deep venous thrombosis was 19%, with pulmonary embolism occurring in 5% [79]. In a large series of 1735 lung resection patients, early fatal acute cardiopulmonary failure occurred in 26 patients. Autopsy in 20 of these patients demonstrated pulmonary embolism in 19 [80]. In patients with shock due to massive pulmonary emboli, the mortality is in excess of 30% [81]. As thoracic surgery patients usually have at least two major risk factors for deep venous thrombosis (malignancy and major surgery), prophylaxis should include both sequential compression devices applied to the calves and low-dose subcutaneous heparin or low-molecular-weight heparin.

Signs and symptoms of pulmonary embolism include dyspnea, tachypnea, arterial hypoxemia, pulmonary hypertension, right ventricular failure, and shock. Lung perfusion scanning with technetium 99 m-labeled albumin combined with ventilation scanning with xenon 133 can demonstrate areas of ventilation-perfusion mismatch, although this test is of limited use when there is preexisting lung disease or recent lung surgery. Current use of lung perfusion scanning is only in patients with renal insufficiency, anaphylaxis to intravenous contrast, or pregnancy [82]. Spiral computed tomography (CT) can demonstrate pulmonary emboli and is noninvasive, quicker, and easier to perform than ventilation-perfusion scanning [83, 84]. While the gold standard for detection of pulmonary emboli is pulmonary angiography, in many centers spiral CT has essentially eliminated the need for this more invasive test. Postoperative patients with low risk PE are not candidates for thrombolytic therapy, but therapeutic heparinization is usually safe if initiated at least 24–48 h after surgery. In cases of sub-massive and massive embolism, surgical embolectomy or catheter-directed therapy with no- or low-dose thrombolytic may be considered [85, 86].

Pulmonary Edema

The etiology of pulmonary edema after thoracic surgery may be cardiogenic or non-cardiogenic. Increased hydrostatic pressure in the pulmonary vasculature, as might be associated with left ventricular dysfunction or excessive intravenous fluid administration, may lead to cardiogenic pulmonary edema. Increased permeability of the alveolar capillary membranes, as occurs with the acute respiratory distress syndrome (ARDS), leads to non-cardiogenic pulmonary edema.

Postpneumonectomy pulmonary edema (PPE) is a particularly severe form of pulmonary edema that can occur after pneumonectomy and is associated with a high mortality. Resection of lesser amounts of lung tissue (i.e., wedge resection) is not associated with this entity [87]. Patients with PPE develop a low-pressure, high-protein pulmonary edema indicating endothelial damage is present [88]. An increase in endothelial permeability has been demonstrated by measuring the pulmonary accumulation of intravenously administered technetium 99 m-labeled albumin after pneumonectomy [89].

The etiology of PPE remains unclear but is likely multifactorial. Risk factors that have been associated with PPE include the side of operation, with right pneumonectomy having a higher risk than left, perioperative fluid overload (>2 L intravenous fluid administration), and higher tidal volumes during one lung ventilation (10 ml/kg) [90–92]. Other potential etiologies include the use of fresh frozen plasma intraoperatively, oxygen toxicity, serum cytokines, and mediastinal lymphatic damage.

The development of pulmonary edema after lung transplantation was initially termed the pulmonary reimplantation response but is now referred to as primary graft dysfunction

(PGD), representing a complex, incompletely understood multifactorial syndrome resulting from both donor and recipient factors and possible perioperative management strategies [93, 94]. Various risk factors have been identified; however, those patients, most consistently at risk, are characterized by a pre-transplant diagnosis of pulmonary hypertension, sarcoidosis, a donor history of smoking, and the need for cardiopulmonary bypass [95]. It appears both the endothelium and epithelium of the donor lungs are targets [94]. The syndrome occurs in approximately 20% of patients and is associated with a 23% absolute risk in mortality at 1 year [93]. Use of ECMO rather than cardiopulmonary bypass during surgery appears to be at least somewhat protective [96], but treatment is otherwise supportive as no specific preventative or therapeutic measures have been clearly shown to reduce the incidence or severity.

Pneumothorax

Following thoracotomy the surgeon usually places two chest tubes into the operative hemithorax. One chest tube is placed inferiorly to preferentially drain blood and fluids and a second tube superiorly to preferentially vent air. Pneumothorax may develop postoperatively if a chest tube is inadvertently kinked, clamped off, or dislodged. While a small leak may cause little or no symptoms, a large, undrained air leak can result in a "tension pneumothorax" with a shift of the trachea and mediastinum to the contralateral side. The increase in intrathoracic pressure causes a decrease in venous return to the right heart and can result in cardiovascular collapse. Pneumothorax may also occur on the nonoperative side as result of rupture of a pulmonary cyst or bulla if excessive airway pressures develop during mechanical (especially one lung) ventilation. Inadvertent and unrecognized surgical entry into the pleura of the nonoperative side may cause pneumothorax, as may inadvertent lung puncture during placement of central venous catheters, or intrapleural catheters for postoperative analgesia. Confirmatory imaging of a pneumothorax can be achieved with the use of ultrasound, particularly with the use of m-mode, as discussed in Chap. 28.

Definitive treatment of a pneumothorax is placement of a chest tube, usually in the fourth or fifth intercostal space between the anterior and mid-axillary lines. In the case of tension pneumothorax, a needle thoracostomy is often performed first by placing a large bore, i.e., 14 gauge, venous catheter above the third rib in the midclavicular line. This effectively converts the tension pneumothorax to a simple pneumothorax. While there is some advocacy for needle decompression to be placed at the same location as a chest tube, there is no definitive data, and there is trauma literature citing increased incidence of catheter kinking/dislodgement in this location [97].

Persistent Air Leaks and Bronchopleural Fistula

Persistent air leaks are reported to occur in 4–20% of pulmonary resections, prolonging and complicating the postoperative course [98]. Bronchopleural fistula is associated with a large air leak from the lung and results from disruption of a bronchial stump or tracheobronchial anastomosis. The initial sign is often a dramatic increase in air leak noticed in the chest tube drainage chamber. If the air leak exceeds the capacity of the chest tube to evacuate the air, there will be a persistent pneumothorax. In large bronchopleural fistulas, respiratory insufficiency may ensue. Positive-pressure ventilation poses a significant problem as the majority of tidal volume escapes into the pleural space and chest tube through the lower-resistance bronchopleural fistula. Pneumonectomy, residual tumor in the bronchial stump, hyperglycemia, hypoalbuminemia, postoperative mechanical ventilation, preoperative steroid use, COPD, and low-predicted postoperative FEV_1 have all been reported as risk factors for the development of bronchopleural fistulas [99].

Although definitive treatment of large leaks requires surgical correction, temporary ventilator management may include placement of a double-lumen endotracheal tube to allow differential lung ventilation (see below). Alternatively, a bronchial blocker may be used on the affected side to limit flow to that side. Smaller air leaks may be treated with endobronchial substances or devices. The use of endobronchial valves (Fig. 54.5), placed via bronchoscopy, has had reasonable success [100, 101].

Aspiration of Gastric Contents

In the thoracic surgery population, the risk of aspiration of gastric contents is increased in patients presenting with esophageal disease. Intraoperative aspiration will lead to a pulmonary injury causing edema and inflammation, leading to hypoxemia. Aspiration pneumonitis is one of the causes of acute respiratory distress syndrome (ARDS), the management of which is discussed below. Not well recognized is the risk of a relatively small-volume aspiration in patients extubated after more than 48 h after thoracic surgery in general and in particular after lung transplantation [102]. In the latter population, a study using fiber-optic endoscopy demonstrated aspiration in the majority of single and double lung transplantation patients [103]. These patients should be evaluated for swallowing competence and risk of aspiration before oral intake is initiated postoperatively and be watched closely for signs of aspiration.

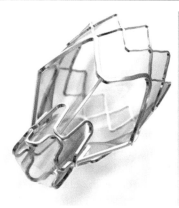

Zephyr EBV®
(Picture courtesy of Pulmonx,
Radwood City, CA)

Spiration IBV®
(Picture courtesy of Olympus Respiratory
America, Radmond, WA)

Fig. 54.5 Example of the two commercially available, one-way valves used in the management of persistent air leaks following lung resection and/or lung volume reduction surgery. The valves are composed of a self-expanding framework of nitinol. Both pictured models are available in Europe, currently only the Spiration IBV has FDA approval for humanitarian use in the United States. Left: Zephyr EBV ® (endobronchial valve). (Picture courtesy of Pulmox, Redwood city, CA), Right, Spiration IBV ® (intrabronchial valve). (Picture courtesy of Olympus Respiratory America, Redmond, WA) [100, 101]

Torsion of Residual Lobe

Torsion of a residual lobe of the lung around its bronchus may complicate lobectomy. The loss of lung tissue on the surgical side may allow abnormal movement of the residual lung tissue, most commonly the right middle lobe and the lingula. In addition to the intrapulmonary shunt that develops secondary to occlusion of the affected bronchus, blood supply to the affected lobe is compromised and can lead to infarction.

The diagnosis can be suspected by the onset of respiratory distress or failure in association with the appearance of a collapsed or abnormal lobe on the chest radiograph, which does not respond to the usual therapies for atelectasis. The diagnosis can then be confirmed by bronchoscopy. Definitive therapy consists of surgical correction of the torsion, which should be performed urgently if infarction of the lobe is to be prevented.

Neurologic Injuries

While rare following thoracic surgery, neurologic injuries may occur which can lead to pulmonary insufficiency in the postoperative period. Damage to a phrenic nerve can occur following thoracotomy, especially if extensive dissection into the mediastinum is necessary to remove a tumor. A patient with good pulmonary reserve usually tolerates unilateral phrenic nerve palsy. In a patient with baseline compromised pulmonary status, such as advanced chronic obstructive pulmonary disease, unilateral phrenic nerve paralysis will lead to difficulty in weaning from mechanical ventilation. Bilateral phrenic nerve paralysis will lead to pulmonary insufficiency in any patient. The diagnosis is suggested by elevated hemidiaphragm on postoperative chest film. It can be confirmed by observing paradoxical motion of the affected hemidiaphragm under fluoroscopy.

Recurrent laryngeal nerve injury may be seen following extensive hilar lymph node dissection. The left recurrent laryngeal nerve is at greater risk of injury due to its more caudal course. Unilateral injury is generally well tolerated, but bilateral injury can cause significant stridor following extubation secondary to spasm of the vocal cord adductor muscles.

Mechanical Ventilation After Thoracic Surgery

Table 54.6 summarizes the common reasons to continue mechanical ventilation into the postoperative period after thoracic surgery. Many of these relative indications are common to major surgery of all types and reflect planning to "stabilize" a patient after major stress. Preoperative and intraoperative discussion with the surgical team allow for appropriate arrangements to be made in advance regarding care in the postanesthesia care unit ("PACU") or intensive care unit (ICU).

Two major issues in early postoperative mechanical ventilation after thoracic surgery are (1) concern for bronchial anastomoses after lung resection and (2) leaving tracheal tubes that are designed for intraoperative lung isolation. Regarding bronchial anastomoses, there is always a concern that positive airway pressures may expose the patient to increased risk of bronchial anastomotic leaks or disruption. This must be balanced with the need for oxygenation (which

Table 54.6 Relative indications for mechanical ventilation after thoracic surgery

Preoperative
Preoperative mechanical ventilation
Predicted low postoperative FEV1 (<30% predicted)
Esophagogastrectomy or thoracoabdominal aneurysm repair
Intraoperative
Prolonged intraoperative course
Massive fluid administration or transfusion
Hypothermia
Cardiac failure
Surgical complication
Need for postoperative lung isolation (air leak, drainage)
Need for postoperative chest wall immobilization/stabilization
Immediate postoperative
Incomplete recovery of neuromuscular function
Inadequate respiratory drive (excessive opioid administration)
Requirement for >50% fiO_2
Visible respiratory distress

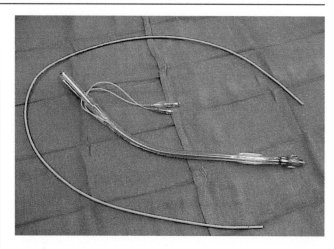

Fig. 54.6 Long tube changer for use with double-lumen tracheal tubes (Cook Medical). A double-lumen tube is illustrated with the tube changer curved around it; the tube changer is more than twice the length of the double-lumen tube

may require positive end-expiratory pressure [PEEP]) and adequate minute ventilation for elimination of CO_2. The clinical goal is to avoid elevated airway pressures by reducing the delivered tidal volume or by using pressure limited modes of ventilation where possible (see below). There are no publications defining the "safe" upper limit of positive airway pressure after lung resection; however, common sense dictates that lower airway pressures are safer.

Double-lumen or specialty tubes which incorporate a bronchial blocker have small inner diameters related to their outer diameter, making tracheal/airway toilet difficult and imposing additional work of breathing when this is demanded of the patient. In addition, PACU and ICU nurses and respiratory therapists are usually unfamiliar with such tubes. Unless there is a need to continue lung isolation postoperatively (e.g., persistent large air leak, draining infection), it is desirable to replace such specialty tubes with single-lumen tubes before leaving the operating room. In those patients with difficult airways or those who have/are expected to have oral or airway edema, clinical judgment must be used; the above mentioned problems may be a necessary evil in the face of potential loss of the airway. While long tube exchanging devices for double lumen tubes are available (Fig. 54.6), use of these does not guarantee the ability to readvance a single lumen tube through a very edematous or difficult airway. It may be prudent to plan to change the tube at a later time/date.

Preoperative Indications for Postoperative Mechanical Ventilation

Patients coming to the operating room already ventilated for any reason are unlikely to tolerate extubation immediately after their procedure. Withdrawal of mechanical ventilation should be done in a gradual, controlled manner, and the operating room is not a suitable place for this process. Patients with poor predicted postoperative FEV_1 (less than 30% predicted) are at the highest risk for immediate postoperative respiratory failure (see Chap. 2). These patients may benefit from a staged withdrawal of mechanical ventilation, while other physiology is assured to be optimal (cardiac, endocrine, renal), and normothermia and analgesia are achieved. Specific major procedures that are usually associated with *elective* postoperative mechanical ventilation for at least 24 h include esophagectomy or esophagogastrectomy and thoracic or thoracoabdominal aortic aneurysm repair [104, 105]. Apart from the extent and duration of surgery, these latter procedures are associated with extended periods of one-lung ventilation, and the operative-side lung is often contused or partially atelectatic despite having been re-inflated at the end of surgery. This leads to hypoxemia and increased work of breathing.

Intraoperative Indications for Postoperative Mechanical Ventilation

Unanticipated operative complications may lead to circumstances that are unfavorable to immediate postoperative extubation. Foremost among these indications are any complications or conditions that lead to difficulty in obtaining adequate oxygenation or CO_2 elimination intraoperatively. Other factors that need to be considered in relation to the list in Table 54.1 are underlying comorbid conditions, age, and time of day (availability of experts in ventilator and airway management). A period of elective postoperative mechanical ventilation permits stabilization of organ systems (e.g., volume status, cardiac function, coagulation/

hemostasis control), while oxygenation and ventilation are assured. Withdrawal of mechanical ventilation can be done in a staged and controlled manner without the pressure of time that exists in the operating room. The list of relative indications in Table 54.6 must be tempered with clinical judgment throughout, and at the end of the procedure, continued discussion of the plan with the surgical team can facilitate a smooth transition from the operating room to the PACU or ICU.

Immediate Postoperative Indications for Mechanical Ventilation

As in any surgical patient, circumstances may arise or become evident at the end of thoracic surgery that prevent extubation. Foremost among these are inadequate neuromuscular function as assessed objectively by nerve stimulation or clinically by weakness and inadequate spontaneous respirations (low rate in association with high end-tidal or arterial CO_2 concentration). In the case of iatrogenic muscle weakness due to an aminosteroid, non-depolarizing muscle relaxant, sugammadex is a viable reversal option in the absence of contraindications [106, 107].

While the aforementioned complications must be resolved before extubation, of greater concern are problems with oxygenation (e.g., requirement of >50% FiO_2 to achieve a SpO_2 >90%), ventilation (inadequate CO_2 elimination despite tachypnea), and visible respiratory distress. Inadequate pain control may contribute to these findings; however, they may also represent a physiologic derangement likely to require more than a few minutes for resolution. Specific blood gas criteria or respiratory measures are frequently quoted as indicating a need for mechanical ventilation; however, in the rapidly changing situation at the end of surgery, it is difficult to apply such criteria. A *clinical judgment* must be made to assist or control ventilation for an additional period, usually requiring the patient also be (re)sedated. At this time a call to the PACU or ICU should be made with a request for a mechanical ventilator and sedative infusion(s). A chest radiograph and arterial blood gas analysis should be performed at the earliest opportunity.

In addition to permitting the administration of high, known concentrations of oxygen, positive-pressure ventilation with positive end-expiratory pressure (PEEP) via a tracheal tube assists oxygenation by opening/expanding partially collapsed alveoli and perhaps opening some fully collapsed ones. Positive end-expiratory pressure or PEEP improves oxygenation in pulmonary edema and acute lung injury both by these mechanisms and by redistributing (but not reducing) lung water [108, 109]. Increasing the fraction of inspired oxygen (FiO_2) will improve arterial oxygenation by increasing transport in those areas that are absorbing O_2.

True shunt will respond only to re-expansion of collapsed segments or reduction of the size of the shunt. This may require bronchoscopy and can be aided by PEEP. Thus, failure of oxygenation is treated with increasing the FiO_2 and/or increasing the mean airway pressure.

Usually the work by the respiratory muscles to ventilate the lungs requires only a few percent of total body oxygen consumption, but this may be several times higher in the postoperative patient and higher still in acute respiratory failure [110]. Mechanical ventilation also takes over the work of breathing for the patient in distress and guarantees alveolar ventilation. Thus, mechanical ventilation with PEEP treats both components of acute respiratory failure.

Ventilatory Modes

Modern mechanical ventilators used in critical care and now present on anesthesia machines are very sophisticated microprocessor controlled devices that sense and interact with the patient (see Chap. 22). This is in stark contrast to the traditional anesthesia ventilator that has three controls: respiratory rate, tidal volume, and inspiratory flow rate delivering only *volume-cycled*, controlled mandatory ventilation (CMV). Modern ICU ventilators offer a variety of interactive modes, as well as pressure or volume-cycled breaths. Many devices administer noninvasive ventilation (NIV), using a specially designed facial or nasal mask (Fig. 54.4a) to deliver either CPAP or "BIPAP" which is analogous to pressure support ventilation with PEEP.

Noninvasive Ventilation

Traditionally, NIV is either CPAP or pressure support with PEEP (BIPAP) provided via a face mask rather than a tracheal tube. There has been recent interest in the addition of high-flow nasal cannula (HFNC) to this category. As will be discussed below, there is some preliminary data to support the prophylactic use of NIV. However, it is still currently thought of as more of a rescue strategy.

We ventilate our lungs by drawing gas in with our respiratory muscles: during spontaneous inspiration, airway pressure (P_{aw}) is negative with respect to the atmosphere, and during expiration P_{aw} is positive. Spontaneous breathing in this way, with a positive rather than atmospheric baseline pressure, is CPAP (Fig. 54.7). Strictly speaking this is not a mode of ventilation as there is no inspiratory assist. This mode of support is usually used to improve oxygenation in patients who do not have ventilatory failure, as it helps increase the FRC and reduces atelectasis. It may allow spontaneous breathing to occur at a more compliant part of the pressure-volume relationship of the thorax, reducing the

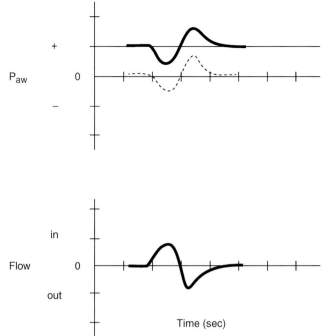

Fig. 54.7 Airway pressure and gas flow during a spontaneous breath through a CPAP mask/circuit. The pressures and flows mirror those for a spontaneous breath (dashed line), but the baseline pressure is elevated. Paw, airway pressure

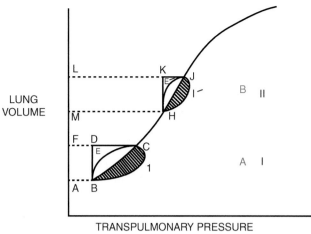

TRANSPULMONARY PRESSURE

Fig. 54.8 Pressure-volume loops illustrated at two different lung volumes, representing tidal volume at reduced lung volume and FRC as might occur with postoperative atelectasis (**a**) and the same tidal volume at normal lung volume and FRC (**b**). The solid sigmoidal line is the elastic pressure-volume curve for the lung and chest wall. Application of CPAP can reopen atelectatic portions of the lung and move tidal breathing up the pressure-volume relationship of the lung and chest wall from A to B, both improving gas exchange and reducing the work of breathing (transpulmonary pressure required to generate same tidal volume)

work of breathing [111] (Fig. 54.8). CPAP can be provided by a continuous high-flow circuit or can be delivered through a microprocessor-controlled ventilator that senses effort (airway pressure or flow) and responds accordingly. In the former case, the airway pressure varies slightly during the respiratory cycle; however, the high level of flow and built in reservoir prevents large swings in pressure. In the latter case, the flow is delivered in response to the sensor, attempting always to meet the patient's demands and to achieve the preset level of CPAP.

An enhancement of CPAP is BIPAP, which provides inspiratory assistance. This mode of NIV can be used in the treatment of acute respiratory failure as well as the treatment of hypoxemia. It has been shown to prevent intubation in several medical and surgical populations including thoracic surgery [112]. Several postoperative studies of CPAP and BIPAP have demonstrated benefit and no harm. Squadrone et al. performed a large multicenter trial on patients who had undergone upper abdominal surgery. Patients with a PaO2/FiO2 ratio <300 mm Hg were randomized to receive CPAP with an FiO2 of 0.5 vs. a face mask with FiO2 of 0.5. Patients receiving CPAP had a lower incidence of reintubation and pneumonia [113]. Another study by Kindgen-Milles looked at post-extubation CPAP in patients who underwent open thoracoabdominal aneurysm repair. The patients who received CPAP post-extubation had better oxygenation, fewer pulmonary complications, and shorter hospital stay

compared to the controls [114]. In a report of 690 patients undergoing lung resection, Lefebvre et al. reported a 16% incidence of respiratory failure, 85% of whom were successfully managed with NIV alone [115]. Perrin et al. used NIV pre- and postoperatively and demonstrated a reduction in pulmonary complications after lung resection, Rocco et al. prevented reintubation in 18/21 patients with respiratory failure after lung transplantation, and Michelet et al. showed similar benefits in patients who developed respiratory failure after esophagectomy [116–118].

Though comprised of small studies, there is increasing evidence supporting the use of heated and humidified, high-flow nasal cannula (HFNC) as an alternative first-line therapy in the treatment of respiratory failure in the cardiothoracic surgery population. HFNC delivers O_2 of concentrations from 0.2 to 1.0 at rates of up to 60 lpm and in the process may generate P_{aw} of 3–5 cm H_2O. It is believed this mode of delivery can decrease the work of breathing, decrease respiratory rate, increase end-expiratory lung volumes, decrease dead space, and reduce the need for intubation [119–122].

It is clear that use of CPAP and BIPAP can both prevent and treat respiratory failure after surgery, can avoid the need for intubation, reduce respiratory complications, and decrease length of stay. However, despite evidence to the contrary, there is still some concern for the integrity of surgical anastomoses in the setting of positive-pressure ventilation. This is one of the ways in which HFNC represents a more attractive alternative as it generates significantly lower P_{aw} pressures compared to CPAP and BiPAP while offering equivalent benefits. Additionally HFNC may provide a more comfortable option, especially for patients who won't tolerate a tight-fitting mask covering their nose and/or face. Though there is data to support its safety, the use of CPAP/BiPAP in the setting of fresh anastomoses is still a commonly stated concern. Given the seemingly equivalent efficacy of HFNC, it is a reasonable first option given the low level of increased airway pressures. Other benefits include full visual access to a patient's face further allaying concerns regarding aspiration and evolving mental status changes.

There are limitations to any mode of NIV. It is not appropriate for patients who cannot cooperate or for those with excessive secretions, hemoptysis, or vomiting who are unable to protect their airway. Table 54.7 lists contraindications [112]. Success requires patience and expertise on the part of the respiratory therapist and usually slow, incremental adjustments to inspiratory and/or expiratory pressures in the case of CPAP/BiPAP or flow rate and oxygen content in the case of HFNC. When using CPAP/BiPAP, the presence of a nasogastric tube may introduce a leak which cannot be managed, and peak airway pressures (i.e., actual pressure during inspiration) should never exceed 25 cm H_2O. No mode of noninvasive ventilation is a long-term ventilator strategy, and it is vital that clear endpoints delineating either success or failure should be kept in mind. If the patient is not clearly improving over a trial period of no more than 1–2 days, then a move to tracheal intubation or tracheotomy should be considered.

Table 54.7 Noninvasive ventilation (NIV) after thoracic surgery

Possible indications
  Prevention of pulmonary dysfunction after lung resection
  Treatment of respiratory failure (short term) after lung resection and lung transplant
Contraindications
  CNS
    Decreased level of consciousness
    Severe agitation or encephalopathy
    Uncooperative patient
    Inability to protect airway
  Cardiorespiratory
    Cardiac or respiratory arrest
    Cardiac instability
    Severe respiratory failure
  Copious secretions or hemoptysis
  Gastrointestinal
    Vomiting/gastric distension
    Upper GI bleeding
  Other
    Facial trauma or other condition preventing facemask application (high-flow nasal cannula may be an option in this instance)
    Multiple organ failure

Lung-Protective Ventilation

The principles of "lung-protective ventilation" discussed in Chap. 21 should be adhered to when a decision is made to continue or initiate mechanical ventilation in the postoperative period. If the patient is an appropriate candidate, NIV as described above should be seriously considered when a patient who has already been extubated requires oxygenation and/or ventilation assistance beyond what can be offered through facemask oxygen. If mechanical ventilation must be provided through a tracheal tube, appropriate levels of inspiratory pressure and PEEP should be selected. While many strong opinions exist regarding specific modes of ventilation, the ARDSnet trial (referred to below) demonstrated an outcome benefit in acute respiratory distress syndrome (ARDS) by employing tidal volumes of 5–8 ml/kg of predicted body weight using assist-control (volume cycled) ventilation and appropriate levels of PEEP. Either pressure or volume modes can be employed so long as delivered tidal volumes are in this range and airway pressures are not excessive. Pressure modes have the advantage of achieving a similar tidal volume with lower peak airway pressure; however, this has not been shown to translate into an outcome benefit. Table 54.8 summarizes the principles of lung-protective ventilation.

The many possible causes of postoperative respiratory failure have been discussed above. In some circumstances these inciting and predisposing factors can be resolved or compensated for by the patient in the first hours or day after surgery, as the acute stress of surgery subsides and effective analgesic techniques are in place. Mechanical ventilation can then be withdrawn rapidly and uneventfully. In other patients the interaction of preexisting functional and pulmonary status, surgical stress, and postoperative complications described above may lead to a more prolonged need for ventilatory assistance. In a small percentage of patients, acute lung injury (ALI) or acute respiratory distress syndrome (ARDS) may occur.

Table 54.8 Principles of "lung-protective" ventilation

Ventilator mode	Volume assist-control most often reported
Tidal volume (ml/kg of predicted body weight)	5–7 (lower is better)
Plateau pressure (cm of water)	<30
Ratio of duration of inspiration to expiration	1:1–1:3
Ventilator rate (breaths/min)	Set to achieve pH > 7.3
Bicarbonate infusion	As needed if pH goal cannot be achieved
Oxygenation goal	PaO_2 > 55 mmHg or SpO_2 > 88%
PEEP	As needed to achieve oxygenation goal (titrated upward with fiO_2)*

*See Ref. [138] for protocol describing incremental adjustments of fiO_2 and PEEP

Acute Respiratory Distress Syndrome

The Berlin criteria, published in 2012, outline the current standard for acute respiratory distress syndrome (ARDS) classification. In brief, the 2012 Berlin criteria describe ARDS as a state of increased pulmonary vascular permeability and loss of aerated lung tissue resulting from an acute, diffuse, and inflammatory lung injury. These updated guidelines differ from the previously accepted definition as delineated by the American-European consensus conference on ARDS by stratifying the severity of ARDS based on the arterial partial pressure of oxygen/fraction of inspired oxygen, or P/F ratio, and removing the designation of acute lung injury (ALI) [123, 124]. Specific requirements regarding timing, chest imaging, origin of edema and oxygenation, as well as differences from the previous guidelines are outlined in Table 54.9.

ARDS can be induced by direct insults to the lung such as aspiration of gastric contents, pulmonary infection, or contusion but is more commonly associated with indirect causes such as sepsis syndrome and severe trauma, pancreatitis, or massive transfusion. The latter causes are typically referred to as "extrapulmonary." Mortality implications are similar with direct pulmonary injury or extrapulmonary causes [125, 126]. It is uncommon to see the diffuse infiltrates that characterize ARDS immediately after surgery; such a finding on the postoperative radiograph is more likely to represent hydrostatic edema due to fluid overload or left-sided cardiac failure. Hydrostatic pulmonary edema may be radiographically indistinguishable from ARDS, at least in the early stages.

Direct injury to the lung as a result of surgery, or indirect effects from other organ system dysfunctions, trauma of sur-gery, or multiple transfusions may initiate the pathophysiology leading to ARDS in thoracic surgery patients. In a six-year review (1991–1997) of all pulmonary resections done at the Royal Brompton Hospital in London, England, the combined incidence of ALI and ARDS was 3.9%. The overall mortality from ARDS is approximately 50%, although recent data suggests a decline over the last 10 years; in the review from the Royal Brompton Hospital, ALI/ARDS was associated with 72.5% of the mortality [127]. Patients with the syndrome typically go on to have other organ dysfunctions, developing the multiple organ dysfunction syndrome or "MODS" [128]. In fact, most patients who succumb do so of non-respiratory organ failures [129]. The MODS syndrome occurs in approximately 15% of ICU patients and is responsible for 80% of ICU deaths [130]. Rather than the severity of gas exchange abnormality in ARDS, other patient-specific factors such as preexisting organ system dysfunction, increasing age, and the presence of sepsis are more predictive of mortality. As more systems become involved in the MODS, mortality increases exponentially. Patients who survive ARDS are likely to have relatively intact pulmonary function within 6–12 months, although health-related quality of life is reduced [131]. If the lung injury in ARDS does not resolve in 7–10 days, it may progress to fibrosis and finally to obliteration of the pulmonary capillary bed with pulmonary hypertension.

Therapy of ARDS

Despite more than 30 years of research into causes and treatment of ALI and ARDS, it remains a clinical syndrome with elusive etiology. A great deal of progress has been made in

Table 54.9 Definition of ARDS

	Berlin criteria (current)			AECC (previous)	
	Mild	Moderate	Severe	ALI	ARDS
Timing	Within 1 week of new or progressive respiratory symptoms with or without a known insult			Acute onset	
Oxygenation	200 mmHg < P/F <= 300 mmHg[a]	100 mmHg < P/F <= 200 mmHg[a]	P/F <= 100 mmHg[a]	P/F < 300 mmHg[b]	P/F < 200 mmHg[b]
Imaging	Bilateral opacities not otherwise explained by effusions, lobar/lung collapse, or nodules			Bilateral infiltrates on CXR	
Etiology of edema	Respiratory failure that cannot be fully explained by cardiac failure or fluid overload[c]			Not addressed	
Pulmonary artery wedge pressure	Removed from criteria			<18 mmHg or no evidence of elevated LAP	

Table 54.9 Comparison of previous vs. current criteria in the diagnosis of ARDS. Note that the Berlin criteria clarify onset period, no longer recognize ALI, have introduced more granularity when differentiating grade of ARDS, clarified imaging criteria, added a requirement for the etiology of pulmonary edema, and removed the requirement for a measured pulmonary artery wedge pressure measurement [123, 124]
ALI acute lung injury, *ARDS* acute respiratory distress syndrome, *AECC* American-European consensus conference, *P/F* ratio of arterial oxygen to inspired oxygen, *CXR* chest X-ray, *LAP* left atrial pressure, *PEEP* positive end-expiratory pressure
[a]With PEEP> = 5 cm H_2O
[b]Regardless of PEEP level
[c]Objective assessment preferred if no risk to patient

understanding the pathophysiology; however, the earliest events which trigger the inflammation and damage of lung tissue continue to be explored. Therapy targeting these early events, and pharmacotherapy in general, has been disappointing. A variety of pharmacological agents including prostaglandins, surfactant, inhaled nitric oxide (NO), and corticosteroids have failed to demonstrate an outcome benefit [132–135]. Current treatment of ARDS is therefore "supportive," attempting to provide vital organ support without further damaging the lungs and providing an environment for healing. As a pulmonary dilator, inhaled NO can reduce pulmonary artery pressure without causing systemic hypotension and improves oxygenation by augmenting blood flow to ventilated alveoli, but these benefits have failed to improve survival.

Mechanical Ventilation with PEEP

Perhaps one of the most surprising outcomes of the intense research into ARDS has been the gradual realization that the mainstay of therapy itself – mechanical ventilation – could worsen, and in some animal models actually *cause*, lung injury. More than 25 years ago, ventilation with high volumes and pressures was shown to cause pulmonary edema in animal models [136]. Further studies documented such injury in a variety of animal models and settings and in particular the worsening of existing injury with high volumes. Inflammatory markers are elevated when high volumes are used to ventilate patients with ARDS, and survival from the syndrome can be improved by using small (6–8 ml/kg vs 10–12 ml/kg) tidal volumes [137]. The "ARDSnet" trial funded by the National Heart, Lung, and Blood Institute in the United States, and performed by the "ARDS network" of institutions, documented a mortality reduction from almost 40% to 31% by simply using a smaller tidal volume to achieve a "plateau pressure" of <30 cm H_2O, in association with a protocolized strategy for FiO_2, PEEP, and management of acid-base disorders [138]. This approach to ventilation, as described above, has been termed "lung protective." An overview of the protocol is given in Table 54.8, and the full protocol can be found at HYPERLINK http://www.ardsnet.org www.ardsnet.org [138]. Evidence from this trial, other clinical and laboratory studies, and now a number of perioperative studies as described in Chap. 21 have resulted in a general move to the use of smaller tidal volumes in all ventilated patients, both in the OR and the ICU.

Collapse and re-expansion of alveoli with each respiratory cycle can cause injury, and this can be reduced or prevented by adequate levels of PEEP [139]. Determining the optimal level of PEEP has concerned clinicians for more than 25 years and continues to be a dilemma. In 1975 Suter et al. coined the phrase "best PEEP" in relating the PEEP level to oxygen delivery to the tissues [140]. These investigators found that although increasing levels of PEEP usually

resulted in better oxygenation of the arterial blood, as the intrathoracic pressure rose above a certain level, the cardiac output and hence oxygen delivery declined. In recent years, while taking this latter concept into consideration, there has been a greater interest in finding the level of PEEP that keeps the most alveoli open, ventilating only on the compliant portion of the pressure-volume relationship of the lung. The theoretical goal is to use adequate PEEP such that ventilation occurs above the "lower inflection point" of the pressure-volume relationship as shown in Fig. 54.9, which may prevent potentially traumatic repeated closing and opening of alveoli in atelectatic areas of the lung. At the same time, a tidal volume that inflates to below the upper inflection point should be employed, preventing trauma from overdistension [141]. This requires some measure of the pressure-volume relationship which may not always be possible. In a follow-up study to the ARDSnet trial, a randomized trial of lower vs. higher PEEP was performed. In this study the PEEP was increased more rapidly in the high PEEP group, usually exceeding 12 cm H_2O; there was no influence in outcome [142]. A more recent meta-analysis suggests that higher PEEP (>10 cm H_2O) may provide a small benefit, especially when lung injury is more severe [143]. It may be that higher levels are most useful in patients where there is a clear beneficial effect in terms of improved oxygenation and compliance.

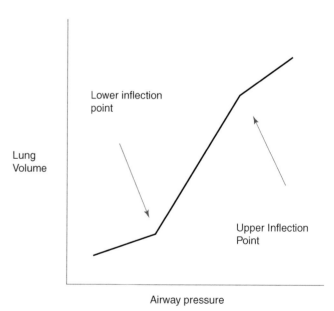

Fig. 54.9 Inspiratory pressure-volume relationship of the respiratory system in a patient with ARDS. Ideally ventilation should occur at a lung volume represented by the middle section of the curve where the lung is most compliant. If ventilation occurs at a lung volume overlapping either the lower inflection point or upper inflection point, ventilator-induced trauma may occur. In the former case, this is due to repeated opening and closing of alveoli due to inadequate level of PEEP; in the latter it is overdistending of already fully inflated alveoli

As the practice of using reduced tidal volumes has increased, two clinical problems have become apparent. The first is the need for high respiratory rates to achieve normal arterial CO_2 levels and sometimes failing to achieve the latter. The phrase "permissive hypercapnia" has been coined, meaning that a higher than normal CO_2 level is tolerated in order to protect the lung from high tidal volume ventilation [144]. Either the respiratory acidosis is tolerated or a bicarbonate infusion can be used to restore the pH toward normal. In the ARDSnet trial, a pH of 7.30 was tolerated; in other studies even lower levels have been accepted. The second problem is that despite relatively high PEEP levels, the use of small tidal volumes may result in gradual collapse of alveoli and worsened oxygenation. This has led to the investigation of "recruitment" maneuvers such as intermittent application of high levels of airway pressure, analogous to the old concept of sighs. There is some data to suggest such recruitment maneuvers can improve oxygenation in ARDS and potentially decrease ICU mortality. However, there is no effect on in-hospital and 28-day mortality [145, 146].

Positive intrathoracic pressure may have an impact on cardiac performance. With relatively compliant lungs, positive pressure created by the ventilator is transmitted to the entire thoracic cavity and may affect the preload and afterload to the heart. If cardiac function is normal, the predominant effect is a reduction in venous return leading to a decrease in cardiac output. As discussed above, "best PEEP" is the level at which the increase in oxygenation of the blood was not offset by a reduction in cardiac output [140]. Where there is left ventricular dysfunction and elevated filling pressure, the reduction in preload may reduce ventricular distension and improve cardiac performance. In addition, making the intrathoracic cavity positive with respect to the rest of the body reduces the afterload to the left ventricle (Fig. 54.10) [147].

Right ventricular function may be adversely affected by high levels of PEEP (e.g., >10 cm H_2O). The right ventricle is a thin-walled cavity that normally generates relatively low pressures (e.g., 25 mm Hg systolic). High levels of PEEP required to oxygenate the blood may increase the impedance to right ventricular ejection, causing right ventricular dilatation and a decrease in contractility [148]. In patients who have undergone pulmonary resection, in particular pneumonectomy, the right ventricle is already "stressed" by needing to pump the normal cardiac output through a reduced pulmonary vascular tree. Overdistension of the right ventricle may distort the interventricular septum, interfering with left ventricular filling [149]. In centers with appropriate experience

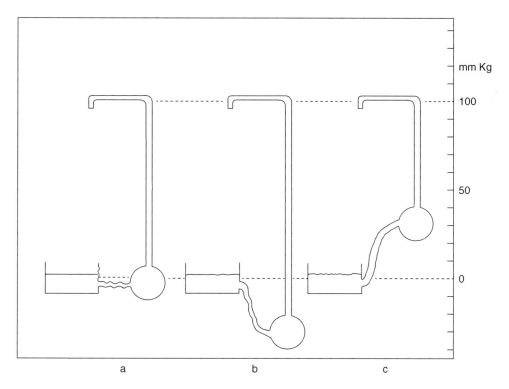

Fig. 54.10 Diagrammatic representation of the effects of respiratory-induced changes in pleural pressure on right ventricular inflow and left ventricular outflow. At end-expiration (**a**) the venous reservoir empties at normal pressure into the heart which generates normal systemic pressure. With deep inspiration (**b**) venous inflow is augmented because the intrathoracic pressure (location of the heart) is made negative; at the same time, the heart must generate a higher pressure to achieve a normal systemic pressure outside of the thorax. During expiration (**c**) venous inflow is reduced at the same time as left ventricular afterload is reduced. This illustrates the mechanism of the beneficial effects of positive intrathoracic pressure (positive-pressure ventilation, PEEP) in patients with heart failure

and expertise, echocardiographic assessment of ventricular function, pulmonary artery catheterization, or cardiac output measurement by "stand-alone" devices may be useful to determine the effect of mechanical ventilation on cardiac performance.

Another undesirable feature of positive-pressure ventilation is the creation or worsening of "autoPEEP," where partially obstructed airways prevent complete emptying of the alveoli during expiration. This results in continued gas flow and airway pressure above baseline (i.e., atmospheric or applied level of PEEP) at the end of expiration. Application of additional PEEP can "match" the autoPEEP and reduce the patient effort required to initiate a spontaneous breath or trigger a machine breath. If, however, a rapid respiratory rate is set on the ventilator and/or lung pathology causes reduced expiratory flow rates not permitting the lung to fully empty with expiration, autoPEEP is worsened with positive-pressure ventilation.

Prone Position

In 1974, Bryan proposed the dorsal regions of the lung would receive improved ventilation in the prone position during mechanical ventilation [150]. Since that time a variety of publications have demonstrated his theory correct. Both animal and human studies have demonstrated improved matching of ventilation to perfusion, as well as overall better distribution of blood flow and transpleural pressures gradients [151, 152]. An elegant study demonstrated the dramatic effects of prone positioning on regional lung density with serial CT scanning [153]. Previously, the majority of studies, including meta-analyses of the prone position in the setting of ALI and ARDS, demonstrated an improvement in oxygenation, a reduction in ventilator-associated pneumonia but no effect on survival [154]. However, the PROSEVA study group published a randomized controlled trial in 2013 showing a significant reduction in 28-day and 90-day mortality when prone positioning was applied within 36 h of diagnosis and for a minimum of 12–18 h daily in the subset of patients classified as having severe ARDS [155]. While this data is promising, it's generalizability to the post-surgical population is unclear, and for the subset of patients with recent sternotomy or abdominal incisions, its use is contraindicated [156].

Alternate Modes of Ventilation

A variety of modes of ventilation including inverse ratio (where inspiration is longer than expiration), airway pressure release ventilation (APRV, spontaneous breathing at high airway pressure, with intermittent release), high-frequency oscillatory ventilation (HFOV, very small tidal volume and high frequency), and high-frequency percussive ventilation (HFPV, high-frequency "stacking" breaths resulting in lower-frequency convective breaths) have been described and evaluated in small clinical studies. Inverse ratio ventilation and APRV are modes available on commercial ventilators; HFOV and HFPV require specialized ventilators. All of these modes have been used to improve oxygenation and/or ventilation, and with the exception of HFOV, there is a paucity of outcome studies [157]. The OSCILLATE [158] and OSCAR [159] trials were randomized controlled studies investigating some preliminary data suggesting the early use of HFOV may prove beneficial in ALI/ARDS. The OSCAR trial showed no mortality benefit, and the OSCILLATE trial showed a trend toward harm that led to its early termination.

Inhaled Pulmonary Vasodilators

As mentioned above, early trials of inhaled nitric oxide and prostaglandins failed to demonstrate an outcome benefit in adults with ARDS from a variety of causes. A few reports of the use of inhaled milrinone exist but not in the context of prolonged use for ARDS. Despite the lack of benefit found in early trials, clinicians, anxious to find benefit, have continued to use and study these agents as they do usually result in at least a transient improvement in oxygenation and may provide "temporization" before starting more invasive treatment such as ECMO. Unfortunately, however, recent meta-analyses continue to demonstrate a lack of benefit and now suggest possibly an increased risk of renal impairment with nitric oxide [160] and systemic hypotension with inhaled prostaglandin [161].

Extracorporeal Membrane Oxygenation (ECMO)

Experience with extracorporeal membrane oxygenation in adults, as reported by the Extracorporeal Life Support Organization (ELSO), has resulted in a renewed interest in this mode of therapy for ARDS. In their 2008 registry report, survival to hospital discharge or transfer in adults where ECMO was initiated for respiratory failure was an impressive 51%; the latest data from the same registry shows 66% survived ECMO and 59% survived to discharge or transfer [162]. Similarly, in a report of 22 patients receiving ECMO for primary graft dysfunction after lung transplantation, the survival was 54% at 1 year [163]. The use of ECMO in severe respiratory failure has increased significantly since 2010 asa result of the publication of two large trials in 2009, and improvements in the circuitry, oxygenators and nonpulsatile pumps. These trials demonstrated positive results with ARDS due to viral pneumonia [164] and in a broader group of patients with ARDS transported to a specialty center for treatment [165]. It has been suggested that patients with a potentially reversible cause of respiratory failure and a P/F ratio of <100 should be referred to an ECMO center, and when this ratio drops below 70, this should be considered an indication to institute ECMO [166].

The greatest use of ECMO in thoracic surgery patients is for the lung transplant population. In patients awaiting transplantation but whose end-stage lung disease is not compatible with adequate ventilation or oxygenation, ECMO can provide life support until donor lungs are available. Intraoperatively, in patients who cannot tolerate one-lung anesthesia or the surgical manipulations preparing for implantation of new lungs, ECMO is now a well-established supportive therapy. For those patients with donor lung dysfunction (most commonly PGD, described above), postoperative ECMO support can be employed until the donor lungs have recovered adequately to support respiration.

For other thoracic surgery patients developing severe postoperative respiratory failure and ARDS, the role of ECMO is less well established with very little supportive literature. Nevertheless if patients are failing conventional ventilator support as described above and appear to be appropriate candidates for ECMO, this form of treatment should be considered. The reader is referred to Chap. 55 for a more detailed consideration of ECMO therapy.

Complications of Mechanical Ventilation

Trauma to the Lungs or Tracheobronchial Tree

Damage to the lung parenchyma as a consequence of mechanical ventilation is discussed above. In thoracic surgery patients, the potential risk of suture line or bronchial stump disruption as a result of positive airway pressure has also been referred to. Suture line disruption can cause catastrophic pneumothorax or respiratory failure or may result in chronic air leak, bronchopleural fistula, and infection. Avoidance of intubation and positive-pressure ventilation are certainly desirable, but not always possible. As discussed above a trial of HFNC when appropriate, the use of pressure-limited modes of ventilation and the use of small tidal volumes if volume-controlled modes are used may help avoid high pressures. Auriant et al. suggested that noninvasive ventilation could reduce the mortality in acute respiratory failure after pneumonectomy [167].

Ventilator-Associated Pneumonia

One of the most serious complications associated with mechanical ventilation is pneumonia. Ventilator-associated pneumonia (VAP) is defined as pneumonia developing >48 h after initiating mechanical ventilation with absence prior to intubation. The reported incidence varies from 8 to 28% of patients receiving mechanical ventilation for more than 48 h, which is approximately three- to tenfold the incidence of pneumonia in non-intubated hospitalized patients [168–171]. Current reporting techniques use the relationship between number of ventilator days and incidence of pneumonia, with surgical units experiencing 9–10 pneumonias per 1000 ventilator days [172]. The mortality is reported from 24% to 50% and can be up to 76% in specific settings with high-risk pathogens. Resistant organisms comprise an ever-increasing proportion of hospital-acquired infections, including VAP [173].

Diagnosis

VAP should be suspected when there is a new or changing infiltrate on chest X-ray and at least two of the following criteria: abnormal temperature (>38 °C or <36 °C), abnormal white blood cell count (>10,000, <4000, or with >10% immature cells), and purulent sputum [174]. The 2016 IDSA guidelines recommend noninvasive sampling, such as endotracheal aspiration, with semiquantitative cultures over quantitative cultures of either invasive sampling, such as bronchoalveolar lavage (BAL), protected specimen brush, and mini-BAL or noninvasive sampling. It is however a weak recommendation that would require extensive discussion among all interested parties in a given institution [175].

Most important is the early initiation of appropriate institution-based empiric broad-spectrum antibiotics. Failure to adequately treat, from the earliest possible opportunity, is associated with worsened outcome. The presence of resistant organisms in the institution or specific ICU determines which agents should be chosen at the outset.

Prevention

Prevention of VAP is a priority in modern intensive care. This has given rise to the concept of the ventilator or VAP "bundle" – a variety of care processes either known or believed to reduce the risk of acquiring VAP [176]. These measures include elevation of the head of the bed to 30 degrees to reduce aspiration risk, oral rinse with antiseptic solution to reduce bacterial load, daily withdrawal of sedation, and daily spontaneous breathing trials to facilitate removal of the endotracheal tube. Prophylaxis for stress ulcers and deep venous thrombosis are often included in the "bundle." Continuous aspiration of subglottic secretions (CASS) has been evaluated with the goal of preventing aspiration. CASS requires a specialized ETT with a second lumen allowing a suction catheter proximal to the endotracheal tube cuff. Bouza et al. were able to demonstrate a reduction in VAP in patients treated with CASS [177]. Coating an endotracheal tube with silver has also been investigated and is theoretically attractive because of silver's broad-spectrum antimicrobial activity. An investigation by Kollef et al. with silver-coated endotracheal tubes was able to demonstrate a reduction in the incidence of VAP [178].

Withdrawal of Mechanical Ventilation

Many factors play into the decision to withdraw ventilatory support, the first being adequate control or resolution of the condition which lead to the need for ventilation. In the postoperative thoracic surgery patient, this may simply be correction of acute issues such as pain control, fluid status, and temperature. If gas exchange has been the principal issue, then ability of the patient to achieve acceptable pH, pCO_2 and pO_2 or saturation must be assessed. In general, the need for positive-pressure ventilation with more than 50% oxygen and/or 5–8 cm H_2O of PEEP to obtain a paO_2 of 60 mmHg or saturation of >90% suggests that oxygenation will not be adequate without ventilatory support. Similarly, elevated pCO_2 in association with decreased pH suggests either oversedation or inadequate ventilatory capacity. Medical problems that may contribute to respiratory failure (e.g., heart failure) should be stable or controlled, and the patient should be responsive and able to clear secretions. Requirement for frequent (e.g., more than every 2 h) suctioning, fever, or significant inotropic or vasopressor therapy all suggests the patient may not be ready for withdrawal of respiratory support. Once these considerations have been addressed, a "physiological" assessment needs to be performed to see if the patient is able to breathe spontaneously without distress. The most common of these is the "rapid shallow breathing index" where the patient is allowed to breathe without support for a few minutes and the index is computed by dividing the breathing frequency by the tidal volume. An index of >100 strongly predicts failure of a longer duration spontaneous breathing trial (SBT); a value of less than this does not necessarily predict success [179].

Analogous to the startling revelation that a relatively modest change in ventilator management (reduced tidal volume with adequate PEEP) leads to improved survival in ARDS, performing a 30–120 min SBT on appropriate patients through a "T-piece" or with low-level CPAP and/or pressure support identifies a large number of patients who are ready to be extubated. Two large trials indicated that clinicians did not recognize that discontinuing support would be possible in more than 2/3 of the patients who were successfully identified with an SBT [180, 181]. These studies found that a SBT reduced the duration of mechanical ventilation when compared to other techniques such as gradual withdrawal of IMV or pressure support. The report of a consensus meeting suggested that a 30–120 min SBT is the "major diagnostic test to determine whether patients can be

Table 54.10 The spontaneous breathing trial

Indication: Daily assessment of readiness to separate from mechanical ventilation
Criteria to perform
At least partial resolution of underlying condition(s) leading to respiratory failure
Conventional ventilation mode (volume or pressure)
Absence of respiratory distress
Sedation infusions withdrawn (daily withdrawal) and patient responsive
No CNS contraindications (e.g., elevated intracranial pressure)
$SpO_2 > 88\%$ with $fiO_2 < 0.5$ and PEEP < 8
Minimal cardiovascular support (e.g., inotropes/pressors) not increasing
Rapid shallow breathing index (RSBI) < 100[a] in first minutes of trial
Criteria for failure
Clinical
Change in mental status, usually agitation/anxiety
Visible distress such as diaphoresis, increasing effort
Objective
Decreasing SpO_2 (below 88%) or increasing end-tidal CO_2
Increasing tachypnea (>35 breaths/min)
Increasing tachycardia (>140/min) or other dysrhythmia and/or hypertension
RSBI[a] increasing to >100
Blood gas if drawn with $SaO_2 < 88\%$; $PaCO_2 > 10$ mm above baseline and pH < 7.32

[a]Respiratory rate (breaths/min) divided by tidal volume (in liters), with no support or 5 cm pressure support/5 cm PEEP)

successfully extubated" [182]. Psychological support, encouragement, and physical presence of a caregiver at the bedside for at least the early part of the trial are essential. Criteria for performing an SBT are summarized in Table 54.10.

Spontaneous breathing trials also identify patients who are *not* ready for withdrawal of ventilator support; Table 54.10 lists criteria for failure of a SBT. Of those patients who fail an initial trial, most will eventually succeed in the following week. A daily SBT identifies these patients. There will be a small percentage of patients who require prolonged care and possibly require transfer to a "weaning facility" or "long-term acute care" (LTAC) facility. When a patient fails an SBT, the reasons for failure need to be carefully examined. They may include inadequate resolution of the primary or underlying problem, weakness (e.g., nutritional depletion), or inadequate recovery from sedation to name a few. Between SBTs, patients should be supported with a mode of ventilation, which requires spontaneous but non-fatiguing efforts by the patient as atrophy and weakness of respiratory muscles develop within less than 24 h of complete ventilatory rest [183]. Malnutrition is increasingly recognized as a contributor to weakness in ventilated patients, and some form of nutrition needs to be addressed in the patient who requires mechanical ventilation for more than a few days.

Daily interruptions of sedative infusions decrease the duration of mechanical ventilation [184]. This is best accomplished by use of a sedation protocol, which has also been shown to reduce the duration of mechanical ventilation [185–187]. A significant issue in the ventilated patient is delirium, which is multifactorial (e.g., pain, sleep deprivation, polypharmacy) and may be associated more with benzodiazepines than other sedative drugs. When it occurs, delirium is associated with significantly worsened outcome [188].

Extubation

Separate from weaning and the requirement for ventilatory assistance, readiness for extubation requires its own assessment. The patient must be awake and cooperative, able to cough and clear secretions, and the airway must be patent. In a study by Khamiees et al., poor cough strength and increased amounts of respiratory secretions were synergistic in predicting extubation failure [189]. While there is no perfect way of assessing airway patency, a "cuff-leak" test can be performed in a subjective or objective manner. For the former, the clinician simply deflates the cuff on the tube and listens for audible air leak during either spontaneous breathing or with positive-pressure ventilation. Absence of an audible leak suggests airway edema and the potential for post-extubation obstruction. This is more likely with prolonged intubation, trauma, obesity, or female gender [190]. The test can be quantified by measuring the volume lost during volume-controlled ventilation although another group of investigators did not find the test useful in surgical patients [191, 192]. If a cuff test of any kind suggests minimal or absent air leak, but a decision is made to proceed with extubation, a "tube changer" should be used to allow urgent reintubation.

Tracheotomy

When the period of mechanical ventilation is likely to be more than 7–10 days, there are several reasons why tracheotomy is a favored approach. First and possibly most important, it allows for a greater degree of comfort by removing the transoral or transnasal tube and associated holding device or tape. This alone can result in a reduced need for sedation. By introducing a permanent path into the airway, the need for physical restraint is reduced, and the patient can be mobilized (e.g., to a chair) with less risk and greater ease. The patient may be able to swallow liquid or solid food at an earlier stage and may be able to speak during periods when they are off the ventilator (with the use of a one-way "Passy-Muir" valve). Replacement of the relatively long transoral or transnasal tube with a much shorter tracheotomy tube reduces the imposed airways resistance and facilitates removal of secretions [193]. In patients projected to need ventilation >2 weeks, Rumbak et al. demonstrated early tracheotomy resulted in lower mortality, fewer cases of VAP, fewer accidental extubations, and less time spent on mechanical ventilation than a late tracheotomy strategy [194]. A recent study failed to demonstrate a benefit in terms of VAP with early tracheotomy performed at 6–8 days vs. later tracheotomy at 13–15 days; other trials have failed to demonstrate a benefit in terms of speed of weaning [195]. In the thoracic surgery patient, the surgeon may prefer to perform his/her own surgical tracheotomy in the operating room; however, there are now many studies attesting to the safety and cost savings of bedside percutaneous tracheotomy [196, 197]. In many of these studies, intensivists performed the tracheotomy in medical ICUs.

Clinical Case Discussion

A 65-year-old male is in the postanesthesia care unit (PACU) after undergoing open right upper lobectomy for squamous cell carcinoma. He has a long history of smoking, and his preoperative room air saturation was 91%. He is tachypneic, slightly lethargic, and complaining of pain; his peripheral saturation reading is 88%, and he is receiving 100% oxygen by face mask. His blood pressure is 160/100 and heart rate 105/min.

Questions

1. What are the likely diagnoses?
2. Which (if any) diagnostic tests should be obtained?
3. Which treatment modalities should be employed, and in what order?

Answers

1. Residual neuromuscular blockade, pain with splinting and resultant low tidal volume, and mechanical complications such as pneumothorax or lobar atelectasis are all possibilities, alone or in combination. Pulmonary edema as a result of cardiac disease and/or volume overload is also possible.
2. Objective assessment of neuromuscular function should be made. The lungs should be auscultated, and a portable chest radiograph should be obtained to determine if edema or a mechanical problem is present. An arterial blood gas (ABG) should be obtained to determine pCO_2 and pH.

3. Application of HFNC, CPAP, or BIPAP may acutely relieve respiratory distress and improve oxygenation if the patient is cooperative. An inhaled bronchodilator may be indicated if the patient is known to have a response and/or if rhonchi or wheezing are audible. Treatment of pain may be important but may also reduce respiratory drive. Appropriate intervention should be made for a mechanical problem.

The chest radiograph demonstrates partial collapse of the right lower lobe, and the patient becomes agitated with the application of BIPAP. The blood pressure is now 180/110, and the saturation remains between 85 and 90%. The ABG shows a pO_2 of 55 mmHg, pCO_2 of 60 mmHg, and pH of 7.25.

Question

1. What should be done now?

Answer

1. The blood gas confirms a diagnosis of respiratory failure of both oxygenation and ventilation. Lobar atelectasis may be resolved with vigorous coughing and "physiotherapy" maneuvers such as percussion, postural drainage, and positive-pressure breathing; however, in this acute setting of an agitated patient unable to tolerate noninvasive positive pressure, most likely intubation is required. In addition, early postoperative lobar atelectasis may be due to retained secretions and is an indication for fiber-optic bronchoscopy. In this patient bronchoscopy will require intubation.

The patient is intubated uneventfully, and bronchoscopy is performed where significant tenacious secretions are aspirated from the right bronchus intermedius. The arterial saturation rises to 95% on 100% fiO_2.

Questions

1. What ventilator settings should be used?
2. Should the patient be prepared for extubation?
3. Should broad-spectrum antibiotics be employed?

Answers

1. This patient is at risk for ventilator-induced lung injury due to underlying disease, pulmonary surgery, and now a postoperative pulmonary complication (see Chapter [Denham Ward]). He should be managed with a lung-protective strategy which includes appropriate PEEP (usually 5–10 cm H_2O) and a tidal volume of 5–7 ml/kg of predicted body weight. The goal is a "plateau" pressure of 30 cm H_2O or less. Ideally a ventilator mode which allows spontaneous efforts should be used. As lobar atelectasis was present before the bronchoscopy, a "recruitment maneuver" should be considered.

2. Assessment for ventilator wean and extubation is a clinical judgment based on a variety of factors. If the patient is easy to ventilate and oxygenate and appears otherwise well-recovered from the complication, then sedation may be withdrawn, a physiologic assessment for rapid shallow breathing made, and a spontaneous breathing trial (SBT) performed. As the patient has a peripheral saturation of only 95% on 100% oxygen, it is more likely he will need a period of positive-pressure ventilation with PEEP before meeting oxygenation requirements for an SBT.

3. If the patient was not hospitalized before surgery, then the likely pathogens in his sputum are "community acquired." The local experience will dictate which antibiotic should be considered, in addition to or instead of the usual surgical prophylaxis. If the patient is an inpatient or was recently hospitalized, then antibiotics appropriate for the hospital experience (such as vancomycin for methicillin-resistant *Staphylococcus aureus*) should be considered. Pneumonia, and especially ventilator-associated pneumonia (VAP), is associated with a high mortality, but there are no data regarding the administration of "prophylactic" antibiotics in a situation such as this. It may be more prudent to obtain a lower airway sample for culture, stay with the usual perioperative prophylaxis, and initiate appropriate antibiotics if a pulmonary infection appears to be developing.

References

1. Hirschler-Schulte CJ, Hylkema BS, Meyer RW. Mechanical ventilation for acute postoperative respiratory failure after surgery for bronchial carcinoma. Thorax. 1985;40(5):387–90.
2. Busch E, et al. Pulmonary complications in patients undergoing thoracotomy for lung carcinoma. Chest. 1994;105(3):760–6.
3. Stephan F, et al. Pulmonary complications following lung resection: a comprehensive analysis of incidence and possible risk factors. Chest. 2000;118(5):1263–70.
4. Wada H, et al. Thirty-day operative mortality for thoracotomy in lung cancer. J Thorac Cardiovasc Surg. 1998;115(1):70–3.
5. Harpole DH Jr, et al. Prognostic models of thirty-day mortality and morbidity after major pulmonary resection. J Thorac Cardiovasc Surg. 1999;117(5):969–79.
6. Harpole DH, et al. Prospective analysis of pneumonectomy: risk factors for major morbidity and cardiac dysrhythmias. Ann Thorac Surg. 1996;61(3):977–82.
7. Kane RD, Rasanene J. Hypoxemia. In: Kirby RR, Gravenstein N, editors. Clinical anesthesia practice. Philadelphia: WB Saunders Company; 1994. p. 782.
8. West JB. Pulmonary pathophysiology, the essentials. 3rd ed. Baltimore: Williams and Wilkins; 1977.

9. Hagen PT, Scholz DG, Edwards WD. Incidence and size of patent foramen ovale during the first 10 decades of life: an autopsy study of 965 normal hearts. Mayo Clin Proc. 1984;59(1):17–20.

10. Dewan NA, et al. Persistent hypoxemia due to patent foramen ovale in a patient with adult respiratory distress syndrome. Chest. 1986;89(4):611–3.

11. Vaughn GC, Downs JB. Perioperative pulmonary function, assessment, and intervention. Anesthesiol Rev. 1990;17:19–24.

12. Arozullah AM, et al. Multifactorial risk index for predicting postoperative respiratory failure in men after major noncardiac surgery. The National Veterans Administration Surgical Quality Improvement Program. Ann Surg. 2000;232(2):242–53.

13. Dales RE, et al. Preoperative prediction of pulmonary complications following thoracic surgery. Chest. 1993;104(1):155–9.

14. Cywinski JB, et al. Predictors of prolonged postoperative endotracheal intubation in patients undergoing thoracotomy for lung resection. J Cardiothorac Vasc Anesth. 2009;23(6):766–9.

15. Cagini L, et al. B-type natriuretic peptide following thoracic surgery: a predictor of postoperative cardiopulmonary complications. Eur J Cardiothorac Surg. 2014;46:e74–80.

16. Smetana GW. Preoperative pulmonary evaluation. N Engl J Med. 1999;340(12):937–44.

17. Epstein SK, et al. Predicting complications after pulmonary resection. Preoperative exercise testing vs a multifactorial cardiopulmonary risk index. Chest. 1993;104(3):694–700.

18. McCracken JL et al: Diagnosis and management of asthma in adults: a review. JAMA 2017;318(3):279–90.

19. Landreneau RJ, et al. Acute and chronic morbidity differences between muscle-sparing and standard lateral thoracotomies. J Thorac Cardiovasc Surg. 1996;112(5):1346–50; discussion 1350–1.

20. Ginsberg RJ, et al. Modern thirty-day operative mortality for surgical resections in lung cancer. J Thorac Cardiovasc Surg. 1983;86(5):654–8.

21. Imperatori A, et al. Peri-operative complications of video-assisted thoracoscopic surgery (VATS). Int J Surg. 2008;6(Suppl 1):S78–81.

22. Flores RM, Alam N. Video-assisted thoracic surgery lobectomy (VATS), open thoracotomy, and the robot for lung cancer. Ann Thorac Surg. 2008;85(2):S710–5.

23. Villamizar NR, et al. Thoracoscopic lobectomy is associated with lower morbidity compared with thoracotomy. J Thorac Cardiovasc Surg. 2009;138(2):419–25.

24. Dylewski MR, Ohaeto AC, Pereira JF. Pulmonary resection using a total endoscopic robotic video-assisted approach. Semin Thorac Cardiovasc Surg. 2011;23:36–42. (description of pilot of robotic surgeries).

25. Kent M, et al. Open, video-assisted thoracic surgery, and robotic lobectomy: review of a national database. Ann Thorac Surg. 2014;97:236–44.

26. Cooper JD, et al. Results of 150 consecutive bilateral lung volume reduction procedures in patients with severe emphysema. J Thorac Cardiovasc Surg. 1996;112(5):1319–29; discussion 1329–30.

27. Naunheim KS, et al. Predictors of operative mortality and cardiopulmonary morbidity in the National Emphysema Treatment Trial. J Thorac Cardiovasc Surg. 2006;131(1):43–53.

28. Fujimoto T, et al. Long-term results of lung volume reduction surgery. Eur J Cardiothorac Surg. 2002;21(3):483–8.

29. Fishman A, Fessler H, Martinez F, RJ MK Jr, Naunheim K, Piantadosi S, Weinmann G, Wise R, National Emphysema Treatment Trial Research Group. Patients at high risk of death after lung-volume-reduction surgery. N Engl J Med. 2001;345(15):1075–83.

30. Drachman DB. Myasthenia gravis (first of two parts). N Engl J Med. 1978;298(3):136–42.

31. Eisenkraft JB, et al. Predicting the need for postoperative mechanical ventilation in myasthenia gravis. Anesthesiology. 1986;65(1):79–82.

32. Moore KH, et al. Thymoma: trends over time. Ann Thorac Surg. 2001;72(1):203–7.

33. Karl RC, et al. Factors affecting morbidity, mortality, and survival in patients undergoing Ivor Lewis esophagogastrectomy. Ann Surg. 2000;231(5):635–43.

34. Ellis FH Jr, et al. Esophagogastrectomy for carcinoma of the esophagus and cardia: a comparison of findings and results after standard resection in three consecutive eight-year intervals with improved staging criteria. J Thorac Cardiovasc Surg. 1997;113(5):836–46; discussion 846–8

35. Alexiou C, et al. Surgery for esophageal cancer in elderly patients: the view from Nottingham. J Thorac Cardiovasc Surg. 1998;116(4):545–53.

36. Bailey SH, et al. Outcomes after esophagectomy: a ten-year prospective cohort. Ann Thorac Surg. 2003;75(1):217–22. discussion 222

37. Atkins BZ, et al. Reducing hospital morbidity and mortality following esophagectomy. Ann Thorac Surg. 2004;78(4):1170–6. discussion 1170-6

38. Money SR, et al. Risk of respiratory failure after repair of thoracoabdominal aortic aneurysm. Am J Surg. 1994;168(2):152–5.

39. Svensson LG, et al. A prospective study of respiratory failure after high-risk surgery on the thoracoabdominal aorta. J Vasc Surg. 1991;14(3):271–82.

40. Etz CD, et al. Pulmonary complications after descending thoracic and thoracoabdominal aortic aneurysm repair: predictors, prevention, and treatment. Ann Thorac Surg. 2007;83(2):S870–6; discussion S890–2.

41. Woo SW, Berlin D, Hedley-Whyte J. Surfactant function and anesthetic agents. J Appl Physiol. 1969;26(5):571–7.

42. Duggan M, Kavanagh BP. Pulmonary atelectasis: a pathogenic perioperative entity. Anesthesiology. 2005;102(4):838–54.

43. Loring SH, Butler JP. Gas exchange in body cavities. In: Farhi LE, Tenney SM, editors. Handbook of physiology, section 3. Bethesda: American Physiological Society; 1987. p. 283–95.

44. Joyce CJ, Baker AB, Kennedy RR. Gas uptake from an unventilated area of lung: computer model of absorption atelectasis. J Appl Physiol. 1993;74(3):1107–16.

45. Uzieblo M, et al. Incidence and significance of lobar atelectasis in thoracic surgical patients. Am Surg. 2000;66(5):476–80.

46. van Kaam AH, et al. Reducing atelectasis attenuates bacterial growth and translocation in experimental pneumonia. Am J Respir Crit Care Med. 2004;169(9):1046–53.

47. Byrd RB, Burns JR. Cough dynamics in the post-thoracotomy state. Chest. 1975;67(6):654–7.

48. Meyers JR, et al. Changes in functional residual capacity of the lung after operation. Arch Surg. 1975;110(5):576–83.

49. Shapiro BA, Peruzzi WT. Respiratory care. In: Miller RD, editor. Anesthesia. New York: Churchill-Livingstone; 2000. p. 2407.

50. Bastin R, et al. Incentive spirometry performance. A reliable indicator of pulmonary function in the early postoperative period after lobectomy? Chest. 1997;111(3):559–63.

51. Overend TJ, et al. The effect of incentive spirometry on postoperative pulmonary complications: a systematic review. Chest. 2001;120(3):971–8.

52. Freitas ER, et al. Incentive spirometry for preventing pulmonary complications after coronary artery bypass graft. Cochrane Database Syst Rev. 2007;(3):CD004466.

53. Guimaraes MM, et al. Incentive spirometry for prevention of postoperative pulmonary complications in upper abdominal surgery. Cochrane Database Syst Rev. 2009;(3):CD006058.

54. Gosselink R, et al. Incentive spirometry does not enhance recovery after thoracic surgery. Crit Care Med. 2000;28(3):679–83.

55. Agostini P, et al. Effectiveness of incentive spirometry in patients following thoracotomy and lung resection including those at high risk for developing pulmonary complications. Thorax. 2013;68:580–5.

56. Tyson AF, et al. The effect of incentive spirometry on postoperative pulmonary function following laparotomy: a randomized clinical trial. JAMA Surg. 2015;150(3):229–36.

57. Stock MC, et al. Prevention of postoperative pulmonary complications with CPAP, incentive spirometry, and conservative therapy. Chest. 1985;87(2):151–7.

58. Ferreyra GP, et al. Continuous positive airway pressure for treatment of respiratory complications after abdominal surgery: a systematic review and meta-analysis. Ann Surg. 2008;247(4):617–26.

59. Tobias JD. Noninvasive ventilation using bilevel positive airway pressure to treat impending respiratory failure in the postanesthesia care unit. J Clin Anesth. 2000;12(5):409–12.

60. Yamazaki S, et al. Intrapleural cough pressure in patients after thoracotomy. J Thorac Cardiovasc Surg. 1980;80(4):600–4.

61. Rodgers A, et al. Reduction of postoperative mortality and morbidity with epidural or spinal anaesthesia: results from overview of randomised trials. BMJ. 2000;321(7275):1493.

62. Mourisse J, et al. Epidural bupivacaine, sufentanil or the combination for post-thoracotomy pain. Acta Anaesthesiol Scand. 1992;36(1):70–4.

63. Davies RG, Myles PS, Graham JM. A comparison of the analgesic efficacy and side-effects of paravertebral vs epidural blockade for thoracotomy--a systematic review and meta-analysis of randomized trials. Br J Anaesth. 2006;96(4):418–26.

64. Khalil KG, et al. Operative intercostal nerve blocks with long-acting bupivacaine liposome for pain control after thoracotomy. Ann Thorac Surg. 2015;100:2013–8.

65. Pepe PE, Marini JJ. Occult positive end-expiratory pressure in mechanically ventilated patients with airflow obstruction: the auto-PEEP effect. Am Rev Respir Dis. 1982;126(1):166–70.

66. Tashkin DP, Cooper CB. The role of long-acting bronchodilators in the management of stable COPD. Chest. 2004;125(1):249–59.

67. Wise RA, Tashkin DP. Optimizing treatment of chronic obstructive pulmonary disease: an assessment of current therapies. Am J Med. 2007;120(8 Suppl 1):S4–13.

68. Celli BR, MacNee W. Standards for the diagnosis and treatment of patients with COPD: a summary of the ATS/ERS position paper. Eur Respir J. 2004;23(6):932–46.

69. Slattery DM, et al. Bronchoscopically administered recombinant human DNase for lobar atelectasis in cystic fibrosis. Pediatr Pulmonol. 2001;31(5):383–8.

70. Quidaciolu F, et al. Use of minitracheostomy in high-risk pulmonary resection surgery. Results of a comparative study. Minerva Chir. 1994;49(4):315–8.

71. Issa MM, et al. Prophylactic minitracheostomy in lung resections. A randomized controlled study. J Thorac Cardiovasc Surg. 1991;101(5):895–900.

72. Balkan ME, et al. Clinical experience with minitracheostomy. Scand J Thorac Cardiovasc Surg. 1996;30(2):93–6.

73. Inagawa G, et al. Tracheal obstruction caused by minitracheostomy. Intensive Care Med. 2000;26(11):1707.

74. Pue CA, Pacht ER. Complications of fiberoptic bronchoscopy at a university hospital. Chest. 1995;107(2):430–2.

75. Ferdinand B, Shennib H. Postoperative pneumonia. Chest Surg Clin N Am. 1998;8(3):529–39, viii.

76. Nan DN, et al. Nosocomial infection after lung surgery: incidence and risk factors. Chest. 2005;128(4):2647–52.

77. Luna CM, et al. Impact of BAL data on the therapy and outcome of ventilator-associated pneumonia. Chest. 1997;111(3):676–85.

78. Dupont H, et al. Impact of appropriateness of initial antibiotic therapy on the outcome of ventilator-associated pneumonia. Intensive Care Med. 2001;27(2):355–62.

79. Ziomek S, et al. Thromboembolism in patients undergoing thoracotomy. Ann Thorac Surg. 1993;56(2):223–6; discussion 227.

80. Kalweit G, et al. Pulmonary embolism: a frequent cause of acute fatality after lung resection. Eur J Cardiothorac Surg. 1996;10(4):242–6; discussion 246–7.

81. Wood KE. Major pulmonary embolism: review of a pathophysiologic approach to the golden hour of hemodynamically significant pulmonary embolism. Chest. 2002;121(3):877–905.

82. Hope WW, et al. Postoperative pulmonary embolism: timing, diagnosis, treatment, and outcomes. Am J Surg. 2007;194(6):814–8; discussion 818–9.

83. Velmahos GC, et al. Spiral computed tomography for the diagnosis of pulmonary embolism in critically ill surgical patients: a comparison with pulmonary angiography. Arch Surg. 2001;136(5):505–11.

84. Mullins MD, et al. The role of spiral volumetric computed tomography in the diagnosis of pulmonary embolism. Arch Intern Med. 2000;160(3):293–8.

85. Yakar A, et al. Cardiac findings of pulmonary thromboembolism by autopsy: a review of 48 cases. Med Sci Monit. 2016;22:1265–73. (CDT for PE in post-surgical patients).

86. McCabe JM, et al. Usefulness and safety of ultrasound-assisted catheter-directed thrombolysis for submassive pulmonary emboli. Am J Cardiol. 2015;115(6):821–4.

87. van der Werff YD, et al. Postpneumonectomy pulmonary edema. A retrospective analysis of incidence and possible risk factors. Chest. 1997;111(5):1278–84.

88. Turnage WS, Lunn JJ. Postpneumonectomy pulmonary edema. A retrospective analysis of associated variables. Chest. 1993;103(6):1646–50.

89. Waller DA, et al. Pulmonary endothelial permeability changes after major lung resection. Ann Thorac Surg. 1996;61(5):1435–40.

90. Fernandez-Perez ER, et al. Intraoperative tidal volume as a risk factor for respiratory failure after pneumonectomy. Anesthesiology. 2006;105(1):14–8.

91. Zeldin RA, et al. Postpneumonectomy pulmonary edema. J Thorac Cardiovasc Surg. 1984;87(3):359–65.

92. Parquin F, et al. Post-pneumonectomy pulmonary edema: analysis and risk factors. Eur J Cardiothorac Surg. 1996;10(11):929–32; discussion 933.

93. Diamond JM, Lee JC, Kawut SM, et al. Clinical risk factors for postoperative graft dysfunction after lung transplantation. Am J Respir Crit Care Med. 2013;187:527–34.

94. Hamilton BCS, Kukreja J, Ware LB, Matthay MA. Protein biomarkers associated with primary graft dysfunction following lung transplantation. Am J Physiol Lung Cell Mol Physiol. 2017;312:L531–41.

95. Aguilar PR, Hachem R. Long term impact of primary graft dysfunction after lung transplantation. Clin Res Pulmonol. 2015;3(1):1026.

96. Nazarnia S, Subramaniam K. Pro: Veno-arterial extracorporeal membrane oxygenation (ECMO) should be used routinely for bilateral lung transplantation. J Cardiothorac Vasc Anesth. 2016; PMID: 27591909. https://doi.org/10.1053/j.jvca.2016.06.015.

97. Beckett A, et al. Needle decompression for tension pneumothorax in tactical combat casualty care: do catheters placed in the midaxillary line kink more often than those in the midclavicular line? J Trauma. 2011;71:S408–12.

98. Shekar K, et al. Bronchopleural fistula: an update for intensivists. J Crit Care. 2010;25(1):47–55.

99. Algar FJ, et al. Prediction of early bronchopleural fistula after pneumonectomy: a multivariate analysis. Ann Thorac Surg. 2001;72(5):1662–7.

100. Gkegkes ID, et al. Endobronchial valves in treatment of persistent air leaks: a systematic review of clinical evidence. Med Sci Monit. 2015;21:432–8.

101. Dooms CA, et al. Bronchial valve treatment for pulmonary air leak after anatomical lung resection for cancer. Eur Respir J. 2014;43:1142–8.

102. Ajemian MS, et al. Routine fiberoptic endoscopic evaluation of swallowing following prolonged intubation: implications for management. Arch Surg. 2001;136(4):434–7.

103. Atkins BZ, et al. Assessing oropharyngeal dysphagia after lung transplantation: altered swallowing mechanisms and increased morbidity. J Heart Lung Transplant. 2007;26(11):1144–8.

104. Schilling MK, et al. Role of thromboxane and leukotriene B4 in patients with acute respiratory distress syndrome after oesophagectomy. Br J Anaesth. 1998;80(1):36–40.

105. Engle J, et al. The impact of diaphragm management on prolonged ventilator support after thoracoabdominal aortic repair. J Vasc Surg. 1999;29(1):150–6.

106. Nag K, et al. Sugammadex: a revolutionary drug in neuromuscular pharmacology. Anesth Essays Res. 2013;7(3):302–6.

107. Sacan O, et al. Sugammadex reversal of rocuronium-induced neuromuscular blockade: a comparison with neostigmine-glycopyrrolate and edrophonium-atropine. Anesth Analg. 2007;104(3):569–74.

108. Gattinoni L, et al. Regional effects and mechanism of positive end-expiratory pressure in early adult respiratory distress syndrome. JAMA. 1993;269(16):2122–7.

109. Malo J, Ali J, Wood LD. How does positive end-expiratory pressure reduce intrapulmonary shunt in canine pulmonary edema? J Appl Physiol. 1984;57(4):1002–10.

110. Field S, Kelly SM, Macklem PT. The oxygen cost of breathing in patients with cardiorespiratory disease. Am Rev Respir Dis. 1982;126(1):9–13.

111. Katz JA, Marks JD. Inspiratory work with and without continuous positive airway pressure in patients with acute respiratory failure. Anesthesiology. 1985;63(6):598–607.

112. Jaber S, Chanques G, Jung B. Postoperative noninvasive ventilation. Anesthesiology. 2010;112(2):453–61.

113. Squadrone V, et al. Continuous positive airway pressure for treatment of postoperative hypoxemia: a randomized controlled trial. JAMA. 2005;293(5):589–95.

114. Kindgen-Milles D, et al. Nasal-continuous positive airway pressure reduces pulmonary morbidity and length of hospital stay following thoracoabdominal aortic surgery. Chest. 2005;128(2):821–8.

115. Lefebvre A, et al. Noninvasive ventilation for acute respiratory failure after lung resection: an observational study. Intensive Care Med. 2009;35(4):663–70.

116. Michelet P, et al. Non-invasive ventilation for treatment of postoperative respiratory failure after oesophagectomy. Br J Surg. 2009;96(1):54–60.

117. Rocco M, et al. Non-invasive pressure support ventilation in patients with acute respiratory failure after bilateral lung transplantation. Intensive Care Med. 2001;27(10):1622–6.

118. Perrin C, et al. Prophylactic use of noninvasive ventilation in patients undergoing lung resectional surgery. Respir Med. 2007;101(7):1572–8.

119. Stephan F, et al. High-flow nasal oxygen vs noninvasive positive airway pressure in hypoxemic patients after cardiothoracic surgery. JAMA. 2015;313(23):2331–9.

120. Corley A, et al. Oyxgen delivery through high-flow nasal cannulae increase end-expiratory lung volume and reduce respiratory rate in post-cardiac surgical patients. Br J Anaesth. 2011;107(6):998–1004.

121. Roca O, et al. Humidified high flow nasal cannula supportive therapy improves outcomes in lung transplant recipients readmitted to the intensive care unit because of acute respiratory failure. Transplantation. 2015;99:1092–8.

122. Roca O, et al. Current evidence for the effectiveness of heated and humidified high flow nasal cannula supportive therapy in adult patients with respiratory failure. Crit Care. 2016;20(1):109.

123. The ARDS Definition Task Force. Acute respiratory distress syndrome the Berlin definition. JAMA. 2012;307(23):2526–33.

124. Bernard GR, et al. The American-European Consensus Conference on ARDS. Definitions, mechanisms, relevant outcomes, and clinical trial coordination. Am J Respir Crit Care Med. 1994;149(3 Pt 1):818–24.

125. Agarwal R, et al. Is the mortality higher in the pulmonary vs the extrapulmonary ARDS? A meta analysis. Chest. 2008;133(6):1463–73.

126. Kutlu CA, et al. Acute lung injury and acute respiratory distress syndrome after pulmonary resection. Ann Thorac Surg. 2000;69(2):376–80.

127. Zambon M, Vincent JL. Mortality rates for patients with acute lung injury/ARDS have decreased over time. Chest. 2008;133(5):1120–7.

128. Khadaroo RG, Marshall JC. ARDS and the multiple organ dysfunction syndrome. Common mechanisms of a common systemic process. Crit Care Clin. 2002;18(1):127–41.

129. Ferring M, Vincent JL. Is outcome from ARDS related to the severity of respiratory failure? Eur Respir J. 1997;10(6):1297–300.

130. Deitch EA. Multiple organ failure. Pathophysiology and potential future therapy. Ann Surg. 1992;216(2):117–34.

131. McHugh LG, et al. Recovery of function in survivors of the acute respiratory distress syndrome. Am J Respir Crit Care Med. 1994;150(1):90–4.

132. Peter JV, et al. Corticosteroids in the prevention and treatment of acute respiratory distress syndrome (ARDS) in adults: meta-analysis. BMJ. 2008;336(7651):1006–9.

133. Agarwal R, et al. Do glucocorticoids decrease mortality in acute respiratory distress syndrome? A meta-analysis. Respirology. 2007;12(4):585–90.

134. Adhikari NK, et al. Effect of nitric oxide on oxygenation and mortality in acute lung injury: systematic review and meta-analysis. BMJ. 2007;334(7597):779.

135. Adhikari N, Burns KE, Meade MO. Pharmacologic therapies for adults with acute lung injury and acute respiratory distress syndrome. Cochrane Database Syst Rev. 2004;(4):CD004477.

136. Webb HH, Tierney DF. Experimental pulmonary edema due to intermittent positive pressure ventilation with high inflation pressures. Protection by positive end-expiratory pressure. Am Rev Respir Dis. 1974;110(5):556–65.

137. Ranieri VM, et al. Effect of mechanical ventilation on inflammatory mediators in patients with acute respiratory distress syndrome: a randomized controlled trial. JAMA. 1999;282(1):54–61.

138. The Acute Respiratory Distress Syndrome Network. Ventilation with lower tidal volumes as compared with traditional tidal volumes for acute lung injury and the acute respiratory distress syndrome. N Engl J Med. 2000;342(18):1301–8.

139. Levy MM. Optimal peep in ARDS. Changing concepts and current controversies. Crit Care Clin. 2002;18(1):15–33, v–vi.

140. Suter PM, Fairley B, Isenberg MD. Optimum end-expiratory airway pressure in patients with acute pulmonary failure. N Engl J Med. 1975;292(6):284–9.

141. Roupie E, et al. Titration of tidal volume and induced hypercapnia in acute respiratory distress syndrome. Am J Respir Crit Care Med. 1995;152(1):121–8.

142. Brower RG, et al. Higher versus lower positive end-expiratory pressures in patients with the acute respiratory distress syndrome. N Engl J Med. 2004;351(4):327–36.

143. Phoenix SI, et al. Does a higher positive end expiratory pressure decrease mortality in acute respiratory distress syndrome? A systematic review and meta-analysis. Anesthesiology. 2009;110(5):1098–105.

144. Hickling KG, Joyce C. Permissive hypercapnia in ARDS and its effect on tissue oxygenation. Acta Anaesthesiol Scand Suppl. 1995;107:201–8.

145. Fan E, et al. Recruitment maneuvers for acute lung injury: a systematic review. Am J Respir Crit Care Med. 2008;178(11):1156–63.

146. Hodgson C, et al. Recruitment manoeuvres for adults with acute respiratory distress syndrome receiving mechanical ventilation. Cochrane Database Syst Rev. 2016;(11):CD006667.

147. McGregor M. Current concepts: pulsus paradoxus. N Engl J Med. 1979;301(9):480–2.

148. Biondi JW, et al. The effect of incremental positive end-expiratory pressure on right ventricular hemodynamics and ejection fraction. Anesth Analg. 1988;67(2):144–51.

149. Sibbald WJ, Driedger AA. Right ventricular function in acute disease states: pathophysiologic considerations. Crit Care Med. 1983;11(5):339–45.

150. Bryan AC. Conference on the scientific basis of respiratory therapy. Pulmonary physiotherapy in the pediatric age group. Comments of a devil's advocate. Am Rev Respir Dis. 1974;110(6 Pt 2):143–4.

151. Pappert D, et al. Influence of positioning on ventilation-perfusion relationships in severe adult respiratory distress syndrome. Chest. 1994;106(5):1511–6.

152. Mure M, et al. Regional ventilation-perfusion distribution is more uniform in the prone position. J Appl Physiol. 2000;88(3):1076–83.

153. Gattinoni L, et al. Body position changes redistribute lung computed-tomographic density in patients with acute respiratory failure. Anesthesiology. 1991;74(1):15–23.

154. Sud S, et al. Effect of mechanical ventilation in the prone position on clinical outcomes in patients with acute hypoxemic respiratory failure: a systematic review and meta-analysis. CMAJ. 2008;178(9):1153–61.

155. Guerin C, for the PROSEVA Study Group, et al. Prone positioning in severe acute respiratory distress syndrome. N Engl J Med. 2013;368:2159–68.

156. Henderson WR, et al. Does prone positioning improve oxygenation and reduce mortality in patients with acute respiratory distress syndrome? Can Respir J. 2014;21(4):213–5.

157. Esan A, et al. Severe hypoxemic respiratory failure: part 1--ventilatory strategies. Chest. 2010;137(5):1203–16.

158. Ferguson ND, for the OSCILLATE Trial Investigators and the Canadian Critical Care Trials Group, et al. High-frequency oscillation in early acute respiratory distress syndrome. N Engl J Med. 2013;368:795–805.

159. Young D, for the OSCAR Study Group, et al. High-frequency oscillation for acute respiratory distress syndrome. N Engl J Med. 2013;368:806–13.

160. Gebistorf F, Karam O, Wetterslev J, Afshari A. Inhaled nitric oxide for acute respiratory distress syndrome (ARDS) in children and adults. Cochrane Database Syst Rev. 2016;(6):CD002787. https://doi.org/10.1002/14651858.CD002787.pub3.

161. Fuller BM, Mohr NM, Skrupky L, et al. The use of inhaled prostaglandins in patients with ARDS. Chest. 2015;147(6):1510–22.

162. Extracorporeal life support registry report (international summary). Ann Arbor: Extracorporeal Life Support Organization; 2008. p. 30.

163. Wigfield CH, et al. Early institution of extracorporeal membrane oxygenation for primary graft dysfunction after lung transplantation improves outcome. J Heart Lung Transplant. 2007;26(4):331–8.

164. Sidebotham D, et al. Extracorporeal membrane oxygenation for treating severe cardiac and respiratory disease in adults: part 1--overview of extracorporeal membrane oxygenation. J Cardiothorac Vasc Anesth. 2009;23(6):886–92.

165. Peek GJ, Mugford M, Tiruvoipati R, for the CESAR trial, et al. Efficacy and economic assessment of conventional ventilatory support versus extracorporeal membrane oxygenation for severe adult respiratory failure (CESAR): a multicentre randomized controlled trial. Lancet. 2009;374:1351–63.

166. Davies A, Jones D, Bailey M, Australia and New Zealand Extracorporeal Membrane Oxygenation (ANZ ECMO) Influenza Investigators, et al. Extracorporeal membrane oxygenation for 2009 influenza A(H1N1) acute respiratory distress syndrome. JAMA. 2009;302(17):1888–95.

167. Auriant I, et al. Noninvasive ventilation reduces mortality in acute respiratory failure following lung resection. Am J Respir Crit Care Med. 2001;164(7):1231–5.

168. Hospital-acquired pneumonia in adults: diagnosis, assessment of severity, initial antimicrobial therapy, and preventive strategies. A consensus statement, American Thoracic Society, 1995. Am J Respir Crit Care Med. 1996;153(5):1711–25.

169. Monitoring hospital-acquired infections to promote patient safety--United States, 1990–1999. MMWR Morb Mortal Wkly Rep. 2000;49(8):149–53.

170. Chastre J, Fagon JY. Ventilator-associated pneumonia. Am J Respir Crit Care Med. 2002;165(7):867–903.

171. Vincent JL, et al. The prevalence of nosocomial infection in intensive care units in Europe. Results of the European Prevalence of Infection in Intensive Care (EPIC) Study. EPIC International Advisory Committee. JAMA. 1995;274(8):639–44.

172. National Nosocomial Infections Surveillance System, Division of Healthcare Quality Promotion, National Center for Infectious Diseases, Centers for Disease Control and Prevention, Public Health Service, US Department of Health and Human Services: Atlanta. http://www.cdc.gov/ncidod/dhqp/pdf/nnis/2004NNISreport.pdf.

173. DiCocco JM, Croce MA. Ventilator-associated pneumonia: an overview. Expert Opin Pharmacother. 2009;10(9):1461–7.

174. A randomized trial of diagnostic techniques for ventilator-associated pneumonia. N Engl J Med. 2006;355(25):2619–30.

175. Management of adults with hospital-acquired and ventilator-associated pneumonia: 2016 clinical practice guidelines by the Infectious Diseases Society of America and the American Thoracic Society. Clin Infect Dis. 2016;63:1–51.

176. Resar R, et al. Using a bundle approach to improve ventilator care processes and reduce ventilator-associated pneumonia. Jt Comm J Qual Patient Saf. 2005;31(5):243–8.

177. Bouza E, et al. Continuous aspiration of subglottic secretions in the prevention of ventilator-associated pneumonia in the postoperative period of major heart surgery. Chest. 2008;134(5):938–46.

178. Kollef MH, et al. Silver-coated endotracheal tubes and incidence of ventilator-associated pneumonia: the NASCENT randomized trial. JAMA. 2008;300(7):805–13.

179. Brochard L, Thille AW. What is the proper approach to liberating the weak from mechanical ventilation? Crit Care Med. 2009;37(10 Suppl):S410–5.

180. Esteban A, et al. A comparison of four methods of weaning patients from mechanical ventilation. Spanish Lung Failure Collaborative Group. N Engl J Med. 1995;332(6):345–50.

181. Brochard L, et al. Comparison of three methods of gradual withdrawal from ventilatory support during weaning from mechanical ventilation. Am J Respir Crit Care Med. 1994;150(4):896–903.

182. Boles JM, et al. Weaning from mechanical ventilation. Eur Respir J. 2007;29(5):1033–56.

183. Levine S, et al. Rapid disuse atrophy of diaphragm fibers in mechanically ventilated humans. N Engl J Med. 2008;358(13):1327–35.

184. Kress JP, et al. Daily interruption of sedative infusions in critically ill patients undergoing mechanical ventilation. N Engl J Med. 2000;342(20):1471–7.

185. Brook AD, et al. Effect of a nursing-implemented sedation protocol on the duration of mechanical ventilation. Crit Care Med. 1999;27(12):2609–15.

186. Ostermann ME, et al. Sedation in the intensive care unit: a systematic review. JAMA. 2000;283(11):1451–9.

187. Jacobi J, et al. Clinical practice guidelines for the sustained use of sedatives and analgesics in the critically ill adult. Crit Care Med. 2002;30(1):119–41.

188. Ely EW, et al. Delirium as a predictor of mortality in mechanically ventilated patients in the intensive care unit. JAMA. 2004;291(14):1753–62.

189. Khamiees M, et al. Predictors of extubation outcome in patients who have successfully completed a spontaneous breathing trial. Chest. 2001;120(4):1262–70.

190. MacIntyre NR, et al. Evidence-based guidelines for weaning and discontinuing ventilatory support: a collective task force facilitated by the American College of Chest Physicians; the American Association for Respiratory Care; and the American College of Critical Care Medicine. Chest. 2001;120(6 Suppl): 375S–95S.

191. Miller RL, Cole RP. Association between reduced cuff leak volume and postextubation stridor. Chest. 1996;110(4):1035–40.

192. Engoren M. Evaluation of the cuff-leak test in a cardiac surgery population. Chest. 1999;116(4):1029–31.

193. Lin MC, et al. Pulmonary mechanics in patients with prolonged mechanical ventilation requiring tracheostomy. Anaesth Intensive Care. 1999;27(6):581–5.

194. Rumbak MJ, et al. A prospective, randomized, study comparing early percutaneous dilational tracheotomy to prolonged translaryngeal intubation (delayed tracheotomy) in critically ill medical patients. Crit Care Med. 2004;32(8):1689–94.

195. Terragni PP, et al. Early vs late tracheotomy for prevention of pneumonia in mechanically ventilated adult ICU patients: a randomized controlled trial. JAMA. 2010;303(15):1483–9.

196. Freeman BD, et al. A meta-analysis of prospective trials comparing percutaneous and surgical tracheostomy in critically ill patients. Chest. 2000;118(5):1412–8.

197. Freeman BD, et al. A prospective, randomized study comparing percutaneous with surgical tracheostomy in critically ill patients. Crit Care Med. 2001;29(5):926–30.

Postoperative Management of Respiratory Failure: Extracorporeal Ventilatory Therapy

55

Vera von Dossow, Maria Deja, Bernhard Zwissler, and Claudia Spies

Abbreviations

ACT	Activated clotting time
aPTT	Activated partial thromboplastin time
ARDS	Acute respiratory distress syndrome
BIPAP	Bi-level positive airway pressure
CO	Cardiac output
CO_2	Carbon dioxide
CPAP	Continuous positive airway pressure
DLB	Double-lumen single bicaval cannula
$ECCO_2R$	Extracorporeal carbon dioxide removal
ECMO	Extracorporeal membrane oxygenation
F_IO_2	Inspiratory oxygen concentration
HFOV	High-frequency oscillation ventilation
HITT	Heparin-induced thrombocytopenia
LV	Left ventricular
PALI	Post-thoracotomy acute lung injury
PBW	Predicted body weight
PEEP	Positive end-expiratory pressure
PMP	Polymethylpentene
RAS	Renin-angiotensin system
RV	Right ventricular
VA	Veno-arterial
VJI	Vena jugularis interna
VV	Veno-venous

V. von Dossow (✉)
Department of Anesthesiology, Ludwig-Maximilians Universität München, Klinikum Großhadern, Munich, Germany

Heart and Diabetes Center Bad Oeynhausen, Ruhr-University Bochum, Bochum, Germany
e-mail: vvondossow@hdz-nrw.de

B. Zwissler
Department of Anesthesiology, Ludwig-Maximilians Universität München, Klinikum Großhadern, Munich, Germany
e-mail:bernhard.zwissler@med.uni-muenchen.de

M. Deja · C. Spies
Department of Anesthesiology and Intensive Care Medicine, Charité-University Medicine Berlin, Berlin, Germany
e-mail: maria.deja@charite.de; claudia.spies@charite.de

Key Points

- The use of extracorporeal ventilatory support in patients with ARDS after thoracic surgery requires an interdisciplinary approach.
- In case of severe postoperative ARDS (paO_2/F_IO_2 <80 mmHg), ECMO therapy is appropriate if the organ failure is thought to be reversible with therapy and rest during ECMO.
- In case of partial respiratory support with severe hypercapnia ($PaCO_2 \geq 70$ mmHg) and the need of high peak pressures, $ECCO_2R$ technique might be indicated to allow the institution of ultra-protective lung ventilation strategies.
- The concept of "awake ECMO" should be the first choice in order to detect early neurological deficits.
- Early spontaneous breathing is considered desirable as it is known to facilitate reduction of airway pressures.

Introduction

Thoracic surgery represents a challenge for anesthesia and requires a high level of human and material resources. Therefore, accurate knowledge of the pathophysiology is essential not only for the intraoperative management but also for the postoperative follow-up care [1]. Perioperative complications can have a relevant effect on patient outcome. Despite major advances in thoracic surgery, the anesthetic management as well as postoperative care, post-thoracotomy acute lung injury (PALI) is responsible for the vast majority of respiratory-related deaths after thoracic surgery [2]. This might be associated with severe hypoxemia and/or severe hypercapnia. The clinical presentation is an acute respiratory distress syndrome (ARDS)

© Springer Nature Switzerland AG 2019
P. Slinger (ed.), *Principles and Practice of Anesthesia for Thoracic Surgery*, https://doi.org/10.1007/978-3-030-00859-8_55

according to the Berlin definition in 2012 [3], which includes an acute onset of symptoms within 1 week, changing of the PaO_2/F_IO_2 ratio to require a specific minimum amount of positive end-expiratory pressure (PEEP), a classification into three degrees (mild [200–300], moderate [<200], severe [<100]) depending on the PaO_2/F_IO_2 ratio, and infiltrates on the chest radiograph. It is well-known that patients undergoing thoracic surgery have a higher risk for developing postoperative ARDS compared with other types of surgery [2]. The incidence rate of post-thoracotomy ARDS is 4–14% in patients undergoing lung resection [4–6]. Mortality rates range from 1% to 3% after lobectomy and from 4% to 9% after pneumonectomy [6]. Nosocomial pneumonia, post-perfusion lung, and post-pneumonectomy pulmonary edema are the most frequent complications with the clinical presentation of ARDS [6]. The pathogenesis of ARDS implies a multiple-hit sequence of various triggering factors, which results in endothelial inflammatory response (e.g., oxidative stress and surgery-induced inflammation). Currently, the renin-angiotensin system (RAS) has been highlighted and is thought to contribute to the increased vascular permeability. Angiotensin-converting enzyme (ACE) is a key enzyme of the RAS that converts inactive angiotensin I to the vasoactive angiotensin II. ACE has been found on the surface of lung endothelial cells. Angiotensin II is a potent fibrogenic factor [7, 8]. In addition the endothelial glycocalyx as an integral part of the vascular endothelium of the alveolo-capillary membrane seems to play a major role of acute lung injury with the clinical manifestation of inflammation, capillary leak, and edema formation. Experimental data demonstrated rapidly induced degradation, pulmonary endothelial glycocalyx degradation, and an activation of endothelial heparanase as well as activation of endothelial adhesion molecules and increased adhesion of neutrophils after endotoxinemia [9]. Fluid overload, ischemia-reperfusion injury, and TRALI are important trigger factors for degradation of pulmonary endothelial glycocalyx in the pathogenesis of ARDS in patients after thoracic surgery [2]. The clinical manifestation is inflammation, capillary leak, and edema formation. Furthermore, breakdown of endothelial glycocalyx in the context of one-lung ventilation is known to be one major risk factor of PALI. Therefore, the knowledge of these risk factors and understanding of the mechanisms of post-thoracotomy ARDS enable anesthesiologists to implement lung-"protective" ventilatory strategies in thoracic surgery.

In addition, ruptures or fistulas of the bronchial tree after pulmonary surgery are reported with an incidence of 1.5–28% [10]. Inflammatory diseases seem to be an important risk factor for the development of bronchial fistulas [10]. Mechanically ventilated patients with bronchopleural fistulas and the clinical presentation of ARDS with the need of positive-pressure ventilation are at a considerable risk of compromising surgical repair and of increased mortality [11]. This underlines the importance of lung-"protective" ventilation strategies as a major goal in these high-risk patients.

In case that lung-"protective" ventilation strategy is not successful, extracorporeal ventilator therapy, the concept of so-called lung rest might be indicated. This chapter provides a summary of the available different options of extracorporeal ventilatory therapy and cannulation techniques for short-term support of adult patients with post-thoracotomy ARDS.

Lung-Protective Ventilatory Strategies

Lung-Protective Ventilation

The lung-"protective" ventilatory strategy includes the use of low tidal volumes, positive expiratory pressure (PEEP), and limitation of the maximum inspiratory pressure [12, 13] which has a tremendous impact on outcome: The lower the level of maximum inspiratory pressure, the better the patient's outcome [12]. According to the American Thoracic Society Guidelines (2017), mechanical ventilation strategies include a limitation of tidal volumes (4–8 ml/kg predicted body weight (PBW)) and inspiratory pressures (plateau pressure $\leq$ 30 cm H_2O). Low-tidal-volume ventilation might reduce the relative risk of death [14]. In addition, the driving pressure (ΔP = plateau pressure – PEEP) has been demonstrated to be a better outcome predictor in ARDS patients than tidal volume or plateau pressure [15, 16].

Extracorporeal Ventilatory Therapy in ARDS Patients

Despite the increasing applications of extracorporeal ventilatory therapy in ARDS patients, there is still limited evidence supporting its use [14]. This is based on recent published studies that compared treatment of ARDS patients with and without extracorporeal ventilatory therapy and did not find significant differences in mortality [14, 17]. Therefore, additional evidence is necessary to define a clear and consistent recommendation for extracorporeal ventilatory therapy in patients with ARDS.

In contrast to the abovementioned guideline recommendation, the first reported successful extracorporeal membrane oxygenation (ECMO) use was in a 24-year-old man supported on veno-arterial (VA) ECMO therapy for 75 h with severe ARDS and aortic repair due to a motorcycle accident. This case was reported by Hill et al. 1972 and includes the concept of "lung rest" reducing peak airway pressures from 60 cm H_2O to 35–40 cm H_2O [18, 19]. In contrast, the authors of the following NIH adult ECMO study concluded that ECMO therapy can support gas exchange but did not increase the probability of long-term survival in patients with severe ARDS [20, 21]. Several major limitations of this study were a prolonged ventilation prior ECMO therapy (mean of 9.6 days) with high tidal volumes indicating already damaged lungs and the use of VA ECMO in all patients with the need of full heparinization. Therefore the concept of "lung rest" with ECMO as an effective strategy to support adult patients with ARDS was not appreciated. In addition, this study did not represent modern practice of ECMO therapy such as veno-venous (VV) ECMO, low-dose or even no heparinization, ultra-protective ventilation with extracorporeal carbon dioxide (CO_2) removal ($ECCO_2R$), as well as the concept of "spontaneous breathing and awake ECMO" [13, 17, 22–27].

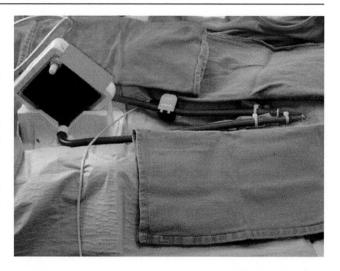

Fig. 55.1 The iLA device is shown between a patient's legs during placement with femoral cannulations. The patient's body is to the right, out of the photograph. The inflow to the device is from the femoral artery (near cannula), and the return is via the femoral vein (far cannula)

Separation of Ventilation and Oxygenation (Concept "Lung Rest")

ARDS patients with severe hypoxemia usually require high PEEP levels which might be associated with limited CO_2 elimination. Therefore, ultra-protective ventilation strategies are impossible due to severe hypercapnia. The clinical consequence is systemic and cerebral vasodilatation, cardiovascular depression, arrhythmia, and pulmonary vasoconstriction with an increase in pulmonary arterial pressure. Acute pulmonary hypertension is associated with increases in RV afterload and subsequent acute cor pulmonale which is associated with an increased mortality [28, 29].

This means that, in such situations of severe hypoxemia and/or hypercapnia, patients are at high risk of death due to lack of response to conservative treatment. Therefore, ECMO therapy is indicated if the disease is potentially reversible. Different kinds of extracorporeal ventilator support are available: Whereas VV ECMO predominantly is used for patients with refractory hypoxia, the extracorporeal CO_2 removal ($ECCO_2R$ or pumpless interventional lung assist (iLA); see Fig. 55.1) allows ultra-protective ventilation technique in case of severe hypercapnia and acidosis [30]. The decoupling of ventilation and oxygenation allows for several ventilation strategies: All strategies have sufficient PEEP level in common to achieve an almost complete recruitment of the lung at minimal pressure amplitude. Whether continuous positive airway pressure (CPAP) with spontaneous breathing, bi-level positive airway pressure (BIPAP) with a low respiratory frequency and a reduced peak airway pressure, or high-frequency oscillation ventilation (HFOV) is applied should be decided for each individual case [27].

Extracorporeal Membrane Oxygenation (ECMO)

Indications

The most frequent causes of hypoxemia and/or hypercapnia after thoracic surgery refractory to conventional lung-"protective" ventilatory and medical treatment include:

- Nosocomial infection
- Post-pneumonectomy edema
- Post-perfusion edema
- Primary graft failure (lung transplantation)
- Bronchopleural fistula: Most cases of bronchopleural fistulas occur early after surgery are difficult to treat and are associated with a high mortality [31]. Achieving adequate ventilation is often difficult in these patients, particularly if single-lung ventilation has to be achieved [11]. Differential ventilation using a double-lumen endotracheal tube and jet ventilation has been the traditional options. VV ECMO is an alternative therapeutic option as bridge for successful surgical repair of bronchopleural fistulas.
- Tracheal resection: Use of ECMO allows rapid weaning of the patient from the ventilator.

The institution of ECMO is appropriate if the organ failure is thought to be reversible with the concept of "lung rest" on ECMO (see Table 55.1). If underlying lung pathology does not recover, ECMO might be instituted as bridging for transplant [34].

Contraindications to ECMO therapy may include premorbid conditions and those related to the current treatment.

Table 55.1 ECMO indication

$PaO_2/F_IO_2 < 70-80$ mmHg; pH < 7.2, Murray Score > 3 [33]
Unresponsiveness to optimal medical conservative management (adapted to Fig. 55.2, [32])
Treatment algorithm for ARDS
Low tidal volume
Plateau pressure $\leq 28-30$ cm H_2O
High PEEP level as possible depending on the surgical intervention
Prone positioning
Neuromuscular blockers
Adjunctive therapies (nitrous oxide, almitrine)

Adapted from Ref. [32] with kind permission from Field House publishing

Active intracranial bleeding is an absolute contraindication. However, all other bleeding complications are relative contraindications.

Technical Aspects of ECMO

Bioengineering, physiology, and pharmacology converge in the intensive care unit. Mechanical devices for monitoring and treatment are essential for the application of physiologic principles and management. Extracorporeal circulation is the ultimate example of this complex interaction.

Cardiopulmonary bypass technology was developed to provide circulatory and respiratory support during cardiac surgery. In the 1960s and 1970s, a number of creative physicians conceived the possibility of employing this technology to support patients with life-threatening cardiac or respiratory failure. The challenge was to provide extracorporeal circulation for a period sufficiently long (i.e., days or weeks) to allow intrinsic healing of the diseased heart and lungs. The various systems that provide these periods of long-term extracorporeal life support are known collectively as ECMO. The development of ECMO technology in the last 10 years provides a variety of options for the multidisciplinary teams who are involved in the management of ARDS patients.

ECMO implies the diversion of blood from a major systemic vessel through a gas exchange device (membrane oxygenator) and back to a major blood vessel. Current devices used for ECMO continue to undergo progressive modifications by their manufactures. These developments include biocompatible circuits, new gas exchange devices, improved pumps, sophisticated computer controlled, and servo-regulated pump systems. The primary goal is to provide patient safety and to improve outcome.

Temporary ECMO support in respiratory and/or heart failure will deliver adequate tissue perfusion through blood circulation and tissue gas exchange. The system mechanically pumps blood through the patient's vasculature delivering oxygen and removing carbon dioxide. It has to be mentioned that there is a variety of different circuits depending on the patient's size and the kind of disease pathology.

There are several important considerations regarding ECMO circuits [35]:

- ECMO circuits should be kept simple in order to provide patient safety.
- Long ECMO tubes increase the foreign surface and increases the priming volume with blood or crystalloids. Resistance through tubes increases with the length of tubing and can cause turbulence and stress on blood elements inducing clot formation. Furthermore, multiple connectors can cause turbulences with the risk of clot formation.
- Membrane oxygenators are used in combination with a pump to supply up to 5–7 L/min support. A roller or occlusive pump operates on the principal of positive fluid displacement. This pump has two rollers and pulls blood from the patient's right atrium and pushes the fluid forward in a fixed length and diameter of tubing with creation of pressure and flows into the oxygenator and then into the patient's system. Newer improved roller pumps with coated circuits have reduced the risk of hemolysis caused by centrifugal pumps.
- Oxygenator. The oxygenator is a critical component of the ECMO circuit. The blood leaves the pump into the oxygenator or the heat exchanger depending which type is used. Moreover, plasma-leakage-resistant oxygenators have enabled the safe use of ECMO for much longer periods of time without changing the oxygenator [36].

VV ECMO

ECMO can be inserted in a VV configuration which provides complete respiratory support and oxygenation (in case of respiratory failure not responding to mechanical ventilation) or either be used as VA configuration (providing both respiratory and cardiac support). The incidence of right ventricular (RV) failure remains high with 25% in ARDS patients [37, 38]. In most cases hemodynamic instability due to RV failure might be resolved with VV ECMO (normoxemia, normocapnia, low tidal volumes, lower plateau pressures, and subsequent reduced pulmonary vascular resistance). However, in the presence of concomitant left ventricular (LV) dysfunction, the use of VA ECMO is indicated [39].

ECMO Cannulation

The femoral and internal jugular veins should be assessed by ultrasound to detect venous thrombosis and to determine the diameter of the vessels. This is important to decide the size of the cannulas. The size of the cannula is the determining factor for the blood flow in the ECMO circuit. The insertion of the largest cannula should be attempted [39].

Cannulation of the internal jugular vein with ultrasound guidance is highly recommended as evidence-based practice [40, 41]. In addition, ultrasound guidance is helpful for all types of vascular access. The preferred technique is the percutaneous approach with the Seldinger technique into femoral and jugular vessels. Percutaneous insertion is associated with less bleeding complication as well as a lower risk of infection.

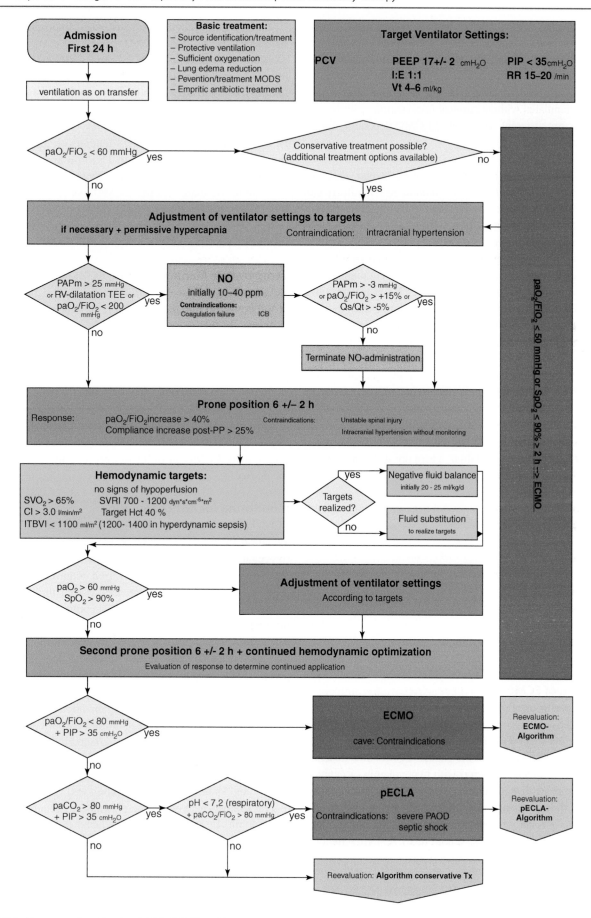

Fig. 55.2 Treatment algorithm for ARDS: ECMO and iLA. (Deja et al. [32], with kind permission from Field House publishing)

The largest possible venous cannula should be used to maximize flow. For adults, the intravascular venous catheters may be 20 French or larger. The cannulas are usually heparin or "bio" coated in order to reduce the risk of clot formation. In case of successful weaning from ECMO, the patient is usually decannulated without surgical intervention.

There are different types of VV ECMO depending on the cannulation sites:

- *The conventional femoro- to internal (vena jugularis interna (VJI)) "double" vein cannulation*: It has the risk of recirculation due to the fact that the reinjection flow is directed to the drainage port. Therefore, at least 15 cm is recommended between the two cannulas to decrease recirculation. Larger cannulas allow lower pump speeds, less negative venous pressures, and reduced recirculation.
- *Recirculation*: Reinjected oxygenated blood is withdrawn by the drainage venous cannula without passing the systemic circulation with decreased ECMO effectiveness.
- *Bilateral femoral cannulation*: This access is a second-line approach in case that VJI is technically not possible.
- Many centers use the *double-lumen single bicaval cannula (DLB)* in the internal jugular: Blood is withdrawn from the inferior vena cava through one port, circulated through the membrane oxygenator and returned to the right atrium through a second port in the same double-lumen catheter. This minimizes recirculation. There are different sizes of DLB available (27 Fr: 4.5 l/min; 31 Fr: 5 L/min).

The effectiveness of VV ECMO in supporting oxygenation depends on several factors:

- Blood flow
- Patient's cardiac output (CO)
- Metabolic demand
- Oxygen fraction in the sweep gas
- Surface area of the membrane
- Recirculation amount within the circuit

Initiation of ECMO

For VV perfusion, flow is initiated at 10–15 ml/kg/min and advanced over 10–15 min to a maximum of 100–150 mL/kg/min. For optimal oxygenation, the VV ECMO flow should reach at least 60% of CO of the patient. ECMO flow depends on volume load and will drop with hypovolemia or cannula malposition, but hypervolemia is not necessary and could be harmful by increasing lung edema. Hypovolemia usually manifests as negative pressure upstream to the blood pump ("kicking" or "chatter" of the venous tube). A slight reduction in flow may be helpful [39].

From a gas exchange point of view, hypoxia is treated by increasing both the ECMO flow rate and inspiratory oxygen concentration (F_1O_2) of the ECMO circuit, not by altering the F_1O_2 and PEEP on the ventilator. Attempts should be made to wean the F_1O_2 on the ventilator and maintain a lung-protective strategy with low plateau pressures, low tidal volumes, and adequate PEEP. Elimination rate of CO_2 depends on gas flow over the membrane. Gas flows up to 15 l/min are necessary in patients without CO_2 elimination by the lungs. CO_2 control should be made via the ECMO gas flow through the membrane, not by altering the respiratory rate on the ventilator to avoid further ventilator-induced acute lung injury.

Temperature Management on ECMO

Because heat is lost through the evaporation of water as blood flows through the artificial lung, it is often necessary to warm the patient on ECMO. Although normothermia can be maintained through use of external warming devices, it is usually more efficient to warm the extracorporeal blood before infusion. In most ECMO centers, heat exchangers are routinely used. At times the heat exchanger may also be used to cool the patient to a preset temperature in order to affect a decrease of oxygen consumption. The heat exchanger should be placed in-line after the artificial lung during ECMO in order to optimize the efficiency of the device.

Monitoring for Anticoagulation

ECMO patients require only a low level of systemic anticoagulation to prevent clotting of the cannulas, tubing, and oxygenator because current devices are coated with heparin. The level of systemic heparinization required is not definitely known, although an activated partial thromboplastin time (aPTT) of 50–70 s and a platelet count >80 × 10 9/L are reasonable [36]. In high-flow systems of about 4–7 l/min, an aPTT above 50 s is sufficient to prevent clotting. Regular measurement of clotting profile, platelet count, and hemoglobin should be performed as least twice per day [42, 43]. This is in accordance with the target guidelines of the Extracorporeal Life Support Organization (ELSO) [36]. Activated clotting time (ACT) should be kept between 160 and 200 s, fibrinogen levels >1.5–4 g/l, and INR <1.8; <1.5 in case of bleeding.

Hemolysis is another well-recognized complication of ECMO and should be routinely monitored. This is done by regular (daily) checking of the plasma-free hemoglobin and haptoglobin. In case of heparin-induced thrombocytopenia (HIT), argatroban seems to be an adequate alternative for anticoagulation during ECMO [36, 43].

Complications

Bleeding and Thrombosis

Hemostatic perturbations are common in patients with ECMO and contribute significantly to morbidity and mortality [44]. This includes thrombosis and excessive bleeding caused by coagulopathy [44]. Thrombosis in ECMO patients occurs in periods of low-flow or inadequate circuit anticoagulation. Clots can be found in the whole circuit at the sites of stasis and turbulent flow [36]. In case of bleeding, continuous activation of the contact and fibrinolytic systems by the circuit as well as consumption and dilution of factors occurs within minutes of initiation of ECMO. Platelets adhere to surface fibrinogen and are activated. As a consequence, platelet aggregation causes platelet count drop. Correction by platelet transfusion produces only a temporary increase. There might be significant platelet dysfunction despite regular platelet transfusions. Furthermore, prolonged duration of ECMO exacerbates these negative effects [44]. The thromboelastogram (TEG) can measure the integrity of platelet activity [17, 36]. The level of heparinization required is still under debate [43]. Often the level of anticoagulation must be reduced in case of bleeding. Most of the newer ECMO circuits are heparin-bonded, and therefore minimal or no heparinization can be accepted for a number of hours until complete control of bleeding.

Cerebral Hemorrhage and Infarction

Changes in cerebral blood flow and the use of heparin may contribute to both hemorrhagic and nonhemorrhagic intracranial lesions. Lidegran and colleagues [45] reported intracranial lesions (bleeding, infarction) within the first 7 days after ECMO initiation in 37% of studied patients. ECMO survivors carry a high risk of brain injury with subsequent functional deficit [46]. Neurological events in patients with ECMO occur frequently. Intracranial bleeding is the most frequent and occurs early, and it is associated with an increased mortality [47]. In addition, ECMO therapy itself can cause cerebral injury. The cannulation itself, together with creation of solid and gaseous microemboli during perfusion, may cause cerebral injury. Arterial emboli may occur in connection with retrograde arterial cannulation, and even careful cannulation with the Seldinger technique may cause thrombus formation.

This implicates an adequate neurological management: According to international guidelines, the patient on ECMO should be awake to interact with care providers and family [36]. Adequate analgesia and delirium monitoring according to the "pain, agitation, and delirium" (PAD) guidelines should be the standard [48]. This is also of gaining importance with respect to early detection of new neurological deficits caused by cerebral infarction or hemorrhage. Therefore, oversedation should be avoided, and this has a valuable impact on outcome [48]. Spontaneous breathing as a part of a "lung-protective strategy" by decreasing intrapulmonary shunt and intrathoracic pressures, as well as improving organ perfusion, should be achieved as early as possible. Furthermore, after thoracic surgery this is beneficial in protecting surgical bronchial reconstruction as well as in preventing of bronchial fistulas and bronchial suture dehiscence [1, 11].

Weaning of ECMO

ECMO support is reduced as the lungs recover. The chest X-ray will demonstrate the improvement of the lungs. Once ECMO flow is reduced to 1 L/min and in case of stable arterial blood gases (see Table 55.2), the patient is ready to trial off ECMO for at least 2 h [32, 35, 36, 49].

Extracorporeal Carbon Dioxide Removal (ECCO$_2$R)

ECCO$_2$R is a technique of partial respiratory support which allows ultra-protective ventilation strategies. It removes CO$_2$ from the blood through a low blood flow (0.4–1 l/min) extracorporeal circuit. The major limitation is that it has no effect on oxygenation. An arterial or venous access cannula is necessary to drain blood, a membrane lung and a return venous cannula. Different heparin-coated cannulas are available to be inserted via Seldinger technique percutaneously via a femoral-femoral access.

New developments in extracorporeal technologies are gaining interest, and various kinds of ECCO$_2$R devices are available from different manufactures. They range from systems such as the Decap system (Hemodec, Salerno, Italy)

Table 55.2 ECMO weaning criteria (Fig. 55.3)

F$_I$O$_2$ < 0.4–0.6
PaO$_2$ > 60–80 mmHg
PaCO$_2$ 30–45 mmHg
Target ventilator settings
BIPAP: PEEP according to maximize saturation, PIP < 30 cm H$_2$O, Vt: 4–8 ml/kg
RR spontaneous ~ 5 breath/min
Procedure
Reducing blood flow 0.5 l/min every 12 h to minimal blood flow of 1.0 l/min
PaCO$_2$ < 60 mmHg, reducing gas flow and F$_I$O$_2$ over membrane
ECMO trial off, gas flow 1 l/min over 2 h; criteria fulfilled, discontinue ECMO

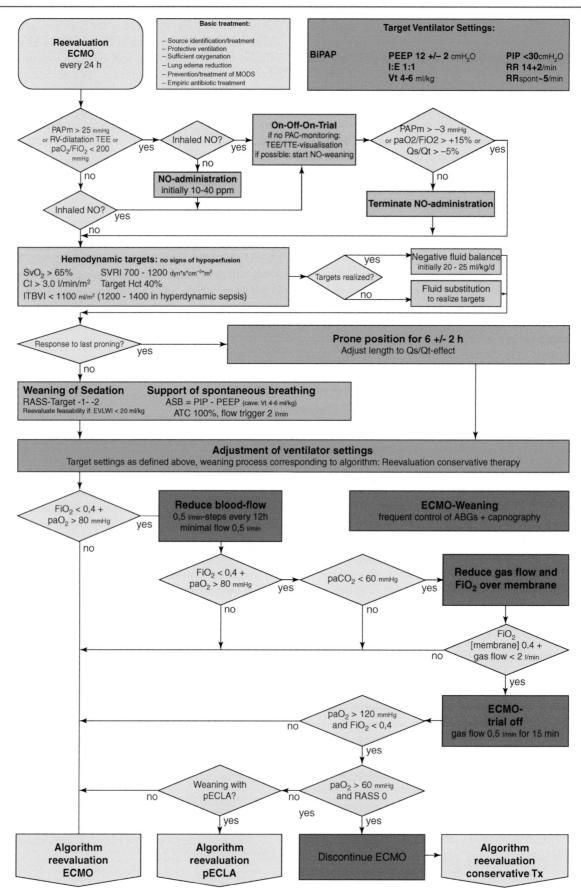

Fig. 55.3 Treatment algorithm for ARDS: ECMO and iLA. (Deja et al. [32], with kind permission from Field House publishing)

that has a dual purpose of renal replacement and $ECCO_2R$ to partial extracorporeal support systems such as the pumpless iLA (Hechingen, Germany) device [50, 51].

The pumpless iLA membrane ventilator marketed by Novalung GmbH is a low-gradient device. It is a pumpless arteriovenous shunt with CO_2 elimination as primary function owing to the arterial inflow blood. The principle is simple diffusion. Blood flows over the exterior surface (1.5 m^2) of the device fibers, and the ventilating gas (O_2 sweep) flows inside these fibers. The iLA consists of a plastic gas exchange module with diffusion membranes made from polymethylpentene (PMP). The PMP fibers are woven into a complex configuration of hollow fibers. Gas transfer takes place without direct contact with blood. In addition, the blood-contacting PMP membrane surface is treated with a heparin coating to provide a biocompatible and non-thrombogenic surface [52]. The iLA is a low pressure-gradient device designed to operate without a mechanical pump. Based on this principle, adequate means arterial blood pressure is mandatory. The preferred access sites are the femoral vessels by percutaneous cannulation using Seldinger's technique (see Fig. 55.1). Used in this configuration, usually about 20% of the cardiac output (1–2 L/min) runs through the iLA, driven by the left ventricle, and mixes with the remaining 80% of the CO in the venous vasculature. One limitation of this device is that patients with primarily an oxygenation disorder may not benefit sufficiently from the pumpless iLA mode in terms of oxygenation; however CO_2 elimination is usually not a problem.

The blood enters the device through the inlet connector. The blood flows into the blood distributing chamber. Any microsized air bubbles that may have entered the device are removed through the de-airing ports. The blood flows into the main chamber where gas exchange takes place. The oxygen- and CO_2-depleted blood is returned to the patient via the blood outflow [50]. Two de-airing membranes are integrated at the top apex on both sides of the device. These de-airing membranes allow gas bubbles but not liquids to cross. In addition, they facilitate priming and de-airing of the device and are also used to eliminate any air trapped in the device during support. An oxygen supply is connected to the gas inflow connector; the lower gas outflow connector is open to the atmosphere and is the site where gas is exhausted from the device [53].

The Decap^{tm} system combines renal replacement with $ECCO_2R$. The so-called Hemolung (ALung Technologies, Pittsburgh, PA, USA) achieves efficient CO_2 removal with flows of 400–600 ml/min similar to renal replacement [54].

Indications for $ECCO_2R$

There are two major indications (see Table 55.3): It can be applied to give the injured or diseased lung a chance to heal

Table 55.3 Criteria for iLA indication and weaning iLA

iLA indication (Fig. 55.2)
$PaCO_2 > 80$ mmHg + PIP > 30 cm H_2O + pH <7.2 (respiratory) + $PaO_2/F_1O_2 > 80$ mmHg
Weaning of iLA/Main criteria (Fig. 55.4)
Richmond Agitation and Sedation Score (RASS) 0/−1
$F_1O_2 < 0.4$
$PaCO_2 < 60$ mmHg
Target ventilator settings
BIPAP: PEEP according to maximize saturation, PIP < 30 cm H_2O, Vt: 4–8 ml/kg, Spontaneous breathing
Procedure
Reducing O_2 flow iLA in steps of 1 l/min
iLA O_2-flow <2 l/min: iLA 6 h without gas flow
iLA trial off: criteria fulfilled: discontinue iLA

Adapted to Ref. [32] with kind permission from Field House publishing, (Fig. 55.4)

("bridge to recovery") or in an end-stage lung disease, and it might be used as a bridge to lung transplantation, i.e., in patients with pulmonary hypertension [53, 55]. In this context the device has been implanted with main pulmonary artery and vein cannulations during sternotomy (see Fig. 55.5). It has been possible to wean several patients with ventilatory and RV failure from iLA and positive-pressure ventilation while waiting for lung transplantation (see Fig. 55.6).

The use of iLA in addition to lung-protective ventilation has been reported in one center to have a high survival rate (84%) in a series patients with severe post lung resection ARDS [56]. The iLA can be used for CO_2 removal in cases of severe hypercapnia and respiratory acidosis in order to avoid the injury of mechanical ventilation. Bein et al. [57] studied, in a single center study, 90 patients with ARDS supported with the pumpless iLA and reported a survival rate (weaning of iLA) of 41%. The iLA has been used in patients with bronchopleural fistulas after lung surgery [11] and with chest trauma (lung contusion) [58], or as a bridge to lung transplant [53]. However, apart from these small randomized studies and case reports, no outcome data are currently available, and additional evidence is necessary to define clear and consistent recommendations.

Complications

Ischemic complications of the lower limb were reported to be associated with the large cannulation size for the arterial cannulation (17 French) initially used for iLA [29, 57]. As smaller cannulae (13 and 15 F) have become available, the ischemic complication rate has markedly decreased. *It is not recommended to use 17 F cannulae for femoral arterial cannulation.* Advantages of iLA are avoiding all the complications related to a mechanical pump, reduced blood-contact surfaces, and relatively easy clinical management.

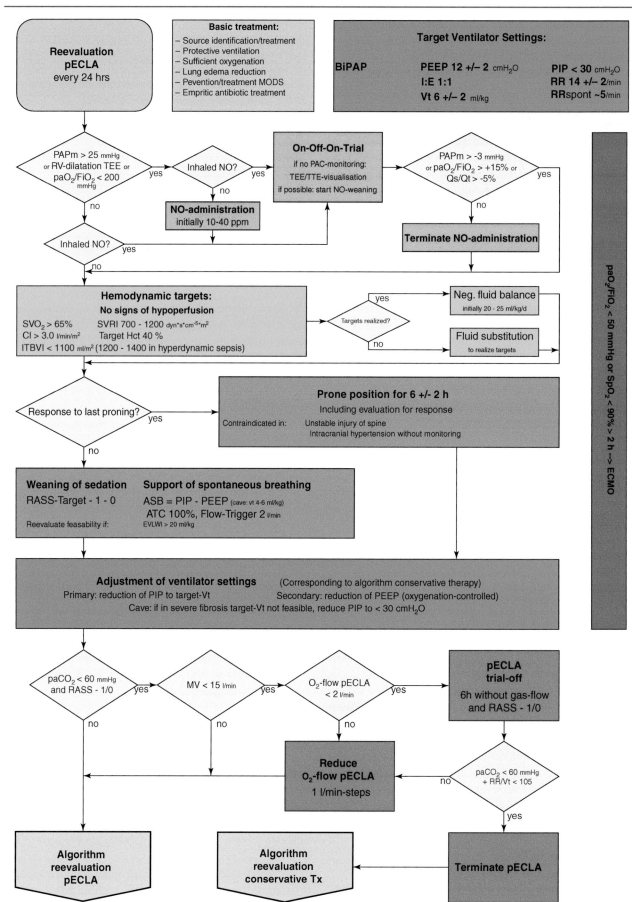

Fig. 55.4 Treatment algorithm for ARDS: ECMO and iLA. (Deja et al. [32], with kind permission from Field House publishing)

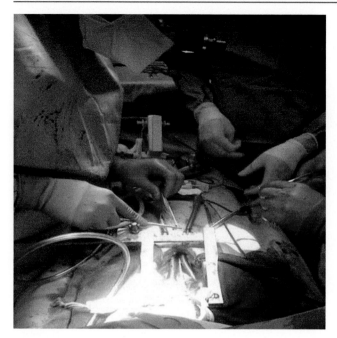

Fig. 55.5 Intrathoracic implantation of interventional lung assists cannulae during sternotomy in a patient with pulmonary hypertension, seen from anesthesiologist's perspective. The iLA device can be seen between the patient's legs. The inflow cannula to the device is on the left side of the incision, placed into the main pulmonary artery. The return cannula, to the right, is into the right upper pulmonary vein. The surgeon is placing a mediastinal drain between the cannulae prior to closing the incision

Disadvantages are the lack of control of blood flow, which is determined by the arteriovenous pressure gradient and the limited oxygen transfer capacity.

Multimodal Therapeutic Approach

Weaning of Sedation
Daily interruption of sedative drugs significantly reduces the duration of mechanical ventilation and the length of stay in the intensive care unit [48]. This should be considered in all patients requiring extracorporeal ventilator support. Moreover, it is important with respect to the early detection of new neurological deficits caused by cerebral infraction or hemorrhage. Therefore, the recommendations of the PAD guideline should be the standard [59].

The concept of the "awake patient" on ECMO is preferred for most patients on ECMO.

Early Spontaneous Breathing
"Spontaneous breathing" as a part of a "lung-protective strategy" by decreasing intrapulmonary shunt and intrathoracic pressures as improving organ perfusion should be achieved as early as possible [11, 32]. Especially after thoracic surgery this is beneficial to protect surgical bronchial reconstruction and to prevent bronchial fistulas as well as bronchial suture dehiscence [11].

Clinical Case Discussion

Case: A 17-year-old male sustained multiple traumas with a traumatic tracheal rupture (approximately 8–10 cm length on the pars membranacea) and bilateral severe lung contusions after a fall of 7 m height (Fig. 55.7). Tracheal rupture as well as mediastinal emphysema was diagnosed on the immediate CT scan. Chest tubes were inserted on both sides due to pneumothoraces. Fiber-optic bronchoscopy was immediately performed in order to position the endotracheal tube as near as possible to the carina. After this intervention, the subcutaneous emphysema decreased. However, within a few hours the patient developed severe ARDS due to its lung contusions (pressure-controlled ventilation; paO_2/F_IO_2 ratio < 200; PEEP, 15 cm H_2O; PIP, 35 cm H_2O).

Tracheal rupture affected the whole tracheal wall with protrusion of mediastinal structures into the lumen; therefore a surgical repair was indicated. The anesthesia team will need to decide if the patient will tolerate the proposed procedure and, if so, then what management strategies can be used to improve the perioperative outcome.

Questions

- Will the patient tolerate the operative procedure without extracorporeal lung assist?
- What specific anesthetic considerations are related to patient's disease?
- How to plan anesthesia and operative procedure in an interdisciplinary approach?
- In this situation of severe ARDS (paO_2/F_IO_2 ratio < 200; PEEP, 15–17 cm H_2O; PIP, 35 cm H_2O), the patient would not tolerate the thoracic surgical procedure under one-lung ventilation without the risk of developing severe hypoxemia and hypercapnia.
- Anesthetic considerations include perioperative difficult airway management (placement of a double-lumen tube?), intraoperative hypoxia and hypercapnia during one-lung ventilation, and postoperative airway management to prevent tracheal suture dehiscence.
- Preoperative management: Conservative treatment strategy with prone positioning, restrictive volume therapy, and nitric oxide administration before the surgical intervention was performed. However, oxygenation index did not increase with prone positioning. Therefore, intraoperative anesthetic management was planned as follows:
  - Preoperative initiation of VV ECMO (femoral veins on both sides 23 F), 4–5 L/min blood flow
  - Apneic oxygenation with PEEP, 10 mmHg, or no ventilation with full ECMO blood flow (advantage: optimal surgical conditions)
  - Airway management: tracheostomy with insertion of an uncuffed tracheostomy tube

Fig. 55.6 A patient with pulmonary hypertension has been weaned from ECMO and mechanical ventilation with a transthoracic implantation of an iLA device. The device can be seen on the side of the patient's bed

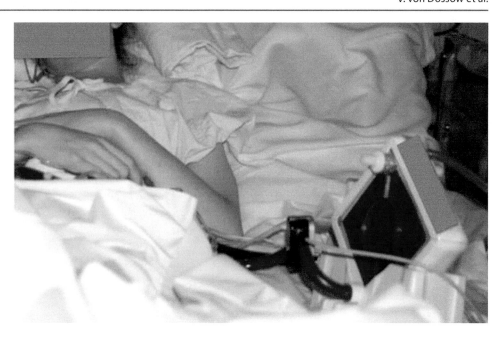

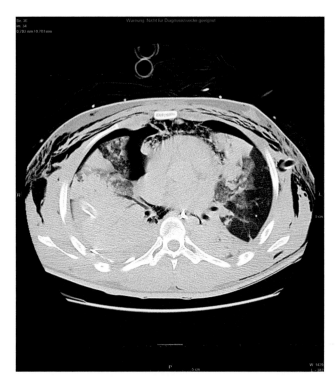

Fig. 55.7 CT scan thorax of a male patient with severe ARDS and traumatic tracheal rupture, mediastinal emphysema

- Postoperative management:
  - Prone positioning should be considered due to lung de-recruitment after lung surgery if there is a clinically relevant increase in oxygenation (re-evaluate every 24 h).
  - ECMO therapy in patients with ARDS improves outcome of some patients.

- Early spontaneous breathing reduces ventilation pressures and prevents tracheal suture dehiscence.
- Daily sedation vacation to detect neurological deficits in patients with ECMO therapy as early as possible.

References

1. Kammerer T, Speck E, von Dossow V. Anesthesia in thoracic surgery. Anaesthesist. 2016;65(5):397–412.
2. Brettner F, von Dossow V, Chappell D. The endothelial glycocalyx and perioperative lung injury. Curr Opin Anaesthesiol. 2017;30(1):36–41.
3. Force ADT, Ranieri VM, Rubenfeld GD, Thompson BT, Ferguson ND, Caldwell E, et al. Acute respiratory distress syndrome: the Berlin definition. JAMA. 2012;307(23):2526–33.
4. Alam N, Park BJ, Wilton A, Seshan VE, Bains MS, Downey RJ, et al. Incidence and risk factors for lung injury after lung cancer resection. Ann Thorac Surg. 2007;84(4):1085–91. discussion 91.
5. Ruffini E, Parola A, Papalia E, Filosso PL, Mancuso M, Oliaro A, et al. Frequency and mortality of acute lung injury and acute respiratory distress syndrome after pulmonary resection for bronchogenic carcinoma. Eur J Cardiothorac Surg. 2001;20(1):30–6. discussion 6–7.
6. Dulu A, Pastores SM, Park B, Riedel E, Rusch V, Halpern NA. Prevalence and mortality of acute lung injury and ARDS after lung resection. Chest. 2006;130(1):73–8.
7. Igic R, Behnia R. Properties and distribution of angiotensin I converting enzyme. Curr Pharm Des. 2003;9(9):697–706.
8. Wang R, Alam G, Zagariya A, Gidea C, Pinillos H, Lalude O, et al. Apoptosis of lung epithelial cells in response to TNF-alpha requires angiotensin II generation de novo. J Cell Physiol. 2000;185(2):253–9.
9. Schmidt EP, Yang Y, Janssen WJ, Gandjeva A, Perez MJ, Barthel L, et al. The pulmonary endothelial glycocalyx regulates neutrophil adhesion and lung injury during experimental sepsis. Nat Med. 2012;18(8):1217–23.
10. Lois M, Noppen M. Bronchopleural fistulas: an overview of the problem with special focus on endoscopic management. Chest. 2005;128(6):3955–65.

11. Hommel M, Deja M, von Dossow V, Diemel K, Heidenhain C, Spies C, et al. Bronchial fistulae in ARDS patients: management with an extracorporeal lung assist device. Eur Respir J. 2008;32(6):1652–5.

12. Hager DN, Krishnan JA, Hayden DL, Brower RG, Network ACT. Tidal volume reduction in patients with acute lung injury when plateau pressures are not high. Am J Respir Crit Care Med. 2005;172(10):1241–5.

13. Terragni PP, Del Sorbo L, Mascia L, Urbino R, Martin EL, Birocco A, et al. Tidal volume lower than 6 ml/kg enhances lung protection: role of extracorporeal carbon dioxide removal. Anesthesiology. 2009;111(4):826–35.

14. Fan E, Brodie D, Slutsky AS. Fifty years of research in ARDS. Mechanical ventilation during extracorporeal support for acute respiratory distress syndrome. For now, a necessary evil. Am J Respir Crit Care Med. 2017;195(9):1137–9.

15. Amato MB, Meade MO, Slutsky AS, Brochard L, Costa EL, Schoenfeld DA, et al. Driving pressure and survival in the acute respiratory distress syndrome. N Engl J Med. 2015;372(8):747–55.

16. Costa EL, Slutsky AS, Amato MB. Driving pressure as a key ventilation variable. N Engl J Med. 2015;372(21):2072.

17. Peek GJ, Mugford M, Tiruvoipati R, Wilson A, Allen E, Thalanany MM, et al. Efficacy and economic assessment of conventional ventilatory support versus extracorporeal membrane oxygenation for severe adult respiratory failure (CESAR): a multicentre randomised controlled trial. Lancet. 2009;374(9698):1351–63.

18. Hill JD, O'Brien TG, Murray JJ, Dontigny L, Bramson ML, Osborn JJ, et al. Prolonged extracorporeal oxygenation for acute post-traumatic respiratory failure (shock-lung syndrome). Use of the Bramson membrane lung. N Engl J Med. 1972;286(12):629–34.

19. Hill JD, De Leval MR, Fallat RJ, Bramson ML, Eberhart RC, Schulte HD, et al. Acute respiratory insufficiency. Treatment with prolonged extracorporeal oxygenation. J Thorac Cardiovasc Surg. 1972;64(4):551–62.

20. Zapol WM, Snider MT, Hill JD, Fallat RJ, Bartlett RH, Edmunds LH, et al. Extracorporeal membrane oxygenation in severe acute respiratory failure. A randomized prospective study. JAMA. 1979;242(20):2193–6.

21. Zapol WM. What future for ECMO? Int J Artif Organs. 1979;2(5):231–2.

22. Kolla S, Awad SS, Rich PB, Schreiner RJ, Hirschl RB, Bartlett RH. Extracorporeal life support for 100 adult patients with severe respiratory failure. Ann Surg. 1997;226(4):544–64. discussion 65-6.

23. Kolla S, Crotti S, Lee WA, Gargulinski MJ, Lewandowski T, Bach D, et al. Total respiratory support with tidal flow extracorporeal circulation in adult sheep. ASAIO J. 1997;43(5):M811–6.

24. Gattinoni L, Pesenti A, Mascheroni D, Marcolin R, Fumagalli R, Rossi F, et al. Low-frequency positive-pressure ventilation with extracorporeal CO2 removal in severe acute respiratory failure. JAMA. 1986;256(7):881–6.

25. Morris AH, Wallace CJ, Menlove RL, Clemmer TP, Orme JF Jr, Weaver LK, et al. Randomized clinical trial of pressure-controlled inverse ratio ventilation and extracorporeal CO2 removal for adult respiratory distress syndrome. Am J Respir Crit Care Med. 1994;149(2 Pt 1):295–305.

26. Hoechter DJ, von Dossow V, Winter H, Muller HH, Meiser B, Neurohr C, et al. The Munich lung transplant group: intraoperative extracorporeal circulation in lung transplantation. Thorac Cardiovasc Surg. 2015;63(8):706–14.

27. Linden V, Palmer K, Reinhard J, Westman R, Ehren H, Granholm T, et al. High survival in adult patients with acute respiratory distress syndrome treated by extracorporeal membrane oxygenation, minimal sedation, and pressure supported ventilation. Intensive Care Med. 2000;26(11):1630–7.

28. Morimont P, Batchinsky A, Lambermont B. Update on the role of extracorporeal CO(2) removal as an adjunct to mechanical ventilation in ARDS. Crit Care. 2015;19:117.

29. Camporota L, Barrett N. Current applications for the use of extracorporeal carbon dioxide removal in critically ill patients. Biomed Res Int. 2016;2016:9781695.

30. Damas P, Frippiat F, Ancion A, Canivet JL, Lambermont B, Layios N, et al. Prevention of ventilator-associated pneumonia and ventilator-associated conditions: a randomized controlled trial with subglottic secretion suctioning. Crit Care Med. 2015;43(1):22–30.

31. Khan NU, Al-Aloul M, Khasati N, Machaal A, Leonard CT, Yonan N. Extracorporeal membrane oxygenator as a bridge to successful surgical repair of bronchopleural fistula following bilateral sequential lung transplantation: a case report and review of literature. J Cardiothorac Surg. 2007;2:28.

32. Deja M, Hommel M, Weber-Carstens S, Moss M, von Dossow V, Sander M, et al. Evidence-based therapy of severe acute respiratory distress syndrome: an algorithm-guided approach. J Int Med Res. 2008;36(2):211–21.

33. Aokage T, Palmer K, Ichiba S, Takeda S. Extracorporeal membrane oxygenation for acute respiratory distress syndrome. J Intensive Care. 2015;3:17.

34. Marasco SF, Lukas G, McDonald M, McMillan J, Ihle B. Review of ECMO (extra corporeal membrane oxygenation) support in critically ill adult patients. Heart Lung Circ. 2008;17(Suppl 4):S41–7.

35. Banfi C, Pozzi M, Siegenthaler N, Brunner ME, Tassaux D, Obadia JF, et al. Veno-venous extracorporeal membrane oxygenation: cannulation techniques. J Thorac Dis. 2016;8(12):3762–73.

36. Peek GJ. In: Annich GM, editor. Adult respiratory ECMO. 4th ed: ELSO; 2012. p. 309–20.

37. Boissier F, Katsahian S, Razazi K, Thille AW, Roche-Campo F, Leon R, et al. Prevalence and prognosis of cor pulmonale during protective ventilation for acute respiratory distress syndrome. Intensive Care Med. 2013;39(10):1725–33.

38. Bouferrache K, Vieillard-Baron A. Acute respiratory distress syndrome, mechanical ventilation, and right ventricular function. Curr Opin Crit Care. 2011;17(1):30–5.

39. Banfi C, Pozzi M, Brunner ME, Rigamonti F, Murith N, Mugnai D, et al. Veno-arterial extracorporeal membrane oxygenation: an overview of different cannulation techniques. J Thorac Dis. 2016;8(9):E875–E85.

40. Lamperti M, Bodenham AR, Pittiruti M, Blaivas M, Augoustides JG, Elbarbary M, et al. International evidence-based recommendations on ultrasound-guided vascular access. Intensive Care Med. 2012;38(7):1105–17.

41. Troianos CA, Hartman GS, Glas KE, Skubas NJ, Eberhardt RT, Walker JD, et al. Guidelines for performing ultrasound guided vascular cannulation: recommendations of the American Society of Echocardiography and the Society of Cardiovascular Anesthesiologists. J Am Soc Echocardiogr. 2011;24(12):1291–318.

42. Beiderlinden M, Treschan T, Gorlinger K, Peters J. Argatroban in extracorporeal membrane oxygenation. Artif Organs. 2007;31(6):461–5.

43. Oliver WC. Anticoagulation and coagulation management for ECMO. Semin Cardiothorac Vasc Anesth. 2009;13(3):154–75.

44. Nair P, Hoechter DJ, Buscher H, Venkatesh K, Whittam S, Joseph J, et al. Prospective observational study of hemostatic alterations during adult extracorporeal membrane oxygenation (ECMO) using point-of-care thromboelastometry and platelet aggregometry. J Cardiothorac Vasc Anesth. 2015;29(2):288–96.

45. Lidegran MK, Mosskin M, Ringertz HG, Frenckner BP, Linden VB. Cranial CT for diagnosis of intracranial complications in adult and pediatric patients during ECMO: clinical benefits in diagnosis and treatment. Acad Radiol. 2007;14(1):62–71.

46. Risnes I, Wagner K, Nome T, Sundet K, Jensen J, Hynas IA, et al. Cerebral outcome in adult patients treated with extracorporeal membrane oxygenation. Ann Thorac Surg. 2006;81(4):1401–6.

47. Luyt CE, Brechot N, Demondion P, Jovanovic T, Hekimian G, Lebreton G, et al. Brain injury during venovenous extracorporeal membrane oxygenation. Intensive Care Med. 2016;42(5):897–907.

48. Barr J, Fraser GL, Puntillo K, Ely EW, Gelinas C, Dasta JF, et al. Clinical practice guidelines for the management of pain, agitation, and delirium in adult patients in the intensive care unit. Crit Care Med. 2013;41(1):263–306.

49. Deja M, Hommel M, Goldmann A, Pille C, von Dossow V, Lojewski C, et al. Lung diseases--multimodal adult respiratory distress syndrome(ARDS)--therapy requires evidence-based studies with clear criteria of results. Anasthesiol Intensivmed Notfallmed Schmerzther. 2008;43(11–12):756–7.

50. Fischer S, Hoeper MM, Tomaszek S, Simon A, Gottlieb J, Welte T, et al. Bridge to lung transplantation with the extracorporeal membrane ventilator Novalung in the veno-venous mode: the initial Hannover experience. ASAIO J. 2007;53(2):168–70.

51. Ruberto F, Pugliese F, D'Alio A, Perrella S, D'Auria B, Ianni S, et al. Extracorporeal removal CO2 using a venovenous, low-flow system (Decapsmart) in a lung transplanted patient: a case report. Transplant Proc. 2009;41(4):1412–4.

52. Meyer A, Struber M, Fischer S. Advances in extracorporeal ventilation. Anesthesiol Clin. 2008;26(2):381–91. viii.

53. Fischer S, Hoeper MM, Bein T, Simon AR, Gottlieb J, Wisser W, et al. Interventional lung assist: a new concept of protective ventilation in bridge to lung transplantation. ASAIO J. 2008;54(1):3–10.

54. Cove ME, MacLaren G, Federspiel WJ, Kellum JA. Bench to bedside review: extracorporeal carbon dioxide removal, past present and future. Crit Care. 2012;16(5):232.

55. Fischer S, Bohn D, Rycus P, Pierre AF, de Perrot M, Waddell TK, et al. Extracorporeal membrane oxygenation for primary graft dysfunction after lung transplantation: analysis of the Extracorporeal Life Support Organization (ELSO) registry. J Heart Lung Transplant. 2007;26(5):472–7.

56. Iglesias M, Martinez E, Badia JR, Macchiarini P. Extrapulmonary ventilation for unresponsive severe acute respiratory distress syndrome after pulmonary resection. Ann Thorac Surg. 2008;85(1):237–44. discussion 44.

57. Bein T, Weber F, Philipp A, Prasser C, Pfeifer M, Schmid FX, et al. A new pumpless extracorporeal interventional lung assist in critical hypoxemia/hypercapnia. Crit Care Med. 2006;34(5):1372–7.

58. Brederlau J, Anetseder M, Wagner R, Roesner T, Philipp A, Greim C, et al. Pumpless extracorporeal lung assist in severe blunt chest trauma. J Cardiothorac Vasc Anesth. 2004;18(6):777–9.

59. Barr J, Fraser GL, Puntillo K, Ely EW, Gelinas C, Dasta JF, et al. Clinical practice guidelines for the management of pain, agitation, and delirium in adult patients in the intensive care unit: executive summary. Am J Health Syst Pharm. 2013;70(1):53–8.

Cardiovascular Adaptations and Complications

Alessia Pedoto and David Amar

Key Points

- Changes in *right ventricular anatomy and function* can occur at several stages of lung resection, starting after induction of general anesthesia and positioning, followed by one-lung ventilation and surgical dissection. Compensatory mechanisms may not occur in patients with advanced COPD who are at risk of developing long-term complications. Several tests are available during the intraoperative period to evaluate right heart function, and their merits are reviewed.

- *Supraventricular arrhythmias* are a common complication after thoracic surgery, depending on the extent of the dissection. Atrial fibrillation is the most common postoperative rhythm disturbance after lung resection. Several pathophysiologic mechanisms as well as prophylactic and/or therapeutic maneuvers have been proposed. Older age and intrapericardial procedures are among the risk factors that strongly correlate with this condition.

- *Acute coronary syndrome* after thoracic surgery is rare but is associated with a high risk of death. Patients at risk are the ones with preoperative coronary artery disease and abnormal exercise testing. There are no clear recommendations on the role of preoperative cardiac catheterization and coronary revascularization.

- *Cardiac failure* can result from either right or left heart dysfunction and can be transient or long standing. Symptoms may be subtle at rest and become evident during exertion. *Cardiac hernia-*

tion is a rare complication that may occur after intrapericardial pneumonectomy and is associated with a high mortality rate. Clinical and electrocardiographic signs are very nonspecific, and treatment is surgical.

- *Mediastinal shift* is the result of changes in the post-pneumonectomy space. A high index of suspicion is needed for the diagnosis, which can present with severe hemodynamic compromise or respiratory symptoms. *Post-pneumonectomy syndrome* may occur in the late postoperative period. It is characterized by an extreme mediastinal shift which causes dynamic compression of the distal airway and respiratory insufficiency. Treatment is surgical.

Introduction

Lung resection, especially if extensive, can cause acute and chronic changes in the anatomy and function of the right heart. This can be the result of either transient or sustained pressure or volume overload, reduction in contractility, cardiomyopathy, or arrhythmias [1], especially in the presence of pre-existing abnormalities [2]. The right heart is very sensitive to increases in afterload [3]. Acute increase in pulmonary arterial pressures (PAP) can lead to a significant decrease in right ventricular (RV) output with subsequent RV failure. Secondary left ventricular (LV) compression can cause systemic hypotension, with right coronary artery (RCA) hypoperfusion and possible right myocardial ischemia [4]. The right heart has recently been recognized as an active mediator, rather than a passive conduit, that can contribute to perioperative morbidity [5]. Any pathology associated with pulmonary hypertension and chronic hypoxia (such as end-stage COPD or connective tissue interstitial lung disease) can cause baseline right

A. Pedoto (✉) · D. Amar
Department of Anesthesiology and Critical Care Medicine, Memorial Sloan Kettering Cancer Center, New York, NY, USA
e-mail: pedotoa@mskcc.org

Table 56.1 Causes of right ventricular failure [6]

Pressure overload	Left heart failure (most common)
	Pulmonary embolus (common)
	Pulmonary hypertension
	Right ventricular outflow tract obstruction
	Peripheral pulmonary stenosis
	Double chamber right ventricle
	Systemic right ventricle
Volume overload	Tricuspid regurgitation
	Pulmonary regurgitation
	Atrial septal defect
	Anomalous pulmonary venous return
	Sinus of Valsalva rupture in the right atrium
	Coronary artery fistula in the right atrium or right ventricle
	Carcinoid syndrome
	Rheumatic valvulitis
Ischemia/infarction	Right ventricular myocardial ischemia
Intrinsic myocardial processes	Cardiomyopathy and heart failure
	Arrhythmogenic right ventricular dysplasia
	Sepsis
Inflow limitation	Tricuspid stenosis
	Superior vena cava stenosis
Congenital defects	Ebstein's anomaly
	Tetralogy of Fallot
	Transposition of the great vessels
	Double outlet right ventricle with mitral atresia
Pericardial disease	Constrictive pericarditis

ventricular dysfunction (see Table 56.1) [6]. Known etiology includes induction of general anesthesia, institution of one-lung ventilation and lateral decubitus, manipulation of the pulmonary circulation, or triggering of the inflammatory response [7]. While cardiac adaptations occur with time after lung resection, cardiac complications, especially arrhythmias, are commonly seen in the immediate postoperative period before patient discharge.

Cardiac Adaptation

Cardiac adaptation can occur in the immediate intraoperative period, after induction of general anesthesia and positioning or in the postoperative phase.

Intraoperative Changes in Right Ventricular Function and Anatomy Related to One-Lung Ventilation and Positioning

Pulmonary arterial pressures can increase after induction of general anesthesia, as a consequence of positive pressure ventilation, placement of the patient in the lateral decubitus, opening of the chest, and initiation of one-lung ventila-

tion (OLV) [8, 9]. Mediastinal shift and gravity-related changes in pulmonary perfusion and hypoxic vasoconstriction can also contribute to higher pulmonary arterial pressure. In patients with normal pulmonary vascular compliance, an increase in right cardiac output can compensate for the higher afterload without significant changes in pulmonary arterial pressures. This may not occur in patients with advanced COPD, or obstructive sleep apnea, even in the presence of baseline right ventricular hypertrophy [7], theoretically making this population at higher risk for intra- and postoperative cardiac complications. Pre-existing significant pulmonary hypertension can worsen during OLV or clamping of the pulmonary artery. Ligation of the main pulmonary artery during pneumonectomy (right more than left) or lung transplantation in patients with severe COPD can cause acute right heart overload and consequent dilation followed by ischemia or arrhythmias, either intra- or postoperatively [10, 11]. A temporary slow "clamp test" of the pulmonary artery can be done intraoperatively to evaluate the clinical and echocardiographic response of the right heart to acute shifting of blood to the remaining pulmonary circulation [12]. However, this maneuver rarely changes the intraoperative management, since the results may be difficult to observe or interpret as soon as the clamp is applied.

If there are any intraoperative concerns of potential hemodynamic instability or right heart dysfunction, transesophageal echocardiography (TEE) has become a first-line diagnostic tool, replacing *pulmonary arterial catheter data* [13]. This information may influence the clinical decision in patients undergoing lung transplantation on when to initiate cardiopulmonary bypass or help evaluate the response to fluid or vasoactive treatment [14]. While TEE is a valuable "real-time" tool to assess left ventricular function, its role in investigating the right ventricular function is less clear. Despite the superficial location of the right heart, its irregular and asymmetric shape makes the motion and volume calculations much more difficult and less detailed than the left side when 2-D echo is used [5]. The advent of 3-D imaging has improved the quality of the right heart exam, in assessing structural changes and hemodynamic parameters [5, 15]. 3-D techniques have demonstrated a good resolution for the study of RV volumes and a good correlation with thermodilution data [15]. The main disadvantage still remains the costs and need for vendor-specific software. In case of high suspicion for perioperative right heart dysfunction, such as in patients with a predicted postoperative FEV_1 less than 40%, detailed preoperative testing becomes extremely important and is highly recommended [16]. In non-transplant patients, there is little evidence that routine TEE influences outcome [14].

Acute and Late Phase Changes in Right Ventricular Anatomy After Lung Resection

Intraoperative increases in resting pulmonary arterial pressure and pulmonary vascular resistance are usually proportional to the extent of the resection [17] and tend to normalize in the immediate postoperative period. However, aging is associated with a slow decline in right ventricular function, suggesting adaptive or reactive processes that can lead to right ventricular hypertrophy [8]. Changes in right ventricular ejection fraction have been described during exercise and depend on the level of exertion [18]. Compensatory mechanisms are more efficient during moderate exercise, with a fixed right ventricular stroke volume at maximal exertion which is independent from the increase in the workload and the time from surgery [8]. The extent of the resection and the compensatory volume expansion of the remaining lung can cause changes in the mediastinal anatomy with a rotation of the heart in the chest cavity, affecting the left ventricular function. Changes in filling and contraction have been observed. The degree of compensation after lung resection seems to be age dependent [8].

Lung surgery is currently the most common treatment for nonmetastatic resectable lung cancer and is part of a multimodal approach with chemotherapy and radiation [19]. Currently, surgical candidates are much older and with more extensive comorbidities, perhaps due to the combination of an aging population and improvement in surgical and anesthesia techniques [20]. Pre-existing cardiac and pulmonary diseases are common factors that may significantly influence the postoperative course and increase mortality rates [20]. The use of minimally invasive techniques, often relying on pneumo-capnothorax to expedite lung collapse, may cause acute changes in pulmonary pressures and right heart function. Severe pulmonary hypertension (mean pulmonary arterial pressure >45 mmHg) has been demonstrated only in 3.7% of patients with lung disease [21], despite a long smoking history and the presence of variable degrees of COPD in some patients. Ninety percent of patients with FEV_1 less than 50% have mean pulmonary arterial pressures of about 20 mmHg, and only 5% may have values greater than 35 mmHg [22].

Several studies have investigated postoperative right ventricular function (see Table 56.2 [7]), but the results are difficult to compare due to small sample sizes and extremely variable methodology. Some agreement exists among studies in patients after pneumonectomy that show a mild increase in pulmonary arterial systolic pressure, right ventricular diastolic volume or systolic pressure on transthoracic echocardiography [7], and CT scan exams [17]. These changes occurred in the second postoperative day and may persist after 4 years [7], suggesting an evolution of the cardiovascular response over time [8]. An increase in both afterload and catecholamine tone after clamping the pulmonary artery may lead to an increase in diastolic volume, pulmonary arterial systolic pressure, and mild tricuspid regurgitation which is observed on 2-D echocardiography. Most of the studies showed an increased incidence of tachyarrhythmias after pneumonectomy, which was transient in most cases and not associated with either heart failure or long-term complications [7]. Despite all these observed changes, there was no effect on 30-day mortality rates.

Cardiac Complications

Supraventricular Tachyarrhythmias (Atrial Fibrillation, Atrial Flutter, and Supraventricular Tachycardia)

Supraventricular tachyarrhythmias occur in approximately 4–25% of patients undergoing noncardiac thoracic surgery [28, 29]. Age of 60 years and older [30] and intrapericardial pneumonectomy [31] remain the most important risk factors. An elevated white blood cell count on postoperative day 1 [32] and an elevated perioperative N-terminal-pro-B-type natriuretic peptide (NT-pro-BNP) [33] and BNP [33–35] have also been suggested as possible predicting biomarkers, with a higher sensitivity when associated with older age [36]. Male gender, extent of surgical resection but not surgical approach or laterality, left ventricular early transmitral velocity/mitral annular early diastolic velocity (E/e') [36], increased trans mitral flow deceleration time, and left diastolic volume index [37] on echocardiography were also reported as potential risk factors for POAF. The combination of multiple risk factors such as gender, age, BNP, and extent of lung volume to be resected can be used as criteria to select high-risk patients who would benefit from a preoperative echocardiographic exam [36] and postoperative arrhythmia prophylaxis [38–41].

Atrial fibrillation (AF) is the most common rhythm disturbance, followed by supraventricular tachycardia (SVT), atrial flutter, and premature ventricular contractions (PVCs). The diagnosis is usually made on the second postoperative day (with a range of 1–7 days), and its duration is usually self-limited. Postoperative atrial fibrillation (POAF) has a good response to pharmacological cardioversion with approximately 85% resolved within 24 h from onset [30, 42–44].

Sustained ventricular tachyarrhythmias are quite rare after lung resection [28, 45]. Non-sustained ventricular tachycardia (more than three consecutive beats but <30 s) has an incidence of 0.5–1.5% and can occur in the first 96 h after lung resection, especially in patients with preoperative

Table 56.2 Summary of the literature analyzing right ventricular changes after lung surgery. All the studies listed are prospective in nature

Study	Time of the study	Type of surgery	Study	Results Lobectomy pneumonectomy		Exclusion	Comments
Venuta [23]	4 years	Lobe (N = 36) Pneumonectomy (N = 15)	TTE	No changes.	↑RVDD ↑PASP moderate TVI	FEV₁ < 60%, h/o MI, angina, valvular ds, AF, cardiac surgery	Mild increase in PASP and RVDV not clinically significant to cause RVH
Foroulis [24]	6 months	Lobe (N = 17) Pneumonectomy (N = 35)	TTE	↑PASP, ↑RVDD ↑TR	↑↑PASP ↑↑RVDD ↑↑TR	Postoperative BPF, empyema, respiratory failure, MI	Small study, higher PASP in pneumonectomy patients at 6 months (R > L cases), with higher incidence of postoperative AF and SVT requiring treatment, attributed to RV dilatation
Amar [25]	1 month	Pneumonectomy (N = 70)	TTE		No changes in R and L atrial diameter, EF, TR and RVSP	AF, lung resection, lesser operations, unresectable	Study to evaluate role of diltiazem and digoxin on AF Echo done as part of their follow-up
Amar [26]	1 week	Lobe (N = 47) Pneumonectomy (N = 39)	TTE	↑HR	↑RSVP ↑HR	Wedge, prior thoracic surgery Non-sinus rhythm	RVSP of 31, not affecting RV systolic function unless respiratory failure occurs
Kowalewski [10]	2 days	Lobe (N = 9) Pneumonectomy (N = 22)	TTE	No changes	↑RVEDV ↓RVEF ↑ SVT		Not very accurate and nonstandard right heart volumes calculations which can underestimate large volumes. RVEF usually underestimates the true value by echo due to RV geometry
Smulders [27]	5 years	Pneumonectomy (N = 15)	MRI		R side = cardiac lateral shift. ↓RVEDV, nl LV function L side = rotation, nl RVEDV, ↓LVEF ↑HR, ↓SV		No signs of RVH at 5 years
Katz [11]	Intraoperative	Lung transplantation (N = 32)	TEE	Immediate ↓PAP (systolic+mean), and ↓RV size post transplantation, normalization of septal geometry in severe pulmonary HTN (↓RVED area)			CPB used in all cases of severe pulmonary HTN

Abbreviations: *N* number of cases, *TTE* transthoracic echocardiography, *RVDD* right midventricular diastolic diameter, *PASP* pulmonary arterial systolic pressures, *TVI* tricuspid valve insufficiency, *FEV₁* forced expiratory volume at 1 s, *MI* myocardial infarction, *AF* atrial fibrillation, *RVDV* right ventricular diastolic volume, *RVH* right ventricular hypertrophy, *TR* tricuspid regurgitation, *BPF* bronchopleural fistula, *SVT* supraventricular tachycardia, *RV* right ventricle, *R* right, *L* left, *EF* ejection fraction, *RVSP* right ventricular systolic pressure, *RVEDV* right ventricular end-diastolic volume, *RVEF* right ventricular ejection fraction, *MRI* magnetic resonance imaging, *LV* left ventricle, *SV* stroke volume, *TEE* transesophageal echocardiography, *PAP* pulmonary arterial pressure, *HR* heart rate, *HTN* hypertension, *CPB* cardiopulmonary bypass

left bundle branch block [46]. It is rarely associated with hemodynamic instability requiring treatment at any time. There is no association with age, other clinical factors, or core temperature upon arrival to PACU. On multivariate analysis, an independent association seems to exist between non-sustained ventricular tachycardia and POAF, possibly due to vagal withdrawal or irritation and/or a surge in sympathetic activity. These findings differ from the cardiac surgical literature, where the presence of postoperative ventricular tachycardia often leads to poor outcome [28].

POAF can be an isolated complication within the first week after surgery or associated with respiratory or infectious disease [30]. It is typically transient and reversible and seems to affect individuals with an electrophysiologic substrate for arrhythmias present before or as a result of surgery [29, 47]. Despite the good prognosis, POAF is associated with a 1.7% risk of developing cerebrovascular accidents if persistent [38, 48]. Thromboembolic events can occur within 24–48 h from the onset of sustained POAF and may have devastating sequelae. If sinus rhythm fails to be restored within this time frame, anticoagulation should be considered weighing the risk of postoperative bleeding [28]. The most recent American Heart Association (AHA) guidelines on management of AF unrelated to surgery provide similar recommendations for which antithrombotic medications one should employ in postoperative patients depending on the patient's risk (i.e., presence of a prosthetic valve, etc., prior cerebrovascular accidents, or no risk factors) [49].

Several mechanisms have been proposed to explain POAF, but the most consistent factors other than age have been prior history of paroxysmal AF and extent of resection. Aging per se has been associated with loss of about 90% of normal sinus nodal fibers and remodeling of the atrial myocardium, with changes in the sinoatrial and atrioventricular nodal conduction, as well as an increased sensitivity to catecholamine activity, especially after surgical trauma in the area [38, 45]. Triggering of an inflammatory response with activation of the complement system and several pro-inflammatory cytokines has also been suggested as a contributing factor for POAF in this age population [50]. This thought is supported by a doubling in white blood cell (WBC) count observed in patients older than 60 years of age on postoperative day 1, which is associated with a threefold increase in the odds of developing POAF [32]. Catecholamine-induced leukocytosis via α- and β_2-receptor activation is a known phenomenon which could in part explain this finding. The use of thoracic epidural analgesia as a modality to cause sympathectomy and prevent POAF has led to disappointing results [51], maybe due to the high individual variability of sympathetic blockade. Stretching or inflammation of the pulmonary veins, hilar manipulation, and mediastinal shift may be additional contributing factors [47]. Positive inotropic agents, i.e., dopamine, as well as anemia, fever, hypoglycemia, postoperative ischemia, and surgical complications, are all aggravating factors [42, 52].

Presenting symptoms of rapid POAF include dyspnea, palpitations, dizziness, syncope, respiratory distress, and hypotension [38, 45]. Although pulmonary embolism or myocardial ischemia and electrolyte abnormality are commonly included in the differential diagnosis they are rarely proven [53]. According to the AHA guidelines, transthoracic echocardiography should be part of the workup for new-onset POAF to rule out any structural disease, if such information is not already available [40]. Similarly, the AHA guidelines do not recommend "ruling out" pulmonary embolism, thyrotoxicosis, or myocardial ischemia if there are no accompanying clinical signs or symptoms.

Postoperative arrhythmia is indirectly associated with higher morbidity [45]. It also can be a direct cause of death in the presence of heart failure or prolonged hypotension [40, 54]. Length of hospital stay and costs are increased in patients with arrhythmias, highlighting the importance of prevention when possible [36, 45, 54]. In most cases, POAF

Table 56.3 Proposed risk factors for supraventricular tachyarrhythmias [28, 30, 43, 45, 47]

Age > 60
Male gender
History of paroxysmal atrial fibrillation
Prolonged P wave duration
Preoperative HR > 72 bpm
Elevated BNP level
Increased WBC count on POD 1
Intrapericardial procedure

Abbreviations: *HR* heart rate, *bpm* beats per minute, *BNP* brain natriuretic peptide, *WBC* white blood cell count, *POD* postoperative day

resolves prior to hospital discharge with a complete resolution at 6 weeks from surgery [38, 45]. Patients are considered at risk for postoperative supraventricular arrhythmias if they have two or more of the risk factors listed in Table 56.3, and, if so, they may be started on pharmacological prophylaxis either preoperatively or in the immediate postoperative period. Several regimens are available to prevent or treat atrial tachyarrhythmias.

Role of Medications Used for Treatment and Prevention

Rate Control Agents

β-blockers are antiarrhythmic agents with cardioprotective effects. As prophylactic agents, they counteract the effects of the high sympathetic tone that occurs after surgery, which may enhance patient susceptibility to dysrhythmias. β-Blockers inhibit intracellular calcium influx via a second messenger have a membrane stabilizing effect and inhibit the renin-angiotensin-aldosterone system [40, 55]. Their respiratory side effects become particularly important after lung resection since nonselective β-blocker can cause bronchospasm and worsen pulmonary function in the postoperative period. Pulmonary edema has been described as a potential side effect [56], as well as hypotension and bradycardia. Moreover, in patients on chronic β-blockers, withdrawal may lead to rebound tachycardia and related complications due to an upregulation of the β receptors [57]. The β-blocker length of stay study (BLOS) analyzed the effects of β-blockers after cardiac surgery used as prophylactic agents in patients both naïve and already taking β-blockers [58]. The goal was to prevent POAF and possibly decrease the length of stay in the hospital and ICU. Patients already on a β-blocker had a small decrease in the incidence of POAF, but their hospital length of stay was increased. This was attributed to the development of adverse cardiac and pulmonary effects. The Perioperative Ischemic Evaluation (POISE) trial showed that aggressive β-blockade in patients at risk or with atherosclerotic disease can reduce postoperative myocardial infarction and even POAF but at the cost of an increase in mortality related to cerebrovascular events in patients who had hypotension and decreased cerebral perfusion [59]. These findings have been consistent with other trials using lower doses of β-blockers, which questioned the safety of this strategy [60]. The AATS 2014 guidelines do not recommend the use of β-blockers in patients who are not already taking the medication [40].

The *calcium channel blockers* verapamil and diltiazem are both prophylactic and therapeutic agents for the treatment of POAF. They decrease intracellular calcium entry by directly blocking the L-type calcium channel and slowing the sinoatrial automaticity and atrioventricular nodal conduction [55]. This class of drugs seems to reduce pulmonary vascular resistance and right ventricular pressure as well, making this an attractive option after major lung resection [56]. Hypotension is one of the major side effects, especially with verapamil, and one of the most common reasons to stop these medications. Calcium channel blockers cause a 40% decrease of postoperative myocardial infarction rates and a 45% reduction of ischemia when used in the cardiac surgical population [56]. Diltiazem is superior to digoxin when used to prevent POAF after intrapericardial or standard pneumonectomy [25]. However, both drugs have equal effect on postoperative ventricular ectopy, echocardiographic changes in right ventricular function, and hospital length of stay. In the largest study to prevent POAF in thoracic surgical patients, diltiazem was safe and effective in reducing the rate of POAF of almost 50% [61]. When administered as a bolus followed by a continuous infusion, diltiazem controls the ventricular rate in about 90% of patients with recent onset of POAF, with an onset of action of 2–7 min [40].

Amiodarone is a sodium-potassium-calcium channel blocker and a β-adrenergic inhibitor. It has been demonstrated to be the most effective prophylactic agent after major lung resection when started in the immediate postoperative period [41]. It is often used to maintain sinus rhythm after electrical cardioversion in the general population. An intravenous bolus followed by a continuous infusion has a similar effect to intravenous diltiazem and digoxin. Its onset is of about 4 h with a 24 h duration of the effect [40]. As a prophylactic agent, it works best when administered 1 week prior to cardiac surgery [62]; however the precise mechanism of action is unknown [63]. The sodium-calcium-potassium channel blockade causes an increase in the duration of the action potential and the refractory period in the cardiac tissue. As a result, hypotension, bradycardia, and QT prolongation can be significant, especially in patients with congestive heart failure and left ventricular dysfunction [52]. Other side effects seen with prolonged oral use include hypo- or hyperthyroidism, hepatic and neurotoxicity, and prolongation of warfarin half-life [63]. However, pulmonary toxicity remains the main concern of amiodarone therapy after lung resection [40, 56]. It can occur at lower dosages and can manifest as chronic interstitial pneumonitis, bronchiolitis obliterans,

adult respiratory distress syndrome (ARDS), or a solitary lung mass [52]. In a very small prospective randomized study, Van Mieghem et al. [64] examined the role of amiodarone prophylaxis on POAF after lung resection. When compared to verapamil, there was no difference in the rate of POAF at the interim analysis. However the study was stopped prematurely due to an increased incidence of ARDS in the amiodarone group, which was 7.4% in the patients who had a right pneumonectomy versus 1.6% for other types of lung resections. This was associated with higher mortality rates and occurred despite using standard intravenous regimens and having therapeutic plasma concentrations. Two mechanisms were proposed: an indirect one, by increasing inflammatory mediators, and a direct one, by causing direct damage to the cells and subsequent fibrosis. Independently from the etiology, their recommendation was to avoid amiodarone after lung resection. By surgically decreasing the amount of lung parenchyma available, standard doses of amiodarone can account for higher pulmonary concentrations of the drug which may reach toxic levels. These results were not confirmed by later studies, when amiodarone was used for a short time period [28]. Tisdale et al. [65] randomized 130 patients undergoing anatomical lung resection, demonstrating a decreased incidence of AF in the amiodarone group (13.8% versus 32.3% in the control), with no difference in respiratory or cardiac complications. The lack of double blinding and the selection bias represented by a high rate of exclusion of cases of intraoperative AF were the main limitations for this study. Riber et al. [66] confirmed these results in a similar patient population. Amiodarone significantly decreased the incidence of POAF, with a good rate control and lack of symptoms in patients who developed POAF while receiving the medication. Overall, amiodarone and diltiazem seem to have similar efficacy in preventing POAF after major lung resection [28]. The main indication for amiodarone use still remains as a second-tier drug for POAF refractory to rate control drugs or as a therapeutic agent for POAF coupled with preexcitation conduction abnormalities, such as Wolff-Parkinson-White syndrome [40]. Monitoring serum concentrations is not necessary; however it is recommended to maintain the total cumulative dose less than 2150 mg given over 48–72 h [40].

Prophylactic *digitalization* to prevent POAF is not recommended any longer since there are no proven benefits but potential side effects [67]. The main mechanism of action is by enhancing vagal stimulation at the atrioventricular node, thus decreasing ventricular response during atrial arrhythmias [57]. There is also an inhibition of the sympathetic response which is unrelated to the increase in cardiac output and a binding of the myocardial sodium-potassium ATPase channel, blocking its transport [68]. The increase in intracellular sodium and subsequent calcium concentrations promote cardiac contractility. Digoxin does not seem to restore normal sinus rhythm in patients with chronic atrial fibrillation, and as a single agent it does not adequately control the ventricular response unless given at very high doses [67] or when combined with β-blockers or calcium channel blockers [68]. Calcium channel blockers have demonstrated to have better results in preventing POAF with fewer side effects [25]. Superior results are seen when digoxin is used in patients with chronic atrial fibrillation and heart failure with systolic dysfunction [67]. The onset after intravenous administration of 0.5–0.75 mg bolus is between 30 min and 2 h. AF rate control is usually achieved with further doses of 0.25 mg iv every 2–6 h to a maximum of 1.25–1.75 mg [40]. Digitalis toxicity and the difficulty in assessing proper plasma levels remain the main limiting factors for its use [43]. However, no difference in mortality was reported when chronic digoxin was compared with beta-blocker or calcium channel blockers [69]. Digoxin should be avoided in patients with renal insufficiency, electrolyte disturbances (hypokalemia, hypomagnesemia, and hypercalcemia), acute coronary syndromes, and thyroid disorders.

Rhythm Control Medications

Sotalol is a class III antiarrhythmic medication with significant activity as a nonselective β-blocker and a potassium channel blocker. Potassium current blockade prolongs both the action potential and the QT interval, predisposing to ventricular dysrhythmias such as torsades de pointes [57]. This can occur at both therapeutic and toxic dosages [55]. Due to the renal excretion, its use is contraindicated in patients with a creatinine clearance less than 46 ml/min. As with other β-blockers, sotalol is effective in decreasing POAF but does not reduce hospital length of stay or postoperative morbidity. Bradycardia can be significant enough to warrant discontinuation [47]. According to the American College of Cardiology recommendations, sotalol may be harmful if used to pharmacologically cardiovert atrial fibrillation [40]. Unfortunately, most of the data on this medication come from the cardiac surgical population [53], with no studies in the noncardiac population [40].

Magnesium is indicated in case of hypomagnesemia. The data on the use of magnesium are mainly from the cardiac surgical literature and are conflicting. One randomized controlled study done in 200 patients undergoing cardiopulmonary bypass surgery showed a decreased incidence of POAF when magnesium sulfate was administered for prophylaxis [70]. However, several other trials in similar surgical populations have given conflicting results on the benefits of magnesium and POAF prophylaxis, with the only agreement to maintain magnesium levels within normal values [57]. Compared to β-blockers and amiodarone, magnesium is inferior in preventing POAF [71]. Except in patients with acute renal failure, magnesium has a relatively safe profile.

Statins (3-hydroxy-3-methylglutaryl coenzyme-A reductase inhibitors) have been shown to suppress electrical remodeling and prevent POAF in animal models [52]. They are powerful lipid lowering drugs highly effective in preventing coronary artery disease [40]. Studies conducted in hypercholesterolemic patients on statins undergoing coronary artery bypass grafting (CAGB) showed a decrease in postoperative major cardiac events [72]. This effect was potentiated by simultaneously taking β-blockers [73]. The main benefits of statins seem to occur when these drugs are started in the preoperative period. When administered 1 week prior to on pump CABG, they decreased the incidence of POAF, as well as hospital length stay [47, 73]. After major lung resection, patients already on statins prior to surgery showed a threefold decrease probability of developing POAF [74] and overall complications [75]. One possible explanation seems to be related to their anti-inflammatory or antioxidant mechanism. Observational studies conducted in patients undergoing major lung resection have reported an increase in C-reactive protein and interleukin 6 in the postoperative period [76]. Atorvastatin (40 mg PO) started 7 days prior to lung resection and continued for 7 postoperative days in statin-naïve patients undergoing elective anatomical lung resection was associated with a decrease in hospital complications [75].

Angiotensin-converting enzyme inhibitors (ACEIs) and angiotensin receptor blockers (ARBs) have been suggested to reduce the incidence of POAF in patients with coexisting heart failure and systolic left ventricular dysfunction, but not in cases associated with systemic hypertension [77]. They may also play a role in maintaining sinus rhythm after electrical cardioversion. The data in the literature has focused on the role of these drugs on the outcome in chronic AF patients. The prophylactic use of ACEIs/ARBs to prevent POAF remains quite controversial. Losartan prevented POAF better than metoprolol when used in the postoperative period after major lung resection (6% vs 12%) [39]. Inhibition of the renin-angiotensin-aldosterone system seems to attenuate left atrial dilatation and atrial fibrosis and contributes in slowing conduction in animal studies, all factors that can trigger and maintain reentry circuits. These effects seem to be potentiated in patients with chronic heart failure when β-blockers are added [47].

Novel Medications

N-Acetylcysteine has successfully been used to decrease POAF and all-cause mortality after cardiac surgery alone or in combination with other agents [78, 79]. The mechanism of action seems to be related to its antioxidant properties, by stimulating glutathione production. Inclusion of cysteine in the perfusate of isolated rat hearts has been shown to confer significant cardioprotection and improved preservation of ATP and glutathione [80]. Other proposed mechanisms include inhibition of the renin-angiotensin system and/or atrial remodeling [78]. There are no current studies in the literature on the role of NAC in thoracic noncardiac surgery.

Vernakalant is an atrial-selective sodium-potassium channel blocker approved for pharmacological cardioversion of recent onset AF. Vernakalant has a better conversion rates than amiodarone but similar to propafenone and flecainide with less side effects [81]. Its main advantage is the rapid onset (10–15 min) and the high success rate after one dose [81]. Hypotension, especially in patients with heart failure, bradycardia, QT prolongation, and torsade de pointes are the most common side effects. Vernakalant is not effective in cardioverting atrial flutter or AF lasting more than 7 days [81]. While it is approved for clinical use in Europe, it is still under FDA investigation in the USA.

Olprinone is a specific phosphodiesterase III inhibitor with inotropic and vasodilating effects, commonly used to treat heart failure. It is also a bronchodilator. When administered prophylactically in patients after lung resection [82], it decreased the incidence of POAF, lowering the BNP and WBC levels without affecting the hemodynamics. It is usually given as a continuous infusion for 1 day, with duration of action up to 7 days. Suggested mechanisms include pulmonary vasodilatation with unloading of the right ventricle, positive chronotropism, and inhibition of the inflammatory response. In the USA this medication is approved for research use only.

Human atrial natriuretic peptide is a peptide hormone synthesized by the atria and available as treatment option for heart failure. It inhibits the sympathetic nervous system and the renin-angiotensin-aldosterone axis, leading to cardioprotective effects. A prophylactic 3-day infusion has been associated with a decrease in POAF, WBC, and CRP but no significant changes in blood pressures in patients with COPD undergoing lung resection [83]. The effect seems to be lasting up to a month after the infusion is stopped. This medication is routinely used in Japan.

Role of Postoperative Chemical and Electrical Cardioversion

Chemical and electrical cardioversion: restoration of sinus rhythm is recommended in patients who have stable AF but are symptomatic, when the duration is longer than 24 h and when anticoagulation may cause postoperative bleeding [84]. Several medications are available for cardioversion, with the greatest success rate when started within 7 days from the onset [85]. Drugs commonly used for chemical cardioversion of POAF include flecainide, dofetilide, propafenone, and ibutilide [28]. Ibutilide is available in the iv form, and it has been shown to have modest success in converting acute AF after cardiac surgery. However, it is associated with polymorphic ventricular tachycardia in up to 2% of patients,

especially in the presence of electrolyte abnormality [85]. In the presence of QT prolongation, hypokalemia and low ejection fraction can trigger ventricular tachycardia. Single oral doses of flecainide (300 mg) or propafenone (600 mg) seem to be safe, cardioverting 91% and 76% of cases, respectively, within 8 h from the onset of AF. To be eligible for this class of medications, patients must be free from cardiac structural disease, such as left ventricular hypertrophy, mitral valve disease, coronary artery disease, or heart failure [86]. Potential side effects include ventricular tachycardia, heart failure, and conversion to atrial flutter with rapid ventricular response [85].

Electrical cardioversion is used to treat AF in case of hemodynamic instability, including symptomatic profound hypotension, myocardial ischemia or infarction, and/or heart failure [40]. The success rate is about 67–94% [52]. Biphasic DC cardioversion has higher success rates than monophasic, using a current around 100–200 J and in a synchronized mode. Higher energy can be used for patients with high body mass index, prolonged AF, or left atrial enlargement. Deep sedation is recommended. Bradycardia (more common in patients on antiarrhythmics prior to cardioversion), ventricular tachyarrhythmias (when the shock is applied during repolarization), hypotension, pulmonary edema (probably due to myocardial stunning), and embolism are all potential complications. Electrolytes should be checked and normalized before cardioversion. In case of digitalis toxicity and hypokalemia, cardioversion should be avoided due to the high incidence of ventricular fibrillation. In this setting, low currents and prophylactic lidocaine should be used. Pacing capabilities should be readily availbale, since bradycardia can be profound to the point of asystole [52]. If the duration of the AF is less than 48 h, cardioversion can be done prior to anticoagulation [40]. After the 48 h mark, anticoagulation is recommended if not contraindicated by the surgical procedure. Whether intravenous heparin should be started and then followed by a 4 weeks cycle of oral anticoagulants is unclear. Common practice is to start patients on oral anticoagulants such as warfarin or the novel anticoagulant drugs [10].

Acute Coronary Syndrome

Myocardial ischemia may occur transiently after lung resection and present as an electrocardiographic finding in 3.8% of patients, while infarction can occur in 0.2–0.9% of the cases [29, 87–89]. The diagnosis of symptomatic perioperative myocardial infarct is associated with a 30–50% risk of death [90]. The incidence increases in the presence of preoperative coronary artery disease and abnormal exercise testing. Patients are at the highest risk during the first 3 postoperative days, when a high degree of monitoring is suggested.

Nonspecific diffuse ST segment changes may be present after intrapericardial resection due to direct mechanical injury [91]. Mediastinal shift can also cause dynamic EKG abnormalities in the postoperative period. An increase in troponin may be observed in all these scenarios.

There are no definite recommendations for preoperative invasive testing or interventions. Most of the decision-making should be based on the clinical presentation [92]. In patients at high risk (such as the ones with unstable angina, uncompensated chronic heart failure, arrhythmias, and severe valvular disease), cardiac catheterization is highly recommended if followed by coronary artery revascularization, when necessary [53, 93]. Patients with and without pre-existing cardiac disease have a similar incidence of postoperative major adverse cardiac events (MACE) after thoracoscopic lung resection [94]. However the former have higher incidence of atrial fibrillation and 30-day postoperative mortality. Preoperative angina is associated with a higher incidence of postoperative adverse cardiac events (such as MI or cardiac arrest) [95]. According to the latest AHA-ACC recommendations [90], if the risk of reinfarction is high for at least 2 months after an MI, CABG but not percutaneous coronary intervention (PCI) may decrease that risk. If patients require revascularization, elective surgery needs to be postponed, with the dilemma of how long to wait, as in the case of cancer where there is potential disease progression [96]. Cardiac stents, especially drug-eluting ones, represent a significant problem due to the prolonged need for anticoagulation. Stopping dual antiplatelet therapy (aspirin and clopidogrel) is associated with a high risk of stent thrombosis, while continuing it leads to an increased risk of intra and postoperative bleeding and precludes regional anesthetic techniques [97]. The duration of the anticoagulation is usually based upon the type of stent: bare-metal stents commonly require 4–6 weeks, while in the presence of drug-eluting stent 12 months are recommended for elective procedures and 6 for urgent cases [90]. The risk of stent thrombosis is higher for drug-eluting stents, especially if the stent is long, at a bifurcation, if the revascularization is incomplete, or if the patient has history of diabetes or heart failure [98]. A non-randomized observational prospective study done in noncardiac surgery patients who had cardiac stents placed within a year from surgery found a 44.7% rate of postoperative cardiac complications and a 4.7% mortality rate [99]. Dual antiplatelet therapy was stopped on average 3 days prior to surgery and substituted with intravenous unfractionated heparin or subcutaneous enoxaparin. Most of the complications occurred within the first 35 days from the stent placement and were cardiac in nature. Bleeding was not a significant variable. This data was not confirmed by another small prospective observational study done in 16 patients undergoing major lung resection 4 weeks after coronary angioplasty or PCI [100]. Dual antiplatelet therapy was given

for 4 weeks and interrupted 5 days prior to surgery when it was bridged with low molecular weight heparin. No MI or deaths were reported. Despite the absence of randomization, these studies stress several important points. Once the antiplatelet treatment is stopped, low molecular weight heparin should be used (heparin alone is insufficient); all non-life-saving procedures should be postponed at least for 6–12 weeks from the stent placement, and aspirin should be continued up to the day of surgery [101, 102]. The protective effects against MACE in the immediate postoperative period outweigh the lower risk of postoperative bleeding [101]. Prophylactic revascularization (CABG versus PCI) does not seem to add further benefits over optimal medical treatment in patients with cardiac risk undergoing elective major vascular surgery [90, 96]. Long-term survival as well as myocardial infarction, death, and hospital length of stay seems to be unchanged. However, CABG is associated with less postoperative myocardial infarctions and decreased hospital length of stay when compared to PCI, probably because of better revascularization [103]. According to the American College of Cardiology, revascularization should be reserved for patients with unstable angina or advanced coronary artery disease [90]. If revascularization is needed before surgery, bare-metal stents [90] or balloon angioplasty [102] are the preferred options due to their lower risk of thrombosis. In both cases, elective surgery needs to be appropriately delayed to prevent graft or stent thrombosis.

Heart Failure and Cardiac Herniation

Heart failure can occur after major lung resection as a result of right- or left-sided dysfunction. *Right heart failure* can result from changes either in contractility or afterload. Unfortunately, most of the studies investigating the changes in right ventricular function after lung resection are small and found minor and transient differences when compared to the preoperative period. In the first 2 postoperative days, there is a reversible increase in right ventricular end-diastolic volume [53], as well as a mild increase in pulmonary arterial pressures and pulmonary vascular resistance [104]. While postoperative changes in pulmonary arterial pressures, central venous pressures, and pulmonary vascular resistance seem to be subtle at rest, they may become significant during exercise. Changes in right ventricular function are usually able to compensate at rest, but they may fail during exercise, leading to pulmonary hypertension [53]. When transthoracic echocardiography has been used to evaluate right ventricular function after pneumonectomy, it has shown only a mild increase in pulmonary arterial pressure which is not associated with ventricular dysfunction [26]. Other possible causes of right ventricular failure, although rare, include pulmonary embolism and cardiac herniation. *Left side heart failure* is usually a consequence of right heart dysfunction, either by decreasing left ventricular preload or shifting the interventricular septum [3, 53]. Acute ischemia and valvular disease may also be contributing factors. *Cardiac herniation*, a rare complication after pneumonectomy, may be responsible for both right and left heart failure. It occurs more commonly after intrapericardial pneumonectomy, right more than left, and leads to a 50% mortality rate [53]. Herniation can be secondary to an incomplete surgical closure of the pericardium or the breakdown of a pericardial patch [105]. One main contributing factor includes an increase in intrathoracic pressure, such as with coughing or sudden increase in peak airway pressures during mechanical ventilation [29]. Changes in position, with the operative side being dependent, positive pressure ventilation, rapid lung re-expansion, or suction on the chest tube are all other possible causes. Symptoms depend on the side of the herniation. Right-sided cases present with superior vena cava syndrome, due to kinking of the superior vena cava and decreased right ventricular filling, with subsequent hypotension, tachycardia, and shock. Left-sided cases present with arrhythmias and ischemia, causing myocardial infarction, hypotension, and ventricular fibrillation if left untreated [106]. This appears to be related to less cardiac rotation, with subsequent pericardial compression on the myocardium. Clinical presentation and electrocardiographic findings are fairly nonspecific in suggesting the diagnosis, stressing the role of chest radiography and a high index of suspicion. Treatment is surgical, with repositioning of the heart and placement of a patch. In order to minimize hemodynamic instability, the patient should be kept on the lateral decubitus with the operative side up [105].

Mediastinal Shift and Post-pneumonectomy Syndrome

Mediastinal shift can occur intraoperatively or in the postoperative period as a result of changes in the post-pneumonectomy space. At the end of surgery, once the chest is closed, some surgeons evacuate the air and fluid that fill the empty space aiming to bring the mediastinum back to midline. Excessive fluid drainage can lead to ipsilateral mediastinal shift and contralateral lung expansion, with decreased venous return and significant hypotension [107]. Rapid accumulation of fluid in the pneumonectomy space (such as hemo- or chylothorax) can cause contralateral shift, with secondary compression of the remaining lung [29]. A high index of clinical suspicion, careful monitoring of the hemodynamics, and communication with the surgical team are needed to prevent hemodynamic collapse. When excessive fluid accumulates in this space, contralateral mediastinal shift occurs, leading to compression of the remaining lung

and secondary respiratory insufficiency. This is seen more often in the postoperative period, and the use of intracavitary pressures monitoring can guide the drainage of the excess fluid if needed [107]. CT scan studies have shown obliteration of the post-pneumonectomy space with fluid over time, elevation of the hemidiaphragm, and expansion of the contralateral lung [108]. In case of extreme mediastinal shift, dynamic compression of the distal airway can occur, leading to the so-called post-pneumonectomy syndrome [29, 109, 110]. This is a rare and late complication, which can occur at a median of 7 years from surgery. It is more common in females and children and with right-sided procedures (even though it has been described for left cases as well) [111]. It manifests with decreased exercise tolerance, exertional respiratory insufficiency, stridor, and recurrent infections. Respiratory symptoms are caused by dynamic compression of the distal trachea and left mainstem bronchus against the spinal column and the left pulmonary artery, secondary to the severe mediastinal shift to the right. Treatment involves the use of airway stents as a temporary measure or thoracotomy and repositioning of the mediastinum via Lucite plastic balls, Silastic implants, or saline-filled prosthesis [111] (see also Chap. 41). In the rare event of *cardiac arrest* (3–7%), close chest compression is ineffective [29]. As a result of the mediastinal shift, the heart cannot be compressed between the sternum and the vertebral bodies, requiring an emergency thoracotomy and open cardiac massage. In the case of intrapericardial dissection, chest compression can cause cardiac herniation.

Conclusion

In the last few decades, a significant improvement in the surgical and anesthetic techniques has made pneumonectomy and anatomical lung resection safer. The introduction of enhanced recovery pathways, minimally invasive surgical techniques, the use of short-acting anesthetics, and a multimodal analgesic approach have all contributed to decrease the incidence of postoperative complications. Fast-track strategies and careful selection of patients undergoing lung resection procedures have also played an important role in postoperative and long-term outcome. Better utilization of step down and acute postoperative care units have decreased the rate of ICU admissions, saving costs. Since the average age of patients requiring lung resection is increasing, anesthesiologists and surgeons will be facing more complex cases, due to the presence of multiple comorbidities. Careful preoperative workup customizing the type of surgery as well as planning for in-hospital and post discharge rehabilitation options will prove to be essential for decreasing even further the possible complications and improving the overall care.

Clinical Case Discussion

A 65-year-old-man with squamous cell cancer of the right upper lobe underwent a right intrapericardial pneumonectomy. Surgery was 150 min and uneventful. Estimated blood loss was 700 cc, and 700 cc of ringer's lactate was used during the case. Urinary output was 100 cc. The patient was extubated in the operating room at the end of the case. A thoracic epidural was used intraoperatively, and the patient was comfortable in PACU. As part of the postoperative blood work, troponin levels were checked, and the first set was 1.66 (1.07 and 0.52 the second and the third one). ST segment elevations transiently occurred on POD 1 in correspondence to a fourth troponin of 1.55.

On POD 2, subcutaneous emphysema was noted on the right chest wall, neck, and eye. While walking, he had an episode of desaturation and tachycardia. Chest X-ray is shown (see Fig. 56.1). Electrocardiogram showed rapid SVT, with hypotension (HR = 128, BP = 88/45). The patient was transferred to the ICU where he was intubated. He slowly became hemodynamically unstable, requiring multiple pressors.

Questions

What are common cardiac complications after lung resection?

1. Arrhythmias (atrial fibrillation, atrial flutter, and supraventricular tachycardia (SVT))
2. Ischemia and acute coronary syndrome
3. Heart failure and cardiac herniation
4. Mediastinal shift and post-pneumonectomy syndrome

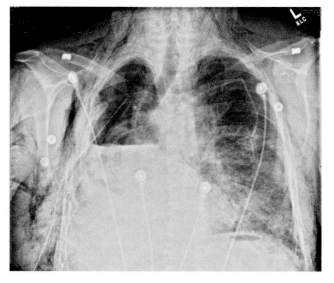

Fig. 56.1 Radiographic changes on postoperative day 2

Specifically

1. *Arrhythmias*: Who is at risk (suggested pathophysiology, role of WBC and inflammatory response, BNP levels)? What we can do to prevent it (rate or rhythm control? Preoperative medications?)? How do we treat postoperatively (medications vs cardioversion)? Risks/side effects of the treatment.
2. *Acute coronary syndrome*: What are known risk factors? Is preoperative stenting better than medical treatment in a patient with a positive stress test? What is the treatment? How does it affect mortality?
3. *Cardiomegaly/ cardiac failure*: Who is at risk (role of the extent of dissection, preoperative risk factors)? How does it affect mortality?
4. *Mediastinal shift*: Why does this happen (extent of dissection)? How common is cardiac herniation? What is the pathophysiology and the diagnosis?

Back to the Case

The intraoperative course was uneventful, despite a more extensive procedure than scheduled. The patient suffered transient ischemia in the PACU (ST changes on EKG and elevated troponin) that was managed medically and resolved. On POD 2, he had both respiratory and hemodynamic symptoms while ambulating.

The CXR at that time showed massive subcutaneous emphysema on the side of surgery, extending to the neck; a post-pneumonectomy cavity filled with fluid and a mediastinal shift toward the operative side; and an opacification of the left lung base. These are all surgical complications that may not be easily preventable, despite a high degree of alertness and aggressive postoperative physical therapy and pulmonary toileting.

In most cases isolated cardiac complications after pneumonectomy can be successfully treated with medications or invasive procedures. Respiratory complications are more difficult to prevent and manage, especially if the onset is quick. In this case scenario, hypoxemia developed very quickly and was so severe to require reintubation and transfer to the ICU for further care. A repeat CXR (Fig. 56.2) after intubation shows a significant worsening of the left base opacification. Ideally treatment should follow a diagnosis. However, in practice, patients may be clinically too unstable for transport to the imaging suite. Supportive measures become the mainstay of therapy. In this case, the need for vasopressor continued to increase and the degree of hypoxia to worsen. The patient suffered a secondary cardiac arrest and expired on POD 2.

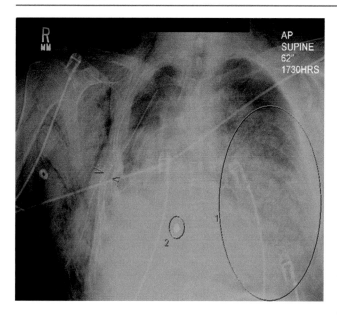

Fig. 56.2 Worsening of the left base opacification

References

1. Harjola VP, et al. Contemporary management of acute right ventricular failure: a statement from the Heart Failure Association and the Working Group on Pulmonary Circulation and Right Ventricular Function of the European Society of Cardiology. Eur J Heart Fail. 2016;18(3):226–41.

2. Ho SY, Nihoyannopoulos P. Anatomy, echocardiography, and normal right ventricular dimensions. Heart. 2006;92(Suppl 1):i2–13.

3. Gordon C, Collard CD, Pan W. Intraoperative management of pulmonary hypertension and associated right heart failure. Curr Opin Anaesthesiol. 2010;23(1):49–56.

4. Szabo G, et al. Adaptation of the right ventricle to an increased afterload in the chronically volume overloaded heart. Ann Thorac Surg. 2006;82(3):989–95.

5. Bartels K, et al. Update on perioperative right heart assessment using transesophageal echocardiography. Semin Cardiothorac Vasc Anesth. 2014;18(4):341–51.

6. Haddad F, et al. Right ventricular function in cardiovascular disease, part II: pathophysiology, clinical importance, and management of right ventricular failure. Circulation. 2008;117(13):1717–31.

7. Pedoto A, Amar D. Right heart function in thoracic surgery: role of echocardiography. Curr Opin Anaesthesiol. 2009;22(1):44–9.

8. Heerdt PM, Malhotra J. The right ventricular response to lung resection. In: Slinger PD, editor. Progress in thoracic anesthesiology. Baltimore: Lippincott Williams & Wilkins; 2004. p. 221–46.

9. Xu WY, et al. Effects of sevoflurane and propofol on right ventricular function and pulmonary circulation in patients undergone esophagectomy. Int J Clin Exp Pathol. 2014;7(1):272–9.

10. Kowalewski J, et al. Right ventricular morphology and function after pulmonary resection. Eur J Cardiothorac Surg. 1999;15(4):444–8.

11. Katz WE, et al. Immediate effects of lung transplantation on right ventricular morphology and function in patients with variable degrees of pulmonary hypertension. J Am Coll Cardiol. 1996;27(2):384–91.

12. Sugarbaker DJ, Haywood-Watson RJ, Wald O. Pneumonectomy for non–small cell lung cancer. Surg Oncol Clin N Am. 2016;25(3):533–51.

13. Marik PE. Obituary: pulmonary artery catheter 1970 to 2013. Ann Intensive Care. 2013;3(1):38.

14. Ashes C, Roscoe A. Transesophageal echocardiography in thoracic anesthesia: pulmonary hypertension and right ventricular function. Curr Opin Anesthesiol. 2015;28(1):38–44.

15. Tan CO, Harley I. Perioperative transesophageal echocardiographic assessment of the right heart and associated structures: a comprehensive update and technical report. J Cardiothorac Vasc Anesth. 2014;28(4):1100–21.

16. Slinger PD, Johnston MR. Preoperative assessment: an anesthesiologist's perspective. Thorac Surg Clin. 2005;15(1):11–25.

17. Rauch M, et al. Cardiovascular computed tomography findings after pneumonectomy: comparison to lobectomy. Acad Radiol. 2017;24(7):860–6.

18. D'Ascenzi F, et al. Right ventricular remodelling induced by exercise training in competitive athletes. Eur Heart J Cardiovasc Imaging. 2016;17(3):301–7.

19. Tam K, Daly M, Kelly K. Treatment of locally advanced non–small cell lung cancer. Hematol Oncol Clin North Am. 2017;31(1):45–57.

20. Pedoto A, Heerdt PM. Postoperative care after pulmonary resection: postanesthesia care unit versus intensive care unit. Curr Opin Anaesthesiol. 2009;22(1):50–5.

21. Galiè N, et al. 2015 ESC/ERS guidelines for the diagnosis and treatment of pulmonary hypertension the joint task force for the diagnosis and treatment of pulmonary hypertension of the European Society of Cardiology (ESC) and the European Respiratory Society (ERS): endorsed by: Association for European Paediatric and Congenital Cardiology (AEPC), International Society for Heart and Lung Transplantation (ISHLT). Eur Heart J. 2016;37(1):67–119.

22. Zangiabadi A, De Pasquale CG, Sajkov D. Pulmonary hypertension and right heart dysfunction in chronic lung disease. Biomed Res Int. 2014;2014:739674.

23. Venuta F, et al. Long-term Doppler echocardiographic evaluation of the right heart after major lung resections. Eur J Cardiothorac Surg. 2007;32(5):787–90.

24. Foroulis CN, et al. Study on the late effect of pneumonectomy on right heart pressures using Doppler echocardiography. Eur J Cardiothorac Surg. 2004;26(3):508–14.

25. Amar D, et al. Effects of diltiazem versus digoxin on dysrhythmias and cardiac function after pneumonectomy. Ann Thorac Surg. 1997;63(5):1374–81; discussion 1381–2.

26. Amar D, et al. Value of perioperative Doppler echocardiography in patients undergoing major lung resection. Ann Thorac Surg. 1996;61(2):516–20.

27. Smulders SA, et al. Cardiac function and position more than 5 years after pneumonectomy. Ann Thorac Surg. 2007;83(6):1986–92.

28. Amar D. Prevention and management of perioperative arrhythmias in the thoracic surgical population. Anesthesiol Clin. 2008;26(2):325–35, vii.

29. Groth SS, Burt BM, Sugarbaker DJ. Management of complications after pneumonectomy. Thorac Surg Clin. 2015;25(3):335–48.

30. Roselli EE, et al. Atrial fibrillation complicating lung cancer resection. J Thorac Cardiovasc Surg. 2005;130(2):438–44.

31. Dancewicz M, Kowalewski J, Peplinski J. Factors associated with perioperative complications after pneumonectomy for primary carcinoma of the lung. Interact Cardiovasc Thorac Surg. 2006;5(2):97–100.

32. Amar D, et al. Leukocytosis and increased risk of atrial fibrillation after general thoracic surgery. Ann Thorac Surg. 2006;82(3):1057–61.

33. Cardinale D, et al. Increased perioperative N-terminal pro-B-type natriuretic peptide levels predict atrial fibrillation after thoracic surgery for lung cancer. Circulation. 2007;115(11):1339–44.

34. Nojiri T, et al. Predictive value of B-type natriuretic peptide for postoperative atrial fibrillation following pulmonary resection for lung cancer. Eur J Cardiothorac Surg. 2010;37(4):787–91.

35. Amar D, et al. Brain natriuretic peptide and risk of atrial fibrillation after thoracic surgery. J Thorac Cardiovasc Surg. 2012;144(5):1249–53.

36. Iwata T, et al. Risk factors predictive of atrial fibrillation after lung cancer surgery. Surg Today. 2016;46(8):877–86.

37. Brecher O, et al. Preoperative echocardiographic indices of diastolic dysfunction and brain natriuretic peptide in predicting postoperative atrial fibrillation after noncardiac surgery. Anesth Analg. 2017;124(4):1099–104.

38. Amar D. Postoperative atrial fibrillation: is there a need for prevention? J Thorac Cardiovasc Surg. 2016;151(4):913–5.

39. Cardinale D, et al. Prevention of atrial fibrillation in high-risk patients undergoing lung cancer surgery: the PRESAGE trial. Ann Surg. 2016;264(2):244–51.

40. Frendl G, et al. 2014 AATS guidelines for the prevention and management of perioperative atrial fibrillation and flutter for thoracic surgical procedures. Executive summary. J Thorac Cardiovasc Surg. 2014;148(3):772–91.

41. Riber LP, Larsen TB, Christensen TD. Postoperative atrial fibrillation prophylaxis after lung surgery: systematic review and meta-analysis. Ann Thorac Surg. 2014;98(6):1989–97.

42. Vaporciyan AA, et al. Risk factors associated with atrial fibrillation after noncardiac thoracic surgery: analysis of 2588 patients. J Thorac Cardiovasc Surg. 2004;127(3):779–86.

43. Foroulis CN, et al. Factors associated with cardiac rhythm disturbances in the early post-pneumonectomy period: a study on 259 pneumonectomies. Eur J Cardiothorac Surg. 2003;23(3):384–9.

44. Bobbio A, et al. Postoperative outcome of patients undergoing lung resection presenting with new-onset atrial fibrillation managed by amiodarone or diltiazem. Eur J Cardiothorac Surg. 2007;31(1):70–4.

45. Haverkamp WW. Post-thoracotomy dysrhythmia. Curr Opin Anaesthesiol. 2016;29(1):26–33.

46. Amar D, Zhang H, Roistacher N. The incidence and outcome of ventricular arrhythmias after noncardiac thoracic surgery. Anesth Analg. 2002;95(3):537–43, table of contents.

47. Mayson SE, et al. The changing face of postoperative atrial fibrillation prevention: a review of current medical therapy. Cardiol Rev. 2007;15(5):231–41.

48. Gialdini G, et al. Perioperative atrial fibrillation and the long-term risk of ischemic stroke. JAMA. 2014;312(6):616–22.

49. Wijeysundera DN, et al. Perioperative Beta blockade in noncardiac surgery: a systematic review for the 2014 ACC/AHA guideline on perioperative cardiovascular evaluation and management of patients undergoing noncardiac surgery. Circulation. 2014;130:1–37.

50. Amar D. Post-thoracotomy atrial fibrillation. Curr Opin Anesthesiol. 2007;20(1):43.

51. Ahn HJ, et al. Thoracic epidural anesthesia does not improve the incidence of arrhythmias after transthoracic esophagectomy. Eur J Cardiothorac Surg. 2005;28(1):19–21.

52. Crawford TC, Oral H. Cardiac arrhythmias: management of atrial fibrillation in the critically ill patient. Crit Care Clin. 2007;23(4):855–72. vii

53. Karamichalis JM, Putnam JB Jr, Lambright ES. Cardiovascular complications after lung surgery. Thorac Surg Clin. 2006;16(3):253–60.

54. Ivanovic J, et al. Incidence, severity and perioperative risk factors for atrial fibrillation following pulmonary resection. Interact Cardiovasc Thorac Surg. 2014;18(3):340–6.

55. DeWitt CR, Waksman JC. Pharmacology, pathophysiology and management of calcium channel blocker and beta-blocker toxicity. Toxicol Rev. 2004;23(4):223–38.

56. Sedrakyan A, et al. Pharmacologic prophylaxis for postoperative atrial tachyarrhythmia in general thoracic surgery: evidence from randomized clinical trials. J Thorac Cardiovasc Surg. 2005;129(5):997–1005.

57. Bradley D, et al. Pharmacologic prophylaxis: American College of Chest Physicians guidelines for the prevention and management of postoperative atrial fibrillation after cardiac surgery. Chest. 2005;128(2 Suppl):39S–47S.

58. Connolly SJ, et al. Double-blind, placebo-controlled, randomized trial of prophylactic metoprolol for reduction of hospital length of stay after heart surgery: the Beta-Blocker Length of Stay (BLOS) study. Am Heart J. 2003;145(2):226–32.

59. Group, P.S., et al. Effects of extended-release metoprolol succinate in patients undergoing non-cardiac surgery (POISE trial): a randomised controlled trial. Lancet. 2008;371(9627):1839–47.

60. Fleisher LA, Poldermans D. Perioperative beta blockade: where do we go from here? Lancet. 2008;371(9627):1813–4.

61. Amar D, et al. Effects of diltiazem prophylaxis on the incidence and clinical outcome of atrial arrhythmias after thoracic surgery. J Thorac Cardiovasc Surg. 2000;120(4):790–8.

62. Mitchell LB, et al. Prophylactic oral amiodarone for the prevention of arrhythmias that begin early after revascularization, valve replacement, or repair: PAPABEAR: a randomized controlled trial. JAMA. 2005;294(24):3093–100.

63. Zimetbaum P. Amiodarone for atrial fibrillation. N Engl J Med. 2007;356(9):935–41.

64. Van Mieghem W, et al. Amiodarone and the development of ARDS after lung surgery. Chest. 1994;105(6):1642–5.

65. Tisdale JE, et al. A randomized trial evaluating amiodarone for prevention of atrial fibrillation after pulmonary resection. Ann Thorac Surg. 2009;88(3):886–93; discussion 894–5.

66. Riber LP, et al. Amiodarone significantly decreases atrial fibrillation in patients undergoing surgery for lung cancer. Ann Thorac Surg. 2012;94(2):339–44; discussion 345–6.

67. Tamargo J, Delpon E, Caballero R. The safety of digoxin as a pharmacological treatment of atrial fibrillation. Expert Opin Drug Saf. 2006;5(3):453–67.

68. Gheorghiade M, Adams KF Jr, Colucci WS. Digoxin in the management of cardiovascular disorders. Circulation. 2004;109(24):2959–64.

69. Gheorghiade M, et al. Lack of evidence of increased mortality among patients with atrial fibrillation taking digoxin: findings from post hoc propensity-matched analysis of the AFFIRM trial. Eur Heart J. 2013;34(20):1489–97.

70. Toraman F, et al. Magnesium infusion dramatically decreases the incidence of atrial fibrillation after coronary artery bypass grafting. Ann Thorac Surg. 2001;72(4):1256–61; discussion 1261–2.

71. Zhao B-C, et al. Prophylaxis against atrial fibrillation after general thoracic surgery: trial sequential analysis and network meta-analysis. Chest. 2017;151(1):149–59.

72. Thielmann M, et al. Lipid-lowering effect of preoperative statin therapy on postoperative major adverse cardiac events after coronary artery bypass surgery. J Thorac Cardiovasc Surg. 2007;134(5):1143–9.

73. Patti G, et al. Randomized trial of atorvastatin for reduction of postoperative atrial fibrillation in patients undergoing cardiac surgery: results of the ARMYDA-3 (Atorvastatin for Reduction of MYocardial Dysrhythmia After cardiac surgery) study. Circulation. 2006;114(14):1455–61.

74. Amar D, et al. Statin use is associated with a reduction in atrial fibrillation after noncardiac thoracic surgery independent of C-reactive protein. Chest. 2005;128(5):3421–7.

75. Amar D, et al. Beneficial effects of perioperative statins for major pulmonary resection. J Thorac Cardiovasc Surg. 2015;149(6):1532–8.

76. Amar D, et al. Inflammation and outcome after general thoracic surgery. Eur J Cardiothorac Surg. 2007;32(3):431–4.

77. Healey JS, et al. Prevention of atrial fibrillation with angiotensin-converting enzyme inhibitors and angiotensin receptor blockers: a meta-analysis. J Am Coll Cardiol. 2005;45(11):1832–9.

78. Liu XH, Xu CY, Fan GH. Efficacy of N-acetylcysteine in preventing atrial fibrillation after cardiac surgery: a meta-analysis of published randomized controlled trials. BMC Cardiovasc Disord. 2014;14:52.

79. Ozaydin M, et al. Metoprolol vs. carvedilol or carvedilol plus N-acetyl cysteine on post-operative atrial fibrillation: a randomized, double-blind, placebo-controlled study. Eur Heart J. 2013;34(8):597–604.

80. Shackebaei D, et al. Mechanisms underlying the cardioprotective effect of L-cysteine. Mol Cell Biochem. 2005;277(1–2):27–31.

81. Savelieva I, Graydon R, Camm AJ. Pharmacological cardioversion of atrial fibrillation with vernakalant: evidence in support of the ESC guidelines. Europace. 2014;16(2):162–73.

82. Nojiri T, et al. A double-blind placebo-controlled study of the effects of olprinone, a specific phosphodiesterase III inhibitor, for preventing postoperative atrial fibrillation in patients undergoing pulmonary resection for lung cancer. Chest. 2015;148(5):1285–92.

83. Nojiri T, et al. Low-dose human atrial natriuretic peptide for the prevention of postoperative cardiopulmonary complications in chronic obstructive pulmonary disease patients undergoing lung cancer surgery. Eur J Cardiothorac Surg. 2013;44(1):98–103.

84. Lomivorotov VV, et al. New-onset atrial fibrillation after cardiac surgery: pathophysiology, prophylaxis, and treatment. J Cardiothorac Vasc Anesth. 2016;30(1):200–16.

85. January CT. AHA/ACC/HRS guideline for the management of patients with atrial fibrillation: a report of the American College of Cardiology/American Heart Association Task Force on practice guidelines and the Heart Rhythm Society. Circulation (New York, NY). 2014;130(23):e199–267.

86. Amar D. Postthoracotomy atrial fibrillation. Curr Opin Anaesthesiol. 2007;20(1):43–7.

87. Martin J, et al. Morbidity and mortality after neoadjuvant therapy for lung cancer: the risks of right pneumonectomy. Ann Thorac Surg. 2001;72(4):1149–54.

88. Boffa DJ, et al. Data from The Society of Thoracic Surgeons General Thoracic Surgery database: the surgical management of primary lung tumors. J Thorac Cardiovasc Surg. 2008;135(2):247–54.

89. Allen MS, et al. Morbidity and mortality of major pulmonary resections in patients with early-stage lung cancer: initial results of the randomized, prospective ACOSOG Z0030 trial. Ann Thorac Surg. 2006;81(3):1013–9; discussion 1019–20.

90. Fleisher LA. ACC/AHA guideline on perioperative cardiovascular evaluation and management of patients undergoing non cardiac surgery: a report of the American College of Cardiology/American Heart Association Task Force on Practice Guidelines. Circulation (New York, NY). 2014;130(24):e278–333.

91. Vasic N, et al. Acute "Pseudoischemic" ECG abnormalities after right pneumonectomy. Case Rep Surg. 2017;2017:4.

92. Jaroszewski DE, et al. Utility of detailed preoperative cardiac testing and incidence of post-thoracotomy myocardial infarction. J Thorac Cardiovasc Surg. 2008;135(3):648–55.

93. Kristensen SD, et al. 2014 ESC/ESA guidelines on non-cardiac surgery: cardiovascular assessment and management: the Joint Task Force on non-cardiac surgery: cardiovascular assessment and management of the European Society of Cardiology (ESC) and the European Society of Anaesthesiology (ESA). Eur Heart J. 2014;35(35):2383–431.

94. Sandri A, et al. Coronary artery disease is associated with an increased mortality rate following video-assisted thoracoscopic lobectomy. J Thorac Cardiovasc Surg. 2017;154(1):352–7.

95. Pandey A, et al. Effect of preoperative angina pectoris on cardiac outcomes in patients with previous myocardial infarction undergoing major noncardiac surgery (Data from ACS-NSQIP). Am J Cardiol. 2015;115(8):1080–4.

96. McFalls EO, et al. Coronary-artery revascularization before elective major vascular surgery. N Engl J Med. 2004;351(27):2795–804.

97. Spahn DR, et al. Coronary stents and perioperative anti-platelet regimen: dilemma of bleeding and stent thrombosis. Br J Anaesth. 2006;96(6):675–7.

98. Albaladejo P, et al. Perioperative management of antiplatelet agents in patients with coronary stents: recommendations of a French Task Force. Br J Anaesth. 2006;97(4):580–2.

99. Vicenzi MN, et al. Coronary artery stenting and non-cardiac surgery--a prospective outcome study. Br J Anaesth. 2006;96(6):686–93.

100. Voltolini L, et al. Lung resection for non-small cell lung cancer after prophylactic coronary angioplasty and stenting: short- and long-term results. Minerva Chir. 2012;67(1):77–85.

101. Oscarsson A, et al. To continue or discontinue aspirin in the perioperative period: a randomized, controlled clinical trial. BJA: Br J Anaesth. 2010;104(3):305–12.

102. Banerjee S, et al. Use of antiplatelet therapy/DAPT for post-PCI patients undergoing noncardiac surgery. J Am Coll Cardiol. 2017;69(14):1861–70.

103. Ward HB, et al. Coronary artery bypass grafting is superior to percutaneous coronary intervention in prevention of perioperative myocardial infarctions during subsequent vascular surgery. Ann Thorac Surg. 2006;82(3):795–800; discussion 800–1.

104. Reed CE, Spinale FG, Crawford FA Jr. Effect of pulmonary resection on right ventricular function. Ann Thorac Surg. 1992;53(4):578–82.

105. Slinger P. Update on anesthetic management for pneumonectomy. Curr Opin Anaesthesiol. 2009;22(1):31–7.

106. Mehanna MJ, et al. Cardiac herniation after right pneumonectomy: case report and review of the literature. J Thorac Imaging. 2007;22(3):280–2.

107. Wolf AS, et al. Managing the pneumonectomy space after extrapleural pneumonectomy: postoperative intrathoracic pressure monitoring. Eur J Cardiothorac Surg. 2010;37(4):770–5.

108. Biondetti PR, et al. Evaluation of post-pneumonectomy space by computed tomography. J Comput Assist Tomogr. 1982;6(2):238–42.

109. Bedard EL, Uy K, Keshavjee S. Postpneumonectomy syndrome: a spectrum of clinical presentations. Ann Thorac Surg. 2007;83(3):1185–8.

110. Shen KR, et al. Postpneumonectomy syndrome: surgical management and long-term results. J Thorac Cardiovasc Surg. 2008;135(6):1210–6; discussion 1216–9.

111. Jung JJ, et al. Management of post-pneumonectomy syndrome using tissue expanders. Thorac Cancer. 2016;7(1):88–93.

Post-thoracic Surgery Patient Management and Complications

Jean Y. Perentes and Marc de Perrot

Key Points

- Chest drains can usually be removed postthoracotomy when the air leak has stopped and drainage is <400 mL/day.
- The majority of thoracic surgical patients are at high risk for postoperative venous thromboembolism.
- Postthoracotomy blood loss via the chest drains requires reexploration if it meets or exceeds 1 L in 1 h or 200 mL/h for 2 h.
- The risk of post-thoracic surgery hemorrhage is increased in patients with a previous thoracotomy, following decortication or surgery for infectious causes.
- Lobar torsion most often occurs in the right middle lobe following a right upper lobectomy.

General Principles of Postoperative Care

In thoracic surgery, perhaps more than in any other surgical field, "an ounce of prevention is worth a pound of cure." To obtain best results in perioperative care after pulmonary pro-

cedures, this care begins before the procedure and does not end until long after the patient leaves the hospital.

Preoperative Preparation

Preoperative Teaching

To achieve the best participation in a patient's postoperative care, the patient and family should be as fully informed as possible. When both patient and family know what to expect, they are better prepared to deal with the problems as they arise. The surgeon should have frank and open discussions with the patient and family concerning the anticipated outcome and expected postoperative problems, along with the usual measures to combat those problems. Such discussions help the patient and family understand that the postoperative course may not be smooth and that aggressive measures may be required to achieve ultimate recovery. According to Wright et al., the most common problems delaying discharge from the hospital include inadequate pain control, prolonged air leak, severe nausea, fever, physical weakness, and arrhythmias [1] (Table 57.1).

Preoperative Pulmonary Exercise and Training

The role of pulmonary rehabilitation is more controversial. In 1979, Gracey et al. [2] studied 157 patients who were

Electronic Supplementary Material The online version of this chapter (https://doi.org/10.1007/978-3-030-00859-8_57) contains supplementary material, which is available to authorized users.

J. Y. Perentes
Department of Thoracic Surgery, University of Toronto, Toronto General Hospital, Toronto, ON, Canada

Department of Thoracic Surgery, University Hospital of Lausanne, Lausanne, Switzerland

M. de Perrot (✉)
Department of Thoracic Surgery, University of Toronto, Toronto General Hospital, Toronto, ON, Canada
e-mail: marc.deperrot@uhn.ca

Table 57.1 Common reasons for delay in discharge

Cause	Percentage
Inadequate pain control	28
Prolonged air leak	19
Severe nausea	17
Fever	16
Physical weakness	12
Atrial arrhythmia	7

Adapted from Wright et al. [1]

about to undergo a major operation. They administered a standard pulmonary preparation program used at that time and found that complications were significantly reduced but also that postoperative pulmonary complications were related to the extent of the operation. In 1999, Debigare et al. [3] studied the preparation for lung volume reduction procedures for severe emphysema. Because many patients traveled a great distance, the investigators devised a home exercise training program that included incentive spirometry, muscle exercises, and aerobic training. It began with a detailed teaching and follow-up and was ensured through weekly phone calls and a diary filled out by each patient. As a result, there was a significant increase in the 6-min walk test, quality-of-life perception, peak work rate, peak oxygen consumption, endurance time, and muscle strength; it was therefore concluded that such training was beneficial when time permits a delay in the timing of the operation. This time delay may however not always be an option in patients with malignancy. In 2016, Licker and colleagues [4] randomized 151 operable lung cancer patients to usual care or to a high-intensity interval training (HIIT) program performed during the waiting period of 27 days. While the HITT program improved the 6-min walk distance and the peak oxygen consumption, the program did not reduce the occurrence of postoperative complications. However, the incidence of pulmonary complications in the HIIT group was decreased due to lesser atelectasis as was the stay of patients in the postanesthesia care unit.

Smoking

Smoking cessation has always been considered an important issue in preparation for an operation. However, the evidence shows that the effects of cigarette smoking linger long after cessation and that inordinately long preoperative delays would be necessary to achieve any significant improvement. The Lung Health Study Research Group has published many reports concerning the effects of smoking cessation. Anthonisen et al. [5] reported the results of one of the aforementioned group's studies involving individuals with documented early chronic obstructive pulmonary disease (COPD) who stopped smoking; they experienced improvement of lung function, with the greatest benefit being noted in the first year. No conclusions can be drawn concerning the early effects of smoking cessation, because the investigators' first observation point was 3 months after intervention. Despite the lack of firm evidence, it is still recommended that patients quit smoking for as long as possible prior to operation. Some data suggest that cessation of smoking could potentially lead to higher postoperative complications. This is based on the fact that patients have increased secretions early after cessation [6]. However, in 2005, Barrera [7] studied smokers

undergoing thoracotomy at Memorial Sloan Kettering Cancer Center. They found no difference in pulmonary complications among recent quitters vs. continuing smokers. Only patients with >60 packs per year and those with a significantly reduced diffusion capacity had a higher risk for postoperative pneumonia in that series. The investigators concluded that it was safe to quit at any time before operation. Similar findings were observed in a recent case-control study of patients undergoing lung cancer surgery that had stopped smoking up to 16 weeks prior to surgery or that were still active smokers. No difference in their postoperative course was observed [8].

Anticoagulant and Anti-aggregant Medication

Preoperative medications should be continued up to the time of operation. The only exceptions are anticoagulant medications. Patients on warfarin (Coumadin), therapeutic doses of low-molecular-weight heparin, or direct oral anticoagulation (DOAC) should stop their medications prior to the procedure. Regarding antiplatelet therapies, their management is more controversial. Noncardiac surgery is associated to major vascular complications of which the most common is myocardial infarction. Surgery is thought to enhance platelet activation which can favor coronary artery thrombosis, in particular in patients with pre-existing cardiac disease or recent angioplasty procedures. Low-dose aspirin was found to prevent myocardial infarction and major vascular events in a meta-analysis involving over 110,000 patients [9]. However, a recent prospective randomized controlled trial in 10,000 patients failed to show that aspirin continuation/initiation could prevent major cardiovascular events, while it caused more postoperative bleeding events [10]. Interestingly, this study was focused on patients at risk for major vascular events but excluded those with recent coronary angioplasties. The latter is a high-risk category of patients, particularly in the context of drug-eluted stents, for which the perioperative antiplatelet therapy management remains a challenge. In the context of thoracic surgery, retrospective and prospective data suggest that aspirin or clopidogrel monotherapy continuation is safe (no added bleeding complications) and preferable to their discontinuation (more myocardial infarction events) [11, 12]. However, if timing or risk of stent occlusion remains a concern, it was demonstrated that thoracic surgery in the context of dual antiplatelet therapy was possible although causing more postoperative bleeding requiring re-interventions with no added mortality [11]. It is our practice to recommend patients to stay on aspirin at the time of their surgery and to switch dual antiplatelet therapy to aspirin alone when possible. We feel this is associated to a decreased risk of postoperative cardiac complications. The use of aspirin has not been associated with increased risk of bleeding in our experience. In the context of high-risk patients with drug-eluted stents, surgery can be performed on clopidogrel therapy or even dual aspirin/clopidogrel therapy with a higher risk of bleeding and re-intervention. A careful evaluation and discussion between the thoracic surgeon, the anesthetist, and the cardiologist are necessary to tailor antiplatelet therapy to the surgical and cardiologic risk.

Postoperative Management

Postoperative Pain Management

Surgical interventions involving incisions to the pleural cavity are known to cause severe pain in patients. It is also clearly established that a good postoperative pain management limits patient morbidity as well as their risk for chronic thoracodynia. The gold standard for thoracic surgery has long been epidural analgesia. It was shown to be effective in controlling pain but also has some drawbacks including a failure rate of up to 12%, a risk for epidural infection or bleeding, and clear contraindications in patients with degenerative arthritis to the spine. Alternative analgesic approaches have been described including opioid administration (intravenous, subcutaneous, and oral), wound infiltration by local anesthetics, and nerve block infiltration.

In open thoracic surgery, the epidural remains the most used approach with good pain management and tolerance. The development of VATS has changed this paradigm: given the small incisions, the fissureless approaches, and minimal drainage time, alternative analgesia protocols were developed including intercostal nerve blockade and continuous wound infiltration in combination with oral opioids with very good results. Currently, clinical trials are testing the use of liposomal local anesthetics that were shown to have longer-lasting effects and to allow more limited use of opioids in the postoperative phase [13, 14]. These have shown interesting results in VATS and open surgery. These intercostal blocks can be applied via direct visualization of each intercostal space placing an anesthetic depot (Supplementary Video 57.1).

Pain management must be tailored to each patient and to the procedure. It is essential that patients can stay active, mobilize, and do their chest physiotherapy to avoid atelectasis and infection. We favor epidural anesthesia for open approaches and intercostal nerve blockade for thoracoscopic procedures.

Respiratory Care

Oxygen is administered as needed during the postoperative period. Chest physiotherapy has been demonstrated to be effective in preventing postoperative pulmonary complications and is considered routine postoperative care for patients undergoing thoracotomy. It is also well established that early mobilization has beneficial effects on the pulmonary outcome by improving basal lobe ventilation and respiratory work and thus limiting complications. We favor early mobilization even in patients that are still intubated or on some forms of respiratory support/ECMO (Fig. 57.1). Many patients with hypoxemia benefit more from physiotherapy to increase functional residual capacity and PaO_2 than from further increases in the fraction of inspired oxygen (FiO_2). Excessive oxygen administration has potential drawbacks despite the short-term margin of safety it can provide. Increased alveolar oxygen tension promotes atelectasis as the oxygen is rapidly absorbed. Drying of secretions, even by humidified gases, can increase difficulty with coughing and clearance of mucus. Patients with COPD may have chronic carbon dioxide retention. Supplemental oxygen will tend to exacerbate hypercapnia in these patients. Therefore, in patients who have an elevated $PaCO_2$ preoperatively, oxygen saturation is maintained at 90% or less, preserving the hypoxic drive to breathe.

Early application of continuous positive airway pressure (CPAP) may prevent the need for intubation and mechanical ventilation in patients with hypoxemia by reducing atelectasis and, therefore, improving oxygenation. Clearing of secretions is very important after thoracic operations, especially after tracheal resections. In our institution, we liberally use bronchoscopy and have a small bronchoscopy suite available on the thoracic surgery ward 24 h/day. Patients can be cleared of secretions daily if their cough is ineffective.

Intravenous Fluids

Lung manipulation and collapse may impair pulmonary lymphatic drainage and increase extravascular lung water due to the disruption of the alveolar-capillary membrane. Because of this, patients undergoing pulmonary resections should not receive excessive fluid replacement, and standard fluid management used in other types of surgical patients needs to be moderated. Excessive fluids can result in pulmonary edema, decreased alveolar gas permeability, decreased pulmonary compliance, atelectasis, and hypoxia. A recent study identified more than 0.7 mL/kg/min of crystalloid administration as a risk for pulmonary complications following anatomical resections [15]. One particularly high-risk situation is the postpneumonectomy patient where fluid management was shown to be crucial to avoid postoperative pulmonary edema. An adult should receive not less than 1000 mL of fluids per day. If there are no previous deficits or current complications, the typical amount of liquid ingested by an adult is 2–3.5 L/day. Two liters per day should maintain an adequate

Fig. 57.1 Early mobilization in postoperative patients even when requiring ventilator support or extracorporeal membrane oxygenation

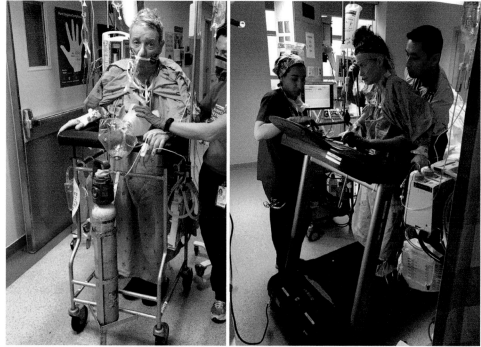

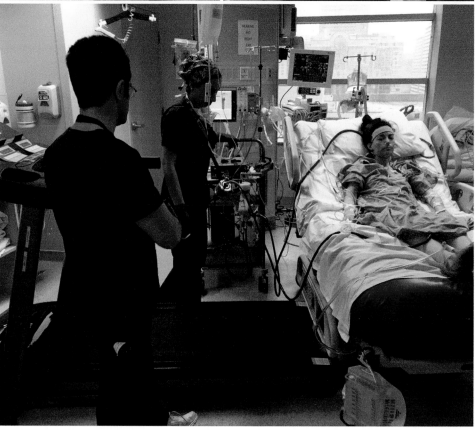

diuretic range (1000 mL) and cover requirements for Na^+, K^+, and Cl^-. In special circumstances, such as after pneumonectomy or lung volume reduction surgery, more extreme fluid restriction (<1.5 L) may be advised. Attention needs to be given to how much fluid is provided with medications. Urine output and serum creatinine must be monitored very carefully, and medications need to be reviewed to reduce or eliminate other nephrotoxins, such as nonsteroidal anti-inflammatory agents (NSAIDs) or angiotensin-converting enzyme inhibitors [16–18].

Chest Drainage System

Surgeons have several different options for draining the chest. For open thoracic surgery, most surgeons will place two #28 Fr chest tubes, one anteriorly and one posteriorly in the chest. For VATS, the practice has evolved, and most surgeons place only one #28 Fr chest tube. The tubes are attached to a drainage system that permits one-way drainage only, with a portion of the device set up to collect fluid. These devices use a variety of valves or liquid to establish a one-way system. All of the collection systems are designed to provide suction on the tubes if the surgeon desires. In the past, all chest tubes were placed on suction at −20 cm H_2O. In recent years, the advisability of the ubiquitous use of suction has been questioned. Several investigators, like Cerfolio and Wain and their respective coworkers, contend that if the lung is fully expanded with the tube on no suction, the patient will do well. Hence, there is currently more individual preference concerning chest tube suction. In our institution, suction at −20 cm H_2O is preferred at least for 24 h and a chest X-ray showing a fully expanded lung the next day. Exceptions are patients with significant emphysema or pneumonectomy or after volume reduction surgery. When pleural apposition is not realistically achievable, suction can potentially prolong the air leak in these patients. In the past years, new devices were developed to allow chest tube suction without the requirement of a wall suction (Fig. 57.2). These devices were shown to favor patient mobility and recovery. In addition, it was demonstrated that fluid and air output digital monitoring was favorable for chest tube removal decision-making [19, 20].

A special consideration with respect to chest drainage is after pneumonectomy. Traditional water-seal devices allow egress of air out from the pleural cavity but not for its return. This can lead to progressive mediastinal shift after pneumonectomy. There are several possible solutions. A chest drain need not be left at all, if the risk of bleeding is minimal. The mediastinum can be balanced by removing a few hundred milliliters of air as the thoracotomy is being closed, by means of a red rubber catheter. In addition, a needle thoracocentesis can be performed in the recovery room after the postoperative chest radiograph is reviewed. If bleeding is sufficient to require drainage, a balanced pneumonectomy chest drainage system is available. This device allows air both in and out, to keep the pleural space within a preset range. Alternatively, a traditional system may be used but clamped and only intermittently opened, although this approach is vulnerable to missteps by the inexperienced staff.

Regardless of the types of chest tubes and the use of suction, the drainage tubes must be assessed at least daily for patency, function, air leakage, and drainage. Inspection of the tube and drainage system for clots or blockages assures patency. Obstructions are removed by "milking" or "stripping" the tubing. This is accomplished by occluding the tubing and pulling it away from the patient to produce a local suction effect. If this does not work, a balloon-tipped catheter may be passed up the tubing to remove the clot, or a suction catheter may be used for the same purpose. A functioning tube is the one that shows variation in the fluid within it when the patient breathes quietly. This may be observed while talking with the patient at the bedside.

Good respiratory variation indicates proper functioning of the tube. Limited changes in the level of the fluid in those drainage systems with a water column may indicate partial blockage. The tubing should be placed so that it does not coil, leaving low points to collect fluid. Such collections impede fluid flow and may cause positive pressure to build up in the tubing and back up into the patient. Air leakage is assessed by observing the water-seal chamber on the drainage device. Air leakage should be assessed on and off suction at quiet respiration. The patient is then asked to cough, and the chamber is observed. Several grading systems have been devised. In general, air leaks should be characterized by the force necessary to produce the air leak and the amount of the air leak. The smallest leak is an intermittent one produced on inspiration only, and the largest one is a continuous air leak. Newer devices being evaluated currently display the amount of air leak digitally. Drainage should be measured twice daily, at least, so that an estimate can be made concerning whether the rate of fluid drainage is increasing or decreasing. Nurses usually record the drainage in 12-h shifts and provide a total daily drainage. In addition, the character of the drainage should be noted. Change in the character of the fluid from sanguineous to serous is usually a good sign. Change from serous to purulent indicates potential empyema and a change to "milky" secretion a chylothorax. In planning the removal of a chest tube, the drainage must decrease to levels acceptable to the surgeon. Although exact numbers are not scientifically demonstrated, the amount is usually 200–400 mL/day or less. Chest tubes and drainage systems are intended to keep the lung expanded and prevent the development of a space. Once air leakage ceases and drainage has decreased to acceptable levels, the system has performed its function and should be removed. In an age of cost containment, this could be any time after the operation and usually is 2–4 days after a lobectomy. The development of VATS has improved the postoperative course and chest tube management. Fissureless techniques and careful air leak prevention now allow patients to have their chest tubes removed as early as 4 h after surgery.

We routinely use a preplaced U stitch to approximate the wound edges after chest tube removal. The chest tube is removed quickly during a breath hold at the end of expiration. The wound borders are brought together, and a wound dressing is applied. A chest radiograph must be obtained after to evaluate for adequate pulmonary reexpansion.

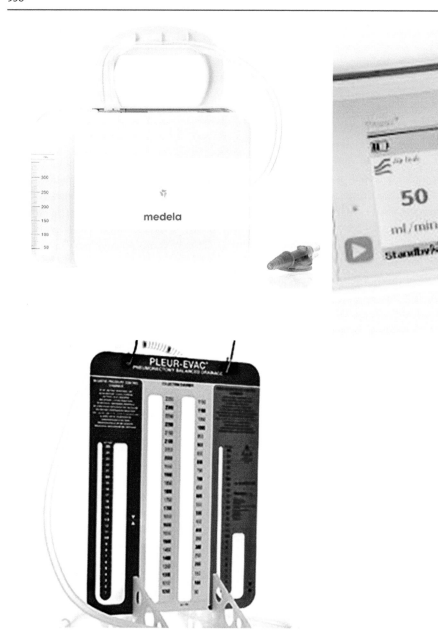

Fig. 57.2 Medela Thopaz device: a suction device with no need for wall suction. This device also has a screen showing fluid and air outputs over time. Some studies have suggested patient mobility could be enhanced with these devices. On the far right, a device for the manage-ment of postpneumonectomy pleural shift is shown. There are two water columns: a positive and a negative pressure column that favors a slow shift of the mediastinum to the side of the pneumonectomy

Postoperative Nutrition

The majority of patients start enteral nutrition in the evening of the day of surgery or the next day, unless they are hemodynamically unstable. Most patients tolerate limited postoperative nutrition for a week. Often overlooked is the early use of laxatives and stool softeners, which should be started on the first day with oral diet. Reduction of narcotics as tolerated, adequate oral hydration, and early ambulation help to overcome constipation.

Prevention of Venous Thromboembolism

Measures to prevent postoperative venous thromboembolism should be implemented in patients undergoing thoracic surgical procedures. The best method of prophylaxis is a low-dose fractionated or unfractionated heparin. Pneumatic compression devices are also used in some patients, although their role has never been formally demonstrated in randomized controlled trials. The risk for venous thromboembolic disease may be stratified according to patient and procedural factors.

Table 57.2 Classification of risk levels for postoperative thromboembolism

Thromboembolic event (%)

Risk level	Calf vein thrombosis	Proximal vein thrombosis	Clinical pulmonary embolism	Fatal pulmonary embolism	Successful prevention strategies
Low					
Uncomplicated minor surgery in patients aged <40 years with no clinical risk factors	2	0.4	0.2	0.0002	No specific prophylaxis, early mobilization
Moderate					
Any surgery in patients aged 40–60 years with no additional risk factors; major surgery in patients aged <40 years with no additional risk factors; minor surgery in patients with risk factors	10–20	2–4	1–2	0.1–0.4	LDUH (q12h), LMWH (≤3400 U daily), GCS or IPC
High					
Major surgery in patients aged >60 years without additional risk factors or patients aged 40–60 years with additional risk factors; patients with myocardial infarction; medical patients with risk factors	20–40	4–8	2–4	0.4–1.0	LDUH (q8h), LMWH (>3400 U daily), or IPC
Highest					
Major surgery in patients aged >40 years with prior venous thromboembolism, malignant disease, or hypercoagulable state; patients with elective major lower extremity orthopedic surgery, hip fracture, stroke, multiple trauma, or spinal cord injury	40–80	10–20	4–10	0.2–5.0	LMWH (>3400 U daily), fondaparinux, oral VKAs (INR, 2–3), or IPC/ GCS + LDUH/LMWH

Adapted from Geerts et al. [23]

LDUH low-dose unfractionated heparin, *LMWH* low-molecular-weight heparin, *GCS* graduated compression stockings, *IPC* intermittent pneumatic compression, *VKA* vitamin K antagonist

The majority of patients undergoing thoracic operation fit the high-risk category, as defined in Table 57.2. These patients have a calf thrombosis rate of 20–40%, a pulmonary embolus rate of 2–4%, and a fatality rate of 0.4–1.0%. In 2006, Mason et al. found a 7.4% incidence of postoperative venous thromboembolism among patients undergoing pneumonectomy for malignancy [21]. In 2007, the American Society of Clinical Oncology guidelines recommended that patients with cancer who will have a thoracotomy or laparoscopy lasting >30 min should receive pharmacologic thromboprophylaxis with either fractionated or unfractionated heparin. Prophylaxis should begin preoperatively or as early as possible in the postoperative period. A combined regimen of pharmacologic and mechanical prophylaxis may improve efficacy among the patients at highest risk. A recent survey among Canadian thoracic surgery centers has shown consensus in the practice of deep venous thrombosis prevention surgery [22].

General Complications of Thoracotomy

Pneumonia

Although the incidence is low, between 2.2% and 6%, pneumonia postthoracotomy contributes to significant morbidity. Risk factors include preoperative hospital stay, immunocompromised status, procedure (pneumonectomy > lobec-

tomy), pulmonary reserve, smoking, and atelectasis. Atelectasis is a common complication after pulmonary surgery, fortunately most is platelike or linear, hence subsegmental, and has little consequence in a patient with adequate pulmonary reserve. However, segmental or lobar atelectasis may cause significant problems. Risk factors include poor cough, usually a result of poor pain control, impaired pulmonary function, chest wall instability, and/or sleeve resection.

Prevention is the best treatment. Chest physiotherapy with vibratory percussion, frequent spirometry exercises, and ambulation is key for prevention. Adequate pain control is also of paramount importance to prevent pneumonia. Whenever pneumonia is suspected, sputum cultures or BAL, if a bronchoscopy is performed, should be obtained, and broad-spectrum antibiotic therapy should be started. Clinical signs of pneumonia are a productive cough, fever, and/or an elevation in the white blood cell count. Radiographic findings often lag behind, especially in dehydrated patients.

Atrial Fibrillation

Arrhythmias are one of the most frequent complications after thoracic surgery. They require immediate management and often prolong the hospital stay. Because atrial arrhythmias are more common (ventricular arrhythmias are rare after thoracotomy), their management is specifically discussed here.

The incidence of atrial tachyarrhythmias ranges from 3.8% to 37% after thoracic surgery, with atrial fibrillation (AF) being the most common arrhythmia [24]. It is commonly associated with respiratory complications. In a study by Bobbio et al. in 2007, there was a 30% incidence of AF in patients with either sputum retention, atelectasis, or pneumonia [25].

Many studies have been performed on the prevention of supraventricular tachyarrhythmias in patients undergoing lung resection. In a prospective randomized double-blind trial, Jakobsen et al. showed that the administration of oral metoprolol initiated preoperatively and continued postoperatively decreased the incidence of AF from 40% to 6.7% [26]. In another trial, administration of magnesium sulfate starting the day of operative resection also resulted in a decrease in the incidence of AF from 26.7% to 10.7% [27]. Prophylactic oral amiodarone, when given before cardiac surgery, was shown to be cost-effective and safe and might be a reasonable preventive strategy in thoracic or other noncardiac surgical patients [28]. The use of amiodarone has however been associated with acute lung injury in rare cases and must be used with caution after lung resection [29, 30]. There are currently no consensus guidelines for the prevention of atrial fibrillation that are specific to thoracic surgical patients.

Dunning et al. on behalf of the European Association for Cardiothoracic Surgery Audit and Guidelines Committee published guidelines and suggested a treatment algorithm for postsurgical AF [31]. Once the diagnosis of an atrial tachyarrhythmia has been established, the first priority is to assess the patient's hemodynamic stability. In addition, one should maintain oxygenation, assess fluid balance, and assess the serum potassium. If the patient experiences syncope or if the blood pressure is less than 80 mmHg systolic, the options are chemical conversion, typically with amiodarone IV or synchronous electrical cardioversion. For electrical conversion, the first shock is typically delivered at 200 J, with subsequent shocks at 300 and 360 J, respectively.

If the patient is hemodynamically stable, one should achieve control over the ventricular rate to allow better ventricular filling and an optimal ejection fraction. In our institution, once the electrolytes (potassium, magnesium, and calcium) are corrected, metoprolol would be the first choice except in patients with COPD and asthma. In this case, our first choice is diltiazem. Amiodarone is usually a second choice in patients who are hemodynamically stable because of its potential pulmonary toxicity. Once rate control has been achieved, the medication may be changed to equivalent doses of oral medication over the next 24 h. Myocardial ischemia should be ruled out by electrocardiography. The natural history of postoperative atrial tachyarrhythmias is self-termination. Therefore, usually nothing more than a day or two of rate control is required. If the patient spontaneously converts to normal sinus rhythm over the next 24 h, the medi-

cation can be discontinued, and no further treatment is required.

If, however, the patient remains in a rate-controlled fibrillation or flutter beyond 24 h, cardioversion can be attempted after echocardiography is performed to exclude the presence of intracardiac thrombus. Amiodarone has become the most popular drug for cardioversion, particularly since it is relatively safe in patients with depressed ventricular function. If the patient converts to sinus rhythm, the oral antiarrhythmic drug should be continued for at least 30 days after surgery.

If the arrhythmia persists for more than 48 h, the patient should be anticoagulated with heparin and then maintained on warfarin or DOAC. Typically, if patients are discharged from the hospital in rate-controlled AF with adequate anticoagulation, they will spontaneously convert to sinus rhythm as outpatients. If, however, they remain in AF beyond 30 postoperative days, they should be offered outpatient electrical cardioversion provided that they have remained therapeutically anticoagulated.

Pleural Space Problems

It is important to have the remaining lung fully expanded to fill the chest cavity following thoracotomy. If this, for any reason, fails to happen, the space between the lung and the chest wall will fill with fluid. This might be the seed for an empyema. A postoperative space problem may occur when atelectasis of the underlying lung occurs or when an air leak from the lung leads to a persistent air space.

Air Leak

Not all patients have an air leak after pulmonary resection. In fact, many patients having a thoracoscopic wedge resection have no air leak. However, many patients having a lobectomy, segmentectomy, or a complicated wedge resection will leave the operating room with a leak. The STS Thoracic Surgery Database defined prolonged air leak as lasting >5 days. By August 2008, the database had recorded a total of 15,178 lobectomies. Of these patients, 9.6% had prolonged leaks. This complication was the second in frequency only after arrhythmia.

Factors increasing the incidence of a prolonged air leak include emphysema, bilobectomy compared to lobectomy, poor chest tube placement, and neglecting operative techniques that help prevent air leaks. These techniques include pleural tents, fissureless surgery, buttressed stapled lines, and checking for air leaks before closing.

However, if significant air leaks occur postoperatively, management varies. The old dictum of "no space, no problem" is a good one to keep in mind. When this is the case, the patient rarely requires intervention. When the lung does not fill the entire cavity and there is a significant air leak, a bronchopleural fistula (BPF) should be taken into consideration.

A BPF is defined as a communication between a bronchus and the pleural space and is therefore different from an alveolopleural fistula. The latter usually seals spontaneously with time, which is not the case for a BPF. Most commonly, a BPF occurs following a right lower bilobectomy or pneumonectomy. This may be due to the lack of coverage of the bronchial stump by the remaining upper lobe because of the posterior-inferior position of the stump. In other types of lobectomy, the bronchial stump is well covered by the remaining lobes. Technical factors are responsible for fistulas occurring in the early postsurgical period. The most frequent errors are inappropriate suturing/stapling and ischemia produced by excessive dissection of the bronchus prior to closure. Prevention is the easiest way to manage BPF. Local tissue pedicle flaps such as pleura, azygos vein, pericardial fat, and intercostal muscle can be used to cover pneumonectomy or bilobectomy stumps. Treatment options for BPF are briefly discussed in section "Empyema."

For patients with complete lung expansion and a prolonged air leak, the first question is whether the lung will stay expanded without suction and if the chest tube output is considered small. If both of these criteria are met, the chest tube can be connected to a Heimlich valve or a similar device, and the patient can be discharged with a close follow-up as an outpatient. This is a good strategy in patients having lung volume reduction surgery, a decidedly sick population with significant underlying lung disease [32]. Alternatively, on rare occasions, there is the possibility of chest tube removal, even with a small air leak. Such a maneuver should be preceded by a trial of tube clamping for up to 6 h prior to removal. If the patient develops pulmonary symptoms, such as shortness of breath or hypoxia, or develops a pneumothorax, the tube can be unclamped and the procedure repeated in another day. If the patient remains asymptomatic and no pneumothorax develops, the tube may be removed. A period of observation for 6–24 h is recommended prior to discharge.

Empyema

Empyema complicating lung resections is an uncommon but morbid and too often deadly sequela, particularly after pneumonectomy. Postsurgical empyema accounts for 20% of all cases of empyema. It most frequently follows a pneumonectomy, occurring in 2–7% of patients with a higher incidence for right pneumonectomy, and it may occur in 1–3% of patients after lobectomy [33]. The incidence of empyema after pulmonary resection varies with the indications for the resection (inflammatory or neoplastic disease), with or without preoperative radiation.

Table 57.3 Factors that increase the risk of development of postsurgical empyema

Delay in diagnosis
Improper choice of antibiotics
Loculation or encapsulation by a dense inflammatory reaction
Presence of a bronchopleural fistula
Foreign body in the pleural space
Chronic infection
Entrapment of the lung by thick visceral peel
Inadequate previous drainage or premature removal of a chest tube

Although empyema may occur at any time postoperatively, even years later, most empyema develops in the early postoperative period. The pleural space may be contaminated at the time of pulmonary resection with the development of a bronchopleural or esophagopleural fistula or from blood-borne sources. After pulmonary resection that is less than a pneumonectomy, an empyema occurs more often when the pleural space is incompletely filled by the remaining lung. Risk factors for empyema are summarized in Table 57.3.

Symptoms and signs vary, but the possibility of an empyema must be considered in any patient with clinical features of infection after pulmonary resection. Expectoration of serosanguineous fluid and purulent discharge from the wound or the drain sites is almost always diagnostic. On radiography of the chest, usually a pleural opacity is seen, with or without a fluid level, when resection has been less than a pneumonectomy. After pneumonectomy, a decrease in the fluid level early postoperatively, or the appearance of a new fluid level when the pneumonectomy site was uniformly opaque, strongly suggests an infected pleural space with BPF. The pleural space should be immediately drained to prevent any contamination of the contralateral lung through the BPF, and a bronchoscopy should be performed to determine the size and location of the defect in the bronchial stump. The timing of surgical intervention and the type of operative procedure undertaken to treat the BPF are tailored to the individual patient (Fig. 57.3).

General treatment principles of postresectional empyema with or without a BPF include surgical drainage by closed chest tube insertion and institution of appropriate antibiotic therapy. Once adequate drainage has been established and the remaining lung fills the chest without significant space and there is no underlying BPF, the course of management can be determined, usually within 10–14 days. If the patient has a persistent space without a BPF, the management depends on the size of the space.

Smaller spaces can be sterilized by irrigation with the appropriate antibiotic solution or fibrinolytic agents. Once the daily amount of drainage is <100 mL/day and no further collapse of the remaining lung develops if the tube is opened to atmospheric pressure, the tube can simply be removed, or

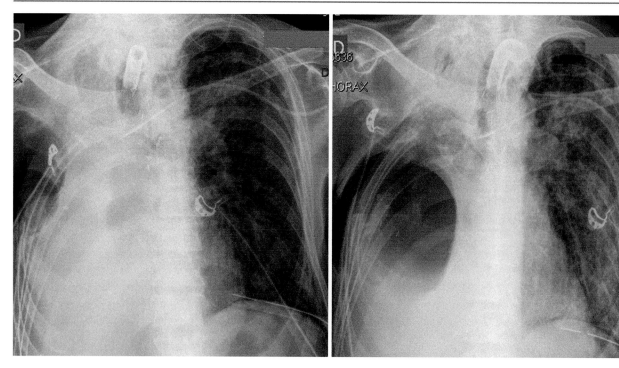

Fig. 57.3 Diagnosis and initial management of postpneumonectomy bronchopleural fistula (BPF). (**a**) A chest X-ray 30 days after the right pneumonectomy with the fluid level filling the entire thorax. At this time, the patient presented with a new onset of coughing. As initial treatment, a chest tube was inserted to drain the chest cavity and protect the left lung. A bronchoscopy and CT scan confirmed the bronchopleural fistula

closed drainage can be changed to open drainage by cutting it close to the chest wall. The tube is then shortened at the rate of about 1 in. per week or until granulation tissue and fibrosis lead to its spontaneous expulsion from the pleural space. In certain cases, if the residual space is seen as too big, two approaches have been described: a single-stage muscle flap closure of the remaining cavity can be performed and a tailored and limited thoracoplasty; both approaches have the aim to occlude the residual space [34]. Larger spaces are more of a challenge and can be managed by an open drainage or, more recently, by an intrathoracic vacuum-assisted closure device approaches (Fig. 57.4). In this context, the aim is to favor chest cavity healing by promoting secondary granulation. The advantage of the VAC therapy is that chest wall integrity is maintained. Once this and microbial control are achieved, chest wall closure can be considered. The Clagett window can also be a definitive alternative in patients with bad nutritional status that are too weak to undergo more consequent procedures [35, 36].

A postpneumonectomy empyema is associated with a BPF in approximately 40% of patients [37]. Significant factors contributing to the development of a BPF after pneumonectomy are induction chemo/radiotherapy, a right pneumonectomy, heavily calcified bronchial stump, positive surgical margin with cancer, and the need for postoperative mechanical ventilation [38]. This can happen early in the postoperative course, usually by days 7–10, but can also

manifest months after surgery. Initial goals in the treatment are the prevention of contamination of the contralateral lung by closed tube drainage of the infected pleural cavity, taking into consideration that the mediastinum takes about 14 days until it is stable post pneumonectomy, institution of antibiotics, and a bronchoscopy.

If no BPF is present, two approaches have been described: the modified Clagett's procedure and the VAC therapy. The modified Clagett's procedure consists in inserting a second small chest tube into the second intercostal space, and a continuous inflow-outflow irrigation system is established through the pleural cavity. The irrigant is based on antibiotic sensitivities to the pleural drainage. This method achieves sterilization of the space in approximately 50% of patients. If the method is successful and the return irrigant is negative by culture on 3 consecutive days after 2 weeks of irrigation, the chest tubes can be removed, and pleural fluid is allowed to reaccumulate to fill the remaining space. If this method fails, a Clagett window can be performed. Recently, VAC therapy or negative pressure dressings using iodine-soaked sponges have been described to accelerate granulation and favor infection control and pleural healing.

In patients with a BPF and postpneumonectomy empyema, reinforcement of the bronchial stump with a healthy tissue flap (pericardial fat, intercostal muscle, etc.) should be achieved. If the fistula closes, one can attempt the aforementioned modified Clagett's sterilization of the cavity. In the

Fig. 57.4 Application of a VAC device in a pleural cavity. The mediastinum is protected with gauze or white foam, and the black foam is formed as to mold the pleural cavity. Two suction devices are placed to favor drainage. (Illustrations from Perentes et al. [35])

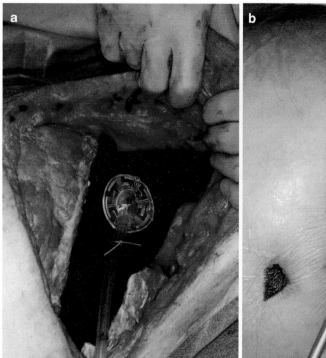

patient in whom the BPF persists, the fistula and space are then managed by transposition of muscle flaps into the empyema space; this can be any extrathoracic muscle such as serratus anterior, latissimus dorsi, pectoralis major, or omentum. If the patient remains critically ill and unstable, a Clagett window is ideal for long-term open drainage and irrigation. After the cavity is clean with granulating tissue, it can be closed. In other cases, acceleration of pleural healing can be achieved with VAC therapy that allows chest cavity closure after a mean period of 2 weeks [35, 36].

Nerve Injury

Injury to the recurrent laryngeal nerve can occur during right- or left-sided thoracic surgery procedures. The left nerve is far more in danger to be injured than is the right. Its position under the aortic arch makes it susceptible to injury during any procedure in this area. The nerve is, on occasion, "sacrificed" intentionally, if radical resection for a tumor known to involve the vagus nerve is required. The incidence ranges somewhere between 4% and 45% according to the type of procedure performed [39].

The patients with injury to the recurrent laryngeal nerve generally present in the postoperative phase with a weak and whispery voice, although cord edema in the very early postextubation period may mask the hoarseness. However, patients with palsy or paresis of the recurrent nerve have symptoms lasting well beyond the postoperative period. Those with paresis may describe a normal voice in the morning that becomes weaker over the course of the day. This may result in a weak cough or aspiration after drinking, leading to poor pulmonary physiotherapy and recurrent pneumonia. At laryngoscopy, adduction of the affected vocal cord will be absent or sluggish. Treatment involves determining the extent of injury and whether the injury is transient or permanent. A thorough evaluation of the significance of the cord should be done by fiber-optic evaluation of swallowing and sensation. To assist with pulmonary physiotherapy and decrease the risk of aspiration, medialization laryngoplasty may be suggested. This can be done with the aid of autologous fat, Gelfoam, collagen, or polytetrafluoroethylene (PTFE). These are usually temporary solutions. A permanent solution involves medialization of the vocal cord by thyroplasty [40].

Injury to the phrenic nerve can occur in both open and thoracoscopic pulmonary resections. The most common causes are adherence of the lung to the pericardium or injuries occurring during performance of resection of anterior mediastinal tumors, resection of superior sulcus tumors, repair of thoracic outlet syndrome, or right-sided mediastinal lymph node dissection. Such injuries may be temporary or permanent. In a spontaneously breathing patient, the diagnosis can be easily made by a chest radiographs demonstrating elevation of the affected hemidiaphragm. If the patient requires postoperative ventilation, this radiographic finding might not be present due to positive-pressure ventilation keeping the diaphragm in a fairly normal position. Depending on the severity of their underlying pulmonary disease, these patients may be difficult to wean from the ventilator. Phrenic nerve palsy can contribute to significant postoperative morbidity and symptoms according to the underlying pulmonary status of the patient. Diaphragmatic plication is indicated for symptomatic relief of dyspnea [41].

Postoperative Hemorrhage

The incidence of significant postoperative bleeding after a pulmonary resection requiring at least four units of packed red blood cells was identified to be 2.9% after lobectomy and 3.0% after pneumonectomy [42]. Chest tube output exceeding 1000 mL over 1 h or persistent bleeding over 200 mL/h for 2 h after a pulmonary resection mandates reexploration, assuming that the coagulation parameters are corrected. Bleeding may occur from mediastinal or bronchial vessels (23%), intercostal vessels (17%), or a pulmonary vessel (17%); in the majority of cases (41%), no source of the hemorrhage is identified [43]. Such troublesome postoperative bleeding is particularly prone to occur if there has been a previous thoracotomy, a decortication of parietal and visceral "peel" due to empyema or resections for inflammatory disease such as old tuberculosis or aspergillosis. With multiple bleeding sites present on the chest wall, it might be necessary for the surgeon to pack the pleural space for a period of time prior to closure of the thoracotomy. This may be particularly useful when the remaining lung fails to fill the pleural space or after pneumonectomy.

Chylothorax

A chylothorax is diagnosed when a "milky" effusion is drained through the chest tube once the patient is on enteral intake. However, if the patient has been fasting after resection, the characteristic creamy color of the effusion may not be noted. In this case, a persistent high chest tube output for unknown reason makes this diagnosis suspicious. The incidence of chylothorax after pulmonary resection is between 0.04% and 2% [44]. Etiologies include aggressive mediastinal lymph node dissection with incomplete ligation of lymphatic channels or direct injury to the thoracic duct [45]. The diagnosis is made by sending the pleural fluid for analysis. A triglyceride level > 110 mg/dL, a lymphocyte count >90%, and the presence of chylomicrons help to confirm the diagnosis [46].

A trial of conservative management is initially recommended, with the objective of adequately draining the pleural space, reexpanding the remaining lung, and keeping the patient fasting. The patient should be strictly NPO and be fed by parenteral nutrition. Occasionally medium-chain triglyceride (MCT) diet has been successfully used to stop the leak. Waiting for 7 days is normally advocated. It is generally agreed that a continuous chyle leak in excess of ≥1 L/day in a patient with complete cessation of oral intake is an indication for reoperation. Attempts at direct repair of the lymphatic injury often fail because of the difficulty of identifying and suturing the injury. Operative ligation of the thoracic duct low in the right chest is appropriate, and the success of thoracic duct ligation is 91%. Other options have been described for the management of chylothorax after pulmonary resection. The current most popular one includes interventional radiology embolization of the chyle leak which has shown interesting results. Other options when the leak cannot be controlled include pleuroperitoneal shunt that has resulted in the resolution of chylothorax in some series [47]. Another option, rarely used because of the technical difficulty, includes the use of a pleural-venous shunt [48].

Torsion of a Residual Lobe

The lobes of the lung are usually held in their position by the other lobes, the inferior pulmonary ligament, and incomplete fissures. After lobectomy these structures no longer exist. In particular, the middle lobe and lingula are most susceptible for torsion following a right upper lobectomy or a lingula-sparing left upper lobectomy, respectively. Lobar torsion typically presents early in the postoperative period with fever, tachycardia, and loss of breath sounds on the affected side. Often the clinical picture is not impressive. Chest X-ray can demonstrate atelectasis of the torsed lobe. Bronchoscopy should be done urgently to make the diagnosis, followed by urgent surgical exploration. The bronchoscopy will show a fish-mouth orifice to the lobe, which easily admits the bronchoscope. If the torsion is discovered early enough, the lobe may be preserved by untwisting the hilum. Most often, however, lobectomy is required. The incidence of lobar torsion after pulmonary resection is between 0.09% and 0.3% [49]. Lobar torsion of the middle lobe after a right upper lobectomy accounted for 70% of the cases in the literature. To prevent this complication, fixation of the middle lobe with the lower lobe may be performed in situations where the oblique fissure is complete.

Postpneumonectomy Syndrome

In a small number of patients undergoing pneumonectomy, mediastinal shift and rotation toward the empty hemithorax may cause pulmonary symptoms. This typically occurs in children or young adults. Along with the shift of the mediastinal contents, there is overdistension and herniation of the remaining lung. This results in dynamic airway compression of the left main bronchus between the left pulmonary artery and aorta after a right pneumonectomy or compression of the right main bronchus between the right pulmonary artery and the thoracic spine after left pneumonectomy. The overall incidence is not clear. Patients typically present with dyspnea, stridor, and recurring pneumonia, which may occur weeks to years after pneumonectomy. Diagnosis is made from chest radiographs, computed tomography scans, and bronchoscopy under conscious sedation demonstrating dynamic obstruction of the bronchus. Repositioning of the mediastinum and placement of a saline-filled tissue expander in the postpneumonectomy space is the treatment of choice [50].

Cardiac Herniation

Cardiac herniation rarely occurs but can be fatal in certain circumstances and therefore requires a high degree of suspicion. If the pericardium is opened widely or removed, the heart is held in place by the lungs on both sides. If a major portion of the lung is removed, the heart finds a space in which it may herniate. On the right side, herniation can be life-threatening in a matter of minutes because both venae cavae would be strangulated by a 180° rotation of the heart into the right pleural space. On the left side, the heart is freely suspended by the major vessels, and the risk of inflow and outflow occlusion is not present. A greater problem is a moderate-sized defect in the pericardium through which the heart can herniate and subsequently become compromised by postoperative edema (Fig. 57.5).

To avoid these scenarios, a simple closure of the pericardial defect can be performed for smaller lesions, while larger defects should be closed with a fenestrated mesh [51]. Simple suture closure of larger defects may lead to cardiac constriction.

The diagnosis of cardiac herniation might not be easy to make, especially for left-sided herniation. Symptoms include the sudden onset of low cardiac output and signs of central venous obstruction. If time is available, a chest radiograph will be diagnostic. Management of these patients includes emergent operative intervention with reduction of the car-

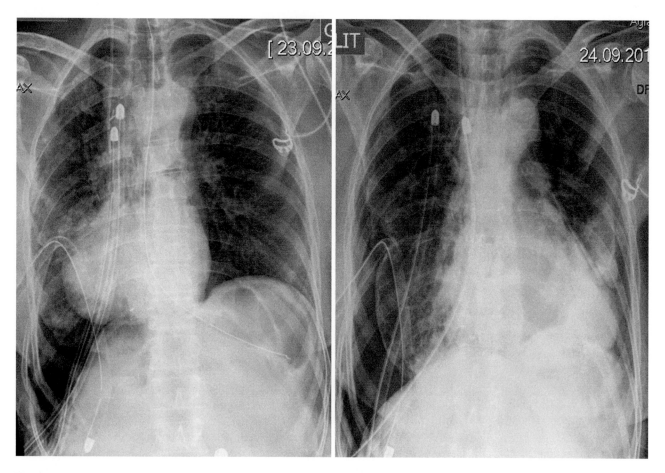

Fig. 57.5 Case of a cardiac herniation following an extensive pleurectomy decortication with pericardial and diaphragmatic resection. Only the diaphragm was reconstructed given the lung was left in place. However, the lung did not expand well because of an important air leak. In the recovery room, the patient developed tachycardia and hypotension. An X-ray showed right-sided cardiac herniation. The patient improved when put on the left decubitus. A re-intervention with pericardial mesh placement stabilized the situation

diac hernia and patch closure of the defect using PTFE. Since PTFE is watertight, fenestrations must be created.

Clinical Case Discussion

A 70-year-old female has a right completion pneumonectomy and partial excision of the right chest wall for non-small cell lung cancer. Thirty years before, the patient had a right upper lobectomy for tuberculosis. The patient is 52 kg and 160 cm, FEV 1 = 64%, DLCO = 60%, V/Q scan perfusion L:R is 65:35, good exercise tolerance, Hb is 124 g/dL, and other laboratory examinations including transthoracic echocardiography are normal. The anesthetic is with a combined T4–T5 thoracic epidural and general anesthesia. The operative duration is 4 h. The blood loss is 500 mL. The patient receives 1 L of Ringer's lactate and 500 mL of synthetic isotonic colloid intravenously during the case. One R chest drain is placed and connected to an underwater-seal drainage system without suction. The patient is extubated in the operating room awake and comfortable and transferred to the recovery room in a stable condition: heart rate 90/min, BP 100/50, CVP 4 mmHg, and urine output 30 mL/h. The thoracic epidural infusion is bupivacaine 0.1% with 15 μg/mL hydromorphone at 5 cc/h.

After 2 h in the recovery room, the patient's HR has gradually increased to 110, the BP has decreased to 90/50, CVP remains 4 mmHg, and the urine output has fallen to 15 mL/h. Repeat Hb is 103 g/dL. The chest tube is fluctuating normally with respiration, and there has been no significant drainage from the right chest. The patient receives repeat boluses of 500 mL Ringer's lactate ×2 intravenously. One hour later, the hemodynamics have not improved; she has a demonstrable sensory block from T2 to T10 without motor block. The thoracic epidural infusion is decreased to 2 mL/h. One hour later, the patient is complaining of five out of ten incisional pain, and there is no demonstrable sensory or motor block. The HR is 115/min, BP 78/50, CVP 4, Hb 98 g/dL, and urine output 10 mL/kg. Arterial blood gases are normal. What is the most appropriate next step?

1. Transfuse 500 mL of colloid.
2. Discontinue the epidural and begin intravenous PCA opioid analgesia.
3. Repeat the chest X-ray.
4. Obtain an ECG.
5. Obtain CT contrast pulmonary angiography.
6. Return to the operating room for cardiac herniation.

The most important postpneumonectomy complication to rule out in this context is cardiac herniation (see also Chap. 41) since it is so treatable and so lethal if not treated promptly. Cardiac herniation after a right pneumonectomy is most likely to present as a sudden onset of severe life-threatening

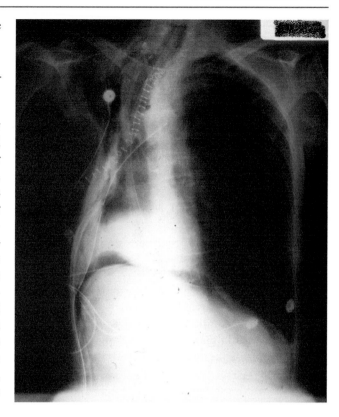

Fig. 57.6 Chest X-ray of a 70-year-old female 4 h post-op. After a right completion pneumonectomy and partial excision of the chest wall. The chest drain was connected to an underwater-seal drainage system which allowed the development of an excessive negative intrathoracic pressure causing a complete shift of the mediastinum to the right lateral chest wall and a compromise of the venous return to the heart

hypotension. That is not the presentation in this case, so there is time to confirm the diagnosis. The repeat chest X-ray 4 h post-op is shown in Fig. 57.6. An unrelieved negative pressure has developed in the right chest due to the one-way valve effect of the underwater-seal chest drain. The mediastinal shift to the right created symptoms equivalent to a herniation with compromise of the venous return to the right heart. The tip of the CVP catheter was at the SVC-right atrial junction and thus was downstream from the venous inflow obstruction and accurately reflected the decreased filling pressures of the right heart, but not the systemic venous volume. The mediastinum was "balanced" by injecting 500 mL of air into the right chest tube which was then clamped (Fig. 57.7). The patient's hemodynamics rapidly returned to normal, the epidural infusion was increased to control the pain, and the chest drain was removed the next day.

The presence of a functioning, normally fluctuating, chest drain in this patient makes the possibility of a tension pneumothorax or massive hemorrhage into the operative hemithorax very unlikely. Epidural local anesthetic overdosing is unlikely with the regression of the sensory block. Myocardial ischemia and pulmonary embolus must be considered in the differential diagnosis of postoperative hypotension but are

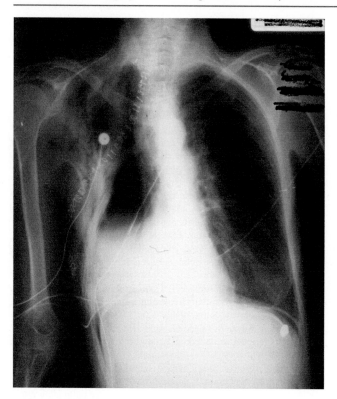

Fig. 57.7 Chest X-ray of the same patient after 500 mL of air was injected via the chest drain which was then clamped. The mediastinum has been "balanced" which relieved the obstruction of venous inflow to the right heart and allowed the hemodynamics to return to normal

not specific complications related to pneumonectomy. The different options for chest drain management after a pneumonectomy are explained in section "Chest Drainage System."

References

1. Wright CD, Wain JC, Grillo HC, Moncure AC, Macaluso SM, Mathisen DJ. Pulmonary lobectomy patient care pathway: a model to control cost and maintain quality. Ann Thorac Surg. 1997;64(2):299–302.
2. Gracey DR, Divertie MB, Didier EP. Preoperative pulmonary preparation of patients with chronic obstructive pulmonary disease: a prospective study. Chest. 1979;76(2):123–9.
3. Debigare R, Maltais F, Whittom F, Deslauriers J, LeBlanc P. Feasibility and efficacy of home exercise training before lung volume reduction. J Cardpulm Rehabil. 1999;19(4):235–41.
4. Licker M, Karenovics W, Diaper J, Fresard I, Triponez F, Ellenberger C, et al. Short-term preoperative high-intensity interval training in patients awaiting lung cancer surgery: a randomized controlled trial. J Thorac Oncol. 2017;12(2):323–33.
5. Anthonisen NR, Connett JE, Kiley JP, Altose MD, Bailey WC, Buist AS, et al. Effects of smoking intervention and the use of an inhaled anticholinergic bronchodilator on the rate of decline of FEV1. The Lung Health Study. JAMA. 1994;272(19):1497–505.
6. Nakagawa M, Tanaka H, Tsukuma H, Kishi Y. Relationship between the duration of the preoperative smoke-free period and the incidence of postoperative pulmonary complications after pulmonary surgery. Chest. 2001;120(3):705–10.
7. Barrera R, Shi W, Amar D, Thaler HT, Gabovich N, Bains MS, et al. Smoking and timing of cessation: impact on pulmonary complications after thoracotomy. Chest. 2005;127(6):1977–83.
8. Rodriguez M, Gomez-Hernandez MT, Novoa N, Jimenez MF, Aranda JL, Varela G. Refraining from smoking shortly before lobectomy has no influence on the risk of pulmonary complications: a case-control study on a matched populationdagger. Eur J Cardiothorac Surg. 2017;51(3):498–503.
9. Antithrombotic Trialists C, Baigent C, Blackwell L, Collins R, Emberson J, Godwin J, et al. Aspirin in the primary and secondary prevention of vascular disease: collaborative meta-analysis of individual participant data from randomised trials. Lancet. 2009;373(9678):1849–60.
10. Devereaux PJ, Mrkobrada M, Sessler DI, Leslie K, Alonso-Coello P, Kurz A, et al. Aspirin in patients undergoing noncardiac surgery. N Engl J Med. 2014;370(16):1494–503.
11. Cerfolio RJ, Minnich DJ, Bryant AS. General thoracic surgery is safe in patients taking clopidogrel (Plavix). J Thorac Cardiovasc Surg. 2010;140(5):970–6.
12. Brichon PY, Boitet P, Dujon A, Mouroux J, Peillon C, Riquet M, et al. Perioperative in-stent thrombosis after lung resection performed within 3 months of coronary stenting. Eur J Cardiothorac Surg. 2006;30(5):793–6.
13. Khalil KG, Boutrous ML, Irani AD, Miller CC 3rd, Pawelek TR, Estrera AL, et al. Operative intercostal nerve blocks with Long-acting bupivacaine liposome for pain control after thoracotomy. Ann Thorac Surg. 2015;100(6):2013–8.
14. Parascandola SA, Ibanez J, Keir G, Anderson J, Plankey M, Flynn D, et al. Liposomal bupivacaine versus bupivacaine/epinephrine after video-assisted thoracoscopic wedge resection dagger. Interact Cardiovasc Thorac Surg. 2017;24(6):925–30.
15. Mizuno Y, Iwata H, Shirahashi K, Takamochi K, Oh S, Suzuki K, et al. The importance of intraoperative fluid balance for the prevention of postoperative acute exacerbation of idiopathic pulmonary fibrosis after pulmonary resection for primary lung cancer. Eur J Cardiothorac Surg. 2012;41(6):e161–5.
16. Bjerregaard LS, Moller-Sorensen H, Hansen KL, Ravn J, Nilsson JC. Using clinical parameters to guide fluid therapy in high-risk thoracic surgery. A retrospective, observational study. BMC Anesthesiol. 2015;15:91.
17. Hamaji M, Keegan MT, Cassivi SD, Shen KR, Wigle DA, Allen MS, et al. Outcomes in patients requiring mechanical ventilation following pneumonectomy. Eur J Cardiothorac Surg. 2014;46(1):e14–9.
18. Matot I, Dery E, Bulgov Y, Cohen B, Paz J, Nesher N. Fluid management during video-assisted thoracoscopic surgery for lung resection: a randomized, controlled trial of effects on urinary output and postoperative renal function. J Thorac Cardiovasc Surg. 2013;146(2):461–6.
19. Gilbert S, McGuire AL, Maghera S, Sundaresan SR, Seely AJ, Maziak DE, et al. Randomized trial of digital versus analog pleural drainage in patients with or without a pulmonary air leak after lung resection. J Thorac Cardiovasc Surg. 2015;150(5):1243–9.
20. Shoji F, Takamori S, Akamine T, Toyokawa G, Morodomi Y, Okamoto T, et al. Clinical evaluation and outcomes of digital chest drainage after lung resection. Ann Thorac Cardiovasc Surg. 2016;22(6):354–8.
21. Mason DP, Quader MA, Blackstone EH, Rajeswaran J, DeCamp MM, Murthy SC, et al. Thromboembolism after pneumonectomy for malignancy: an independent marker of poor outcome. J Thorac Cardiovasc Surg. 2006;131(3):711–8.
22. Agzarian J, Linkins LA, Schneider L, Hanna WC, Finley CJ, Schieman C, et al. Practice patterns in venous thromboembolism (VTE) prophylaxis in thoracic surgery: a comprehensive Canadian Delphi survey. J Thorac Dis. 2017;9(1):80–7.

23. Geerts WH, Pineo GF, Heit JA, Bergqvist D, Lassen MR, Colwell CW, et al. Prevention of venous thromboembolism: the seventh ACCP conference on antithrombotic and thrombolytic therapy. Chest. 2004;126(3 Suppl):338S–400S.

24. Rena O, Papalia E, Oliaro A, Casadio C, Ruffini E, Filosso PL, et al. Supraventricular arrhythmias after resection surgery of the lung. Eur J Cardiothorac Surg. 2001;20(4):688–93.

25. Bobbio A, Caporale D, Internullo E, Ampollini L, Bettati S, Rossini E, et al. Postoperative outcome of patients undergoing lung resection presenting with new-onset atrial fibrillation managed by amiodarone or diltiazem. Eur J Cardiothorac Surg. 2007;31(1):70–4.

26. Jakobsen CJ, Bille S, Ahlburg P, Rybro L, Hjortholm K, Andresen EB. Perioperative metoprolol reduces the frequency of atrial fibrillation after thoracotomy for lung resection. J Cardiothorac Vasc Anesth. 1997;11(6):746–51.

27. Terzi A, Furlan G, Chiavacci P, Dal Corso B, Luzzani A, Dalla VS. Prevention of atrial tachyarrhythmias after non-cardiac thoracic surgery by infusion of magnesium sulfate. Thorac Cardiovasc Surg. 1996;44(6):300–3.

28. White CM, Giri S, Tsikouris JP, Dunn A, Felton K, Reddy P, et al. A comparison of two individual amiodarone regimens to placebo in open heart surgery patients. Ann Thorac Surg. 2002;74(1):69–74.

29. Kolokotroni SM, Toufektzian L, Harling L, Bille A. In patients undergoing lung resection is it safe to administer amiodarone either as prophylaxis or treatment of atrial fibrillation? Interact Cardiovasc Thorac Surg. 2017;24(5):783–8.

30. Spartalis M, Tzatzaki E, Schizas D, Spartalis E. eCommentAmiodarone-induced pulmonary toxicity in patients with atrial fibrillation undergoing lung resection. Interact Cardiovasc Thorac Surg. 2017;24(5):788.

31. Dunning J, Treasure T, Versteegh M, Nashef SA, Audit E, Guidelines C. Guidelines on the prevention and management of de novo atrial fibrillation after cardiac and thoracic surgery. Eur J Cardiothorac Surg. 2006;30(6):852–72.

32. McKenna RJ Jr, Fischel RJ, Brenner M, Gelb AF. Use of the Heimlich valve to shorten hospital stay after lung reduction surgery for emphysema. Ann Thorac Surg. 1996;61(4):1115–7.

33. Deschamps C, Bernard A, Nichols FC 3rd, Allen MS, Miller DL, Trastek VF, et al. Empyema and bronchopleural fistula after pneumonectomy: factors affecting incidence. Ann Thorac Surg. 2001;72(1):243–7. discussion 8

34. Fournier I, Krueger T, Wang Y, Meyer A, Ris HB, Gonzalez M. Tailored thoracomyoplasty as a valid treatment option for chronic postlobectomy empyema. Ann Thorac Surg. 2012;94(2):387–93.

35. Perentes JY, Abdelnour-Berchtold E, Blatter J, Lovis A, Ris HB, Krueger T, et al. Vacuum-assisted closure device for the management of infected postpneumonectomy chest cavities. J Thorac Cardiovasc Surg. 2015;149(3):745–50.

36. Saadi A, Perentes JY, Gonzalez M, Tempia AC, Wang Y, Demartines N, et al. Vacuum-assisted closure device: a useful tool in the management of severe intrathoracic infections. Ann Thorac Surg. 2011;91(5):1582–9.

37. Cerfolio RJ. The incidence, etiology, and prevention of postresectional bronchopleural fistula. Semin Thorac Cardiovasc Surg. 2001;13(1):3–7.

38. Hollaus PH, Setinek U, Lax F, Pridun NS. Risk factors for bronchopleural fistula after pneumonectomy: stump size does matter. Thorac Cardiovasc Surg. 2003;51(3):162–6.

39. Krasna MJ, Forti G. Nerve injury: injury to the recurrent laryngeal, phrenic, vagus, long thoracic, and sympathetic nerves during thoracic surgery. Thorac Surg Clin. 2006;16(3):267–75. vi

40. Schneider B, Schickinger-Fischer B, Zumtobel M, Mancusi G, Bigenzahn W, Klepetko W, et al. Concept for diagnosis and therapy of unilateral recurrent laryngeal nerve paralysis following thoracic surgery. Thorac Cardiovasc Surg. 2003;51(6):327–31.

41. Simansky DA, Paley M, Refaely Y, Yellin A. Diaphragm plication following phrenic nerve injury: a comparison of paediatric and adult patients. Thorax. 2002;57(7):613–6.

42. Harpole DH Jr, DeCamp MM Jr, Daley J, Hur K, Oprian CA, Henderson WG, et al. Prognostic models of thirty-day mortality and morbidity after major pulmonary resection. J Thorac Cardiovasc Surg. 1999;117(5):969–79.

43. Sirbu H, Busch T, Aleksic I, Lotfi S, Ruschewski W, Dalichau H. Chest re-exploration for complications after lung surgery. Thorac Cardiovasc Surg. 1999;47(2):73–6.

44. Kutlu CA, Sayar A, Olgac G, Akin H, Olcmen A, Bedirhan MA, et al. Chylothorax: a complication following lung resection in patients with NSCLC – chylothorax following lung resection. Thorac Cardiovasc Surg. 2003;51(6):342–5.

45. Haniuda M, Nishimura H, Kobayashi O, Yamanda T, Miyazawa M, Aoki T, et al. Management of chylothorax after pulmonary resection. J Am Coll Surg. 1995;180(5):537–40.

46. Agrawal V, Doelken P, Sahn SA. Pleural fluid analysis in chylous pleural effusion. Chest. 2008;133(6):1436–41.

47. Murphy MC, Newman BM, Rodgers BM. Pleuroperitoneal shunts in the management of persistent chylothorax. Ann Thorac Surg. 1989;48(2):195–200.

48. Itkin M, Kucharczuk JC, Kwak A, Trerotola SO, Kaiser LR. Nonoperative thoracic duct embolization for traumatic thoracic duct leak: experience in 109 patients. J Thorac Cardiovasc Surg. 2010;139(3):584–9; discussion 9-90.

49. Cable DG, Deschamps C, Allen MS, Miller DL, Nichols FC, Trastek VF, et al. Lobar torsion after pulmonary resection: presentation and outcome. J Thorac Cardiovasc Surg. 2001;122(6):1091–3.

50. Shen KR, Wain JC, Wright CD, Grillo HC, Mathisen DJ. Postpneumonectomy syndrome: surgical management and long-term results. J Thorac Cardiovasc Surg. 2008;135(6):1210–6; discussion 6-9.

51. Sugarbaker DJ, Jaklitsch MT, Bueno R, Richards W, Lukanich J, Mentzer SJ, et al. Prevention, early detection, and management of complications after 328 consecutive extrapleural pneumonectomies. J Thorac Cardiovasc Surg. 2004;128(1):138–46.

Troubleshooting Chest Drains

Hadley K. Wilson, Emily G. Teeter, Lavinia M. Kolarczyk, Benjamin Haithcock, and Jason Long

Introduction and Relevance

Chest tubes are the gold standard for the drainage of the pleural and pericardial spaces. They are used to treat a variety of conditions including pneumothorax, pleural effusion, and postoperative evacuation of air and fluid. There are a number of types and sizes of chest tubes available ranging from 6 Fr to 40 Fr. This chapter will discuss the indications for chest tube placement and removal as well as the best uses for different types of chest tubes. Lastly, we will address complications associated with chest tube placement as well as special situations such as bronchopleural fistula, postpneumonectomy chest tubes, abrupt changes in chest tube output, and clamping chest tubes.

Indications and Physiology

Normal pulmonary physiology relies on the generation of negative intrapleural pressure by the contraction of the diaphragm to draw air into the distal airways for gas exchange. Any accumulation of air or fluid in the pleural space may disrupt this process and may prevent sufficient pulmonary expansion and diffusion of carbon dioxide and oxygen. In the case of penetrating thoracic trauma, the negative intra-

pleural pressure leads to the influx of air into the pleural space down a pressure gradient from positive atmospheric pressure to the negative intrapleural pressure. Fluid collections in the pleural space obstruct appropriate expansion of the lung parenchyma by mass effect and lead to collapse of the affected lung. A combination of both air and fluid in the pleural cavity can also produce collapse of the lung if not adequately drained. Postoperatively the anticipation of inflammatory pleural fluid, blood, and air prompts placement of chest tubes at the time of thoracic and cardiac surgery. Any symptomatic accumulation of air or fluid in the pleural space is an indication for chest tube placement. The goals of pleural drainage are sufficient evacuation of any air or fluid to promote normal pulmonary function and biomechanics. The presence of air or serous, exudative, purulent, sanguinous, or chylous fluid is integral in determining the type of pleural drain placed. Regardless of the pleural contents, all drains are connected to a collection system that allows evacuation of pleural contents and prevents entrance of air or fluid from outside the thorax [1].

Chest Tubes and Insertion

There are many different chest tubes available for evacuation of air and fluid from the pleural cavity ranging in size from 6 Fr to 40 Fr (Figs. 58.1 and 58.2). Chest tubes are constructed of a variety of synthetic materials including polyvinyl chloride and silicone. It is simplest to think about chest tubes in terms of large bore (>=20 Fr) and small bore (<20 Fr) chest tubes. French (Fr) measures the external diameter of the tube. Every French unit is equivalent to 1/3 millimeter, making a 3 Fr tube equivalent to 1 millimeter external diameter. Poiseuille's law shows that even small increases in diameter will drastically increase flow of air and fluid through the chest tube, thus giving large bore chest tubes a considerable advantage. For that reason conventional large bore chest tubes are the mainstay of pleural drainage. Small

H. K. Wilson (✉)
Department of Surgery, Division of Cardiothoracic Surgery, UNC Hospitals, Chapel Hill, NC, USA
e-mail: Hadley.wilson@unchealth.unc.edu

E. G. Teeter · L. M. Kolarczyk
Department of Anesthesiology, University of North Carolina at Chapel Hill, Chapel Hill, NC, USA

B. Haithcock
Department of Surgery, Department of Anesthesiology, University of North Carolina at Chapel Hill, Chapel Hill, NC, USA

J. Long
Department of Surgery, University of North Carolina Hospitals, Chapel Hill, NC, USA

© Springer Nature Switzerland AG 2019
P. Slinger (ed.), *Principles and Practice of Anesthesia for Thoracic Surgery*, https://doi.org/10.1007/978-3-030-00859-8_58

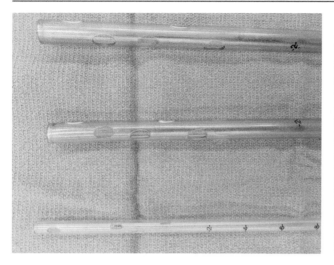

Fig. 58.1 From top to bottom: 36 Fr, 32 Fr, 20 Fr conventional chest tubes

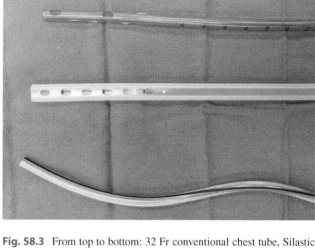

Fig. 58.3 From top to bottom: 32 Fr conventional chest tube, Silastic chest tube, 24 Fr Blake drain

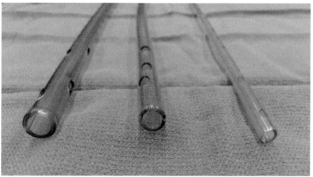

Fig. 58.2 The bore size of conventional chest tubes, from left to right: 36 Fr, 32 Fr, 20 Fr

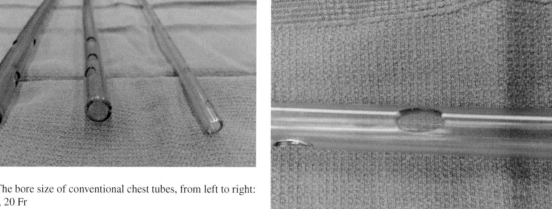

Fig. 58.4 Sentinel hole of conventional chest tube

bore chest tubes, however, are gaining popularity and have been shown to be quite effective and less painful in select situations such as spontaneous pneumothorax or simple pleural effusion [1–8]. Small bore chest tubes include flexible silicone drains such as the Blake drain (Ethicon, Inc., Somerville, NJ), pigtail catheters, and indwelling pleural catheters (Fig. 58.3). Despite their ease and growing popularity, small bore chest tubes are not suitable for loculated or complex pleural effusions, hemothorax, or trauma [3]. In those situations a large bore chest tube should be used to prevent clogging of the tube and inadequate drainage [9].

Chest Tube Insertion Techniques

While large bore chest tubes provide effective drainage of a wide range of pleural collections, they are associated with patient discomfort during insertion and while in place [6]. Large bore chest tubes range in size from 20 Fr to 40 Fr and have a series of side holes at their proximal end and a radi-

opaque marker (Figs. 58.4 and 58.5). The most distal of these side holes is referred to as the sentinel hole. It interrupts the radiopaque marker and is easily visualized on chest radiograph. Large bore chest tubes can be inserted by both blunt dissection and trocar techniques [9]. In the blunt dissection technique, the patient is positioned either with the ipsilateral arm extended over the head or abducted. The affected side is prepped and draped using chlorhexidine or betadine solution anterior to the midaxillary line, posterior to the pectoral groove, and anterior to the latissimus at the level of the third to fifth intercostal space. The clinician should always include the nipple in the prepped and draped area to maintain landmarks during insertion. While adhering to standard sterile technique, generous amounts of local anesthetic should be used to anesthetize first the skin and then the subcutaneous tissue. The needle is then advanced until the rib is encountered, and then the periosteum is anesthetized by injecting

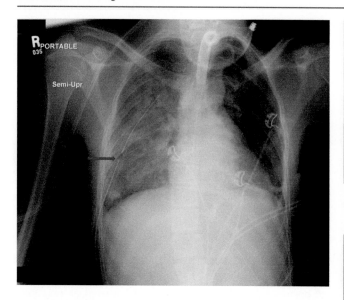

Fig. 58.5 Conventional chest tube sentinel hole on chest radiograph, arrow marks sentinel hole well within chest cavity

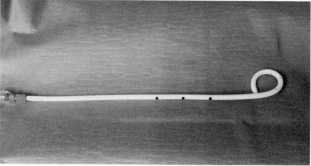

Fig. 58.6 Pigtail catheter

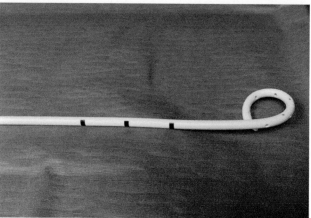

Fig. 58.7 Side holes and markings on pigtail catheter

local anesthetic at this level. The needle may then be directed superiorly, and while aspirating on the syringe, it may be advanced over the superior aspect of the rib. Once air or fluid is encountered, the clinician is sure that they are in the pleural space. Local anesthetic is then injected as the needle is withdrawn to anesthetize the pleura. Once the area for insertion is prepped, draped, and appropriately anesthetized, an approximately 2–3 cm incision (or large enough to insert a finger into the chest) is made in the skin. The subcutaneous tissues are dissected using a blunt instrument such as Kelly forceps or tonsil forceps until the rib and intercostal muscle are encountered. At this point, the clinician palpates the rib with the instrument and advances over the superior aspect of the rib to avoid the neurovascular bundle. Slow, steady, and controlled pressure is applied in the intercostal space just superior to the rib until the instrument penetrates the pleural cavity. On entry into the pleura, the forceps is gently spread, and a rush of air, fluid, or both should be noted. The clinician then inserts a finger into the pleural cavity and sweeps around the entry site to ensure there are no adhesions or attachments to the chest wall. This will reduce the risk of damaging lung tissue when the tube is inserted into the pleural space [6, 10]. The chest tube can then be inserted next to a finger in the pleural cavity to guide the tube posteriorly and to the apex for air. If pleural fluid is the problem being treated, the chest tube may be placed more inferiorly and directed more posteriorly to drain accumulating fluid. Alternatively, it is acceptable to grasp the tip of the chest tube with the Kelly forceps to better direct the chest tube into the chest. Once the tube is in the pleura, the Kelly forceps are released, and the tube is advanced to the desired location as described previously. The tube should then be connected to a water seal collection system and the collection system placed below the level of the lung. There are many ways to secure the chest tube to the skin; however a single interrupted suture is commonly placed using heavy permanent suture and the free ends wrapped around the tube and tied to the chest tube tight enough to notice a slight crimp in the tubing to prevent dislodgement [6]. The tube can then be dressed using 4 × 4 gauze and tape. Once the chest tube is in place, chest x-ray is performed to ensure adequate position. The sentinel hole must be in the thorax to provide adequate drainage and prevent the entry of air into the thoracic cavity.

Small bore chest tubes (less than 20 Fr) may be considered first-line therapy for simple pleural effusions or pneumothorax [3]. Small bore conventional chest tubes are inserted in the same manner as the large bore chest tubes described above. Pigtail catheters are small in caliber and have a series of side holes at the proximal end, but do not have a radiopaque marker. Instead these catheters have markings on the tubes themselves to guide the tube to the adequate depth (Figs. 58.6, 58.7, and 58.8). Pigtail catheters may be inserted using anatomic landmarks or using ultrasound guidance. If using ultrasound guidance, a pocket of fluid is first identified, and then that area is prepped, draped, and anesthetized as described above. If not using ultrasound guidance, the clinician may use chest percussion to delineate the level

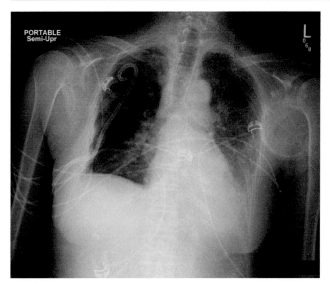

Fig. 58.8 Pigtail on chest radiograph

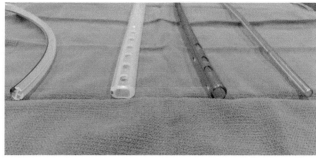

Fig. 58.9 Bores of different chest tubes from left to right: 24 Fr Blake drain, Silastic drain, 32 Fr conventional chest tube, 20 Fr conventional chest tube

of fluid in the thoracic cavity, and that area is then prepped, draped, and anesthetized as described above. Regardless of whether ultrasound is used, a 10 cc syringe with a large bore needle is advanced just superior to the rib in the area of interest, aspirating as the clinician advances. Once fluid or air is encountered, the clinician should stop advancing and remove the syringe. A wire is then inserted into the large bore needle. The needle can then be withdrawn over the wire, taking care to leave the wire in place within the pleural cavity. Using an 11 blade scalpel, a puncture incision is made along the wire large enough to accommodate the chest tube and the dilator. The chest tube with dilator inside is then advanced over the wire with slow steady pressure until all side holes are within the pleural space. The wire and dilator are then removed leaving the tube in place. The tube should then be connected to a water seal collecting system and the collecting system placed on the floor next to the patient.

Postsurgical Chest Drains

Following surgical procedures of the chest, tube thoracostomy is the gold standard for evacuation of accumulated postoperative fluid and air. Large bore chest tubes are commonly used to drain both the pericardial and pleural spaces following open heart surgery and are nearly always placed following esophageal and lung surgery.

Postoperative chest tubes are inserted in the same fashion as conventional large bore chest tubes; however, in the operating room, the surgeon benefits from direct visualization of the chest tube placement. Following pulmonary resections, the conditions in the pleural space change. Postoperative blood, pleural fluid, and air accumulate in the pleural space. Because of the body's natural position and gravity, fluid

tends to collect posteriorly and inferiorly, while air collects anteriorly and superiorly [7]. For these reasons, the mainstay of postoperative chest drainage has been to place two chest tubes: one anteriorly to evacuate air and one posteriorly to evacuate fluid [7]. The decision of the type, location, and number of chest tubes is largely based upon surgeon preference [7, 11]. The placement of two chest tubes after surgery is thought to reduce atelectasis, hemothorax, and inadequate lung re-expansion. One study showed that a single chest tube is as effective at draining the pleural space after thoracic surgery as two chest tubes [12]. Furthermore this study demonstrated that a single chest tube is, not surprisingly, far less painful than two chest tubes, likely aiding in patient participation in pulmonary rehabilitation [12]. A recent meta-analysis showed a statistically significant decrease in pain and length of stay with a single chest tube vs two chest tubes following lobectomy [13]. A consensus paper from the European Society of Thoracic Surgeons, American Association of Thoracic Surgeons, and Society of Thoracic Surgeons found no benefit to using two chest tubes and likely decreased pain using only one chest tube after non-cardiac thoracic surgery [14]. Based on the above studies, the use of a single conventional large bore chest tube is safe, effective, and likely less painful after lung resection. In the case of empyema or hemothorax requiring decortication, two or more chest tubes are left given the high risk for air leak and need to fully drain the pleura and expand the lung. Right angle chest tubes may be used to drain the space posterior and anterior to the diaphragm depending on the location of the collections found at the time of surgery [15].

There is much debate about the type of chest tube that should be placed following lung resections. The traditional practice has been to use large bore semirigid chest tubes postoperatively; however recent studies suggest that smaller bore flexible drains such as the Blake drain (Ethicon, Inc., Somerville, NJ) may be safe and effective [8, 16] (Figs. 58.3, 58.9, and 58.10). Flexible, spiral, fluted silicone drains were shown to decrease pain scores and provide adequate drainage without significant difference from standard large bore

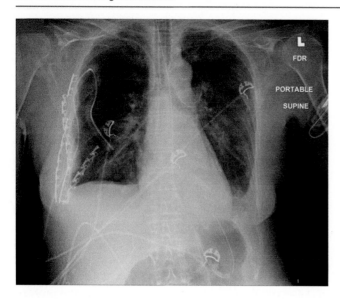

Fig. 58.10 Chest radiograph of flexible Silastic drain in right chest after rib fracture fixation

chest tubes after pulmonary resection [16]. The drains in this study were placed to −20 mmHg suction postoperatively, although they do not describe when if ever the drains in either the small flexible drain group or conventional chest tube group were placed to water seal. Another study showed that the Blake drain (Blake drain Ethicon, Inc., Somerville, NJ) was adequate for evacuation of fluid but only when placed to suction [8]. Additionally the Blake drains used in this study were inferior to conventional large bore semirigid chest tubes for the evacuation of air when air leakage occurred [8]. One case report describes life-threatening hemothorax not detected due to occlusion of a Blake drain which ultimately required return to the operating room for control of hemorrhage [17]. The consensus document from the European Society of Thoracic Surgeons, American Association of Thoracic Surgeons, and Society of Thoracic Surgeons agreed that flexible spiral fluted silicone drains are likely safe and effective but the evidence is weak and needs to be further studied [14].

Another area of great debate is the use of suction to increase negative pressure in the collection system (and thus drainage) to improve re-expansion of the lung. Suction is commonly used to re-expand the lung postoperatively and obliterate residual airspace, thereby preventing symptomatic collapse of the surgical lung. There is relatively little data to substantiate the use of suction. A prospective randomized trial from Poland sought to answer this question and found that nonsuction had improved drainage volume, shorter duration of chest tube, and decreased air leakage compared to suction drainage [18]. There were more residual air spaces noted in the nonsuction group; however these were largely asymptomatic and clinically insignificant [18]. Cerfolio et al. showed in 2001 that in the case of persistent air leak, nonsuction drainage was superior [19]. This

is likely due to the decreased negative pressure applied upon the leaking pulmonary tissue, thus drawing less air through the wound allowing proper healing. Large randomized trials are lacking for this question, and further studies are required to further elucidate the benefits of suction and nonsuction chest drainage. Suction for 24 h postoperatively followed by conversion to water seal on postoperative day 1 appears to be safe and effective for management of postsurgical chest tubes [18].

Regarding cardiac surgery, both the pleura and the pericardium are routinely drained postoperatively. If the pleura is violated during the dissection, a single chest tube is commonly placed in the pleural space. The type and number of chest tubes placed in the pericardium is debated. Le and colleagues found no advantage to using multiple pericardial chest tubes over a single pericardial chest tube following cardiac surgery [20]. Additionally there was no increase in bleeding or return to the operating room for cardiac tamponade [20]. Frankel et al. showed no difference in small Silastic pericardial drains vs conventional large bore chest tubes in patients undergoing coronary artery bypass grafting [4]. In this study there was no significant increase in risk of bleeding or cardiac tamponade in the group randomized to Silastic drains. Additionally patients with Silastic drains were more easily mobilized than the group with conventional large bore chest tubes [4]. A randomized trial studying delayed removal of Silastic mediastinal drains, and early removal of conventional chest tubes confirmed there was no difference in bleeding or cardiac tamponade between traditional chest tubes and Silastic chest tubes [2]. The literature on this topic suggests that a single chest tube is as effective at draining the pericardial space postoperatively as two chest tubes. Furthermore, the more comfortable Silastic tubes seem to be as safe and effective as conventional large bore chest tubes but possibly afford the patient less pain and earlier mobility [2].

Indwelling Pleural Catheters

In patients with malignant pleural effusions, recurrent fluid accumulation is a significant burden to patients which may cause crippling dyspnea and poor quality of life in a group of patients who already have a short life expectancy [21]. There are several ways to treat malignant pleural effusion including repeat thoracentesis, pleurodesis, and indwelling pleural catheters. Indwelling pleural catheters can be inserted on an outpatient basis and provide patients with a long-term solution to recurrent dyspnea [22]. The PleurX catheter is one type of indwelling pleural silicone catheter with fenestrations used for drainage of pleural fluid [22].

To insert a PleurX catheter, the skin over the 7th to 8th intercostal space is prepped using chlorhexidine solution and anesthetized at the entry site of the catheter extending 5 cm to the exit site of the catheter. The pleural space is accessed in the same manner as the Seldinger technique described above. Once the wire is well within the pleural cavity, the introducer sheath can be removed, and a 1 cm incision is made over the wire using an 11 blade scalpel. A second 1–2 cm incision is made 5 cm laterally at an exit site that will be comfortable and feasible for the patient. The PleurX catheter is then connected to the tunneling device, and the catheter is tunneled from the exit site to come out of the skin at the entry site. The catheter is pulled through until the polyester cuff is under the skin approximately 1 cm from the exit incision. The 12 Fr dilator is then advanced over the wire and into the pleural space. Next the 16 Fr dilator and peel-away introducer are advanced over the guide wire until the peel-away introducer is flush with the skin. The dilator and wire are then removed as a unit, and the surgeon uses a finger to occlude the peel-away dilator to prevent air from entering the pleura. The PleurX catheter can then be threaded through the peel-away introducer until it is entirely within the pleural space and not kinked. At this point the peel-away introducer may be cracked and peeled away taking care not to remove the PleurX catheter. The entry site incision is then closed, and the PleurX catheter is then secured to the skin at the exit site using a single interrupted suture that is wrapped and tied around the catheter [22]. Occlusion rates of the PleurX catheter are <5% and infection rates are <3% [23]. The patient may then use this catheter to drain pleural fluid at home to relieve dyspnea using a suction canister and appropriate tubing. BD recommends not draining more than 1500 cc of pleural fluid on initial placement to prevent re-expansion pulmonary edema. Once the pleural catheter is in place, it should be drained daily to improve symptoms and increase the rate autopleurodesis where formation of adhesions between visceral and parietal pleura obliterates the pleural space and prevents fluid accumulation [24]. Patients undergoing indwelling pleural catheter placement have shorter hospital stays and equal relief from dyspnea compared to patients undergoing talc pleurodesis [21].

Drainage Collection Systems

Playfair described the first reported case of underwater drainage for empyema in 1875 [25]. A child developed empyema and failed multiple aspiration attempts, ultimately resulting in abscess formation. The surgeon placed a flexible drainage tube in the affected thorax and placed the distal end of this tube under water in a container placed under the patient's bed. This technique led to rapid resolution of the empyema and convalescence of the sick child. With the chest tube's distal end submerged, the risk of air entering the pleural cavity is quite low; however, the outflow of both fluid and air is still permitted [26]. The depth of the column of water in which the tube is placed determines the hydrostatic pressure that must be overcome to evacuate air and fluid from the

chest. During the negative pressure generated in inspiration, some of this fluid may be drawn back into the tube and introduce nonsterile contents into the pleura. If the water level is low enough, then the entire column may be drawn up the tube during deep inspiration and subsequently air may be drawn into the pleural space. For this reason the column of water must be sufficiently high that a deep inspiration will not draw all of the water into the tubing. Increased thoracic pressure such as coughing overcomes the hydrostatic pressure generated by the column of water allowing the exit of air and fluid from the pleural space [26]. Furthermore, there is significant dead space in a pleural collection system created by the volume of the tubing and collection chamber. As the dead space increases, so does the work of the patient to expel air and fluid from the pleural cavity. The single-bottle model was abandoned as increased fluid accumulation increased resistance to flow. The two-bottle system solved this problem allowing fluid to collect in the first bottle, while air was collected in the second bottle. The increase in tubing, however, increased resistance, and the addition of a third bottle to the system facilitated the use of suction to decrease resistance to flow. The application of suction to the collection system maintains a constant subatmospheric pressure to facilitate drainage and reduce the work of the patient [26]. The drainage system should not normally be placed to suction greater than −10 or −20 mmHg as this may exert too much force on the lung resulting in injury [27]. Additionally if a patient has an air leak, higher levels of suction may cause changes in expiratory ventilation volumes by drawing more air through the air leak. Higher levels of suction are available up to −40 mmHg but should only be reserved for patients in whom an expanding pneumothorax does not respond to lower levels of suction [28]. There are many varieties of pleural drainage collecting systems available. For hospitalized patients these systems all consist of a collecting chamber, a water seal, and a vacuum port for the application of suction.

Digital pleural drainage systems such as the DigiVent™ allow the precise measurement of air leakage and graphical representation of daily changes that may be used to monitor progress and alter treatment [29]. The digital collection system is both safe and effective and does not require a battery to permit successful drainage of the thorax. Digital systems have been used to detect the presence of air leaks not seen on traditional analog pleural collection systems [30]. In one study the digital pleural collection system reduced the time that chest tubes were in place compared to analog pleural collection systems [30]. With further research digital collection systems could improve our detection and management of air leaks in post-thoracic surgery patients.

For patients who have a persistent air leak after lung resection, smaller collection systems are used to facilitate in discharging the patient home with chest tube still in place. Generally, these systems consist of a one-way valve with or without a reservoir that allows the patient to go home safely while the air leak has time to heal [31]. Determining when to remove the chest tube and time to follow up is discussed later in this chapter.

Drainage Volume

Chest tube output is extremely useful in guiding clinical decision-making. The quantity and quality of chest tube output can be indicative of the underlying problem in a patient requiring tube thoracostomy. Whether the output is sanguinous, serous, chylous, purulent, gastric, or a combination of these, it will determine the next therapeutic decision. In trauma, a moderate hemothorax of 500–1200 mL of initial bloody output can be safely monitored if drainage resolves after chest tube placement. If the initial output is greater than 1200 mL of blood or the output continues at a rate of >200 mL/h with no signs of slowing, emergency thoracotomy or thoracoscopy is indicated [15]. In postoperative patients, chest tube output of >200 mL/h of blood for 4 h warrants further investigation and coagulopathy workup. Reoperation can be avoided if the coagulopathy is corrected; however, if there is retained hemothorax or ongoing bleeding, it should be evaluated by thoracoscopy or thoracotomy [15].

Air Leak

Following thoracic surgical procedures, patients may have an alveolar-pleural fistula or a connection between the small airways and pleural space that leads to an "air leak." By definition an air leak is a connection between airways distal to the segmental bronchi and the pleural space [15]. An air leak is identified in the water seal chamber as bubbles rising through the fluid and can be quantified using digital collection systems [28] (Fig. 58.11). Air leaks can also be present as the result of a malfunction in the tubing or connections of the chest tube system. If the chest tube is clamped proximal to the connection of the chest tube and collecting tubing and the air leak persists, then it is likely the result of a poor connection and air is being sucked around the tubing and into the collection system. For this reason, if an air leak is present, all connections must be checked and verified to be adequate. The incidence of air leak in lung resection patients postoperatively is 20–25% [15]. Most air leaks resolve in the first 2–3 days; however, a prolonged air leak is defined as an air leak that persists on postoperative day 4. By this definition, the incidence of prolonged air leak is approximately 5% [15]. The risk factors for air leak are surgery for emphysema, bilobectomy, and malposition of the chest tube [15]. The incidence of air leaks may be reduced by pleural tents, buttressing of staple lines using pericardium, fissureless surgery

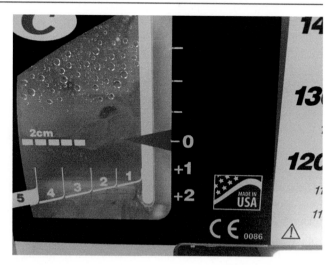

Fig. 58.11 Air leak visible as air rushing through the number 1 hole with bubbles in the water seal chamber

and ensuring the absence of air leak prior to closure [15]. Additionally, patients who had poor pulmonary function tests and had undergone neoadjuvant therapy were at a significantly higher risk of air leak than their counterpart likely secondary to friable tissue and poor wound healing [32]. Cerfolio developed a classification system for air leaks in 2002 that describes an air leak both qualitatively based on when it occurs during the respiratory cycle and quantitatively by the size of the air leak [28]. The largest type of air leak is a continuous air leak which is present during inspiration and expiration, Type C. This type of air leak can be indicative of bronchopleural fistula and is seen usually in intubated patients. Inspiratory phase air leaks occur when patients are mechanically ventilated, Type I. Air leaks that occur exclusively during expiratory phase are very common after pulmonary resection and are a smaller type of air leak, Type E. The smallest and by far the most common type of air leak is one that is not present during inspiration or expiration but only noticed during forced expiration such as coughing, Type FE. To quantify the air leak, the physician requires a drainage system equipped with an air leak meter. These are commercially available and quite common. The air leak meter has a series of small chambers starting at 1 (smallest) and going as high as 7 (largest chamber). Larger leaks will be seen bubbling in the higher-numbered chambers, while smaller leaks will be seen in the lower-numbered chambers. By this classification system, Cerfolio has defined a spectrum of air leaks, the largest of which would be classified as a continuous 7, or C7, and the smallest of which would be classified as a forced expiratory 1, or FE1 [28]. The best treatment for air leak is to place chest tubes to water seal [32]. If the patient has large growing residual air space, increasing subcutaneous emphysema or hypoxia, then the tube should be placed to suction [32]. Patients with prolonged air leak may be discharged with chest tube in place connected to a one-way valve such as a Heimlich valve or similar device. Patients can then have their chest tube safely removed at 2-week follow-up visit [32]. The specific criteria for chest tube removal will be discussed later in this chapter.

Complications of Insertion

The standard of care in pleural effusion, pneumothorax, and post-thoracic surgery patients is effective drainage of the pleural space with chest tubes. While this is a common and safe procedure, it is not without risks. The most serious complication is damaging surrounding organs such as the lung, heart, diaphragm, esophagus, stomach, liver, and spleen [27]. Intercostal artery, diaphragm, phrenic nerve, and sympathetic chain injuries may occur as well [33]. Most of these complications occur during insertion with the trocar method, and for this reason, trocars are not the first choice for chest tube placement [34]. On average complications can be seen in up to 5–10% of tube thoracostomy placements and are mainly related to tube malposition and other technical complications [33] (Fig. 58.12). Malposition of the chest tube in the subcutaneous tissues will prevent the function of the chest tube. Risk factors for subcutaneous chest tube insertion are obesity, rib fractures, and hasty insertion [33].

Re-expansion pulmonary edema is the accumulation of alveolar fluid secondary to rapid expansion of a collapsed lung [35]. The mechanism of this phenomenon is not entirely understood; however, it is thought that a decrease in surfactant production, while the lung is collapsed, and release of inflammatory cytokines and increased hydrostatic pressure after re-expansion all contribute. The main risk factor for

developing re-expansion pulmonary edema is a lung that has been collapsed for greater than 3 days. The treatment is supportive and symptoms may persist for up to 1 week [35]. To prevent re-expansion pulmonary edema, it is probably safe to remove less than 1500 mL of fluid during a single thoracic drainage procedure. Larger volumes require careful clinical monitoring, and suction should not exceed −20 mmHg [35].

If chest tubes are left in place for too long, empyema may develop requiring thoracotomy or thoracoscopy for evacuation and has been shown to range from 2% to 5% [33, 36, 37]. Risk factors for developing empyema after chest tube placement are increased duration of chest tube and retained hemothorax [33]. Other risk factors for empyema development after tube thoracostomy are prolonged ICU stay, pulmonary contusion, and need for laparotomy. The treatment of empyema is intravenous administration of antibiotics and surgical evacuation.

Other rare complications exist such as pleurocutaneous fistula or retained portion of catheter. A pleurocutaneous fistula is a rare problem in which a tract between the skin and pleural space develops after chest tube removal. Pleurocutaneous fistulas may heal spontaneously or require surgical intervention. Retained catheter is rare but requires thoracoscopy or thoracotomy for removal [33].

Chest Tube Removal and Thresholds

There are mixed opinions regarding when to remove a chest tube. The two main factors that contribute to the decision to remove a chest tube are quantity of liquid output and the presence or absence of an air leak. Chest tubes may be removed on suction or water seal for trauma patients [21]. In pulmonary resections, the chest tube is placed to suction on the day of surgery to aid in expansion of the lung and fill the space created during resection. On postoperative day 1, patients may be transitioned to water seal [38]. Patients frequently develop pleural effusion after lung resection, and this can prevent timely discharge of patients if they are otherwise suitable for discharge. In patients with more than one chest tube, the anterior and apical chest tube should be removed last as this tube will evacuate air more effectively and prevent post-removal pneumothorax [1]. It has been shown that chest tubes may be safely removed with an output of 450 mL or less of nonchylous drainage per day [39]. Another study showed that after VATS lobectomy, chest tubes may be safely removed with up to 500 mL of fluid output per day [40]. It is possible that it is safe to remove chest tubes with higher levels of output; however, there is currently no evidence to support this.

The issue of when to remove a chest tube becomes more complicated if the patient has an air leak. As mentioned above, most air leaks will resolve within 1–2 days postoperatively. For those that do not resolve, Cerfolio and colleagues have detailed

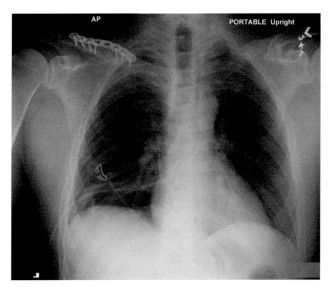

Fig. 58.12 Right chest tube placed into the mediastinum

an algorithm to guide physicians [32]. Patients undergoing pulmonary resections other than pneumonectomy who had persistent air leak at 3 days had their tubes attached to an outpatient collection device and discharged with prophylactic cephalexin 500 mg daily until their follow-up in 2 weeks (approximately 3 weeks postop). All of the chest tubes were safely removed from patients with persistent air leak even in the presence of pneumothorax [32]. As long as residual air space on chest radiograph was asymptomatic and not expanding and there was no increase in subcutaneous emphysema, these chest tubes could be removed 2 weeks after discharge with prophylactic antibiotics continued as long as the chest tube was in place [32]. The reason for why the lung does not collapse after 2 weeks with persistent air leak is not well understood. It is possible that sufficient adhesions have formed at 2 weeks to prevent the collapse of the lung [32]. It is unknown how long a chest tube can safely remain in place, but the chest tube should be removed as soon as possible to prevent development of empyema. Chest tubes may safely remain in place in the case of prolonged air leak up to 3 weeks after placement [32].

Using the correct technique to remove a chest tube is important to prevent a post-removal pneumothorax. All patients should have their chest tubes removed while performing a Valsalva, and an occlusive dressing using petroleum gauze should be placed over the incision and held firmly in place during the removal of the tube. The tube should be pulled at end expiration—the patient should be asked to fully and forcibly exhale, and then perform a Valsalva. At the end of expiration and during a Valsalva, the chest tube may be withdrawn rapidly with one hand, while the other hand holds the occlusive dressing in place over the incision [41]. This technique was shown to be more effective at reducing post-pull pneumothorax compared to the removal of chest tubes at the end of maximal inspiration [41]. Patients with extensive COPD and low forced expiratory volume in 1 s are at higher risk for developing post-pull pneumothorax [41].

Follow-up chest x-ray after chest tube removal is routinely performed. In post-thoracic surgery patients, it is important to assess an enlarging pneumothorax after placing to water seal and after removal of the chest tubes [38, 39]. In trauma patients, however, chest x-rays only for symptomatic patients have been shown to be as effective at identifying pathology as routine chest x-ray and result in fewer interventions in trauma patients [42, 43].

Special Situations

Bronchopleural Fistula

A bronchopleural fistula is a connection between a segmental or more proximal bronchus and the pleural space. It is crucial to differentiate bronchopleural fistula from alveolar-pleural fistula as the treatment is drastically different. The incidence of bronchopleural fistula is 1.6–2.7% following pulmonary resection, and it is increased in patients who have undergone neoadjuvant therapy owing to their friable tissues and poor wound healing [15]. Bronchopleural fistula most commonly occurs after pneumonectomy, but it is also seen in lobectomy or segmentectomy. Patients at higher risk for bronchopleural fistula are those who have undergone radiation, are immunocompromised, or have diabetes. Surgically speaking a long bronchial stump, injury to arterial supply of the bronchus, and leaving lymph nodes on the bronchus all increase patient risk for bronchopleural fistula. Bronchopleural fistula will present with continuous air leak that was not present previously. When a bronchopleural fistula is suspected, the patient should undergo bronchoscopy. Most moderate to large bronchopleural fistulae are easily diagnosed on bronchoscopy. If there is no sign of bronchopleural fistula on bronchoscopy, and a high suspicion for bronchopleural fistula persists, the patient should undergo xenon ventilation scan. This study will demonstrate xenon escaping the bronchus and entering the pleural space and chest tube. If a bronchopleural fistula is identified, reoperation and flap or omentum coverage will be required [15].

Post-pneumonectomy Chest Tubes

After pneumonectomy, the patient has a large empty space that will ultimately be occupied by fluid. Postoperatively there is great debate about whether or not to leave a chest. The goal of a chest tube is to return the mediastinum to a normal position. After pneumonectomy the mediastinum will be forced away from the operative side by the entry of air into the pleural space. This may compress the remaining lung and can even compromise venous return. If the mediastinum is not balanced appropriately, this could lead to cardiopulmonary collapse. Balancing the mediastinal space may be performed with needle aspiration or a chest tube placed to water seal with half the water volume and never to suction. Air may be removed with aspiration until resistance is noted. The benefit of a chest tube in this unique situation is early recognition of potentially fatal bleeding or bronchial stump breakdown. The chest tube is typically removed in 12–24 h to prevent infection [15]. Ultimately, it is up to the surgeon whether to leave a chest tube after pneumonectomy, and an experienced team is required to monitor the patient postoperatively.

Abrupt Changes in Chest Tube Output

An abrupt decrease in chest tube output may be an ominous sign and should prompt clinical correlation to assure no undrained enlarging collections are present. It may signal that the space is inadequately drained, and dangerous accumulation of fluid or air may result. Pericardial effusion, cardiac tamponade, and tension pneumothorax could all be the result of a chest tube that stops draining. Clark reports the case of a clogged chest tube that led to massive hemothorax requiring repeat operation [17]. Abrupt increase in chest tube output may signal new bleeding if the output is bloody or other problems including chylothorax, bronchopleural fistula, or anastomotic leak.

Clamping Chest Tubes

Some centers will clamp chest tubes as a test to identify occult air leak prior to chest tube removal. In this strategy, the tube is clamped, and follow-up chest radiograph is performed to evaluate for collapse of the affected lung. It has been shown to be safe and beneficial to prevent premature removal with follow-up x-ray in 6 h [44]. In the case of massive hemothorax, it has been suggested that clamping a chest tube prior to the operating room might improve patient survival and help tamponade the bleeding. There is little data to support this strategy, and it has been shown that clamping a chest tube in massive hemothorax will not decrease the volume of blood lost. Instead clamping the chest tube in massive hemothorax will lead to increased compression of the lung and worsened gas exchange [45]. Chest tubes should therefore not be clamped in the case of massive hemothorax, and the patient should be taken emergently to the operating room and resuscitated as needed.

Summary

Chest tubes are an integral part of cardiothoracic surgery, and the well-being of patients depends on their appropriate management. In this chapter we discussed the types of chest tubes, how they are inserted, collection systems, drainage volumes, air leaks, chest tube removal, and special situations including bronchopleural fistula, post-pneumonectomy chest tubes, abrupt changes in chest tube output, and when a chest tube may need to be clamped.

All chest tubes should be connected to a water seal collection system, and suction may be applied if needed. Chest tubes are not without complications; however, they are generally very safe in the hands of an experienced clinician, and serious complications are exceedingly rare. Chest tubes can be safely removed when there is no air leak and their liquid output is less than 450 mL for the previous 24 h. Patients who have an alveolar-pleural fistula, or air leak, should have chest tubes placed to water seal as soon as clinically feasible, and these leaks will normally resolve in 2–3 days. Patients with a prolonged air leak may be discharged with an outpatient collection system, and their chest tubes may be removed safely at 2-week follow-up if there is no expanding pneumothorax, increasing subcutaneous emphysema, or change in respiratory status.

Bronchopleural fistula should not be confused with alveolar-pleural fistula as the management of the former is operative and the latter is typically nonoperative. Patients undergoing pneumonectomy may have a chest tube placed in the space previously occupied by their lung to balance the mediastinum, and they should never be placed to suction. Abrupt changes in chest tube output may represent obstruction in the chest tube or hemorrhage and should be further evaluated. Chest tubes should never be clamped in the setting of massive hemothorax as this will result in increased compression of the lung and decreased oxygenation. It is safe to clamp chest tubes as a diagnostic test for occult air leak.

Over the last 20 years, our knowledge of chest tube management has significantly improved, thanks to a number of publications seeking to provide evidence-based guidelines to substantiate clinical experience and assist in decision-making. Further study is still needed to further define the role of small bore chest tubes in patients after cardiothoracic surgery, output thresholds for chest tube removal, and the need for suction.

References

1. Venuta F, Diso D, Anile M, Rendina E, Onorati I. Chest tubes. Thorac Surg Clin. 2017;27(1):1–5.
2. Moss E, Miller C, Jensen H, Basmadjian A, Bouchard D, Carrier M, et al. A randomized trial of early versus delayed mediastinal drain removal after cardiac surgery using silastic and conventional tubes. Interact Cardiovasc Thorac Surg. 2013;17(1):110–5.
3. Cooke D, David E. Large-bore and small-bore chest tubes. Thorac Surg Clin. 2013;23(1):17–24.
4. Frankel T, Hill P, Stamou S, Lowery R, Pfister A, Jain A, et al. Silastic drains vs conventional chest tubes after coronary artery bypass. Chest. 2003;124(1):108–13.
5. Havelock T, Teoh R, Laws D, Gleeson F. Pleural procedures and thoracic ultrasound: British Thoracic Society pleural disease guideline 2010. Thorax. 2010;65(Suppl 2):i61–76.
6. McElnay P, Lim E. Modern techniques to insert chest drains. Thorac Surg Clin. 2017;27(1):29–34.
7. Filosso P, Sandri A, Guerrera F, Roffinella M, Bora G, Solidoro P. Management of chest drains after thoracic resections. Thorac Surg Clin. 2017;27(1):7–11.
8. Sakakura N, Fukui T, Mori S, Hatooka S, Yokoi K, Mitsudomi T. Fluid drainage and air evacuation characteristics of Blake and conventional drains used after pulmonary resection. Ann Thorac Surg. 2009;87(5):1539–45.
9. Filosso P, Sandri A, Guerrera F, Ferraris A, Marchisio F, Bora G, et al. When size matters: changing opinion in the management of pleural space—the rise of small-bore pleural catheters. J Thorac Dis. 2016;8(7):E503–10.
10. Miller K, Sahn S. Chest tubes* indications, technique, management and complications. Chest. 1987;91(2):258–64.
11. Kim S, Khalpey Z, Daugherty S, Torabi M, Little A. Factors in the selection and management of chest tubes after pulmonary lobectomy:

results of a national survey of thoracic surgeons. Ann Thorac Surg. 2016;101(3):1082–8.

12. Alex J, Ansari J, Bahalkar P, Agarwala S, Ur Rehman M, Saleh A, et al. Comparison of the immediate postoperative outcome of using the conventional two drains versus a single drain after lobectomy. Ann Thorac Surg. 2003;76(4):1046–9.

13. Zhou D, Deng X, Liu Q, Chen Q, Min J, Dai J. Single chest tube drainage is superior to double chest tube drainage after lobectomy: a meta-analysis. J Cardiothorac Surg. 2016;11(1):88.

14. Brunelli A, Beretta E, Cassivi S, Cerfolio R, Detterbeck F, Kiefer T, et al. Consensus definitions to promote an evidence-based approach to management of the pleural space. A collaborative proposal by ESTS, AATS, STS, and GTSC. Eur J Cardiothorac Surg. 2011;40(2):291–7.

15. Pearson F, Patterson G. Pearson's thoracic & esophageal surgery. 1st ed. Philadelphia: Churchill Livingstone/Elsevier; 2008.

16. Terzi A, Feil B, Bonadiman C, Lonardoni A, Spilimbergo I, Pergher S, et al. The use of flexible spiral drains after non-cardiac thoracic surgery. A clinical study. Eur J Cardiothorac Surg. 2005;27(1):134–7.

17. Clark G, Licker M, Bertin D, Spiliopoulos A. Small size new silastic drains: life-threatening hypovolemic shock after thoracic surgery associated with a non-functioning chest tube. Eur J Cardiothorac Surg. 2007;31(3):566–8.

18. Gocyk W, Kużdżal J, Włodarczyk J, Grochowski Z, Gil T, Warmus J, et al. Comparison of suction versus nonsuction drainage after lung resections: a prospective randomized trial. Ann Thorac Surg. 2016;102(4):1119–24.

19. Cerfolio R, Bass C, Katholi C. Prospective randomized trial compares suction versus water seal for air leaks. Ann Thorac Surg. 2001;71(5):1613–7.

20. Le J, Buth K, Hirsch G, Légaré J. Does more than a single chest tube for mediastinal drainage affect outcomes after cardiac surgery? Can J Surg. 2015;58(2):100–6.

21. Davies H, Mishra E, Kahan B, Wrightson J, Stanton A, Guhan A, et al. Effect of an indwelling pleural catheter vs chest tube and talc pleurodesis for relieving dyspnea in patients with malignant pleural effusion. JAMA. 2012;307(22):2383.

22. PleurX™ Resources – BD [Internet]. Carefusion.com. 2017 [cited 22 April 2017]. Available from: http://www.carefusion.com/our-products/interventional-specialties/drainage/about-the-pleurx-drainage-system/pleurx-resources.

23. Warren W, Kim A, Liptay M. Identification of clinical factors predicting Pleurx® catheter removal in patients treated for malignant pleural effusion☆. Eur J Cardiothorac Surg. 2008;33(1):89–94.

24. Wahidi M, Reddy C, Yarmus L, Feller-Kopman D, Musani A, Shepherd R, et al. Randomized trial of pleural fluid drainage frequency in patients with malignant pleural effusions. The ASAP trial. Am J Respir Crit Care Med. 2017;195(8):1050–7.

25. Playfair. Reports of medical and surgical practice in the Hospitals of Great Britain. BMJ. 1875;2(769):396–7.

26. Kam A, O'Brien M, Kam P. Pleural drainage systems. Anaesthesia. 1993;48(2):154–61.

27. Henry M, Arnold T, Harvey J. BTS guidelines for the management of spontaneous pneumothorax. Thorax. 2003;58(Supplement 2):ii39–52.

28. Cerfolio R. Chest tube management after pulmonary resection. Chest Surg Clin N Am. 2002;12(3):507–27. Sargeant J, Hoffa J. Pleural Drainage System. US; 4,439,189, 1984.

29. Dernevik L, Belboul A, Rådberg G. Initial experience with the world's first digital drainage system. The benefits of recording air leaks with graphic representation. Eur J Cardiothorac Surg. 2007;31(2):209–13.

30. Cerfolio R, Bryant A. Results of a prospective algorithm to remove chest tubes after pulmonary resection with high output. J Thorac Cardiovasc Surg. 2008;135(2):269–73.

31. Brunelli A, Varela G, Refai M, Jimenez M, Pompili C, Sabbatini A, et al. A scoring system to predict the risk of prolonged air leak after lobectomy. Ann Thorac Surg. 2010;90(1):204–9.

32. Cerfolio R, Minnich D, Bryant A. The removal of chest tubes despite an air leak or a pneumothorax. Ann Thorac Surg. 2009;87(6):1690–6.

33. Mao M, Hughes R, Papadimos T, Stawicki S. Complications of chest tubes: a focused clinical synopsis. Curr Opin Pulm Med. 2015;21(4):376–86.

34. John M, Razi S, Sainathan S, Stavropoulos C. Is the trocar technique for tube thoracostomy safe in the current era?: Table 1. Interact Cardiovasc Thorac Surg. 2014;19(1):125–8.

35. Stawicki S, Sarani B, Braslow B. Reexpansion pulmonary edema. OPUS 12 Sci. 2008;2(2):29–31.

36. Chan L, Reilly K, Henderson C, Kahn F, Salluzzo R. Complication rates of tube thoracostomy. Am J Emerg Med. 1997;15(4):368–70.

37. Helling T, Gyles N, Eisenstein NC, Soracco C. Complications following blunt and penetrating injuries in 216 victims of chest trauma requiring tube thoracostomy. J Trauma Inj Infect Crit Care. 1989;29(10):1367–70.

38. Cerfolio R, Bryant A. The benefits of continuous and digital air leak assessment after elective pulmonary resection: a prospective study. Ann Thorac Surg. 2008;86(2):396–401.

39. Cerfolio R, Bryant A. The management of chest tubes after pulmonary resection. Thorac Surg Clin. 2010;20(3):399–405.

40. Bjerregaard L, Jensen K, Petersen R, Hansen H. Early chest tube removal after video-assisted thoracic surgery lobectomy with serous fluid production up to 500 ml/day. Eur J Cardiothorac Surg. 2013;45(2):241–6.

41. Cerfolio R, Bryant A, Skylizard L, Minnich D. Optimal technique for the removal of chest tubes after pulmonary resection. J Thorac Cardiovasc Surg. 2013;145(6):1535–9.

42. McCormick J, O'Mara M, Papasavas P, Caushaj P. The use of routine chest x-ray films after chest tube removal in postoperative cardiac patients. Ann Thorac Surg. 2002;74(6):2161–4.

43. Sepehripour A, Farid S, Shah R. Is routine chest radiography indicated following chest drain removal after cardiothoracic surgery? Interact Cardiovasc Thorac Surg. 2012;14(6):834–8.

44. Funk G, Petrey L, Foreman M. Clamping thoracostomy tubes: a heretical notion? Baylor Univ Med Proc. 2009;22(3):215–7.

45. Ali J, Qi W. Effectiveness of chest tube clamping in massive hemothorax. J Trauma Inj Infect Crit Care. 1995;38(1):59–63.

Pain Management After Thoracic Surgery

59

Stephen H. Pennefather, Clare Paula-Jo Quarterman, Rebecca Y. Klinger, and George W. Kanellakos

Abbreviations

AAGBI	Association of Anaesthetists of Great Britain and Ireland
ACTH	Adrenocorticotropic hormone
ADH	Antidiuretic hormone
ASRA	American Society of Regional Anesthesia and Pain Medicine
COX	Cyclooxygenase
ESA	European Society of Anaesthesiology
FEV$_1$	Forced expiratory volume in 1 second
FRC	Functional residual capacity
FVC	Forced vital capacity
HR	Heart rate
IL	Interleukin
IM	Intramuscular
IV	Intravenous
IV-PCA	Intravenous patient-controlled analgesia
NMDA	N-methyl-D-aspartate
NSAIDs	Nonsteroidal anti-inflammatory drugs
PFTs	Pulmonary function tests
TENS	Transcutaneous nerve stimulation
TNFα	Tumor necrosis factor alpha
V/Q	Ventilation/perfusion ratio
VATS	Video-assisted thoracoscopic surgery

Electronic Supplementary Material The online version of this chapter (https://doi.org/10.1007/978-3-030-00859-8_59) contains supplementary material, which is available to authorized users.

S. H. Pennefather
Department of Anesthesia, Liverpool Heart and Chest Hospital, Liverpool, Merseyside, UK

C. P.-J. Quarterman (✉)
Department of Anaesthesia, Liverpool Heart and Chest NHS Foundation Trust, Liverpool, Merseyside, UK
e-mail: clare.quarterman@lhch.nhs.uk

R. Y. Klinger
Department of Anesthesiology, Duke University Medical Center, Durham, NC, USA

G. W. Kanellakos
Department of Anesthesia, Pain Management & Perioperative Medicine, Dalhousie University, Halifax, NS, Canada

Key Points

- Thoracic surgery can cause significant pain and suffering. Poor pain relief can increase pulmonary complications and mortality.
- Pain after thoracic surgery is generated from multiple structures and is transmitted via a number of afferent pathways. Factors that affect pain postoperatively can be divided into patient factors, analgesic technique, and surgical approach.
- An aggressive multimodal analgesic strategy is advised to control the acute pain associated with thoracic surgery, allowing the clinician to minimize reliance on opioid-based drugs and the side effects they are associated with.
- Paravertebral catheters and thoracic epidural analgesia are widely used for thoracotomies and both have advantages and disadvantages. Recent studies suggest a similar quality of pain relief between the two approaches but a preferable side effect profile where paravertebral analgesia is utilized.
- Ultrasound guidance is increasingly used to guide paravertebral block and catheter placement. There are a number of approaches described.
- Serratus anterior and erector spinae plane blocks have recently been introduced as alternatives to traditional intercostal, epidural, and paravertebral regional anesthetic techniques for post-thoracotomy analgesia.
- Opioid-tolerant patients pose a particular challenge. Maintenance opioid should be continued perioperatively to avoid withdrawal symptoms. A multimodal technique involving regional blocks and supplemented with non-opioid analgesics is advised.

© Springer Nature Switzerland AG 2019
P. Slinger (ed.), *Principles and Practice of Anesthesia for Thoracic Surgery*, https://doi.org/10.1007/978-3-030-00859-8_59

Introduction

A posterolateral thoracotomy is among the most painful incisions, and thus unsurprisingly patients can, and sometimes do, suffer considerable pain in the postoperative period if analgesia is not managed appropriately [1]. Poorly treated post-thoracotomy pain greatly reduces patient satisfaction and quality of life, leads to longer hospitalization times, and is associated with greater costs [2].

The surgical wound is subject to continuous movement as the patient breathes and ventilation is adversely affected. Inspiration stretches the injured structures initiating a reflex contraction of the expiratory muscles. Splinting of the injured hemithorax occurs to limit the distraction of the injured structures. Similarly, the usually passive expiration becomes active. Thoracic surgery creates a restrictive pulmonary function pattern, leading to a reduction to approximately 40% of baseline measurements of forced vital capacity (FVC), forced expiratory volume in 1 s (FEV_1), and functional residual capacity (FRC). Where the FRC falls below the closing capacity, airway closure and atelectasis may develop with a consequent area of ventilation perfusion mismatch [3]. Deep inspiration is limited by pain; forced expiratory flow is thus further reduced and effective coughing impaired. Sputum clearance is often adversely affected. Inadequate pain control can also reduce the patient's ability to cooperate with postoperative physiotherapy and remobilization, all contributing to an increased incidence of hypoxemia. Acute pain is also associated with a significant increase in circulating catecholamine levels, catabolic hormone release, and overall sympathetic tone. This can lead to tachycardia, increased blood pressure, hyperglycemia, and raised serum lactate and is thought to therefore contribute to the increased risk of myocardial ischemia in the perioperative period [4–7] (Table 59.1).

Effective analgesia can reverse some of these changes and improve pulmonary function post-thoracotomy. There are, however, many other causes for the deterioration in pulmonary function that occurs post-thoracotomy. To date it has not been possible to determine with any accuracy the relative importance of pain in the etiology of this (Table 59.2).

Ultimately, it is advised that a multimodal approach to analgesia after thoracic surgery is considered for all patients. Multimodal analgesia, also frequently known as balanced analgesia, involves the use of more than one modality of pain control or class of drug in order to achieve a synergistic effect, while minimizing adverse effects [10].

Pathophysiology of Post-Thoracotomy Pain

The pathogenesis of post-thoracotomy pain is complex. Nociceptive receptors are stimulated by the skin incision, division and retraction of the muscles, and retraction and

Table 59.1 Consequences of inadequate acute pain control

System	Physiological change	Consequence
Pulmonary	Decreased lung compliance, atelectasis, hypoventilation and splinting, V/Q mismatch, reduced FRC	Hypoxia and hypercarbia
Cardiovascular	Increased HR, preload, afterload, and myocardial oxygen consumption	Increased risk of myocardial ischemia
Endocrine	Increased catecholamine, ACTH, aldosterone, ADH, angiotensin, and glucagon secretion	Free water retention, hyperglycemia, catabolic state
Hematological	Increased blood viscosity, platelet function, altered coagulation pathways, and fibrinolysis	Hypercoagulability, increased risk of thromboembolism, and thromboembolic events
Immunological	Impaired cell-mediated immune function	Increased risk of infection
Gastrointestinal	Reduced gastric emptying and gut motility	Nausea, vomiting, ileus
Urological	Increased sympathetic outflow	Urinary retention

Reproduced with permission, Doan et al. [8]

Table 59.2 Causes for deterioration in pulmonary function post-thoracotomy

Lung tissue resection
Hemorrhage and edema in residual lung tissue
Distortion in bronchial architecture with resultant lobar collapse
Gastric and abdominal distension
Increased airway resistance
Impaired mucociliary clearance
Residual effects of anesthesia
Pain-related changes in lung mechanics
Diaphragmatic dysfunction

Reproduced with permission, Pennefather and Russell [9]

sometimes fracture of ribs. In addition, ligaments may be stretched, costochondral joints dislocated, and intercostal nerves injured, causing further pain. The incised pleura are frequently irritated by partial surgical stripping, chest drains, and residual pleural blood; the resulting inflammatory responses activate further nociceptors. The central transmission of these multiple nociceptive signals amplifies pain transmission and increases pain perception through central sensitization (Fig. 59.1).

There are a number of mechanisms for transmitting pain generated post-thoracotomy to the sensorium. Stimuli from the chest wall and costal and peripheral diaphragmatic pleura are transmitted via the intercostal nerves. The phrenic nerve supplies sensory branches to the mediastinal

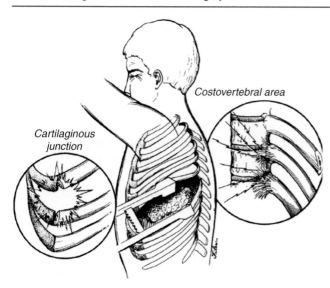

Fig. 59.1 Sites of thoracotomy incisional trauma. Direct injury to ribs and neurovascular intercostal bundles along with injuries to anterior and posterior intercostal articulations during a thoracotomy. (Reproduced with permission, Landreneau et al. [11])

Table 59.3 Components of a clinical pathway for acute pain management

Preoperative
Staff education
Patient education
Optimize outpatient analgesic
Identify potentially challenging patients during preoperative assessment
Day of surgery and intraoperative
Patient education
Multimodal analgesic approach
Postoperative
Prompt commencement of regional infusions
Regular non-opioid analgesia
Use of rescue analgesia on a PRN basis
Protocolized early mobilization and physiotherapy

Reproduced with permission, Doan et al. [8]

pleura, fibrous pericardium, parietal layer of the serous pericardium, and diaphragmatic dome pleura. In addition, the vagus nerve contains somatic and visceral afferent nerve fibers, and blockade of the vagus nerve has been advocated during thoracic surgery [12]. The sympathetic nerves may play a role in transmitting pain from the lung and mediastinum. It has been suggested that stretching of the brachial plexuses and distraction of the shoulder contributes to the generation of ipsilateral shoulder pain in some patients [13].

Factors Influencing Pain After Thoracic Surgery

Preoperative Preparedness and Use of Perioperative Clinical Pathways

Well-informed patients may experience less pain [14], so patients should receive a full explanation of the proposed analgesic technique and its likely effects, including its limitations, potential side effects, and complications. Patients can also be educated regarding how to deal with pain postoperatively [15]. Enhanced recovery programs consist of a series of perioperative interventions, often presented in the form of a patient pathway, that together aim to reduce the impact of surgery on the patient. Through a reduction in the incidence of complications and by encouraging a return to normal function as soon as possible, the patient and institution benefit in terms of improved patient satisfaction and reduced length of hospital stay [16, 17]. Pain management is an integral part of an enhanced recovery pathway and has

been considered in terms of preoperative day of surgery and postoperative components (Table 59.3). The preoperative component of this includes education of staff regarding the importance of good pain management, education of patients regarding their expectations surrounding pain and pain control, optimizing patients with preexisting pain issues, and identifying patients in whom pain control perioperatively may be more challenging, requiring early input and support from a multidisciplinary acute pain team [8]. One study showed that where preoperative pain management education was provided, there was a lower rate of analgesic consumption [15]. Education programs included instruction on pain and management methods and advice on how to express feelings and concerns and on the importance of anxiety control.

Opioid Tolerance

Opioid-tolerant patients presenting for thoracic surgery include patients with malignant diseases receiving opioids for pain, a rapidly increasing group of patients with nonmalignant disease receiving opioids chronically for pain management, opioid-dependent substance abusers, and former addicts on long-term maintenance programs. There is some evidence to suggest that the use of a strong opioid for just 2 weeks may precipitate an increased opioid requirement during the perioperative period [18]. Achieving good postoperative analgesia in patients who are chronically receiving opioids is frequently difficult. There is evidence to suggest that opioid-tolerant patients have longer hospital admissions and a higher all-cause 30-day readmission rate [19]. This group of patients may experience more postoperative pain, manifesting as higher pain scores that take a longer to fall postoperatively. Patients should, when practical, be involved in the plans for their postoperative pain management, and their care should be individualized.

Preemptive Analgesia

The concept of preemptive analgesia was first suggested by Crile [20] although modern clinical interest is largely the result of basic science research done by Woolf [21]. Preemptive analgesia is antinociceptive treatment started before the noxious stimulus that aims to prevent the establishment of altered central processing of sensory input that amplifies postoperative pain [22]. Preemptive analgesia aims to decrease acute postoperative pain, even after the analgesic effects of the preemptive drugs have worn off, and to inhibit the development of chronic postoperative pain. Potential candidates for patients undergoing a thoracotomy include pre-incisional thoracic epidurals, paravertebral blocks, NMDA antagonists, gabapentin, and systemic opioids. Although the results of clinical studies to support the concept of initiating the pain treatment prior to the injury are conflicting, there is widespread belief in the concept among clinicians. A 2002 systematic review of preemptive analgesia for postoperative pain relief found no evidence of benefit for the preemptive administration of systemic opioids, nonsteroidal anti-inflammatory drugs (NSAIDs), or ketamine and little evidence of benefit with continuous epidural analgesia [23]. A 2005 systemic review on the impact of preemptive epidural analgesia on pain after thoracotomy concluded that preemptive thoracic epidural analgesia was associated with a reduction in acute pain but no reduction in chronic post-thoracotomy pain [24].

Sex

A considerable amount of work has been undertaken in an attempt to determine the influence of the sex of the patient on the pain experienced after surgery. Female patients report pain to be more severe, frequent, and diffuse than male patients with similar disease processes [25]. A meta-analysis of the influence of sex differences in the perception of noxious experimental stimuli found that females were less tolerant of noxious stimuli than males [26]. The difference in pain perception between males and females decreases with age [27, 28], has not been found by all investigators, and is usually only moderately large. Social gender roles have a significant influence on pain tolerance levels [28], are sometimes difficult to differentiate from the sex of the patient, and may account for some of the differences in pain tolerance between the sexes. Coping strategies also influence patient's pain tolerance; catastrophizing is associated with an increased sensitivity to experimental pain [29]. Women are more likely to catastrophize and this may help account for the differences in pain tolerance between the sexes [30]. Anesthetists should be aware of the different responses male and female patients have to pain but as yet no specific recommendation with respect to treatment can be made.

Age

A recent systematic review found young age to be a significant predictor of postoperative pain [31]. The pharmacokinetics of analgesic drugs can be affected by aging, and the elderly are considered to be more sensitive to systemic opioids [32]. Similarly, there is a positive correlation between age and thoracic epidural spread with elderly patients requiring about 40% less epidural solution [33, 34]. It has also been suggested that age blunts peripheral nociceptive function decreasing pain in some contexts [35] although this is not the experience of at least one aging author.

Psychological Factors

Pain is a sensory and emotional experience and thus is influenced by psychological factors. It has been suggested that anxiety lowers pain thresholds [36]. Preoperative anxiety has been shown to be a predictor of more severe postoperative pain in studies of patients undergoing a variety of surgeries including thoracic surgery [31, 37]. Good preoperative communication with the patient and the development of rapport will facilitate reducing the anxiety by reassurance and, if appropriate, anxiolytics [31]. A depressive mood preoperatively [38] and neuroticism [39] have also been found to be predictors of more severe postoperative pain. There may be a relationship between preoperative depression and the development of chronic pain [40]. Cognitive factors can also influence pain perception. Catastrophizing, a multidimensional construct with elements of rumination, magnification, and helplessness, has emerged as one of the most reliable predictors of heightened pain experience [29]. Cognitive behavioral strategies may have a role in managing patients who catastrophize about pain [31].

Surgical Approach

Sternotomy

The sternum is usually internally fixed with steel wire after a sternotomy. Bone movement during respiration is thus minimal and the postoperative pain usually only moderate. However, wide or inexpert distraction of the sternum may fracture the sternum and strain or even disrupt the anterior or posterior intercostal articulations with the potential to considerably increase the postoperative pain experienced.

Video-Assisted Thoracoscopic Surgery

With video-assisted thoracoscopic (VAT) surgery, the extent of the surgical incision is limited, and early postoperative pain can be reduced [41] when compared to thoracotomy. These benefits may be reduced by the use of larger-diameter instruments, multiple ports, and/or the twisting of surgical instruments against the ribs causing injury to the intercostal nerves and bruising or even fracturing of the ribs. This approach is therefore still associated with significant postoperative pain and, with this, impairment of respiratory function with associated respiratory complications. There is also a similar incidence in the development of chronic postsurgical pain. Control of acute pain in this surgical group should therefore not be overlooked or underestimated [8].

Open Thoracotomy

Posterolateral Incision

Posterolateral incision is the classic approach to a thoracotomy as it provides good surgical access and can easily be extended if required. It does, however, involve the cutting of some of the major chest wall muscles and is considered one of the most painful surgical incisions. There is some evidence that internal fixation of divided ribs reduces postoperative pain [42].

Muscle-Sparing Incision

Many surgeons now use one or more of the many muscle-sparing incisions that have been described. A popular approach is the axillary muscle-sparing incision, the skin incision for which extends vertically downward from the axilla with obvious cosmetic advantages. Although muscle-sparing incisions were initially reported to produce less perioperative pain [43–45], most studies have not supported this [46, 47]. Muscle-sparing incisions may result in less chronic post-thoracotomy pain [48] particularly where techniques involve free dissection of the costal nerve bundle to

avoid injury through the use of retractors [49]. Wider rib retraction is frequently required for muscle-sparing thoracotomies to compensate for the reduced field of view [47]. Wider retraction may increase the risk of rib fractures, distraction of the posterior costovertebral joints, and damage to the intercostal nerves, all of which can increase post-thoracotomy pain.

Anterior Incision

Anterior incisions are used to provide access for some cardiac and anterior mediastinal procedures. Exposure for lung surgery is, however, limited particularly on the left because of the heart. Rib resections are frequently performed with this incision to improve surgical access. Postoperative pain depends in part on the extent of the excision and the extent of surgical retraction but is similar to that after a posterolateral thoracotomy. Intercostal nerve blocks are particularly effective with this approach because the incision does not involve any part of the chest supplied by the posterior cutaneous nerves which arise from the dorsal rami and are not blocked by an intercostal nerve block.

Transverse Sternothoracotomy

Transverse sternothoracotomy (clamshell) incisions (Fig. 59.2) provide excellent surgical exposure of both chest cavities and the mediastinum and were in the past used for cardiac surgery. This incision results in significant postoperative pain, and its use is now largely limited to lung transplantation, complex cardiopulmonary surgery, and complex mediastinal tumors [50]. Postoperative pain control can be challenging with this incision.

Fig. 59.2 Schematic view of a clamshell incision. (Reproduced with permission, Macchiarini et al. [50])

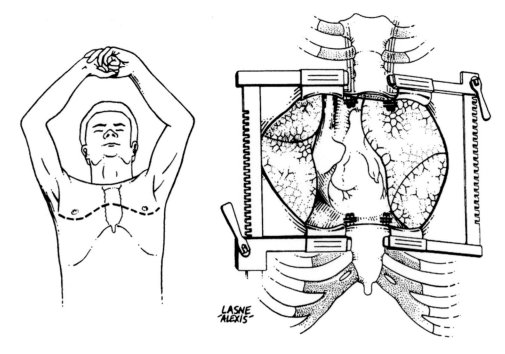

LASNE ALEXIS

Analgesic Drugs and Techniques

The afferent signaling leading to the perception of pain is complex, and therefore there are numerous potential targets that can be pursued to achieve adequate analgesia (Fig. 59.3). By targeting more than one pathway simultaneously, there can be a synergistic effect and better quality analgesia.

Acute post-thoracotomy pain management aims to reduce the patient's pain as much as possible but to do so safely. In practice, most patients undergoing thoracic surgery can be safely and effectively managed using a multimodal approach including thoracic epidural analgesia, paravertebral blocks, or systemic opioids supplemented when appropriate by other systemic analgesics.

Systemic Opioids

Systemic opioids were used in the past as the mainstay of post-thoracotomy analgesia; however, the pain control achieved was often poor and frequently accompanied by a range of detrimental side effects including respiratory depression, nausea, vomiting, constipation, and changes in cognition [8]. It is now appreciated that for open thoracotomies, systemic opioids are best administered as part of a multimodal strategy including a regional technique.

Titration of systemic opioids post-thoracotomy is needed if the balance between the beneficial effects and detrimental effects is to be achieved. In comparison to IM opioids, IV-PCA systems provide superior analgesia [52] and improve patient satisfaction [53]. In part this is because IV-PCA systems accommodate patient variation in postoperative opioid requirement [54], the halving of opioid requirements approximately every 24 h postoperatively [55], and the small group of patients that experience minimal postsurgery pain [1]. Several studies support the view that regional techniques are superior to systemic analgesia alone. A meta-analysis published in 1998 found that compared to systemic opioids, epidural local anesthetic significantly reduced the incidence of pulmonary complications after surgery [56] and patients undergoing thoracotomy with IV-PCA have been shown to have a lower FVC and FEV_1 postoperatively when compared with thoracic epidural [57]. This finding was not, however, supported by a systematic review published in 2008 [58], potentially because of improvements in the administration of systemic opioids in later studies included in the second review. Studies have suggested that acute exposure to opioids can lead to the development of acute opioid tolerance in patients previously opioid naïve [59]. Exposure to higher doses of opioids intraoperatively has been associated with increased postoperative pain, as demonstrated by a higher opioid requirement [60].

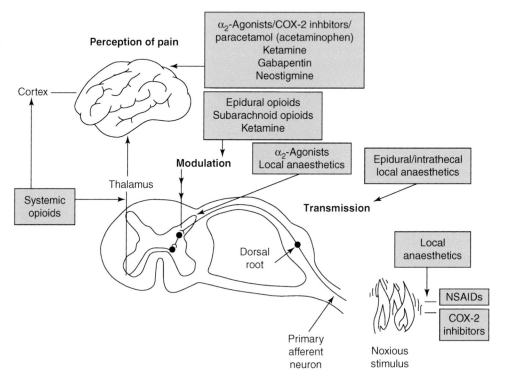

Fig. 59.3 Action of analgesics at various sites of the pain pathway. COX = cyclooxygenase. (Reproduced with permission, Pyati and Gan [51])

Non-opioid Analgesic Drugs

Nonsteroidal Anti-inflammatory Drugs

Prostaglandins have a role in pain perception. NSAIDs block the synthesis of prostaglandins by inhibiting the enzyme cyclooxygenase (COX). NSAIDs reduce the inflammatory response to surgical trauma, have a peripheral non-prostaglandin analgesic effect [61], and act centrally [62] in part by inhibiting prostaglandin synthesis in the spinal cord [63]. The side effects of NSAIDs are well known and include gastrointestinal mucosal damage [64] and renal tubular and platelet dysfunction [65]. The amount, if any, of NSAID-mediated increased bleeding after thoracotomy has not been established, although studies after tonsillectomy suggest that the increased bleeding is probably minimal [66]. In normal adults the risk of renal toxicity secondary to NSAIDs is estimated to be between 1:1000 and 1:10,000 [67]. Patients particularly at risk, however, include elderly patients undergoing major surgery [68, 69], patients with preexisting renal failure, and hypovolemic patients as they are more dependent upon the vasodilatory effects of prostaglandins to ensure maintenance of effective renal perfusion [70]. These risk factors are often present in patients scheduled for thoracic surgery. There is a concern that NSAID-mediated reductions in inflammation may reduce the efficacy of a surgically performed pleurodesis. For more than 25 years, NSAIDs have been used to control post-thoracotomy pain [71]. NSAIDs have been shown to significantly improve pain control in patients receiving systemic opioids post-thoracotomy [72, 73]. For patients receiving thoracic epidural analgesia post-thoracotomy, there is conflicting evidence for the benefit of NSAIDs. Early studies did not show a significant reduction in pain scores in [74]. Latter studies with COX-2 inhibitors did show significantly reduced pain scores [75, 76]. NSAIDs may be effective in controlling the ipsilateral shoulder pain post-thoracotomy in patients receiving thoracic epidural analgesia [77, 78], although research in this area has been limited.

COX-2 Inhibitors

Different isoenzymes of the cyclooxygenase enzyme exist including COX-1 and COX-2 [79]. The COX-1 isoenzyme has physiological functions, while the COX-2 isoenzyme is induced during inflammation. NSAIDs vary in their selectivity for inhibiting these cyclooxygenase isoenzymes. Some are selective cyclooxygenase 2 inhibitors and are termed COX-2 inhibitors. These agents have a lower risk of causing serious upper gastrointestinal side effects and cause less platelet inhibition than the nonselective NSAIDs. There is some evidence that COX-2 inhibitors may limit the develop-

ment of acute opioid tolerance [80]. Senard et al. [75] found significantly reduced pain scores at rest and during coughing and improved patient satisfaction where thoracic epidural was combined with the COX-2 inhibitor celecoxib.

There are concerns about the detrimental effects of COX-2 inhibitors and NSAIDs on bone growth [81, 82]. In 2004/2005, two COX-2 inhibitors (rofecoxib and valdecoxib) were withdrawn because of concerns that there was an increased risk of cardiovascular thrombotic complications when these agents were taken daily for long periods. Subsequent studies support this finding as being a COX-2 and nonselective NSAID class effect [83, 84] likely due to the vasoconstrictive and pro-thrombotic effects associated with COX-2 inhibition and reduced prostacyclin production [70]. Caution is required if these drugs are to be administered regularly over long periods. The safety of COX-2 inhibitors in the perioperative setting is controversial. For patients undergoing CABG on cardiopulmonary bypass, there is an increased risk of cardiovascular thrombotic events in patients receiving the selective COX-2 inhibitors parecoxib and valdecoxib [85, 86]. A study of a variety of non-cardiac surgical procedures including thoracic surgery did not show an increased incidence of cardiovascular thrombotic events in patients receiving the same selective COX-2 inhibitors [87]. The cardiovascular risk between agents varies, for example, the NSAID naproxen has a lower cardiovascular risk profile than diclofenac [88]. Intravenous parecoxib 40 mg, administered preoperatively then every 12 h for 3 days following surgery in addition to patient-controlled epidural analgesia (PCEA), has been associated with significantly reduced pain scores at rest and after coughing, along with a suggestion of a reduced incidence of chronic pain, although further studies are required to confirm this [76]. Intravenous parecoxib administered in addition to paravertebral infusion with ropivacaine has shown similar positive results [89]. The level of cardiovascular risk associated with the short-term perioperative use of COX-2 and NSAIDs remains controversial. For individual patients, their cardiovascular risk factors and the risks of alternative drugs or analgesic techniques need to be considered.

Acetaminophen

Acetaminophen, perhaps the safest of the non-opioid analgesic agents, acts centrally by inhibiting prostaglandin synthesis potentially through weak COX-2 and COX-3 suppression [70, 90] and possibly via the serotoninergic system [91]. Acetaminophen may also have peripheral anti-inflammatory actions [92]. Acetaminophen can be administered through several routes, orally, rectally, and more recently intravenously. The intravenous preparation is significantly more costly to administer than via the oral or rectal route. Use of intravenous acetaminophen following median sternotomy for cardiac surgery was associated with reduced pain scores, but not opioid consumption [93]. Propacetamol, a prodrug that is hydrolyzed to acetaminophen by plasma esterases, can be administered intravenously and has been shown to decrease morphine consumption after spinal [94] and cardiac surgery [95] although a reduction in morphine consumption after cardiac surgery was not shown in an earlier study, possibly because of the methodology [96]. The recent Cochrane review [97] found that a single dose of intravenous paracetamol or propacetamol provided 4 h of effective analgesia in significantly more patients than placebo. A meta-analysis found that after major surgery, adding acetaminophen to morphine PCA reduced the morphine consumption by 20% but did not decrease the incidence of morphine-related adverse effects [98] (Fig. 59.4).

More recently, the clinical effectiveness of orally versus intravenously administered acetaminophen have been compared. Following major joint surgery, a first perioperative intravenous dose of acetaminophen has been associated with improved pain scores in the first 4 h after surgery compared to oral administration. At all time periods after this, there was no difference in the effectiveness of the oral or intravenous preparation in terms of pain score or opioid consumption [99]. Regular rectal acetaminophen has been shown to reduce the severity of ipsilateral post-thoracotomy shoulder pain [100]. When administered rectally the dosage should exceed the oral dose by 50%, and account should be taken of its slower onset [101]. There is some evidence that the effects of acetaminophen and NSAIDs are additive [102, 103]. Unlike NSAIDs and COX-2 inhibitors, acetaminophen at clinical doses has few contraindications or side effects. It is considered safe for patients at risk of renal failure [101]. Acetaminophen is frequently administered post-thoracotomy [104].

NMDA Antagonists

The involvement of glutamate, an excitatory neurotransmitter acting via the N-methyl-D-aspartate (NMDA) receptor, in nociception makes this an attractive target for both acute and chronic pain management strategies. Activation of the NMDA glutamate receptor has been heavily implicated in the process of central sensitization, also known as "wind up," which has then been linked to the transition from acute to chronic pain and the states of hyperalgesia and allodynia [105]. Ketamine, an anesthetic with analgesic properties, is a noncompetitive antagonist of the phencyclidine site of the NMDA receptor but additionally has been demonstrated to display some anti-inflammatory and anti-hyperalgesic properties. In recent years, there has been renewed interest in the use of small doses of ketamine as an adjuvant to postoperative analgesia. NMDA receptor antagonists enhance opioid-induced analgesia and can limit the development of opioid tolerance and opioid-induced hyperalgesia [105–107]. Small doses of ketamine have been shown to have opioid-sparing effects after abdominal surgery [108], but results after thoracic surgery are dependent upon the other modalities of analgesia utilized. A meta-analysis [109] assessing the effectiveness of IV-PCA morphine with the addition of ketamine concluded this to be a safe technique associated with improved pain scores, reduced morphine consumption, and potentially an improvement in respiratory function, as demonstrated by one double-blind study suggesting an improved early postoperative FEV_1 [110]. Where ketamine was administered as a single IV dose at induction of anesthesia, there was evidence of reduced opiate requirement for 48 h postoperatively [111]. Where ketamine infusion has been used perioperatively and for the first 24 h postoperatively, pain control in the immediate postoperative period was improved but with no impact upon the incidence of chronic post-thoracotomy pain [112]. The incidence of hallucinations associated with intravenous ketamine is low. One study involving a ketamine/morphine IV-PCA within the general surgical population reported an incidence of hallucinations of 6.2%, with half of these patients requiring dose reduction or cessation of treatment [113]. In all cases where treatment was stopped, hallucinations resolved within 1–2 h.

Use of IV or epidural ketamine as an adjunct to epidural analgesia has also been considered. While one group found that adding a low-dose IV infusion of ketamine to thoracic

Study or sub-category	N	Treatment Mean (SD)	N	Control Mean (SD)	VVMD (random) 95% CI	Weight %	VVMD (random) 95% CI
Fletcher 1997	15	30.00 (4.00)	15	33.00 (3.00)		24.39	−3.00 (−5.53, −0.47)
Hernandez 2001	21	22.00 (10.00)	21	41.00 (10.00)		20.23	−19.00 (−25.05, −12.95)
Mimoz 2001	38	36.00 (22.00)	38	45.00 (19.00)		15.86	−9.00 (−18.24, 0.24)
Peduto 1998	42	12.10 (9.90)	47	20.10 (12.80)		22.00	−8.00 (−12.73, −3.27)
Schug 1998	28	50.28 (40.10)	33	59.49 (42.30)		6.29	−9.21 (−29.92, 11.50)
Siddik 2001	20	61.10 (23.00)	20	66.70 (20.00)		11.23	−5.60 (−18.96, 7.76)
Total (95% CI)	164		174			100.00	−8.97 (−14.95, −2.99)

Test for heterogeneity: Chi^2 = 24.33, df = 5 (P = 0.0002), I^2 = 79.4%
Test for overall effect: Z = 2.94 (P = 0.003)

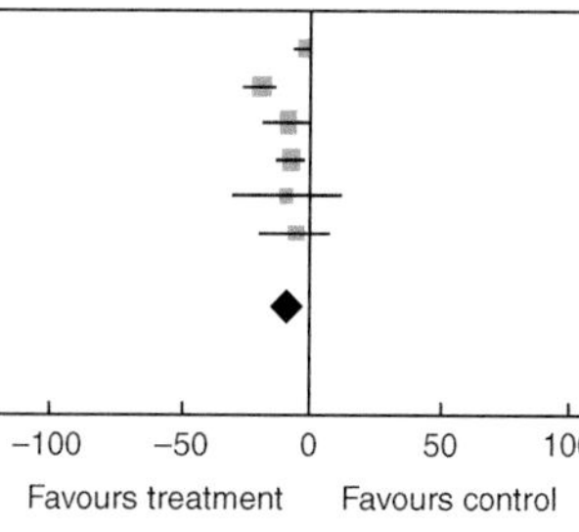

−100   −50   0   50   100
Favours treatment   Favours control

Fig. 59.4 Effect of acetaminophen on postoperative morphine consumption during the first 24 h after major surgery. (Reproduced with permission, Remy et al. [98])

epidural analgesia improved early post-thoracotomy analgesia [114], this finding has not been reproduced more recently
by other groups who found no difference [115, 116], although
the quality of analgesia produced by effective thoracic epidurals in these studies may negate the additional impact of
ketamine. Both the IV and epidural routes of administration
have been shown to be of benefit in the management of postoperative pain, but with no significant differences in efficacy
between the two routes [105]. Ultimately, the literature
appears to support a benefit for postoperative use of ketamine
in some patients, particularly those without a thoracic epidural or chronically receiving high-dose opioids. Side effects
of ketamine include increased secretions and dysphoria,
although the use in low doses is generally well tolerated. At
the authors' institution, ketamine is sometimes administered
either by infusion or orally where analgesia with more conventional means proves challenging (Table 59.4).

Gabapentinoids

Gabapentin, 1-(aminomethyl)cyclohexane acetic acid, is an
anticonvulsant drug that is effective in treating neuropathic
pain [125] and postherpetic neuralgia [126]. Gabapentin
may act through a number of mechanisms. The most likely
site of its antinociceptor effect is thought to be by binding to
the $\alpha_2\delta$ subunit of voltage-dependent calcium channels
[127]. The absorption of gabapentin is dose dependent.
There is some evidence that gabapentin reduces early postoperative pain scores and reduces opioid consumption in the
first 24 h for patients undergoing a variety of surgical procedures [123, 128]. Gabapentin has been administered as a
single preoperative oral dose ranging from 300 to 1200 mg
and as multiple perioperative doses [122]. A single preoperative dose of gabapentin 600 mg in conjunction with epidural analgesia had no impact upon acute pain experienced
postoperatively or the incidence of chronic pain 3 months
later [129]. Administration of gabapentin as a preoperative
1200 mg bolus dose followed postoperatively by 600 mg
12-hourly in conjunction with IV-PCA led to improved
analgesia, lower morphine consumption, and improvement
in postoperative pulmonary function [130]. In a placebo-
controlled study, gabapentin did not decrease ipsilateral
shoulder pain in patients receiving thoracic epidural analgesia [131]. Overall evidence currently suggests that gabapentin, if used, should be administered as a multidose regime
over the perioperative period rather than a single preoperative dose [123, 124], but more studies to ascertain the most
efficacious dose and duration of treatment are required.
Gabapentin is sedative and anxiolytic [132], and therefore
the doses of other premedication drugs used should be
adjusted accordingly, and the risk of postoperative sedation
should not be overlooked.

Table 59.4 Adult analgesic regimes

Technique	Dose	Comment
Paravertebrals		
Lower-dose regime		
Loading dose	0.3 mL kg^{-1} 0.25% levobupivacaine	Higher-dose regime produces improved analgesia and pulmonary function [117]
Maintenance	0.1 mL kg^{-1} h^{-1} 0.25% levobupivacaine	
High-dose regime		
Loading dose	20 mL 0.5% levobupivacaine	
Maintenance	0.1 mL kg^{-1} h^{-1} 0.5% levobupivacaine	
Intrathecal opioids	Morphine 200 µg + sufentanil 20 µg [118] or morphine 500 µg + sufentanil 50 µg [119]	
Thoracic epidural		
Levobupivacaine Or	0.1%	Titrate to effect
Ropivacaine	0.15%	Reduce rate by 40% for elderly
with		
Fentanyl	4–5 µg mL^{-1} or	
Sufentanil	1 µg mL^{-1} or	
Hydromorphine	10–25 µg mL^{-1} [120]	
Bolus	7 mL	
Infusion	7 mL h^{-1}	
Intercostal nerve blocks		
Injection sites T3–T7	0.25% Levobupivacaine with epinephrine 1:200,000 3–5 mL per site	Use repeated doses or continuous infusion [58]. Associated with rapid absorption of local anesthetic
Ketamine		
For intravenous supplementation of epidural analgesia	0.05 mg kg^{-1} h^{-1} [114]	
Without epidural analgesia		
Bolus	0.25–0.5 mg kg^{-1} [[121], authors' institution]	
Infusion Oral	1–6 µg kg^{-1} min^{-1} continued for few days [[121], authors' institution] 10 mg TDS, titrated to 25 mg TDS according to effect [author's institution]	
Gabapentin	300–1200 mg orally 1–2 h preoperatively [122] followed by 100–300 mg OD to TDS titrated according to effect [author's institution]	Where gabapentin is used, it is recommended as part of a multidose regime over the perioperative period, not solely preoperatively [123, 124]

Pregabalin is a structural analogue of γ-aminobutyric acid and probably acts via the same mechanism as gabapentin to exert an anticonvulsant, anti-hyperalgesic, and anxiolytic effect more potent than that of gabapentin [133]. Meta-analyses [133, 134] and reviews [135, 136] revealed the considerable heterogeneity of the patient populations studied, dosing regime, and timing of administration in the trials. Possibly as a consequence, pain intensity was not consistently altered. Many studies involved surgeries in which low pain severity would be expected and therefore whether pregabalin would significantly reduce the pain associated with thoracic surgery is not clear [135]. Two studies, one using a single preoperative dose of pregabalin [137] and the second using a single preoperative dose followed by twice daily dosing for 2 postoperative days in patients undergoing coronary artery bypass grafting [138], suggested a reduction in postoperative pain scores. There is a suggestion of a lower incidence of nausea and vomiting where pregabalin is used, but a greater incidence of visual disturbance, dizziness, headache, and sedation. More studies addressing use of pregabalin following thoracic surgery are required in order to make any recommendation.

α₂ Adrenergic Agonists

Clonidine and dexmedetomidine are α_2 adrenergic receptor agonists that have an analgesic effect without concomitant respiratory depression, although they do cause central sedation, an effect for which they are more frequently prescribed in the intensive care unit [139]. They have been shown to reduce sympathetically mediated pain but are also associated with hypotension and bradycardia – clonidine to a greater degree than dexmedetomidine [140]. IV dexmedetomidine 4 mcg kg^{-1} added to sufentanil IV-PCA led to a significant improvement in pain scores at rest and during coughing for the first 48 h after surgery, with lower sufentanil requirement and greater patient satisfaction in the group receiving dexmedetomidine [141]. Comparison of clonidine administered as a single intravenous bolus dose of 3 mcg kg^{-1} prior to induction of anesthesia with placebo demonstrated a reduction in pain scores in the immediate postoperative period in the clonidine group and a reduced fentanyl requirement over the first 24 h, but the study period did not extend beyond this [142]. There is limited data on the usage of α_2 adrenergic receptor agonists during thoracic surgery, but the studies conducted so far suggest that there may be a benefit, particularly in patients that are unable to undergo regional analgesic techniques or are already taking large doses of opioid medications. The additional sedating effects and propensity to hypotension and bradycardia, although not recorded as causing significant adverse effects in the studies discussed, should not be overlooked.

Glucocorticoids

Thoracotomy induces a significant pro-inflammatory response, with marked increases in pro-inflammatory mediators including IL-6 and IL-8 that correlate positively with the extent of dynamic pain experienced by the patient [143]. Glucocorticoids have many actions including analgesic, anti-emetic, antipyretic, and anti-inflammatory effects. Reduced prostaglandin production by the inhibition of phospholipase and COX-2 isoenzymes is believed to be the major pathway for the analgesic effect. There is also some evidence that administration decreases presynaptic release of neurotransmitters and causes production of kynurenic acid, an NMDA antagonist [144, 145]. Dexamethasone is a soluble glucocorticoid and has been shown to produce a dose-dependent opioid-sparing effect [146] in a general surgical setting and has been particularly effective in reducing pain scores with dynamic movement [147, 148]. The onset of analgesia is slower than traditional analgesics but appears to last longer and has been reported to last for up to 7 days [149]. Although these effects have been produced with a single dose of dexamethasone within the range of 10–40 mg with few reported serious side effects, more recent studies have shown similar effectiveness with smaller doses. Dexamethasone has also been suggested as an effective adjunct to prolong the duration of peripheral nerve blocks for orthopedic surgery [150] and paravertebral blocks for nephrectomy [151]. The use of both 8 mg of IV and 4 mg of perineural dexamethasone significantly prolonged the duration of intercostal nerve blocks used for VATS surgery and led to improved pain scores at 24 h [152]. The data also suggested reduced pain scores, reduced opioid consumption, and better PFTs where more than one route of administration was used. No trials reported any adverse outcomes related to the perineural administration of dexamethasone although, in animal models, high doses have been associated with neuronal cell death [153]. Risks of glucocorticoid use include gastric irritation, impaired wound healing, impaired glucose homeostasis, and sodium retention. The optimal dose that balances the advantages against these, and other, risks has yet to be defined, and further research, particularly in the setting of thoracic surgery, is required. If there are no contraindications to glucocorticoid use, selected patients may benefit from a single 8–16 mg dose of dexamethasone as part of a multimodal analgesia regime.

Non-pharmacologic Techniques

Transcutaneous Nerve Stimulation

Transcutaneous nerve stimulation (TENS) was developed to utilize the gate theory to reduce pain [154] via modulation of nociceptive signals from the spinal cord and the release of endogenous opioids [155]. Patients treated with TENS have also been found to have significantly reduced levels of circulating inflammatory cytokines IL-6, IL-8, and TNFα [156]. An initial meta-analysis published in 1996 of the effectiveness of TENS in acute postoperative pain found little evidence for effectiveness in adequately randomized studies [157]. In contrast, TENS was considered by the original authors to be effective in most of the nonrandomized studies analyzed [157]. A more recent meta-analysis [158] of 11 randomized controlled trials assessing of the use of TENS in patients undergoing thoracotomy concluded that, when compared to placebo, TENS did effectively modulate pain when combined with other pharmacological methods and was associated with an improvement in FVC. TENS therefore appears to be a safe and effective complementary analgesic technique, but only in the context of a primarily pharmacological approach.

Cryoanalgesia

While the chest is open, the intercostal nerves can be blocked transiently from 1 to 4 days or even for up to 6 months in some cases by the application of a cryoprobe. The analgesia is inferior to thoracic epidural fentanyl [159] and the technique is associated with an increased incidence of chronic post-thoracotomy pain [160]. Cryoanalgesia is now rarely used to provide post-thoracotomy analgesia and cannot be recommended.

Regional Techniques

Over the years, a large number of regional techniques, and drugs to deliver via these regional techniques, have been developed and used to control post-thoracotomy pain. Unfortunately, no technique has emerged that is safe, effective, and applicable to all patients. Until the early 1980s, systemic opioids formed the mainstay of post-thoracotomy analgesia in the West. Thoracic epidurals were introduced into clinical practice for post-thoracotomy analgesia in the mid-1970s [161, 162] and had become the gold standard of post-thoracotomy analgesia by the mid-1990s [163]. Somatic paravertebral blocks are now gaining acceptance as an alternative method for providing post-thoracotomy analgesia. A number of factors have led to the increased use of somatic paravertebral blocks. The risks associated with the perioperative use of epidural analgesia are becoming clearer and are perhaps greater than previously thought [164, 165]. More patients are presenting for thoracic surgery on multiple antiplatelet agents sometimes with intracoronary stents in situ. While dual antiplatelet therapy is known to be a contraindi-

cation to thoracic epidural analgesia [166], the risk of discontinuing antiplatelet agents perioperatively is now quantifiable [167–169].

There are an ever-increasing number of studies comparing effectiveness of, and outcomes after, thoracic epidural analgesia or paravertebral block. The Cochrane review [170], published in 2016, comparing paravertebral block and thoracic epidural analgesia concluded that paravertebral blockade was as effective as thoracic epidural in controlling acute pain, both at rest and after coughing or physiotherapy for at least the first 48 h. Paravertebral blockade had a better minor complication profile than thoracic epidural with a significantly lower incidence of hypotension, nausea, vomiting, pruritis, and urinary retention. There was no difference in incidence of major complications, length of hospital stay, or 30-day mortality between the two groups although the group did comment that a larger randomized control trial would be beneficial. They were unable to comment on the incidence of chronic pain following the two techniques. Numerous other studies [171–176] have supported the view that continuous paravertebral infusion provides an acceptable degree of analgesia following thoracotomy comparable to epidural analgesia and superior to wound infiltration, intercostal block, and intravenous opioids. This can then be improved further via a multimodal approach. El-Sayed et al. [177] also reported no difference in the incidence of postoperative respiratory complications, unplanned readmission to the intensive care unit, or in-hospital mortality in a retrospective analysis of a large case series. With this in mind, and given the rare but potentially catastrophic complication profile of the thoracic epidural, the use of paravertebral blockade in thoracic anesthesia is increasingly appealing.

Consent for Regional Analgesia

Recent guidance [178] issued by the Association of Anaesthetists of Great Britain and Ireland (AAGBI) clearly states that clinicians have a professional obligation to ensure that patients fully understand what is going to happen to them and what they should therefore expect during the course of their treatment. In order to preserve patient autonomy and obtain informed consent prior to any procedure, including regional analgesic techniques, it is essential that the patient be given a comprehensive explanation of what the procedure will entail, the benefits, the limitations, the potential side effects, and the risks, along with a discussion of the relative merits of alternative strategies. It is the duty of the clinician to ensure that this information is understood and that the patient is given an opportunity to ask questions. A 2015 landmark ruling in the United Kingdom (Montgomery v Lanarkshire Health Board [179]) stated that a doctor should provide information on all "material risks" to the patient, where materiality is defined as "…whether a reasonable person in the patient's position would be likely to attach significance to the risk, or the doctor should reasonably be aware that the particular patient would be likely to attach significance to it." This followed a trend of openness that has been evolving over many years, leading to a marked change in practice. Most anesthetists now, for example, take specific consent for thoracic epidural analgesia [180].

Local Anesthetic Patches

Lidocaine 5% patches contain 700 mg lidocaine in an aqueous base held on a 10 cm by 14 cm soft adhesive patch. They are positioned and are placed 5–7 cm from the incision over the intact skin. The quantity of lidocaine absorbed is related to the duration of application and the total skin area covered [181]. Their use is approved by the FDA for the treatment of neuropathic pain syndrome and postherpetic neuralgia. As yet there is little validated evidence regarding their effectiveness in thoracic surgery, but a recent meta-analysis [181] and study assessing their use after robotic cardiac valve surgery [182] found no improvement in pain scores, morphine consumption, or length of hospital stay associated with their use. Currently therefore their routine use cannot be recommended.

Continuous Wound Infiltration Catheters

Randomized studies have shown that delivering local anesthetic into the wound via catheters placed prior to closure can improve resting and dynamic pain scores [183], reduce postoperative opioid use [183, 184], may reduce wound edema [185], and improve recovery of FEV_1 and FVC [183]. Where continuous wound infusion of local anesthetic was utilized in addition to morphine IV-PCA, there was a reduction in levels of systemic inflammatory markers [183]. The catheter was positioned at the end of surgery so that it lay between the pericostal sutures, in close proximity to the intercostal nerve and the deep surface of the serratus muscle, and it has been postulated that this catheter position, deeper than in other studies, was crucial to its success. Despite a continuous slow rise in serum local anesthetic concentration throughout the 48 h study period, levels remained within a safe range, and there were no complications associated with the technique [183], although for patients receiving continuous paravertebral infusions, the potential for local anesthetic toxicity makes use inappropriate. For patients receiving thoracic epidural analgesia, this technique is usually unnecessary. It could, however, be considered for patients not scheduled to receive local anesthetic infusions by other routes for postoperative pain control. A particular advantage of this technique is the ability to utilize it in surgeries where paravertebral catheter cannot be placed, such as pleurectomy or chest wall resection.

Intercostal Nerve Blocks

The spinal nerves divide into a dorsal and ventral ramus. The upper 11 thoracic ventral rami form the intercostal nerve which runs forward between the ribs in the intercostal spaces. Each intercostal nerve gives off a lateral cutaneous branch that pierces the intercostal muscles proximal to the posterior axillary line to supply the lateral aspect of the chest wall. It is important therefore the intercostal nerves are blocked posterior to the posterior axillary line to ensure that the lateral cutaneous branches and thus the lateral aspect of the chest wall are blocked. The thoracic dorsal rami pass backward close to the vertebrae to supply the cutaneous innervation to the back. The dorsal rami are not blocked by an intercostal nerve block. This limits the effectiveness of intercostal nerve blocks for posterolateral thoracotomies (Fig. 59.5).

The intercostal nerves can easily be blocked under direct vision, while the chest is open, but because of the relatively short half-life of most local anesthetics, repeated percutaneous blocks are usually required. The intercostal nerves consistently lie in a plane deep to the internal intercostal muscle although there is considerable variability in the position of intercostal nerves within the intercostal space. Small (5 ml) bolus of local anesthetic deposited in the correct plane will block the appropriate intercostal nerve. Larger doses may also block adjacent intercostal nerves by spreading medially to the paravertebral space or directly to the adjacent spaces (Fig. 59.6).

The systemic uptake of local anesthetic from the highly vascular intercostal space is rapid and the dose of local anesthetic administered by this route needs to be appropriately limited. Intercostal nerve blocks significantly reduce postoperative pain and analgesic requirements post-thoracotomy [187].

Interpleural Blocks

In healthy human adults, the two layers of the pleura have a surface area of about 0.2 m^2, are separated by a distance of 10–20 µm, and contain approximately 10 mL of pleural fluid [186]. The deposition of local anesthetic between the parietal and visceral pleura, with the aim of producing an ipsilateral somatic block of multiple thoracic dermatomes, constitutes an interpleural block and was originally described by Kvalheim and Reiestad [188]. Unfortunately, the terminology used in the literature to describe this block can be confusing; some authors use the term intrapleural block [189] and others pleural block [190]. The issue is further confused

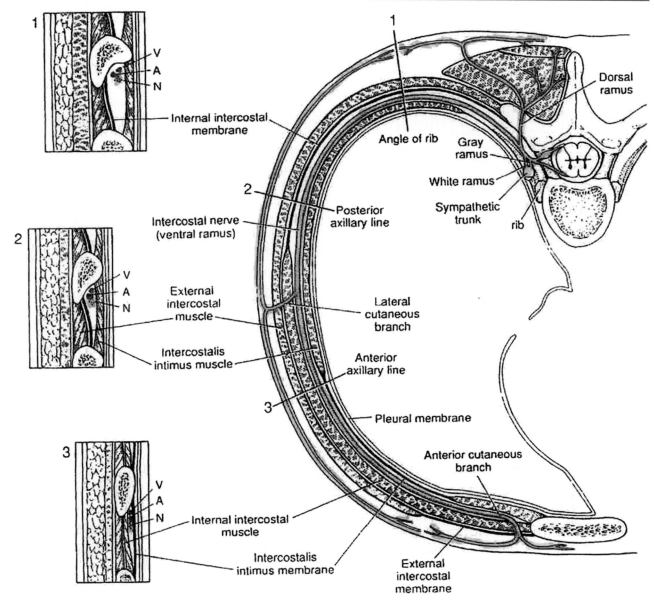

Fig. 59.5 Anatomy of intercostal nerve and space. (Reproduced with permission from Dravid and Paul [186])

when the term interpleural block is used to describe a paravertebral block [191]. Although studies have consistently shown interpleural blocks to be effective for pain relief after cholecystectomy, most studies of patients undergoing a thoracotomy have shown interpleural blocks to be ineffective [192]. The widespread of local anesthetic within the normally small (10 mL) pleural space is aided by surface tension forces, and this probably accounts for the effectiveness of interpleural blocks after cholecystectomy. After thoracotomy, the volume of the pleural space is much larger and contains blood and air. The effect of surface tension forces is reduced and the spread of local anesthetics is limited and principally via gravity. Dilution of the administered local anesthetic by interpleural blood [193] and the loss of local anesthetic into the chest drains [194] further reduce the efficacy of this technique. A possible role for interpleural bupivacaine, administered post-thoracotomy via the basal chest drain to reduce local diaphragmatic irritation from the basal chest drain, was explored in a double-blind study. Interpleural local anesthetic administered by this route was found to be ineffective [195]. Large doses of local anesthetic are frequently required in order for the block to be effective, and therefore, given the vascular nature of the pleural space, systemic absorption can be considerable and high plasma levels of local anesthetics have been reported. The block is also of limited duration and may impair function of the ipsilateral diaphragm [70]. Interpleural blocks are not recommended for post-thoracotomy analgesia in adults [58].

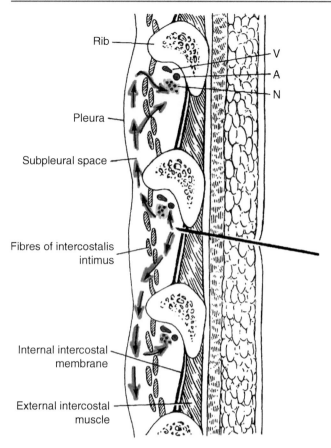

Rib

V

A

N

Pleura

Subpleural space

Fibres of intercostalis
intimus

Internal intercostal
membrane

External intercostal
muscle

Fig. 59.6 Intercostal nerve block. Showing spread of local anesthetic to adjacent spaces (arrows). (Reproduced with permission from Dravid and Paul [186])

Serratus Anterior Plane Blocks

Introduction

Several novel regional analgesic strategies for surgery involving the chest wall have been described in the past several years. These chest wall blocks all involve the ultrasound-guided deposition of local anesthetic in a plane between the thoracic musculature. Like the transversus abdominis plane (TAP) block of the abdomen, these are truncal field blocks that rely on volume-based spread of local anesthetic within intermuscular planes to target multiple nerves. Currently, one of the most relevant of these chest wall blocks to thoracic surgery is the serratus anterior plane block (SAPB).

The SAPB was first described in 2013 by Blanco and colleagues [196] who also described the Pecs I and II blocks, which have found use in anterior chest wall procedures including breast surgery. Blanco based the SAPB on an examination of the thoracic anatomy that revealed two potential spaces, one superficial and one deep to the serratus anterior muscle. Injection of local anesthetic into either of these spaces was postulated to provide analgesia of the lateral hemithorax by blocking the intercostal nerves along with the thoracodorsal and long thoracic nerves. In their 2013 paper, Blanco and colleagues noted that the SAPB provided paresthesia of the hemithorax from approximately T2 to T9 in four healthy volunteers. While the dermatomal distribution was consistent regardless of position of the block above or below the serratus muscle, the duration of the block tended to be approximately twice as long when the local anesthetic was injected above the serratus muscle. Magnetic resonance imaging of gadolinium injected along with the local anesthetic indicated that injection superficial to serratus tended to spread more posteriorly, while injection deep to serratus spread both anteriorly and posteriorly along the chest wall in supine subjects.

SAPB in Clinical Practice

Following Blanco's description of the SAPB in 2013, several papers have been published describing the clinical use of this block. Many of these have focused on breast surgery, but applications related to thoracic surgery are growing. Kunhabdulla and colleagues described a case in which a SAPB with catheter was used to provide successful analgesia in a patient with fractures of ribs 4–7 following a motor vehicle accident [197]. Shortly thereafter, Madabushi and colleagues [198] reported the successful use of a SAPB with catheter for analgesia following thoracotomy for esophagectomy in a patient in whom the preoperatively placed thoracic epidural could not be used due to hypotension related to early sepsis. In this case, the SAPB catheter provided adequate analgesia for a total of 6 days without complications. Okmen and colleagues published a case report on the use of a SABP with catheter placed preoperatively to provide analgesia after a wedge resection performed via thoracotomy for lung malignancy [199]. Subsequently, this group published a retrospective study comparing the use of intravenous patient-controlled analgesia (PCA) with morphine to the use of PCA morphine plus SAPB for the management of post-thoracotomy pain [200]. In this study of 40 patients, the authors found that patients who received the SAPB in addition to PCA morphine have significantly lower visual analogue scale pain scores at 6, 12, and 24 h after surgery compared to the group that received only PCA morphine. Importantly, morphine consumption was significantly lower in the group that also received the SAPB, although the actual difference in morphine consumption between groups was relatively small.

Research on the use of the SAPB in thoracic surgery is ongoing, and it remains unclear whether this block alone is sufficient to provide analgesia after thoracic surgery. The most success has been achieved with the placement of a catheter at the time of the block to provide a continuous infusion of local anesthetic. The existing evidence indicates that the SAPB is a useful adjunct and may reduce overall opioid consumption as part of a multimodal approach to pain management after chest wall procedures. It may be particularly useful for anterior thoracic incisions and may be useful as a bilateral block for sternotomy pain.

Technique

The technique for performing the SAPB was described by Blanco and colleagues [196]. This block is performed under ultrasound guidance using a linear transducer. Positioning of the patient is flexible, depending on provider preference. The SAPB was originally described with the subjects positioned supine but has also been reported in the sitting position. Our preference for thoracic surgical procedures is to perform this block after the induction of anesthesia and once the patient is positioned in the lateral decubitus position as this positioning offers the best access to the lateral thorax. The block should be performed at the level of the fifth rib in the midaxillary line. At this level, the serratus anterior muscle should be identified overlying the ribs, with the latissimus dorsi muscle lying superior to the serratus muscle. Intercostal muscles can be identified between the ribs, and below them lies the pleura. Figure 59.7a demonstrates the relevant ultrasound anatomy. Needle insertion can be performed in-plane or out-of-plane, depending on provider preference. As described above, the SAPB can be achieved by injecting local anesthetic either above or below the serratus muscle, with equivalent analgesic spread with both techniques. Our preference is to perform the block below the serratus muscle as the plane between the latissimus and serratus muscles can be difficult to develop in some patients. Furthermore, the sub-serratus approach allows for a definitive target – touching the surface of the rib with the needle virtually guarantees that the local anesthetic will spread below the serratus muscle. Blanco originally described the use of 0.4 mL/kg of 0.125% levobupivacaine. We typically perform this block with 20 mL of either 0.25% bupivacaine or 0.2% ropivacaine with 1:400,000 epinephrine. Figure 59.7b demonstrates spread of local anesthetic beneath the serratus muscle both cranial and caudal to the injection site over the fifth rib. A catheter may be left in this plane after the initial injection to provide a continuous infusion of local anesthetic. Of note, due to the proximity of the block site to the pleura and the intercostal neurovascular bundle, care must be taken to avoid insertion of the needle below the rib surface as pneumothorax and intrathoracic bleeding are possible complications. Figure 59.8 shows the in-plane approach to SAPB.

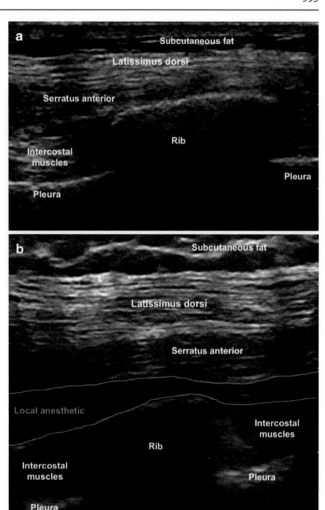

Fig. 59.7 (**a**) Anatomy seen with a linear transducer positioned over the fifth rib in the midaxillary line. Ribs are identified as rectangular structures with curved hyperechoic edges and posterior acoustic shadow. Approximately 0.5 cm deep to the rib edge lies the hyperechoic pleura, which should be seen to "slide" with respiration. The serratus anterior muscle can be identified as a thin strip of muscle overlying the ribs. Above the serratus muscle lies the latissimus dorsi muscle, and overlying the latissimus dorsi is subcutaneous fat and tissue. (**b**) Following injection of local anesthetic deep to the serratus muscle, the local anesthetic can be seen to spread both cranial and caudal to the rib in the plane developed between the ribs/intercostal muscles and the serratus muscle (outlined in blue). This block was performed using the out-of-plane technique, which is why the needle cannot be readily seen in this image

Paravertebral Blocks

Paravertebral blocks were introduced into clinical practice in 1906 [201] and were then largely abandoned before being reintroduced in 1979 [202]. There has now been substantial experience in the use of thoracic paravertebral block for thoracic surgery, and their safety has been established.

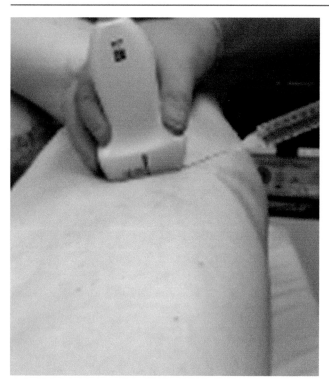

Fig. 59.8 The in-plane approach to the serratus anterior plane block. With the patient in the lateral position and the ipsilateral arm extended anteriorly, the ultrasound transducer probe is placed over the fifth rib in the midaxillary line. The needle is guided onto the rib deep to the serratus anterior muscle

Paravertebral blocks may be performed as so-called "single-shot" blocks, with introduction of a single dose of long-acting local anesthetic, or may take the form of a continuous block, via placement of a catheter allowing local anesthetic infusion. Continuous thoracic paravertebral blocks can provide excellent post-thoracotomy analgesia, and a number of studies have shown that the analgesia is comparable to that provided by thoracic epidurals but with fewer complications such as urinary retention, hypotension, nausea, vomiting, and pruritis [203–206] and less perioperative hemodynamic instability [174].

Anatomy

The paravertebral space is a potential space. At the thoracic level, the paravertebral space is a wedge-shaped area bounded posteriorly by the costotransverse ligaments, transverse processes, and necks of the ribs (Fig. 59.9). Medially it is bound by the vertebral bodies, discs, and intervertebral foramina, through which there is communication with the epidural space. The anterior border of the space is formed by the parietal pleura. Lateral to the tips of the transverse processes, the paravertebral space is continuous with the intercostal neurovascular space (Fig. 59.10).

The paravertebral space is contiguous with the paravertebral spaces above and below. The caudal boundary is formed by the psoas major muscle [208]; the cranial boundary is, however, not well defined [207]. The thoracic paravertebral space is divided into an anterior subpleural paravertebral compartment and a posterior subendothoracic paravertebral compartment by the endothoracic fascia which is the deep fascia of the thorax [207] (Figs. 59.10 and 59.11). Contained within the paravertebral space are the dorsal and ventral rami of the spinal nerves, the gray and white rami communicans, and the sympathetic chain. The intercostal nerves (ventral ramus) are devoid of a fascial sheath within the paravertebral space making them highly susceptible to local anesthetic block at this site [209] and therefore where performed at this level result in ipsilateral blockade of sympathetic nerves and thoracic dermatomes [210].

Methods of Performing Paravertebral Blocks

There are several approaches described to access the paravertebral space, and they can be broadly divided into those performed preoperatively using landmark or ultrasound-guided techniques and those performed intraoperatively under direct vision. When blocks are performed in the awake patient, the patient may be positioned either sitting or in the lateral decubitus position. When performed after induction of anesthesia, the anesthetized patient is generally positioned in the lateral decubitus position, with the side to be blocked uppermost. Generally, blocks should be performed at the level of the intended incision(s). Hutchins et al. [219] describe, for thoracoscopic surgery, performing blocks and inserting catheters at T5/6 for upper/middle lobe surgery and T6/7 for lower lobe surgery because of the more caudal position of the ports.

Landmark Methods

Perhaps the most widely used landmark technique is the one described by Eason and Wyatt [202], involving loss of resistance upon "walking off" a transverse process (Fig. 59.7). A Tuohy needle is inserted 3 cm lateral to the cranial edge of a spinous process at the appropriate level. The needle is then advanced perpendicular to the skin until contact is made with the underlying transverse process. If contact with bone is not made at the expected depth, the needle is withdrawn and then readvanced slowly, while fanning it in the sagittal plane, until contact with bone is made. The needle is then walked off the cranial edge of the transverse process and advanced slowly until a loss of resistance, less complete than that in the epidural space, is encountered, usually after a further 1 cm. This is frequently preceded by a subtle click as the costo-

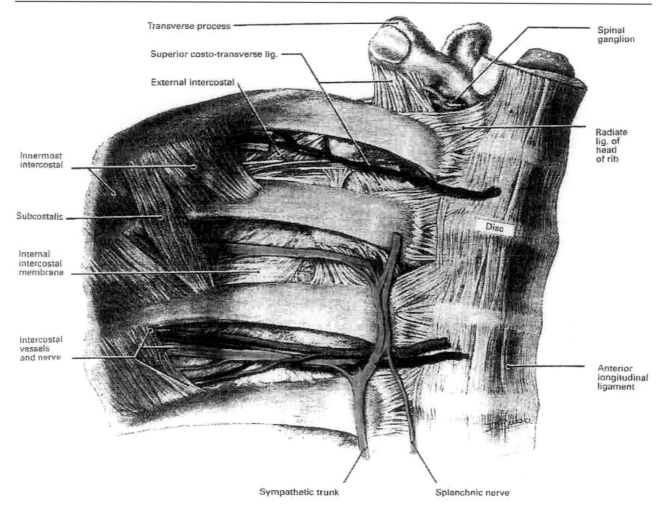

Fig. 59.9 Posterior relations of the thoracic paravertebral space. (Reproduced with permission, Murphy [193])

Fig. 59.10 Anatomy of the thoracic paravertebral space. (Reproduced with permission, Karmakar et al. [207])

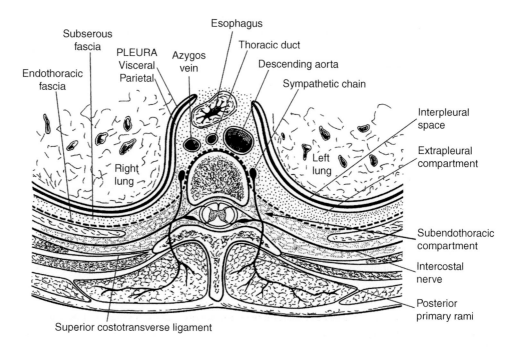

Fig. 59.11 Sagittal section through the paravertebral space showing a needle that has been walked off the transverse process. (Reproduced with permission, Karmakar [207])

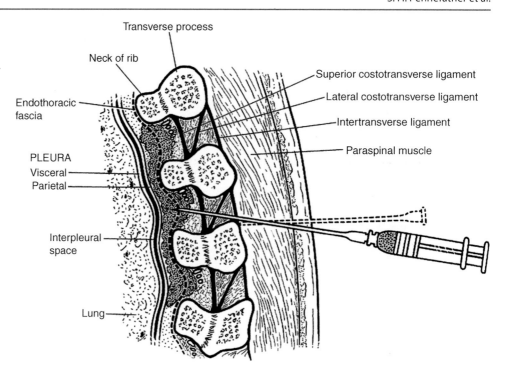

Transverse process

Neck of rib

Superior costotransverse ligament

Lateral costotransverse ligament

Intertransverse ligament

Paraspinal muscle

Endothoracic fascia

PLEURA
Visceral
Parietal

Interpleural space

Lung

transverse ligament is penetrated. In adults, after aspiration to confirm the needle is extravascular, approximately 20 mL of an appropriate local anesthetic (e.g., 0.25% levobupivacaine) is administered. Where placement of a catheter for continuous infusion is planned, the initial injection of a bolus of local anesthetic serves to open up the paravertebral space before threading an epidural catheter. Consideration may be given to adding a small quantity of dye to the local anesthetic administered, so correct placement of the block can be confirmed visually at subsequent thoracoscopy or thoracotomy.

An alternative technique whereby the paravertebral space is approached from an intercostal space has been described [211]. A Tuohy needle is positioned posteriorly over a rib at the appropriate level about 8 cm lateral to the head of that rib and advanced until contact is made with the rib. The needle is then orientated so the bevel is pointing medially and the tip is angulated 45° cephalad and 60° medial to the sagittal plane. The needle tip is then walked off the inferior border of the rib while maintaining this orientation and advanced a few millimeters until loss of resistance confirms that the intercostal neurovascular space has been entered. After aspirating to confirm the needle is extravascular, approximately 5 mL of 0.25% levobupivacaine is injected to open up the intercostal neurovascular space. An epidural catheter is then inserted into the Tuohy needle and advanced into the intercostal neurovascular space. The orientation of the needle directs the catheter along the intercostal neurovascular space toward the paravertebral space. The catheter is inserted about 8 cm into the intercostal space so the tip lies in the paravertebral space [211].

Ultrasound-Guided Methods

Percutaneous thoracic paravertebral blocks are technically simple to perform but have a failure rate of up to 10%. The use of ultrasound guidance may result in reduced failure rates. Ultrasound-guided thoracic paravertebral blockade can be divided into in-plane techniques where the long axis of the needle is visualized in its entirety as it traverses the plane of ultrasound toward the target and out-of-plane techniques where the needle enters the skin away from the probe and across the scanning plane, allowing it to be visualized in its short axis only. The approach may either be in the transversal or sagittal plane. Blocks described are most frequently performed using a linear ultrasound transducer and the accompanying images reflect this. Some groups advocate using micro-convex array transducers to allow better imaging of deeper structures [212]. Correct identification of landmarks is essential for all techniques, although their appearance will differ according to the orientation of the transducer. Krediet et al. [213] published a detailed description of the ultrasonographic anatomy of the paravertebral space and its neighboring tissues. Their descriptions have been used to illustrate the approaches that follow, but as with other regional techniques, there are many other methods advocated by experienced groups [214–217].

The spinous and transverse processes are easily identifiable as rounded, hyperechoic structures with areas of acoustic shadowing stretching anteriorly and are frequently the starting point for any ultrasound-guided approach [218].

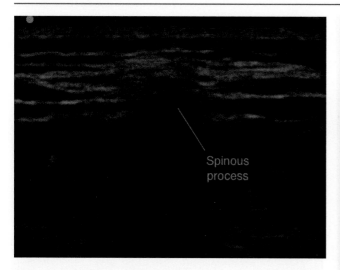

Fig. 59.12 Ultrasound image showing the central spinous process, a starting point for many ultrasound-guided paravertebral blocks

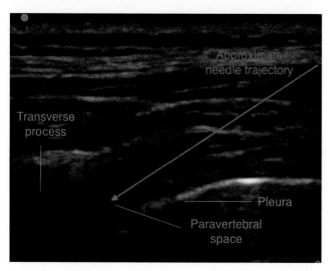

Fig. 59.13 Ultrasound image showing the view of the paravertebral space obtained with the transducer in a transversal orientation and the approximate trajectory of a needle in order to perform a paravertebral block at this level

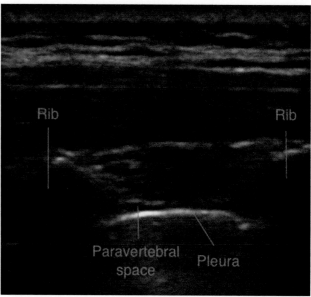

Fig. 59.14 Ultrasound image showing the view of the paravertebral space with the ultrasound transducer in the sagittal plane at the level of the ribs

In-plane thoracic paravertebral blockade [210, 213] commences with identification of the spinous process within the midline (Fig. 59.12), with the probe oriented in a transverse direction. The probe is then slowly moved laterally, until the transverse process can be identified with the parietal pleura visible as a hyperechoic line moving with respiration (Fig. 59.13). The image can be refined by gradual angulation of the probe in cephalad or caudad directions, in order to acquire an uninterrupted view between adjacent ribs. In this position, the paravertebral space can be obscured by the shadow of the transverse process, although its lateral continuation, the intercostal space, can usually be seen [213]. By gradually moving the transducer caudally, the paravertebral space can be visualized more clearly (Fig. 59.13). The pari-etal pleura lying more laterally on the screen and parallel to the ultrasound beam is a bright, hyperechoic structure visible at levels T2 to T10. As its border is followed medially, the structure fades as it becomes more perpendicular to the ultrasound beam [213]. The paravertebral space is identified through its proximity to the transverse process and lung pleura. Once identified, the needle is inserted from a lateral to medial direction in a trajectory similar to that shown in Fig. 59.9, under ultrasound guidance throughout until the tip lies within the paravertebral space.

Another approach involves passage of a needle out-of-plane to perform the block and commences with identification of the paravertebral space with ultrasound as described above. The needle is then inserted from a point 1 cm caudal to the ultrasound transducer and is advanced with a slight craniocaudal angulation so that the tip of the needle can be visualized reaching the desired target and the local anesthetic can be injected under direct vision with the characteristic movement of the pleura.

A further approach to the paravertebral block involves positioning of the ultrasound transducer in the sagittal, rather than transversal, plane [213]. Understandably, the ultrasound anatomy will be markedly different. The paravertebral space can be identified and the block can be performed in several positions as the probe is manipulated. The ultrasound transducer should begin at a position approximately 5 cm from the midline in the sagittal plane and is then slowly moved medially to allow identification of landmarks. The ribs will be visualized initially as areas of acoustic shadow, and the hyperechogenic line of the pleura with movement with respiration should be easily recognizable (Fig. 59.14). Between

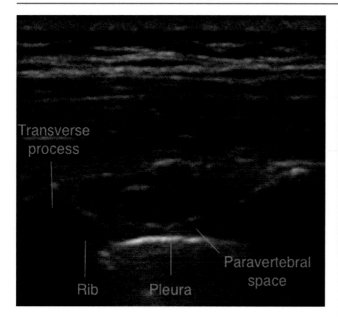

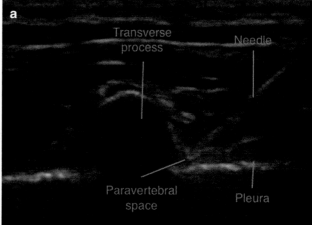

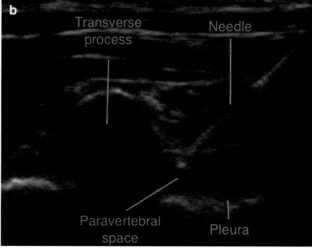

Fig. 59.15 Ultrasound image showing the view of the paravertebral space with the ultrasound transducer in the sagittal plane at the level of the costotransverse junction

two ribs, the paravertebral space can be visualized, surrounded by anteriorly, the innermost intercostal muscle and pleura; posteriorly, the external intercostal muscle and intercostal membrane; medially, the membrane of the innermost intercostal muscle; and laterally, the costotransverse joint. At this point, the block can be performed by inserting the needle in-plane on the inferior aspect of the transducer with the tip directed in a cephalad direction to reach the space between the internal intercostal membrane and the pleura. This provides a similar needle tip location to the first block described in this section, but it has been suggested that this approach may require a greater number of attempts before a successful result is achieved.

As the ultrasound transducer is slowly moved medially, the transverse processes gradually appear, and the costotransverse joint is visualized at a point approximately 3–4 cm from the midline. Between the two joints, the multifidus and rotator muscles can be seen, with the superior costotransverse ligament posterior to them, the paravertebral space lying posterior to this, and the pleura lying most anterior (Fig. 59.15). By rotating the probe slightly into a cephalomedial/caudolateral orientation, the space between the transverse process and rib opens. Introduction of the block needle in-plane from the caudal aspect of the transducer allows passage between the rib and transverse process, through the superior costotransverse ligament into the paravertebral space. As with other approaches, anterior movement of the pleura is confirmatory of correct needle position.

A final approach to the block involves continued medial movement of the ultrasound probe. The rib now lies almost directly anterior to the transverse process with a narrow

Fig. 59.16 (a) Ultrasound image showing transverse view of a needle approaching the paravertebral space and (b) movement of the pleura anteriorly with injection of local anesthetic

space between adjacent transverse process/rib groups. The pleura here will be more parallel to the ultrasound beam and is therefore much less visible. To perform a paravertebral block at this location, the ultrasound probe will be approximately 2.5 cm lateral to the midline so that the space between two adjacent transverse processes is central. Using an in-plane approach from either the caudal or cranial end of the transducer, the needle can be seen to pass into the space with anterior movement of the pleura on injection ultimately confirming correct placement. Alternatively, the needle can be inserted out-of-plane so that the tip contacts the transverse process. The block from here is blind, as the needle is walked off the transverse process and advanced a further 1–1.5 cm, potentially with a loss of resistance as the costotransverse ligament is pierced. Anterior movement of the pleura on injection can still be seen if the needle is positioned correctly, as demonstrated in Fig. 59.16a, b.

Krediet et al. [213] give an interesting and detailed summary regarding the choice of ultrasound approach and the direction of needle insertion, in-plane or out-of-plane. The paravertebral space changes in size being 2–2.5 cm in diameter at a position 1–2 cm from the midline to being only 0.5 cm in diameter where it is approached most laterally for an intercostal approach. From a point of view of avoiding accidental pleural puncture, it would seem that the margin of error is significantly larger with the more medial approaches.

The choice of needle for injection is dependent upon the type of intended block. Where passage of an epidural catheter to allow continuous infusion is required, a Touhy needle must be employed. Where a "single-shot" block is being performed, while a Touhy needle can still be used, utilizing a specialist regional block needle with features that increase echogenicity to optimize needle identification may lead to a more successful block placement. Regardless of the choice of needle, the techniques for accessing the paravertebral space are unchanged. The needle is introduced until the tip is seen to lie within the paravertebral space. A loss of resistance may be palpable, as with a landmark approach, as the space is entered. Injection of local anesthetic should lead to an obvious anterior movement of the parietal pleura. If this is not seen, the needle tip should be repositioned. Where a catheter is to be inserted, there is a recommendation that it be passed no more than 2 cm past the end of the needle where there is a lateral to medial approach, to limit the likelihood of epidural migration of the catheter tip [213, 219].

In thoracoscopic surgery where a catheter is not to be used, multi-injection approaches have been advocated with a perception that this may lead to greater dispersement of local anesthetic and therefore a more effective block than a single-injection approach. Cowie et al. [210] performed a cadaveric study comparing spread of local anesthetic containing contrast dye, between a single-injection approach with 20 mL and a dual-injection technique involving two 10 mL boluses. Spread of contrast evaluated via dissection found no difference between the two approaches regarding paravertebral spread of the injected fluid, although the dual-injection technique led to involvement of a greater number of intercostal segments. The degree to which the eventual success of the block could be attributed to enhanced intercostal involvement is not clear. A study in patients undergoing thoracoscopic surgery [220] compared a single injection at T6 with a multi-injection technique involving five injections from T4 to T8. Postoperative pain scores, morphine consumption, times to first mobilization, and time to hospital discharge were comparable between the groups. While this trial reported no complications relating to the blocks, the risk of a complication is likely to be larger where multiple injections are performed, and therefore multiple injections cannot, at present, be recommended.

The association between the location of local anesthetic injection and clinical effect can be inconsistent. Assessment of local anesthetic spread following a single ultrasound-

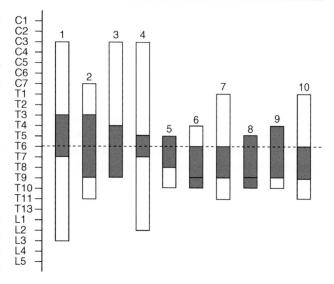

Fig. 59.17 Analysis of the spread of local anesthetic solution (full boxes) and sensory evaluation (open boxes) of left thoracic paravertebral blocks in ten healthy volunteers. (Reproduced with permission, Marhofer et al. [221])

guided injection within the paravertebral space of healthy volunteers using magnetic resonance imaging [221] showed a median spread to involve a total of five vertebral levels but a sensory distribution that was considerably greater and variable, involving a median of approximately ten dermatomes (Fig. 59.17). Spread outside of the paravertebral space was detected in 40% of cases with 25% showing evidence of spread into the epidural space.

It is probable that ultrasound-guided paravertebral blocks will improve with the refinement of the described approaches and evolution of new techniques. Use of three-dimensional ultrasound may improve success by allowing more accurate identification of the paravertebral space, but as yet this is only in the experimental phase [218].

Open Methods

Placement of a paravertebral catheter via a percutaneous approach has been shown to be challenging and the eventual position of the catheter tip is unpredictable. The position of paravertebral catheters placed with ultrasound guidance in cadavers has been assessed [210]. Only 60% of catheters were positioned as intended. 20% had passed into the prevertebral space anterior to the vertebral bodies, 15% lay posterior to the vertebral bodies within soft tissue, and 5% were within the epidural space. Therefore, although it is possible to place catheters percutaneously into the paravertebral space, it may be more appropriate for the surgeon to insert the catheter into the paravertebral space under direct vision while the chest is open. Direct placement facilitates clear advancement of the catheter along the paravertebral space to create a narrow longitudinal pocket that may block sufficient dermatomes to provide adequate analgesia.

Direct placement techniques may require some surgical preplanning. The posterior extent of the incision needs to be limited to allow sufficient room for the paravertebral catheter. In particular, it is important to preserve enough pleura posterior to the surgical incision. Direct placement techniques were initially undertaken at the end of surgery immediately prior to closure to reduce the risk of inadvertent catheter dislodgement. However, at least in the author's institution, they are now frequently positioned prior to lung resection to allow time for adequate spread of the local anesthetic within the paravertebral space. The direct placement of catheter into the paravertebral space at the end of surgery was first popularized by Sabanathan et al. [222]. They described a technique whereby a catheter is inserted via a Tuohy needle. The catheter is inserted percutaneously medial to the posterior edge of the thoracotomy incision to emerge between the angle of the ribs into the chest cavity. The parietal pleura two spaces above and below the incision is peeled back medially to expose the intercostal nerves taking care not to perforate the pleura. The catheter is then positioned to lie against the angles of the exposed ribs before the parietal pleura is reattached to the posterior aspect of the wound. The authors later reported an improvement in their technique [223]. After reflecting back the parietal pleura to the vertebral bodies as before, a small incision is made in the endothoracic fascia and the catheter is passed into the subendothoracic paravertebral compartment and advanced cranially for a few centimeters, aided if necessary by blunt dissection. The hole in the endothoracic fascia is then closed by a suture (Fig. 59.18).

Another technique used in the author's institution is for the surgeon to insert a Tuohy needle percutaneously, under direct vision, into the paravertebral space one or two segments caudal to the thoracotomy incision. A catheter is then introduced through the Tuohy needle and advanced 10 cm or more cranially in the paravertebral space. This requires careful manipulation of the Tuohy needle and catheter to ensure it advances in the correct direction and damage to the overlying pleura is avoided. The other end of the catheter is then tunneled subcutaneously to limit the risk of inadvertent dislodgement. For patients undergoing video-assisted surgery, video-assisted surgical placement of a catheter is possible [224] (see Video 59.1).

Insertion of paravertebral catheters under thoracoscopic guidance before thoracotomy in order to allow administration of local anesthetic prior to skin incision and ahead of disturbing the parietal pleura have been described [225] conducted. A randomized, double-blind study comparing thoracic epidural analgesia with surgically placed paravertebral analgesia suggested paravertebral analgesia to be superior in terms of

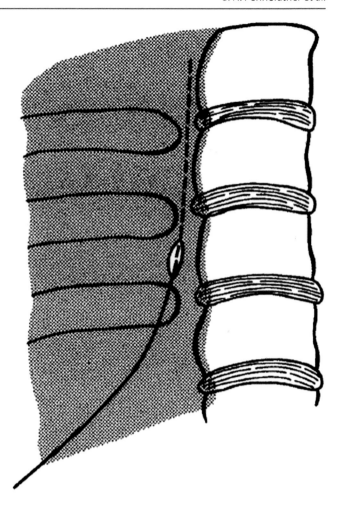

Fig. 59.18 A technique for performing paravertebral blocks. The endothoracic fascia (stippled) is exposed by raising the parietal pleura from the posterior chest wall. A catheter is inserted deep to the endothoracic fascia through a small hole created in the fascia. (Reproduced with permission, Berrisford and Sabanathan [223])

pain scores at rest and when coughing but also measurements of FEV_1 and oxygen saturation in ambient air [226].

Management of Paravertebrals

Single-shot paravertebral injections using currently available local anesthetic preparations have been shown to last between 6 and 24 h. Comparison of a single-shot approach with IV opioids to IV opioids alone for thoracoscopic surgery found pain scores to be significantly lower in those receiving the paravertebral block [227]. Improved pain scores, decreased opioid requirements, and improved results of lung function tests 4 h postoperatively have been shown with use of a preemptive single-shot paravertebral block over surgically placed single-shot intercostal blocks [228]. Preoperative single-shot paravertebral analgesia for patients undergoing thoracoscopic surgery was associated with a lower total opioid consumption, less nausea and vomiting, and improved pain scores in recovery and at 24 h both at rest and with movement [229]. Comparison of a single-shot surgically performed intercostal block with continuous paravertebral infusion in patients undergoing thoracoscopic surgery [219] found no significant difference in pain score or opioid consumption in the first 24 h after surgery although in the 24–48 h time period, patients with a paravertebral catheter had significantly lower pain scores, had lower opioid requirements, and overall had a significantly higher level of patient-reported satisfaction with their pain control compared to the group receiving intercostal blocks.

The overall suggestion is that, in patients undergoing thoracoscopic surgery, a paravertebral block is preferable to intravenous analgesia alone. The relatively short duration of action of clinically available local anesthetics makes single bolus paravertebral blocks inappropriate for most post-thoracotomy patients. These patients are best treated by establishing a PVB with a bolus of local anesthetic and then maintaining the block with a catheter placed in the paravertebral space. Ultra-long-acting local anesthetic agents are being developed. Placement of these agents in the paravertebral space may, in the future, make single bolus paravertebral blocks practical, reducing the risks of local anesthetic toxicity and block failure secondary to catheter displacement. Consideration has been given to the use of adjuncts to prolong the duration of action of a paravertebral block. Clonidine, epinephrine, dexamethasone, and dexmedetomidine have been used with anecdotal reports of blocks with a duration of up to 6 days and lower pain scores [150, 230, 231]. As yet there have been no good quality randomized controlled trials to formally assess effectiveness and therefore the use of such adjuncts cannot be routinely recommended.

The appropriate management of paravertebrals (drug choice, rate, adjuvant and administration technique) has not yet been established and further work is required to optimize the efficacy and safety of this technique. A review and meta-regression analysis [117] found that a higher bupivacaine dose (890–990 mg per 24 h) predicted lower pain scores and faster recovery of pulmonary function compared to lower dose (325–472.5 mg) without a significant difference in the rate of local anesthetic toxicity. A recent randomized prospective study [232] suggested no difference in effectiveness between intermittent bolus dosing and continuous local anesthetic infusion.

The use of safer local anesthetic, such as levobupivacaine, vigilance for signs and symptoms of local toxicity (e.g., confusion), the addition of adrenaline to the solution, and reducing the infusion rate for elderly or frail patients may all be appropriate steps to reduce the incidence of toxicity with the use of paravertebrals. A typical dosing regimen for an adult patient might be 0.3 mL kg^{-1} initial bolus of 0.25% levobupivacaine followed by a 0.1 mL kg^{-1} h^{-1} infusion of 0.25% levobupivacaine (Table 59.4).

Duration of catheter placement and use will be guided by the individual patient. Studies range from 3 days to a maximum duration of insertion of 7 days [219, 226].

Advantages of Paravertebral Analgesia

Paravertebral block is a relatively simple technique that is easy to learn, has few contraindications, and has a low incidence of complications. In addition, the open technique enables paravertebral catheters to be safely inserted in anesthetized patients, for example, where a VAT procedure is converted to an open thoracotomy. Impaired coagulation is a relative contraindication to the percutaneous insertion of paravertebral blocks and catheters, but open placement under direct vision is relatively safe and can be recommended. Hypotension, urinary retention, pruritis, nausea, and vomiting are less frequent postoperatively with paravertebral blocks and infusions than with thoracic epidurals [170, 203]. In the author's institution, paravertebral analgesia is associated with earlier mobilization and shorter length of hospital stay than thoracic epidural [177].

Limitations and Complications of Paravertebral Blocks

To provide effective analgesia in the affected somatic dermatomes, post-thoracotomy paravertebral blocks may need to cover up to ten segments. It may take a number of hours for local anesthetic to spread sufficiently along the paravertebral space, and as a result early postoperative analgesia may be poor unless supplemented initially by other analgesic agents or techniques. Absolute contraindications are generally limited to local and systemic infection, allergy to local anesthetics, and the presence of tumor at intended injection site. Relative contraindications include severe coagulopathy, severe respiratory disease where there is dependence upon intercostal muscles for ventilation, ipsilateral diaphragmatic paresis, and severe spinal deformities such as kyphosis or scoliosis or conditions where there may be dilated intercostal vessels, such as with aortic coarctation or thoracic aneurysm [233]. Complications that have been reported include inadvertent pleural puncture, pulmonary hemorrhage, inadvertent dural puncture, hypotension, ipsilateral Horner's syndrome, nerve injury, and central nervous system local anesthetic toxicity. The incidence of these complications is low, but the available published data does not enable an exact incidence to be quoted to patients [207].

The large volume of local anesthetic required and rapid uptake of local anesthesia from the vessel-rich paravertebral space mean that local anesthetic toxicity is a concern. The toxic plasma concentration of bupivacaine is described as between 2 and 4.5 mg L⁻¹ by different groups [234], and mean plasma concentrations have been shown to exceed the threshold for central nervous system toxicity 48 h after commencing a 0.1 mL kg⁻¹ h⁻¹ infusion of 0.5% bupivacaine [235]. In a separate study of patients receiving paravertebral 0.5% bupivacaine at this rate, 7% of patients developed temporary confusion attributed to bupivacaine accumulation [236], and there have been case reports of patients in whom systemic local anesthetic toxicity related to a paravertebral infusion have occurred [237]. As a result, cumulative administered dose must be considered, and a maximum administration not to exceed 2 mg kg⁻¹ in a 4 h period is advocated [237]. Until recently, there has been no specific treatment available for local anesthetic toxicity. There is now a growing body of evidence from animal studies and case reports that lipid emulsion given intravenously improves outcome. It is therefore recommended that lipid emulsion is available wherever patients receive large doses of local anesthetic such as for a paravertebral block. The management of local anesthetic toxicity-induced cardiovascular collapse should involve CPR as per standard protocols followed by the consideration to administer a lipid emulsion [238, 239].

Erector Spinae Plane Blocks

The erector spinae plane (ESP) block is a recently described ultrasound-guided block for both acute and chronic post-thoracotomy pain. It may, in fact, be a variant of the paravertebral block. Cadaveric investigation has shown that injection of 20 mL of solution into the fascial plane deep to the erector spinae muscle at the level of the T5 transverse process can result in a spread of injectate from C7 to T8 vertebral levels [240]. This block has been described for post-thoracotomy analgesia rescue in a case of failed epidural analgesia in a patient receiving prophylactic anticoagulation [241]. The benefit of an ESP block over a paravertebral block may be the more obvious endpoint for an ESP block as the needle tip contacts the transverse process of the vertebra. The spread of local anesthetic, dosing, and the clinical effects seem very similar to a paravertebral block. The place of this block in the armamentarium of the anesthesiologist remains to be determined. It has not been studied in a controlled fashion vs. paravertebral or epidural analgesic techniques.

Technique (See Figs. 59.19 and 59.20)

An ultrasound-visible regional anesthetic needle (e.g., 8 cm, 17 gauge) is inserted using an in-plane approach in a superior to inferior fashion to contact the transverse process of the appropriate thoracic vertebra deep to the anterior fascia of the erector spinae muscle. A total of 20–25 ml of local anesthetic

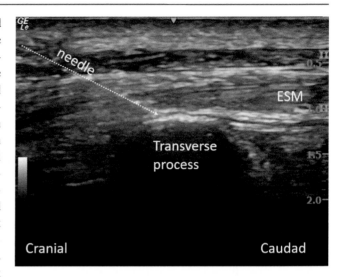

Fig. 59.19 Erector spinae plane block. The ultrasound probe is placed lateral to the spinous process (line S) to obtain a parasagittal view of the tip of the targeted transverse process (TP) with overlying erector spinae muscle (ESM). The block needle (dotted arrow) is advanced in a cranial-caudal direction to contact the TP. (Photo courtesy of KJ Chin Medicine Professional Corporation)

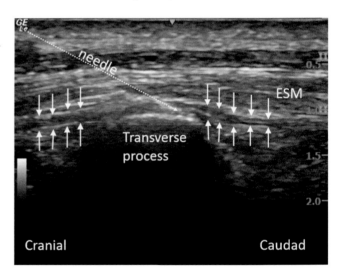

Fig. 59.20 Erector spinae plane block. Correct needle tip position is signaled by linear spread of local anesthetic (solid arrows) deep to the erector spinae muscle (ESM) and superficial to the transverse process. (Photo courtesy of KJ Chin Medicine Professional Corporation)

solution (e.g., 0.2% ropivacaine) is administered in 5 ml aliquots under direct vision. A catheter is then passed 5 cm distal to the tip of the needle, and an infusion of 5–8 ml/h is begun.

Intrathecal Analgesia

The lumbar administration of subarachnoid opioids is an infrequently used technique that may have a wider role in providing post-thoracotomy analgesia. The use of intrathecal morphine to provide operative analgesia was first described in 1979 [242]. Since then a number of studies have reported the use of intrathecal opioids for post-thoracotomy analgesia [243–245]. The intrathecal route of opioid delivery is 100 times more potent than the equivalent intravenous dose [246]. The onset time and degree of rostral spread of intrathecal opioids depend in part on their lipid solubility [247]. The most hydrophilic opioids, such as morphine, exhibit a greater degree of intrathecal spread and are therefore more likely to cause respiratory depression. This is in comparison to a more lipophilic drug, such a fentanyl or sufentanil, that is less prone to spread and therefore exhibits fewer respiratory side effects [70]. With intrathecal sufentanil, for example, the onset of analgesia is very rapid, whereas morphine has a slower onset but longer duration of action. Combinations of morphine and sufentanil have therefore been used to provide post-thoracotomy analgesia. In one study, morphine 200 μg was combined with sufentanil 20 μg [118]; in another study, morphine 500 μg was combined with sufentanil 50 μg [119]; both studies reported good early analgesia. Side effects of intrathecal opioids include nausea, vomiting, pruritus, urinary retention, and delayed respiratory depression. Respiratory depression of a severity requiring treatment with an antagonist such as naloxone occurs in 0.2–1% of patients receiving neuraxial opioids [248]. The lumbar epidural space is easy to locate making it an attractive technique in patients with, for example, fixed spinal deformities. The combination of low-dose intrathecal morphine and a paravertebral block via a directly placed catheter has been suggested as an alternative to epidural analgesia post-thoracotomy [249].

Epidural Analgesia

Epidural injections via the sacral hiatus in dogs were described in 1901 [250]. The interspinous approach for epidural anesthesia in clinical surgery was demonstrated in 1921 [251] and an article in 1933 by Dogliotti popularized epidural anesthesia [252]. Post-thoracotomy thoracic epidural analgesia was introduced into clinical practice in the mid-1970s for high-risk procedures [161, 162], by the mid-1980s it was being used by some for routine surgery [253], and by the 1990s it had become the mainstay of post-thoracotomy analgesia in many high-volume Western units [104]. The widespread use of thoracic epidural for routine post-thoracotomy analgesia occurred because it provides effective, reliable post-thoracotomy analgesia, had been shown in a meta-analysis to reduce post-thoracotomy pulmonary complications [56], and was believed by many to improve the outcome after thoracic surgery.

Lumbar Epidural Analgesia

Lumbar epidural insertion is an easier and more familiar technique for most anesthesiologists, and also because of the absence of an underlying spinal cord, lumbar epidurals are probably safer than thoracic epidurals. Lumbar epidural hydrophilic opioids are effective and were once used by a number of units to provide post-thoracotomy analgesia. Their widespread use declined when a meta-analysis showed that, unlike epidural local anesthetics, epidural opioids did not reduce the incidence of postoperative pulmonary complications [56]. Late respiratory depression is also a potential problem with epidural hydrophilic opioids. As a result of synergistic antinociceptive interactions, mixtures of local anesthetics and opioids are now usually used to provide post-thoracotomy analgesia [180]. Epidural mixtures of segmentally acting lipophilic opioids and local anesthetics are best administered at the dermatomal level of the surgical incision. For thoracic procedures, this equates to a thoracic epidural. If the mixture is administered by a lumbar epidural away from the incision, larger volumes are required, greater hemodynamic instability results, and achieving good analgesia is more difficult. Lumbar epidurals are not now generally used for providing post-thoracotomy analgesia; however, in the occasional patient in whom attempts at placing a thoracic epidural are unsuccessful, a lumbar epidural may be appropriate. It is also a technique worth considering in the rare circumstance in which it is considered appropriate to insert an epidural in an anesthetized patient.

Thoracic Epidural Analgesia

Technique of Insertion

After inserting a venous cannula and positioning the patient in either the lateral or sitting position, depending largely on operator preference, a wide area of the back is prepped with alcoholic chlorhexidine or an alternative antiseptic solution. At least two applications are recommended. The initial application should be with a sponge or similar material to abrade the superficial layers of the skin. Care should be taken to ensure that epidural drugs and equipment are not contaminated by the antiseptic used as all antiseptics are potentially neurotoxic. Similarly, the antiseptic solution used should be allowed to dry before commencing epidural insertion. The vertebral spinous processes are at their most oblique in the mid-thoracic region. At this level, the tip of the spinous process is a landmark for the intervertebral space below the next vertebrae.

For the midline approach, a local anesthetic wheal is raised over the appropriate vertebral interspace. A Tuohy needle is then inserted immediately above the palpable tip of the lower spinous process and advanced at the oblique cephalad angle determined by the obliquity of the spinous processes at this particular level. The angle of insertion may need adjustment if contact is made with a spinous process. For the paramedian approach, a local anesthetic wheal is raised about 1 cm lateral to the palpable tip of the appropriate spinous process. A Tuohy needle is then inserted through this wheal perpendicular to all the planes. When contact is made with bone (lamina), the needle is withdrawn to the skin and angulated about 45° cephalad and 10° medial before being reinserted to the original depth. The needle is then gradually advanced into the epidural space. If contact is again made with the lamina, it may be necessary to walk the needle up the lamina to find the epidural space. After the tip of the Touhy needle has been in contact with bone, it is advisable to ensure that the needle remains patent by gently reinserting the trocar before readvancing the needle.

Identifying the epidural space at the thoracic level can be more difficult than at the lumbar level since the ligamentum flavum may be thinner and less resistant to an epidural needle at higher levels. Several alternatives to the traditional loss-of-resistance technique have been described such as the hang-

ing-drop technique [254]. A technique to identify the thoracic epidural space using pressure waveform analysis has been recently described. After initial identification of the epidural space with a loss-of-resistance technique, 5 ml of saline is injected through the Tuohy needle and a flushed sterile tubing attached at one end to a pressure transducer at the level of the patient's heart then attached to the proximal hub of the needle (see Fig. 59.21) [255]. A false loss of resistance can be distinguished from the actual epidural space with a high predictive value by the absence of an arterial waveform.

It is known that during insertion epidural catheters do not follow a predictable course in the epidural space [256]. The optimal length of epidural catheter to leave in the epidural space is thus a balance between insufficient length resulting in catheter migration out of the space and excessive length resulting in technical failure because of malpositioning of the catheter tip. In a prospective analysis of postoperative epidural failure by computed tomography epidurography during which 4 cm of epidural catheter was left in the epidural space, 25% of the epidurals failed. The major cause of epidural failure was dislodgement of the epidural catheter out of the epidural space [257]. Four centimeter of catheter is probably insufficient for thoracic epidurals that are to remain in situ for a few days; 5–6 cm may be more appropriate [258]. Migration of the catheter out of the epidural space can be reduced by appropriate fixation with adhesive dressings (see Fig. 59.22), tunneling, or suturing. The author recommends suturing of the catheter to the skin.

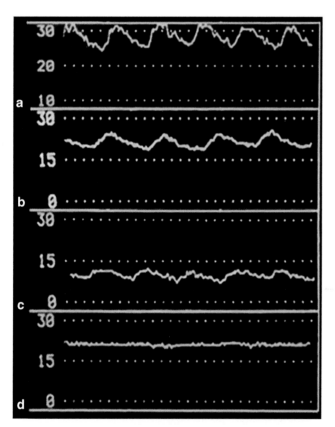

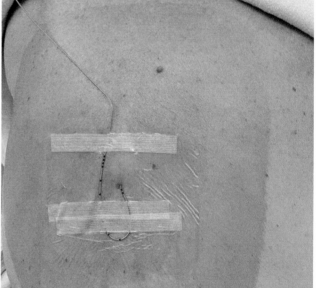

Fig. 59.21 Epidural space pressure tracings in mmHg from four different patients. The presence of an arterial-form tracing (**a–c**) was highly correlated with subsequent successful epidural analgesia. An absent arterial-form tracing (**d**) had a high sensitivity for subsequent failure of epidural analgesia. (Reproduced with permission from Leurcharusmee et al. [255])

Fig. 59.22 A technique of fixation of a thoracic epidural catheter to minimize catheter migration is demonstrated. The catheter is initially secured by sterile adhesive strips and is then covered by a sterile occlusive see-through skin dressing. The entire dressing is then covered by a large opaque adhesive elastic bandage which has a small observation window placed over the site of the skin puncture

Epidural Solutions

High concentrations of unsupplemented thoracic epidural local anesthetics can provide effective post-thoracotomy analgesia, but the incidence of hypotension is high [259], while lower concentrations are less effective. Because the synergistic antinociceptive interactions of epidural local anesthetics and opioids [260] enable the amount of each drug to be minimized reducing the incidence and severity of the associated side effects, mixtures of local anesthetics and opioids are now routinely used to provide post-thoracotomy analgesia [171, 180]. Although there is probably no epidural mixture that is optimal for all patients, a mixture of 4 µg mL^{-1} of fentanyl in 0.125% bupivacaine is close to the optimal [261–263]. The newer local anesthetic agents (levobupivacaine and ropivacaine) are less toxic than bupivacaine and give comparable results [264], and although relatively small amounts are administered epidurally, we now use 4 µg mL^{-1} of fentanyl in 0.125% levobupivacaine.

The analgesic effects of epidural opioid and local anesthetic mixtures are improved by epinephrine. Vasoconstriction of epidural vessels with reduced systemic uptake of epidural opioids is thought to be the major cause of this potentiation. The α_2 adrenergic action of epinephrine in the substantia gelatinosa may also contribute to the improved analgesia [265]. Potential cord ischemia as a result of excessive vasoconstrictive has limited the use of epidural epinephrine. Clonidine, another α_2 adrenergic agonist, is moderately lipid soluble and rapidly crosses the blood-brain barrier. The sedation associated with its systemic use has limited its systemic usage for analgesic purposes. The half-life of clonidine within the epidural space is about 30 min and when combined with epidural opioids clonidine improves analgesia and reduces opioid requirements and side effects [266, 267]. However, in a study using an optimization model to find the best epidural combination of fentanyl, bupivacaine, and clonidine to administer after laparotomy, the addition of clonidine did not significantly improve analgesia [261]. Epidural clonidine is not widely used to provide post-thoracotomy analgesia [180], although the addition of clonidine should be considered for patients who are particularly sensitive to the systemic effects of epidural opioids.

Magnesium which may act as a NMDA receptor antagonist is another adjuvant agent that has been given epidurally. In one study, epidural blocks were supplemented with 50 mg magnesium sulfate. Compared to controls patients receiving magnesium had a decreased requirement for rescue analgesia [268]. Another study has also shown a reduction in local anesthetic and opioid requirement where magnesium was administered IV concomitantly with epidural at a rate of 10 mg kg^{-1} h^{-1} for the first 24 h [269]. Epidural administration of magnesium is not currently recommended.

The extent of the sensory block after the administration of epidural anesthetics varies considerably between individuals. A number of factors are known to affect the spread of the sensory block during thoracic epidural analgesia including the level at which the epidural is sited. For high thoracic epidurals, the direction of spread is mainly caudal; for low thoracic epidurals, the spread is mainly cranial; and for mid-thoracic epidurals, the spread is almost equally distributed [33, 270]. The total extent of the spread, however, is not significantly different at these three sites [33, 270]. While administering an epidural solution via a high thoracic epidural, it may be appropriate to avoid neck flexion to further limit the potentially harmful cranial spread of the epidural solution [271]. Although widely believed and apparently logical, there is little evidence that the extent of thoracic epidural spread is related to the height of the patient [33]. Similarly, for adult patients weight does not appear to correlate with the extent of thoracic epidural spread [33]. There is, however, a positive correlation between the patient's age and the thoracic epidural spread, with elderly patients requiring about 40% less epidural solution [33, 34]. For younger patients, we usually administer a ~7 mL epidural bolus of a mixture containing 4 µg mL^{-1} of fentanyl in 0.125% levobupivacaine via a mid-thoracic catheter and then infuse the epidural solution at ~7 mL h^{-1}. For elderly patients, we reduce both the bolus and infusion rate by about 40% (Table 59.4 and Fig. 59.23).

Impact of Thoracic Epidural Analgesia

Thoracic epidurals provide excellent early post-thoracotomy analgesia and are widely regarded as the "gold standard" for post-thoracotomy pain relief. Given the low doses of local anesthetic and opioid administered via a thoracic epidural, the option remains to administer additional analgesia if required in the form of other local anesthetic infusions, e.g., into wound catheters [8].

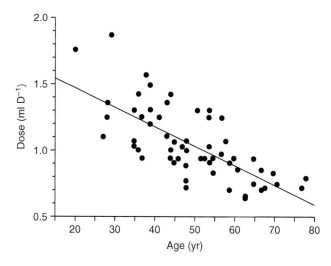

Fig. 59.23 Relationship between age and epidural dose requirements of 2% mepivacaine in thoracic epidural analgesia. D Dermatome. (Reproduced with permission, Hirabayashi and Shimizu [34])

Improvement of Postoperative Diaphragmatic Dysfunction

Prolonged diaphragmatic dysfunction has been shown to occur after thoracic [272] and upper abdominal [273] surgery. Diaphragmatic contractility is not impaired [274, 275], and the diaphragmatic dysfunction is thought to be secondary to reflex inhibition of the phrenic nerve as a result of stimulation of afferents in the viscera, diaphragm, and chest wall [274]. Pain is not considered to be a major mediator of this dysfunction [276]. Thoracic epidural local anesthetics have been shown to improve diaphragmatic function after upper abdominal surgery [277]. Epidural opioids are not effective [273]. Thoracic epidural local anesthetics have not been shown to improve the impaired diaphragmatic segmental shortening after thoracotomy, but other ventilatory parameters did improve. However, as epidural local anesthetics can alter other respiratory muscle functions, the improvement in diaphragmatic function may have been masked [272]. Thoracic epidural analgesia may directly affect FRC post-thoracotomy as an increase in FRC occurs in healthy humans receiving thoracic epidural analgesia [278].

Incidence of Cardiovascular Complications

Cardiovascular complications contribute significantly to post-thoracotomy morbidity and mortality. Thoracic epidural local anesthetics can block the sympathetic nerve fibers to the heart and have been used to treat refractory angina [279, 280]. Thoracic epidural analgesia can also dilate constricted coronary arteries and improve the hemodynamic stability of patients undergoing thoracic surgery. When compared to lumbar epidural analgesia, there is a lower incidence of hypotension and bradycardia where thoracic epidurals are used [281]. These changes have the potential to reduce myocardial ischemia. A meta-analysis of patients undergoing various surgeries has confirmed this potential and shows that epidural analgesia reduces postoperative myocardial infarctions by 40%; thoracic epidural analgesia is superior to lumbar epidural analgesia in this respect [282]. There is some evidence that thoracic epidural local anesthetics reduce the incidence of supraventricular arrhythmias [283], which occur in 20–30% of post-thoracotomy patients [284, 285] and are associated with an increased mortality [286, 287]. More recently however, a post hoc analysis of data collected during the POISE trial [288] has advised caution regarding the use of neuraxial analgesia in patients deemed particularly high risk of cardiovascular morbidity as use of thoracic epidural with general anesthesia was associated with a threefold increase in the risk of the trial primary composite outcome (cardiovascular death, nonfatal myocardial infarction, or nonfatal cardiac arrest) versus general anesthesia alone. While this was a post hoc analysis, clinicians should bear this is mind when considering and consenting for thoracic epidural analgesia in patients with significant cardiovascular disease.

Thoracic Epidurals and Outcome

The mortality from lung cancer surgery has decreased over the last few decades, and this reduction in post-thoracotomy mortality has been attributed, in part, to improvements in postoperative analgesia. There are a number of possible mechanisms whereby thoracic epidural analgesia may reduce respiratory complications post-thoracotomy. These include better preservation of FRC, improved mucociliary clearance, reduction of inhibitory effects on the diaphragm, less pain, nausea and sedation and better collaboration with physiotherapy. Although transferable evidence and early analysis found that when compared with systemic analgesia, thoracic epidural analgesia reduced postoperative pulmonary complications [56], later quantitative analyses have not shown this reduction [58]. Similarly, although thoracic epidurals may decrease perioperative myocardial infarctions [282] and reduce the incidence of thromboembolic events [289, 290], there are no prospective studies showing thoracic epidurals improve survival after thoracotomy. A meta-analysis of randomized controlled studies did show reduced mortality with neuraxial blocks after surgery, but much of this effect was after orthopedic surgery [291]. Following an initial prospective randomized study [292] that suggested no mortality benefit associated with epidural analgesia for major abdominal surgery, a more recent meta-analysis identified a 40% reduction in mortality after major abdominal surgery where epidural analgesia was employed [293]. A large prospective study is still required to determine if post-thoracotomy outcome is improved with thoracic epidural analgesia.

Limitations and Adverse Effects

The reported rates of epidural failure vary. Although successful catheter placement rates of 99% and subsequent technical failure rates of <1% have been reported [294], some audits have reported a 30–50% failure rate [295] and a recent meta-analysis reported a 15% thoracic epidural failure rate [203]. Thoracic epidurals are considered technically more difficult to insert than lumbar epidurals; however, the dural perforation rate has been found to be lower during thoracic epidural insertion (0.9%) than during lumbar epidural insertion (3.4%) [294].

The use of enhanced recovery protocols within thoracic surgery is increasing in popularity as they have been shown to be associated with reduced complication rates and duration of hospital stay. Use of epidural analgesia and their associated adverse effects can impact upon recovery, despite high-quality pain control, and therefore their use is less attractive given the other options available [17]. Respiratory depression is a concern with epidural opioids particularly hydrophilic opioids. The incidence is related to the type and dose of the epidural opioids used. A Swedish study also found that age >70 years and the administration of additional opioids by other routes were risk factors for the development of respiratory depression [296]. However, the reported incidence of respiratory depression with fentanyl local anesthetic epidurals of 0.3% [297] is no higher than the incidence of respiratory depression when opioids are administered by other routes. Drug errors whereby the wrong drug is administered epidurally have been reported [298] but fortunately are rare and should be reduced further by using dedicated epidural delivery systems.

The reported incidence of serious complications has varied although an estimate of 0.0007% is often quoted. The Third National Audit Project, the largest prospective study of complications after central neuraxial blocks, has helped clarify the incidence of serious complications associated with epidurals [164, 165]. This confirmed that overall (perioperative, obstetric, pediatric, and chronic pain) central nerve blocks were associated with a very low (0.007%) incidence of major complications. The incidence of major complication after epidurals inserted perioperatively was, however, much higher at 0.02%. The most frequent complications were epidural hematomas [165]. This incidence of major complications after perioperative epidurals is almost the same as that incidence reported in an earlier Swedish study [299].

Urinary Retention

Urinary retention is a well-known complication of epidural opioid use [300]. The mechanisms for this include inhibition of sacral parasympathetic outflow and inhibition of the pontine micturition center [301]. Epidural morphine-mediated reduction in detrusor muscle function is antagonized by naloxone [302], and in post-hysterectomy patients naloxone can reverse bladder dysfunction without reversing epidural morphine analgesia [303]. When given to post-thoracotomy patients receiving thoracic fentanyl bupivacaine epidural analgesia, naloxone reversed the analgesic effects of the epidural without reducing the need for urinary catheterization [304] and so is not recommended.

Gastric Emptying

The excellent early analgesia provided by thoracic epidural analgesia enables most patients to resume their normal diet and oral medications a few hours post-thoracotomy. The rate-limiting step for the absorption of most orally adminis-

tered drugs is gastric emptying. Gastric emptying is variably affected by anesthesia and surgery [305–307]. Epidural opioids can result in gastric hypomobility. Branches of the T6–T10 sympathetic nerves innervate the stomach [308] and sympathetic blockade of these nerves could hasten gastric emptying. Gastric emptying has been shown to be normal in patients receiving bupivacaine epidural analgesia post-cholecystectomy [307] although for post-thoracotomy patients receiving a fentanyl bupivacaine epidural, there is some evidence that gastric emptying is delayed for >48 h [309]. A recent Cochrane review [310] concluded that, following a meta-analysis of recent studies, epidural analgesia, following abdominal surgery either with or without the addition of an opioid, was associated with a faster return of gastric motility when compared to an opioid-based analgesic regimen such as an IV-PCA. Delayed gastric emptying should therefore be assumed to occur in any situation where an opioid is employed and may be better in the context of epidural versus intravenously administered opioid but may overall be associated with reflux or regurgitation and altered effects of orally administered drugs. Dexmedetomidine has also been added to epidural solutions in colonic surgery as an alternative to morphine. In one study [311] the use of epidural dexmedetomidine in addition to levobupivacaine was associated with similar pain scores and additional analgesic requirements, but there was a suggestion of improved gastric motility in the group receiving dexmedetomidine, along with a reduced incidence of nausea, vomiting, and pruritis.

Hypotension

Hypotension is a common occurrence during thoracic epidural analgesia. It is important to appreciate the differences between hypotension due to a lumbar versus mid-thoracic epidural sympathetic blockade. With lumbar neuraxial blockade, hypotension is primarily due to systemic vasodilation, decreasing cardiac preload and afterload. The hypotension due to thoracic epidural blockade occurs for these two previous reasons and also due to blockade of the cardiac sympathetic supply, interfering with the heart's ability to increase contractility. Unlike treatment of hypotension during lumbar blockade, hypotension during thoracic epidural blockade will have a limited response to increases of preload and afterload and so requires treatment with a β-adrenergic or mixed agonist (e.g., ephedrine, dopamine, etc.) to increase contractility and restore cardiac output [312]. One meta-analysis [313] has suggested that use of thoracic epidural analgesia in the context of one-lung ventilation may reduce hypoxic pulmonary vasoconstriction through this mechanism, causing an increase in shunt fraction and reduction in partial pressure of oxygen (P_aO_2) and mixed arterial oxygen saturation (S_aO_2).

Neuraxial Block and Coagulation

The risk of an epidural inserted for post-thoracotomy analgesia resulting in a permanent injury or death is approximately 0.02%. Epidural hematomas account for most of this morbidity [164, 165]. Anticoagulants and antiplatelet agents can further increase the risk of vertebral canal hematoma [314, 315] and may increase the risk of epidural abscesses by causing small hematomas that become secondarily infected. All patients receiving thoracic epidural analgesia and patients who have undergone unsuccessful attempts at epidural catheter placement should be monitored regularly for symptoms and signs of vertebral canal hematoma, specifically back pain, motor or sensory changes, and urinary retention, if not catheterized. Of these, motor block is the most reliable sign and most sensitive prognostic indicator [316]. Vertebral canal hematomas occurring in the perioperative period have a poor outcome. Where there is a clinical suspicion of epidural hematoma, intervention should be planned urgently with diagnostic imaging, e.g., magnetic resonance imaging (MRI), and surgical intervention, e.g., decompressive laminectomy [317].Due to the rarity of spinal epidural hematoma, case reports and expert opinion, not scientific evidence from controlled trials, provide the mainstay of recommendations for epidural analgesia in patients receiving antithrombotic medications. This is particularly true for thromboprophylaxis [317, 318]. Recommendations by the European Society of Anaesthesiology (ESA) [317] and the American Society of Regional Anesthesia and Pain Medicine (ASRA) [166] are based upon the known pharmacology of the individual agents in the context of normal physiology, case reports, clinical series, and risk factors for surgical bleeding. Reduced renal or hepatic clearance due to use of other medications or underlying pathology may impact this and increase the risk of bleeding [317]. One suggestion has been to use the rule of not performing a neuraxial block or removing an epidural catheter until the time from the last dose of anticoagulant is equal to $2 - T_{1/2}$ h (where $T_{1/2}$ takes into account the renal and hepatic function of the individual patient) in order to achieve the optimum risk/benefit ratio leaving 25% pharmacodynamic efficacy or the rule of $5 - T_{1/2}$ h in high-risk patients or where there is a drug with limited clinical experience to leave 3.125% [319]. Where cessation of anticoagulant treatment is not possible or deemed to be of high risk to the patient, neuraxial analgesia should be abandoned and alternative plans should be made.

Heparin and Thromboprophylaxis

Subcutaneous unfractionated heparin is effective in reducing the incidence of thromboembolic complications [166, 320]. There are a limited number of case reports of vertebral canal hematoma associated with neuraxial blockade in patients receiving subcutaneous unfractionated heparin published in the literature [321–323], and therefore subcutaneous heparin in patients with thoracic epidurals in situ appears safe [324]. If subcutaneous heparin is continued for greater than 4–5 days, a platelet count is recommended prior to removal of the epidural catheter as heparin-induced thrombocytopenia may occur [325]. Low molecular weight heparins have different biochemical and pharmacological properties to unfractionated heparin including anti-Xa activity [166] and the fact that their effect cannot easily be reverse with protamine. Routine anti-Xa monitoring is not, at present, recommended when planning neuraxial anesthesia or analgesia [325]. The half-life of anticoagulant activity following the administration of a dose of subcutaneous low molecular weight heparin is considerably longer than that following a subcutaneous dose of unfractionated heparin, allowing once daily dosage. In the late 1990s, there were reports of more than 40 cases of vertebral canal hematoma in patients following neuraxial blockade in the United States. This may have been the result of the North American guidelines recommending twice daily dosage, meaning there was effectively no "safe" time in which to perform a block or remove an epidural catheter. Similar clusters of cases of hematoma were not reported in Europe despite extensive experience of regional blockade concurrent with low molecular weight heparin thromboprophylaxis [326, 327]. This is thought to represent the once daily dosage employed in Europe. However, despite this neuraxial blockade in the presence of low molecular weight heparin, thromboprophylaxis is more risky than with unfractionated heparin, especially for epidural catheter techniques [166].

Removal of epidural catheters should not be performed until at least 4 h after cessation of unfractionated heparin administration and after confirmation that the coagulation profile has normalized [317]. If a bloody puncture occurs, the ESA recommends that low-dose anticoagulation be avoided for 1–2 h and full heparinization for 6–12 h [317], while the ASRA recommends waiting for 24 h until LMWH are used [325]. Where low molecular weight heparin is administered prophylactically, clinicians should wait at least 12 h from the previous dose before performing neuraxial blockade or removing an epidural catheter and should wait until 2–4 h after catheter removal to give a further dose [317, 325]. For a treatment dose of LMWH, at least 24 h should pass between the last dose and neuraxial block or catheter removal. Treatment can be restarted 2–4 h after catheter removal [317]. This guidance is issued in the context of normal renal function and therefore the impact of the reduced renal function must be taken into account when planning any neuraxial block.

Fondaparinux

Fondaparinux is a synthetic pentasaccharide factor Xa inhibitor that is similar in structure to the low molecular weight heparins [325]. Where fondaparinux is used at prophylactic doses, the last dose should have been administered at least 36 h prior to neuraxial block or catheter insertion or removal and ideally 3–4 days prior to minimize risk. Following removal of an epidural catheter, at least 24 h should pass before the next dose is administered [328]. This advice is given in the context of a single-needle atraumatic needle pass, and therefore where the procedure proves to be more complicated, ongoing use of fondaparinux should be avoided [325]. Where fondaparinux is administered in treatment doses (5–10 mg per day), neuraxial block should not be performed due to the risks of accumulation of effect [317].

Warfarin

When thoracic epidural analgesia is planned, warfarin should be discontinued at least 4–5 days preoperatively. The INR should be within normal limits prior to placing the epidural catheter to ensure adequate levels of active vitamin K-dependent clotting factors. Hemostasis may not be adequate even with an INR of 1.3 [166] since, in the first 1–3 days after cessation of treatment, a return to normal levels of factor VII leads to a relatively normal INR despite still low levels of factor II and X leading to potential ongoing coagulopathy [325]. Warfarin therapy should ideally not be reinstituted until after removal of the epidural catheter and the INR should be <1.4 prior to catheter insertion or removal. The clinician should not overlook the potential use of bridging anticoagulation during the period of warfarin cessation, and these agents must also be taken into account when planning neuraxial blockade.

NOACs: Novel Oral Anticoagulants

This group includes drugs such as rivaroxaban, dabigatran, and apixaban. They are increasing in popularity due to their fixed dose administration, reduced need for monitoring, and more favorable pharmacokinetics and pharmacodynamics [319]. Dabigatran is a prodrug that acts through reversible inhibition of free and clot-bound thrombin. The most recent ASRA guidance states that clinicians should wait a minimum of 4–5 days to perform neuraxial block or remove an epidural catheter and that the next dose should not be administered until 6 h later. Rivaroxaban and apixaban are orally administered direct inhibitors of factor Xa. For rivaroxaban, with prophylactic doses of <10 mg per day, 22–26 h between the last dose and neuraxial block or catheter removal is

advised. Further doses should not be administered until 4–6 h after catheter removal. Where patients are taking apixaban (prophylactic dose, 2.5 mg BD), 3–5 days should pass between the last dose and neuraxial block or catheter removal. The next dose after catheter removal should not be administered until 6 h later [328]. It must be reiterated that this advice is in the context of normal renal function, and therefore in other circumstances, the use of neuraxial blockade should be considered more cautiously.

Antiplatelet Medications

There is considerable variability in patient responses to antiplatelet agents. The increased risk in individual patients may therefore be difficult to quantify, although female sex, advanced age, and a history of easily bruising can signify an increased risk. The role of near-patient testing of platelet function prior to neuraxial block needs to be established.

NSAIDs (Including Aspirin)

NSAIDs appear not to increase the risk of vertebral canal hematoma in patients undergoing neuraxial blockade [166, 325, 329, 330]. Concurrent administration of other hemostasis altering medications does, however, appear to increase the risk of bleeding [166], especially in the case of aspirin. This includes heparin for postoperative thromboprophylaxis [315, 318] and thienopyridine drugs [317]. Thus, if feasible, aspirin should be discontinued 5–7 days prior to surgery if central neuraxial blockade and heparin-based DVT prophylaxis are planned. Where aspirin is co-administered with other drugs that impact coagulation, neuraxial analgesia should usually be avoided [325].

Thienopyridine Derivatives

These include clopidogrel and ticlopidine. They are potent antiplatelet agents causing irreversible inhibition of ADP-induced platelet aggregation and platelet fibrinogen-binding inhibition. Clopidogrel should be discontinued at least 7 days and ticlopidine at least 10–14 days prior to neuraxial blockade [166, 317].

Platelet Glycoprotein IIb/IIIa Inhibitors

This group of drugs includes abciximab and tirofiban and acts through inhibition of platelet aggregation [319]. While platelet function should normalize following a dose of abciximab after 24–48 h and following cessation of tirofiban infusion within 4–8 h, performance of neuraxial blockade should not occur until the clinician is confident that platelet function has normalized [319].

Herbal (Alternative) Medication

Up to 50% of surgical patients may be taking herbal medications preoperatively although many do not volunteer this information. Although herbal drugs by themselves probably pose no significant added risk, garlic, ginseng, and gingko have raised concern because they are associated with thrombocytopenia, inhibition of platelet aggregation, and interaction with vitamin K antagonists. There may be a small increased risk of an epidural hematoma if patients receive heparin for thromboembolism prophylaxis [166, 318]. It is probably wise to actively seek a history of such herbal therapy usage and discontinue it 7 days preoperatively.

Coronary Stents

An increasing number of patients with coronary artery stents in situ and receiving antiplatelet drugs are presenting for thoracic surgery. After insertion patients receiving bare metal stents require aspirin and clopidogrel for at least 4 weeks. Patients receiving drug-eluting stents require aspirin and clopidogrel for at least 12 months. All patients with stents in situ require aspirin for life [167, 169, 331]. Dual antiplatelet therapy is a contraindication to epidural analgesia [166]. Although discontinuing clopidogrel ≥7 days preoperatively while continuing aspirin may make thoracic epidural feasible, the premature discontinuation of one antiplatelet agent markedly increases the risk of acute perioperative stent thrombosis with significant cardiac morbidity and mortality [167–169]. Aspirin therapy should rarely be interrupted [169]. The planned duration of postoperative epidural analgesia is also relevant as antiplatelet therapy should be recommenced as soon as possible post-procedure as delays may expose the patient to an unacceptable risk of stent thrombosis [167].

Techniques for Specific Situations

Sternotomy

A sternotomy can be used to provide access for a range of surgical procedures including the resection of anterior mediastinal tumors. At closure the divided sternum is usually internally fixed with wire. This fixation restricts bone movement and limits pain. Adequate post-sternotomy analgesia can usually be achieved with a morphine IV-PCA system supplemented when appropriate by non-opioid analgesics.

Local anesthetic wound infiltration can reduce opioid consumption [332] and should be considered. Continuous wound infiltration via deep and/or subcutaneous catheters may be more effective, but evidence of effectiveness is limited, with some studies showing no benefit [333]. Thoracic epidurals can provide very effective post-sternotomy analgesia and have previously been used to provide analgesia following cardiac surgery, where one meta-analysis [334] showed a reduced incidence of arrhythmias, respiratory complications including atelectasis and pneumonia, duration of tracheal intubation, and visual analogue scores. Despite this however there was no clinically significant improvement in overall mortality. The catheter should be sited at a higher level (T3/T4) than for a thoracotomy (T6/T7) and any paresthesia of the medial surface of the arms detected early, to enable a timely reduction in the epidural infusion rate to limit the risk of bilateral phrenic nerve blocks. Thoracic epidural analgesia should be considered for patients with poor lung function undergoing bilateral pulmonary procedures via a sternotomy (e.g., volume reduction surgery). A parasternal local anesthetic block can reduce opioid requirements [335] and could be considered in patients with poor lung function in whom epidural anesthesia is contraindicated.

Video-Assisted Surgery

The limited incision may limit postoperative pain, but several studies support that, particularly where VATS lobectomy is performed, there is frequently at least a moderate level of postoperative pain [336, 337]. Despite this fact, many feel that this less invasive surgery may still require a less invasive form of analgesia [338]. One review article concluded that thoracic epidural analgesia did not exhibit a significant effect on pain scores when compared to other modalities and, given the potential side effects, suggested less invasive techniques may be preferable [339]. The appropriate analgesia depends in part on the nature of the surgery undertaken. Thoracic epidural analgesia may be advantageous in patients undergoing minimally invasive esophagectomies [340], whereas paravertebral blocks, either single shot or ideally with a catheter for ongoing infusion, potentially in combination with an IV-PCA system may be appropriate for patients undergoing VAT lung resections. Minimal analgesia may be required after VAT pleural biopsies or sympathectomies, and a single-shot paravertebral block along with a basic analgesic regime may be more than adequate.

Open Thoracotomy

A large number of pain management techniques have been described for open thoracotomy patients. These have included the administration of local anesthetics, opioids, and other drugs to provide intercostal nerve blocks [186–188], interpleural blocks [194–197], paravertebral blocks [236, 341, 342], lumbar epidural analgesia [343–345], thoracic epidural analgesia [161, 162, 255, 262, 263], intrathecal analgesia [118, 119, 242–245], and systemic analgesia [58]. In addition, the non-pharmacological techniques of cryoanalgesia [159, 160] and TENS [346–352] have been used. Good post-thoracotomy pain control is difficult to achieve without regional anesthesia and it is recommended that a regional anesthetic technique be used as part of a multimodal analgesic regimen to provide post-thoracotomy analgesia. Apart from paravertebral blocks, all other regional analgesic techniques are inferior to thoracic epidural analgesia [58]; the choice of regional anesthetic technique is usually between thoracic epidural analgesia and a paravertebral block. In practice both techniques have advantages in particular patients and the acquisition of expertise in both techniques is recommended. For patients with borderline predicted postoperative lung function, good early analgesia and the ability to cooperate with lung recruitment maneuvers immediately postoperatively may be critical. A retrospective analysis of one institute's data showed that a preoperative FEV_1 of less than 60% predicted was an independent risk factor for the development of post-thoracotomy pulmonary complications and mortality. The use of thoracic epidural analgesia was associated with reduced pulmonary complications and a reduced mortality in patients with an $FEV_1 < 60\%$, although no patients were reported to have received a paravertebral block [353] (Fig. 59.24). A prospective 1-year observational study of pneumonectomies in the United Kingdom found epidural analgesia to be a significant associate of poor outcome [354].

For patients with good pulmonary function undergoing limited lung resection, early analgesia may be less critical and paravertebral analgesia may enable earlier mobilization and shorten hospital stays. For most patients, the decision is less clear-cut, and consideration of the relative risks and benefits of the two techniques should be made for the particular patient (Table 59.5). For patients for whom neither thoracic epidural or paravertebral blocks is appropriate, consideration should be given to the use of intercostal nerve blocks or preoperative intrathecal opioids.

Esophageal Surgery

With a perioperative mortality of approximately 3% and an incidence of major morbidity of up to 30%, esophagectomy is one of the highest-risk thoracic surgical procedures [355]. Postoperative pain can be very severe after open esophageal surgery, and thoracic epidural analgesia is usually used to provide postoperative analgesia for these patients. In nonran-

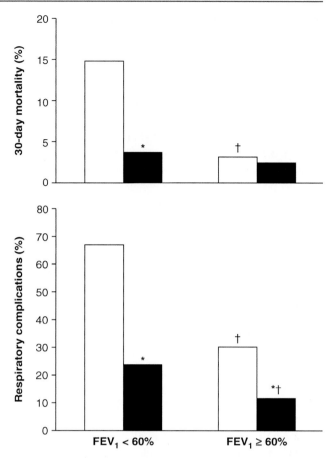

Fig. 59.24 Thirty-day mortality rate (top) and incidence of respiratory complications (bottom) according to preoperative FEV1 (<60% or ≥60%) and type of analgesic regimen: without thoracic epidural analgesia (white bars) or with thoracic epidural analgesia (black bars). *$p < 0.05$, compared with group without thoracic epidural analgesia; †$p < 0.05$, compared with group FEV1 ≥ 60%. (Reproduced with permission, Licker et al. [353])

Table 59.5 Factors influencing choice of paravertebral block or thoracic epidural

Favors thoracic epidural	Favors paravertebral block
Poor PFTs	Good PFTs
Extensive lung resection	Limited lung resection
Chest wall involvement	Sepsis
Nonsteroidal anti-inflammatory drugs (NSAIDs) contraindicated	Impaired coagulation
Patient preference	Patient preference
	Fixed spinal deformity
	Anesthetized patient

domized studies comparing systemic opioids with epidural analgesia after open esophageal surgery, patients receiving epidural analgesia had fewer respiratory complications [356, 357], spent less time in intensive care [356, 358], and had a lower mortality [356, 359, 360] potentially secondary to a reduction in the systemic pro-inflammatory response [357]. Thoracic epidurals may decrease the incidence of anastomotic leakage post-esophagectomy [357, 361]. Ischemia at the anastomotic end of the newly formed gastric tube is a major cause of anastomotic leaks post-esophagectomy [362]. A relationship between low Doppler determined blood flow at the anastomotic site and subsequent anastomotic leakage has been shown [363]. Although intraoperative epidural boluses can cause hypotension and reduced blood flow to the anastomotic end of the gastric tube [364], a study using continuous postoperative thoracic epidurals found epidurals to be associated with minimal hypotension and an increased distal conduit blood flow [365]. We recommend that "anesthesiologists should be cautious in accepting intra-operative hypotension secondary to epidural administration in patients undergoing esophagectomy" [364]. For patients undergoing a minimally invasive esophagectomy, some groups have utilized the combination of an IV-PCA system, bilateral paravertebral blocks, and non-opioid analgesics. There is conflicting evidence regarding the influence of epidural analgesia on mortality, with some describing an increased mortality in patients undergoing minimally invasive esophagectomy without a thoracic epidural [340] and others identifying no difference in overall mortality or incidence of disease recurrence [357]. Expert groups tend to advocate the use of a thoracic epidural for all patients scheduled to undergo an esophagectomy in order to limit the postoperative inflammatory response and provide high-quality pain control [366, 367]. For patients undergoing open esophageal surgery in whom epidural analgesia is inappropriate or contraindicated, consideration should be given to the use of a continuous paravertebral block as they have been reported to provide reasonable analgesia when supplemented by systemic analgesics [368].

Shoulder Pain

Ipsilateral shoulder pain is common in patients receiving effective thoracic epidural analgesia and occurs occasionally in patients receiving paravertebral blocks, but is rare in patients not receiving nerve blocks for post-thoracotomy analgesia. The reported incidence of ipsilateral shoulder pain varies from 37 to 97% [77, 131, 200, 369–371] and can lead to significantly impaired respiratory and physical function postoperatively. This shoulder pain is often described by patients as an ache, usually of moderate to severe intensity which may fluctuate over the course of the day [371], and lasts for 3–4 days postoperatively [372]. While shoulder pain may follow both open and thoracoscopic surgeries, the overall incidence appears to be higher following thoracotomy and with longer duration of surgery [373].

Early explanations of this shoulder pain were that it was related to the transection of a major bronchus although no mechanism was suggested [77]. Other early explanations included stretching of the brachial plexus or the shoulder joint as a result of the intraoperative positioning and distraction of the posterior thoracic ligaments by surgical retractors [13]. The location of the pain varies and has been reported in differing locations from posterior shoulder, deltoid, and lateral third of the clavicle, although all locations share innervation with the diaphragm [374], leading to a further hypothesis regarding the etiology of referred pain. Several studies have helped clarify the pathogenesis of this pain, with one group recently suggesting multiple contributing etiologies. In a prospective observational study [371], pain was classified as either referred or musculoskeletal, where patients with evidence of muscle tenderness in the painful area, reproducible shoulder pain on palpation of muscles in other areas, or aggravation of pain on movement of the shoulder were placed in the latter group. In 55% of patients, shoulder pain was deemed to be of musculoskeletal origin and was found to be of greater intensity than in the 45% of patients where pain was classified as referred. In a few patients with ipsilateral post-thoracotomy shoulder pain and an apical chest drain extending to the apex of the chest cavity, withdrawal of the chest drain by a few centimeters relieves the pain. This implies that irritation of the apical pleura by the chest drain is another cause of ipsilateral post-thoracotomy shoulder pain.

Management of ipsilateral shoulder pain following thoracic surgery proves challenging. The pain is resistant to epidural boluses [78] and intravenous opioids [369]. Preoperative gabapentin [131] is similarly ineffective. A double-blind study of patients who had developed ipsilateral post-thoracotomy shoulder pain, in which patients were given either bupivacaine or saline to block the suprascapular nerve, found that blocking the suprascapular nerve did not affect the incidence of pain [370]. A placebo-controlled study of the administration of bupivacaine through the basal drain to anesthetize the diaphragmatic pleura found that bupivacaine was not effective in reducing ipsilateral post-thoracotomy shoulder pain [200]. A placebo-controlled study in which the periphrenic fat pad, at the level of the diaphragm, was infiltrated with either lidocaine or saline intraoperatively reduced the early incidence of ipsilateral post-thoracotomy shoulder pain from 85% to 33% [369] (Fig. 59.25).

This marked reduction in the incidence of ipsilateral post-thoracotomy shoulder pain with phrenic nerve infiltration was confirmed in a later study [376]. The phrenic nerve must therefore be importantly involved in the pathogenesis of ipsilateral post-thoracotomy shoulder pain. The phrenic nerve supplies sensory branches to the mediastinal pleura, the fibrous pericardium, the parietal layer of the serous pericar-

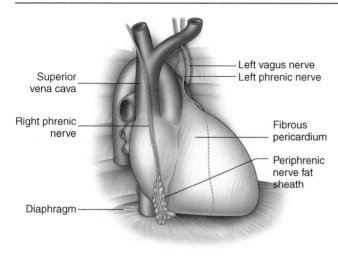

Fig. 59.25 Diagram to illustrate the site of the periphrenic nerve fat sheath for phrenic nerve blocks. (Modified with permission from Gosling et al. [375] in Scawn et al. [369])

dium, and the pleura related to the central part of the diaphragm. In many patients, the likely explanation of ipsilateral post-thoracotomy shoulder pain is irritation of the pericardium, mediastinal, and diaphragmatic pleural surfaces resulting in pain referred to the shoulder via the phrenic nerve.

Effective treatment options for ipsilateral post-thoracotomy shoulder pain therefore include acetaminophen [100], nonsteroidal anti-inflammatory agents [77, 78], direct intraoperative phrenic nerve blocks [369, 376], and indirect postoperative phrenic nerve blocks [377, 378]. The use of acetaminophen orally, rectally, or intravenously to treat ipsilateral post-thoracotomy shoulder pain is recommended. Rectal acetaminophen is safe and moderately effective [100] although personal experience suggests intravenous acetaminophen to be more effective. NSAIDs are effective in controlling ipsilateral post-thoracotomy shoulder pain [77, 78] and personal experience suggests that they are more effective than acetaminophen. The well-known side effects of NSAIDs are, however, a particular concern in the often old and debilitated patients who have undergone thoracic surgery and the risks should be assessed before their use. Intraoperative phrenic nerve blocks are effective. The short duration of effect with lidocaine [369] can be extended by the use of ropivacaine [376], but patient selection is important as the resultant unilateral diaphragmatic paresis can further impair ventilation. Phrenic nerve blocks should be considered for patients in whom postoperative pulmonary function is not a concern and for patients undergoing a pneumonectomy. In post-pneumonectomy patients, the unilateral loss of diaphragmatic function has limited effects on ventilation and may have an additional benefit of helping to reduce the pneumonectomy space. Postoperative interscalene brachial plexus blocks have been shown to be effective in treating ipsilateral post-thoracotomy shoulder pain in case reports

[377] and in a prospective study [378]. The phrenic nerve block that is a side effect of interscalene brachial plexus block [379] almost certainly explains the block's effectiveness. As a result of the potential complications associated with this block, we recommend that interscalene brachial plexus blocks be considered only in patients with severe ipsilateral post-thoracotomy shoulder pain and adequate pulmonary reserve. Although a stellate ganglion block may be effective in treating ipsilateral post-thoracotomy shoulder pain [380], its use for this purpose is not recommended.

Opioid-Tolerant Patients

Continuous opioid exposure results in a rightward shift of the dose-response curve to opioids, resulting in patients requiring increased amounts of opioid to obtain the same pharmacological effect. It is a predictable pharmacological adaptation [381]. The degree of opioid tolerance is related to the dosage, duration, and type of opioid administered. Opioid tolerance occurs when higher doses of opioids are required to achieve adequate analgesia due to desensitizing of signaling via the opioid receptor [60], decreased opioid receptor density [382], upregulation of cyclic adenosine monophosphate [383], and neural adaptation [384]. Activation of NMDA receptors plays an important role in the development of opioid tolerance [385]. Opioid-tolerant patients are relatively pain intolerant [386] and may have greater difficulty in coping with acute pain [387].

The principles of treatment are similar for all groups, but opioid substance abusers may present additional challenges due to their psychological problems, dependency on other substances (e.g., alcohol), concomitant infectious diseases (e.g., tuberculosis, human immunodeficiency virus), and the use of antagonist drugs which may affect the delivery of anesthesia. A thorough history should be taken to ascertain the location and characteristics of their chronic pain condition, along with the route and usual daily dose of opioids. Patients should be encouraged to continue their usual analgesic regime up until the time of surgery and where able in the perioperative period [60]. For patients scheduled for major surgery where oral intake is likely to be disrupted, an equivalent intravenous dose of morphine should be estimated. Unfortunately, variability in the pharmacokinetics, pharmacodynamics, route of administration, and daily opioid consumption can make estimating a morphine equivalent dose difficult. Abrupt cessation of opioids can result in an acute opioid withdrawal syndrome and should be avoided. Naltrexone, a long-acting competitive opioid antagonist used to help prevent relapse in detoxified former opioid-dependent patients and in alcohol addiction, should be discontinued a few days before surgery if possible. Where it has been administered via a depot injection, since the antagonism lasts approximately 30 days, surgery should be delayed until after this time if possible [60]. Similarly, buprenorphine, a partial mu agonist, is frequently stopped approximately 3 days prior to surgery in order to allow the full mu agonist effect of other strong opioids to take effect [388].

This group of patients benefit greatly from a multimodal approach to pain management and the use of non-opioid drugs must be carefully considered. Acetaminophen, either via the oral or intravenous route, is a beneficial adjunct along with oral or intravenous NSAIDs if there are no contraindications. Ketamine has been suggested to reverse morphine tolerance and therefore return its effectiveness in animal models and the use of ketamine orally, as an intravenous infusion alone or as part of an IV-PCA regime may contribute to better pain control. Clonidine, dexmedetomidine, and the gabapentinoids have also been suggested as useful adjuncts [388].

Most patients undergoing open thoracic surgery benefit from the addition of a regional anesthetic technique. Thoracic epidurals can provide excellent post-thoracotomy analgesia in opioid-tolerant patients, and their use should therefore be considered. The use of a lipophilic opioid local anesthetic mixture is recommended. Lipophilic opioid local anesthetic mixtures have been shown to provide pain control that is superior to morphine local anesthetic mixtures in opioid-tolerant patients, perhaps because analgesic effects are exerted at lower receptor occupancy [389, 390]. An alternative for patients scheduled to receive significant amounts of opioids by other routes is the use of a plain local anesthetic epidural solution. Where thoracic epidural use is inappropriate, a catheter-based paravertebral technique is recommended.

For a few patients, parental opioids may be the most appropriate means of providing postoperative analgesia. Despite earlier concerns of increasing addiction and manipulative behavior, the use of intravenous IV-PCA systems to control pain in substance abusers is now generally considered acceptable, if this system is used appropriately. Increasing opioid dose in order to overcome tolerance is an inadequate strategy as frequently there is minimal improvement in pain control but a marked increase in the incidence of opioid-related side effects, such as sedation, respiratory depression, ileus, and a paradoxical worsening of pain perception [60, 391]. Predicting the postoperative opioid requirement for opioid-dependent patients is difficult. For opioid-naïve patients receiving an IV-PCA for post-thoracotomy analgesia, a background opioid infusion is usually not appropriate. Opioid-dependent patients however may require a background infusion and are likely to require higher doses in addition to their preoperative regime. Opioid rotation can be considered as sometimes changing the agent may lead to an overall reduction in the total dose required.

Swenson et al. noted that during drug administration, there is initially a disparity between the plasma concentration and the concentration of the drug at its site of action (effect site concentration). They describe a method of determining the effect site concentration of fentanyl at the threshold of respiratory depression in individual patients using simulation software and a fentanyl infusion. After determining the effect site concentration of fentanyl at the threshold for respiratory depression, an hourly fentanyl administration rate that will result in 30% of this effect site concentration is calculated. Utilizing an intravenous PCA system, half of this calculated fentanyl dose can be administered as a background infusion, while the remaining 50% is programmed for demand administration as boluses with a 15-min lockout period. They recommend that the regimen be reviewed at 4-hourly intervals and adjustments made based on the number of demand boluses administered, the level of conscious, and the respiratory rate [392].

Methadone, a NMDA receptor antagonist which can activate α adrenergic receptors and a different range of μ receptors subtypes to morphine, is regarded as the intravenous PCA opioid of choice for opioid-dependent patients by some authors [393]. Consideration should be given to using a methadone IV-PCA system in opioid-dependent patients whose postoperative pain is refractory to large doses of systemic morphine. A single dose of opioid has been shown to cause activation of NMDA receptors [394]. In animal studies where ketamine was administered, reversal of morphine intolerance and consequent improved opioid effectiveness has been shown [395]. The administration of a low-dose ketamine infusion should be considered particularly in patients for whom regional anesthetic techniques are not planned. The literature suggests that for opioid-tolerant patients, an intraoperative bolus of ketamine ($\sim$0.25 mg kg^{-1}) should be followed by an intravenous infusion ($\sim$2 μg kg^{-1} min^{-1}) continued for a few days [121]. Although adding ketamine to morphine delivered via an IV-PCA has been described [110], this is not recommended in opioid-tolerant patients because the large and unpredictable opioid requirement may result in the administration of excessive doses of ketamine with the associated psychotropic side effects [121].

Conclusion

Pain control after surgery is central to the anesthetic management of patients undergoing thoracic surgery. The provision of good postoperative analgesia is of itself important and is regarded by some as the core business of anesthesia and a fundamental human right [396]. Effective analgesia can reduce pulmonary complications and mortality [353]. It is unlikely that a single technique will optimally fulfill these objectives for all patients, and therefore a balanced, multimodal approach should be used. Analgesia should be tailored to the specific patient undergoing a specific procedure and aim to minimize mortality, patient suffering, pulmonary complications, and other morbidity. Experience with a wide range of analgesic techniques is helpful as it enables the implementation of an appropriate technique. For open thoracotomies, most patients are best managed by a combination of regional analgesia and opioids, sometimes supplemented with non-opioid analgesics.

There is no role for interpleural blocks or cryoanalgesia in adults. Lumbar epidural analgesia, intrathecal opioids, or intercostal nerve blocks should usually be considered only if neither thoracic epidural analgesia nor paravertebral blocks are possible. At present the dilemma for thoracic anesthetists and their patients scheduled to undergo a thoracotomy is the choice between thoracic epidural analgesia and paravertebral block. It has been well established that thoracic epidurals produce excellent post-thoracotomy analgesia. Thoracic epidurals are, however, associated with a risk of permanent injury and the most frequent disabling complications are epidural hematomas [165]. Paravertebral blocks and infusions have been shown to produce equivalent analgesia but with a preferable side effect profile. An increasing number of patients presenting for thoracic surgery are receiving drugs that affect coagulation, not all of which are prescribed. Current anticoagulant and antiplatelet medication increases the risk of epidural by an unquantified amount. Impaired coagulation is less of a contraindication to thoracic paravertebrals, particularly when they are inserted under direct vision. Serious complications are rare with paravertebrals and therefore paravertebral blocks, as "single shots" and with catheters to allow continuous infusion, are growing in popularity. In the future, the development of clinically useable ultra-long-acting local anesthetics might enable significant further advances to be made in the provision of post-thoracotomy analgesia.

Case Study

A 64-year-old man has been admitted following a 2-week history of productive cough, lethargy, and collapse. He was initially treated for a community-acquired pneumonia with intravenous antibiotics, but serial chest x-rays and a CT scan have shown a cavitating lesion in the right upper lobe and a loculated pleural collection, likely to represent an empyema. Attempts have been made to drain the collection percutaneously but they have been unsuccessful, and he is scheduled to undergo open drainage of the empyema with decortication. Past medical history includes chronic obstructive pulmonary disease. He is a current heavy smoker and has been for more than 40 years.

Clinical examination reveals a slim man with a respiratory rate of 22 breaths per minute, heart rate 110 beats per minute, blood pressure 120/64, and a temperature 101 °F.

Full blood count shows a Hb 87 g/dl, WCC 23.0 $\times 10^9$ L^{-1}, neutrophil count 20.3 $\times 10^9$ L^{-1}, platelet count 637 $\times 10^9$ L^{-1}, and CRP 180 mgL^{-1}. His renal function and clotting screen are normal. Pulmonary function tests show an FVC of 74% predicted, FEV$_1$ of 43% predicted, and DLCO of 45% predicted.

Questions

What regional analgesic techniques could be employed here?

– Epidural and intrathecal analgesia are not advised in the presence of an active infection.
– Paravertebral catheter techniques are similarly best avoided in the presence of active infection.
– Intraoperative paravertebral blocks are unlikely to be effective because of the disruption of the anatomical planes by infection and surgery.
– Intercostal nerve blocks and local anesthetic wound infiltration should be considered.

Describe the analgesic agents that could be utilized.

A multimodal analgesic approach should be considered for this patient in the absence of contraindications:

– Regular IV acetaminophen 1 g QDS
– NSAID – nonselective or COX-2, this could commence intravenously postoperatively and then continue via either an IV or oral route
– Gabapentin – for example, 100–300 mg pre-op and then 100–300 mg titrated OD to TDS
– IV-PCA morphine
– Ketamine – may be administered via intravenous infusion or orally
– Clonidine or dexmedetomidine via infusion

References

1. Loan WB, Morrison JD. The incidence and severity of postoperative pain. Br J Anaesth. 1967;39(9):695–8.
2. Stadler M, Schlander M, Braeckman M, Nguyen T, Boogaerts JG. A cost-utility and cost-effectiveness analysis of an acute pain service. J Clin Anesth. 2004;16(3):159–67.
3. Nosotti M, Baisi A, Mendogni P, Palleschi A, Tosi D, Rosso L. Muscle sparing versus posterolateral thoracotomy for pulmonary lobectomy: randomised controlled trial. Interact Cardiovasc Thorac Surg. 2010;11(4):415–9.
4. Holte K, Kehlet H. Effect of postoperative epidural analgesia on surgical outcome. Minerva Anestesiol. 2002;68(4):157–61.
5. Kehlet H. Effect of pain relief on the surgical stress response. Reg Anesth. 1996;21(6 Suppl):35–7.
6. Sorkin LS, Wallace MS. Acute pain mechanisms. Surg Clin North Am. 1999;79(2):213–29.
7. Liu S, Carpenter RL, Neal JM. Epidural anesthesia and analgesia. Their role in postoperative outcome. Anesthesiology. 1995;82(6):1474–506.
8. Doan LV, Augustus J, Androphy R, Schechter D, Gharibo C. Mitigating the impact of acute and chronic post-thoracotomy pain. J Cardiothorac Vasc Anesth. 2014;28(4):1048–56.
9. Pennefather SHR, G.N. Postthoracotomy analgesia. In: Slinger PD, editor. Progress in thoracic anesthesia A society of cardiovascular anesthesiologists monograph. Philadelphia: Lippincott Williams and Wilkins; 2004.
10. Buvanendran A, Kroin JS. Multimodal analgesia for controlling acute postoperative pain. Curr Opin Anaesthesiol. 2009;22(5):588–93.
11. Landreneau RJ, Mack MJ, Hazelrigg SR, Naunheim K, Dowling RD, Ritter P, et al. Prevalence of chronic pain after pulmonary resection by thoracotomy or video-assisted thoracic surgery. J Thorac Cardiovasc Surg. 1994;107(4):1079–85. discussion 85-6.
12. Macintosh RRM, W.W. Anaesthetics research in wartime. Med Times. 1945:253–5.

13. Mark JB, Brodsky JB. Ipsilateral shoulder pain following thoracic operations. Anesthesiology. 1993;79(1):192. author reply 3.

14. Egbert LD, Battit GE, Welch CE, Bartlett MK. Reduction of postoperative pain by encouragement and instruction of patients. A study of Doctor-Patient rapport. N Engl J Med. 1964;270:825–7.

15. Kol E, Alpar SE, Erdogan A. Preoperative education and use of analgesic before onset of pain routinely for post-thoracotomy pain control can reduce pain effect and total amount of analgesics administered postoperatively. Pain Manag Nurs. 2014;15(1):331–9.

16. Scarci M, Solli P, Bedetti B. Enhanced recovery pathway for thoracic surgery in the UK. J Thorac Dis. 2016;8(Suppl 1):S78–83.

17. Gimenez-Mila M, Klein AA, Martinez G. Design and implementation of an enhanced recovery program in thoracic surgery. J Thorac Dis. 2016;8(Suppl 1):S37–45.

18. Twycross RG. Choice of strong analgesic in terminal cancer: diamorphine or morphine? Pain. 1977;3(2):93–104.

19. Gulur P, Williams L, Chaudhary S, Koury K, Jaff M. Opioid tolerance--a predictor of increased length of stay and higher readmission rates. Pain Physician. 2014;17(4):E503–7.

20. Crile GW. The kinetic theory of shock and its prevention through anoci-association (shockless operation). Lancet. 1913;182(4688):7–16.

21. Woolf CJ. Evidence for a central component of post-injury pain hypersensitivity. Nature. 1983;306(5944):686–8.

22. Kissin I. Preemptive analgesia. Anesthesiology. 2000;93(4):1138–43.

23. Moiniche S, Kehlet H, Dahl JB. A qualitative and quantitative systematic review of preemptive analgesia for postoperative pain relief: the role of timing of analgesia. Anesthesiology. 2002;96(3):725–41.

24. Bong CL, Samuel M, Ng JM, Ip-Yam C. Effects of preemptive epidural analgesia on post-thoracotomy pain. J Cardiothorac Vasc Anesth. 2005;19(6):786–93.

25. Hurley RW, Adams MC. Sex, gender, and pain: an overview of a complex field. Anesth Analg. 2008;107(1):309–17.

26. Riley JL 3rd, Robinson ME, Wise EA, Myers CD, Fillingim RB. Sex differences in the perception of noxious experimental stimuli: a meta-analysis. Pain. 1998;74(2–3):181–7.

27. Pickering G, Jourdan D, Eschalier A, Dubray C. Impact of age, gender and cognitive functioning on pain perception. Gerontology. 2002;48(2):112–8.

28. Gijsbers K, Nicholson F. Experimental pain thresholds influenced by sex of experimenter. Percept Mot Skills. 2005;101(3):803–7.

29. Sullivan MJ, Rodgers WM, Kirsch I. Catastrophizing, depression and expectancies for pain and emotional distress. Pain. 2001;91(1–2):147–54.

30. Keefe FJ, Lefebvre JC, Egert JR, Affleck G, Sullivan MJ, Caldwell DS. The relationship of gender to pain, pain behavior, and disability in osteoarthritis patients: the role of catastrophizing. Pain. 2000;87(3):325–34.

31. Ip HY, Abrishami A, Peng PW, Wong J, Chung F. Predictors of postoperative pain and analgesic consumption: a qualitative systematic review. Anesthesiology. 2009;111(3):657–77.

32. Bellville JW, Forrest WH Jr, Miller E, Brown BW Jr. Influence of age on pain relief from analgesics. A study of postoperative patients. JAMA. 1971;217(13):1835–41.

33. Yokoyama M, Hanazaki M, Fujii H, Mizobuchi S, Nakatsuka H, Takahashi T, et al. Correlation between the distribution of contrast medium and the extent of blockade during epidural anesthesia. Anesthesiology. 2004;100(6):1504–10.

34. Hirabayashi Y, Shimizu R. Effect of age on extradural dose requirement in thoracic extradural anaesthesia. Br J Anaesth. 1993;71(3):445–6.

35. Perry F, Parker RK, White PF, Clifford PA. Role of psychological factors in postoperative pain control and recovery with patient-controlled analgesia. Clin J Pain. 1994;10(1):57–63. discussion 82-5.

36. Rhudy JL, Meagher MW. Fear and anxiety: divergent effects on human pain thresholds. Pain. 2000;84(1):65–75.

37. Bachiocco V, Morselli-Labate AM, Rusticali AG, Bragaglia R, Mastrorilli M, Carli G. Intensity, latency and duration of post-thoracotomy pain: relationship to personality traits. Funct Neurol. 1990;5(4):321–32.

38. Caumo W, Schmidt AP, Schneider CN, Bergmann J, Iwamoto CW, Adamatti LC, et al. Preoperative predictors of moderate to intense acute postoperative pain in patients undergoing abdominal surgery. Acta Anaesthesiol Scand. 2002;46(10):1265–71.

39. Bisgaard T, Klarskov B, Rosenberg J, Kehlet H. Characteristics and prediction of early pain after laparoscopic cholecystectomy. Pain. 2001;90(3):261–9.

40. Tasmuth T, Estlanderb AM, Kalso E. Effect of present pain and mood on the memory of past postoperative pain in women treated surgically for breast cancer. Pain. 1996;68(2–3):343–7.

41. Landreneau RJ, Hazelrigg SR, Mack MJ, Dowling RD, Burke D, Gavlick J, et al. Postoperative pain-related morbidity: video-assisted thoracic surgery versus thoracotomy. Ann Thorac Surg. 1993;56(6):1285–9.

42. Iwasaki A, Hamatake D, Shirakusa T. Biosorbable poly-L-lactide rib-connecting pins may reduce acute pain after thoracotomy. Thorac Cardiovasc Surg. 2004;52(1):49–53.

43. Bethencourt DM, Holmes EC. Muscle-sparing posterolateral thoracotomy. Ann Thorac Surg. 1988;45(3):337–9.

44. Ginsberg RJ. Alternative (muscle-sparing) incisions in thoracic surgery. Ann Thorac Surg. 1993;56(3):752–4.

45. Fry WA. Thoracic incisions. Chest Surg Clin N Am. 1995;5(2):177–88.

46. Khan IH, McManus KG, McCraith A, McGuigan JA. Muscle sparing thoracotomy: a biomechanical analysis confirms preservation of muscle strength but no improvement in wound discomfort. Eur J Cardiothorac Surg. 2000;18(6):656–61.

47. Ochroch EA, Gottschalk A, Augoustides JG, Aukburg SJ, Kaiser LR, Shrager JB. Pain and physical function are similar following axillary, muscle-sparing vs posterolateral thoracotomy. Chest. 2005;128(4):2664–70.

48. Benedetti F, Vighetti S, Ricco C, Amanzio M, Bergamasco L, Casadio C, et al. Neurophysiologic assessment of nerve impairment in posterolateral and muscle-sparing thoracotomy. J Thorac Cardiovasc Surg. 1998;115(4):841–7.

49. Lee JI, Kim GW, Park KY. Intercostal bundle-splitting thoracotomy reduces chronic post-thoracotomy pain. Thorac Cardiovasc Surg. 2007;55(6):401–2.

50. Macchiarini P, Ladurie FL, Cerrina J, Fadel E, Chapelier A, Dartevelle P. Clamshell or sternotomy for double lung or heart-lung transplantation? Eur J Cardiothorac Surg. 1999;15(3):333–9.

51. Pyati S, Gan TJ. Perioperative pain management. CNS Drugs. 2007;21(3):185–211.

52. Boulanger A, Choiniere M, Roy D, Boure B, Chartrand D, Choquette R, et al. Comparison between patient-controlled analgesia and intramuscular meperidine after thoracotomy. Can J Anaesth. 1993;40(5 Pt 1):409–15.

53. Ballantyne JC, Carr DB, Chalmers TC, Dear KB, Angelillo IF, Mosteller F. Postoperative patient-controlled analgesia: meta-analyses of initial randomized control trials. J Clin Anesth. 1993;5(3):182–93.

54. Bullingham RE. Optimum management of postoperative pain. Drugs. 1985;29(4):376–86.

55. Bullingham RE. Postoperative pain. Postgrad Med J. 1984;60(710):847–51.

56. Ballantyne JC, Carr DB, deFerranti S, Suarez T, Lau J, Chalmers TC, et al. The comparative effects of postoperative analgesic therapies on pulmonary outcome: cumulative meta-analyses of randomized, controlled trials. Anesth Analg. 1998;86(3):598–612.

57. Bauer C, Hentz JG, Ducrocq X, Meyer N, Oswald-Mammosser M, Steib A, et al. Lung function after lobectomy: a randomized, double-blinded trial comparing thoracic epidural ropivacaine/sufentanil and intravenous morphine for patient-controlled analgesia. Anesth Analg. 2007;105(1):238–44.

58. Joshi GP, Bonnet F, Shah R, Wilkinson RC, Camu F, Fischer B, et al. A systematic review of randomized trials evaluating regional techniques for postthoracotomy analgesia. Anesth Analg. 2008;107(3):1026–40.

59. Guignard B, Bossard AE, Coste C, Sessler DI, Lebrault C, Alfonsi P, et al. Acute opioid tolerance: intraoperative remifentanil increases postoperative pain and morphine requirement. Anesthesiology. 2000;93(2):409–17.

60. Wenzel JT, Schwenk ES, Baratta JL, Viscusi ER. Managing opioid-tolerant patients in the perioperative surgical home. Anesthesiol Clin. 2016;34(2):287–301.

61. Romsing J, Moiniche S, Ostergaard D, Dahl JB. Local infiltration with NSAIDs for postoperative analgesia: evidence for a peripheral analgesic action. Acta Anaesthesiol Scand. 2000;44(6): 672–83.

62. Bjorkman RL, Hedner T, Hallman KM, Henning M, Hedner J. Localization of the central antinociceptive effects of diclofenac in the rat. Brain Res. 1992;590(1–2):66–73.

63. Vanegas H, Schaible HG. Prostaglandins and cyclooxygenases [correction of cycloxygenases] in the spinal cord. Prog Neurobiol. 2001;64(4):327–63.

64. Hawkey CJ. Non-steroidal anti-inflammatory drugs and peptic ulcers. BMJ. 1990;300(6720):278–84.

65. Souter AJ, Fredman B, White PF. Controversies in the perioperative use of nonsteroidal antiinflammatory drugs. Anesth Analg. 1994;79(6):1178–90.

66. Moiniche S, Romsing J, Dahl JB, Tramer MR. Nonsteroidal anti-inflammatory drugs and the risk of operative site bleeding after tonsillectomy: a quantitative systematic review. Anesth Analg. 2003;96(1):68–77. table of contents.

67. Myles PS, Power I. Does ketorolac cause postoperative renal failure: how do we assess the evidence? Br J Anaesth. 1998;80(4): 420–1.

68. Appadurai IR, Power I. NSAIDS in the postoperative period. Use with caution in elderly people. BMJ. 1993;307(6898):257.

69. Gibson P, Weadington D, Winney RJ. NSAIDS in the post-operative period. Clinical experience confirms risk. BMJ. 1993;307(6898):257–8.

70. Bottiger BA, Esper SA, Stafford-Smith M. Pain management strategies for thoracotomy and thoracic pain syndromes. Semin Cardiothorac Vasc Anesth. 2014;18(1):45–56.

71. Keenan DJ, Cave K, Langdon L, Lea RE. Comparative trial of rectal indomethacin and cryoanalgesia for control of early postthoracotomy pain. Br Med J (Clin Res Ed). 1983;287(6402): 1335–7.

72. Pavy T, Medley C, Murphy DF. Effect of indomethacin on pain relief after thoracotomy. Br J Anaesth. 1990;65(5):624–7.

73. Rhodes M, Conacher I, Morritt G, Hilton C. Nonsteroidal antiinflammatory drugs for postthoracotomy pain. A prospective controlled trial after lateral thoracotomy. J Thorac Cardiovasc Surg. 1992;103(1):17–20.

74. Bigler D, Moller J, Kamp-Jensen M, Berthelsen P, Hjortso NC, Kehlet H. Effect of piroxicam in addition to continuous thoracic epidural bupivacaine and morphine on postoperative pain and lung function after thoracotomy. Acta Anaesthesiol Scand. 1992;36(7):647–50.

75. Senard M, Deflandre EP, Ledoux D, Roediger L, Hubert BM, Radermecker M, et al. Effect of celecoxib combined with thoracic epidural analgesia on pain after thoracotomy. Br J Anaesth. 2010;105(2):196–200.

76. Ling XM, Fang F, Zhang XG, Ding M, Liu QA, Cang J. Effect of parecoxib combined with thoracic epidural analgesia on pain after thoracotomy. J Thorac Dis. 2016;8(5):880–7.

77. Burgess FW, Anderson DM, Colonna D, Sborov MJ, Cavanaugh DG. Ipsilateral shoulder pain following thoracic surgery. Anesthesiology. 1993;78(2):365–8.

78. Barak M, Ziser A, Katz Y. Thoracic epidural local anesthetics are ineffective in alleviating post-thoracotomy ipsilateral shoulder pain. J Cardiothorac Vasc Anesth. 2004;18(4):458–60.

79. Goppelt-Struebe M. Regulation of prostaglandin endoperoxide synthase (cyclooxygenase) isozyme expression. Prostaglandins Leukot Essent Fatty Acids. 1995;52(4):213–22.

80. Troster A, Sittl R, Singler B, Schmelz M, Schuttler J, Koppert W. Modulation of remifentanil-induced analgesia and postinfusion hyperalgesia by parecoxib in humans. Anesthesiology. 2006;105(5):1016–23.

81. Einhorn TA. Cox-2: Where are we in 2003? - The role of cyclooxygenase-2 in bone repair. Arthritis Res Ther. 2003;5(1):5–7.

82. Glassman SD, Rose SM, Dimar JR, Puno RM, Campbell MJ, Johnson JR. The effect of postoperative nonsteroidal anti-inflammatory drug administration on spinal fusion. Spine (Phila Pa 1976). 1998;23(7):834–8.

83. Graham DJ, Campen D, Hui R, Spence M, Cheetham C, Levy G, et al. Risk of acute myocardial infarction and sudden cardiac death in patients treated with cyclo-oxygenase 2 selective and non-selective non-steroidal anti-inflammatory drugs: nested case-control study. Lancet. 2005;365(9458):475–81.

84. Hippisley-Cox J, Coupland C. Risk of myocardial infarction in patients taking cyclo-oxygenase-2 inhibitors or conventional non-steroidal anti-inflammatory drugs: population based nested case-control analysis. BMJ. 2005;330(7504):1366.

85. Ott E, Nussmeier NA, Duke PC, Feneck RO, Alston RP, Snabes MC, et al. Efficacy and safety of the cyclooxygenase 2 inhibitors parecoxib and valdecoxib in patients undergoing coronary artery bypass surgery. J Thorac Cardiovasc Surg. 2003;125(6):1481–92.

86. Nussmeier NA, Whelton AA, Brown MT, Langford RM, Hoeft A, Parlow JL, et al. Complications of the COX-2 inhibitors parecoxib and valdecoxib after cardiac surgery. N Engl J Med. 2005;352(11):1081–91.

87. Nussmeier NA, Whelton AA, Brown MT, Joshi GP, Langford RM, Singla NK, et al. Safety and efficacy of the cyclooxygenase-2 inhibitors parecoxib and valdecoxib after noncardiac surgery. Anesthesiology. 2006;104(3):518–26.

88. Joshi GP, Gertler R, Fricker R. Cardiovascular thromboembolic adverse effects associated with cyclooxygenase-2 selective inhibitors and nonselective antiinflammatory drugs. Anesth Analg. 2007;105(6):1793–804. table of contents.

89. Argiriadou H, Papagiannopoulou P, Foroulis CN, Anastasiadis K, Thomaidou E, Papakonstantinou C, et al. Intraoperative infusion of S(+)-ketamine enhances post-thoracotomy pain control compared with perioperative parecoxib when used in conjunction with thoracic paravertebral ropivacaine infusion. J Cardiothorac Vasc Anesth. 2011;25(3):455–61.

90. Flower RJ, Vane JR. Inhibition of prostaglandin synthetase in brain explains the anti-pyretic activity of paracetamol (4-acetamidophenol). Nature. 1972;240(5381):410–1.

91. Tjolsen A, Lund A, Hole K. Antinociceptive effect of paracetamol in rats is partly dependent on spinal serotonergic systems. Eur J Pharmacol. 1991;193(2):193–201.

92. Honore P, Buritova J, Besson JM. Aspirin and acetaminophen reduced both Fos expression in rat lumbar spinal cord and inflammatory signs produced by carrageenin inflammation. Pain. 1995;63(3):365–75.

93. Mamoun NF, Lin P, Zimmerman NM, Mascha EJ, Mick SL, Insler SR, et al. Intravenous acetaminophen analgesia after cardiac sur-

gery: a randomized, blinded, controlled superiority trial. J Thorac Cardiovasc Surg. 2016;152(3):881–9. e1.

94. Hernandez-Palazon J, Tortosa JA, Martinez-Lage JF, Perez-Flores D. Intravenous administration of propacetamol reduces morphine consumption after spinal fusion surgery. Anesth Analg. 2001;92(6):1473–6.

95. Cattabriga I, Pacini D, Lamazza G, Talarico F, Di Bartolomeo R, Grillone G, et al. Intravenous paracetamol as adjunctive treatment for postoperative pain after cardiac surgery: a double blind randomized controlled trial. Eur J Cardiothorac Surg. 2007;32(3):527–31.

96. Lahtinen P, Kokki H, Hendolin H, Hakala T, Hynynen M. Propacetamol as adjunctive treatment for postoperative pain after cardiac surgery. Anesth Analg. 2002;95(4):813–9. table of contents.

97. McNicol ED, Ferguson MC, Haroutounian S, Carr DB, Schumann R. Single dose intravenous paracetamol or intravenous propacetamol for postoperative pain. Cochrane Database Syst Rev. 2016;5:CD007126.

98. Remy C, Marret E, Bonnet F. Effects of acetaminophen on morphine side-effects and consumption after major surgery: meta-analysis of randomized controlled trials. Br J Anaesth. 2005;94(4):505–13.

99. Politi JR, Davis RL 2nd, Matrka AK. Randomized prospective trial comparing the use of intravenous versus oral acetaminophen in total joint arthroplasty. J Arthroplast. 2017;32(4):1125–7.

100. Mac TB, Girard F, Chouinard P, Boudreault D, Lafontaine ER, Ruel M, et al. Acetaminophen decreases early post-thoracotomy ipsilateral shoulder pain in patients with thoracic epidural analgesia: a double-blind placebo-controlled study. J Cardiothorac Vasc Anesth. 2005;19(4):475–8.

101. Dahl V, Raeder JC. Non-opioid postoperative analgesia. Acta Anaesthesiol Scand. 2000;44(10):1191–203.

102. Montgomery JE, Sutherland CJ, Kestin IG, Sneyd JR. Morphine consumption in patients receiving rectal paracetamol and diclofenac alone and in combination. Br J Anaesth. 1996;77(4):445–7.

103. Seymour RA, Kelly PJ, Hawkesford JE. The efficacy of ketoprofen and paracetamol (acetaminophen) in postoperative pain after third molar surgery. Br J Clin Pharmacol. 1996;41(6):581–5.

104. Cook TM, Riley RH. Analgesia following thoracotomy: a survey of Australian practice. Anaesth Intensive Care. 1997;25(5):520–4.

105. Moyse DW, Kaye AD, Diaz JH, Qadri MY, Lindsay D, Pyati S. Perioperative ketamine administration for thoracotomy pain. Pain Physician. 2017;20(3):173–84.

106. Mao J, Price DD, Mayer DJ. Mechanisms of hyperalgesia and morphine tolerance: a current view of their possible interactions. Pain. 1995;62(3):259–74.

107. Celerier E, Rivat C, Jun Y, Laulin JP, Larcher A, Reynier P, et al. Long-lasting hyperalgesia induced by fentanyl in rats: preventive effect of ketamine. Anesthesiology. 2000;92(2):465–72.

108. Guillou N, Tanguy M, Seguin P, Branger B, Campion JP, Malledant Y. The effects of small-dose ketamine on morphine consumption in surgical intensive care unit patients after major abdominal surgery. Anesth Analg. 2003;97(3):843–7.

109. Mathews TJ, Churchhouse AM, Housden T, Dunning J. Does adding ketamine to morphine patient-controlled analgesia safely improve post-thoracotomy pain? Interact Cardiovasc Thorac Surg. 2012;14(2):194–9.

110. Michelet P, Guervilly C, Helaine A, Avaro JP, Blayac D, Gaillat F, et al. Adding ketamine to morphine for patient-controlled analgesia after thoracic surgery: influence on morphine consumption, respiratory function, and nocturnal desaturation. Br J Anaesth. 2007;99(3):396–403.

111. Fiorelli A, Mazzella A, Passavanti B, Sansone P, Chiodini P, Iannotti M, et al. Is pre-emptive administration of ketamine a significant adjunction to intravenous morphine analgesia for controlling postoperative pain? A randomized, double-blind, placebo-controlled clinical trial. Interact Cardiovasc Thorac Surg. 2015;21(3):284–90.

112. Duale C, Sibaud F, Guastella V, Vallet L, Gimbert YA, Taheri H, et al. Perioperative ketamine does not prevent chronic pain after thoracotomy. Eur J Pain. 2009;13(5):497–505.

113. Sveticic G, Eichenberger U, Curatolo M. Safety of mixture of morphine with ketamine for postoperative patient-controlled analgesia: an audit with 1026 patients. Acta Anaesthesiol Scand. 2005;49(6):870–5.

114. Suzuki M, Haraguti S, Sugimoto K, Kikutani T, Shimada Y, Sakamoto A. Low-dose intravenous ketamine potentiates epidural analgesia after thoracotomy. Anesthesiology. 2006;105(1):111–9.

115. Tena B, Gomar C, Rios J. Perioperative epidural or intravenous ketamine does not improve the effectiveness of thoracic epidural analgesia for acute and chronic pain after thoracotomy. Clin J Pain. 2014;30(6):490–500.

116. Joseph C, Gaillat F, Duponq R, Lieven R, Baumstarck K, Thomas P, et al. Is there any benefit to adding intravenous ketamine to patient-controlled epidural analgesia after thoracic surgery? A randomized double-blind study. Eur J Cardiothorac Surg. 2012;42(4):e58–65.

117. Kotze A, Scally A, Howell S. Efficacy and safety of different techniques of paravertebral block for analgesia after thoracotomy: a systematic review and metaregression. Br J Anaesth. 2009;103(5):626–36.

118. Mason N, Gondret R, Junca A, Bonnet F. Intrathecal sufentanil and morphine for post-thoracotomy pain relief. Br J Anaesth. 2001;86(2):236–40.

119. Liu N, Kuhlman G, Dalibon N, Moutafis M, Levron JC, Fischler M. A randomized, double-blinded comparison of intrathecal morphine, sufentanil and their combination versus IV morphine patient-controlled analgesia for postthoracotomy pain. Anesth Analg. 2001;92(1):31–6.

120. Gottschalk A, Cohen SP, Yang S, Ochroch EA. Preventing and treating pain after thoracic surgery. Anesthesiology. 2006;104(3):594–600.

121. Carroll IR, Angst MS, Clark JD. Management of perioperative pain in patients chronically consuming opioids. Reg Anesth Pain Med. 2004;29(6):576–91.

122. Kong VK, Irwin MG. Gabapentin: a multimodal perioperative drug? Br J Anaesth. 2007;99(6):775–86.

123. Chang CY, Challa CK, Shah J, Eloy JD. Gabapentin in acute postoperative pain management. Biomed Res Int. 2014;2014:631756.

124. Zakkar M, Frazer S, Hunt I. Is there a role for gabapentin in preventing or treating pain following thoracic surgery? Interact Cardiovasc Thorac Surg. 2013;17(4):716–9.

125. Serpell MG. Neuropathic pain study g. Gabapentin in neuropathic pain syndromes: a randomised, double-blind, placebo-controlled trial. Pain. 2002;99(3):557–66.

126. Rowbotham M, Harden N, Stacey B, Bernstein P, Magnus-Miller L. Gabapentin for the treatment of postherpetic neuralgia: a randomized controlled trial. JAMA. 1998;280(21):1837–42.

127. Maneuf YP, Gonzalez MI, Sutton KS, Chung FZ, Pinnock RD, Lee K. Cellular and molecular action of the putative GABA-mimetic, gabapentin. Cell Mol Life Sci. 2003;60(4):742–50.

128. Mathiesen O, Moiniche S, Dahl JB. Gabapentin and postoperative pain: a qualitative and quantitative systematic review, with focus on procedure. BMC Anesthesiol. 2007;7:6.

129. Kinney MA, Mantilla CB, Carns PE, Passe MA, Brown MJ, Hooten WM, et al. Preoperative gabapentin for acute post-thoracotomy analgesia: a randomized, double-blinded, active placebo-controlled study. Pain Pract. 2012;12(3):175–83.

130. Omran AFM, A.E. A randomized study of the effects of gabapentin versus placebo on post-thoracotomy pain and pulmonary function. Egypt J Anaesth. 2005;21:277–81.

131. Huot MP, Chouinard P, Girard F, Ruel M, Lafontaine ER, Ferraro P. Gabapentin does not reduce post-thoracotomy shoulder pain: a randomized, double-blind placebo-controlled study. Can J Anaesth. 2008;55(6):337–43.

132. Menigaux C, Adam F, Guignard B, Sessler DI, Chauvin M. Preoperative gabapentin decreases anxiety and improves early functional recovery from knee surgery. Anesth Analg. 2005;100(5):1394–9. table of contents.

133. Zhang J, Ho KY, Wang Y. Efficacy of pregabalin in acute postoperative pain: a meta-analysis. Br J Anaesth. 2011;106(4): 454–62.

134. Mishriky BM, Waldron NH, Habib AS. Impact of pregabalin on acute and persistent postoperative pain: a systematic review and meta-analysis. Br J Anaesth. 2015;114(1):10–31.

135. Baidya DK, Agarwal A, Khanna P, Arora MK. Pregabalin in acute and chronic pain. J Anaesthesiol Clin Pharmacol. 2011;27(3):307–14.

136. Singla NK, Chelly JE, Lionberger DR, Gimbel J, Sanin L, Sporn J, et al. Pregabalin for the treatment of postoperative pain: results from three controlled trials using different surgical models. J Pain Res. 2015;8:9–20.

137. Ziyaeifard M, Mehrabanian MJ, Faritus SZ, Khazaei Koohpar M, Ferasatkish R, Hosseinnejad H, et al. Premedication with oral pregabalin for the prevention of acute postsurgical pain in coronary artery bypass surgery. Anesth Pain Med. 2015;5(1):e24837.

138. Joshi SS, Jagadeesh AM. Efficacy of perioperative pregabalin in acute and chronic post-operative pain after off-pump coronary artery bypass surgery: a randomized, double-blind placebo controlled trial. Ann Card Anaesth. 2013;16(3):180–5.

139. Kernan S, Rehman S, Meyer T, Bourbeau J, Caron N, Tobias JD. Effects of dexmedetomidine on oxygenation during one-lung ventilation for thoracic surgery in adults. J Min Access Surg. 2011;7(4):227–31.

140. Wahlander S, Frumento RJ, Wagener G, Saldana-Ferretti B, Joshi RR, Playford HR, et al. A prospective, double-blind, randomized, placebo-controlled study of dexmedetomidine as an adjunct to epidural analgesia after thoracic surgery. J Cardiothorac Vasc Anesth. 2005;19(5):630–5.

141. Dong CS, Zhang J, Lu Q, Sun P, Yu JM, Wu C, et al. Effect of Dexmedetomidine combined with sufentanil for post- thoracotomy intravenous analgesia:a randomized, controlled clinical study. BMC Anesthesiol. 2017;17(1):33.

142. Samantaray A, Rao MH, Chandra A. The effect on post-operative pain of intravenous clonidine given before induction of anaesthesia. Indian J Anaesth. 2012;56(4):359–64.

143. Talbot RM, McCarthy KF, McCrory C. Central and systemic inflammatory responses to thoracotomy - potential implications for acute and chronic postsurgical pain. J Neuroimmunol. 2015;285:147–9.

144. Hong D, Byers MR, Oswald RJ. Dexamethasone treatment reduces sensory neuropeptides and nerve sprouting reactions in injured teeth. Pain. 1993;55(2):171–81.

145. Marek P, Ben-Eliyahu S, Vaccarino AL, Liebeskind JC. Delayed application of MK-801 attenuates development of morphine tolerance in rats. Brain Res. 1991;558(1):163–5.

146. Jokela RM, Ahonen JV, Tallgren MK, Marjakangas PC, Korttila KT. The effective analgesic dose of dexamethasone after laparoscopic hysterectomy. Anesth Analg. 2009;109(2):607–15.

147. Kardash KJ, Sarrazin F, Tessler MJ, Velly AM. Single-dose dexamethasone reduces dynamic pain after total hip arthroplasty. Anesth Analg. 2008;106(4):1253–7. table of contents.

148. Hval K, Thagaard KS, Schlichting E, Raeder J. The prolonged postoperative analgesic effect when dexamethasone is added to a nonsteroidal antiinflammatory drug (rofecoxib) before breast surgery. Anesth Analg. 2007;105(2):481–6.

149. Bisgaard T, Klarskov B, Kehlet H, Rosenberg J. Preoperative dexamethasone improves surgical outcome after laparoscopic cholecystectomy: a randomized double-blind placebo-controlled trial. Ann Surg. 2003;238(5):651–60.

150. Rasmussen SB, Saied NN, Bowens C Jr, Mercaldo ND, Schildcrout JS, Malchow RJ. Duration of upper and lower extremity peripheral nerve blockade is prolonged with dexamethasone when added to ropivacaine: a retrospective database analysis. Pain Med. 2013;14(8):1239–47.

151. Tomar GS, Ganguly S, Cherian G. Effect of perineural dexamethasone with bupivacaine in single space paravertebral block for postoperative analgesia in elective nephrectomy cases: a double-blind placebo-controlled trial. Am J Ther. 2017;24:e713–7.

152. Maher DP, Serna-Gallegos D, Mardirosian R, Thomas OJ, Zhang X, McKenna R, et al. The combination of IV and perineural dexamethasone prolongs the analgesic duration of intercostal nerve blocks compared with IV dexamethasone alone. Pain Med. 2016;18:1152–60.

153. Williams BA, Hough KA, Tsui BY, Ibinson JW, Gold MS, Gebhart GF. Neurotoxicity of adjuvants used in perineural anesthesia and analgesia in comparison with ropivacaine. Reg Anesth Pain Med. 2011;36(3):225–30.

154. Melzack R, Wall PD. Pain mechanisms: a new theory. Science. 1965;150(3699):971–9.

155. Rodriguez-Aldrete D, Candiotti KA, Janakiraman R, Rodriguez-Blanco YF. Trends and new evidence in the management of acute and chronic post-thoracotomy pain-an overview of the literature from 2005 to 2015. J Cardiothorac Vasc Anesth. 2016;30(3):762–72.

156. Fiorelli A, Morgillo F, Milione R, Pace MC, Passavanti MB, Laperuta P, et al. Control of post-thoracotomy pain by transcutaneous electrical nerve stimulation: effect on serum cytokine levels, visual analogue scale, pulmonary function and medication. Eur J Cardiothorac Surg. 2012;41(4):861–8. discussion 8.

157. Carroll D, Tramer M, McQuay H, Nye B, Moore A. Randomization is important in studies with pain outcomes: systematic review of transcutaneous electrical nerve stimulation in acute postoperative pain. Br J Anaesth. 1996;77(6):798–803.

158. Sbruzzi G, Silveira SA, Silva DV, Coronel CC, Plentz RD. Transcutaneous electrical nerve stimulation after thoracic surgery: systematic review and meta-analysis of 11 randomized trials. Rev Bras Cir Cardiovasc. 2012;27(1):75–87.

159. Gough JD, Williams AB, Vaughan RS, Khalil JF, Butchart EG. The control of post-thoracotomy pain. A comparative evaluation of thoracic epidural fentanyl infusions and cryo-analgesia. Anaesthesia. 1988;43(9):780–3.

160. Muller LC, Salzer GM, Ransmayr G, Neiss A. Intraoperative cryoanalgesia for postthoracotomy pain relief. Ann Thorac Surg. 1989;48(1):15–8.

161. Griffiths DP, Diamond AW, Cameron JD. Postoperative extradural analgesia following thoracic surgery: a feasibility study. Br J Anaesth. 1975;47(1):48–55.

162. Shuman RL, Peters RM. Epidural anesthesia following thoracotomy in patients with chronic obstructive airway disease. J Thorac Cardiovasc Surg. 1976;71(1):82–8.

163. Cook TM, Eaton JM. Epidural analgesia after thoracotomy: United Kingdom practice. Eur J Anaesthesiol. 1997;14(1):108–11.

164. Cook TM, Counsell D, Wildsmith JA. Royal College of Anaesthetists Third National Audit P. Major complications of central neuraxial block: report on the Third National Audit Project of the Royal College of Anaesthetists. Br J Anaesth. 2009;102(2):179–90.

165. Counsell D. Complications after perioperative central neuraxial blocks. The Third National Audit Project (NAP3) Major complications of central neuraxial blocks in the United Kingdom. London: Royal College of Anaesthetists; 2009. p. 101–11.

166. Horlocker TT, Wedel DJ, Benzon H, Brown DL, Enneking FK, Heit JA, et al. Regional anesthesia in the anticoagulated patient: defining the risks (the second ASRA Consensus Conference on Neuraxial Anesthesia and Anticoagulation). Reg Anesth Pain Med. 2003;28(3):172–97.

167. Howard-Alpe GM, de Bono J, Hudsmith L, Orr WP, Foex P, Sear JW. Coronary artery stents and non-cardiac surgery. Br J Anaesth. 2007;98(5):560–74.

168. Chassot PG, Delabays A, Spahn DR. Perioperative antiplatelet therapy: the case for continuing therapy in patients at risk of myocardial infarction. Br J Anaesth. 2007;99(3):316–28.

169. Newsome LT, Weller RS, Gerancher JC, Kutcher MA, Royster RL. Coronary artery stents: II. Perioperative considerations and management. Anesth Analg. 2008;107(2):570–90.

170. Yeung JH, Gates S, Naidu BV, Wilson MJ, Gao SF. Paravertebral block versus thoracic epidural for patients undergoing thoracotomy. Cochrane Database Syst Rev. 2016;2:CD009121.

171. Grider JS, Mullet TW, Saha SP, Harned ME, Sloan PA. A randomized, double-blind trial comparing continuous thoracic epidural bupivacaine with and without opioid in contrast to a continuous paravertebral infusion of bupivacaine for post-thoracotomy pain. J Cardiothorac Vasc Anesth. 2012;26(1):83–9.

172. Scarfe AJ, Schuhmann-Hingel S, Duncan JK, Ma N, Atukorale YN, Cameron AL. Continuous paravertebral block for post-cardiothoracic surgery analgesia: a systematic review and meta-analysis. Eur J Cardiothorac Surg. 2016;50(6):1010–8.

173. Scarci M, Joshi A, Attia R. In patients undergoing thoracic surgery is paravertebral block as effective as epidural analgesia for pain management? Interact Cardiovasc Thorac Surg. 2010;10(1):92–6.

174. Pintaric TS, Potocnik I, Hadzic A, Stupnik T, Pintaric M, Novak JV. Comparison of continuous thoracic epidural with paravertebral block on perioperative analgesia and hemodynamic stability in patients having open lung surgery. Reg Anesth Pain Med. 2011;36(3):256–60.

175. Fortier S, Hanna HA, Bernard A, Girard C. Comparison between systemic analgesia, continuous wound catheter analgesia and continuous thoracic paravertebral block: a randomised, controlled trial of postthoracotomy pain management. Eur J Anaesthesiol. 2012;29(11):524–30.

176. Daly DJ, Myles PS. Update on the role of paravertebral blocks for thoracic surgery: are they worth it? Curr Opin Anaesthesiol. 2009;22(1):38–43.

177. Elsayed H, McKevith J, McShane J, Scawn N. Thoracic epidural or paravertebral catheter for analgesia after lung resection: is the outcome different? J Cardiothorac Vasc Anesth. 2012;26(1):78–82.

178. Yentis SM, Hartle AJ, Barker IR, Barker P, Bogod DG, Clutton-Brock TH, et al. AAGBI: Consent for anaesthesia 2017: Association of Anaesthetists of Great Britain and Ireland. Anaesthesia. 2017;72(1):93–105.

179. Montgomery vs Lanarkshire Health Board. UKSC. 2015;11.

180. Pennefather SH, Gilby S, Danecki A, Russell GN. The changing practice of thoracic epidural analgesia in the United Kingdom: 1997-2004. Anaesthesia. 2006;61(4):363–9.

181. Bai Y, Miller T, Tan M, Law LS, Gan TJ. Lidocaine patch for acute pain management: a meta-analysis of prospective controlled trials. Curr Med Res Opin. 2015;31(3):575–81.

182. Vrooman B, Kapural L, Sarwar S, Mascha EJ, Mihaljevic T, Gillinov M, et al. Lidocaine 5% patch for treatment of acute pain after robotic cardiac surgery and prevention of persistent incisional pain: a randomized, placebo-controlled. Double-Blind Trial Pain Med. 2015;16(8):1610–21.

183. Fiorelli A, Izzo AC, Frongillo EM, Del Prete A, Liguori G, Di Costanzo E, et al. Efficacy of wound analgesia for controlling post-thoracotomy pain: a randomized double-blind studydagger. Eur J Cardiothorac Surg. 2016;49(1):339–47.

184. Liu SS, Richman JM, Thirlby RC, Wu CL. Efficacy of continuous wound catheters delivering local anesthetic for postoperative analgesia: a quantitative and qualitative systematic review of randomized controlled trials. J Am Coll Surg. 2006;203(6):914–32.

185. Hahnenkamp K, Theilmeier G, Van Aken HK, Hoenemann CW. The effects of local anesthetics on perioperative coagulation, inflammation, and microcirculation. Anesth Analg. 2002;94(6):1441–7.

186. Dravid RM, Paul RE. Interpleural block - part 1. Anaesthesia. 2007;62(10):1039–49.

187. Dryden CM, McMenemin I, Duthie DJ. Efficacy of continuous intercostal bupivacaine for pain relief after thoracotomy. Br J Anaesth. 1993;70(5):508–10.

188. Kvalheim LR, Reiestad F. Intrapleural catheter in the management of postoperative pain. Anesthesiology. 1984;61:A231.

189. Miguel R, Smith R. Intrapleural, not interpleural, analgesia. Reg Anesth. 1991;16(5):299.

190. Baumgarten RK. Intrapleural, interpleural, or pleural block? Simpler may be better. Reg Anesth. 1992;17(2):116.

191. Murphy DF. Interpleural analgesia. Br J Anaesth. 1993;71(3):426–34.

192. Schneider RF, Villamena PC, Harvey J, Surick BG, Surick IW, Beattie EJ. Lack of efficacy of intrapleural bupivacaine for postoperative analgesia following thoracotomy. Chest. 1993;103(2):414–6.

193. Kambam JR, Hammon J, Parris WC, Lupinetti FM. Intrapleural analgesia for post-thoracotomy pain and blood levels of bupivacaine following intrapleural injection. Can J Anaesth. 1989;36(2):106–9.

194. Broome IJ, Sherry KM, Reilly CS. A combined chest drain and intrapleural catheter for post-thoracotomy pain relief. Anaesthesia. 1993;48(8):724–6.

195. Pennefather SH, Akrofi ME, Kendall JB, Russell GN, Scawn ND. Double-blind comparison of intrapleural saline and 0.25% bupivacaine for ipsilateral shoulder pain after thoracotomy in patients receiving thoracic epidural analgesia. Br J Anaesth. 2005;94(2):234–8.

196. Blanco R, Parras T, McDonnell JG, Prats-Galino A. Serratus plane block: a novel ultrasound-guided thoracic wall nerve block. Anaesthesia. 2013;68(11):1107–13.

197. Kunhabdulla NP, Agarwal A, Gaur A, Gautam SK, Gupta R, Agarwal A. Serratus anterior plane block for multiple rib fractures. Pain Physician. 2014;17(5):E651–3.

198. Madabushi R, Tewari S, Gautam SK, Agarwal A, Agarwal A. Serratus anterior plane block: a new analgesic technique for post-thoracotomy pain. Pain Physician. 2015;18(3):E421–4.

199. Okmen K, Okmen BM, Uysal S. Serratus anterior plane (SAP) block used for thoracotomy analgesia; a case report. Korean J Pain. 2016;29:189–92.

200. Okmen K, Okmen BM. The efficacy of serratus anterior plane block in analgesia for thoracotomy: a retrospective study. J Anesth. 2017;31(4):579–85.

201. Sellheim H. Verh Dtch Ges Gynak 1906;176.

202. Eason MJ, Wyatt R. Paravertebral thoracic block-a reappraisal. Anaesthesia. 1979;34(7):638–42.

203. Davies RG, Myles PS, Graham JM. A comparison of the analgesic efficacy and side-effects of paravertebral vs epidural blockade for thoracotomy--a systematic review and meta-analysis of randomized trials. Br J Anaesth. 2006;96(4):418–26.

204. Ding X, Jin S, Niu X, Ren H, Fu S, Li Q. A comparison of the analgesia efficacy and side effects of paravertebral compared with epidural blockade for thoracotomy: an updated meta-analysis. PLoS One. 2014;9(5):e96233.

205. Baidya DK, Khanna P, Maitra S. Analgesic efficacy and safety of thoracic paravertebral and epidural analgesia for thoracic surgery: a systematic review and meta-analysis. Interact Cardiovasc Thorac Surg. 2014;18(5):626–35.

206. Okajima H, Tanaka O, Ushio M, Higuchi Y, Nagai Y, Iijima K, et al. Ultrasound-guided continuous thoracic paravertebral block

provides comparable analgesia and fewer episodes of hypotension than continuous epidural block after lung surgery. J Anesth. 2015;29(3):373–8.

207. Karmakar MK. Thoracic paravertebral block. Anesthesiology. 2001;95(3):771–80.

208. Lonnqvist PA, Hildingsson U. The caudal boundary of the thoracic paravertebral space. A study in human cadavers. Anaesthesia. 1992;47(12):1051–2.

209. Nunn JF, Slavin G. Posterior intercostal nerve block for pain relief after cholecystectomy. Anatomical basis and efficacy. Br J Anaesth. 1980;52(3):253–60.

210. Cowie B, McGlade D, Ivanusic J, Barrington MJ. Ultrasound-guided thoracic paravertebral blockade: a cadaveric study. Anesth Analg. 2010;110(6):1735–9.

211. Burns DA, Ben-David B, Chelly JE, Greensmith JE. Intercostally placed paravertebral catheterization: an alternative approach to continuous paravertebral blockade. Anesth Analg. 2008;107(1):339–41.

212. Taketa Y, Fujitani T, Irisawa Y, Sudo S, Takaishi K. Ultrasound-guided thoracic paravertebral block by the paralaminar in-plane approach using a microconvex array transducer: methodological utility based on anatomical structures. J Anesth. 2017;31(2):271–7.

213. Krediet AC, Moayeri N, van Geffen GJ, Bruhn J, Renes S, Bigeleisen PE, et al. Different approaches to ultrasound-guided thoracic paravertebral block: an illustrated review. Anesthesiology. 2015;123(2):459–74.

214. Renes SH, Bruhn J, Gielen MJ, Scheffer GJ, van Geffen GJ. In-plane ultrasound-guided thoracic paravertebral block: a preliminary report of 36 cases with radiologic confirmation of catheter position. Reg Anesth Pain Med. 2010;35(2):212–6.

215. Riain SCO, Donnell BO, Cuffe T, Harmon DC, Fraher JP, Shorten G. Thoracic paravertebral block using real-time ultrasound guidance. Anesth Analg. 2010;110(1):248–51.

216. Ben-Ari A, Moreno M, Chelly JE, Bigeleisen PE. Ultrasound-guided paravertebral block using an intercostal approach. Anesth Analg. 2009;109(5):1691–4.

217. Shibata Y, Nishiwaki K. Ultrasound-guided intercostal approach to thoracic paravertebral block. Anesth Analg. 2009;109(3):996–7.

218. Karmakar MK, Li X, Li J, Hadzic A. Volumetric three-dimensional ultrasound imaging of the anatomy relevant for thoracic paravertebral block. Anesth Analg. 2012;115(5):1246–50.

219. Hutchins J, Sanchez J, Andrade R, Podgaetz E, Wang Q, Sikka R. Ultrasound-guided paravertebral catheter versus intercostal blocks for postoperative pain control in video-assisted thoracoscopic surgery: a prospective randomized trial. J Cardiothorac Vasc Anesth. 2017;31(2):458–63.

220. Kaya FN, Turker G, Mogol EB, Bayraktar S. Thoracic paravertebral block for video-assisted thoracoscopic surgery: single injection versus multiple injections. J Cardiothorac Vasc Anesth. 2012;26(1):90–4.

221. Marhofer D, Marhofer P, Kettner SC, Fleischmann E, Prayer D, Schernthaner M, et al. Magnetic resonance imaging analysis of the spread of local anesthetic solution after ultrasound-guided lateral thoracic paravertebral blockade: a volunteer study. Anesthesiology. 2013;118(5):1106–12.

222. Sabanathan S, Smith PJ, Pradhan GN, Hashimi H, Eng JB, Mearns AJ. Continuous intercostal nerve block for pain relief after thoracotomy. Ann Thorac Surg. 1988;46(4):425–6.

223. Berrisford RG, Sabanathan SS. Direct access to the paravertebral space at thoracotomy. Ann Thorac Surg. 1990;49(5):854.

224. Soni AK, Conacher ID, Waller DA, Hilton CJ. Video-assisted thoracoscopic placement of paravertebral catheters: a technique for postoperative analgesia for bilateral thoracoscopic surgery. Br J Anaesth. 1994;72(4):462–4.

225. Yamauchi Y, Isaka M, Ando K, Mori K, Kojima H, Maniwa T, et al. Continuous paravertebral block using a thoracoscopic catheter-insertion technique for postoperative pain after thoracotomy: a retrospective case-control study. J Cardiothorac Surg. 2017;12(1):5.

226. Raveglia F, Rizzi A, Leporati A, Di Mauro P, Cioffi U, Baisi A. Analgesia in patients undergoing thoracotomy: epidural versus paravertebral technique. A randomized, double-blind, prospective study. J Thorac Cardiovasc Surg. 2014;147(1):469–73.

227. Vogt A, Stieger DS, Theurillat C, Curatolo M. Single-injection thoracic paravertebral block for postoperative pain treatment after thoracoscopic surgery. Br J Anaesth. 2005;95(6):816–21.

228. Matyal R, Montealegre-Gallegos M, Shnider M, Owais K, Sakamuri S, Shakil O, et al. Preemptive ultrasound-guided paravertebral block and immediate postoperative lung function. Gen Thorac Cardiovasc Surg. 2015;63(1):43–8.

229. Amlong C, Guy M, Schroeder KM, Donnelly MJ. Out-of-plane ultrasound-guided paravertebral blocks improve analgesic outcomes in patients undergoing video-assisted thoracoscopic surgery. Local Reg Anesth. 2015;8:123–8.

230. Goravanchi F, Kee SS, Kowalski AM, Berger JS, French KE. A case series of thoracic paravertebral blocks using a combination of ropivacaine, clonidine, epinephrine, and dexamethasone. J Clin Anesth. 2012;24(8):664–7.

231. Dutta V, Kumar B, Jayant A, Mishra AK. Effect of continuous paravertebral dexmedetomidine administration on intraoperative anesthetic drug requirement and post-thoracotomy pain syndrome after thoracotomy: a randomized controlled trial. J Cardiothorac Vasc Anesth. 2017;31(1):159–65.

232. Fibla JJ, Molins L, Mier JM, Hernandez J, Sierra A. A randomized prospective study of analgesic quality after thoracotomy: paravertebral block with bolus versus continuous infusion with an elastomeric pump. Eur J Cardiothorac Surg. 2015;47(4):631–5.

233. Tighe SQMG, Rajadurai N. Paravertebral block. Contin Educ Anaesth Crit Care Pain. 2010;10:133–7.

234. Karmakar MK, Ho AM, Law BK, Wong AS, Shafer SL, Gin T. Arterial and venous pharmacokinetics of ropivacaine with and without epinephrine after thoracic paravertebral block. Anesthesiology. 2005;103(4):704–11.

235. Berrisford RG, Sabanathan S, Mearns AJ, Clarke BJ, Hamdi A. Plasma concentrations of bupivacaine and its enantiomers during continuous extrapleural intercostal nerve block. Br J Anaesth. 1993;70(2):201–4.

236. Richardson J, Sabanathan S, Jones J, Shah RD, Cheema S, Mearns AJ. A prospective, randomized comparison of preoperative and continuous balanced epidural or paravertebral bupivacaine on post-thoracotomy pain, pulmonary function and stress responses. Br J Anaesth. 1999;83(3):387–92.

237. Fagenholz PJ, Bowler GM, Carnochan FM, Walker WS. Systemic local anaesthetic toxicity from continuous thoracic paravertebral block. Br J Anaesth. 2012;109(2):260–2.

238. Ireland AoAoGBa. Guidelines for the management of severe local anaesthetic toxicity 2010. Available from: https://www.aagbi.org/sites/default/files/la_toxicity_2010_0.pdf.

239. Resuscitation Council (UK) Adult Advanced Life Support 2015. Available from: https://www.resus.org.uk/resuscitation-guidelines/adult-advanced-life-support/.

240. Chin KJ, Malhas L, Perlas A. The erector spinae plane block provides visceral abdominal analgesia in bariatric surgery, a report of 3 cases. Reg Anesth Pain Med. 2017;42(3):372–6.

241. Forero M, Rajarathinam M, Adhikary S, Chin KJ. Continuous erector spinae plane block for rescue analgesia in thoracotomy after epidural failure: a case report. A&A Case Reports. 2017;8:254–6.

242. Samii K, Feret J, Harari A, Viars P. Selective spinal analgesia. Lancet. 1979;1(8126):1142.

243. Neustein SM, Cohen E. Intrathecal morphine during thoracotomy, Part II: Effect on postoperative meperidine requirements and pulmonary function tests. J Cardiothorac Vasc Anesth. 1993;7(2):157–9.

244. Liu M, Rock P, Grass JA, Heitmiller RF, Parker SJ, Sakima NT, et al. Double-blind randomized evaluation of intercostal nerve blocks as an adjuvant to subarachnoid administered morphine for post-thoracotomy analgesia. Reg Anesth. 1995;20(5):418–25.

245. Sudarshan G, Browne BL, Matthews JN, Conacher ID. Intrathecal fentanyl for post-thoracotomy pain. Br J Anaesth. 1995;75(1):19–22.

246. Gustafsson LL, Wiesenfeld-Hallin Z. Spinal opioid analgesia. A critical update. Drugs. 1988;35(6):597–603.

247. Cousins MJ, Mather LE. Intrathecal and epidural administration of opioids. Anesthesiology. 1984;61(3):276–310.

248. Liu SS, Block BM, Wu CL. Effects of perioperative central neuraxial analgesia on outcome after coronary artery bypass surgery: a meta-analysis. Anesthesiology. 2004;101(1):153–61.

249. Dango S, Harris S, Offner K, Hennings E, Priebe HJ, Buerkle H, et al. Combined paravertebral and intrathecal vs thoracic epidural analgesia for post-thoracotomy pain relief. Br J Anaesth. 2013;110(3):443–9.

250. Sicard A. Les injections medicamenteuses extra-durales par voie sacrococcygienne. Compt Rend Soc De Biol. 1901;53:396–8.

251. Pages F. Anesthesia metamerica. Rev Esp Chir. 1921;3:3–30.

252. Dogliotti AM. A new method of block: segmental peridural spinal anesthesia. Am J Surg. 1933;20:107–18.

253. Logas WG, El-Baz N, El-Ganzouri A, Cullen M, Staren E, Faber LP, et al. Continuous thoracic epidural analgesia for postoperative pain relief following thoracotomy: a randomized prospective study. Anesthesiology. 1987;67(5):787–91.

254. Hoffmann VL, Vercauteren MP, Vreugde JP, et al. Posterior epidural space depth: safety of the loss of resistance and hanging drop techniques. Br J Anaesth. 1999;83:807–9.

255. Leurcharusmee P, Arnuntasupakul V, Chora De La Garza D, et al. Reliabilty of waveform analysis as an adjunct to loss of resistance for thoracic epidural blocks. Reg Anesth Pain Med. 2015;40:694–7.

256. Muneyuki M, Shirai K, Inamoto A. Roentgenographic analysis of the positions of catheters in the epidural space. Anesthesiology. 1970;33(1):19–24.

257. Motamed C, Farhat F, Remerand F, Stephanazzi J, Laplanche A, Jayr C. An analysis of postoperative epidural analgesia failure by computed tomography epidurography. Anesth Analg. 2006;103(4):1026–32.

258. Konigsrainer I, Bredanger S, Drewel-Frohnmeyer R, Vonthein R, Krueger WA, Konigsrainer A, et al. Audit of motor weakness and premature catheter dislodgement after epidural analgesia in major abdominal surgery. Anaesthesia. 2009;64(1):27–31.

259. Conacher ID, Paes ML, Jacobson L, Phillips PD, Heaviside DW. Epidural analgesia following thoracic surgery. A review of two years' experience. Anaesthesia. 1983;38(6):546–51.

260. Kaneko M, Saito Y, Kirihara Y, Collins JG, Kosaka Y. Synergistic antinociceptive interaction after epidural coadministration of morphine and lidocaine in rats. Anesthesiology. 1994;80(1):137–50.

261. Curatolo M, Schnider TW, Petersen-Felix S, Weiss S, Signer C, Scaramozzino P, et al. A direct search procedure to optimize combinations of epidural bupivacaine, fentanyl, and clonidine for postoperative analgesia. Anesthesiology. 2000;92(2):325–37.

262. Mahon SV, Berry PD, Jackson M, Russell GN, Pennefather SH. Thoracic epidural infusions for post-thoracotomy pain: a comparison of fentanyl-bupivacaine mixtures vs. fentanyl alone. Anaesthesia. 1999;54(7):641–6.

263. Tan CN, Guha A, Scawn ND, Pennefather SH, Russell GN. Optimal concentration of epidural fentanyl in bupivacaine 0.1% after thoracotomy. Br J Anaesth. 2004;92(5):670–4.

264. Cok OY, Eker HE, Turkoz A, Findikcioglu A, Akin S, Aribogan A, et al. Thoracic epidural anesthesia and analgesia during the perioperative period of thoracic surgery: levobupivacaine versus bupivacaine. J Cardiothorac Vasc Anesth. 2011;25(3):449–54.

265. Niemi G, Breivik H. Epinephrine markedly improves thoracic epidural analgesia produced by a small-dose infusion of ropivacaine, fentanyl, and epinephrine after major thoracic or abdominal surgery: a randomized, double-blinded crossover study with and without epinephrine. Anesth Analg. 2002;94(6):1598–605. table of contents.

266. Eisenach JC, De Kock M, Klimscha W. Alpha(2)-adrenergic agonists for regional anesthesia. A clinical review of clonidine (1984-1995). Anesthesiology. 1996;85(3):655–74.

267. Neil MJ. Clonidine: clinical pharmacology and therapeutic use in pain management. Curr Clin Pharmacol. 2011;6(4):280–7.

268. Mohammad W, Mir SA, Mohammad K, Sofi K. A randomized double-blind study to evaluate efficacy and safety of epidural magnesium sulfate and clonidine as adjuvants to bupivacaine for postthoracotomy pain relief. Anesth Essays Res. 2015;9(1):15–20.

269. Gupta SD, Mitra K, Mukherjee M, Roy S, Sarkar A, Kundu S, et al. Effect of magnesium infusion on thoracic epidural analgesia. Saudi J Anaesth. 2011;5(1):55–61.

270. Visser WA, Liem TH, van Egmond J, Gielen MJ. Extension of sensory blockade after thoracic epidural administration of a test dose of lidocaine at three different levels. Anesth Analg. 1998;86(2):332–5.

271. Lee CJ, Jeon Y, Lim YJ, Bahk JH, Kim YC, Lee SC, et al. The influence of neck flexion and extension on the distribution of contrast medium in the high thoracic epidural space. Anesth Analg. 2007;104(6):1583–6. table of contents.

272. Fratacci MD, Kimball WR, Wain JC, Kacmarek RM, Polaner DM, Zapol WM. Diaphragmatic shortening after thoracic surgery in humans. Effects of mechanical ventilation and thoracic epidural anesthesia. Anesthesiology. 1993;79(4):654–65.

273. Simonneau G, Vivien A, Sartene R, Kunstlinger F, Samii K, Noviant Y, et al. Diaphragm dysfunction induced by upper abdominal surgery. Role of postoperative pain. Am Rev Respir Dis. 1983;128(5):899–903.

274. Dureuil B, Viires N, Cantineau JP, Aubier M, Desmonts JM. Diaphragmatic contractility after upper abdominal surgery. J Appl Physiol (1985). 1986;61(5):1775–80.

275. Torres A, Kimball WR, Qvist J, Stanek K, Kacmarek RM, Whyte RI, et al. Sonomicrometric regional diaphragmatic shortening in awake sheep after thoracic surgery. J Appl Physiol (1985). 1989;67(6):2357–68.

276. Polaner DM, Kimball WR, Fratacci MD, Wain JC, Zapol WM. Thoracic epidural anesthesia increases diaphragmatic shortening after thoracotomy in the awake lamb. Anesthesiology. 1993;79(4):808–16.

277. Manikian B, Cantineau JP, Bertrand M, Kieffer E, Sartene R, Viars P. Improvement of diaphragmatic function by a thoracic extradural block after upper abdominal surgery. Anesthesiology. 1988;68(3):379–86.

278. Warner DO, Warner MA, Ritman EL. Human chest wall function during epidural anesthesia. Anesthesiology. 1996;85(4):761–73.

279. Richter A, Cederholm I, Jonasson L, Mucchiano C, Uchto M, Janerot-Sjoberg B. Effect of thoracic epidural analgesia on refractory angina pectoris: long-term home self-treatment. J Cardiothorac Vasc Anesth. 2002;16(6):679–84.

280. Gramling-Babb P, Miller MJ, Reeves ST, Roy RC, Zile MR. Treatment of medically and surgically refractory angina pectoris with high thoracic epidural analgesia: initial clinical experience. Am Heart J. 1997;133(6):648–55.

281. Sagiroglu G, Meydan B, Copuroglu E, Baysal A, Yoruk Y, Altemur Karamustafaoglu Y, et al. A comparison of thoracic or lumbar patient-controlled epidural analgesia methods after thoracic surgery. World J Surg Oncol. 2014;12:96.

282. Beattie WS, Badner NH, Choi P. Epidural analgesia reduces postoperative myocardial infarction: a meta-analysis. Anesth Analg. 2001;93(4):853–8.

283. Oka T, Ozawa Y, Ohkubo Y. Thoracic epidural bupivacaine attenuates supraventricular tachyarrhythmias after pulmonary resection. Anesth Analg. 2001;93(2):253–9. 1st contents page.

284. Oka T, Ozawa Y. Correlation between intraoperative hemodynamic variability and postoperative arrhythmias in patients with pulmonary surgery. Masui. 1999;48(2):118–23.

285. Ritchie AJ, Bowe P, Gibbons JR. Prophylactic digitalization for thoracotomy: a reassessment. Ann Thorac Surg. 1990;50(1):86–8.

286. Krowka MJ, Pairolero PC, Trastek VF, Payne WS, Bernatz PE. Cardiac dysrhythmia following pneumonectomy. Clinical correlates and prognostic significance. Chest. 1987;91(4):490–5.

287. von Knorring J, Lepantalo M, Lindgren L, Lindfors O. Cardiac arrhythmias and myocardial ischemia after thoracotomy for lung cancer. Ann Thorac Surg. 1992;53(4):642–7.

288. Leslie K, Myles P, Devereaux P, Williamson E, Rao-Melancini P, Forbes A, et al. Neuraxial block, death and serious cardiovascular morbidity in the POISE trial. Br J Anaesth. 2013;111(3):382–90.

289. Modig J, Borg T, Karlstrom G, Maripuu E, Sahlstedt B. Thromboembolism after total hip replacement: role of epidural and general anesthesia. Anesth Analg. 1983;62(2):174–80.

290. Sharrock NE, Cazan MG, Hargett MJ, Williams-Russo P, Wilson PD Jr. Changes in mortality after total hip and knee arthroplasty over a ten-year period. Anesth Analg. 1995;80(2):242–8.

291. Rodgers A, Walker N, Schug S, McKee A, Kehlet H, van Zundert A, et al. Reduction of postoperative mortality and morbidity with epidural or spinal anaesthesia: results from overview of randomised trials. BMJ. 2000;321(7275):1493.

292. Rigg JR, Jamrozik K, Myles PS, Silbert BS, Peyton PJ, Parsons RW, et al. Epidural anaesthesia and analgesia and outcome of major surgery: a randomised trial. Lancet. 2002;359(9314):1276–82.

293. Popping DM, Elia N, Van Aken HK, Marret E, Schug SA, Kranke P, et al. Impact of epidural analgesia on mortality and morbidity after surgery: systematic review and meta-analysis of randomized controlled trials. Ann Surg. 2014;259(6):1056–67.

294. Giebler RM, Scherer RU, Peters J. Incidence of neurologic complications related to thoracic epidural catheterization. Anesthesiology. 1997;86(1):55–63.

295. Wheatley RG, Schug SA, Watson D. Safety and efficacy of postoperative epidural analgesia. Br J Anaesth. 2001;87(1):47–61.

296. Gustafsson LL, Schildt B, Jacobsen K. Adverse effects of extradural and intrathecal opiates: report of a nationwide survey in Sweden. Br J Anaesth. 1982;54(5):479–86.

297. Liu SS, Allen HW, Olsson GL. Patient-controlled epidural analgesia with bupivacaine and fentanyl on hospital wards: prospective experience with 1,030 surgical patients. Anesthesiology. 1998;88(3):688–95.

298. Shanker KB, Palkar NV, Nishkala R. Paraplegia following epidural potassium chloride. Anaesthesia. 1985;40(1):45–7.

299. Moen V, Dahlgren N, Irestedt L. Severe neurological complications after central neuraxial blockades in Sweden 1990-1999. Anesthesiology. 2004;101(4):950–9.

300. Bromage PR, Camporesi EM, Durant PA, Nielsen CH. Nonrespiratory side effects of epidural morphine. Anesth Analg. 1982;61(6):490–5.

301. Yaksh TL. Spinal opiate analgesia: characteristics and principles of action. Pain. 1981;11(3):293–346.

302. Rawal N, Mollefors K, Axelsson K, Lingardh G, Widman B. An experimental study of urodynamic effects of epidural morphine and of naloxone reversal. Anesth Analg. 1983;62(7):641–7.

303. Husted S, Djurhuus JC, Husegaard HC, Jepsen J, Mortensen J. Effect of postoperative extradural morphine on lower urinary tract function. Acta Anaesthesiol Scand. 1985;29(2):183–5.

304. Wang J, Pennefather S, Russell G. Low-dose naloxone in the treatment of urinary retention during extradural fentanyl causes excessive reversal of analgesia. Br J Anaesth. 1998;80(4):565–6.

305. Goldhill DR, Whelpton R, Winyard JA, Wilkinson KA. Gastric emptying in patients the day after cardiac surgery. Anaesthesia. 1995;50(2):122–5.

306. Petring OU, Dawson PJ, Blake DW, Jones DJ, Bjorksten AR, Libreri FC, et al. Normal postoperative gastric emptying after orthopaedic surgery with spinal anaesthesia and i.m. ketorolac as the first postoperative analgesic. Br J Anaesth. 1995;74(3):257–60.

307. Thorn SE, Wattwil M, Naslund I. Postoperative epidural morphine, but not epidural bupivacaine, delays gastric emptying on the first day after cholecystectomy. Reg Anesth. 1992;17(2):91–4.

308. Bonica JJ. Autonomic innervation of the viscera in relation to nerve block. Anesthesiology. 1968;29(4):793–813.

309. Guha A, Scawn ND, Rogers SA, Pennefather SH, Russell GN. Gastric emptying in post-thoracotomy patients receiving a thoracic fentanyl-bupivacaine epidural infusion. Eur J Anaesthesiol. 2002;19(9):652–7.

310. Jorgensen H, Wetterslev J, Moiniche S, Dahl JB. Epidural local anaesthetics versus opioid-based analgesic regimens on postoperative gastrointestinal paralysis, PONV and pain after abdominal surgery. Cochrane Database Syst Rev. 2000;(4):CD001893.

311. Zeng XZ, Lu ZF, Lv XQ, Guo YP, Cui XG. Epidural Co-administration of dexmedetomidine and levobupivacaine improves the gastrointestinal motility function after colonic resection in comparison to co-administration of morphine and levobupivacaine. PLoS One. 2016;11(1):e0146215.

312. Lundberg JF, Martner J, Raner C, Winso O, Biber B. Dopamine or norepinephrine infusion during thoracic epidural anesthesia? Differences in hemodynamic effects and plasma catecholamine levels. Acta Anaesthesiol Scand. 2005;49(7):962–8.

313. Li XQ, Tan WF, Wang J, Fang B, Ma H. The effects of thoracic epidural analgesia on oxygenation and pulmonary shunt fraction during one-lung ventilation: an meta-analysis. BMC Anesthesiol. 2015;15:166.

314. Horlocker TT, Wedel DJ. Neurologic complications of spinal and epidural anesthesia. Reg Anesth Pain Med. 2000;25(1):83–98.

315. Stafford-Smith M. Impaired haemostasis and regional anaesthesia. Can J Anaesth. 1996;43(5 Pt 2):R129–41.

316. Meikle J, Bird S, Nightingale JJ, White N. Detection and management of epidural haematomas related to anaesthesia in the UK: a national survey of current practice. Br J Anaesth. 2008;101(3):400–4.

317. Kozek-Langenecker SA. Neuraxial anaesthesia and anticoagulant and analgesic agents: The ESA guidelines: European Society of Anaesthesia; 2010.

318. Gogarten W, van Aken H, Riess H. German guidelines on regional anaesthesia and thromboembolism prophylaxis. Anaesthesiol Intensivmed. 2007;48:124–9.

319. Li J, Halaszynski T. Neuraxial and peripheral nerve blocks in patients taking anticoagulant or thromboprophylactic drugs: challenges and solutions. Local Reg Anesth. 2015;8:21–32.

320. Collins R, Scrimgeour A, Yusuf S, Peto R. Reduction in fatal pulmonary embolism and venous thrombosis by perioperative administration of subcutaneous heparin. Overview of results of randomized trials in general, orthopedic, and urologic surgery. N Engl J Med. 1988;318(18):1162–73.

321. Vandermeulen EP, Van Aken H, Vermylen J. Anticoagulants and spinal-epidural anesthesia. Anesth Analg. 1994;79(6):1165–77.

322. Greaves JD. Serious spinal cord injury due to haematomyelia caused by spinal anaesthesia in a patient treated with low-dose heparin. Anaesthesia. 1997;52(2):150–4.

323. Sandhu H, Morley-Forster P, Spadafora S. Epidural hematoma following epidural analgesia in a patient receiving unfractionated heparin for thromboprophylaxis. Reg Anesth Pain Med. 2000;25(1):72–5.

324. Liu SS, Mulroy MF. Neuraxial anesthesia and analgesia in the presence of standard heparin. Reg Anesth Pain Med. 1998;23(6 Suppl 2):157–63.

325. Horlocker TT, Wedel DJ, Rowlingson JC, Enneking FK, Kopp SL, Benzon HT, et al. Regional anesthesia in the patient receiving anti-thrombotic or thrombolytic therapy: American Society of Regional Anesthesia and Pain Medicine Evidence-Based Guidelines (Third Edition). Reg Anesth Pain Med. 2010;35(1):64–101.

326. Bergqvist D, Lindblad B, Matzsch T. Low molecular weight heparin for thromboprophylaxis and epidural/spinal anaesthesia--is there a risk? Acta Anaesthesiol Scand. 1992;36(7):605–9.

327. Tryba M, Wedel DJ. Central neuraxial block and low molecular weight heparin (enoxaparine): lessons learned from different dosage regimes in two continents. Acta Anaesthesiol Scand Suppl. 1997;111:100–4.

328. Narouze S, Benzon HT, Provenzano DA, Buvanendran A, De Andres J, Deer TR, et al. Interventional spine and pain procedures in patients on antiplatelet and anticoagulant medications: guidelines from the American Society of Regional Anesthesia and Pain Medicine, the European Society of Regional Anaesthesia and Pain Therapy, the American Academy of Pain Medicine, the International Neuromodulation Society, the North American Neuromodulation Society, and the World Institute of Pain. Reg Anesth Pain Med. 2015;40(3):182–212.

329. CLASP: a randomised trial of low-dose aspirin for the prevention and treatment of pre-eclampsia among 9364 pregnant women. CLASP (Collaborative Low-dose Aspirin Study in Pregnancy) Collaborative Group. Lancet. 1994;343(8898):619–29.

330. Horlocker TT, Bajwa ZH, Ashraf Z, Khan S, Wilson JL, Sami N, et al. Risk assessment of hemorrhagic complications associated with nonsteroidal antiinflammatory medications in ambulatory pain clinic patients undergoing epidural steroid injection. Anesth Analg. 2002;95(6):1691–7. table of contents.

331. Newsome LT, Kutcher MA, Royster RL. Coronary artery stents: Part I. Evolution of percutaneous coronary intervention. Anesth Analg. 2008;107(2):552–69.

332. Kocabas S, Yedicocuklu D, Yuksel E, Uysallar E, Askar F. Infiltration of the sternotomy wound and the mediastinal tube sites with 0.25% levobupivacaine as adjunctive treatment for postoperative pain after cardiac surgery. Eur J Anaesthesiol. 2008;25(10):842–9.

333. Magnano D, Montalbano R, Lamarra M, Ferri F, Lorini L, Clarizia S, et al. Ineffectiveness of local wound anesthesia to reduce postoperative pain after median sternotomy. J Card Surg. 2005;20(4):314–8.

334. Ziyaeifard M, Azarfarin R, Golzari SE. A review of current analgesic techniques in cardiac surgery. Is epidural worth it? J Cardiovasc Thorac Res. 2014;6(3):133–40.

335. McDonald SB, Jacobsohn E, Kopacz DJ, Desphande S, Helman JD, Salinas F, et al. Parasternal block and local anesthetic infiltration with levobupivacaine after cardiac surgery with desflurane: the effect on postoperative pain, pulmonary function, and tracheal extubation times. Anesth Analg. 2005;100(1):25–32.

336. Nagahiro I, Andou A, Aoe M, Sano Y, Date H, Shimizu N. Pulmonary function, postoperative pain, and serum cytokine level after lobectomy: a comparison of VATS and conventional procedure. Ann Thorac Surg. 2001;72(2):362–5.

337. McKenna RJ Jr, Houck W, Fuller CB. Video-assisted thoracic surgery lobectomy: experience with 1,100 cases. Ann Thorac Surg. 2006;81(2):421–5. discussion 5-6.

338. Kamiyoshihara M, Nagashima T, Ibe T, Atsumi J, Shimizu K, Takeyoshi I. Is epidural analgesia necessary after video-assisted thoracoscopic lobectomy? Asian Cardiovasc Thorac Ann. 2010;18(5):464–8.

339. Steinthorsdottir KJ, Wildgaard L, Hansen HJ, Petersen RH, Wildgaard K. Regional analgesia for video-assisted thoracic surgery: a systematic review. Eur J Cardiothorac Surg. 2014;45(6):959–66.

340. Zingg U, McQuinn A, DiValentino D, Esterman AJ, Bessell JR, Thompson SK, et al. Minimally invasive versus open esophagectomy for patients with esophageal cancer. Ann Thorac Surg. 2009;87(3):911–9.

341. Perttunen K, Nilsson E, Heinonen J, Hirvisalo EL, Salo JA, Kalso E. Extradural, paravertebral and intercostal nerve blocks for post-thoracotomy pain. Br J Anaesth. 1995;75(5):541–7.

342. Matthews PJ, Govenden V. Comparison of continuous paravertebral and extradural infusions of bupivacaine for pain relief after thoracotomy. Br J Anaesth. 1989;62(2):204–5.

343. Coe A, Sarginson R, Smith MW, Donnelly RJ, Russell GN. Pain following thoracotomy. A randomised, double-blind comparison of lumbar versus thoracic epidural fentanyl. Anaesthesia. 1991;46(11):918–21.

344. Haak-van der Lely F, van Kleef JW, Burm AG, Bovill JG. An intra-operative comparison of lumbar with thoracic epidural sufentanil for thoracotomy. Anaesthesia. 1994;49(2):119–21.

345. Thomson CA, Becker DR, Messick JM Jr, de Castro MA, Pairolero PC, Trastek VF, et al. Analgesia after thoracotomy: effects of epidural fentanyl concentration/infusion rate. Anesth Analg. 1995;81(5):973–81.

346. Stratton SA, Smith MM. Postoperative thoracotomy. Effect of transcutaneous electrical nerve stimulation on forced vital capacity. Phys Ther. 1980;60(1):45–7.

347. Rooney SM, Jain S, Goldiner PL. Effect of transcutaneous nerve stimulation on postoperative pain after thoracotomy. Anesth Analg. 1983;62(11):1010–2.

348. Warfield CA, Stein JM, Frank HA. The effect of transcutaneous electrical nerve stimulation on pain after thoracotomy. Ann Thorac Surg. 1985;39(5):462–5.

349. Stubbing JF, Jellicoe JA. Transcutaneous electrical nerve stimulation after thoracotomy. Pain relief and peak expiratory flow rate--a trial of transcutaneous electrical nerve stimulation. Anaesthesia. 1988;43(4):296–8.

350. Benedetti F, Amanzio M, Casadio C, Cavallo A, Cianci R, Giobbe R, et al. Control of postoperative pain by transcutaneous electrical nerve stimulation after thoracic operations. Ann Thorac Surg. 1997;63(3):773–6.

351. Erdogan M, Erdogan A, Erbil N, Karakaya HK, Demircan A. Prospective, randomized, placebo-controlled study of the effect of TENS on postthoracotomy pain and pulmonary function. World J Surg. 2005;29(12):1563–70.

352. Solak O, Turna A, Pekcolaklar A, Metin M, Sayar A, Solak O, et al. Transcutaneous electric nerve stimulation for the treatment of postthoracotomy pain: a randomized prospective study. Thorac Cardiovasc Surg. 2007;55(3):182–5.

353. Licker MJ, Widikker I, Robert J, Frey JG, Spiliopoulos A, Ellenberger C, et al. Operative mortality and respiratory complications after lung resection for cancer: impact of chronic obstructive pulmonary disease and time trends. Ann Thorac Surg. 2006;81(5):1830–7.

354. Powell ES, Pearce AC, Cook D, Davies P, Bishay E, Bowler GM, et al. UK pneumonectomy outcome study (UKPOS): a prospective observational study of pneumonectomy outcome. J Cardiothorac Surg. 2009;4:41.

355. Raymond DP, Seder CW, Wright CD, Magee MJ, Kosinski AS, Cassivi SD, et al. Predictors of major morbidity or mortality after resection for esophageal cancer: a society of thoracic surgeons general thoracic surgery database risk adjustment model. Ann Thorac Surg. 2016;102(1):207–14.

356. Cense HA, Lagarde SM, de Jong K, Omloo JM, Busch OR, Henny Ch P, et al. Association of no epidural analgesia with postoperative morbidity and mortality after transthoracic esophageal cancer resection. J Am Coll Surg. 2006;202(3):395–400.

357. Li W, Li Y, Huang Q, Ye S, Rong T. Short and long-term outcomes of epidural or intravenous analgesia after esophagectomy: a propensity-matched cohort study. PLoS One. 2016;11(4): e0154380.

358. Smedstad KG, Beattie WS, Blair WS, Buckley DN. Postoperative pain relief and hospital stay after total esophagectomy. Clin J Pain. 1992;8(2):149–53.

359. Whooley BP, Law S, Murthy SC, Alexandrou A, Wong J. Analysis of reduced death and complication rates after esophageal resection. Ann Surg. 2001;233(3):338–44.

360. Watson A, Allen PR. Influence of thoracic epidural analgesia on outcome after resection for esophageal cancer. Surgery. 1994;115(4):429–32.

361. Michelet P, D'Journo XB, Roch A, Papazian L, Ragni J, Thomas P, et al. Perioperative risk factors for anastomotic leakage after esophagectomy: influence of thoracic epidural analgesia. Chest. 2005;128(5):3461–6.

362. Page RD, Shackcloth MJ, Russell GN, Pennefather SH. Surgical treatment of anastomotic leaks after oesophagectomy. Eur J Cardiothorac Surg. 2005;27(2):337–43.

363. Ikeda Y, Niimi M, Kan S, Shatari T, Takami H, Kodaira S. Clinical significance of tissue blood flow during esophagectomy by laser Doppler flowmetry. J Thorac Cardiovasc Surg. 2001;122(6):1101–6.

364. Al-Rawi OY, Pennefather SH, Page RD, Dave I, Russell GN. The effect of thoracic epidural bupivacaine and an intravenous adrenaline infusion on gastric tube blood flow during esophagectomy. Anesth Analg. 2008;106(3):884–7. table of contents.

365. Michelet P, Roch A, D'Journo XB, Blayac D, Barrau K, Papazian L, et al. Effect of thoracic epidural analgesia on gastric blood flow after oesophagectomy. Acta Anaesthesiol Scand. 2007;51(5):587–94.

366. Durkin C, Schisler T, Lohser J. Current trends in anesthesia for esophagectomy. Curr Opin Anaesthesiol. 2017;30(1):30–5.

367. Bartels K, Fiegel M, Stevens Q, Ahlgren B, Weitzel N. Approaches to perioperative care for esophagectomy. J Cardiothorac Vasc Anesth. 2015;29(2):472–80.

368. Kelly FE, Murdoch JA, Sanders DJ, Berrisford RG. Continuous paravertebral block for thoraco-abdominal oesophageal surgery. Anaesthesia. 2005;60(1):98–9.

369. Scawn ND, Pennefather SH, Soorae A, Wang JY, Russell GN. Ipsilateral shoulder pain after thoracotomy with epidural analgesia: the influence of phrenic nerve infiltration with lidocaine. Anesth Analg. 2001;93(2):260–4. 1st contents page.

370. Tan N, Agnew NM, Scawn ND, Pennefather SH, Chester M, Russell GN. Suprascapular nerve block for ipsilateral shoulder pain after thoracotomy with thoracic epidural analgesia: a double-blind comparison of 0.5% bupivacaine and 0.9% saline. Anesth Analg. 2002;94(1):199–202. table of contents.

371. Blichfeldt-Eckhardt MR, Andersen C, Ording H, Licht PB, Toft P. Shoulder pain after thoracic surgery: type and time course, a prospective cohort study. J Cardiothorac Vasc Anesth. 2017;31(1):147–51.

372. MacDougall P. Postthoracotomy shoulder pain: diagnosis and management. Curr Opin Anaesthesiol. 2008;21(1):12–5.

373. Bunchungmongkol N, Pipanmekaporn T, Paiboonworachat S, Saeteng S, Tantraworasin A. Incidence and risk factors associated with ipsilateral shoulder pain after thoracic surgery. J Cardiothorac Vasc Anesth. 2014;28(4):979–82.

374. Yousefshahi F, Predescu O, Colizza M, Asenjo JF. Postthoracotomy ipsilateral shoulder pain: a literature review on characteristics and treatment. Pain Res Manag. 2016;2016:3652726.

375. Gosling JAH, Harris PF, Humpherson JR. Atlas of human anatomy. London: Churchill Livingstone; 1985.

376. Danelli G, Berti M, Casati A, Bobbio A, Ghisi D, Mele R, et al. Ipsilateral shoulder pain after thoracotomy surgery: a prospective, randomized, double-blind, placebo-controlled evaluation of the efficacy of infiltrating the phrenic nerve with 0.2%wt/vol ropivacaine. Eur J Anaesthesiol. 2007;24(7):596–601.

377. Ng KP, Chow YF. Brachial plexus block for ipsilateral shoulder pain after thoracotomy. Anaesth Intensive Care. 1997;25(1):74–6.

378. Barak M, Iaroshevski D, Poppa E, Ben-Nun A, Katz Y. Low-volume interscalene brachial plexus block for post-thoracotomy shoulder pain. J Cardiothorac Vasc Anesth. 2007;21(4):554–7.

379. Urmey WF, McDonald M. Hemidiaphragmatic paresis during interscalene brachial plexus block: effects on pulmonary function and chest wall mechanics. Anesth Analg. 1992;74(3):352–7.

380. Garner L, Coats RR. Ipsilateral stellate ganglion block effective for treating shoulder pain after thoracotomy. Anesth Analg. 1994;78(6):1195–6.

381. Mitra S, Sinatra RS. Perioperative management of acute pain in the opioid-dependent patient. Anesthesiology. 2004;101(1):212–27.

382. Bohn LM, Gainetdinov RR, Lin FT, Lefkowitz RJ, Caron MG. Mu-opioid receptor desensitization by beta-arrestin-2 determines morphine tolerance but not dependence. Nature. 2000;408(6813):720–3.

383. Nestler EJ, Aghajanian GK. Molecular and cellular basis of addiction. Science. 1997;278(5335):58–63.

384. Nestler EJ. Molecular basis of long-term plasticity underlying addiction. Nat Rev Neurosci. 2001;2(2):119–28.

385. Mayer DJ, Mao J, Holt J, Price DD. Cellular mechanisms of neuropathic pain, morphine tolerance, and their interactions. Proc Natl Acad Sci U S A. 1999;96(14):7731–6.

386. Compton P, Charuvastra VC, Kintaudi K, Ling W. Pain responses in methadone-maintained opioid abusers. J Pain Symptom Manag. 2000;20(4):237–45.

387. Laulin JP, Celerier E, Larcher A, Le Moal M, Simonnet G. Opiate tolerance to daily heroin administration: an apparent phenomenon associated with enhanced pain sensitivity. Neuroscience. 1999;89(3):631–6.

388. Shah S, Kapoor S, Durkin B. Analgesic management of acute pain in the opioid-tolerant patient. Curr Opin Anaesthesiol. 2015;28(4):398–402.

389. de Leon-Casasola OA, Lema MJ. Epidural sufentanil for acute pain control in a patient with extreme opioid dependency. Anesthesiology. 1992;76(5):853–6.

390. de Leon-Casasola OA, Lema MJ. Epidural bupivacaine/sufentanil therapy for postoperative pain control in patients tolerant to opioid and unresponsive to epidural bupivacaine/morphine. Anesthesiology. 1994;80(2):303–9.

391. Rapp SE, Ready LB, Nessly ML. Acute pain management in patients with prior opioid consumption: a case-controlled retrospective review. Pain. 1995;61(2):195–201.

392. Swenson JD, Davis JJ, Johnson KB. Postoperative care of the chronic opioid-consuming patient. Anesthesiol Clin North Am. 2005;23(1):37–48.

393. Fitzgibbon DR, Ready LB. Intravenous high-dose methadone administered by patient controlled analgesia and continuous infusion for the treatment of cancer pain refractory to high-dose morphine. Pain. 1997;73(2):259–61.

394. Larcher A, Laulin JP, Celerier E, Le Moal M, Simonnet G. Acute tolerance associated with a single opiate administration: involvement of N-methyl-D-aspartate-dependent pain facilitatory systems. Neuroscience. 1998;84(2):583–9.

395. Shimoyama N, Shimoyama M, Inturrisi CE, Elliott KJ. Ketamine attenuates and reverses morphine tolerance in rodents. Anesthesiology. 1996;85(6):1357–66.

396. Barrington MJ, Scott DA. Do we need to justify epidural analgesia beyond pain relief? Lancet. 2008;372(9638):514–6.

Long-Acting Local Anesthetics for Analgesia Following Thoracic Surgery

60

Wendell H. Williams III, Jagtar Singh Heir, and Anupamjeet Kaur Sekhon

Key Points
- Though optimal pain management for thoracic surgery can be quite challenging considering the numerous contributing mechanisms, a comprehensive pain management strategy can improve overall patient safety and satisfaction.
- Local anesthetics work by inhibiting membrane depolarization along neurons by binding to the alpha subunit of intracellular voltage-gated sodium channels; they may also possess some degree of antagonism toward the potassium (K+) and calcium (Ca2+) channels and NMDA receptors.
- Liposomal bupivacaine, a novel slow-release local anesthetic formulation, encapsulates the local anesthetic by utilizing an innovative delivery system known as DepoFoam®. The bilayered lipid septa provide a stable and reliable platform for the prolonged release of medications (72–96 h) without alteration to its molecular structure.
- Liposomal bupivacaine does not diffuse through tissues in the same manner as conventional bupivacaine. Consequently, meticulous infiltration technique is imperative to ensure best results regardless of regional technique. Decreased spread means more injections are needed in closer proximity than with traditional bupivacaine.
- The bupivacaine contained in liposomal bupivacaine is free-base bupivacaine form, distinct from bupivacaine HCl, salt form of bupivacaine. Providers should be cognizant of the fact that different formulations of bupivacaine are not bioequivalent even if the milligram dosage is the same.
- Alternatives to systemic opioids and thoracic epidurals include regional techniques such as the paravertebral, intercostal, phrenic, intrapleural, serratus anterior plane, as well as local wound infiltration.
- Combining minimally invasive surgery with multimodal, regional, and pharmacological approaches to analgesia can provide a higher level of postoperative analgesia while reducing undesired side effects of narcotic usage, such as nausea, vomiting, constipation, and respiratory depression.
- Novel long-acting local anesthetic such as liposomal bupivacaine offer a promising analgesic solution, but further studies are warranted to better understand the efficacy and long-term safety profile of these newer local anesthetics.
- This chapter reviews the localized regional techniques currently used at the University of Texas MD Anderson Cancer Center.

Introduction

Surgery remains the cornerstone therapy for early-stage lung and esophageal cancers. It is expected that the number of thoracic procedures for lung and esophageal disease will increase in the future [1]. Optimal pain management can be very challenging after thoracic surgery for multiple reasons. There are numerous mechanisms that contribute to the pain a patient experiences: disruption of the skin and muscles, ligamentous damage, and rib fractures and dislocations, as well

W. H. Williams III (✉) · J. S. Heir
The University of Texas MD Anderson Cancer Center, Department of Anesthesiology and Perioperative Medicine, Houston, TX, USA
e-mail: whwilliams@mdanderson.org

A. K. Sekhon
Detar Family Medicine Residency Program, Texas A&M University College of Medicine, Victoria, TX, USA

© Springer Nature Switzerland AG 2019
P. Slinger (ed.), *Principles and Practice of Anesthesia for Thoracic Surgery*, https://doi.org/10.1007/978-3-030-00859-8_60

as chest tube and shoulder pain from diaphragmatic irritation and positioning. Not only is inadequate pain control significant for humanitarian reasons, it is also linked to increased pulmonary and extrapulmonary complications [2]. The risks of pulmonary complications can be mitigated by appropriate pain management [3]. The literature has shown that early postoperative pain is predictive of long-term pain after thoracotomy. Providers have responded by incorporating aggressive pain management strategies to decrease the high incidence of chronic pain within this vulnerable patient population [4]. The healthcare costs of chronic pain developing from acute pain can represent a significant financial burden for the patient, as well as the community. In fact, some researchers have estimated that the lifetime economic costs of a single 30-year-old patient suffering from chronic pain will reach one million US dollars [5]. For much of the modern era of medicine, postoperative pain management has been primarily accomplished by systemic opioids. Following thoracic surgery, intravenous opioids alone are often insufficient to adequately control pain and have been supplemented with the application of local anesthetics using various regional techniques.

Local anesthetics work by inhibiting the signal propagation along neurons by binding to the alpha subunit of intracellular voltage-gated sodium channels. Neurons utilize the sodium-potassium pump (Na + K+ ATPase) to maintain a negative resting potential difference of -60 to -70 mV through active transport and passive diffusion of ions [6]. The sodium-specific channels are membrane-bound proteins, made up of alpha and beta subunits that exist in three states: resting (nonconducting), open (conducting), and inactivated (nonconducting). Local anesthetics inhibit the action potential necessary to propagate signals along neurons by blocking the influx of sodium needed for membrane depolarization. Secondarily, local anesthetics may possess some degree of antagonism toward the potassium (K+) and calcium (Ca2+) channels, as well as NMDA receptors. By inhibiting the propagation of peripheral nociceptive signals, regional and local anesthesia have the potential to reduce or eliminate postoperative pain as well as mitigate the endocrine and metabolic response to surgery.

Techniques for the administration of local anesthetics to block nociception include (1) surgical site infiltration (single injection or catheter), (2) peripheral nerve blocks (single injection or catheter), and (3) neuraxial anesthesia. With the advent of liposomal local anesthetic agents, it is now possible for thoracic anesthesiologists to tailor or combine regional techniques to suit specific surgical scenarios. Significant pain reduction can be achieved for several days with single-shot injections of multiple, distinct, even unplanned surgical sites without the dependence on perineural catheters. This chapter reviews the history of local anesthetics from the coca leaf to liposomal bupivacaine, the methodology behind specific regional blocks for thoracic surgery, and how the development of long-acting, liposomal anesthetics may improve our ability to manage postoperative thoracic pain.

History of Local Anesthetics

Origins in the Americas

Derived from shrubs of the genus *Erythroxylum* native to Central and South America, the coca leaf held an important social, religious, and medicinal role of the Incan people from as far back as 1900 B.C. [7]. Initially reserved for the aristocracy, coca's use became widespread following the fall of the Incan empire in 1532. From that time until the dawn of the twentieth century, most scientists championed its energizing and euphoric properties while neglecting its other effects. The full potential for medical cocaine wasn't realized until 1880, when Russian physician Basil von Anrep of the University of Würzburg recommended its use as a surgical anesthetic based on numerous experiments upon animals and himself. It was Viennese ophthalmologist Carl Koller (1857–1944) who performed the first operation using local anesthetic on a patient with glaucoma on September 11, 1884. The impact of his work was instantaneous and global, with over 60 publications concerning local anesthesia using cocaine in the United States and Canada by the end of 1885 [8] (Table 60.1).

Synthetic Anesthetics

By the turn of the twentieth century, the potential toxicity and addictive properties of cocaine were well established, and a search for the ideal local anesthetic had begun. In 1904, German chemist Alfred Einhorn (1856–1917) patented novocaine and 17 other para-aminobenzoic derivatives which are now collectively known as ester group local anesthetics [9]. Novocaine, or alternatively named procaine, had its own limitations. Like all ester-based anesthetics, novocaine was limited by a relatively low potency and strong association with hypersensitivity and anaphylaxis among patients and healthcare workers [10]. The serious deficiencies of the ester group anesthetics encouraged the development of another group of anesthetics.

In 1946, Nils Löfgren and Bengt Lundquist developed a xylidine derivative they called "lidocaine," whose chemical composition was distinct from novocaine and was found to be more potent and safer, with little allergenic potential [11]. Bupivacaine, mepivacaine, and most of the other amide

Table 60.1 Important dates in the history of local anesthetics

Date	Subject	Event
1900 B.C.	Incan empire	Oldest known use of coca
A.D. 1532	Fall of Incan empire	Endemic use of coca among many people in Central and South America
1653	Spanish Jesuit father Bernabé Cobo	First documentation of local anesthetic properties of coca leaf
1860	German chemist Albert Niemann	Isolates active compound in coca leaf, names it "cocaine"
1868	Peruvian Thomas Moreno y Maïz	First experimental studies on cocaine as anesthetic in animal models
1880	Russian physician Basil von Anrep of University of Würzburg	Based on studies on animals and himself, Von Anrep recommends cocaine as surgical anesthetic
September 11, 1884	Viennese ophthalmologist Carl Koller	Performs first operation using local anesthetic on a patient with glaucoma
November 1884	William Burke or William Halsted and Richard Hall	First nerve blocks performed
1898	August Bier of Kiel, Germany	Performed first spinal blocks for surgery using cocaine
1904	German chemist Alfred Einhorn	Patents novocaine and 17 other ester group local anesthetics
1905	Hugo Sellheim of Leipzig	Performed first thoracic paravertebral block
1946	Nils Löfgren and Bengt Lundquist	Developed xylidine derivative named "lidocaine," first amide group local anesthetic and foundation for other amide anesthetics
1957	Longer-acting amide anesthetics developed	Mepivacaine and bupivacaine first synthesized
1965		Bupivacaine first introduced into the market
1996		Less toxic enantiomer of mepivacaine named "ropivacaine" released to market
1999		Less toxic enantiomer of bupivacaine named "levobupivacaine" released to market
2011	Liposomal bupivacaine	First multivesicular liposomal local anesthetic approved by FDA

group anesthetics would be introduced over the next half century. Amide anesthetics possess an aromatic head which is linked to a hydrocarbon chain by an amide bond rather than an ester. This results in amide anesthetics being more stable and hence less prone to causing allergic reactions as compared to ester anesthetics. As a butyl group homologue of mepivacaine, bupivacaine was initially discarded as it was found to be four times more toxic. Since its introduction in 1965, the nature of the central nervous system (CNS) and

cardiac toxicity linked to bupivacaine has been well chronicled. The discovery of mepivacaine's optically active isomers, and the extensive study of their decreased toxicology, led to the selection and development of a pure S-(-) enantiomer ropivacaine in 1996. Levobupivacaine, the S-(-) enantiomer of bupivacaine, was approved by the FDA in 1999 [12] (Table 60.2).

Current Long-Acting Local Anesthetics

Although there are a number of amino-amide anesthetics currently available, two of the most commonly used in the United States include bupivacaine and ropivacaine. Due to their longer duration of action, they have been the most common choice for the prevention and treatment of postsurgical pain by local infiltration, peripheral nerve blocks, as well as epidural and spinal anesthesia. For bupivacaine, the typical concentration ranges from 0.0625% to 0.5%. The alteration in concentration allows for a differential blockade in terms of various degrees of sensory and/or motor blockade. Lower concentrations of local anesthetic allow sensory blockade, while increasing higher concentrations provide motor blockade. The potential for cardiotoxicity with bupivacaine use is usually sufficiently mitigated by appropriate measures taken to minimize systemic absorption. Most adverse reactions are linked to direct vascular injection and infiltration of areas at higher risk of absorption or to slow metabolic degradation by the liver. Treatment of overdose or inadvertent intravascular injection has been reported in both animal and human case reports with intralipid, an intravenous lipid emulsion whose prompt administration can reverse even life-threatening cardiotoxicity. Though the precise mechanism for reversal is unclear, it is possible that the addition of the intralipid acts as a reservoir "sink" which creates a gradient that draws the lipophilic toxins away from the affected tissues. Lipid emulsions may also work by overriding the inhibition of mitochondrial carnitine-acylcarnitine translocase which provide fuel for the myocardium [13–16].

As an alternative to bupivacaine with a greater safety margin, ropivacaine was found to have less cardiotoxicity and possess better sensorimotor dissociation at lower doses. In practice, this results in greater motor sparing than bupivacaine at lower doses. Typical concentrations for ropivacaine are 0.1–1%. The onset and duration of action for ropivacaine are similar to bupivacaine though the former has less variability secondary to its more homogenous composition [17]. As with all non-liposomal local anesthetics, the duration of action has been limited by the redistribution of the anesthetic away from the targeted site.

Table 60.2 Common long-acting local anesthetics and LB

Anesthetic	Max dose	Onset (min)	Duration of anesthesia (h)	Duration of analgesia (h)
2% lidocaine (HCO3 + epinephrine)	7 mg/kg	10–20	2–5	3–8
0.5% ropivacaine	0.3 mg/kg	15–30	4–8	5–12
0.75% ropivacaine	0.3 mg/kg	10–15	5–10	6–24
0.5% bupivacaine (+ epinephrine)	0.3 mg/kg	15–30	5–15	6–30
13.3% liposomal bupivacaine (LB)	266 mg	[a]Variable Analgesia 5 min; anesthesia 30–45+ min	[a]Variable	[a]Variable Up to 72 h
13.3% LB (+ 0.25% bupivacaine HCl up to 50% liposomal dose)	266 mg and 150 mg, respectively	[a]Variable Analgesia 5 min; anesthesia ~30 min	[a]Variable	[a]Variable Up to 72 h

[a]Data on LB directly compared to other amide local anesthetics is limited. Many components may contribute to variable block duration of LB including site of injection, use for local infiltration vs. nerve blockade, technique of injection, and amount of dilution. Most studies have used LB for local infiltration and did not objectively measure sensory block over the entire block duration. There is limited information on the use of LB for regional anesthesia as the primary anesthetic to assess onset and duration of anesthesia

Liposomal Bupivacaine and the Introduction of a New Class of Anesthetics

The most recent development in the evolution of local anesthetics may represent an attractive alternative in the management of postoperative pain. Liposomal bupivacaine (LB), a novel slow-release local anesthetic formulation, encapsulates the local anesthetic by utilizing an innovative delivery system known as DepoFoam®. These multivesicular liposomes consist of hundreds of water-filled polyhedral compartments which are separated by biocompatible, biodegradable, lipid-based vesicles ranging in size between 10 and 30 μm. The bilayered lipid septa provide a stable and reliable platform for the prolonged release of medications. The local anesthetic is encapsulated by DepoFoam® without alteration to its molecular structure and is steadily released over 72–96 h [18–21] (Fig. 60.1).

Safety

The safety of LB appears to be comparable to other local anesthetic agents. Initial studies by Bramlett et al. found when comparing LB to bupivacaine, both formulations were safe and well tolerated with a low incidence of adverse events [22]. Golf et al., based on application during bunionectomy, found that LB provided superior analgesia and was well tolerated and safe with a slightly higher incidence of medication-related adverse events, most notably postoperative nausea and vomiting [23]. Gorfine et al. concluded in their study of patients undergoing hemorrhoidectomy that a 300 mg formulation of LB was safe [24]. The effect of LB on QTc interval was studied by Naseem et al. who demonstrated that doses up to 750 mg did not cause significant prolongation [25]. Although initial studies evaluating the safety and efficacy were done with patients in soft tissue and orthopedic models, a recent

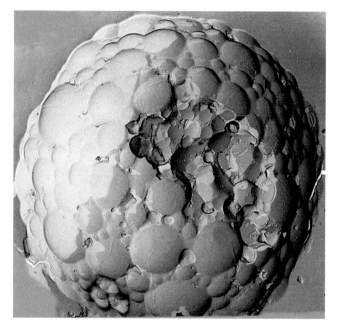

Fig. 60.1 DepoFoam EM. Scanning electron microscopy of EXPAREL® (bupivacaine liposome injectable suspension) with the DepoFoam® technology ©*Pacira Pharmaceuticals, Inc. All Rights Reserved. Used Under License*

review evaluated six randomized controlled double-blind trials in adult patients that used a single dose of LB for postoperative pain control in a more diverse group of surgical patients. Essentially, this review concluded that LB when used in therapeutic doses was well tolerated, had a higher safety margin, and showed a favorable safety profile compared to bupivacaine and control groups [26]. A Cochrane meta-analysis of liposomal bupivacaine for use in local wound infiltration (10 reports, 1377 participants) also found it to have a comparable safety profile to bupivacaine HCL [27].

Preparation and Application

LB is manufactured as a single-use 20 ml vial, which is 1.3% formulation containing a total of 266 mg of bupivacaine. The bupivacaine contained in LB is a free-base bupivacaine form which differs from other frequently used amide-type, bupivacaine-based local anesthetics which contain the salt form of bupivacaine, bupivacaine HCl. Therefore, 266 mg of bupivacaine free base is chemically the molar equivalent to 300 mg of bupivacaine HCl. Providers should be cognizant of the fact that different formulations of bupivacaine are not bioequivalent even if the milligram dosage is the same. Therefore, it is not possible to convert dosing between LB and other formulations.

Liposomal agents should be injected slowly with frequent aspiration to check for the blood and minimize the risk of intravascular injection. It is important to recognize that LB does not diffuse through tissues in the same manner as conventional bupivacaine. Consequently, meticulous infiltration technique is imperative to ensure best results regardless of regional technique. For surgical site injections, that means using a deep tissue infiltration technique with continuous injection of the anesthetic from the fascia to dermis. Decreased spread means more injections are needed in closer proximity than with traditional bupivacaine. Many surgeons in clinical practice often expand the volume of the injectate up to a total volume of 300 mL with either normal saline (0.9%) for injection or lactated Ringer's solution. Volumes used in clinical practice range from 20 to 300 mL (diluted) depending on the size of the surgical site. The onset of action is longer than with conventional bupivacaine as a natural consequence of the slow release of the anesthetic from the liposomes. The addition of normal bupivacaine HCL to the LB at a ratio that does not exceed 1:2 can hasten the onset of sensory blockade. The addition of greater amounts of bupivacaine or the combination of LB with other unapproved anesthetics or agents can cause the premature breakdown of the liposomal matrix and potentially a dangerous uncontrolled release of the anesthetic.

Contraindications and Precautions

LB is contraindicated in obstetrical paracervical block anesthesia. Although LB has not been used in paracervical blocks, the use of bupivacaine HCl with this technique has resulted in fetal bradycardia and death; hence, it should not be used in this type of block. Furthermore, the manufacturer cautions that there is a potential risk of severe life-threatening adverse effects associated with the administration of bupivacaine; therefore, LB should be administered in a setting where trained personnel and equipment are available to promptly treat patients who show evidence of neurological or cardiac toxicity. Care should be exercised to avoid accidental intravascular injection of LB. Multiple reports have reported convulsions and cardiac arrest following accidental intravas-cular injection of bupivacaine and other amide-containing products.

The aforementioned studies have shown that LB is a promising drug formulation which can potentially improve the postoperative pain control in surgical patients. However, further studies are needed in both larger patient populations and wider array of patient populations to enhance the current level of knowledge of the drug's advantages and disadvantages and define the areas of best application. Until recently there had been only two studies, both limited by their retrospective nature, on the efficacy and safety of this liposomal formulation in thoracic patients.

Regional Anesthetic Techniques for Thoracic Surgery

Thoracic Epidural Anesthesia

The infusion of local anesthetics, typically bupivacaine or ropivacaine, into the epidural space has been considered the "gold standard" for optimal pain management in postoperative pain after thoracotomy; however, this technique may not be feasible for a number of reasons: contraindications such as those patients with certain antithrombotic agents, systemic heparinization, or local and systemic infection who possess an elevated risk for epidural hematoma or abscess, respectively. Thoracic epidural anesthesia (TEA) has also been shown to have a high incidence of failure, with rates as high as 32% having been reported in the literature [28, 29]. The efficacy of the thoracic epidural is highly operator dependent, and successful catheter placement can be influenced by many factors, such as the patient's body habitus, patient positioning, and anatomical variations. The undesirable side effects of epidural anesthesia, the resultant bilateral sympathectomy, and epidural opioid exposure are numerous and can include postoperative hypotension, decreased pulmonary function, urinary retention, and pruritus [30–32]. Pain management strategies have continued to evolve, and some research has begun to suggest a shift away from systemic opioids and thoracic epidurals toward regional nerve blockade with lower rates of adverse events [33].

Shift Toward More Peripheral Regional Techniques

Alternatives to thoracic epidural have been described with variable success, including techniques which target the paravertebral, intercostal, phrenic, intrapleural, serratus anterior plane, in addition to local wound infiltration. The most enduring argument which supports the continued use

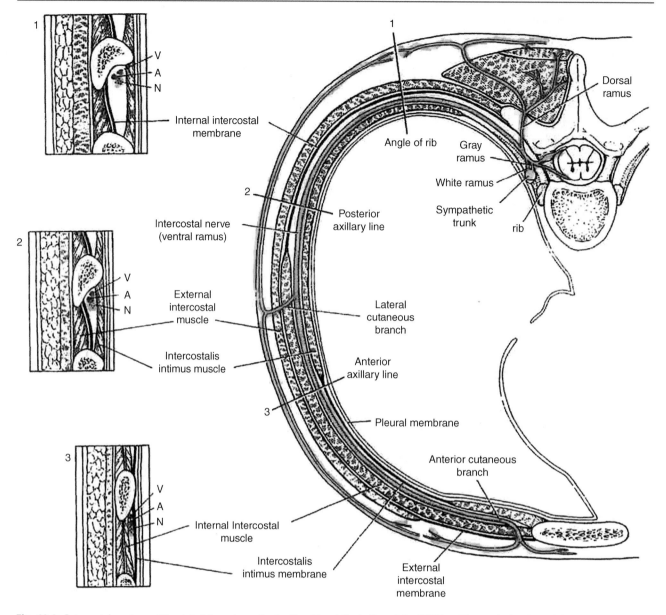

Fig. 60.2 Intercostal anatomy. (Reprinted from Anaesthesia, Dravid and Paul, Copyright (2007), with permission from John Wiley and Sons. (Dravid and Paul [108]))

of thoracic epidurals is its ability to provide analgesia for several days. In contrast, the efficacy of single-shot administration of local anesthetic has naturally been limited to the duration of action for the applied local anesthetic. Anesthesia providers have attempted to prolong the analgesic benefit by utilizing other additives such as corticosteroids, epinephrine, and clonidine or by combining different local anesthetics to the anesthetic with variable success [34]. Perineural catheters can also continuously infuse local anesthetic and thus prolong the duration of regional techniques; however, there are conflicting reports about their ability to appropriately control postoperative thoracotomy pain. Plausible reasons for these conflicting

reports are these catheters require greater technical expertise and are prone to migration, kinking, occlusion, and infection [35–38].

At the University of Texas MD Anderson Cancer Center, our pain management strategy for thoracic procedures has undergone a major change over the last few years. For the better part of the last two decades, we have utilized epidurals for postoperative pain management in patients having thoracic surgery. With the introduction and refinement of regional techniques such as paravertebral and intercostal blocks, surgical preference has more often favored the use of these more peripheral blocks in lieu of epidurals specifically for thoracic procedures.

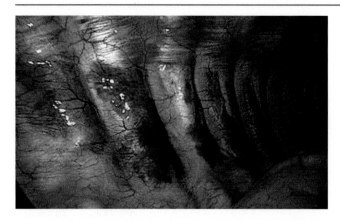

Fig. 60.3 Rice block methylene blue. Posterior intercostal block with LB and methylene blue. Thoracoscopic visualization allows accurate injection of LB into the intercostal space without violation of the parietal pleura. Note that the site of injection is at the level of the innermost intercostal muscles and that the drug tracks medially to the paravertebral space. Methylene blue was added to the LB for purposes of illustrating the extent of subpleural spread only. (Reprinted from The Annals of Thoracic Surgery, D Rice, Copyright (2015), with permission from Elsevier. (Rice et al. [109]))

Thoracic Paravertebral Blockade (Please See Figs. 59.5 and 59.6 from Chap. 59)

First introduced by Hugo Sellheim in 1905, thoracic paravertebral blockade (TPVB) fell out of favor during most of the twentieth century until its reintroduction by Eason and Wyatt in 1979. TPVB has continued to evolve with the use of various landmark techniques and adjuncts such as pressure sensors, fluoroscopy, nerve stimulators and, most recently, ultrasound-guidance. The resultant ipsilateral, segmental, somatic, and sympathetic blockade has become increasingly popular in the treatment of acute and chronic pain [39]. For patients undergoing thoracotomy, several large meta-analyses have concluded that when compared with TEA, TPVB has comparable analgesic benefit, levels of cortisol stress markers, and frequency of major complications but with improved preservation of lung function and significantly less hypotension, nausea and vomiting, pruritus, urinary retention and block failure [40–43].

In the treatment of post-thoracotomy pain, TPVB has traditionally been limited in reliability and duration. Using landmark-based techniques, TPVB has commonly been described as easy to learn and safe though failure and complication rates can be as high as 10% and 5%, respectively [44–47]. The advancement of ultrasound-guided techniques allows for the placement of local anesthetic with greater precision and reliability [48, 49]. Prior to LB, the duration of single-injection TPVB was generally limited to less than 24 h. Despite the correct needle tip position by ultrasound-guided techniques, catheter migration into the adjacent prevertebral, epidural, intercostal, and pleural space remains problematic (see Fig. 60.2) [50]. When

compared to percutaneous TPVB, catheters inserted surgically have generally been even less reliable though techniques are quite variable with some institutional success being greater than others [36].

The combination of ultrasound-guided techniques and LB has the potential to substantially improve the reliability, duration, and therefore the practicality of the TPVB in treating post-thoracotomy pain. While the potential for TPVB and LB seems promising, there is currently insufficient data to evaluate the efficacy, safety, and practicality of utilizing LB for TPVB in thoracic surgery. At least one study found that local wound infiltration with LB was similar if not superior to TPVB with conventional bupivacaine following reconstructive breast surgery [51]. With the advent of very long-acting anesthetics, the utility of the TPVB is uncertain. Further studies on post-thoracotomy patients are needed which directly compare the use of LB and TPVB versus other more peripheral regional techniques, such as intercostal nerve blocks, before conclusions can be drawn on the future role of TPVB in thoracic surgery.

Intercostal Nerve Block

Although epidural LB use has been described as apparently being safe in healthy volunteers, more specifically, other than two retrospective studies, LB's safety and efficacy have not been studied in thoracic surgical population. At our institution, posterior intercostal blocks with LB have replaced TEA as the preferred technique for postoperative analgesia in thoracic surgery, with patients reporting lower pain scores and using less opioids (Fig. 60.3).

Depending upon the surgical approach, a five-level posterior intercostal block is either done under direct visualization for open procedures or with thoracoscopic guidance for video-assisted thoracoscopic or robotic-assisted thoracoscopic procedures. Specifically, after the skin has been infiltrated with 1–2 ml of LB, a 12 mm camera thoracoscopy port is introduced at the appropriate site. Using a 22G spinal needle, the surgeon advances the needle over the superior edge of the rib approximately 5–7 cm lateral to the anatomic midline. Meticulous technique is used to advance the spinal needle to the innermost intercostal muscle without disrupting the parietal pleura. This is extremely important so that the local anesthetic remains confined to the intercostal space and is not lost to the pleural space. Typically this injection entails a 2 ml injection of LBs over the superior edges of ribs 6 through 10, but obviously the location of injection can be tailored toward other surgical sites [52]. The remaining volume of LB is injected at the remaining port sites or surgical wounds. Thoracoscopic visualization can significantly enhance the accurate injection into the intercostal space without interrupting the parietal space as local anesthetic can

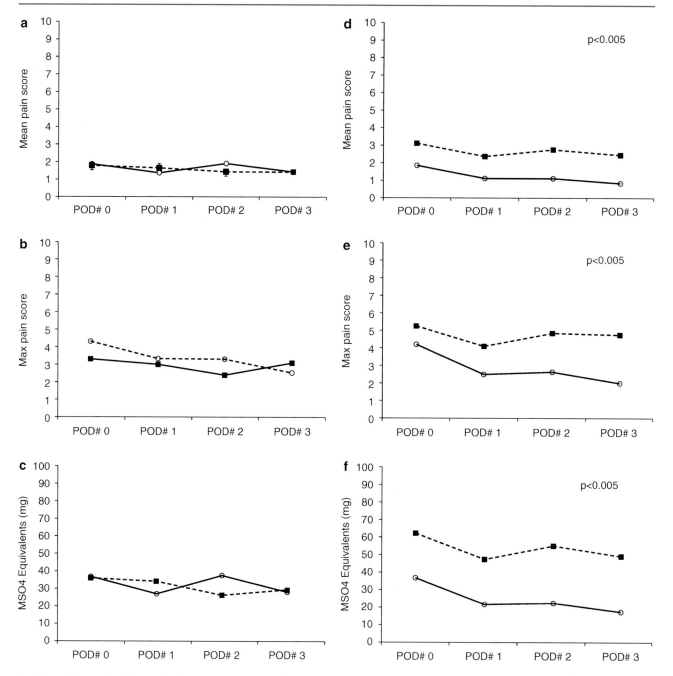

Fig. 60.4 Rice results. The results from one comparison of posterior intercostal block with LB vs. TEA with bupivacaine HCl. Pain scores and narcotic requirements for patients who received (A–C) LB or (D–F) thoracic epidural analgesia. The dashed lines indicate thoracotomy; the solid lines indicate minimally invasive surgery. Wilcoxon signed-rank test. (Max maximum, MSO4 morphine sulfate, POD postoperative day). (Reprinted from The Annals of Thoracic Surgery, D Rice, Copyright (2015), with permission from Elsevier. (Rice et al. [109]))

then egress out. Trainees can more easily appreciate the appropriate injection and demarcation of the intercostal space if 2 ml of methylene blue are added to the local injection solution (see Fig. 60.4).

With respect to the local anesthetic solution used for intercostal blocks, many institutions use 0.5% bupivacaine as local anesthetic, although some use 0.25% bupivacaine or 1% lidocaine [53–67]. The rate of infusion is generally 5–7 mL/h for an average-sized adult which typically helps establish five-level dermatomal analgesia to pinprick unilaterally.

Wanting to cover a larger surgical area, surgeons at our institution initially mixed LB with normal saline to create a larger volume to be injected into the surgical site; however, according to the updated prescribing information for LB, some of the surgeons now also utilize 0.25% bupivacaine combined with LB when performing intercostal blocks. According to the updated prescribing information, it is feasible to administer bupivacaine HCl with LB; however, this may impact the pharmacokinetic and/or physicochemical properties of LB, and this effect is concentration dependent [68]. Therefore, bupivacaine HCl and LB may be administered simultaneously in the same syringe, and bupivacaine HCl may be injected immediately prior to LB as long as the bioequivalent ratio of the dose of bupivacaine HCl solution to LB does not exceed 1:2. The typical 266 mg vial of LB may be coadministered with 150 mg of bupivacaine HCl. The toxic effects of these drugs are additive, and their administration should be used with caution including monitoring for neurologic and cardiovascular effects related to toxicity [68]. Although our institution like many other institutions mixes local anesthetics in clinical practice with the intent of getting faster onset and longer duration of local anesthetics, it should be kept in mind that mixing various local anesthetics at times can lead to variable onset, duration, and unpredictable potency. Likewise, mixing of different formulations of local anesthetics with their respective concentrations and volumes can increase the chances of drug error. Furthermore, despite having negative aspiration, usage of recommended dosage and avoidance of intravascular injections, no currently available method of monitoring can prevent local anesthetic toxicity; therefore, it is incumbent upon the anesthesia provider to be steadfastly vigilant and maintain preparation to treat systemic toxicities that may manifest unexpectedly.

Direct Interpleural Anesthesia

Although first described in 1984, interpleural blockade via the introduction of local anesthetic in between the parietal and visceral pleura has not gained widespread usage [69]. An epidural catheter is placed in the pleural space through a 16 Tuohy needle after the patient is placed in the lateral position with the operative side up. The site of insertion is in the eighth intercostal space approximately 8–10 cm from the posterior anatomic midline with the needle being introduced at 30–40° angle to the skin. The bevel of the Tuohy needle is faced upward as the needle is advanced over the rib and as the parietal pleura is entered. The plunger of the syringe may move passively inward due to the negative pressure in the pleural space during inspiration. A multi-orificed epidural catheter is then advanced 5–6 cm into the pleural space, and after negative aspiration, local anesthetic can then be injected.

Typically, bupivacaine is rebolused in intermittent boluses at either 4, 6, or 8 h; however, there are institutions which use a constant infusion of bupivacaine [56, 70–79].

The block's potential for several different types of complications has limited its use. For instance, the most common complication is that of a pneumothorax described in 2% of the patients [80]. Other complications described include pleural effusions, Horner's syndrome, infection, catheter displacement or rupture, and even toxic symptoms when the local anesthetic is absorbed systemically. More recently, phrenic nerve paralysis has been described as an additional complication [81]. Patient position, particularly when a patient is sitting upright, as well as site of lowest chest tube placement most likely influences the pooling of local anesthetic near the diaphragm. The decrease in forced vital capacity, especially if done bilaterally or in patients with compromised respiratory function, can further worsen respiratory status. This impairment in pulmonary function from diaphragmatic weakness is a plausible explanation for the significantly worse pulmonary function with interpleural analgesia when compared with paravertebral analgesia [56].

Serratus Plane (SAP) Block

Distal to the lateral cutaneous branches of the intercostal nerve, sensory divisions pass through the muscles of the chest. With ultrasound guidance, the practitioner can achieve analgesia of different regions of the chest by injecting local anesthetic between those muscle layers. Injection between pectoralis major and minor, the so-called Pecs I and II blocks, achieves somatic blockade of the anterior chest. Injection of anesthetic superficial to the serratus anterior muscle adjacent to the fourth and fifth intercostal spaces along the midaxillary line results in anesthesia of the lateral chest. The size of distribution is related to the volume of the injectate. With the injection of 20 ml, the area of sensory deficit covers from the scapula to the nipple, T4–T9. The initial study was small and simply demonstrated the application of the block and the subsequent sensory block and spread of local anesthetic by MRI [82]. The utility of the SAP block for thoracic surgery has yet to be determined. It has been noted that the SAP block likely doesn't cover the posterior primary rami, the anterior cutaneous branches of the intercostal nerve and afferents of the autonomic nervous systems [83, 84].

The SAP block may be best suited for procedures with anterolateral incisions such as anterior muscle-sparing thoracotomy or anterolateral thoracotomy, though these may need to be supplemented with local wound infiltration as the incision approaches the limits of sensory blockade. The block did not extend past the inferior angle of the scapula, so this block may not be appropriate for posterior muscle-sparing thoracotomy, as is common at our institution, or thoracoscopic surgery with more posterior incision sites. It may be useful as a rescue technique for patients with a failed thoracic epidural or those experiencing pain at the chest tube site. One such case has already been reported in a patient status post esophagectomy whose epidural had failed the pain was successfully treated by the SAP block with catheter-based infusion [85]. Little research to date has validated this technique for surgery in comparison with other approaches.

Local Surgical Site Infiltration

The rationale for wound infiltration with local anesthetics is to target the most proximal and selective site responsible for the perception of pain, the peripheral nociceptors. With direct infiltration into the surgical site, the local anesthetic can simply and effectively provide analgesia for a variety of surgical procedures. Furthermore, infiltration in this manner is usually not associated with severe side effects such as local toxicity, wound infection, and impaired wound healing [86, 87]. Long-acting amide local anesthetics such as bupivacaine and ropivacaine have been shown to provide superior pain control over opioids and are commonly used in the postoperative period for infiltrative, regional, and neuraxial blocks [88–90]. Until recently, the duration of analgesia with infiltration into the surgical site in single doses was limited by the specific local anesthetic used. As mentioned earlier, LB diffuses within tissue less than conventional local anesthetics. A dose can be diluted to make large volumes that can then be injected using a deep infiltration technique. At our institution, some surgeons have found increased success by injecting LB invanvoverlapping, crosshatch fashion as a means to avoid patchy block (Table 60.3).

Table 60.3 Administration of liposomal bupivacaine (LB)

Original preparation	13.3% LB in 20 cc vial
Maximum dose of LB	266 mg
Maximum dilution	Up to 1:14 ratio with normal saline (NS), down to concentration of 0.89% OR 20 cc LB diluted with 280 cc NS for total volume of 300 cc
Coadministration with bupivacaine HCl	May be mixed with bupivacaine HCl only; for above dilution, up to 150 mg (60 cc of 0.25% bupivacaine HCl) may be substituted for NS
[a]Examples of preparations used for thoracic surgery at MD Anderson Cancer Center	20 cc undiluted LB given at the time of incision for intercostal blocks or diluted with 30 cc 0.25% bupivacaine HCl to cover additional sites
[a]Examples of preparations used for larger surgical site infiltrations at MD Anderson Cancer Center	20 cc LB with 30 cc of 0.25% bupivacaine HCl and 50 cc of N or 20 cc LB with 60 cc of 0.25%

[a]At our institution, practice patterns vary widely based on surgical service, individual provider, and procedure

Phrenic Nerve Block and Other Blocks Targeting Ipsilateral Shoulder Pain (ISP)

The significance of post-thoracotomy ipsilateral shoulder pain (ISP) differs from incisional thoracotomy pain in quality, location, etiology, and treatment. It is a common occurrence, affecting up to 85% of patients following thoracic surgery [91, 92]. The pain can be severe despite the well-functioning TEA. The exact distribution of pain is variable but lies within the C4–C5 dermatomes, sharing a common innervation with the phrenic nerve. The duration of pain typically lasts for hours but can persist for days or longer, with some patients experiencing chronic pain more than 6 months after surgery [93, 94].

Etiology

ISP is correlated with the extent of pleural disruption, size of thoracotomy incision, transection of major bronchial airways, patient BMI, and length of surgery [95, 96]. Currently, no pharmacological or regional treatment exists which can completely eradicate or prevent the pain. ISP is considered a type of pain that is usually referred from the afferents of the phrenic nerve. Originating from the third, fourth, and fifth cervical nerve roots, the phrenic nerve contains sensory, motor, and sympathetic fibers. It provides the only afferents to the diaphragm and afferents for the pleura and pericardium of the thorax as well as the diaphragmatic peritoneum. ISP is most commonly thought to be the result of phrenic nerve impulses brought on by intraoperative pleural irritation by intrathoracic dissection, bronchial transection, and chest tube placement.

The precise etiology of post-thoracotomy ISP remains debatable. While targeted phrenic blockades are usually effective, they are not universally effective at eliminating ISP for all patients. A series of case reports concluded that there may be a dual etiology of ISP wherein some patients' pain is caused by phrenic nerve afferents, while other patients' ISP is from direct shoulder ligament strain [95]. In one study, suprascapular block performed postoperatively had no effect on patient's pain [97]. When compared directly to peri-phrenic diaphragmatic fat pad infiltration, suprascapular nerve block was significantly less effective at preventing ISP [93]. This suggests that ISP is not related to the strain of the acromioclavicular or glenohumeral joints for most patients unless localizing signs of musculoskeletal shoulder pain are present [95, 98].

Though representing a minority of patients with ISP, patients presenting with pain localized to the shoulder, elicited with palpation or movement, benefited from suprascapular nerve block 85% of the time [98]. Unlike the interscalene nerve, the suprascapular is not adjacent to the phrenic and therefore is not associated with concomitant phrenic blockade and diaphragmatic palsy.

Treatment

NSAIDs such as intravenous diclofenac or ketorolac can be effective in reducing ISP, but they are not universally effective and should be used with caution in certain patient populations such as those with chronic renal insufficiency [99]. Neither standard TEA nor intrapleural infusion is typically effective at preventing ISP; however, lower rates have been associated with epidural catheter placement above T5 [100, 101]. Higher thoracic catheters may provide enough local anesthetic spread for a sensory blockade of phrenic nerve afferents. The resultant hypotension and decreased pulmonary function from higher epidural blocks may limit this approach in patients with low cardiopulmonary reserve.

Scawn, Pennefather, and colleagues demonstrated that injection of lidocaine into the diaphragmatic periphrenic fat pad at the end of surgery reduced the incidence of ISP for up to 2 h [91]. The injection of ropivacaine 0.2% provided a relatively selective sensory blockade which significantly reduced the incidence (32% vs. 64%) and delayed the median onset (36 vs. 16 h) of ISP with no difference in postoperative arterial blood gases [102]. It has been suggested that targeting of the phrenic nerve at alternative locations, such as the periphrenic fat pad around the hilum, may affect the efficacy of the block, but such variations have not been validated and require further study [103].

Others have shown that post-thoracotomy ISP can be significantly reduced by interscalene nerve blockade. Barak et al. employed an interscalene block with bupivacaine to reduce ISP though the effect was limited to less than 24 h [104]. The exact mechanism of pain relief from interscalene block is unclear because of the high incidence of simultaneous phrenic nerve blockade despite the use of relatively low volumes of local anesthetic and ultrasound guidance [105]. The same is true for supraclavicular nerve block which also has a high rate of simultaneous phrenic nerve involvement. The use of an ultrasound-guided supraclavicular approach to perform a targeted phrenic nerve block with ropivacaine had a 65% relative rate reduction of ISP in patients undergoing lobectomy or pneumonectomy [106]. A phrenic nerve catheter was placed, but the ISP was most severe on the day of surgery. There was no difference in rescue analgesics used on postoperative day 1. By specifically targeting the phrenic nerve for blockade, the block may more effectively reduce ISP without as much of the associated upper extremity motor weakness.

Phrenic nerve blockade is not without risks. Hemidiaphragm phrenic nerve palsy results in a decrease in vital capacity, forced expiratory volume per second, and maximum inspiratory flow [105]. These effects are well tolerated even for those with preexisting pulmonary disease but may cause respiratory distress in patients with contralateral diaphragm dysfunction. Long-acting local anesthetics such as LB should therefore be used with caution in this patient population. The use of catheter-based ropivacaine, or the development of liposomal ropivacaine, may have the advantage of more selective sensory blockade and therefore less phrenic nerve palsy.

Many of these studies utilized the relatively short-acting lidocaine, and no studies to date have evaluated agents with a duration of action exceeding 24 h. The use of short-acting agents has potentially limited the benefits of decreased ISP. The duration of ISP is variable however, and the use of long-acting agents may not be beneficial for many patients. Further prospective studies are needed to directly compare the safety and efficacy of the aforementioned techniques and to determine whether long-acting modalities such as catheter-based infusions or liposomal amide anesthetics are beneficial. Until then, practitioners should use their clinical judgment to devise a treatment strategy for ISP that is most appropriate for their patient population.

Conclusion

In summation, it is well recognized that optimal pain management for thoracic surgery remains challenging given the multiple mechanisms that contribute to postoperative pain. Combining minimally invasive surgery with multimodal, multidisciplinary regional and pharmacological approaches to analgesia can mitigate pain and suffering by acting at various levels of the nervous system. This holistic and comprehensive pain management strategy can improve overall patient safety and satisfaction by providing a higher level of postoperative analgesia while reducing the undesired side effects of narcotic usage, such as nausea, vomiting, constipation, and respiratory depression. Furthermore, improving postoperative pain control can impact hospital stay, reduce the rates of postsurgical complications and readmissions, prevent opioid dependence, and, potentially, reduce mortality [107]. At our institution, we have successfully incorporated long-acting local anesthetics into surgery-specific, evidence-based treatment protocols which utilize multimodal analgesia such as nonsteroidal anti-inflammatory drugs, N-methyl-D-aspartate (NMDA) antagonists, and peripheral nerve blocks. Although novel long-acting local anesthetic such as LB has created excitement among providers and may represent a significant advancement in the evolution of local anesthesia, it should be remembered that they are not a panacea but rather a component of a comprehensive pain strategy. Moreover, given the limited number of case reports and studies available specifically in the thoracic surgery population, further studies are warranted to better understand not only the efficacy but also the long-term safety profile of long-acting local anesthetics such as LB.

Case Discussion

A 75-year-old female is scheduled for a right VATS requiring multiple wedges due to metastatic colon cancer. Past medical history is significant for obesity (BMI 47 kg/m^2), hypertension, stable coronary artery disease which is medically managed, and obstructive sleep apnea for which patient uses CPAP nightly. Patient stopped smoking 2 weeks ago but has a 100 pack-year smoking history. The patient received tramadol XR 300 mg PO and celecoxib 200 mg PO as part of her ERAS preemptive regimen. Pregabalin was held to avoid postoperative sedation given her history of sleep apnea. Additionally, the surgeon performed a deep tissue injection at the incision sites using a total of 40 cc of a solution made of 20 ml of 1.3% LB mixed with 20 ml of 0.9% sterile normal saline. During the course of the surgery, vigorous surgical bleeding required conversion to open thoracotomy incision. As the surgery is concluding, patient is administered 1 mg of hydromorphone for tachypnea. The patient wakes up in extreme pain from the thoracotomy incision site.

1. How could the risk of insufficient local anesthetic coverage been decreased in this case?
   (a) The LB should be diluted in order to achieve an adequate volume to cover the planned surgical sites along with the most common contingencies. A maximum ratio of 14:1 normal saline to LB can be used to achieve a volume of 300 ml though typical amounts are in the range of 40–80 ml. As mentioned previously, bupivacaine HCl is the only local anesthetic not contraindicated in patients receiving LB. The bupivacaine HCl to LB ratio should not exceed 1:2 which corresponds with a maximum dose of 150 mg bupivacaine HCl for 266 mg LB. Best practice would be to administer a portion of the diluted LB around the time of incision to manage intraoperative pain (within 4 hrs after preparation in a syringe) and to inject the remainder of the solution upon surgical closure.
2. What additional medications can be utilized in combination with LB?
   (a) Other analgesics such as intravenous acetaminophen, dexmedetomidine, ketamine, ketorolac, and narcotics are safe to administer following LB administration. At our institution, ketorolac is routinely given to our thoracic surgery patients during skin closure provided patient does not have contraindications such as compromised renal function and high risk for postoperative bleeding. Other local anesthetics such as lidocaine are absolutely contraindicated in a patient who has received liposomal bupivacaine.
3. Are there any additional regional blocks which can be used in the setting of LB usage?

   (a) At our institution, we do not administer any local anesthetics, including bupivacaine HCl, for several days following the use of LB. That said, it may be safe to administer an appropriately low dose of bupivacaine HCl by TEA, TPVB, or intercostal block in the case of a failed LB surgical site injection. There is insufficient evidence to date on the use of regular bupivacaine HCl to supplement missed pain areas in the setting of the recent administration of LB. Though risk of bupivacaine toxicity from a slow-release LB is probably low, it is difficult to know how high free bupivacaine concentrations may rise in the setting of intravascular injection or in combination with bupivacaine HCl administered by other regional techniques. The risk benefit analysis has to be considered by the providing anesthesiologist for the given patient and situation.
4. What if the surgeon initially administered LB by five-level posterior intercostal nerve block? The thoracotomy incision and chest tube site are well covered by the block, and the patient has minimal pain upon emergence. The patient is taken to the PACU, and the blood pressure is noted to be 85/55 mmHg with a heart rate of 55 bpm.
   (a) Depending on the site of injection and volume of injectate, significant spread of local anesthetic can occur from the intercostal space to the TPVS and epidural space. Consequently, relative hypotension and bradycardia can occur in the setting of posterior intercostal blockade with LB. At our institution, this presentation is most common following esophagectomy when the posterior intercostal blocks are performed within a few centimeters of the TPVS. Correctable causes of hypotension such as relative hypovolemia and cardiac dysfunction should be ruled out. If the patient is comfortable without signs or symptoms of cardiac or respiratory distress, a colloid is usually given as the blood pressure often will have some response to volume expansion even in the setting of minimal blood loss. With continued monitoring and expectant management, the relative hypotension usually resolves within the first 6-24 h following surgery.

References

1. Siegel R, DeSantis C, Virgo K, Stein K, Mariotto A, Smith T, et al. Cancer treatment and survivorship statistics, 2012. CA Cancer J Clin. 2012;62(4):220–41.
2. Richardson J, Sabanathan S, Shah R. Post-thoracotomy spirometric lung function: the effect of analgesia. A review. J Cardiovasc Surg. 1999;40:445–56.
3. Ballantyne JC, Carr DB, de Ferranti S, Suarez T, Lau J, Chalmers TC, et al. The comparative effects of postoperative analgesic therapies on pulmonary outcome: cumulative meta-analyses of randomized, controlled trials. Anesth Analg. 1998;86:598–612.

4. Bayman EO, Parekh KR, Keech J, Selte A, Brennan TJ. A prospective study of chronic pain after thoracic surgery. Anesthesiol. 2017;126:938–51.

5. Apfelbaum JL, Chen C, Mehta SS, Gan TJ. Postoperative pain experience: results from a national survey suggest postoperative pain continues to be undermanaged. Anesth Analg. 2003;97(2): 534–40.

6. Butterworth J, Mackey D, Wasnick J. Morgan & Mikhail's Clinical anesthesiology. 5th ed. New York [etc.]: McGraw-Hill Education/Medical; 2013.

7. Biondich AS, Joslin JD. Coca: high altitude remedy of the ancient Incas. Wilderness Environ Med. 2015;26(4):567–71.

8. Calatayud J, González A. History of the development and evolution of local anesthesia since the coca leaf. Anesthesiol. 2003;98(6):1503–8.

9. Link WJ. Alfred Einhorn, Sc. D: inventor of novocaine. Dent Radiog Photog. 1959;32(1):20.

10. Guptill AE. Novocain as a skin irritant. Dent Cosmos. 1920;62:1460–1.

11. Löfgren N, Lundquist B. Studies on local anaesthetics: II. Svenks Kem Tidskr. 1946;58:206–17.

12. Ruetsch Y, Bönibc T, Borgeatac A. From cocaine to ropivacaine: the history of local anesthetic drugs. Curr Top Med Chem. 2001;1(3):175–82.

13. Weinberg GL, VadeBoncouer T, Ramaraju GA, Garcia-Amaro MF, Cwik MJ. Pretreatment or resuscitation with a lipid infusion shifts the dose-response to bupivacaine-induced asystole in rats. Anesthesiol. 1998;88(4):1071–5.

14. Weinberg G, Ripper R, Feinstein DL, Hoffman W. Lipid emulsion infusion rescues dogs from bupivacaine-induced cardiac toxicity. Reg Anesth Pain Med. 2003;28(3):198–202.

15. Rosenblatt M, Abel M, Fischer G, Itzkovich C, Eisenkraft J. Successful use of a 20% lipid emulsion to resuscitate a patient after a presumed bupivacaine-related cardiac arrest. Anesthesiology. 2006;105(1):217–8.

16. Litz R, Popp M, Stehr S, Koch T. Successful resuscitation of a patient with ropivacaine-induced asystole after axillary plexus block using lipid infusion. Anaesthesia. 2006;61(8):800–1.

17. Klein SM, Greengrass RA, Steele SM, D'Ercole FJ, Speer KP, Gleason DH, et al. A comparison of 0.5% bupivacaine, 0.5% Ropivacaine, and 0.75% Ropivacaine for interscalene brachial plexus block. Anesth Analg. 1998;87(6):1316–9.

18. Angst MS, Drover DR. Pharmacology of drugs formulated with DepoFoam®: a sustained release drug delivery system for parenteral administration using multivesicular liposome technology. Clin Pharmacokinet. 2006;45(12):1153–76.

19. Lambert WJ, Los K. In: Rathbone MJ, et al., editors. Modified-release drug delivery technology. Volume 2. 2nd ed. New York: Informa Healthcare; 2008. p. 207–14.

20. Bergese S, Onel E, Portillo J. Evaluation of DepoFoam® bupivacaine for the treatment of postsurgical pain. Pain Manag. 2011;1(6):539–47.

21. Chahar P, Cummings KC III. Liposomal bupivacaine: a review of a new bupivacaine formulation. J Pain Res. 2012;5:257–64.

22. Bramlett K, Onel E, Viscusi E, Jones K. A randomized, double-blind, dose-ranging study comparing wound infiltration of DepoFoam® bupivacaine, an extended-release liposomal bupivacaine, to bupivacaine HCl for postsurgical analgesia in total knee arthroplasty. Knee. 2012;19(5):530–6.

23. Golf M, Daniels S, Onel E. A phase 3, randomized, placebo-controlled trial of DepoFoam®® bupivacaine (extended-release bupivacaine local analgesic) in bunionectomy. Adv Ther. 2011;28(9):776.

24. Gorfine S, Onel E, Patou G, Krivokapic Z. Bupivacaine extended-release liposome injection for prolonged postsurgical analgesia in patients undergoing hemorrhoidectomy: a multicenter, randomized, double-blind, placebo-controlled trial. Dis Colon Rectum. 2011;54(12):1552–9.

25. Naseem A, Harada T, Wang D, Arezina R, Lorch U, Onel E, et al. Bupivacaine extended release liposome injection does not prolong QTc interval in a thorough QT/QTc study in healthy volunteers. J Clin Pharmacol. 2012;52(9):1441–7.

26. Portillo J, Kamar N, Melibary S, Quevedo E, Bergese S. Safety of liposome extended-release bupivacaine for postoperative pain control. Front Pharmacol. 2014;5:90.

27. Hamilton TW, Athanassoglou V, Mellon S, Strickland LH, Trivella M, Murray D, Pandit HG. Liposomal bupivacaine infiltration at the surgical site for the management of postoperative pain. Cochrane Database Syst Rev. 2017;2:CD011419.

28. Rodgers A, Walker N, Schug S, McKee A, Kehlet H, van Zundert A, et al. Reduction of postoperative mortality and morbidity with epidural or spinal anaesthesia: results from overview of randomised trials. BMJ. 2000;321(7275):1493.

29. Rigg J, Jamrozik K, Myles P, Silbert B, Peyton P, Parsons R, et al. Epidural anaesthesia and analgesia and outcome of major surgery: a randomised trial. Lancet. 2002;359(9314):1276–82.

30. Leslie K, Myles P, Devereaux P, Williamson E, Rao-Melancini P, Forbes A, et al. Neuraxial block, death and serious cardiovascular morbidity in the POISE trial. Br J Anaesth. 2013;111(3):382–90.

31. de Leon-Casasola OA, Parker B, Lema MJ, Harrison P, Massey J. Postoperative epidural bupivacaine-morphine therapy experience with 4,227 surgical cancer patients. Anesthesiology. 1994;81(2):368–75.

32. Ready LB. Acute pain: lessons learned from 25,000 patients. Reg Anesth Pain Med. 1999;24(6):499–505.

33. Practice guidelines for acute pain management in the perioperative setting: an updated report by the American Society of Anesthesiologists Task Force on Acute Pain Management. Anesthesiol. 2012;116:248–73.

34. Goravanchi F, Kee SS, Kowalski AM, Berger JS, French KE. A case series of thoracic paravertebral blocks using a combination of ropivacaine, clonidine, epinephrine, and dexamethasone. J Clin Anesth. 2012;24(8):664–7.

35. Allen M, Halgren L, Nichols F, Cassivi S, Harmsen W, Wigle D, et al. A randomized controlled trial of bupivacaine through Intracostal catheters for pain management after thoracotomy. Ann Thorac Surg. 2009;88(3):903–10.

36. Helms O, Mariano J, Hentz J, Santelmo N, Falcoz P, Massard G, et al. Intra-operative paravertebral block for postoperative analgesia in thoracotomy patients: a randomized, double-blind, placebo-controlled study. Eur J Cardiothorac Surg. 2011;40:902–6.

37. Gebhardt R, Mehran RJ, Soliz J, Cata JP, Smallwood AK, Feeley TW. Epidural versus ON-Q local anesthetic infiltrating catheter for post-thoracotomy pain control. J Cardiothorac Vasc Anesth. 2013;27:423–6.

38. Detterbeck FC. Efficacy of methods of intercostal nerve blockade for pain relief after thoracotomy. Ann Thorac Surg. 2005;80:1550–9.

39. Eason MJ, Wyatt R. Paravertebral thoracic block-a reappraisal. Anaesthesia. 1979;34:638–42.

40. Yeung JH, Gates S, Naidu BV, Wilson MJ, Gao SF. Paravertebral block versus thoracic epidural for patients undergoing thoracotomy. Cochrane Database Syst Rev. 2016;2:CD009121.

41. Baidya DK, Khanna P, Maitra S. Analgesic efficacy and safety of thoracic paravertebral and epidural analgesia for thoracic surgery: a systematic review and meta-analysis. Interact Cardiovasc Thorac Surg. 2014;18(5):626–35.

42. Scarci M, Joshi A, Attia R. In patients undergoing thoracic surgery is paravertebral block as effective as epidural analgesia for pain management? Interact Cardiovasc Thorac Surg. 2010;10(1):92–6.

43. Matyal R, Montealegre-Gallegos M, Shnider M, Owais K, Sakamuri S, Shakil O, et al. Preemptive ultrasound-guided paravertebral block and immediate postoperative lung function. Gen Thorac Cardiovasc Surg. 2015;63(1):43–8.

44. Karmaker MK. Thoracic paravertebral block. Anesthesiol. 2001;95:771–80.

45. Richardson J, Vowden P, Sabanathan S. Bilateral paravertebral analgesia for major abdominal vascular surgery: a preliminary report. Anaesthesia. 1995;50:995–8.

46. Coveney E, Weltz CR, Greengrass R, Iglehart JD, Leight GS, Steele SM, et al. Use of paravertebral block anesthesia in the surgical management of breast cancer: experience in 156 cases. Ann Surg. 1998;227:496–501.

47. Lönnqvist PA, MacKenzie J, Soni AK, Conacher ID. Paravertebral blockade. Failure rate and complications. Anaesthesia. 1995;50(9):813–5.

48. Krediet AC, Moayeri N, van Geffen GJ, Bruhn J, Renes S, Bigeleisen PE, et al. Different approaches to ultrasound-guided thoracic paravertebral block: an illustrated review. Anesthesiol. 2015;123(2):459–74.

49. Denny NM. Editorial I: location, location, location! Ultrasound imaging in regional anaesthesia. Br J Anaesth. 2005;94(1):1–3.

50. Luyet C, Meyer C, Herrmann G, Hatch GM, Ross S, Eichenberger U. Placement of coiled catheters into the paravertebral space. Anaesthesia. 2012;67(3):250–5.

51. Abdelsattar JM, Boughey JC, Fahy AS, Jakub JW, Farley DR, Hieken TJ, et al. Comparative study of liposomal bupivacaine versus paravertebral block for pain control following mastectomy with immediate tissue expander reconstruction. Ann Surg Oncol. 2016;23(2):465–70.

52. Nunn JF, Slavin G. Posterior intercostal nerve block for pain relief after cholecystectomy. Anatomical basis and efficacy. Br J Anaesth. 1980;52:253–60.

53. Bilgin M, Akcali Y, Oguzkaya F. Extrapleural regional versus systemic analgesia for relieving post thoracotomy pain: a clinical study of bupivacaine compared with metamizol. J Thorac Cardiovasc Surg. 2003;126:1580–3.

54. Watson DS, Panian S, Kendall V, Maher DP, Peters G. Pain control after thoracotomy: bupivacaine versus lidocaine in continuous extrapleural intercostal nerve blockade. Ann Thorac Surg. 1999;67:825–9.

55. Sabanathan S, Smith PJ, Pradhan GN, Hashimi H, Eng JB, Mearns AJ. Continuous intercostal nerveblock for pain relief after thoracotomy. Ann Thorac Surg. 1988;46:425–6.

56. Richardson J, Sabanathan S, Mearns AJ, Shah RD, Goulden C. A prospective, randomized comparison of interpleural and paravertebral analgesia in thoracic surgery. Br J Anaesth. 1995;75:405–8.

57. Mozell EJ, Sabanathan S, Mearns AJ, Bickford-Smith PJ, Majid MR, Zografos G. Continuous extrapleural intercostal nerve block after pleurectomy. Thorax. 1991;46:21–4.

58. Kaiser AM, Zollinger A, De Lorenzi D, Largiader F, Weder W. Prospective, randomized comparison of extrapleural versus epidural analgesia for post thoracotomy pain. Ann Thorac Surg. 1998;66:367–72.

59. Deneuville M, Bisserier A, Regnard JF, Chevalier M, Levasseur P, Herve P. Continuous intercostal analgesia with 0.5% bupivacaine after thoracotomy: a randomized study. Ann Thorac Surg. 1993;55:381–5.

60. Richardson J, Sabanathan S, Jones J, Shah RD, Cheema S, Mearns AJ. A prospective, randomized comparison of preoperative and continuous balanced epidural or paravertebral bupivacaine on post-thoracotomy pain, pulmonary function and stress responses. Br J Anaesth. 1999;83:387–92.

61. Barron DJ, Tolan MJ, Lea RE. A randomized controlled trial of continuous extra-pleural analgesia post-thoracotomy: efficacy and choice of local anaesthetic. Eur J Anaesthesiol. 1999;16:236–45.

62. Majid AA, Hamzah H. Pain control after thoracotomy: an extrapleural tunnel to provide a continuous bupivacaine infusion for intercostal nerve blockade. Chest. 1992;101:981–4.

63. Perttunen K, Nilsson E, Heinonen J, Hirvisalo EL, Salo JA, Kalso E. Extradural, paravertebral and intercostal nerve blocks for post-thoracotomy pain. Br J Anaesth. 1995;75:541–7.

64. Richardson J, Sabanathan S, Eng J, et al. Continuous intercostal nerve block versus epidural morphine for post thoracotomy analgesia. Ann Thorac Surg. 1993;55:377–80.

65. Debreceni G, Molnar Z, Szelig L, Molnar TF. Continuous epidural or intercostal analgesia following thoracotomy: a prospective randomized double-blind clinical trial. Acta Anaesthesiol Scand. 2003;47:1091–5.

66. Matthews PJ, Govenden V. Comparison of continuous paravertebral and extradural infusions of bupivacaine for pain relief after thoracotomy. Br J Anaesth. 1989;62:204–5.

67. Sullivan E, Grannis FW Jr, Ferrell B, Dunst M. Continuous extrapleural intercostal nerve block with continuous infusion of lidocaine after thoracotomy: a descriptive pilot study. Chest. 1995;108:1718–23.

68. [Internet]. 2017 [cited 31 May 2017]. Available from: https://www.exparel.com/hcp/pdf/EXPAREL_Prescribing_Information.pdf.

69. Kvalheim L, Reiestad F. Interpleural catheter in the management of postoperative pain. Anesthesiol. 1984;61:A231.

70. Mann LJ, Young GR, Williams JK, Dent OF, McCaughan BC. Intrapleural bupivacaine in the control of post thoracotomy pain. Ann Thorac Surg. 1992;53:449–54.

71. Scheinin B, Lindgren L, Rosenberg PH. Treatment of post thoracotomy pain with intermittent instillations of intrapleural bupivacaine. Acta Anaesthesiol Scand. 1989;33:156–9.

72. Schneider RF, Villamena PC, Harvey J, Surick BG, Surick IW, Beattie EJ. Lack of efficacy of intrapleural bupivacaine for postoperative analgesia following thoracotomy. Chest. 1993;103:414–6.

73. Francois T, Blanloeil Y, Pillet F, Moren J, Mazoit X, Geay G, et al. Effect of interpleural administration of bupivacaine or lidocaine on pain and morphine requirement after esophagectomy with thoracotomy: a randomized, double-blind and controlled study. Anesth Analg. 1995;80:718–23.

74. Ferrante FM, Chan VW, Arthur GR, Rocco AG. Interpleural analgesia after thoracotomy. Anesth Analg. 1991;72:105–9.

75. Silomon M, Claus T, Huwer H, Biedler A, Larsen R, Molter G. Interpleural analgesia does not influence post thoracotomy pain. Anesth Analg. 2000;91:44–50.

76. Miguel R, Hubbell D. Pain management and spirometry following thoracotomy: a prospective, randomized study of four techniques. J Cardiothorac Vasc Anesth. 1993;7:529–34.

77. Symreng T, Gomez MN, Rossi N. Intrapleural bupivacaine v saline after thoracotomy: effects on pain and lung function—a double-blind study. J Cardiothorac Anesth. 1989;3:144–9.

78. Tartiere J, Samba D, Lefrancois C, et al. Intrapleural bupivacaine analgesia after thoraco-abdominal incision for oesophagectomy. Eur J Anaesthesiol. 1991;8:145–9.

79. Brockmeier V, Moen H, Karlsson BR, Fjeld NB, Reiestad F, Steen PA. Interpleural or thoracic epidural analgesia for pain after thoracotomy. A double blind study. Acta Anaesthesiol Scand. 1993;38:317–21.

80. Strømskag KE, Minor B, Steen PA. Side effects and complications related to interpleural analgesia: an update. Acta Anaesthesiol Scand. 1990;34:473–7.

81. Lander GR. Interpleural analgesia and phrenic nerve paralysis. Anaesthesia. 1993;48:315–6.

82. Blanco R, Parras T, McDonnell JG, Prats-Galino A. Serratus plane block: a novel ultrasound-guided thoracic wall nerve block. Anaesthesia. 2013;68(11):1107–13.

83. Tighe SQ, Karmakar MK. Serratus plane block: do we need to learn another technique for thoracic wall blockade? Anaesthesia. 2013;68(11):1103–6.

84. Conacher ID. Pain relief after thoracotomy. Br J Anaesth. 1990;65:806–12.

85. Madabushi R, Tewari S, Gautam SK, Agarwal A, Agarwal A. Serratus anterior plane block: a new analgesic technique for post-thoracotomy pain. Pain Physician. 2015;18(3):E421–4.

86. Scott NB. Wound infiltration for surgery. Anaesthesia. 2010;65:67–75.

87. Gupta A. Wound infiltration with local anaesthetics in ambulatory surgery. Curr Opin Anesthesiol. 2010;23(6):708–13.

88. Ersayli DT, Gurbet A, Bekar A, Uckunkaya N, Bilgin H. Effects of perioperatively administered bupivacaine and bupivacaine-methylprednisolone on pain after lumbar discectomy. Spine. 2006;31(19):2221–6.

89. Kuthiala G, Chaudhary G. Ropivacaine: a review of its pharmacology and clinical use. Indian J Anaesth. 2011;55(2):104–10.

90. Sakai N, Inoue T, Kunugiza Y, Tomita T, Mashimo T. Continuous femoral versus epidural block for attainment of 120° knee flexion after total knee arthroplasty: a randomized controlled trial. J Arthroplasty. 2013;28(5):807–14.

91. Scawn NDA, Pennefather SH, Soorae A, Wang JYY, Russell GN. Ipsilateral shoulder pain after thoracotomy with epidural analgesia: the influence of phrenic nerve infiltration with lidocaine. Anesth Analg. 2001;93(2):260–4.

92. Yousefshahi F, Predescu O, Colizza M, Asenjo JF. Postthoracotomy ipsilateral shoulder pain: a literature review on characteristics and treatment. Pain Res Manag. 2016;2016:3652726.

93. Martinez-Barenys C, Busquets J, de Castro PE, Garcia-Guasch R, Perez J, Fernandez E, et al. Randomized double-blind comparison of phrenic nerve infiltration and suprascapular nerve block for ipsilateral shoulder pain after thoracic surgery. Eur J Cardiothorac Surg. 2011;40(1):106–12.

94. Stammberger U, Steinacher C, Hillinger S, Schmid RA, Kinsbergen T, Weder W. Early and long-term complaints following video-assisted thoracoscopic surgery: evaluation in 173 patients. Eur J Cardiothorac Surg. 2000;18:7–11.

95. Bamgbade OA, Dorje P, Adhikary GS. The dual etiology of ipsilateral shoulder pain after thoracic surgery. J Clin Anesth. 2007;19(4):296–8.

96. Bunchungmongkol N, Pipanmekaporn T, Paiboonworachat S, Saeteng S, Tantraworasin A. Incidence and risk factors associated with ipsilateral shoulder pain after thoracic surgery. J Cardiothorac Vasc Anesth. 2014;28(4):991–4.

97. Tan N, Agnew NM, Scawn ND, Pennefather SH, Chester M, Russell GN. Suprascapular nerve block for ipsilateral shoulder pain after thoracotomy with thoracic epidural analgesia: a double-blind comparison of 0.5% bupivacaine and 0.9% saline. Anesth Analg. 2002;94(1):199–202.

98. Saha S, Brish EL, Lowry AM, Boddu K. In select patients, ipsilateral post-thoracotomy shoulder pain relieved by suprascapular nerve block. Am J Ther. 2011;18(4):309–12.

99. Burgess FW, Anderson DM, Colonna D, Sborov MJ, Cavanaugh DG. Ipsilateral shoulder pain following thoracic surgery. Anesthesiol. 1993;78:365–8.

100. Pennefather SH, Akrofi ME, Kendall JB, Russell GN, Scawn NDA. Double-blind comparison of intrapleural saline and 0.25% bupivacaine for ipsilateral shoulder pain after thoracotomy in patients receiving thoracic epidural analgesia. Br J Anaesth. 2005;94(2):234–8.

101. Misiołek H, Karpe J, Copik M, Marcinkowski A, Jastrzębska A, Szelka A, et al. Ipsilateral shoulder pain after thoracic surgery procedures under general and regional anesthesia - a retrospective observational study. Kardiochir Torakochirurgia Pol. 2014;11(1):44–7.

102. Danelli G, Berti M, Casati A, Bobbio A, Ghisi D, Mele R, et al. Ipsilateral shoulder pain after thoracotomy surgery: a prospective, randomized, double-blind, placebo-controlled evaluation of the efficacy of infiltrating the phrenic nerve with 0.2% wt/vol ropivacaine. Eur J Anaesthesiol. 2007;24(7):596–601.

103. Rychlik IJ, Burnside N, McManus K. The phrenic nerve infiltration for ipsilateral shoulder pain. Eur J Cardiothorac Surg. 2012;41(3):716.

104. Barak M, Iaroshevski D, Poppa E, Ben-Nun A, Katz Y. Low-volume interscalene brachial plexus block for post-thoracotomy shoulder pain. J Cardiothorac Vasc Anesth. 2007;21(4):554–7.

105. Bergmann L, Martini S, Kesselmeier M, Armbruster W, Notheisen T, Adamzik M, et al. Phrenic nerve block caused by interscalene brachial plexus block: breathing effects of different sites of injection. BMC Anesthesiol. 2015;16:45.

106. Blichfeldt-Eckhardt MR, Laursen CB, Berg H, Holm JH, Hansen LN, Ørding H, et al. A randomised, controlled, double-blind trial of ultrasound-guided phrenic nerve block to prevent shoulder pain after thoracic surgery. Anaesthesia. 2016;71(12):1441–8.

107. White PF, Kehlet H. Improving postoperative pain management: what are the unresolved issues? Anesthesiol. 2010;112:220–5.

108. Dravid RM, Paul RE. Interpleural block – Part 1. Anaesthesia. 2007;62(10):1039–49.

109. Rice DC, Cata JP, Mena GE, Rodriguez-Restrepo A, Correa AM, Mehran RJ. Posterior intercostal nerve block with LB: an alternative to thoracic epidural analgesia. Ann Thorac Surg. 2015;99(6):1953–60.

Chronic Post-thoracotomy Pain

Peter MacDougall

Introduction

Entry to the human chest cavity has long been fraught with challenges for the anesthesiologist, the surgeon, and the patient. As we know, from the discussions in this text, these challenges include a multitude of physiologic perturbations before, during, and after the surgery. In addition to the overt physiologic changes, chronic pain may present an ongoing challenge for the patient. In this chapter we will review the complex phenomenon of chronic post – thoracotomy pain (CPTP), its incidence and prevalence, causes as we know them, prevention and treatment and what the future may hold.

As we will see, there has really been a perfect storm that has led us to this point. It can be traced back more than 70 years to the end of the Second World War. Thousands of young men and women returned home from fighting and working to support the war effort. They produced the largest cohort of children in history – the baby boomers. That generation, in turn, became the most prosperous, most educated, and most longest lived group of people in human history. At the same time, advances in surgical treatment and anesthetic care combined to increase the number of illnesses successfully treated with surgery. As this generation grew older, they also developed sequela of long life in the form of chronic illnesses. Many of these would, in turn, require such surgical treatment. We are still learning of the sometimes unexpected consequences of these surgeries.

Chronic pain after surgery has been recognized as a sequela of surgery for more than two decades. Crombie and colleagues in 1998 [1] initially described the scope of the problem and reviews over the next 10–15 years [2, 3] highlighted this condition. All forms of surgery can be viewed as an injury and such injury creates the risk of a chronic pain syndrome [1–17]. Rates of chronic pain from different types of surgery range from as high as 85% after amputation to as low as 6% after cesarean section [2, 3]. Chronic pain after surgery may range in intensity from minor to such severity

P. MacDougall (✉)

Department of Anesthesia and Family Medicine, Queen Elizabeth II Health Sciences Centre, Halifax, NS, Canada

e-mail: pmacdougall@toh.ca

that it interferes with the persons' daily activity and their ability to return to their baseline level of function [2]. A large cross-sectional population study of more than 12,000 people in Norway reported a prevalence of moderate to severe chronic postsurgical pain in 18% of those reporting surgery more than 3 months earlier [16]. Similarly, a large prospective observational study in Europe followed patients for 12 months [17] and reported overall rates of moderate to severe chronic pain after surgery at 6 months was 16% falling to 11.8% at 12 months. An important finding in the latter study was the decline over time of the rate of chronic postsurgical pain. Given the aging of our population and concomitant increasing numbers of people having surgery, the impact of such a complication cannot be ignored. As we will discuss, the impact of chronic pain on cost, function, and risk of morbidity and mortality is significant.

As noted, chronic pain after surgery is a frequent occurrence. It can be a complication of surgery in any body region and outranks trauma as a cause of ongoing pain [1]. Surgeries most commonly associated with significant rates of CPSP include breast surgery, limb amputation, thoracic surgery, cardiac surgery, abdominal surgery, and hernia surgery [2–17]. The impact of the sequelae of surgery cannot be overstated. While many of these surgeries are increasingly common as we age and have an impact on our ability to function with increasing age, some such as hernia surgery are more common in younger people and may have a much broader effect by preventing a young person from working and contributing to society. Perhaps of greater immediacy are recent findings that chronic pain is significantly related to suicidal ideation [18, 19]. Suicidal ideation was noted to be more closely related to the chronicity of the pain and psychological factors rather than the intensity of the pain or instability to incapacitate the person. Most of the factors related to suicidal ideation were modifiable risk factors [19]. Therefore, chronic pain is more than an inconvenience. It is a potentially modifiable, life-threatening condition.

Characteristics and Prevalence of Chronic Post-thoracotomy Pain

Chronic pain after thoracotomy has been described as one of the most intense post-operative forms of pain. This pain has been described most commonly in the area of the thoracotomy scar [20, 21]. It may also be found in the ipsilateral pectoral area, scapula, and the ipsilateral arm and shoulder [20]. It is usually described as a burning or numbness over the incision site [20–22]. Pain is also described as a cutting, drawing or tender pain [23]. The pain may be constant or intermittent in nature and is often exacerbated by such factors as lifting heavy objects. It has also been described as responsive to damp weather or rapid changes in weather [20, 21].

Of the pain experienced by those with chronic pain, neuropathic pain is the most devastating form. Characterized by burning, lancinating, sharp, or dysesthetic pain, it is the culmination of changes resulting in peripheral and central sensitization [24–26]. Maguire and colleagues [27] were among the first to report symptoms of neuropathic pain in CPTP. They reported that the prevalence of individual neuropathic symptoms varied from 35% to 85% among patients with CPTP. Steegers et al. [28] studied the type of pain experienced by those having CPTP and noted that half of the patients with CPTP had neuropathic components to their pain. Of those with CPTP, 23% had definite neuropathic pain, and 30% of patients with CPTP had some component of neuropathic pain. Similar results were noted by Hopkins et al. [29]. They reported that of patients with CPTP, 30% had neuropathic symptoms only and overall almost 55% had pain and neuropathic symptoms. Mongardon et al. [30] noted that approximately 26% of patients with pain 1 year after thoracotomy had neuropathic symptoms. These studies highlight the severity of the pain suffered by a significant portion of those with CPTP.

A number of studies have examined the prevalence of CPTP after thoracic surgery. One of the earliest and most influential studies in this area was that of Katz et al. [31] who demonstrated that up to 50% of patients had long-term pain after thoracotomy. Further studies have confirmed the high rate of chronic pain after thoracotomy [20, 21, 27, 28, 30–36]. Over the years the rate of CPTP has remained surprisingly constant at about 50%. Studies of the impact of less invasive video-assisted thoracoscopy have produced variable results. Steegers et al. [28] reported a slightly higher rate of CPTP in patients having VATS versus those having open thoracotomy (47% vs 40%). More recently Shanthanna et al. [36] reported rates of CPTP of 35% and 54% for VATS and open thoracotomy respectively. Hopkins et al. [29] reported a rate of CPTP among patients having VATS or thoracotomy at 45.3% and 54.7% respectively. This difference did not reach statistical significance. Ochroch et al. [37] reported a 21% rate of CPTP after muscle-sparing thoracotomy with aggressive epidural analgesia. This group [38] reported a similar rate in a study of muscle-sparing vs posterolateral thoracotomy with aggressive epidural analgesia. Peng et al. [39] reported a CPTP rate of 24.9% after 3 months. It is worth noting that although the rate of CPTP appears to hover at about 50%, the rate of severe CPTP is much lower, reported recently at 7–8% 1 year after surgery [27, 35].

The time course of CPTP does not appear to be static. A number of reports have indicated that the prevalence of CPTP gradually decreases over time [27, 39–41]. In addition, the intensity of the pain seems to gradually decrease over time [29, 35]. Studies tracking patients for a number of years indicate that surviving patients tend to gradually improve with respect to the impact of pain on their lives [37,

41]. This does not seem to be true, however, of neuropathic pain [39]. Of particular interest is a report by Hetmann et al. [35]. This study followed 97 patients for 12 months after thoracotomy. While they report that the rate of CPTP is approximately 50% at 6 and 12 months, they note that of the patients not reporting pain at 6 months 20% reported pain at 12 months and of those who reported pain at 6 months 11% did not report pain at 12 months. These results suggest that there are processes continuing well after surgery that contribute to CPTP.

The Impact of Chronic Post-thoracotomy Pain on Function

Chronic pain has significant impact on our society as a whole. Stewart et al. [42] estimated that common pain conditions in the USA were responsible for $62.2 billion per year in losses from lost productivity. This impact is not limited to the wealthy countries as Jackson et al. [43] demonstrated that chronic pain contributed significantly to the global burden of disease in countries with low and middle incomes. Chronic pain in this setting was, not surprisingly, more prevalent in the elderly persons and in workers. Further, a survey of chronic pain in Europe and Israel, countries with robust economies, indicated that almost 1/5 persons suffer from moderate to severe chronic pain [44]. Of those, 21% were also diagnosed with depression, 61% were less able or unable to work, and 60% visited their physician 2–9 times in the preceding 6 months. Fletcher et al. [17] used telephone and e-mail to review more than 3000 patient s in 11 European countries after surgery. Chronic postsurgical pain was reported as moderate in 9.6% and severe in 2.2% of respondents. It is evident that the social and financial burden of this illness is large and likely to grow as the population ages.

The impact of CPTP on individual function is also significant. Chronic pain affects nearly every aspect of daily life. It interferes with the ability of the patient to sleep, work, and interact with others. As such, it has a profound impact upon family life, emotional health, and relationships with friends and co-workers. A number of studies have investigated the impact of this pain condition on function after surgery [20, 37, 38, 45–48]. Persons with chronic pain have lower rates of self-rated health and indicators of increased morbidity and mortality [46–48]. It may also be related to abnormal immune function and changes in stress regulatory mechanisms in the hypothalamic-pituitary-adrenal axis [49–51]. It is closely associated with depression, and there is evidence that suicide risk is significantly increased in persons with chronic pain. Tang and Crane [18] reported that persons with chronic pain have a significantly increased risk of death by suicide. This risk is further borne out by a recent study demonstrating greater risk of suicidal ideation among patients with chronic pain [19].

In 1999 Pertunnen et al. [20] studied 111 patients following thoracotomy and noted that half of patients were having difficulties with normal daily life 12 months after surgery. They also noted that 25–30% of patients had sleep disturbances. Hopkins et al. [29] studied patients who underwent both open thoracotomy and VATS and assessed pain, neuropathic symptoms, symptom distress, mental health symptoms, and quality of life. Patients with CPTP were significantly younger than those without CPTP (average age 65 vs 71 yrs). Patients with CPTP had more symptom distress and lower quality of life [29]. Kinney et al. [52] examined 110 patients involved in a study of preoperative gabapentin for acute post-operative pain 3 months after thoracotomy. Of those 68% had pain at 3 months, and 16% were continuing to use opioid analgesics. The pain group reported lower scores in physical functioning, bodily pain, and vitality. Similar data was also reported by Maguire et al. [27]. Of more than 600 patients queried, 45% reported that pain was their most significant problem, 40% stated that it limited their daily activities, and 40% continued to take analgesic medications. The presence of a neuropathic component to the pain was also noted to lead to worse outcomes [27].

The factors which play a role in the development of disability related to pain and the risk of suicidality related to chronic pain have been examined. Katz et al. [33] utilized a number of pain and disability measurement devices to examine these factors. They determined that pain intensity and emotional numbing predicted pain disability at 6 months after surgery. Later results suggest that over time there is a decoupling of pain intensity and pain disability over the ensuing 6 months. Their results also suggest that pain disability is more closely related to post-operative factors than to preoperative factors or acute movement-related pain. Racine et al. [19] studied suicidality-related chronic pain. They determined that male gender, longer pain duration, high anger levels, feelings of helplessness, greater pain magnification, and being more depressed were significantly independent predictive factors of suicidal ideation. Feelings of better mental health were related to a reduced risk of suicidality. These findings were particularly interesting as many of the negative predictive factors are potentially modifiable [19].

Factors Influencing the Development of Chronic Post-thoracotomy Pain

Pain Before and After Surgery

In the search for factors that may predict long-term pain, pain prior to surgery is clearly associated with the development of chronic post-operative pain states [6, 12, 13, 34, 35, 38, 53–57]. A relationship between preoperative pain and chronic post-operative pain has been demonstrated in hysterectomy [55, 56], post-amputation pain [12, 13], herniorrhaphy [6, 14, 54], and CPTP [34, 35]. Hoofwijk et al. [58] studied more than 900 patients having surgery. Acute post-operative pain, preoperative pain, and preoperative analgesic use were identified as predictive of chronic post-operative pain. Hetmann et al. [35] studied 170 patients undergoing thoracotomy and noted that preoperative pain and dispositional optimism were predictive of CPTP. This group reported again [34] on 97 patients undergoing thoracotomy. They reported that 50% of those reporting CPTP at 6 months and 48% of those reporting CPTP at 12 months had preoperative pain. Niraj et al. [59] reviewed the records of more than 500 patients and followed with a questionnaire and telephone review. Poorly controlled pain was a key predictor chronic pain at 6 months. These results are supported by the findings of Kinney et al. [60]. In a database study of 66 patients presenting to a tertiary care, pain clinic indicated that those patients who used more opioid in the immediate post-operative period were more likely to have CPTP.

Genetic Factors

Since Watson and Crick first identified the double helix in the 1950s, there has been a tremendous increase in our understanding of the genetics of human illness. The last decade has seen some of that attention turn to the enigma of pain. Genetic variability may affect pain in many ways. These may include the susceptibility to pain, how pain is manifested, and how it is treated. Variants of the catecholamine-O-methyltransferase (COMT) gene have been demonstrated in a number of studies to be linked to the risk of developing pain [58, 61–63]. George et al. [62, 63] have demonstrated that a link between psychosocial constructs such as pain catastrophizing and genetic variability can be predictive of pain outcomes after shoulder surgery. They also identified pain-modifying genetic variants, KCNS1, ADRB2, and GCH1, linked to preoperative kinesophobia, post-operative depression, and anxiety, respectively. Polymorphisms in this gene have been shown to be related to back, but not leg, pain intensity in persons undergoing discectomy [64, 65].

Genetic variability can affect the way that we respond to treatment in a number of ways. The pharmacodynamics and pharmacokinetics of pain treatment are governed by our genetic makeup. Opioid medications are the most studied drugs in relation to pain. Genetic polymorphism can have an effect on transport of the drug across cell membranes [66]. Fentanyl, methadone, and morphine transports into the brain are affected by polymorphism in the ABCB1 gene. Metabolism of prodrugs such as codeine and tramadol are affected by variability in the type of CYP2D6 expressed in the liver [61, 66–68]. Expression of the CP2D6 variants determines the amount of active drug produced by the liver.

Expression of the μ-opioid receptor, a product of the OPRM1 gene is related to the response to opioid medications. A number of studies have demonstrated that this gene is highly variable [58, 66, 68]. This variability is correlated with pain response to opioids and also to the susceptibility to dependence.

These are but a few examples of genetic variability playing a role in the development of pain and the treatment of pain. Much more work is necessary, but the science of pharmacogenomics, targeting drugs to individual genotypes, is growing rapidly. Ultimately, this will allow us to be able to predict who is likely to have pain after surgery, how best to treat it, and who may develop dependence on the medications use to treat the pain.

Anesthetic Factors

Anesthesia has at its heart the prevention of pain in the surgical and perioperative period. Song et al. [69] conducted a prospective, randomized, controlled trial of TIVA vs inhalation anesthesia for 366 patients undergoing thoracotomy. They found a significant difference in CPTP at 3 and 6 months. No difference was noted in acute pain. Although these findings are compelling, the results have not been repeated in other settings.

Post-operative pain control has been identified as a factor in the development of long-term pain after surgery [31, 40, 70]. Several options are available for management of acute post-operative pain. These include regional anesthetic techniques such as thoracic epidural analgesia (TEA), paravertebral blockade (PVB), intercostal blockade, and serratus anterior plane blockade (SAP). Intravenous patient-controlled analgesia (PCA) and oral analgesics are commonly utilized in the perioperative period. Adjunct pain management may involve such modalities as transcutaneous electrical nerve stimulation (TENS).

A recent Cochrane review of pharmacotherapy for prevention of chronic pain after surgery reported that there was modest support for the use of ketamine [71]. Similarly, McNicol et al. [72], in a meta-analysis of studies of ketamine for the prevention of chronic postsurgical pain, found only a modest effect of ketamine in reducing chronic pain after surgery. Interestingly, this result was only present in studies of intravenous and not epidural ketamine [72]. In a randomized controlled trial of S(+) ketamine in the perioperative period, Mendola et al. [73] demonstrated an improvement in perioperative pain control, but this did not translate into reduced rates of CPTP.

Other medications have also been evaluated for efficacy in preventing acute and chronic pain after thoracotomy. Gabapentin was studied in a randomized trial of 120 patients

[52] and reported to have no significant effect on acute or chronic post-thoracotomy pain. However, a small randomized study of 50 patients compared pregabalin for 2 days beginning in the perioperative period with as needed diclofenac [74]. This study reported a significant reduction in CPTP at 24 weeks. Similarly, a small trial of intravenous dexketoprofen with TEA prior to surgery was reported to show an improvement in perioperative acute pain and pain at 3 and 6 months [75]. Another small study of anti-inflammatory effects on CPTP was reported by Ling [76]. They studied the use of intravenous parecoxib in the perioperative period in conjunction with TEA. They report that CPTP, both incisional and evoked, is significantly reduced at 3 and 12 months. These studies indicate that there may be merit to further trials of pharmacologic means to prevent CPTP.

Most patients undergoing thoracotomy have a regional anesthetic. The most common of the techniques for managing acute pain is TEA, typically placed between T5 and T8. Paravertebral catheters may be placed either by the surgeon under direct vision or by the anesthesiologist with the aid of ultrasound. A number of recent meta-analyses comparing these techniques have been published including a Cochrane review [77–79]. These studies concluded that the two techniques provided similar pain relief in the post-operative period and that PVB may have somewhat lower risk of side effects such as hypotension and urinary retention. It is not clear whether this is due to the technique or dose of medication used in the different blocks. None of the studies reported on the impact of these techniques on CPTP.

A number of small studies have evaluated the effect of TEA on CPTP [37, 80–82]. These studies have examined initiation of epidural analgesia before and after thoracotomy incision [37, 38, 80–82]. Different analgesic regimens were studied as were different methods of administering TEA [80, 82]. The effects of TEA on CPTP were varied. A meta-analysis of the effects of preemptive TEA on post-thoracotomy pain did not find sufficient evidence to state that preemptive TEA reduced CPTP. A later Cochrane review by Andrae and Andrae [83] reviewed studies including 250 patients. They concluded that there was evidence to suggest that the use of TEA or regional analgesia reduces the risk of CPTP in one in every three to four patients. Although the methodology of the studies was not strong and the studies were small, the use of TEA or regional anesthesia should be considered for all patients undergoing thoracotomy.

Surgical Factors

Access to the chest cavity can be accomplished in a number of ways as noted in earlier chapters. Surgical methods include the standard posterolateral thoracotomy (PLT), muscle-sparing thoracotomy (MLT), antero-axillary thora-

cotomy (AAT) and video-assisted thoracoscopic surgery (VATS). Each method brings with it a unique set of challenges. A number of studies have compared posterolateral and muscle-sparing thoracotomy techniques to determine their impact on perioperative outcomes [84]. Nosotti et al. [85] in a large randomized controlled trial demonstrated that post-operative pain outcome was similar but those with PLT used more opioids via patient-controlled analgesia than the MLT group. There was no difference in CPTP between the groups. Pain decreased in both groups over 3 years of follow-up, with 20% of patients reporting pain at that time. Noromi et al. [86] compared AAT and PLT on post-operative pain. In as study of 51 patients, they noted patients having AAT with significantly less pain in the perioperative and at 3- and 6-month follow-up. Axillary MLT was compared to standard PLT in two studies [37, 38]. Data from the initial study was re-examined and published separately [38]. The incidence of CPTP did not vary based on the type of incision. Similarly, a study of 101 patients undergoing MLT or PLT by Athanassiadi et al. [87] did not demonstrate a difference in the quantity of pain at 2 months. Unfortunately, the incidence of CPTP was not reported. Elshiekh and colleagues [84] reviewed evidence comparing MLT and PLT. They determined that MLT techniques may provide an advantage in return to mobility but that there was no clear evidence that pain was improved although there did seem to be an inverse relationship between incision length and post-thoracotomy pain.

The last decade has seen VATS or variations thereof become standard surgical approaches. The procedure is minimally invasive and performed through a series of ports or a combination of ports and mini-thoracotomy incisions. Early studies of VATS suggested that pain following VATS may be related to the type of surgery. Rates of CPTP varied widely from almost zero to more than 61% [4, 88–91]. Two early studies of VATS procedures for benign disease reported an initial rate of CPTP at 20% after a mean follow-up of 34 months declining to 12.5% after 10 years. Early studies of VATS for oncologic disease reported much higher rates of CPTP [4, 92]. More recent studies have compared VATS to anterolateral thoracotomy [93], limited thoracotomy [94], and video-assisted minimal thoracotomy [41, 95] reflecting a shift in surgical practice to less invasive techniques. Yamashita et al. [95] reported that VATS patients had earlier surgical recovery and less post-operative pain as evidenced by less analgesic use than those in the VATS-assisted minimal thoracotomy group. Unfortunately, CPTP rates were not reported. Noromi et al. [94] compared VATS lobectomy to a limited thoracotomy for segmentectomy and wide thoracotomy for segmentectomy. Chronic pain, as assessed by the need for analgesics at 3 months, was reported as 4%, 1%, and 6% respectively. These differences were not statistically significant. VATS was compared to ALT by Bendixen and colleagues [93]. They report that more patients report moderate to severe pain after ALT than VATS at 1 year. The proportion of patients with moderate to severe pain showed a time-dependent decline over the study period. Thus, while the data remains limited and heterogeneous in outcome measures, there appears to be a trend indicating that less invasive forms of surgery reduce the long-term pain associated with chest surgery.

To understand more clearly the impact of shifts in surgical practice on chronic pain, it is important to acknowledge that factors beyond the type of incision may play a role in the development of CPTP. As the surgeon accesses the chest through a thoracotomy incision, the ribs are spread using a rib spreader. This compresses the neurovascular bundle on the cranial rib. During a VATS procedure, the neurovascular bundle may be compressed by instrument ports or directly by the instruments. At the end of surgery, during rib closure, there is risk of compression of the neurovascular bundle as the ribs are approximated. Traditional intercostal suture techniques bring the suture from the superior edge of the cranial rib and through the intercostal muscle inferior to the caudad rib. This risks entrapment and compression of the neurovascular bundle as the sutures are tightened to approximate the rib. Finally, traction on the intercostal nerve occurs as the ribs are spread and the nerve is stretched along the arc of the rib. Injury by compression, traction, or entrapment of the nerve is thought to be the central injury responsible for post-thoracotomy neuropathic pain.

Early reports of the effect of nerve injury studied the superficial abdominal reflexes (in part, mediated by the inferior intercostal nerves) and indicated a strong correlation between the absence of these reflexes and the intensity of post-thoracotomy pain including CPTP in the setting of PLT [96]. Subsequent studies of these reflexes in the setting of PLT and MLT demonstrated that the absence of abdominal reflexes and increased tactile threshold for electrical stimulation were highly correlated to the intensity of CPTP [97]. However, interoperative studies of intercostal nerve motor-evoked potentials demonstrated nerve injury during thoracotomy, but did not correlate to CPTP [98, 99]. In addition to the impact of the thoracotomy or VATS incision, chest drains are also placed through small thoracotomy incisions. Wildgaard et al. [100] reported post-thoracotomy pain and sensory changes at the site of chest drains in a long-term follow-up study. Similarly, Peng et al. [39] noted a significant correlation between CPTP and prolonged presence of chest drains.

A number of studies have begun to address the issue of neurovascular bundle compression on opening and closing of the chest wall. Mongardon [30] reported that the number of chest drains was positively correlated with the development of CPTP suggesting that nerve compression from the chest drain may contribute to the problem. Cerfolio and colleagues [101] studied a technique of intracostal sutures and

demonstrated a significant reduction in CPTP. Studies of intercostal muscle flaps, either pedicled or non-pedicled, and nerve-sparing suture techniques [102–108] to prevent compression of the intercostal nerve during rib spreading and at rib closure, demonstrate a reduction in CPTP. However, neurectomy does not appear to provide protection against CPTP. In a parallel-group randomized controlled trial of 161 patients undergoing ALT, Koryllos and colleagues [109] evaluated the effect of a paravertebral neurectomy on CPTP. No difference was found in neuropathic pain after 4 months of follow-up. Garcia-Tirado and Rieger-Reyes [110] reviewed methods of reducing impact of opening and closure techniques on post-thoracotomy pain. They conclude that there is good evidence to indicate that mechanisms to prevent entrapment of the intercostal nerve on closure reduce post-thoracotomy pain, both acute and chronic.

Neuroinflammation, the infiltration of active immune cells into the peripheral or central nervous system, may be a significant mediator of chronic pain. Astrocytes and microglial cells infiltrate the peripheral or central nervous system in response to injury and secrete inflammatory cytokines and chemokines such as TNF and interleukin 1β [111, 112]. In light of the evidence that reducing the compression of the intercostal nerve reduces risk of chronic pain after thoracotomy, it is reasonable to hypothesize that CPTP may be related to neuroinflammation in the intercostal nerve and associated dorsal root ganglion. Certainly data demonstrating sensory changes after thoracotomy [100, 113, 114] are consistent with this hypothesis. Novel therapies with bone marrow stromal cells that modulate neuroinflammation are now at the stage of animal testing [112]. Recent studies of intrathecal injection of these cells resulted in long-term relief of experimental neuropathic pain from peripheral nerve injury [112]. Further, animal studies of intrathecal administration of DNA decoys that inhibit the production of early growth factor response protein 1 (EGR1) in the dorsal root ganglion reduce the acute and chronic pain after experimental nerve injury in rats [115].

The concept of neuroinflammation as a factor contributing to CPTP may be further supported by studies characterizing the neuropathic pain. Neuropathic pain is a result of nerve injury leading to peripheral or central sensitization. Wildegaard and colleagues [100, 113, 114] and Hetmann et al. [34] studied the sensory changes after thoracotomy and VATS. Neurophysiological studies of post-thoracotomy patients suggested nerve injury is common in patients with and without CPTP but it seems to be more severe in those with CPTP [114]. Quantitative sensory testing after VATS did not demonstrate a significant difference in nerve injury between those with and without CPTP suggesting that other factors may be involved in the CPTP after VATS. A similar study of chest drain sites also demonstrated sensory indicating nerve injury both in patients with and without CPTP [100] and that these changes were related to late nerve injury. Hetmann et al. [34], in a multimodal study of post-thoracotomy pain at 6 and 12 months after surgery, noted that patient self-exploration for sensory changes indicated that 40–60% of patients had some kind of sensory disturbance at 6 months. This declined to 20–50% at 12 months. Sensory disturbances in this study were strongly associated with CPTP. Of considerable interest in this study was the identification of patients who had no pain at 6 months but reported pain at 12 months.

In addition to the concept of neuroinflammation at the level of individual nerves, a number of studies have identified psychological factors that seem to increase the risk of CPTP [33, 35]. Li and Hu [51] reviewed studies of stress regulation on pain the hypothalamic-pituitary-adrenal axis and pain chronification. In addition to changes in the HPA axis, the shift from acute to chronic pain involves changes in a number of areas of the brain. Li and Hu [51] bring these together in a unifying theory of the role of stress regulation on pain chronification. These studies suggest that CPTP, like many other postsurgical pain conditions, is multifactorial in nature and involves changes from the periphery to the central nervous system.

Prevention of Chronic Post-thoracotomy Pain

Management of chronic pain conditions including CPTP differs from acute pain conditions in that the goals are prevention first followed by long-term management. Acute pain states, by their nature, are limited in time and typically have a declining course over that time. Deductive reasoning would suggest that identification of contributing factors should provide a clear path to prevention of CPTP. However, the reality is proving to be more complex. It seems that there are a number of factors that are related to the development of CPTP but clear causality from a single factor has not yet been demonstrated.

As noted previously, in acute pain and preoperative pain, preoperative analgesic use has been identified as a predictor of chronic postsurgical pain including CPTP in number of studies [31, 35, 39, 40, 58–60]. Additionally, psychological states seem to have a predictive relationship with CPTP. Hetmann et al. [35] demonstrated that dispositional optimism was correlated with CPTP at 12 months. Katz et al. [33] reported a relationship between emotional numbing and CPTP at 6 and 12 months. Each of these conditions may be amenable to identification in the preoperative period and modifiable.

Interestingly, an epidemiological study of 189 patients undergoing thoracotomy identified a relationship between CPTP and inhaled β-agonist use [116]. The use of inhaled

β-agonist medications in the perioperative period was an independent predictor of CPTP. These results suggest that further study is warranted to more clearly elucidate the relationship between β-agonist medications and CPTP.

Perioperative medication administration to prevent chronic post-operative pain is attractive in its relative simplicity. Humble et al. [117] conducted a systematic review of therapeutic interventions aimed at preventing chronic postsurgical pain. Gabapentinoids reduced chronic pain after mastectomy but were not effective as a single dose to prevent CPTP. Venlafaxine reduced chronic pain after mastectomy as did EMLA and intravenous lidocaine. Preoperative pregabalin was studied in patients undergoing thoracotomy [118]. CPTP was more common in the pregabalin group although those in the pregabalin group had lower pain scores and less neuropathic symptoms.

Age and gender have been implicated as predictors in a number of postsurgical pain conditions [5, 6]. Younger patients have a greater likelihood of developing postsurgical pain after herniorrhaphy [15, 119]. The effect of age is not consistent across studies of CPTP. Some studies have demonstrated an inverse relationship between age and the risk of development of CPTP [9, 27, 41] with that risk declining by about 2% per year of age [27]. Others have found no relationship between age and risk of CPTP [16, 35]. Similarly, the effect of gender on CPTP is not yet certain. Some studies have reported that women have a greater risk of developing CPTP after thoracic surgery [40, 45]. A large study of persistent postsurgical pain in the general population in Norway failed to find a correlation between age and gender with persistent pain states [16]. Similarly, Hetmann et al. [35] did not find a correlation with gender and CPTP. However, Ochroch et al. [45] in a study designed to study the effect of gender on CPTP reported that women were more likely to have pain 49 weeks after thoracotomy and that the pain would be of greater intensity. This study also noted that older patients suffered less CPTP. However, the study was small and the sample size may be a complicating factor.

Granot [120] reviewed studies of static and dynamic responses to pain perception as predictors of acute and chronic post-operative pain. A number of studies of static pain parameters (tolerance, pain threshold, suprathreshold nociceptive stimuli) have been conducted and demonstrate variable predictive capability for acute and chronic post-operative pain [120–122]. Yarnitsky et al. [122] evaluated the diffuse noxious inhibitory control (DNIC) system in patients preparing for thoracotomy. They reported that those persons who have an efficient DNIC are less likely to develop CPTP than those with a less efficient DNIC. This study is measurable preoperatively and may provide a means to predict those with a propensity to develop CPTP and allow appropriate intervention.

Active attempts to predict and prevent chronic postsurgical pain are now becoming reality. Tawfic et al. [123] reviewed the known predictive factors for chronic postsurgical pain. They advocated for active preoperative risk factor identification, patient preparation, optimization of anesthetic and surgical techniques, and careful attention to management of acute pain. They also suggested that high-risk patients have an individualized discharge plan to manage persistent pain early. These interventions should include appropriate use of perioperative multimodal analgesia and TEA or regional analgesia as these have been identified as having benefit on CPTP [83]. Pharmacologic intervention with anti-inflammatory medications and pregabalin may also be efficacious for CPTP prevention [74–76]. Careful surgical attention should be paid to prevention of nerve injury during the procedure. Institutions are now beginning to develop perioperative programs to prevent chronic postsurgical pain. Such a program has been reported [124, 125]. The transitional pain service is an inter-professional program to identify and manage patients who may develop chronic pain after surgery. The effect of this program and others like it will ultimately determine key methods to reduce and mitigate chronic post-operative pain syndromes.

Management of Chronic Post-thoracotomy Pain

Treatment of CPTP begins with assessment of the type and cause of the pain. As with any form of chronic pain, it is important to search for reversible causes of CPTP. Foremost among these in patients with CPTP after cancer surgery is the search for recurrence of tumor. This is true at all visits after thoracotomy. Tumor recurrence may be heralded by onset of new pain or change in existing pain. Treatment for the pain of tumor recurrence differs from that of chronic non-cancer pain and may include chemotherapy, radiation, or further surgical intervention.

Patients presenting post-operatively to surgical clinics or to their primary care practitioner should be evaluated for post-operative pain at each visit. Ideally, the first post-operative visit with the primary care provider would be part of surgical planning. In the first 2–4 weeks after surgery patients should receive appropriate analgesic therapy for their pain. This may include antiepileptic medications, tricyclic antidepressants, or opioids. Opioids should be prescribed carefully and consideration given to tapering and withdrawal after 4–6 weeks. Patients with pain persisting beyond 3 months should be referred to an inter-professional pain clinic.

Once it is established that the pain is not from tumor or other reversible cause such as occult rib fracture or lung herniation [126], it is important to characterize the pain to determine and identify any neuropathic component. A number of screening tools exist to assist in the diagnosis of neuropathic pain [127]. Use of one of the tools on a regular basis may assist in the development of a comprehensive treatment plan.

A number of guidelines have been developed to treat neuropathic pain [128–132]. These guidelines provide advice on pharmacologic treatment. Treatments typically begin with the use of tricyclic antidepressants, SSRI antidepressants, and antiepileptics, as first- and second-line treatment. Opioids and cannabinoids are considered third line in treatment of neuropathic pain. Topical medications such as capsaicin cream or topical lidocaine [132, 133] may be of benefit. Treatment with other medications including compounded topical medications may be undertaken collaboration with specialist pain management providers. In a small subset of patients, pharmacologic treatment will be inadequate to manage the pain sufficiently to allow the patient to function well. A recent report of reprogramming of an indwelling spinal cord stimulator providing relief for CPTP [134] provides promise of a long-term therapy for those with intractable pain after thoracotomy.

Other treatments that have begun to show promise in the treatment of CPTP include transcutaneous electrical nerve stimulation (TENS). The use of this therapy was reviewed by Freynet and Falcoz [135]. It has been demonstrated to have positive effects both in the immediate perioperative setting [136, 137] and in the management of CPTP [135]. Acupuncture treatment in the setting of chronic pain was the subject of a recent meta-analysis [138]. They examined its use in osteoarthritis, musculoskeletal pain, and headache and found that relief obtained from the intervention may be sustained for many months. Acupuncture has not been evaluated for CPTP. Case reports of botulinum toxin for use in mitigating CPTP have indicated that this treatment for CPTP provided relief for at least 12 weeks [139, 140]. It is not known how long the effect may last or whether it can be repeated. This treatment merits further study.

Treatment of CPTP may require trials of a variety of therapies to determine the optimal treatment for each patient. Optimal treatment of CPTP will often involve multiple professions and disciplines. Overall treatment can be summarized as follows:

- Early post-operative assessment of pain to rule out reversible factors
- Treatment with non-opioid medications such as antiepileptic medications antidepressants, and tricyclic antidepressants
- Judicious use of opioids carefully monitored for effect and dosage
- Referral to an inter-professional pain management clinic
- Topical lidocaine, capsaicin, or compounded medications

- Minimally invasive interventions such as TENS, botulinum toxin, and acupuncture
- Invasive strategies including spinal cord stimulation

Clinical Case Discussion

Mrs. VP is a 49-year-old woman referred to the Pain Management Centre by her family physician with a complaint of right-sided chest pain in the area of her thoracotomy scar. She had undergone a VATS right upper lobe lobectomy for Stage I non-small cell lung carcinoma 6 months earlier.

Past Medical/Surgical History

Mrs. VP has a history of 30 pack years of smoking, having quit 2 years prior to her surgery. She has hypertension and diabetes mellitus Type II managed by diet therapy. Her preoperative medications included hydrochlorothiazide 12.5 mg and daily ASA 82 mg.

Perioperative Course

Her interoperative course was uneventful and mediastinal lymph node biopsies were negative. She had a paravertebral block placed by the surgeon at the end of surgery. Her pain was well controlled, and she was started on oral analgesics 24 h after surgery. The paravertebral catheter was removed at day 3 after surgery as were her chest tubes. She was discharged home on day 5. Nursing notes recorded an average pain score of 5/10 at discharge.

First Visit

At the time of presentation, she described a burning, stabbing pain in the area of the thoracotomy scar. Recent chest radiograph and CT scan were negative for recurrent malignancy. She rated the pain as an average of 5/10. She stated that "good days" brought a pain level of 4/10, and "bad days" brought pain at a level of 7–8/10. She had considerably more bad days than good. The pain radiated to the scapula and anterior chest wall. Her sleep was interrupted by the pain, and she was unable to return to her work as a cashier. Treatment at the time of presentation consisted of two acetaminophen 325 mg/oxycodone 5 mg combination tablets four times daily.

Examination revealed allodynia in the area of the scar. The wound appeared to have healed otherwise well. No other abnormalities were noted.

A diagnosis of post-thoracotomy chronic pain with neuropathic features was made, and an inter-professional treatment plan was discussed. The treatment plan was as follows:

1. The patient was referred for rehabilitation physiotherapy and acupuncture. TENS therapy was explained, and written instructions were provided along with a prescription for a TENS unit and pads.
2. She was started on nortriptyline 25 mg qhs. Recommendations were made to her primary care provider to start gabapentin at 300 mg qhs, increasing to 600–1800 mg every 8 h..
3. She was referred to the local pain self-management program, consisting of physiotherapy, occupational therapy, psychology, diet therapy, and vocational therapy.
4. A follow-up appointment was made for 6 months.

Second Visit

Mrs. VP reported mild improvement with the pharmacotherapy regimen and TENS therapy. She continued to have significant burning pain over the thoracotomy site interfering with her ability to return to full function. A prescription for a trial of acupuncture and a compounded topical medication was provided.

Third Visit

Mrs. VP returned to the Pain Management Centre 3 months later. She had minimal relief from her acupuncture. The topical medication was effective for a few hours only. She asked if there was anything more permanent that could be done. A trial of neurostimulation was scheduled.

Fourth Visit

The trial of neurostimulation was successful reducing pain to a level of 1–2/10. A permanent stimulator had been placed. Mrs. VP was discharged from the Pain Management Centre to the care of her family physician. She follows up periodically for management of the neurostimulator.

References

1. Crombie IK, Davies HT, Macrae WA. Cut and thrust: antecedent surgery and trauma among patients attending a chronic pain clinic. Pain. 1998;76(1–2):167.
2. Macrae WA. Chronic pain after surgery. Br J Anaesth. 2001; 87(1):88.

3. Macrae WA. Chronic post-surgical pain: 10 years on. Br J Anaesth. 2008;101(1):77.

4. Burke S, Shorten G. When pain after surgery doesn't go away …. Biochem Soc Trans. 2009;37(1):318.

5. Eisenberg E. Post-surgical neuralgia. Pain. 2004;111(1–2):3.

6. Kehlet H, Jensen T, Woolf C. Persistent postsurgical pain: risk factors and prevention. Lancet. 2006;367(9522):1618.

7. Vilholm OJ, Cold S, Rasmussen L, Sindrup SH. Sensory function and pain in a population of patients treated for breast cancer. Acta Anaesthesiol Scand. 2009;53(6):800.

8. Poleshuck E, Katz J, Andrus C, Hogan L, Jung B, Kulick D, et al. Risk factors for chronic pain following breast cancer surgery: a prospective study. J Pain. 2006;7(9):626.

9. Steegers MA, Wolters B, Evers AW, Strobbe L, Wilder-Smith OH. Effect of axillary lymph node dissection on prevalence and intensity of chronic and phantom pain after breast cancer surgery. J Pain. 2008;9(9):813.

10. Amichetti M, Caffo O. Pain after quadrantectomy and radiotherapy for early-stage breast cancer: incidence, characteristics and influence on quality of life. Results from a retrospective study. Oncology. 2003;65(1):23.

11. Flor H. Phantom-limb pain: characteristics, causes, and treatment. Lancet Neurol. 2002;1(3):182.

12. Nikolajsen L, Jensen TS. Phantom limb pain. Br J Anaesth. 2001;87(1):107.

13. Jensen TS, Krebs B, Nielsen J, Rasmussen P. Immediate and long-term phantom limb pain in amputees: incidence, clinical characteristics and relationship to pre-amputation limb pain. Pain. 1985;21(3):267.

14. Aasvang EK, Bay-Nielsen M, Kehlet H. Pain and functional impairment 6 years after inguinal herniorrhaphy. Hernia. 2006;10(4):316.

15. Aasvang E, Kehlet H. Chronic postoperative pain: the case of inguinal herniorrhaphy. Br J Anaesth. 2005;95(1):69.

16. Johansen A, Romundstat L, Nielsen CS, Schirmer H, Stubhaug A. Persistent postsurgical pain in a general population: prevalence and predictors in the Tromso study. Pain. 2012;153:1390–6.

17. Fletcher D, Stamer UM, Pogatzki-Zahn E, Zaslansky R, Tanase NV, Perruchoud C, et al. Chronic postsurgical pain in Europe. An observational study. Eur J Anaesthesiol. 2015;32:725–34.

18. Tang NKY, Crane C. Suicidality in chronic pain: a review of the prevalence, risk factors and psychological links. Psychol Med. 2006;36(5):575.

19. Racine M, Sanchez-Rodriguez E, Galan S, Tome-Pires C, Sole E, Jensen MP, et al. Factors associated with suicidal ideation in patient with chronic non-cancer pain. Pain Med. 2017;18:283–93.

20. Perttunen K, Tasmuth T, Kalso E. Chronic pain after thoracic surgery: a follow-up study. Acta Anaesthesiol Scand. 1999;43(5):563.

21. Dajczman E, Gordon A, Kreisman H, Wolkove N. Long-term post-thoracotomy pain. Chest. 1991;99(2):270.

22. Hazelrigg S, Cetindag I, Fullerton J. Acute and chronic pain syndromes after thoracic surgery. Surg Clin North Am. 2002;82(4):849.

23. Kalso E, Perttunen K, Kaasinen S. Pain after thoracic surgery. Acta Anaesthesiol Scand. 1992;36(1):96.

24. Baron R. Neuropathic pain: a clinical perspective. Handb Exp Pharmacol. 2009;194:3.

25. O'Connor A. Neuropathic pain: quality-of-life impact, costs and cost effectiveness of therapy. PharmacoEconomics. 2009;27(2):95.

26. Costigan M, Scholz J, Woolf C. Neuropathic pain: a maladaptive response of the nervous system to damage. Annu Rev Neurosci. 2009;32:1.

27. Maguire MF, Ravenscroft A, Beggs D, Duffy JP. A questionnaire study investigating the prevalence of the neuropathic component of chronic pain after thoracic surgery. Eur J Cardiothorac Surg. 2006;29(5):800.

28. Steegers MAH, Snik DM, Verhagen AF, van der Drift MA, Wilder-Smith OHG. Only half of the chronic pain after thoracic surgery shows a neuropathic component. J Pain. 2008;9(10):955.

29. Hopkins KG, Hoffman LA, Dabbs ADV, Ferson PF, King L, Dudjak LA, et al. Postthoracotomy pain syndrome following surgery for lung cancer: symptoms and impact on quality of life. J Adv Pract Oncol. 2015;6:121–32.

30. Mongardon N, Pinton-Gonnet C, Szekely B, Michel-Cherqui M, Dreyfus J-F, Fischler M. Assessment of chronic pain after thoracotomy: a 1 year prevalence study. Clin J Pain. 2011;27:167–81.

31. Katz J, Jackson M, Kavanagh BP, Sandler AN. Acute pain after thoracic surgery predicts long-term post-thoracotomy pain. Clin J Pain. 1996;12(1):50.

32. Pluijms WA, Steegers MAH, Verhagen AFTM, Scheffer GJ, Wilder-Smith OHG. Chronic post-thoracotomy pain: a retrospective study. Acta Anaesthesiol Scand. 2006;50(7):804.

33. Katz J, Asmundson GJG, McRae K, Halket E. Emotional numbing and pain intensity predict the development of pain disability up to one year after lateral thoracotomy. Eur J Pain. 2009;13(8):870.

34. Hetmann F, Kongsgaard UE, Sandvik L, Schoou-Bredal I. Post-thoracotomy pain syndrome and sensory disturbances following thoracotomy at 6 and 12 month follow-ups. J Pain Res. 2017;10:663–8.

35. Hetmann F, Kongsgaard UE, Sandvik L, Schou-Bredal I. Prevalence and predictors of persistent post-surgical pain 12 months after thoracotomy. Acta Anaesthesiol Scand. 2015;59:740–8.

36. Shanthanna H, Aboutouk D, Poon E, Cheng J, Finley C, Paul J, Thabane L. A retrospective study of open thoracotomies versus thoracoscopic surgeries for persistent postthoracotomy pain. J Clin Anesth. 2016;35:215–20.

37. Ochroch EA, Gottschalk A, Augostides J, Carson K, Kent L, Malayaman N, et al. Long-term pain and activity during recovery from major thoracotomy using thoracic epidural analgesia. Anesthesiology. 2002;97(5):1234.

38. Ochroch EA, Gottschalk A, Augoustides J, Aukburg S, Kaiser L, Shrager J. Pain and physical function are similar following axillary, muscle-sparing vs posterolateral thoracotomy. Chest. 2005;128(4):2664.

39. Peng Z, Li H, Zhang C, Qian X, Feng Z, Zhu S. A retrospective study of chronic post-surgical pain following thoracic surgery: prevalence, risk factors, incidence of neuropathic component, and impact on quality of life. PLoS One. 2014;9:1–7.

40. Gotoda Y, Kambara N, Sakai T, Kishi Y, Kodama K, Koyama T. The morbidity, time course and predictive factors for persistent post-thoracotomy pain. Eur J Pain. 2001;5(1):89.

41. Gottschalk A, Ochroch EA. Clinical and demographic characteristics of patients with chronic pain after major thoracotomy. Clin J Pain. 2008;24(8):708.

42. Stewart W, Ricci J, Chee E, Morganstein D, Lipton R. Lost productive time and cost due to common pain conditions in the US workforce. JAMA. 2003;290:2443.

43. Jackson T, Thomas S, Stabile V, Shotwell M, Han X, McQueen K. A systematic review and meta-analysis of the global burden of chronic pain without clear etiology in low and middle-income countries: trends in heterogeneous data and a proposal for new assessment methods. Anesth Analg. 2016;123:739–48.

44. Breivik H, Collett B, Ventafridda V, Cohen R, Gallacher D. Survey of chronic pain in Europe: prevalence, impact on daily life and treatment. Eur J Pain. 2006;10:287–333.

45. Ochroch EA, Gottschalk A, Troxel AB, Farrar JT. Women suffer more short and long-term pain than men after major thoracotomy. Clin J Pain. 2006;22(5):491.

46. Mossey JM, Shapiro E. Self-rated health: a predictor of mortality among the elderly. Am J Public Health. 1982;72(8):800.

47. Kaplan GA, Goldberg DE, Everson SA, Cohen RD, Salonen R, Tuomilehto J, et al. Perceived health status and morbidity and mortality: evidence from the Kuopio ischaemic heart disease risk factor study. Int J Epidemiol. 1996;25(2):259.

48. Idler EL, Benyamini Y. Self-rated health and mortality: a review of twenty-seven community studies. J Health Soc Behav. 1997;38(1):21.
49. Liebeskind JC. Pain can kill. Pain. 1991;44(1):3.
50. Watkins LR, Maier SF. Immune regulation of central nervous system functions: from sickness responses to pathological pain. J Intern Med. 2005;257(2):139.
51. Li X, Hu L. The role of stress regulation on neuroplasticity in pain chronicfication. Neural Plast. 2016. https://doi.org/10.1155/2016/6402942.
52. Kinney MO, Hooten WM, Cassivi SD, Allen MS, Passe MA, Hanson AC, et al. Chronic post-thoracotomy pain and health-related quality of life. Ann Thorac Surg. 2012;93:1242–7.
53. Wildgaard K, Ravn J, Kehlet H. Chronic post-thoracotomy pain: a critical review of pathogenic mechanisms and strategies for prevention. Eur J Cardiothorac Surg. 2009;36:170–80.
54. Perkins FM, Kehlet H. Chronic pain as an outcome of surgery. A review of predictive factors. Anesthesiology. 2000;93(4):1123.
55. Brandsborg B, Nikolajsen L, Hansen C, Kehlet H, Jensen T. Risk factors for chronic pain after hysterectomy: a nationwide questionnaire and database study. Anesthesiology. 2007;106(5):1003.
56. Brandsborg B, Dueholm M, Nikolajsen L, Kehlet H, Jensen T. A prospective study of risk factors for pain persisting 4 months after hysterectomy. Clin J Pain. 2009;25(4):263.
57. Gerbershagen HJ, Ozgur E, Dagtekin O, Straub K, Hahn M, Heidenreich A, et al. Postoperative pain as a risk factor for chronic post-surgical pain – six month follow-up after radical prostatectomy. Eur J Pain. 2009;13:1054–61.
58. Hoofwijk DMN, van Reij RRI, Rutten BP, Kenis G, Buhre WF, Joosten EA. Genetic polymorphisms and their association with the prevalence and severity of chronic postsurgical pain: a systematic review. BJA. 2016;117:708–19.
59. Niraj G, Kelkar A, Kaushik V, Tang Y, Fleet D, Tait F, et al. Audit of postoperative pain management after open thoracotomy and the incidence of chronic postthoracotomy pain in more than 500 patients at a tertiary center. J Clin Anesth. 2017;36:174–7.
60. Kinney MA, Jacob AK, Passe MA, Mantilla CB. Increased risk of postthoracotomy pain syndrome in patients with prolonged hospitalization and increased postoperative opioid use. Pain Res Treat. 2016. https://doi.org/10.1155/2016/7945145.
61. Diatchenko L, Slade G, Nackley A, Bhalang K, Sigurdsson A, Belfer I, et al. Genetic basis for individual variations in pain perception and the development of a chronic pain condition. Hum Mol Genet. 2005;14(1):135.
62. George SZ, Wallace MR, Wright T, Moser MW, Greenfield WH, Sack BK. Evidence for a biopsychosocial influence on shoulder pain: catastrophizing and catechol-O-methyltransferase (COMT) diplotype predict clinical pain ratings. Pain. 2008;136:53–61.
63. George SZ, Wu SS, Wallace MR, Moser MW, Wright TW, Farmer KW, et al. Biopsychosocial influence on shoulder pain: influence of genetic and psychological combinations on twelve-month postoperative pain and disability outcomes. Arthritis Care Res. 2016;11:1671–80.
64. Rut M, Machoy-Mokrynska A, Reclawowicz D, Sloniewski P, Kurzawski M, Drozdzik M, et al. Influence of variation in the catechol-O-methyltransferase gene on the clinical outcome after lumbar spine surgery for one-level symptomatic disc disease: a on 176 cases. Acta Neurochir. 2014;156:245–52.
65. Tegeder I, Costigan M, Griffin R, Abele A, Belfer I, Schmidt H, et al. GTP cyclohydrolase and tetrahydrobiopterin regulate pain sensitivity and persistence. Nat Med. 2006;12(11):1269.
66. Jannetto PJ, Bratanow NC. Pain management in the 21st century: utilization of pharmacogenomics and therapeutic drug monitoring. Expert Opin Drug Metab Toxicol. 2011;7:745–52.
67. Ltsch J, Geisslinger G, Tegeder I. Genetic modulation of the pharmacological treatment of pain. Pharmacol Ther. 2009;124(2):168.
68. Lloyd RA, Hotham E, Hall C, Williams M, Suppiah V. Pharmacogenomics and patient treatment parameters to opioid treatment in chronic pain: a focus on morphine, oxycodone, tramadol and fentanyl. Pain Med. 2016;0:1–19.
69. Song J-G, Shin JW, Lee EH, Choi DK, Bang JY, Chin JH, Choi IC. Incidence of post-thoracotomy pain: a comparison between total intravenous anaesthesia and inhalation anaesthesia. Eur J Cardio-Thor Surg. 2012;41:1078–82.
70. Searle RD, Simpson MP, Simpson KH, Milton R, Bennett MI. Can chronic neuropathic pain following thoracic surgery be predicted during the post-operative period? Interact Cardiovasc Thorac Surg. 2009;9:999–1002.
71. Chaparro LE, Smith SA, Moore RA, Wiffen PJ, Gilron I. Pharmacotherapy for the prevention of chronic pain after surgery in adults. Cochrane Database Syst Rev. 2013;7:CD008307.
72. McNicol ED, Schumann R, Haroutounian S. A systematic review and meta-analysis of ketamine for the prevention of persistent post-surgical pain. Acta Anaesthesiol Scand. 2014;58:1199–213.
73. Mendola C, Cammarota G, Netto R, Cecci G, Pisterna A, Ferrante D, et al. S(+)-ketamine for control of perioperative pain and prevention of post thoracotomy pain syndrome: a randomized, double-blind study. Minerva Anestesiol. 2012;78:757–66.
74. Mishra A, Nar AS, Bawa A, Kaur G, Bawa S, Kaur G, Bawa S, Mishra S. Pregabalin in chronic post-thoracotomy pain. J Clin Diagn Res. 2013;7:1659–61.
75. Comez M, Celik M, Dostbil A, Aksoy M, Ahiskalioglu A, Erdem AF, et al. The effect of pre-emptive dexketoprofen + thoracal epidural on the chronic post-thoracotomy pain. Int J Clin Exp Med. 2015;8:8101–7.
76. Ling X-M, Fang F, Zhang X-G, Ding M, Xue QA, Cang J. Effect of parecoxib combined with thoracic epidural analgesia on pain after thoracotomy. J Thorac Dis. 2016;8:880–7.
77. Baidya DK, Khanna P, Maitra S. Analgesic efficacy and safety of thoracic paravertebral and epidural analgesia for thoracic surgery: a systematic review and meta-analysis. Interact Cardiovasc Thorac Surg. 2014;18:626–36.
78. Ding X, Jin S, Niu X, Ren H, Fu S, Li Q. A comparison of the analgesia efficacy and side effects of paravertebral compared with epidural blockade for thoracotomy: an updated meta-analysis. PLoS One. 2016;9:e96233.
79. Yeung JHY, Gates S, Naidu BV, Wilson MJA, Gao Smith F. Parvertebral block versus thoracic epidural for patients undergoing thoracotomy. Cochrane Database Syst Rev. 2016;2:CD009121.
80. Senturk M, Ozcan P, Talu G, Kiyan E, Camci E, Ozyalin S, et al. The effects of three different analgesia techniques on long-term postthoracotomy pain. Anesth Analg. 2002;94(1):11.
81. Tiippana E, Nilsson E, Kalso E. Post-thoracotomy pain after thoracic epidural analgesia: a prospective follow-up study. Acta Anaesthesiol Scand. 2003;47(4):433.
82. Obata H, Saito S, Fujita N, Fuse Y, Ishizaki K, Goto F. Epidural block with mepivacaine before surgery reduces long-term post-thoracotomy pain. Can J Anesth. 1999;46(12):1127.
83. Andrae MH, Andrae DA. Local anaesthetics and regional anaesthesia for preventing chronic pain after surgery. Cochrane Database Syst Rev. 2012;10:CD007105.
84. Elshiekh MAF, Lo TTH, Shipolini AR, McCormack DJ. Does muscle-sparing thoracotomy as opposed to posterolateral thoracotomy result in better recovery. Interact Cardiovasc Thorac Surg. 2013;16:60–7.
85. Nosotti M, Baisi A, Mendogni P, Palleschi A, Tosi D, Rosso L. Muscle sparing versus posterolateral thoracotomy for pulmonary lobectomy: randomized controlled trial. Interact Cariovasc Thorac Surg. 2010;11:415–9.
86. Nomori H, Horio H, Fuyuno G, Kobayashi R. Non-serratus-sparing antero-axillary thoracotomy with disconnection of anterior rib cartilage: improvement in postoperative pulmonary function and pain in comparison to posterolateral thoracotomy. Chest. 1997;111(3):572.

87. Athanassiadi K, Kakaris S, Theakos N, Skottis I. Muscle-sparing versus posterolateral thoracotomy: a prospective study. Eur J Cardiothorac Surg. 2007;31(3):496.

88. Furrer M, Rechsteiner R, Eigenmann V, Signer C, Althaus U, Ris HB. Thoracotomy and thoracoscopy: postoperative pulmonary function, pain and chest wall complaints. Eur J Cardiothorac Surg. 1997;12(1):82.

89. Stammberger U, Steinacher C, Hillinger S, Schmid RA, Kinsbergen T, Weder W. Early and long-term complaints following video-assisted thoracoscopic surgery: evaluation in 173 patients. Eur J Cardiothorac Surg. 2000;18(1):7.

90. Bertrand PC, Regnard JF, Spaggiari L, Levi JF, Magdeleinat P, Guibert L, et al. Immediate and long-term results after surgical treatment of primary spontaneous pneumothorax by VATS. Ann Thorac Surg. 1996;61(6):1641.

91. Hutter J, Miller K, Moritz E. Chronic sequels after thoracoscopic procedures for benign diseases. Eur J Cardiothorac Surg. 2000;17(6):687.

92. Handy JR, Asaph JW, Douville EC, Ott GY, Grunkemeier GL, Wu Y. Does video-assisted thoracoscopic lobectomy for lung cancer provide improved functional outcomes compared with open lobectomy? Eur J Cardiothorac Surg. 2010;37:451–5.

93. Bendixen M, Jergensen OD, Kronborg C, Andersen C, Licht PB. Postoperative pain and quality of life after video assisted thoracoscopic surgery or anterolateral thoracotomy for early stage lung cancer: a randomized controlled trial. Lancet Oncol. 2016;17:836–44.

94. Noromi H, Cong Y, Sugimura H. Limited thoracotomy for segmentectomy: a comparison of postoperative pain with thoracoscopic lobectomy. Surg Today. 2016;46:1243–8.

95. Yamashita Y, Mukaida H, Harada H, Tsubokawa N. Post-thoracotomy pain and long-term survival associated with video-assisted thoracic surgery lobectomy methods for clinical T1N0 lung cancer: a patient -oriented, prospective cohort study. Eur J Cardo-Thor Surg. 2013;44:e71–6.

96. Benedetti F, Amanzio M, Casadio C, Filosso PL, Molinatti M, Oliaro A, et al. Postoperative pain and superficial abdominal reflexes after posterolateral thoracotomy. Ann Thorac Surg. 1997;64(1):207.

97. Benedetti F, Vighetti S, Ricco C, Amanzio M, Bergamasco L, Casadio C, et al. Neurophysiologic assessment of nerve impairment in posterolateral and muscle-sparing thoracotomy. J Thorac Cardiovasc Surg. 1998;115(4):841.

98. Rogers ML, Henderson L, Mahajan RP, Duffy JP. Preliminary findings in the neurophysiological assessment of intercostal nerve injury during thoracotomy. Eur J Cardiothorac Surg. 2002;21(2):298.

99. Maguire MF, Latter JA, Mahajan R, Beggs FD, Duffy JP. A study exploring the role of intercostal nerve damage in chronic pain after thoracic surgery. Eur J Cardiothorac Surg. 2006;29(6):873.

100. Wildgaard K, Ringsted TK, Ravn J, Werner MU, Kehlet H. Late sensory changes following chest drain insertion during thoracotomy. Acta Anaesthesiol Scand. 2013;57:776–83.

101. Cerfolio RJ, Price TN, Bryant AS, Sale Bass C, Bartolucci AA. Intracostal sutures decrease the pain of thoracotomy. Ann Thorac Surg. 2003;76(2):407.

102. Cerfolio RJ, Bryant AS, Patel B, Bartolucci AA. Intercostal muscle flap reduces the pain of thoracotomy: a prospective randomized trial. J Thorac Cardiovasc Surg. 2005;130(4):987.

103. Cerfolio RJ, Bryant AS, Maniscalco LM. A nondivided intercostal muscle flap further reduces pain of thoracotomy: a prospective randomized trial. Ann Thorac Surg. 2008;85(6):1901.

104. Hong K, Bae M, Han S. Subcostal closure technique for prevention of postthoracotomy pain syndrome. Asian Cardiovasc Thorac Ann. 2016;24:681–6.

105. Lu Q, Han Y, Cao W, Lei J, Wan Y, Fang Z, et al. Comparison of non-divided intercostal muscle flap and intercostal nerve cryo-analgesia treatments for post-oesophagectomy neuropathic pain control. Eur J Cardiothorac Surg. 2013;43:e64–70.

106. Visagan R, McCormack DJ, Shipolini AR, Jarral OA. Are intracostal sutures better than pericostal sutures for closing a thoracotomy? Interact Cardiovasc Thorac Surg. 2012;14:807–15.

107. Allama AM. Intercostal muscle flap for decreasing pain after thoracotomy: a prospective randomized trial. Ann Thorac Surg. 2010;89:195–9.

108. Koop O, Gries A, Eckert S, Ellermeier S, Hoksch B, Branscheid D, Beshay M. The role of intercostal nerve preservation in pain control after thoracotomy. Eur J Cardiothorac Surg. 2013;43:808–12.

109. Koryllos A, Althaus A, Poels M, Joppich R, Lefering R, Wappler F, et al. Impact of paravertebral neurectomy on post thoracotomy pain syndrome after thoracotomy in lung cancer patients: a randomized controlled trial. J Thorac Dis. 2016;8:2427–33.

110. Garcia-Tirado J, Rieger-Reyes C. Suture techniques of the intercostal space in thoracotomy and their relationship with post thoracotomy pain: a systematic review. Arch Bronconeumol. 2012;48:22–8.

111. Ji R-R, Xu Z-Z, Gao Y-J. Emerging targets in neuroinflammation-driven chronic pain. Nat Rev. 2014;13:533–48.

112. Huh Y, Ji R-R, Chen G. Neuroinflammation, bone marrow stem cells, and chronic pain. Front Immunol. 2017;8:1–9.

113. Wildgaard K, Ringsted TK, Hansen HJ, Petersen RH, Werner MU, Kehlet H. Quantitative sensory testing of persistent pain after video-assisted thoracic surgery lobectomy. Br J Anaesth. 2012;108:126–33.

114. Wildgaard K, Ringsted TK, Aasvang EK, Ravn J, Werner MU, Kehlet H. Neurophysiological characterization of persistent post-thoracotomy pain. Clin J Pain. 2012;28:136–42.

115. Mamet J, Klukinov M, Yaksh TL, Malkmus SA, Williams S, Harris S, et al. Single intrathecal administration of the transcription factor decoy AYX1 prevents acute and chronic pain after incisional, inflammatory or neuropathic injury. Pain. 2014;155:322–33.

116. Salvat E, Schweitzer B, Massard G, Meyer N, de Blay F, Muller A, Barrot M. Effects of β2 agonists on post-thoracotomy pain incidence. Eur J Pain. 2015;19:1428–36.

117. Humble SR, Dalton AJ, Li L. A systematic review of therapeutic interventions to reduce acute and chronic post-surgical pain after amputation, thoracotomy or mastectomy. Eur J Pain. 2015;19:451–65.

118. Brulotte V, Ruel MM, Lavontaine E. Impact of pregabalin on the occurrence of postthoracotomy pain syndrome: a randomized trial. Reg Anesth Pain Med. 2015;40:262–9.

119. Poobalan A, Bruce J, Smith WCS, King P, Krukowski Z, Chambers WA. A review of chronic pain after inguinal herniorrhaphy. Clin J Pain. 2003;19(1):48.

120. Granot M. Can we predict persistent postoperative pain by testing preoperative experimental pain? Curr Opin Anaesthesiol. 2009;22(3):425.

121. Weissman-Fogel I, Granovsky Y, Crispel Y, Ben-Nun A, Best L, Yarnitsky D, et al. Enhanced presurgical pain temporal summation response predicts post-thoracotomy pain intensity during the acute postoperative phase. J Pain. 2009;10(6):628.

122. Yarnitsky D, Crispel Y, Eisenberg E, Granovsky Y, Ben-Nun A, Sprecher E, et al. Prediction of chronic post-operative pain: pre-operative DNIC testing identifies patients at risk. Pain. 2008;138(1):22.

123. Tawfic Q, Kumar K, Pirani Z, Armstrong K. Prevention of chronic post-surgical pain: the importance of early identification of risk factors. J Anesth. 2017. http://doi.10.1007/s00540-017-2339-x.

124. Katz J, Weinrib A, Fashler SR, Katznelzon R, Shah BR, Ladak SSJ, et al. The Toronto General Hospital Transitional Pain Service: development and implementation of a multidisciplinary program to prevent chronic postsurgical pain. J Pain Res. 2015;8:695–702.

125. Clarke H, Poon M, Weinrib A, Katznelson R, Wentlandt K, Katz J. Preventive analgesia and novel strategies for the prevention of chronic post-surgical pain. Drugs. 2015;75:339–51.

126. DiMarco AF, Oca O, Renston JP. Lung herniation. A cause of chronic chest pain following thoracotomy. Chest. 1995;107(3):877.

127. Bennett M, Attal N, Backonja M, Baron R, Bouhassira D, Freynhagen R, et al. Using screening tools to identify neuropathic pain. Pain. 2007;127(3):199.

128. O'Connor A, Dworkin R. Treatment of neuropathic pain: an overview of recent guidelines. Am J Med. 2009;122(10 Suppl):S22.

129. Saarto T, Wiffen PJ. Antidepressants for neuropathic pain. Cochrane Database Syst Rev. 2007;4:CD005454.

130. Attal N, Cruccu G, Haanp M, Hansson P, Jensen TS, Nurmikko T, et al. EFNS guidelines on pharmacological treatment of neuropathic pain. Eur J Neurol. 2006;13(11):1153.

131. Dworkin R, O'Connor A, Backonja M, Farrar J, Finnerup N, Jensen T, et al. Pharmacologic management of neuropathic pain: evidence-based recommendations. Pain. 2007;132(3):237.

132. Neuropathic pain – pharmacological management. The pharmacological management of neuropathic pain in adults in non-specialist settings. NICE clinical guideline 173. 2013. http://guidance.nice.org.uk/CG173.

133. Sansone P, Passavanti MB, Fiorelli A, Aurilio C, Colella U, De Nardis L, et al. Efficacy of the topical 5% lidocaine medicated plaster in the treatment of chronic post-thoracotomy neuropathic pain. Pain Manag. 2017;7:189–96.

134. Knezevic NN, Rana MV, Czarnocki P, Anantamongkol U. Reprogramming of in situ spinal cord stimulator for covering newly developed postthoracotomy pain. J Clin Anesth. 2015;27:411–5.

135. Freynet A, Falcoz P. Is transcutaneous electrical nerve stimulation effective in relieving postoperative pain after thoracotomy? Interact Cardiovasc Thorac Surg. 2010;10(2):283.

136. Solak O, Tuma A, Pekcolaklar A, Metin M, Sayar A, Solak O, Gurses A. Transcutaneous electric nerve stimulation for the treatment of postthoracotomy pain: a randomized prospective study. Thorac Cardiovasc Surg. 2007;55:182–5.

137. Fiorelli A, Morgillo F, Milione R, Pace MC, Passavanti MB, Laperuta P, Aurilio C, Santini M. Control of post-thoracotomy pain by transcutaneous electrical nerve stimulation: effect on serum cytokine levels, visual analogue scale, pulmonary function and medication. Eur J Cardiothorac Surg. 2012;41:861–8.

138. MacPherson H, Vertosick EA, Foster NE, Lewith G, Linde K, Sherman KJ, et al. The persistence of effects of acupuncture after a course of treatment: a meta-analysis of patients with chronic pain. Pain. 2017;158:784–93.

139. Fabregat G, Asensio-Samper JM, Palmisani S, Villanueva-Perez VL, De Andres J. Subcutaneous botulinum toxin for chronic post-thoracotomy pain. Pain Pract. 2013;13:233–4.

140. Rashid S, Fields AR, Baumrucker SJ. Subcutaneous botulinum toxin injection for post-thoracotomy pain syndrome in palliative care: a case report. Am J Hosp Palliat Med. 2018;35:511–3.

Index